THE ADULT KNEE

Knee Arthroplasty

SECOND EDITION

THE ADULT KNEE

Knee Arthroplasty

SECOND EDITION

Harry E. Rubash, MD, FAOA

Chief Emeritus
Orthopaedic Surgcry
Massachusetts General Hospital
Edith M. Ashley Distinguished Professor
Harvard Medical School
Boston, Massachusetts

Robert L. Barrack, MD

Charles and Joanne Knight
Distinguished Professor
Department of Orthopaedic Surgery
Washington University School of Medicine
St. Louis, Missouri

Aaron G. Rosenberg, MD

Professor
Department of Orthopedic Surgery
Rush Medical College
Chicago, Illinois

Hany S. Bedair, MD

Medical Director, Kaplan Joint Center
Newton-Wellesley Hospital
Newton, Massachusetts
Department of Orthopaedic Surgery
Massachusetts General Hospital
Harvard Medical School
Boston, Massachusetts

James I. Huddleston III, MD

Associate Professor of Orthopaedic Surgery
Adult Reconstruction Division Director
Department of Orthopaedic Surgery
Stanford University Medical Center
Stanford, California

Brett R. Levine, MD, MS

Associate Professor
Department of Orthopaedics
Rush University Medical Center
Service Line Director
Edward-Elmhurst Health
Chicago, Illinois

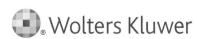 Wolters Kluwer

Philadelphia · Baltimore · New York · London
Buenos Aires · Hong Kong · Sydney · Tokyo

Director, Medical Practice: Brian Brown
Senior Development Editor: Stacey Sebring
Marketing Manager: Phyllis Hitner
Production Project Manager: Sadie Buckallew
Design Coordinator: Holly McLaughlin
Editorial Coordinator: Dave Murphy
Manufacturing Coordinator: Beth Welsh
Prepress Vendor: TNQ Technologies

2nd edition

9 8 7 6 5 4 3 2 1

Printed in China

Library of Congress Cataloging-in-Publication Data

ISBN-13: 978-1-975114-68-8

Cataloging in Publication data available on request from publisher.

shop.lww.com

To my sons Adam and Toby.
You were my inspiration and joy
when you were growing up and I cannot be more proud
of the outstanding young professionals and caring
young men you have become.
R.L.B.

To my wife, Kari for her love, support, and friendship
that we have shared over the years; to my children Kylie
and AJ who always keep me going and proved inspiration
and strength on a daily basis; to my parents Nate and Noreen
for their constant love and support; and in the memory of my grandmother,
Dorothy, who may be gone but will never be forgotten.
B.R.L.

To Heather, and our three children Riley, Sage, and Sam for allowing me
the time to devote to this important project.
J.I.H.

To my teachers and mentors who taught me the skills of our craft.
To my residents and fellows, who have allowed me to become part of
their professional lives. To my patients, who have entrusted me with
their most precious possession, their health. I am truly humbled.
Most importantly to my wife Naglaa and daughters Emelle
and Layla, who bring the greatest joy into my life. Finally,
to all those who have contributed to the second edition
of *The Adult Knee* and who have made this the premier
textbook on the topic. I am grateful to have been a part
of this outstanding team.
H.B.

To my lovely wife Kimberly, for more than four decades of love,
friendship, support, and joy!
H.E.R.

CONTRIBUTORS

Matthew P. Abdel, MD
Professor of Orthopedic Surgery
Mayo Clinic College of Medicine
Consultant
Department of Orthopedic Surgery
Mayo Clinic
Rochester, Minnesota

Vinay K. Aggarwal, MD
Assistant Professor
Department of Orthopaedic Surgery
NYU Langone Medical Center
New York, New York

Vignesh K. Alamanda, MD
Fellow in Adult Reconstruction
Hospital for Special Surgery
New York, New York

Hassan Alosh, MD
Beaumont Orthopedic Institute
Royal Oak, Michigan

Hiba K. Anis, MD
Clinical Research Fellow
Department of Orthopaedic Surgery
Cleveland Clinic Foundation
Cleveland, Ohio

David W. Anderson, MD, MS
Adult Reconstruction
Department of Orthopedic Surgery
Kansas City Joint Replacement at Menorah Medical
    Center
Overland Park, Kansas

Jean-Noël A. Argenson, MD, PhD
Professor and Chairman of Orthopedic Surgery
Director Institute for Locomotion
Aix-Marseille University
Marseille, France

David C. Ayers, MD
Professor and Chair
Department of Orthopedics and Rehabilitation
University of Massachusetts Medical School
Worcester, Massachusetts

David Backstein, MD, MEd, FRCSC
Associate Professor, Surgery
Head, Division of Orthopaedics
Granovsky Gluskin Chair in Complex Hip & Knee
    Reconstruction
Sinai Health System
University of Toronto
Toronto, Ontario, Canada

Matthew D. Beal, MD
Vice-Chair for Education
Department of Orthopaedic Surgery
Associate Professor of Orthopaedic Surgery
Residency Program Director
Department of Orthopaedic Surgery
Northwestern University
Chicago, Illinois

Hany S. Bedair, MD
Medical Director, Kaplan Joint Center
Newton-Wellesley Hospital
Newton, Massachusetts
Department of Orthopaedic Surgery
Massachusetts General Hospital
Harvard Medical School
Boston, Massachusetts

Nicholas A. Bedard, MD
Assistant Professor
Department of Orthopedics & Rehabilitation
University of Iowa
Iowa City, Iowa

Alex Beletsky, BS
Medical Student
University of California
San Diego School of Medicine
San Diego, California

Keith R. Berend, MD
President and CEO White Fence Surgical Suites
Senior Partner JIS Orthopedics
New Albany, Ohio

Richard A. Berger, MD
Assistant Professor
Department of Orthopaedics
Rush University Medical Center
Chicago, Illinois

Daniel J. Berry, MD
L.Z. Gund Professor of Orthopedic Surgery
Department of Orthopedic Surgery
Mayo Clinic
Rochester, Minnesota

James R. Berstock, MBChB, MRCS, FRCS (T&O), MD, PGCert Med Ed
Department of Orthopaedics
University of British Columbia
Vancouver, British Columbia, Canada

Kevin Bigart, MD
Fellow
Department of Orthopaedic Surgery
Midwest Orthopaedics at Rush
Chicago, Illinois
Parkview Orthopaedic Group
Palos Heights, Illinois

Sourabh Boruah, PhD
Research Fellow
Orthopaedic Surgery
Massachusetts General Hospital
Boston, Massachusetts

Matthew L. Brown, MD
Department of Orthopaedic Surgery
St. Lukes University Health Network
Bethlehem, Pennsylvania

Robert H. Brophy, MD
Professor
Department of Orthopaedic Surgery
Washington University School of Medicine
St. Louis, Missouri

James A. Browne, MD
Alfred R. Shands Associate Professor of Orthopaedic
    Surgery
Department of Orthopaedic Surgery
University of Virginia
Charlottesville, Virginia

Alissa J. Burge, MD
Director of Fellowship Research
Assistant Attending Radiologist
Department of Radiology and Imaging
Hospital for Special Surgery
New York, New York
Assistant Professor of Radiology
Weill Medical College of Cornell University
New York, New York
Assistant Scientist
Magnetic Resonance Imaging Research
Hospital for Special Surgery
New York, New York

Joost A. Burger, MD
Research Fellow
Department of Orthopedic Surgery, Sports Medicine,
    and Shoulder Service
Hospital for Special Surgery
New York, New York

Andrew D. Carbone, MD
Department of Orthopedic Surgery
Mount Sinai Health System
New York, New York

Charles S. Carrier, MD
Harvard Combined Orthopaedic Residency Program
Boston, Massachusetts

Laura K. Certain, MD, PhD
Assistant Professor
Division of Infectious Diseases
University of Utah
Salt Lake City, Utah

Antonia F. Chen, MD, MBA
Associate Professor
Department of Orthopaedic Surgery
Harvard University
Brigham and Women's Hospital
Boston, Massachusetts

Zlatan Cizmic, MD
Orthopaedic Resident
Wayne State University
Detroit, Michigan

Brian J. Cole, MD, MBA
Professor and Associate Chairman
Department of Orthopaedic Surgery
Rush University Medical Center
Chicago, Illinois

Clifford W. Colwell Jr, MD
Medical Director
Shiley Center for Orthopaedic Research and Education
    at Scripps Clinic
La Jolla, California

P. Maxwell Courtney, MD
Assistant Professor of Orthopaedic Surgery
Rothman Institute at Thomas Jefferson University
Philadelphia, Pennsylvania

David A. Crawford, MD
Orthopedic Surgeon
JIS Orthopedics
New Albany, Ohio

William M. Cregar, MD
Resident Physician
Department of Orthopaedic Surgery
Rush University Medical Center
Chicago, Illinois

Lawrence S. Crossett, MD
Associate Clinical Professor
Department of Orthopaedic Surgery
University of Pittsburgh Medical Center
Pittsburgh, Pennsylvania

Fred D. Cushner, MD
Assistant Clinical Professor
Department of Orthopedics
Hospital for Special Surgery
New York, New York

Ivan De Martino, MD
Attending
Orthopaedic and Traumatology Division
Fondazione Universitaria Policlinico Universitario
  Agostino Gemelli IRCCS
Catholic University of the Sacred Heart
Rome, Italy

Douglas A. Dennis, MD
Orthopaedic Surgeon
Colorado Joint Replacement
Centura Health Physician Group
Denver, Colorado

Matthew E. Deren, MD
Assistant Professor
Department of Orthopedics and Rehabilitation
University of Massachusetts Medical School
Worcester, Massachusetts

Matthew J. Dietz, MD
Associate Professor
Department of Orthopaedics
West Virginia University School of Medicine
Morgantown, West Virginia

Malcolm E. Dombrowski, MD
Resident
Department of Orthopaedic Surgery
University of Pittsburgh Medical Center
Pittsburgh, Pennsylvania

Joseph O. Ehiorobo, MD
Clinical Research Fellow
Department of Orthopaedic Surgery
Northwell Health
New York, New York

Shane C. Eizember, MD
Resident
Harvard Combined Orthopaedic Residency Program
Harvard Medical School
Boston, Massachusetts

Jacob M. Elkins, MD, PhD
Assistant Professor
Department of Orthopedics
Department of Biomedical Engineering
University of Iowa
Iowa City, Iowa

C. Anderson Engh Jr, MD
Orthopaedic Surgeon
Anderson Orthopaedic Clinic
Alexandria, Virginia

Mary Kate Erdman, MD
Resident Physician
Department of Orthopaedic Surgery
Keck School of Medicine of the University of Southern
  California
Los Angeles, California

John G. Esposito, MD, MSc, FRCS(C)
Instructor in Orthopaedic Surgery
Department of Orthopaedic Surgery
Massachusetts General Hospital
Harvard Medical School
Boston, Massachusetts

Patricia D. Franklin, MD, MPH, MBA
Professor
Co-Director, Measurement and Outcomes Hub
Department of Medical Social Sciences
Northwestern University Feinberg School of Medicine
Chicago, Illinois

Kevin B. Fricka, MD
Orthopaedic Surgeon
Anderson Orthopaedic Clinic
Alexandria, Virginia

James E. Feng, MD, MS
Orthopaedic Resident
Beaumont Health
Royal Oak, Michigan

David W. Fitz, MD
Adult Reconstruction Fellow
Massachusetts General Hospital
Department of Orthopaedic Surgery
Harvard Medical School
Boston, Massachusetts

Timothy E. Foster, MD
Associate Professor
Department of Orthopaedic Surgery
Tufts University School of Medicine
Boston, Massachusetts

Nicholas B. Frisch, MD, MBA
Orthopaedic Surgeon
Department of Orthopaedic Surgery
Ascension Providence Rochester Hospital
Rochester, Michigan

Jiri Gallo, MD, PhD
Professor and Chair
Department of Orthopaedics
Faculty of Medicine and Dentistry, Palacky University,
   University Hospital
Olomouc, Czech Republic

Donald S. Garbuz, MD, MHSc, FRCS
Professor and Head
Division of Lower Limb Reconstruction
Department of Orthopaedics
University of British Columbia
Vancouver, British Columbia, Canada

Kevin L. Garvin, MD
Professor and Chair
Department of Orthopaedic Surgery and Rehabilitation
University of Nebraska Medical Center
Omaha, Nebraska

J. Joseph Gholson, MD
Fellow Physician
Department of Orthopaedics
Instructor in Orthopaedic Surgery
Rush University Medical Center
Chicago, Illinois

Nicholas J. Giori, MD, PhD
Professor
Department of Orthopedic Surgery
Stanford University
Chief of Orthopaedic Surgery
Palo Alto Veteran Affairs Health Care System
Palo Alto, California

Stuart B. Goodman, MD, PhD, FRCSC, FACS, FBSE, FICORS
Robert L. and Mary Ellenburg Professor of Surgery,
Professor, Department of Orthopaedic Surgery and
   (by courtesy) Bioengineering
Stanford University Medical Center Outpatient Center
Redwood City, California

Allan E. Gross, MD, FRCSC, O.Ont
Professor of Surgery
Faculty of Medicine
University of Toronto Orthopaedic Surgeon
Mount Sinai Hospital
Bernard I. Ghert Family Foundation
Chair Lower Extremity Reconstruction
Granovsky Gluskin Division of Orthopaedics
Mount Sinai Hospital
Toronto, Ontario, Canada

Anthony P. Gualtieri, MD
Resident Physician
Department of Orthopedic Surgery
NYU Langone Orthopedic Hospital
New York, New York

Kenneth Gustke, MD
Florida Orthopaedic Institute
Clinical Professor of Orthopaedic Surgery
University of South Florida College of Medicine
Tampa, Florida

Nadim James Hallab, PhD
Department of Orthopedic Surgery
Rush University
Chicago, Illinois

John L. Hamilton, MD, PhD
Post-doctorate Researcher
Department of Orthopaedics
Rush University Medical Center
Chicago, Illinois

Arlen D. Hanssen, MD
Emeritus Professor of Orthopedic Surgery
Department of Orthopedic Surgery
Mayo Clinic
Rochester, Minnesota

Ryan E. Harold, MD
Resident Physician
Department of Orthopaedic Surgery
Northwestern University
Chicago, Illinois

Nathanael Heckmann, MD
Assistant Professor
Department of Orthopaedic Surgery
Adult Reconstruction Division
Keck Medicine of the University of Southern California
Los Angeles, California

Kelly J. Hendricks, MD
Adult Reconstruction
Department of Orthopedic Surgery
Kansas City Joint Replacement at Menorah Medical
    Center
Overland Park, Kansas

James I. Huddleston III, MD
Associate Professor
Department of Orthopaedic Surgery
Stanford University
Palo Alto, California

Kevin Hug, MD
Clinical Instructor
Department of Orthopaedic Surgery
Stanford University
Stanford, California

Shazaan F. Hushmendy, MD
Assistant Clinical Professor
Central Orthopedic Group
Plainview, New York

Ugonna N. Ihekweazu, MD
Adult Reconstruction & Joint Replacement Surgery
Fondren Orthopedic Group/Texas Orthopedic Hospital
Houston, Texas

Paul M. Inclan, MD
Orthopedic Surgery Resident
Department of Orthopedic Surgery
Washington University
St. Louis, Missouri

Richard Iorio, MD
Richard D. Scott, MD Distinguished Chair in
    Orthopaedic Surgery
Chief of Adult Reconstruction and Total Joint
    Replacement
Vice Chairman of Clinical Effectiveness
Brigham and Women's Hospital
Boston, Massachusetts

Joshua J. Jacobs, MD
William A. Hark, MD, Susanne G. Swift Professor &
    Chair
Department of Orthopaedic Surgery
Rush University Medical Center
Chicago, Illinois

Toufic R. Jildeh, MD
Resident Physician
Department of Orthopaedic Surgery
Henry Ford Health System
Detroit, Michigan

Joseph A. Karam, MD
Assistant Professor
Department of Orthopaedic Surgery
The University of Illinois at Chicago
Chicago, Illinois

Michael A. Kelly, MD
Chairman, Department of Orthopaedic Surgery and
    Physical Medicine/ Rehabilitation, Hackensack
    University Medical Center
Clinical Professor, Hackensack-Meridian Health School
    of Medicine at Seton Hall University
Hackensack University Medical Center
Hackensack, New Jersey

Mick P. Kelly, MD
Resident
Department of Orthopedic Surgery
Rush University Medical Center
Chicago, Illinois

Milad Khasian, MS
Doctoral Candidate
Department of Mechanical, Aerospace, and Biomedical
    Engineering
The University of Tennessee
Knoxville, Tennessee

Yair D. Kissin, MD, FAAOS
Vice Chairman
Department of Orthopaedics and Sports Medicine
Hackensack University Medical Center
Assistant Clinical Professor
Rutgers University and Hackensack-Meridian Health
    School of Medicine at Seton Hall University
Hackensack, New Jersey

Lindsay T. Kleeman-Forsthuber, MD
Orthopaedic Surgeon
Colorado Joint Replacement
Denver, Colorado

Michael A. Kolosky, DO
Medical Director
Musculoskeletal Department
North Shore Physicians Group | Partners Healthcare
Beverly, Massachusetts

Richard D. Komistek, PhD
Fred M. Roddy Professor
Department of Mechanical, Aerospace, and Biomedical
    Engineering
The University of Tennessee
Knoxville, Tennessee

Paul F. Lachiewicz, MD
Consulting Professor
Department of Orthopaedic Surgery
Duke University Medical Center
Attending Surgeon
Durham Veterans Affairs Medical
Durham, North Carolina

Michael T. LaCour, PhD
Research Assistant Professor
Department of Mechanical, Aerospace, and Biomedical
  Engineering
The University of Tennessee
Knoxville, Tennessee

Brent A. Lanting, MD, FRCSC, MSc
Associate Professor
Department of Surgery
The University of Western Ontario
London, Ontario, Canada

Darin J. Larson, MD
Orthopaedic Surgery Resident
Department of Orthopaedic Surgery and Rehabilitation
University of Nebraska Medical Center
Omaha, Nebraska

Cameron K. Ledford, MD
Adult Reconstruction
Department of Orthopedic Surgery
Kansas City Joint Replacement at Menorah Medical
  Center
Overland Park, Kansas

Brett R. Levine, MD, MS
Associate Professor
Rush University Medical Center
Department of Orthopaedics
Chicago, Illinois
Service Line Director
Elmhurst Memorial Hospital
Elmhurst, Illinois

Guoan Li, PhD
Associate Professor
Harvard Medical School
Director
Orthopaedic Bioengineering Research Center
Newton-Wellesley Hospital
Newton, Massachusetts

Jay R. Lieberman, MD
Professor and Chairman
Department of Orthopaedic Surgery
Keck School of Medicine University of Southern
  California
Los Angeles, California

Adolph V. Lombardi Jr, MD, FACS
President
Joint Implant Surgeons, Inc.
New Albany, Ohio
Clinical Assistant Professor
Department of Orthopaedics
The Ohio State University Wexner Medical Center
Columbus, Ohio

Jess H. Lonner, MD
Attending Orthopaedic Surgeon
Rothman Orthopaedic Institute
Professor of Orthopaedic Surgery
Sidney Kimmel Medical College of Thomas Jefferson
  University
Philadelphia, Pennsylvania

Steven J. MacDonald, MD, FRCSC
Professor
Department of Surgery
The University of Western Ontario
London, Ontario, Canada

Noah T. Mallory, Pre-medical Year-4
Research Intern
Joint Implant Surgeons, Inc.
New Albany, Ohio

Niv Marom, MD
Clinical Fellow
Sports Medicine Institute
Hospital for Special Surgery
New York, New York

Bassam A. Masri, MD, FRCSC
Professor and Head
Department of Orthopaedics
University of British Columbia
Vancouver, British Columbia, Canada

Matthew J. Matava, MD
Professor and Chief of Sports Medicine
Department of Orthopedic Surgery
Washington University
St. Louis, Missouri

John B. Meding, MD
The Center for Hip and Knee Surgery
St. Francis Hospital
Mooresville, Indiana

Christopher M. Melnic, MD
Clinical Instructor
Massachusetts General Hospital / Newton-Wellesley
  Hospital
Department of Orthopaedic Surgery
Harvard Medical School
Boston, Massachusetts

R. Michael Meneghini, MD
Professor
Department of Orthopaedic Surgery
Indiana University School of Medicine
Indianapolis, Indiana

Tom Minas, MD, MS
Professor of Orthopedics
Emeritus Harvard Medical School
Director
Cartilage Repair Center
The Paley Orthopedic and Spine Institute
St. Mary's Hospital
West Palm Beach, Florida

Robert M. Molloy, MD
Vice Chairman
Director of Adult Reconstruction
Department of Orthopaedic Surgery
Cleveland Clinic Foundation
Cleveland, Ohio

Michael A. Mont, MD
Chief of Joint Reconstruction
Vice President of Strategic Initiatives
Department of Orthopaedic Surgery
Northwell Health
New York, New York

Jessica Morton, MD
Resident
Department of Orthopedic Surgery
NYU Langone Orthopedic Hospital
NYU Langone Health
New York, New York

Brett Mulawka, MD
Adult Reconstruction Fellow
Massachusetts General Hospital
Department of Orthopaedic Surgery
Harvard Medical School
Boston, Massachusetts

Orhun Muratoglu, PhD
Professor, Orthopaedic Surgery
Harvard Medical School
Alan Gerry Scholar
Director
Harris Orthopaedics Laboratory
Director
Technology Implementation Research Center
Massachusetts General Hospital
Boston, Massachusetts

Trevor G. Murray, MD
Staff Orthopaedic Surgeon
Department of Orthopaedic Surgery
Cleveland Clinic Foundation
Cleveland, Ohio

Denis Nam, MD, MSc
Associate Professor
Department of Orthopaedic Surgery
Rush University Medical Center
Chicago, Illinois

Neal B. Naveen, BS
Research Fellow
Department of Orthopaedic Surgery
Rush University Medical Center
Chicago, Illinois

Arbi Nazarian, MD
Clinical Instructor
Orthopedic Surgery
University California San Francisco, Fresno
Fresno, California

Sandra B. Nelson, MD
Associate Physician
Massachusetts General Hospital
Assistant Professor
Harvard Medical School
Division of Infectious Diseases
Massachusetts General Hospital
Boston, Massachusetts

Stephen J. Nelson, MD
Connecticut Orthopaedics
Hamden, Connecticut

Richard Nicolay, MD
Resident Physician
Department of Orthopaedic Surgery
Northwestern University
Chicago, Illinois

Takahiro Ogura, MD
Sports Medicine and Joint Center
Funabashi Orthopaedic Hospital
Chiba, Japan

Jason H. Oh, MD
Assistant Professor
Department of Orthopaedic Surgery
Zucker School of Medicine at Hofstra University
Lenox Hill Hospital, Northwell Orthopaedic Institute
New York, New York

Kelechi R. Okoroha, MD
Assistant Professor
Department of Orthopaedic Surgery
Henry Ford Health System
Detroit, Michigan

Matthieu Ollivier, MD, PhD
Associate Professor
Institute of Movement
Marseille, France

Michael J. O'Malley, MD
Assistant Professor
Department of Orthopaedic Surgery
University of Pittsburgh
Pittsburgh, Pennsylvania

Ebru Oral, PhD
Associate Professor
Harris Orthopaedic Laboratory
Massachusetts General Hospital
Department of Orthopaedic Surgery
Harvard Medical School
Boston, Massachusetts

Mark Oyer, MD
Resident Physician
Department of Orthopaedic Surgery
Northwestern University
Chicago, Illinois

Jorge A. Padilla, MD
Division of Adult Reconstructive Surgery
    Department of Orthopaedic Surgery
NYU Langone Health NYU
Langone Orthopedic Hospital
New York, New York

Wayne G. Paprosky, MD
Professor
Department of Orthopaedic Surgery
Rush University Medical Center
Chicago, Illinois

Nancy L. Parks, MS
Biomedical Engineer
Anderson Orthopaedic Research Institute
Alexandria, Virginia

Ronak M. Patel, MD
Resident
Department of Orthopaedic Surgery
Washington University School of Medicine
St. Louis, Missouri

Andrew D. Pearle, MD
Chief of Sports Medicine and Associate Attending
    Orthopedic Surgeon
Department of Orthopedic Surgery, Sports Medicine,
    and Shoulder Service
Hospital for Special Surgery
New York, New York

Christopher E. Pelt, MD, FAAOS
Associate Professor, Orthopaedic Surgery
Chief Value Officer, Inpatient Orthopaedics
Medical Director of Orthopaedic & Trauma Unit
Adult Reconstruction Division
University of Utah Department of Orthopaedics
Salt Lake City, Utah

Kevin I. Perry, MD
Assistant Professor
Department of Orthopedic Surgery
Mayo Clinic
Rochester, Minnesota

Hollis G. Potter, MD
Chairman
Attending Radiologist
Department of Radiology and Imaging
Hospital for Special Surgery
Professor of Radiology
Weill Medical College of Cornell University
The Coleman Chair
Magnetic Resonance Imaging Research
Hospital for Special Surgery
New York, New York

Robin A. Pourzal, PhD
Assistant Professor
Department of Orthopedic Surgery
Rush University Medical Center
Chicago, Illinois

Shannon Powers, DO
Primary Care Sports Medicine Fellow
Rush University Medical Center
Chicago, Illinois

Mark D. Price, MD, PhD
Assistant Professor
Department of Orthopedic Surgery
Harvard Medical School
Boston, Massachusetts

Fernando J. Quevedo Gonzalez, PhD
Instructor
Department of Biomechancis
Hospital for Special Surgery
New York, New York

Zhitao Rao, MD
Associate Professor
Department of Orthopaedic Surgery
Tongji Hospital of Tongji University School of Medicine
Shanghai, China

Kevin A. Raskin, MD
The Orthopaedic Oncology Service
Department of Orthopaedic Surgery
Massachusetts General Hospital
Assistant Professor of Orthopaedic Surgery
    Harvard Medical School
Program Director
Fellowship in Orthopaedic Oncology
Boston, Massachusetts

Scott A. Rodeo, MD
Professor of Orthopaedic Surgery
Sports Medicine Institute
Hospital for Special Surgery
Weill Cornell Medical College
New York, New York

Pakdee Rojanasopondist, BA
Clinical Research Coordinator
Harris Orthopaedics Laboratory
Massachusetts General Hospital
Boston, Massachusetts

Aaron G. Rosenberg, MD
Professor
Department of Orthopedic Surgery
Rush Medical College
Chicago, Illinois

Harry E. Rubash, MD, FAOA
Chief Emeritus
Orthopaedic Surgery
Massachusetts General Hospital
Edith M. Ashley Distinguished Professor
Harvard Medical School
Boston, Massachusetts

Hayeem Rudy, BA
Clinical Research Fellow
Department of Orthopedic Surgery
NYU Langone Health
New York, New York

Karim G. Sabeh, MD
Clinical Fellow in Adult Reconstruction
Division of Orthopaedic Surgery
Massachusetts General Hospital
Harvard Medical School
Boston, Massachusetts

Alex J. Sadauskas, MD
Research Fellow
Department of Orthopaedics
Rush University Medical Center
Chicago, Illinois

Axel Schmidt, MD
Hopital Sainte marguerite APHM
Marseille, France

Blake J. Schultz, MD
Resident
Department of Orthopaedic Surgery
Stanford University
Palo Alto, California

Ran Schwarzkopf, MD, MSc
Associate Professor
Department of Orthoapedic Surgery
NYU Langone Orthopaedic Hospital
NYU Langone Health
New York, New York

Eric S. Schwenk, MD
Associate Professor
Department of Anesthesiology
Sidney Kimmel Medical College at Thomas Jefferson
    University
Philadelphia, Pennsylvania

Giles R. Scuderi, MD, FACS
Associate Professor
Department of Orthopaedic Surgery
Zucker School of Medicine at Hofstra/Northwell
Hempstead, New York

Peter K. Sculco, MD
Assistant Attending Orthopedic Surgeon
Department of Orthopaedic Surgery
The Stavros Niarchos Foundation Complex Joint
    Reconstruction Center
Hospital for Special Surgery
New York, New York

Thomas P. Sculco, MD
Surgeon in Chief Emeritus
Hospital for Special Surgery
New York, New York

Robert A. Sershon, MD
Orthopaedic Surgeon
Anderson Orthopaedic Clinic
Alexandria, Virginia

Roshan P. Shah, MD, JD
Assistant Professor of Orthopaedic Surgery
Columbia University Medical Center
New York, New York

Humza S. Shaikh, MD
Surgical Resident
Department of Orthopaedic Surgery
University of Pittsburgh Medical Center
Pittsburgh, Pennsylvania

Raj K. Sinha, MD, PhD
President
STAR Orthpaedics
Palm Desert, California

James Slover, MD, MS
Professor
Department of Orthopedic Surgery
NYU Langone Health
New York, New York

Nipun Sodhi, MD
Resident
Department of Orthopaedic Surgery
Northwell Health
New York, New York

Taylor M. Southworth, BS
Research Fellow
Department of Orthopaedic Surgery
Rush University Medical Center
Chicago, Illinois

Bryan D. Springer, MD
OrthoCarolina Hip and Knee Center
Fellowship Director
Professor, Department of Orthopedic Surgery
Atrium Musculoskeletal Institute
Charlotte, North Carolina

James B. Stiehl, MD, MBA
Founder
Stiehl Tech, LLC
Salem, Illinois

Vanni Strigelli, MD
Orthopedic Surgeon
Department of Surgery
Valdisieve Hospital
Florence, Italy

Patrick K. Strotman, MD
Department of Orthopaedic Surgery
University of Virginia
Charlottesville, Virginia

Dale Rick Sumner, PhD
The Mary Lou Bell McGrew Presidential Professor for
    Medical Research and Chair
Department of Cell and Molecular Medicine
Rush University
Chicago, Illinois

E. Grant Sutter, MD, MS
Adult Reconstruction Surgeon
Department of Orthopaedic Surgery
Northwestern Medicine Regional Medical Group
Warrenville, Illinois

Stephanie Swensen, MD
Clinical Fellow
Sports Medicine Institute
Hospital for Special Surgery
New York, New York

Tracy M. Tauro, BS, BA
Research Fellow
Department of Orthopaedic Surgery
Rush University Medical Center
Chicago, Illinois

Shankar Thiagarajah, MB ChB, FRCS (Tr&Orth), PhD
Consultant Trauma and Orthopaedic Surgeon
Doncaster and Bassetlaw Teaching Hospitals
University of Sheffield
Yorkshire, United Kingdom

Robert W. Tracey, MD, CDR MC USN
Adult Reconstruction Surgeon
Department of Orthopedic Surgery
Walter Reed National Military Medical Center
Bethesda, Maryland

Kenneth L. Urish, MD, PhD
Associate Professor
Magee Bone and Joint Center
Department of Orthopaedic Surgery
University of Pittsburgh
Pittsburgh, Pennsylvania

Andrew O. Usoro, MD
Resident Physician
Department of Orthopedic Surgery
Harvard Medical School
Boston, Massachusetts

Venus Vakhshori, MD
Resident Physician
Department of Orthopaedic Surgery
Keck School of Medicine of the University of Southern
    California
Los Angeles, California

Douglas VanderBrook, MD
Adult Reconstruction Fellow
Lenox Hill Hospital/ Northwell
New York, New York

Kartik M. Varadarajan, PhD
Assistant Professor
Orthopaedic Surgery
Massachusetts General Hospital
Boston, Massachusetts

Jonathan M. Vigdorchik, MD
Assistant Professor of Orthopedic Surgery
Adult Reconstruction and Joint Replacement
Hospital for Special Surgery
New York, New York

Tyler J. Vovos, MD
Department of Orthopaedic Surgery
Duke University Medical Center
Durham, North Carolina

Christopher S. Wahal, MD
Assistant Professor
Department of Anesthesiology
Sidney Kimmel Medical College at Thomas Jefferson
    University
Philadelphia, Pennsylvania

Carl B. Wallis, MD
Orthopaedic Institute of Henderson
Henderson, Nevada

Lucian C. Warth, MD
Assistant Professor
Department of Orthopaedic Surgery
Indiana University School of Medicine
Indianapolis, Indiana

Ray C. Wasielewski, MD, MS
Medical Director
Bone and Joint Center
Grant Medical Center
OhioHealth Columbus Ohio
Adjunct Professor of Materials
Aerospace, Biomedical and Materials Engineering
University of Tennessee
Knoxville, Tennessee

Richard A. Wawrose, MD
Resident
Department of Orthopaedic Surgery
University of Pittsburgh Medical Center
Pittsburgh, Pennsylvania

Kathleen Weber, MD, MS
Assistant Professor
Department of Orthopedic Surgery
Rush University Medical Center
Chicago, Illinois

Geoffrey Westrich, MD
Professor of Clinical Orthopedic Surgery
Adult Reconstruction and Joint Replacement Service
Hospital for Special Surgery/Cornell University
New York, New York

Leo A. Whiteside, MD
Director
Missouri Bone and Joint Center
Director
Missouri Bone and Joint Research Foundation
St. Louis, Missouri

Markus A. Wimmer, PhD
Professor
Department of Orthopedic Surgery
Rush University Medical Center
Chicago, Illinois

Timothy M. Wright, PhD
F. M. Kirby Chair
Department of Biomechanics
Hospital for Special Surgery
New York, New York

Adam B. Yanke, MD, PhD
Assistant Professor
Department of Orthopaedic Surgery
Rush University Medical Center
Chicago, Illinois

Caleb M. Yeung, MD
Resident
Harvard Combined Orthopaedic Residency Program
Harvard Medical School
Boston, Massachusetts

Qidong Zhang, MD
Associate Professor
Department of Orthopaedic Surgery
China-Japan Friendship Hospital
Peking Union Medical College
Beijing, China

Jason P. Zlotnicki, MD
Chief Resident
Department of Orthopaedic Surgery
University of Pittsburgh
Pittsburgh, Pennsylvania

PREFACE

This second edition of *The Adult Knee* follows its predecessor by more than 15 years. During this time, the authors completed two updates of *The Adult Hip* and we were determined to complete a second edition of *The Adult Knee*.

We continue to see tremendous technical, diagnostic, and philosophical changes in the treatment of diseases of the adult knee. Thus, we planned another comprehensive, balanced, well-illustrated reference text on the adult knee; an area that is clearly the core of many orthopaedic surgeons' practice worldwide. In planning this book, we again elected not to include fractures or pediatrics and omitted topics related to the treatment of athletic knee injuries, where numerous texts are available.

So, we strive to provide in-depth coverage of the adult knee as it relates to knee pathology and both surgical and nonsurgical treatment. Although comprehensive in nature, we have principally stressed the technical and practical information that is critical to today's orthopaedic surgeons' practice.

The Adult Knee is a complete source for orthopaedic surgeons, arthroplasty fellows, and residents, as well as medical students, researchers, or anyone with an interest in adult knee surgery. The text is presented in one volume with 11 sections. Section I includes a wonderful and comprehensive view of the history and important milestones in total knee arthroplasty. This is followed by Section II which covers surgical anatomy, knee pain, arthritis, alignment, kinematics, and the all-important materials in total knee arthroplasty.

Sections III, IV, and V cover clinical science, patellofemoral disorders, and alternatives to arthroplasty for total knee arthroplasty. The largest section in the book, Section VI, covers the expansive topics in primary total knee arthroplasty, including new discussions on episodes of care and outpatient surgeries. After a complete review of complications of total knee arthroplasty and the important topic of revision total knee arthroplasty, we conclude the major didactic sections on the management of an infected total knee replacement.

Finally, Section XI covers the future perspectives in total knee replacement.

A text of this breadth and depth is often best judged by the authors who contributed to its creation. Again, we are pleased and honored to assemble today's leading experts in the field of total knee arthroplasty and are indebted to their excellent contributions and their lasting friendships. This group of international authors represents the finest in the field—opinion leaders, clinician scientists, and basic scientists, all of whom are dedicated to improving the lives of our patients by providing the very best research and clinical evaluation of treatments and disorders of the adult knee.

The senior authors of this text have enlisted a group of outstanding rising stars in the field of knee arthroplasty as editors. We have asked them to continue the tradition of this text into the future. We hope that *The Adult Knee* is comprehensive, informative, and the go-to resource serving readers for years to come.

H.B.
R.B.
J.H.
B.R.L.
A.R.
H.R.

CONTENTS

SECTION 7
Perioperative Management in Total Knee Replacement
Editor: JAMES I. HUDDLESTON III

SECTION 8
Complications of Total Knee Replacement
Editors: BRETT R. LEVINE, HANY S. BEDAIR

Historical Perspectives

SECTION **1**

AARON G. ROSENBERG

BRETT R. LEVINE

chapter 1

Total Knee Arthroplasty: Milestones

Matthew L. Brown, MD | Clifford W. Colwell Jr, MD

Advances in anesthesia, materials, and antisepsis allowed surgeons to begin contemplating and ultimately performing operations on joints, with most early surgeries being débridement or resection for infection, most commonly tuberculosis, arthritis, or deformity. Anthony White is credited with performing the first resection arthroplasty of the knee in 1821 at Westminster Hospital, London.[1] In 1861, Ferguson performed the first knee resection for an indication of primary arthritis.[2] These early resection arthroplasties initially provided pain relief but failed due to either recurrent instability with excessive bone resection or arthrofibrosis/arthrodesis with inadequate bone excision. Surgeons sought to address the shortcomings of resection arthroplasty by experimenting with other techniques, including prosthetic replacement and interposition arthroplasty.

Professor Themistocles Gluck was an innovative surgeon working in Berlin in the 1880s who developed new ideas for intramedullary treatment of fractures and large bone defects as well as for the replacement of damaged joints. Gluck also theorized and experimented with: the transplantation of allograft tissues to reconstruct damaged tissues,[3,4] fracture fixation using steel plates and screws,[4] various compounds to be used as a bone cement—including copper amalgam, plaster of Paris, pumice, and other materials,[4,5] and with various prosthetic materials for suitability in reconstructing tissue defects in humans—including silk, cat cut, aluminum, wood, glass, and ivory.[3,4] His initial knee replacement consisted of ivory tibial and femoral components that relied on intramedullary fixation and were linked together with a hinged joint (**Fig. 1-1**).[3] Gluck proposed fixating his implants with a combination of press-fit into the meta-diaphyseal bone with possible augmentation via screw fixation using nickel-plated steel screws or ivory pegs that interlocked the host bone to the intramedullary portion of the ivory components.[3] On May 20, 1890, Dr Gluck implanted his hinged ivory prosthesis to replace the joint of a 17-year-old girl whose knee had been destroyed by tuberculosis.[4] These replacements were reported to be successful over short-term follow-up but ultimately failed secondary to chronic infection, which is not surprising given the implantation into joints infected with tuberculosis. Although many of Dr Gluck's ideas would become foundational for modern knee arthroplasty, his contemporaries paid little attention to his theories and his ideas were largely abandoned until the mid-20th century when Judet, Walldius, and others redeveloped and ultimately implanted versions of a hinged knee prosthesis.

INTERPOSITION ARTHROPLASTY

Verneuil is recognized as performing the first interpositional arthroplasty of the knee in 1863 when he inserted a flap of joint capsule between the distal femur and proximal tibia.[6,7] The clinical outcomes of this initial interpositional arthroplasty are unknown. Others continued to develop and experiment with interpositional arthroplasty utilizing various materials, including fascia lata, muscle, chromicized pig bladder, silk, gutta percha, magnesium, gold, silver, rubber, cellophane, nylon, and other materials. Dr John D. Murphy, working at Rush Medical College and Northwestern Medical College in Chicago during the first decades of the 20th century, conducted experiments with interposition of local tissues, pedunculated fascia and fat, into ankylosed joints and reported on the histologic appearance of these tissues in animal models as well as performing interpositional arthroplasty in various joints of human patients.[8,9] Dr Willis C. Campbell, practicing in Memphis, was also a proponent of interpositional arthroplasty and published widely on his technique, including indications, surgical technique, postoperative protocols, and outcomes (**Fig. 1-2**).[10] Campbell reported on 12 cases and the majority of patients were purported to have reasonable results with most patients achieving near full extension and flexion from 50° to 90°.[10] Duncan C. McKeever, working in Houston, Texas, experimented with cellophane interpositional arthroplasty in the 1940s, but results were unsatisfactory. John G. Kuhns and associates at the Robert B. Brigham Hospital in Boston reported on their experience with interpositional arthroplasty utilizing various synthetic materials.[7] Their initial attempts to interpose "malleable, nonoxidized metallic sheets" proved unsuccessful, and they ultimately settled on the use of nylon interposition. The authors reported complications that included motion less than 60°, pain, re-ankylosis, infection, worsening arthritis, and others; however, they did report satisfactory results in 58 patients and unsatisfactory in 12 patients treated with their nylon interposition technique.[7] Although interpositional arthroplasty, particularly with transfer of local autogenous tissues, provided encouraging outcomes over short-term follow-up, these

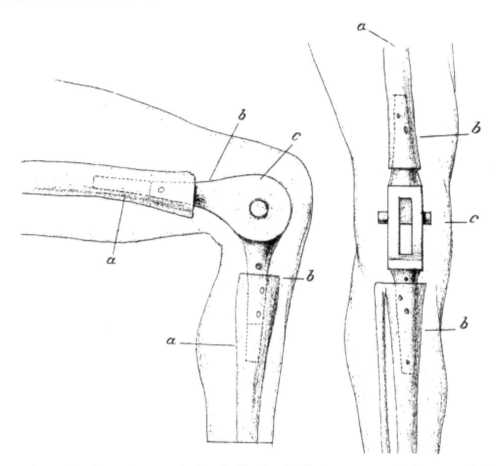

FIGURE 1-1   Diagram of hinged ivory knee replacement developed by Themistocles Gluck. *a,* appears to be femur and tibia bone; *b,* femoral and tibial components; *c,* hinge. (From Gluck T. The classic: report on the positive results obtained by the modern surgical experiment regarding the suture and replacement of defects of superior tissue, as well as the utilization of re-absorbable and living tamponade in surgery. *Clin Orthop Relat Res.* 2011;469:1528-1535.)

procedures were ultimately subject to degradation of the interpositional material, which later authors attributed to recurrence of pain and instability, and these procedures were unable to correct mechanical deformity.

HEMIARTHROPLASTY

Dissatisfied with results of soft-tissue interpositional arthroplasty and taking inspiration from Smith-Petersen's technique of vitallium cup arthroplasty in the hip, surgeons began to design devices for hemiarthroplasty in the knee. Dr Campbell, in conjunction with his colleague Dr Harold B. Boyd, developed a vitallium prosthesis to resurface the distal femur in much the same way Campbell had resurfaced the distal femur with his soft-tissue interposition. The size of the implant required was estimated preoperatively using radiographs and was then fabricated for each patient. The prosthesis was affixed to the distal femur utilizing two flanges that hooked to the posterior condyles and then a vitallium screw inserted through the device into the anterior distal femur.[11] Boyd implanted the first vitallium distal femoral hemiarthroplasty in 1938 and Campbell published a preliminary report of the technique in 1940, which he had performed on two patients.[12] The results of the initial two vitallium

distal femoral hemiarthroplasties were disappointing, with both patients achieving only limited motion postoperatively. The work of Boyd, Campbell, and Smith-Petersen would ultimately lead to the development of the femoral prosthesis used at the Massachusetts General Hospital, which included a stem for intramedullary fixation attached to the femoral resurfacing portion of the prosthesis that was intended to provide increased stability. The implant would become known as the MGH prosthesis (**Fig. 1-3**).

Charles C. Townley, who spent the majority of his career in private practice in Port Huron, Michigan, developed a tibial hemiarthroplasty in 1951.[11,13] Townley's stainless steel tibial plate was asymmetric to match medial and lateral plateaus, necessitating a right and left prosthesis, was available in three sizes, and was fixed with screws to the anterior tibia. Among the initial 39 cases, 19 had follow-up of at least 2 years (range 2 to 9 years) and 14 (74%) were reported to have satisfactory results ("minimal or no pain and with useful motion").[11]

McKeever, not satisfied with the cellophane interpositional arthroplasty, developed a metallic, monoblock prosthesis to resurface either the lateral or medial tibial plateau (**Fig. 1-4**).[14,15] The prosthesis was first implanted in April 1952.[14] Several authors have reported mid- to

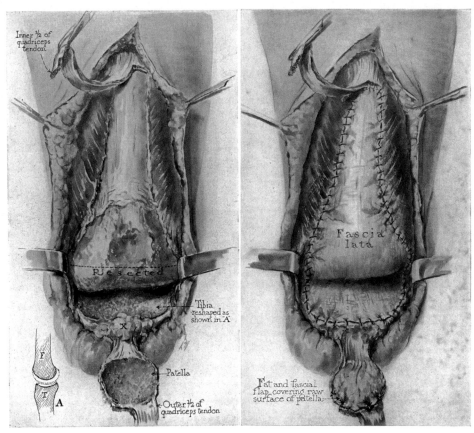

FIGURE 1-2 Illustration depicting Dr Willis C. Campbell's technique of resection and interposition arthroplasty for the treatment of painful knee joint. (From Campbell WC. Arthroplasty of the knee. *Ann Surg.* 1924;80:88-102.)

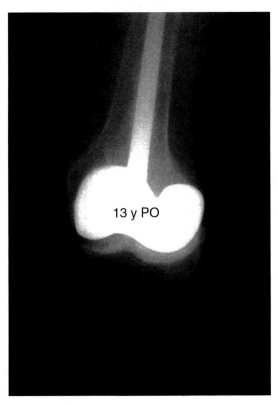

13 y PO

FIGURE 1-3 Radiograph of Massachusetts General Hospital (MGH) prosthesis, which was a stemmed femoral hemiarthroplasty.

long-term follow-up of the McKeever unicompartmental hemiarthroplasty and results were good to excellent in approximately 70% of knees.[15,16]

McKeever also developed a patellar prosthesis and reported his results in 1955.[17] His prosthesis was made of vitallium and came in three sizes, and fixation was achieved using two lips that captured the bony patella and augmented with a transfixion screw. McKeever reported using his prosthesis in 40 patients and reported 4 failures due to infection but no mechanical failures; however, the follow-up time was not specified.[17] Harrington reported long-term results of the McKeever patellar prosthesis in a cohort of 28 patients with minimum 4-year follow-up (range 4 to 16 years) and reported excellent results in 17 of the 28 patients at 5-year follow-up.[18]

HINGED KNEE PROSTHESES

During the 1940s and 1950s, as surgeons in the United States were developing metallic hemiarthroplasty options, those working in Europe were reconsidering the concepts for hinged knee replacement first described by Themistocles Gluck some 70 years earlier. Judet and colleagues reported on their hinged knee replacement in 1947[19] and Magnoni followed with his own report shortly after in 1949.[20] Throughout the 1950s the

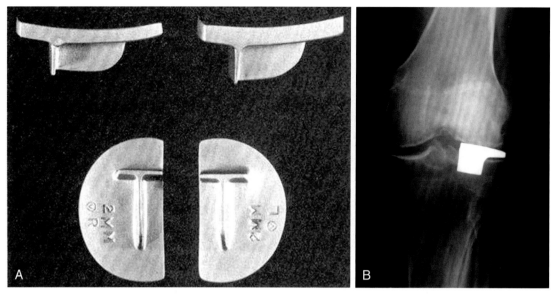

FIGURE 1-4   Clinical photograph **(A)** and radiograph **(B)** of McKeever tibial plateau prosthesis. (From Springer BD, Scott RD, Sah AP, Carrington R. McKeever hemiarthroplasty of the knee in patients less than 60 years old. *J Bone Joint Surg Am*. 2006;88:366-371.)

concept of a hinged knee prosthesis were refined and further developed by Dr Börje Walldius and colleagues working at the Karolinska Institute in Stockholm, Sweden.[21-23] Walldius developed his initial hinged knee prosthesis using an acrylic material called Bonoplex for the femoral and tibial components, which were then linked by a stainless steel axel.[21] The articular portions of the femur and tibia required 38 mm bone resection, which was made perpendicular to the long axis of the bone. Fixation relied on a long intramedullary stem and two small pegs inserted in the cancellous medullary bone; cement was not used. Walldius reported reasonable success in his initial 32 knees (26 patients): 75% achieving pain relief and average motion of 84°, 4 required arthrodesis, and 2 required amputation.[22] Walldius reported 8-year follow-up for his initial 64 knees (51 patients) and 74% were either "very good" or "good."[23] He went on to describe modifications to his original prosthesis, which included changing the prosthesis from acrylic to vitallium due to problems with fracture, reducing the central articular height to 28 mm, and shortening the supplementary fixation pins to avoid conflict with cortical bone (**Fig. 1-5**).[23]

The Walldius hinged prosthesis was appealing for several reasons. Its high degree of constraint enabled correction of large deformities about the knee and eliminated the need to retain soft-tissue structures about the knee, including the cruciate or collateral ligaments. This simplified the operative technique and it was relatively straightforward to achieve appropriate alignment. Significant drawbacks included its large size and high degree of constraint. The size of the endoprosthesis required significant bone resection that limited future salvage options, and infection was a prominent concern given the large amount of retained foreign material

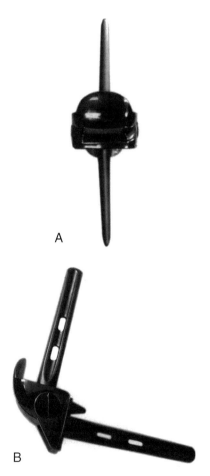

FIGURE 1-5   Photograph showing the Walldius hinged knee replacement.

and resulting dead space between host tissues and the implant. The high degree of constraint resulted in significant force transmission to the implant–bone interface and led to bone destruction and ultimately loosening

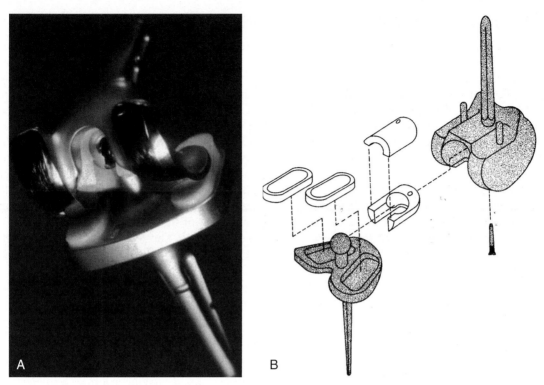

FIGURE 1-6 **A:** Photograph showing the spherocentric knee. **B:** Diagram depicting the spherocentric knee. (B from Matthews LS, Sonstegard DA, Kaufer H. The spherocentric knee. *Clin Orthop Relat Res*. 1973;94:234-241.)

of fixation. Shiers,[24] Young,[25] and others designed and implanted hinged knee prostheses; however, these did not achieve widespread usage.

The Guepar hinged prosthesis was developed by a group of surgeons in Paris in the late 1960s and early 1970s. The designing surgeons focused on six design principles: (1) minimal prosthetic bulk in width (avoid superficial soft tissues) and height (preserve bone), (2) avoid flexion limitation by contact between the two parts, (3) obtain "rolling" of the tibia under the femur in flexion, (4) preserve patellar motion, (5) dampen component-component contact in extension, and (6) reestablish normal knee axis by incorporating a valgus tilt to the femoral stem.[26] The prosthesis incorporated a posteriorized hinge toward achieving rolling of the tibia and silastic thrusters to absorb impact between components.[26] Clinically, the Guepar prosthesis performed quite well. Insall and others at the Hospital for Special Surgery (HSS) compared results from their experience with four different prosthetic designs, which they indicated for varying degrees of deformity and instability. The prostheses studied included a unicondylar prosthesis, two surface replacement prostheses (the Duocondylar and the Geometric), and the Guepar hinge. The Guepar was implanted in knees with the worst preoperative deformity and function and yielded the best postoperative function and had the lowest overall complication rate, but the authors noted that the Guepar prosthesis had the highest infection rate and was the most difficult prosthesis to effectively salvage.[27]

In 1973, Larry Matthews and colleagues at the University of Michigan reported on the spherocentric knee, which they designed to address problems with previous hinged designs.[28] Previous hinged designs allowed motion only in the sagittal plane, with no motion in the coronal (varus/valgus) or axial plane (internal rotation/external rotation), which provided stability but placed increased force on the bone implant interface, leading to bone resorption and implant loosening. Another problem was metal-to-metal stops at terminal flexion and extension, which again provided stability but led to loosening and wear debris. Recognizing that polyethylene wear remained problematic, modularity was then incorporated into the design. The spherocentric knee included stemmed tibial and femoral components that were cemented into the bone; the tibial component included a central metal sphere in the intercondylar region and posterior to the midline of the femur and two tracks along the plateaus to accommodate polyethylene runners in which the femoral condyles would track. The femoral component incorporated a variable radius femoral condyle to provide gradual deceleration at extremes of motion, and the intercondylar notch contained a housing for the polyethylene component that captured the tibial sphere (**Fig. 1-6**). The authors reported on the longer-term outcome of their prosthesis and reported 5% infection rate, 11% loosening rate, 15% reoperation rate, and 32% incidence of radiolucent lines at an average 8-year follow-up.[29]

RESURFACING KNEE PROSTHESES

The 1960s saw the recognition that the polymethylmeth-acrylate (PMMA) bone cement and high-density poly-ethylene utilized successfully by Sir John Charnley in hip arthroplasty might be incorporated into designs for knee arthroplasty. Dr Frank Gunston, a Canadian who had per-formed a fellowship with John Charnley, developed the first cemented surface knee replacement without a hinge in 1968 in Wrightington Hospital in Lancashire, England.[30] The polycentric knee arthroplasty consisted of two inde-pendent stainless steel runners to resurface the distal femoral condyles that articulated with high-density poly-ethylene tracks implanted into slots in the proximal tibia (**Fig. 1-7**).[30] All components were affixed to the bone uti-lizing PMMA cement. The articular surface was designed to permit both rocking and gliding movements in the sag-ittal plane as well as 20° of rotation in the axial plane. The cement fixation and allowance for axial rotation were both designed to disperse forces at the bone–implant inter-face. The initial experience with this prosthesis and tech-nique in 22 knees (20 patients) was reportedly successful for pain relief and motion.[30] Gunston's polycentric knee was implanted in larger numbers at the Mayo Clinic and there were 35 complications among the initial 450 cases, including 9 infections, 7 dislocations, 6 fractures, 6 VTEs, 4 skin necrosis events, and 4 cases of loose prosthetic com-ponents.[31] Ten-year results revealed a 34% failure rate.[32]

The 1970s saw two distinct design philosophies arise as surgeons and engineers sought to improve on designs for condylar total knee replacement. The anatomic camp generally sought to maintain soft-tissue structures about the knee and design the prosthesis around these soft tis-sues. The functional camp sought to design the prosthe-sis to substitute for the function of soft-tissue structures, which would permit a simplified surgical technique.

ANATOMIC APPROACH

Professor Toshio Kodama and Sumiki Yamamoto, work-ing at Okayama University Medical School, designed a prosthesis they called the Mark I, which was first implanted in 1970.[33] The femoral component was a mod-ified Sbarbaro femoral condyle mold that incorporated an anterior flange for patellar tracking, and was made of COP alloy (Cr, Ni, Co, Mo, P).[33] The tibial component was minimally constrained with a cutout to preserve both cruciate ligaments.[33] The Mark I utilized no cement.[33] A subsequent iteration of the Mark I increased constraint between the femur and tibia, which prevented poste-rior sliding of the tibia and restricted flexion if the PCL was retained.[33] The Mark I was implanted in 43 knees. Yamamoto visited Freeman in 1974, and design alter-ations following this visit led to the Mark II prosthesis, which remained noncemented but reverted to less con-straint between the femur and tibia to allow some rota-tory motion in flexion but to restrict it in extension.[33]

Theodore Waugh, MD, PhD, working with colleagues at the University of California at Irvine (UCI), developed the UCI total knee replacement and reported early results in 1973.[34] The design incorporated a single cobalt-chrome femoral component consisting of two "J" shaped runners, designed to mimic the instant center of rotation of the human knee, connected by a thin piece of metal anteriorly. The tibial component was horseshoe shaped to facilitate preservation of the cruciate ligaments and was made from ultra-high-density polyethylene. Intermediate results for 103 knees indicated most patients (78%) improved but mechanical complications occurred in 17.4%.[35]

Dr Townley, not completely satisfied with results from his tibial hemiarthroplasty technique and recognizing failures with hinged total knee replacements, developed the Townley anatomic total knee and reported its use in

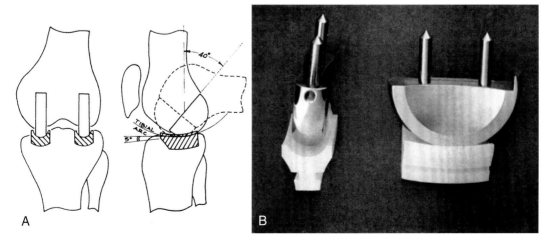

FIGURE 1-7 Dr Frank Gunston developed the polycentric knee arthroplasty, which is credited with being the first cemented surface knee replace-ment. Panel A is a schematic drawing of the prosthesis. Panel B is a photograph of a femoral and tibial component; the system was designed to resurface both the medial and lateral compartment of the knee; it was not intended for unicompartmental knee arthroplasty. (From Gunston FH. Polycentric knee arthroplasty. Prosthetic simulation of normal knee movement. *J Bone Joint Surg Br.* 1971;53:272-277.)

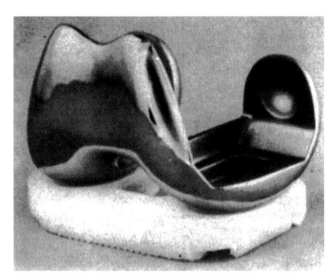

FIGURE 1-8 Photograph showing the Townley anatomic total knee. Similar to other early anatomic designs, it preserved the cruciate ligaments and had concave tibial geometry to match the femoral condyles. The anterior portion of the femoral component, for the first time, was designed to provide an articular surface for the patella, rather than simply connect the two femoral condyles. (From Townley C, Hill L. Total knee replacement. *Am J Nurs.* 1974;74:1612-1617.)

1974 (**Fig. 1-8**).[36] The femoral component for the first time incorporated an anterior flange designed not only to connect the condyles but to provide an articular surface for the patella. The all-polyethylene tibial component was again cut out to preserve both cruciates and had a dished articular surface conforming to the femoral condyles, and the undersurface was corrugated to facilitate PMMA interdigitation.[36]

Seedhom and colleagues developed the Leeds knee following an anatomic approach.[37] The femoral prosthesis, attempting to replicate native anatomy, was asymmetric, with the medial condyle employing a J curve and the lateral condyle designed with a relatively uniform radius.[37] It was manufactured in three sizes. The polyethylene tibial component consisted of two disks connected anteriorly; the disks incorporated a dished design to replicate the menisci and the degree of dishing was modified with subsequent designs to facilitate increased motion. Results of the Leeds knee were never published by the surgeons.[38]

The Duocondylar prosthesis was developed at HSS in New York City with major contributions from surgeon Chitranjan Ranawat and engineer Peter Walker.[39] It was first implanted in December 1971. The cobalt-chrome femoral component consisted of condylar surfaces closely replicating the normal knee connected with an anterior bar, each condyle had a peg affixed to the back for augmented fixation with PMMA.[39] The femoral component came in two sizes. The tibia was resurfaced with two independent polyethylene implants, which were dovetailed on the undersurface to facilitate cementation into the tibial bone.[39] The tibial articular geometry was designed to permit sagittal plane motion without limit but had an upward curvature toward the intercondylar notch to provide some

stability in the coronal and axial planes.[39] The tibial components were affixed to a jig to maintain alignment with the femoral component during implantation. Ranawat described contraindications for the duocondylar prosthesis, which included sagittal plane instability, fixed coronal plane subluxation, hyperextension greater than 10°, and flexion contracture greater than 25°. Initial results were acceptable, but failure modes included instability and tibial loosening and led to a 5.5% revision rate at 3-year follow-up.[40] The Duocondylar prosthesis was subsequently modified to create the Duopatellar prosthesis, which included an anterior flange on the femoral component, a patellar resurfacing, and a single-piece tibial polyethylene component with increased conformity and a large fixation peg.[41,42] Although initially satisfied with the Duopatellar prosthesis, Ranawat ultimately favored the Total Condylar Prosthesis, which was developed at the HSS contemporaneous with the Duopatellar. In 1974 Ranawat and Walker traveled to Boston to present the Duopatellar and Total Condylar Prosthesis to a group of surgeons at MGH in Boston who had experience with the Duocondylar prosthesis but were dissatisfied with nearly 20% of patients with residual patellofemoral symptoms; the MGH surgeons included Bill Harris, Bill Jones, Clement Sledge, Richard Scott, and others.[43] The Boston contingent, given their considerable experience and overall good results with the McKeever hemiarthroplasty, preferred retention of the PCL and favored the Duopatellar prosthesis and it was first implanted in Boston in 1974.[42,43] The initial experience over short-term follow-up with the Duopatellar prosthesis in Boston was good, with a 2.8% revision rate among which half were for patella problems (pain, tracking, fracture) and another third were for aseptic tibial loosening.[42] The Duopatellar prosthesis was subsequently modified in Boston over the next 7 years and would come to be called the Robert Brent Brigham Hospital (RBBH) knee; modifications included a deepened and valgus aligned trochlea, extension of the posterior condyles, incorporation of a one-piece tibial component with central stem to improve fixation (they would later incorporate a metal-backed monoblock tibial component), and flattening of the tibial polyethylene in the coronal plane to allow femoral rollback in flexion.[42]

Clement Sledge and Frederick Ewald, among other surgeons working at the Robert Brent Brigham Hospital in Boston, worked with Peter Walker, who had left HSS to work as an engineer for Howmedica, to develop the Kinematic knee system, which was a modification of the RBBH knee and was first implanted by Ewald in 1978.[42,44] Results at 10-year follow-up were generally good with 96% survivorship, but loosening of the patellar component was problematic.[45] The Kinematic knee would evolve into the Kinemax knee, which modified the articular geometry to increase contact area.[46] The Kinemax knee demonstrated acceptable midterm results with survivorship of 99% at 5 years and 97% after 9 years.[46] Other surgeons working in Boston, including Richard D. Scott and

Thomas S. Thornhill, who had previously worked on the Kinematic team, would go on to develop the cruciate-sparing Press Fit Condylar (PFC) knee system in conjunction with Johnson & Johnson.[47] Most current cruciate-sparing total knee prostheses have origins in these systems designed in Boston.

FUNCTIONAL APPROACH

During the late 1960s and early 1970s three different teams were simultaneously but independently developing total knee systems utilizing a functional approach: (1) Freeman and Swanson at Imperial College London Hospital (ICLH prosthesis), (2) Insall, Ranawat, and Walker at HSS in New York (Total Condylar Prosthesis), and (3) a consortium of US surgeons from Mayo Clinic, Harvard, Johns Hopkins, UCLA, and The Doctor's Hospital in Texas (Geometric Total Knee Prosthesis).

Surgeon Michael Freeman and engineer SAV Swanson developed the Freeman-Swanson (ICLH) knee prosthesis while working at Imperial College London Hospital between February 1966 and April 1970, when it was first implanted.[48,49] Freeman had previously used the MGH stemmed femur articulating against two Macintosh-type tibial polyethylene components.[50] This construct proved unsatisfactory for several reasons, including technical difficulty aligning components, impingement on the intercondylar eminence leading to limited motion, and reliance on cruciate ligaments, often of questionable competency, for stability. Several tenets guided prosthetic development: (1) minimal bone resection to implant the procedure to facilitate salvage procedures should the implant fail, (2) minimize risk of component loosening by limiting constraint between femoral and tibial components, providing a gradual mechanism to limit hyperextension, using bone cement fixation over broad bony surfaces to reduce stress at the bone-prosthesis interface, and selecting a low-friction bearing surface, (3) minimizing wear debris and making the wear debris as innocuous as possible, (4) minimize or eliminate reliance on the cruciate ligaments for mechanical function of the prosthesis, and (5) desire to make the femoral component a good articular surface for the patella or resurfacing posterior patellar surface.[48,49] Freeman and Swanson settled on a "roller in trough" design concept. They also developed specialized instruments for the first time to aid with implantation of their prosthesis. The authors reported good short-term results for their initial 69 arthroplasties using the Freeman-Swanson (ICLH) prosthesis.[49] Freeman and Sculco reported that the ICLH (Freeman-Swanson) prosthesis could successfully be used to treat arthritic knees with significant deformity (valgus >25°, varus >20°, or flexion contracture >30°) that previously required a hinged prosthesis.[51] Longer-term follow-up would reveal problems including tibial component subsidence, excessive polyethylene wear, configuration of the patellofemoral joint, alignment, and stability difficulties.[52]

The Geometric Total Knee prosthesis was first implanted in 1971.[53,54] The prosthesis was designed by a consortium of surgeons in conjunction with Howmedica, which manufactured the prosthesis. The surgeon consortium included Mark B. Coventry from the Mayo Clinic, Gerald A.M. Finerman from University of California at Los Angeles, Lee H. Riley from Johns Hopkins, Roderick H. Turner from Harvard, and Jackson E. Upshaw from The Doctor's Hospital in Texas[53] The femoral component was made from vitallium and had symmetric, single-radius condyles connected by a central crossbar. The femur had fixation lugs for the medial and lateral condyle and also had depressions in the anterior and posterior portions of the condyle for augmented cement fixation.[53] The tibia was constructed of high-density polyethylene with two concave tibial plateau units connected with an anterior bridge to allow preservation of the cruciate ligaments and minimize bone resection. The tibial articular geometry was concave, which the designers intended to "prevent movement in the anteroposterior and lateral planes when the units are mated but slight rotation of the tibia about the femur is permitted."[53] The designers specifically commented that "a specific indication for the geometric knee is varus or valgus deformity associated with loss of bone."[53]

In the early 1970s, a team working at the HSS in New York City that included surgeons John Insall and Chitranjan Ranawat, along with engineer Peter Walker, developed the Total Condylar Prosthesis. This was the result of a modification of the previous HSS designs, the Duocondylar and Duopatellar. Interestingly, John Insall and Michael Freeman attended Cambridge together and maintained a close personal relationship throughout their lives and discussed design concepts for knee prostheses professionally.[38,50] The HSS team reported on their initial clinical experience implanting the Total Condylar Prosthesis in 1976 (**Fig. 1-9**).[55] Based on prior experience with total knee replacement at HSS, including both hinge and surface replacement designs, the team identified three major problems they hoped to address with their new prosthesis. First, the patellofemoral joint remained a source of pain when unresurfaced and previous experience with patellectomy proved unacceptable. Second, tibial component fixation was poor, with frequent radiolucent lines and component loosening. Third, they felt surgical techniques to implant previous prostheses provided insufficient accuracy, especially with greater deformity. Fourth, they felt that hinged designs did not provide an adequate solution given problems stating, "the disadvantages of hinges are well known."[55] The total condylar prosthesis included a cobalt chromium femur with a so-called J curve intended to provide conformity in extension but allow rotation and anteroposterior translation in flexion. The femur also was designed with an anterior flange to articulate with the native patella or with an optional patella "dome." The all-polyethylene tibia featured a large keel shaped to fit against the posterior cortex of the

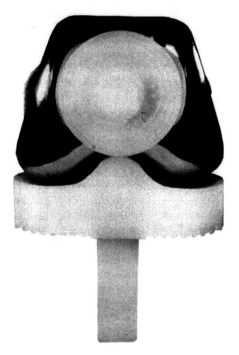

FIGURE 1-9 Photograph showing the total condylar knee.

tibia designed to enhance fixation. The tibial surface was designed with "cup" shaped articulations for the femoral condyles with a median intercondylar eminence to enhance stability. Incorporating the keel and intercondylar eminence required excision of both cruciate ligaments, which the authors felt superfluous given the stability afforded by the cupping and intercondylar eminence. Excising the cruciates provided greater ability to correct deformity and improve exposure of the tibia and femur to facilitate use of new instruments to accurately implant the components, which Insall considered paramount for successful prosthetic function and longevity.[56] The published technique included references to using spacers to check for equal flexion and extension spaces and ligament releases to achieve a balanced knee.[55] Targeted tibial component position was 90° to the mechanical axis of the tibia in the coronal and sagittal planes; these targets were achieved within 5° in 99% and 92% of cases, respectively.[55] Targeted femoral component position was 5° valgus on the anteroposterior radiograph and 90° to the femoral shaft on the lateral radiograph; these targets were achieved within 5° in 82% and 73% of cases, respectively.[55] The authors reported encouraging results at 3- to 5-year follow-up with 198 of 220 knees having an excellent or good result,[57] which exceeded their previously reported experience with other prosthetic designs.[27]

In 1978, Dr Insall, working with engineer Albert Burstein at HSS, introduced a modified total condylar prosthesis that he called the posterior stabilized condylar prosthesis and would later become known as the Insall-Burstein Posterior Stabilized (IBPS) prosthesis.[58] The IBPS was developed to address two specific concerns with the total condylar knee: (1) laxity in flexion/posterior

subluxation and (2) limited motion (90° on average)/difficulties climbing stairs.[58] The IBPS maintained many features of the total condylar prosthesis but incorporated a central polyethylene spine on the articular side of the tibial component and a cam mechanism on the femoral component. As the tibial spine engaged the femoral cam, the tibia was pushed forward, creating femoral rollback. The tibial spine was not designed to provide any varus–valgus stability. The tibial component was all-polyethylene. The IBPS knee was implanted in a cohort of 118 knees between 1978 and 1979, and results at 2- to 4-year follow-up exceeded a cohort of patients implanted with the total condylar prosthesis in terms of function and motion and demonstrated no difference in radiolucent lines.[58] Over longer-term follow-up, 9 to 12 years, the IBPS knee also demonstrated better functional outcomes and similar survivorship compared to a similar cohort implanted with the total condylar prosthesis.[59] Laboratory research indicated that a metal-backed tibial component better optimized load transmission at the bone–prosthesis interface, and by November 1980 the first metal-backed tibial monoblock component was implanted.[59]

As prosthesis design continued to be refined, concepts from the functional and anatomic approaches blended; however, two separate techniques coalesced around the fate of the posterior cruciate ligament (PCL). Proponents of posterior cruciate retaining (CR) designs suggested that retaining the PCL when performing TKA provides increased proprioception[60-64] and a more normal gait pattern.[65-67] Supporters of posterior cruciate sacrificing (PS) designs posit that sacrifice of the PCL provides increased knee range of motion[68-71] and more predictable femoral rollback[68,72,73] and is technically easier to achieve a balanced knee. A Cochrane meta-analysis found no significant difference between CR and PS designs in terms of motion.[74] As implant designs continue to evolve, with most companies now offering multiple polyethylene designs to mate with the tibial baseplate, surgeons could fine-tune the arthroplasty construct. Recently, published data suggest that this historic argument may be a moot point, as good results may be obtained with PCL retention with congruent bearings[75] as well as with PCL sacrifice with a CR femur and appropriate polyethylene design.[76-78]

CEMENTLESS FIXATION

In the late 1970s, David Hungerford, a surgeon working at Johns Hopkins, began developing a prosthesis and surgical techniques to perform TKA utilizing osseointegration for fixation. Dr Hungerford observed relatively high rates of failure with surface replacement prostheses and felt that the bone–cement interface would not survive the high stresses of the knee over the long term and biologic fixation, being a "living entity," would be able to respond to physiologic stresses.[79,80] He also noted that cement application devascularized adjacent cancellous bone due to the exothermic polymerization reaction, which resulted in the bone–cement interface being separated by a layer of fibrous tissue, rcgardless of the quality of the cement technique employed.[79,80] Cementless fixation would also eliminate the possibility of retained cement debris as a cause for third-body wear within the joint and provide the theoretical advantage of preservation of bone stock if revision were later required.[79,80]

The Porous-Coated Anatomic (PCA) knee prosthesis was designed to provide fixation without cement utilizing a porous surface on all three components comprised of sintered chrome cobalt beads with average pore size of 425 microns and porosity of 35% (**Fig. 1-10**).[79] The femoral component was asymmetric with medial and lateral condyles having different radius of curvature and resulted in 7 mm of lateral posterior condyle being replaced compared to 8.5 mm on the medial posterior femoral condyle to facilitate external rotation of the tibia in flexion.[79] The condyles were flattened in the coronal plane to increase contact area with the tibia.[79,80] There were porous coated lugs on the medial and lateral aspects. The tibia was asymmetric and designed for cementless or cemented fixation. The cementless baseplate had cobalt-chrome porous coat beads similar to the femur and medial and lateral fixation pegs with 30° posterior slope and required supplemental fixation with a molly bolt or vitallium screw anteriorly.[79] The polyethylene incorporated asymmetric plateaus; the medial plateau was more conforming than the lateral plateau and both were relatively flat in the coronal plane to increase surface contact area.[79,80] The patellar component was shaped anatomically with medial and lateral facets and was metal-backed for cementless fixation.[79] The PCA prosthesis was designed for cementless implantation but could also be cemented if desired. The authors recommended cement fixation if any movement or rocking of components was noted intraoperatively, recognizing the importance of precise bone cuts to provide initial implant stability to permit osseointegration rather than fibrous ingrowth.[79,80] The importance of precise bone cuts led the authors to develop the Universal Total Knee Instrumentation System, which relied on long, extramedullary alignment rods to position cutting blocks.[79] The technique attempted to reproduce normal coronal plane alignment, which the authors described as 3° valgus; this was achieved by making coronal cuts of 3° varus at the tibia and 9° valgus at the distal femur.[79]

Hungerford and colleagues reported early results for 63 TKAs (56 patients) performed using the PCA prosthesis and follow-up was available for 46 TKAs (41 patients) (range 4 to 25 months, mean 12 months). Radiographic lucency was not seen on any femoral or patellar components but was occasionally seen in zones 15 and 19 (medial and lateral) of the tibia.[80] The authors initially utilized cementless fixation selectively, but by the end of their initial experience they reported utilizing cementless fixation in greater than 90% of patients indicated for TKA at their institution. Longer-term follow-up data demonstrated high failure rates. One study reported only 77% survivorship at 6-year follow-up; all failures were attributed to the tibial component, although the authors did not routinely resurface the patella.[81] In addition to problems with tibial fixation, longer-term follow-up revealed problems with the design and manufacturing of the polyethylene implanted with the PCA.[82,83] The nonconforming geometry exposed the bearing to the highest contact pressures and the polyethylene was heat-treated, leaving it vulnerable to surface delamination.[82,83] There were also problems related to aseptic loosening and wear of the metal-backed patella.[84]

Several recent systematic reviews and meta-analyses have reported equivalent survivorship between cementless and cemented TKA at medium- to longer-term follow-up.[85-88]

More recent attempts at cementless total knee arthroplasty have utilized highly porous metal designs that seek to more closely mimic human trabecular bone and provide improved ingrowth surface. However, despite encouraging survivorship data, there has not been high-quality data published to suggest cementless TKA improves outcomes compared to cemented TKA.[89,90] At the time of this writing (2019) cementless fixation in TKA appears promising but has not yet shown any definitive advantages compared to cemented TKA, which remains the gold standard.

MOBILE BEARING

Mobile bearing in knee arthroplasty started in the late 1970s with the work of surgeon John Goodfellow and engineer John O'Connor, working at the Nuffield Orthopaedic Centre, Oxford, England. Goodfellow and O'Connor described the competing issues regarding bearing surface geometry.[91] Conforming geometries (round on round) provided mechanical stability and increased surface area of bearing contact to minimize contact pressures but did so at the expense of altered knee kinematics and transmitting forces to the bone–implant interface that might increase risk for loosening. A nonconforming tibiofemoral geometry (round on flat) did not impose kinematic conflict and attempted to minimize force transmission to the bone–implant interface

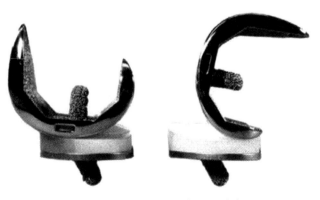

FIGURE 1-10   Porous-coated anatomic knee.

but provided less joint stability and had a small surface area of bearing contact that led to high pressure and wear. Their innovative solution was to utilize mobile "washers" that conformed to the femoral surface and were free to move along the tibia.[91] This design included a so-called meniscal bearing, which utilized a polyethylene insert dished on the femoral surface and flat on the tibial surface that allowed the polyethylene component to translate in the sagittal plane (anterior/posterior) along the tibial tray.[91]

Buechel, a surgeon working at the University of Medicine and Dentistry New Jersey (UMDNJ), and engineer M.J. Pappas developed the New Jersey Low-Contact-Stress (LCS) knee replacement system to incorporate the principles of mobile bearing for TKA (**Fig. 1-11**). The system was diverse and incorporated components for unicompartmental, bicruciate retaining, posterior cruciate retaining, and posterior cruciate sacrificing arthroplasty. The rotating platform design was intended for use in the absence of the posterior cruciate ligament. The rotating platform design incorporated a polyethylene with conforming articular geometry and a stem that fit into the tibial baseplate that allowed axial motion but no sagittal or coronal translation of the polyethylene.[92] The design was intended to provide simultaneously for low contact stress via conforming articular geometry and to minimize stresses to the bone–implant interface via axial mobility at the polyethylene–tibial baseplate interface. This axial mobility would provide additional benefits of accommodating a certain degree of surgical component malalignment and allowing the surgeon freedom to rotate the tibial baseplate to achieve maximal bony coverage of the tibia.[92,93] The system would be made available for both cemented and cementless fixation. The design was subject to the unique failure method of dislocation of the rotating platform, which the authors noted occurred in 1.2% of cases in a multicenter trial.[93]

The concept of mobile bearing in knee arthroplasty was developed to achieve several goals, including stress-reduction at the tibial implant–bone interface, decreased

polyethylene wear at the interface between the femur and polyethylene insert, and to provide improved kinematics. Mobile bearing designs also resulted in unique problems, the most serious of which include bearing dislocation. Systematic reviews have failed to demonstrate any difference in outcomes between fixed-bearing and mobile bearing TKA designs.[94-96]

ALTERNATIVE MATERIALS IN TKA

Despite significant advancements in TKA, failures persist. Registry and long-term follow-up data suggest that aseptic loosening remains a significant mechanism of TKA failure.[97,98] Given this, surgeons and implant manufacturers have sought to develop alternative bearing surfaces to address this problem. Ceramic on polyethylene as a bearing couple has shown significant promise for low rates of wear.[99,100] In addition to addressing wear-related concerns, these systems were also developed to be metal-free or nickel-free, which has advantages in patients with metal sensitivity, which are reported in approximately 10% to 20% of patients.[101] Concerns with ceramics in TKA include brittleness with increased risk or fracture[102,103] and concerns for increased risk of debonding at the cement–implant interface.[104-106] A recent systematic identified 14 published studies including 1438 TKAs (1245 patients) and reported survival rate of 98% at 5 years and 95% at 20-year follow-up.[107] All studies included ceramic femoral prosthesis (alumina, zirconia, zirconia/niobium, alumina/zirconia, or alumina/yttria) and either metal or ceramic tibial baseplate. Further investigation of ceramics in TKA is necessarily prior to widespread adoption of these technologies.

ADVANCES IN PERIOPERATIVE CARE

Venous thromboembolism (VTE) represents a relatively common complication following TKA. Fortunately, however, life-threatening VTE is relatively an uncommon event. VTE prophylaxis following TKA has evolved over time as surgeons and other providers have sought to balance the risk of perioperative bleeding complications, including need for transfusion and wound complications, against the competing interest of preventing life-threatening VTE. Heparin, enoxaparin, and warfarin were traditionally used for VTE prophylaxis. These agents typically required monitoring and injection and were associated with bleeding and wound complications. Newer oral agents have been developed that typically do not require monitoring and have indications for VTE prophylaxis: examples include apixaban, rivaroxaban, dabigatran, and others. Concerns with these newer oral agents included bleeding and wound healing problems and lack of or inconvenient reversal agent. Aspirin (ASA) has been demonstrated effective to prevent serious VTE events and lower risk of major bleeding compared to other agents.[108,109] Clinical practice guidelines have

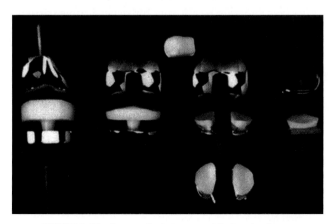

FIGURE 1-11   Low-contact-stress mobile bearing knee.

recently recognized ASA as a chemotherapeutic agent for VTE prophylaxis following major orthopedic surgery, which includes TXA.[110] Recent work supports an expanding role for ASA in TKA. ASA demonstrated equal efficacy to prevent VTE in high-risk patients compared to more potent agents[111] and a separate study suggested that ASA use following TKA provided an all-cause mortality benefit.[112] Low-dose ASA (81 mg BID) has recently been shown to be safe and effective following TKA.[113]

Tranexamic acid (TXA) is a synthetic derivative of the amino acid lysine (4-aminoethyl cyclohexane carboxylic acid) that reversibly blocks lysine binding sites on plasminogen molecules, which reduces the conversion of plasminogen to plasmin and stabilizes fibrin clots.[114,115] TXA has been shown effective in reducing blood loss and transfusion rate following TKA without increasing the rates of VTE.[116] TXA may be administered intravenously, orally, or topically and these various routes of administration appear equally effective.[116,117] The optimal dosing strategy for TXA has evolved and recent evidence suggests that a single 1 g dose is effective.[118]

Rehabilitation following TKA is important to achieve optimal outcomes. Protocols should seek to maximize patient safety and functional outcomes while minimizing cost and inconvenience for patients. Early protocols prescribed bed rest and a Robert Jones dressing for up to 1 week postoperatively followed by gradual motion. Continuous passive motion (CPM) machines were widely utilized in the past to get the operative knee moving; however, these devices are no longer used routinely given the absence of data demonstrating any advantage to early active motion.[119] More recently, there has been interest in developing therapy protocols without direct involvement of formal physical therapy (PT). Patients were typically guided through therapy with a PT, either with home therapy or with outpatient therapy; however, there has been increased interest in home-based therapy protocols without direct involvement of a physical therapist due to concerns over cost, convenience, and patient preference. Randomized controlled trials (RCTs) have shown that supervised home-based programs provide equivalent outcomes to formal outpatient PT protocols.[120,121] Additionally, investigators have also demonstrated that therapy administered via Web-based protocols can be effective.[122-124]

In the past decade, new anesthesia and analgesic techniques have been introduced for TKA patients. Opioids have been the historic gold standard for pain management but are associated with a host of adverse effects[125-128] and a growing recognition of the potential for abuse. Multimodal analgesia protocols have been developed to mitigate pain while simultaneously decreasing narcotic usage, minimize adverse medication effects, and maximize patient function. Protocols typically utilize preoperative peripheral nerve blockade, intraoperative periarticular injection, and various medications in the postoperative setting. The adductor canal blockade was developed to block the saphenous nerve in the adductor (Hunter's) canal,[129] which blocks the majority of sensory nerves to the knee but preserves quadriceps function more than lumbar plexus and femoral nerve blocks.[130,131] Periarticular injections have been of interest to surgeons and many different cocktails for injection has been used. Liposomal bupivacaine gained significant interest as a means to provide prolonged analgesia at the surgical site, but evidence regarding the benefits of liposomal bupivacaine has been conflicting and inconclusive and to date there is no evidence supporting its superiority to other techniques.[132-134]

Hospital length of stay (LOS) following TKA has decreased over the past decade as a result of improvements in care pathways as highlighted above as well as patient preferences and pressure from payers. Minimizing LOS following TKA has been shown to improve patient outcomes, reduce infection rates, and be cost-effective.[135-137] The natural extension of this trend toward reduced LOS following TKA has been same-day surgery, which has proven successful in specific settings.[138,139]

FUTURE OUTLOOK

The innovators of total knee arthroplasty have collectively brought us to the current situation where TKA provides a reliable procedure to alleviate pain and improve function for patients with degenerative joint disease (DJD) of the knee. Demand for TKA will continue to grow as the population ages and patients desire to remain active throughout their lives. Estimates suggest that by the year 2030 the demand for TKA will be 3.5 million procedures annually.[140] Despite significant advances in total knee arthroplasty, a small subset of patients remain dissatisfied following TKA. As surgeons, engineers, and implant manufacturers seek to improve outcomes, they have focused on robotics, computer navigation systems, surgical techniques (kinematic vs. mechanical alignment), and implant refinement. To date, there has not been significant evidence that any of these evolving innovations translate to provide improved patient outcomes. In addition to improvements in TKA, researchers are continuing to seek biologic treatments for degenerative cartilage lesions—as greater understanding of the human genome, stem cells, and three-dimensional printing technologies continues to improve, it is likely that the future of care for DJD of the knee will incorporate these technologies.

REFERENCES

1. Anthony White (Obituary). *Lancet.* 1849;1:324.
2. Ferguson M. Excision of the knee joint: recovery with a false joint and a useful limb. *Med Times Gaz.* 1861;1:601.
3. Gluck T. The classic: report on the positive results obtained by the modern surgical experiment regarding the suture and replacement of defects of superior tissue, as well as the utilization of reabsorbable and living tamponade in surgery. *Clin Orthop Relat Res.* 2011;469:1528-1535.

4. Eynon-Lewis NJ, Ferry D, Pearse MF. Themistocles Gluck: an unrecognised genius. *BMJ*. 1992;305:1534-1536.

5. Brand RA, Mont MA, Manring MM. Biographical sketch: Themistocles Gluck (1853-1942). *Clin Orthop Relat Res*. 2011;469:1525-1527.

6. Verneuil A. De la creation d'une fausse articulation par section ou resection partielle de 1'os maxillaire inferieur, comme moyen de remedier a 1'ankylose vraie ou fausse de la machoire inferieure. *Arch Gen Med*. 1860;15:174.

7. Kuhns JG, Potter TA, Hormell RS, Elliston WA. Nylon membrane arthroplasty of the knee in chronic arthritis. *J Bone Joint Surg Am*. 1953;35-A:929-936.

8. Murphy JB. The classic: ankylosis: arthroplasty—clinical and experimental. *Clin Orthop Relat Res*. 2008;466:2573-2578.

9. Murphy JB. Arthroplasty. *Ann Surg*. 1913;57:593-647.

10. Campbell WC. Arthroplasty of the knee. *Ann Surg*. 1924;80:88-102.

11. Townley CO, Marmor L. The classic: articular-plate replacement arthroplasty for the knee joint. *Clin Orthop Relat Res*. 2005;440:9-12.

12. Campbell WC. Interposition of vitallium plates in arthroplasties of the knee. Preliminary report. By Willis C. Campbell, 1940. *Clin Orthop Relat Res*. 1988;226:3-5.

13. Pritchett JW. Obituary: Charles O. Townley, MD, 1916-2006. *Clin Orthop Relat Res*. 2009;467:308-309.

14. McKeever DC, Pickett JC. The classic: tibial plateau prosthesis. *Clin Orthop Relat Res*. 1985;192:3-12.

15. Springer BD, Scott RD, Sah AP, Carrington R. McKeever hemiarthroplasty of the knee in patients less than sixty years old. *J Bone Joint Surg Am*. 2006;88:366-371.

16. Scott RD, Joyce MJ, Ewald FC, Thomas WH. McKeever metallic hemiarthroplasty of the knee in unicompartmental degenerative arthritis. Long-term clinical follow-up and current indications. *J Bone Joint Surg Am*. 1985;67:203-207.

17. McKeever DC, Sherk HH. The classic: patellar prosthesis. *Clin Orthop Relat Res*. 2005;440:13-21.

18. Harrington KD. Long-term results for the McKeever patellar resurfacing prosthesis used as a salvage procedure for severe chondromalacia patellae. *Clin Orthop Relat Res*. 1992;279:201-213.

19. Judet J, Judet R. Essais de prosthese osteso-articulaire. *Presse Med*. 1947;55:302.

20. Magnoni DJ. Genou en resin acrylique. *Rev Chir Orthop Reparatrice Appar Mot*. 1949;35:556.

21. Walldius B. Arthroplasty of the knee joint employing an acrylic prosthesis. *Acta Orthop Scand*. 1953;23:121-131.

22. Walldius B. Arthroplasty of the knee using an endoprosthesis. *Acta Orthop Scand Suppl*. 1957;24:1-112.

23. Walldius B. Arthroplasty of the knee using an endoprosthesis. 8 years' experience. *Acta Orthop Scand*. 1960;30:137-148.

24. Shiers LG. Arthroplasty of the knee; preliminary report of new method. *J Bone Joint Surg Br*. 1954;36-B:553-560.

25. Young HH. Use of a hinged vitallium prosthesis for arthroplasty of the knee. A preliminary report. *J Bone Joint Surg Am*. 1963;45:1627-1642.

26. Mazas FB. Guepar total knee prosthesis. *Clin Orthop Relat Res*. 1973;94:211-221. doi:10.1097/00003086-197307000-00026.

27. Insall JN, Ranawat CS, Aglietti P, Shine J. A comparison of four models of total knee-replacement prostheses. *J Bone Joint Surg Am*. 1976;58:754-765.

28. Matthews LS, Sonstegard DA, Kaufer H. The spherocentric knee. *Clin Orthop Relat Res*. 1973;94:234-241. doi:10.1097/00003086-197307000-00028.

29. Matthews LS, Goldstein SA, Kolowich PA, Kaufer H. Spherocentric arthroplasty of the knee. A long-term and final follow-up evaluation. *Clin Orthop Relat Res*. 1986;205:58-66.

30. Gunston FH. Polycentric knee arthroplasty. Prosthetic simulation of normal knee movement. *J Bone Joint Surg Br*. 1971;53:272-277.

31. Bryan RS, Peterson LF, Combs JJ. Polycentric knee arthroplasty. A preliminary report of postoperative complications in 450 knees. *Clin Orthop Relat Res*. 1973;94:148-152.

32. Lewallen DG, Bryan RS, Peterson LF. Polycentric total knee arthroplasty. A ten-year follow-up study. *J Bone Joint Surg Am*. 1984;66:1211-1218.

33. Yamamoto S. Total knee replacement with the Kodama-Yamamoto knee prosthesis. *Clin Orthop Relat Res*. 1979;(145):60-67.

34. Waugh TR, Smith RC, Orofino CF, Anzel SM. Total knee replacement: operative technic and preliminary results. *Clin Orthop Relat Res*. 1973;94:196-201.

35. Evanski PM, Waugh TR, Orofino CF, Anzel SH. UCI knee replacement. *Clin Orthop Relat Res*. 1976;120:33-38.

36. Townley C, Hill L. Total knee replacement. *Am J Nurs*. 1974;74:1612-1617.

37. Seedhom BB, Longton EB, Dowson D, Wright V. Designing a total knee prosthesis. *Eng Med*. 1972;1:28-32.

38. Robinson RP. The early innovators of today's resurfacing condylar knees. *J Arthroplasty*. 2005;20:2-26.

39. Ranawat CS, Shine JJ. Duo-condylar total knee arthroplasty. *Clin Orthop Relat Res*. 1973;94:185-195. doi:10.1097/00003086-197307000-00023.

40. Ranawat CS, Insall J, Shine J. Duo-condylar knee arthroplasty: hospital for special surgery design. *Clin Orthop Relat Res*. 1976;(120):76-82.

41. Sledge CB, Ewald FC. Total knee arthroplasty experience at the Robert Breck Brigham hospital. *Clin Orthop Relat Res*. 1979;145:78-84.

42. Scott RD. Duopatellar total knee replacement: the Brigham experience. *Orthop Clin North Am*. 1982;13:89-102.

43. Ranawat CS. History of total knee replacement. *J South Orthop Assoc*. 2002;11:218-226.

44. Ewald FC, Jacobs MA, Miegel RE, Walker PS, Poss R, Sledge CB. Kinematic total knee replacement. *J Bone Joint Surg Am*. 1984;66:1032-1040.

45. Malkani AL, Rand JA, Bryan RS, Wallrichs SL. Total knee arthroplasty with the kinematic condylar prosthesis. A ten-year follow-up study. *J Bone Joint Surg Am*. 1995;77:423-431.

46. Back DL, Cannon SR, Hilton A, Bankes MJ, Briggs TW. The Kinemax total knee arthroplasty. Nine years' experience. *J Bone Joint Surg Br*. 2001;83:359-363.

47. Scott RD, Thornhill TS. Posterior cruciate supplementing total knee replacement using conforming inserts and cruciate recession. Effect on range of motion and radiolucent lines. *Clin Orthop Relat Res*. 1994;309:146-149.

48. Freeman MA, Swanson SA, Todd RC. Total replacement of the knee design considerations and early clinical results. *Acta Orthop Belg*. 1973;39:181-202.

49. Freeman MA, Swanson SA, Todd RC. Total replacement of the knee using the Freeman-Swanson knee prosthesis. *Clin Orthop Relat Res*. 1973;94:153-170. doi:10.1097/00003086-197307000-00020.

50. Freeman MA, Levack B. British contribution to knee arthroplasty. *Clin Orthop Relat Res*. 1986;210:69-79.

51. Freeman MA, Sculco T, Todd RC. Replacement of the severely damaged arthritic knee by the ICLH (Freeman-Swanson) arthroplasty. *J Bone Joint Surg Br*. 1977;59:64-71.

52. Freeman MA, Todd RC, Bamert P, Day WH. ICLH arthroplasty of the knee: 1968-1977. *J Bone Joint Surg Br*. 1978;60-B: 339-344.

53. Coventry MB, Finerman GA, Riley LH, Turner RH, Upshaw JE. A new geometric knee for total knee arthroplasty. *Clin Orthop Relat Res*. 1972;83:157-162.

54. Riley LH. Geometric total knee replacement. Operative considerations. *Orthop Clin North Am*. 1973;4:561-573.

55. Insall J, Ranawat CS, Scott WN, Walker P. Total condylar knee replacment: preliminary report. *Clin Orthop Relat Res*. 1976;120:149-154.

56. Scuderi GR, Scott WN, Tchejeyan GH. The Insall legacy in total knee arthroplasty. *Clin Orthop Relat Res.* 2001;392:3-14. doi:10.1097/00003086-200111000-00002.

57. Insall J, Scott WN, Ranawat CS. The total condylar knee prosthesis. A report of two hundred and twenty cases. *J Bone Joint Surg Am.* 1979;61:173-180.

58. Insall JN, Lachiewicz PF, Burstein AH. The posterior stabilized condylar prosthesis: a modification of the total condylar design. Two to four-year clinical experience. *J Bone Joint Surg Am.* 1982;64:1317-1323.

59. Stern SH, Insall JN. Posterior stabilized prosthesis. Results after follow-up of nine to twelve years. *J Bone Joint Surg Am.* 1992;74:980-986.

60. Nelissen RG, Hogendoorn PC. Retain or sacrifice the posterior cruciate ligament in total knee arthroplasty? A histopathological study of the cruciate ligament in osteoarthritic and rheumatoid disease. *J Clin Pathol.* 2001;54:381-384.

61. Martins GC, Camanho G, Rodrigues MI. Immunohistochemical analysis of the neural structures of the posterior cruciate ligament in osteoarthritis patients submitted to total knee arthroplasty: an analysis of thirty-four cases. *Clinics.* 2015;70:81-86.

62. Del Valle ME, Harwin SF, Maestro A, Murcia A, Vega JA. Immunohistochemical analysis of mechanoreceptors in the human posterior cruciate ligament: a demonstration of its proprioceptive role and clinical relevance. *J Arthroplasty.* 1998;13:916-922.

63. Simmons S, Lephart S, Rubash H, Borsa P, Barrack RL. Proprioception following total knee arthroplasty with and without the posterior cruciate ligament. *J Arthroplasty.* 1996;11:763-768.

64. Schultz RA, Miller DC, Kerr CS, Micheli L. Mechanoreceptors in human cruciate ligaments. A histological study. *J Bone Joint Surg Am.* 1984;66:1072-1076.

65. Andriacchi TP, Galante JO, Fermier RW. The influence of total knee-replacement design on walking and stair-climbing. *J Bone Joint Surg Am.* 1982;64:1328-1335.

66. Kelman GJ, Biden EN, Wyatt MP, Ritter MA, Colwell CW. Gait laboratory analysis of a posterior cruciate-sparing total knee arthroplasty in stair ascent and descent. *Clin Orthop Relat Res.* 1989;248:21-25; discussion 25-6.

67. Dorr LD, Ochsner JL, Gronley J, Perry J. Functional comparison of posterior cruciate-retained versus cruciate-sacrificed total knee arthroplasty. *Clin Orthop Relat Res.* 1988;236:36-43.

68. Yoshiya S, Matsui N, Komistek RD, Dennis DA, Mahfouz M, Kurosaka M. In vivo kinematic comparison of posterior cruciate-retaining and posterior stabilized total knee arthroplasties under passive and weight-bearing conditions. *J Arthroplasty.* 2005;20:777-783.

69. Li N, Tan Y, Deng Y, Chen L. Posterior cruciate-retaining versus posterior stabilized total knee arthroplasty: a meta-analysis of randomized controlled trials. *Knee Surg Sports Traumatol Arthrosc.* 2014;22:556-564.

70. Matsumoto T, Muratsu H, Kubo S, Matsushita T, Kurosaka M, Kuroda R. Intraoperative soft tissue balance reflects minimum 5-year midterm outcomes in cruciate-retaining and posterior-stabilized total knee arthroplasty. *J Arthroplasty.* 2012;27:1723-1730.

71. Jiang C, Liu Z, Wang Y, Bian Y, Feng B, Weng X. Posterior cruciate ligament retention versus posterior stabilization for total knee arthroplasty: a meta-analysis. *PLoS One.* 2016;11:e0147865.

72. Dennis DA, Komistek RD, Colwell CE, et al. In vivo anteroposterior femorotibial translation of total knee arthroplasty: a multicenter analysis. *Clin Orthop Relat Res.* 1998;356:47-57.

73. Straw R, Kulkarni S, Attfield S, Wilton TJ. Posterior cruciate ligament at total knee replacement. Essential, beneficial or a hindrance? *J Bone Joint Surg Br.* 2003;85:671-674.

74. Verra WC, van den Boom LGH, Jacobs W, Clement DJ, Wymenga AAB,Nelissen RGHH. Retention versus sacrifice of the posterior cruciate ligament in total knee arthroplasty for treating osteoarthritis. *Cochrane Database Syst Rev.* 2013;(10):CD004803. doi:10.1002/14651858.CD004803.pub3.

75. Stronach BM, Adams JC, Jones LC, Farrell SM, Hydrick JM. The effect of sacrificing the posterior cruciate ligament in total knee arthroplasties that use a highly congruent polyethylene component. *J Arthroplasty.* 2019;34:286-289.

76. Parsley BS, Conditt MA, Bertolusso R, Noble PC. Posterior cruciate ligament substitution is not essential for excellent postoperative outcomes in total knee arthroplasty. *J Arthroplasty.* 2006;21:127-131.

77. Sathappan SS, Wasserman B, Jaffe WL, Bong M, Walsh M, Di Cesare PE. Midterm results of primary total knee arthroplasty using a dished polyethylene insert with a recessed or resected posterior cruciate ligament. *J Arthroplasty.* 2006;21:1012-1016.

78. Dion C, Howard J, McAuley J. Does recession of the posterior cruciate ligament influence outcome in total knee arthroplasty? *J Arthroplasty.* 2019;34:2383-2387.

79. Hungerford DS, Kenna RV, Krackow KA. The porous-coated anatomic total knee. *Orthop Clin North Am.* 1982;13:103-122.

80. Hungerford DS, Kenna RV. Preliminary experience with a total knee prosthesis with porous coating used without cement. *Clin Orthop Relat Res.* 1983;176:95-107.

81. Moran CG, Pinder IM, Lees TA, Midwinter MJ. Survivorship analysis of the uncemented porous-coated anatomic knee replacement. *J Bone Joint Surg Am.* 1991;73:848-857.

82. Wright TM, Rimnac CM, Stulberg SD, et al. Wear of polyethylene in total joint replacements. Observations from retrieved PCA knee implants. *Clin Orthop Relat Res.* 1992;276:126-134.

83. Collier JP, Mayor MB, McNamara JL, Surprenant VA, Jensen RE. Analysis of the failure of 122 polyethylene inserts from uncemented tibial knee components. *Clin Orthop Relat Res.* 1991;273:232-242.

84. Firestone TP, Teeny SM, Krackow KA, Hungerford DS. The clinical and roentgenographic results of cementless porous-coated patellar fixation. *Clin Orthop Relat Res.* 1991;273:184-189.

85. Mont MA, Pivec R, Issa K, Kapadia BH, Maheshwari A, Harwin SF. Long-term implant survivorship of cementless total knee arthroplasty: a systematic review of the literature and meta-analysis. *J Knee Surg.* 2014;27:369-376.

86. Zhou K, Yu H, Li J, Wang H, Zhou Z, Pei F. No difference in implant survivorship and clinical outcomes between full-cementless and full-cemented fixation in primary total knee arthroplasty: a systematic review and meta-analysis. *Int J Surg.* 2018;53:312-319.

87. Hu B, Chen Y, Zhu H, Wu H, Yan S. Cementless porous tantalum monoblock tibia vs cemented modular tibia in primary total knee arthroplasty: a meta-analysis. *J Arthroplasty.* 2017;32:666-674.

88. Franceschetti E, Torre G, Palumbo A, et al. No difference between cemented and cementless total knee arthroplasty in young patients: a review of the evidence. *Knee Surg Sports Traumatol Arthrosc.* 2017;25:1749-1756.

89. Fricka KB, McAsey CJ, Sritulanondha S. To cement or not? Five-year results of a prospective, randomized study comparing cemented vs cementless total knee arthroplasty. *J Arthroplasty.* 2019;34:S183-S187.

90. Boyle KK, Nodzo SR, Ferraro JT, Augenblick DJ, Pavlesen S, Phillips MJ. Uncemented vs cemented cruciate retaining total knee arthroplasty in patients with body mass index greater than 30. *J Arthroplasty.* 2018;33:1082-1088.

91. Goodfellow J, O'Connor J. The mechanics of the knee and prosthesis design. *J Bone Joint Surg Br.* 1978;60-B:358-369.

92. Buechel FF, Pappas MJ. The New Jersey low-contact-stress knee replacement system: biomechanical rationale and review of the first 123 cemented cases. *Arch Orthop Trauma Surg.* 1986;105:197-204.

93. Buechel FF, Pappas MJ. New Jersey low contact stress knee replacement system. Ten-year evaluation of meniscal bearings. *Orthop Clin North Am.* 1989;20:147-177.

94. Fransen BL, van Duijvenbode DC, Hoozemans MJM, Burger BJ. No differences between fixed- and mobile-bearing total knee arthroplasty. *Knee Surg Sports Traumatol Arthrosc.* 2017;25:1757-1777.

95. Hofstede SN, Nouta KA, Jacobs W, et al. Mobile bearing vs fixed bearing prostheses for posterior cruciate retaining total knee arthroplasty for postoperative functional status in patients with osteoarthritis and rheumatoid arthritis. *Cochrane Database Syst Rev.* 2015;(2):CD003130. doi:10.1002/14651858.CD003130.pub3.

96. Sappey-Marinier E, de Abreu FGA, O'Loughlin P, et al. No difference in patellar position between mobile-bearing and fixed-bearing total knee arthroplasty for medial osteoarthritis: a prospective randomized study. *Knee Surg Sports Traumatol Arthrosc.* 2019. doi:10.1007/s00167-019-05565-5.

97. Sharkey PF, Lichstein PM, Shen C, Tokarski AT, Parvizi J. Why are total knee arthroplasties failing today—has anything changed after 10 years? *J Arthroplasty.* 2014;29:1774-1778.

98. Abdel MP, Ledford CK, Kobic A, Taunton MJ, Hanssen AD. Contemporary failure aetiologies of the primary, posterior-stabilised total knee arthroplasty. *Bone Joint J.* 2017;99-B:647-652.

99. Bizot P, Hannouche D, Nizard R, Witvoet J, Sedel L. Hybrid alumina total hip arthroplasty using a press-fit metal-backed socket in patients younger than 55 years. A six- to 11-year evaluation. *J Bone Joint Surg Br.* 2004;86:190-194.

100. Hamadouche M, Boutin P, Daussange J, Bolander ME, Sedel L. Alumina-on-alumina total hip arthroplasty: a minimum 18.5-year follow-up study. *J Bone Joint Surg Am.* 2002;84:69-77.

101. Frigerio E, Pigatto PD, Guzzi G, Altomare G. Metal sensitivity in patients with orthopaedic implants: a prospective study. *Contact Dermatitis.* 2011;64:273-279.

102. Traina F, De Fine M, Di Martino A, Faldini C. Fracture of ceramic bearing surfaces following total hip replacement: a systematic review. *BioMed Res Int.* 2013;2013:157247.

103. Howard DP, Wall PDH, Fernandez MA, Parsons H, Howard PW. Ceramic-on-ceramic bearing fractures in total hip arthroplasty: an analysis of data from the National Joint Registry. *Bone Joint J.* 2017;99-B:1012-1019.

104. Bergschmidt P, Bader R, Ganzer D, et al. Ceramic femoral components in total knee arthroplasty - two year follow-up results of an international prospective multi-centre study. *Open Orthop J.* 2012;6:172-178.

105. Kumahashi N, Uchio Y, Kitamura N, Satake S, Iwamoto M, Yasuda K. Biomechanical comparison of the strength of adhesion of polymethylmethacrylate cement to zirconia ceramic and cobalt-chromium alloy components in a total knee arthroplasty. *J Orthop Sci.* 2014;19:940-947.

106. Lionberger D, Conlon C, Wattenbarger L, Timothy JW.. Unacceptable failure rate of a ceramic-coated posterior cruciate-substituting total knee arthroplasty. *Arthroplast Today.* 2019;5:187-192.

107. Xiang S, Zhao Y, Li Z, Feng B, Weng X. Clinical outcomes of ceramic femoral prosthesis in total knee arthroplasty: a systematic review. *J Orthop Surg Res.* 2019;14:57.

108. An VVG, Phan K, Levy YD, Bruce WJM. Aspirin as thromboprophylaxis in hip and knee arthroplasty: a systematic review and meta-analysis. *J Arthroplasty.* 2016;31:2608-2616.

109. Wilson DGG, Poole WEC, Chauhan SK, Rogers BA. Systematic review of aspirin for thromboprophylaxis in modern elective total hip and knee arthroplasty. *Bone Joint J.* 2016;98-B:1056-1061.

110. Falck-Ytter Y, Francis CW, Johanson NA, et al. Prevention of VTE in orthopedic surgery patients. Antithrombotic therapy and prevention of thrombosis, 9th ed: American College of Chest Physicians Evidence-Based Clinical Practice Guidelines. *Chest.* 2012;141:e278S-e325S.

111. Tan TL, Foltz C, Huang R, et al. Potent anticoagulation does not reduce venous thromboembolism in high-risk patients. *J Bone Joint Surg Am.* 2019;101:589-599.

112. Rondon AJ, Shohat N, Tan TL, Goswami K, Huang RC, Parvizi J. The use of aspirin for prophylaxis against venous thromboembolism decreases mortality following primary total joint arthroplasty. *J Bone Joint Surg Am.* 2019;101:504-513.

113. Faour M, Piuzzi NS, Brigati DP, et al. Low-dose aspirin is safe and effective for venous thromboembolism prophylaxis following total knee arthroplasty. *J Arthroplasty.* 2018;33:S131-S135.

114. Dunn CJ, Goa KL. Tranexamic acid: a review of its use in surgery and other indications. *Drugs.* 1999;57:1005-1032.

115. Nilsson IM. Clinical pharmacology of aminocaproic and tranexamic acids. *J Clin Pathol Suppl.* 1980;14:41-47.

116. Zhang L-K, Ma J-X, Kuang M-J, et al. The efficacy of tranexamic acid using oral administration in total knee arthroplasty: a systematic review and meta-analysis. *J Orthop Surg Res.* 2017;12:159.

117. Xie J, Hu Q, Huang Q, Ma J, Lei Y, Pei F. Comparison of intravenous versus topical tranexamic acid in primary total hip and knee arthroplasty: an updated meta-analysis. *Thromb Res.* 2017;153:28-36.

118. Wilde JM, Copp SN, McCauley JC, Bugbee WD. One dose of intravenous tranexamic acid is equivalent to two doses in total hip and knee arthroplasty. *J Bone Joint Surg Am.* 2018;100:1104-1109.

119. Harvey LA, Brosseau L, Herbert RD. Continuous passive motion following total knee arthroplasty in people with arthritis. *Cochrane Database Syst Rev.* 2010;(3):CD004260. doi:10.1002/14651858.CD004260.pub2.

120. Han ASY, Nairn L, Harmer AR, et al. Early rehabilitation after total knee replacement surgery: a multicenter, noninferiority, randomized clinical trial comparing a home exercise program with usual outpatient care. *Arthritis Care Res.* 2015;67:196-202.

121. Ko V, Naylor J, Harris I, Crosbie J, Yeo A, Mittal R. One-to-one therapy is not superior to group or home-based therapy after total knee arthroplasty: a randomized, superiority trial. *J Bone Joint Surg Am.* 2013;95:1942-1949.

122. Fleischman AN, Crizer MP, Tarabichi M, et al. 2018 John N. Insall Award: Recovery of knee flexion with unsupervised home exercise is not inferior to outpatient physical therapy after TKA: a randomized trial. *Clin Orthop Relat Res.* 2019;477:60-69.

123. Russell TG, Buttrum P, Wootton R, Jull GA. Internet-based outpatient telerehabilitation for patients following total knee arthroplasty: a randomized controlled trial. *J Bone Joint Surg Am.* 2011;93:113-120.

124. Jiang S, Xiang J, Gao X, Guo K, Liu B. The comparison of telerehabilitation and face-to-face rehabilitation after total knee arthroplasty: a systematic review and meta-analysis. *J Telemed Telecare.* 2018;24:257-262.

125. Horlocker TT, Kopp SL, Pagnano MW, Hebl JR. Analgesia for total hip and knee arthroplasty: a multimodal pathway featuring peripheral nerve block. *J Am Acad Orthop Surg.* 2006;14:126-135.

126. Block BM, Liu SS, Rowlingson AJ, Cowan AR, Cowan JA Jr, Wu CL. Efficacy of postoperative epidural analgesia: a meta-analysis. *J Am Med Assoc.* 2003;290:2455-2463.

127. Wheeler M, Oderda GM, Ashburn MA, Lipman AG. Adverse events associated with postoperative opioid analgesia: a systematic review. *J Pain.* 2002;3:159-180.

128. Rathmell JP, Pino CA, Taylor R, Patrin T, Viani BA. Intrathecal morphine for postoperative analgesia: a randomized, controlled, dose-ranging study after hip and knee arthroplasty. *Anesth Analg.* 2003;97:1452-1457.

129. van der Wal M, Lang SA, Yip RW. Transsartorial approach for saphenous nerve block. *Can J Anaesth.* 1993;40:542-546.

130. Jaeger P, Nielsen ZJK, Henningsen MH, Hilsted KL, Mathiesen O, Dahl JB. Adductor canal block versus femoral nerve block and quadriceps strength: a randomized, double-blind, placebo-controlled, crossover study in healthy volunteers. *Anesthesiology.* 2013;118:409-415.

131. Kwofie MK, Shastri UD, Gadsden JC, et al. The effects of ultrasound-guided adductor canal block versus femoral nerve block on quadriceps strength and fall risk: a blinded, randomized trial of volunteers. *Reg Anesth Pain Med.* 2013;38:321-325.

132. Barrington JW, Emerson RH, Lovald ST, Lombardi AV, Berend KR. No difference in early analgesia between liposomal bupivacaine injection and intrathecal morphine after TKA. *Clin Orthop Relat Res.* 2017;475:94-105.

133. Kuang M-J, Du Y, Ma J-X, He W, Fu L, Ma X-L. The efficacy of liposomal bupivacaine using periarticular injection in
total knee arthroplasty: a systematic review and meta-analysis.
J Arthroplasty. 2017;32:1395-1402.

134. Sun H, Huang Z, Zhang Z, Liao W. A meta-analysis comparing liposomal Bupivacaine and traditional periarticular injection for pain control after total knee arthroplasty. *J Knee Surg.*
2019;32:251-258.

135. Berger RA, Kusuma SK, Sanders SA, Thill ES, Sporer SM. The feasibility and perioperative complications of outpatient knee arthroplasty. *Clin Orthop Relat Res.* 2009;467:1443-1449.

136. Kim S, Losina E, Solomon DH, Wright J, Katz JN. Effectiveness
of clinical pathways for total knee and total hip arthroplasty: literature review. *J Arthroplasty.* 2003;18:69-74.

137. Poultsides LA, Triantafyllopoulos GK, Sakellariou VI, Memtsoudis
SG, Sculco TP. Infection risk assessment in patients undergoing
primary total knee arthroplasty. *Int Orthop.* 2018;42:87-94.

138. Hoeffel DP, Daly PJ, Kelly BJ, Giveans MR. Outcomes of the first
1,000 total hip and total knee arthroplasties at a same-day surgery
center using a rapid-recovery protocol. *J Am Acad Orthop Surg
Glob Res Rev.* 2019;3:e022.

139. Shah RR, Cipparrone NE, Gordon AC, Raab DJ, Bresch JR, Shah
NA. Is it safe? Outpatient total joint arthroplasty with discharge
to home at a freestanding ambulatory surgical center. *Arthroplast
Today.* 2018;4:484-487.

140. Kurtz S, Ong K, Lau E, Mowat F, Halpern M. Projections of primary and revision hip and knee arthroplasty in the United States
from 2005 to 2030. *J Bone Joint Surg Am.* 2007;89:780-785.

chapter 2

Surgical Anatomy of the Knee

E. Grant Sutter, MD, MS | Robert W. Tracey, MD, CDR MC USN | Ray C. Wasielewski, MD, MS

INTRODUCTION

An understanding of normal knee anatomy is paramount to successful total knee arthroplasty (TKA). The complex relationships of joint articulation to the periarticular muscles and ligaments about the knee allow for normal function in the nonpathologic knee. If preservation of these relationships is maintained and optimized in TKA, near-normal function is also possible in the pathologic knee. A comprehensive review of these interrelationships is studied and developed in this chapter.

EMBRYOLOGY

The morphologic development of the knee and its ligaments has been extensively studied,[1] and has shed light on the structure and function of the knee joint cavity and the tibiofibular joint anatomy.

The femur is ossified from five discrete centers: (1) the shaft, (2) the head, (3) the distal femur including the condyles, (4) the greater trochanter, and (5) the lesser trochanter. The shaft begins to ossify during the seventh week of development and is fully ossified at birth. The center of ossification for the distal femur appears during the ninth month of intrauterine life. The epiphysis of the femur begins to ossify at the age of 13 weeks and finally fuses with the shaft at the age of approximately 17.5 years in males and at 13 years in females, plus or minus 2 years.

The tibia is formed from three ossification centers, arising from (1) the body, (2) the proximal end, and (3) the distal end. The center for the tibial shaft appears in the seventh week of intrauterine life. The proximal epiphysis begins to ossify at week 13 and joins the body at approximately 17 years in males and 15 years in females.

The fibula also has three centers of ossification. One center appears in the middle of the shaft at approximately 8 weeks of intrauterine life with only the distal end still being cartilaginous at birth. A proximal tibiofemoral zone is present as early as week 9 of development. Ossification of this proximal end begins in the fourth year in males and early in the third year in females. The proximal epiphysis fuses during the eighteenth year in males and at 15.5 years in females. Variations in an individual's development may alter the fusion times by several years.

The patella begins its ossification in the 14th week of development and arises from a single ossification center that becomes apparent early in the third year of

life in males and at approximately 2.5 years in females. Ossification is usually complete by approximately the 13th year in males and the 10th year in females.

The cruciate ligaments begin to develop in the eighth week, with the posterior cruciate being the first to be distinguishable. With the development of the meniscofemoral ligament of Wrisberg in week 10, the cruciate ligament system is complete. The lateral collateral ligament (LCL) begins to organize in week 8 and the medial collateral in week 9, both being well developed by week 10. Organization of the menisci begins in week 8, but they are not clearly distinguishable until week 9. By week 10, the meniscal horns become attached to the anterior and posterior aspects of the upper tibial surface. The patellar ligaments begin to form as a continuation of the developing quadriceps muscle in week 8 of development. As development proceeds, the fibers of the tendon extend across the superficial aspect of the patella to the tibial tubercle. By week 9, the quadriceps muscle is visible, as is the mesenchymal tissue, which gives rise to the patellar fat pad and ligament in week 11 and 12, respectively. During week 13, the organization of the joint ligaments is mostly complete. Formation of the suprapatellar bursa in week 14 finalizes joint development.

BONES OF THE KNEE

Femur

The femur is the longest and strongest bone in the body. Its shaft is nearly cylindrical and fairly uniform in caliber; however, an extremely variable bow can often be present. The caliber is important when using intramedullary referencing for femoral arthroplasty, particularly when stem fixation of the femoral component is desired. Marker balls used on the preoperative radiographs are recommended in cases in which the canal diameter is needed. Bowing, when excessive, can affect the radiographic measurements used in TKA. Long-cassette anteroposterior and lateral radiographs are most accurate in assessing the femur when concerns are present.[2,3]

The distal aspect of the femur broadens approximately threefold into the medial and lateral condyles. All but the sides of these condyles are articular. The inferior, posterior oblong-shaped portions of the condyles articulate smoothly with the tibial plateau, whereas the central, anterior surface between the condyles articulates with the facets of the patella. The inferior, oblong surfaces of the condyles are separated by the intercondylar fossa, which houses the cruciate ligaments. These ligaments can be damaged and tension altered by osteophyte formation in patients with osteoarthritis.[4] The intercondylar fossa is especially deep posteriorly and is separated by a ridge from the popliteal surface of the femur superiorly.[5] This surface, bounded by the two supracondylar ridges where the gastrocnemius muscles originate, is in contact with the popliteal artery. The bone in the deep intracondylar fossa is hard and unyielding. Therefore, if cutting this posterior bone for the box resection to house a cam-post mechanism of a posterior-stabilized knee, the correct depth is critical to prevent condylar fracture during implant impaction. The lateral condyle has a greater posterior excursion than the medial so that internal rotation of the femoral cuts during TKA seldom results in notching of the posterior femur except in cases of excessive component downsizing or rotation. Because there is little deformation of the posterior condyles in the arthritic varus knee, a posterior condylar line can be used as a guide to estimate femoral implant rotation, as will be discussed later.[6] The medial condylar surface is longer than that of the lateral and is flatter anteriorly and more curved posteriorly. In the sagittal plane, the radius of curvature of both condyles is greatest posteriorly as mentioned, but the larger medial condyle is slightly more symmetric.[7] Rotation can affect the apparent size of the condyles on radiographs.[8]

The contact surface for the patella is derived mostly from the lateral condyle. The anterior extensions (rises) of both condyles form a fossa for the patella to sit in extension. The lateral rise is the greatest. Therefore, with external rotation of the femoral cut (to improve patellar tracking in TKA), more lateral bone is taken from the anterior femur, increasing the likelihood of notching laterally. The lateral condyle is broader than the medial condyle, and in the frontal plane, the lateral condyle is slightly shorter than the medial, giving rise to the valgus angulation of the distal femur (this is why the distal femoral cutting guide will typically rest against the medial femoral condyle and not the lateral). With weight-bearing, however, the two condyles rest on the horizontal plane of the tibial condyles, and the shaft of the femur inclines downward and inward. This inclination is the result of the greater breadth of the body at the pelvis than at the knees.

The epicondyles of the femur bulge above and within the curvature of the condyles. The medial epicondyle is more prominent and provides attachment for the tibial collateral ligament and also remains the insertion point for the adductor magnus muscle at the adductor tubercle. Behind this tubercle, the bony surface is roughened and provides the origin of the medial head of the gastrocnemius muscle. The lateral epicondyle gives rise to the fibular collateral ligament and the lateral head of the gastrocnemius. In addition, the plantaris muscle arises

posteriorly. Immediately below the lateral epicondyle and bordering the articular surface of the condyle is an oblique groove that houses the tendon of the popliteus muscle.

Berger et al. found that the surgical epicondylar axis—defined as the line connecting the lateral epicondylar prominence and the medial sulcus of the medial epicondyle—was a useful reference for the rotational orientation of the femoral component during primary or revision TKA when the posterior condylar surfaces could not be used.[9] Similarly, using magnetic resonance imaging (MRI), the transepicondylar axis was found to be a reliable rotational landmark[6] and is approximately 6° externally rotated relative to the posterior condyles in both normal and varus knees (with no medial condylar posterior bone loss). More recently, Miller et al. found that femoral component rotation parallel to the surgical epicondylar axis maximized patellar tracking within the femoral sulcus and minimized tibiofemoral wear motion and that these benefits were less reproducible when using the posterior condylar axis as a reference.[10]

Femoral bony landmarks can also be used to estimate the joint line, an important consideration in primary and revision knee surgery. Absolute distances have been previously published; however, these have been shown to vary depending on bone size and gender. Therefore, more recent studies have focused on anatomic ratios. Servien et al. found that the normalized ratios between the distance from the medial and lateral epicondyle to the respective distal condyle articular surface and the femoral width were 0.34 and 0.28, respectively.[11] Importantly, these values did not vary with gender. Re-creating an anatomic joint line is important in both primary and revision surgery as alteration can potentially lead to patella baja/alta, flexion-extension mismatch, and midflexion instability.

Tibia

The proximal tibia is expanded to receive the condyles of the femur. The shaft of the bone flares out into lateral and medial buttresses, which form the medial and lateral condyles. The tibia is the weight-bearing bone of the leg, whereas the fibula serves for muscular attachments and for completion of the ankle joint. The superior articular surface of the tibia presents two facets. The medial facet is oval in shape and has a slight concavity. The lateral facet is nearly round, and although concave from side to side, it is convex in front. The rims of these facets are in contact with the medial and lateral menisci, but the central portions receive the condyles of the femur. A femorotibial offset exists, with the center of the femur being medial and anterior to the center of the tibia.[12] If this offset is present preoperatively, a posterior-stabilized knee design with a cam-post mechanism may be the prudent option to resist this intrinsic deformity and to prevent it from occurring postoperatively. An intercondylar eminence with two tubercles arises between the two articular facets. The articular surfaces continue on to the adjacent sides of the medial and lateral intercondylar tubercles. Anterior to the intercondylar eminence is the anterior intercondylar area, which provides attachment for the anterior horns of the medial and lateral menisci and the anterior cruciate ligament (ACL). The posterior intercondylar area is a broad groove that separates the posterior aspects of the condyles. The posterior cruciate ligament (PCL) originates in the posterior intercondylar area approximately 1 cm inferior to the joint line and a few millimeters lateral to the center of the lateral intercondylar tubercle.[13] From its origin, the PCL travels anterior and slightly medial, where it is joined by a cord from the lateral meniscus (the posterior meniscofemoral ligament, or *ligament of Wrisberg*) to attach to the medial condyle of the femur. When exposing the tibia during a cruciate-retaining TKA, care must be taken not to sever the PCL. In addition, tibial cuts that are excessively deep or posteriorly sloped may violate the origin of the PCL. The posterior intercondylar area also gives attachment to the posterior horns of the medial and lateral menisci. Anteriorly, the two condylar surfaces blend in a triangular area that leads distally to the tibial tuberosity. This anterior tibial triangle has large vascular foramina and is sharply marked at its borders by oblique lines where the fascia lata attaches. The tibial tuberosity is smooth superiorly and rough inferiorly for the termination of the patellar ligament. The proximal aspect of the rough area identifies the safe level of resection that will not harm the patellar tendon insertion. Posteriorly, the medial condyle is marked by a transverse groove that accommodates the insertion of the tendon of the semimembranosus muscle. The rough medial surface of the condyle gives attachment to the tibial collateral ligament. The lateral condyle has a nearly circular facet on its posteroinferior surface for articulation with the head of the fibula. Anterior to this facet, at the junction of the anterior and lateral surfaces of the condyle, is an oblique line on which the iliotibial band (ITB) attaches.

The body of the tibia is expanded at its extremities but is otherwise fairly uniform in size. In cross section, it is triangular, with medial, lateral, and posterior surfaces and having anterior, medial, and interosseous borders. The anterior border (crest), just distal to the tibial tubercle, is subcutaneous and prominent. It is slightly sinuous, beginning at the lateral margin of the tuberosity proximally and moving medially distally. Therefore, the midline of the tibia for extramedullary alignment during TKA is found just distal to the tubercle, where the crest has moved medially. The intramedullary canal relative to the proximal tibial plateau is such that a rod placed down the tibia will exit slightly medially within the plateau. At its upper medial portion, the tibia provides for the attachment of the tibial collateral ligament and the more medial fibers of the popliteus muscle. The soleus muscle arises from the middle one-third of the medial border.

The interosseous border is on the fibular side of the tibia and is sharp throughout its length. Superiorly, it begins below and anterior to the facet for the head of the fibula and provides, throughout its length, for the attachment of the interosseous membrane.

The medial surface of the body of the tibia is smooth and convex. Its upper one-third receives the insertions of the sartorius, gracilis, and semitendinosus muscles. The distal two-thirds of the medial surface are subcutaneous. Gerdy tubercle is the proximal, most lateral prominence. The fascia lata can refer pain from the hip to this region in cases of severe trochanteric bursitis. The lateral surface has a shallow groove in its upper two-thirds, which provides the origin of the tibialis anterior muscle. The lateral parapatellar approach in TKA usually requires release to this point during lateral exposure and anterior subluxation of the patella.

The most prominent marking on the posterior surface of the tibia is the soleal line. Beginning behind the facet for the head of the fibula, this line extends obliquely downward across the back of the tibia. The triangular area above this line gives insertion to the popliteus muscle. The soleal line itself serves for the attachment of the popliteus fascia and as origin for the soleus muscle. Occasionally, release along this line is necessary to increase the medial flexion gap.

The tibia slopes posteriorly, but with great variability, generally angling in a range of 5° to 10° from the intramedullary canal. The bone trabeculae are aligned relatively perpendicular to this slope orientation but are greatly affected by osteoarthritic changes. Studies have demonstrated the variables affecting bone strength after arthroplasty.[14,15] Posterior angulation matching the anatomic angulation is likely to optimize the strength of the underlying bone.[16] However, when a deep tibial cut is made at a less than anatomic angulation, more distal fixation should be considered to meet the load-bearing needs of TKA.

Recent hypotheses and studies suggest that knee kinematics is described as two simultaneous rotations occurring about fixed axes. Knee flexion and extension occur about an optimal flexion axis in the femur, whereas tibial internal and external rotations occur about a longitudinal rotation axis in the tibia. Churchill et al. found that the transepicondylar axis closely approximated the optimal flexion axis.[17] According to Matsumoto et al., the axis location for tibial rotation remained approximately in the area between the two cruciate ligament insertions throughout the range of flexion. However, the axis did change with changes in cruciate ligament tension and surrounding soft tissues.[18]

Similar to the femur discussed above, proximal tibia bony landmarks can be used to estimate the joint line. Using MRI, Servien et al. determined that the tibial tubercle was a reliable landmark for reference, especially when using anatomic ratios. Specifically, the ratio of the distance between the tibial tubercle and the joint line to the anteroposterior width of the tibia at the level of the tubercle was 0.50 in both males and females. Similarly, femoral width can also be used, as the ratio of the distance between the tubercle and the anterior tibial joint level to femoral width was 0.27.[11]

Fibula

The fibula is a long, slender bone that lies parallel and lateral to the tibia. It does not participate in weight-bearing, but rather serves for muscle and tendon attachment and provides stability at the ankle distally. The head of the fibula is knob-like, and superiorly, slanted toward the tibia, is the almost circular articular surface, which participates in the tibiofibular articulation. Violation of this joint during TKA is usually noted by the appearance of articular cartilage in the posterior lateral corner of the resected tibial surface and occurs most frequently with an excessively deep tibial resection. At the posterolateral limit of the articular facet, the apex of the head projects upward and provides attachment to the fibular collateral ligament of the knee joint. The tendon of the biceps femoris muscle attaches to the lateral aspect of the head of the fibula. The circumference of the head is rough and has anterior and posterior tubercles, which provide attachment for the proximal-most fibers of the peroneus longus muscle and upper fibers of the soleus muscle, respectively.

The joint between the circular facet on the head of the fibula and a similarly shaped surface on the posterolateral aspect of the underside of the lateral condyle of the tibia can be nearly flat or slightly grooved and may be transverse or oblique. Movement is slight at this joint. The articular capsule is attached at the margins of the facets on the tibia and the fibula and is strengthened by accessory ligaments anteriorly and posteriorly. The anterior ligament of the head of the fibula consists of fibrous bands that pass obliquely from the front of the head of the fibula to the front of the lateral condyle of the tibia. The posterior ligament is a single broad band that runs obliquely between the head and the back of the lateral tibial condyle. The tendon of the popliteus muscle crosses it. The subpopliteal recess of the synovial cavity of the knee joint occasionally communicates here with the cavity of the tibiofibular articulation. The joint receives its arterial supply from the lateral inferior genicular and anterior recurrent tibial arteries. Nerves to the articulation are derived from the common peroneal nerve, the nerve to the popliteus muscle, and the anterior tibial recurrent nerve.

The interosseous membrane of the leg extends between the interosseous borders of the tibia and the fibula and consists largely of fibers that pass from the tibia laterally and inferiorly toward the fibula. The upper margin of the membrane does not reach the tibiofibular articulation, and the anterior tibial vessels pass over the upper edge of the membrane to the anterior compartment of the leg.

Patella

The patella is a largest sesamoid bone in the body, developed in the tendon of the quadriceps femoris muscle. It articulates against the anterior articular surface of the distal femur. It holds the patellar tendon off the distal femur, thus improving the angle of approach of the tendon to its distal insertion on the tibial tuberosity, increasing the moment arm of the force vector generated by the quadriceps muscle. The anterior surface of the patella is convex and is vertically striated by the tendon fibers. The superior border is thick and gives attachment to the tendinous fibers of the rectus femoris and vastus intermedius muscles. The lateral and medial borders are thinner and receive the tendinous fibers of the vastus lateralis and vastus medialis muscles, respectively. These two borders converge inferiorly to the pointed lower pole of the patella, which gives attachment to the patellar ligament. During arthroplasty, a deep patellar cut may violate this inferior pole. Although a deep cut may yield a larger patellar surface for arthroplasty, it does so to the detriment of patellar thickness and strength. On the other hand, it may allow for slightly inferior positioning of the patella button, helpful in decreasing component loading at higher flexion angles.[19] Also, if the patella is thinned to 10 mm, the lower pole contributes to the overall fixation surface, thus creating a larger, more circular shape for fixation of a larger size button. Thus, this cut must be carefully performed to optimize strength and surface diameter.

The articular surface of the patella has a smooth, oval shape that is greater in the medial to lateral direction. This shape allows for medialization of the patellar component if sized to the smaller superoinferior dimension. The surface is divided into two facets by a vertical ridge that occupies the patellar groove on the articular surface of the femur. The lateral facet is broader and deeper than the medial facet. These patellar facets correspond to convex areas on the patellar groove of the femur. The anterior femoral sulcus has medial and lateral ridges, with the lateral being the highest.

KNEE JOINT STRUCTURES

The knee joint is required to function as a weight-bearing joint in which there is free motion in one primary plane combined with considerable stability. Support for the weight of the body on the vertical apposed ends of the two long bones is secured at the knee joint by the twofold to threefold expansion of the bearing surfaces of the femur and tibia optimized by the intervening menisci. Additionally, internal structures that reinforce and support joint function include the cruciate ligaments, the capsule, the synovial membrane, and the bursae (**Figs. 2-1 to 2-5**).

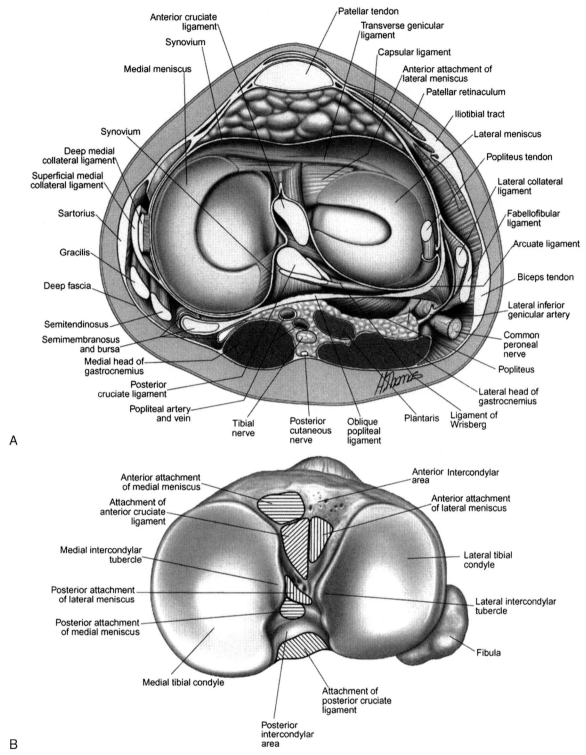

FIGURE 2-1 **A:** Cross section of knee joint at level of menisci, superior view. The medial meniscus is larger than the lateral and more ovoid in shape and closely adhered to the medial tibial condyle. Thus, it is more commonly torn, injured, or entrapped. The lateral meniscus is smaller and more circular but covers a greater proportion of the surface area of the tibial condyle than does the medial. The lateral meniscus is more mobile and more loosely attached to the tibial condyle. Thus, it is less likely to become injured. Note that the anterior cruciate ligament and posterior cruciate ligament are lined by synovium, are intra-articular structures that lie outside the joint capsule, and cross as the limbs of an X. Ligament of Wrisberg is an extension of the lateral meniscus that joins or runs alongside the posterior cruciate ligament to attach the medial condyle of the femur. The "bare area" on the lateral side of the lateral meniscus houses the popliteus tendon and represents the safe level of excision of the lateral meniscus during total knee arthroplasty. The lateral inferior genicular artery runs along the margin of the lateral meniscus. **B:** Superior aspect of proximal tibia. The anterior attachment of the medial meniscus is directly anterior to the attachment of the anterior cruciate ligament. The posterior attachment of the medial meniscus is anterior to the origin of the posterior cruciate ligament. The anterior attachment of the lateral meniscus is adjacent and lateral to the attachment of the anterior cruciate ligament. The posterior attachment of the lateral meniscus is directly anterior to the posterior attachment of the medial meniscus. Note that the anterior and posterior attachments of the lateral meniscus are in close proximity, allowing for more mobility and flexibility, making it less prone to injury. The posterior cruciate ligament originates in the posterior intercondylar area approximately 1 cm inferior to the joint line.

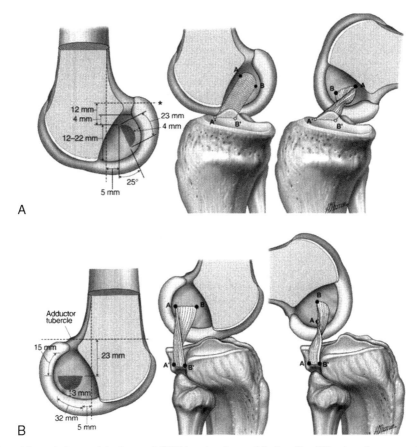

FIGURE 2-2   A: Lateral view of the anterior cruciate ligament (ACL) in extension and flexion. The ACL arises from a rough, nonarticular area anterior to the intercondylar eminence of the tibia and extends upward and backward to the posteromedial aspect of the lateral femoral condyle. Line A to A' represents the anteromedial band. Line B to B' represents the posterolateral bulk. In extension, the posterolateral bulk is taut. In flexion, the anteromedial band is tight, and the posterolateral bulk is relatively relaxed. Thus, via its two bands, the ACL prevents anterior displacement of the proximal tibia in the full range of motion. Note the measurements of the superior attachment. The asterisked line represents the level of the adductor tubercle. **B:** Lateral view of the posterior cruciate ligament (PCL) in extension and flexion. The PCL arises from the posterior intercondylar area approximately 1 cm distal to the joint line. It travels upward and forward along the medial border of the ACL to attach to the lateral side of the medial condyle of the femur. In flexion, the bulk of the PCL tightens, and in extension, it is relaxed. The PCL prevents posterior displacement of the proximal tibia. Note the measurements for the superior attachment of the PCL. The horizontal dashed line is at the level of the adductor tubercle.

Menisci

The menisci are crescent-shaped wedges of fibrocartilage that rest on the peripheral aspects of the articular surfaces of the proximal tibia. They function to effectively deepen the medial and lateral tibia fossae for articulation with the condyles of the femur. They are thickest at their external margins and taper to thin, unattached edges as they progress inwardly. The menisci are attached along the outer edges of the condyles of the tibia and behind its intercondylar eminence (**Fig. 2-1B**). The superior surfaces are slightly concave to accommodate the condyles of the femur, thus providing greater surface area contact. The medial meniscus is larger than the lateral and more ovoid in shape. Anteriorly, it is thin and pointed at its attachment in the anterior intercondylar area of the tibia directly in front of the ACL. Posteriorly, it is broadest, attaching in the corresponding posterior fossa, anterior to the origin of the PCL. The lateral meniscus is smaller and more circular, covering a greater proportion of the tibial surface than does the medial meniscus. Its anterior horn is attached in the anterior intercondylar area, posterior and

lateral to the insertion of the ACL. Posteriorly, it terminates in the posterior intercondylar area, anterior to the termination of the medial meniscus. The lateral meniscus is weakly attached around the margin of the lateral condyle of the tibia. In addition, it lacks attachment where it is crossed and notched by the popliteus tendon. This "bare area" is easily identified during TKA and provides a reference for the surgeon as to the safe depth of lateral meniscal excision, thus helping to prevent injury to the lateral inferior geniculate artery during excision of the anterior margin. Near its posterior attachment, the lateral meniscus frequently sends off a collection of fibers, the posterior meniscofemoral ligament (ligament of Wrisberg), which either joins or lies behind the PCL. This ligament ends in the medial condyle of the femur, immediately behind the attachment of the PCL. Occasionally, an anterior meniscofemoral ligament is also present, with a similar but anterior relationship to the PCL. The lateral meniscus is thus loosely attached to the tibia and has frequent attachment to the femur. Therefore, it tends to translate with the lateral femoral condyle during flexion of the knee.

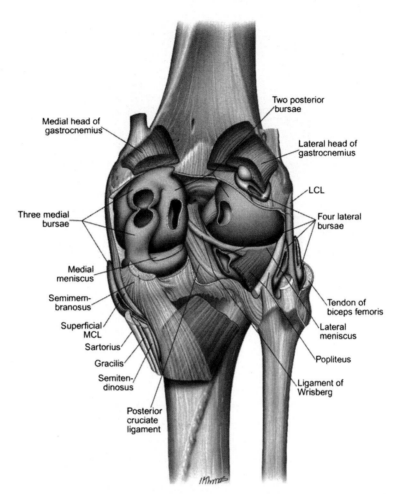

FIGURE 2-3 Bursae of the knee joint, posterior view. The popliteus muscle and medial and lateral heads of the gastrocnemius muscle are cut to show underlying bursae. Four lateral bursae: (1) the inferior subtendinous bursa separating the tendon of the biceps femoris from the fibular collateral ligament, (2) the bursa between the tendon of the popliteus tendon and the fibular collateral ligament, (3) the subpopliteal bursa separating the popliteus muscle from the lateral femoral condyle, and (4) the subtendinous bursa under the tendon of origin of the lateral head of the gastrocnemius muscle. Three medial bursae: (1) the bursa anserina separates the sartorius, gracilis, and semitendinosus tendons from the tibial collateral ligament; (2) the bursa of the semimembranosus muscle separating it from the tibia; and (3) the subtendinous bursa under tendon of origin of the medial head of the gastrocnemius. Two large posterior bursae: (1) the bursa separating the medial head of the gastrocnemius muscle from the capsule, which generally communicates with the knee joint and (2) the bursa separating the lateral head of the gastrocnemius muscle from the capsule, which occasionally communicates with the knee joint. The bursae of the medial and lateral heads of the gastrocnemius muscle are frequent locations of collection of wear debris in failed total knee arthroplasties because of their frequent communication with the knee joint. LCL, lateral collateral ligament; MCL, medial collateral ligament.

In contrast, the medial mensicus is less mobile with capsular attachments to the tibia (coronary ligament) and femur (meniscofemoral ligament) and is intimate with the deep portion of the medial collateral ligament (MCL) at its periphery. Therefore, when excising the medial meniscus during arthroplasty procedures, care must be taken not to disrupt the MCL at the medial periphery. Finally, the convex, anterior margin of the lateral meniscus is connected to the anterior horn of the medial meniscus by the transverse genicular ligament.

Cruciate Ligaments

The cruciate ligaments are strong, rounded cords that lie within the capsule of the knee joint and cross each other like the limbs of an X (**Fig. 2-1**A). They are named *anterior* and *posterior* based on their relationships to the intercondylar eminence of the proximal tibia (**Fig. 2-1**B). The ACL arises from a rough, nonarticular area anterior to the intercondylar eminence of the tibia and extends upward and backward to the posteromedial aspect of the lateral femoral condyle (**Fig. 2-2**A). In extension, the posterolateral bulk is taut, whereas in flexion, the anteromedial band is tight and the posterolateral bulk is relatively relaxed.[20] The PCL arises from the area posterior to the tibial eminence and travels upward and forward along the medial border of the ACL to attach to the lateral aspect of the medial condyle of the femur (**Figs. 2-1B** and **2-2B**). In flexion, the bulk of the PCL tightens, and in extension, it is relaxed (**Fig. 2-2**B). The ACL prevents anterior displacement of the tibia, and the PCL restricts posterior displacement.

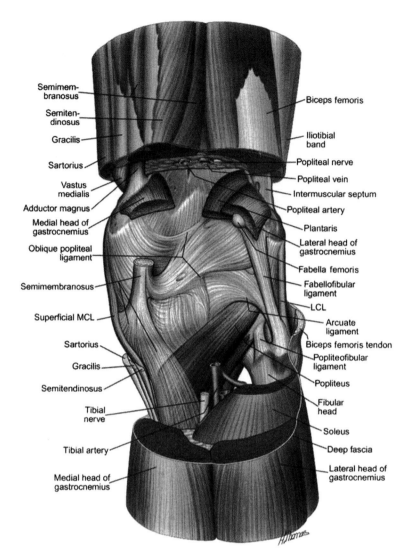

Semimem-
branosus

Semiten-
dinosus

Gracilis

Sartorius

Vastus
medialis

Adductor magnus

Medial head of
gastrocnemius

Oblique popliteal
ligament

Semimembranosus

Superficial MCL

Sartorius

Gracilis

Semitendinosus

Tibial
nerve

Tibial artery

Medial head of
gastrocnemius

Biceps femoris

Iliotibial
band

Popliteal nerve

Popliteal vein

Intermuscular septum

Popliteal artery

Plantaris

Lateral head of
gastrocnemius

Fabella femoris

Fabellofibular
ligament

LCL

Arcuate
ligament

Biceps femoris tendon

Popliteofibular
ligament

Popliteus

Fibular
head

Soleus

Deep fascia

Lateral head of
gastrocnemius

FIGURE 2-4 Articular capsule of the knee joint, posterior view. The vertical fibers of the posterior capsule are inseparable from the ligaments and aponeuroses, which appose and reinforce them. The heads of the gastrocnemius and plantaris muscles are cut to expose underlying capsule. The vertical fibers of the capsule are attached superiorly to the femur and inferiorly to the tibia. The oblique popliteal ligament is an extension of the tendon of the semimembranosus muscle and reinforces the posterior capsule. It travels in the superolateral direction to attach to the lateral femoral condyle. The arcuate popliteal ligament reinforces the lower, lateral section of the posterior knee joint. It arises from the back of the head of the fibula, arches upward and medial over the tendon of the popliteus muscle, then spreads out over the posterior surface of the joint. LCL, lateral collateral ligament; MCL, medial collateral ligament.

Synovial Membrane and Cavity

The articular cavity of the knee is the largest joint space of the body. The cavity includes the space between and around the tibial and femoral condyles but also extends proximally, behind the patella, to include the femoropatellar articulation, and further into the suprapatellar bursa, which lies between the tendon of the quadriceps femoris muscle and the femur, where it communicates freely. The synovial membrane lines the articular capsule and reflects onto the bones as far as the edges of their articular surfaces. It also follows the suprapatellar bursa and extends to the sides of the patella under the aponeurosis of the vastus muscles. The synovial membrane covers the recesses that lie behind the posterior areas of each femoral condyle. At the superior-most portion of the medial recess, the bursa under the medial head of the gastrocnemius muscle occasionally opens into the joint cavity. In the subpopliteal recess, the cavity and the synovium lining extend beyond the capsule to lie against the tendon of the popliteus muscle. The synovial membrane also covers the cruciate ligament except where the PCL is attached to the back of the capsule. Thus, the cruciate ligaments are intra-articular structures that lie outside the capsule. The infrapatellar fat pad, which lies below the patella, represents an anterior section of the median septum of tissues that, with the cruciate ligaments, separate the two tibiofemoral articulations. The fat pad is often taut after eversion of the patella during a medial parapatellar approach in TKA. Release of the infrapatellar synovium to the level of the lateral meniscus

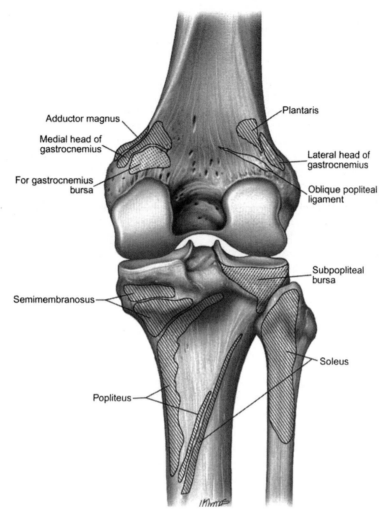

FIGURE 2-5   Sites of attachment of posterior muscles and ligaments of the knee.

can significantly decrease tension when the patella is everted. From the synovial surface of the infrapatellar fat pad, a vertical fold frequently passes toward the cruciate ligaments and attaches to the intracondylar fossa of the femur anterior to the ACL and lateral to the PCL. From the medial and lateral borders of the articular surface of the patella, the synovial membrane projects into the interior joint and curls around to attach adjacent to the cartilage of the medial and lateral femoral condyles.

Knee Joint Bursae

Because almost all tendons at the knee lie parallel to the bones and pull lengthwise across the joint, bursae are numerous (**Fig. 2-3**). The suprapatellar bursa lies between the quadriceps tendon and the anterior femur. Three other bursae are associated with the patella and its ligament. The prepatellar bursa, located between the skin and the anterior surface of the patella, allows free movement of the skin over the patella during flexion and extension. The subcutaneous infrapatellar bursa lies between the patellar

tendon and the overlying skin. The prepatellar and subcutaneous infrapatellar bursae may become inflamed as a result of direct trauma to the front of the knee or through activities like repetitive or prolonged kneeling. The deep infrapatellar bursa, located between the patellar ligament and the tibial tuberosity, is separated from the synovial cavity of the joint by the infrapatellar fat pad and helps to reduce friction between the patellar ligament and the tibial tuberosity.

Lateral to the joint, the inferior subtendinous bursa of the biceps femoris muscle lies between the tendon of this muscle and the fibular collateral ligament. The subpopliteal bursa (recess of the synovial membrane) lies between the tendon of the popliteus muscle and the lateral femoral condyle. Another bursa may separate the popliteus tendon from the fibular collateral ligament, or the membrane of the subpopliteal recess may wrap around the tendon to separate them. Also belonging to this lateral group is the subtendinous bursa of the lateral head of the gastrocnemius muscle, which lies beneath the tendon of origin of this muscle and occasionally communicates with the knee joint.

Medially, the bursa anserina lies deep to the pes anserinus tendons (sartorius, gracilis, and semitendinosus muscles), and separates them from the tibial collateral ligament. The bursa of the semimembranosus muscle lies between the muscle and the tibia. The subtendinous bursa of the medial head of the gastrocnemius muscle underlies the tendon of the origin of the medial head, separating it from the femur. With the knee flexed, the gastrocnemio-semimembranosus bursa communicates with the knee joint, and this communication closes with knee extension.[21] Posteriorly, there are two large bursae associated with the medial and lateral heads of the gastrocnemius muscle. The bursa of the lateral head of the gastrocnemius separates the muscle from the joint capsule and occasionally communicates with the knee joint. The bursa of the medial head of the gastrocnemius underlies the medial head, separating it from the joint capsule, and generally communicates with the knee joint. This bursa is the most common site of occurrence of a Baker cyst (in patients with rheumatoid arthritis) or for the collection of substantial debris and synovial fluid extravasation around the failed TKA with osteolysis.

Capsule

The articular capsule of the knee joint is inseparable from the ligaments and aponeuroses apposed to it. Posteriorly, its vertical fibers arise from the femoral and tibial condyles and the intercondylar fossa of the femur and are covered by the oblique popliteal ligament (**Fig. 2-4**). Inferiorly, the capsule attaches to the tibial condyles and the borders of the menisci. External ligaments that reinforce the capsule are the fascia lata and the iliotibial tract; the medial patellar and lateral patellar retinacula; and the patellar, oblique popliteal, and arcuate popliteal ligaments.

The aponeurotic tendons of the vastus medialis and vastus lateralis muscles are attached to the medial and lateral margins of the patella, down to the level of the attachment of the patellar ligament. The tendons expand over the sides of the capsule as the medial patellar and lateral patellar retinacula. They insert on the front of the tibial condyles and onto the oblique lines of the condyles as far around as the sides of the collateral ligaments. Medially, the retinaculum blends with the periosteum of the shaft of the tibia. Laterally, it blends with the iliotibial tract. Superficial to the retinacula, the fascia lata covers the front and sides of the knee joint. It descends to attach to the tibial tuberosity, and at the level of the oblique lines of the condyles, it overlies and blends with the patellar retinacula. On the lateral side, its strong iliotibial tract attaches to the oblique line of the lateral condyle and to the head of the fibula. Medially, the fascia lata is thinner and sends some longitudinal fibers inferiorly to blend with the fibrous expansion of the sartorius muscle.

The ligamentum patellae is a strong, flat band attached superiorly to the inferior pole of the patella and inferiorly to the tibial tuberosity and is actually a continuation of the tendon of the quadriceps femoris running over the anterior surface of the patella. The ligament inserts somewhat obliquely on the tibia, the lateral portion carries distally several centimeters farther than the medial portion. This longer lateral insertion may provide some protection against patellar tendon dehiscence when exposing the knee via the medial parapatellar approach. A deep infrapatellar bursa intervenes between the ligament and the bone immediately superior to the insertion. A large subcutaneous infrapatellar bursa is developed in the subcutaneous tissue over the ligament.

The oblique popliteal ligament is a posterior reinforcement of the capsule provided by the tendon of the semimembranosus muscle. As the tendon inserts into the groove on the posterior aspect of the medial condyle of the tibia (**Fig. 2-5**), it sends an oblique expansion laterally and superiorly across the posterior surface of the capsule toward the lateral condyle of the femur. Large foramina for vessels and nerves perforate the oblique popliteal ligament, and the popliteal artery lies against it. The arcuate popliteal ligament strengthens the lower, lateral section of the knee joint posteriorly and arises from the back of the head of the fibula, arching upward and medially over the tendon of the popliteus muscle and then spreading out over the posterior surface of the joint.

THREE LAYERS OF THE MEDIAL AND LATERAL KNEE

Warren and Marshall divided the medial retinacular complex from superficial to deep into three principal layers—(1) layer I, the deep crural fascia; (2) layer II, the superficial medial collateral ligament (SMCL) and variable anterior structures; and (3) layer III, the joint capsule proper.[22] In similar fashion, the layers of the lateral side of the knee have also been characterized. An understanding of these layers will assist in the medial[23,24] and lateral[24,25] dissection necessary for knee joint exposure of the varus and valgus knee, respectively. Additionally, an understanding of these complex layers will facilitate maximal preservation of the structures within, thus optimizing knee joint stability and function. **Fig. 2-6** illustrates these complex layers in cross section. **Figs. 2-7 to 2-10** further illustrate the relationships discussed below.

Layers of the Medial Knee

Layer I

Layer I, the deep crural fascia, is the most superficial, residing just deep to the subcutaneous tissues. The medial and posteromedial fascia of this layer invests the sartorius and medial gastrocnemius muscles, respectively (**Fig. 2-7**). It can be separated from the underlying superficial medial collateral (layer II) by sharp dissection. Posteriorly, this fascia supports the popliteal vessels, neural structures, and

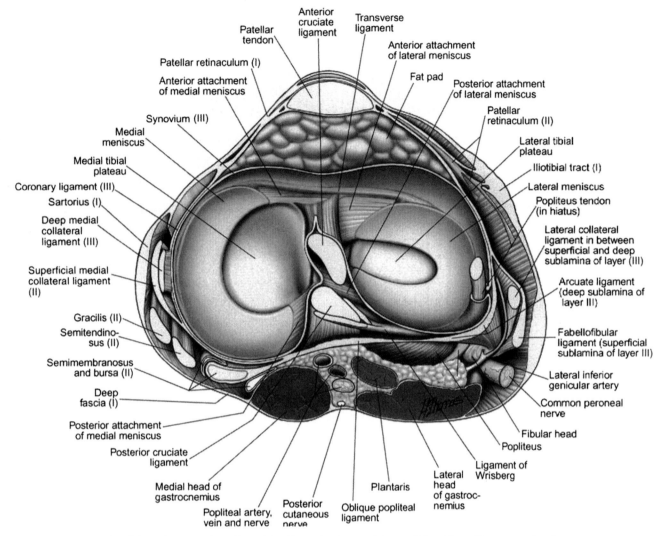

FIGURE 2-6 Cross section of knee joint illustrating layers of the medial and lateral knee, superior view.

the lateral head of the gastrocnemius muscle. Anteriorly, layer I joins layer II to form the medial patellar retinaculum (**Fig. 2-6**). Anteriorly and superiorly, the crural fascia is continuous with the overlying fascia of the vastus medialis muscle. Anteriorly and distally, the sartorius muscle inserts into the crural fascia of layer I, joining the periosteum as it inserts on the tibia. Between layer I and the deeper layer II, the gracilis and semitendinosus muscles course to their variable attachment on the pes anserinus.[26] The tendons, which are fused approximately 3 cm from their insertion point, are firmly adherent to the sartorius muscle in this layer.

Layer II

The components of layer II are the SMCL, the medial patellofemoral ligament (MPFL) and the patellotibial ligament. These component ligaments together are called the *medial retinacular complex* and form an inverted triangle with a central fascial deficiency (**Fig. 2-8A**). Interestingly, a similar inverted triangle is found in this layer posterior to the SMCL, having a similar deficient area.[27]

The principal component of layer II is the superficial portion of the MCL (SMCL), whose parallel fibers clearly define the plane of this layer. This ligament is composed of a vertically oriented anterior component and an obliquely oriented posterior component (**Fig. 2-8A**). The most proximal and distal extents of layer II are defined where the vertical component of the SMCL inserts onto the femur and tibia, respectively. The proximal insertion of the SMCL is at the medial femoral epicondyle approximately 5 cm above the tibiofemoral joint line (**Fig. 2-8B**). The distal attachment is at the medial aspect of the tibial metaphysis, 6 to 8 cm distal to the joint line, and posterior to the sartorius, semitendinosus, and gracilis tendons.[26] The fiber arrangement is such that in extension, the posterior margin of the SMCL is tense while the anterior border is relatively relaxed.[23] Therefore, the posterior portion of the SMCL should be selectively released first to balance a medial contracture of the extension gap. The more anterior portion of the vertical component of the SMCL should be released to address flexion contractures in the medial compartment. When releasing the SMCL,

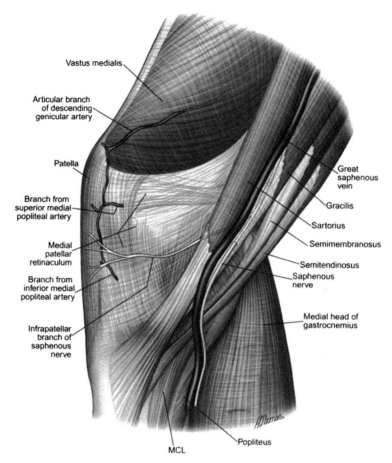

Vastus medialis

Articular branch
of descending
genicular artery

Patella

Branch from
superior medial
popliteal artery

Medial
patellar
retinaculum

Branch from
inferior medial
popliteal artery

Infrapatellar
branch of
saphenous
nerve

MCL

Great
saphenous
vein

Gracilis

Sartorius

Semimembranosus

Semitendinosus
Saphenous
nerve

Medial head of
gastrocnemius

Popliteus

FIGURE 2-7 Layer I of the medial knee—the deep crural fascia. Layer I is the most superficial medial layer of the knee, residing just deep to the subcutaneous tissues. The medial deep crural fascia invests the sartorius muscle. Distally, the sartorius inserts onto the fascia. The posteromedial fascia invests the medial head of the gastrocnemius muscle. Note that the great saphenous vein runs between the tendons of the sartorius and gracilis muscles. Posteriorly, the fascia invests the popliteal vessels and neural structures (not shown). Anteriorly, layer I joins layer II to form the medial patellar retinaculum. Anterosuperiorly, the fascia is continuous with the fascia of the vastus medialis muscle. The tendons of the gracilis and semitendinosus muscles run deep to layer I. MCL, medial collateral ligament.

care should be taken not to release the anterior pes anserinus attachment so that its contribution to dynamic joint stability is maintained.

The fibers of the oblique portion of the SMCL arise just posterior to the proximal attachment of the vertical fibers of the SMCL and extend distally in a posterooblique fashion to fuse with layer III, where it closely attaches to the posterior edge of the medial meniscus. This conjoined structure, known as the *posterior oblique ligament* (POL), receives additional fibers from the semimembranosus tendon sheath and the synovial sheath before attaching to the posteromedial aspect of the knee. The POL envelops the femoral condyle in a structure termed the *oblique popliteal ligament*. The oblique fibers that fan out and blend into the posteromedial capsule become slack when the knee is flexed. However, after complete release of the MCL, these fibers may help support the medial flexion gap. Hughston and Barrett described this posterior complex, stating that the POL–semimembranosus–medial meniscus complex is the primary deterrent to anteromedial instability of the knee.[28]

The MPFL arises from the adductor tubercle of the femur (**Fig. 2-8B**) and travels forward toward the patella, deep to layer I. It inserts on the proximal half of the medial aspect of the patella. With some variability, the fibers travel distally to the vastus medialis, joining the plane of layer I as they form the parapatellar retinaculum. The fibers of the MPFL fuse with layer I at their patellar insertion, invest the fascia of the quadriceps tendon, and merge with the fibers of the vastus medialis obliquus (VMO). The MPFL is one of the most important structures in the medial retinacular complex, as it serves as the primary deterrent to lateral patellar subluxation.

The patellotibial ligament arises from the tibia near the attachments of the gracilis and semitendinosus muscles and courses in an anterior, proximal direction to fuse with layer I. It then inserts into the inferior aspect of the patella and the contiguous patellar tendon (**Fig. 2-6**).

Layer III

Layer III, the joint capsule proper, is the deepest layer and consists of three ligaments: (1) the deep portion of the MCL, (2) coronary ligament (with its meniscofemoral

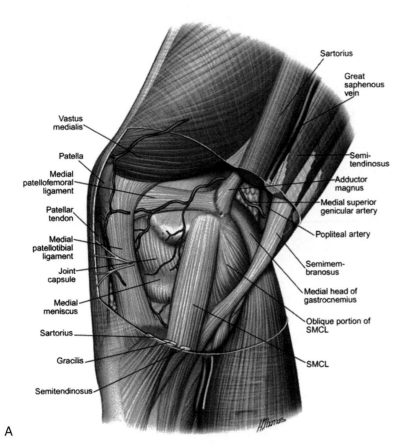

A

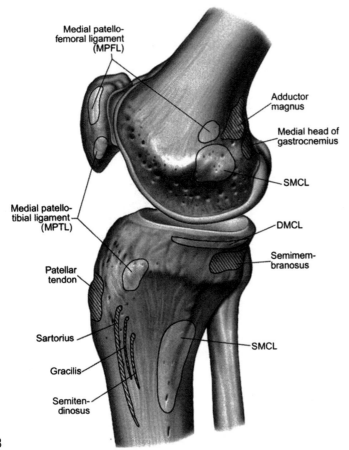

B

FIGURE 2-8   A: Layer II of the medial knee—the medial retinacular complex. Layer II, the medial retinacular complex, lies deep to layer I and is made of the superficial medial collateral ligament (SMCL), the medial patellofemoral ligament (MPFL), and the medial patellotibial ligament (MPTL). Layer I and superficial muscles are cut away to view layer II. The ligaments of the medial retinacular complex form an inverted triangle with a central fascial deficiency. The SMCL is divided into two portions: a vertically oriented anterior component and an obliquely oriented posterior component. The superior and inferior points of attachment of the vertical portion of the SMCL define the extents of layer II. The fibers of the oblique portion of the SMCL arise just posterior to the proximal attachment of the vertical fibers of the SMCL and extend distally in a posterooblique fashion to fuse with layer III to become the posterior oblique ligament (not shown). The MPFL arises from the adductor tubercle of the medial femoral condyle and travels to the patella, where it fuses with layer I at the patellar insertion. The MPFL is a key structure preventing lateral subluxation of the patella. The MPTL arises from the tibia near the insertion of the muscles of the pes anserinus. It travels superiorly to fuse with layer I at the insertion on the inferior aspect of the patella and the patellar tendon. **B:** Sites of attachment of the ligaments of layer II and muscles of the medial knee. The proximal insertion of the SMCL is at the medial femoral epicondyle approximately 5 cm above the tibiofemoral joint line. The distal attachment is at the medial aspect of the tibial metaphysis, 6 to 8 cm distal to the joint line and posterior to the sartorius, semitendinosus, and gracilis tendons. The MPFL ligament arises from the adductor tubercle on the medial femoral epicondyle superior to the proximal attachment of the SMCL. It travels anteriorly to variable attachments on the proximal half of the medial edge of the patella. The PTL arises near the insertion of the pes anserinus and travels superiorly to attach to the inferior margin of the patella. DMCL, deep portion of the medial collateral ligament.

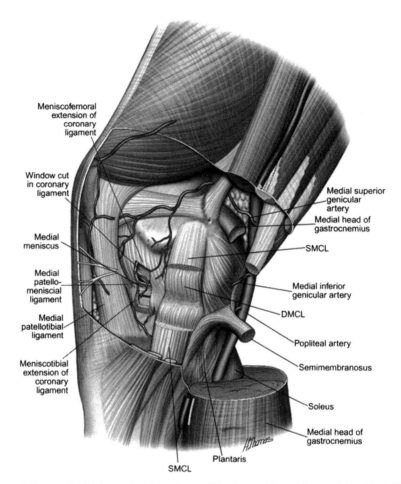

FIGURE 2-9   Layer III of the medial knee—the joint capsule—is made up of the deep portion of the medial collateral ligament (DMCL), the coronary ligament with its meniscofemoral and meniscotibial extensions, and the medial patellomeniscal ligament. The superficial medial collateral ligament (SMCL) has been cut to view the underlying DMCL. The DMCL is actually composed of fibrous extensions of the underlying medial meniscus and of fibers from the meniscofemoral and meniscotibial extensions of the coronary ligament. The window cuts into the coronary ligament exposing the medial meniscus and articular surfaces beneath. The ligaments of layer III are closely interdigitating and are difficult to distinguish from the underlying medial meniscus. Thus, care must be taken when resecting the medial meniscus to not violate the superficial and deep portions of the medial collateral ligament.

and meniscotibial extensions), and (3) medial patellomeniscal ligament (**Fig. 2-9**). Anteriorly, this layer is thin and is continuous with the capsule of the suprapatellar recess that extends to the margin of the patella. Beneath the vertical component of the SMCL, the capsule thickens, forming the deep MCL. This deep collateral ligament is composed of fibers from the adjacent meniscal rim and from the meniscofemoral and meniscotibial extensions of the coronary meniscal ligament. On MRI scan, it is difficult to distinguish the outer margin of the meniscus from the capsule and deep portion of the MCL, thus indicating their close interdigitation.[29] The meniscotibial and meniscofemoral extensions of the coronary meniscal ligament can be seen as low-signal-intensity structures deep to the SMCL, often with fat interposed between their attachment sites and layer II. Care must be taken when resecting the medial meniscus so that the integrity of the MCL is not compromised, particularly in the valgus knee with medial laxity.

Layers of the Lateral Knee

The lateral aspect of the knee is a complex arrangement of tendons, ligaments, and muscles that provide static and dynamic stabilization of the anterolateral, lateral, and posterolateral aspects of the knee based on their location and function.[30] The lateral structures of the knee have similarly been divided into three layers.[31]

Layer I

Layer I, the most superficial layer, is composed of the ITB and its anterior expansion and the biceps femoris and its posterior expansion (**Fig. 2-10A**), these being interconnected by fascia. Eventually, layer I becomes continuous with the prepatellar bursa anteriorly, while covering the popliteal fossa posteriorly. At their extremes, the components of layer I merge with layer I of the medial knee (**Fig. 2 6**).

The ITB, or iliotibial band, is formed proximally from the fascia investing the tensor fascia lata, the gluteus

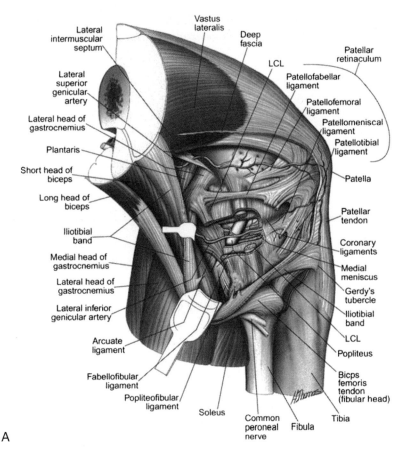

Lateral intermuscular septum
Vastus lateralis
Deep fascia
Patellar retinaculum
LCL
Patellofabellar ligament
Lateral superior genicular artery
Patellofemoral ligament
Patellomeniscal ligament
Lateral head of gastrocnemius
Patellotibial ligament
Plantaris
Patella
Short head of biceps
Long head of biceps
Patellar tendon
Iliotibial band
Coronary ligaments
Medial head of gastrocnemius
Medial meniscus
Lateral head of gastrocnemius
Gerdy's tubercle
Lateral inferior genicular artery
Iliotibial band
LCL
Arcuate ligament
Popliteus
Fabellofibular ligament
Biceps femoris tendon (fibular head)
Popliteofibular ligament
Soleus
Common peroneal nerve
Fibula
Tibia

A

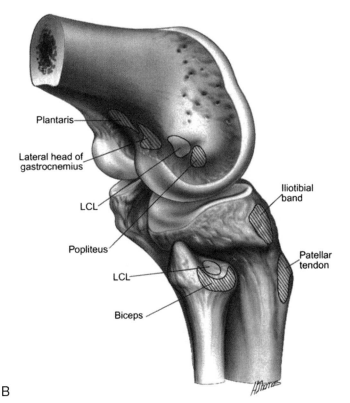

Plantaris
Lateral head of gastrocnemius
Iliotibial band
LCL
Popliteus
Patellar tendon
LCL
Biceps

B

FIGURE 2-10   A: Three layers of the lateral knee. Note that three windows have been cut in all three layers of the lateral knee to illustrate the location of these structures. Layer I of the lateral knee—the most superficial layer—is composed of the iliotibial band with its anterior expansion and the fascia of the biceps femoris with its posterior expansion, along with an intervening fascia. The iliotibial band connects to the femur at the linea aspera via the intermuscular septum, forming a posterior sling that assists the anterior cruciate ligament in preventing posterior displacement of the femur in near full extension. The iliotibial band is continuous with the crural fascia of the knee and attaches anterolaterally to the patella, patellar ligament, and tibial tuberosity, thus contributing to the anterolateral stability of the knee. Layer II of the lateral knee includes the retinaculum of the quadriceps muscles anteriorly and the patellofemoral and patellomeniscal ligaments posteriorly. The main components of layer III include the joint capsule, the fabellofibular ligament, and the arcuate complex. The joint capsule splits into the superficial and deep sublaminae. The lateral collateral ligament (LCL) and the inferior lateral geniculate artery lie between these two sublaminae. The fabellofibular ligament is part of the superficial sublamina, and the arcuate complex is part of the deep sublamina. The window cut in the coronary ligament shows the tendon of the popliteus muscle deep to it on the way to its femoral attachment. **B:** Attachment sites of the ligaments and muscles of the lateral knee. Observe the insertion of iliotibial band at Gerdy tubercle. The tendon of the biceps femoris muscle is split into two parts by the lateral collateral ligament and inserts on the lateral aspect of the head of the fibula, on the lateral condyle of the tibia, and in the deep fascia of the lateral aspect of the leg.

maximus, and the gluteus medius muscles. It continues distally to attach to the linea aspera of the femur via the lateral intermuscular septum and to the lateral tubercle of the tibia (*Gerdy tubercle*), thus reinforcing the anterolateral aspect of the knee joint (**Fig. 2-10B**). Continuous with the crural fascia in the region of the knee, it attaches anteriorly to the patella, the patellar ligament, and the tibial tuberosity. Medially and laterally, it attaches to the condyles of the tibia and to the head of the fibula and, reinforced by tendinous fibers of the vastus muscles, forms the retinacula of the patella. The crural fascia is strengthened in the region of the knee by expansions of the tendons of the sartorius, gracilis, semitendinosus, and biceps femoris muscles.

Although there are muscular connections to the ITB, it is essentially a passive structure at the knee joint because contraction of either the tensor fascia lata or the gluteus maximus muscles does not produce appreciable excursion of the distal ITB. The ITB appears to be relatively taut regardless of position of the hip joint or knee joint, although it falls anterior to the knee joint axis in extension and posterior to the axis in flexion.[32,33] In the valgus knee, it often must be released to balance lateral joint contracture.[24,25] In the lateral parapatellar approach, the ITB is released as part of the exposure, often sufficient to balance the valgus knee.[34] The ITB's fibrous connections to the biceps femoris and vastus lateralis muscles through the lateral intermuscular septum form a sling behind the lateral femoral condyle, assisting the ACL in preventing posterior displacement of the femur when the tibia is fixed and the knee joint is near extension. The ITB sends fibers from its anterior margin to attach to the patella, forming an iliopatellar band that may be implicated in abnormal lateral forces on the patella (**Fig. 2-10A**).

Layer II

Layer II is made up of the retinaculum of the quadriceps muscles anteriorly and the patellofemoral and patellomeniscal ligaments posteriorly (**Fig. 2-10A**). As part of this layer, the patellar retinaculum has attachments at the lateral intermuscular septum, the iliotibial tract of layer I, the fabella, the lateral meniscus, and the lateral tubercle of the tibia. Layer I and layer II are adherent to each other in a line at the lateral margin of the patella (**Fig. 2-6**).

Layer III

The main components of layer III, the deepest layer, are (1) the joint capsule, (2) the fabellofibular ligament, and (3) the arcuate complex. This layer is attached inferiorly and superiorly to the edges of the tibia and femur, respectively (**Fig. 2-6**). The capsular attachment at the lateral meniscus is called the *coronary ligament*. Internal to this layer, the popliteus tendon passes through a hiatus in the coronary ligament along the lateral border of the lateral meniscus to its attachment on the femur. The superior and inferior fascicles of the lateral meniscus border this popliteal tendon tunnel. This area has been studied to differentiate pathologic from anatomic consideration related to its complex structure.[35]

The joint capsule splits into two sublaminae at the anterolateral knee at the 2 o'clock position (viewing caudad in the right knee from above) (**Fig. 2-6**). The more anterior, superficial sublamina includes the fabellofibular ligament. The more posterior, deep sublamina includes the arcuate ligament. This split creates an interval that contains the LCL and the inferior lateral geniculate artery. The inferior lateral geniculate artery enters this interval between the LCL and the deep capsular sublamina to run along the periphery of the lateral meniscus. Thus, great care must be exercised when removing the lateral meniscus, particularly when using the lateral parapatellar approach, as this artery is the vascular supply to the fat pad pedicle.

The fabellofibular ligament of the more superficial sublamina and the arcuate ligament of the deep sublamina both insert on the apex of the head of the fibula at the fibular styloid. The anterior, superficial lamina travels posteriorly and ends at the posterior border of the fabellofibular ligament. The phylogenetically newer deep sublamina passes from the coronary ligaments to the arcuate ligament. The arcuate ligament fans out medially over the popliteus muscle to join the oblique popliteal ligament. Significant variations in layer III have been described.[34]

KNEE JOINT MUSCLES AND STABILITY

Knee Flexors

Seven muscles flex the knee: (1) semimembranosus, (2) semitendinosus, (3) biceps femoris, (4) sartorius, (5) gracilis, (6) popliteus, and (7) gastrocnemius muscles. The semitendinosus, semimembranosus, and the biceps femoris muscles are known collectively as the *hamstrings*, and all originate on the ischial tuberosity of the pelvis. All of the knee flexors, except for the short head of the biceps femoris and the popliteus, are two joint muscles (i.e., crossing the hip and the knee). As two joint muscles, their ability to produce effective force can be influenced by the relative position of the two joints over which they pass. Four of the flexors (popliteus, gracilis, semimembranosus, and semitendinosus muscles) medially rotate the tibia on the fixed femur, whereas the biceps femoris is a lateral rotator of the tibia.

The *semitendinosus muscle* arises from the lower and medial impression on the ischial tuberosity in common with the long head of the biceps femoris muscle. Its tendon forms the medial margin of the popliteal fossa, then curves around the medial condyle of the tibia, and inserts as part of the pes anserinus into the upper medial surface of the tibia (**Fig. 2-8B**). Along with the gracilis, it is separated from the more posteriorly located tibial collateral ligament of the knee joint by a bursa. Two branches of the tibial division of the sciatic nerve (L4 - S3) usually innervate the muscle. The upper branch, frequently also supplying the long head of the biceps femoris muscle, enters the middle one-third of the semitendinosus muscle on its deep surface. The lower branch splits to enter the deep surface of the distal half of the semitendinosus muscle and the distal third of the semimembranosus muscle.

The *semimembranosus muscle* originates from the upper and lateral impression on the tuberosity of the ischium by a long, flat tendon that lies beneath the proximal half of the semitendinosus muscle. This tendon, which adheres proximally to the tendon of the adductor magnus anteriorly and to the tendons of the biceps femoris and semitendinosus muscles posteriorly, descends to the middle of the muscle. The tendon of the insertion of the semimembranosus ends primarily in the horizontal groove on the posteromedial aspect of the medial condyle of the tibia (**Fig. 2-5**). Fibrous expansions of the tendon reach the lateral condyle of the femur (via fusion with the oblique popliteal ligament of the knee joint), the fascia of the popliteus muscle, and the tibial collateral ligament. Some fibers of the semimembranosus muscle attach to the medial meniscus, thus assisting in knee flexion by facilitating posterior motion of the medial meniscus during active knee flexion. As mentioned, the semimembranosus muscle is innervated by a branch of the tibial division of the sciatic nerve, which subsequently splits to send limbs to the semitendinosus and semimembranosus muscles. This branch divides into several small nerves that enter the deep surface of the muscle at approximately its midpoint.

The *biceps femoris* is a combination of one preaxial muscle (the long head) and one postaxial muscle (the short head). The *long head* arises from the lower and medial impression on the ischial tuberosity in conjunction with the semitendinosus muscle. The *short head* arises from the lateral aspect of the linea aspera (from the middle of the shaft of the femur down to its bifurcation) and from the lateral intermuscular septum. The muscle fibers join the tendon of the long head to form a heavy, round tendon that constitutes the lateral margin of the popliteal fossa. At the knee, the tendon is split into two parts by the fibular collateral ligament and inserts on the lateral aspect of the head of the fibula, the lateral condyle of the tibia, and in the deep fascia of the lateral aspect of the leg (**Fig. 2-10B**). The biceps femoris tendon may also be attached to the ITB and retinacular fibers of the lateral joint capsule. These attachments imply that the biceps femoris has a stabilizing role at the posterolateral aspect of the joint. The short head of the biceps femoris does not cross the hip joint and therefore has a unique action at the knee joint. The biceps femoris, as a combined muscle, has double innervation. The long head usually receives two branches of the tibial division of the sciatic nerve. One branch innervates the upper one-third, and the other, the middle one-third of the deep surface of the muscle. The nerve to the short head is a branch of the common peroneal division of the sciatic nerve (L4 - S2). It enters the superficial surface of the muscle near its lateral margin.

The semitendinosus, semimembranosus, and the biceps femoris muscles (hamstrings) flex the knee and extend the thigh. Because the muscles usually produce a combined action, maximal excursion at one joint (e.g., extension of the thigh) limits the movement at the other joint to less than maximal. Therefore, they work most effectively at the knee joint if they are lengthened over a flexed hip. With the body in the prone position, active knee flexion forces the hamstring muscles to shorten over both the hip (which will be extended) and over the knee. The hamstrings will weaken as knee flexion proceeds because the muscle group is approaching maximum contractile shortening, while the tension in the rectus femoris is increasing.

Supplemented by the almost vestigial plantaris muscle, the two heads of the *gastrocnemius muscle* and the soleus muscle form the triceps surae. The larger *medial head* takes origin from the rough area of the posterior popliteal surface of the femur immediately above the medial femoral condyle (**Fig. 2-5**). The *lateral head* arises from an impression superior and lateral to the superior edge of the lateral femoral condyle and from the distal end of the lateral supracondylar line of the femur (**Fig. 2-5**). Frequently, severe flexion contractures will require the release of not only the posterior capsule but also the subperiosteal origins of these muscles as dissection is carried proximal to the femoral metaphysis. Both heads also receive fibers from the back of the capsule of the knee joint, and a bursa lies deep to each tendon of origin. The bursa of the medial head frequently opens into the knee joint and may also communicate with the bursa deep to the tendon of the semimembranosus muscle.[21] Because of these communications, wear debris in failed TKAs is frequently found in these bursae. Extending distally approximately two-thirds of the length of the muscle, aponeurotic bands cover the outer margins and posterior surfaces of the two heads and provide further attachment for the muscular fibers. The muscle fibers from both heads end distally in the calcaneal tendon, which inserts into the calcaneus. Except for the plantaris muscle, the gastrocnemius is the only muscle at the knee that crosses both the ankle and knee joints. The gastrocnemius makes a relatively small contribution to knee flexion but is effective in preventing knee joint hyperextension. It contributes substantially by resisting the very large extension torque at the knee joint during the hyperextension point in the gait cycle. Thus, the gastrocnemius appears to be more a dynamic stabilizer at the knee joint. The medial and lateral heads of the gastrocnemius are each innervated by separate branches of the tibial division of the sciatic nerve that branch at the popliteal fossa.

The *plantaris muscle* has a short, fleshy belly that arises from the lateral supracondylar line of the femur above the origin of the lateral head of the gastrocnemius (**Fig. 2-5**) and the oblique popliteal ligament. Its belly ends in a long, slender tendon that descends between the gastrocnemius and soleus muscles and then along the medial border of the calcaneal tendon to insert into the calcaneus.

The plantaris muscle is innervated by a branch of the tibial division of the sciatic nerve.

The *sartorius muscle* arises superiorly from the anterior superior spine of the ilium and crosses the femur to insert into the anteromedial surface of the tibial shaft posterior to the tibial tuberosity (**Fig. 2-8B**). Variations in distal attachment of the sartorius muscle are not uncommon in contradistinction to those of the underlying gracilis and semitendinosus muscles.[26] Usually, it is a potential flexor and medial rotator of the tibia. When attached just anterior to its more usual location, it may fall anterior to the knee joint axis, serving as a mild knee joint extensor rather than as a flexor. The sartorius is the only flexor to be innervated by the femoral nerve (L2 - 4).

The *gracilis muscle* arises from the medial one-half of the inferior pubic ramus near the pubic symphysis. It travels superficially along the medial aspect of the thigh distally to the medial knee. At the knee it tapers into a thin tendon positioned between the tendons of the sartorius and the semitendinosus muscles. The tendon of the gracilis inserts into the anteromedial aspect of the tibia with the semitendinosus and sartorius muscles as part of the pes anserinus ("goose's foot"). These muscles collectively insert anterior and proximal to the insertion of the SMCL (**Fig. 2-8B**). The gracilis flexes the knee joint and produces slight medial rotation of the tibia. The three muscles of the pes anserinus appear to function effectively as a group to stabilize the medial aspect of the knee joint. Thus, the SMCL and deep MCL should be released instead of the pes anserinus when addressing varus contractures to preserve stability. The gracilis is the only knee flexor to be innervated by the obturator nerve (L2 - 4), receiving branches at its medial third from the anterior branch.

The other one joint knee flexor (in addition to the short head of the biceps femoris mentioned above) is the *popliteus muscle*. This muscle originates on the posterolateral aspect of the lateral femoral condyle and attaches on the medial aspect of the tibia (**Fig. 2-5**). It receives medial fibers from the posterior capsular ligaments and the lateral semilunar cartilage.[35] The popliteus is a flat, triangular muscle that lies in the floor of the inferior part of the popliteal fossa. The tendon passes between the lateral meniscus and the capsule of the knee joint and has a bursa that regularly communicates with the cavity of the joint (subpopliteal recess). The muscle inserts into the back of the tibia above the soleal line and into the fascia covering the soleus muscle (**Fig. 2-5**). The popliteus muscle is innervated by a branch of the tibial nerve that winds around the lower border of the muscle to enter its deep surface.

The popliteus flexes the leg at the knee and rotates it medial, thus serving as a medial rotator of the tibia on the femur. The popliteus muscle may play a role in initiating unlocking of the knee because it reverses the direction of automatic rotation that occurs in the final stages of knee extension. Also, in cases of osteoarthritis of the knee,

where lateral tibial subluxation relative to the femur is evident on anteroposterior weight-bearing radiographs, the popliteus may be contracted. In these cases, its release should be considered. However, the popliteus may stabilize the lateral flexion gap and should be one of the last structures released in cases of valgus knee deformity, as a flexion gap laxity can be created.[25,36] The popliteus muscle is commonly attached to the lateral meniscus, as the semimembranosus muscle is commonly attached to the medial meniscus. Because both the semimembranosus and the popliteus are knee flexors, activity in these muscles will not only generate a flexion torque, but also will actively augment the posterior movement of the two menisci on the tibial condyles that occurs during knee flexion as the femur begins its rolling motion. Although the menisci will move posteriorly on the tibial condyle even during passive flexion, the assistance of the semimembranosus and popliteus muscles reinforces the movement and minimizes the chance that the menisci will become entrapped, thus limiting knee flexion.

Knee Extensors

The four extensors of the knee are known collectively as the *quadriceps femoris muscle*. The only portion of the quadriceps that crosses two joints is the *rectus femoris*, which originates on the anterior inferior iliac spine. The vastus intermedius, vastus lateralis, and vastus medialis muscles originate on the femur and merge into a common quadriceps tendon. The fibers of the quadriceps tendon continue distally as the patellar ligament. The patellar ligament runs from the apex of the patella, across the anterior surface of the patella, to insert into the proximal portion of the tibial tubercle. The vastus medialis and vastus lateralis also insert directly into the medial and lateral aspects of the patella by way of the retinacular fibers of the joint capsule. Expansions of the aponeuroses of the vastus muscles insert into the condyles of the tibia as the medial and lateral retinacula of the patella.

The VMO serves as an important dynamic stabilizer of the patella.[37] The VMO portion of the vastus medialis overlies the superior aspect of the MPFL in layer II of the medial knee and is therefore not part of the medial retinacular complex. But, cephalad to the MPFL, the VMO tapers into its aponeurosis, which fuses with layer II of the medial retinacular complex near its insertion into the superior-medial patella. Because this insertion is divided during the medial parapatellar approach to the knee, careful reapproximation after arthroplasty is necessary to reestablish its important function of dynamic stabilization.

The vastus lateralis obliquus muscle on the lateral side of the knee may have important significance in the evolution of soft tissue pain and chondromalacia in patients with patellofemoral malalignment.[38] Great variability can exist in the anatomic orientation of its fibers and insertion, contributing a variable lateral force vector on the patella.[39] A lateral release of this structure will allow for medial stabilization of the patella.

Knee Joint Stabilization

The supporting structures of the knee contribute to knee joint stability based on their function and location. Categorizing structures as either static or dynamic further differentiates their functional contribution to stability. The static stabilizers include passive structures such as the joint capsule and various ligaments and other associated structures such as the menisci, the coronary ligaments, and the meniscopatellar and patellofemoral ligaments. Ligaments that are static stabilizers include the MCL and LCL, the ACL and PCL, the oblique popliteal and arcuate ligaments, and the transverse ligament. Because the ITB is considered to be a passive force at the knee in spite of its muscular connections, it is best categorized as a static stabilizer. The *dynamic stabilizers* of the knee include the following muscles and aponeuroses: (1) quadriceps femoris and extensor retinaculum, (2) pes anserinus (semitendinosus, sartorius, and gracilis muscles), (3) popliteus, (4) biceps femoris, and (5) semimembranosus. The supporting structures of the knee joint that are located on the anteromedial, medial, and posteromedial aspects of the knee are medial compartment structures. Structures located in the same respective areas on the lateral aspect stabilize lateral compartment structures (**Fig. 2-6**).

The contribution that both muscles and ligaments make to stability in an actual knee is dependent on joint position of the knee and surrounding joints, the magnitude and direction of force, and the availability of reinforcing structures to resist forces if the primary restraints become incompetent. Many knee joint structures can contribute to stability in all directions under specific normal or abnormal conditions. The variations among individuals (and between knees in the same individuals) also can contribute to significant variation. Therefore, the following summary should be considered a generalization with the aforementioned considerations.

Anterior/Posterior Stability

Anterior/posterior stability of the knee is provided by static and dynamic stabilizers and lateral and medial compartment structures. The contribution of the ligaments to anterior/posterior stability was discussed in Cruciate Ligaments. Some stabilizers, however, are particularly critical and bear reiteration of their function. The extensor retinaculum, which is composed of fibers from the quadriceps femoris, fuses with fibers of the joint capsule to provide dynamic support for the anteromedial and anterolateral aspects of the knee. The medial and lateral heads of the gastrocnemius reinforce the medial and lateral aspects of the posterior capsule. The popliteus is considered to be a particularly important posterolateral stabilizer, complementing the function of the PCL. The ACL and the hamstrings work in a complementary manner to resist forces that are attempting to displace the tibia anteriorly or shear the femur posteriorly.[40] Such forces are exemplified by the pull of the quadriceps and by the effect of the ground reaction force on the tibia when the heel hits the ground.[32] Kaplan placed particular emphasis on the semimembranosus muscle, contending that the knee could not be stable in flexion unless this structure and its multiple connections remain intact.

The role of the patella itself cannot be ignored when examining anterior/posterior stability of the knee. The patella prevents the femur from sliding forward off the tibia, actually serving as an extension of the tibia connected by an elastic tendon. This combination of patella and tibia creates a cradling effect on the femur.

Medial/Lateral Stability

Medial/lateral stability at the knee is provided for by static and dynamic soft tissue structures and by the tibial tubercles and menisci when the knee is in full extension. The knee is reinforced on its medial and lateral aspects by the collateral ligaments. The collaterals clearly play a critical role in resisting varus/valgus stresses, especially in the more extended knee. The tibial collateral ligament is a strong, flat band that extends from the tubercle on the medial condyle of the femur to the medial condyle of the tibia and to the medial surface of its shaft. It is the primary restraint to valgus angulation at the knee. The inferior genicular blood vessels pass between them and the capsule of the joint. Its deeper fibers end on the condyle and are attached to the medial meniscus. Care should thus be taken when excising the medial meniscus so as not to violate the substance of the MCL. The fibular collateral ligament is a rounded cord approximately 5 cm long and is the primary restraint to varus angulation at the knee. Superiorly, it is attached to the tubercle on the lateral epicondyle of the femur superior and posterior to the groove for the popliteus muscle. It ends inferiorly approximately 1 cm inferior to the apex of the head of the fibula on the lateral surface. The tendon of the popliteus muscle passes deep to the fibular collateral ligament, and the tendons of the long and short heads of the biceps femoris muscle split on either side of its lower attachment. Although the collateral ligament is frequently contracted and in need of release in the valgus knee, the popliteus stabilizes the lateral compartment in flexion and should seldom be released.

Both cruciate ligaments also contribute medial/lateral stability, although the magnitude and balance of the contribution vary with many factors. As knee flexion increases, the dynamic stability provided by the musculature such as the muscles of the pes anserinus on the medial aspect of the knee become increasingly important. Laterally, the iliotibial tract, LCL, popliteus tendon, and biceps tendon form a quadruple complex that contributes to stability. The posterolateral capsule is particularly important to varus stability in extension, whereas the popliteus is a major stabilizer in 0° to 90° of flexion.[41] The menisci are particularly important to medial/lateral stability because the knee remains stable in full extension regardless of sectioning of ligamentous structures. Removing both menisci would appear to have its greatest effect in stabilization during varus and valgus stresses.[42]

Restoration of appropriate medial/lateral laxity remains an important principle for TKA and knowing normal collateral ligament laxity in both extension and flexion is fundamental to intraoperatively balancing. Deep quantified the normal varus and valgus laxity in extension and 15° flexion in 267 knees in patients aged 19 to 35 years. Total varus valgus laxity in full extension was 7.7° and at 15° flexion measured 14.8°. He also found that females had greater valgus laxity in both full extension and 15° flexion. Additionally, the mean femorotibial mechanical axis was 1.7° varus in men compared to 0.8° varus in women.[43] Tokuhara et al. assessed varus valgus laxity in 90° flexion using MRI in 20 healthy patients with a mean age of 27.2 years and found medial gap opening of 2.1 ± 1.1 mm and lateral gap opening of 6.7 ± 1.9 mm. They concluded that the tibiofemoral flexion gap is not rectangular and the lateral gap has significantly more laxity.[44]

Rotational Stability

The complex nature of rotational stabilization of the knee makes it particularly difficult to isolate certain structures as being major contributors. It would appear, however, that the role of the passive mechanisms predominates over the dynamic mechanisms. The cruciates are most often credited with rotational stability of the joint, especially in the extended knee.[45] In the posterior cruciate–sacrificing TKA, these main rotational stabilizers are gone, requiring the femoral tibial congruency or cam-post mechanism to resist rotational forces. Credit is also given to the MCL and LCL, posteromedial capsule, posterolateral capsule, and the popliteus tendon by investigators exploring rotational stability under varied conditions.[46]

Patellofemoral Function

The patellofemoral joint is restrained by a transverse group and a longitudinal group of stabilizers. The position of the patella and its mobility will be determined by the relative tension in these two stabilizing systems. In the extended knee, the patella sits on the femoral sulcus. Medial/lateral stability in extension rests solely on active and passive tension in the structures around the patella. During flexion, as the patella begins sliding down the femoral condyles and is drawn into the intercondylar notch (at approximately 20° of flexion), the resulting patellofemoral compression contributes to medial/lateral stability.

The transverse stabilizers of the patella are the medial and lateral patellar retinacula, which join the vastus medialis and lateralis muscles directly to the patella, respectively. Several investigators have described medial and lateral patellofemoral ligaments that may be part of or blend with the retinacular fibers.

The longitudinal stabilizers of the patella are the patellar tendon inferiorly and the quadriceps tendon superiorly. The patellotibial ligaments are thickenings of the capsule anteriorly that extend from the inferior border of the patella distally to the anterior coronary ligaments and anterior margins of the tibia on each side of the patellar tendon. The longitudinal structures stabilize the patella through the patellofemoral compression that occurs with flexion. The compression is essentially absent in the extended knee, leaving the patella relatively unstable in this knee joint position. When extension is exaggerated, as in genu recurvatum, the pull of the quadriceps muscle and patellar ligament may actually distract the patella from the femoral sulcus, further aggravating the instability of the patella. Both the transverse and the longitudinal structures along with the configuration of the intercondylar notch will influence patellar tracking within the femoral sulcus.

KNEE MOTION

The active movements of the knee joint are customarily described as flexion, extension, medial rotation, and lateral rotation. The flexion and extension at this ginglymus joint differ from those of a true hinge, as the axis around which movement occurs is not fixed, but translates upward and forward during extension and backward and downward during flexion.

With the foot fixed on the ground, the last 30° of extension is associated with medial rotation of the femur. Compared with the medial femoral condyle, the articular surface of the smaller lateral femoral condyle is rounder and flattens more rapidly anteriorly. Consequently, it approaches a more fully congruent relationship with its apposed tibiomeniscal surface some 30° before full extension has been obtained. Full congruence laterally is obtained (rather than blocked) by deformation of the anterior horn of the meniscus as the lateral condyle passes progressively up the sloping anterior surface of the lateral tibial condyle. To achieve full extension, the lagging medial compartment must medially rotate about a fixed vertical axis while moving backward in an arc.

There is a progressive increase in the passive mechanisms that resist further extension. In full extension, parts of both cruciate ligaments, the collateral ligaments, the posterior capsular and oblique posterior ligament complex, and the skin and fascia are all taut. There is also passive or active tension in the hamstrings and gastrocnemius muscles and the ITB. In addition, the anterior parts of the menisci are compressed between the femoral condyles and the tibia. Because the menisci are no longer present in TKA, the articular surfaces must replace this function by conformity and congruence. Depending on knee design type and subsequent cruciate ligament resection, this function is replaced by the sagittal geometry, cam-post mechanism, and/or soft tissue tension. An appropriately sized implant spacer must be placed back into the extension gap to tense the periarticular structures and prevent recurvatum.

With the foot on the ground, the beginning of flexion from the fully extended position requires lateral rotation of the femur to "unlock" the knee joint. Although an opposite interplay of the meniscal, articular, and ligamentous structures is involved, evidence indicates the importance of the popliteus muscle. It pulls downward and posterior on its attachment to the lateral condyle of the femur, helping the greater rollback in this compartment that occurs with flexion. Via its meniscal attachment, it pulls on the posterior horn of lateral meniscus. In this way, while rollback and posterior motion of the menisci occur in both compartments, the greater motions laterally can be facilitated.

Flexion is checked by the tension in the quadriceps mechanism, the anterior sections of the capsule, and the PCL and by compression of the soft tissue structures in the popliteal fossa. Following TKA, retained posterior meniscal horns, posterior osteophytes, posterior soft tissue calcifications, and/or oversized implant spacers can create posterior compression significant enough to severely limit flexion.

ARTERIES

The arteries to the knee joint and surrounding structures are supplied by the large femoral and popliteal arteries (**Fig. 2-11**). The femoral artery enters the lower limb by passing deep to the inguinal ligament and into the femoral triangle. The artery then sends off the large profunda femoris, which dives deep into the thigh. Immediately after splitting off the femoral artery, the profunda femoris gives rise to the lateral circumflex femoral artery. The descending branch of this artery travels down the thigh to contribute to knee circulation and periarticular anastomoses. The femoral artery proper continues its more superficial course, giving off muscular branches to the vastus medialis and lateralis, which allow for their use as muscle flaps for coverage of wounds about the knee.[47] Immediately superior to its entrance through the adductor hiatus in the distal thigh (where it becomes the popliteal artery), the femoral artery gives rise to the descending genicular artery. This artery immediately divides into the saphenous branch and the articular branch, which contributes to knee circulation and periarticular anastomoses (**Fig. 2-12**). The saphenous branch pierces the fascia of the adductor canal to pass between the tendons of the gracilis and sartorius muscles along with the saphenous

nerve. With the nerve, the artery perforates the fascia lata and supplies the skin and the superficial tissues in the upper medial aspect of the leg. The saphenous artery forms the basis for a medial knee fasciocutaneous flap for use in central wound coverage.[48-52] The articular branch descends in the substance of the vastus medialis muscle, anterior to the adductor magnus tendon, to the medial side of the knee. It supplies branches to the vastus medialis muscle and anastomoses with the medial superior genicular and the anterior recurrent tibial arteries. A branch passes laterally over the patellar surface of the femur, supplies the knee joint, and anastomoses with the descending branch of the lateral circumflex femoral and lateral superior genicular arteries.

At the apex of the femoral triangle, the femoral artery enters the adductor (Hunter) canal at the junction of the middle and distal thirds of the femur. At the adductor hiatus, in the tendon of the adductor magnus muscle, the femoral artery passes into the popliteal space and becomes the popliteal artery (**Fig. 2-11**). It descends through the popliteal space and is separated from the intercondylar fossa of the femur by fat, the POL, and the popliteus fascia distal to the joint line (from superior to inferior). The popliteal artery is the deepest of the vascular structures in the popliteal fossa, lying deep to the popliteal vein and the tibial nerve (most superficial). During its course through the popliteal fossa, it gives off multiple branches that supply the knee joint and musculature (discussed in Geniculate Vessels and Knee Anastomoses). Opposite the lower border of the popliteus muscle, the popliteal artery ends by dividing into the anterior tibial and posterior tibial arteries. Some variability may occur at this bifurcation.[53]

The anterior tibial artery is a division of the popliteal artery at the lower border of the popliteus muscle. It passes forward into the anterior compartment of the leg between the two origins of the tibialis posterior muscle, above the upper margin of the interosseous membrane. Immediately after entering the anterior compartment, the anterior tibial artery gives off the anterior tibial recurrent artery, which ascends among the deep fibers of the tibialis anterior muscle. It then branches over the front and sides of the knee joint. Participating in the patellar plexus, it anastomoses with the genicular branches of the popliteal artery and with the descending genicular branches of the femoral artery. The posterior tibial recurrent artery usually arises from the anterior tibial artery in the posterior compartment of the leg before it traverses the interosseous membrane. It ascends between the popliteus muscle and the back of the knee, supplies the popliteus muscle and the tibiofibular joint, and anastomoses with the lateral inferior geniculate artery.

With medial or posterior proximal knee dissections, the popliteal artery can be injured, particularly in its less mobile position within the hiatus. It can be indirectly injured with fixing of a bulk allograft, during

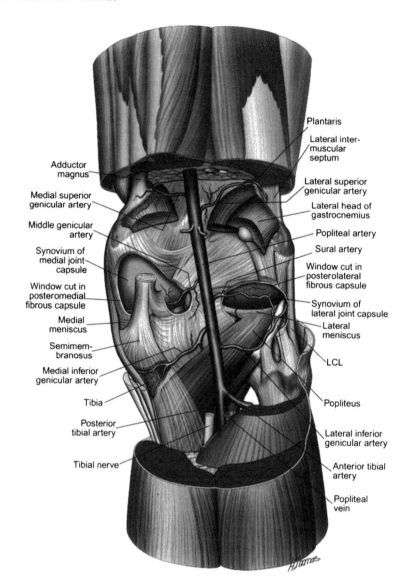

FIGURE 2-11   Branches of the popliteal artery in the popliteal fossa. The artery is separated from the intercondylar fossa of the femur by fat, the posterior oblique ligament, and the popliteus fascia (from superior to inferior). The popliteal vein lies interposed between the artery and the tibial nerve (not shown). Musculature is cut away to observe the deep fossa. During its course through the popliteal fossa, the artery gives rise to many muscular branches and five genicular branches. From proximal to distal, they are as follows: lateral superior genicular, medial superior genicular, middle genicular, sural, lateral inferior genicular, and medial inferior genicular. Near the inferior margin of the popliteus muscle, the popliteal artery ends in two branches: the anterior tibial artery and the posterior tibial artery. The anterior tibial artery crosses into the anterior compartment above the superior border of the interosseous membrane. LCL, lateral collateral ligament.

replacement of the distal femoral, or with cerclage wire fixation of periprosthetic fractures. The popliteal artery can be directly injured with extensive posterior release when addressing a severe flexion contracture, if dissection is not directly on bone. Rarely, a saw can penetrate the popliteus muscle and injure the vessel during tibial preparation. Warrington et al. concluded that the safest knee position is between 60° and 90° of flexion based on a mean posterior popliteal artery movement of 3.15 mm in 45 knees using color-flow duplex imaging. Interestingly, these results were not observed in knees that had undergone a previous knee arthroplasty.[54] Although flexing the knee is frequently protective, in one study, MRI evaluation showed the artery moved closer to the posterior knee joint with flexion.[55] Another study utilized duplex

ultrasonography in 100 knees and demonstrated that the popliteal artery actually moved closer to the posterior tibial surface at 1 to 1.5 cm below the joint line in 24% and at 1.5 to 2 cm below the joint line in 15%.[56] Additionally, a smaller study of 40 patients undergoing TKA showed a small but significant difference between preoperatively measured distances in flexion and extension where extension showed a slightly larger posterior movement away from the tibia.[57]

Geniculate Vessels and Knee Anastomoses

The extensive *anastomoses* about the knee joint effectively link the femoral artery proximally with the popliteal and anterior and posterior tibial arteries distally.[58]

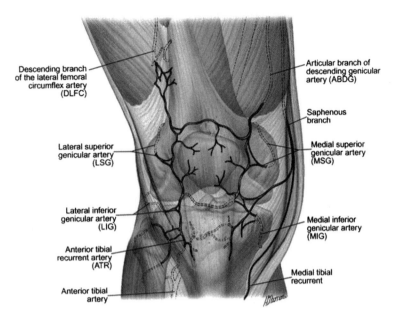

FIGURE 2-12 Vascular anastomoses of the peripatellar ring. Note the seven vessels of the peripatellar ring: the ABDG, the MSG, the MIG, the ATR, the LIG, the LSG, and the DLFC.

The popliteal vessel contributes the middle linkage to this potential collateral circulation through its genicular vessels. During its course through the popliteal fossa, the popliteal artery gives off many muscular branches and genicular arteries.[5] From proximal to distal they are as follows: (1) lateral superior genicular, (2) medial superior genicular, (3) middle genicular, (4) sural, (5) lateral inferior genicular, and (6) medial inferior genicular. All hug the skeletal plane, with nothing intervening except the popliteus tendon, which is crossed by the lateral inferior genicular artery (**Fig. 2-11**).

The *lateral superior genicular artery* is given off proximal to the lateral condyle of the femur. It passes laterally against the origin of the plantaris muscle followed by the origin of the lateral head of the gastrocnemius muscle. Lying deep to the tendon of the biceps femoris muscle, the artery winds anteriorly around the femur immediately above the lateral femoral condyle. It supplies a superficial branch to the vastus lateralis muscle. It then anastomoses with the descending branch of the lateral circumflex femoral and the lateral inferior genicular arteries (**Fig. 2-12**). Its deep branch supplies the knee joint and forms an anastomotic arch across the front of the femur with the descending genicular and the medial superior genicular arteries (see the discussion of the peripatellar ring [PPR] below). Despite its considerable size, its sacrifice during lateral release to realign the patella does not significantly impact patella blood supply as ascertained by bone scan.[59] However, its ligation may be a reason for problems with the viability of lateral skin flaps, giving rise to the statement that the lateral-most incision should be chosen for TKA. This artery in conjunction with popliteal perforators supplies cutaneous circulation to the distal lateral thigh and forms the basis for the fasciocutaneous flap in this region.[60-62]

The *medial superior genicular artery* courses medially on the medial head of the gastrocnemius muscle anterior to the tendons of the semimembranosus and semitendinosus muscles. It has two branches, one of which perforates through the medial intramuscular septum to supply the vastus medialis muscle. This vessel is easily injured (and it often retracts and is difficult to ligate) with extensive elevation of the vastus medialis off of the medial intramuscular septum for exposure during a subvastus approach.[63] It can also be injured with division of the fibers of the vastus medialis during the midvastus approach. This branch anastomoses with the descending genicular and the medial inferior genicular arteries (**Fig. 2-12**). The other branch supplies the knee joint and, through the anastomotic arch across the femur, anastomoses with the lateral superior genicular artery.

The *middle genicular artery* is an unpaired branch that arises from the anterior aspect of the popliteal artery opposite the back of the knee joint. It pierces the POL and supplies the posterior capsule and the intracapsular cruciate ligaments and posterior horns of the menisci. An intraosseous branch of this vessel is found when elevating the cruciate ligaments off of their femoral attachments in the notch as the first step in a subperiosteal posterior capsular dissection.

The *sural arteries* are usually two large muscular branches that enter the proximal aspects of the heads of the gastrocnemius to send branches to this muscle, the plantaris, and the upper aspect of the soleus. They also send proximal unnamed muscular branches to the lower end of the hamstring muscles and cutaneous branches to the skin over the popliteal fossa. One cutaneous branch descends along the middle of the back of the calf with the lesser saphenous vein. The sural arteries are the vascular pedicle for a gastrocnemius flap used for wound coverage about the knee.[64]

The *lateral inferior genicular artery* passes across the popliteus muscle anterior to the lateral head of the gastrocnemius and the plantaris muscle. As it courses laterally over the arcuate popliteal ligament, it often divides into two branches. One branch turns anterior at the side of the knee, lying deep to the fibular collateral ligament just lateral to the lateral meniscus at the level of the joint line. This vessel can be easily injured when removing the lateral meniscus at the region anterior to the popliteal hiatus, with an excessively deep lateral dissection. This anatomic relationship of the vessel to the lateral meniscus is particularly important when using the lateral parapatellar approach, as the lateral inferior geniculate is the predominant vascular supply for the fat pad flap.[34] One should leave the lateral meniscus attached to this pedicle as the lateral meniscus is being separated from its attachment on the lateral tibia. The branches of the lateral inferior genicular artery anastomose with the lateral superior genicular, the medial inferior genicular, and the anterior and recurrent tibial arteries (**Fig. 2-12**).

The *medial inferior genicular artery* passes medial along the upper border of the popliteus muscle, anterior to the medial head of the gastrocnemius muscle. On the medial side of the knee, two fingerbreadths distal to the joint line, the artery runs deep to the tibial collateral ligament. At the anterior border of the ligament, branches ascend to anastomose with the descending genicular and medial superior genicular arteries. Other branches pass across the tibia under the patellar ligament and anastomose with the lateral inferior genicular and the anterior recurrent tibial arteries.

The PPR is supplied by seven vessels: (1) the articular branch of the descending genicular, (2) the medial superior geniculate, (3) the medial inferior geniculate, (4) the anterior tibial recurrent, (5) the lateral inferior geniculate, (6) the lateral superior geniculate, and (7) the descending branch of the lateral femoral circumflex artery.[48,65,66] The transverse suprapatellar portion of the PPR is supplied medially by the articular branch of the descending genicular and medial superior geniculate arteries and laterally by the lateral superior geniculate and descending branch of the lateral femoral circumflex arteries. Therefore, a medial parapatellar approach only interrupts the medial contributions from the articular branch of the descending genicular and medial superior geniculate. And, if the peripatellar dissection leaves an adequate sleeve of tissue (1 cm), the vertical limb of the PPR is left intact.[67] The transverse infrapatellar portion of the PPR passes deep to the patellar tendon and is supplied by the lateral inferior geniculate, medial inferior geniculate, and anterior tibial recurrent arteries. Of note, these vessels are protected if the portion of the fat pad that lies against the undersurface of the patella tendon is left intact. However, in the lateral parapatellar approach, as the fat pad is elevated from the undersurface of the tendon, this limb is interrupted, whereas the more significant inferior lateral geniculate is preserved. The interosseus blood supply to the patella from the PPR and anterior cortical perforating vessels is such that a patellar component with a central peg is most likely to jeopardize its vascularity (in contrast to a component with peripheral pegs only).[68]

VEINS

At a variable level in the popliteal fossa, the union of the venae comitantes of the anterior tibial, posterior tibial, and peroneal arteries forms the popliteal vein. It is usually a single vein that ascends through the popliteal fossa superficial to the popliteal artery and deep to tibial nerve. The vein is bound to the artery by a dense fascial sheath and lies somewhat medial to the artery inferiorly but against its lateral side above the knee joint. A single popliteal vein is to be expected with certainty only above a point approximately 5 cm above the level of the knee joint.[69] Three or four bicuspid valves prevent backflow in the vein, one valve being consistently found just distal to the adductor hiatus. The popliteal vein becomes continuous with the femoral vein at the adductor hiatus.

The popliteal vein is a common site of deep venous thrombosis, especially in the TKA patient. The intima of the vein may be injured during manipulation of the knee in surgery. This, combined with postsurgical immobility and a hypercoagulable state (Virchow triad), greatly predisposes the patient to deep venous thrombosis.

NERVES

Muscle and Knee Joint Innervation

The nerves of significance to the knee joint in TKA are from branches of the obturator and femoral nerves of the lumbar plexus and the tibial and common peroneal nerves from the sacral plexus.

The *obturator nerve* is a preaxial nerve that arises from the anterior branches of lumbar plexus nerves two, three, and four and descends along the medial border of the psoas muscle, entering the thigh through the obturator canal, where it divides into an anterior and a posterior branch at the level of the obturator externus muscle. The posterior branch descends behind the adductor brevis muscle and under the muscular fascia of the adductor magnus and supplies the obturator externus and adductor magnus muscles and at times the adductor brevis muscle. The posterior branch continues through the substance of the adductor magnus and ends in an articular branch to the knee joint. This articular branch accompanies the popliteal artery in the popliteal fossa, where it penetrates the oblique popliteal ligament to supply the posterior aspect of the knee joint. This innervation may be the anatomic reason for hip pain referred to the knee.

The *femoral nerve* is a postaxial nerve formed by the posterior branches of the second, third, and fourth lumbar nerves. It passes under the inguinal ligament, entering the femoral triangle where the terminal muscular, articular, and cutaneous branches arise. Muscular branches supply the pectineus, sartorius, and quadriceps femoris muscles. Three or four articular branches from the femoral nerve reach the knee joint. A continuation of the muscular branch to the vastus lateralis muscle penetrates the joint capsule on its anterior aspect. A second articular branch, the *medial retinacular nerve*, is a filament derived from the lower branch to the vastus medialis muscle and accompanies the descending genicular artery to enter the knee joint on its medial side. This nerve may be important in medial retinacular pain.[70] Selective block of the femoral nerve and its knee joint afferents can help determine the correct etiology of medial patella knee pain.[71] Third, the nerve to the articularis genu muscle also supplies the joint. A fourth articular branch sometimes arises from the *saphenous nerve* (the terminal branch of the femoral nerve), which is particularly important because of its frequent involvement in neuromas after TKA. The cutaneous branches, the anterior femoral cutaneous nerve and the saphenous nerve, are discussed in Cutaneous Innervation.

The *sciatic nerve* is derived from the sacral plexus (L4 - S3) and is made up of the *tibial* (medial) and *common peroneal* (lateral) nerves contained within a common connective tissue sheath. The tibial division is formed from the anterior branches of L4 through S3. The common peroneal division of the sciatic is formed from the posterior branches of nerves L4 through S2. The tibial and common peroneal nerves supply the muscles of the leg. The tibial nerve distributes to the muscles of both the superficial and deep portions of the posterior (preaxial) compartment of the leg and the common peroneal nerve to those of the anterior and lateral (postaxial) compartments. The superficial peroneal supplies the peroneus longus and brevis muscles of the lateral compartment and the deep peroneal the muscles of the anterior compartment.

The tibial nerve is the larger of the two divisions of the sciatic nerve. Separating from the common peroneal nerve at the proximal aspect of the popliteal fossa, the tibial nerve runs vertically through the fossa directly under the popliteal fascia. As it courses distally, it passes between the heads of the gastrocnemius and under the soleus muscle. Three articular branches arise in the popliteal fossa and accompany the medial superior genicular, medial inferior genicular, and middle genicular arteries to the knee joint. Also arising here are the medial sural cutaneous nerve and muscular branches to the plantaris, soleus, popliteus, and both gastrocnemius muscles. The muscular branch to the popliteus muscle also supplies articular branches to the knee and to the tibiofibular articulation.

While still in combination with the tibial nerve in the sciatic nerve, the common peroneal nerve gives a muscular branch to the short head of the biceps femoris muscle and an articular branch to the knee joint. The nerve to the short head of the biceps femoris muscle (L5 - S2) arises

from the lateral side of the common peroneal division of the sciatic in the middle one-third of the thigh and enters the superficial surface of the muscle near its lateral margin. This nerve continues to the knee as an articular branch. In the popliteal fossa, it divides into proximal and distal branches that accompany the lateral superior genicular and lateral inferior genicular arteries to the knee joint.

The common peroneal nerve separates from the tibial portion of the sciatic nerve at the apex of the popliteal fossa. In the popliteal fossa, the nerve gives off the lateral sural cutaneous and the peroneal communicating branches. It then follows the tendon of the biceps femoris muscle along the upper lateral margin of the popliteal fossa to the back of the head of the fibula. At this point, considerable restriction in nerve mobility can occur,[72] necessitating release when significant scarring or contracture is present (severe valgus or flexion contractures).[73] Deep tibial resection to levels below the head of the fibula can violate the nerve. Visualization of the cartilage of the tibiofibular joint after resection of the tibia can alert one to this possibility. The nerve then winds around the neck of the bone, passes deep to the peroneus longus muscle, and divides into the *superficial peroneal* and *deep peroneal nerves*. Just proximal to its terminal division, the *recurrent articular branch* arises and continues forward through the fibers of the peroneus longus and extensor digitorum longus muscles. Ascending with the anterior tibial recurrent artery, the *recurrent articular nerve* supplies the uppermost fibers of the tibialis anterior, the tibiofibular articulation, and the knee joint. The superficial peroneal nerve arises between the peroneus longus muscle and the neck of the fibula. It descends in the anterior intermuscular septum, supplying branches to the peroneus longus and peroneus brevis muscles and cutaneous twigs to the skin of the lower aspect of the front of the leg. The deep peroneal nerve also arises from the division of the common peroneal nerve between the peroneus longus muscle and the neck of the fibula. It continues anteriorly and distally to join the anterior tibial artery in its distal descent at its lateral margin.

Cutaneous Innervation

The infrapatellar branch of the saphenous nerve and other cutaneous nerves around the knee have recently been investigated because of their frequent association with neuromas after TKA.[74] Their successful ablation has also been discussed.[71] These same cutaneous nerves are valuable in supplying subcutaneous fascial pedicle flaps, providing sensate coverage of knee wounds.[75] Therefore, study of cutaneous innervation about the knee region bears consideration. The cutaneous innervation of the knee region is derived from the femoral, obturator, tibial, and common peroneal nerves (**Fig. 2-13**). The *cutaneous branch* of the obturator nerve, the *anterior cutaneous nerve*, and the *saphenous nerve* originate from lumbar

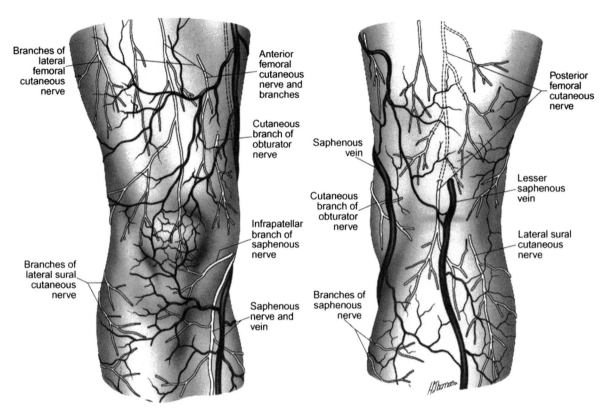

FIGURE 2-13   Cutaneous innervation of the knee. The cutaneous innervation of the knee region is derived from the femoral, obturator, tibial, and common peroneal nerves.

plexus nerves. The *posterior femoral cutaneous nerve* and *sural nerve* are from the sacral plexus nerves.

The anterior cutaneous branches of the femoral nerve are multiple and descend vertically over the quadriceps femoris muscle, becoming cutaneous by piercing the fascia lata at varying points. A proximal branch pierces the fascia lata near the apex of the femoral triangle and follows the greater saphenous vein. A medial branch distributes filaments to the skin and the subcutaneous tissue of the distal two-thirds of the medial thigh. The distal branch communicates, in the middle one-third of the thigh, with the saphenous and obturator nerves. It pierces the fascia lata in the lower one-third of the thigh and ramifies over the medial aspect of the knee, participating in the patellar plexus.

The cutaneous branch of the obturator nerve is a variable offshoot of the anterior branch of the obturator nerve. It communicates variably with the anterior cutaneous and saphenous branches of the femoral nerve and also has variable size. When present, it is distributed to the skin of the distal one-third of the medial thigh.

The saphenous nerve is the terminal branch of the femoral nerve. Arising from the femoral nerve in the femoral triangle, it crosses the adductor canal, piercing its distal fascial covering, and accompanies the saphenous branch of the descending genicular artery. A branch arising in the adductor canal communicates with the cutaneous branch of the obturator nerve and the anterior cutaneous branch of the femoral nerve. An *infrapatellar branch* pierces the sartorius muscle and fascia lata to exit the medial side of the knee. It curves downward below the patella and over the medial condyle of the tibia to the front of the knee and the upper part of the leg. It forms the patellar plexus along with communicating branches of the anterior cutaneous branch of the femoral nerve and branches of the lateral femoral cutaneous nerve. The infrapatellar branch of the saphenous nerve has been implicated in many cases of knee pain after knee surgery.[71,76-78] This nerve is almost exactly in the location of the inferior medial parapatellar portal for knee arthroscopy.[77]

The posterior femoral cutaneous nerve is a branch of both the anterior and posterior divisions of the sacral plexus. The nerve descends in the posterior midline of the thigh deep to the fascia lata, giving off small branches from both sides that individually pierce the fascia lata. They distribute to the skin of the back of the thigh and over the popliteal fossa. The posterior femoral cutaneous nerve finally pierces the fascia lata to end as one or two cutaneous branches over the calf.

The *lateral sural cutaneous nerve* is a branch of the common peroneal nerve that arises in the popliteal fossa. It pierces the deep fascia over the lateral head of the gastrocnemius muscle and distributes to the skin and the subcutaneous connective tissue on the posterolateral aspect of the proximal two-thirds of the leg.

CONCLUSION

In summary, the adult knee is a complex joint with unique anatomy and mechanics. Knowledge of the normal structures and their relationships is critical to understand the injury and pathology as well as treatment, both conservative and surgical.

REFERENCES

1. Mérida-Velasco JA, Sánchez-Monntesinos I, Espín-Ferra J, et al. Development of the human knee joint ligaments. *Anat Rec.* 1997;248:259-268.
2. Swanson KE, Stocks GW, Warren PD, et al. Does axial limb rotation affect the alignment measurements in deformed limbs?. *Clin Orthop.* 2000;371:246-252.
3. Jiang C, Insall JN. Effect of rotation on the axial alignment of the femur. *Clin Orthop.* 1989;248:50-56.
4. Good L, Odensten M, Gillquist J. Intercondylar notch measurements with special reference to anterior cruciate ligament surgery. *Clin Orthop.* 1991;263:185-278.
5. Pansky B. *Review of Gross Anatomy.* 4th ed. New York: MacMillian; 1979:437.
6. Matsuda S, Matsuda H, Miyagi T, et al. Femoral condyle geometry in the normal and varus knee. *Clin Orthop.* 1998;349:183-188.
7. Elias SG, Freeman MAR, Gokcay EI. A correlative study of the geometry and anatomy of the distal femur. *Clin Orthop.* 1990;260:98-103.
8. Highenboten CL, Jackson A, Aschliman M, et al. The estimation of femoral condyle size. *Clin Orthop.* 1989;246:225-233.
9. Berger RA, Rubash HE, Seel MJ, et al. Determining the rotational alignment of the femoral component in total knee arthroplasty using the epicondylar axis. *Clin Orthop.* 1993;286:40-47.
10. Miller MC, Berger RA, Petrella AJ, et al. Optimizing femoral component rotation in total knee arthroplasty. *Clin Orthop.* 2001;392:38-45.
11. Servien E, Viskontas D, Guiffre BM, et al. Reliability of bony landmarks for restoration of the joint line in revision knee arthroplasty. *Knee Surg Sports Traumatol Arthrosc.* 2008;16:263-269.
12. Eckhoff DG, Aukennan R. Femorotibial offset. A morphologic feature of the natural and arthritic knee. *Clin Orthop.* 1999;368:162-165.
13. Racanelli JA, Drez D Jr. Posterior cruciate ligament tibial attachment anatomy and radiographic landmarks for tibial tunnel placement in PCL reconstruction. *Arthroscopy.* 1994;10:546-549.
14. Hvid I. Trabecular bone strength at the knee. *Clin Orthop.* 1988;227:210-220.
15. Finlay JB, Bourne RB, Kraemer WJ, et al. Stiffness of bone underlying the tibial plateaus of osteoarthritic and normal knees. *Clin Orthop.* 1989;247:193-201.
16. Hofmann AA, Bachus KN, Wyatt RWB. Effect of the tibial cut on subsidence following total knee arthroplasty. *Clin Orthop.* 1991;261:63-69.
17. Churchill DL, Incavo SJ, Johnson CC, et al. The transepicondylar axis approximates the optimal flexion axis of the knee. *Clin Orthop.* 1998;356:111-118.
18. Matsumoto H, Seedhom BB, Suda Y, et al. Axis location of tibial rotation and its change with flexion angle. *Clin Orthop.* 2000;371:178-182.
19. Lee TQ, Budoff JE, Glaser FE. Patellar component positioning in total knee arthroplasty. *Clin Orthop.* 1999;366:274-281.
20. Girgis FG, Marshall JL, Monojem A. The cruciate ligaments of the knee joint. Anatomical, functional and experimental analysis. *Clin Orthop.* 1975;106:216-231.
21. Rauschning W. Anatomy and function of the communication between knee joint and popliteal bursae. *Ann Rheum Dis.* 1980;39:354-358.
22. Warren LF, Marshall JL. The supporting structures and layers on the medial side of the knee. *J Bone Joint Surg Am.* 1979;61:56-62.
23. Whiteside LA, Saeki K, Mihalko W. Functional medial ligament balancing in total knee arthroplasty. *Clin Orthop.* 2000;380:45-57.
24. Matsueda M, Gengerke TR, Murphy M, et al. Soft tissue release in total knee arthroplasty. *Clin Orthop.* 1999;366:264-273.
25. Whiteside LA. Selective ligament release in total knee arthroplasty of the knee in valgus. *Clin Orthop.* 1999;367:130-140.
26. Ivey M, Prud'homme J. Anatomic variations of the pes anserinus: a cadaver study. *Orthopedics.* 1993;16:601-606.
27. Fischer RA, Arms SW, Johnson RJ, et al. The functional relationship of the posterior oblique ligament to the medial collateral ligament of the human knee. *Am J Sports Med.* 1985;13:390-397.
28. Hughston JC, Barrett GR. Acute anteromedial rotatory instability. Long-term results of surgical repair. *J Bone Joint Surg Am.* 1983;65:145-153.
29. Loredo R, Hodler J, Pedowitz R, et al. Posteromedial corner of the knee: MR imaging with gross anatomic correlation. *Skeletal Radiol.* 1999;28:305-311.
30. Recondo JA, Salvador E, Villanúa JA, et al. Lateral stabilizing structures of the knee: functional anatomy and injuries assessed with MR imaging. *RadioGraphics.* 2000;20:S91-S102.
31. Seebacher JR, Inglis AE, Marshall JL, et al. The structure of the posterolateral aspect of the knee. *J Bone Joint Surg Am.* 1982;64:536-541.
32. Kaplan EB. Some aspects of functional anatomy of the human knee joint. *Clin Orthop.* 1962;23:18-29.
33. Kaplan EB. The iliotibial tract: clinical and morphologic significance. *J Bone Joint Surg Am.* 1958;40:817-832.
34. Keblish PA. The lateral approach to the valgus knee. *Clin Orthop.* 1991;271:52-62.
35. Cohn AK, Mans DB. Popliteal hiatus of the lateral meniscus. *Am J Sports Med.* 1979;7:221-226.
36. Mihalko WM, Miller CM, Krackow ICA. Total knee arthroplasty ligament balancing and gap kinematics with posterior cruciate ligament retention and sacrifice. *Am J Orthop.* 2000;29:610-616.
37. Goh JC, Lee PY, Bose K. A cadaver study of the function of the oblique part of vastus medialis. *J Bone Joint Surg Br.* 1995;77:225-231.
38. Hallisey MJ, Doherty N, Bennett WF, et al. Anatomy of the junction of the vastus lateralis tendon and the patella. *J Bone Joint Surg Am.* 1987;1994:545-549.
39. Weinstabl R, Scharf W, Firbas W. The extensor apparatus of the knee joint and its peripheral vasti: anatomic investigation and clinical relevance. *Surg Radiol Anat.* 1989;11:17-22.
40. Feagin JA, Lambert KL. Mechanisms of injury and pathology of the anterior cruciate ligament injuries. *Orthop Clin North Am.* 1985;16:41-45.
41. Nielsen S, Rasmussen O, Ovesen J, et al. Rotatory instability of cadaver knees after transection of collateral ligaments and capsule. *Arch Orthop Trauma Surg.* 1984;103:165-169.
42. Markolf KL, Barger WL, Shoemaker SC, et al. Role of joint load in knee stability. *J Bone Joint Surg Am.* 1981;63:570-585.
43. Deep K. Collateral ligament laxity in knees: what is normal?. *Clin Orthop Relat Res.* 2014;472:3426-3431.
44. Tokuhara Y, Kadoya Y, Nakagawa S. The flexion gap in normal knees. An MRI study. *J Bone Joint Surg Br.* 2004;86B1:1133-1136.
45. Fukubaya T, Torzilli PA, Sherman MF, et al. An in vitro biomechanical evaluation of anterior-posterior motion of the knee. Tibial displacement, rotation, and torque. *J Bone Joint Surg Am.* 1982;64:258-264.
46. Lipke JM, Janecki CJ, Nelson CL, et al. The role of incompetence of the anterior cruciate and lateral ligaments in anterolateral and anteromedial instability. A biomechanical study of cadaver knees. *J Bone Joint Surg Am.* 1981;63:954-960.
47. Swartz WM, Ramasastry SS, McGill JR, et al. Distally based vastus lateralis muscle flap for coverage of wounds about the knee. *Plast Reconstr Surg.* 1987;80:255-262.
48. Colombel M, Mariz Y, Dahhan P, et al. Arterial and lymphatic supply of the knee integuments. *Surg Radiol Anat.* 1998;20:35-40.

49. Lin S, Lai C, Chiu Y, et al. Adipofascial flap of the lower leg based on the saphenous artery. *Br J Plast Surg*. 1996;49:390-395.

50. Ballmer FT, Masquelet AC. The reversed-flow medio-distal fasciocutaneous island thigh flap: anatomic basis and clinical applications. *Surg Radiol Anat*. 1998;20:311-316.

51. Whetzel TP, Barnard MA, Stokes RB. Arterial fasciocutaneous vascular territories of the lower leg. *Plast Reconstr Surg*. 1997;100:1172-1182.

52. Tsai C, Lin S, Lai C, et al. Reconstruction of the upper leg and knee with a reversed flow saphenous island flap based on the medial inferior genicular artery. *Ann Plast Surg*. 1995;35:480-484.

53. Colbom GL, Lumsden AB, Taylor BS, et al. The surgical anatomy of the popliteal artery. *Am Surg*. 1994;60:238-246.

54. Warrington WJ, Charnley GJ, Harries SR, et al. The position of the popliteal artery in the arthritic knee. *J Arthroplast*. 1999;14:800-802.

55. Smith PN, Gelinas J, Kennedy K, et al. Popliteal vessels in knee surgery. *Clin Orthop*. 1999;367:158-164.

56. Shetty AA, Tindall AJ, Qureshi F, et al. The effect of knee flexion on the popliteal artery and its surgical significance. *J Bone Joint Surg Br*. 2003;85-B:218-222.

57. Eriksson K, Bartlett J. Popliteal artery-tibial plateau relationship before and after total knee replacement: a prospective ultrasound study. *Knee Surg Sports Traumatol Arthrosc*. 2010;18:967-970.

58. Shim S, Leung G. Blood supply of the knee joint. *Clin Orthop*. 1986;208:119-125.

59. Ritter MA, Keating EM, Faris PM. Clinical, roentgenographic, and scintigraphic results after interruption of the superior lateral genicular artery during total knee arthroplasty. *Clin Orthop*. 1989;248:145-151.

60. Laitung JKG. The lower posterolateral thigh flap. *Br J Plast Surg*. 1989;42:133-139.

61. Hallock GG. Salvage of total knee arthroplasty with local fasciocutaneous flaps. *J Bone Joint Surg Am*. 1990;72:1236-1239.

62. Hayashi A, Maruyama Y. The lateral genicular artery flap. *Ann Plast Surg*. 1990;24:310-317.

63. Hofmann AA, Plaser RL, Murdock LE. Subvastus (southern) approach for primary total knee arthroplasty. *Clin Orthop*. 1991;269:70-77.

64. Greenberg B, LaRossa D, Lotke PA, et al. Salvage of jeopardized total-knee prosthesis: the role of the gastrocnemius muscle flap. *Plast Reconstr Surg*. 1989;83:85-89.

65. Kirschner MH, Menck J, Nerlich A, et al. The arterial blood supply of the human patella. Its clinical importance for the operating technique in vascularized knee joint transplantations. *Surg Radiol Anat*. 1997;19:345-351.

66. Brick GW, Scott RD. Blood supply to the patella. Significance in total knee arthroplasty. *Arthroplasty*. 1989;4 suppl:S75-S79.

67. Kayler DE, Lyttle D. Surgical interruption of patellar blood supply by total knee arthroplasty. *Clin Orthop*. 1988;229:221-227.

68. Bonutti PM, Miller BG, Cremens MJ. Intraosseous patellar blood supply after medial parapatellar arthrotomy. *Clin Orthop*. 1998;352:202-214.

69. Farrah J, Saharay M, Georgiannos SN, et al. Variable venous anatomy of the popliteal fossa demonstrated by duplex scanning. *Dermatol Surg*. 1998;24:901-903.

70. Fulkerson JP, Tennant R, Jaivin JS, et al. Histologic evidence of retinacular nerve injury associated with patellofemoral malalignment. *Clin Orthop*. 1985;197:196-205.

71. Dellon AL, Mont MA, Mullick T, et al. Partial denervation for persistent neuroma pain around the knee. *Clin Orthop*. 1996;329:216-222.

72. Diop M, Ndiaye A, Dia A, et al. Anatomic study via dissection of the common fibular nerve: etiopathogenic consideration. *Morphologie*. 1997;81:9-12.

73. Asp JPL, Rand JA. Peroneal nerve palsy after total knee arthroplasty. *Clin Orthop*. 1990;261:233-237.

74. Horner G, Dellon AL. Innervation of the human knee joint and implications for surgery. *Clin Orthop*. 1994;301:221-226.

75. Masquelet AC, Romana MC, Wolf G. Skin island flaps supplied by the vascular axis of the sensitive superficial nerves: anatomic study and clinical experience in the leg. *Plast Reconstr Surg*. 1992;89:1115-1121.

76. Tenet TD, Birch NC, Holmes MJ, et al. Knee pain and the infrapatellar branch of the saphenous nerve. *J R Soc Med*. 1998;91:573-575.

77. Tifford CD, Spero L, Luke T, et al. The relationship of the infrapatellar branches of the saphenous nerve to arthroscopy portals and incisions for anterior cruciate ligament surgery. An anatomic study. *Am J Sports Med*. 2000;28:562-567.

78. Nahabedian MY, Johnson CA. Operative management of neuromatous knee pain: patient selection and outcome. *Ann Plast Surg*. 2001;46:15-22.

chapter 3

Anesthesia for Total Knee Replacement

Christopher S. Wahal, MD | Eric S. Schwenk, MD

INTRODUCTION

Total knee arthroplasty (TKA) is one of the most common operations performed in the United States with over 700,000 being performed annually.[1] With an aging population, the number of TKAs performed annually per capita is expected to increase by 150% by the year 2050.[2] Additionally, there is a greater push to decrease length of stay in the setting of rising healthcare costs. Complicating the matter is the intense and complex postoperative pain experienced after TKA, often considered one of the most painful orthopedic procedures.[3] For these reasons, the importance of a multifaceted approach to pain as well as an anesthetic allowing for a rapid recovery is paramount to any TKA operative pathway.

PREOPERATIVE PHASE

One of the most important aspects of any operative pathway is the setting of realistic expectations for patients who are undergoing TKA. Educating patients and realistic goal setting typically begin with information provided on a pamphlet or website. Education then continues at the preoperative visit in the surgeon's office, followed by preadmission testing when available, and lastly completed by the anesthesia team prior to surgery. At some institutions, the process has been streamlined by combining these visits.

Ideally, preadmission testing visits occur 3 to 4 weeks prior to the actual date of surgery. This allows the preoperative team to optimize the patient and intervene on any risk factors which could lead to increased perioperative morbidity. Modifiable risk factors include but are not limited to smoking, anemia, diabetic control, BMI, and significant opioid tolerance. Anemia has been shown to independently increase risk of infection, increase length of stay, and lead to a greater than twofold increase in mortality for noncardiac surgery.[4]

Preoperative testing not only allows for medical optimization, but it also allows for a detailed explanation of the anesthetic plan to be delivered to the patient as well as what to expect after surgery, reducing anxiety. High levels of stress and anxiety have shown to both inhibit wound healing and extend hospital length of stay.[5] Alternatively, patients who have been mentally prepared for surgery with realistic expectations experience improved outcomes. Preemptive cognitive and behavioral interventions have shown to both increase the response to and decrease the consumption of analgesics and reduce postoperative pain.[6] Even with the use of a multimodal analgesic regimen in combination with a regional anesthetic, patients should still expect to have discomfort in the immediate postoperative period. Telling patients that "you won't have any pain" does them a disservice and is unrealistic. Patient expectations can even have an impact on a patient's discharge destination (e.g., home versus a rehab facility or skilled nursing facility), where they have shown to be both an independent and strong predictor.[7]

Preoperative anesthetic evaluation begins with a complete history and physical to identify any specific medical conditions which could result in a challenging intraoperative and postoperative course. Patients are encouraged to stay well hydrated prior to surgery and may continue clear liquids until 2 hours prior to surgery. The opioid-tolerant patient deserves special attention. When compared to opioid-naïve patients, opioid-tolerant patients undergoing total hip arthroplasty had a longer length of stay, used more opioids, and were more likely to still be on opioids 6 weeks postoperatively.[8] There is a dearth of evidence with respect to weaning opioids prior to total joint arthroplasty (TJA). One study showed improved functional outcomes in TJA patients who successfully weaned opioid use by at least 50% compared to patients who did not wean.[9] However, there is no evidence comparing different opioid weaning strategies prior to TKR. It would be prudent to allow at least several weeks for patients to reduce opioid doses, especially if they are doing it on their own schedules. If weaning is not possible or desired, patients who are taking chronic opioids should be given their normal dose, whether it be immediate acting or sustained release, in addition to "as-needed" doses for breakthrough pain on the day of surgery. However, we recommend that multimodal nonopioid analgesics form the foundation of perioperative analgesia with opioids being reserved for severe pain not effectively treated with other agents. It is essential that a multidisciplinary discussion between the anesthesiologist and orthopedic surgeon take place to develop a postoperative plan. Adjustments to standard orders and pathways are often necessary. Opioid tolerance has been shown to be an independent predictor of increased length of stay and greater 30-day readmission rates.[10] Additionally, high pain trajectories postoperatively have also been shown to increase emergency room visits and readmission rates.[11] The consultation of an inpatient pain service, if available, may speed up discharge in these patients and help to prevent readmission for pain-related reasons.

The administration of analgesics prior to surgical incision is known as preemptive analgesia. The goal of preemptive analgesia is twofold: help limit opioid use and prevent peripheral and central sensitization that occurs with tissue trauma associated with surgery. In theory, through the administration of analgesics prior to surgical incision, the production of inflammatory mediators can be attenuated. Typically, inflammatory mediators generated from tissue trauma sensitize nerve fibers which can lead to nonpainful stimuli being perceived as painful (allodynia) and eventually be the genesis of chronic postsurgical pain.[12] Targets of specific analgesics use for TKA patients are shown in **Fig. 3-1**. The idea that preemptive analgesia can prevent sensitization remains controversial. The following sections will review some commonly used analgesics and available clinical evidence for their use.

MULTIMODAL AGENTS

Acetaminophen

Acetaminophen is one of the most common oral medications used to treat postoperative pain. While it has been available as an analgesic since the 1950s, its mechanism of action has still not been fully elucidated. Studies have shown it inhibits prostaglandins at a central level via the cyclooxygenase (COX) pathway, acts as a nitric oxide pathway inhibitor, acts on cannabinoid receptors, as well as modulates descending serotonergic pathways in the spinal cord.[13] Despite being available over the counter, it is an effective analgesic and has been shown to have similar efficacy to intramuscular morphine 10 mg in treating moderate to severe pain.[14] Additionally, it is generally well tolerated and has been extensively used both as an analgesic as well as an antipyretic for decades resulting in a well-known safety profile. When total daily dose is kept at or below 4 g, the risk for acute hepatotoxicity is rare, and its safety has also been confirmed in those with chronic liver disease.[15] Acetaminophen has shown to decrease morphine use by up to 33% as well as provide

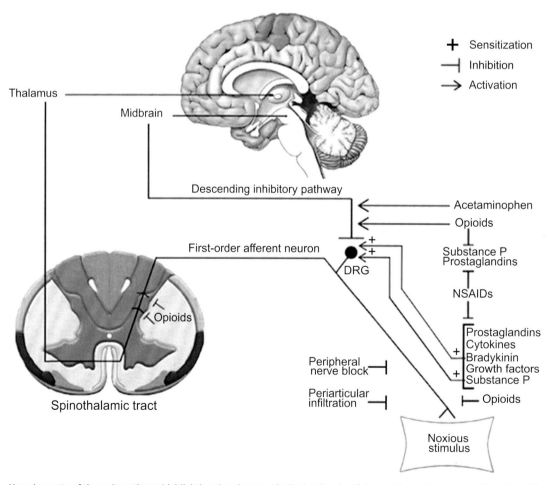

FIGURE 3-1 Key elements of the pain pathway highlighting the pharmacological rationale of the multimodal approach. Note the different but complementary sites of action, producing the desired synergistic analgesic effects. DRG, dorsal root ganglion; NSAIDs, nonsteroidal anti-inflammatory drugs. (Halawi M, Grant S, Bolognesi M. Multimodal analgesia for total joint arthroplasty. *Orthopedics*. 2015;38:e616-e625. Reprinted with permission from SLACK Incorporated.)

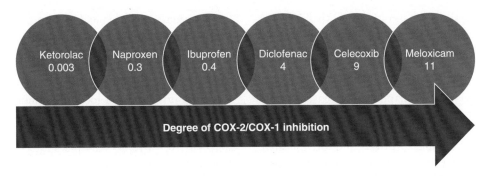

FIGURE 3-2 Commonly used nonsteroidal anti-inflammatory drugs ordered in increasing ratio of COX-2 to COX-1 inhibition. Number represents the 80% inhibitory concentration ratios of COX-2 relative to COX-1 in human whole blood assays.[82]

more effective pain control when compared to placebo.[16] An additional benefit of decreased postoperative nausea and vomiting (PONV) has also been shown.[17]

The Food and Drug Administration (FDA) recommends keeping the total daily dose of acetaminophen under 4 g.[18] We recommend a scheduled dose of 650 to 1000 mg every 6 hours. While combination formulas (i.e., oxycodone/acetaminophen) are available, it is our experience that separating combination analgesics into their individual components will lead to more consistent administration of the nonopioid agents.

An IV formulation of acetaminophen has been available in the United States since being approved by the FDA in 2010. Proposed benefits of an IV formulation are pharmacokinetic data showing the IV formulation leads to higher concentration in the cerebral spinal fluid in the first 6 hours of therapy.[19] However, the daily cost difference between 4 g of IV acetaminophen and 4 g of the PO formulation is substantial ($43 vs. $0.10), which has slowed its adoption.[20] Additionally, none of the limited number of randomized controlled trials evaluating the IV formulation versus the oral formulation in total joint arthroplasty has showed any significant differences in opioid consumption, pain scores, or length of stay.[21-23]

Nonsteroidal Anti-inflammatory Drugs

Nonsteroidal anti-inflammatory drugs (NSAIDs) are another class of highly effective nonopioid analgesics which have been extensively used to treat pain for centuries. Their mechanism of action, inhibition of the synthesis of prostaglandins, was first described in 1971.[24] They work by inhibiting the enzymes COX-1 and COX-2, which are responsible for the conversion of arachidonic acid to both prostaglandins and thromboxane A2.[24] When formed, prostaglandins, specifically prostaglandin E2 (PGE2), play a role in central sensitization, which can lower pain thresholds. The COX-1 isoform is expressed in most tissues, while the COX-2 isoform is normally found only in the brain and kidneys. However, production of COX-2 is induced when tissues are damaged and cytokines and growth factors are released. The prostaglandins that are produced sensitize tissues leading to increased levels of pain.[25]

NSAIDs are used not only for their analgesic properties but also their anti-inflammatory and antipyretic effects. Despite their prevalent use, all prescription NSAIDs do carry a warning from the FDA due to their risk of gastrointestinal bleeding, cardiovascular side effects (increased risk of stroke and myocardial infarction), and risk of acute kidney injury.[26] NSAIDs are categorized into either nonselective or COX-2–selective agents, the latter of which were designed to reduce the risks associated with nonselective NSAIDs, such as gastrointestinal bleeding and platelet dysfunction.[27]

Despite being categorized as "nonselective NSAIDs," each drug varies in its selectivity for the COX-1 and COX-2 isoforms. Some commonly used NSAIDs and their degree of COX-2/COX-1 inhibition are displayed in **Fig. 3-2**. While no specific NSAID has been shown to provide superior analgesia, COX-2–selective drugs may be more desirable due to their more limited side effect profile. Celecoxib is the only FDA-approved COX-2–selective medication currently available in the United States. COX-2 inhibitors have been shown to reduce opioid consumption, pain, vomiting, and sleep disturbances as well as improve knee range of motion after TKA when used in addition to epidural anesthesia.[28]

Gabapentinoids

Gabapentinoids, which consist of gabapentin and pregabalin, work by binding to the alpha-2-delta subunit of voltage-gated calcium channels and prevent the release of neurotransmitters. They work at both the level of the brain and dorsal horn of the spinal cord, where they decrease excitatory signaling. Both medications are renally cleared and doses need to be adjusted in patients with chronic kidney disease. Absorption between the two medications differs. With escalating doses of gabapentin, its absorption decreases. Pregabalin, on the other hand, is absorbed both more rapidly and in a linear fashion with escalating doses, leading to maximum plasma concentrations being achieved more quickly than with gabapentin.[29] Gabapentin has been available for over a decade longer than pregabalin, leading to a much larger wealth of studies evaluating gabapentin.

A recent meta-analysis of six studies with 859 TKA patients evaluated gabapentin versus placebo and found gabapentin resulted in statistically significant decreased opioid use at 12, 24, and 48 hours as well as decreased incidence of pruritis.[30] Another meta-analysis evaluating all types of surgery found gabapentin decreased opioid use and improved pain scores for the first 24 hours after surgery while also leading to decreased incidence of postoperative nausea, vomiting, pruritis, and preoperative anxiety while increasing patient satisfaction.[31] In addition to the benefits seen in the immediate postoperative period, long-term benefits have also been observed. A 2-week course of pregabalin initiated on the day of surgery led to a decreased incidence in chronic neuropathic pain when compared to placebo (0% vs. 8.7% and 0% vs. 5.2% at 3 and 6 months, respectively) in TKA patients.[32]

While numerous positive studies have been performed, there are some studies showing conflicting results. In a study comparing pregabalin to placebo in TKA patients who also received a femoral nerve block, epidural, oxycodone-paracetamol, and meloxicam, there was no difference in pain at rest or with ambulation, but the addition of pregabalin did result in a higher rate of sedation and decreased satisfaction.[33] Additionally, the incidence of sedation and dizziness with these medications is not insignificant and special attention should be paid to the elderly population.[31] Despite these concerns, gabapentinoids provide several benefits in the TKA patient and we recommend their perioperative use. Dosing suggestions for common oral multimodal analgesics are provided in **Table 3-1**.

INTRAOPERATIVE PHASE

Anesthesia Techniques

The goal when choosing an anesthetic technique is to optimize operating conditions while also improving outcomes such as pain, PONV, and patient satisfaction. The decision is often based on the anesthesiologist's, surgeon's, and patient's preferences; patient comorbidities and contraindications; and institutional protocols. The two most common options for TKA are neuraxial and general anesthesia.

Neuraxial anesthesia includes both spinal anesthesia as well as epidural anesthesia. Spinal anesthesia involves the injection of a local anesthetic directly into the intrathecal space, while epidural anesthesia often involves the placement of a catheter into the epidural space, which is subsequently dosed with a local anesthetic. Recent database studies have shown numerous benefits of spinal anesthesia compared to general anesthesia. One such study from 2013 of over 14,000 patients showed spinal anesthesia was associated with lower rates of wound infections (0.68% vs. 0.92%), blood transfusions, and complications in addition to decreased operating time and hospital length of stay.[34] These differences were again noted, with the exception of operating time, in another large database study of 1236 patients from 2017.[35]

There are numerous choices for local anesthetic as well as opioid additives used during spinal anesthesia. The most commonly used local anesthetics are 0.5% isobaric bupivacaine, 0.5% hyperbaric bupivacaine, and 0.75% hyperbaric bupivacaine. Typical doses range from 7.5 to 15 mg of bupivacaine for a primary TKA, with larger doses being used for longer surgical times. Lower doses have been shown to be effective; for example, one study evaluating the optimal intrathecal dose of 0.5% isobaric bupivacaine for fast-track TKA found an ED95 of 5 mg.[36] In addition to local anesthetics, opioids can also be administered intrathecally with the spinal anesthesic. Intrathecal morphine has been used effectively to treat pain associated with major orthopedic surgery for a number of years.[37,38] It has been shown to provide similar postoperative analgesia to a single injection femoral nerve block in TKA patients.[39] The use of intrathecal opioids, especially morphine, comes with the drawback of increased side effects such as sedation, pruritis, nausea, vomiting, urinary retention, and delayed respiratory depression which can last for up to 24 hours. In healthy volunteers, doses as low as 200 mg have shown to produce respiratory depression.[40] Due to the increased incidence of side effects with intrathecal morphine, we utilize a local anesthetic only spinal for our TKA patients.

Possible complications of neuraxial anesthesia include epidural/spinal hematomas. While these consequences can be devastating, they are very rare, with

TABLE 3-1	**Recommended Dosing for Commonly Used Multimodal Oral Analgesics**		
Medication	**Preoperative Dose (mg)**	**Route of Administration**	**Postoperative Dose**
Acetaminophen	1000	PO/IV	650-1000 mg every 6 hours
Celecoxib	400	PO	200-400 mg every 12 hours
Gabapentin	300	PO	300-1200 mg every 8-12 hours
Ketorolac	15-30	PO/IV	15-30 mg every 6 hours, max of seven doses
Meloxicam	7.5-15	PO	7.5-15 mg every 24 hours
Pregabalin	75	PO	75-150 mg every 12 hours

rates of epidural hematoma in obstetric patients being as low as 1:168,000.[41] In the orthopedic population they may be slightly higher; one study evaluated 100,027 patients undergoing THA or TKA under neuraxial anesthesia and revealed spinal hematoma in 7 of the patients, all of whom were on medications which impaired coagulation.[42]

One complicating factor which has become more prevalent in recent years is the introduction of novel oral anticoagulants (NOACs). Each NOAC has different pharmacokinetic properties and must therefore be stopped at varying times prior to placement of neuraxial anesthesia. Complicating matters further, some medications such as dabigatran are cleared renally, leading to different clearance times based on creatinine clearance.[43] For a list of some newer and older anticoagulants as well as antiplatelet agents with their suggested cessation times prior to neuraxial anesthesia, see **Table 3-2**.

Despite numerous benefits associated with neuraxial anesthesia, there are a few downsides, including decreased time to ambulation and increased risk of urinary retention postoperatively. In recent years, there has been an increased push for ambulatory total joint arthroplasty. General anesthesia may be preferable for some patients, especially patients planned for same-day discharge, as it may allow for earlier ambulation. Current published ambulatory protocols that use general anesthesia utilize a laryngeal mask airway.[44,45]

To summarize, evidence suggests neuraxial anesthesia may be associated with improved outcomes in TKA. However, the decision on neuraxial or general anesthesia should be based on surgeon, anesthesiologist, and patient factors to provide the patient with the best surgical and postoperative outcomes.

Dexamethasone

Systemic corticosteroids are frequently given to patients undergoing surgical procedures as prophylaxis against PONV. In addition to this benefit, corticosteroids have also shown to provide analgesic benefits in a variety of surgical procedures. Analgesic benefits are typically seen at higher doses (>0.1 mg/kg) compared to antiemetic doses (4 mg).[46] The analgesic benefits provided have been shown to be particularly useful in TJA. One such study from 2013 of 120 patients who underwent TJA compared three groups: placebo versus one dose of dexamethasone 10 mg prior to surgery versus one dose of dexamethasone 10 mg prior to surgery and one dose of dexamethasone 10 mg on postop day 1. They showed dexamethasone decreased risk of PONV, decreased VAS pain scores, and decreased length of stay, with the additional dose on post-op day 1 providing further benefits of decreased opioid use and VAS pain scores on post-op day 2.[47]

Recent meta-analyses have evaluated the use of high-dose dexamethasone in the setting of TKA. These have shown a reduction in postoperative pain scores and opioid use over the first 48 hours postoperatively.[48,49] A major concern regarding the use of perioperative corticosteroids is increased blood glucose levels leading to an increased risk of prosthetic joint infection (PJI). There does not appear to be a higher rate of PJI in patients receiving dexamethasone versus those who do not.[50] Additionally, while diabetic patients are at higher risk for PJI, the addition of dexamethasone does not appear to further increase this risk.[51] Evidence suggests most patients, including diabetics, benefit from perioperative dexamethasone. Despite this, the benefits and risks of dexamethasone for the diabetic patient should be weighed and the decision should ultimately be a joint decision between the surgeon and anesthesiologist.

Tranexamic Acid

TKA is associated with considerable blood loss, and acute postoperative anemia is not uncommon in this population, with patients experiencing a mean hemoglobin drop of 3.0 ± 1.2 g/dL.[52] Tranexamic acid (TXA) is an antifibrinolytic agent which has greatly reduced the frequency of blood transfusion in total joint arthroplasty.[53] It can be given in multiple forms: as an oral medication prior to surgery, an intravenous medication during surgery, or as a topical medication during surgery. Practice guidelines were published in 2019 by the American Association of Hip and Knee Surgeons, American Society of Regional Anesthesia and Pain Medicine, American Academy of Orthopaedic Surgeons, Hip Society, and Knee Society

TABLE 3-2 Recommended Minimal Cessation Time Before Neuraxial Anesthesia for Some Common Anticoagulants[43]

Drug	When to Stop Drug	Special Considerations
Aspirin	N/A	There are no restrictions with aspirin use and neuraxial anesthesia
Apixaban	72 h	n/a
Clopidogrel	5-7 d	n/a
Dabigatran	3-5 d	3 d for CrCl > 80 mL/min 4 d for CrCl from 50 to 79 mL/min 5 days for CrCl of 30-49 mL/min
Enoxaparin (therapeutic dosing)	24 h	n/a
Rivaroxaban	72 h	n/a
Ticagrelor	5-7 d	n/a
Warfarin	5 d	Normal INR

to help guide intraoperative management. They did not find any method of administration (topical, oral, IV) was superior at reducing blood loss. Additionally, if giving IV TXA, they recommend giving it prior to incision and found no difference in blood loss when the dose was repeated. They found no evidence of an increased risk of venous thromboembolism (VTE) in patients with a history of one when TXA was administered. Some clinicians have concerns regarding administration of TXA to patients with a history of VTE, myocardial infarction, cerebrovascular accident, transient ischemic attack, and vascular stent placement despite known mechanism as a fibrin clot stabilizer. These guidelines recommend administration of TXA to these patients.[54]

POSTOPERATIVE ANALGESIA

Pain management after TKA is a complex problem. Historically, epidural analgesia was used, which ensured the sciatic, obturator, and femoral nerves were anesthetized, and thus resulted in very good pain control. While epidural local anesthetics and/or opioids can provide excellent pain control, side effects including decreased time to ambulation, postoperative hypotension, and urinary retention have limited the use of epidurals in modern TKA. For this reason, the use of epidural analgesia is typically reserved for exceptional situations such as complex revision surgery or opioid-tolerant patients. The use of peripheral nerve blocks and/or periarticular infiltration has replaced the use of epidurals at most institutions. An overview of the most common nerve blocks and injections in TKA, and the evidence behind them, will be reviewed in the following section.

Local Infiltration Analgesia

Local infiltration analgesia (LIA) includes a local anesthetic with or without adjuvants such as epinephrine, ketorolac, opioids, and other medications. The technique first gained traction after Busch et al[55] published a prospective RCT comparing LIA plus PCA to PCA alone for postoperative pain control after TKA. They showed a significant reduction in morphine consumption for 24 hours postoperatively, improved VAS pain scores, and improved VAS patient satisfaction scores in the LIA group.[55] LIA typically consists of a large volume of injectate consisting of several components (60 to 100 mL).[55-57] The local anesthetic mixture is typically administered to the posterior capsule, collateral ligaments, capsular incision, quadriceps tendon, and subcutaneous tissues.[58] Evidence for LIA compared to placebo was recently analyzed in a meta-analysis performed by Jiang et al. They found lower VAS scores at 6, 24, and 48 hours; less opioid consumption at 24 and 48 hours; greater knee ROM at 24, 48, and 72 hours; and fewer opioid-related side effects.[59]

LIA using long-acting liposomal bupivacaine, which was designed to last for 72 hours, has been a heavily researched topic. There have been conflicting results with some studies showing improved pain control and less opioid consumption compared to plain bupivacaine, while others have shown no difference.[60,61] A meta-analysis published in 2017 by Kuang et al[62] included 11 studies and showed there was no advantage in terms of VAS scores, range of motion, total amount of opioid consumption, postoperative nausea, ambulation distance, or LOS when comparing liposomal bupivacaine to plain bupivacaine for LIA. Due to the significantly higher cost of liposomal bupivacaine compared to plain bupivacaine, current evidence does not support its regular use in LIA.

Femoral Nerve Block

Historically, the femoral nerve block (FNB) was the most commonly used peripheral nerve block for TKA. FNB is easy to perform with nerve stimulation, allowing the block to become popularized prior to the introduction of ultrasound guidance for peripheral nerve blocks, and the femoral nerve is responsible for most of the sensation to the knee. Additionally, a perineural catheter can be inserted which could extend the analgesia over the immediate postoperative period. FNB has been shown to decrease opioid consumption, improve pain scores with activity, and reduce incidence of opioid consumption when compared to PCA.[63] The use of continuous femoral nerve block (CFNB) has been compared to single injection FNB, and there have been mixed results. Salinas et al showed CFNB significantly improve mean VAS scores at rest, with walking, and decrease opioid use on post-op days 1 and 2.[64] However, in a meta-analysis by Paul et al published in 2010, they found no benefit of CFNB as compared to single injection.[63] FNB has also been compared to epidural analgesia and has been shown to provide similar pain relief. A recent Cochrane review which evaluated 47 RCTs which included 2710 patients showed no difference in pain relief between FNB and epidural analgesia, with FNB patients having a higher rate of satisfaction and lower incidence of nausea.[65]

Despite providing very good analgesia, FNB does come with the disadvantage of quadriceps weakness, which increases the risk of falling in the postoperative period. Varying concentrations of local anesthetic have been evaluated with hopes of decreasing quadriceps weakness, but lower concentrations have not been shown to lead to less weakness.[66,67] A retrospective analysis of 707 primary TKA patients over the course of 3 years showed 19 (2.7%) patients with CFNB experienced falls.[68] For this reason, the use of a knee immobilizer while ambulating with a femoral nerve block is often recommended and has even become a hospital policy at some facilities.

Adductor Canal Nerve Block

Concerns of fall risks with FNB led to the development of the adductor canal block (ACB). The ACB is commonly performed lower in the leg, at the midpoint between the anterior superior iliac spine and patella, although other locations in the thigh have been studied.[69] ACB is primarily a sensory block, anesthetizing the saphenous nerve and the nerve to the vastus medialis, and provides sensory blockade to the anteromedial aspect of the knee.[70] The ACB has shown to maintain quadriceps strength compared to FNB both in healthy volunteers as well as TKA patients.[71,72] From an analgesic standpoint, Kim et al. showed the ACB provides noninferior pain control to the FNB at 8, 24, and 48 hours in a noninferiority trial.[71] Additionally, a meta-analysis of six studies involving 408 patients comparing FNB and ACB revealed similar VAS pain scores at 4, 24, and 48 hours.[73] The use of continuous adductor canal block (CACB) is also of great interest. Elkassabany et al[74] compared single injection ACB to CACB for 24- and 48-hour infusions and found that significantly less patients in the CACB cohort experienced severe pain on POD 1 (21% vs. 12%). Further studies are needed to determine the optimal length of time for CACB.

ACB is also used in conjunction with LIA, and the combination of the two has been shown to be beneficial. One such study showed single-injection ACB plus LIA had lower worst pain scores and more pain relief at 24 hours after anesthesia compared to LIA alone.[75] A meta-analysis of three studies involving 337 patients of studies comparing ACB and LIA to LIA alone showed the combination of ACB and LIA led to longer distances walked on POD 1.[76]

Interspace Between the Popliteal Artery and Posterior Capsule of the Knee Block

Even with the use of FNB or ACB, patients often report posterior knee pain, likely from the terminal branches of the popliteal plexus from the tibial branch of the sciatic nerve and posterior division of the obturator nerve (**Fig. 3-3**). Common practice typically avoids sciatic nerve due to concerns for falls and inhibiting work with physical therapy. For this reason, the iPACK (interspace between the popliteal artery and posterior capsule of the knee) block was developed to target the nerve branches to the posterior capsule while maintaining motor function. Cadaveric dye studies have revealed the iPACK injection reliably stained the articular branches supplying the posterior capsule of the knee.[77] Addition of the iPACK injection to a multimodal analgesic pathway including an ACB led to decreased lowest pain scores when compared to ACB and multimodal analgesia alone.[78] The combination of LIA, iPACK, and ACB has been shown to provide better satisfaction and reduced opioid consumption in TKA patients when compared to LIA alone.[79] Evidence indicates the iPACK injection could be a beneficial addition to regional anesthesia

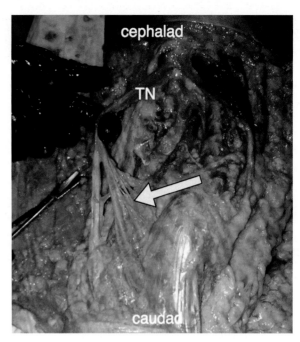

FIGURE 3-3 The popliteal plexus in a cadaver dissection. The web-like plexus (arrow) is seen coming off the tibial nerve (TN) before supplying the posterior capsule and soft tissues of the knee joint. (Reproduced from Kumar L, Kumar AH, Grant S, Gadsden J. Updates in enhanced recovery pathways for total knee arthroplasty. *Anesthesiol Clin.* 2018;36(3):375-386, Copyright Elsevier (2018).)

and/or a LIA regimen, but further studies are needed to evaluate the efficacy of the iPACK block including studies comparing it to placebo.

Postoperative Multimodal Analgesia

In the postoperative phase, it is essential to continue the multimodal analgesia regimen as outlined previously in the chapter while the patient is hospitalized. The optimal duration of therapy for the components of multimodal analgesia is unknown. It has been suggested that NSAIDs and acetaminophen be continued for at least 2 weeks after surgery, with a goal of reducing the inflammation associated with the surgery.[80] Duration of therapy for gabapentinoids is a more difficult question, as some patients experience significant side effects such as sedation. Some studies only continue them while the patient is in the hospital,[81] while others continued for 14 days postoperatively.[32,33] We recommend continuing them at least while the patient is hospitalized. In addition to these medications, most patients will require an opioid on an as-needed basis, especially prior to physical therapy. Common opioids and their dosing are described in **Table 3-3**. We strongly recommend a bowel regimen be continued as long as the patient is taking opioids. A typical combination includes both a stool softener, such as docusate, and a promotility agent, such as senna. For patients who develop postoperative ileus, a peripherally acting mu-receptor opioid antagonist may be considered, such as alvimopan, methylnaltrexone, or naloxegol.

TABLE 3-3 Recommended Dosing for Commonly Used Opioid Analgesics

Medication	Dose (mg)	Route of Administration	Dose Frequency
Oxycodone	5-10	PO	As needed every 4-6 h
Tramadol	50-100	PO	As needed every 4-6 h
Hydromorphone	2-4	PO	As needed every 3-4 h
Hydromorphone	0.25-0.5	IV	As needed for breakthrough pain, 3 doses daily

CONCLUSION

Anesthesia and postoperative pain management for TKA are complicated topics which continue to evolve. While multimodal analgesic pathways help to ensure a timely recovery with adequate pain relief, care still needs to be individualized to consider numerous patient factors. The use of regional anesthesia and LIA have been shown to improve recovery and the surgical experience. Surgical and anesthetic considerations need to be balanced to provide the patient with the overall best perioperative experience. By doing so, care can be individualized for the patient while still adhering to evidence-based practices, and outcomes will be optimized.

REFERENCES

1. Kurtz S, Ong K, Lau E, Mowat F, Halpern M. Projections of primary and revision hip and knee arthroplasty in the United States from 2005 to 2030. *J Bone Joint Surg Am.* 2007;89(4):780-785.
2. Inacio MCS, Paxton EW, Graves SE, Namba RS, Nemes S. Projected increase in total knee arthroplasty in the United States – an alternative projection model. *Osteoarthr Cartil.* 2017;25(11):1797-1803.
3. Gerbershagen HJ, Aduckathil S, van Wijck AJM, Peelen LM, Kalkman CJ, Meissner W. Pain intensity on the first day after surgery: a prospective cohort study comparing 179 surgical procedures. *Anesthesiology.* 2013;118(4):934-944.
4. Beattie WS, Karkouti K, Wijeysundera DN, Tait G. Risk associated with preoperative anemia in noncardiac surgery: a single-center cohort study. *Anesthesiology.* 2009;110(3):574-581.
5. Carr DB, Goudas LC. Acute pain. *Lancet.* 1999;353(9169):2051-2058.
6. Kiecolt-Glaser JK, Page GG, Marucha PT, MacCallum RC, Glaser R. Psychological influences on surgical recovery. Perspectives from psychoneuroimmunology. *Am Psychol.* 1998;53(11):1209-1218.
7. Halawi MJ, Vovos TJ, Green CL, Wellman SS, Attarian DE, Bolognesi MP. Patient expectation is the most important predictor of discharge destination after primary total joint arthroplasty. *J Arthroplasty.* 2015;30(4):539-542.
8. Pivec R, Issa K, Naziri Q, Kapadia BH, Bonutti PM, Mont MA. Opioid use prior to total hip arthroplasty leads to worse clinical outcomes. *Int Orthop.* 2014;38(6):1159-1165.
9. Nguyen LC, Sing DC, Bozic KJ. Preoperative reduction of opioid use before total joint arthroplasty. *J Arthroplasty.* 2016;31(9 suppl):282-287.
10. Gulur P, Williams L, Chaudhary S,Koury K, Jaff M. Opioid tolerance–a predictor of increased length of stay and higher readmission rates. *Pain Physician.* 2014;17(4):E503-E507.
11. Hernandez-Boussard T, Graham LA, Desai K, et al. The fifth vital sign: postoperative pain predicts 30-day readmissions and subsequent emergency department visits. *Ann Surg.* 2017;266(3):516-524.
12. Woolf CJ, Chong MS. Preemptive analgesia–treating postoperative pain by preventing the establishment of central sensitization. *Anesth Analg.* 1993;77(2):362-379.
13. Koh W, Nguyen KP, Jahr JS. Intravenous non-opioid analgesia for peri- and postoperative pain management: a scientific review of intravenous acetaminophen and ibuprofen. *Korean J Anesthesiol.* 2015;68(1):3-12.
14. Bandolier. *The Oxford League Table of Analgesic Efficacy.* [Webpage] [cited 2019 August 1]. Available at http://www.bandolier.org.uk/booth/painpag/Acutrev/Analgesics/Leagtab.html. Accessed September 2, 2019.
15. Rumack BH. Acetaminophen hepatotoxicity: the first 35 years. *J Toxicol Clin Toxicol.* 2002;40(1):3-20.
16. Sinatra RS, Jahr JS, Reynolds LW, Viscusi ER, Groudine SB, Payen-Champenois C. Efficacy and safety of single and repeated administration of 1 gram intravenous acetaminophen injection (paracetamol) for pain management after major orthopedic surgery. *Anesthesiology.* 2005;102(4):822-831.
17. Apfel CC, Turan A, Souza K, Pergolizzi J, Hornuss C. Intravenous acetaminophen reduces postoperative nausea and vomiting: a systematic review and meta-analysis. *Pain.* 2013;154(5):677-689.
18. Larson AM. Acetaminophen hepatotoxicity. *Clin Liver Dis.* 2007;11(3):525-548, vi.
19. Singla NK, Parulan C, Samson R, et al. Plasma and cerebrospinal fluid pharmacokinetic parameters after single-dose administration of intravenous, oral, or rectal acetaminophen. *Pain Pract.* 2012;12(7):523-532.
20. Yeh YC, Reddy P. Clinical and economic evidence for intravenous acetaminophen. *Pharmacotherapy.* 2012;32(6):559-579.
21. O'Neal JB, Freiberg AA, Yelle MD, et al. Intravenous vs oral acetaminophen as an adjunct to multimodal analgesia after total knee arthroplasty: a prospective, randomized, double-blind clinical trial. *J Arthroplasty.* 2017;32(10):3029-3033.
22. Westrich GH, Birch GA, Muskat AR, et al. Intravenous vs oral acetaminophen as a component of multimodal analgesia after total hip arthroplasty: a randomized, blinded trial. *J Arthroplasty.* 2019;34(7S):S215-S220.
23. Politi JR, Davis RL II, Matrka AK. Randomized prospective trial comparing the Use of intravenous versus oral acetaminophen in total joint arthroplasty. *J Arthroplasty.* 2017;32(4):1125-1127.
24. Candido KD, Perozo OJ, Knezevic NN. Pharmacology of acetaminophen, nonsteroidal antiinflammatory drugs, and steroid medications: implications for anesthesia or unique associated risks. *Anesthesiol Clin.* 2017;35(2):e145-e162.
25. Kidd BL, Urban LA. Mechanisms of inflammatory pain. *Br J Anaesth.* 2001;87(1):3-11.
26. FDA. *FDA strengthens warning that non-aspirin nonsteroidal antiinflammatory drugs (NSAIDs) can cause heart attacks or strokes.* 2015 [cited 2019 June 15]; Drug Safety Communication. Available at https://www.fda.gov/media/92768/download. Accessed September 2, 2019.
27. Funk CD, FitzGerald GA. COX-2 inhibitors and cardiovascular risk. *J Cardiovasc Pharmacol.* 2007;50(5):470-479.
28. Buvanendran A, Kroin JS, Tuman KJ, et al. Effects of perioperative administration of a selective cyclooxygenase 2 inhibitor on pain management and recovery of function after knee replacement: a randomized controlled trial. *J Am Med Assoc.* 2003;290(18):2411-2418.
29. Bockbrader HN, Wesche D, Miller R, Chapel S, Janiczek N, Burger P. A comparison of the pharmacokinetics and pharmacodynamics of pregabalin and gabapentin. *Clin Pharmacokinet.* 2010;49(10):661-669.

30. Han C, Li XD, Jiang HQ, Ma JX, Ma XL. The use of gabapentin in the management of postoperative pain after total knee arthroplasty: a PRISMA-compliant meta-analysis of randomized controlled trials. *Medicine (Baltimore)*. 2016;95(23):e3883.

31. Doleman B, Heinink TP, Read DJ, Faleiro RJ, Lund JN, Williams JP. A systematic review and meta-regression analysis of prophylactic gabapentin for postoperative pain. *Anaesthesia*. 2015;70(10):1186-1204.

32. Buvanendran A, Kroin JS, Della Valle CJ, Kari M, Moric M, Tuman KJ. Perioperative oral pregabalin reduces chronic pain after total knee arthroplasty: a prospective, randomized, controlled trial. *Anesth Analg*. 2010;110(1):199-207.

33. YaDeau JT, Lin Y, Mayman DJ, et al. Pregabalin and pain after total knee arthroplasty: a double-blind, randomized, placebo-controlled, multidose trial. *Br J Anaesth*. 2015;115(2):285-293.

34. Pugely AJ, Martin CT, Gao Y, Mendoza-Lattes S, Callaghan JJ. Differences in short-term complications between spinal and general anesthesia for primary total knee arthroplasty. *J Bone Joint Surg Am*. 2013;95(3):193-199.

35. Park YB, Chae WS, Park SH, Yu JS, Lee SG, Yim SJ. Comparison of short-term complications of general and spinal anesthesia for primary unilateral total knee arthroplasty. *Knee Surg Relat Res*. 2017;29(2):96-103.

36. van Egmond JC, Verburg H, Derks EA, et al. Optimal dose of intrathecal isobaric bupivacaine in total knee arthroplasty. *Can J Anaesth*. 2018;65(9):1004-1011.

37. Grace D, Bunting H, Milligan KR, Fee JPH. Postoperative analgesia after co-administration of clonidine and morphine by the intrathecal route in patients undergoing hip replacement. *Anesth Analg*. 1995;80(1):86-91.

38. Sites BD, Beach M, Biggs R, et al. Intrathecal clonidine added to a bupivacaine-morphine spinal anesthetic improves postoperative analgesia for total knee arthroplasty. *Anesth Analg*. 2003;96(4):1083-1088.

39. Sites BD, Beach M, Gallagher JD, Jarrett RA, Sparks MB, Lundberg CJF. A single injection ultrasound-assisted femoral nerve block provides side effect-sparing analgesia when compared with intrathecal morphine in patients undergoing total knee arthroplasty. *Anesth Analg*. 2004;99(5):1539-1543.

40. Bailey PL, Rhondeau S, Schafer PG, et al. Dose-response pharmacology of intrathecal morphine in human volunteers. *Anesthesiology*. 1993;79(1):49-59; discussion 25A.

41. Ruppen W, Derry S, McQuay H, Moore RA. Incidence of epidural hematoma, infection, and neurologic injury in obstetric patients with epidural analgesia/anesthesia. *Anesthesiology*. 2006;105(2):394-399.

42. Pumberger M, Memtsoudis SG, Stundner O. An analysis of the safety of epidural and spinal neuraxial anesthesia in more than 100,000 consecutive major lower extremity joint replacements. *Reg Anesth Pain Med*. 2013;38(6):515-519.

43. Horlocker TT, Vandermeulen E, Kopp SL, Gogarten W, Leffert LR, Benzon HT. Regional anesthesia in the patient receiving antithrombotic or thrombolytic therapy: american society of regional anesthesia and pain medicine evidence-based guidelines (fourth edition). *Reg Anesth Pain Med*. 2018;43(3):263-309.

44. Gondusky JS, Choi L, Khalaf N, Patel J, Barnett S, Gorab R. Day of surgery discharge after unicompartmental knee arthroplasty: an effective perioperative pathway. *J Arthroplasty*. 2014;29(3):516-519.

45. Hoeffel DP, Daly PJ, Kelly BJ, Giveans MR. Outcomes of the first 1,000 total hip and total knee Arthroplasties at a same-day surgery center using a rapid-recovery protocol. *J Am Acad Orthop Surg Glob Res Rev*. 2019;3(3):e022.

46. Salerno A, Hermann R. Efficacy and safety of steroid use for postoperative pain relief. Update and review of the medical literature. *J Bone Joint Surg Am*. 2006;88(6):1361-1372.

47. Backes JR, Bentley JC, Politi JR, Chambers BT. Dexamethasone reduces length of hospitalization and improves postoperative pain and nausea after total joint arthroplasty: a prospective, randomized controlled trial. *J Arthroplasty*. 2013;28(8 suppl):11-17.

48. Li X, Xu G, Xie W, Ma S. The efficacy and safety of dexamethasone for pain management after total knee arthroplasty: a systematic review and meta-analysis. *Int J Surg*. 2018;53:65-71.

49. Zhou G, Ma L, Jing J, Jiang H. A meta-analysis of dexamethasone for pain management in patients with total knee arthroplasty. *Medicine (Baltimore)*. 2018;97(35):e11753.

50. Richardson AB, Bala A, Wellman SS, Attarian DE, Bolognesi MP, Grant SA. Perioperative dexamethasone administration does not increase the incidence of postoperative infection in total hip and knee arthroplasty: a retrospective analysis. *J Arthroplasty*. 2016;31(8):1784-1787.

51. Godshaw BM, Mehl AE, Shaffer JG, Meyer MS, Thomas LC, Chimento GF. The effects of peri-operative dexamethasone on patients undergoing total hip or knee arthroplasty: is it safe for diabetics?. *J Arthroplasty*. 2019;34(4):645-649.

52. Park JH, Rasouli MR, Mortazavi SMJ, Tokarski AT, Maltenfort MG, Parvizi J. Predictors of perioperative blood loss in total joint arthroplasty. *J Bone Joint Surg Am*. 2013;95(19):1777-1783.

53. Fillingham YA, Ramkumar DB, Jevsevar DS, et al. The efficacy of tranexamic acid in total hip arthroplasty: a network meta-analysis. *J Arthroplasty*. 2018;33(10):3083-3089 e4.

54. Fillingham YA, Ramkumar DB, Jevsevar DS, et al. Tranexamic acid in total joint arthroplasty: the endorsed clinical practice guides of the American Association of Hip and Knee Surgeons, American Society of Regional Anesthesia and Pain Medicine, American Academy of Orthopaedic Surgeons, Hip Society, and Knee Society. *Reg Anesth Pain Med*. 2019;44(1):7-11.

55. Busch CA, Shore BJ, Bhandari R, et al. Efficacy of periarticular multimodal drug injection in total knee arthroplasty. A randomized trial. *J Bone Joint Surg Am*. 2006;88(5):959-963.

56. Kelley TC, Adams MJ, Mulliken BD, Dalury DF. Efficacy of multimodal perioperative analgesia protocol with periarticular medication injection in total knee arthroplasty: a randomized, double-blinded study. *J Arthroplasty*. 2013;28(8):1274-1277.

57. Parvataneni HK, Shah VP, Howard H, Cole N, Ranawat AS, Ranawat CS. Controlling pain after total hip and knee arthroplasty using a multimodal protocol with local periarticular injections: a prospective randomized study. *J Arthroplasty*. 2007;22(6 suppl 2):33-38.

58. Moucha CS, Weiser MC, Levin EJ. Current strategies in anesthesia and analgesia for total knee arthroplasty. *J Am Acad Orthop Surg*. 2016;24(2):60-73.

59. Jiang J, Teng Y, Fan Z, Khan MS, Cui Z, Xia Y. The efficacy of periarticular multimodal drug injection for postoperative pain management in total knee or hip arthroplasty. *J Arthroplasty*. 2013;28(10):1882-1887.

60. Collis PN, Hunter AM, Vaughn MDD, Carreon LY, Huang J, Malkani AL. Periarticular injection after total knee arthroplasty using liposomal bupivacaine vs a modified ranawat suspension: a prospective, randomized study. *J Arthroplasty*. 2016;31(3):633-636.

61. Webb BT, Spears JR, Smith LS, Malkani AL. Periarticular injection of liposomal bupivacaine in total knee arthroplasty. *Arthroplast Today*. 2015;1(4):117-120.

62. Kuang MJ, Du Y, Ma J-x, He W, Fu L, Ma X-l. The efficacy of liposomal bupivacaine using periarticular injection in total knee arthroplasty: a systematic review and meta-analysis. *J Arthroplasty*. 2017;32(4):1395-1402.

63. Paul JE, Arya A, Hurlburt L, et al. Femoral nerve block improves analgesia outcomes after total knee arthroplasty: a meta-analysis of randomized controlled trials. *Anesthesiology*. 2010;113(5):1144-1162.

64. Salinas FV, Liu SS, Mulroy MF. The effect of single-injection femoral nerve block versus continuous femoral nerve block after total knee arthroplasty on hospital length of stay and long-term functional recovery within an established clinical pathway. *Anesth Analg*. 2006;102(4):1234-1239.

65. Chan EY, Fransen M, Parker DA, Assam PN, Chua N. Femoral nerve blocks for acute postoperative pain after knee replacement surgery. *Cochrane Database Syst Rev*. 2014;(5):CD009941.

66. Bauer M, Wang L, Onibonoje OK, et al. Continuous femoral nerve blocks: decreasing local anesthetic concentration to minimize quadriceps femoris weakness. *Anesthesiology*. 2012;116(3):665-672.

67. Charous MT, Madison SJ, Suresh PJ, et al. Continuous femoral nerve blocks: varying local anesthetic delivery method (bolus versus basal) to minimize quadriceps motor block while maintaining sensory block. *Anesthesiology*. 2011;115(4):774-781.

68. Pelt CE, Anderson AW, Anderson MB, Van Dine C, Peters CL. Postoperative falls after total knee arthroplasty in patients with a femoral nerve catheter: can we reduce the incidence?. *J Arthroplasty*. 2014;29(6):1154-1157.

69. Abdallah FW, Mejia J, Prasad GA, et al. Opioid- and motor-sparing with proximal, mid-, and distal locations for adductor canal block in anterior cruciate ligament reconstruction: a randomized clinical trial. *Anesthesiology*. 2019;131(3):619-629.

70. Lund J, Jenstrup MT, Jaeger P, Sørensen AM, Dahl JB. Continuous adductor-canal-blockade for adjuvant post-operative analgesia after major knee surgery: preliminary results. *Acta Anaesthesiol Scand*. 2011;55(1):14-19.

71. Kim DH, Lin Y, Goytizolo EA, et al. Adductor canal block versus femoral nerve block for total knee arthroplasty: a prospective, randomized, controlled trial. *Anesthesiology*. 2014;120(3):540-550.

72. Jaeger P, Nielsen ZJ, Henningsen MH, Hilsted KL, Mathiesen O, Dahl JB. Adductor canal block versus femoral nerve block and quadriceps strength: a randomized, double-blind, placebo-controlled, crossover study in healthy volunteers. *Anesthesiology*. 2013;118(2):409-415.

73. Hussain N, Ferreri TG, Prusick PJ, et al. Adductor canal block versus femoral canal block for total knee arthroplasty: a meta-analysis: what does the evidence suggest?. *Reg Anesth Pain Med*. 2016;41(3):314-320.

74. Elkassabany NM, Cai LF, Badiola I, et al. A prospective randomized open-label study of single injection versus continuous adductor canal block for postoperative analgesia after total knee arthroplasty. *Bone Joint J*. 2019;101-B(3):340-347.

75. Goytizolo EA, Lin Y, Kim DH, et al. Addition of adductor canal block to periarticular injection for total knee replacement: a randomized trial. *J Bone Joint Surg Am*. 2019;101(9):812-820.

76. Ma J, Gao F, Sun W, Guo W, Li Z, Wang W. Combined adductor canal block with periarticular infiltration versus periarticular infiltration for analgesia after total knee arthroplasty. *Medicine (Baltimore)*. 2016;95(52):e5701.

77. Tran J, Giron Arango L, Peng P, Sinha SK, Agur A, Chan V. Evaluation of the iPACK block injectate spread: a cadaveric study. *Reg Anesth Pain Med*. 2019;44:689-694.

78. Kandarian B, Indelli PF, Sinha S, et al. Implementation of the IPACK (Infiltration between the Popliteal Artery and Capsule of the Knee) block into a multimodal analgesic pathway for total knee replacement. *Korean J Anesthesiol*. 2019;72(3):238-244.

79. Kim DH, Beathe JC, Lin Y, et al. Addition of infiltration between the popliteal artery and the capsule of the posterior knee and adductor canal block to periarticular injection enhances postoperative pain control in total knee arthroplasty: a randomized controlled trial. *Anesth Analg*. 2019;129(2):526-535.

80. Kopp SL, Børglum J, Buvanendran A, et al. Anesthesia and analgesia practice pathway options for total knee arthroplasty: an evidence-based review by the American and European Societies of Regional Anesthesia and Pain Medicine. *Reg Anesth Pain Med*. 2017;42(6):683-697.

81. Paul JE, Nantha-Aree M, Buckley N, et al. Randomized controlled trial of gabapentin as an adjunct to perioperative analgesia in total hip arthroplasty patients. *Can J Anaesth*. 2015;62(5):476-484.

82. Wright JM. The double-edged sword of COX-2 selective NSAIDs. *Can Med Assoc J*. 2002;167(10):1131-1137.

Basic Science

HARRY E. RUBASH

SECTION **2**

chapter 4

Meniscus, Tendons, and Ligaments: Pathophysiology

Andrew O. Usoro, MD | Michael A. Kolosky, DO | Mark D. Price, MD, PhD

The menisci are two crescent-shaped fibrocartilaginous structures found on the medial and lateral aspects of the knee. The menisci enable effective articulation between the concave femoral condyles and the relatively flat tibial plateau.[1,2] In cross section, they are triangular in shape starting with a thick peripheral rim, and then thinning to the central margin. The undersurface or inferior portion of the meniscus is convex, whereas the superior surface is more concave, mirroring the tibial and femoral articular surfaces, respectively. Each meniscus is made up of three sections: the anterior horn, meniscal body, and posterior horn; and the menisci are anchored to the subchondral tibial bone of the tibia through insertional fibers at the anterior and posterior horns called the meniscal roots. The anterior horns of the medial and lateral menisci are connected via a dense fibrous band called the anterior intermeniscal ligament in 50% to 90% of the population[3-5] (**Fig. 4-1**).

MEDIAL MENISCUS

The medial meniscus is a C-shaped structure that is larger in radius compared to the lateral meniscus and covers roughly 50% of the medial tibial surface.[2,6] The anterior horn has a robust attachment to the tibia near the intercondylar fossa anterior to the anterior cruciate ligament (ACL).[2] The posterior horn whose cross-sectional area is larger than the anterior horn is anchored to the tibial plateau at the posterior intercondylar fossa, just anterior to the attachments of the posterior cruciate ligament (PCL) and posterior to the lateral meniscal root.[2] Its entire peripheral border is attached to the tibial condylar ridge through the coronary ligament. Further anchoring the medial meniscus is its contiguous insertion to the deep medial collateral and capsular ligaments at the body, and to the posteromedial complex (posterior oblique ligament, oblique popliteal ligament, and semimembranosus tendon) at the posterior horn.[1] There are no attachments to the capsule or fat pad at the anterior horn.[7] The sum of these attachments is what accounts for the decreased mobility of the medial meniscus when compared to the lateral with the degree of movement in one study measured at 3 and 9 mm, respectively.[8,9]

LATERAL MENISCUS

Covering nearly 70% of the underlying lateral tibial plateau, the lateral meniscus is almost uniformly circular and in contrast to the medial meniscus, it is smaller and considerably more mobile, due to significantly fewer capsular and ligamentous attachments.[6,8,10,11] The anterior horn of the lateral meniscus is attached to the intercondylar fossa, just lateral to the broad attachment site of the ACL. The posterior horn emanates just posterior to the lateral tibial spine and is in very close proximity to the broad PCL footprint.[2] Unique to the lateral meniscus are two meniscofemoral ligaments that attach the meniscus to the medial femoral condyle. Individually, their existence within the knee is roughly 70%, whereas their prevalence found together is significantly lower at 4%.[12-15] These fibrous bands are known as the ligament of Wrisberg and Humphrey and straddle the PCL posterior and anterior, respectively.[13] Aiding in the mobility of the lateral meniscus is the lack of stout tibial and capsular attachments at the popliteal hiatus.[14] The intra-articular portion of the popliteus tendon can be identified at the hiatus located between the posterolateral border of the lateral meniscus and the posterior knee capsule, aptly named the popliteal hiatus.[16] Providing some stability to this area are the superior and inferior popliteomeniscal fascicules, which secure the posterolateral meniscus to the posterior joint capsule.[14,16,17] Without these attachments, the lateral meniscus may become hypermobile and could require meniscocapsular repair.

MENISCUS STRUCTURE

The menisci are predominantly water (72%), collagen (22%), and other organic matter organized into a dense extracellular matrix.[18] The extracellular matrix is composed primarily of collagen, glycosaminoglycans, and other adhesion molecules.[12,19-21] The primary glycosaminoglycans involved are dermatan sulfate (20% to 30%), chondroitin-6 sulfate (40%), chondroitin-4 sulfate (10% to 20%), and keratan sulfate (15%).[21,22] The highest concentration of these glycosaminoglycans can be found in the weight-bearing portion, along the inner half of the meniscus, and in the anterior and posterior horns. The

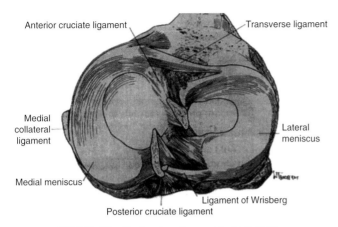

FIGURE 4-1   Meniscal anatomy and attachments.

hydrophilic properties of the glycosaminoglycans play an important role and allow for water absorption and retention throughout the meniscus.[23] The influx of water is paramount for the meniscal maintenance of structure while under compression during weight bearing. The degree of meniscal hydration is determined by the balance between the total swelling pressure and the constraining forces such as the Donnan osmotic pressure, defined as the extracellular osmotic pressure attributable to extracellular cations attached to the negatively charged surrounding proteoglycans. This additional pressure within meniscal tissue allows for increased resistance against compression loading. Consequently, the meniscus is able to maintain its structure without water extrusion during normal weight bearing. Additionally, due to small pore size within the meniscus, significant hydraulic pressures are required to force fluid outside the meniscal issue. Thus, the menisci are able to maintain their innate structure without water loss despite routine compression during weight bearing.[21,24,25] Aggrecan is the major proteoglycan in the meniscus and largely responsible for this effect and its viscoelastic properties. Biglycan and decorin constitute the main smaller proteoglycans. As the meniscus transitions toward the inner free margin, the density of proteoglycans increases in order to allow for changes in the stress felt in the outer versus inner meniscus. Adhesion glycoproteins, primarily fibronectin, thrombospondin, and type VI collagen, link the extracellular matrix and provide structural support.[23,26,27]

Type 1 collagen is the main component of the extracellular matrix and varies in response to the region of the meniscus. It is collagen that is responsible for the tensile strength of the meniscus, which varies with age, injury, or pathologic condition.[18,23,28] In the peripheral third of the meniscus, type I collagen accounts for 80% of the total collagen. This number dramatically drops to 40% in the avascular inner meniscal margin.[29] There are noted to be smaller amounts of type II, III, IV, VI, and XIII collagen throughout the meniscus as well. In the deeper layers of the meniscus, collagen fibers are oriented circumferentially, parallel to the meniscal peripheral

border. Superficially, radially oriented "tie" fibers are woven between the circumferential fibers to add structural integrity and prevent longitudinal tearing.[30-32] These radial fibers prevent radial extrusion and allow the meniscus to maintain its structure during normal weight bearing of the knee.[30,32] Radial tie fibers are more abundant in the posterior horn and decrease in concentration through the body, toward the anterior horn.[32-34] Thus, in the meniscus, compressive force is transduced into a circumferentially directed tensile stress (known as the *hoop stress*) that is supported by the circumferential cross-linked collagen fibers.[35,36] At the inner third of the meniscus, the collagen fibrils become heavily cross-linked by hydroxylpyridinium aldehydes in order to resist shear forces of the tibiofemoral articulation. Collagen type II (60%), glycosaminoglycans, and aggrecan predominate, leading to smaller fiber bundles and a structure more similar to articular cartilage[37] (**Figs. 4-2** and **4-3**).

The meniscus is sparsely populated with cells that are responsible for producing and maintaining the extracellular matrix. Early in development, the cells of the meniscus have a similar morphology with regional variations throughout the meniscus. These primary meniscal cells are categorized into two types: fibroblast-like cells with a fusiform appearance and chondrocyte-like cells with an ovoid appearance, found in the deep zones of the meniscus. They communicate with other cells via long cellular extensions.[1,2,38] Cells in the inner, avascular portion of the meniscus resemble chondrocytes in morphology, whereas cells in the outer periphery are more fibroblastic in appearance and again account for the various stresses found in the different zones of the meniscus.[1,38-40] Additionally, these cells are multipotent and are capable of trilineage differentiation (chondrogenic, adipogenic, and osteogenic).[19] Because of their lack of proximity to each other and to the vascular supply of the meniscus, nutrition is obtained through diffusion.

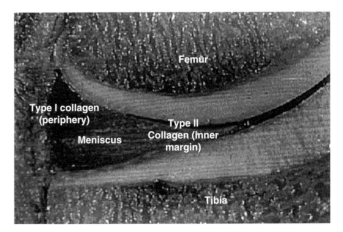

FIGURE 4-2   Microscopic view of meniscal collagen transition from peripheral type I collagen (dark) to inner margin type II collagen (light).

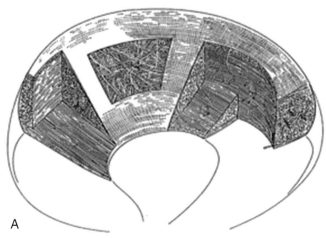
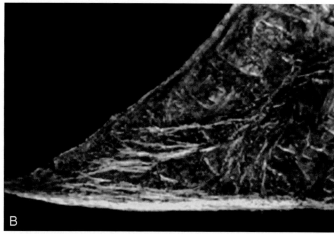

FIGURE 4-3 Biomechanical properties of the meniscus. **A:** Cross-sectional fiber patterns of the meniscus. **B:** Cross-sectional cut of meniscus. Note varying orientations of meniscal fibers. (Modified from Bullough PG, Munuera L, Murphy J, et al. The strength of the menisci of the knee as it relates to their fine structure. *J Bone Joint Surg Br*. 1970;52:564-567, with permission).

Vascular Supply

The vascular supply to the medial and lateral menisci originates predominantly from the lateral and medial geniculate vessels (both with inferior and superior branches). Branches from these vessels give rise to a perimeniscal capillary plexus within the synovial and capsular tissue. This plexus is a tree-like network of vessels that supply the peripheral border of the meniscus throughout the synovial and capsular attachments. These vessels are oriented in a predominantly circumferential pattern with radial branches directed toward the center of the joint in a gradient fashion with the central most zone of the meniscus being avascular.[41,42] Multiple studies have shown that the depth of peripheral vascular penetration is ~10% to 30% of the width of the menisci[42-45] (**Fig. 4-4**). Completing the vascular circuit are endoligamentous vessels arising from the anterior and posterior horns of the menisci forming terminal loops. The remaining portion of the menisci receive their necessary nourishment from the synovial fluid through diffusion and mechanical pumping (joint motion) similar to that of articular cartilage[42,46] (**Fig. 4-5**). With the varying degrees of vascularity throughout the menisci, zones were created for easier classification and ultimately treatment. The "red–red" zone, named for its rich blood supply, is the peripheral third of the meniscus and consists of a high concentration of vascular channels, leading to its high healing potential. The middle third, known as the "red–white" zone, has less predictable healing after injury due to the intermediate density of vascular channels. Injuries in this zone tend to require ancillary procedures such as trephination, synovial abrasion, and a fibrin clot to increase vascularity. The "white–white" zone or inner third of the meniscus is named for its complete avascularity and demonstrates a poor healing potential.[44] To provide nutrition to the inner periphery, knee range of motion assists with the passive diffusion of synovial fluid, which is the only method to obtain nutrition to this region of the meniscus[47] (**Fig. 4-6**).

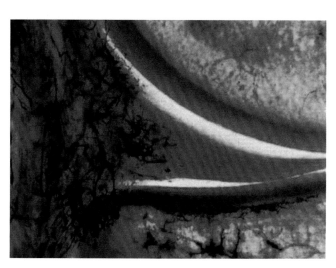

FIGURE 4-4 Vascularity of the meniscus. Note the avascular inner third and highly vascular peripheral third.

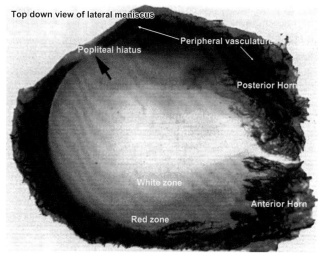

FIGURE 4-5 Vascularity of the meniscus. Note the highly vascular periphery, anterior and posterior horns.

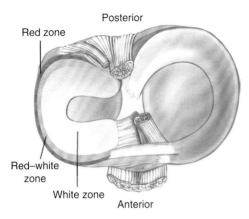

Posterior

Red zone

Red–white zone

White zone

Anterior

FIGURE 4-6 Relation of meniscus tear location to healing. (From Wiesel S. *Operative Techniques in Orthopedic Surgery*. Philadelphia: Wolters Kluwer; 2015.)

Neurology

The central and medial portion of the tibiofemoral joint (and the meniscal tissue located therein) receives innervation from posterior articular branches of the posterior tibial nerve and terminal branches of the obturator and femoral nerves. The lateral meniscus and knee capsule receive innervation via the recurrent peroneal branch of the common peroneal nerve.[48] These fibers follow the blood supply and are found primarily in the peripheral vascular zone covering the outer third of the meniscus as well as the anterior and posterior horns.[45] The middle and inner third are innervated to a lesser degree. Three particular mechanoreceptors, Ruffini endings, Pacinian, and Golgi tendon organs, have been identified within the meniscus and may contribute to pain and proprioception during knee motion.[49] These neural elements are important in deformation and pressure, tension changes, and neuromuscular inhibition, respectively, which may attribute for pain experienced after meniscal injury.[48,50]

Biomechanical Properties

Once thought to be vestigial structures of the knee, the menisci serve many roles including secondary stabilization, proprioception, and load sharing of the tibiofemoral joint.[51] The mechanism by which the menisci transmit load between the femur and tibia has been studied extensively. Biomechanical studies have demonstrated that approximately 50% to 70% of load acting on the extended knee joint is transmitted through the meniscus. This increases up to 85% in flexion.[52] Also, during flexion the articular contact area is observed to decrease in size and shift posteriorly on the tibial plateau, placing more stress across the posterior horns.[53] Throughout weight bearing, the femoral condyles provide an axial force, pushing the menisci away from the center of the joint, creating temporary radial meniscal extrusion and compression of the menisci.[31] As the menisci become circumferentially displaced, tension among the meniscal fibers increases (hoop stress), thus

creating a shock absorption–like effect of the tibiofemoral joint. Keeping the menisci located under the femur and not completely displacing are the strong tibial, meniscofemoral, and capsular attachment sites previously discussed.[37]

The menisci play an essential role in decreasing contact stresses throughout the knee joint. The biomechanics of how meniscus distributes contact stress have been extensively studied, through studies that examine knees that undergo partial or total meniscectomy. When a simulated total medial meniscectomy is performed, the tibiofemoral contact area decreases by 50% to 70%. This decrease was accompanied by a 100% increase in both peak pressure and pressure gradient at the edges of the contact area.[37] Furthermore, this increase expands to 200% to 300% in the lateral compartment after a total lateral meniscectomy and sees a modest 40% to 50% decrease in contact area. With increasing compressive load, the contact stress rose more rapidly and to a significantly higher peak in the absence of menisci.[54] Several cadaver studies of meniscectomies observed increased contact pressure of up to 80% to 90%, which increased with progressive larger amounts of meniscal resection.[55-57] Moreover, resection of 75% of the posterior horn may increase contact stresses similar to those who undergo complete meniscectomy.[54] Notably, a partial meniscectomy of the lateral meniscus leads to higher contact stresses due to the convex–convex relationship between the lateral femoral condyle and the lateral tibial plateau.[10,11] With partial meniscectomy, the remaining peripheral rim of tissue continues to transmit a portion of the load although it should be noted that even with these meniscal-sparing procedures, contact stresses rise dramatically to upward of 350% with as little as 15% tissue resection[58] (**Fig. 4-7**). Therefore, it is these changes in meniscal tensile properties that allow for more evenly distributed load bearing across the knee joint. These increases in contact pressures may lead to early cartilage wear and may contribute to the early onset of osteoarthritis.

In addition to the circumferential tensile forces seen across the meniscus, the menisci also see shear forces that vary depending on the articulation angle of the joint. As the knee moves through extension into flexion, the femoral condyles translate posteriorly onto the tibia as part of the femoral roll back phenomenon.[59-61] The varying femoral condyle geometry as it moves through its arc of motion requires that the menisci change shape and slide relatively to the tibia. In extension, the menisci lie anterior–posterior, whereas in flexion, they lie more medial–lateral. Therefore, one of the important biomechanical properties of menisci is the low shear modulus, or modulus of rigidity which allows the surface of menisci to adapt easily to the changing geometry in the joint as it moves through its arc of motion. An increasing density of proteoglycans toward the inner regions of the menisci helps accommodate the changing stress throughout the meniscus.

It is therefore clear that the menisci play an essential role in load transmission. Additionally, the meniscus serves as

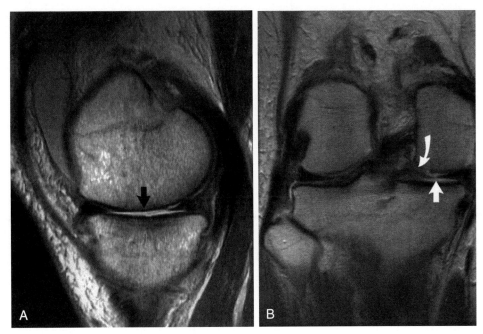

FIGURE 4-7 Increased contact stress of the articular cartilage with reactive signal changes within the chondral surface.

a secondary stabilizer of the knee. Although they are not primary stabilizers, they can assist in this role when the ACL's function as a primary restraint is compromised. When the ACL has been transected, the meniscus aids to resist anterior translation of the tibia.[62] This effect is primarily due to the posterior horn of the medial meniscus, which acts as a wedge between the femur and tibia to prevent anterior tibial translation.[63,64] Prior data suggest a 58% increase in anterior tibial translation with meniscectomy when tested in ACL-deficient knees.[65,66] The lateral meniscus also plays a significant role as a secondary stabilizer of the knee. While its role in sagittal translation is limited (likely due to the increased mobility of the lateral meniscus in this plane), it is much more significant in axial rotation of the knee. In particular, internal tibial rotation dramatically increases in dual ACL- and lateral meniscal–deficient knees. During a pivoting injury resulting in an ACL rupture, the lateral meniscus experiences significant shear forces due to this unstable rotary moment.[67] This may explain the increased incidence of lateral meniscus tears in acute ACL injury. Even in the intact knee, the menisci appear to play an important role in rotary stability, providing additional and more subtle control of position and alignment beyond that provided by the primary restraints.[68,69] It is therefore clear that the menisci play a key role in knee stability as well as load transmission.

INJURIES

According to the American Academy of Orthopaedic Surgeons, arthroscopic knee surgery accounted for 636,000 cases per year in the United States as of 1999.[25,70] Of these cases, treatment of meniscal injuries was the most commonly performed procedure and can account for upward of 20% of all procedures performed at some surgery centers.[71] As one of the most common orthopedic injuries regardless of patient age, meniscal injury can greatly range in the degree of physical impairment. While the meniscus demonstrates amazingly resilient properties, injury may still occur if tension, compression, or shear forces exceed the strength of the meniscal matrix. Through improved understanding of etiology through epidemiologic data, we know that risk and prevalence is affected by age, activity level, gender, and patient comorbidities.[72-74] Men are four times as likely to sustain a meniscal tear. Sports that require cutting and pivoting at various knee flexion angles such as basketball, soccer, gymnastics, football, wrestling, and skiing generate the highest risk for meniscal injury. Furthermore, lateral meniscal tears are less common than medial across all cohorts in an isolated setting.[72,74]

When clinically assessing for meniscal injury, a thorough and detailed history and physical are key. Clinical symptoms of catching, locking, pain, swelling, buckling, and decreased motion are some of the more common symptoms encountered. Pain is localized to the joint line of the affected side and unlike acute traumatic tears, degenerative tears are not associated with an acute effusion, but more intermittent symptoms and generalized discomfort. Provocative tests such as joint line tenderness to palpation, McMurray, Apley grind, and Thessaly test are used to help improve the physical exam diagnostic accuracy.[75] Of these tests, Thessaly test has repeatedly demonstrated in the literature low false-positive and false-negative results with accuracy in the 95% range.[76] While isolated meniscal pathology can be accurately diagnosed with history and physical examination alone, plain radiographs and MRI should still be obtained to rule out other pathology, check mechanical alignment, and confirm the suspected diagnosis. Plain radiographs should include weight-bearing AP, Rosenberg, lateral, and merchant views. If there is suspicion for malalignment of the lower extremity, full-length standing, long cassette films should be obtained. MRI, the diagnostic imaging modality of choice for soft tissue pathology, has greatly improved the ability to diagnose a meniscal injury with an 88% sensitivity and a 94% accuracy.[77,78] Normal meniscal structure will uniformly have low signal intensity throughout on both fat-suppressed and fast spin-echo images. If a nonfocal high signal is noted within the meniscal structure but does not extend to the meniscal surface, this is indicative of intrasubstance degeneration or grade I meniscal signal. Grade II is a focal linear high signal that again does not extend to the articular surface. Finally, grade III is a linear high-grade signal that extends to either the superior or inferior meniscal surface.[79] In addition, blunting of the free margin of the meniscus is highly indicative of meniscal tear with a displaced fragment. Of particular note, it is also essential to view the meniscus in the sagittal, coronal, and axial planes to evaluate for displaced meniscal fragments in the gutters or intercondylar notch. For example, a displaced bucket-handle medial meniscal tear will take on the appearance of a "double PCL" on sagittal images as the displaced fragment runs in parallel with the native PCL creating a mirror image (**Fig. 4-8**).

With the rise in the aging population, we have also seen an increase in prevalence of asymptomatic meniscal pathology. Previous studies have demonstrated that there is a 5.6% incidence of asymptomatic meniscal tears in a younger patient population (mean age of 35).[80] As the population increases, these incidental findings increase as

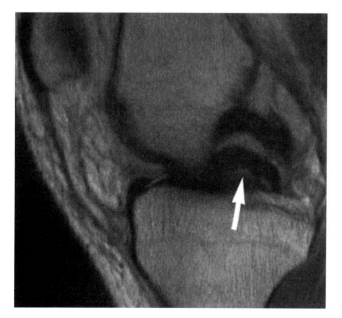

FIGURE 4-8 "Double PCL" sign with the arrow pointing to the displaced medial meniscal bucket-handle tear.

well. At an average age of 65, the prevalence is an astonishing 76%.[81] In the setting of concomitant injury, specifically an ACL tear, there is a 57% and 36% prevalence of lateral and medial meniscal tear, respectively. Of these, the lateral meniscus is more commonly identified in acute ACL injuries, whereas medial meniscal injuries are more common with chronic ACL tears.[82]

DEGENERATIVE TEAR

Degenerative meniscal tears are very commonplace and may be attributed to normal aging of the knee. They occur more commonly in older people and in addition to aging, may be related to intrinsic collagen breakdown and "wear and tear" of the knee joint.[23,83] Over time, degenerative changes seen in the meniscus include decreased cellular density, mucoid degeneration with disruption of collagen fiber orientation, and the appearance of acellular zones. Oftentimes, degenerative meniscal tears occur in the setting of potential osteoarthritis of the knee.[84-87] In patients with osteoarthritis, 70% to 90% are noted to have concomitant degenerative meniscal pathology.[18,23]

Degenerative tears are typically horizontal-cleavage or complex tears with frayed, macerated edges. Degenerative tears may be unstable and complex or simple and stable. Cells in the superficial meniscus layer can be hyperplastic, and the collagenous bundles are separated by degenerative mucoid changes. In stable tears, there may be minimal meniscal displacement and patients may be asymptomatic. As a result, degenerative meniscal tears are often noted as incidental findings when advanced imaging of the knee is obtained.[23,85]

The hallmark of degeneration of the meniscus is loss of proteoglycan and collagen from the meniscus extracellular matrix.[18,88-90] Two specific classes of degradative enzymes, metalloproteinases (MMPs) and aggrecanases (ADAMTS), are primarily responsible for degradation of meniscal extracellular matrix proteins. As a result, many studies have utilized these two proteins as potential biomarkers for meniscal degeneration.[91-93] Specifically, elevated levels of MMP-1, MMP-2, MMP-3, and MMP-13 have been associated with meniscal injury and development of osteoarthritis.[18]

ACUTE TEAR

Acute traumatic meniscal tears are frequently associated with sports-related activities. The healthy meniscus often splits vertically and in line with the orientation of the circumferentially oriented collagen fibers (i.e., longitudinal tear, bucket-handle tear) or perpendicular to the long axis (radial tears).[94] This leads to decreased biomechanical function of the knee joint. In addition, these tears may be associated with concomitant ligamentous injury and knee instability. Therefore, traumatic tears may disrupt the normal meniscal structure and biomechanical advantage

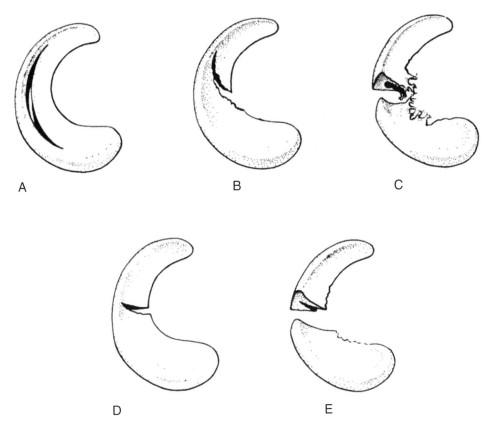

FIGURE 4-9   Meniscal classification based on tear pattern. **A:** Vertical longitudinal. **B:** Oblique. **C:** Degenerative. **D:** Transverse (radial). **E:** Horizontal.

of hoop stresses, leading to increased contact forces and abnormal loading of cartilage. Meniscal tears can be classified according to their tear pattern. The main categories of acute meniscal tears include vertical longitudinal, radial, horizontal, and oblique tears (**Fig. 4-9**).

Vertical longitudinal tears are oriented between the collagen fibers circumferentially around the meniscus, perpendicular to the tibial plateau and parallel to the long axis of the meniscus (**Fig. 4-10**). They occur more often in younger patients, noted more frequently medially in isolated cases or commonly in the lateral meniscus when in association with ACL tears. Because these tears occur between circumferential collagen fibers, the biomechanics of the knee joint may not be disrupted and patients may be asymptomatic if the tear is not displaced. However, extensive longitudinal (bucket-handle) tears can cause mechanical locking if the central portion of the meniscus is displaced.[95,96]

Radial tears are vertical tears, which often occur at the junction of the posterior and middle third and from the inner free margin toward the periphery. The posteromedial meniscus is the most common site of injury due to its decreased concentration of radial tie fibers and therefore decreased tensile strength.[34,62] Radial tears are most often traumatic and occur in a younger population. Biomechanically, these tears often happen with excessive forces that traumatically separate the anterior and posterior portions of the meniscus, stretching the inner periphery and causing a transverse tear. Bedi demonstrated that cutting the meniscus radially from the inner radius, up to 60% of the width, resulted in no significant change in the contact pressure on the tibial plateau.[97] In contrast, if the radial tear extends into the middle and peripheral thirds, significant increases in peak compartment pressures are noted.[97] Because radial tears traverse

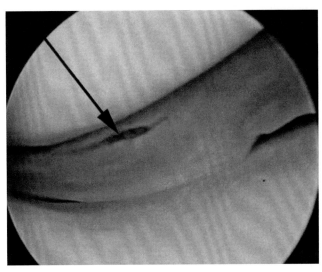

FIGURE 4-10   Arrow pointing to longitudinal tear of the meniscus.

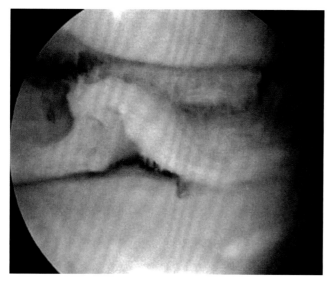

FIGURE 4-11 Complex meniscal tear with horizontal, oblique, and degenerative component.

perpendicular to the orientation of the collagen fibrils, these tears disrupt the ability of menisci to evenly distribute their natural hoop stresses associated with weight bearing.[98] Thus radial meniscal tears inherently alter the biomechanics of the meniscus.

Horizontal tears are oriented parallel to the tibial plateau, dividing the meniscus into superior and inferior segments. Though they may occur in all ages, they are more common in middle-aged patients and are often associated with meniscal cyst formation. Horizontal tears occur most commonly in the posterior horn of the medial meniscus. Similar to radial tears, horizontal tears occur due to shear stresses across the superior and inferior portions of the meniscus that separate the upper and lower portions of the meniscus. More often however, horizontal tears are associated with degenerative meniscal tears (**Fig. 4-11**). Tears may be confined within the meniscus itself (type II signal) or may extend to the inner and outer periphery.[99]

Similar to radial tears, oblique tears most commonly occur at the junction of the posterior and middle body of the meniscus due to the decreased concentration of radial tie fibers. These tears are often unstable and can create mechanical symptoms including locking and catching and/or pain from meniscocapsular irritation.[47] Oblique tears occur within the inner periphery of the meniscus. In addition, due to their oblique orientation across the meniscus, these tears also disrupt the natural distribution of hoop stresses across the knee.[96]

RELATION OF TEAR LOCATION TO HEALING

The vascular supply to the meniscus determines its potential for repair. After injury, the meniscus is capable of a reparative process similar to that seen in other connective tissues. Within the peripheral vascular zone, a fibrin hematoma forms due to the perimeniscal capillary plexus. This hematoma is rich in inflammatory cells and growth factors such as platelet-derived growth factor and transforming growth factor-β, allowing for the recruitment and proliferation of differentiated mesenchymal cells. The peripheral lesion eventually fills with cellular fibrous scar tissue that is eventually penetrated by the perimeniscal capillary plexus. Vasculature from the perimeniscal capillary plexus penetrates this scar tissue providing an inflammatory response. After several months, this scar tissue matures into normal-appearing fibrocartilage dominated by type I collagen. Conversely, the inner two-thirds resemble more of a hyaline cartilage with type II collagen and proteoglycans.[100-102]

The current concept of healing potential includes meniscal zones that are delineated by the availability of blood supply. As previously discussed, the meniscal zones of injury can be defined as the red–red, red–white, and white–white zones. Tears that are closer to the free margin of the meniscus, defined as those in the white–white zone, have poor blood supply and therefore a lower ability to heal than those tears located on the periphery (red–red zone). Over time, an age-related decrease in vascularity occurs, thus shrinking the available red–red zone, causing decreasing meniscal healing potential as one ages.[44,103]

TENDON

Normal Structure and Function

Anatomy

Tendons are soft connective tissues that are composed of closely packed, parallel collagen fiber bundles. Tendons play an essential role in the musculoskeletal system by transferring tensile loads from muscle to bone in order to enable joint motion and stabilization. Tendons can be divided into two large groups: those that function to transmit loads (i.e., patellar and Achilles tendon) and those that mainly transmit motion (e.g., flexor tendons). This section discusses tendon anatomy, biomechanics, and their associated pathophysiology.

Tendon Structure

The elemental unit of a tendon is a fiber that is composed of a bundle of collagen fibrils and cells that comply a well-organized extracellular matrix (ECM).[104] These collagen molecules organize themselves via intermolecular cross-links into parallel organized collagen fibrils, which are responsible for the crimp and wave-like appearance of the tendon.[105] These fibrils are arranged longitudinally into collagen fibers, bundles of fibers called fascicles, and then finally the tendon unit itself[105] (**Fig. 4-12**). Each tendon fiber is surrounded by a thin reticular network of tissue called the endotenon.

Macroscopically the tendon unit is covered by epitenon, which functions to reduce friction with adjacent tissues and ensure each tendon's vascular, lymphatic,

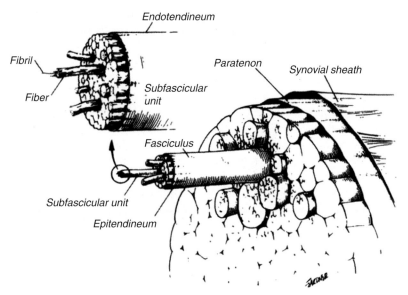

FIGURE 4-12 Tendon microstructure.

and nerve supply.[106] In some tendons, the epitenon is surrounded by loose areolar tissue called the paratenon that functions as an elastic sheath throughout which the tendon can slide.[106] This hierarchical macrostructure of the tendon lies parallel to the long axis of the tendon, making it ideal to transmit large tensile mechanical loads.[107]

Tendons are primarily composed of type I collagen, which accounts for 65% to 80% of the dry tendon mass.[104] Further studies have demonstrated that there exist a number of varying collagen types, including collagen type II within cartilaginous zones, collagen type III in reticular fibers of blood vessels, collagen type V in vascular membranes, collagen type IV in capillary membranes, collagen type X in the mineralized fibrocartilage within the osteotendinous junction as well as collagen type XII, XIV, and XV as fibril-associated collagens.[104,108,109] Type V collagen serves as a regulator of collagen fibril diameter.[110] Type III collagen is important for tendon healing due to its ability to create rapid cross-links to enhance injury site repair.[110] Type XII collagen provides lubrication between collagen fibers.[111] These varying amounts of collagen help optimize tendon function.

Alongside collagen, proteoglycans and glycoproteins play an important role in tendon function and composition. Proteoglycans and glycoproteins (1% to 5%), elastin (2%), and inorganic molecules (0.2%) are components of the extracellular matrix. Via their glycosaminoglycan (GAG) side chains, proteoglycans bind to form cross-links between collagen fibrils in a parallel alignment.[104] This allows for structural integrity as well as diminished friction during tendon movement. Several proteoglycans have been implicated as important to normal tendon function including decorin, fibromodulin, aggrecan, and lumican. Decorin is responsible for direct binding and cross-linking collagen fibrils and facilitates fibrillar slippage.[37,112] Aggrecan allows for rapid diffusion

of water-soluble molecules and cell migration. Elastin is another important molecule responsible for elastic stretch and recoil and regulates interactions between cells and the ECM.[37]

In addition to the structural components, there are many types of cells within the tendon. Tendons have a varied cellular makeup. The most prevalent cell is the tenocyte, though tendon cellular makeup includes chondrocytes, synovial cells, and vascular cells.[66] Tenocytes are fibroblastic-like and are interspersed within the collagen fiber bundles.[66] Mature tendon cells modulate activity based on their long, thin cytoplasmic projections that allow for intercellular communication via gap junctions.[113] Importantly they are largely responsible for extracellular matrix maintenance and production of collagen, fibronectin, and proteoglycan accordingly in order to maintain its structure.[37,114] More recently, the discovery of a tendon progenitor cell, named the tendon stem cell (TSC), has been found to be critically important in tendon maintenance, repair, and regeneration.[104] This is thought to be due to their ability to differentiate into tenocytes as needed depending on associated pathology or injury.[104] Decreasing quantities of TSC as seen in association with aging or tendinopathy may be responsible for subsequent tendon degradation.[115] Many studies have examined the potential use of stem cell therapy for the treatment of tendinopathy, but the results largely remain preclinical.[106,114,116]

Tendon Blood Supply

The blood supply of the tendon originates from three different sites: the myotendinous junction, osteotendinous junction, and the tendon sheaths. The main vascular supply of the tendon comes from the paratenon, where a vascular network is able to penetrate the epitenon and reach the endotendon sheet.[117] At the myotendinous junction, the vascular supply to the muscle flows directly to the proximal third of the tendon. The sparse blood supply from the osteotendinous junction is restricted to the tendon insertion site.[118] The selective nature of the tendinous vascularity leads to "watershed" areas that are susceptible to injury. Other sources of nutrition include passive diffusion through synovial fluid, which is an essential mechanism of nutrient delivery in flexor tendons of the hand.[66] Although vascular flow is varied, nutrients are able to penetrate throughout the length of the tendon. Because the metabolic activity of tendon is relatively slow, its vascularity and capacity to heal is lower than other soft tissues.[113,116]

Tendon Junctional Anatomy

The enthesis, which directly inserts into bone, is a composite that allows for transition from tendon to bone through four zones: tendon ECM, fibrocartilage, mineralized fibrocartilage, and finally bone.[119] This gradual change is essential to avoid rupture between the two tissues when faced with a mechanical load.[118] In the zone of uncalcified cartilage, chondrocytes and cartilage matrix lie in between bundles of collagen fibers that are originating from the tendon portion.[118] As the tendon musculature approaches, chondrocytes become increasingly numerous and are arranged in short rows.[118] As the bone is approached along the tendon, bundles of collagen fibers are seen at the osteochondral junction.[118] Insertion of tendon into bone is via two mechanisms: direct and indirect.[118,119] Direct insertion occurs when the tendon fibrils directly attach onto bone through zones of fibrocartilage and progressive transition to bone. Indirect insertion occurs when the superficial fibrils insert into the periosteum and deeper fibrils insert onto bone directly. Tendons attached to the end of long bones generally attach to bones directly through fibrocartilage. However, the amount of fibrocartilage transition can vary from muscle to muscle.[118] In tendons that attach particularly close to the articular surface (such as the rotator cuff in the humeral head) the uncalcified cartilage becomes continuous with the articular cartilage.[118] Biomechanical stress caused by muscle contraction on bone promotes further development of the tendon–bone interface. At the other end of the tendinous unit is the myotendinous junction. This is the weakest component of the functional muscle unit. A complexion of GAGs, fibronectin, laminin, tenascin, and collagen fibrils of varying size help comprise this transition zone and absorb shock during muscle contraction.[115]

BIOMECHANICS

The biomechanics of tendons have been widely studied, with the key to tendon tensile stiffness coming from its collagen makeup.[66] The unique structure and composition of tendons afford them their characteristic mechanical behavior, which is reflected by a typical stress–strain curve consisting of regions. The first region, the toe region, in the stress–strain curve is when the tendon strain is less than 2%. This region represents the "stretching out" of crimped tendon fibrils due to mechanical loading on the tendon.[66,120] With increased strain, the stress–strain curve enters a linear region where the strain is less than 4%, or less than the physiological upper limit of tendon strain. In this region, tendon fibrils are oriented in the direction of mechanical load. The slope of this linear region is termed the Young modulus of the tendon, representing tendon stiffness.[66,120,121] When the strain reaches past 4%, microscopic tearing of the tendon occurs, resulting in microtear failure of the tendon.[66] When strain reaches 8% to 10%, macroscopic tearing of tendon fibers occur, leading to tendon rupture.[66]

Tensile stiffness of tendons across the human body varies, allowing for varying mechanical properties. In addition to their significant stiffness, tendons are also viscoelastic, meaning that their mechanical behavior is dependent on the rate of mechanical strain.[122,123] Viscoelasticity makes tendons more deformable at low strain rates but less deformable across high strain rates.[120,121] Thus, tendons experiencing low strain rates absorb more mechanical energy but are less effective in carrying mechanical loads. On the other hand, tendons experiencing high strain rates become much stiffer, and therefore more effective at transmitting high muscular loads to bone. The viscoelastic properties of tendons are likely related to tendon makeup, including collagenous proteins, water, and the associated reactions between proteoglycans and collagen.[122,123] Importantly, tendons are capable of adapting to variations in mechanical loading.[107]

Several studies demonstrate the benefit that appropriate mechanical loads play to tendon mechanobiology, leading to an increased anabolic effect.[124-127] With appropriate tensile loading, the three-dimensional orientation of tendon fibers becomes more organized in response to tensile load, thus increasing tensile tendon stiffness. On the other hand, excessive mechanical loads are catabolic, creating ECM breakdown.[128] Concurrently, tendon disuse leads to ECM breakdown and tendon atrophy, as seen by a decrease in anabolic activities, but an increase in catabolic activities of the tendon matrix.[106] Macroscopically, this results in significant changes to tendon cell shape, cell number, and collagen fiber alignment.[106] Physiologic mechanical loading is also necessary for tendon repair and rehabilitation.[125,126] Thus, physiologic mechanical loading directly relates to tendon structure and homeostasis.

INJURIES

While tendons vary across the human body, these tendons can see varying changes in their tensile properties over time. Moreover, aging significantly affects the mechanical properties of tendons: the Young modulus of human patellar tendons from young donors (29 to 50 years old) was on average 600 MPa, whereas that of the same

SECTION 2 / BASIC SCIENCE

tendons from older donors (64 to 93 years old) was on average 504 MPa.[66] The prescribed mechanism is the alteration in tendon metabolism, increasing the susceptibility for microdamage and the prevalence of degenerative changes.[129] Additionally, excessive mechanical loads can lead to tendon injury and degeneration.

Patterns of Injury

Tendon injuries can be roughly divided into two types: acute and degenerative tears. As previously described, acute injuries occur when the stress–strain curve of the tendon reaches 8% to 10%. Degenerative tears occur due to chronic tendinopathy and currently can be organized into three main mechanisms: (1) mechanical overuse, (2) vascularization, and (3) aging.[129,130] Tendons have the capacity to remodel and adapt through a careful balance of collagen synthesis against metalloproteinase activity and breakdown. This mechanobiological adaptation modifies the mechanical strength and viscoelastic properties of the tendon, decreasing its stress-susceptibility, leading to higher load resistances.[129] Nevertheless, repetitive activities can cause an undue strain on the tendon over time. Over time, repetitive tensile loading under the tendon injury threshold can lead to an accumulation of microdamage, elevating the risk for tendinopathy or rupture. As a result of microdamage, scattered vascular in-growth, including necrotic capillaries, contributes to vascular compromise. This leads to local tissue hypoxia, which is considered a risk for degeneration and tendinopathy.[37]

DEGENERATION

From a cellular level, tendon degeneration can be described as a failure of the matrix adaptation and remodeling due to an imbalance between matrix decomposition and synthesis caused by a variety of stresses and mechanical loads.[131] The imbalance of metalloproteinases and the tissue inhibitors of metalloproteinases is considered an important role in the degenerative process. Recent studies have improved our understanding of the degenerative process. Increased levels of collagen III to collagen I have been implicated in the degenerative process as well as increased levels of fibronectin, tenascin C, GAGs, disintegrin, and biglycan. Additionally, increased levels of MMP-1, MMP-9, MMP-19, MMP-25, and TIMP-1 were thought to be related to tendon degeneration.[37]

Macroscopically, chronic tendon pain is thought to be a degenerative process as opposed to an inflammatory process.[66,104,130] With overuse, repetitive tensile forces outside the range of physiologic loading can lead to microdamage, which only further makes it more susceptible to injury. This cycle, in turn, leads to increased microdamage. As a result of this microdamage, scattered vascular in-growth, including damaged microcapillaries, leads to local tissue hypoxia, further leading to decreased healing potential.[66,104,128] Age is also associated with tendon degeneration, likely due to decreased proliferation and tendon metabolism that naturally occurs over time. It may be characterized by increased cellular senescence, decreasing blood flow, and enhanced lipid formation, though the exact mechanism through aging remains yet to be understood completely.[66,130] Associated factors include weaker vasculature, which may lead to overall decreased healing capacity[129] (**Fig. 4-13**).

TENDON HEALING AND REPAIR

Tendons possess the capacity for self-repair through intrinsic tendon stem cells and surrounding ECM. This process is dictated by three different stages: (1) the initial tissue inflammation, (2) cell proliferation, and (3) ECM remodeling.[131] During the inflammatory phase, vascular

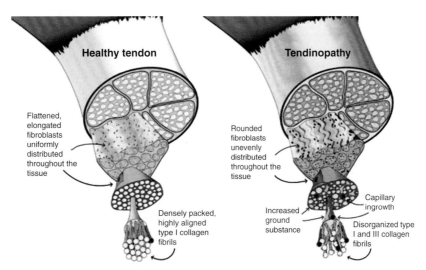

FIGURE 4-13 Degeneration of the tendon. (From Mead MP, Gumucio JP, Awan TM, et al. Pathogenesis and management of tendinopathies in sports medicine. *Transl Sports Med.* 2018;1(1):5-13. Copyright © 2018 American Association of Physicists in Medicine. Reprinted by permission of John Wiley & Sons, Inc).

permeability increases and an influx of inflammatory cells, including platelets, neutrophils, and erythrocytes attracted by pro-inflammatory cytokines, enter the healing site. These cells, in turn, produce more cytokines and growth factor that lead to proliferation of macrophages and resident tendon fibroblasts. Components of the ECM, primarily type III collagen, are synthesized by surrounding fibroblasts.[132] Mesenchymal cells enter the area of injury and are able to differentiate into fibroblasts.[132] The inflammatory phase is evident until the eight to tenth day of injury.[133]

After this, the beginning of the proliferation stage is indicated by the abundance of ECM component production, such as proteoglycan and collagen. These products are initially arranged randomly within the ECM. Collagen, primarily type I, synthesis begins within the first week and reaches maximum level after about 4 weeks.[134] Procollagen is initially synthesized by resident and migratory fibroblasts, which is eventually converted into type 1 collagen and released into the extracellular matrix in random orientation.[115] TGF-β plays an important role in the production of procollagen.[135] At this stage, there is also a significant influx of water and an increase in cellularity.[130]

The final stage, ECM remodeling, takes place over a lengthy period of time. The initial portion of ECM remodeling takes place as consolidation, where there is a decrease in cellularity and matrix production.[130] At this stage, the tissue becomes increasingly fibrous through the replacement of collagen type III to collagen type I. Collagen fibers then begin to organize themselves longitudinally, helping to restore tendon stiffness.[136] Subsequently, tendons enter the maturation phase, which consists of collagen fibril cross-linking and increasing collagen production.[137] The strength of the healing tendon increases as the collagen becomes stabilized by cross-links and the fibrils assemble into fibers.[137] During the maturation phase, the mechanical strength of the healing tendon increases as a result of remodeling and reorganization of the fiber architecture.[137]

A number of growth factors play a role as powerful regulators during the remodeling phase. These include platelet-derived growth factors (PDGF-BB), basic fibroblast growth factor (bFGF), transforming growth factor beta (TGF-β), and vascular endothelial growth factor (VEGF), which vary dramatically throughout tendon healing and help promote fibroblast proliferation and collagen remodeling.[104,115] PDGF promotes the expression of growth factors along with stimulation of cell proliferation and collagen synthesis.[138] bGFG increases cell proliferation and may aid in wound healing.[139] VEGF is known to promote angiogenesis and has been shown to be expressed by many cells at the site of injury.[140] Despite extensive study on the varying growth factors, no major breakthrough regarding clinically improving tendon healing through growth factor modulation has been made.

LIGAMENT

Normal Structure and Function

Anatomy

Ligaments are broad fibrous bands that span two or more bones and perform a crucial role in the stability of joints. The ligamentous complex or unit is composed of a proximal osseous insertion, the substance of the ligament or capsular thickening, and the distal osseous insertion.[141,142] When we further examine the molecular structure, we see that the ligament is composed of various arrays of collagen, elastic fibers, glycoproteins, and adhesion molecules.[143] Type I collagen, the major component, accounts for 90% of the collagen content found in ligaments, followed by type III (3% to 10%), and the rest varying degrees of type IV, V, and VI.[144] Individual collagen fibrils ranging from 40 to 150 nm in diameter are grouped to form a fiber, which are then grouped into fascicles. These fibrils are oriented parallel to the line of tension they are expected to resist.[145,146] Together, the fascicles combine to form the ligament bundle. Some ligaments will have more than one collagen fibril bundle. An example of this is the ACL and PCL whose various bundles become taut at different points throughout the range of motion of the knee. Similar to tendons, ligaments are composed of stable and unstable fibrillar collagen cross-links that allow for increased structural stability. Unique to the ligamentous structure is that the collagen bundles exhibit a wave or crimp pattern under light microscopic examination. It is hypothesized that this wave pattern may allow for mild elongation of the ligament without damage.[147] Elastin sheets, while limited in their gross amount contributing to the overall makeup of the ligament (less than 5%), play a vital role in allowing for the structure to undergo some deformation without rupturing, and then returning to its original form once the load is removed.[148] Maintaining this microscopic megastructure are proteoglycans. Similar to tendons, articular cartilage, and menisci, ligaments contain two classes of proteoglycans: large, containing chondroitin and keratan sulfate, and small, containing dermatan sulfate. These proteoglycans work together, filling the ligamentous structure with water between the collagen fibrils for stability, organization, and nutritional demands of the ligament.[149,150] Rounding out the overall ligament structure are scattered blood vessels and nerve fibers similar to that of mechanoreceptors that tend to run in parallel with matrix collagen fibers.[141,151]

Supporting this extracellular matrix (ECM) are fibroblasts. Their role is to help form and maintain the ECM as their presence varies in activity and density along the ligament. Many of these cells are spindle shaped and are located between the collagen fibrils. Because these cells sparsely populate the tissue and reside some distance from vascularity, they must depend on diffusion of nutrients and metabolites through the tissue fluid which contributes roughly 60% of the wet weight of the ligament.[149,152]

Aiding the fibroblasts are noncollagenous proteins, such as fibronectin, that appear to maintain and organize the macromolecular framework of the ECM and possibly influence cellular function. By comparison, ligaments are more metabolically active than tendons, as shown by a higher content of DNA within intrinsic ligament cells in comparison to tendoblasts. This is hypothesized to be due to the fact that ligaments, in comparison to tendons, have a higher need for adaptive remodeling due to functional demands.[141,145]

Bony Insertion Anatomy

Generally, ligaments insert to bone via two mechanisms: direct and indirect. An example of direct insertion is the femoral origin of the ACL. Here, fibers attach to the bone via sharply defined regions. The thin superficial aspect of the ligamentous collagen fibers becomes continuous with the periosteum at the insertion. The rest of the insertion occurs through the deep collagen fibers that directly penetrate the cortex of the osseous surface at a right angle. The transition of ligament insertion occurs through four different zones: ligament, fibrocartilage, mineralized fibrocartilage, and bone.[118,142,143,145,152] For indirect insertions (such as the tibial insertion of the MCL), superficial fibers are attached to the periosteum, while the deeper fibers are directly attached to the bone at acute angles via Sharpey fibers. Oftentimes these areas of insertion cover more osseous surface area than their direct counterparts. Additionally, type II, IX, X, XI, and XIV collagen have all been identified at the insertion site.[37]

Biomechanics

Type I collagen is the primary constituent of ligaments and, like tendons, is responsible for the tensile strength of ligaments. Additionally, ligaments are composed of type II, III, IX, X, XI, and XIV collagen, and it is the varying combinations of these constituents that impart the varying mechanical properties of ligaments seen across the human body.[144,153] Ligaments, biomechanically, are best suited to transfer load from bone to bone along the longitudinal direction of the ligament. Thus, force application in a linear direction with the collagen fiber orientation results in a greater proportion of collagen fibril recruitment, resulting in higher tensile strength.[147] But perhaps the most well-known responsibility of the ligament is the resistance of forces perpendicular to their long axis, providing stability to the joint.

Stress–strain dynamics are vital to proper material function based on application. For ligaments and tendons, the curve begins with a low-stiffness toe region followed by a higher stiff linear portion.[148] As the ligament begins to stretch, elongation of the ligament occurs due to straightening of the "crimped" collagen fibrils. Allowing for ligaments to maintain smooth movements of joints under normal, physiologic circumstances and to restrain excessive joint displacement under high loads, the number of ligament fiber bundles utilized increases with load. Past this linear curve, the ligament starts to reach physiologic failure, leading to microtears and eventually, complete ligament rupture[147] (**Figs. 4-14** and **4-15**).

As mentioned earlier, ligaments rely on their fluid composition to help maintain their viscoelastic and structural properties. The phenomenon of ligamentous preconditioning occurs when fluid is extruded during initial force applied to the ligament, resulting in greater stiffness and hysteresis energy loss. This is replenished during inactivity. Affecting the ligaments resilience to stress and strain are location, skeletal maturity, age, immobilization, and stress exposure.[147,154] In the skeletally immature, ligaments tend to fail by bony avulsion versus the skeletally mature who tend to fail at the mid-substance. With age, water content and collagen synthesis decrease similar to that of articular and meniscal cartilage, thereby leading to a weaker and more frail ligament.[155,156] With immobilization, histologic changes occur throughout the course of the ligament and most notably at the insertion site where osteoclastic subperiosteal bone resorption weakens the

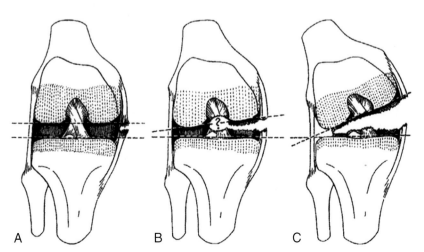

FIGURE 4-14 Valgus force resulting in MCL rupture **(A)**. Increasing valgus force resulting in progressive ligamentous damage. Possible cruciate injury **(B)**. MCL and cruciate injury **(C)**.

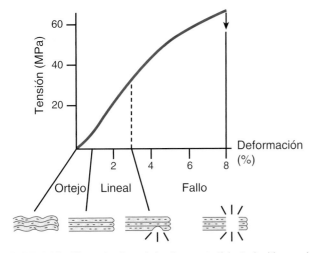

FIGURE 4-15 Biomechanics of the ligament. (Adapted with permission from Butler DL, Grood ES, Noyes FR, Zernicke RE. Biomechanics of ligaments and tendons. *Exerc Sport Sci Rev.* 1978;6:125-181.)

direct ligamentous attachment. Additionally, the cellular metabolism becomes altered with prolonged immobilization, leading to a more catabolic state.[156]

INJURIES

A cascade of inflammatory, cytokine, and regenerative mediators are released in response to ligamentous injury. At the time of injury, damaged cells and blood vessels result in an acute inflammatory period lasting 48 to 72 hours. During this time, cytokines and other growth factors (TGF-β and platelet-derived growth factor) are released, promoting vascular dilation and permeability and leading to swelling of the affected ligament and surrounding tissue.[145] At the specific site of injury, a hematoma forms as platelets bind to fibrillar collagen creating the initial scaffold for vascular and fibroblastic proliferation. Shortly after initial injury, polymorphonuclear leukocytes and monocytes appear in the clot to assist with the removal necrotic tissue and cellular debris. As the site of injury begins to clear of nonviable tissue, chemotactic factors released from newly formed capillaries helps to recruit and stimulate the proliferation of fibroblasts. Within 2 to 3 days, fibroblasts have begun to replace the clot with a disorganized fibrous matrix of type III collagen, water, and glycosaminoglycans.[157,158] Eventually, the ligament enters the remodeling phase where disorganized type III collagen is replaced with organized type I collagen that is synthesized to form tightly packed bundles. As the fibroblasts and macrophages decrease in activity, the matrix becomes more organized with collagen fibrils growing in size and concentration. Inversely, water and proteoglycans decrease. The majority of remodeling phase lasts from a couple of weeks to 4 to 6 months after injury but has been noted to continue at some level for years. Nearing the end of the remodeling phase, the uninjured ligament returns to normal histologic appearance, whereas the site of injury is characterized as scar. This scar tissue is weaker than the native ligament due to increased concentrations of type III, V, and VI collagen; decreased cross-links; and comparatively increased amounts of glycosaminoglycans.[159,160]

Intra-articular ligament tears, however, have a different biologic mechanism of repair, and oftentimes are not able to be healed primarily, leading to several studies questioning the difference in biological healing of extra-articular versus intra-articular ligament tears.[145,161] Structural differences (e.g., fiber orientation, and crimp patter), cellular differences (i.e., fibroblast shape), and differences in blood supply may play a role in the ability of intra-articular ligaments to heal. An example of this is the inability of the ruptured ACL to heal. At the time of rupture, the acutely torn ends of the ACL rapidly degenerate due to high collagenase activity, thus increasing the distance of repair required and destabilizing any collagen matrix trying to form.[162]

Additional factors affecting a ligament's ability to heal are the size of the injury, location, and ligament type. As previously mentioned, intracapsular ligaments have a lower propensity to heal compared to their extracapsular counterparts due to synovial fluid interposition, blood supply, structural, and cellular differences. Avoidance of widely separated ruptured ligament ends minimizes the volume of repair tissue needed and maximizes the length of normal ligamentous tissue. Furthermore, as noted during the discussion on immobilization, some loading of the healing ligament can promote healing, but excessive stresses will only delay or prevent healing.[157]

Degenerative Tears

Age remains a significant factor in chronic degeneration. Histologically, ligaments become more disorganized with increasing age. Cystic changes, disorientation of collagen fibers, and mucoid degeneration are all seen with ligament degeneration. This has been most widely studied in the ACL. Additionally, with age comes a decrease in collagen fibril diameter and a corresponding increase in smaller fibrils, suggesting a reduced biomechanical capacity.[67,163]

Intra- Versus Extra-articular Ligament Injury

There has been extensive study analyzing the differences between intra- and extra-articular ligament healing, none more so than the ACL and MCL. A study performed by Murray et al. discovered that the ruptured ACL undergoes four histologic phases: inflammation, epiligamentous regeneration, proliferation, and remodeling.[164] Interestingly during this study, they observed that at the time of injury, the ruptured ends of the ligament were covered with alpha-smooth muscle actin-expressing synovial cell layer that, they propose, inhibits the healing response and even direct repair.[165] The structures of the ACL and MCL are also different. The collagen fibrils of the MCL are larger as well as the concentration of subfascicles within the larger fibril. This in turn creates more surface area and possibly more microscopic contact between the torn ends of the ligament.[154,165] Unfortunately, MCL fibroblasts also proliferate more rapidly than those of the ACL. Differences in response to various cytokines such as integrin expression are a key component to the upregulation of fibroblastic proliferation. On the surface of the MCL fibroblasts, there are an increased number of active integrins during the healing phase of the MCL when compared to the ACL. mRNA for procollagen is increased in the MCL as well.[154,166]

REFERENCES

1. Fox AJ, Wanivenhaus F, Burge AJ, Warren RF, Rodeo SA. The human meniscus: a review of anatomy, function, injury, and advances in treatment. *Clin Anat.* 2015;28(2):269-287.
2. Fox AJ, Bedi A, Rodeo SA. The basic science of human knee menisci: structure, composition, and function. *Sports Health.* 2012;4(4):340-351.
3. Abraham AC, Donahue TL. From meniscus to bone: a quantitative evaluation of structure and function of the human meniscal attachments. *Acta Biomater.* 2013;9(5):6322-6329.
4. Aydingöz U, Kaya A, Atay OA, Oztürk MH, Doral MN. MR imaging of the anterior intermeniscal ligament: classification according to insertion sites. *Eur Radiol.* 2002;12(4):824-829.
5. de Abreu MR, Chung CB, Trudell D, Resnick D. Anterior transverse ligament of the knee: MR imaging and anatomic study using clinical and cadaveric material with emphasis on its contribution to meniscal tears. *Clin Imaging.* 2007;31(3):194-201.
6. Bloecker K, Wirth W, Hudelmaier M, Burgkart R, Frobell R, Eckstein F. Morphometric differences between the medial and lateral meniscus in healthy men – a three-dimensional analysis using magnetic resonance imaging. *Cells Tissues Organs.* 2012;195(4):353-364.
7. Miller M, Thompson S, et al. *DeLee & Drez's Orthopaedic Sports Medicine*; 1991:1047-1072.
8. Thompson WO, Thaete FL, Fu FH, Dye SF. Tibial meniscal dynamics using three-dimensional reconstruction of magnetic resonance images. *Am J Sports Med*, 1991;19(3):210-215; discussion 215-6.
9. Kapandji I. *The Physiology of the Joints.* Edinburgh: Livingstone; 1987.
10. Fukubayashi T, Kurosawa H. The contact area and pressure distribution pattern of the knee. A study of normal and osteoarthrotic knee joints. *Acta Orthop Scand.* 1980;51(6):871-879.
11. Alford JW, Lewis P, Kang RW, Cole BJ. Rapid progression of chondral disease in the lateral compartment of the knee following meniscectomy. *Arthroscopy.* 2005;21(12):1505-1509.
12. Kohn D, Moreno B. Meniscus insertion anatomy as a basis for meniscus replacement: a morphological cadaveric study. *Arthroscopy.* 1995;11(1):96-103.
13. Wan AC, Felle P. The menisco-femoral ligaments. *Clin Anat.* 1995;8(5):323-326.
14. Gupte CM, Smith A, McDermott ID, Bull AMJ, Thomas RD, Amis AA. Meniscofemoral ligaments revisited. Anatomical study, age correlation and clinical implications. *J Bone Joint Surg Br.* 2002;84(6):846-851.
15. Shahriaree H. Menisci. In: Shahriaree H, ed. *O'Connor's Textbook of Arthroscopic Surgery.* 2nd ed. Philadelphia: J.B. Lippincott; 1992.
16. Simonian PT, Sussmann PS, Wickiewicz TL, et al. Popliteomeniscal fasciculi and the unstable lateral meniscus: clinical correlation and magnetic resonance diagnosis. *Arthroscopy.* 1997;13(5):590-596.
17. Johnson DL, Swenson TM, Livesay GA, Aizawa H, Fu FH, Harner CD. Insertion-site anatomy of the human menisci: gross, arthroscopic, and topographical anatomy as a basis for meniscal transplantation. *Arthroscopy.* 1995;11(4):386-394.
18. Cook JL, Kuroki K, Stoker AM, Monibi FA, Roller BL. Meniscal biology in health and disease. *Connect Tissue Res.* 2017;58(3-4):225-237.
19. Ghadially FN, Lalonde JM, Wedge JH. Ultrastructure of normal and torn menisci of the human knee joint. *J Anat.* 1983;136(pt 4):773-791.
20. Ghadially FN, Thomas I, Yong N, Lalonde JM. Ultrastructure of rabbit semilunar cartilages. *J Anat.* 1978;125(pt 3):499-517.
21. Herwig J, Egner E, Buddecke E. Chemical changes of human knee joint menisci in various stages of degeneration. *Ann Rheum Dis.* 1984;43(4):635-640.
22. Habuchi H, Yamagata T, Iwata H, Suzuki S. The occurrence of a wide variety of dermatan sulfate-chondroitin sulfate copolymers in fibrous cartilage. *J Biol Chem.* 1973;248(17):6019-6028.
23. Melrose J, Fuller ES, Little CB. The biology of meniscal pathology in osteoarthritis and its contribution to joint disease: beyond simple mechanics. *Connect Tissue Res.* 2017;58(3-4):282-294.
24. Lai WM, Hou JS, Mow VC. *Triphasic theory for the swelling properties of hydrated charged soft biological tissues.* In: *Biomechacnis of Diarthrodial Joints.* New York: Springer-Verlag; 1990:283-312.
25. Proctor CS, Schmidt MB, Whipple RR, Kelly MA, Mow VC. Material properties of the normal medial bovine meniscus. *J Orthop Res.* 1989;7(6):771-782.
26. Nakano T, Dodd CM, Scott PG. Glycosaminoglycans and proteoglycans from different zones of the porcine knee meniscus. *J Orthop Res.* 1997;15(2):213-220.
27. McDevitt CA, Webber RJ. The ultrastructure and biochemistry of meniscal cartilage. *Clin Orthop Relat Res.* 1990;(252):8-18.
28. Fithian DC, Kelly MA, Mow VC. Material properties and structure-function relationships in the menisci. *Clin Orthop Relat Res.* 1990;(252):19-31.
29. Cheung HS. Distribution of type I, II, III and V in the pepsin solubilized collagens in bovine menisci. *Connect Tissue Res.* 1987;16(4):343-356.
30. Andrews SH, Rattner JB, Abusara Z, et al. Tie-fibre structure and organization in the knee menisci. *J Anat.* 2014;224(5):531-537.
31. Andrews SHJ, Adesida AB, Abusara Z, Shrive NG. Current concepts on structure-function relationships in the menisci. *Connect Tissue Res.* 2017;58(3-4):271-281.
32. Skaggs DL, Warden WH, Mow VC. Radial tie fibers influence the tensile properties of the bovine medial meniscus. *J Orthop Res.* 1994;12(2):176-185.
33. Bullough PG, Munuera L, Murphy J, Weinstein AM. The strength of the menisci of the knee as it relates to their fine structure. *J Bone Joint Surg Br.* 1970;52(3):564-567.
34. Skaags DL, Mow VC. Function of the radial rie fibers in the meniscus. *Trans Orthop Res Soc.* 1994;12(2):176-185.
35. Messner K, Gao J. The menisci of the knee joint. Anatomical and functional characteristics, and a rationale for clinical treatment. *J Anat.* 1998;193(pt 2):161-178.
36. Eyre DR, Wu JJ. Collagen of fibrocartilage: a distinctive molecular phenotype in bovine meniscus. *FEBS Lett.* 1983;158(2):265-270.
37. Yoon JH, Halper J. Tendon proteoglycans: biochemistry and function. *J Musculoskelet Neuronal Interact.* 2005;5(1):22-34.
38. Melrose J, Smith S, Cake M, Read R, Whitelock J. Comparative spatial and temporal localisation of perlecan, aggrecan and type I, II and IV collagen in the ovine meniscus: an ageing study. *Histochem Cell Biol.* 2005;124(3-4):225-235.
39. Benjamin M, Ralphs JR. Biology of fibrocartilage cells. *Int Rev Cytol.* 2004;233:1-45.
40. Verdonk PC, Forsyth RG, Wang J, et al. Characterisation of human knee meniscus cell phenotype. *Osteoarthr Cartil.* 2005;13(7):548-560.

41. Arnoczky SP. Gross and vascular anatomy of the meniscus and its role in meniscal healing, regeneration and remodeling. In: Mow VC, Arnoczky SP, Jackson DW, eds. *Knee Meniscus: Basic and Clinical Foundations*. New York, NY: Raven Press; 1992:1-14.

42. Danzig L, Resnick D, Gonsalves M, Akeson WK. Blood supply to the normal and abnormal menisci of the human knee. *Clin Orthop Relat Res*. 1983;(172):271-276.

43. Arnoczky SP, Warren RF. Microvasculature of the human meniscus. *Am J Sports Med*. 1982;10(2):90-95.

44. Kimura M, Shirakura K, Hasegawa A, Kobuna Y, Niijima M. Second look arthroscopy after meniscal repair. Factors affecting the healing rate. *Clin Orthop Relat Res*. 1995;(314):185-191.

45. Gray JC. Neural and vascular anatomy of the menisci of the human knee. *J Orthop Sports Phys Ther*. 1999;29(1):23-30.

46. Meyers E, Zhu W, Mow V. Viscoelastic properties of articular cartilage and meniscus. In: Nimni M, ed. *Collagen: Chemistry, Biology and Biotechnology*. Boca Raton, FL: CRC; 1988.

47. Maak TG, Rodeo SA. Meniscal injuries. In: Miller MD, Thompson SR, eds. *Delee & Drez's Orthopaedic Sports Medicine*. 4th ed. Philadelphia, PA: Elsevier Saunders; 1996.

48. Kennedy JC, Alexander IJ, Hayes KC. Nerve supply of the human knee and its functional importance. *Am J Sports Med*. 1982;10(6):329-335.

49. Assimakopoulos AP, Katonis PG, Agapitos MV, Exarchou EI. The innervation of the human meniscus. *Clin Orthop Relat Res*. 1992;(275):232-236.

50. Zimny ML. Mechanoreceptors in articular tissues. *Am J Anat*. 1988;182(1):16-32.

51. Sutton JB. *Ligaments: Their Nature and Morphology*. 2nd ed. London: HK Lewis; 1987.

52. Ahmed AM, Burke DL. In-vitro measurement of static pressure distribution in synovial joints–Part I: tibial surface of the knee. *J Biomech Eng*. 1983;105(3):216-225.

53. Maquet PG, Van de Berg AJ, Simonet JC. Femorotibial weight-bearing areas. Experimental determination. *J Bone Joint Surg Am*. 1975;57(6):766-771.

54. Lee SJ, Aadalen KJ, Malaviya P, et al. Tibiofemoral contact mechanics after serial medial meniscectomies in the human cadaveric knee. *Am J Sports Med*. 2006;34(8):1334-1344.

55. Jones RS, Keene G, Learmonth D, et al. Direct measurement of hoop strains in the intact and torn human medial meniscus. *Clin Biomech*. 1996;11(5):295-300.

56. Kurosawa H, Fukubayashi T, Nakajima H. Load-bearing mode of the knee joint: physical behavior of the knee joint with or without menisci. *Clin Orthop Relat Res*. 1980;(149):283-290.

57. Baratz ME, Fu FH, Mengato R. Meniscal tears: the effect of meniscectomy and of repair on intraarticular contact areas and stress in the human knee. A preliminary report. *Am J Sports Med*. 1986;14(4):270-275.

58. Seedholm BB, Hargreaves DJ. Transmission of the load in the knee joint with special reference to the role of the menisci. Part II: experimental results, discussion and conclusions. *Eng Med*. 1979;8(4):220-228.

59. Gilbert S, Chen T, Hutchinson ID, et al. Dynamic contact mechanics on the tibial plateau of the human knee during activities of daily living. *J Biomech*. 2014;47(9):2006-2012.

60. Zhou T. Analysis of the biomechanical characteristics of the knee joint with a meniscus injury. *Healthc Technol Lett*. 2018;5(6):247-249.

61. Bursac P, Arnoczky S, York A. Dynamic compressive behavior of human meniscus correlates with its extra-cellular matrix composition. *Biorheology*. 2009;46(3):227-237.

62. Allen CR, Wong EK, Livesay GA, et al. Importance of the medial meniscus in the anterior cruciate ligament-deficient knee. *J Orthop Res*. 2000;18(1):109-115.

63. Bedi A, Maak T, Musahl V, et al. Effect of tibial tunnel position on stability of the knee after anterior cruciate ligament reconstruction: is the tibial tunnel position most important?. *Am J Sports Med*. 2011;39(2):366-373.

64. Shoemaker SC, Markolf KL. The role of the meniscus in the anterior-posterior stability of the loaded anterior cruciate-deficient knee. Effects of partial versus total excision. *J Bone Joint Surg Am*. 1986;68(1):71-79.

65. Levy IM, Torzilli PA, Gould JD, Warren RF. The effect of lateral meniscectomy on motion of the knee. *J Bone Joint Surg Am*. 1989;71(3):401-406.

66. Wang JH, Guo Q, Li B. Tendon biomechanics and mechanobiology–a minireview of basic concepts and recent advancements. *J Hand Ther*. 2012;25(2):133-140; quiz 141.

67. Scranton PE, Farrar EL. Mucoid degeneration of the patellar ligament in athletes. *J Bone Joint Surg Am*. 1992;74(3):435-437.

68. Amiri S, Cooke D, Kim IY, Wyss U. Mechanics of the passive knee joint. Part 1: the role of the tibial articular surfaces in guiding the passive motion. *Proc Inst Mech Eng H*. 2006;220(8):813-822.

69. Musahl V, Citak M, O'Loughlin PF, Choi D, Bedi A, Pearle AD. The effect of medial versus lateral meniscectomy on the stability of the anterior cruciate ligament-deficient knee. *Am J Sports Med*. 2010;38(8):1591-1597.

70. Praemer A, Furner S, Rice DP. *Musculoskeletal Conditions in the United States*. Park Ridge, IL: American Academy of Orthopaedic Surgeons; 1999.

71. Renstrom P, Johnson RJ. Anatomy and biomechanics of the menisci. *Clin Sports Med*. 1990;9(3):523-538.

72. Baker BE, Peckham AC, Pupparo F, Sanborn JC. Review of meniscal injury and associated sports. *Am J Sports Med*. 1985;13(1):1-4.

73. Hede A, Jensen DB, Blyme P, Sonne-Holm S. Epidemiology of meniscal lesions in the knee. 1,215 open operations in Copenhagen 1982-84. *Acta Orthop Scand*. 1990;61(5):435-437.

74. Metcalf MH, Barrett GR. Prospective evaluation of 1485 meniscal tear patterns in patients with stable knees. *Am J Sports Med*. 2004;32(3):675-680.

75. Fowler PJ, Lubliner JA. The predictive value of five clinical signs in the evaluation of meniscal pathology. *Arthroscopy*. 1989;5(3):184-186.

76. Karachalios T, Hantes M, Zibis AH, et al. Diagnostic accuracy of a new clinical test (the Thessaly test) for early detection of meniscal tears. *J Bone Joint Surg Am*. 2005;87(5):955-962.

77. Kocher MS, DiCanzio J, Zurakowski D, Micheli LJ. Diagnostic performance of clinical examination and selective magnetic resonance imaging in the evaluation of intraarticular knee disorders in children and adolescents. *Am J Sports Med*. 2001;29(3):292-296.

78. Mackenzie R, Dixon AK, Keene GS, Hollingworth W, Lomas DJ, Villar RN. Magnetic resonance imaging of the knee: assessment of effectiveness. *Clin Radiol*. 1996;51(4):245-250.

79. De Smet AA, Norris MA, Yandow DR, Quintana FA, Graf BK, Keene JS. MR diagnosis of meniscal tears of the knee: importance of high signal in the meniscus that extends to the surface. *AJR Am J Roentgenol*. 1993;161(1):101-107.

80. LaPrade RF, Burnett QM, Veenstra MA, Hodgman CG. The prevalence of abnormal magnetic resonance imaging findings in asymptomatic knees. With correlation of magnetic resonance imaging to arthroscopic findings in symptomatic knees. *Am J Sports Med*. 1994;22(6):739-745.

81. Bhattacharyya T, Gale D, Dewire P, et al. The clinical importance of meniscal tears demonstrated by magnetic resonance imaging in osteoarthritis of the knee. *J Bone Joint Surg Am*. 2003;85(1):4-9.

82. Spindler KP, Schils JP, Bergfeld JA, et al. Prospective study of osseous, articular, and meniscal lesions in recent anterior cruciate ligament tears by magnetic resonance imaging and arthroscopy. *Am J Sports Med*. 1993;21(4):551-557.

83. Howell R, Kumar NS, Patel N, Tom J. Degenerative meniscus: pathogenesis, diagnosis, and treatment options. *World J Orthop*. 2014;5(5):597-602.

84. Englund M, Guermazi A, Lohmander SL. The role of the meniscus in knee osteoarthritis: a cause or consequence?. *Radiol Clin North Am*. 2009;47(4):703-712.

85. Englund M, Roemer FW, Hayashi D, Crema MD, Guermazi A. Meniscus pathology, osteoarthritis and the treatment controversy. *Nat Rev Rheumatol.* 2012;8(7):412-419.

86. Englund M, Guermazi A, Lohmander LS. The meniscus in knee osteoarthritis. *Rheum Dis Clin North Am.* 2009;35(3):579-590.

87. Englund M. The role of the meniscus in osteoarthritis genesis. *Rheum Dis Clin North Am.* 2008;34(3):573-579.

88. Lopez-Franco M, López-Franco O, Murciano-Antón MA, et al. Meniscal degeneration in human knee osteoarthritis: in situ hybridization and immunohistochemistry study. *Arch Orthop Trauma Surg.* 2016;136(2):175-183.

89. Lopez-Franco M, Gomez-Barrena E. Cellular and molecular meniscal changes in the degenerative knee: a review. *J Exp Orthop.* 2018;5(1):11.

90. McAlinden A, Dudhia J, Bolton MC, Lorenzo P, Heinegård D, Bayliss MT. Age-related changes in the synthesis and mRNA expression of decorin and aggrecan in human meniscus and articular cartilage. *Osteoarthr Cartil.* 2001;9(1):33-41.

91. Lohmander LS, Brandt KD, Mazzuca SA, et al. Use of the plasma stromelysin (matrix metalloproteinase 3) concentration to predict joint space narrowing in knee osteoarthritis. *Arthritis Rheum.* 2005;52(10):3160-3167.

92. Tchetverikov I, Ronday HK, Van El B, et al. MMP profile in paired serum and synovial fluid samples of patients with rheumatoid arthritis. *Ann Rheum Dis.* 2004;63(7):881-883.

93. Tchetverikov I, Lohmander LS, Verzijl N, et al. MMP protein and activity levels in synovial fluid from patients with joint injury, inflammatory arthritis, and osteoarthritis. *Ann Rheum Dis.* 2005;64(5):694-698.

94. Pavlov H, Ghelman B, Vigorita VJ. *Atlas of the Knee Menisci.* New York, NY: Appleton-Century-Crofts; 1983.

95. Fitzgibbons RE, Shelbourne KD. "Aggressive" nontreatment of lateral meniscal tears seen during anterior cruciate ligament reconstruction. *Am J Sports Med.* 1995;23(2):156-159.

96. Ciccotti MG, Shields CL, El Attrache NS. Meniscectomy. In: Fu FH, Harner CD, Vince KG, eds. *Knee Surgery.* Baltimore: Williams & Wilkins; 1994.

97. Bedi A, Kelly NH, Baad M, et al. Dynamic contact mechanics of the medial meniscus as a function of radial tear, repair, and partial meniscectomy. *J Bone Joint Surg Am.* 2010;92(6):1398-1408.

98. Harper KW, Helms CA, Lambert HS, Higgins LD. Radial meniscal tears: significance, incidence, and MR appearance. *AJR Am J Roentgenol.* 2005;185(6):1429-1434.

99. Lu KH. Arthroscopic meniscal repair and needle aspiration for meniscal tear with meniscal cyst. *Arthroscopy.* 2006;22(12):1367.e1-4.

100. Arnoczky SP, McDevitt CA. The meniscus: structure, function, repair, and replacement. In: Buckwalter JA, Einhorn TA, Simon SR, eds. *Orthopedic Basic Science: Biology and Biomechanics of the Musculoskeletal System.* Rosemont, IL: American Academy of Orthopedic Surgeons; 2000.

101. Spindler KP, Mayes CE, Miller RR, Imro AK, Davidson JM. Regional mitogenic response of the meniscus to platelet-derived growth factor (PDGF-AB). *J Orthop Res.* 1995;13(2):201-207.

102. Tanaka T, Fujii K, Kumagae Y. Comparison of biochemical characteristics of cultured fibrochondrocytes isolated from the inner and outer regions of human meniscus. *Knee Surg Sports Traumatol Arthrosc.* 1999;7(2):75-80.

103. Periera H, Silva-Correia J, Oliveira J, Reis L. The meniscus: basic science. In: Verdonk R, Espregueira-Mendes J, Monllau JC, eds. *Meniscal Transplantation.* Vol 119. Springer. ISAKOS Booklets; 2013:7-14.

104. Wu F, Nerlich M, Docheva D. Tendon injuries: basic science and new repair proposals. *EFORT Open Rev.* 2017;2(7):332-342.

105. Hulmes DJ. Building collagen molecules, fibrils, and suprafibrillar structures. *J Struct Biol.* 2002;137(1-2):2-10.

106. James R, Kesturu G, Balian G, Chhabra AB. Tendon: biology, biomechanics, repair, growth factors, and evolving treatment options. *J Hand Surg Am.* 2008;33(1):102-112.

107. Wang JH. Mechanobiology of tendon. *J Biomech.* 2006;39(9):1563-1582.

108. Fukuta S, Oyama M, Kavalkovich K, Fu FH, Niyibizi C. Identification of types II, IX and X collagens at the insertion site of the bovine achilles tendon. *Matrix Biol.* 1998;17(1):65-73.

109. Fukushige T, Kanekura T, Ohuchi E, Shinya T, Kanzaki T. Immunohistochemical studies comparing the localization of type XV collagen in normal human skin and skin tumors with that of type IV collagen. *J Dermatol.* 2005;32(2):74-83.

110. Birk DE, Mayne R. Localization of collagen types I, III and V during tendon development. Changes in collagen types I and III are correlated with changes in fibril diameter. *Eur J Cell Biol.* 1997;72(4):352-361.

111. Niyibizi C, Visconti CS, Kavalkovich K, Woo SL. Collagens in an adult bovine medial collateral ligament: immunofluorescence localization by confocal microscopy reveals that type XIV collagen predominates at the ligament-bone junction. *Matrix Biol.* 1995;14(9):743-751.

112. Zhang G, Ezura Y, Chervoneva I, et al. Decorin regulates assembly of collagen fibrils and acquisition of biomechanical properties during tendon development. *J Cell Biochem.* 2006;98(6):1436-1449.

113. Benjamin M, Kaiser E, Milz S. Structure-function relationships in tendons: a review. *J Anat.* 2008;212(3):211-228.

114. Tomasek JJ, Gabbiani G, Hinz B, Chaponnier C, Brown RA. Myofibroblasts and mechano-regulation of connective tissue remodelling. *Nat Rev Mol Cell Biol.* 2002;3(5):349-363.

115. Leong DJ, Sun HB. Mesenchymal stem cells in tendon repair and regeneration: basic understanding and translational challenges. *Ann N Y Acad Sci.* 2016;1383(1):88-96.

116. Jósza L, Lehto MUK, Järvinen M, Kvist M, Réffy A, Kannus P. A comparative study of methods for demonstration and quantification of capillaries in skeletal muscle. *Acta Histochem.* 1993;94(1):89-96.

117. Zantop T, Tillmann B, Petersen W. Quantitative assessment of blood vessels of the human Achilles tendon: an immunohistochemical cadaver study. *Arch Orthop Trauma Surg.* 2003;123(9):501-504.

118. Benjamin M, Toumi H, Ralphs JR, Bydder G, Best TM, Milz S. Where tendons and ligaments meet bone: attachment sites ('entheses') in relation to exercise and/or mechanical load. *J Anat.* 2006;208(4):471-490.

119. Benjamin M, McGonagle D. Entheses: tendon and ligament attachment sites. *Scand J Med Sci Sports.* 2009;19(4):520-527.

120. Maganaris CN. Tensile properties of in vivo human tendinous tissue. *J Biomech.* 2002;35(8):1019-1027.

121. Maganaris CN, Paul JP. In vivo human tendon mechanical properties. *J Physiol.* 1999;521(pt 1):307-313.

122. Purslow PP, Wess TJ, Hukins DW. Collagen orientation and molecular spacing during creep and stress-relaxation in soft connective tissues. *J Exp Biol.* 1998;201(pt 1):135-142.

123. Elliott DM, Robinson PS, Gimbel JA, et al. Effect of altered matrix proteins on quasilinear viscoelastic properties in transgenic mouse tail tendons. *Ann Biomed Eng.* 2003;31(5):599-605.

124. Kjaer M. Role of extracellular matrix in adaptation of tendon and skeletal muscle to mechanical loading. *Physiol Rev.* 2004;84(2):649-698.

125. Kjaer M, Langberg H, Miller BF, et al. Metabolic activity and collagen turnover in human tendon in response to physical activity. *J Musculoskelet Neuronal Interact.* 2005;5(1):41-52.

126. Kjaer M, Magnusson P, Krogsgaard M, et al. Extracellular matrix adaptation of tendon and skeletal muscle to exercise. *J Anat.* 2006;208(4):445-450.

127. Kjaer M, Langberg H, Heinemeier K, et al. From mechanical loading to collagen synthesis, structural changes and function in human tendon. *Scand J Med Sci Sports.* 2009;19(4):500-510.

128. Maganaris CN, Narici MV, Almekinders LC, Maffulli N. Biomechanics and pathophysiology of overuse tendon injuries: ideas on insertional tendinopathy. *Sports Med.* 2004;34(14):1005-1017.

129. Sharma P, Maffulli N. Biology of tendon injury: healing, modeling and remodeling. *J Musculoskelet Neuronal Interact.* 2006;6(2):181-190.

130. Sharma P, Maffulli N. Tendon injury and tendinopathy: healing and repair. *J Bone Joint Surg Am.* 2005;87(1):187-202.

131. Thomopoulos S, Parks WC, Rifkin DB, Derwin KA. Mechanisms of tendon injury and repair. *J Orthop Res.* 2015;33(6):832-839.

132. Gelberman RH, Steinberg D, Amiel D, Akeson W. Fibroblast chemotaxis after tendon repair. *J Hand Surg Am.* 1991;16(4):686-693.

133. Hope M, Saxby TS. Tendon healing. *Foot Ankle Clin.* 2007;12(4):553-567, v.

134. Voleti PB, Buckley MR, Soslowsky LJ. Tendon healing: repair and regeneration. *Annu Rev Biomed Eng.* 2012;14:47-71.

135. Chang J, Most D, Stelnicki E, et al. Gene expression of transforming growth factor beta-1 in rabbit zone II flexor tendon wound healing: evidence for dual mechanisms of repair. *Plast Reconstr Surg.* 1997;100(4):937-944.

136. Abrahamsson SO. Matrix metabolism and healing in the flexor tendon. Experimental studies on rabbit tendon. *Scand J Plast Reconstr Surg Hand Surg Suppl.* 1991;23:1-51.

137. Fessel G, Wernli J, Li Y, Gerber C, Snedeker JG. Exogenous collagen cross-linking recovers tendon functional integrity in an experimental model of partial tear. *J Orthop Res.* 2012;30(6):973-981.

138. Nakamura N, Shino K, Natsuume T, et al. Early biological effect of in vivo gene transfer of platelet-derived growth factor (PDGF)-B into healing patellar ligament. *Gene Ther.* 1998;5(9):1165-1170.

139. Chang J, Most D, Thunder R, et al. Molecular studies in flexor tendon wound healing: the role of basic fibroblast growth factor gene expression. *J Hand Surg Am.* 1998;23(6):1052-1058.

140. Zhang F, Liu H, Stile F, et al. Effect of vascular endothelial growth factor on rat Achilles tendon healing. *Plast Reconstr Surg.* 2003;112(6):1613-1619.

141. Buckwalter JA, Maynard JA, Vailas AC. Skeletal fibrous tissues: tendon, joint capsule, and ligament. In: Albright JA, Brand RA, eds. *The Scientific Basis of Orthopaedics.* Norwalk, CT: Appleton & Lange; 1987.

142. Woo SLY, Maynard J, Butler D. Ligament, Tendon, and joint capsule insertions into bone. In: Woo SLY, Buckwalter JA, eds. *Injury and Repair of Musculoskeletal Soft Tissues.* Park Ridge, IL: American Academy of Orthopedic Surgeons; 1988.

143. Benjamin M, Ralphs JR. Tendons and ligaments–an overview. *Histol Histopathol.* 1997;12(4):1135-1144.

144. Amiel D, Frank C, Harwood F, Fronek J, Akeson W. Tendons and ligaments: a morphological and biochemical comparison. *J Orthop Res.* 1984;1(3):257-265.

145. Woo SL, Debski RE, Zeminski J, et al. Injury and repair of ligaments and tendons. *Annu Rev Biomed Eng.* 2000;2:83-118.

146. el Hawary R, Stanish WD, Curwin SL. Rehabilitation of tendon injuries in sport. *Sports Med.* 1997;24(5):347-358.

147. Butler DL, Grood ES, Noyes FR, Zernicke RE. Biomechanics of ligaments and tendons. *Exerc Sport Sci Rev.* 1978;6:125-181.

148. Nakamura N, Rodeo S, et al. Physiology and pathophysiology of musculoskeletal tissues. In: Miller MD, Thompson SR, eds. *DeLee & Drez's Orthopaedic Sports Medicine.* 4th ed. Philadelphia, PA: Elsevier Saunders; 2014:3-19.

149. Frank C, Shrive N, Hiraoka H, et al. Optimisation of the biology of soft tissue repair. *J Sci Med Sport.* 1999;2(3):190-210.

150. Schaefer L, Iozzo RV. Biological functions of the small leucine-rich proteoglycans: from genetics to signal transduction. *J Biol Chem.* 2008;283(31):21305-21309.

151. Barrack RL, Skinner HB. The sensory function of knee ligaments. In: Daniel DM, Akeson WH, O'Connor JJ, eds. *Knee Ligaments: Structure, Function, Injury, and Repair.* New York: Raven Press; 1990.

152. Cooper RR, Misol S. Tendon and ligament insertion. A light and electron microscopic study. *J Bone Joint Surg Am.* 1970;52(1):1-20.

153. Rodeo SA, Arnoczky SP, Torzilli PA, Hidaka C, Warren RF. Tendon-healing in a bone tunnel. A biomechanical and histological study in the dog. *J Bone Joint Surg Am.* 1993;75(12):1795-1803.

154. Amiel D, Kuiper SD, Wallace CD, Harwood FL, Vandeberg JS. Age-related properties of medial collateral ligament and anterior cruciate ligament: a morphologic and collagen maturation study in the rabbit. *J Gerontol.* 1991;46(4):B159-B165.

155. Shadwick RE. Elastic energy storage in tendons: mechanical differences related to function and age. *J Appl Physiol.* 1990;68(3):1033-1040.

156. Walsh S, Frank C, Shrive N, Hart D. Knee immobilization inhibits biomechanical maturation of the rabbit medial collateral ligament. *Clin Orthop Relat Res.* 1993;(297):253-261.

157. Buckwalter JA, Cruess R. Healing of musculoskeletal tissues. In: Rockwood CA, Green DP, eds. *Fractures.* Philadelphia, PA: J.B. Lippincott; 1991.

158. Leadbetter WB. Cell-matrix response in tendon injury. *Clin Sports Med.* 1992;11(3):533-578.

159. Letson AK, Dahners LE. The effect of combinations of growth factors on ligament healing. *Clin Orthop Relat Res.* 1994;(308):207-212.

160. Hildebrand KA, Frank CB. Scar formation and ligament healing. *Can J Surg.* 1998;41(6):425-429.

161. Woo SL, Vogrin TM, Abramowitch SD. Healing and repair of ligament injuries in the knee. *J Am Acad Orthop Surg.* 2000;8(6):364-372.

162. Amiel D, Kleiner JB, Roux RD, Harwood FL, Akeson WH. The phenomenon of "ligamentization": anterior cruciate ligament reconstruction with autogenous patellar tendon. *J Orthop Res.* 1986;4(2):162-172.

163. Amiel D, Ishizue KK, Harwood FL, Kitabayashi L, Akeson WH. Injury of the anterior cruciate ligament: the role of collagenase in ligament degeneration. *J Orthop Res.* 1989;7(4):486-493.

164. Murray MM, Spindler KP, Ballard P, et al. Enhanced histologic repair in a central wound in the anterior cruciate ligament with a collagen-platelet-rich plasma scaffold. *J Orthop Res.* 2007;25(8):1007-1017.

165. Murray MM, Martin SD, Martin TL, Spector M. Histological changes in the human anterior cruciate ligament after rupture. *J Bone Joint Surg Am.* 2000;82(10):1387-1397.

166. Rodeo SA, Suzuki K, Deng XH, Wozney J, Warren RF. Use of recombinant human bone morphogenetic protein-2 to enhance tendon healing in a bone tunnel. *Am J Sports Med.* 1999;27(4):476-488.

chapter 5

Knee Arthritis: Pathology and Progression

John L. Hamilton, MD, PhD I Brett R. Levine, MD, MS

INTRODUCTION

Arthritis is a general term used to describe inflammation or degeneration of a particular joint. In general, osteoarthritis (OA) is a specific form of arthritis with an underlying pathological pathway and progressive pattern that is associated with a multifactorial degenerative process. Alternatively, other forms of arthritis, such as rheumatoid arthritis (RA) and associated conditions, are primarily mediated by an inflammatory condition that leads to degeneration of the afflicted joint; as a whole these conditions are grouped together using a catch-all phrase, termed inflammatory arthropathies. In the United States alone, over 50 million adults have some form of diagnosed arthritis, which is projected to increase 49% by 2040.[1] In the United States, arthritis is a leading cause of work disability.[2]

The knee is commonly involved in various types of arthritic conditions. The knee joint is a modified hinge joint that predominately allows flexion and extension but also permits slight internal and external rotation; it is composed of three compartments, which include the medial tibiofemoral, lateral tibiofemoral, and patellofemoral joint. In the context of arthritis within the knee joint, pathology at multiple tissues should be considered, including but not limited to the cartilage, bone, and synovium. Pathological changes at multiple tissue types contribute to the knee joint pain, dysfunction, and subsequent impaired mobility experienced by individuals with arthritis. There are over 100 forms of arthritis and related diseases; this chapter will discuss the pathologic pathways of progression and clinical presentation of the types of arthritis most commonly found within the knee.

OSTEOARTHRITIS

Epidemiology

Osteoarthritis (OA) is the most common form of arthritis, and the knee is the most commonly affected joint. In the United States, it is estimated that there is nearly a 50% chance of developing symptomatic knee OA in any given individual's lifetime.[3] There are a number of modifiable and nonmodifiable risk factors that contribute to the increased risk associated with the development and progression of OA. OA is predominately found in adults of older age, and the incidence of knee involvement increases with each decade as we age.[4] Studies have investigated the role of aging in OA development and have found that aging can affect cellular processes at articular chondrocytes including elevated oxidative stress, reduced repair response, and increased catabolic matrix metalloproteinase activity.[5,6] Furthermore, aging can affect all tissues at the joint including muscle and ligaments, which can further influence mechanical loading.

Younger adults who develop OA often have a history of a prior knee injury, and this type of OA is subclassified as posttraumatic OA (PTOA). Injuries can include acute damage to the cartilage, bone, ligament, and/or meniscus. In general, these injuries can result in the initiation of an inflammatory cascade, which can help facilitate OA development.[7] Furthermore, trauma can cause acute and irreparable cartilage damage, and chondrocyte cell death can occur at the articular surface. Acute traumatic events can also lead to sustained upregulation of catabolic and inflammatory cytokine signaling.[7] Damage that occurs at the knee as a result from the trauma can result in mechanical instability. Altered mechanical influences can lead to altered transduction of biochemical signaling molecules. These mechanically transduced signals can lead to increased expression of catabolic cytokines and mediators and stimulate cartilage degeneration, synovial inflammation, and bone remodeling, with subsequent joint degeneration over time.[8]

Individuals with obesity, defined as a BMI>30 kg/m^2, have an increased incidence of OA and develop OA earlier.[9,10] Coggon et al. found that obesity can lead to a 6.8 times greater risk of developing knee OA.[11] Obesity can increase mechanical loading at the joint and will accentuate these abnormal forces in the setting of mechanical axis deviations. However, mechanical influences are not the only mechanism for increased OA risk. There is an increased risk of OA in non–weight bearing joints, such as the hands, with obesity.[12] Another potential mechanism through which obesity can contribute to OA pathogenesis is by facilitating low-grade chronic inflammation through secretion of adipose-derived cytokines, called adipokines.[10]

Hereditary influences can play a role in OA development. Rare genetic mutations encoding structural collagens found in articular cartilage can result in premature

OA; these rare mutations can cause OA in early adolescence and affect multiple joints.[13,14] Twin studies have demonstrated that, even with adjustment for age, sex, and BMI, there is an association of genetic heritability in terms of knee structure, cartilage volume, and radiographic progression of OA.[15] Genome-wide association studies have compared control and OA populations and have identified over 80 gene mutations or single nucleotide polymorphisms associated with OA; many of the genes encode important components of the cartilage matrix or are important signaling molecules for articular cartilage and joint maintenance.[5]

Gender seems to play a role in knee OA, with a greater prevalence found in women as compared to men.[16] Women often present with more advanced stages of OA and have higher reported pain and disability.[17,18] Isolated patellofemoral OA is also more prevalent in women as compared to men.[18] Potential reasons for the gender difference in women include anatomic and kinematic differences and increased incidence of ACL injuries. Postmenopausal women have a particular increased risk of OA, which has been suggested to be related to decreased estrogen. Estrogen receptors have been identified at the articular cartilage.[19,20] However, assessment of what role and significance estrogen plays in OA pathology and progression is ongoing. **Table 5-1** summarizes major influences on the development of OA.

The classification of OA can be primary or secondary. Primary OA implies an unknown or idiopathic attributable cause to OA development. Secondary OA signifies development of OA due to known injury or disease. Posttraumatic OA and obesity can be considered as secondary causes of OA. Congenital and developmental diseases, calcium deposition diseases, other bone and joint disorders, endocrine disorders, and other miscellaneous diseases such as neuropathic arthropathy can lead to the development of secondary OA.[21] **Table 5-2** summarizes secondary causes of OA. While there is an extensive list of secondary causes of OA, these pathologies can precipitate OA by previously characterized mechanism of OA development, such as altered biomechanical influences, inflammation and catabolic cytokines signaling, and altered remodeling and changes in the bone architecture.

TABLE 5-1 Major Influences on Knee Osteoarthritis Development

INFLUENCES
• Aging
• Previous trauma/injury
• Obesity
• Hereditary/genetic
• Gender (women)

TABLE 5-2 Causes of Secondary Knee Osteoarthritis (OA)

SECONDARY KNEE OA	
Posttraumatic OA	Bone and joint disorders
Obesity	Avascular necrosis
Congenital developmental diseases	Rheumatoid arthritis
Unequal lower extremity length	Gouty arthritis
Extreme valgus/varus deformity	Septic arthritis
Bone dysplasia	Paget disease
Genetic and metabolic diseases	Endocrine diseases
Hemochromatosis	Diabetes mellitus
Ochronosis	Acromegaly
Gaucher disease	Hypothyroidism
Hemoglobinopathy	Hyperparathyroidism
Ehlers–Danlos disease	Neuropathic arthropathy (Charcot joint)
Calcium deposition disorders	
Calcium pyrophosphate deposition disease	Frostbite
	Kashin–Beck disease
Apatite arthropathy	Caisson disease

Reproduced with permission from Altman R, et al. Development of criteria for the classification and reporting of osteoarthritis. Classification of osteoarthritis of the knee. Diagnostic and Therapeutic Criteria Committee of the American Rheumatism Association. *Arthritis Rheum*. 1986.

Symptoms

A primary complaint of individuals seeking knee OA treatment is pain. The pain is often described as exacerbated with activity and relieved with rest and characterized as a deep, dull ache. In certain cases the pain can be isolated to a single compartment of the knee but is more often diffuse in nature. With advanced disease, pain can occur at rest, resulting in difficulty falling and staying asleep. With chronic OA, pain-related psychological stress can occur.[22] Symptoms of joint stiffness can occur in individuals with OA, and this is often described as short-lived stiffness that occurs after inactivity. Furthermore, degeneration of the joint can lead to a range of mechanical symptoms such as joint instability, buckling, or giving away. At the knee joint, reduced movement, deformity, contractures, effusion, and crepitus can occur.[22]

There are number of different methods to quantify the severity of symptoms in knee OA, which are often used to assess responsiveness to surgical or nonsurgical interventions. The most commonly used patient-reported questionnaire for OA of the knee is the Western Ontario and McMaster Universities Osteoarthritis (WOMAC) index. In the WOMAC index, symptoms of OA are classified into three sections: pain, stiffness, and physical function.

The severity of pain is rated during various positions, times, and movements; these five-items include walking, stair climbing, sleeping at night, rest, and standing. Items of morning stiffness as well as stiffness occurring later in the day after sitting, lying, or resting are evaluated. There are 17 items related to impairments in physical function; these impairments include descending and ascending stairs; rising from sitting, standing, walking on a flat surface; getting in and out of car; going shopping; putting on and taking off socks; rising from bed; lying in bed; getting in and out of bath; sitting; getting on and off toilet; and heavy and light domestic duties. Each individual item is scored, and the severity of OA symptoms can be characterized using these 24 items and 3 sections. Higher scores overall or within individual sections can be used to quantify severity of OA symptoms.[23]

Physical Exam and Diagnosis

Physical exam of individuals with suspected knee OA should include the following: body height/weight and body mass index (BMI), joint range of motion, location of joint tenderness, skin integrity, adjacent joint assessment, muscle strength, ligament stability, gait pattern, and alignment of the lower limbs in standing and walking.[22] Increased body weight and BMI are independent risk factors for OA. Restricted joint range of motion, crepitus with movement of the joint, or pain with active or passive movement of the joint can be seen in OA. Physical exam findings can show tenderness that is more classically located over the joint line. Along the joint line, bone deformity and osteophytes may be palpated. Visual deformity of the knees may be found—most often varus deformity. Patients may have instability at the knee joint and altered gait. Furthermore, muscle atrophy, weakness, contracture/lag, or joint effusions can be found.[22]

Radiographs can be insensitive to the earliest pathologic features of OA, and absence of radiographic findings should not be used for definitive exclusion of the presence of OA.[22] Furthermore, radiographic evidence of OA does not confirm pain at the knee is generated from the arthritic process rather than other pathology, such as for instance pes anserine bursitis.[22,24] In general, the diagnosis of OA is made on history and physical exam, and radiography is used to confirm clinical suspicion and rule out alternative diagnoses. Plain radiographs are commonly used to aid in the diagnosis of OA and can show features including joint space narrowing, osteophytes, subchondral sclerosis, and cysts.

Laboratory findings are not used to aid in the diagnosis of OA, as they are generally expected to be relatively normal. Synovial fluid analysis at the knee in individuals with OA will predominantly demonstrate that the fluid is classified as "noninflammatory," which is designated to synovial fluid containing less than 2000 leukocytes per milliliter (ml). Normal synovial fluid is classified as a leukocyte count of less than 200 leukocytes per mL. Most individuals with OA at a joint will have synovial fluid with less than 500 leukocytes per mL.[25]

Imaging

A common classification system used to describe the radiographic evidence and severity of OA is the Kellgren and Lawrence (KL) scale. Using this scale, radiography of the knee joint can be classified into five grades: 0 (none), 1 (doubtful OA), 2 (minimal OA), 3 (moderate OA), 4 (severe OA). A grade of 0 represents a normal knee joint; grade 1 demonstrates doubtful joint space narrowing and possible marginal osteophyte formation; grade 2 represents possible narrowing of the joint space with definite marginal osteophyte formation; grade 3 represents definite joint space narrowing, moderate marginal osteophyte formation, some sclerosis, and possible deformity of bony ends; grade 4 demonstrates large marginal osteophyte formation, severe joint space narrowing, marked subchondral bone sclerosis, and definite deformity of bone ends.[26-28] **Fig. 5-1** demonstrates knee radiographic images corresponding to the KL classification scale.

When radiographically assessing the knee, there are three compartments to consider: medial tibiofemoral joint, lateral tibiofemoral joint, and patellofemoral joint. Often two or more of the compartments are affected. In some instances, patellofemoral or medial/lateral tibiofemoral joint OA can occur in isolation. With joint space narrowing, the narrowing is usually asymmetric, typically having greater effect on the medial tibiofemoral joint and/or patellofemoral joint. One criticism of classifications systems, such as the KL system, is often a lack of description and assessment of patellofemoral joint OA.[26] However, the KL system, for instance, can be used to assess patellofemoral joint OA alone.[29]

Conventional radiography (standard knee series includes an AP, lateral, Skiers, Merchant, and mechanical axis views of the affected limb) is the gold standard imaging approach used to assess and aid in the diagnosis of OA. However, MRI, while not necessary in the diagnosis of OA, can detect additional secondary changes in OA not seen on radiography. MRI can detect joint fluid changes, ligamentous and meniscal damage, cartilage morphology, bone marrow edema, effusion, and synovitis/synovial thickening.[30] Therefore, MRI can serve to provide greater understanding of OA within the knee, affording greater details on the mechanism and pathology of OA. The enhanced detail seen with an MRI may serve as an important investigative tool in regard to OA pathology and progression. MRI of the knee can also be used to rule out isolated causes of knee pain outside of OA including but not limited to ligamentous and meniscal damage, bursitis, iliotibial band syndrome, chondral and osteochondral defects, or avascular necrosis not seen on plain radiography.[22]

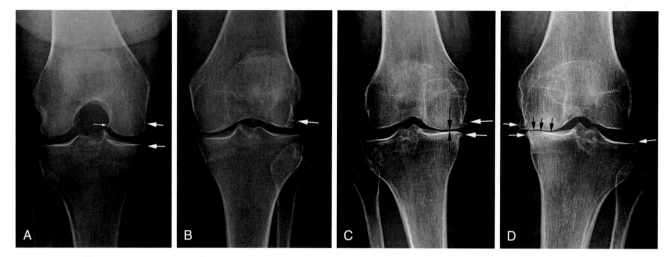

FIGURE 5-1   Radiographic images of the knee representative of the Kellgren and Lawrence (KL) scale for classification of OA severity. KL = 0, normal-appearing knee joint (not shown in the image); **A:** KL = 1 (doubtful OA), doubtful joint space narrowing and possible marginal osteophyte formation; **B:** KL = 2 (minimal OA), possible narrowing of the joint space with definite marginal osteophyte formation; **C:** KL = 3 (moderate OA), definite joint space narrowing, moderate marginal osteophyte formation, some sclerosis, and possible deformity of bony ends; **D:** KL = 4 (severe OA), severe joint space narrowing, large marginal osteophyte formation, marked subchondral bone sclerosis, and definite deformity of bony ends. White arrows show osteophyte formation. Black arrows show joint space narrowing. (Reproduced with permission from Hayashi D, et al. Imaging for osteoarthritis. 2016.)

Pathophysiology and Progression

Greater emphasis is now placed in classifying OA as a "whole joint" disease; therefore, consideration of the cartilage, bone, synovium, ligaments, and surrounding soft tissues are packaged as part of the pathophysiology. In the early pathogenesis of OA, it has been debated whether changes in the cartilage occur before bone or changes in the bone occur before cartilage. Extensive evidence in both human and animal studies suggests that remodeling of the subchondral bone is evident at the preradiography stage of OA and can potentially influence worsening of cartilage loss.[31] Early adaptations of the subchondral bone such as increased thickness and stiffness can result in increased load transfer to the overlying cartilage.[32] The capacity of chondrocytes to respond to altered mechanical loads and their capacity for a repair response is rather limited in comparison to the underlying subchondral bone. During the course and progression of OA, it is likely that there are parallel and distinct changes in the cartilage and subchondral bone, which are responding to similar biomechanical signals.[33]

An early change seen at the cartilage in OA is surface fibrillation. Hydrophilic proteoglycans within the collagen network of cartilage attract water and aid in the "shock absorbing" properties of cartilage. As the collagen network loosens and breaks down, there is an initial swelling of the cartilage matrix through these hydrophilic interactions. Chondrocytes are the only cell type present within cartilage; they are relatively quiescent but aid in homeostasis of the cartilage through anabolic and catabolic activities. Likely due to matrix loss during OA progression, chondrocytes respond by proliferating and forming clusters. Aiding in the cartilage degeneration at the chondrocyte level is an

upregulation of catabolic proteinases and ultimately cell death. Proteolytic enzymes degrading the cartilage can also be produced from the synovium. Some of the chondrocytes undergo a shift to a hypertrophic phenotype that have increased cytoplasm area and characteristically express type X collagen and matrix metalloproteinase (MMP)-13 and can undergo apoptosis.[34]

Endochondral ossification aids in the degeneration of the adult articular cartilage in OA. During OA development, a proportion of hyaline articular chondrocytes undergo a hypertrophic phenotype; these cells can aid in calcifying the surrounding matrix. During OA progression, there is expansion of the region of the calcified cartilage which is evidence by tidemark duplication. The tidemark is the boundary between the calcified and noncalcified cartilage. Blood vessels penetrate from the subchondral bone into the calcified cartilage and to some degree in OA the normally avascular noncalcified hyaline cartilage. These blood vessels carry osteo/chondroclasts, which resorb the surrounding calcified matrix and carry progenitor cells that lay down new bone into the calcified and hyaline cartilage, leading to cartilage thinning.[33,35-38] **Fig. 5-2** demonstrates cartilage degeneration, tidemark duplication, and vascular invasion during the course of OA development.

Bone marrow lesions (BMLs) can be found on MRI in individuals with OA, and their presence has been linked with pain and cartilage degeneration. Evidence of BMLs can occur before radiographic evidence of cartilage degeneration. The lesions have been further associated with knee malalignment and increased mechanical loading.[39] BMLs can be characterized histologically by areas of fat necrosis and local marrow fibrosis and occur in regions of microfractures of the trabecular bone.[40] Subchondral

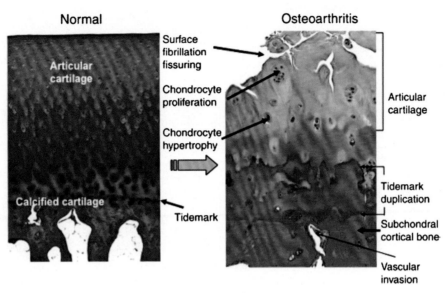

FIGURE 5-2   Histologic cross-section of a normal knee joint and joint affected by end-stage OA. During OA development, there are surface fibrillation, chondrocyte proliferation and cell death, increased chondrocyte hypertrophy, tidemark duplication, vascular invasion, and subsequent endochondral ossification. (Reproduced with permission from Goldring MB, et al. *Osteoarthritis and the Immune System.* 2nd ed. Academic Press; 2016.)

bone cysts are found in focal areas of bone damage and necrosis. While the appearance of subchondral bone cysts has often been described as a cardinal feature of OA, they are not part of the KL OA classification—potentially for good reason. In one study, utilizing assessment of 806 plain radiographs of patients with knee OA who had failed a trial of conservative management and were planned for total knee arthroplasty, evidence of joint space narrowing was found in 99.5% of the radiographs, osteophytes in 98.1%, subchondral bone sclerosis in 88.3%, and subchondral bone cysts were found in 30.6% of the radiographs.[41] Subchondral bone remodeling overall is increased in OA, and this remodeling can give rise to sclerotic or osteoporotic features of bone in the same individual. Regions of increased mechanical loading can have increased bone formation ultimately giving rise to sclerosis. However, as bone remodeling occurs in OA progression, other areas of bone may experience influences such as stress shielding, yielding an osteoporotic phenotype.[42]

Based on the KL scale, osteophyte formation increases with radiographic progression of OA, and, indeed, joint space narrowing is highly associated with the presence of osteophytes.[43] Of important note, osteophyte formation can begin during early development of OA. It has been questioned whether osteophyte formation is either a functional adaptation or a pathologic phenomenon. In knee joints with an ACL tear, osteophyte formation can limit anterior and posterior translation of the femur on the tibia. Furthermore, while marginal osteophytes can cause fixed deformity at the knee, they can also reduce varus–valgus instability in osteoarthritic knees; this reduction in instability is presumed to occur through osteophytes reducing collateral ligament pseudolaxity by directly pressing against the ligaments.[44,45] Cells that give rise to

osteophytes are mesenchymal stem cells or precursor cells derived from the periosteum and the synovium. In general these cells undergo chondrogenesis, and the cartilage scaffolding that arises undergoes endochondral ossification.[45] The triggers of osteophyte formation are not completely understood but likely result from a combination of mechanical and biochemical stimuli. Growth factors belonging to the TGFβ superfamily can induce osteophyte formation *in vivo*.[45]

Pathologic changes at the synovium such as increased synovial volume on MRI correlates with disease severity of knee OA by the Kellgren–Lawrence scale.[46] Synovial thickening and inflammatory changes are seen in approximately 50% of patients with OA on arthroscopy, and the presence of synovitis is associated with more severe chondropathy.[47,48] Features of synovial inflammation include hypervascularization, synovial lining hyperplasia, proliferation of hypertrophic or hyperemic villi, and fibrosis.[48,49] The synovium contains macrophage-like synovial cells. These cells can phagocytose products of cartilage breakdown, and in return are stimulated to release pro-inflammatory and catabolic mediators. This chronic low-grade inflammation can result in the hypertrophy, hyperemia, fibrosis, and hypervascularization/angiogenesis seen at the synovium; angiogenesis can perpetuate further inflammation, and the pro-inflammatory and catabolic mediators released by the synovium can further perpetuate cartilage breakdown.[48,49] Inflammation can also result in increased microvascular permeability and effusion of the joint. **Fig. 5-3** demonstrates microscopic assessment of synovial pathology during OA progression.

Mechanical influences play a major role in OA development. These mechanical influences in OA pathology are more intricate than simply "wear and tear," as altered biomechanics can influence downstream biochemical

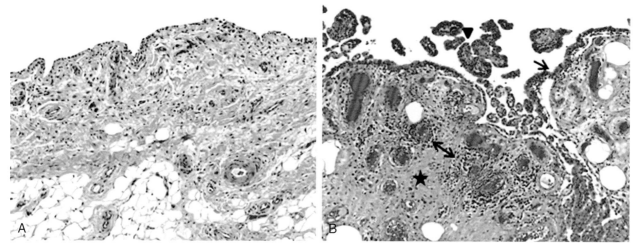

FIGURE 5-3 Representative synovial histopathology observed in osteoarthritis. Panel **(A)** depicts normal appearing synovial membrane with a thin lining layer and loose connective tissue subintimal layer. The section in panel **(B)** demonstrates synovial lining hyperplasia (arrow), villous hyperplasia (arrowhead), fibrosis (star), and perivascular mononuclear cell infiltrates (double-headed arrow) which are histopathologic features often observed in OA. (Reproduced with permission from Scanzello CR, Goldring SR. The role of synovitis in osteoarthrisits pathogenesus. *Bone.* 2012.)

signaling pathways. For instance, mechanical overloading can be sensed by chondrocytes, which can ultimately result in upregulation of mediators of chondrocyte apoptosis (nitric oxide and reactive oxygen species), proteases (MMP-1, 3, 8, 13 and ADAMTS-4, 5), as well as inflammatory cytokines (IL-1, TNF-α, and PGE$_2$), leading to cartilage destruction.[50] Mechanical stimulation sensed by osteocytes can lead to a series of events including decreased production of sclerostin, a negative regulator of osteoblast activity; this decreased production can enhance bone formation.[51,52] One study found that OA subchondral bone osteocytes have decreased production of sclerostin, which may be responsible for facilitating increased bone volume in OA.[53]

In the process of OA development, there is a coordination of degeneration among tissues. As previously discussed, cartilage breakdown products can result in synovial inflammation, and inflammatory cytokines and proteases produced at the synovium can be transmitted through the synovial fluid and influence cartilage breakdown. Pathologic changes in the cartilage and bone can influence one another through changes in biomechanical properties. Furthermore, there is a potential for crosstalk of signaling molecules between the cartilage and bone through defects, channels, and vasculature between the subchondral bone and cartilage. Therefore, signaling molecules and proteins involved in the pathogenesis of OA produced at the cartilage can affect the subchondral bone, and signaling molecules produced at the subchondral bone can affect the cartilage.[54-61]

The development of OA involves pathology at multiple different tissues at the knee joint. OA development is a result of biomechanical influences and biochemical signaling processes that occur over years resulting in progressive joint degeneration. The mechanisms of joint degeneration in OA is not completely understood. Forms

of inflammatory arthritis, such as RA, have a more robust inflammatory component leading to joint destruction, which will be discussed further below.

RHEUMATOID ARTHRITIS

Epidemiology

Rheumatoid arthritis (RA) is an autoimmune disease that affects roughly 1% of the population. It is associated with progressive disability, systemic complications, and early death.[62] The cause of RA is not completely understood but involves interaction between genotype, environmental triggers, and chance.[63] Twin studies have demonstrated that genetic factors account for approximately 60% of the variation in disease liability.[64] Differences in human leukocyte antigen (HLA)-DRB1 alleles is one potential genetic factor in RA susceptibility.[65] A number of environmental triggers have been suggested to increase RA risk in genetically susceptible individuals. Women who take oral contraceptives appear to have a lower risk for RA, while women with subfertility and immediately postpartum after first pregnancy appear to have an increased risk of RA.[65] Approximately 70% of individuals with RA are females.

Additional environmental triggers that have been associated with RA development include viral (Epstein–Barr and parvovirus) and bacterial (*Proteus* and *Mycoplasma*) infections, heat shock proteins, stressors such as physical or emotional trauma, smoking, air pollution, insecticides, silica exposure, obesity, or differences in the gastrointestinal microbiome.[65] These environmental–gene interactions can potentially trigger self-protein citrullination, loss of tolerance to self-proteins, production of autoantibodies against citrullinated peptides such as anti-citrullinated protein antibody (ACPA), and production of autoantibody rheumatoid factor (RF), and trigger a cascade of events leading to a chronic inflammatory response.[63,66]

Symptoms

Rheumatoid arthritis classically presents as a polyarticular disease. Joint most commonly involved include the wrists, proximal interphalangeal, metacarpophalangeal, and metatarsophalangeal joints; the distal interphalangeal joints and spinal joints are usually spared. Large joints such as the hip, knee, and shoulder can also be involved. Joints are often affected in a bilateral symmetric pattern. Joint pain, swelling, and stiffness at the joint can occur. Joint symptoms often develop over weeks to months and can be accompanied by systemic symptoms such as weakness, fatigue, anorexia; furthermore, multiple organs such as the heart and lung can be affected.[67] Unlike OA, morning stiffness is prolonged often lasting more than an hour. Rheumatoid nodules, which are lumps of inflammatory tissue that are often nontender and only occasionally painful, can be found at joints—most often over bony prominences such as tip of the elbow or interphalangeal joints but also at locations such as the knee and back of the heel as well as other diverse sites of the body including internal organs.

Physical Exam and Diagnosis

Classic exam findings of the affected joint include swelling, bogginess, tenderness, and warmth; these findings can be associated with synovitis/inflammation and effusion. There can be atrophy of muscles near the affected joint, and weakness of the involved joint can be out of proportion to tenderness.[67] In 2010, the American College of Rheumatology and European League Against Rheumatism put forward joint classification criteria for RA. The classification criteria for RA include scoring four sections: number of small and/or large joints that are involved, serologic marker and quantity of RF and ACPA, normal or abnormal acute phase reactants CRP and ESR, and duration of symptoms. These sections are scored, and a higher score indicates a higher probability of an RA diagnosis and RA severity. This classification system is a revision of the 1987 American College of Rheumatology classification criteria, and the 2010 classification system was designed as an effort to diagnose/categorize RA earlier in patients. The new criteria do not include the presence of RA nodules, radiographic evidence of erosive changes, which are more common in advanced RA. Furthermore, symmetric arthritis is not a criterion under 2010 guidelines, allowing for an asymmetric presentation. These classification criteria are designed for formally diagnosing RA and following RA in research trials. In the general clinical setting, RA may be diagnosed at the best judgment of the health care practitioner with all available background even with lack of scoring on these classification criteria indicating RA.[67,68] While not necessary for diagnosis, affected joints in RA and other forms of inflammatory arthritis will demonstrate a synovial fluid white cell count ranging from 2000 to 50,000 per mL with absence of crystals, and the fluid will be sterile.

Imaging

The most commonly performed imaging modality in patients with RA is radiography. Radiography may be able to detect soft tissue thickening, which is a combination of synovial thickening, tenosynovitis, and joint effusion. Joint space widening may be seen as one of the earliest radiographic abnormalities. This widening is transient and related to synovial thickening and effusion. A combination of localized inflammation, disuse of the affected joint, and later steroid administration may lead to osteopenia seen on radiographs in OA. Bony erosions on radiograph indicate a more severe and progressed staged of RA; these erosions traditionally occur between the periosteal synovial membrane insertion, the bone, and the cartilage; furthermore, subchondral bone cysts can be found underlying the cartilage. Additional deformities in the late stage of RA seen on radiograph include marked joint destruction (and joint space narrowing), alignment deformities, and stress fractures.[69,70] Unlike OA, joint space narrowing in the three compartments of the knee is relatively uniform in all three compartments, and osteophyte formation is not associated with RA. **Fig. 5-4** demonstrates traditional radiographic features of RA of the knee. Radiographs for suspected RA at the knee can serve additional uses; they can be used as a baseline and be used to evaluate disease progression over time, and they can serve to rule out alternative diagnoses, such as gout or calcium pyrophosphate disease.[70] Radiography is limited in its utility to detect early changes in RA; it provides only indirect evidence of synovial inflammation; furthermore, it can be insensitive in detecting early bone changes.[71] MRI and ultrasound can be used to detect some of these early changes and also be able to provide a greater detailed assessment of the cartilage, tendon, synovium, and bone. MRI and ultrasound can detect bone marrow edema, tenosynovitis, and bursitis and provide better characterization of bony erosions and synovitis; these imaging modalities can provide greater sensitivity in detecting these changes as compared to clinical exam and conventional radiography.[72] In the setting of knee pain with minimal detectable changes on radiography, MRI and ultrasound may be used to rule in or rule out alternative sources of knee symptoms.

Pathophysiology and Progression

The appearance of autoantibodies, including ACPAs and RF, can be present in the serum greater than 10 years before clinical arthritis.[73] Autoantibodies are suggested to be mediators of stimulating synovial and joint

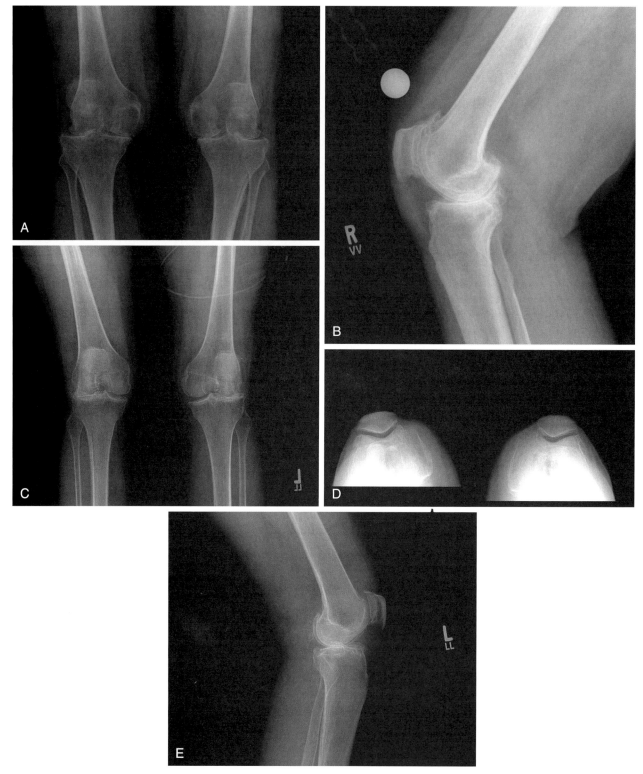

FIGURE 5-4 Radiographic representation depicting features of inflammatory arthritis. AP (**A**) and lateral (**B**) of bilateral knees with psoriatic arthritis. AP (**C**), Merchant (**D**), and lateral (**E**) of valgus knees in a patient with rheumatoid arthritis.

inflammation. Mechanisms through which synovial and joint inflammation is suggested to be triggered include (1) immune complex deposition along vessel walls, which may induce vasculitis, (2) autoantibody or immune complex deposition into the synovial tissue, (3) entrance of autoantibodies directly into the synovial space and binding of specific antigens in the cartilage. Chronic synovitis can occur through perpetual activation of cytokine pathways, neoangiogenesis, and inflammatory cell recruitment and activity.[74,75]

Structural damage to the cartilage in RA can occur through a number of different mechanisms. The major contributor to cartilage damage is suggested to be the RA synovium. The RA synovium has increased expression of MMPs and ADAMTSs that degrade the cartilage matrix, as well as has increased expression of inflammatory cytokines, which can inundate the synovial fluid.[63] Synovial effusions can occur within the joint space, which contain inflammatory cells such as neutrophils and can have a high protein content. The synovium itself can invade the edge of the cartilage; this in part is mediated by inflammatory destruction of the cartilage and invasion of hypertrophic synovium (also known as pannus).

Bone erosion is associated with prolonged and increased inflammation. Increased expression of cytokines from the synovium such as TNF-α and IL-1 can stimulate increased expression of macrophage colony–stimulating factor and receptor activator of NF-κB ligand (RANKL), which increases osteoclast differentiation and activity at the periosteal surface.[63] These erosions occur at a region called the bare area, which is where the synovial membrane inserts into the periosteum. Destruction of this subchondral bone can occur simultaneously to degradation and synovial invasion of cartilage, and pannus invasion can occur in the bone as well. The pathogenesis of subchondral bone erosions itself can further result in degeneration in the overlying cartilage.[66] While synovitis is a major trigger for bone erosions, osteitis of the intertrabecular space or bone marrow edema (assumed to represent inflammation within the bone) can also correlate with development of bone erosions.[76] Subchondral cysts can also develop which is also stimulated by inflammatory activity.[77] In general, inflammation stimulates osteoclast precursor cell migration, osteoclastogenesis, and osteoclast function; therefore, features of bone loss are a common phenomenon in RA and other forms of inflammatory arthritis.[78]

JUVENILE IDIOPATHIC ARTHRITIS

Juvenile idiopathic arthritis (JIA) is a term used to categorize development of inflammatory arthritis that occurs before the age of 16. Diagnosis of JIA requires persistence of arthritis for at least 6 weeks. JIA has a prevalence of 16 to 150 per 100,000 population and is the most common childhood chronic rheumatic disease.[79] The International League of Associations of Rheumatology have proposed a classification system for the various types of JIA: systemic arthritis, oligoarthritis, polyarthritis (RF negative), polyarthritis (RF positive), psoriatic arthritis, enthesis-related arthritis (ERA), and undifferentiated.[80] Oligoarthritis commonly involves the knees or ankles of preschool-aged girls and is the most common JIA subtype; it involves one to four affected joints within 6 months of onset. Polyarthritis involves five or more joints with 6 months of onset and can be RF negative and RF positive. RF positive polyarthritis often involves small joints of the hands and has a symmetric distribution and is often found in adolescent girls. RF negative polyarthritis can have a more variable presentation.[81]

Systemic arthritis affects one or more joints that is found with or preceded by 2 weeks of fevers that have been daily for at least 3 days. One of the following symptoms is also found: transitory rash, generalized lymphadenopathy, hepato- or splenomegaly, or serositis. ERA is classified as arthritis and enthesitis, or arthritis or enthesitis with additional features. Enthesitis involves inflammation of tendon insertion points. It commonly affects joints of the lower extremities in boys older than 8 years. Enthesitis is linked with inflammatory bowel disease and ankylosing spondylitis. Psoriatic arthritis involves a variable presentation of arthritis symptoms with one or two of the following: dactylitis, nail pitting or onycholysis, or psoriasis in a first-degree relative. If the symptoms of arthritis fit into none or at least two of the other categories, it can be classified as undifferentiated.[81]

SERONEGATIVE SPONDYLOARTHROPATHIES

Seronegative spondyloarthropathies (SpAs) are spectrum of inflammatory arthritides; they are called seronegative because these conditions are usually negative for RF. These disorders commonly affect the spine and peripheral joints, including the knee. There is a correlation between the prevalence of SpA and prevalence of HLA-B27 gene in a given population. The prevalence of SpA is estimated to be 0.5% to 1.9% worldwide. SpA can include but not limited to the following: ankylosing spondylitis (AS), psoriatic arthritis (PsA), inflammatory bowel disease (IBD)-associated arthritis, reactive arthritis (formerly Reiter syndrome; ReA), and undifferentiated SpA. AS involves primarily the sacroiliac joints and the axial skeleton. It can include oligoarthritis including the knees, hips, and shoulders; enthesopathy; and anterior uveitis.[82] PsA is an inflammatory joint disease that can present with arthritis, enthesitis, dactylitis, axial involvement, psoriatic nail dystrophy, and psoriasis.[83]

Individuals with IBD can have articular involvement with a prevalence ranging between 17% and 39%. It can be characterized by involvement of axial joints but also can be associated with peripheral arthritis with features such as synovitis, dactylitis, and/or enthesopathy.[84,85] ReA is classified as a sterile synovitis that develops from an infection typically associated with the genitourinary or gastrointestinal tract.[86] The triad of nongonococcal postinfectious arthritis, urethritis, and conjunctivitis is a classic description of ReA; however, this triad is found in only a minority of cases.[87] Undifferentiated SpA does not fit the criteria for other forms of seronegative SpA. It can present with back pain, enthesitis, peripheral arthritis, and extra-skeletal manifestations such as dactylitis and fatigue. Often undifferentiated SpA will be later classified as another form of arthritis, such as rheumatoid arthritis, ankylosing spondylitis, psoriatic arthritis, or degenerative joint disease.[88]

OTHER INFLAMMATORY ARTHROPATHIES

The crystal-induced arthropathies include gout and pseudogout. Gout is the result of accumulation of monosodium urate (MSU) crystals at the joint while pseudogout (also known as calcium pyrophosphate deposition disease) is the result of calcium pyrophosphate crystal deposition at the joint. Clinical presentation of gout and pseudogout can include asymmetric monoarticular or polyarticular inflammation that can occur for acute onset and duration. Gout and pseudogout can precipitate erosions and joint destruction. Synovial fluid leukocyte concentration for gout, pseudogout, and most inflammatory arthritis is generally between 2000 and 50,000 cells/mL. Synovial fluid analysis of gout can demonstrate negatively birefringent needle-like crystals, while analysis of pseudogout can show weakly positively birefringent rhomboid crystals. Evidence of chondrocalcinosis on x-ray is commonly found at the affected joint in patients with pseudogout. Clinical manifestations of gout and pseudogout can present similarly to septic arthritis. Septic arthritis is most commonly found at the knee. Synovial fluid analysis in septic arthritis will demonstrate elevated leukocyte count, often exceeding 50,000 cells/mL, and Gram stain can often reveal staphylococcal or gram-negative bacteria.

Connective tissue diseases, such as lupus, can cause inflammatory arthritis at the knee. However, often as is the case with lupus, other systemic and extra-skeletal manifestations will be present. Lyme disease is related to the *Borrelia burgdorferi* spirochete and can cause Lyme arthritis, characterized by recurrent attacks of swelling in large joints in particular. Lyme disease–associated arthritis is characteristically a late stage manifestation of Lyme disease. The *B. burgdorferi* spirochete can invade the joint causing an inflammatory arthritis, which can eventually lead to joint destruction over time.[89]

CONCLUSION

Arthritis encompasses a broad range of conditions that can affect the knee joint. These conditions include OA, RA, JIA, seronegative spondyloarthropathies (i.e., AS, PsA, IBD-associated arthritis, reactive arthritis), crystal-induced arthritides (gout and pseudogout), septic arthritis, Lupus-associated arthritis, and Lyme disease–associated arthritis. In general, OA is distinct from the other forms of arthritis discussed, as it is classified as "noninflammatory." While inflammatory pathways are involved in pathology and progression in OA, the level of inflammation is comparatively reduced in OA, and disease progression in OA is a multifactorial process that also involves noninflammatory pathways in disease

progression. In general, knee joint pathology and progression from various forms of inflammatory arthritis can be reduced by directly inhibiting inflammatory pathways. In inflammatory arthropathies, synovial and bone pathology can often be improved by inhibition of inflammatory mediators. Cartilage, however, has a limited intrinsic ability of self-repair, and once significant damage has occurred, cartilage will not be able to repair itself over time. Understanding the pathophysiology of arthritic conditions will aid in making the correct diagnosis and initiating the appropriate treatment options for each individual disorder.

REFERENCES

1. Hootman JM, Helmick CG, Barbour KE, Theis KA, Boring MA. Updated projected prevalence of self-reported doctor-diagnosed arthritis and arthritis-attributable activity limitation among US adults, 2015-2040. *Arthritis Rheumatol.* 2016;68(7):1582-1587. doi:10.1002/art.39692. PubMed PMID: 27015600.
2. Theis KA, Roblin DW, Helmick CG, Luo R. Prevalence and causes of work disability among working-age U.S. adults, 2011-2013, NHIS. *Disabil Health J.* 2018;11(1):108-115. doi:10.1016/j.dhjo.2017.04.010. PubMed PMID: 28476583.
3. Murphy L, Schwartz TA, Helmick CG, et al. Lifetime risk of symptomatic knee osteoarthritis. *Arthritis Rheum.* 2008;59(9):1207-1213. doi:10.1002/art.24021. PubMed PMID: 18759314; PMCID: 4516049.
4. Felson DT, Naimark A, Anderson J, Kazis L, Castelli W, Meenan RF. The prevalence of knee osteoarthritis in the elderly. The Framingham Osteoarthritis Study. *Arthritis Rheum.* 1987;30(8):914-918. PubMed PMID: 3632732.
5. Chen D, Shen J, Zhao W, et al. Osteoarthritis: toward a comprehensive understanding of pathological mechanism. *Bone Res.* 2017;5:16044. doi:10.1038/boneres.2016.44. PubMed PMID: 28149655; PMCID: PMC5240031.
6. Lotz M, Loeser RF. Effects of aging on articular cartilage homeostasis. *Bone.* 2012;51(2):241-248. doi:10.1016/j.bone.2012.03.023. PubMed PMID: 22487298; PMCID: PMC3372644.
7. Lieberthal J, Sambamurthy N, Scanzello CR. Inflammation in joint injury and post-traumatic osteoarthritis. *Osteoarthritis Cartilage.* 2015;23(11):1825-1834. doi:10.1016/j.joca.2015.08.015. PubMed PMID: 26521728; PMCID: PMC4630675.
8. Buckwalter JA, Anderson DD, Brown TD, Tochigi Y, Martin JA. The roles of mechanical stresses in the pathogenesis of osteoarthritis: implications for treatment of joint injuries. *Cartilage.* 2013;4(4):286-294. doi:10.1177/1947603513495889. PubMed PMID: 25067995; PMCID: PMC4109888.
9. Sowers MR, Karvonen-Gutierrez CA. The evolving role of obesity in knee osteoarthritis. *Curr Opin Rheumatol.* 2010;22(5):533-537. doi:10.1097/BOR.0b013e32833b4682. PubMed PMID: 20485173; PMCID: 3291123.
10. King LK, March L, Anandacoomarasamy A. Obesity & osteoarthritis. *Indian J Med Res* 2013;138:185-193. PubMed PMID: 24056594; PMCID: PMC3788203.
11. Coggon D, Reading I, Croft P, McLaren M, Barrett D, Cooper C. Knee osteoarthritis and obesity. *Int J Obes Relat Metab Disord.* 2001;25(5):622-627. doi:10.1038/sj.ijo.0801585. PubMed PMID: 11360143.
12. Oliveria SA, Felson DT, Cirillo PA, Reed JI, Walker AM. Body weight, body mass index, and incident symptomatic osteoarthritis of the hand, hip, and knee. *Epidemiology.* 1999;10(2):161-166. PubMed PMID: 10069252.
13. Snead MP, Yates JR. Clinical and molecular genetics of stickler syndrome. *J Med Genet* 1999;36(5):353-359. PubMed PMID: 10353778; PMCID: PMC1734362.

14. Kannu P, Bateman JF, Randle S, et al. Premature arthritis is a distinct type II collagen phenotype. *Arthritis Rheum*. 2010;62(5):1421-1430. doi:10.1002/art.27354. PubMed PMID: 20131279.

15. Valdes AM, Spector TD. Genetic epidemiology of hip and knee osteoarthritis. *Nat Rev Rheumatol*. 2011;7(1):23-32. doi:10.1038/nrrheum.2010.191. PubMed PMID: 21079645.

16. Srikanth VK, Fryer JL, Zhai G, Winzenberg TM, Hosmer D, Jones G. A meta-analysis of sex differences prevalence, incidence and severity of osteoarthritis. *Osteoarthritis Cartilage*. 2005;13(9):769-781. doi:10.1016/j.joca.2005.04.014. PubMed PMID: 15978850.

17. Debi R, Mor A, Segal O, et al. Differences in gait patterns, pain, function and quality of life between males and females with knee osteoarthritis: a clinical trial. *BMC Musculoskeletal Disorders*. 2009;10:127. doi:10.1186/1471-2474-10-127. PubMed PMID: 19825163; PMCID: PMC2765955.

18. McAlindon TE, Snow S, Cooper C, Dieppe PA. Radiographic patterns of osteoarthritis of the knee joint in the community: the importance of the patellofemoral joint. *Ann Rheum Dis*. 1992;51(7):844-849. PubMed PMID: 1632657; PMCID: PMC1004766.

19. Richmond RS, Carlson CS, Register TC, Shanker G, Loeser RF. Functional estrogen receptors in adult articular cartilage: estrogen replacement therapy increases chondrocyte synthesis of proteoglycans and insulin-like growth factor binding protein 2. *Arthritis Rheum*. 2000;43(9):2081-2090. doi:10.1002/1529-0131(200009)43:9<2081::AID-ANR20>3.0.CO;2-I. PubMed PMID: 11014360.

20. Hame SL, Alexander RA. Knee osteoarthritis in women. *Curr Rev Musculoskelet Med*. 2013;6(2):182-187. doi:10.1007/s12178-013-9164-0. PubMed PMID: 23471773; PMCID: PMC3702776.

21. Altman R, Asch E, Bloch D, et al. Development of criteria for the classification and reporting of osteoarthritis. Classification of osteoarthritis of the knee. Diagnostic and Therapeutic Criteria Committee of the American Rheumatism Association. *Arthritis Rheum*. 1986;29(8):1039-1049. PubMed PMID: 3741515.

22. Hunter DJ, McDougall JJ, Keefe FJ. The symptoms of osteoarthritis and the genesis of pain. *Med Clin N Am*. 2009;93(1):83-100, xi. doi:10.1016/j.mcna.2008.08.008. PubMed PMID: 19059023.

23. Bellamy N, Buchanan WW, Goldsmith CH, Campbell J, Stitt LW. Validation study of WOMAC: a health status instrument for measuring clinically important patient relevant outcomes to antirheumatic drug therapy in patients with osteoarthritis of the hip or knee. *J Rheumatol*. 1988;15(12):1833-1840. PubMed PMID: 3068365.

24. Hannan MT, Felson DT, Pincus T. Analysis of the discordance between radiographic changes and knee pain in osteoarthritis of the knee. *J Rheumatol*. 2000;27(6):1513-1517. PubMed PMID: 10852280.

25. Hinton R, Moody RL, Davis AW, Thomas SF. Osteoarthritis: diagnosis and therapeutic considerations. *Am Fam Physician*. 2002;65(5):841-848. PubMed PMID: 11898956.

26. Kohn MD, Sassoon AA, Fernando ND. Classifications in brief: Kellgren-Lawrence classification of osteoarthritis. *Clin Orthop Relat Res*. 2016;474(8):1886-1893. doi:10.1007/s11999-016-4732-4. PubMed PMID: 26872913; PMCID: PMC4925407.

27. Kellgren JH, Lawrence JS. Radiological assessment of osteoarthrosis. *Ann Rheum Dis*. 1957;16(4):494-502. PubMed PMID: 13498604; PMCID: PMC1006995.

28. Hayashi D, Roemer FW, Guermazi A. Imaging for osteoarthritis. *Ann Phys Rehabil Med*. 2016;59(3):161-169. doi:10.1016/j.rehab.2015.12.003. PubMed PMID: 26797169.

29. Heng HY, Bin Abd Razak HR, Mitra AK. Radiographic grading of the patellofemoral joint is more accurate in skyline compared to lateral views. *Ann Transl Med*. 2015;3(18):263. doi:10.3978/j.issn.2305-5839.2015.10.33. PubMed PMID: 26605309; PMCID: PMC4630554.

30. Shapiro LM, McWalter EJ, Son MS, Levenston M, Hargreaves BA, Gold GE. Mechanisms of osteoarthritis in the knee: MR imaging appearance. *J Magn Reson Imaging : JMRI*. 2014;39(6):1346-1356. doi:10.1002/jmri.24562. PubMed PMID: 24677706; PMCID: PMC4016127.

31. Neogi T. Clinical significance of bone changes in osteoarthritis. *Ther Adv Musculoskelet Dis*. 2012;4(4):259-267. doi:10.1177/1759720X12437354. PubMed PMID: 22859925; PMCID: PMC3403249.

32. Radin EL, Rose RM. Role of subchondral bone in the initiation and progression of cartilage damage. *Clin Orthop Relat Res*. 1986;213:34-40. PubMed PMID: 3780104.

33. Goldring SR. Alterations in periarticular bone and cross talk between subchondral bone and articular cartilage in osteoarthritis. *Ther Adv Musculoskelet Dis*. 2012;4(4):249-258. doi:10.1177/1759720X12437353. PubMed PMID: 22859924; PMCID: 3403248.

34. Goldring MB. Articular cartilage degradation in osteoarthritis. *HSS J*. 2012;8(1):7-9. doi:10.1007/s11420-011-9250-z. PubMed PMID: 23372517; PMCID: PMC3295961.

35. Hamilton JL, Nagao M, Levine BR, Chen D, Olsen BR, Im HJ. Targeting VEGF and its receptors for the treatment of osteoarthritis and associated pain. *J Bone Miner Res*. 2016;31(5):911-924. doi:10.1002/jbmr. 2828. PubMed PMID: 27163679; PMCID: 4863467.

36. Nagao M, Hamilton JL, Kc R, et al. Vascular endothelial growth factor in cartilage development and osteoarthritis. *Sci Rep*. 2017;7(1):13027. doi:10.1038/s41598-017-13417-w. PubMed PMID: 29026147; PMCID: PMC5638804.

37. Goldring MB, Dayer J-M, Goldring SR. Osteoarthritis and the immune system. In: Lorenzo J, Horowitz MC, Choi Y, Takaynagi H, Schett G, eds. *Osteoimmunology*. 2nd ed. Academic Press; 2016:257-269.

38. Mapp PI, Walsh DA. Mechanisms and targets of angiogenesis and nerve growth in osteoarthritis. *Nat Rev Rheumatol*. 2012;8(7):390-398. doi:10.1038/nrrheum.2012.80. PubMed PMID: 22641138.

39. Hayashi D, Englund M, Roemer FW, et al. Knee malalignment is associated with an increased risk for incident and enlarging bone marrow lesions in the more loaded compartments: the MOST study. *Osteoarthritis Cartilage*. 2012;20(11):1227-1233. doi:10.1016/j.joca.2012.07.020. PubMed PMID: 22874524; PMCID: PMC3448813.

40. Taljanovic MS, Graham AR, Benjamin JB, et al. Bone marrow edema pattern in advanced hip osteoarthritis: quantitative assessment with magnetic resonance imaging and correlation with clinical examination, radiographic findings, and histopathology. *Skelet Radiol*. 2008;37(5):423-431. doi:10.1007/s00256-008-0446-3. PubMed PMID: 18274742.

41. Audrey HX, Abd Razak HR, Andrew TH. The truth behind subchondral cysts in osteoarthritis of the knee. *Open Orthop J*. 2014;8:7-10. doi:10.2174/1874325001408010007. PubMed PMID: 24533038; PMCID: PMC3924209.

42. Favero M, Giusti A, Geusens P, et al. OsteoRheumatology: a new discipline? *RMD Open*. 2015;1(suppl 1):e000083. doi:10.1136/rmdopen-2015-000083. PubMed PMID: 26557384; PMCID: PMC4632147.

43. Boegard T, Rudling O, Petersson IF, Jonsson K. Correlation between radiographically diagnosed osteophytes and magnetic resonance detected cartilage defects in the patellofemoral joint. *Ann Rheum Dis*. 1998;57(7):395-400. PubMed PMID: 9797565; PMCID: PMC1752672.

44. Pottenger LA, Phillips FM, Draganich LF. The effect of marginal osteophytes on reduction of varus-valgus instability in osteoarthritic knees. *Arthritis Rheum*. 1990;33(6):853-858. PubMed PMID: 2363739.

45. van der Kraan PM, van den Berg WB. Osteophytes: relevance and biology. *Osteoarthritis Cartilage*. 2007;15(3):237-244. doi:10.1016/j.joca.2006.11.006. PubMed PMID: 17204437.

46. Krasnokutsky S, Belitskaya-Levy I, Bencardino J, et al. Quantitative magnetic resonance imaging evidence of synovial proliferation is associated with radiographic severity of knee osteoarthritis. *Arthritis Rheum*. 2011;63(10):2983-2991. doi:10.1002/art.30471. PubMed PMID: 21647860; PMCID: PMC3183134.

47. Ayral X, Pickering EH, Woodworth TG, Mackillop N, Dougados M. Synovitis: a potential predictive factor of structural progression of medial tibiofemoral knee osteoarthritis – results of a 1 year longitudinal arthroscopic study in 422 patients. *Osteoarthritis Cartilage.* 2005;13(5):361-367. doi:10.1016/j.joca.2005.01.005. PubMed PMID: 15882559.

48. Sellam J, Berenbaum F. The role of synovitis in pathophysiology and clinical symptoms of osteoarthritis. *Nat Rev Rheumatol.* 2010;6(11):625-635. doi:10.1038/nrrheum.2010.159. PubMed PMID: 20924410.

49. Scanzello CR, Goldring SR. The role of synovitis in osteoarthritis pathogenesis. *Bone.* 2012;51(2):249-257. doi:10.1016/j.bone.2012.02.012. PubMed PMID: 22387238; PMCID: 3372675.

50. Bader DL, Salter DM, Chowdhury TT. Biomechanical influence of cartilage homeostasis in health and disease. *Arthritis.* 2011;2011:979032. doi:10.1155/2011/979032. PubMed PMID: 22046527; PMCID: PMC3196252.

51. Hemmatian H, Bakker AD, Klein-Nulend J, van Lenthe GH. Aging, osteocytes, and mechanotransduction. *Curr Osteoporos Rep.* 2017;15(5):401-411. doi:10.1007/s11914-017-0402-z. PubMed PMID: 28891009; PMCID: PMC5599455.

52. Robling AG, Niziolek PJ, Baldridge LA, et al. Mechanical stimulation of bone in vivo reduces osteocyte expression of Sost/sclerostin. *J Biol Chem.* 2008;283(9):5866-5875. doi:10.1074/jbc.M705092200. PubMed PMID: 18089564.

53. Jaiprakash A, Prasadam I, Feng JQ, Liu Y, Crawford R, Xiao Y. Phenotypic characterization of osteoarthritic osteocytes from the sclerotic zones: a possible pathological role in subchondral bone sclerosis. *Int J Biol Sci.* 2012;8(3):406-417. doi:10.7150/ijbs. 4221. PubMed PMID: 22419886; PMCID: PMC3303142.

54. Imhof H, Sulzbacher I, Grampp S, Czerny C, Youssefzadeh S, Kainberger F. Subchondral bone and cartilage disease: a rediscovered functional unit. *Invest Radiol.* 2000;35(10):581-588. PubMed PMID: 11041152.

55. Findlay DM, Kuliwaba JS. Bone-cartilage crosstalk: a conversation for understanding osteoarthritis. *Bone research.* 2016;4:16028. doi:10.1038/boneres.2016.28. PubMed PMID: 27672480; PMCID: PMC5028726.

56. Arkill KP, Winlove CP. Solute transport in the deep and calcified zones of articular cartilage. *Osteoarthritis Cartilage.* 2008;16(6):708-714. doi:10.1016/j.joca.2007.10.001. PubMed PMID: 18023368.

57. O'Hara BP, Urban JP, Maroudas A. Influence of cyclic loading on the nutrition of articular cartilage. *Ann Rheum Dis.* 1990;49(7):536-539. PubMed PMID: 2383080; PMCID: PMC1004145.

58. Zhang L, Gardiner BS, Smith DW, Pivonka P, Grodzinsky AJ. On the role of diffusible binding partners in modulating the transport and concentration of proteins in tissues. *J Theor Biol.* 2010;263(1):20-29. doi:10.1016/j.jtbi.2009.11.023. PubMed PMID: 20005880.

59. Zhang L, Gardiner BS, Smith DW, Pivonka P, Grodzinsky A. The effect of cyclic deformation and solute binding on solute transport in cartilage. *Arch Biochem Biophys.* 2007;457(1):47-56. doi:10.1016/j.abb.2006.10.007. PubMed PMID: 17107655.

60. Wang B, Zhou X, Price C, Li W, Pan J, Wang L. Quantifying load-induced solute transport and solute-matrix interaction within the osteocyte lacunar-canalicular system. *J Bone Miner Res.* 2013;28(5):1075-1086. doi:10.1002/jbmr. 1804. PubMed PMID: 23109140; PMCID: PMC3593787.

61. Priam S, Bougault C, Houard X, et al. Identification of soluble 14-3-3 as a novel subchondral bone mediator involved in cartilage degradation in osteoarthritis. *Arthritis Rheum.* 2013;65(7):1831-1842. doi:10.1002/art.37951. PubMed PMID: 23552998.

62. Firestein GS. Evolving concepts of rheumatoid arthritis. *Nature.* 2003;423(6937):356-361. doi:10.1038/nature01661. PubMed PMID: 12748655.

63. McInnes IB, Schett G. The pathogenesis of rheumatoid arthritis. *N Engl J Med.* 2011;365(23):2205-2219. doi:10.1056/NEJMra1004965. PubMed PMID: 22150039.

64. MacGregor AJ, Snieder H, Rigby AS, et al. Characterizing the quantitative genetic contribution to rheumatoid arthritis using data from twins. *Arthritis Rheum.* 2000;43(1):30-37. doi:10.1002/1529-0131(200001)43:1<30::AID-ANR5>3.0.CO;2-B. PubMed PMID: 10643697.

65. Silman AJ, Pearson JE. Epidemiology and genetics of rheumatoid arthritis. *Arthritis Res.* 2002;4(suppl 3):S265-S272. doi:10.1186/ar578. PubMed PMID: 12110146; PMCID: PMC3240153.

66. Guo Q, Wang Y, Xu D, Nossent J, Pavlos NJ, Xu J. Rheumatoid arthritis: pathological mechanisms and modern pharmacologic therapies. *Bone Res.* 2018;6:15. doi:10.1038/s41413-018-0016-9. PubMed PMID: 29736302; PMCID: PMC5920070.

67. Majithia V, Geraci SA. Rheumatoid arthritis: diagnosis and management. *Am J Med.* 2007;120(11):936-939. doi:10.1016/j.amjmed.2007.04.005. PubMed PMID: 17976416.

68. Arnett FC, Edworthy SM, Bloch DA, et al. The American Rheumatism Association 1987 revised criteria for the classification of rheumatoid arthritis. *Arthritis Rheum.* 1988;31(3):315-324. PubMed PMID: 3358796.

69. Vyas S, Bhalla AS, Ranjan P, Kumar S, Kumar U, Gupta AK. Rheumatoid arthritis revisited - advanced imaging review. *Pol J Radiol.* 2016;81:629-635. doi:10.12659/PJR.899317. PubMed PMID: 28105245; PMCID: PMC5223782.

70. Teh J, Ostergaard M. What the rheumatologist is looking for and what the radiologist should know in imaging for rheumatoid arthritis. *Radiol Clin North Am.* 2017;55(5):905-916. doi:10.1016/j.rcl.2017.04.001. PubMed PMID: 28774454.

71. Boutry N, Morel M, Flipo RM, Demondion X, Cotten A. Early rheumatoid arthritis: a review of MRI and sonographic findings. *AJR Am J Roentgenol.* 2007;189(6):1502-1509. doi:10.2214/AJR.07.2548. PubMed PMID: 18029892.

72. Freeston JE, Bird P, Conaghan PG. The role of MRI in rheumatoid arthritis: research and clinical issues. *Curr Opin Rheumatol.* 2009;21(2):95-101. doi:10.1097/BOR.0b013e32832498f0. PubMed PMID: 19339918.

73. Wegner N, Lundberg K, Kinloch A, et al. Autoimmunity to specific citrullinated proteins gives the first clues to the etiology of rheumatoid arthritis. *Immunol Rev.* 2010;233(1):34-54. doi:10.1111/j.0105-2896.2009.00850.x. PubMed PMID: 20192991.

74. Arend WP, Firestein GS. Pre-rheumatoid arthritis: predisposition and transition to clinical synovitis. *Nat Rev Rheumatol.* 2012;8(10):573-586. doi:10.1038/nrrheum.2012.134. PubMed PMID: 22907289.

75. Cope AP, Schulze-Koops H, Aringer M. The central role of T cells in rheumatoid arthritis. *Clin Exp Rheumatol.* 2007;25(5 suppl 46):S4–S11. PubMed PMID: 17977483.

76. Haavardsholm EA, Boyesen P, Ostergaard M, Schildvold A, Kvien TK. Magnetic resonance imaging findings in 84 patients with early rheumatoid arthritis: bone marrow oedema predicts erosive progression. *Ann Rheum Dis.* 2008;67(6):794-800. doi:10.1136/ard.2007.071977. PubMed PMID: 17981915.

77. Ostrowska M, Maslinski W, Prochorec-Sobieszek M, Nieciecki M, Sudol-Szopinska I. Cartilage and bone damage in rheumatoid arthritis. *Reumatologia.* 2018;56(2):111-120. doi:10.5114/reum.2018.75523. PubMed PMID: 29853727; PMCID: PMC5974634.

78. Zerbini CAF, Clark P, Mendez-Sanchez L, et al, Bone Structure Working G. Biologic therapies and bone loss in rheumatoid arthritis. *Osteoporos Int.* 2017;28(2):429-446. doi:10.1007/s00198-016-3769-2. PubMed PMID: 27796445.

79. Ravelli A, Martini A. Juvenile idiopathic arthritis. *Lancet.* 2007;369(9563):767-778. doi:10.1016/S0140-6736(07)60363-8. PubMed PMID: 17336654.

80. Petty RE, Southwood TR, Manners P, et al, International League of Associations for R. International League of Associations for Rheumatology classification of juvenile idiopathic arthritis: second revision, Edmonton, 2001. *J Rheumatol.* 2004;31(2):390-392. PubMed PMID: 14760812.

81. Sheybani EF, Khanna G, White AJ, Demertzis JL. Imaging of juvenile idiopathic arthritis: a multimodality approach. *RadioGraphics.* 2013;33(5):1253-1273. doi:10.1148/rg.335125178. PubMed PMID: 24025923.

82. Dakwar E, Reddy J, Vale FL, Uribe JS. A review of the pathogenesis of ankylosing spondylitis. *Neurosurg Focus.* 2008;24(1):E2. doi:10.3171/FOC/2008/24/1/E2. PubMed PMID: 18290740.

83. Coates LC, Helliwell PS. Psoriatic arthritis: state of the art review. *Clin Med.* 2017;17(1):65-70. doi:10.7861/clinmedicine.17-1-65. PubMed PMID: 28148584.

84. Peluso R, Di Minno MN, Iervolino S, et al. Enteropathic spondyloarthritis: from diagnosis to treatment. *Clin Dev Immunol.* 2013;2013:631408. doi:10.1155/2013/631408. PubMed PMID: 23690825; PMCID: PMC3649644.

85. Peluso R, Manguso F, Vitiello M, Iervolino S, Di Minno MN. Management of arthropathy in inflammatory bowel diseases. *Ther Adv Chronic Dis.* 2015;6(2):65-77. doi:10.1177/2040622314563929. PubMed PMID: 25729557; PMCID: PMC4331233.

86. Colmegna I, Cuchacovich R, Espinoza LR. HLA-B27-associated reactive arthritis: pathogenetic and clinical considerations. *Clin Microbiol Rev.* 2004;17(2):348-369. PubMed PMID: 15084505; PMCID: PMC387405.

87. Parker CT, Thomas D. Reiter's syndrome and reactive arthritis. *J Am Osteopath Assoc.* 2000;100(2):101-104. PubMed PMID: 10732393.

88. Thabet MM, Huizinga TW, van der Heijde DM, van der Helm-van Mil AH. The prognostic value of baseline erosions in undifferentiated arthritis. *Arthritis Res Ther.* 2009;11(5):R155. doi:10.1186/ar2832. PubMed PMID: 19832979; PMCID: PMC2787272.

89. Smith BG, Cruz AI Jr, Milewski MD, Shapiro ED. Lyme disease and the orthopaedic implications of lyme arthritis. *J Am Acad Orthop Surg.* 2011;19(2):91-100. PubMed PMID: 21292932; PMCID: PMC3656475.

chapter 6

Lower Extremity Alignment

Shane C. Eizember, MD | Caleb M. Yeung, MD | Hany S. Bedair, MD |
John G. Esposito, MD, MSc, FRCS(C)

ANATOMY AND BIOMECHANICS OF THE KNEE

The anatomy and geometry of the knee is uniquely suited for its motion and offers both static and dynamic stability, allowing it to withstand many multiples of our body weight during daily activities.

The femur, tibia, and patella make up the tibiofemoral and patellofemoral joints of the knee. The femoral condyles are rounded, especially posteriorly, and have a posterior offset relative to the femoral shaft, allowing for deep flexion.[1,2] The medial condyle is larger and more circular in comparison to the lateral condyle and has a more uniform radius of curvature, allowing it to remain mostly stationary during knee flexion while the lateral condyle translates posteriorly, creating the posterior femoral rollback. This crucially allows the distal femur to externally rotate and promotes patellar engagement with the trochlear groove during knee flexion. Anteriorly, the condyles flatten and merge, forming the trochlear groove and centrally to form the intercondylar notch.[1,3]

The articular surface of the tibia, also known as the tibial plateau, is asymmetric like the distal femur, conferring stability to the knee. In the coronal plane, the tibial plateau has a slight inward tilt that matches the medial to lateral asymmetry of the femoral condyles. In the sagittal plane, the plateaus are slightly posterior in relation to the tibial shaft axis and usually have a posterior slope. One study analyzing MRIs found that for males the medial tibial slope ranged from −3° to 10° (average 3.7) and the lateral tibial slope ranged from 0° to 9° (average 5.4). In females the medial tibial slope ranged from 0° to 10° (average 5.9) and the lateral tibial slope ranged from 1° to 14° (average 7.0).[4] The tibial slopes are variable between different sexes and population and depend on the imaging and reference axis used. The more increased lateral tibial plateau slope enhances the posterior rollback.

Additional congruence between the femoral condyles and the medial and lateral tibial surfaces is granted by the menisci, which also behave as loading and stabilizing gaskets.[1,4-6] The medial and lateral menisci increase the effective joint surface, reducing contact forces by dissipating axial load into hoop stress. The medial tibial plateau is larger and more concave and is effectively deepened by its meniscus anchored along the tibial margins.[6] In contrast, the lateral tibial plateau is smaller and more convex, with a centrally fixed lateral meniscus that remains more mobile on the periphery to accommodate the posterior rollback of the lateral condyle.[7]

The ligaments of the knee also play an important role in motion and stability. The medial and lateral collateral ligaments offer stability to varus and valgus stresses in the coronal plane. The superficial MCL is the major medial stabilizer, while the LCL provides lateral stability. The anterior and posterior cruciate ligaments provide stability to anteroposterior stresses in the sagittal plane. In ACL-deficient knees, the tibia subluxates anteriorly leading to cartilage wear in the posterior-medial aspect of the knee compared to the anterior-medial aspect. In PCL-deficient knees, the tibia subluxates posteriorly interfering with the proper posterior rollback and thus terminal flexion.

During normal gait, 60% to 70% of weightbearing forces in the stance phase pass through the medial compartment of the knee. Small changes in alignment lead to significant changes in load distribution in each compartment, which may predispose to or accelerate arthritis.[8-10]

Restoration of lower extremity alignment with proper TKA component alignment normalizes the distribution forces across the implant. Malpositioned components change the load distribution in the compartments and predispose to early failures.[11,12]

KNEE MOTION

Motion patterns of the knee are complex. The knee primarily flexes and extends but also rotates in the axial plane (internal–external rotation) and the coronal plane (varus–valgus rotations).[13] Although the knee is believed to have two rotation axes in the sagittal plane,[14] several studies recommend assessing knee motion in the sagittal plane by a line connecting the medial and lateral epicondyles—the transepicondylar line (TEL).[3,4,14,15] When viewed parallel to the TEL, the posterior projections of the femoral condyle are two concentric circular outlines with the larger medial outline reflecting the larger radius of curvature of the medial femoral condyle (**Fig. 6-1**). The flexion–extension gap, the area between the TEL and tibial joint surface, remains constant throughout flexion and allows for constant tension on the collateral ligaments (**Fig. 6-2**).[16]

As the knee flexes, the tibia shifts slightly from varus to valgus and also internally rotates (femur externally rotates).[17] The internal–external rotation of the tibia with

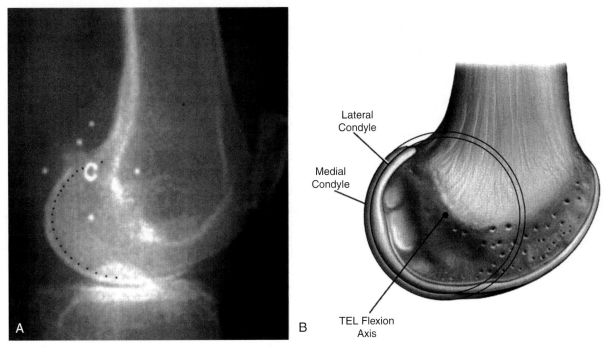

FIGURE 6-1 **A:** Lateral radiograph of a knee when viewed along the transepicondylar line (TEL). The medial and lateral femoral condyle curves are concentric posteriorly, the medial having a slightly larger radius of curvature. **B:** Diagrammatic portrayal of this perspective.

respect to the femur occurs about the tibia's long axis (**Fig. 6-3A**).[14,15,18] The rotation of the tibia during flexion and extension is accommodated by the medial and lateral asymmetry in the tibiofemoral joint described previously.[1,6] The medial compartment has a concave tibial surface and a more immobile meniscus in comparison to the convex tibial surface, which has a more mobile meniscus in the lateral compartment. This results in less posterior translation of the medial tibiofemoral contact point in comparison with the lateral tibiofemoral contact point, resulting in tibial internal rotation (femoral external rotation) during knee flexion (**Fig. 6-3B**).[1,15,17,18] This rotation totals approximately 30° over the entire flexion–extension arc. When the knee reaches full flexion, the lateral tibiofemoral contact point has translated posteriorly to the edge of the tibial surface with 30° of external

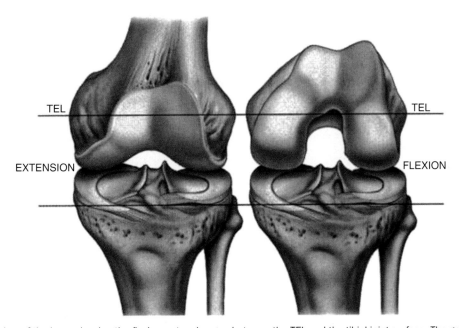

FIGURE 6-2 Frontal view of the knee showing the flexion–extension gap between the TEL and the tibial joint surface. The gap is filled by the "articular material" (distal condyles, proximal tibia, menisci, and cruciate ligament). The gap size is constant throughout range of motion which serves to maintain tension in the collateral ligaments, whose origins lie on the TEL.

MEDIAL   LATERAL

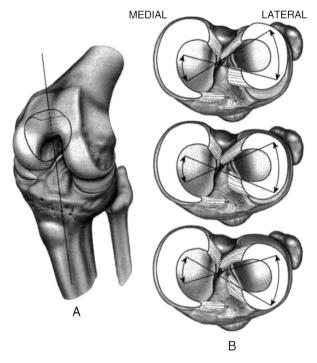

A

B

FIGURE 6-3 Illustrations of axial rotation occurring between the tibia and the femur during flexion and extension. **A:** The tibia rotates about an axis that passes through the tibial plateau at a point just medial to the center. **B:** The medial displacement of the axis is due to the concavity of the medial plateau which limits excursion relative to the medial condyle. In the lateral compartment, the convex plateau surface allows greater anterior–posterior excursion, further facilitated by the more mobile lateral meniscus.

rotation and 5° of valgus rotation.[19] Variation in the anteroposterior translations of the tibiofemoral contact points in different studies can be explained by different anatomic references, activity, and foot positions.[19]

Patellofemoral kinematics are also affected with knee flexion and extension. In stance, while the knee is extended, the patella lies proximal and lateral to the trochlear groove. As the knee flexes, the femur begins to externally rotate and the patella enters the trochlear groove and tracks along the groove.[20] The patella itself also begins to flex as it moves distally with knee flexion, causing the patellofemoral contact point to move distally.[21,22] At terminal flexion, the patella sinks between the two femoral condyles, making contact with each (**Fig. 6-4**).[2] The patella's flexion–extension motion is about an axis located transversely to the femoral condyle, slightly anterior and distal to the TEL (**Fig. 6-4**).[3,20] Patellofemoral kinematics is altered by femoral and tibial tubercle variations as well as ligamentous laxity.[23-26]

LOWER EXTREMITY AXES

There is significant variation in lower extremity alignment. Individual differences in height and bone morphology, including degenerative changes, affect knee alignment. The mechanical axis of the lower extremity is determined by drawing a line from the center of the femoral head to the center of the ankle.[27] In normal limbs, the mechanical axis usually passes through the medial tibial spine but is also dependent on height and pelvic width as noted above. The mechanical axis can be subdivided into the femoral mechanical axis and the tibial mechanical axis. The femoral mechanical axis is measured from the center of the femoral head to the center of the intercondylar notch of the distal femur. The tibial mechanical axis is measured from the center of the proximal tibia to the center of the ankle.

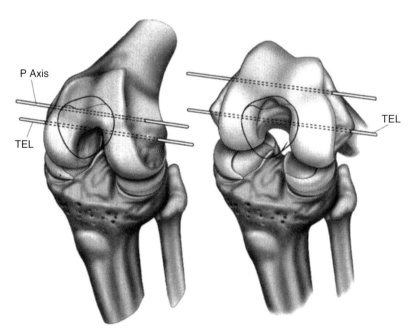

P Axis

TEL

TEL

FIGURE 6-4 Oblique illustrations of partial and deep knee flexion, showing the transverse axes of motion for the tibia (TEL) and patella (P axis). In full knee flexion, the patella becomes the most flexed with respect to the femoral axis.

Normal
Alignment

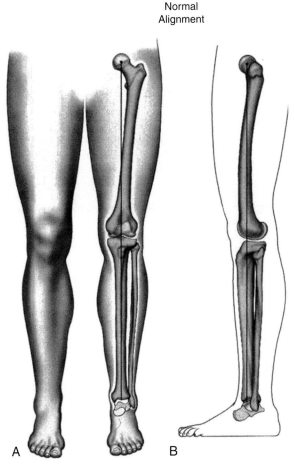

FIGURE 6-5   Frontal **(A)** and lateral **(B)** aspects of the lower limbs with depiction of the femur and tibia and their mechanical (load) axes. The reference points are hip center, knee center, and ankle center.

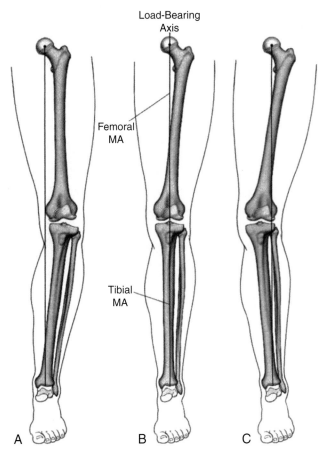

FIGURE 6-6   Frontal illustration of limb alignment: varus **(A)**, neutral **(B)**, and valgus **(C)**. In the neutral knee, the knee center is located on the load axis. In the other conditions, the knee is off-center, displaced either laterally (varus) or medially (valgus) of the load axis. MA, mechanical axis.

The anatomic axis of the lower extremity is based on the relationship of the intramedullary canals of the femur and tibia.[27] The anatomic axis of the femur is created by a line drawn proximal to distal in the intramedullary canal bisecting the femur in half. The angle between the anatomical and mechanical axis of the femur is usually 5° to 7°. The anatomic axis of tibia is created by a line drawn proximal to distal in the intramedullary canal bisecting the tibia in half. The anatomic axis and mechanical axis of the tibia are often the same, though the anatomic axis can vary if there are bony angular deformities.

KNEE ALIGNMENT

Knee alignment is described as the orientation of the thigh (femur) with the leg (tibia, fibula, and ankle). It can be further described in the coronal and sagittal perspectives (**Fig. 6-5**).

In the coronal view, while standing, the ground reaction force passes from the hindfoot through the ankle joint to the center of the hip. When the knee is well aligned, it is centered on this load-bearing axis (LBA). Coronal malalignment occurs when the knee center deviates significantly from the LBA. The varus knee deviates laterally with the respect to the LBA, overloading the medial tibiofemoral compartment, while the valgus knee deviates medially, overloading the lateral compartment (**Fig. 6-6**).[10,28-31] This can bias locations of osteoarthritis based on the particular compartment of the joint that sees this increased load.

In the sagittal view, the knee center is slightly posterior to the LBA. Genu recurvatum results when the knee center is located significantly posterior to the LBA, creating a hyperextension deformity. By contrast, a flexion contracture results in a knee center which is anterior to the LBA (**Fig. 6-7**).

ASSESSING ALIGNMENT

Radiographic assessment of knee alignment is best made with AP and lateral weightbearing views.[10,25,28,29] Complete alignment of the limb requires inclusion of the hip, knee, and ankle using a full-length radiograph (such

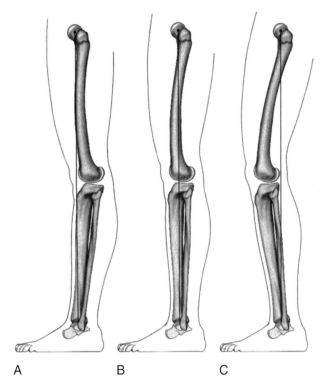

A   B   C

FIGURE 6-7 Lateral illustration of limb alignment: hyperextension deformity **(A)**, neutrally aligned limb **(B)**, and flexion deformity **(C)**. In the neutral limb, the bone contact points are almost coincident with the load axis. The knee center is well behind the load axis in the hyperextended knee and is anterior to the axis in a flexion deformity.

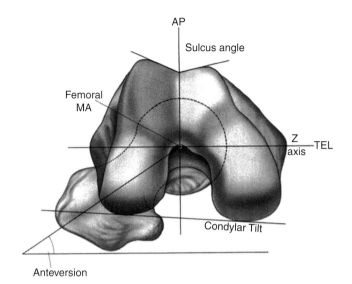

FIGURE 6-8 Axial view of the distal femur, showing the condylar orientation relative to the TEL superimposed on the femoral mechanical axis (MA). The approach recommended is to use the TEL as the reference axis to define the angles of femoral anteversion, condylar tilt, patella tilt, and sulcus. AP, anteroposterior.

as a standard 36-inch cassette) or from digitally stitched images.[25,31,32] To minimize variability and rotation errors, the knee should be positioned with the flexion plane facing straight ahead rather than basing this off of the patella facing ahead due to the variability of the latter.[25,29] To assess patellar orientation, axial (Merchant) views should be obtained, and the TEL be used as a reference (**Fig. 6-8**).[4,24,33] A CT scan may also be used to assess rotational variation.[34]

ANGULAR COMPONENTS OF CORONAL ALIGNMENT

The coronal alignment of the femur, tibia, and patella is described using their angular orientation with respect to their mechanical axis. The components of coronal alignment are shown in **Fig. 6-9**. The mechanical axis of the femur passes from the femoral head to the knee center. The mechanical axis of the tibia passes from the center of the tibia to the center of the ankle.[4,35] The angle between these axes is the hip-knee-ankle (HKA) angle. When the knee is ideally aligned, the knee is centered on the LBA and the HKA angle is 0.

The HKA angle has three components

1. Condylar–hip (CH) angle: the angle of the femoral condylar tangent with respect to the femoral mechanical axis

2. Plateau–ankle (PA) angle: the angle of the tibial plateau tangent with respect to the tibial mechanical axis

3. Condylar–plateau (CP) angle: the angle between the femoral and tibial joint surface tangents

The relationship between these angles is HKA angle = (CH angle + PA angle) + CP angle.[36,37]

The HKA angle is expressed as degrees of deviation from linearity (i.e. 180° yields a HKA angle of 0), and both the CH angle and PA angle are expressed as degrees of deviation from 90°.[29,37] By convention, negative angles indicate varus while positive angles indicate valgus.

The femoral and tibial mechanical axes normally lie in neutral alignment (HKA angle = 0°). **Table 6-1** shows the mean HKA angles and standard deviation of asymptomatic adults from several different studies. HKA angles are known to be higher in young males when compared to females and the angle is closer to 0 in asymptomatic adults compared younger groups.[10,30,38] Nonetheless, the HKA angle is dependent on age, gender, and other factors with a relatively large standard deviation, with "normal alignment" comprising a range of HKA angles.

The Q-angle defines patellar alignment relative to the anterior–superior iliac spine and the tibial tubercle. In asymptomatic adults, the Q-angle is 11 ± 6° (**Fig. 6-10**).[25,39] As the tibial tubercle position can be variable, this also leads to a range of normal Q-angles.[35] In the valgus knee, the Q-angle is increased and the forces on the patella tend to lateralize it. However, in the osteoarthritic varus knee, a lateral shift of the patella is often seen with concomitant wear in the lateral patellofemoral compartment.[26] This is thought to be due to a developmental abnormality involving rotation of the distal femur or proximal tibia.

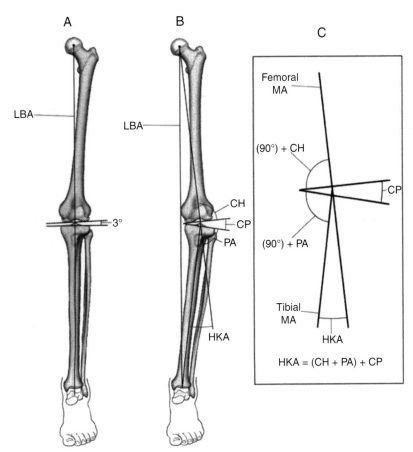

FIGURE 6-9   Frontal limb alignment angles. In the neutrally aligned limb **(A)**, the femoral and tibial mechanical axes are coincident with the load-bearing axis (LBA), and the joint surfaces are inclined inward approximately 3°. In the varus limb **(B)**, the mechanical axes intersect laterally to the LBA, forming a varus (negative) hip-knee-ankle (HKA) angle. The joint surface components of the HKA angle **(C)** are the condylar–hip (CH) and plateau–ankle (PA) angles (each measured as increments beyond 90°) and condylar–plateau (CP) angle. By convention, varus angles are negative (−) and valgus angles are positive (+). The HKA angle is equal to the sum of the angles (CH angle + PA angle) + CP angle. MA, mechanical axis.

Additional terms used to describe the coronal alignment in limb deformity are noted in **Fig. 6-11**.[31,40,41]

ANGULAR COMPONENTS OF SAGITTAL ALIGNMENT

The roundedness of the femoral condyles and their posterior offset from the axis of the femoral shaft present additional complexities with regard to definitions of alignment. The angle between the femoral axis and the femoral articular marginal line joining the anterior and posterior margins of the condylar profile is the posterior distal femoral angle (PDFA). The average PDFA is 83°

with a normal range of 79° to 87° (**Fig. 6-12A**).[42] An alternative definition is to describe the roof of the intercondylar notch by a line (Blumensaat's line) and to measure the angle between it and the femoral axis (**Fig. 6-12B**).

The sagittal alignment of the tibia is defined by a line from the anterior to posterior articular margins in reference to the mechanical axis.[35] Both compartments have a posterior tilt of 7° ± 3.5°.[35]

OSTEOTOMIES AND COMPONENT PLACEMENT

Alignment Goals

There is significant potential for error during component implantation when considering the femoral, tibial, and patellar components of a TKA and the combined degrees of freedom they each may have in flexion–extension, proximal–distal positioning, varus–valgus tilt, internal–external rotation, anterior–posterior translation, and medial–lateral translation.

Three principle cuts are made to align and balance the TKA: the proximal tibial cut, the distal femoral cut, and

TABLE 6-1 **Lower Limb Alignment of Asymptomatic Adults: Mean Hip-Knee-Ankle (HKA)**		
Study	**HKA angle (°)**	**Standard deviation (°)**
Moreland et al[28]	−1.3	2.0
Hsu et al[10]	−1.2	2.2
Cooke et al[29]	−1.0	2.8

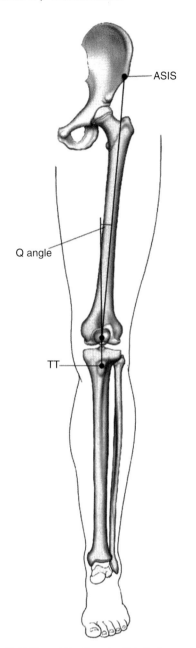

FIGURE 6-10 Definition of the Q angle. This is the angle of intercept of lines connecting the patella center proximally to the anterior superior iliac spine (ASIS) and distally to the tibial tubercle (TT).

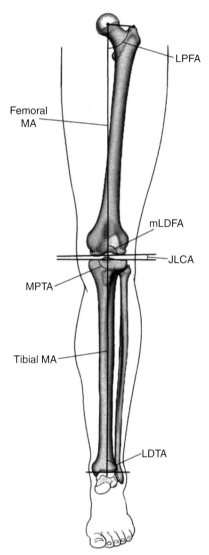

FIGURE 6-11 Frontal alignment parameters commonly used in the correction of limb lengthening and deformity. The lateral proximal femoral angle (LPFA) is between the line joining the trochanteric tip to the femoral head center and the femoral mechanical axis (MA) measured laterally. The mechanical lateral distal femoral angle (mLDFA) is measured laterally as the angle that the condylar tangent makes with the femoral MA (this is equivalent to the condylar–hip angle shown in **Fig. 6-9**). The medial proximal tibial angle (MPTA) is measured medially as the tibial plateau tangent to the tibial MA (equivalent to the plateau–ankle angle shown in **Fig. 6-9**). The joint line convergence angle (JLCA) is measured as the intercept of the condylar and tibial articular tangents (this is equivalent to the condylar–plateau angle in **Fig. 6-9**). At the ankle, the lateral distal tibial angle (LDTA) is measured laterally as the intercept of the tibial articular plafond with the tibial MA.

the anterior and posterior femoral condylar cuts (**Fig. 6-13**). The distal femur cut sets the axial alignment while the anterior and posterior femoral condylar cuts determine the rotational alignment. Standardized techniques and instrumentation allow the surgeon to create reproducible and accurate bone cuts that restore the mechanical (or kinematic) axis of the limb.

Restoring limb alignment to neutral is the primary goal of TKA. It is believed that the tibiofemoral alignment should be restored to approximately 6° ± 2° of valgus, though this varies depending on conditions such as preoperative alignment, obesity, and surrounding ligament sufficiency. Although the average knee has a 3° varus tilt

in the tibia, a transverse cut is commonly preferred. The resultant femur is then cut in 4° to 7° of valgus.

Two techniques are used to integrate the tibial and femoral cuts: the measured resection technique and the tension gap (i.e. gap balancing) technique.

The measured resection technique restores knee anatomy by replacing what is removed. For example, if 10 mm of the proximal tibia is resected, 10 mm of combined thickness of the tibial tray and polyethylene liner are used

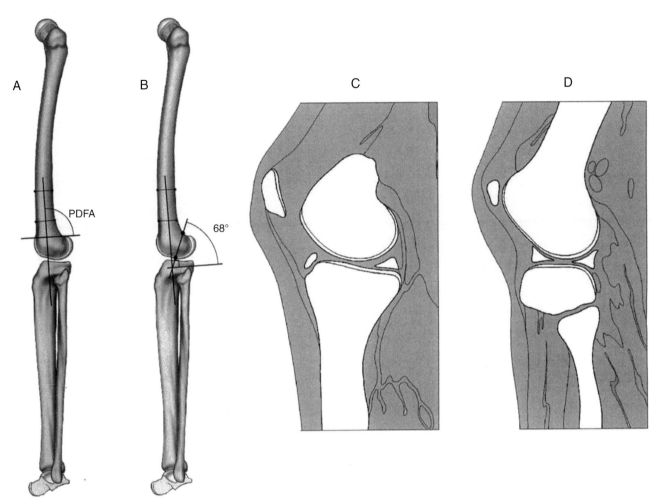

FIGURE 6-12 Lateral perspectives of knee alignment. **A:** Condylar orientation—the angle between the proximal condylar articular line and the femoral anatomic axis, known as the posterior distal femoral angle (PDFA). **B:** Condylar orientation—the angle of intercept between Blumensaat's line (line describing the roof of the intercondylar notch) and the femoral anatomic axis. **C:** Sagittal knee section tracing through the medial compartment, showing the concave articulating surface of the medial plateau. **D:** Sagittal knee tracing through the lateral compartment showing the convex surface of the lateral plateau. The posterior slope of the tibial plateau surfaces may be defined by lines connecting the anterior to posterior articular margins and measuring their angle of intersection with the tibial mechanical axis.

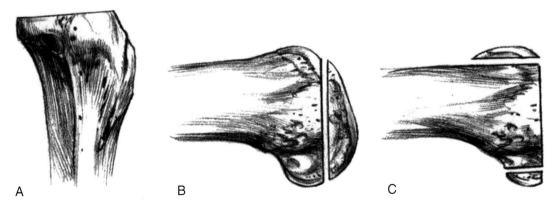

FIGURE 6-13 Three osteotomy cuts determine the alignment of the knee: the proximal tibia **(A)**, distal femur **(B)**, and the anterior and posterior cuts of the distal femur **(C)**.

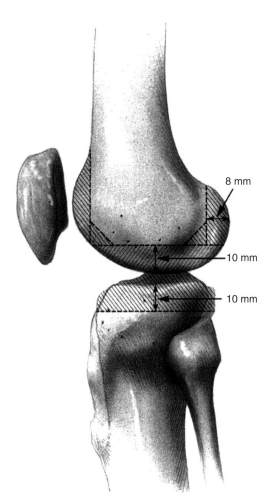

FIGURE 6-14 The measured resection technique removes as much bone and cartilage as to be replaced by the thickness of the arthroplasty components.

to restore the anatomy. Posterior and distal femoral condylar resections are made to match the thickness of the implant (**Fig. 6-14**).

The tension gap technique is based on the initial tibial resection. Equal rectangular gaps in 90° of flexion and full extension are created. Femoral external rotation (posterior condylar cut) and femoral valgus (distal femoral cut) are determined during tensioning so that equal rectangular gaps are created. Care must be taken to ensure that an accurate tibial cut, removal of surrounding osteophytes, and proper soft-tissue balancing are performed, as the accuracy of the subsequent flexion–extension gaps will otherwise be affected (**Fig. 6-15**).

Tibial Osteotomy

Instruments are used to make the proximal tibial cut.[43] These instruments are either intramedullary or extramedullary guides that are placed on the tibia to guide this cut. Each has its own benefits and detriments. Prior literature has shown that extramedullary and intramedullary (IM) instruments can be equally effective for performing the

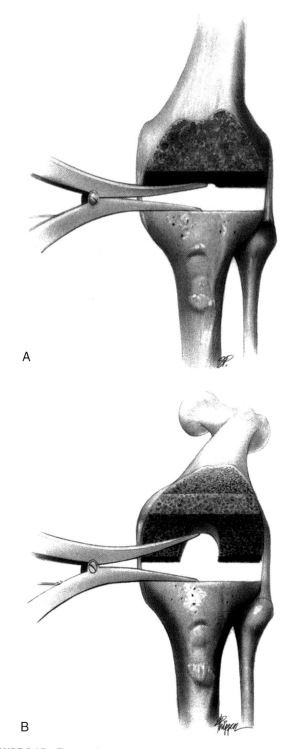

FIGURE 6-15 The tension technique makes a transverse tibial osteotomy first **(A)**, and the femoral osteotomy is determined with tension to make equal rectangular spaces in flexion and extension **(B)**.

tibial osteotomy (**Fig. 6-16**), even in those who are obese with obscured external landmarks.[44] As such, the choice typically is based on surgeon preference.

In the case of extramedullary guides, these are placed parallel to the tibial crest in the coronal plane with the ability to adjust for a posterior slope. Extramedullary

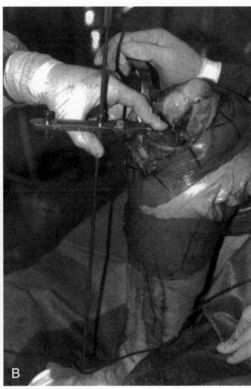

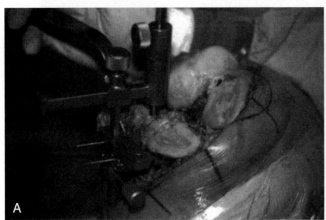

FIGURE 6-16   Intramedullary **(A)** or extramedullary **(B)** guides may be used for the tibial osteotomy.

systems are not affected by deformities of the tibial shaft and avoid the risk of fat embolism that can occur with cannulation of the tibial medullary canal as with intramedullary guides. However, studies have found significant alignment errors can occur with these guides, particularly in those cut perpendicular to the mechanical axis of the tibial shaft in the coronal plane.

Intramedullary guides are applicable for most knees except in those with significant tibial shaft deformity or hardware that obstructs the medullary canal. These guides have telescoping elements that are used to place a cutting block at the desired resection level on the proximal tibia (**Fig. 6-17**). The varus and valgus alignment

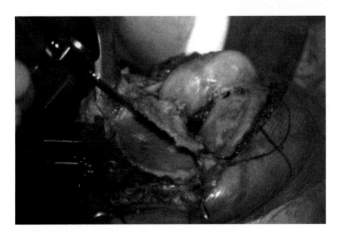

FIGURE 6-17   A tibial cutting block is fixed in place and used to guide the tibial osteotomy.

and posterior slope can be modified with these guides as with the extramedullary guides.

In both systems, a stylus is used to help determine the amount of bone being resected, generally the goal is to remove 10 mm of bone from the less arthritic tibial hemiplateau. As such, in the measured resection technique, the amount of resection should be equal to the tibial component and polyethylene liner as noted above.

Distal Femur Osteotomy

The distal femoral osteotomy is typically made in 4° to 7° of valgus. As with the tibial osteotomy, both extramedullary and intramedullary guides are available. However, prior literature has shown that intramedullary devices typically provide more accurate and reproducible results when compared with extramedullary guides (**Fig. 6-18**).[9,36,44-48] Indeed, one prior study comparing groups of TKA patients in whom extramedullary and intramedullary guides were used found that the distal femoral resection angle was outside the accepted range (4° to 10° of femoral valgus) in 28% of the extramedullary group compared to 14% in the IM group.[44] Joint line orientation was also outside the normal range twice as frequently in the EM group.

Importantly, in the case of femoral intramedullary guides, similar to tibial intramedullary guides, these guides can also result in errors in those with capacious femoral canals or femoral shaft deformity. The guides allow for the adjustment of the distal femur osteotomy to create a 4° to 7° valgus angle.

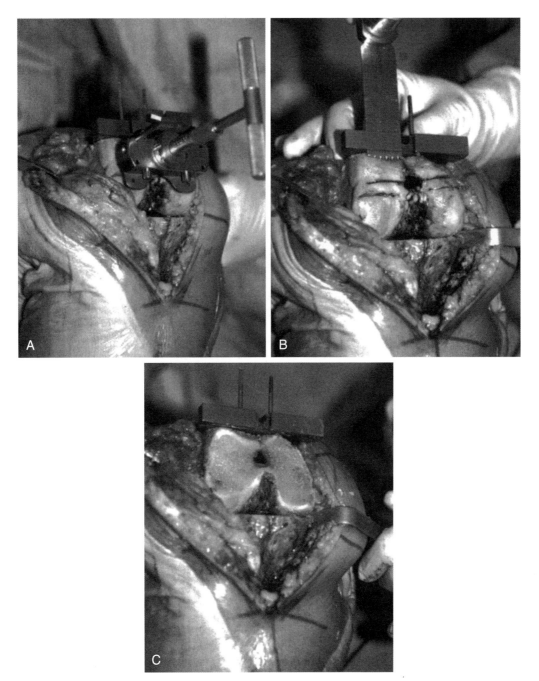

FIGURE 6-18 An intramedullary guide is set at 4° to 6° of valgus and placed into the femur **(A)**. The rod is removed and the osteotomy is performed **(B)**. Distal femur after the osteotomy is performed **(C)**.

Anterior and Posterior Femoral Condylar Cuts

The size of the distal femur is determined by either anterior or posterior referencing. Anterior referencing creates a measured resection with the anterior surface of the femur as a guide (**Fig. 6-19**). A cut at the level of the anterior cortex of the distal femoral shaft is preferred, as a cut above this level can lead to overstuffing the patellofemoral joint, impeding flexion of the knee. It is also important not to overaggressively resect, as excessive resection will lead to notching of the anterior femur which can predispose to fracture at this level.

A disadvantage of anterior referencing occurs when condylar anatomy falls between the standard sizes available in TKA systems. If this occurs, the smaller size implant should typically be selected to avoid overstuffing the patellofemoral joint. In cruciate-retaining knees, anterior referencing effectively elongates the posterior cruciate ligament and should be avoided.

Posterior-referencing, in contrast to anterior referencing, allows for optimization of the posterior condylar cut to maintain the tension of a retained PCL in cruciate-retaining TKAs. As with anterior referencing, knees that fall in between the standard sizes of TKA systems can be problematic. Oversized components again

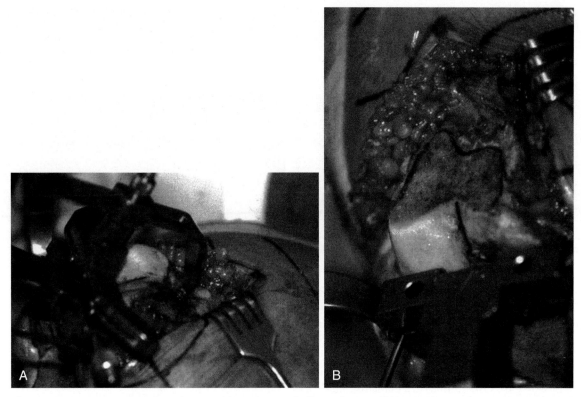

FIGURE 6-19 **A:** Anterior references systems place a guide on the anterior femoral cortex. This generally prevents anterior notching of the femur. **B:** When the appropriate anterior osteotomy has been completed, the contours of the osteotomy should have a bimodal shape referred as the grand piano sign and enough area to receive the anterior flange of the femoral component.

will overstuff the patellofemoral joint while undersizing will result in notching of the femur (**Fig. 6-20**). In PCL-substituting designs, the flexion gap increases by 2 to 3 mm requiring additional resection of the distal femur. Significant flexion of the femoral component can cause impingement on the tibial post.

External rotation of the femoral component is necessary to create a symmetric flexion gap and to facilitate normal patellar tracking.[49,50] Several methods are used to determine femoral component rotation, each which may be prone to inherent errors (**Fig. 6-21**).

1. The transepicondylar axis: a line drawn between the medial and lateral epicondyles.[51] The anatomy however can be difficult to identify (**Fig. 6-22**).
2. Whiteside's line[52,53]: a line in the deepest portion of the trochlea to the center of the intercondylar notch. A line perpendicular to this is the effective degree of femoral component external rotation (**Fig. 6-21**). This can be affected by altered trochlear anatomy such as patellofemoral arthritis.[54]

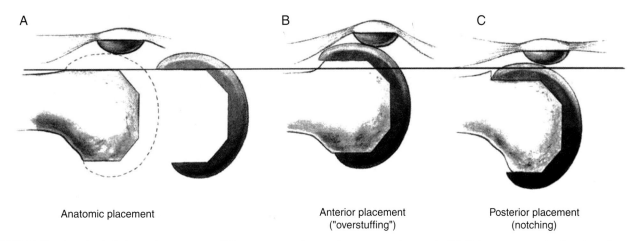

Anatomic placement   Anterior placement
                                             ("overstuffing")

                                             Posterior placement
                                             (notching)

FIGURE 6-20 A perfectly fit femoral component will have contours that conform to normal anatomy (**A**). If the component is placed too far anteriorly, it will lead to overstuffing of the patellofemoral joint (**B**). If it is placed too far posteriorly, it will notch the femur and narrow the flexion gap (**C**).

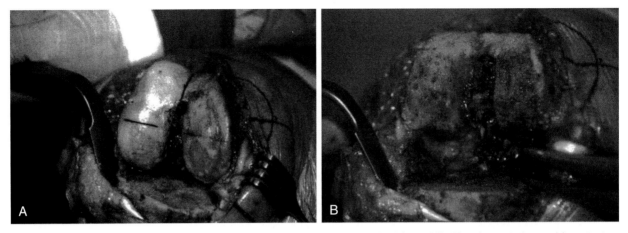

FIGURE 6-21 A knee with a transepicondylar axis and Whiteside's line drawn on the distal femur **(A)**. After the posterior condylar osteotomy, the flexion gap should be rectangular under tension of a laminar spreader **(B)**.

3. Posterior condylar axis: a line drawn between the posterior surface of the medial and lateral condyles with a prefixed 3° external rotation guide. The posterior femoral condyles however can be altered in significant arthritis.

4. Tension gap technique: a spreader is used to tension the flexion gap. Osteotomies are made to establish a symmetric flexion gap with the tibial shaft axis.[55] Again, this can be affected by the initial tibial cut and in those with ligamentous imbalance.

In prior studies, the transepicondylar axis most consistently created a balanced flexion gap when compared with methods based on of Whiteside's line or the posterior condylar axis.[56] In the case of the posterior condylar axis method, it has been demonstrated that the prefixed 3° of external rotation of the posterior condylar axis performed poorly in preoperatively valgus knees.[56,57]

An additional intraoperative check for proper rotation is the "footprint" created by the anterior osteotomy. It should look like a low and high bimodal curve referred as the grand piano sign (**Fig. 6-19B**). Most surgeons will use a combination of these techniques in combination to estimate femoral component rotation.

Patellofemoral tracking is influenced by the rotation of the femoral component.[49,58] External rotation of the femoral component brings the trochlea closer to the center of the patella. Excessive external rotation will also alter the flexion gap. By contrast, internal rotation of the femoral component results in a tight medial flexion gap and patella maltracking. Appropriate rotational alignment is essential in TKA.

ALIGNMENT STRATEGIES IN TKA

There are two alignment strategies in TKA to restore the mechanical axis of the lower extremity: mechanical alignment and kinematic alignment. In both cases, the HKA angle is often the same.

Mechanical alignment in TKA is performed by making the distal femoral cut and the proximal tibial cut perpendicular to their respective mechanical axes. Proponents of

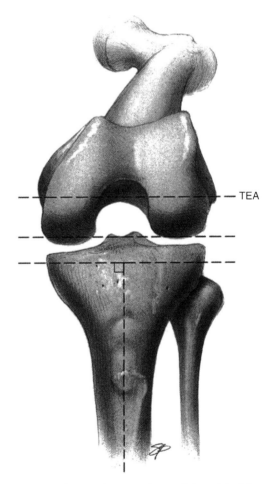

FIGURE 6-22 In flexion, the posterior medial condyle falls approximately 3° (3 mm) below the transepicondylar axis (TEA) than the lateral posterior condyle. The medial tibial plateau is approximately 3° (3 mm) more distal than the lateral tibial plateau. If you make a transverse tibial osteotomy, to maintain a balanced rectangular flexion space, you will resect more bone from the medial posterior condyle.

mechanical alignment believe that restoration of a neutral mechanical axis improves implant durability and function.[27] A prior study demonstrated that when the mechanical axis passed through the middle one-third of the TKA prosthesis, there was a 3% loosening rate compared to a 24% rate when it passed either medially or laterally.[59]

In kinematically aligned TKAs, the distal femoral osteotomy is made in 1° to 2° more valgus and the tibial cut is made in 1° to 2° more varus than in the native knee, leading to preservation of the natural alignment of the knee. Proponents believe that restoring kinematic alignment reestablishes the obliquity and location of the normal, prearthritic joint line and thus improves outcome, function, and satisfaction.[27]

Compared to the coronal alignment, the effects of variance in sagittal alignment of TKAs are not as well studied. Studies however have shown that when femoral components are flexed >3° or when the tibial component is in <0° or >7° of posterior slope, there is a significantly higher failure rate.[60] Therefore it is recommended the surgeon aim to place the femoral component in 0° to 3° of flexion and the tibial component with a posterior slope of 0° to 7°.[61]

CONCLUSION

The knee has multiple layers of complexity that allows for the full range of normal knee motion and function. These complexities must be well-understood in order to effectively reconstitute knee kinematics and motion when performing total knee arthroplasty. Although there are numerous options for individual surgeon preferences with regard to TKA instrumentation and referencing, the underlying principles of knee alignment remain the same across these systems and methods. When employed correctly, TKAs can accurately recapitulate native knee motion and function and can be a highly effective option for the treatment of osteoarthritis or other degenerative conditions of the knee.

REFERENCES

1. Muller W. *The Knee: Form, Function, and Ligament Reconstruction*. Berlin: Springer; 1983.
2. Hefzy MS, Kelly BP, Cooke TDV. Kinematics of the knee joint in deep flexion: a radiographic assessment. *Med Eng Phys*. 1998;20(4):302-307. doi:10.1016/s1350-4533(98)00024-1.
3. Elias SG, Freeman R, Gokcay EI. A correlative study of the geometry and anatomy of the distal femur. *Clin Orthop Relat Res*. 1990;260:98-103. doi:10.1097/00003086-199011000-00018.
4. Yoshioka Y, Siu D, Cooke TD. The anatomy and functional axes of the femur. *J Bone Joint Surg Am*. 1987;69(6):873-880. doi:10.2106/00004623-198769060-00012.
5. Shrive NG, O'Connor JJ, Goodfellow JW. Load-bearing in the knee joint. *Clin Orthop Relat Res*. 1978;131:279-287.
6. DeHaven KE, Arnoczky SP. Meniscus repair: basic science, indications for repair, and open repair. *Instr Course Lect*. 1994;43:65-76.
7. Hashemi J, Chandrashekar N, Gill B, et al. The geometry of the tibial plateau and its influence on the biomechanics of the tibiofemoral joint. *J Bone Joint Surg Am*. 2008;90(12):2724-2734. doi:10.2106/JBJS.G.01358.
8. Harrington IJ. A bioengineering analysis of force actions at the knee in normal and pathological gait. *Biomed Eng*. 1976;11(5):167-172.
9. Harrington IJ. Static and dynamic loading patterns in knee joints with deformities. *J Bone Joint Surg Am*. 1983;65(2):247-259.
10. Hsu RW, Himeno S, Coventry MB, Chao EY. Normal axial alignment of the lower extremity and load-bearing distribution at the knee. *Clin Orthop Relat Res*. 1990;255:215-227.
11. Hsu HP, Garg A, Walker PS, Spector M, Ewald FC. Effect of knee component alignment on tibial load distribution with clinical correlation. *Clin Orthop Relat Res*. 1989;248:135-144.
12. Ritter MA, Faris PM, Keating EM, Meding JB. Postoperative alignment of total knee replacement. Its effect on survival. *Clin Orthop Relat Res*. 1994;299:153-156.
13. Freeman MAR, Pinskerova V. The movement of the knee studied by magnetic resonance imaging. *Clin Orthop Relat Res*. 2003;410:35-43. doi:10.1097/01.blo.0000063598.67412.0d.
14. Hollister AM, Jatana S, Singh AK, Sullivan WW, Lupichuk AG. The axes of rotation of the knee. *Clin Orthop Relat Res*. 1993;290:259-268.
15. Churchill DL, Incavo SJ, Johnson CC, Beynnon BD. The transepicondylar axis approximates the optimal flexion axis of the knee. *Clin Orthop Relat Res*. 1998;356:111-118. doi:10.1097/00003086-199811000-00016.
16. Cooke TDV, Kelly B, Li J. Prosthetic reconstruction of the arthritic knee: considerations for limb alignment, geometry and soft tissue reconstruction. *Knee*. 1998;5(3):165-174. doi:10.1016/s0968-0160(97)10014-x.
17. Mills OS, Hull ML. Rotational flexibility of the human knee due to varus/valgus and axial moments in vivo. *J Biomech*. 1991;24(8):673-690. doi:10.1016/0021-9290(91)90332-h.
18. Asano T, Akagi M, Tanaka K, Tamura J, Nakamura T. In vivo three-dimensional knee kinematics using a biplanar image-matching technique. *Clin Orthop Relat Res*. 2001;388:157-166. doi:10.1097/00003086-200107000-00023.
19. Hamai S, Moro-oka T, Dunbar NJ, Miura H, Iwamoto Y, Banks SA. In vivo healthy knee kinematics during dynamic full flexion. *BioMed Res Int*. 2013;2013:717546. doi:10.1155/2013/717546.
20. Goodfellow J, O'Connor J. The mechanics of the knee and prosthesis design. *J Bone Joint Surg Br*. 1978;60-B(3):358-369. doi:10.1302/0301-620x.60b3.581081.
21. Fujikawa K, Seedhom BB, Wright V. Biomechanics of the patello-femoral joint. Part I: A study of the contact and the congruity of the patello-femoral compartment and movement of the patella. *Eng Med*. 1983;12(1):3-11. doi:10.1243/emed_jour_1983_012_004_02.
22. Ahmed AM, Burke DL, Hyder A. Force analysis of the patellar mechanism. *J Orthop Res*. 1987;5(1):69-85. doi:10.1002/jor.1100050110.
23. Cooke TDV, Chir B, Price N, Fisher B, Hedden D. The inwardly pointing knee. An unrecognized problem of external rotational malalignment. *Clin Orthop Relat Res*. 1990;260:56-60. doi:10.1097/00003086-199011000-00011.
24. Derek T, Cooke V, Allan Scudamore R, Greer W. Axial alignment of the lower limband its association with disorders of the knee. *Oper Tech Sports Med*. 2000;8(2):98-107. doi:10.1053/otsm.2000.6575.
25. Cooke TD, Li J, Scudamore RA. Radiographic assessment of bony contributions to knee deformity. *Orthop Clin North Am*. 1994;25(3):387-393.
26. Harrison MM, Cooke TD, Fisher SB, Griffin MP. Patterns of knee arthrosis and patellar subluxation. *Clin Orthop Relat Res*. 1994;309:56-63.
27. Cherian JJ, Kapadia BH, Banerjee S, Jauregui JJ, Issa K, Mont MA. Mechanical, anatomical, and kinematic axis in TKA: concepts and practical applications. *Curr Rev Musculoskelet Med*. 2014;7(2):89-95. doi:10.1007/s12178-014-9218-y.
28. Moreland JR, Bassett LW, Hanker GJ. Radiographic analysis of the axial alignment of the lower extremity. *J Bone Joint Surg*. 1987;69(5):745-749. doi:10.2106/00004623-198769050-00016.

29. Cooke TD, Scudamore RA, Bryant JT, Sorbie C, Siu D, Fisher B. A quantitative approach to radiography of the lower limb. Principles and applications. *J Bone Joint Surg Br.* 1991;73-B(5):715-720. doi:10.1302/0301-620x.73b5.1894656.

30. Cooke D, Scudamore A, Li J, Wyss U, Bryant T, Costigan P. Axial lower-limb alignment: comparison of knee geometry in normal volunteers and osteoarthritis patients. *Osteoarthr Cartil.* 1997;5(1):39-47. doi:10.1016/s1063-4584(97)80030-1.

31. Paley D, Tetsworth K. Mechanical axis deviation of the lower limbs. Preoperative planning of uniapical angular deformities of the tibia or femur. *Clin Orthop Relat Res.* 1992;280:48-64.

32. Neil MJ, Atupan JB, Panti JPL, Massera RAJ, Howard S. Evaluation of lower limb axial alignment using digital radiography stitched films in pre-operative planning for total knee replacement. *J Orthop.* 2016;13(4):285-289. doi:10.1016/j.jor.2016.06.013.

33. Yoshioka Y, Cooke TDV. Femoral anteversion: assessment based on function axes. *J Orthop Res.* 1987;5(1):86-91. doi:10.1002/jor.1100050111.

34. Fulkerson JP, Shea KP. Disorders of patellofemoral alignment. *J Bone Joint Surg.* 1990;72(9):1424-1429. doi:10.2106/00004623-199072090-00027.

35. Yoshioka Y, Siu DW, Scudamore RA, Cooke TDV. Tibial anatomy and functional axes. *J Orthop Res.* 1989;7(1):132-137. doi:10.1002/jor.1100070118.

36. Siegel JL, Shall LM. Femoral instrumentation using the anterosuperior iliac spine as a landmark in total knee arthroplasty. An anatomic study. *J Arthroplasty.* 1991;6(4):317-320.

37. Sled EA, Sheehy LM, Felson DT, Costigan PA, Lam M, Cooke TDV. Reliability of lower limb alignment measures using an established landmark-based method with a customized computer software program. *Rheumatol Int.* 2011;31(1):71-77. doi:10.1007/s00296-009-1236-5.

38. Glimet T, Massé JP, Ryckewaert A. Radiological study of painless knees in 50 women more than 65 years old. I. Frontal teleradiography in an upright position. *Rev Rhum Mal Osteoartic.* 1979;46(11):589-592.

39. Caylor D, Fites R, Worrell TW. The relationship between quadriceps angle and anterior knee pain syndrome. *J Orthop Sports Phys Ther.* 1993;17(1):11-16. doi:10.2519/jospt.1993.17.1.11.

40. Tetsworth K, Paley D. Malalignment and degenerative arthropathy. *Orthop Clin North Am.* 1994;25(3):367-377.

41. Paley D. *Principles of Deformity Correction.* Berlin Heidelberg: Springer-Verlag; 2002.

42. Jeong C, Noh JH. Clinical and radiological analysis of angular deformity of lower extremities. *J Korean Fract Soc.* 2017;30(3):156. doi:10.12671/jkfs.2017.30.3.156.

43. Dennis DA, Channer M, Susman MH, Stringer EA. Intramedullary versus extramedullary tibial alignment systems in total knee arthroplasty. *J Arthroplasty.* 1993;8(1):43-47.

44. Cates HE, Ritter MA, Keating EM, Faris PM. Intramedullary versus extramedullary femoral alignment systems in total knee replacement. *Clin Orthop Relat Res.* 1993;286:32-39.

45. Teter KE, Bregman D, Colwell CW. The efficacy of intramedullary femoral alignment in total knee replacement. *Clin Orthop Relat Res.* 1995;321:117-121.

46. Engh GA, Petersen TL. Comparative experience with intramedullary and extramedullary alignment in total knee arthroplasty. *J Arthroplasty.* 1990;5(1):1-8.

47. Ritter MA, Campbell ED. A model for easy location of the center of the femoral head during total knee arthroplasty. *J Arthroplasty.* 1988;3(Suppl):S59-S61.

48. Tillett ED, Engh GA, Petersen T. A comparative study of extramedullary and intramedullary alignment systems in total knee arthroplasty. *Clin Orthop Relat Res.* 1988;230:176-181.

49. Anouchi YS, Whiteside LA, Kaiser AD, Milliano MT. The effects of axial rotational alignment of the femoral component on knee stability and patellar tracking in total knee arthroplasty demonstrated on autopsy specimens. *Clin Orthop Relat Res.* 1993;287:170-177.

50. Rhoads DD, Noble PC, Reuben JD, Mahoney OM, Tullos HS. The effect of femoral component position on patellar tracking after total knee arthroplasty. *Clin Orthop Relat Res.* 1990;260:43-51.

51. Stiehl JB, Abbott BD. Morphology of the transepicondylar axis and its application in primary and revision total knee arthroplasty. *J Arthroplasty.* 1995;10(6):785-789.

52. Arima J, Whiteside LA, McCarthy DS, White SE. Femoral rotational alignment, based on the anteroposterior axis, in total knee arthroplasty in a valgus knee. A technical note. *J Bone Joint Surg Am.* 1995;77(9):1331-1334.

53. Whiteside LA, Arima J. The anteroposterior axis for femoral rotational alignment in valgus total knee arthroplasty. *Clin Orthop Relat Res.* 1995;321:168-172.

54. Poilvache PL, Insall JN, Scuderi GR, Font-Rodriguez DE. Rotational landmarks and sizing of the distal femur in total knee arthroplasty. *Clin Orthop Relat Res.* 1996;331:35-46.

55. Stiehl JB, Cherveny PM. Femoral rotational alignment using the tibial shaft axis in total knee arthroplasty. *Clin Orthop Relat Res.* 1996;331:47-55.

56. Olcott CW, Scott RD. A comparison of 4 intraoperative methods to determine femoral component rotation during total knee arthroplasty. *J Arthroplasty.* 2000;15(1):22-26.

57. Akagi M, Yamashita E, Nakagawa T, Asano T, Nakamura T. Relationship between frontal knee alignment and reference axes in the distal femur. *Clin Orthop Relat Res.* 2001;388:147-156.

58. Berger RA, Crossett LS, Jacobs JJ, Rubash HE. Malrotation causing patellofemoral complications after total knee arthroplasty. *Clin Orthop Relat Res.* 1998;356:144-153.

59. Jeffery RS, Morris RW, Denham RA. Coronal alignment after total knee replacement. *J Bone Joint Surg Br.* 1991;73(5):709-714.

60. Kim Y-H, Park J-W, Kim J-S, Park S-D. The relationship between the survival of total knee arthroplasty and postoperative coronal, sagittal and rotational alignment of knee prosthesis. *Int Orthop.* 2014;38(2):379-385. doi:10.1007/s00264-013-2097-9.

61. Gromov K, Korchi M, Thomsen MG, Husted H, Troelsen A. What is the optimal alignment of the tibial and femoral components in knee arthroplasty? *Acta Orthop.* 2014;85(5):480-487. doi:10.3109/17453674.2014.940573.

chapter 7

Knee Kinematics Following Total Knee Arthroplasty

Michael T. LaCour, PhD | Milad Khasian, MS | Douglas A. Dennis, MD | Richard D. Komistek, PhD

Following the logic of the "Forgotten Knee," a common goal of total knee arthroplasty (TKA) is to restore joint functionality as closely as possible to that of a healthy, nonimplanted knee, such that the implant effectively restores overall function to the point where the patient completely forgets they have a replaced knee.[1-3] In an effort to quantify and analyze joint performance to improve overall TKA designs, substantial research has been done to better understand joint mechanics. This research is commonly done under the assumption that "if components are moving correctly, then the device must be performing well."[3]

Simply determining the motion (kinematics) of a TKA is the easy part, as this is just a matter of utilizing proper imaging techniques to extract the desired kinematic parameters. Determining if the components are moving "correctly" is often a debated topic. However, the general consensus is that the motions of a knee following a TKA procedure should closely mimic those of the healthy, nonimplanted knee.[3,4]

OVERVIEW OF KNEE KINEMATICS

A brief overview of the kinematics of the knee will be provided in this section.

A properly constrained knee has three independent degrees of freedom, two rotational and one translational, yielding flexion and extension about the medial/lateral axis, internal and external rotation about the superior/inferior axis, and translational sliding in the anterior and posterior directions. Under certain conditions, it is also possible for the femur to rotate about the anterior/posterior axis, demonstrating a phenomenon of condylar lift-off,[5-7] but this is generally considered abnormal. Other forms of motion of the knee joint are also possible, but these are generally negligible compared to the aforementioned three.

Due to soft-tissue constraints in combination with the bone geometry of the knee, it is generally a safe assumption that the normal knee actually functions as a one degree-of-freedom joint (knee flexion/extension), driven by the quadriceps and hamstring muscle groups, and that other motions are dependent on knee flexion.[3] More specifically, at full extension and in early flexion, the femur

is generally internally rotated with respect to the tibia.[8-10] As the knee begins to flex (such as with a knee bend or squat activity), the femur begins to rotate externally with respect to the tibia.[4,7,11-16] Throughout flexion, both condyles of the femur generally roll or slide posteriorly atop the tibia.[3,7,10,12] However, the lateral condyle moves more posteriorly than the medial condyle, resulting in more of a pivoting pattern about the medial condyle with a roll-back pattern of the lateral condyle, which directly correlates to the external rotation pattern of the femur. In deep flexion, it is possible for both condyles to roll so far posteriorly that they can roll off the edge of the tibial plateau.

The patella bone plays an integral role in transmitting the forces of the quadriceps muscles by increasing the moment arms of the extensor forces and creating a direct link between the quadriceps and the tibial tuberosity. Hence, the patellofemoral joint is an integral part of the knee. Throughout flexion, the patella generally remains in contact with the femur.[17,18] In early- and mid-flexion, there is a single region of contact between the femur and patella as the patella tracks within the trochlear groove of the femur. At deeper angles of flexion (greater than 90°), the patella begins to track between the femoral condyles, dividing the contact area into two separate regions. In general, patellar flexion increases with increasing knee flexion,[17,19-23] but it does so at a lower rate than the femur relative to tibia.

While kinematic evaluations of the nonimplanted knee commonly document posterior translation of the femoral condyles and external rotation of the femur with respect to the tibia with increasing knee flexion, the kinematic patterns of patients having a TKA can vary considerably. Common differences include reduced posterior translation of the femur, paradoxical anterior sliding of the femur, reverse axial rotation patterns of the femur with increasing flexion, occurrences of femoral condylar lift-off, and abnormal patellofemoral mechanics.[4,7,11,24-27]

KINEMATIC ANALYSIS TECHNIQUES

Many different methods have been used to analyze the kinematics of the normal knee and the knee after implantation of total knee arthroplasty. These have included roentgen stereophotogrammetric analyses,[28-33] *in vitro* cadaveric evaluations,[34-36] quasi-dynamic magnetic resonance imaging testing,[13,37,38] noninvasive laboratory motion analysis systems using marker tracking,[14,39-43] and *in vivo* video fluoroscopy.[5,26,44-49] While each of these techniques certainly is valuable in its own way, it is essential to recognize both the advantages and disadvantages of each technique to accurately interpret the results of a specific analysis.

For example, roentgen stereophotogrammetric analyses, although generally highly accurate and precise,[28,29] are also highly invasive and are commonly performed under non–weight-bearing conditions and are quasi-dynamic.[30-33] Cadaveric studies allow for up-close observation of a physical specimen, but they often do not simulate *in vivo* conditions because the actuators used to apply joint loads are unable to accurately reproduce *in vivo* motions. MRI testing is conducted under static, non–weight-bearing conditions, which does not represent what is happening during daily dynamic activity. Additionally, while video marker systems excel in capturing high-speed multibody movement, error analyses of video marker evaluations have suggested these systems can induce significant out-of-plane rotational and translational error, owing to motion between skin markers and underlying osseous structures.[14,50,51] Finally, video fluoroscopy (single-plane and biplanar) and 3D model-fitting techniques have the advantage of being highly accurate when testing under *in vivo*, weight-bearing, fully dynamic conditions, but the subjects generally must perform slower-speed activities.[5,44-49,52]

This chapter summarizes various *in vivo* kinematic analyses of multiple groups of patients implanted with various designs of fixed- and mobile-bearing TKA and compares their *in vivo* knee kinematic patterns to those studies of the normal knee. The specific results found herein were collected using video fluoroscopy and three-dimensional-to-two-dimensional (3D-to-2D) registration techniques. Therefore, more specific information on the employed fluoroscopic analysis techniques is presented below.

FLUOROSCOPIC ANALYSIS METHODS

During fluoroscopic study data collection, subjects perform various activities, such as deep knee bend, gait, chair rise, step up, step down, ramps, leg swings, and more, while the subject's joint is under fluoroscopic surveillance (**Fig. 7-1**). Fluoroscopic studies of the knee are generally conducted in the sagittal plane. Upon completion of the activities, specific frames of interest (for example, specific increments of flexion or specific phases of the gait cycle) are extracted from the fluoroscopic video and exported into preprocessing software for further analysis. Depending on the type of fluoroscopy unit used, the images may experience distortion, which must be corrected. After the images have been properly processed, they can be exported to a model-fitting software program for 3D-to-2D registration.[53-55]

A more recent advancement in fluoroscopic studies is the implementation of robotic tracking fluoroscope system (TFS) units. These units have automated control systems

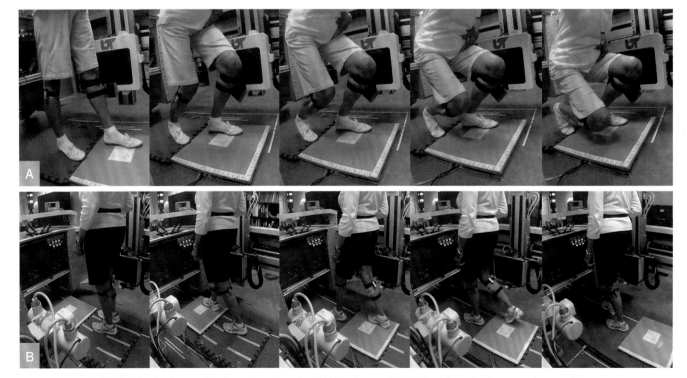

FIGURE 7-1   Subject performing a deep knee bend **(A)** and normal gait **(B)** while under fluoroscopic surveillance.

that (1) allow the entire unit to follow a patient around a room, and (2) allow the x-ray source and detector to move independently from the rest of the unit to keep the knee (or any joint of interest) in the center of the fluoroscopy video. These robotic units allow for fluoroscopic evaluations of more complex activities, such as ramp activities, several stair steps in succession, and multiple gait cycles, all at more natural speeds.[56] Although fluoroscopic studies with TFS units are relatively new, it is hypothesized that these TFS studies will allow patients to conduct activities in a much more natural, unconstrained manner versus traditional C-arm fluoroscopy units, thereby yielding results that more accurately represent a patient's daily activities.[53,56]

Fluoroscopic analysis and 3D-to-2D registration techniques can be utilized on both implanted and nonimplanted knee images. For implanted knees, the component CAD models must be used. For nonimplanted knees, the bone models must be created from CT, MRI, or other imaging methods. In either case, to find the orientation of a desired knee "component" (implanted CAD model or nonimplanted bone model) from an x-ray image, the fluoroscopic space is virtually modeled within a specialized computer program. This program allows the user to virtually recreate the fluoroscopic space between the x-ray source and the image intensifier, and the models of the knee components are virtually placed in the space between the camera and the image (**Fig. 7-2**). This allows the user to superimpose (overlay) the CAD model silhouettes on top of the implant component silhouettes from the x-ray image. By matching a 3D model of the knee component to each fluoroscopic frame of interest from the video, the 3D *in vivo* kinematics can be extracted by interpolating between multiple 2D images (**Fig. 7-3**).[53]

In general, the errors associated with this model-fitting technique are less than 0.5 mm for in-plane translations and 0.5° for rotations.[54] Out-of-plane errors are normally higher. The use of fluoroscopy units with higher frame rates and greater image resolutions will increase the accuracy of the fluoroscopic analyses.

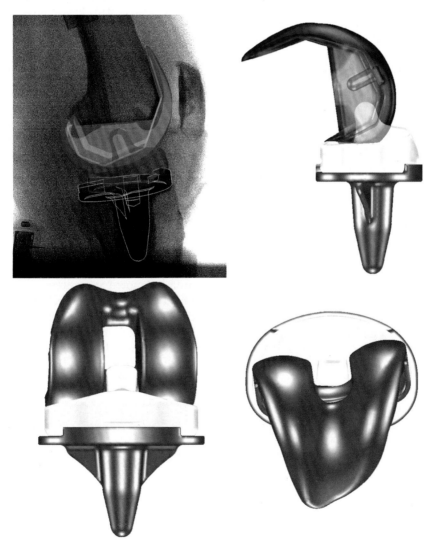

FIGURE 7-2 Example of the three-dimensional model-fitting overlay **(top left)**, the implant component grouped together and rotated to a pure sagittal view **(top right)**, then rotated to a pure frontal view to assess for condylar lift-off **(bottom left)**, and then to a pure top view to assess for axial rotation **(bottom right)**.

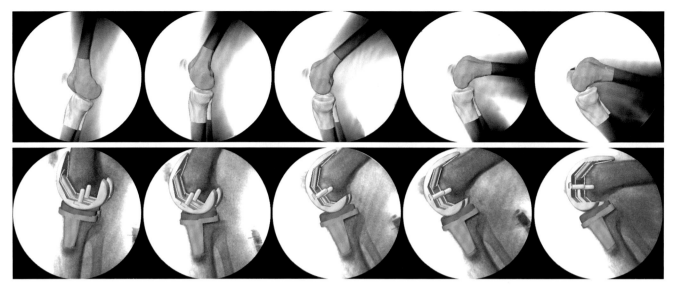

FIGURE 7-3   Discrete 3D kinematic representations for both nonimplanted and implanted knees.

KNEE KINEMATICS

The data presented below include the knee joint kinematics of 491 subjects assessed using video fluoroscopy techniques, consisting of 104 nonimplanted knees, 225 implanted with a fixed-bearing (FB) posterior cruciate retaining (PCR) TKA, 142 featuring an FB posterior stabilized (PS) TKA, and 20 having mobile-bearing (MB) PS TKA. All TKA subjects selected from studies done in our research facility in the past 7 years, featuring modern commercialized knee implants. The average age of subjects was 38.1 (18.1 to 84.2 years, $\sigma = 18.1$ years), 68.1 (43.0 to 85.0 years, $\sigma = 7.7$ years), 67.2 (49.0 to 84.2 years, $\sigma = 7.4$ years), and 66.7 (58.6 to 68.9 years, $\sigma = 2.3$ years) for normal, FB PCR TKA, FB PS TKA, and MB PS TKA respectively, shown in **Table 7-1**.

Deep Knee Bend—Range of Motion

The average maximum weight-bearing flexion was 141.1° (61° to 163°, $\sigma = 21.5$°), 103.0° (46° to 138°, $\sigma = 13.7$°), 103.7° (58° to 140°, $\sigma = 17.9$°), and 114.5° (88° to 140°, $\sigma = 14.4$°) for normal, FB PCR TKA, FB PS TKA, and MB PS TKA, respectively (**Fig. 7-4A**). There are 10 subjects in the

healthy group with maximum weight-bearing flexion less than 100° (**Fig. 7-4B**). These subjects were from a study on patients having TKA on one knee and performing the DKB with their nonimplanted knee. The implanted knee was a limiting factor for these subjects achieving higher knee flexion. Finally, among all groups, 2/104 (1.9%) of non-implanted knees experienced overall reverse axial rotation from full extension to maximum flexion, while this ratio was 55/225 (24.4%) for FB PCR TKAs, 9/142 (6.3%) for FB PS TKAs, and 2/20 (10.0%) for MB PS TKAs.

Deep Knee Bend—Condylar Translation

Throughout flexion, the lowest points on the femoral condyles were tracked and used to calculate the relative motion of the lateral condyle (lateral anteroposterior position, LAP) and the medial condyle (medial anteroposterior position, MAP) relative to the tibial tray. Anterior motion is denoted as positive.

On average, during DKB the lateral condyle translated -21.5 ± 7.2 mm, -1.8 ± 3.5 mm, -7.8 ± 5.1 mm, and -5.8 ± 2.3 mm from full extension to maximum flexion for normal, FB PCR, FB PS, and MB PS groups, respectively. On average the majority of lateral rollback

TABLE 7-1	Demographics Data for Subjects in This Review			
	Healthy	**FB PCR**	**FB PS**	**MB PS**
Parameter	**N = 104**	**N = 225**	**N = 142**	**N = 20**
Gender (female/male)	55/49	91/134	87/55	6/14
Age (y)	38.1 ± 18.1	68.1 ± 7.7	67.2 ± 7.4	66.7 ± 2.3
Height (m)	1.67 ± 0.11	1.71 ± 0.11	1.70 ± 0.11	1.73 ± 0.07
Mass (kg)	71.0 ± 16.6	89.8 ± 17.5	86.1 ± 16.7	82.3 ± 11.1
BMI (kg/m²)	25.2 ± 4.6	30.1 ± 4.9	30.0 ± 5.1	27.3 ± 3.9

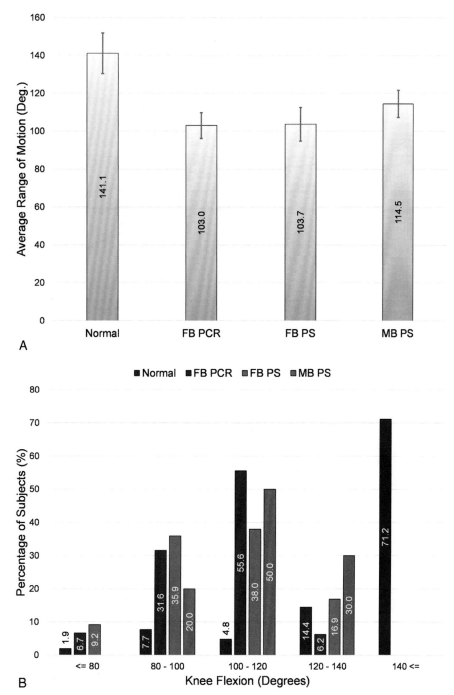

FIGURE 7-4 The average maximum weight-bearing flexion. **A:** The average range of motion for each group. **B:** Percentage of subjects who achieve knee flexion greater than specified.

happened in the first 30° of flexion (**Fig. 7-5B**). For all groups except the FB PCR, between 30° to 90° of flexion a slight lateral rollback was observed. Subjects in the FB PCR group experienced slight anterior sliding during mid-flexion. For subjects achieving more than 90° of flexion, all groups experienced lateral rollback, with subjects in FB PS and MB PS group experiencing the most rollback, which could be because of the cam-post engagement.

Overall, the medial condyle motion is smaller compared to the lateral condyle, and all group averages except for the FB PCR group showed posterior rollback. During DKB, the medial condyle moved −13.8 ± 3.5 mm, 1.3 ± 2.9 mm, −2.6 ± 3.6 mm, and −1.3 ± 2.5 mm from full extension to maximum flexion for normal, FB PCR, FB PS, and MB PS groups, respectively. Normal subjects experienced consistent medial rollback throughout flexion except from 90° to 120° of knee flexion (**Fig. 7-6**). The patterns of medial AP translation for all TKA groups were mixed, generally yielding posterior translation in early flexion, anterior sliding in mid-flexion, and posterior rollback during late flexion.

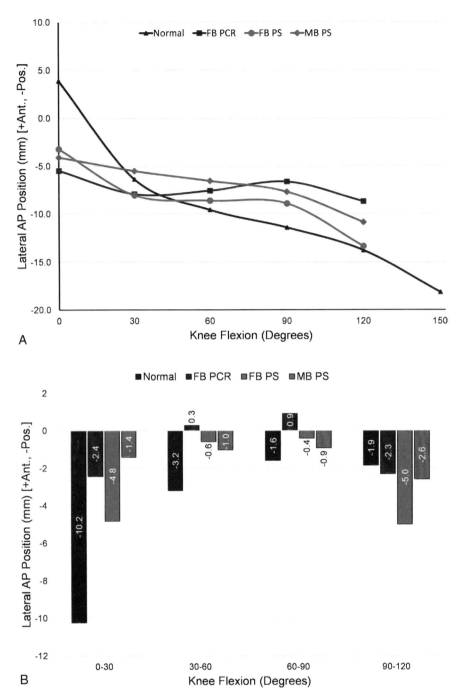

FIGURE 7-5   Average lateral femoral condyle AP position during the DKB activity. **A:** Overall lateral condyle AP motion for each group. **B:** Amount of lateral AP motion broken down by flexion range.

Deep Knee Bend—Axial Rotation

Two different methods were utilized to calculate the axial rotation. For TKA groups, axial rotation was obtained using the low point method by calculating the angle created between the line joining the LAP/MAP points and the mediolateral axis of the tibial tray (external rotation of the femur with respect to the tibia is denoted as positive).[57] For normal subjects, the Grood and Suntay[58] method was used. When comparing these two methods, it is important to note that the low point method calculates

and assumes axial rotation values based on computed contact points, while the Grood and Suntay method calculates axial rotation values based on bone landmarks and coordinate systems. In the case of TKA analyses, the required bony landmarks for Grood and Suntay are often not present. Conversely, for nonimplanted analyses, the lowest point of the condyles is often not the true contact point.

The average axial rotation from full extension to max flexion during DKB was 27.1° ± 12.1°, 3.9° ± 4.9°, 6.6° ± 4.9°, and 5.9° ± 4.4°, for normal, FB PCR, FB PS, and MB

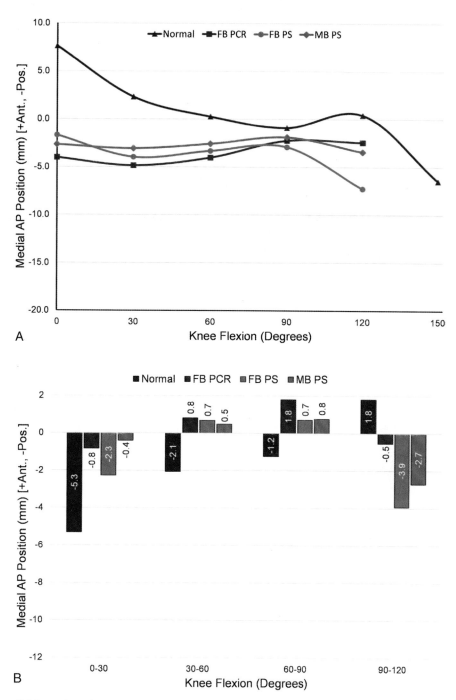

FIGURE 7-6   Average medial femoral condyle AP position during the DKB activity. **A:** Overall medial condyle AP motion for each group. **B:** Amount of medial AP motion broken down by flexion range.

PS subjects, respectively. On average, all group averages generally demonstrated consistent external axial rotation throughout the flexion. The largest axial rotation occurred in the early flexion for the normal group, shown in **Fig. 7-7**.

Gait

The kinematics parameters during gait for 228 patients, 175 implanted with FB PCR TKA and 53 having FB PS TKA, were obtained. The average age was 67.8 ± 7.7 years and 65.3 ± 6.7 years, for FB PCR and FB PS, respectively. These

parameters include LAP, MAP, and axial rotation at ipsilateral heel strike (0%), contralateral toe off (33%), contralateral heel strike (66%), and ipsilateral toe off (100%) (**Table 7-2**). On average, the lateral condyle moved −1.2 ± 2.1 mm and −0.5 ± 2.3 mm throughout gait cycle, while the medial AP translations were 0.0 ± 2.3 mm and −0.3 ± 2.4 mm, for FB PCR and FB PS, respectively. These patterns are similar to what has been reported for normal subjects during walking, where the lateral condyle translates more than the medial condyle during the gait cycle. In 2003, Komistek et al. reported average AP translations for normal subjects of

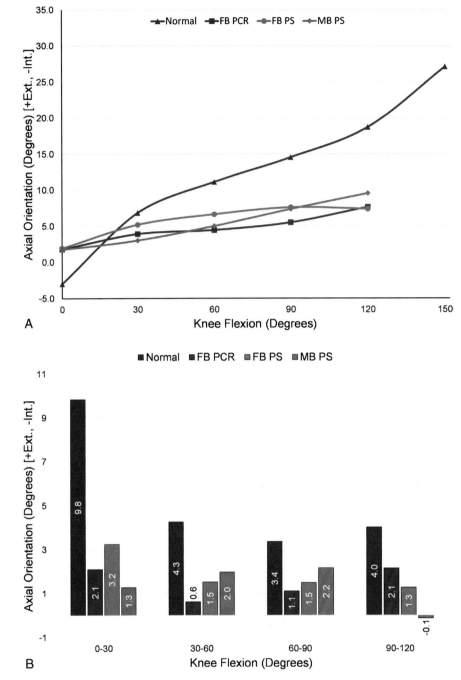

FIGURE 7-7   Average axial rotation of femur with respect to the tibia during the DKB activity. **A:** Overall axial rotation for each group. **B:** Amount of axial rotation broken down by flexion range.

−4.3 mm (−10.3 to −1.9 mm) and −0.9 mm (−0.8 to 6.2 mm) for lateral and medial condyles, respectively.[4] In 2019, Gray et al. also reported greater posterior rollback of the lateral condyle (15.4 mm) than the medial condyle (9.7 mm).[59]

On average from the current data, the axial rotation throughout the entire cycle was 1.1° ± 3.5° and 0.5° ± 2.7°, for FB PCR and FB PS, respectively (**Fig. 7-8**). Similar to condylar motion, axial rotation in TKA patients during gait was smaller relative to normal subjects. In 2003, Komistek et al. reported 4.4° (−1.8° to 7°) of external rotation for normal subjects during level walking.[4]

Chair Rise

The kinematics were assessed during a chair rise activity for 207 patients, 175 having FB PCR and 32 having FB PS, with an average age of 67.8 ± 7.7 years and 60.6 ± 6.3 years, respectively. On average, for the patients who were able to achieve 90° of flexion, the lateral condyle moved 1.4 ± 2.9 mm and 4.0 ± 3.8 mm from 90° of flexion to full extension for FB PCR and FB PS, respectively. Medial condyle translations were −4.0 ± 3.1 mm and −2.1 ± 2.8 mm, for FB PCR and FB PS, respectively. The femur began externally rotated at 90° and then rotated internally with

TABLE 7-2 Average Kinematics During Gait for FB PCR and FB PS

Gait Cycle (%)			LAP (mm)				MAP (mm)				Axial Rotation (°)			
			0	33	66	100	0	33	66	100	0	33	66	100
FB PCR	N = 175	Average	−5.3	−5.9	−6.0	−6.4	−4.4	−5.1	−5.1	−4.7	1.1	1.1	1.3	2.2
		Standard deviation	3.3	3.6	3.4	3.7	3.0	3.2	3.2	3.2	4.2	4.3	3.8	4.6
		Minimum	−14.9	−17.3	−19.5	−20.3	−14.7	−15.4	−16.7	−16.9	−8.2	−9.6	−8.5	−10.4
		Maximum	2.5	5.5	3.0	5.2	2.2	2.0	4.0	4.3	14.7	18.0	17.0	18.7
FB PS	N = 53	Average	−5.8	−6.6	−6.5	−6.3	−4.6	−4.9	−4.7	−4.7	1.6	2.2	2.2	2.1
		Standard deviation	2.6	2.7	2.6	2.7	2.7	2.0	2.1	2.7	4.1	3.9	3.9	4.5
		Minimum	−12.4	−15.1	−15.6	−14.2	−9.0	−8.9	−8.8	−10.2	−6.2	−4.3	−6.1	−5.7
		Maximum	0.7	−0.3	−0.6	−0.4	5.2	1.5	2.1	3.8	11.9	12.5	14.5	13.1

LAP, lateral anteroposterior position; MAP, medial anteroposterior position.

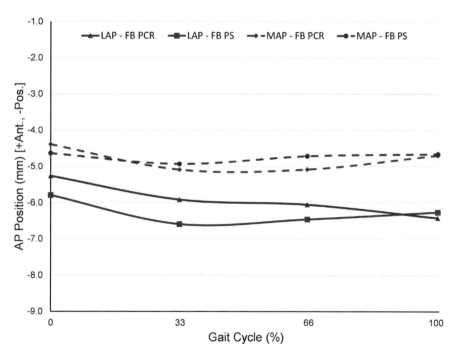

FIGURE 7-8 Tibiofemoral AP position kinematics during gait for FB PCR and FB PS knees.

respect to the tibia by −6.2° ± 4.7° and −7.5° ± 6.0° for FB PCR and FB PS, respectively (**Fig. 7-9**).

Like other activities, the magnitudes of condylar translation and axial rotation during chair rise for TKA patients were smaller compared to normal subjects. In 2003, Komistek et al. reported 16.9 mm and 2.2 mm of lateral and medial condylar rollback for normal subjects, respectively.[4] In the Komistek 2003 study, while the average lateral condyle translation was greater than the average medial condyle translation, one out of the five subjects experienced less translation of the lateral condyle than of the medial condyle, which is opposite the commonly reported pattern. Komistek et al. in 2003[4] and Lafortune et al. in 1992[14] reported 19.4° and 18.3° of internal rotation during chair rise activity for normal subjects, respectively.

Ramp Activities

During an activity where the subjects walked up a ramp (ramp up), the lateral condyle moved posteriorly from start to finish for all three groups, −1.5 ± 1.8 mm, −1.0 ± 2.6 mm, and −2.1 ± 5.0 mm, for normal, FB PCR, and FB PS, respectively. For the medial condyle, normal subjects showed a slight anterior slide, 0.3 ± 1.1 mm, while FB PCR and FB PS subjects showed posterior rollback, −1.7

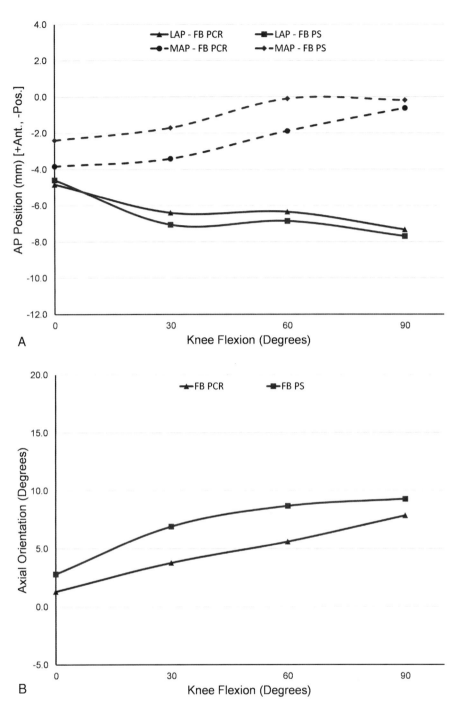

FIGURE 7-9   Tibiofemoral kinematics for all patients during chair rise. **A:** AP position. **B:** Axial rotation. Patients sitting in chair denoted with flexion of 0° and fully extend denoted with 90° of flexion.

± 2.9 mm and −1.1 ± 3.7 mm, respectively (**Fig. 7-10**). Throughout the entire cycle, the femur externally rotates with respect to the tibia for normal and FB PS subjects by 2.4° ± 3.0° and 1.2° ± 3.9°, respectively. However, the FB PCR subjects, the femur showed an internal rotation of −1.0° ± 5.0° (**Fig. 7-11**).

During ramp down, the LAP translations for all three groups are similar in corresponding ranges of the cycle, showing rollback except between contralateral heel strike (66%) and ipsilateral toe off (100%), where anterior sliding was observed for all groups (**Fig.**

7-12). On average, subjects in all groups showed medial rollback, with normal and FB PCR groups having the majority of the rollback between ipsilateral heel strike (0%) and contralateral toe off (33%), while the FB PS group showed the largest rollback between contralateral toe off (33%) and contralateral heel strike (66%) (**Fig. 7-12**). The normal subject showed 4.5° ± 5.1° of axial rotation throughout the entire activity. Subjects in FB PCR and FB PS groups experienced slightly smaller axial rotation values, 1.0° ± 4.5° and 1.7° ± 4.5°, respectively (**Fig. 7-13**).

77

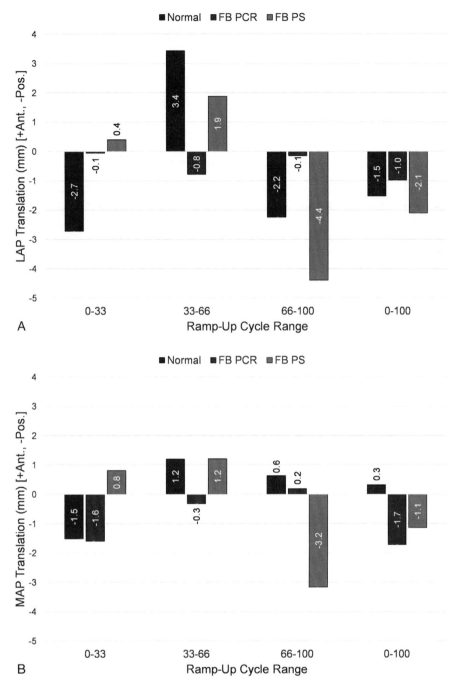

FIGURE 7-10 AP translation during the ramp up activity for different ranges of the ramp-up cycle. **A:** Lateral AP translation. **B:** Medial AP translation.

HIGHLY VARIABLE KNEE KINEMATICS

In vivo, weight-bearing fluoroscopic analyses of various TKA, including the results presented herein, commonly demonstrate numerous kinematic abnormalities when compared to nonimplanted knees.[7,10,12,26,48,52,60-62] For the results presented here, the most prevalent abnormalities include paradoxical anterior femoral translation, reverse axial rotational patterns, and decreased range of motion (ROM). In general, high variability (indicated by high standard deviations) among all groups and all activities designates that, while there are

certainly general patterns that are common, knee kinematics are largely patient-specific and can be highly variable.

This highly variable nature of both nonimplanted and implanted knee kinematics is an extremely important aspect of TKA design. While condylar motion and axial rotation patterns certainly have physical effects on the behavior of the knee, it would be counterproductive to *force* a knee to match a desired pattern. Every human being in the world is different, and therefore every knee in the world is different, and assuming that each knee must match a specific pattern would

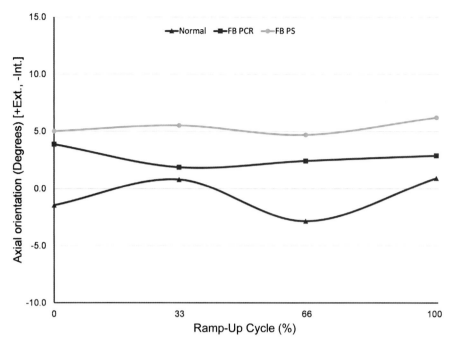

FIGURE 7-11 Average axial rotation of femur with respect to the tibia during the ramp-up activity.

be a mistake. Thus, the prospect of patient-specific implants and surgical jigs quickly becomes appealing. While it is certainly important to understand how specific kinematic patterns affect the overall success of the system, it is more important that we figure out how to let these kinematic patterns be a *result* of a successful TKA instead of a *driver*.

EFFECTS OF CONDYLAR TRANSLATION

Reduced anteroposterior translation when comparing implanted to nonimplanted knees was commonly observed during a DKB maneuver. Posterior femoral rollback (PFR) is greater in PS TKA designs, which is attributed to mechanical engagement of the cam-and-post mechanism of these designs. The cam-and-post mechanism effectively "pushes" the knee posteriorly during deeper flexion, ensuring that PFR is achieved, as opposed to relying on ligament functionality in CR designs. PFR does not appear to be directly related to bearing mobility, as we have observed increased PFR in both fixed- and mobile-bearing PS TKA designs, as long as a cam-and-post mechanism is present.[48,63] Typically, less anteroposterior femorotibial translation occurs during lower flexion activities such as gait.

The anterior translation of the femur on the tibia observed in fluoroscopic investigations has numerous potential negative consequences. First, anterior femoral translation results in a more anterior axis of flexion, lessening maximum knee flexion.[47] Secondly, the quadriceps moment arm is decreased, resulting in reduced quadriceps efficiency. Third, anterior sliding of the femoral component on the tibial polyethylene surface risks accelerated polyethylene wear. Blunn et al.,[64] in a sophisticated laboratory evaluation of polyethylene wear, found dramatically increased polyethylene wear with cyclic sliding, as occurs with paradoxical anterior translation, when compared with compression or rolling because of increased subsurface shear stresses.

Andriacchi et al.[65] reported that the predominant shear force during gait and stair climbing is directed posteriorly on the tibia and is normally resisted by tension in the PCL, preventing anteriorization of the femorotibial contact position. Multiple authors[65-67] have shown that anteroposterior femorotibial translation is related to the integrity of the cruciate ligaments and the mechanics of the extensor mechanism, particularly the direction of pull of the patellar ligament and the degree of knee flexion. At lesser degrees of flexion, the direction of the patellar ligament pull is directed anteriorly, creating an anterior pull on the tibia. This anteriorly directed shear force on the tibia is normally resisted by the anterior cruciate ligament. However, at greater degrees of flexion (more than 45° to 60°), the direction of patellar ligament pull on the tibial changes to posterior. This creates a posterior shear force on the tibia, which normally is resisted by tension in the PCL. This may explain the abnormal posterior contact observed at full extension in some of the TKA designs discussed in this report. At this flexion range, shear stresses on the tibia are directed anteriorly, allowing posterior femorotibial contact to occur because of the absence of the anterior cruciate ligament. Beyond mid-flexion, the shear forces on the tibia are directed posteriorly,

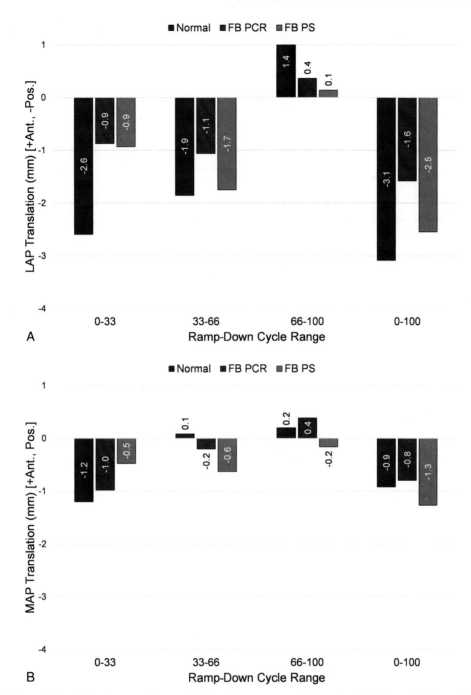

FIGURE 7-12 AP translation during the ramp-down activity for different ranges of the gait cycle. **A:** Lateral AP translation. **B:** Medial AP translation.

allowing anterior translation of femorotibial contact to occur, possibly because of inadequate function and tension in the PCL.[44,45]

Draganich et al.[68] found a similar relationship between femorotibial contact position and cruciate ligament integrity. In a cadaveric analysis, they also observed a posterior shift in femorotibial contact after sectioning of the anterior cruciate ligament. After the addition of PCL sectioning, an anterior shift in femorotibial contact occurred as knee flexion progressed, as was commonly observed in fixed-bearing PCR TKA designs studied in this report.

AXIAL ROTATION OF TKA AND NORMAL KNEES

Overall, axial rotation magnitudes were reduced in all TKA designs when compared to the normal knee, and among TKA types the average axial rotation magnitudes appeared similar. This indicates that, while

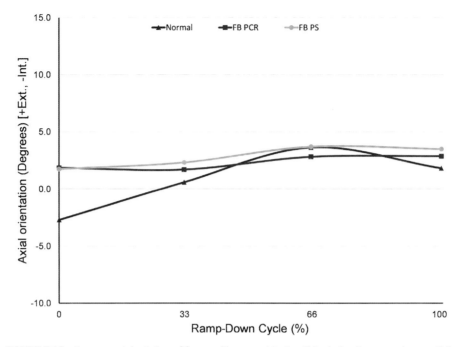

FIGURE 7-13   Average axial rotation of femur with respect to the tibia during the ramp-down activity.

the cam-and-post mechanism does appear to have an impact on medial and lateral condylar motion, it does not appear to be a driver of axial rotation. Depending on design, the lack of rotational conformity between the faces of the cam and post may yield increased stresses on both the cam and the post. In other words, as the knee rotates (or does not rotate) axially, if the femoral cam face is not oriented normal to the post face, then the contact area between the cam and the post will decrease because the cam will make contact with the edge of the post as opposed to the face. This would yield an increase in contact stresses and correspondingly a potential increase in component wear. Conversely, rounded posts may yield less post edge-loading, as the contact area of these designs is not dependent on axial orientation.

Although a positive screw-home rotational pattern from full extension to max flexion was observed in most TKA groups (**Fig.** 7-7), a negative (reverse) screw-home rotational pattern was nonetheless often present for subjects implanted with a TKA, which can adversely affect ROM and patellar stability. Less than 2% of nonimplanted patients experienced negative screw-home pattern, while over 24% of patients with a FB PCR TKA experienced negative patterns. This negative screw-home pattern may be related, at least in part, to abnormal anterior femoral translation that was observed laterally during knee flexion. Negative screw-home axial rotation is potentially detrimental, enhancing the risk of patellofemoral instability due to lateralization of the tibial tubercle if external tibial rotation occurs with increasing knee flexion.

REDUCED RANGE OF MOTION AFTER TKA

Weight-bearing ROM was significantly diminished for all TKA subjects during fluoroscopic analysis, presumably resulting from the complex interaction of dynamic muscle forces, soft-tissue constraints, posterior soft-tissue impingement, and articular congruity. Under passive, non–weight-bearing conditions, the knee seeks a course of least resistance and may not reflect normal, weight-bearing articulated motion. The importance of bearing weight in kinematic evaluations of the knee is supported by the work of Hsieh and Walker,[69] who determined that in the unloaded knee joint, joint laxity is primarily determined by soft-tissue constraints, whereas in the loaded knee joint, the geometric conformity of the joint surfaces is the primary determinant in controlling knee joint laxity. When tested under weight-bearing conditions, patients with a fixed-bearing TKA exhibited slightly lower postoperative ROM than those with mobile-bearing TKA.

Several *in vivo* kinematic studies of TKA have found that PFR is not a predictable phenomenon in the knees of patients implanted with PCR TKA.[31-33,37,44-46,48,52] As discussed previously, the femorotibial contact position in extension is drawn posteriorly. This has been attributed, in part, to the absence of the anterior cruciate ligament, excessive tension in the PCL, or the anteriorly directed pull of the patellar ligament on the tibia within this range of knee flexion, or all.[39,44-46,66,67] With knee flexion, anterior translation of the femur on the tibia has been observed, creating a kinematic pathway opposite that displayed by the normal knee joint. This anterior translation of femorotibial contact with progressive flexion may limit maximum flexion due to anteriorization of the axis of flexion, earlier impingement of the posterior soft tissue structures, and tightening of the extensor mechanism (from anterior femoral displacement). Alternatively, patients implanted with PS TKA demonstrate PFR dictated by interaction of the femoral cam and tibial post mechanism of the PS design, regardless of weight-bearing status.[44-47]

KNEE KINEMATICS AND PATIENT-SPECIFIC TKA

Due to the highly accurate and minimally invasive nature of *in vivo* fluoroscopic analysis techniques, these techniques have become a widely popular joint analysis method in orthopedics today. Fluoroscopic analysis can clearly be used to determine detailed *in vivo* kinematics for both normal and implanted knees, as well as for other joints (including ankles, hip, and shoulders). The results from such studies can be used to infer the importance of the posterior motion of the femoral condyles throughout flexion and how this motion affects both the axial rotation and ROM of the implanted knee.

However, while it is certainly important to keep these kinematic patterns in mind when designing total knee systems, the high levels of variability seen among TKA kinematics must serve as a reminder of the importance of patient-specific implants. While the normal knee may experience kinematic patterns such as "medial pivot" and "lateral rollback," it would be catastrophic to force the implanted knee to adhere to such patterns. Thus, to the best of our ability, it is essential to let the soft tissues be the primary drivers of knee kinematics, while implant geometry remains secondary. If the implants are designed with individual patient needs in mind, and if the systems/surgical techniques are patient-specific and nondestructive enough to maintain soft-tissue integrity, then the "correct" patient-specific kinematics will follow.

A thorough understanding of knee kinematics, along with data gathered from gait laboratories, cadaveric studies, MRIs, and more, can all be used in conjunction to help both surgeons and implant companies develop and improve surgical techniques, surgical instrumentation, and component design, ultimately resulting in improved postoperative outcomes and greater patient satisfaction.[53]

REFERENCES

1. Behrend H, Giesinger K, Giesinger JM, Kuster MS. The "forgotten joint" as the ultimate goal in joint arthroplasty: validation of a new patient-reported outcome measure. *J Arthroplasty.* 2012;27:430-436, e1.
2. Eymard F, Charles-Nelson A, Katsahian S, Chevalier X, Bercovy M. "Forgotten knee" after total knee replacement: a pragmatic study from a single-centre cohort. *Joint Bone Spine.* 2015;82:177-181.
3. Zeller IM. *Parameterization of a Next Generation In-Vivo Forward Solution Physiological Model of the Human Lower Limb to Simulate and Predict Demographic and Pathology Specific Knee Mechanics* [PhD dissertation]. University of Tennessee; 2018.
4. Komistek RD, Dennis DA, Mahfouz MR. In vivo fluoroscopic analysis of the normal human knee. *Clin Orthop Relat Res.* 2003;410:69-81.
5. Dennis DA, Komistek RD, Walker S, Cheal E, Stiehl J. Femoral condylar lift-off in vivo in total knee arthroplasty. *J Bone Joint Surg Br Vol.* 2001;83:33-39.
6. Insall JN, Scuderi GR, Komistek RD, Math K, Dennis DA, Anderson DT. Correlation between condylar lift-off and femoral component alignment. *Clin Orthop Relat Res.* 2002;403:143-152.
7. LaCour MT, Sharma A, Carr CB, et al. Confirmation of long-term in vivo bearing mobility in eight rotating-platform TKAs. *Clin Orthop Relat Res.* 2014;472:2766-2773.
8. Dennis DA, Mahfouz MR, Komistek RD, Hoff W. In vivo determination of normal and anterior cruciate ligament–deficient knee kinematics. *J Biomech.* 2005;38:241-253.
9. Freeman MA, Pinskerova V. The movement of the normal tibio-femoral joint. *J Biomech.* 2005;38:197-208.
10. Sharma A, Komistek RD. Contact mechanics of the human knee. In: Norman Scott W, ed. *Insall & Scott Surgery of the Knee.* 6th ed. Philadelphia, PA: Elsevier, Churchill & Livingstone; 2017.
11. Dennis DA, Komistek RD, Mahfouz MR, Walker SA, Tucker A. A multicenter analysis of axial femorotibial rotation after total knee arthroplasty. *Clin Orthop Relat Res.* 2004;428:180-189.
12. Grieco TF, Sharma A, Dessinger GM, Cates HE, Komistek RD. In vivo kinematic comparison of a bicruciate stabilized total knee arthroplasty and the normal knee using fluoroscopy. *J Arthroplasty.* 2018;33(2):565-571.
13. Johal P, Williams A, Wragg P, et al. Tibio-femoral movement in the living knee. A study of weight bearing and non-weight bearing knee kinematics using "interventional" MRI. *J Biomech.* 2005;38:269-276.
14. Lafortune MA, Cavanagh PR, Sommer HJ III, Kalenak A. Three dimensional kinematics of the human knee during walking. *J Biomech.* 1992;25:347-357.
15. Li G, Zayontz S, DeFrate LE, et al. Kinematics of the knee at high flexion angles: an in vitro investigation. *J Orthop Res.* 2004;22:90-95.
16. Mahfouz MR, Komistek RD, Dennis DA, Hoff WA. In vivo assessment of the kinematics in normal and anterior cruciate ligament-deficient knees. *J Bone Joint Surg Am.* 2004;86-A(suppl 2):56-61.
17. Leszko F, Sharma A, Komistek RD, et al. Comparison of in vivo patellofemoral kinematics for subjects having high-flexion total knee arthroplasty implant with patients having normal knees. *J Arthroplasty.* 2010;25:398-404.
18. Yildirim G, Walker PS, Sussman-Fort J, et al. The contact locations in the knee during high flexion. *Knee.* 2007;14:379-384.
19. Fellows R, Hill N, Gill H, MacIntyre N, Harrison M, Ellis R, Wilson D. Magnetic resonance imaging for in vivo assessment of three-dimensional patellar tracking. *J Biomech.* 2005;38:1643-1652.
20. Heegaard J, Leyvraz P, Kampen A, Rakotomanana L, Rubin P, Blankevoort L. Influence of soft structures on patellar three-dimensional tracking. *Clin Orthop Relat Res.* 1994;299:235.
21. Hinterwimmer S, von Eisenhart-Rothe R, Siebert M, Welsch F, Vogl T, Graichen H. Patella kinematics and patello-femoral contact areas in patients with genu varum and mild osteoarthritis. *Clin Biomech.* 2004;19:704-710.
22. Mahfouz M, Badawi A, Fatah E, Kuhn M, Merkl B. *Reconstruction of 3D patient-specific bone models from biplanar x-ray images utilizing morphometric measurements.* Proc. Int. Conf. on Image Processing, Computer Vision & Pattern Recognition, IPCV. Vol 2. Citeseer; 2006:345-349.
23. Wretenberg P, Nemeth G, Lamontagne M, Lundin B. Passive knee muscle moment arms measured in vivo with MRI. *Clin Biomech.* 1996;11(8):439-446.
24. Dennis DA, Komistek RD, Mahfouz MR, Haas BD, Stiehl JB. Multicenter determination of in vivo knee kinematics after total knee arthroplasty. *Clin Orthop Relat Res.* 2003;416:37-57.
25. Komistek RD, Allain J, Anderson DT, Dennis DA, Goutallier D. In vivo kinematics for subjects with and without an anterior cruciate ligament. *Clin Orthop Relat Res.* 2002;404:315-325.

26. Stiehl JB, Dennis DA, Komistek RD, Crane HS. In vivo determination of condylar lift-off and screw-home in a mobile bearing total knee arthroplasty. *J Arthroplasty*. 1999;14:293-299.
27. Stiehl JB, Dennis DA, Komistek RD, Keblish PA. In vivo kinematic analysis of a mobile bearing total knee prosthesis. *Clin Orthop Relat Res*. 1997;345:60-66.
28. Allen MJ, Hartmann SM, Xacks JM, et al. Technical feasibility and precision of radiostereometric analysis as an outcome measure in canine cemented total hip replacement. *J Orthop Sci*. 2004;9:66-75.
29. Benoit DL, Ramsey DK, Lamontagne M, et al. Effect of skin movement artifact on knee kinematics during gait and cutting motions measured in vivo. *Gait Posture*. 2006;24:152-164.
30. Karrholm J, Brandsson S, Freeman MAR. Tibiofemoral movement 4: changes of axial tibial rotation caused by forced rotation at the weight-bearing knee studied by RSA. *J Bone Joint Surg Br*. 2000;82(8):1201-1203.
31. Karrholm J, Jonsson H, Nilsson KG, et al. Kinematics of successful knee prosthesis during weight-bearing: three dimensional movements and positions of screw axes in the Tricon-M and Miller-Galante designs. *Knee Surg Sports Traumatol Arthrosc*. 1994;2(1):50-59.
32. Nilsson KG, Karrhohn J, Ekelund L. Knee motion in total knee arthroplasty. A roentgen stereophotogrammetric analysis of the kinematics of the Tricon-M knee prosthesis. *Clin Orthop*. 1990;256:147-161.
33. Nilsson KG, Karrholm J, Gadegaard P. Abnormal kinematics of the artificial knee. Roentgen stereophotogrammetric analysis of 10 Miller-Galante and five New Jersey LCS knees. *Acta Orthop Scand*. 1991;62:440-446.
34. Dennis DA, Komistek RD, Kim RH, et al. Gap balancing versus measured resection technique for total knee replacement. *Clin Orthop Relat Res*. 2010;468:102-107.
35. Mahoney OM, Nobel PC, Rhoads DD, et al. Posterior cruciate function following total knee arthroplasty: a biomechanical study. *J Arthroplasty*. 1994;9:569.
36. Oishi CS, Kaufman KR, Irby SE, et al. Effects of patellar thickness on compression and shear forces in total knee arthroplasty. *Clin Orthop*. 1996;331:283-290.
37. Hill PF, Williams VV, Iwaki H, et al. Tibiofemoral movement 2: the loaded and unloaded living knee studied by MRI. *J Bone Joint Surg Br*. 2000;82(8):1196-1200.
38. Iwaki H, Pinskerova V, Freeman MAR. Tibiofemoral movement 1: the shapes and relative movements of the femur and tibia in unloaded cadaver knee. *J Bone Joint Surg Br*. 2000;82(8):1189-1195.
39. Andriacchi TP. Functional analysis of pre- and post-knee surgery. "Total knee arthroplasty and ACL reconstruction." *J Biomech Eng*. 1993;115:575-581.
40. Andriacchi TP, Galante JO, Fernier RS. Patient outcomes following tricompartmental total knee replacement. *JAMA*. 1994;271:1349.
41. Cereatti A, Croce UD, Cappozzo A. Reconstruction of skeletal movement using skin markers: comparative assessment of bone pose estimators. *J Neuroeng Rehabil*. 2006;3:7.
42. Schulz BW, Kimmel WL. Can hip and knee kinematics be improved by eliminating thigh markers? *Clin Biomech*. 2010;25:687-692.
43. Wilson SA, McCann PD, Gotlin RS, et al. Comprehensive gait analysis in posterior-stabilized knee arthroplasty. *J Arthroplasty*. 1996;11:359.
44. Dennis DA, Komistek RD, Colwell CE, et al. In vivo anteroposterior femorotibial translation of total knee arthroplasty: a multicenter analysis. *Clin Orthop*. 1998;356:47-57.
45. Dennis DA, Komistek RD, Hoff WA, et al. In vivo knee kinematics derived using an inverse perspective technique. *Clin Orthop*. 1996;331:107-117.
46. Dennis DA, Komistek RD, Stiehl JB, et al. In vivo condylar lift-off in total knee arthroplasty. *Orthop Trans*. 1997;21:1112.
47. Dennis DA, Komistek RD, Stiehl JB, et al. Range of motion following total knee arthroplasty: the effect of implant design and weight-bearing conditions. *J Arthroplasty*. 1998;13(7):748-752.
48. Haas B, Komistek RD, Dennis DA. In vivo kinematic comparison of posterior cruciate sacrificing and stabilized mobile total bearing knee arthroplasty. Scientific exhibit presented at: 68th Annual Meeting of American Academy of Orthopaedic Surgeons; March 1-4, 2001; San Francisco, CA.
49. Hoff WA, Komistek RD, Dennis DA, et al. A three dimensional determination of femorotibial contact positions under in vivo conditions using fluoroscopy. *J Clin Biomech*. 1998;13:455-470.
50. Akbarshahi M, Schache AG, Fernandez JW, et al. Non-invasive assessment of soft-tissue artifact and its effect on knee joint kinematics during functional activity. *J Biomech*. 2010;43:1292-1301.
51. Garling EH, Kaptein BL, Mertens B, et al. Soft-tissue artifact assessment during step-up using fluoroscopy and skin-mounted markers. *J Biomech*. 2007;40:S18-S24.
52. Stiehl JB, Dennis DA, Komistek RD, et al. In vivo comparison of posterior cruciate retaining and sacrificing mobile bearing total knee arthroplasty. *Am J Knee Surg*. 2000;13(1):13-18.
53. LaCour MT, Komistek RD. Fluoroscopic analysis of total knee replacement. In: Norman Scott W, ed. *Insall & Scott Surgery of the Knee*. 6th ed. Philadelphia, PA: Elsevier, Churchill & Livingstone; 2017.
54. Mahfouz MR, Hoff WA, Komistek RD, et al. A robust method for registration of three-dimensional knee implant models to two dimensional fluoroscopy images. *IEEE Trans Med Imaging*. 2003;22:1561-1574.
55. Mahfouz MR, Hoff WA, Komistek RD, et al. Effect of segmentation errors on 3D-to-2D registration of implant models in x-rays images. *J Biomech*. 2005;38:229-239.
56. Hamel W. Robotic in vivo fluoroscopic arthroplasty evaluations with normal patient movements. *Bone Joint J*. 2013;95-B(suppl 15):S70.
57. Grieco TF, Sharma A, Komistek RD, Cates HE. Single versus multiple-radii cruciate-retaining total knee arthroplasty: an in vivo mobile fluoroscopy study. *J Arthroplasty*. 2016;31:694-701.
58. Grood ES, Suntay WJ. A joint coordinate system for the clinical description of three-dimensional motions: application to the knee. *J Biomech Eng*. 1983;105:136-144.
59. Gray HA, Guan S, Thomeer LT, et al. Three-dimensional motion of the knee-joint complex during normal walking revealed by mobile biplane X-ray imaging. *J Orthop Res*. 2019;37(3):615-630.
60. Kobori M, Komistek RD, Dennis DA, et al. An in vivo determination of patellar kinematics for fixed and mobile bearing TKA in Japanese patients having either a resurfaced or unresurfaced patella. Paper presented at: 68th Annual Meeting American Academy of Orthopaedic Surgeons; March 2001; San Francisco.
61. Oakshott R, Komistek RD, Anderson DT, et al. In vivo passive vs weight-bearing knee kinematics for subjects implanted with a mobile bearing that can freely translate and rotate. Internal report: Rocky Mountain Musculoskeletal Research Laboratory; Denver, CO; 2000.
62. Running D, Komistek RD, Haas BD, et al. Determination of in vivo kinematics for subjects having either a traditional or posterior stabilized mobile bearing TKA. Paper presented at: European Society of Biomechanics; August 2000; Dublin, Ireland.
63. Jones R, Komistek RD, Dennis DA, et al. An In Vivo Kinematic Analysis of the S-ROM PS Rotating Platform Knee Design. Paper presented at: SICOT; April 1999; Sydney, Australia.
64. Blunn GW, Walker PS, Joshi A, et al. The dominance of cyclic sliding in producing wear in total knee replacements. *Clin Orthop*. 1991;273:253-260.
65. Andriacchi TP, Stanwyck TS, Galante JO. Knee biomechanics and total knee replacement. *J Arthroplasty*. 1986;1:211-219.
66. Daniel DM, Stone ML, Barnett P, et al. Use of the quadriceps active test to diagnose posterior cruciate-ligament disruption and measure posterior laxity of the knee. *J Bone Joint Surg Am*. 1988;70:386-391.
67. Van Eijden TM, DeBoer W, Weijs WA. The orientation of the distal part of the quadriceps femoris muscle as a function of the knee flexion-extension angle. *J Biomech*. 1985;18:803-809.
68. Draganich LF, Andriacchi T, Anderson GBJ. Interaction between intrinsic knee mechanics and the knee extensor mechanism. *J Orthop Res*. 1987;5:539-547.
69. Hsieh HH, Walker PS. Stabilizing mechanisms of the loaded and unloaded knee joint. *J Bone Joint Surg Am*. 1976;58:87-93.

chapter 8

Kinematics of the Normal Knee: In Vivo Investigation Using Advanced Imaging Technique

Zhitao Rao, MD | Qidong Zhang, MD | Hany S. Bedair, MD | Timothy E. Foster, MD |
Harry E. Rubash, MD FAOA | Guoan Li, PhD

INTRODUCTION

Accurate knowledge of knee joint kinematics is vital for understanding normal knee joint function and for investigation of knee joint injury/disease mechanisms as well as for development of efficient treatment methods for knee pathology.[1-3] The data on the characteristic motion of the knee is also necessary for design and evaluation of contemporary total knee arthroplasties (TKAs) that aim to restore normal knee function and achieve full range of knee flexion.[4-6] In literature, numerous researches have reported on the investigation of knee joint kinematics using various measurement technologies.[7-11] These include skin/bone marker-based motion analysis systems[7] and imaging-based technologies (including X-ray, CT, MRI, fluoroscopy, etc.).[2,8,9,12-17] In general, these studies have revealed that the knee kinematics is activity- and loading-dependent.[18-20] The femoral condyles were shown to move posteriorly (or called rollback) with knee flexion.[21-23] Further, the femoral condyles were found to rotate externally with knee flexion or described with respect to a long tibial axis located at the medial compartment of the tibial plateau (demonstrating a "medial pivoting" motion) during non–weight-bearing[11,24] or weight-bearing flexion.[25-27] Data of these studies have greatly improved our understanding of physiological motion characters of the knee. These knowledges have also provided guidelines for development of contemporary TKA surgeries.[28,29] For example, rollback and medial pivoting motion during knee flexion have been discussed in various contemporary TKA component designs.[2,4,27]

The knee joint motion (tibiofemoral joint motion in this chapter) is achieved through articulation between the articular surfaces of the distal femur and proximal tibia. It is therefore critically important to examine the articular contact kinematics of the knee during various functional activities. However, traditional motion measurement technologies are limited to measure the intrinsic articular contact biomechanics of the knee during dynamic, functional activities. Recently, we developed a combined MRI and dual fluoroscopic image system (DFIS) technique for accurate investigation of the knee kinematics during various functional knee joint motion.[1,14,30,31] Using this method, a three-dimensional (3D) model of the target knee, including the tibial and femoral bones and corresponding cartilage surfaces, was constructed using the 3D MR images of the knee. The *in vivo* knee motion is then captured using two orthogonally positioned fluoroscopy. Through a 2D to 3D matching algorithm, the *in vivo* knee motion can be reproduced using a series of the 3D knee models, representing accurate 6 degrees of freedom (DOFs) knee kinematics and articular cartilage contact kinematics. In this chapter, we first introduce the combined MRI and DFIS technique and then introduce the data on 6 DOF tibiofemoral joint motion and the articular contact kinematics of the knee during three functional knee activities: treadmill gait (low range knee motion), stair step-up (moderate range of knee motion), and weight-bearing deep flexion (full range of knee motion).

IMAGING TECHNIQUE FOR ACCURATE MEASUREMENTS OF KNEE MOTION

Tibiofemoral Kinematics and Relevant Coordinate Systems

Tibiofemoral kinematics refers to the relative motion of the femur and tibia. Motion of the knee is a synergistic function of many physiological factors around the joint, including the anatomy of the articular surfaces, the passive soft tissues such as ligaments and menisci, and active muscular structures. Cartesian coordinate systems are usually used to describe the relative motions between the tibia and femur (**Fig. 8-1**). The motion or kinematics of the knee can be described in 6 DOFs in 3 principle planes, i.e., sagittal, transverse, and frontal planes, including three translations along the principle axes and three rotations around the principle axes. The rotations are widely referred as internal–external rotation in transverse plane, varus–valgus rotation in frontal plane, and flexion–extension in sagittal plane.

In investigation of TKA kinematics, it is more conventional to use transepicondyle axis (TEA)[32-34] or geometric center axis (GCA)[35,36] to describe femoral condyle motion (**Fig. 8-2**). The condyle motion and the articulating surface contact motion are not equivalent measurements

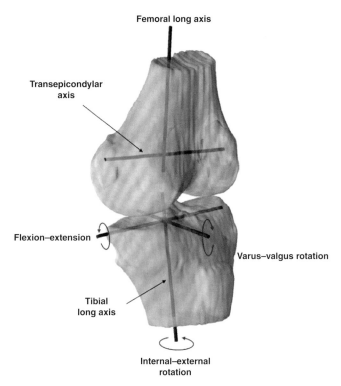

FIGURE 8-1 Cartesian coordinate systems and 6 degrees of freedom (DOFs) motions of the knee joint. (Reproduced from Kozanek M, Van de Velde SK, Gill TJ, Li G. The contralateral knee joint in cruciate ligament deficiency. *Am J Sports Med.* 2008;36(11):2151-2157. Reprinted with permission.)

and cannot be used interchangeably. The *in vivo* knee kinematics represented by the 3D knee models at each flexion angle was combined with the anatomical surface models of the cartilage to determine cartilage contact during various activities (**Fig. 8-3**). The tibial and femoral cartilage surfaces were usually constructed from the MR images of each subject. The method for determination of cartilage contact has been described as the area of overlap of the cartilage models of tibia and femur.[10] The articular contact kinematics is widely represented by an assessment of the positions of the contact point between the two articular surfaces. The contact point was defined as the location where the cartilage contact deformation was maximal in the contact area. To further quantify the geometry of the cartilage contact area, two orthogonal sectional planes, sagittal and coronal, were created at the contact point along the knee motion path. The profiles of the tibial and femoral cartilage in the contact area on these two planes were fitted using circles and the radii were measured (**Fig. 8-4**). For tibial cartilage, if the tibiofemoral cartilage is in a conforming contact, i.e., its curvature was in the same direction of the femoral cartilage, the radius value was defined as positive; if the tibiofemoral cartilage is in a convex contact, i.e., its curvature was in the opposite direction of the femoral cartilage, the radius value of the tibial cartilage was defined as negative.

Coordinate System for Measurement of 6 Degrees of Freedom Kinematics

To calculate the 6 DOF kinematics during various activities, a coordinate system was built for each femur and tibia (**Fig. 8-1**). In the femoral coordinate system, the medial–lateral axis was first defined as the TEA, which passed the most pivot points on the medial and lateral

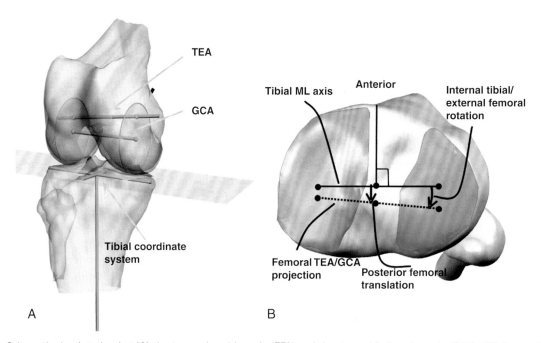

FIGURE 8-2 Schematic drawing showing **(A)** the transepicondylar axis (TEA) and the geometrical center axis (GCA); **(B)** the mediolateral axis connecting the centers of the medial and lateral compartments. (Modified from Li JS, Hosseini A, Cancre L, Ryan N, Rubash HE, Li G. Kinematic characteristics of the tibiofemoral joint during a step-up activity. *Gait Posture.* 2013;38(4):712-716. Reprinted with permission.)

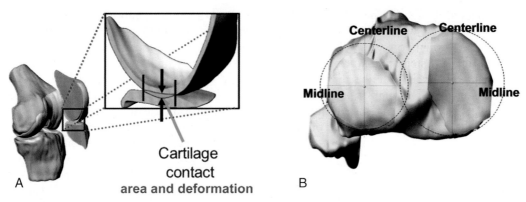

FIGURE 8-3   A: Measurement of cartilage contact area and deformation of the knee joint. **B:** The coordinate system for measurement of cartilage contact locations on the tibial plateau. (Modified from Yin P, Li JS, Kernkamp WA, et al. Analysis of in-vivo articular cartilage contact surface of the knee during a step-up motion. *Clin Biomech.* 2017;49:101-106. Reprinted with permission.)

condyles.[32,34] The mid-point of the axis was defined as the femoral center. The femoral long axis was parallel to the shaft of the femur and passed through the femoral center. The anterior–posterior axis was perpendicular to the other two axes. In the tibial coordinate system, the tibial long axis was defined as the line parallel to the posterior tibial shaft wall. Two circles were created to fit the medial and lateral plateaus separately.[37] The line connecting the centers of these two circles was defined as the medial–lateral axis and the mid-point as the tibial center. The cross product of the medial–lateral axis and the tibial long axis was defined as the anterior–posterior axis of the tibia. In this chapter, we present the data of 6 DOF

knee kinematics, including knee flexion, internal–external tibial rotation, and varus–valgus rotation, as well as anteroposterior translation, medial–lateral translation, and proximal distal translation.[38]

Definitions of TEA/GCA for Measurements of Condylar Motions

The TEA was defined as the line connecting the sulcus of the medial condyle and the lateral condyle prominence,[32-34] whereas the GCA was constructed by fitting maximal circles to the posterior medial and lateral condyles in sagittal plane and by connecting the centers of these circles with a line (**Fig. 8-2**). The center points were defined as the

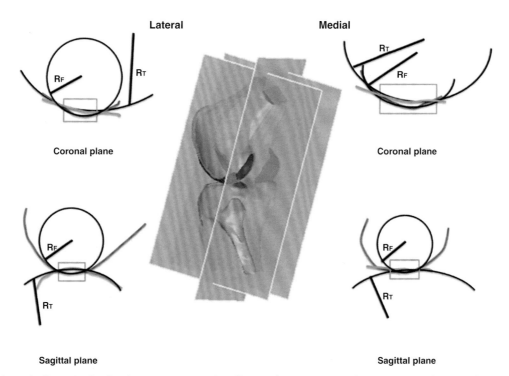

FIGURE 8-4   Schematic diagrams showing the measurement of cartilage surface geometry at the contact areas in the sagittal and coronal planes. (Reproduced from Yin P, Li JS, Kernkamp WA, et al. Analysis of in-vivo articular cartilage contact surface of the knee during a step-up motion. *Clin Biomech.* 2017;49:101-106. Reprinted with permission.)

femoral condyle centers of the GCA. The medial and lateral condyle centers of the TEA were defined as the crossing points of the TEA and the two sagittal circle planes. The anatomical coordinate system of the proximal tibia was established to quantitatively describe the positions of the TEA or GCA on the tibial plateau surfaces. For measurements of the AP translations of TEA and GCA centers, the corresponding points were projected onto the transverse tibial plane.[37]

Coordinate Systems for Cartilage Contact Kinematics/Deformation

Tibial coordinate systems constructed above using two circles to fit the medial and lateral plateaus were applied to describe the motion of the contact points[20,39,40] (**Fig. 8-3B**). The center of each circle was the origin of the coordinate system. The medial–lateral axis (X-axis) for the medial and lateral tibial plateaus was created by drawing a line through the origin of each coordinate system, parallel to the posterior edges of the tibial plateaus. The anterior–posterior axis (Y-axis) for each tibial plateau was created by drawing a line through the origin of the coordinate system perpendicular to the respective medial–lateral axis. The two quadrants nearest the tibial spine were defined as the "inner half," and the remaining quadrants the "outer half."

Dual Fluoroscopic Image System

The dual fluoroscopic imaging system (DFIS) setup (**Fig. 8-5**) is used for dynamic knee joint kinematics analysis.[30] The DFIS consists of two pulse fluoroscopes (BV Pulsera, Philips) that are set to generate 8 ms width X-ray pulses. A subject is free to move within the common imaging zone of the two fluoroscopes (corresponding to a 315 × 315 mm field of view). Various motions can be imaged this way such as treadmill gait, stair step-up, sit-to-stand, lunge, and squat, etc. The knee is imaged simultaneously by the fluoroscopes from two directions. The fluoroscopes took 30 evenly distributed snapshot images per second during dynamic knee joint motion. This procedure records the *in vivo* poses of the knee as a series of two-dimensional (2D) paired fluoroscopic images. The images are then segmented and corrected for distortion. The outlines of the knee structures from the edge detection are manually reviewed and saved. Next, a virtual replica of the DFIS is constructed in a solid modeling software. Two virtual source-intensifier pairs are created in the modeling software to recreate the geometry of the real fluoroscopic system. The outlines of the knee obtained from the DFIS are placed on their respective virtual intensifiers. Three-dimensional (3D) models of the knee are introduced into the virtual system. The tibial and femoral models can be manipulated independently in the virtual environment in 6 DOF and projected onto the virtual imaging intensifiers. If the projection outline matches the actual bony outline captured from the actual knee, the *in vivo* knee position in space is reproduced by the 3D knee models in the computer. In this manner, the knee motion can be represented by a series of 3D knee models reproduced along the motion path. Joint coordinate systems described previously can then be used to determine the 6 DOF knee joint kinematics.[25,31,37,41]

The DFIS technique has been rigorously validated for measurements of *in vivo* knee joint kinematics.[30] It could determine knee position with an accuracy of $0.16° \pm 0.61°$ in rotation and 0.24 ± 0.16 mm in translation when compared to radiostereometric analysis (RSA). The cartilage contact area could be determined with $14\% \pm 11\%$ error of measurement. Finally, the cartilage thickness based on MR meshed models could be constructed with an error of 0.04 ± 0.01 mm (corresponding to a $1.8\% \pm 1.6\%$ difference).

KNEE KINEMATICS DURING FUNCTIONAL ACTIVITIES

In this section, we will introduce the *in vivo* knee biomechanics during three knee motions measured using the DFIS technology. These activities include gait (representing small range of knee motion),[31,37,40] stair step up (representing moderate range of knee motion),[20,42] and weight-bearing maximal flexion (representing large range of knee flexion).[1,19,43] We presented the 6 DOF tibiofemoral motion and the articular contact kinematics of the knee during these motions.

Treadmill Gait

Experiment Design

Using the combined MRI and DFIS technique, we evaluated the *in vivo* tibiofemoral kinematics and the condylar motion of the knee during treadmill gait in eight healthy subjects.[37,40] Six males and two females, aged 32 to 49 years were recruited, with average body mass index (BMI) of 23.5 kg/m². During experiment, each subject practiced the gait on the treadmill for 1 minute at a treadmill speed of 1.5 miles per hour (MPH), i.e., 0.67 m/s (**Fig. 8-6**). Two thin pressure sensors (Force Sensor Resistor [FSR], Interlink Electronics Specifications, Camarillo, CA) were fixed to the bottom of each shoe, recording the heel strike and toe-off of the testing foot and the contralateral foot. Two laser-positioning devices, attached to the fluoroscopes, helped to align the target knee within the field of view of the fluoroscopes during the stance phase. The knee was then imaged during three consecutive strides. After testing, the fluoroscopic images and the 3D MR-based knee model were imported into the modeling software to reproduce the *in vivo* knee positions during the gait. The data include 6 DOF knee kinematics, femoral condyle motions measured using TEA and GCA, and the cartilage contact kinematics.

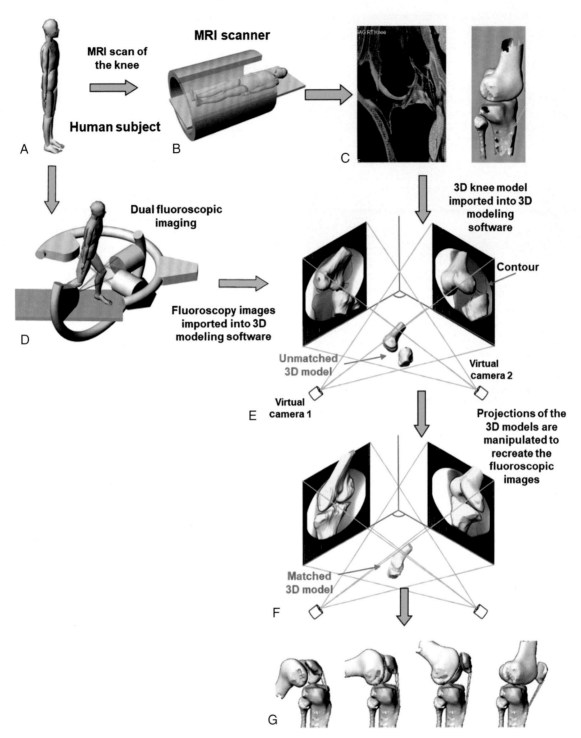

FIGURE 8-5 The overall procedure used to reproduce *in vivo* knee kinematics using the combined dual fluoroscopic–magnetic resonance (MR) imaging technique. Each subject's MR images **(A** and **B)** are used to construct a 3D anatomic knee model **(C)**. Each subject's knees are then imaged from two directions during *in vivo* activities **(D)**. The knee model is manipulated in 6 degrees of freedom to reproduce the knee positions **(E-G)**.

6 Degrees of Freedom Kinematics

The predominant motion of the knee during the stance phase of gait occurred in the sagittal plane (**Fig. 8-7**). The knee was extended at heel strike, flexed during loading response, and reached the first flexion peak of about 8° during early midstance. Thereafter, the knee begun to extend until about 40% of stance phase and remained in slight hyperextension (average 3.5°) throughout midstance. Approximately halfway through the terminal stance, the knee was observed to flex again and the

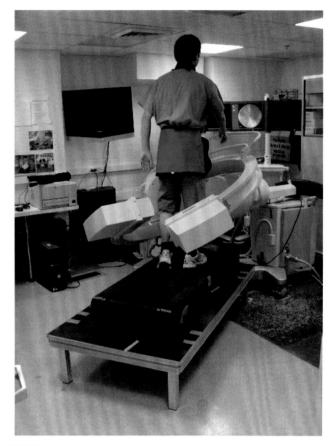

FIGURE 8-6 Each subject performed gait on a treadmill while the knee was scanned by the dual fluoroscopic image system (DFIS). (Reproduced from Kozanek M, Hosseini A, Liu F, et al. Tibiofemoral kinematics and condylar motion during the stance phase of gait. *J Biomech.* 2009;42(12):1877-1884. Reprinted with permission.)

flexion continued throughout the preswing and peaked at toe-off when the stance phase ended. The magnitude of this second flexion peak was on average 36°.

The axial rotation of the knee (internal–external) showed similar pattern to the flexion–extension. At heel strike, the femur was found to be internally rotated on average 1.6°. The femur then rotated externally and reached the first peak of external rotation (average 5°) shortly after opposite toe off, i.e., in early midstance. Direction of the axial rotation was then reversed and the femur was noted to rotate internally throughout midstance until early terminal extension when the rotation reversed again. During the terminal extension and preswing, the femur rotated externally until it reached the second maximum of external rotation at toe-off (average 7.4°).

The pattern of anteroposterior shift (femur relative to tibia) also followed that of flexion–extension. We noted that at heel strike the femur was 2.6 mm posterior to the tibia. The femur then shifted anteriorly during loading response and reached the first peak of anterior shift during early midstance. At this point the femur was on average 0.1 mm posterior to the tibia. The femur then

begun to shift back posteriorly during the midstance. The posterior motion peaked at 50% of stance when it was 4 mm posterior to the tibia. Thereafter its direction reversed and the femur was shifting anteriorly until toe-off when it reached the second maximum and was on average 2.5 mm anterior to the tibia. Therefore, the average excursions in the anteroposterior directions during stance phase were approximately 5 mm.

Femoral Condylar Motion

The motion of medial and lateral femoral condyle with respect to the tibia were measured using both the TEA and the GCA. When measured with the TEA (**Fig. 8-8A**), at heel strike, the medial and lateral condyles were located 3.3 ± 1.1 mm and 1.9 ± 1.0 mm posterior to the mediolateral axis of the tibia, respectively. The anterior motion of the medial condyle during the first half of stance phase peaked at about 20% of stance phase, and the medial condyle then moved posteriorly. The anterior motion of the lateral condyle reversed its direction earlier in the stance phase than the medial condyle (at about 10% of stance). After reaching the first anterior peak, both the medial and the lateral condyles shifted slightly posteriorly to 3.3 ± 0.5 mm and 2.9 ± 0.8 mm at 50% of stance, respectively. Thereafter, the condylar shift was minimal until 75% of stance when both condyles moved anteriorly again until toe-off when the medial condyle was 5.3 anterior and the lateral condyle 0.7 mm posterior to tibia. The range of motion of the medial condyle in the anteroposterior direction (9.7 ± 0.7 mm) was significantly greater than that of the lateral condyle (4.0 ± 1.7 mm, *P* < .01).

Condylar motion demonstrated similar trends when measured with the GCA along motion path during the gait (**Fig. 8-8B**). At heel strike the position of the medial and lateral condyle was 9.3 ± 2.9 and 6.6 ± 3.2 posterior to the mediolateral axis of the tibia. The excursions of the medial condyle (17.4 ± 2.0 mm) were greater than those of the lateral condyle (7.4 ± 6.1 mm, *P* < .01) in the anteroposterior direction.

Cartilage Contact Kinematics

On the medial tibial side, from heel-strike to 20% stance, the location of contact points shifted 2.3 mm anteriorly (**Fig. 8-9**). This was followed by a 2.0 mm posterior shift from 20% to 60% of stance phase. From 60% stance phase to toe-off, contact points moved 4.7 mm anteriorly. With regards to motion in the mediolateral direction, the peak contact first moved 0.4 mm laterally, i.e., toward the intercondylar eminence of the tibia (heel-strike to 20% phase) then 0.5 mm medially (20% to 50% stance phase) and again laterally (1 mm) until toe-off.

On the lateral tibial side, from heel-strike to 80% stance, the contact point moved <1.0 mm anteriorly and 0.7 mm posteriorly, thereafter (**Fig. 8-9**). In the mediolateral direction, the contact point first moved 0.6 mm

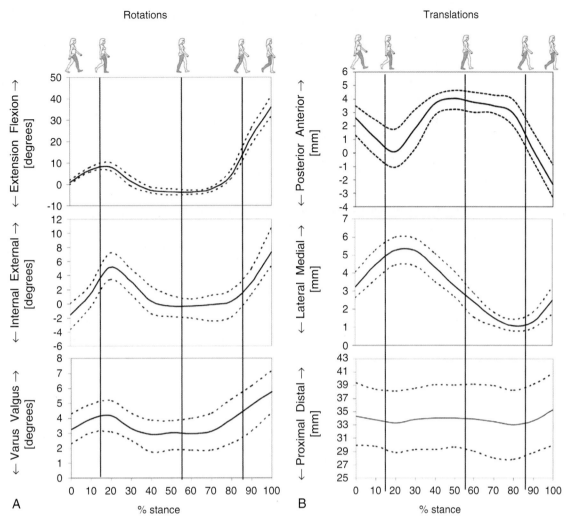

FIGURE 8-7 Schematic diagrams showing the 6 degrees of freedom (DOF) tibiofemoral kinematics of the knee joint during the stance phase of treadmill gait. The figure drawings represent the motion of the tibia relative to the femur. **A:** Rotations; solid lines = contralateral toe-off, ipsilateral heel rise, and contralateral initial contact in extension–flexion, internal–external rotation, and varus–valgus, respectively. **B:** Translations; solid lines = contralateral toe-off, ipsilateral heel rise, and contralateral initial contact in posterior–anterior, lateral–medial, and proximodistal, respectively. Dashed lines = kinematic range (maximal and minimal displacement). The intervals between the solid lines represent loading response, midstance, terminal stance, and preswing, respectively. (Reproduced from Kozanek M, Hosseini A, Liu F, et al. Tibiofemoral kinematics and condylar motion during the stance phase of gait. *J Biomech.* 2009;42(12):1877-1884. Reprinted with permission.)

laterally (heel-strike to 20% stance phase), then 0.9 mm medially (20% to 50% stance phase) and then 0.9 mm laterally again.

Summary

The data of contact location changes during the stance phase of gait were consistent with the 6 DOF tibiofemoral motion patterns.[7,44] The medial femoral condyle moved in a larger range in anteroposterior direction than the lateral femoral condyle using both the TEA and GCA. Throughout the stance phase, the anteroposterior contact excursions in the lateral tibiofemoral compartment (1.6 ± 0.4 mm) were significantly smaller than in the medial compartment (3.6 ± 0.3 mm) (**Fig. 8-9**)

($P < .05$). These data indicate that the knee exhibits "lateral pivoting" motion character during gait motion.

Stair Step-Up

Experiment Design

Twenty-one healthy knees of 21 subjects (age, 34.6 ± 10.4 years; gender, 14 males and 7 females; body height, 1.8 ± 0.1 m; body weight, 80.9 ± 18.1 kg) were recruited. Each subject performed a dynamic step-up (**Fig. 8-10**), and the knee motion was captured using the DFIS.[20] The beginning (0%) of the step-up activity was defined as the initiation of the knee extension motion and the end point (100%) was defined when the subject's knee

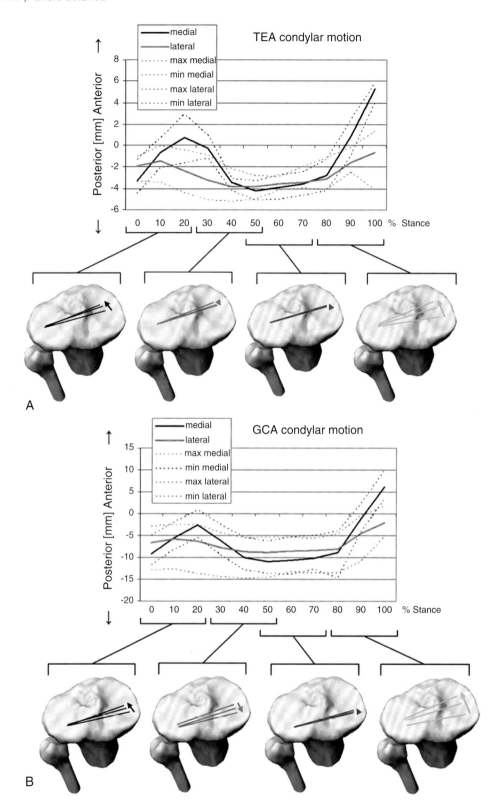

FIGURE 8-8   Motion of the medial and lateral femoral condyle in the anteroposterior direction measured by **(A)** transepicondyle axis (TEA) and **(B)** geometric center axis (GCA) of the femur. The medial femoral condyle made greater excursions than lateral femoral condyle. (Modified from Kozanek M, Hosseini A, Liu F, et al. Tibiofemoral kinematics and condylar motion during the stance phase of gait. *J Biomech*. 2009;42(12):1877-1884. Reprinted with permission.)

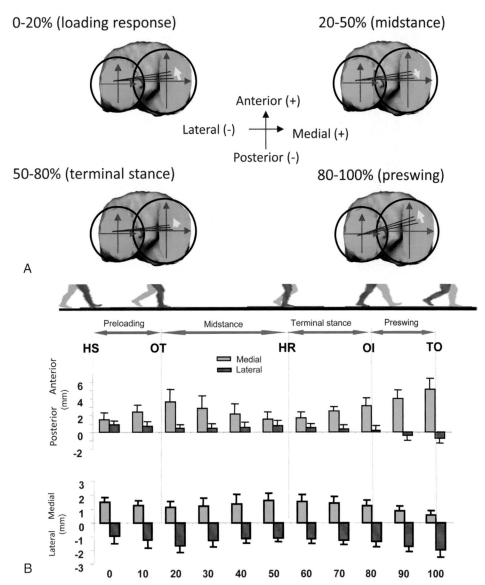

FIGURE 8-9   A: Excursions of the contact points on the tibial plateau. **B:** Anteroposterior and mediolateral kinematics of the contact points on the medial and lateral tibial plateau during the stance phase of gait. (Reproduced from Liu F, Kozanek M, Hosseini A, et al. In vivo tibiofemoral cartilage deformation during the stance phase of gait. *J Biomech*. 2010;43(4):658-665. Reprinted with permission.)

fully extended. The articular cartilage contact kinematics was also investigated on both tibial and femoral cartilage surfaces during a step-up activity.

Condylar Motion

The flexion angles ranged from 54.4 ± 7.1° at initial contact to full extension at the end of the step-up activity. The average time for the activity was 0.8 ± 0.2 seconds. The condylar motion measured using the TEA gradually shifted anteriorly (medial: −5.0 ± 3.5 to −0.1 ± 2.8 mm; lateral: −15.1 ± 3.9 to −10.2 ± 4.3 mm) from beginning to 70% of the activity (**Fig. 8-11**A). The position of the medial condyle remained constant throughout the activity thereafter; however, the lateral condyle continued to move anteriorly to −6.0 ± 4.5 mm. The total excursions of the medial and lateral femoral condyles measured

using the TEA were 12.7 ± 2.9 mm and 14.5 ± 4.0 mm, respectively, and no significant difference was found between the two excursions. The tibia rotated internally 13.3 ± 5.6° at the beginning and externally rotated to 8.3 ± 5.4° at the end of the step-up activity.

The condylar motions measured using the GCA showed an opposite trend between the medial and lateral condyles (**Fig. 8-11**B). The medial condyle moved posteriorly from −5.5 to −8.9 mm while the lateral condyle shifted from −14.7 to −11.0 mm. The total excursions measured using GCA were 11.9 ± 4.1 mm and 11.8 ± 4.1 mm for the medial and lateral femoral condyles, respectively, with no significant difference between them. The axial tibial rotation was measured to be 14.3 ± 5.7° internal rotation at the beginning and was 3.9 ± 5.5° at the end of the step-up activity.

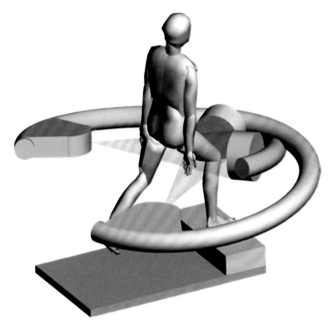

FIGURE 8-10 Schematic drawing showing the step-up activity captured by the dual fluoroscopic image system (DFIS). (Modified from Li JS, Hosseini A, Cancre L, Ryan N, Rubash HE, Li G. Kinematic characteristics of the tibiofemoral joint during a step-up activity. *Gait Posture.* 2013;38(4):712-716. Reprinted with permission.)

6 Degrees of Freedom Kinematics and Contact Kinematics

For contact points on tibial plateau (**Fig. 8-11**C), the contact points started at −1.4 ± 3.1 and −10.1 ± 2.5 mm to the centers of the medial and lateral tibial plateaus, respectively. Both medial and lateral contact points slightly shifted posteriorly from initiation of movement until 30% of the step-up, and then gradually shifted anteriorly until 80% of the step-up motion. Thereafter, the medial contact points moved slightly anteriorly to 1.6 ± 4.2 mm, whereas the lateral contact points continued to shift anteriorly to −5.3 ± 3.0 mm at 100% of the step-up activity. In addition, the total excursions of the medial and lateral contacts were 13.5 ± 3.2 and 10.7 ± 5.0 mm, respectively. No significant difference was found in total excursion between the medial and lateral compartments. In the medial–lateral direction, the translation of the medial contact points during the step-up was within 0.4 mm. The lateral contact point started from −18.7 ± 3.1 mm and then slightly moved medially from −19.0 ± 2.8 to −16.0 ± 3.6 mm between 30% and 100% of the activity.

Characters of Articular Cartilage Contact Surface Geometry

The articular surface geometry at the contact area is an important variable that affects the articular contact behaviors, such as contact stress and knee joint

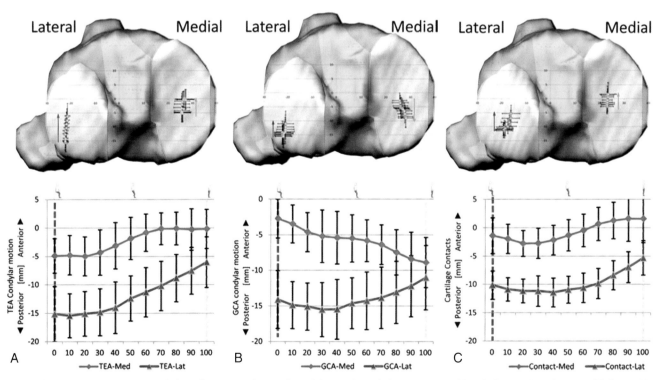

FIGURE 8-11 Anteroposterior translation of contact points and condylar motions during step-up activity. **A:** Transepicondyle axis (TEA) condylar motion. **B:** Geometric center axis (GCA) condylar motion. **C:** Articular cartilage contact points. (Modified from Li JS, Hosseini A, Cancre L, Ryan N, Rubash HE, Li G. Kinematic characteristics of the tibiofemoral joint during a step-up activity. *Gait Posture.* 2013;38(4):712-716. Reprinted with permission.)

stability. Therefore, we investigated the surface geometry at the articular contact areas of the tibiofemoral joint (**Fig. 8-4**) during a dynamic step-up activity in 10 healthy knees.[42]

Using the definition shown in **Fig. 8-4**, the mean sagittal radius of the femur cartilage was larger in the medial side than in the lateral side ($P < .001$) (**Fig. 8-12**). No significant difference was found in the mean coronal radii of the medial and lateral femoral cartilage ($P = .27$). The mean sagittal radius in the tibia cartilage was larger in medial compartment than the lateral compartment ($P < .001$). The average coronal radius in tibia cartilage was smaller in medial compartment than in the lateral compartment ($P < .001$).

Both the medial and lateral compartments exhibited that the convex-to-convex tibiofemoral cartilage contact feature in sagittal plane. This geometric feature of the articular contact area in medial compartment indicates that the femur is less constrained by the tibial cartilage surface geometry in the anteroposterior direction than a convex-to-concave contact in the medial–lateral direction.

Summary

Using the TEA, the femoral condylar motions presented a similar pattern as the contact points throughout the activity. When the GCA was used, the femoral condyle motion pattern was dramatically different. The medial condyle moved anteriorly, while the lateral condyle shifted posteriorly throughout the activity. Selection of coordinate systems changed knee joint kinematics description dramatically. The total excursion of the articular contact points was similar on the medial and lateral tibial surfaces. The knee joint kinematics during the step-up activity did not show the phenomenon of medial-pivoting knee flexion as observed during passive, non–weight-bearing flexion or quasi-static knee joint flexion.[24]

Further, medial and lateral cartilage contact geometries were similar in pattern, but different in dimensions. The convex-to-convex contact feature implies that the dynamic stability of the knee joint could depend on a synergistic interaction of articular contact, mechanical function of the meniscus, ligament constraints (such as the cruciate and collateral ligaments), muscle contractions, and other tissues around the knee joint. Dysfunction of

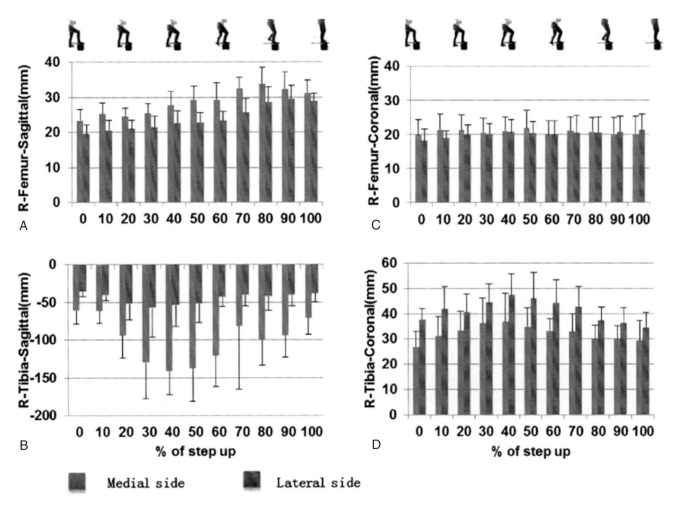

FIGURE 8-12 The radii of the contact areas in both medial and lateral cartilage surfaces in sagittal (**A**) femur and (**B**) tibia cartilages and in coronal (**C**) femur and (**D**) tibia surfaces of the knee. (Reproduced from Yin P, Li JS, Kernkamp WA, et al. Analysis of in-vivo articular cartilage contact surface of the knee during a step-up motion. *Clin Biomech*. 2017;49:101-106. Reprinted with permission).

any of these structural components could cause alteration of articular contact biomechanics of the knee and possibly result in damage to the cartilage. It may provide important insights into the investigation of intrinsic articular contact biomechanics of the knee.

Kinematics of the Knee During Weight-Bearing Deep Flexion

Experiment Design

Eight healthy human knees (age, 23 to 49; 5 males and 2 females; BMI, 19.9 to 29.3 kg/m²) with no history of injuries or chronic pain were recruited to investigate the 6 DOF kinematics and tibiofemoral cartilage contact biomechanics of the knee during weight-bearing flexion from full extension to maximal flexion.[19,43] After MR scanning, each subject performed a quasi-static single-legged lunge from full extension to maximal flexion and measured by the DFIS technique (**Fig. 8-13**). Full extension was defined as the flexion angle of the knee when the subject was standing naturally on one leg with the knee held as straight as possible. The subjects were instructed to hold the knee position for a second while bearing the body weight at each selected flexion angle (~every 15° from full extension to maximal flexion) and allowed to use the contralateral leg and a handrail to keep their body stable if necessary. Flexion angles of the knee were monitored using a goniometer. The DFIS captured the knee position at each target flexion angles. The knee joint position was then reproduced using the 2D-3D matching method.

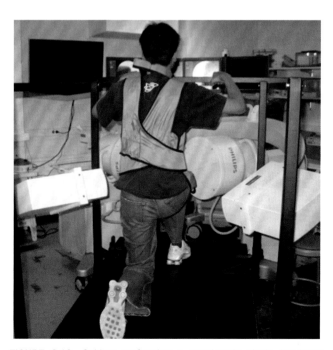

FIGURE 8-13 Subject performing a quasi-static single leg lunge (right knee) in the dual fluoroscopic system. (Reproduced from Qi W, Hosseini A, Tsai TY, Li JS, Rubash HE, Li G. In vivo kinematics of the knee during weight bearing high flexion. *J Biomech.* 2013;46(9):1576-1582. Reprinted with permission.)

After reproducing the knee joint motion, the cartilage contact on the femur and tibia were determined. The 6 DOF condylar motion and cartilage contact kinematics during the weight-bearing knee flexion were quantified along the flexion of the knee.

6 Degrees of Freedom Kinematics

The flexion angles ranged from full extension of −2.9° ± 7.0° to the maximal flexion of 145.3° ± 5.7° during the quasi-static single-legged lunge of this subject group. From full extension to 30° flexion of the knee, the femur moved posteriorly 4.4 ± 3.1 mm; from 30° to 120°, the femur moved 13.3 ± 3.2 mm posteriorly, and from 120° to maximal flexion, the femur moved 7.5 ± 4.3 mm posteriorly (**Fig. 8-14A, Table 8-1**). Posterior femoral excursion in the middle flexion range was significantly larger than those of low and high flexion ranges.

In the medial–lateral direction, the femur moved laterally 1.7 ± 1.1 mm from full extension to 30° of flexion, 0.1 ± 1.7 mm laterally from 30° to 120° of flexion, and 3.8 ± 2.6 mm medially from 120° to maximal flexion (**Fig. 8-14B**). Femoral excursion in medial–lateral direction at high range of flexion was significantly greater compared to that of low and middle flexion ranges.

The tibia rotated internally by 6.1° ± 7.6° (**Fig. 8-14C**) and in varus by 1.7° ± 2.6° from full extension to 30° of flexion (**Fig. 8-14D**). From 30° to 120°, the tibia rotated internally by 2.1° ± 8.2° and in varus by 4.1° ± 3.6°. From 120° to maximal flexion, the tibia internally rotated by 7° ± 6.2° and in valgus by 0.2° ± 3.3°.

Condyle Motion

Both medial and lateral TEA were close to the origin of tibia coordinate system at full extension (−1.6 and −0.7 mm, respectively) and moved posteriorly by 9.2 and 16.4 mm, respectively, at maximum knee flexion (**Fig. 8-15, Table 8-2**). The medial and lateral GCA were posterior to the origin of the tibia coordinate system at full extension (−4.6 and −3.4 mm, respectively). The medial GCA moved slightly anteriorly by 2.6 mm until 45° of knee flexion and posteriorly by 6.1 mm at maximum knee flexion, whereas the lateral GCA moved posteriorly by 11.6 mm from full extension to maximum knee flexion.

Articular Cartilage Contact Motion

In anteroposterior direction, the tibial contact points sharply moved posteriorly both in the medial and lateral compartments from full extension to 30° of knee flexion by 5.1 ± 4.9 mm and 4.9 ± 3.9 mm, respectively (**Fig. 8-16, Table 8-1**). Thereafter, the contact points slightly moved posteriorly by 4.2 ± 1.6 mm in the medial compartment and 5.0 ± 2.9 mm in the lateral compartment from 30° to 120° of flexion. From 120° flexion to maximal flexion, the medial contact point moved 1.9 ± 2.1 mm posteriorly and the lateral contact point moved 4.8 ± 2 mm posteriorly (*P* < .05). Lateral femoral condyle lift at maximal

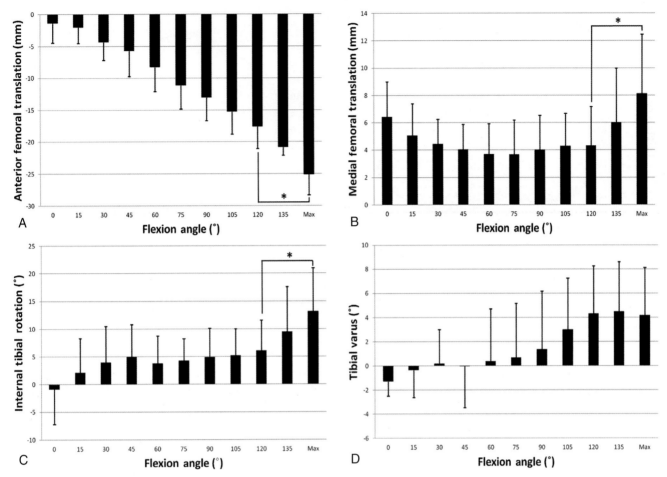

FIGURE 8-14 A: Anterior and **(B)** medial translations; **(C)** internal and **(D)** varus rotations of the tibia relative to femur during the full range of knee flexion (FE: full extension; Max: maximal flexion). Asterisk means a statistically significant. (Modified from Qi W, Hosseini A, Tsai TY, Li JS, Rubash HE, Li G. In vivo kinematics of the knee during weight bearing high flexion. *J Biomech.* 2013;46(9):1576-1582. Reprinted with permission.)

TABLE 8-1   Femoral Translation, Tibial Rotation, and Tibiofemoral Contact Kinematics in Different Flexion Ranges of the Knee (Mean ± SD)

Motions	FE-30°	30°-120°	120°-Max	FE-MaxF
Femoral Anterior Translation (mm)	−4.4 ± 3.1	−13.3 ± 3.2[a]	−7.5 ± 4.3[b]	−25.2 ± 5.0
Femoral Medial Translation (mm)	−1.7 ± 1.1	−0.1 ± 1.7	3.8 ± 2.6[a,b]	2.0 ± 3.4
Tibial Internal Rotation (°)	6.1 ± 7.6	2.1 ± 8.2	7.0 ± 6.2	15.2 ± 9.2
Tibial Varus (°)	1.7 ± 2.6	4.1 ± 3.6	−0.2 ± 3.3[b]	5.6 ± 4.9
Medial A-P Contact (mm)	−5.1 ± 4.9	−4.2 ± 1.6	−1.9 ± 2.1	−11.1 ± 3.3
Lateral A-P Contact (mm)	−4.9 ± 3.9	−5.0 ± 2.9	−4.8 ± 2.0[c]	−14.6 ± 3.7[c]

FE, full extension; MaxF, maximal flexion.
Positive values indicate internal rotation, varus, and anterior and medial translation, whereas negative values indicate external rotation, valgus, and posterior and lateral translation.
[a]Significant difference between the range and the 0° to 30° of flexion angles (P < .05).
[b]Significant difference between the range and the 30° to 120° of flexion angles (P < .05).
[c]Significant difference between the medial and lateral A-P contact positions (P < .05).
Reproduced from Qi W, Hosseini A, Tsai TY, Li JS, Rubash HE, Li G. In vivo kinematics of the knee during weight bearing high flexion. *J Biomech.* 2013;46(9):1576-1582. Reprinted with permission.

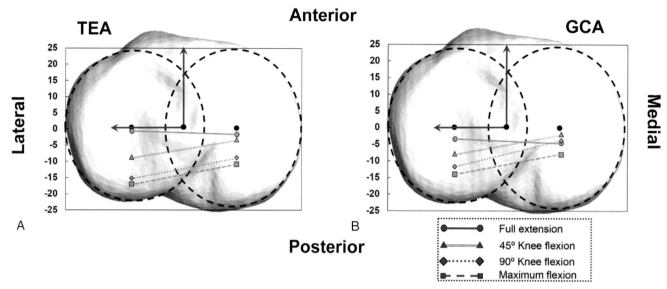

FIGURE 8-15 Average excursion of the femoral condyles measured using the **(A)** transepicondyle axis (TEA) and **(B)** geometric center axis (GCA) during weight-bearing deep flexion. (Modified from Dimitriou D, Tsai TY, Park KK, et al. Weight-bearing condyle motion of the knee before and after cruciate-retaining TKA: in-vivo surgical transepicondylar axis and geometric center axis analyses. *J Biomech*. 2016;49(9):1891-1898.)

TABLE 8-2 Anterior–Posterior Translations of Femoral Condyle During Weight-Bearing Knee Flexion

	Medial Condyle				Lateral Condyle			
	0°-15°	30°-45°	60°-75°	90°-max	0°-15°	30°-45°	60°-75°	90°-max
sTEA AP Translation (mm)	−1.6 to −1.4	−1.8 to −3.3	−5.3 to −7.5	−8.8 to −10.8	−0.7 to −3.6	−6.0 to −8.7	−10.2 to −12.9	−15.2 to −17.0
GCA AP Translation (mm)	−4.6 to −3.1	−2.2 to −2.0	−2.8 to −3.7	−3.9 to −8.1	−3.4 to −5.3	−6.3 to −7.9	−8.3 to −10.0	−11.7 to −14.0

GCA, geometric center axis; TCA, transepicondyle axis.
Modified from Dimitriou D, Tsai TY, Park KK, et al. Weight-bearing condyle motion of the knee before and after cruciate-retaining TKA: in-vivo surgical transepicondylar axis and geometric center axis analyses. *J Biomech*. 2016;49(9):1891-1898. Reprinted with permission.

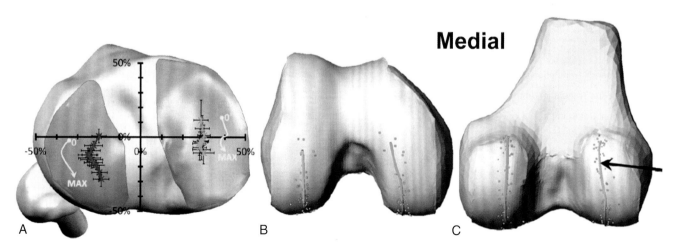

FIGURE 8-16 Tibiofemoral cartilage contact positions on the medial and lateral tibial plateau and femoral condyles at different flexion during weight-bearing deep flexion. **A:** The crosses stand for the mean locations of cartilage contacts during the knee flexion and the error bars are the standard deviation. **B:** Distal view. **C:** Posterior view. The dots on the cartilage stand for the individual contact points of all the subjects and the lines (arrow) shows the average location of the contact. (Modified from Qi W, Hosseini A, Tsai TY, Li JS, Rubash HE, Li G. In vivo kinematics of the knee during weight bearing high flexion. *J Biomech*. 2013;46(9):1576-1582. Reprinted with permission).

flexion was observed in three knees where no cartilage contact was detected at the maximal flexion angles of the knee.

Summary

The data indicated that the kinematics is not uniform along the knee flexion path. It showed that at low flexion angles (FE-30°), the internal tibial rotation increased sharply and the contact points on the medial compartment slightly moved posteriorly more than those on the lateral compartment. The internal tibial rotation maintained a small variation and the similar shift pattern of the contact points in the moderate range of flexion (30° to 120°). In high flexion angles (120° - MaxF), the internal tibial rotation sharply increased again, and the contact point moved less on the medial compartment compared to the lateral compartment. The data indicated that the knee motion cannot be described using one character in the entire range of flexion.

SUMMARY

The tibiofemoral joint biomechanics is critical in transmitting loads, maintaining body alignment, and facilitating locomotor activities. This chapter summarized the data recently measured using the combined MRI and DFIS technique on 6 DOF tibiofemoral kinematics, femoral condylar motion, and articular cartilage contact kinematics of normal knees during treadmill gait, stair step-up, and weight-bearing deep flexion.

Numerous studies have reported the 6 DOF tibiofemoral kinematics during the stance phase of gait (low range knee motion). While the DFIS observed the similar trend in 6 DOF knee kinematics, the DFIS data further revealed that the motion of the medial femoral condyle in the anteroposterior direction were greater than those of the lateral femoral condyle, and the excursions of the contact point in the anteroposterior direction were greater in the medial than in the lateral tibiofemoral compartment. The trend of condylar motion and articular contact biomechanics did not show the reported "medial pivoting" motion character during flexion–extension of the knee.[11,26,45-47] It corroborated the findings of Koo and Andriacchi[44] by showing that the medial condyle makes greater excursions in the transverse plane than the lateral femoral condyle during the stance phase of gait, i.e., the knee may actually have a lateral-pivoting motion pattern in the low flexion angles of the knee (during stance phases of gait).

During the stair step-up activity (moderate range of knee motion), both medial and lateral contact points moved anteriorly on the tibial articular surfaces along the step-up motion path. The total excursions of the articular contact points were similar on the medial and lateral tibial surfaces, similar to the femoral condylar motion measured with TEA. When the GCA was used,

the femoral condylar motion pattern was dramatically different. The medial condyle moved anteriorly, while the lateral condyle shifted posteriorly throughout the activity when GCA was used. Selection of coordinate systems could cause changes in knee joint kinematics description. Interestingly, both medial and lateral compartments were under convex (femur) to convex (tibia) contact in the sagittal plane; the medial tibial articular contact radius was larger than the lateral side. These data could provide new insights into the understanding of dynamic knee stability.

During the weight-bearing deep flexion (full range of knee motion), a continued internal tibial rotation with flexion occurred and the cartilage contact excursion at medial side is smaller at the high flexion range when compared to those at the lateral side. The locations of the tibiofemoral articular cartilage contact points were in the central portion of the medial compartment and in the posterior half of the lateral compartment. This indicated the path dependence of the knee motion during the high flexion of the knee. Yildirim et al[48] reported that at 155° of flexion, the contacts on the femur were at the extreme superior–posterior region of the articular surfaces using a cadaveric testing model. On the medial side, there was also contact between the posterior femoral cortex and the posterior edge of the tibia, which represented an "impingement" of the knee and the lateral femoral condyle lift. These data showed that the posterior impingement between bone and soft tissue may play an important role in the stability of the knee in high flexion.

In summary, these data provide insights into the *in vivo* physiological kinematics of the knee and may be instrumental in the development of TKA that is aimed to reproduce native knee function. In addition to the application of femoral rollback and medial pivoting as kinematic foundations, contemporary TKA techniques may need to consider the articular contact geometry and kinematics of the knee. The data further suggested that there are several points that should be noted in understanding the characteristics of knee kinematics. First, the knee kinematics is greatly activity or loading dependent and should therefore be interpreted in the context of the test modality. Biomechanical studies of the knee, performed *in vitro* or *in vivo*, may report different patterns of knee kinematics. Second, the various coordinate system or measurement definitions of the knee kinematics may directly affect the described characters of the knee motion. Selection of coordinate systems could change the knee joint kinematics description dramatically. Different definitions of the motion axes among the various studies might lead to different conclusions of the knee joint kinematics data. Third, it is important to understand the advantages and disadvantages of the various technologies used for measurements of knee joint kinematics. The main advantages of the combined DFIS and 3D-MRI technique are the high accuracy, relatively low radiation, and noninvasive nature.

This technique could provide information on the *in vivo* motion of the knee, which is valuable for understanding various types of knee pathology and for evaluating the effectiveness of surgical procedures for treatments of diseased knees.

REFERENCES

1. Li G, DeFrate LE, Park SE, Gill TJ, Rubash HE. In vivo articular cartilage contact kinematics of the knee: an investigation using dual-orthogonal fluoroscopy and magnetic resonance image-based computer models. *Am J Sports Med.* 2005;33(1):102-107.
2. Komistek RD, Dennis DA, Mahfouz M. In vivo fluoroscopic analysis of the normal human knee. *Clin Orthop Relat Res.* 2003;410:69-81.
3. Banks SA, Harman MK, Hodge WA. Mechanism of anterior impingement damage in total knee arthroplasty. *J Bone Joint Surg Am.* 2002;84-A(suppl 2):37-42.
4. Fitz W, Sodha S, Reichmann W, Minas T. Does a modified gap-balancing technique result in medial-pivot knee kinematics in cruciate-retaining total knee arthroplasty? A pilot study. *Clin Orthop Relat Res.* 2012;470(1):91-98.
5. Kuroyanagi Y, Mu S, Hamai S, Robb WJ, Banks SA. In vivo knee kinematics during stair and deep flexion activities in patients with bicruciate substituting total knee arthroplasty. *J Arthroplasty.* 2012;27(1):122-128.
6. Moynihan AL, Varadarajan KM, Hanson GR, et al. In vivo knee kinematics during high flexion after a posterior-substituting total knee arthroplasty. *Int Orthop.* 2010;34(4):497-503.
7. Lafortune MA, Cavanagh PR, Sommer HJ III, Kalenak A. Three-dimensional kinematics of the human knee during walking. *J Biomech.* 1992;25(4):347-357.
8. Nakagawa S, Kadoya Y, Todo S, et al. Tibiofemoral movement 3: full flexion in the living knee studied by MRI. *J Bone Joint Surg Br.* 2000;82(8):1199-1200.
9. Stiehl JB, Komistek RD, Dennis DA, Paxson RD, Hoff WA. Fluoroscopic analysis of kinematics after posterior-cruciate-retaining knee arthroplasty. *J Bone Joint Surg Br.* 1995;77(6):884-889.
10. Van de Velde SK, Bingham JT, Gill TJ, Li G. Analysis of tibiofemoral cartilage deformation in the posterior cruciate ligament-deficient knee. *J Bone Joint Surg Am.* 2009;91(1):167-175.
11. Wretenberg P, Ramsey DK, Nemeth G. Tibiofemoral contact points relative to flexion angle measured with MRI. *Clin Biomech.* 2002;17(6):477-485.
12. van Dijk R, Huiskes R, Selvik G. Roentgen stereophotogrammetric methods for the evaluation of the three dimensional kinematic behaviour and cruciate ligament length patterns of the human knee joint. *J Biomech.* 1979;12(9):727-731.
13. Andriacchi TP, Alexander EJ, Toney MK, Dyrby C, Sum J. A point cluster method for in vivo motion analysis: applied to a study of knee kinematics. *J Biomech Eng.* 1998;120(6):743-749.
14. Li G, Wucrz TH, DeFrate LE. Feasibility of using orthogonal fluoroscopic images to measure in vivo joint kinematics. *J Biomech Eng.* 2004;126(2):314-318.
15. You BM, Siy P, Anderst W, Tashman S. In vivo measurement of 3-D skeletal kinematics from sequences of biplane radiographs: application to knee kinematics. *IEEE Trans Med Imaging.* 2001;20(6):514-525.
16. Asano T, Akagi M, Tanaka K, Tamura J, Nakamura T. In vivo three-dimensional knee kinematics using a biplanar image-matching technique. *Clin Orthop Relat Res.* 2001;388:157-166.
17. Sheehan FT, Zajac FE, Drace JE. Using cine phase contrast magnetic resonance imaging to non-invasively study in vivo knee dynamics. *J Biomech.* 1998;31(1):21-26.
18. Moro-oka TA, Hamai S, Miura H, et al. Dynamic activity dependence of in vivo normal knee kinematics. *J Orthop Res.* 2008; 26(4):428-434.
19. Qi W, Hosseini A, Tsai TY, Li JS, Rubash HE, Li G. In vivo kinematics of the knee during weight bearing high flexion. *J Biomech.* 2013;46(9):1576-1582.
20. Li JS, Hosseini A, Cancre L, Ryan N, Rubash HE, Li G. Kinematic characteristics of the tibiofemoral joint during a step-up activity. *Gait Posture.* 2013;38(4):712-716.
21. Bertin KC, Komistek RD, Dennis DA, Hoff WA, Anderson DT, Langer T. In vivo determination of posterior femoral rollback for subjects having a NexGen posterior cruciate-retaining total knee arthroplasty. *J Arthroplasty.* 2002;17(8):1040-1048.
22. Most E, Zayontz S, Li G, Otterberg E, Sabbag K, Rubash HE. Femoral rollback after cruciate-retaining and stabilizing total knee arthroplasty. *Clin Orthop Relat Res.* 2003;410:101-113.
23. Dennis DA, Komistek RD, Colwell CE Jr, et al. In vivo anteroposterior femorotibial translation of total knee arthroplasty: a multi-center analysis. *Clin Orthop Relat Res.* 1998;356:47-57.
24. Iwaki H, Pinskerova V, Freeman MA. Tibiofemoral movement 1: the shapes and relative movements of the femur and tibia in the unloaded cadaver knee. *J Bone Joint Surg Br.* 2000;82(8):1189-1195.
25. DeFrate LE, Sun H, Gill TJ, Rubash HE, Li G. In vivo tibiofemoral contact analysis using 3D MRI-based knee models. *J Biomech.* 2004;37(10):1499-1504.
26. Logan M, Dunstan E, Robinson J, Williams A, Gedroyc W, Freeman M. Tibiofemoral kinematics of the anterior cruciate ligament (ACL)-deficient weightbearing, living knee employing vertical access open "interventional" multiple resonance imaging. *Am J Sports Med.* 2004;32(3):720-726.
27. Schmidt R, Komistek RD, Blaha JD, Penenberg BL, Maloney WJ. Fluoroscopic analyses of cruciate-retaining and medial pivot knee implants. *Clin Orthop Relat Res.* 2003;410:139-147.
28. Ranawat CS. Design may be counterproductive for optimizing flexion after TKR. *Clin Orthop Relat Res.* 2003;416:174-176.
29. Walker PS, Sathasivam S. Design forms of total knee replacement. *Proc Inst Mech Eng H.* 2000;214(1):101-119.
30. Li G, Van de Velde SK, Bingham JT. Validation of a non-invasive fluoroscopic imaging technique for the measurement of dynamic knee joint motion. *J Biomech.* 2008;41(7):1616-1622.
31. Li G, Kozanek M, Hosseini A, Liu F, Van de Velde SK, Rubash HE. New fluoroscopic imaging technique for investigation of 6DOF knee kinematics during treadmill gait. *J Orthop Surg Res.* 2009;4:6.
32. Stiehl JB, Abbott BD. Morphology of the transepicondylar axis and its application in primary and revision total knee arthroplasty. *J Arthroplasty.* 1995;10(6):785-789.
33. Churchill DL, Incavo SJ, Johnson CC, Beynnon BD. The transepicondylar axis approximates the optimal flexion axis of the knee. *Clin Orthop Relat Res.* 1998;356:111-118.
34. Niki Y, Nagai K, Sassa T, Harato K, Suda Y. Comparison between cylindrical axis-reference and articular surface-reference femoral bone cut for total knee arthroplasty. *Knee Surg Sports Traumatol Arthrosc.* 2017;25(12):3741-3746.
35. Eckhoff DG, Bach JM, Spitzer VM, et al. Three-dimensional mechanics, kinematics, and morphology of the knee viewed in virtual reality. *J Bone Joint Surg Am.* 2005;87(suppl 2):71-80.
36. Eckhoff D, Hogan C, DiMatteo L, Robinson M, Bach J. Difference between the epicondylar and cylindrical axis of the knee. *Clin Orthop Relat Res.* 2007;461:238-244.
37. Kozanek M, Hosseini A, Liu F, et al. Tibiofemoral kinematics and condylar motion during the stance phase of gait. *J Biomech.* 2009; 42(12):1877-1884.
38. Grood ES, Suntay WJ. A joint coordinate system for the clinical description of three-dimensional motions: application to the knee. *J Biomech Eng.* 1983;105(2):136.
39. Li G, Moses JM, Papannagari R, Pathare NP, DeFrate LE, Gill TJ. Anterior cruciate ligament deficiency alters the in vivo motion of the tibiofemoral cartilage contact points in both the anteroposterior and mediolateral directions. *J Bone Joint Surg Am.* 2006; 88(8):1826-1834.

40. Liu F, Kozanek M, Hosseini A, et al. In vivo tibiofemoral cartilage deformation during the stance phase of gait. *J Biomech.*
2010;43(4):658-665.

41. Defrate LE, Papannagari R, Gill TJ, Moses JM, Pathare NP, Li G.
The 6 degrees of freedom kinematics of the knee after anterior cru-
ciate ligament deficiency: an in vivo imaging analysis. *Am J Sports
Med.* 2006;34(8):1240-1246.

42. Yin P, Li JS, Kernkamp WA, et al. Analysis of in-vivo articular
cartilage contact surface of the knee during a step-up motion. *Clin
Biomech.* 2017;49:101-106.

43. Dimitriou D, Tsai TY, Park KK, et al. Weight-bearing condyle
motion of the knee before and after cruciate-retaining TKA: in-vivo
surgical transepicondylar axis and geometric center axis analyses.
J Biomech. 2016;49(9):1891-1898.

44. Koo S, Andriacchi TP. The knee joint center of rotation is predominantly on the lateral side during normal walking. *J Biomech.*
2008;41(6):1269-1273.

45. Todo S, Kadoya Y, Moilanen T, et al. Anteroposterior and rotational movement of femur during knee flexion. *Clin Orthop Relat
Res.* 1999;362:162-170.

46. Bingham J, Li G. An optimized image matching method for determining in-vivo TKA kinematics with a dual-orthogonal fluoroscopic imaging system. *J Biomech Eng.* 2006;128(4):588-595.

47. Shefelbine SJ, Ma CB, Lee KY, et al. MRI analysis of in vivo meniscal and tibiofemoral kinematics in ACL-deficient and normal knees.
J Orthop Res. 2006;24(6):1208-1217.

48. Yildirim G, Walker PS, Sussman-Fort J, Aggarwal G, White B,
Klein GR. The contact locations in the knee during high flexion.
Knee. 2007;14(5):379-384.

SECTION 2 / BASIC SCIENCE

chapter 9

Knee Biomechanics and Implant Design

Timothy M. Wright, PhD | Fernando J. Quevedo Gonzalez, PhD

The mechanics and to a large extent the clinical performance of total knee arthroplasty can best be explained by considering design objectives. Replacing diseased and damaged tissues with human-made implants requires that the resulting composite structure restore normal joint function while also transferring large loads across the joint. The implant components themselves must remain well-fixed to the supporting bone and be as wear-resistant as possible to maintain a low-friction articulation and to avoid osteolysis. The challenge in designing an effective knee replacement is that these goals are competing; the optimal solution to reach one goal may be far from optimal to reach another. Ensuring normal joint kinematics, for example, requires articular surfaces that are not overly constrained. However, reduced constraint usually means reduced conformity between the surfaces, which may lead to unacceptably high contact stresses that increase the chance for wear and mechanical loosening of the implant components.

Contemporary knee replacement designs form an array of solutions aimed at reaching the best compromise between these competing objectives. Understanding how a specific design solution affects mechanical performance requires consideration of the functional and structural aspects of the normal knee joint, together with the mechanical principles that control kinematics, load transmission, and wear in a bone–implant system.

LESSONS FROM THE NATURAL KNEE JOINT

Functional Considerations

The primary motion of the knee joint is flexion and extension in the sagittal plane. The kinematics of the femur, tibia, and patella during this activity are determined by the anatomy of the femoral condyles, the tibial plateaus, and the patella; the muscle forces exerted across the joint; and the constraints provided by the cruciate and collateral ligaments. In the sagittal plane, the tibial plateaus are relatively flat, whereas the femoral condyles can each be approximated by two radii, a large radius forming the inferior portion of the condyle that contacts the plateau in extension and a smaller radius forming the posterior portion that contacts in flexion. If load transmission were based only on the bony anatomy, contact between the condyles and the plateaus would occur over a very small area, regardless of joint position, thus producing unacceptably large contact stresses. Fortunately, the menisci and the articular cartilage layers serve as effective load-transmission structures, distributing the joint loads over larger contact areas.

As the knee is flexed, the constraint provided by the posterior cruciate ligament (PCL) causes the femur to roll back on the tibia. The posterior translation combined with the smaller radii of curvature of the femoral condyles contacting the tibia as flexion increases provide the knee with a large range of motion. Rollback also increases the quadriceps moment arm by increasing the distance between the femorotibial contact points and the line of action of the muscle, providing a mechanical advantage for the muscle in resisting further flexion and in extending the knee.[1]

Rollback is asymmetric; femorotibial contact translates more posteriorly on the lateral than on the medial plateau, consistent with internal rotation of the tibia in flexion. The asymmetric rollback with greater translation of the lateral compartment of the knee can also be described as an internal rotation of the tibial relative to the femur. As the knee flexes, the tibia rotates internally guided by the anatomy of the condyles and forces exerted by the soft tissues. However, tibial rotation is quite variable. For example, in a recent study of 19 adult men between the ages of 45 and 75 years, the amount of internal rotation averaged between 11° and 12°, but the standard deviation was 6.6°.[2] The same was true for other activities such as climbing and descending stairs, bowling, and golfing. Similarly, in a study combining fluoroscopy with computed tomography to determine the three-dimensional, *in vivo*, weight-bearing kinematics of five normal knees, wide variations in tibial rotation were found across several activities.[3] For example, during rising from a chair, the average internal rotation was 19°, but the values ranged from 3° to 32° across the five subjects.

The primary motion of the patella with respect to the femur is in the sagittal plane. The kinematics of the natural patella is complex and affected markedly by the internal rotation of the tibia as the knee flexes. The bony anatomy of the patella and of the patellar groove of the femur provides considerable constraint to the patellofemoral joint,[4] but during flexion, subject-specific anatomy combines with soft tissue forces to cause the patella to rotate and translate about all three anatomic axes, including a medial shift by as much as 5 mm as the knee flexes.[5-7] Abnormalities in the way that the patella tracks along the trochlear groove of the distal femur can be the cause of patellofemoral disorders such as pain, instability, and arthritis. The reporting of patellar tracking is affected significantly by how coordinate systems are defined and by the way in which the joint is loaded and moved during testing. The measurement accuracy is important as differences in tracking can be small. Comparison between existing studies is difficult because of differences in methodology. Nonetheless, other than general agreement that the patella translates medially in early knee flexion and then translates laterally, other motions are less consistent and highly variable.[8]

The total resultant force on the distal femur is made up of a component due to patellofemoral contact and a component due to tibiofemoral contact.[1] During normal gait, the contact points between the patella and the femur and between the tibia and the femur move, and the positions and magnitudes of the contact forces change. However, the positions and magnitudes of these forces vary in such a way that the direction of the total resultant force on the tibia remains relatively constant. This is consistent with the need for only small variations in surface curvature of the tibial plateau to maintain equilibrium through joint compression loading.[1]

Knee motions in the medial–lateral plane and in internal and external rotation are considerably smaller than in flexion–extension. Varus and valgus moments are created across the knee joint because of the medial–lateral components of the ground reaction force that occur during daily activities such as walking (**Fig. 9-1**). The knee resists these external moments by redistributing the load transmitted between the two plateaus.[1,9] Little medial–lateral translation is required between the joint surfaces; rather, the compliant nature of the meniscus, articular cartilage, and underlying subchondral bone provide the ability for load redistribution.

When the knee joint experiences varus or valgus moment, the pressure distribution on the two plateaus creates a net contact force acting on the tibia that is in reasonable alignment with the patellar ligament force (**Fig. 9-2**). But in response to a varus moment, for example, increased pressure is produced in the medial compartment of the knee, while pressure is reduced in the lateral compartment (**Fig. 9-3**); in effect, the location of the net contact force shifts to the medial side of the joint. The contact force creates an internal valgus moment about the center of the knee joint that resists the externally applied varus moment. Given the compliant nature of articular cartilage, the amount of joint angulation required to produce such redistribution in the pattern of surface deformation is small, typically less than a degree. Shifting the contact force as a mechanism for resisting varus and valgus moments has its limitations, of course, because the

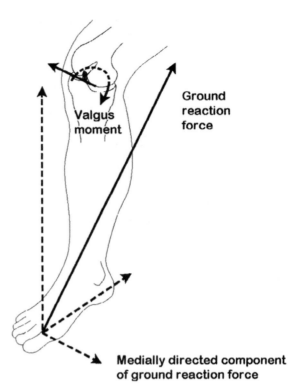

FIGURE 9-1 During the stance phase of gait, the medial component of the ground reaction force generates a varus moment about the knee. This moment is resisted by an internal valgus moment created by the structures at the knee joint. (Adapted from Burstein AH, Wright TM. *Fundamentals of Orthopaedic Biomechanics*. Baltimore: Williams & Wilkins; 1994, Fig. 3-11.)

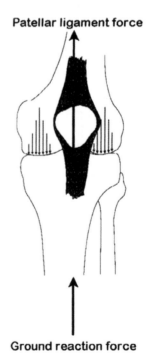

FIGURE 9-2 When the ground reaction force passes through the knee joint, no varus or valgus moment is created. The compressive effect of the force can be resisted by joint contact forces created on the medial and lateral condyles. (Adapted from Burstein AH, Wright TM. *Fundamentals of Orthopaedic Biomechanics*. Baltimore: Williams & Wilkins; 1994, Fig. 3-14.)

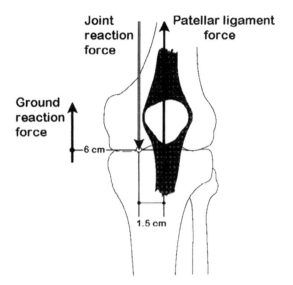

FIGURE 9-3 When the ground reaction force passes medially from the knee (the same conditions as shown in **Fig. 9-1**), the resulting varus moment can be resisted by the valgus moment created by a shift of the contact force to the medial side of the joint. (Adapted from Burstein AH, Wright TM. *Fundamentals of Orthopaedic Biomechanics*. Baltimore: Williams & Wilkins; 1994, Fig. 3-15.)

contact force can shift only as far as the outer edge of the joint. For larger varus or valgus moments, such as when the line of action of the ground reaction force passes at a larger distance from the knee than in normal gait, supplementary mechanisms, such as additional muscle forces, are necessary to generate an adequate resisting moment. However, the moment arms of the muscles about the center of the knee are quite short; because of this mechanical disadvantage, large muscle forces are necessary (**Fig. 9-4**).

With extreme externally applied moments, such as might occur in athletic activities or during a traumatic event, redistribution of joint pressures and additional muscle forces are insufficient to generate a large enough internal resisting moment. In such circumstances, a large angulation of the knee results in lift-off of one condyle and stretching of the collateral ligaments (**Fig. 9-5**). Such extreme conditions place considerable mechanical burden on the knee joint.

The mechanical disadvantage of the muscle and joint contact forces about the knee in resisting externally applied functional loads creates both large muscle forces and large contact forces. Such loads cannot be measured directly in normal knees but loads across the tibiofemoral joint have been measured with instrumented total knee devices implanted in patients. The recorded values of joint load in these patients reached as high as four times body weight between the femur and tibia during normal activities of daily living.[9,10] Large contact forces also occur across the patellofemoral joint. In activities such as stair climbing, a ground reaction force of body weight passes far away from the knee joint (**Fig. 9-6**). To offset the resulting flexion moment, the quadriceps muscle must provide a much larger force than body weight to maintain equilibrium and control joint position. Patellofemoral contact forces exceed three times body weight for these more strenuous activities, but also exceed one and a half times body weight even for level walking.[11,12] In general, contact pressures increase with flexion angle and increase as the quadriceps angle (Q angle) deviates from normal.[9]

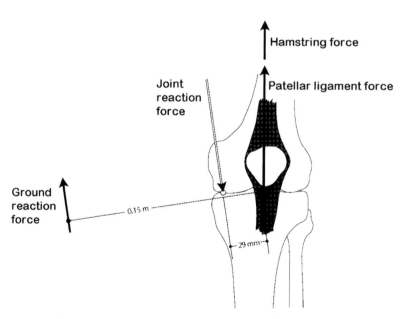

FIGURE 9-4 When the ground reaction force passes a greater distance from the knee (than is shown in **Fig. 9-3**), additional muscle forces act along with the contact force to offset the varus moment. (Adapted from Burstein AH, Wright TM. *Fundamentals of Orthopaedic Biomechanics*. Baltimore: Williams & Wilkins; 1994, Fig. 3-16.)

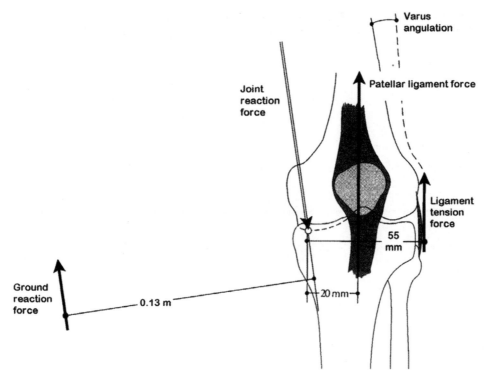

FIGURE 9-5   When the ground reaction force passes too great a distance medially from the knee joint, the joint may open on the lateral side. The resulting stretching of the collateral ligament provides a valgus moment to help offset the varus moment. (Adapted from Burstein AH, Wright TM. *Fundamentals of Orthopaedic Biomechanics*. Baltimore: Williams & Wilkins; 1994, Fig. 3-18.)

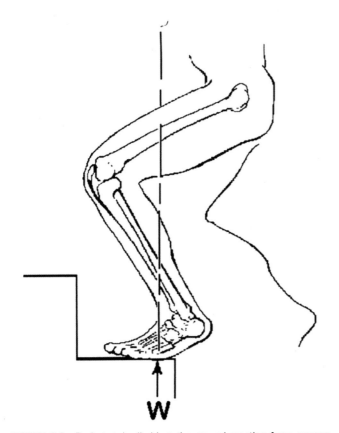

FIGURE 9-6   During stair climbing, the ground reaction force passes far behind the knee joint, creating a large flexion moment about the knee joint. This moment is resisted by the pull of the quadriceps, which in turn generates a large contact force across the patellofemoral joint. W, body weight. (Adapted from a very old In-Training exam, but as far as is known, an original drawing.)

Structural Considerations

Transmission of the joint contact loads into the supporting cancellous bone and then to the metaphyseal cortex dominates the mechanical burden placed on the knee joint. In comparison to these large loads, the additional ligamentous loads placed on the joint are quite small. Consider the tibia, for example. Below the cartilage surface and subchondral bone, the joint loads are borne primarily by cancellous bone, which is quite dense under the tibial plateaus, decreasing distally (**Fig. 9-7**). The denser the cancellous bone, the greater its stiffness and strength,[13] so the greater its load-carrying capacity. Therefore, the density distribution of the cancellous bone provides a map of the load-transmission pathway through the epiphysis.

While the cancellous bone density decreases distally, the density and thickness of the cortical bone forming the outer shell of the proximal tibia increase. The shell is thin and porous near the joint line, with mechanical properties more like that of the cancellous bone in this region,[14] but the shell becomes thicker and denser (and thus stiffer) as the metaphysis is approached. The relative portions of the load carried by the two structures (the cancellous bone and the outer shell) are determined by their relative stiffness. The structure that has the greater stiffness carries more of the load (this concept is explored in more detail later for the case of a knee joint with a total joint replacement). Thus, the axial load is carried almost entirely by the cancellous bone near the joint and is gradually transmitted to the cortical bone as the stiffness of the cancellous bone decreases and the stiffness of the outer shell increases.

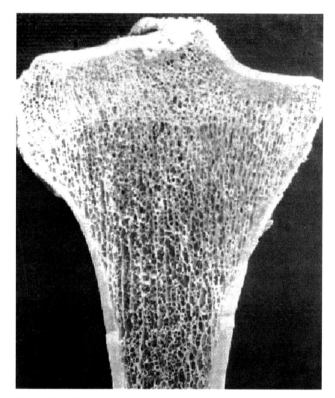

FIGURE 9-7 The structure of the proximal tibia shows dense cancellous bone primarily under the condyles. The architecture of the trabeculae provides a map of the load distribution from the joint surface down to the metaphyseal cortex. (From Hayes WC, Swenson LW Jr, Schurman DJ. Axisymmetric finite element analysis of the lateral tibial plateau. *J Biomech*. 1978;11:21-33, with permission.)

Cancellous bone density and hence its structural mechanical properties also vary with position in the transverse plane of the proximal tibia.[15] The greatest density occurs beneath the central plateaus, the regions in contact with the femoral condyles during most activities of daily living. The lowest density bone is found in the region between the plateaus. This bone has little stiffness or strength, consistent with the low mechanical demand required by this region. Density also varies in the anteroposterior direction, with denser bone often present in the posterior portions of the plateaus, especially on the lateral condyle.[15]

For the distal femur, the cancellous bone is most dense near the joint, immediately beneath the articular surfaces of the condyles, and in the region of the trochlear groove. Both the distribution of density and the orientation of the cancellous bone architecture in the distal femur show that the load is transferred from the dense subchondral bone to the cortical bone of the diaphysis over a relatively short metaphyseal region.[16] As with the tibia, the cortical shell is quite thin near the joint and so adds little to load transmission.

KNEE REPLACEMENT DESIGN

In restoring function by reconstructing a diseased or damaged knee joint, the implant designer must seek adequate kinematics and joint stability while maximizing the implant's longevity in terms of maintaining fixation of the implant components to the surrounding bone and limiting damage and wear to the implant components. Just as the bony anatomy of the natural knee and the mechanical properties of the soft tissues directly control the kinematics, stability, contact forces, and load transmission across the joint, the designer's choices of geometries and materials for the implant determine these same biomechanical traits for the knee replacement. The requirements for adequate function while also achieving adequate long-term fixation and damage resistance can create conflicting design objectives. To make rational choices among knee replacement systems, the surgeon must understand the interplay between competing requirements for total knee replacements and the influence of the implant's design factors on each of these functional requirements.

Most modern total knee replacements consist of a metallic femoral component with a bicondylar convex articular surface that replaces the femoral condyles, a tibial component consisting of a metallic tray and a polyethylene insert to replace the tibial plateaus, and a polyethylene component to resurface the patella. Conceptually speaking, we can divide the process of knee replacement design into (1) the design of the articular surfaces, which determines the kinematics, joint stability, and wear characteristics of the implant and (2) the design of the fixation features, which determines how the load is transferred from the implant to the surrounding bone.

Design of Articular Surfaces

When designing the articular surfaces, the designer must balance the competing objectives of achieving adequate kinematics, like that in the natural knee, ensuring adequate joint stability, and generating low-contact stresses to reduce polyethylene damage and wear.

Kinematics

Knee replacement designs control their main motion, flexion–extension, primarily through the geometry of the femoral condyles and the tibial plateaus in the sagittal plane. Most contemporary total knee designs approximate the anteroposterior geometry of the natural femoral condyles using two radii: a large radius that contacts the plateau near extension and a smaller posterior radius that contacts as the knee flexes. Also known as J-curve, this design differs from single-radius designs that utilize a unique radius of curvature for the femoral condyles in the sagittal plane. Single-radius designs were introduced to improve mid-flexion instability (instability between 30° and 45° of flexion) and to provide a longer extensor moment arm, thus reducing quadriceps forces during extension.[17] Clinical results with single versus J-curve type designs are equivocal with randomized clinical trials that show no difference in clinical or functional outcomes[18,19] and others that show improved outcomes for single-radius designs.[20,21]

The articular geometry of the tibial surface is concave, usually with a larger radius than that of the femoral condyles. The concave shape forces the femoral component to rest in the lowest or most distal point of the tibial articular surface, called the dwell point. However, the larger radius of the tibial surface provides some laxity in the antero-posterior direction, allowing the femoral component to roll back on the tibial component as the knee flexes. In this way, the closer the radius of the femoral and tibial surfaces, the lesser the anteroposterior translation of the femur. Deep-dish (also called ultracongruent) designs are an example of how designers have exploited such radial conformity to constraint anteroposterior translation of the femur by more conforming tibial and femoral surfaces.

The rollback of the femur on the tibia as the knee flexes is ensured by one of two methods. The first method is retention of the PCL so that it provides the same function as in the natural knee; these implants are known as cruciate-retaining (CR) designs. CR designs often use relatively flat surfaces on the plateaus of the tibial component so that the articular surfaces do not constrain the posterior translation created by the pull of the ligament. Flatter surfaces are advantageous for contact stresses when load is transferred through both condyles, but they are at disadvantage when varus–valgus rotations are introduced, as edge loading may occur. Advantages of PCL retention include more natural kinematics and maintenance of the proprioception and load transfer capabilities of the ligament.[22,23] However, the PCL is difficult to balance at surgery and often does not remain functional after knee replacement.[24,25] Furthermore, studies showed that proprioception did not differ whether the ligament was retained or not at knee replacement.[26,27] To ensure proper PCL function after knee replacement, the joint line must remain near its preoperative level or kinematics will be adversely affected. For example, if too thick a tibial component is used, the joint line will be raised, and the PCL will become tight in flexion, adding to the femorotibial contact force and increasing contact stresses and polyethylene wear.[28]

Alternatively, the PCL ligament can be replaced by a geometric constraint to anterior translation of the femoral component through a post-and-cam mechanism; these implants are known as posterior-stabilized (PS) designs. In PS designs, posterior translation of the femur as the knee flexes is ensured by combining a posteriorly positioned dwell point with the post-cam mechanism (**Fig. 9-8**). Before the femoral cam engages the tibial post, the femoral component sits at the dwell point and shows little posterior translation as the knee flexes provided that large compressive loads are applied across the joint, such as would occur during level gait. After post-cam engagement, the cam "pushes" on the post, resulting in posterior rollback of the femur. The flexion angle at which the post and cam engage depends on several factors, including the shape of the tibial and femoral articular surfaces, the surgical placement and orientation of the knee components, and the variations

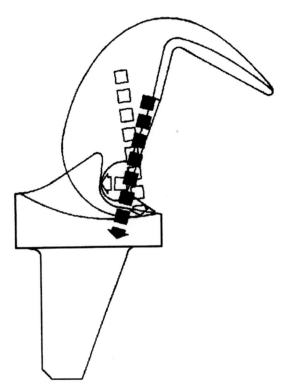

FIGURE 9-8 Posterior-stabilized knee implants replace the function of the posterior cruciate ligament with a mechanism by which a post on the tibial component impacts a cam on the femoral component as the joint flexes. The resultant force on the tibia (the solid dashed arrow) is composed of the joint contact force and the shear force of the cam on the post (two open dashed arrows). (From Insall JN, Lachiewicz PF, Burstein AH. The posterior stabilized condylar prosthesis: a modification of the total condylar design. Two to four-year clinical experience. *J Bone Joint Surg.* 1982;64A:1317-1323, with permission.)

in knee loading among patients and across activities of daily living. Reports from *in vivo* kinematic studies of PS patients showed that cam-post engagement does indeed vary considerably from as little as about 30° of flexion to as much as 90°.[29,30]

Substituting for the PCL provides both range of motion and joint stability and allows for more conforming surfaces without compromising kinematics.[31] Posterior stabilized designs have disadvantages as well. Greater bone must be resected from the femoral intercondylar notch than in CR designs to make room for the cam mechanism. Furthermore, significant wear and even fracture of the polyethylene post can occur because of impingement of the post with the femoral component.[32,33]

Clinical performance and outcome differences between CR and PS designs are generally insignificant. Meta-analysis of randomized clinical trials and comprehensive review of studies directly comparing CR and PS designs have found few differences,[34,35] though both types of studies revealed greater range of motion with PS designs. This difference is likely the result of the controlled rollback that is afforded by the post-cam mechanism, as has been shown in *in vivo* fluoroscopic analyses of patients with CR and PS total knee replacements (**Fig. 9-9**).[36]

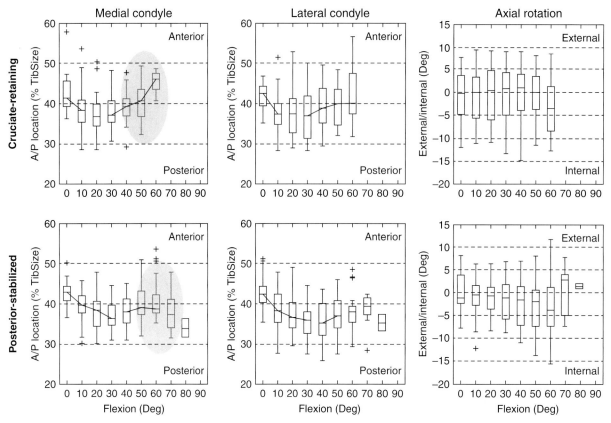

FIGURE 9-9 Similar patterns of anteroposterior translation of the medial femoral condyle on the tibia (left), the lateral condyle (center), and axial rotation (right) for cruciate-retaining and posterior-stabilized knee replacement designs. Note the shaded gray ovals that demonstrate paradoxical anterior displacement of the medial condyle with flexion for the CR knee, while the post-cam mechanism forces the condyle displacement posteriorly with flexion back on the tibia. (From Fantozzi S, Catani F, Ensini A, Leardini A, Giannini S. Femoral rollback of cruciate-retaining and posterior-stabilized total knee replacements: in vivo fluoroscopic analysis during activities of daily living. *J Orthop Res*. 2006;24:2222-2229, with permission.)

High-flexion versions of CR and PS designs incorporate design changes to accommodate flexion typically beyond 135°. These changes include decreasing the femoral condyle radii at mid- and high-flexion, reducing the anterior-central portion of the tibial plateau to avoid patellofemoral impingement and, in the case of PS designs, changes to the cam and post to avoid dislocation as the cam moves toward the top of the intercondylar spine. However, as with CR versus PS designs, meta-analyses of randomized clinical trials revealed that high-flex knee replacements did not appear to confer any benefit as compared to standard designs.[37,38]

Flexion–extension in the natural knee is accompanied by rotational motion in the axial plane. For knee replacements, combining curved surfaces in the anteroposterior direction with curvature in the medial–lateral direction (creating a toroidal shape) is a common method used to provide rotational laxity to knee replacements.[39] Rotational laxity is limited even in the natural knee, so these curved surfaces can be quite, although not completely, conforming in the medial–lateral direction[40] and nonetheless allow sufficient axial rotation. Many designs use a single radius for each condyle of the femoral component and a single, slightly larger radius for each tibial plateau; however, toroidal

geometries have the added advantage of being somewhat forgiving in terms of surgical positioning and orientation. Even if the components are not ideally positioned and oriented with respect to one another, contact between toroidal surfaces provides contact between curved surfaces and hence larger contact areas.

Many current designs use the same two radii in the lateral and medial condyles so that the implant is symmetric about the sagittal plane. However, alterations from symmetric condylar geometries are sometimes included to use the femorotibial surfaces to guide internal rotation of the tibia. The prime example of this approach is the medial pivot design, which forces contact to remain near the center of the medial plateau by incorporating a large, single degree-of-freedom, ball and socket articulation, combined with a much less conforming lateral plateau. More recently, CR designs have employed asymmetric geometries with the lateral distal radius extended posteriorly to further aid natural anteroposterior rollback when the PCL is present.

The other main design approach to guide internal rotation of the tibia is that of mobile-bearing knee replacements. In these designs, the bearing needed for function is separate from the bearing between the articular surfaces.

The former bearing is typically placed between the tibial component and a polished metallic base plate, whereas the latter remains a more conventional bearing between the femoral and tibial components. The mobile nature of the tibial component, whether as a meniscal type bearing, a medial pivot bearing, or a rotating platform, is intended to allow the muscles and ligaments to control and constrain joint motion. Theoretically, this approach provides for normal joint kinematics while also allowing the articular joint surfaces to be more conforming than in a fixed bearing knee, leading to larger contact areas, lower contact stresses, and presumably better wear resistance.[41-43] However, long-term clinical studies with results beyond 10 years of follow-up have found no difference between mobile- and fixed-bearing designs.[44,45] Similarly, a longer-term study (with follow-up from 15 to 18 years) in young active bilateral total knee patients who had received a mobile-bearing design in one knee and a fixed-bearing in the contralateral knee found no superiority of the mobile-bearing total knee prosthesis over the fixed-bearing total knee prosthesis.[46]

The kinematics of the patellofemoral joint is an important part of any total knee replacement design. The need for a large range of motion leads to the same design dilemma as in the femorotibial joint: the need for articular geometries that cause decreased contact areas with flexion coincident with increasing contact forces. Patellar component design alone cannot be expected to provide the necessary constraint for all patients and all activities. Moreover, as with the natural knee joint, the stability of the patellofemoral joint depends on the constraint (or stability) of the femorotibial joint in a total knee replacement. Three general design solutions exist for patellar implants: an anatomic shape intended to provide a conforming patellar track; a spherical, dome shape for the patellar implant intended to eliminate the importance of rotational alignment between the patellar and femoral components; and a mobile bearing intended to have the same rotational advantage as the dome design but with more conforming articular surfaces.

Few well-controlled clinical studies exist to determine the effect of the patella design on clinical outcome. An *in vivo* fluoroscopic study compared the patella kinematics of normal volunteers and total knee patients performing a weight-bearing deep-knee bend from full knee extension to maximum flexion.[47] The total knee patients had received either a dome-shaped or anatomic-shaped patella component. Both patellar component designs exhibited kinematics close to those of the normal patella, with good tracking of the patella in the trochlear groove throughout flexion. Though the patellofemoral contact areas were smaller in the total knee groups than the in the normal group, they were comparable between the two designs.

The kinematics of domed and anatomic patellar components have also been evaluated with computational models in combination with *in vivo* measurements.[48] Twenty total knee patients, half with domed and half with anatomic patellar components, but all with the same femoral and tibial component design, performed two tasks—while the motions of the patella were tracked using stereo radiography. Subject-specific finite element models were used to combine the *in vivo* kinematics with the models to evaluate the effect of patella design on loading and kinematics of the quadriceps mechanism. Though the anatomic design demonstrated kinematics closer to that of natural knees, patient variability and compensation strategies seemed to mask the effect of implant design on functional performance.

Closely matching normal anatomy would appear an obvious goal to maintaining normal function after knee replacement, but reaching this goal intraoperatively relies on surgical skill to achieve both appropriate alignment between the three joint components and adequate soft tissue balance throughout the range of motion. Replacing normal anatomy with a dome-shaped patellar implant bearing against a concave femoral flange does not require the same level of anatomic reconstruction because the curved shapes allow a small amount of surgical and functional misalignment while maintaining curved surfaces in contact with curved surfaces. The primary disadvantage is in flexion in which contact becomes much less conforming, increasing contact stresses in the polyethylene of the patellar implant.[49] Mobile-bearing designs allow very conforming geometries, thus addressing the contact problem.[50] But they require a metal backing that reduces the maximum polyethylene thickness, leading to the potential for excessive wear and loosening (as discussed further in Contact Problems and Implant Wear).

Joint Stability

When adequate ligamentous constraint is present, such as in the case of many primary knee replacements, the designer can emphasize functional (i.e., kinematic) over joint stability (i.e., constraint) requirements. This is the case for designs such as the CR and PS described above, which can be considered low-constraint designs. However, knee replacement systems usually provide multiple options to the surgeon to address the situations of inadequate collateral ligaments and bony deformities, such as might be encountered at difficult primary and many revision surgeries. These implants must provide greater joint stability than a conventional knee replacement. The additional levels of constraint are often gathered under common classifications—PS-plus (or PS constrained), constrained condylar knees, and hinges—even though levels of constraint can differ among the offerings from device manufacturers within any one classification. Increasing constraint between the femoral and tibial component often comes at the cost of higher burden placed in the cement and surrounding bone. As we will describe later, higher constraint usually requires the use of stems to provide additional resistance to varus–valgus moments.[51,52]

PS-plus designs include small modifications to conventional PS designs to increase primarily the varus–valgus constraint. Such modifications often include a wider intercondylar spine, narrower femoral box, or more pronounced lips on the edges of the tibial articulation. Constrained condylar knee replacements provide constraint by a polyethylene central spine on the tibial insert that fits into a mating intercondylar box on the femoral component.[53] The polyethylene spine and the metallic intercondylar box are more conforming than in a PS or PS-plus implant, such that varus–valgus and rotational motions are constrained when contact occurs between the medial and lateral surfaces of the spine and the corresponding surfaces of the box.

Mechanical laboratory testing has been used to examine limitations in the performance of these designs.[54] A robot testing system was used to determine the joint stability in human cadaveric knees as described by the moment versus angular rotation behavior under varus–valgus moments through a range of flexion up to 90°.[55] The primary stabilizing mechanism was found to be the redistribution of the contact force on the bearing surfaces (**Fig. 9-10**). Contact between the tibial post and the femoral box provided a secondary stabilizing mechanism after lift-off of a condyle had occurred. Collateral ligaments provide limited stability because little ligament elongation occurred under such small angular rotations. Compressive loads applied across the knee joint, such as would occur with the application of muscle forces, enhanced the ability of the bearing surfaces to provide resisting internal varus–valgus moment and, thus, reduced the exposure of the tibial post to the external varus–valgus loads.

Retrieved implants can be used to examine the impact of increased constraint on the implant components.

For example, retrieved PS-plus tibial polyethylene inserts were matched to retrieved PS inserts from the same manufacturer according to patient age, body mass index, and length of implantation.[56] By examining the surfaces of the tibial posts and performing laser scanning to establish permanent deformation and wear, PS-plus posts were significantly more damaged than PS posts. Surface deviation was significantly greater in the posterior and medial post regions of the PS-plus inserts. These results suggest that added constraint is accompanied by greater polyethylene surface damage.

In the absence of appropriate soft tissue constraints and in the presence of large bony defects, a mechanical solution is required by which the implant components provide nearly all the constraint and stability to the joint. This situation matches the early days of total knee replacement when highly constrained metal-on-metal hinges were used as primary knee replacements, often with resection of the collateral ligaments.[57] Modern hinged designs incorporate metal-on-polyethylene bushings for joint contact, less conforming "sloppy" hinges accommodating some small degree of translations and rotations between the axle and the bushings, and mobile rotating platforms to provide a degree of rotational freedom.[58] Though considered a salvage procedure, rotating hinge implants have shown good long-term clinical results with a low 4.5% cumulative incidence of revision for aseptic loosening at 10 years.[59] Overall revision rates are considerably higher,[59,60] with major reasons for failure such as periprosthetic fracture and extensor mechanism failure underscoring the mechanical burden caused when the implant transfers all the loads to the adjacent structures.

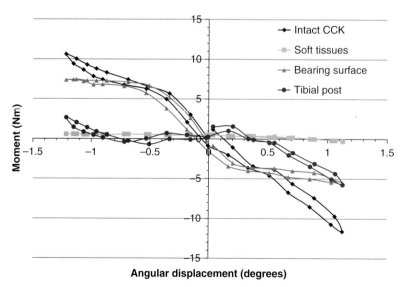

FIGURE 9-10 Relative contribution of the soft tissues (ligaments), the bearing surfaces, and the tibial post–box contact to the varus–valgus constraint of a constrained condylar knee total knee implant at 30° of flexion. (From Wang X, Malik A, Bartel DL, Wright TM, Padgett DE. Load sharing among collateral ligaments, articular surfaces, and the tibial post in constrained condylar knee arthroplasty. *J Biomech Eng*. 2016;138, with permission.)

Contact Problems and Implant Wear

Wear of the ultra-high-molecular-weight polyethylene bearing surfaces in total knee replacements is inevitable. The large stresses created in the material are enough to cause wear damage even in highly conforming designs.[61,62] Surface damage in turn generates polyethylene debris that accumulates in the surrounding joint space and soft tissues. The types of surface damage observed in total knee replacements differ from those seen in more conforming joint implants such as total hip replacements. In total hips, abrasive and adhesive wear dominate, causing burnishing and scratching of the polyethylene surface. These same damage modes occur in total knees but pitting and delamination (damage modes rarely seen in hip replacements) can dominate. Although the resulting wear particles are larger and therefore less active biologically,[63,64] these damage modes can nonetheless release large amounts of debris.

The underlying mechanisms responsible for wear damage remain poorly understood. Abrasive wear occurs at a rate proportional to the product of the contact pressure across the joint (P) and the relative sliding velocity of one surface across the other (V), so that wear rate = $k \times P \times V$, often referred to as the *Archard equation*.[65] The constant, k, depends on several factors, including the properties of the bearing materials and the lubrication conditions, in an unknown manner. Therefore, k must be determined empirically. Nonetheless, with the proper constant, the Archard-type equation has been used successfully to describe abrasive wear in total hip replacements.[65,66]

The mechanism for the pitting and delamination damage that occurs in total knee tibial components is less well understood. The mechanism most likely to be responsible is fatigue.[62,67] Because of the nonconforming nature of knee-bearing surfaces, the contact area between the femoral and tibial components moves over the tibial polyethylene surface during functional activities, creating large repetitive stresses at points along the path of the contact area that fluctuate from tensile to compressive at and near the material's surface. The cyclic nature of these stresses is enough to cause crack initiation and propagation from surface or subsurface defects.[67,68]

As previously discussed when considering kinematics and load transfer, the conformity between the femorotibial articular surfaces affects both the constraint and the contact area (and therefore the stresses associated with wear). Conformity changes in the medial–lateral direction significantly affect both contact stresses (**Fig. 9-11**) and constraint. If the femoral and tibial radii were made the same, the contact area would be maximized, and the stress would be minimized, similar to the situation described earlier for PCL-retaining designs in which the surfaces were flat (completely conforming with both radii equal lo infinity). These surfaces presented no rotational constraint because they were also flat in an anteroposterior direction. Making the femorotibial surfaces completely conforming for a total condylar implant, however, would effectively eliminate rotational laxity because of

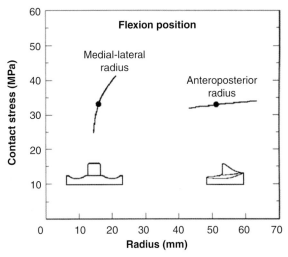

FIGURE 9-11 The contact stress on the surface of a condylar-type polyethylene implant is plotted against the radii of curvature of the implant in the medial–lateral and anteroposterior directions. If all other radii are held constant, the contact stress is not very sensitive to the anteroposterior radius but is markedly affected by the medial–lateral radius. MPa, megapascal. (Adapted from Bartel DL, Bicknell VL, Wright TM. The effect of conformity, thickness, and material on stresses in UHMWPE components for total joint replacement. *J Bone Joint Surg.* 1986;68A:1041-1051.)

the constraint between the medial–lateral and anteroposterior curved surfaces. Torsional loads across the knee joint would be taken entirely by the implant, with increased stresses placed on the fixation interfaces and therefore an increased likelihood for implant loosening.

Appropriate condylar design therefore requires a compromise between two objectives: minimizing contact stresses and providing appropriate kinematics and constraint. The choice of the appropriate balance between radii can be understood by plotting the contact stresses and medial–lateral constraint forces that result from different combinations of radii (**Fig. 9-12**). An analysis of contact stresses leads to a set of lines depicting constant maximum contact stress. A second analysis leads to a set of lines representing constant rotational resistance under joint compressive load. As radii become less equal (moving further away from the 45° line), constraint force decreases while contact stress increases. Using such information, the designer can choose a desired rotational resistance and determine the radii with the least contact stress.

Besides design of the articular surfaces, the contact problem between knee replacement components is also controlled by the mechanical properties of the bearing materials. Materials used for the femoral components (typically cobalt–chromium alloy or oxidized zirconium alloy) are much harder than polyethylene, with elastic moduli more than 200 times greater. The femoral component acts like a rigid indenter pushing against the much softer polyethylene, creating stresses in the polyethylene that dominate the wear behavior. Thus, the elastic modulus of the polyethylene directly influences the contact area and hence the contact stresses.[62]

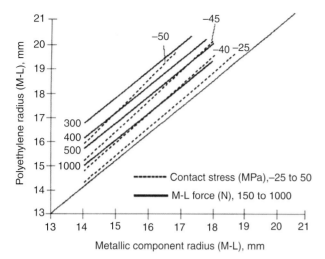

FIGURE 9-12 A completely conforming situation that would exist if the polyethylene radius (vertical axis) was the same as the metallic component radius (horizontal axis) is depicted as the 45° line. As the polyethylene component becomes less conforming, the contact stress increases, while resistance to rotation (depicted by the medial–lateral force required to rotate the components) decreases. Thus, the trade-off between wear and constraint can be examined on a case-by-case basis and for differing conditions (here, the applied load was 3,000 N, the polyethylene thickness was 7 mm, and the medial displacement at which the force was calculated was 0.25 mm). MPa, megapascal. (Adapted from Burstein AH, Wright TM. *Fundamentals of Orthopaedic Biomechanics*. Baltimore: Williams & Wilkins; 1994, Fig. 7-18.)

Modulus increases are a detrimental byproduct of the oxidative degradation experienced by polyethylene after radiation sterilization and continued exposure to air.[69-71] Polymer chain scission, increased cross-links between polymer chains, and reaction of free radicals with oxygen all combine to increase density and hence elastic modulus. Degradation was implicated in severe wear of total knee implants manufactured from polyethylene that had been gamma-sterilized in air (e.g., Refs. 72-76). Those findings led to the introduction of new forms of packaging and sterilization intended to reduce or eliminate the exposure of the components to oxygen prior to implantation. While such efforts showed a reduction in degradation, it was not eliminated, as shown by analyses of retrieved components, which showed increased oxidation with time *in vivo*.[77,78]

The other approach to addressing the wear problem is to change the wear resistance of the polyethylene. The introduction of highly cross-linked polyethylenes, fabricated through the combination of radiation exposure to create the cross-links in the material followed by thermal treatments to quench free radicals,[79,80] has revolutionized total hip replacement surgery. Indeed, clinical results beyond a decade with highly cross-linked acetabular components on total hip replacement have shown low wear rates and no or few cases of osteolysis secondary to polyethylene wear debris (e.g., Refs. 81,82). Highly cross-linked polyethylenes have also been introduced into total knee replacement. Clinical results between highly cross-linked and conventional polyethylenes have generally not shown a superiority for the highly

cross-linked versions,[83,84] though the Australian Orthopaedic Association National Joint Replacement Registry data for these two types of polyethylene does show a reduced cumulative revision rate at 15 years (**Fig. 9-13**).[85] The difference in revision rate when broken down by diagnosis shows the biggest difference in failures due to loosening, suggesting that the improved performance could be due to reduced wear and osteolysis (**Fig. 9-13**).

Analysis of retrieved highly cross-linked knee replacement components has also been used to assess the performance of these new forms of polyethylene. For example, similar *in vivo* oxidation has been reported in sequentially annealed highly cross-linked polyethylene tibial inserts as that found in tibial inserts gamma sterilized in an inert environment for implants retrieved after as long as nine and a half years of service.[86,87] Similar findings of oxidation have been reported for retrieved tibial components fabricated from remelted highly cross-linked polyethylene,[88] even though the remelting process, as opposed to annealing, should have quenched all free radicals from the material. As with the sequentially annealed material, oxidation increased with *in vivo* duration for the remelted polyethylene. Furthermore, in highly loaded regions of the bearing surface, the cross-link density was reduced with time *in vivo*,[86,88,89] suggesting that *in vivo* oxidation is related to material degradation. While the results of retrieval analyses of highly cross-linked polyethylenes have thus far not correlated to poor clinical outcomes, the findings suggest that continued vigilance is warranted as these materials are in use for longer times.

Other material properties, especially fracture toughness, can directly influence the performance of polyethylene knee replacement implants. Pitting and delamination are caused by crack initiation and propagation, phenomena made easier if the toughness of the material is low. Gross failure has been a major concern with the introduction of highly cross-linked polyethylenes for knee components because of the reduced fracture toughness and ductility of these materials over conventional polyethylene.[90,91] Reduction in ductility and strength secondary to oxidative degradation in conventional gamma-irradiated-in-air polyethylene was thought to contribute to several reports of fractured posts in tibial components of PS knee replacement implants (e.g., Ref. 92). The potential for reduced toughness to be detrimental to implant performance is a concern for the introduction of elevated cross-linked polyethylenes into total knee implants.[93] Indeed, cases of post fracture in highly cross-linked polyethylene PS implants have been reported,[94] though no strong evidence exists that the problem has been exacerbated using these new forms of the material.

Design of Fixation

Knee replacements must provide large but confined motions between bones, which results in load transmission across contact areas that can move appreciably across

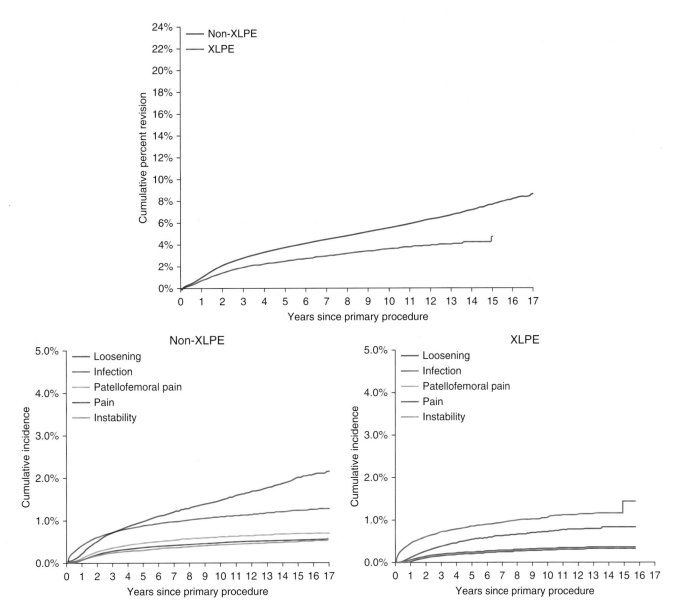

FIGURE 9-13 Registry data in the top plot demonstrate a reduced revision rate of total knee replacements with highly cross-linked polyethylene (XLPE) tibial inserts compared to those with conventional polyethylene (non-XLPE) inserts. The largest contributor to the differences is the reduction in failures related to aseptic loosening, as seen in the bottom plot, which suggests that the improvements in performance are related to reduced wear and osteolysis. (From *AOANJRR Hip, Knee & Shoulder Arthroplasty Annual Report for 2018,* Figures KT43 and KT44, p284. https://aoanjrr. sahmri.com/annual-reports-2018.)

the surfaces of the bones. The combination of moving contact points and large applied loads places considerable mechanical burden on the fixation between the implant components and the surrounding bone. The inability of the fixation to withstand such a burden leads directly to aseptic loosening, a primary reason for failure and the need for revision surgery.[85,95] The two main objectives that the designer must address are as follows: (1) how to achieve stable initial fixation between bone and implant; and (2) how to maximize the longevity of fixation. The latter objective is a trade-off between minimizing loads transferred to the interfaces to avoid mechanical loosening of the implant components and maintaining adequate load transfer to avoid stress shielding, which could also

weaken fixation. Therefore, the surgeon should understand the mechanisms by which implants transfer loads to the bone and how the designer's choices in terms of mode of fixation, fixation features, surface finish, and materials affect the load transfer and the burden placed on the bone–implant system both immediately after surgery and in the long term.

Load Transmission

Load transmission between knee replacement components and the surrounding bone can be divided load transfer and load sharing. Most total knee implants rely on broad areas of contact with adjoining cancellous bone in the distal femur, proximal tibia, and posterior patella. In such a situation, no composite structure is created within which the load can be shared, and direct load transfer between implant and bone occurs. From a mechanical standpoint, the stresses generated in the bone are inversely proportional to the area over which the load is distributed. Therefore, increasing the bone–implant interface area (i.e., by greater coverage) should, in general, contribute to reducing the stresses.

Nonetheless, for most daily activities the load in the proximal tibia is shifted posteriorly and medially. The load on the medial compartment can represent up to 85% of the total load during walking,[96] and it can reach eight times the load on the lateral compartment during activities such as squatting (**Fig. 9-14**).[97] Because of this inhomogeneous load transfer, the area of contact is small and increasing the coverage of the tibial baseplate will reduce the stresses in a less-than-proportional manner. Moreover, because the epiphyseal shell of the proximal tibia is thin and flexible[10] and, therefore, not much stiffer than the intracortical cancellous bone bed itself, extending the coverage to the cortical shell of the proximal tibia provides little advantage in terms of load transfer.

The inhomogeneous load transfer between implant components and bone has two other major implications for bone homeostasis. On the one hand, the high stresses that can be generated in the bone due to load transfer across a small area can overcome the strength of the bone and lead to implant migration[98] and ultimately failure by bone collapse.[99] On the other hand, zones of the bone–implant interface, like the femoral condyles and the trochlear groove, in which the stresses are reduced with respect to the natural knee, are shielded from load and thus are susceptible to bone resorption.[16,100,101]

Another important concept that impacts load transfer is component deformation during load transfer. Tibial components for knee replacements are subject to bending moments created because the area of cancellous bone on the superior surface over which the interface contact force is distributed is larger than the area at the articular surface over which the contact force is distributed (**Fig. 9-15**). Bending moments will cause the implant to deform, which, combined with the inhomogeneous load transfer described above, results in lift-off of the implant if the bone–implant interface cannot withstand tensile loads. The lower the stiffness of the component, the more the tendency for distortion and bending, so total knee implants that are relatively thin (and hence compliant), like monoblock tibial components with three-dimensional porosity for bone ingrowth, will exhibit more dramatic lift-off. On the other hand, the bending effect for a unicondylar implant (**Fig. 9-15**, bottom) is much less than in the total knee case because the plateau is narrow with a much larger thickness-to-width ratio, making the implant in effect stiffer than the total knee implant. The load is transferred across the implant–bone interface in a more uniform manner. Unfortunately, at the edges of the implant an abrupt change in load transfer occurs, causing high shear stresses in the bone. Unicondylar tibial components commonly subside as the bone around the periphery of the interface fails under these large shear loads.[102-104] As we will see later, one of the principal ways by which designers can reduce the magnitude of the lift-off is including supplemental fixation features, such as pegs, keels, or spikes.

As with the femoral component of a total hip replacement, the concept of load sharing is important for

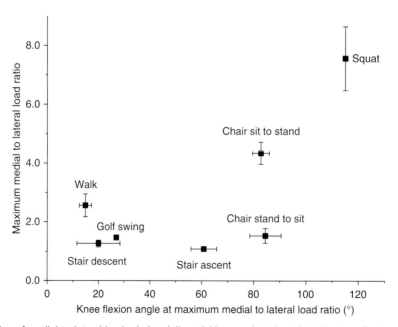

FIGURE 9-14 Maximum ratios of medial to lateral loads during daily activities as plotted against the knee flexion angle at which they occurred during the activity. (From Mundermann A, Dyrby CO, D'lima DD, Colwell C, Andriacchi TP. In vivo knee loading characteristics during activities of daily living as measured by an instrumented total knee replacement. *J Orthop Res.* 2008;26:1197-1172, with permission.)

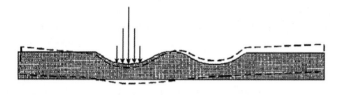

FIGURE 9-15 The distortion that a tibial component undergoes is a function of its material and thickness-to-width ratio. Thin, broad components with a small ratio will distort more than thick, narrow components with a larger ratio. Similarly, flexible components will distort more than stiff components. (Adapted from Burstein AH, Wright TM. *Fundamentals of Orthopaedic Biomechanics*. Baltimore: Williams & Wilkins; 1994, Fig. 7-10.)

understanding the performance of stems in total knee replacement. Load sharing between stem and bone does not result in a gradual transfer of the bending moment; instead, the stem carries part of the load throughout its length (**Fig. 9-16**). Near the stem tip, a more rapid transition occurs, with a large fraction of the moment transmitted to the bone over a short distance. The magnitude of the load carried by each structure (bone and stem) is controlled by its stiffness relative to the other structure. Because stem and bone are in intimate contact, bending the composite structure (consisting of the stem and the bone) produces the same deformation or curvature in the

bone as in the stem. However, the moment required to generate such deformation depends on the stiffness of each component, which is directly proportional to the product of the elastic modulus (E) and the moment of inertia of the cross-section (I). The more rigid structure (i.e., the structure with the higher bending stiffness) will require a larger bending moment to create the same deformation as in the less rigid structure.

As an example, consider a bone with a diaphyseal periosteal diameter (d_{outer}) of 22 mm and endosteal diameter (d_{inner}) of 11 mm (**Fig. 9-17**) with a canal filling cobalt–chrome alloy stem (i.e., 11 mm in diameter). The cobalt–chrome alloy has an elastic modulus roughly 10 times that of cortical bone (E = 200 GPa for the alloy as compared to E = 20 GPa for the bone tissue); however, the moment of inertia of the bone (I_{bone}) is approximately 15 times that of the stem (I_{stem}) because of its larger diameter. Therefore, the stiffness of the bone is 1.5 times that of the stem, and therefore, the bone will carry roughly 60% of the bending moment, and the stem, the remaining 40%. If the same stem were made from titanium alloy, with a modulus (E = 110 GPa) five times higher than the bone, the amount of the total moment carried by the bone would increase to approximately 75%.

Next suppose that the option exists to introduce a 1 mm larger cobalt–chrome stem (12 mm diameter) down the medullary canal, perhaps by reaming more bone from the endosteal surface of the cortex. In such a situation, the relative stiffness of the stem and bone changes significantly, to the point that the two structures now have the same relative bending stiffness, so the percentage of

FIGURE 9-16 A plot of the proportion of the bending moment taken by the stem as part of a stem–bone composite shows that the stem carries a large portion of the load over a considerable distance along its length. (Adapted from Burstein AH, Wright TM. *Fundamentals of Orthopaedic Biomechanics*. Baltimore: Williams & Wilkins; 1994, Fig. 7-4.)

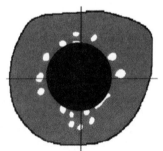

$$I_{bone} \propto d_{outer}^4 - d_{inner}^4 = 22^4 - 11^4 = 2.2 \times 10^5 \text{ mm}^4$$
$$I_{stem} \propto d^4 = 11^4 = 1.46 \times 10^4 \text{ mm}^4$$
$$I_{bone}/I_{stem} = 220000/14600 = 15$$

$$A_{bone} \propto d_{outer}^2 - d_{inner}^2 = 22^2 - 11^2 = 363 \text{ mm}^2$$
$$A_{stem} \propto d^2 = 11^2 = 121 \text{ mm}^2$$
$$A_{bone}/A_{stem} = 363/121 = 3$$

FIGURE 9-17 The cross-sectional properties of a long bone and an intramedullary stem show that while the moment of inertia (I) of the bone is 15 times that of the stem, its area (A) is only three times that of the stem. d, diameter. (Original artwork created by Timothy M. Wright.)

the bending moment carried by the bone and the stem is similar and equal to 50%. Thus, small changes in stem diameter (in the example, it changed by just 10%) can have quite large effects on load sharing, while changes in the stem's modulus (in the example, it changed by 50%) have only moderate effects on the load sharing of the components.

Stems on total knee implants are not always smooth and round, so they can also transmit axial and torsional loads along with bending loads. The transmission of axial and torsional loads is analogous to that of bending moments. For example, if the stem is well coupled to the bone surface by bone cement, the deformation caused by an axial compressive load (i.e., shortening) will be the same in the stem, cement mantle, and bone. As with bending, the amount of axial load required to produce such equal deformation in each structure will be proportional to that structure's stiffness which, in this case, is proportional to the product of the elastic modulus (E) and the area of the cross-section (A).

Consider the same geometry for the stem and the bone used in the bending example (**Fig. 9-17**). The stem still has an elastic modulus 10 times that of the bone tissue, but the area of the bone is only three times greater of the stem. Therefore, the axial stiffness of the bone is 3/10 times that of the stem, so the bone carries 23% of the axial load. Like the bending example, if the stem were made from titanium alloy, the fraction of the load carried by the bone will increase to 38%. Increasing the cobalt–chrome stem's diameter to 12 mm will further decrease the fraction of axial load carried by the bone to 19%. Note that, in this case, changes in stem's diameter have also greater effects than changes in stem's modulus.

In summary, both geometry and material properties directly influence the load sharing between the bone and the implant, such that the more rigid structure carries a larger proportion of the load. Moreover, the relationship between stiffness and the geometry of the structures (i.e., diameter of the stem) is not linear; in the case of bending (**Fig. 9-17**) and torsion, the stiffness depends on the fourth power of the diameter. Therefore, small geometric changes often have great impact in the load sharing between the bone and the implant, compared to changes in material properties.

Modes of Implant Fixation

Two ways exist for achieving a stable link between a knee replacement component and the surrounding bone: cemented and cementless fixation. Cemented knee replacements utilize polymethylmethacrylate (PMMA) as a grout between the component and the adjacent bone to achieve an immediate, stable bone–implant construct. As the implant is pressurized into the bone, the cement grout penetrates the trabeculae of cancellous bone, creating a mechanical interlock.[105,106] Adequate cement penetration into the cancellous bone is paramount for

successful fixation. Postmortem retrieval studies of tibial components for total knee replacement have revealed that cement penetration decreases with time *in vivo*, possibly due to bone remodeling.[107] Furthermore, it was estimated that 3 mm of cement penetration at the time of surgery is enough for long-term fixation.[107] To enhance cement penetration into the cancellous bone, the backside of cemented implants often includes pockets that allow for some level of cement pressurization as the implant is impacted. Failures of cemented implants can be related to debonding at both the implant–cement and bone–cement interfaces.[108] The strength of the cement–implant interface is also affected by the surface roughness of the implants[109] and by the type of cement utilized. For example, the use of high-viscosity cement is increasing among knee replacement surgeons,[110] because it allows for faster mixing and lower waiting times and increases the working and hardening times. Nonetheless, clinical reports show that high-viscosity cement may be at higher risk of early aseptic loosening.[111,112]

Cementless fixation devices rely on bone ingrowth into porous surfaces to ensure long-lasting bonding with the bone. This type of fixation is often thought as bone-preserving because it requires less bone removal than cemented fixation. The principal requirement for bone to grow into the porous surface is low relative motion between the implant and the bone. The maximum bone–implant micromotion for a stable interface that will result in bone ingrowth was quantified in canine bones to be in the range of 20 to 50 μm.[113-115] Similarly, well-fixed porous-coated anatomic medullary locking femoral hip stems retrieved post-mortem had at most 40 μm of relative motion.[116] Conversely, micromotions more than 150 μm result in the formation of fibrous tissue instead of bone tissue.[113,114,116]

The friction coefficient between implant and bone directly impacts the amount of relative motion. Traditional porous surfaces, consisting of a plasma spray or sintered beaded layer over the bulk material of the implant, have friction coefficients around 0.6.[117] Conversely, modern 3D-printed highly porous metallic materials have a structure that more closely mimics that of cancellous bone, with friction coefficients that approach 1.[118] Furthermore, the elastic modulus of these porous materials is close to that of cancellous bone, which has advantages for load transfer to the bone, but can also increase the lift-off of the implant due to bending, as explained earlier in the load transmission section.

The clinical superiority of one mode of fixation over the other is unclear. Radiostereometric analyses showed that although cementless tibial components with highly porous materials exhibit larger initial migration than cemented components, after 3 to 12 months the components stabilize[119-121] with excellent survivorship at 10 years,[122] like that of cemented components.[121] Interestingly, the amount of bone ingrowth required for adequate fixation appears to be low.

For example, for titanium fiber metal coatings in cementless acetabular components, limited human retrieval studies show bone ingrowth typically less than 15%,[123] including retrievals from autopsy cases in which the joint replacements were well functioning prior to death.[124] Similarly, ingrowth into trabecular metal coatings filled only about 4% of the pores of tantalum-coated acetabular components retrieved from total hip patients undergoing revision surgery,[125] like findings of 2% to 5% bone ingrowth into tantalum tibial trays from human total knee retrievals.[126]

Fixation Features

Knee replacement implants often include additional fixation features, such as pegs, spikes, keels, or stems that are utilized to provide other load transfer and load sharing pathways and resistance against rotational moments and shear forces. On the femoral and patellar components of primary knee replacements, the fixation is enhanced almost exclusively with the use of pegs regardless of the mode of fixation (cemented or cementless). In contrast, tibial components exhibit a wider variety of fixation features that often depend on the mode of fixation. Most cemented tibial components include either a central peg, that can be flanged or not, or a keel. Most designs also include the option of augmenting the fixation with short stems. On the other hand, cementless tibial components often include pegs or spikes, placed toward the periphery of the components in areas of good-quality cancellous bone. Although some cementless designs augment their fixation with keels or central stems, these features are usually smaller than for cemented components, as the designer's intent with cementless fixation is to preserve as much bone as possible.

Although these fixation features are capable of acting as load-sharing structures, they are in contact with the cancellous bone in the central region of the proximal tibia. This bone is too low in density and therefore in stiffness to share appreciable load with the peg (**Fig. 9-7**). Conversely, pegs placed directly under the tibial plateaus, like those utilized in certain cementless knee replacements, carry more load than might be expected, especially if the pegs are bonded to the bone.[127,128] The peg and the surrounding dense cancellous bone under the plateau form an effective load-sharing composite structure, so a major portion of the load is transferred through the tray into regions surrounding the relatively high stiffness peg-cancellous bone interface. A problem may commence at the time of implantation, when an interference fit between the peg and the cancellous bone produces considerable residual radial stresses in the bone. Although these stresses might encourage bone ingrowth and provide initial rigid fixation between the peg and the bone, the interference fit relieves stresses between the underside of the metallic tray and the cancellous bone. For porous surfaces intended for bone ingrowth, preferential load transfer through the pegs may lead to lack of bone ingrowth at other regions (**Fig. 9-18**), making the tray susceptible to failure or loosening in these regions.

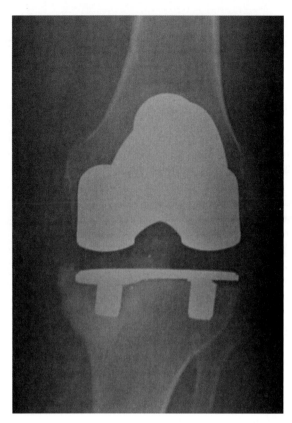

FIGURE 9-18 A well-ingrown lateral peg led to catastrophic failure of a cementless tibial implant with highly porous backing and pegs. (From Meneghini RM, de Beaubien BC. Early failure of cementless porous tantalum monoblock tibial components. *J Arthrop.* 2013;28:1505-1508, with permission.)

Long metallic stems are often included on revision components of total knee replacements to enhance the load transmission under varus–valgus loads, particularly in situations in which higher bending and torsional moments are to be expected due to more highly constrained components (i.e., constrained components to address soft tissue deficiency) or when bone quality is suspect. Stems on total knee implants, provided that they have the length and diameter to contact the cortex, can transmit bending loads, even if they are smooth and round[51]; however, smooth stems cannot transmit axial and torsional loads. An interposed layer of bone cement or a layer of porous coating into which bone has grown is necessary to fix the stem to the bone, allowing load sharing of axial and torsional loads. Similarly, cutting flutes along the length of the stem can transmit torsional loads, but have little capacity to transmit axial loads. Of course, stems are also usually tapered, which further enhances their ability to transfer axial load. Axial and torsional loads are distributed in a similar fashion to that for bending moments. For example, if the stem is well-coupled to the bone surface by cement, the shortening caused by an axial compressive load will be the same in the stem, the cement mantle, and the bone. As with load sharing in bending, the amount of axial load required to produce equal deformation in each structure will be proportional to that structure's stiffness.

Augmentation of Fixation

Surgeons are often faced with bony defects when performing revision or complex primary total knee arthroplasty. Though defects can be addressed with bone cement or bone graft, depending on the location and type of defect, most modern knee replacement systems include metallic augments in the form of wedges and cones or sleeves.[128-131] Wedges bridge the differential height that results from unicompartmental bone loss, effectively creating a flat continuous surface that provides enough support (and thus adequate load transfer) for normal alignment of the components (e.g., aligning the tibial baseplate perpendicular to the tibial mechanical axis). Cones or sleeves are available in a variety of sizes and shapes to address metaphyseal bone loss and to enhance bone–implant stability by maximizing the contact area between implant and bone (thus, improving load transmission). Most cone/sleeve designs include highly porous materials to seek biologic fixation by bone ingrowth, and they allow for some degree of freedom in terms of implant alignment within the augment. Mid-term clinical results have shown that cones and sleeves can achieve stable bone ingrowth.[132,133]

Cones and sleeves are often used in combination with stems; however, it is unclear how the enhanced stability provided by the augment may affect the required stem length. Furthermore, recent clinical results showed that metaphyseal cones were not associated with superior outcomes at short-term follow-up (minimum of 2 years, mean of 3.5 years).[134] Under optimal conditions, cones and sleeves behave as load-sharing structures that can minimize the micromotion between the augment and the surrounding bone.[135] However, concern remains that these augments could cause stress shielding of the bone, as suggested by computational studies.[136] Nonetheless, such stress shielding does not appear to be clinically significant, as the mid-term survivorship with aseptic loosening as the endpoint is greater than 96%.[132,133,137]

REFERENCES

1. Burstein AH, Wright TM. Biomechanics. In: Insall JN, Scott WN, eds. *Surgery of the Knee*. 3rd ed. New York: Churchill Livingstone; 2001:215-231.
2. Pfeiffer JL, Zhang S, Milner CE. Knee biomechanics during popular recreational and daily activities in older men. *Knee*. 2014;21:683-687.
3. Komistek RD, Dennis DA, Mahfouz M. In vivo fluoroscopic analysis of the normal human knee. *Clin Orthop Relat Res*. 2003;410:69-81.
4. Ahmed AM, Duncan NA. Correlation of patellar tracking pattern with trochlear and retropatellar surface topographies. *J Biomech Eng*. 2000;122:652-660.
5. Van Kampen A, Huiskes R. The tree-dimensional tracking pattern of the human patella. *J Orthop Res*. 1990;8:372-382.
6. Rhoads DD, Noble PC, Reuben JD, et al. The effect of femoral component position on patellar tracking after total knee arthroplasty. *Clin Orthop*. 1990;260:43-51.
7. Kaltwasser P, Uematsu O, Walker PS. The patella-femoral joint in total knee replacement. *Trans Orthop Res Soc*. 1987;12:292.
8. Katchburian MV, Bull AM, Shih YF, et al. Measurement of patellar tracking: assessment and analysis of the literature. *Clin Orthop Relat Res*. 2003;412:241-259.
9. Morrison JB. The mechanics of the knee joint in relation to normal walking. *J Biomech*. 1970;3:51-61.
10. Bergmann G, Bender A, Graichen F, et al. Standardized loads acting in knee implants. *PLoS One*. 2014;9:e86035.
11. Reilly DT, Martens M. Experimental analysis of the quadriceps muscle force and patello-femoral joint reaction force for various activities. *Acta Orthop Scand*. 1972;43:126-137.
12. Huberti HH, Hayes WC. Patellofemoral contact pressures. The influence of Q-angle and tendofemoral contact. *J Bone Joint Surg*. 1984;66-A:715-724.
13. Carter DR, Hayes WC. The compressive behavior of bone as a two-phase porous structure. *J Bone Joint Surg*. 1977;59-A:954-962.
14. Murray RP, Hayes WC, Edwards WT, et al. Mechanical properties of the subchondral plate and the metaphyseal shell. *Trans Orthop Res Soc*. 1984;9:197.
15. Hvid I, Hansen SL. Trabecular bone strength patterns at the proximal tibial epiphysis. *J Orthop Res*. 1985;3:464-472.
16. Tissakht M, Ahmed AM, Chan KC. Calculated stress-shielding in the distal femur after total knee replacement corresponds to the reported location of bone loss. *J Orthop Res*. 1996;14:778-785.
17. D'Lima DD, Poole C, Chadha H, et al. Quadriceps moment arm and quadriceps forces after total knee arthroplasty. *Clin Orthop Relat Res*. 2001;392:213-220.
18. Wellman SS, Klement MR, Queen RM. Performance comparison of single-radius versus multiple-curve femoral component in total knee arthroplasty: a prospective, randomized study using the lower quarter y-balance test. *Orthopedics*. 2017;40:e1074-e1080.
19. Hall J, Copp SN, Adelson WS, et al. Extensor mechanism function in single-radius vs multiradius femoral components for total knee arthroplasty. *J Arthroplasty*. 2008;23:216-219.
20. Hamilton DF, Burnett R, Patton JT, et al. Implant design influences patient outcome after total knee arthroplasty: a prospective double-blind randomised controlled trial. *Bone Joint J*. 2015;97-B:64-70.
21. Collados-Maestre I, Lizaur-Utrilla A, Gonzalez-Navarro B, et al. Better functional outcome after single-radius TKA compared with multi-radius TKA. *Knee Surg Sports Traumatol Arthrosc*. 2017;25:3508-3514.
22. Hungerford DS, Kenna RV. Preliminary experience with a total knee prosthesis with porous coating used without cement. *Clin Orthop Relat Res*. 1983;176:95-107.
23. Warren PJ, Olanlokun TK, Cobb AG, et al. Proprioception after knee arthroplasty. The influence of prosthetic design. *Clin Orthop Relat Res*. 1993;297:182-187.
24. Corces A, Lotke PA, Williams JL. Strain characteristics of the posterior cruciate ligament in total knee replacement. *Orthop Trans*. 1989;13:527-528.
25. Incavo SJ, Johnson CC, Beynnon BD, et al. Posterior cruciate ligament strain biomechanics in total knee arthroplasty. *Clin Orthop Relat Res*. 1994;309:88-93.
26. Vandekerckhove PJ, Parys R, Tampere T, et al. Does cruciate retention primary total knee arthroplasty affect proprioception, strength and clinical outcome? *Knee Surg Sports Traumatol Arthrosc*. 2015;23:1644-1652.
27. Götz J, Beckmann J, Sperrer I, et al. Retrospective comparative study shows no significant difference in postural stability between cruciate-retaining (CR) and cruciate-substituting (PS) total knee implant systems. *Int Orthop*. 2016;40:1441-1446.
28. Emodi GJ, Callaghan JJ, Pedersen DR, et al. Posterior cruciate ligament function following total knee arthroplasty: the effect of joint line elevation. *Iowa Orthop J*. 1999;19:82-92.
29. Zingde SM, Leszko F, Sharma A, et al. In vivo determination of cam-post engagement in fixed and mobile-bearing TKA. *Clin Orthop Relat Res*. 2014;472:254-262.

30. Belvedere C, Leardini A, Catani F, et al. In vivo kinematics of knee replacement during daily living activities: condylar and post-cam contact assessment by three-dimensional fluoroscopy and finite element analyses. *J Orthop Res.* 2017;35:1396-1403.

31. Insall JN, Lachiewicz PF, Burstein AH. The posterior stabilized condylar prosthesis: a modification of the total condylar design. Two to four-year clinical experience. *J Bone Joint Surg.* 1982;64-A:1317-1323.

32. Puloski SK, McCalden RW, MacDonald SJ, et al. Tibial post wear in posterior stabilized total knee arthroplasty. An unrecognized source of polyethylene debris. *J Bone Joint Surg.* 2001;83-A:390-397.

33. Mestha P, Shenava Y, D'Arcy JC. Fracture of the polyethylene tibial post in posterior stabilized (Insall Burstein II) total knee arthroplasty. *J Arthroplasty.* 2000;15:814-815.

34. Jiang C, Liu Z, Wang Y, et al. Posterior cruciate ligament retention versus posterior stabilization for total knee arthroplasty: a meta-analysis. *PLoS One.* 2016;11:e0147865.

35. Longo UG, Ciuffreda M, Mannering N, et al. Outcomes of posterior-stabilized compared with cruciate-retaining total knee arthroplasty. *J Knee Surg.* 2018;31:321-340.

36. Fantozzi S, Catani F, Ensini A, et al. Femoral rollback of cruciate-retaining and posterior-stabilized total knee replacements: in vivo fluoroscopic analysis during activities of daily living. *J Orthop Res.* 2006;24:2222-2229.

37. Fu H, Wang J, Zhang W, et al. No clinical benefit of high-flex total knee arthroplasty. A meta-analysis of randomized controlled trials. *J Arthroplasty.* 2015;30:573-579.

38. Luo SX, Su W, Zhao JM, et al. High-flexion vs conventional prostheses total knee arthroplasty: a meta-analysis. *J Arthroplasty.* 2011;26:847-854.

39. Insall JN, Clarke HD. Historic development, classification, and characteristics of knee prostheses. In: Insall JN, Scott WN, eds. *Surgery of the Knee.* 3rd ed. New York: Churchill Livingstone; 2001:1516-1532.

40. Burstein AH, Wright TM. *Fundamentals of Orthopaedic Biomechanics.* Baltimore: Williams & Wilkins; 1994:213-216.

41. Buechel FF, Pappas MJ. The New Jersey low-contact stress knee replacement system: biomechanical rationale and review of the first 123 cemented cases. *Arch Orthop Trauma Surg.* 1986;105:197-204.

42. Minns RJ. The Minns meniscal knee prosthesis: biomechanical aspects of the surgical procedure and a review of the first 165 cases. *Arch Orthop Trauma Surg.* 1989;108:231-235.

43. O'Connor JJ, Goodfellow JW. Theory and practice of meniscal knee replacement: designing against wear. *Proc Inst Mech Eng.* 1996;210:217-222.

44. Abdel MP, Tibbo ME, Stuart MJ, et al. A randomized controlled trial of fixed- versus mobile-bearing total knee arthroplasty: a follow-up at a mean of ten years. *Bone Joint J.* 2018;100-B:925-929.

45. Woolson ST, Epstein NJ, Huddleston JI. Long-term comparison of mobile-bearing vs fixed-bearing total knee arthroplasty. *J Arthroplasty.* 2011;26:1219-1223.

46. Kim YH, Kim JS, Choe JW, et al. Long-term comparison of fixed-bearing and mobile-bearing total knee replacements in patients younger than fifty-one years of age with osteoarthritis. *J Bone Joint Surg.* 2012;94-A:866-873.

47. Sharma A, Grieco TF, Zingde SM, et al. In vivo three-dimensional patellar mechanics: normal knees compared with domed and anatomic patellar components. *J Bone Joint Surg.* 2017;99-A:e18.

48. Ali AA, Mannen EM, Rullkoetter PJ, et al. In vivo comparison of medialized dome and anatomic patellofemoral geometries using subject-specific computational modeling. *J Orthop Res.* 2018;36:1910-1918.

49. Elbert KE, Bartel DL, Wright TM. The effect of conformity on stresses in dome-shaped patellar components. *Clin Orthop Relat Res.* 1995;317:71-75.

50. Buechel FF, Rosa RA, Pappas MJ. A metal-backed, rotating-bearing patellar prosthesis to lower contact stress. An 11-year clinical study. *Clin Orthop Relat Res.* 1989;248:34-49.

51. Rawlinson JJ, Peters LE, Campbell DA, et al. Cancellous bone strains indicate efficacy of stem augmentation in constrained condylar knees. *Clin Orthop Relat Res.* 2005;440:107-116.

52. Rawlinson JJ, Closkey RF Jr, Davis N, et al. Stemmed implants improve stability in augmented constrained condylar knees. *Clin Orthop Relat Res.* 2008;466:2639-2643.

53. Donaldson WF III, Sculco TP, Insall JN, et al. Total condylar III knee prosthesis. Long term follow-up study. *Clin Orthop Relat Res.* 1988;226:21-28.

54. Wright TM, Daellenback K, Rosenthal D, et al. Mechanical performance of constrained total knees. *Ann Biomed Eng.* 1997;25(suppl 1):S-73.

55. Wang X, Malik A, Bartel DL, et al. Load sharing among collateral ligaments, articular surfaces, and the tibial post in constrained condylar knee arthroplasty. *J Biomech Eng.* 2016;138.

56. Konopka J, Weitzler L, Westrich D, et al. The effect of constraint on post damage in total knee arthroplasty: posterior stabilized vs posterior stabilized constrained inserts. *Arthroplast Today.* 2017;4:200-204.

57. Insall JN, Ranawat CS, Aglietti P, et al. A comparison of four models of total knee-replacement prostheses. *J Bone Joint Surg.* 1976;58-A:754-765.

58. Walker PS, Manktelow AR. Comparison between a constrained condylar and a rotating hinge in revision knee surgery. *Knee.* 2001;8:269-279.

59. Cottino U, Abdel MP, Perry KI, et al. Long-term results after total knee arthroplasty with contemporary rotating-hinge prostheses. *J Bone Joint Surg.* 2017;99-A:324-330.

60. Kearns SM, Culp BM, Bohl DD, et al. Rotating hinge implants for complex primary and revision total knee arthroplasty. *J Arthroplasty.* 2018;33:766-770.

61. Bartel DL, Rawlinson JJ, Burstein AH, et al. Stresses in polyethylene components of contemporary total knee replacements. *Clin Orthop Relat Res.* 1995;317:76-82.

62. Bartel DL, Bicknell VL, Wright TM. The effect of conformity, thickness, and material on stresses in ultra-high molecular weight components for total joint replacement. *J Bone Joint Surg.* 1986;68-A:1041-1051.

63. Shanbhag AS, Bailey HO, Hwang DS, et al. Quantitative analysis of ultrahigh molecular weight polyethylene (UHMWPE) wear debris associated with total knee replacements. *J Biomed Mater Res.* 2000;53:100-110.

64. Hirakawa K, Bauer TW, Stulberg BN, et al. Comparison and quantification of wear debris of failed total hip and total knee arthroplasty. *J Biomed Mater Res.* 1996;31:257-263.

65. Maxian TA, Brown TD, Pedersen DR, et al. Three-dimensional sliding/contact computational simulation of total hip wear. *Clin Orthop Relat Res.* 1996;14:668-675.

66. Maxian TA, Brown TD, Pedersen DR, et al. Adaptive finite element modeling of long-term polyethylene wear in total hip arthroplasty. *J Orthop Res.* 1996;333:41-50.

67. Bartel DL, Rimnac CM, Wright TM. Evaluation and design of the articular surface. In: Goldberg V, ed. *Controversies of Total Knee Arthroplasty.* New York: Raven; 1991:61-73.

68. Estupiñán JA, Wright TM, Bartel DL. Simulation predicts location and orientation of initial cracks in UHMWPE in low conformity sliding contact. *Trans Orthop Res Soc.* 2001;26:220.

69. Bostrom MP, Bennet AP, Rimnac CM, et al. The natural history of ultra high molecular weight polyethylene. *Clin Orthop Relat Res.* 1994;309:20-28.

70. Rimnac CM, Klein RW, Betts F, et al. Post-irradiation aging of ultra-high molecular weight polyethylene. *J Bone Joint Surg.* 1994;76-A:1052-1056.

71. Kurtz SM, Rimnac CM, Santner TJ, et al. Exponential model for the tensile true stress-strain behavior of as-irradiated and oxidatively degraded ultra high molecular weight polyethylene. *J Orthop Res.* 1996;14:755-761.

72. Tsao A, Mintz L, McCrae CR, et al. Failure of the porous-coated anatomic prosthesis in total knee arthroplasty due to severe polyethylene wear. *J Bone Joint Surg.* 1993;75-A:19-26.

73. Bohl JR, Bohl WR, Postak PD, et al. The effects of shelf life on clinical outcome for gamma sterilized polyethylene tibial components. *Clin Orthop Relat Res.* 1999;367:28-38.

74. Bell CJ, Walker PS, Abeysundera MR, et al. Effect of oxidation on delamination of ultrahigh-molecular-weight polyethylene tibial components. *J Artrhoplasty.* 1998;13:280-290.

75. Currier BH, Currier JH, Collier JP, et al. Shelf life and in vivo duration. Impacts on performance of tibial bearings. *Clin Orthop Relat Res.* 1997;342:111-122.

76. Williams IR, Mayor MB, Collier JP. The impact of sterilization method on wear in knee arthroplasty. *Clin Orthop Relat Res.* 1998;356:170-180.

77. Medel FJ, Kurtz SM, Hozack WJ, et al. Gamma inert sterilization: a solution to polyethylene oxidation?. *J Bone Joint Surg.* 2009;91-A:839-849.

78. Berry DJ, Currier BH, Mayor MB, et al. Gamma-irradiation sterilization in an inert environment: a partial solution. *Clin Orthop Relat Res.* 2012;470:1805-1813.

79. Muratoglu OK, Bragdon CR, O'Connor DO, et al. A novel method of cross-linking ultra-high-molecular-weight polyethylene to improve wear, reduce oxidation, and retain mechanical properties. Recipient of the 1999 HAP Paul Award. *J Arthroplasty.* 2001;16:149-160.

80. McKellop H, Shen FW, Lu B, et al. Development of an extremely wear-resistant ultra high molecular weight polyethylene for total hip replacements. *J Orthop Res.* 1999;17:157-167.

81. Hopper RH Jr, Ho H, Sritulanondha S, et al. Otto Aufranc Award: crosslinking reduces THA wear, osteolysis, and revision rates at 15-year followup compared with noncrosslinked polyethylene. *Clin Orthop Relat Res.* 2018;476:279-290.

82. Bragdon CR, Doerner M, Martell J, et al. The 2012 John Charnley Award. Clinical multicenter studies of the wear performance of highly crosslinked remelted polyethylene in THA. *Clin Orthop Relat Res.* 2013;471:393-402.

83. Lachiewicz PF, Soileau ES. Is there a benefit to highly crosslinked polyethylene in posterior-stabilized total knee arthroplasty? A Randomized Trial. *Clin Orthop Relat Res.* 2016;474:88-95.

84. Meneghini RM, Ireland PH, Bhowmik-Stoker M. Multicenter study of highly cross-linked vs conventional polyethylene in total knee arthroplasty. *J Arthroplasty.* 2016;31:809-814.

85. AOANJRR Hip, Knee & Shoulder Arthroplasty Annual Report for 2018. https://aoanjrr.sahmri.com/annual-reports-2018. Accessed April 12, 2019.

86. Reinitz SD, Currier BH, Van Citters DW, et al. Oxidation and other property changes of retrieved sequentially annealed UHMWPE acetabular and tibial bearings. *J Biomed Mater Res B Appl Biomater.* 2015;103:578-586.

87. MacDonald DW, Higgs GB, Chen AF, et al. Oxidation, damage mechanisms, and reasons for revision of sequentially annealed highly crosslinked polyethylene in total knee arthroplasty. *J Arthroplasty.* 2018;33:1235-1241.

88. Reinitz SD, Currier BH, Levine RA, et al. Oxidation and other property changes of a remelted highly crosslinked UHMWPE in retrieved tibial bearings. *J Biomed Mater Res B Appl Biomater.* 2017;105:39-45.

89. Liu T, Esposito CI, Burket JC, et al. Crosslink density is reduced and oxidation is increased in retrieved highly crosslinked polyethylene TKA tibial inserts. *Clin Orthop Relat Res.* 2017;475:128-136.

90. Sobieraj MC, Rimnac CM. Ultra high molecular weight polyethylene: mechanics, morphology, and clinical behavior. *J Mech Behav Biomed Mater.* 2009;2:433-443.

91. Ansari F, Ries MD, Pruitt L. Effect of processing, sterilization and crosslinking on UHMWPE fatigue fracture and fatigue wear mechanisms in joint arthroplasty. *J Mech Behav Biomed Mater.* 2016;53:329-340.

92. Mauerhan DR. Fracture of the polyethylene tibial post in a posterior cruciate-substituting total knee arthroplasty mimicking patellar clunk syndrome: a report of 5 cases. *J Arthroplasty.* 2003;18:942-945.

93. Sakellariou VI, Sculco P, Poultsides L, et al. Highly cross-linked polyethylene may not have an advantage in total knee arthroplasty. *HSS J.* 2013;9:264-269.

94. Diamond OJ, Howard L, Masri B. Five cases of tibial post fracture in posterior stabilized total knee arthroplasty using Prolong highly cross-linked polyethylene. *Knee.* 2018;25:657-662.

95. Pitta M, Esposito CI, Li Z, et al. Failure after modern total knee arthroplasty: a prospective study of 18,065 knees. *J Arthroplasty.* 2018;33:407-414.

96. Halder A, Kutzner I, Graichen F, et al. Influence of limb alignment on mediolateral loading in total knee replacement. *J Bone Joint Surg.* 2012;94-A:1023-1029.

97. Mundermann A, Dyrby CO, D'lima DD, et al. In vivo knee loading characteristics during activities of daily living as measured by an instrumented total knee replacement. *J Orthop Res.* 2008;26:1167-1172.

98. Perillo-Marcone A, Ryd L, Johnson K, et al. A combined RSA and FE study of the implanted proximal tibia: correlation of the post-operative mechanical environment with implant migration. *J Biomech.* 2004;37:1205-1213.

99. Fehring TK, Fehring KA, Anderson LA, et al. Catastrophic varus collapse of the tibia in obese total knee arthroplasty. *J Arthroplasty.* 2017;32:1625-1629.

100. van Loon CJ, Oyen WJ, de Waal Malefijt MC, et al. Distal femoral bone mineral density after total knee arthroplasty: a comparison with general bone mineral density. *Arch Orthop Trauma Surg.* 2001;212:282-285.

101. van Lenthe GH, de Waal Malefijt MC, Huiskes R. Stress shielding after total knee replacement may cause bone resorption in the distal femur. *J Bone Joint Surg.* 1997;79-B:117-122.

102. Deshmukh RV, Scott RD. Unicompartmental knee arthroplasty: long-term results. *Clin Orthop Relat Res.* 2001;392:272-278.

103. Lindstrand A, Stenstrom A, Ryd L, et al. The introduction period of unicompartmental knee arthroplasty is critical: a clinical, clinical multicentered, and radiostereometric study of 251 Duracon unicompartmental knee arthroplasties. *J Arthroplasty.* 2000;15:608-616.

104. Squire MW, Callaghan JJ, Goetz DD, et al. Unicompartmental knee replacement. A minimum 15 year followup study. *Clin Orthop Relat Res.* 1999;367:61-72.

105. Jawhar A, Stetzelberger V, Kollowa K, et al. Tourniquet application does not affect the periprosthetic bone cement penetration in total knee arthroplasty. *Knee Surg Sport Traumatol Arthrosc.* 2019;27(7):2071-2081.

106. Goodheart JR, Miller MA, Oest ME, et al. Trabecular resorption patterns of cement-bone interlock regions in total knee replacements. *J Orthop Res.* 2017;35:2773-2780.

107. Miller MA, Goodheart JR, Izant TH, et al. Loss of cement-bone interlock in retrieved tibial components from total knee arthroplasties. *Clin Orthop Relat Res.* 2014;472:304-313.

108. Arsoy D, Pagnano MW, Lewallen DG, et al. Aseptic tibial debonding as a cause of early failure in a modern total knee arthroplasty design. *Clin Orthop Relat Res.* 2013;471:94-101.

109. Pittman GT, Peters CL, Hines JL, et al. Mechanical bond strength of the cement–tibial component interface in total knee arthroplasty. *J Arthroplasty.* 2006;21(6):883-888.

110. Kelly MP, Illgen RL, Chen AF, et al. Trends in the use of high-viscosity cement in patients undergoing primary total knee arthroplasty in the United States. *J Arthroplasty.* 2018;33:3460-3464.

111. Hazelwood KJ, O'Rourke M, Stamos VP, et al. Case series report: early cement–implant interface fixation failure in total knee replacement. *Knee*. 2015;22:424-428.

112. Kopinski JE, Aggarwal A, Nunley RM, et al. Failure at the tibial cement-implant interface with the use of high-viscosity cement in total knee arthroplasty. *J Arthroplasty*. 2016;31:2579-2582.

113. Pilliar RM, Lee JM, Maniatopoulos C. Observations on the effect of movement on bone ingrowth into porous-surfaced implants. *Clin Orthop Relat Res*. 1986;208:108-113.

114. Jasty M, Bragdon C, Burke D, et al. In vivo skeletal responses to porous-surfaced implants subjected to small induced motions. *J Bone Joint Surg*. 1997;79:707-714.

115. Jasty M, Bragdon C, Zalenski E, et al. Enhanced stability of uncemented canine femoral components by bone ingrowth into the porous coatings. *J Arthroplasty*. 1997;12:106-113.

116. Engh CA, O'Connor D, Jasty M, et al. Quantification of implant micromotion, strain shielding, and bone resorption with porous-coated anatomic medullary locking femoral prostheses. *Clin Orthop Relat Res*. 1992;285:13-29.

117. Dammak M, Shirazi-Adl A, Schwartz M, et al. Friction properties at the bone-metal interface: comparison of four different porous metal surfaces. *J Biomed Mater Res*. 1997;35:329-336.

118. Zhang Y, Ahn PB, Fitzpatrick DC, et al. Interfacial frictional behavior; cancellous bone, cortical bone, and a novel porous tantalum biomaterial. *J Musculoskelet Res*. 1999;3:245-251.

119. Dunbar MJ, Wilson DAJ, Hennigar AW, et al. Fixation of a trabecular metal knee arthroplasty component. A prospective randomized study. *J Bone Joint Surg*. 2009;91-A:1578-1586.

120. Wilson DAJ, Richardson G, Hennigar AW, et al. Continued stabilization of trabecular metal tibial monoblock total knee arthroplasty components at 5 years-measured with radiostereometric analysis. *Acta Orthop*. 2012;83:36-40.

121. Henricson A, Nilsson KG. Trabecular metal tibial knee component still stable at 10 years. *Acta Orthop*. 2016;87:504-510.

122. De Martino I, D'Apolito R, Sculco PK, et al. Total knee arthroplasty using cementless porous tantalum monoblock tibial component: a minimum 10-year follow-up. *J Artrhoplasty*. 2016;31:2193-2198.

123. Cook SD, Barrack RL, Thomas KA, et al. Quantitative analysis of tissue growth into human porous total hip components. *J Arthroplasty*. 1988;3:249-262.

124. Pidhorz LE, Urban RM, Jacobs JJ, et al. A quantitative study of bone and soft tissues in cementless porous-coated acetabular components retrieved at autopsy. *J Arthroplasty*. 1993;8:213-225.

125. Hanzlik JA, Day JS; Acknowledged Contributors: Ingrowth Retrieval Study Group. Bone ingrowth in well-fixed retrieved porous tantalum implants. *J Arthroplasty*. 2013;28:922-927.

126. Hanzlik JA, Day JS, Rimnac CM, et al. Is there a difference in bone ingrowth in modular versus monoblock porous tantalum tibial trays? *J Arthroplasty*. 2015;30:1073-1078.

127. Ranawat CS, Johanson NA, Rimnac CM, et al. Retrieval analysis of porous-coated components for total knee replacement: a report of two cases. *Clin Orthop*. 1986;209:244-248.

128. Dawson JM, Bartel DL. Consequences of an interference fit on the fixation of porous-coated tibial components in total knee replacement. *J Bone Joint Surg*. 1992;74-A:233-238.

129. Sculco PK, Abdel MP, Hanssen AD, et al. The management of bone loss in revision total knee arthroplasty: rebuild, reinforce, and augment. *Bone Joint J*. 2016;98-B:120-124.

130. Sheth NP, Bonadio MB, Demange MK. Bone loss in revision total knee arthroplasty: evaluation and management. *J Am Acad Orthop Surg*. 2017;25:348-357.

131. Engh G. *Bone defect classification*. In: *Revision Total Knee Arthroplasty*. Baltimore: Lippincott Williams & Wilkins; 1997:63-120.

132. De Martino I, De Santis V, Sculco PK, et al. Tantalum cones provide durable mid-term fixation in revision TKA. *Clin Orthop Relat Res*. 2015;473:3176-3182.

133. Chalmers BP, Desy NM, Pagnano MW, et al. Survivorship of metaphyseal sleeves in revision total knee arthroplasty. *J Arthroplasty*. 2017;32:1565-1570.

134. Bohl DD, Brown NM, McDowell MA, et al. Do porous tantalum metaphyseal cones improve outcomes in revision total knee arthroplasty? *J Arthroplasty*. 2018;33:171-177.

135. Faizan A, Bhowmik-Stoker M, Alipit V, et al. Development and verification of novel porous titanium metaphyseal cones for revision total knee arthroplasty. *J Arthroplasty*. 2017;32:1946-1953.

136. Paz Quilez M, Seral B, Perez MA. Biomechanical evaluation of tibial bone adaptation after revision total knee arthroplasty: a comparison of different implant systems. *PLoS One*. 2017;12:e0184361.

137. Kamath AF, Lewallen DG, Hanssen AD. Porous tantalum metaphyseal cones for severe tibial bone loss in revision knee arthroplasty: a five to nine-year follow-up. *J Bone Joint Surg*. 2015;97-A:216-223.

chapter 10

Biomechanical and Clinical Aspects of the Stable and Unstable Total Knee Arthroplasty

Kartik M. Varadarajan, PhD | Sourabh Boruah, PhD | Guoan Li, PhD | Harry E. Rubash, MD FAOA

INTRODUCTION

Knee instability continues to be an important cause of revision following total knee arthroplasty (TKA), accounting for 7% to 22% of all revision procedures, and is usually ranked as the fourth or fifth most common cause of revision.[1-5] For example, in the Swedish knee arthroplasty registry, instability accounts for ~15% of revisions and is reported to be the fourth most common reason for revision, after infection, loosening, and patellar complications.[4] Instability accounted for 17.6% of revisions in the 2017 UK national joint registry report and was ranked as the fifth most common reason for revision, behind aseptic loosening, other indications, infection, and pain.[3] In the Australian national joint registry, instability accounted for 7.8% of revisions where primary TKA was performed for osteoarthritis (OA) diagnosis and was the fifth most common reason for revision after loosening, infection, patellar complications, and pain.[1] Mechanical instability may arise from a variety of causes including component failure (fracture, wear, or loosening), bone loss, ligamentous instability, or malalignment.[2,6-8] Component failure is a mode that is distinct from biomechanical instability linked to alignment, implant placement, and soft-tissue–related factors. In this chapter, we will focus on biomechanical instability.

Symptoms of mechanical instability are variable and can range from no symptoms to discomfort, including feeling of insecurity in the knee without frank giving way, abnormal gait (varus/valgus thrust gait, stiff-legged gait, or hyperextension to lock joint during stance phase of walking), difficulty with stairs, recurrent knee swelling, anterior knee pain, or subluxation of the articulation.[2,6] Instability affecting the tibiofemoral joint is generally classified into three main types (in roughly decreasing order of frequency): flexion instability, extension instability, and genu recurvatum. A fourth type, namely, mid-flexion instability has largely been discussed in biomechanical studies and remains controversial in clinical literature. This is in part due to difficulty in recognizing mid-flexion instability clinically. In the following sections, we discuss the clinical presentation, biomechanical features, and mechanisms of each form of instability.

FLEXION INSTABILITY

Clinical Presentation

As suggested by the name, flexion instability refers to a scenario where the knee is stable in extension with full extension permitted, but lax in flexion. It is generally characterized by a flexion gap that is larger than the extension gap. Excessive anterior sliding (>5 to 7 mm) and occasionally posterior tibial sag under gravity are observable at 90° flexion (**Figs. 10-1 and 10-2**).[2,6] Patients with flexion instability may also achieve high degrees of flexion in the hospital post surgery.[9] The excess laxity permits femoral sliding relative to the tibia until its arrest by soft-tissue stabilizers, thus explaining the avoidance of weight-bearing on flexed knee. Challenges experienced by patients with flexion instability include, chronic effusions, swelling and soft-tissue tenderness, difficult rising from a chair, and ascending and descending stairs.[9] Factors contributing to flexion instability include excess tibial slope, reduced posterior femoral offset, distalized joint line, undersized femoral component, and femoral component malrotation in flexion. Late posterior cruciate ligament (PCL) rupture or injury can also lead to flexion instability.[2,6]

Biomechanics of the Native Knee and Stable TKA

Having discussed the clinical presentation and underlying risk factors of flexion instability, the next logical question is what varus–valgus and anteroposterior laxity in flexion should be considered "normal" or acceptable.

In the native knee, varus–valgus laxity in flexion has been reported to range from 1.7° to 5.5° under applied varus–valgus stress, with lateral (varus force) laxity being 0.6° to 3.1° greater than medial (valgus force) laxity (**Table 10-1**). This difference translates to approximately 0.5 to 2.5 mm greater gap opening on the lateral side, assuming an average condylar spacing of 47 mm. Studies in which laxity measurements were performed via application of a distraction force also demonstrate greater laxity on the lateral side in flexion. The difference between

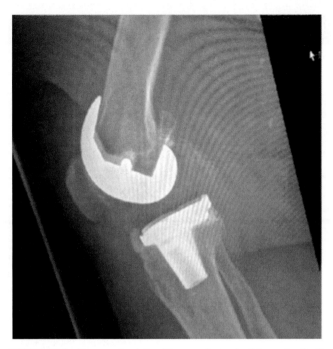

FIGURE 10-1 Preoperative lateral knee radiograph of the patient with flexion instability. (Reprinted with permission from Rajgopal A, Panjwani TR, Rao A, et al. Are the outcomes of revision knee arthroplasty for flexion instability the same as for other major failure mechanisms? *J Arthroplasty.* 2017;32(10):3093-3097.)

lateral versus medial laxity in these studies is reported to be somewhat larger (2 to 4.6 mm) than those involving measurements with the application of varus–valgus stress. The difference in results between the two approaches (distraction versus varus–valgus stress) may result from differences in magnitude of forces, mechanism of joint

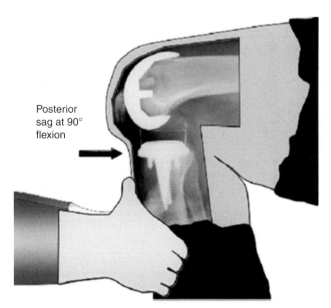

Posterior sag at 90° flexion

FIGURE 10-2 Schematic diagram of clinical examination of patient with flexion instability. (Reprinted with permission from Rajgopal A, Panjwani TR, Rao A, et al. Are the outcomes of revision knee arthroplasty for flexion instability the same as for other major failure mechanisms? *J Arthroplasty.* 2017;32(10):3093-3097.)

opening during distraction versus levering, or constraints applied to the joints during measurement.

In TKA, most surgeons aim for either equal medial and lateral laxity or accept slightly greater laxity on the lateral side. The above discussion about asymmetry in medial versus lateral laxity in the normal knee may be used to establish acceptable thresholds for medial/lateral gap asymmetry in flexion. Resection of the anterior cruciate ligament (ACL) has negligible influence on varus–valgus laxity in flexion, while PCL resection has been shown to increase flexion gap by ~1 to 3 mm.[10-12] Nonetheless, due to the dominant role played by the collateral structures in coronal plane stability,[13] an appropriately balanced cruciate retaining (CR) or posterior substituting (PS) TKA can closely match the varus–valgus laxity of the native knee.[14-17]

With regards to anteroposterior laxity of the native knee, tibial displacement in flexion has been reported to range from 4.7 to 7.7 mm in response to 98-134 N of anterior drawer force (**Table 10-2**). Resection of the ACL, in the native knee or following a bi-cruciate retaining (BCR) TKA, has been shown to lead to substantial increase in anterior tibial laxity in flexion (~4 to 12 mm increase relative to intact condition).[18-20] The effect of ACL resection on posterior tibial laxity is relatively small, reflecting the greater role of the PCL in resisting posterior drawer forces in flexion.[14,20,21]

The effect of ACL resection on flexion stability following conventional CR or PS TKA is somewhat mixed. This is likely related to the restrain provided by the posterior tibial insert lip and the tibiofemoral conformity. For example, Hunt et al. and Stoddard et al. found no differences in anteroposterior (AP) laxity between CR TKA (Triathlon CR and Kinemax CR, Stryker Corp., Mahwah NJ) and native knees.[16,17] Van Damme et al. found slight increase in anterior laxity in flexion for CR TKA (Genesis II CR, Smith & Nephew, London, UK) relative to the native knee (~2.6 mm).[22] In contrast, Halewood et al. noted substantially higher anterior laxity in flexion for CR TKA (Unity Knee, Corin Group, Cirencester, UK), compared to BCR TKA and native knees (~4 to 7 mm greater).[14] However, the differences in posterior tibial laxity between CR, BCR, and native knees at 90° flexion were relatively small.[14] This likely reflects the role of the retained PCL in restraint against posterior drawer. In the PS knee, the PCL substituting post offers a hard restraint against posterior drawer often heard as a click when posterior force is applied. Substantial anterior tibial movement is indicative of flexion instability as in a CR knee.[23]

EXTENSION INSTABILITY

Clinical Presentation

Extension instability can be either symmetric or asymmetric with the latter being more common, and therefore extension instability is also sometimes referred to as varus–valgus or coronal plane instability when patient is

TABLE 10-1 Varus–Valgus Laxity of the Native Knee as Reported in the Literature

Author	Type of Study	Loading Type	Varus/Lateral	Valgus/Medial	Difference (Lateral–Medial)
		EXTENSION LAXITY			
Markolf et al. 1976[13]	Cadaver	Corresponding to 10 Nm	1.25°	1.12°	0.13°
Van Damme et al. 2005[22]	Cadaver	9.8 Nm V/V stress	3.1 mm	2.6 mm	0.5 mm
Salvadore et al. 2018[32]	Cadaver	10 Nm V/V stress	1.84°	1.72°	0.12°
Nowakowski et al. 2012[10]	Cadaver	100 N per compartment distraction	6.9 mm	5.8 mm	1.1 mm
Okazaki et al. 2006[37]	In vivo, age 19-59 y	147 N V/V stress	4.90°	2.40°	2.50°
Heesterbeek et al. 2008[38]	In vivo, avg age 62 y	15 Nm V/V stress	2.80°	2.30°	0.50°
Ishii et al. 2018[39]	In vivo, avg age 26 y	147 N V/V stress	2.00°	3.00°	−1.00°
Deep 2014[40]	In vivo, age 19-35 y	10 Nm	3.10°	4.60°	−1.50°
Lujan et al. 2007[11]	Cadaver	10 Nm valgus		3.82°	
Mayman et al. 2009[41]	Cadaver	100 N per compartment distraction	0.0 mm	0.2 mm	−0.2 mm
		MID-FLEXION LAXITY			
Markolf et al. 1976[13]	Cadaver	Corresponding to 10 Nm	3.26°	3.04°	0.22°
Van Damme et al. 2005[22]	Cadaver	9.8 Nm V/V stress	5.9 mm	5.1 mm	0.9 mm
Salvadore et al. 2018[32]	Cadaver	10 Nm V/V stress	3.92°	3.85°	0.07°
Deep 2014[40]	In vivo, age 19-35 y	10 Nm	6.90°	7.90°	−1.00°
Lujan et al. 2007[11]	Cadaver	10 Nm valgus		5.06°	
Mayman et al. 2009[41]	Cadaver	100 N per compartment distraction	4.0 mm	4.2 mm	−0.2 mm
		FLEXION LAXITY			
Markolf et al. 1976[13]	Cadaver	Corresponding to 10 Nm	4.78°	3.93°	0.85°
Van Damme et al. 2005[22]	Cadaver	9.8 Nm V/V stress	8.1 mm	7.1 mm	1.0 mm
Salvadore et al. 2018[32]	Cadaver	10 Nm V/V stress	5.24°	3.79°	1.45°
Nowakowski et al. 2012[10]	Cadaver	100 N per compartment distraction	9.2 mm	6.9 mm	2.3 mm
Okazaki et al. 2006[37]	In vivo, age 19-59 y	147 N V/V stress	4.8°	1.7°	3.1°
Heesterbeek et al. 2008[38]	In vivo, avg age 62 y	15 Nm V/V stress	3.1°	2.5°	0.6°
Tokuhara et al. 2004[42]	In vivo, age 18-53 y	Not standardized	6.7 mm	2.1 mm	4.6 mm
Lujan et al. 2007[11]	Cadaver	10 Nm valgus		5.66°	
Mayman et al. 2009[41]	Cadaver	100 N per compartment distraction	5.0 mm	2.9 mm	2.1 mm

examined with knee in extension (**Fig. 10-3**).[2,9] Excessive distal femoral or proximal tibial resections can result in symmetric extension instability, while inadequate deformity correction, under release of medial/lateral soft-tissues, damage to medial collateral ligament (MCL) during tibial resection, or aggressive varus–valgus testing could lead to asymmetric instability. In the case of instability arising from excess distal femoral resection, it is recommended to restore the joint line via distal augmentation as opposed to use of a thicker polyethylene insert,

which could lead to patellar overstuffing, flexion tightness, and possibly mid-flexion instability (see section on mid-flexion instability).[2,6]

Biomechanics of the Native Knee and Stable TKA

Normal varus–valgus laxity in extension for the native knee has been reported to range from 1.5° to 5° under varus–valgus stress, with no obvious difference between

TABLE 10-2   Anterior Posterior Laxity of the Native Knee as Reported in the Literature

Author	Type of Study	Loading Type	Anterior	Posterior
EXTENSION LAXITY				
Markolf et al. 1976[13]	Cadaver	Corresponding to 100 N	1.8 mm	1.4 mm
Van Damme et al. 2005[22]	Cadaver	98 N (anterior load on tibia)	3.9 mm	
Okada et al. 2018[18]	Cadaver	±100 N	11.1 mm	
Sim et al. 2011[19]	Cadaver	134 N (anterior tibial load)	4.0 mm	
Halewood et al. 2015[14]	Cadaver	135 N anterior/135 N posterior on tibia	1.5 mm	2.8 mm
Song et al. 2009[20]	In vivo intraop, age 16-57 y	Manual	3.6 mm	2.1 mm
Lujan et al. 2007[11]	Cadaver	100 N	6.9 mm	
MID-FLEXION LAXITY				
Markolf et al. 1976[13]	Cadaver	Corresponding to 100 N	3.8 mm	3.3 mm
Van Damme et al. 2005[22]	Cadaver	98 N (anterior load on tibia)	9.2 mm	
Okada et al. 2018[18]	Cadaver	±100 N	12.5 mm	
Sim et al. 2011[19]	Cadaver	134 N (anterior tibial load)	7.1 mm	
Halewood et al. 2015[14]	Cadaver	135 N anterior/135 N posterior on tibia	2.3 mm	4.6 mm
Song et al. 2009[20]	In vivo intraop, age 16-57 y	Manual	6.7 mm	2.4 mm
Lujan et al. 2007[11]	Cadaver	100 N	8.0 mm	
FLEXION LAXITY				
Markolf et al. 1976[13]	Cadaver	Corresponding to 100 N	2.1 mm	2.3 mm
Van Damme et al. 2005[22]	Cadaver	98 N (anterior load on tibia)	7.7 mm	
Okada et al. 2018[18]	Cadaver	±100 N	7.7 mm	
Sim et al. 2011[19]	Cadaver	134 N (anterior tibial load)	5.3 mm	
Halewood et al. 2015[14]	Cadaver	135 N anterior/135 N posterior on tibia	3.4 mm	1.7 mm
Song et al. 2009[20]	In vivo intraop, age 16-57 y	Manual	4.7 mm	2.2 mm
Lujan et al. 2007[11]	Cadaver	100 N	5.8 mm	

medial versus lateral laxity. While resection of PCL has minimal influence on varus–valgus laxity in extension, resection of ACL has shown to increase VV laxity in extension by 2 to 3 mm.[10,11,13] Nonetheless, an appropriately balanced TKA can closely match the varus–valgus laxity of the native knee,[15-17,22] due to the dominant role of the collaterals in coronal stability.[13]

With regards to anteroposterior laxity of the native knee in extension, anterior tibial displacement has been reported to range from ~4 to 7 mm in response to 98-134 N of force (**Table 10-2**). The ACL plays a significant role in anteroposterior stability, and its resection in the native knee or following BCR TKA was shown to substantially increase anterior tibial laxity in extension (~3 to 7 mm increase).[18-21] ACL resection also increases anteroposterior laxity in CR or PS TKA relative to the native knee (~3 to 7 mm).[14,17] However, this is partly compensated by the high degree of tibiofemoral conformity in extension. This may explain some of the variabilities in the literature. For example, while Halewood et al. and Stoddard et al. reported higher AP laxity in extension for CR TKA relative to native knees,[14,17] Hunt et al. and Van Damme et al. reported minimal differences.[16,22]

GENU RECURVATUM

Genu recurvatum, hyperextension instability, or sagittal plane instability is a rare but challenging condition affecting 0.5% to 1% of patients presenting for TKA (defined as >5° hyperextension deformity) (**Fig. 10-4**).[2,8,9,24] This form of instability is often associated with neuromuscular conditions such as poliomyelitis, Charcot disease, and other conditions where motor imbalances occur. The presence of bony deformities, quadriceps weakness, paralysis, and plantarflexion contracture predisposes the knee to hyperextension and is likely to recur after surgery. In the absence of neuromuscular disease, factors such as previous high tibial osteotomies (due to anterior tibial bone impaction which can lead to anterior tibial slope), valgus deformity with tightened iliotibial band located anterior to knee

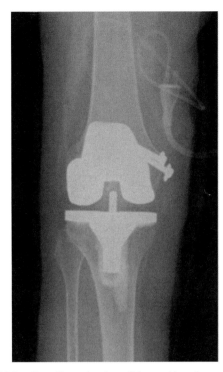

FIGURE 10-3 AP radiograph of an 87-year-old patient treated with open reduction and internal fixation to address intraoperative fracture of the medial femoral condyle and associated risk for asymmetric extension instability. (Reprinted with permission from Cottino U, Sculco PK, Sierra RJ, et al. Instability after total knee arthroplasty. *Orthop Clin North Am*. 2016;47(2):311-316.)

flexion axis, and ligamentous laxity in rheumatoid arthritis patients can lead to genu recurvatum. The missing ACL following TKA may add to the challenge. The ACL has been shown to rapidly tension with hyperextension,[25] with its resection allowing for marked increase in extension.[21]

Possible techniques to address the deformity surgically include tightening of extension gaps (such as by under-resecting distal femur, using a thicker polyethylene, or placing femoral component in flexion), proximal and posterior transfer of the collateral ligament femoral insertions, posterior capsular plication, use of rotating hinged TKA with extension stop, and arthrodesis in severe cases.[2,6,24] In the absence of neuromuscular issues, most cases of genu recurvatum are addressable via standard TKA prosthesis with careful attention to joint balancing with minimal risk of recurrence. The authors always recommend the availability of hinged TKA when addressing this problem (**Fig. 10-5**). Rotating hinged prosthesis with extension stop is an option for patients with severe quadriceps weakness, although concerns have been expressed about possible overloading of the prosthesis bone interface leading to loosening. Permanent postoperative bracing may also be required in these patients. Long-term outcomes of hinged total knee replacement (TKR) prosthesis have been reported to range from 51% to 92.5% at 10 years, with the most common reasons for failure being deep infection and aseptic loosening. While the outcomes appear promising, analysis of the data is particularly complicated by the heterogenous nature of the underlying studies with varying mix of indications, implant types, and definition of complications.[26]

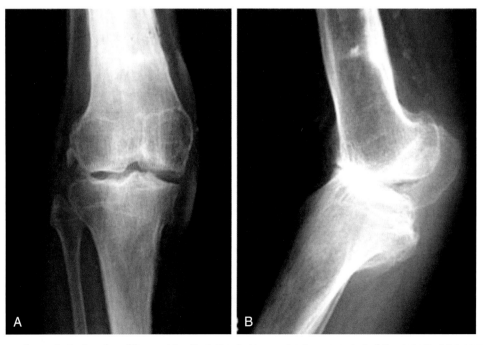

FIGURE 10-4 Preoperative radiographs of an 80-year-old patient showing bone atrophy, narrowing of the anterior joint space, and genu recurvatum. **A:** Anteroposterior view and **B:** passive hyperextension view. (Reprinted with permission from Nishitani K, Nakagawa Y, Suzuki T, et al. Rotating-hinge total knee arthroplasty in a patient with genu recurvatum after osteomyelitis of the distal femur. *J Arthroplasty*. 2007;22(4):630-633.)

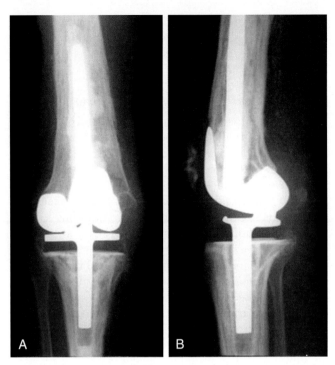

FIGURE 10-5 Postoperative radiographs showing rotating hinged total knee replacement used to treat deformity shown in **Fig. 10-4**. **A:** Anteroposterior and **B:** lateral view. (Reprinted with permission from Nishitani K, Nakagawa Y, Suzuki T, et al. Rotating-hinge total knee arthroplasty in a patient with genu recurvatum after osteomyelitis of the distal femur. *J Arthroplasty*. 2007;22(4):630-633.)

MID-FLEXION INSTABILITY

Clinical Presentation

The term mid-flexion instability refers to a situation where the knee is adequately balanced in extension and at 90° flexion, yet unstable in the intermediate flexion range.

The term was first defined by Martin and Whiteside in a biomechanical study, based on observation of increased laxity in 30° to 60° flexion range following proximal and anterior shift of the femoral component.[27] McPherson et al. describe it as manifesting as a rotational instability under combined external rotation and valgus stress in 45° to 90° knee flexion.[28] Potential risk factors include uncorrected flexion deformity, joint line elevation, and attenuated anterior MCL.[9,27,28] Role of sagittal geometry of the implants has also been suggested. The mechanisms by which these factors could contribute to mid-flexion instability is discussed below.

Tight Posterior Structures

One potential mechanism of mid-flexion instability relates to masking of underlying collateral ligament laxity by the secondary effect of posterior structures.[9] In this scenario, the knee may appear to be well balanced in extension due to tightening of the posterior structures. However, with slight flexion, the restraint from posterior capsule relaxes and the effect of collateral laxity manifests as mid-flexion instability. This situation could also arise from tight or insufficiently released posterior capsule, which is balanced by increased distal femoral resection (**Fig. 10-6**). The increased distal femoral resection allows the knee to extend in the presence of the tight posterior structures. However, this causes femoral component center of rotation to shift proximal relative to the femoral insertion site of the MCL. The increased distal femoral resection relaxes the posterior structures as well as the MCL, thereby allowing the knee to extend. The MCL continues to be in a relaxed state in mid-flexion, which could potentially contribute to mid-flexion instability. Subsequently, the MCL regains tension at 90° flexion as the femoral component continues rotation around its center of rotation.

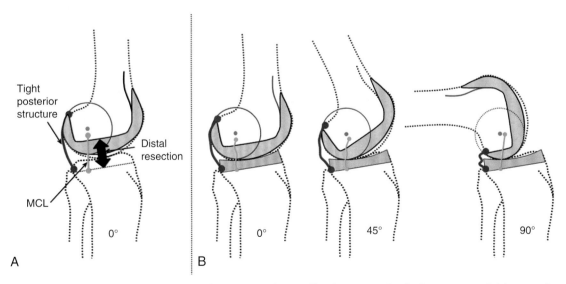

FIGURE 10-6 **A:** Schematic showing increased distal femoral resection to allow knee extension in the presence of tight posterior structures. However, this causes femoral component center of rotation to shift proximal relative to the femoral insertion site of the MCL. **B:** Schematic showing how the raised joint line relaxes the posterior structures, thus allowing for knee extension. Simultaneously the MCL is also relaxed. The MCL continues to be in a relaxed state in mid-flexion which could contribute to mid-flexion instability. Subsequently the MCL regains tension at 90° flexion as the femoral component continues rotation around its center of rotation. MCL, medial collateral ligament.

Elevated Joint Line

Another proposed mechanism of mid-flexion laxity relates to the change in location of femoral component flexion axis relative to axis of ligament isometry.[27,29] Martin and Whiteside observed increased laxity in 30° to 60° flexion range following 5 mm proximal and 5 mm anterior shift of the femoral component.[27] Similar observation was made by Luyckx et al. in a biomechanical study of posterior stabilized implants, where 2 and 4 mm joint line elevation were simulated a with smaller femoral component placed more proximally, together with a thicker insert to compensate on the tibial side.[29] Laxity was increased by 51% to 64% in 30° to 60° flexion range with 2 mm joint line elevation and by 95% to 111% with 4 mm joint line elevation relative to baseline. No significant effects were seen at 0 and 90° flexion.

This mechanism is described schematically in **Fig. 10-7**. The superficial MCL, which is the primary stabilizer on the medial side, shows a relatively isometric behavior with flexion. In the ideal scenario, the ligament insertion center coincides with axis of rotation of the knee, such as when the joint line is restored. However, when the femoral component is moved proximally and anteriorly, the ligament insertion no longer coincides with the femoral component's axis of rotation. Consequently, as the knee moves from extension into mid-flexion, the superficial MCL insertion moves distally relative to the center of rotation, thereby slackening. With further flexion, the MCL tightens, returning to a tensed state matching that in extension. Luyckx et al. also looked at the effect of kinematic versus mechanical alignment in their study and found that the effect of joint line elevation was identical in both alignments.[29] The only difference between the alignments was the resection on the lateral side.

This suggests that the lateral structures contribute less to overall stability in mid-flexion or are not sensitive to joint line elevation to the same degree as the medial structures.

Sagittal Geometry of the Femoral Component

The above discussion on collateral ligament isometry suggests potential role of the femoral (and tibial insert) component geometry in mid-flexion stability. Conceptually, restoration of the medial collateral isometry via a single-radius femoral component design appears to be logical. However, the actual difference in articular surface geometries in the sagittal plane between a multiradius femoral and a single-radius femoral over the primary arc of knee motion (10° to 120° flexion) is likely small compared to the 2 to 5 mm joint line elevation simulated in the biomechanical studies that demonstrated mid-flexion instability. This may explain the lack of differences noted in studies directly comparing stability of multiradius and single-radius femoral designs.[17] It is also important to point out that not all multiradius or single-radius designs are the same. Within multiradius designs, some designs have a more pronounced condylar profile in the mid-flexion range,[17] while others have a less pronounced mid-flexion profile (**Fig. 10-8**). The overlay of femoral component sagittal geometries shown in **Fig. 10-8** demonstrates the variability across designs, which is not accurately reflected by broad terminology such as "single-radius" or "multiradius." Within the so-called single-radius designs, the range of flexion angle over which single radius is employed varies (**Fig. 10-9**). Other newer designs propose a gradually decreasing radius from extension to deeper flexion as the optimal solution over single- or multiradius designs.[30,31]

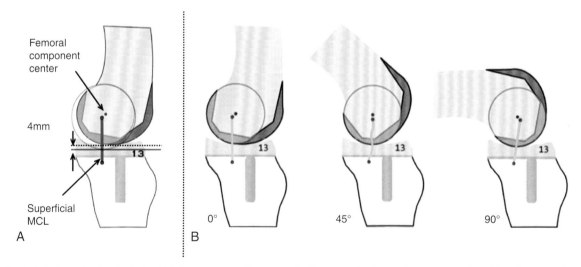

FIGURE 10-7 **A:** Schematic showing raised joint line resulting from use of a 4 mm smaller femoral component placed in a 4 mm proximal position and coupled with a 4 mm thicker polyethylene insert. The raised joint line in turn causes femoral component center of rotation to shift proximal and anterior relative to the femoral insertion site of the superficial MCL. **B:** Schematic showing how an appropriately tensioned MCL at 0° flexion slackens in mid-flexion as the femur rotates around the new femoral center of rotation and subsequently regains tension at 90° flexion. (Reprinted with permission from Luyckx T, Vandenneucker H, Ing LS, et al. Raising the joint line in TKA is associated with mid-flexion laxity: a study in cadaver knees. *Clin Orthop Relat Res.* 2018;476(3):601-611.)

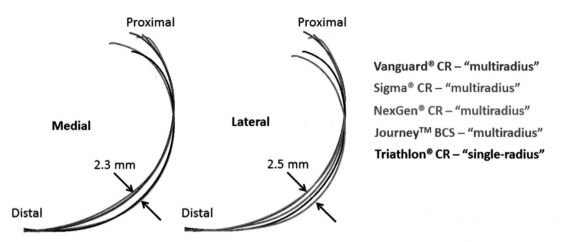

FIGURE 10-8 Overlay of sagittal geometries of four different "multiradius" femoral components and one "single-radius" femoral component. The overlay demonstrates the variability across designs, which is not accurately reflected by broad terminology such as "single-radius" or "multiradius." Vanguard CR, NexGen CR—Zimmer Biomet, Warsaw, IN; Sigma CR—DePuy Synthes, Raynham, MA; Journey BCS—Smith & Nephew, London, UK; Triathlon CR—Stryker, Mahwah, NJ.

Biomechanics of the Native Knee and Stable TKA

Change in varus–valgus stability as a function of knee flexion angle is inherent to the normal knee. Traditional clinical wisdom emphasizes importance of equalizing the flexion and extension gaps. However, it must be realized that the native knee does not demonstrate a constant laxity envelope with flexion. Total varus–valgus laxity increases noticeability from extension to about 30° flexion (~3.5 mm or 4.5°).[13,15,32] At higher flexion, some studies show a constant or gradual increase in laxity through 90° flexion,[13,16,17,22,32] while others show a return to laxity values similar to extension.[15] Therefore, equalization of laxity in extension and flexion may not automatically lead to a matching mid-flexion coronal plane stability. For example, Hino et al. observed greater joint laxity from 10° to 60° flexion in the preoperative knees of TKA patients, compared to the laxities at 0° and 90° flexion. This pattern remained post surgery in both CR and PS TKA patients, in spite of balanced flexion and extension gaps.[15] Minoda et al. observed increased intraoperative joint gap in 30° to 60° flexion range in patients undergoing a mobile-bearing PS TKA, although gap dimensions in extension and flexion were similar.[33] Thus, increased laxity in mid-flexion by itself may not indicate

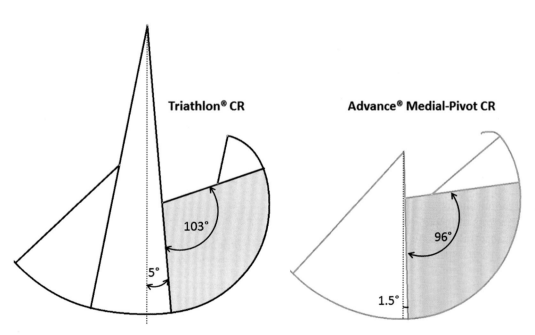

FIGURE 10-9 Comparison of sagittal geometries of "single-radius" femoral component designs from two different manufacturers showing variations in range of flexion angle over which a single radius (shaded portion) is employed. Triathlon CR—Stryker, Mahwah, NJ; Advance Medial-Pivot BCS—MicroPort Orthopedics, Arlington, TN.

mid-flexion instability suggestive of a pathological condition. Substantial increase in mid-flexion laxity over normal values, such as resulting from excess joint line elevation or failure to recognize masked collateral laxity in extension, may be a truer indicator of mid-flexion instability.

The role of the absent ACL also needs to be acknowledged in the discussion of mid-flexion instability. In contrast to the direct contribution of the cruciate ligaments to AP stability, the collaterals and capsular structures contribute to AP stability through the interplay of compressive forces and tibiofemoral conformity. This is particularly relevant in mid-flexion as opposed to 0° or 90° flexion. In extension, the anterior insert lip resists posterior tibial load while the large distal femoral radius maximizes tibiofemoral conformity. In flexion, the PCL in CR TKA or PCL-substituting force in PS TKA resists posterior tibial load; while the posterior insert lip resists anterior tibial load. In contrast, in mid-flexion, the tibiofemoral conformity reduces substantially from extension, and the femoral component has greater distance to traverse before reaching either the anterior or posterior insert lip. At the same time, varus–valgus laxity is inherently lower in mid-flexion as discussed above. In the absence of the native ACL or a distinct mechanism to substitute for its stabilizing role (e.g., through a tibial post or ball-in-socket construct),[34-36] TKA, whether a single- or multiradius design, will have less anteroposterior stability in early flexion than the native knee. For example, Stoddard et al. observed greater anterior drawer displacement relative to the intact knee for both single- and multiradius designs from full extension to 30° flexion compared to native knees.[17] No differences were noted at other flexion angles or in rotational or varus–valgus laxity. Resection of the ACL in the native knee or following BCR TKA has the greatest impact at ~30° flexion, leading to substantial increase in AP tibial laxity (~8 to 14.5 mm increase).[18-20] ACL resection also increases AP laxity in low flexion for conventional TKA relative to the native knee (~2 to 9 mm).[14,17] However, this may be partially compensated for by tibiofemoral conformity.

SUMMARY

Mechanical instability of the tibiofemoral compartment continues to be an important reason for revision of knee arthroplasty, accounting for ~13% (7% to 22%) of all cases. The main forms of instability include flexion instability, extension instability, genu recurvatum, and mid-flexion instability, each with its own unique set of clinical and biomechanical characteristics.

Flexion instability is generally characterized by a flexion gap that is larger than the extension gap, with anterior sliding exceeding 5 to 7 mm, and occasionally posterior tibial sag under gravity. Extension instability is most often asymmetric in nature, arising from undercorrected deformity or soft-tissue imbalance. The absence of the ACL in

contemporary TKA can increase anterior laxity relative to the native knee, in both extension and flexion. However, this effect appears to be mitigated by the higher tibiofemoral conformity in extension and the posterior insert lip in flexion. With regards to coronal stability, the collaterals structures play a more dominant role compared to the cruciate ligaments. Consequently, a well-balanced TKA can achieve varus–valgus and AP stability in both extension and flexion comparable to that of the intact knee, even in the absence of the ACL and PCL. While the data on native knee stability (**Tables 10-1** and **10-2**) can be used to inform thresholds for "normal" or acceptable values for varus–valgus and anteroposterior stability, it should be noted that substantial variations exist across both individual normal knees and well-functioning TKA knees.

Genu recurvatum is an infrequent but challenging complication affecting 0.5% to 1% of patients scheduled to undergo TKA. It is commonly associated with neuromuscular conditions, which can increase the risk of recurrence. While standard TKA prosthesis can be effectively utilized for cases without neuromuscular issues, options such as rotating hinged design seem to be promising for the more challenging cases.

Mid-flexion instability continues to receive greater attention in the clinical community but nonetheless remains poorly understood. It refers to a scenario where the knee is adequately balanced in extension and at 90° flexion but is unstable in the intermediate range. It has also been described as a rotational instability under combined external rotation and valgus stress in 45° to 90° knee flexion. Tight posterior structures and elevation of joint line are the most likely mechanisms of mid-flexion instability. Furthermore, the absence of the ACL likely plays an important and underrecognized role in mid-flexion instability.

REFERENCES

1. Australian Orthopaedic Association National Joint Replacement Registry. 2018 Annual Report. Adelaide, SA: Australia; 2018.
2. Cottino U, Sculco PK, Sierra RJ, et al. Instability after total knee arthroplasty. *Orthop Clin North Am.* 2016;47(2):311-316.
3. National Joint Registry for England W, Northern Ireland and the Isle of Man. 15th Annual Report. United Kingdom: Hemel Hempstead; 2018.
4. Swedish Knee Arthroplasty Register. Annual Report 2017. Lund: Sweden; 2017.
5. Abdel MP, Haas SB. The unstable knee: wobble and buckle. *Bone Joint Lett J.* 2014;96-B(11 suppl A):112-114.
6. Chang MJ, Lim H, Lee NR, et al. Diagnosis, causes and treatments of instability following total knee arthroplasty. *Knee Surg Relat Res.* 2014;26(2):61-67.
7. Wilson CJ, Theodoulou A, Damarell RA, et al. Knee instability as the primary cause of failure following Total Knee Arthroplasty (TKA): a systematic review on the patient, surgical and implant characteristics of revised TKA patients. *Knee.* 2017;24(6):1271-1281.
8. Vince KG, Abdeen A, Sugimori T. The unstable total knee arthroplasty: causes and cures. *J Arthroplasty.* 2006;21(4 suppl 1):44-49.
9. Vince K. Mid-flexion instability after total knee arthroplasty: woolly thinking or a real concern? *Bone Joint J.* 2016;98-B(1 suppl A):84-88.

10. Nowakowski AM, Majewski M, Muller-Gerbl M, et al. Measurement of knee joint gaps without bone resection: "physiologic" extension and flexion gaps in total knee arthroplasty are asymmetric and unequal and anterior and posterior cruciate ligament resections produce different gap changes. *J Orthop Res.* 2012;30(4):522-527.

11. Lujan TJ, Dalton MS, Thompson BM, et al. Effect of ACL deficiency on MCL strains and joint kinematics. *J Biomech Eng.* 2007;129(3):386-392.

12. Schnurr C, Eysel P, Konig DP. Is the effect of a posterior cruciate ligament resection in total knee arthroplasty predictable? *Int Orthop.* 2012;36(1):83-88.

13. Markolf KL, Mensch JS, Amstutz HC. Stiffness and laxity of the knee–the contributions of the supporting structures. A quantitative in vitro study. *J Bone Joint Surg Am.* 1976;58(5):583-594.

14. Halewood C, Traynor A, Bellemans J, et al. Anteroposterior laxity after bicruciate-retaining total knee arthroplasty is closer to the native knee than ACL-resecting TKA: a biomechanical cadaver study. *J Arthroplasty.* 2015;30(12):2315-2319.

15. Hino K, Ishimaru M, Iseki Y, et al. Mid-flexion laxity is greater after posterior-stabilised total knee replacement than with cruciate-retaining procedures: a computer navigation study. *Bone Joint J.* 2013;95-B(4):493-497.

16. Hunt NC, Ghosh KM, Blain AP, et al. How does laxity after single radius total knee arthroplasty compare with the native knee? *J Orthop Res.* 2014;32(9):1208-1213.

17. Stoddard JE, Deehan DJ, Bull AM, et al. The kinematics and stability of single-radius versus multi-radius femoral components related to mid-range instability after TKA. *J Orthop Res.* 2013;31(1):53-58.

18. Okada Y, Teramoto A, Takagi T, et al. ACL function in bicruciate-retaining total knee arthroplasty. *J Bone Joint Surg Am.* 2018 5;100(17):e114.

19. Sim JA, Gadikota HR, Li JS, et al. Biomechanical evaluation of knee joint laxities and graft forces after anterior cruciate ligament reconstruction by anteromedial portal, outside-in, and transtibial techniques. *Am J Sports Med.* 2011;39(12):2604-2610.

20. Song EK, Seon JK, Park SJ, et al. In vivo laxity of stable versus anterior cruciate ligament-injured knees using a navigation system: a comparative study. *Knee Surg Sports Traumatol Arthrosc.* 2009;17(8):941-945.

21. Girgis FG, Marshall JL, Monajem A. The cruciate ligaments of the knee joint. Anatomical, functional and experimental analysis. *Clin Orthop Relat Res.* 1975;(106):216-231.

22. Van Damme G, Defoort K, Ducoulombier Y, et al. What should the surgeon aim for when performing computer-assisted total knee arthroplasty? *J Bone Joint Surg Am.* 2005;87 suppl 2:52-58.

23. Schwab JH, Haidukewych GJ, Hanssen AD, et al. Flexion instability without dislocation after posterior stabilized total knees. *Clin Orthop Relat Res.* 2005;440:96-100.

24. Meding JB, Keating EM, Ritter MA, et al. Genu recurvatum in total knee replacement. *Clin Orthop Relat Res.* 2003;(416):64-67.

25. Markolf KL, Gorek JF, Kabo JM, et al. Direct measurement of resultant forces in the anterior cruciate ligament. An in vitro study performed with a new experimental technique. *J Bone Joint Surg Am.* 1990;72(4):557-567.

26. Kouk S, Rathod PA, Maheshwari AV, et al. Rotating hinge prosthesis for complex revision total knee arthroplasty: a review of the literature. *J Clin Orthop Trauma.* 2018;9(1):29-33.

27. Martin JW, Whiteside LA. The influence of joint line position on knee stability after condylar knee arthroplasty. *Clin Orthop Relat Res.* 1990;(259):146-156.

28. McPherson EJ, Cuckler J, Lombardi AV. Midflexion instability in revision total knee arthroplasty. *Surg Technol Int.* 2008;17:249-252.

29. Luyckx T, Vandenneucker H, Ing LS, et al. Raising the joint line in TKA is associated with mid-flexion laxity: a study in cadaver knees. *Clin Orthop Relat Res.* 2018;476(3):601-611.

30. Clary CW, Fitzpatrick CK, Maletsky LP, et al. The influence of total knee arthroplasty geometry on mid-flexion stability: an experimental and finite element study. *J Biomech.* 2013;46(7):1351-1357.

31. Fitzpatrick C, Clary C, Rullkoetter P. The influence of design on TKR mechanics during activities of daily living. *Orthopaedic Research Society.* 2012;31.

32. Salvadore G, Meere PA, Verstraete MA, et al. Laxity and contact forces of total knee designed for anatomic motion: a cadaveric study. *Knee.* 2018;25(4):650-656.

33. Minoda Y, Nakagawa S, Sugama R, et al. Intraoperative assessment of midflexion laxity in total knee prosthesis. *Knee.* 2014;21(4):810-814.

34. Zumbrunn T, Duffy MP, Rubash HE, et al. ACL substitution may improve kinematics of PCL-retaining total knee arthroplasty. *Knee Surg Sports Traumatol Arthrosc.* 2018;26(5):1445-1454.

35. Pritchett JW. Patients prefer a bicruciate-retaining or the medial pivot total knee prosthesis. *J Arthroplasty.* 2011;26(2):224-228.

36. van Duren BH, Pandit H, Price M, et al. Bicruciate substituting total knee replacement: how effective are the added kinematic constraints in vivo? *Knee Surg Sports Traumatol Arthrosc.* 2012;20(10):2002-2010.

37. Okazaki K, Miura H, Matsuda S, et al. Asymmetry of mediolateral laxity of the normal knee. *J Orthop Sci.* 2006;11(3):264-266.

38. Heesterbeek PJ, Verdonschot N, Wymenga AB. In vivo knee laxity in flexion and extension: a radiographic study in 30 older healthy subjects. *Knee.* 2008;15(1):45-49.

39. Ishii Y, Noguchi H, Sato J, et al. Medial and lateral laxity in knees with advanced medial osteoarthritis. *Osteoarthr Cartil.* 2018;26(5):666-670.

40. Deep K. Collateral ligament laxity in knees: what is normal? *Clin Orthop Relat Res.* 2014;472(11):3426-3431.

41. Mayman D, Plaskos C, Kendoff D, et al. Ligament tension in the ACL-deficient knee: assessment of medial and lateral gaps. *Clin Orthop Relat Res.* 2009;467(6):1621-1628.

42. Tokuhara Y, Kadoya Y, Nakagawa S, et al. The flexion gap in normal knees. An MRI study. *J Bone Joint Surg Br.* 2004;86(8):1133-1136.

43. Rajgopal A, Panjwani TR, Rao A, et al. Are the outcomes of revision knee arthroplasty for flexion instability the same as for other major failure mechanisms? *J Arthroplasty.* 2017;32(10):3093-3097.

44. Nishitani K, Nakagawa Y, Suzuki T, et al. Rotating-hinge total knee arthroplasty in a patient with genu recurvatum after osteomyelitis of the distal femur. *J Arthroplasty.* 2007;22(4):630-633.

chapter 11

Metals

Nadim James Hallab, PhD | Robin A. Pourzal, PhD | Joshua J. Jacobs, MD

Metals are well suited for orthopedic applications by providing appropriate material properties, such as high strength, ductility, fracture toughness, hardness, corrosion resistance, formability, and biocompatibility, necessary for use in load-bearing roles required in fracture fixation and total joint arthroplasty (TJA). Implant alloys were originally developed for maritime and aviation uses in which mechanical properties, such as high strength and corrosion resistance, are paramount. There are three principal metal alloys used in orthopedics and particularly in total joint replacement: (1) titanium (Ti)-based alloys, (2) cobalt (Co)-based alloys, and (3) stainless steel alloys. Alloy-specific differences in strength, ductility, and hardness generally determine which of these three alloys is used for a particular application or implant component. However, it is primarily the high-corrosion resistance of all three alloys that has led to their widespread use as load-bearing orthopedic implant materials. These material properties of metals (Table 11-1) required for load-bearing implant components arise from the nature of the metallic bond, the crystalline microstructure, and the elemental composition of metals.[1-5]

METALLIC BOND

The unique combination of material properties found within orthopedic alloys is the result of the metallic bonds formed between metal atoms. The positively charged nuclei of metal atoms form a crystal lattice structure and are held together in a sea of valence electrons (electrons of the outer orbital shells). The resulting balance between positive and negative charges results in overall neutrality. This freely flowing sea of valence electrons within any metal solid is responsible for the related material properties of high thermal and electrical conductivity. Although the nuclei of metal atoms are held within a sea of electrons, these nuclei are fixed in closely packed crystalline arrays, forming a distinct arrangement. The more closely packed these metal nuclei, the stronger the resultant bonding. The structure of the metal crystals can be broken down to a three-dimensional repeating unit (a unit cell) that generally takes one of three configurations (Fig. 11-1): face-centered cubic (FCC), body-centered cubic (BCC), and hexagonal close packed (HCP). The nondirectionality of the metallic bond allows these unit structures to be stretched, deformed, broken, and reformed, permitting defects (dislocations) to pass through the structure.

Alloying elements can be used to fill the spaces between metal atoms—also known as interstitial elements—or replace the base alloy element within the lattice—also known as substitutional elements. Either way, alloying elements change or distort the basic crystal structure of a metal to alter or enhance the material properties by hindering dislocation movement throughout the lattice (e.g., the addition of 6% aluminum [Al] and 4% vanadium [V] are used to enhance the mechanical properties of Ti).

ALLOY MICROSTRUCTURE

As metals cool from a liquid state, crystals begin to form at nucleation sites within the liquid. These crystals grow, forming a granular structure (or a polycrystalline array). Such crystal grains can be observed microscopically on the surface of a polished metal specimen (Fig. 11-2). The microstructural morphology (grain size, shape, etc.) predominantly determines the mechanical properties of the metal. Finer grain sizes generally result in increased yield strength, fatigue strength, and fracture toughness, thereby decreasing the chances for implant fracture. Insufficient quality control in the manufacture of earlier total hip arthroplasty (THA) stem designs demonstrated that large grain sizes within the stems resulted in decreased fatigue strength, which resulted in fracture of the implants *in vivo*. All the grains within a pure metal have the same crystal structure. This "single phase" of a chemically homogeneous metal can be maintained, in some cases, even after the addition of other metals with similar atomic size. However, if added elements are not of similar size or atomic structure, then additional phases develop. Therefore, in a multiphase metal, there will be two or more distinct types of grains or crystal structures.

Although metal alloys do contain a variety of phases and crystal structures in practice, there are usually only a few dominant phases present. The three aforementioned alloys used in TJA usually exhibit the following phases: Ti-based alloys are a mixture of an alpha-phase (HCP) and a beta-phase (BCC) (Fig. 11-3). Co-based alloys are generally single phase (FCC) after casting, but an HCP structure can be introduced by cold working of the alloy. Additional carbidic or intermetallic hard phases may occur depending on the carbon content and heat treatment. Implant-grade stainless steels are so-called austenitic steels comprised of the FCC phase. The amount of

TABLE 11-1 Approximate Weight Percent of Different Metals Within Orthopedic Alloys

Alloy	Ni	N	Co	Cr	Ti	Mo	Al	Fe	Mn	Cu	W	C	Si	V
Stainless steel														
(ASTM F138)	10.0-15.5	<0.5	*	17-19	*	2-4	*	61-68	*	<0.5	<2.0	<0.06	<1.0	*
CoCrMo alloys														
(ASTM F75)	<2.0	*	61-66	27-30	*	4.5-7.0	*	<1.5	<1.0	*	*	<0.35	<1.0	*
(ASTM F90)	9-11	*	46-51	19-20	*	*	*	<3.0	<2.5	*	14-16	<0.15	<1.0	*
(ASTM F562)	33-37	*	35	19-21	<1	9.0-11.0	*	<1	<0.15	*	*	*	<0.15	*
Ti Alloys														
CPTi (ASTM F67)	*	*	*	*	99	*	*	0.2-0.5	*	*	*	<0.1	*	*
Ti-6Al-4V (ASTM F136)	*	*	*	*	89-91	*	5.5-0.5	*	*	*	*	<0.08	*	3.5-4.5
45TiNi	55	*	*	*	45	*	*	*	*	*	*	*	*	*

*, indicates less than 0.05%; Al, aluminum; ASTM, American Society for Testing and Materials; C, carbon; Co, cobalt; Cr, chromium; Cu, copper; Fe, iron; Mn, manganese; Mo, molybdenum; N, nitrogen; Ni, nickel; Si, silicon; Ti, titanium; V, vanadium; W, tungsten.
Note: Alloy compositions are standardized by the ASTM (Annual book of ASTM standards. ASTM, vol. 13.01).

carbon in the steel is intentionally kept to low concentrations, because it can form additional phases, which may settle at grain boundaries and lower the overall strength of the alloy.[1-8]

CORROSION OF ORTHOPEDIC METAL ALLOYS

All metal alloy implants corrode *in vivo*. When severe, the degradative process may reduce structural integrity of the implant, and the release of corrosion products is potentially toxic to the host or can cause adverse local tissue reaction and subsequent implant failure.[9,10] Electrochemical corrosion of implants includes generalized forms of corrosion uniformly affecting an entire surface and localized forms of corrosion affecting areas of a device relatively shielded from the environment (crevice corrosion) or at seemingly random sites on the surface (pitting corrosion).

Metal corrosion is governed by the thermodynamic driving forces that cause corrosion (oxidation–reduction) reactions and the kinetic barriers that limit the rate of these reactions. The chemical driving force (ΔG) determines whether corrosion will take place under the conditions of interest. If the free energy for oxidation is less than zero, then oxidation is energetically favorable and will take place spontaneously. During corrosion, positive and negative charges (metal ions and electrons, respectively) leave one another for more chemically stable partners. The metal ions generally leave to form an oxide or another more stable ionic compound (or are released into solution), and the electrons are left behind in the metal

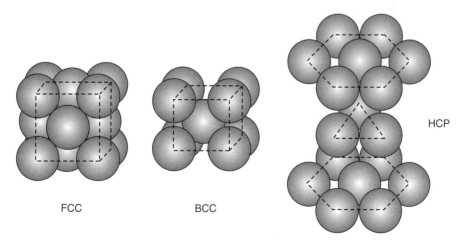

FCC   BCC   HCP

FIGURE 11-1 The three unit cell crystal structures comprising implant alloys. The grains of implant alloys are made up of one or more types of crystal structures that can be broken down to the smallest repeating unit, called a *unit cell*. From left to right the unit cells are termed: face centered cubic (FCC), body centered cubic (BCC) and hexagonal close packed (HCP).

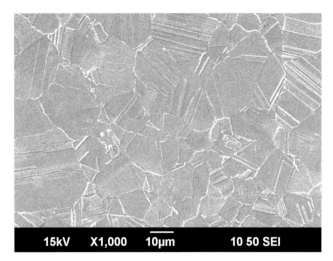

FIGURE 11-2 Scanning electron micrograph of a wrought CoCrMo implant alloy. The alloy sample was polished and etched to visualize the inherent grain structure. The fine microstructure with an average grain size of 3 to 6 µm is typical for this alloy and the reason for its high strength. Also, twin boundaries can be observed within grain which is also a typical occurrence for this alloy. No hard phases can be seen which is typical for the low carbon configuration of this alloy.

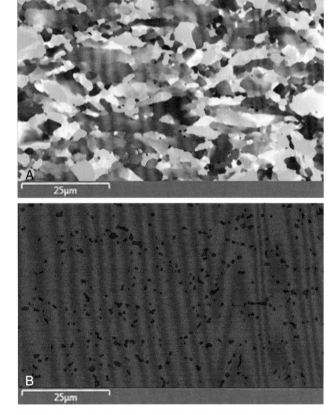

FIGURE 11-3   A: The grain structure of a wrought Ti6Al4V implant alloy visualized by electron backscatter diffraction (EBSD) in a scanning electron microscope. Colors correspond to grains with different crystal orientations. **B:** EBSD phase image of the same area. Red areas correspond to the alpha-phase (HCP) and blue areas indicate the beta-phase (BCC). A beta-content of 5% to 15% is typical for Ti6Al4V alloy used in orthopedic implants.

and undergo other electrochemical reactions on the surface such as the reduction of oxygen or hydrolysis of water. A charge separation across the metal–solution interface contributes to what is known as the *electrical double layer* and creates an electrical potential (much like a capacitor).

The corrosion resistance of implant alloys to this electrochemical driving force is primarily due to the formation of surface barriers that limit implant corrosion. Were it not for the protective barriers that form on the surfaces of implant alloys, vigorous corrosion would take place. Kinetic barriers prevent corrosion by physically limiting the rate at which oxidation and reduction processes can take place. Alloys used in orthopedic implants rely on the formation of passive films to prevent significant electrochemical dissolution from taking place. These films consist of metal oxides that form spontaneously on the surface of metals in such a way that they prevent further transport of metallic ions or electrons, or both, across the film. Passive films must have certain characteristics to limit further oxidation:

- They must be compact (dense) and fully cover the metal surface (contiguous).
- They must have an atomic structure that limits the migration of ions or electrons, or both, across the metal-oxide–solution interface (chemically stable).
- They must be able to remain on the surface of these alloys even under mechanical stress (mechanically sound).
- On bearing surfaces, passive films need to be able to regenerate if abrasive wear or surface fatigues leads to the removal of the passive film (repassivation).

The oxide film will change crystal structure, size, and thickness depending on the conditions of the electrolytic solution (e.g., Co–Cr alloy in serum will form a thin oxide layer (2 to 5 nm) versus the thick oxide layer (10 to 20 nm) formed in nitric acid). Thus, various surface treatments, known as *passivation*, have been used to improve the barrier effect of the oxide film. Typically, such treatments have included a hot 35% nitric acid bath, boiling in distilled water, and anodization. Implant metals are generally passivated using a series of steps that include (1) thorough cleaning using detergent, ultrasound, and heat; (2) cleaning again with ethanol; (3) rinsing in deionized water; (4) treating with a dilute acid solution (e.g., 35% nitric acid); and (5) rinsing and sterilization. However, the development of treatments to optimize the shape, integrity, and protective ability of oxide films of the various implant alloys remains an ongoing process.

One of the current issues associated with implant alloys is the corrosion observed around the modular junction connections of retrieved joint replacement components, which use metal-on-metal conical taper connections (**Fig. 11-4**).[10-12] Dual-modular stems contain additional potential corrosion sites due to neck–stem modularity.[9] Accelerated corrosion can take place in the crevices

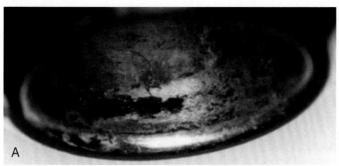
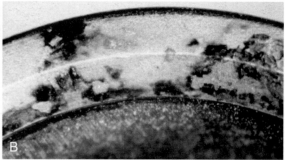

FIGURE 11-4   Retrieved joint replacement components showing corrosion around the metal-on-metal conical taper connections. **A:** Female taper of cobalt-based alloy head showing evidence of corrosion precipitates. **B:** Macrograph of deposits of CrPO$_4$ corrosion products on the rim of a modular cobalt–chrome femoral component. Fretting and crevice corrosion are responsible for generating this type of implant degradation.

formed by these tapers *in vivo* due to (1) the occurrence of micromotion, fretting, and subsequent abrasion of the passive film and (2) the depletion of oxygen. Corrosion has been observed in the Co-based alloy systems used in these modular taper connections through such mechanisms as intergranular corrosion, fretting corrosion, phase boundary corrosion, etching, and selective dissolution of Co.[11,12] Oxide-induced stress corrosion cracking and selective corrosion of the beta-phase have also been observed in Ti alloy stems.[10,13] However, stainless steel alloys generally corrode to a greater extent than Co or Ti alloys (**Table 11-2**).[4,5,14-16]

STAINLESS STEEL ALLOYS

Stainless steels were the first metals to be widely used for orthopedic applications in 1926. However, it was 1943 before American Society for Testing and Materials (ASTM) 304 was developed as a standard implant material. All steels are comprised of Fe and carbon and may contain Cr, nickel (Ni), and molybdenum (Mo). Trace elements such as manganese (Mn), phosphorous, sulfur, and silicon are also present. Carbon and the other alloying elements affect the mechanical properties of steel through alteration of its microstructure.

The form of stainless steel most commonly used in orthopedic practice is designated 316LV (ASTM F138). "316" classifies the material as austenitic, the "L" denotes the low carbon content, and "V," the vacuum under which it is formed. The carbon content must be kept at a low level to prevent carbide (Cr–carbon) accumulation at the grain boundaries. This carbide formation weakens the material by allowing a combination of corrosion and stress to degrade the material at its grain boundaries. In the past, elevated levels of carbon have been associated with the fracture of some orthopedic implants *in vivo*. Mo is added to enhance the corrosion resistance of the grain boundaries, whereas Cr dissipated evenly within the microstructure allows the formation of a Cr oxide (Cr$_2$O$_3$) passive film on the surface of the metal. Stainless steels are surface treated (e.g., in nitric acid) to further promote the growth and thickening of the initial passive oxide film.

TABLE 11-2	Electrochemical Properties of Implant Metals (Corrosion Resistance) in 0.1 M NaCl at pH = 7				
Alloy	**ASTM Designation**	**Density (g/cm³)**	**Corrosion PotenTial (vs. Calomel) (mV)**	**Passive Current Density (mA/cm²)**	**Breakdown Potential (mV)**
Stainless steel	F138	8.0	−400	0.56	200-770
Co-Cr-Mo	F75	8.3	−390	1.36	420
Ti					
CPTi	F67	4.5	−90 to −630	0.72-9.0	>2000
Ti-6Al-4V	136	4.43	−180 to −510	0.9-2.0	>1500
Ti5Al2.5Fe	*	4.45	−530	0.68	>1500
Ni45Ti	*	6.4-6.5	−430	0.44	890

*, no current ASTM standard; Al, aluminum; ASTM, American Society for Testing and Materials; Co, cobalt; CPTi, commercially pure titanium; Cr, chromium; Fe, iron; Mo, molybdenum; NaCl, sodium chloride; Ni, nickel; Ti, titanium; V, vanadium.

Note: The corrosion potential represents the open circuit potential between the metal and a calomel electrode. The more negative the open circuit potential, the more chemically reactive and, thus, the less corrosion resistance. Generally, low current density indicates greater corrosion resistance. The higher the breakdown potential the better (i.e., the more elevated the breakdown potential, the more stable the protective layer).

Alternative Stainless Steels

The addition of Cr to ASTM F138 stainless steel also stabilizes (and thus strengthens) the BCC (ferritic) phase, which is weaker than the more predominant FCC (austenitic) phase. Other added elements, such as silicon and Mn, also serve as stabilizers of the ferrite (BCC) phase. After addition of these ferrite stabilizers, Ni is used to stabilize the austenitic (FCC) phase to produce a uniformity of microstructural strength. Stainless steels can be strengthened by cold working. Although the mechanical properties of stainless steels are generally less desirable than those of the other implant alloys, stainless steels do possess greater ductility indicated quantitatively by a threefold greater "percentage of elongation at fracture" when compared to other implant metals (**Table 11-3**). This aspect of stainless steel has allowed it to remain as

a popular material for cable fixation. However, the superior mechanical properties of Co- and Ti-based alloys for different implant components have led to their dominance in TJA stem and head components.[4,5,15]

The relatively poor corrosion resistance and biocompatibility of stainless steels when compared to Ti and Co-Cr-Mo alloys provide incentive for development of improved stainless steels. New alloys, such as BioDur 108 (Carpenter Technology Corp., Reading PA), attempt to solve the problem of corrosion with an essentially Ni-free austenitic stainless alloy. This steel contains a high nitrogen content to maintain its austenitic structure and boasts improved levels of tensile yield strength, fatigue strength, and improved resistance to pitting corrosion and crevice corrosion as compared to Ni-containing alloys such as type 316L (ASTM F138).

TABLE 11-3 Mechanical Properties of Implant Alloys

Implant Alloy	ASTM Designation	Trade Name and Company (Examples)	Elastic Modulus (GPa)	Yield Strength (MPa)	Ultimate Strength (MPa)	Fatigue Strength (Endurance Limit) (MPa)	Hardness (VHN)	Elongation at Fracture (%)
Stainless steel	F138	Protasul S30—Sulzer	190	792	930	241-820	130-180	43-45
Co-Cr-Mo	F75	Alivium—Biomet CoCrMo—Biomet Endocast SIL—Krupp Francobal—Benoist Girard Orthochrome—DePuy Protasul 2—Sultzer Vinertia—Deloro Vitallium C—Howmedica Vitallium FHS—Howmedica Zimaloy—Zimmer Zimaloy Micrograin—Zimmer	210-253	448-841	655-1277	207-950	300-400	4-14
	F90	Vitallium W—Howmedica	210	448-1606	1896	586-1220	300-400	10-22
	F562	HS251—Haynes Stellite MP35N—Std Pressed Steel Corp.	200-230	300-2000	800-2068	340-520	8-50 (RC)	10-40
	1537	TJA 1537—Allvac Metasul—Sulzer	200-300	960	1300	200-300	41 (RC)	20
Ti								
CPTi	F67	CSTi—Sulzer	110	485	760	300	120-200	14-18
Ti-6Al-4V	136	Isotan—Aesculap Werke Protasul 64WF—Sulzer Tilastin—Waldemar Link Tivaloy 12—Biomet Tivanium—Zimmer	116	897-1034	965-1103	620-689	310	8
Ti5Al2.5Fe	*	*	100-110	780	860	300-725	310	7-13
Ni45Ti	*	Nitinol—Nitinol Medical Technologies	28-110	621-793	827-1172	<200	40-62 (RC)	1-60

*, No current ASTM standard; Al, aluminum; ASTM, American Society for Testing and Materials; Co, cobalt; Cr, chromium; Fe, iron; GPa, gigapascal; Mo, molybdenum; MPa, megapascal; Ni, nickel; RC, Rockwell hardness scale; Ti, titanium; TJA, total joint arthroplasty; V, vanadium; VHN, Vickers hardness number (kg/mm).

COBALT–CHROMIUM ALLOYS

Co-based alloys were developed in 1926, yet it was not until 1929 before they were used in dentistry and 1937 before Co-Cr-Mo alloys were first used in orthopedics (under the trade name Vitallium). The two basic constituents of all Co–Cr alloys are Co (approximately 65%) and Cr (approximately 35%). Co and Cr form a solid solution of large FCC grains. Mo is added primarily as a solid solution strengthener, to decrease the grain size, and thus improve the mechanical properties. Additionally, it was shown that Mo further improves the effectiveness of the oxide passive film that is primarily composed of Cr_2O_3. The homogeneous solid solution of Co, Cr, and Mo is comprised of an FCC (austenitic) crystal. Co-Cr-Mo implant alloys fall into one of two categories: those with Ni and other alloying elements and those without. Of the many Co–Cr alloys available, there are two most commonly used implant alloys (**Table 11-1**): (1) CoCrMo, which is specified in ASTM F75 and F1537 and (2) CoNiCrMo, designated as ASTM F562. Others approved for implant use include one that incorporates tungsten (W) (CoCrNiW, ASTM F90) and another with Fe (CoNiCrMoWFe, ASTM F563). Co-Ni-Cr-Mo alloys that contain large percentages of Ni (25% to 37%) promise increased corrosion resistance, yet raise concerns of possible toxicity or immunogenic reactivity, or both (see Clinical Concerns Regarding Metal Implant Degradation), from released Ni. The biologic reactivity of released Ni from Co-Ni-Cr alloys is the cause for concern under static conditions. Owing to their poor frictional (wear) properties, Co-Ni-Cr alloys are also inappropriate for use in articulating components. Therefore, the dominant implant alloy used for total joint components is CoCrMo alloy.

CoCrMo alloy can be used as either cast (ASTM F75) or wrought (ASTM F1537) alloy. Cast alloys are generally cast into their final shape possibly followed by different heat treatments (e.g., solution annealing, hot isostatical pressing) and surface finishing. This method is especially preferred for implant components with complicated geometries (e.g., femoral condyles in TKRs or femoral stems in THRs). The most common casting method is called investment casting or lost-wax method. The casting processes are carefully controlled, and finished products are evaluated to ensure quality. The grain size and microstructure of cast alloy can vary broadly depending on the manufacturer (**Fig. 11-5**). If cooling is too fast, the formation of large grains will reduce the strength of the component. If cooling is too slow, carbides at grain boundaries will form too thickly, also reducing the strength of the metal.

Wrought alloys are available as bar stock material that implants can be subsequently machined from (e.g., most femoral heads in THRs). Implants made from wrought alloys usually have higher strength compared to cast alloy due to a significantly smaller grain size. The forging process uses repetitive compression between negative volume dies to shape a cast ingot into its final shape. This process is more popularly used in THA (rather than total knee arthroplasty [TKA]) for shaping stems and cups, in which rod-shaped raw material is heated to approximately 900°C, depending on the alloy. During the forging process for implants, the die and the blank are commonly maintained at a constant temperature—isothermal. In this low-speed forming process, the plasticity of the material remains constant throughout the entire forming process. CoCrMo alloy can be further distinguished in low- (<0.05%) and high-carbon alloys (0.2% to 0.4%). The carbon content is related to the formation of carbides. Such hard phases were purposefully introduced to increase the resistance against abrasive wear especially in metal-on-metal total hip replacements. The amount and size of carbide and other intermetallic hard phases also strongly depend on the heat treatment of the alloy (**Fig. 11-5**).[17,18]

The corrosion resistance of Co-Cr-Mo alloys is primarily due to the Cr content within the metal, which results in the formation of a protective passive layer of Cr oxide on the surface of the metal. The hot isostatic pressing processes of the Co-Cr-Mo component creates a more homogeneous microstructure during fabrication, which results in an even distribution of Cr throughout the metal alloy and improved corrosion resistance.

Although Co-Cr-Mo alloys are among the strongest, hardest, and most fatigue resistant of the metals used for joint replacement components, care must be taken to maintain these properties, because the use of finishing treatments can also function to reduce these same properties (**Table 11-2**). For example, sintering of porous coatings onto femoral or tibial components can decrease the fatigue strength of the alloy to 150 MPa.[19-22]

TITANIUM ALLOYS

Ti alloys were developed in the mid-1940s for the aviation industry and were first used in orthopedics around the same time. Two post–World War II alloys, commercially pure Ti (CPTi) and Ti-6Al-4V, remain the two dominant Ti alloys used in implants. CPTi (ASTM F67) is 98% to 99.6% pure Ti. The crystal structure of CPTi is HCP, yet it can be cold worked for further improvement in the mechanical properties. The addition of other elements within a CPTi alloy drastically affects the mechanical properties. For example, the difference between 0.18% and 0.4% oxygen increases the yield strength threefold (from 170 to 450 MPa). Although CPTi is most commonly used in dental applications, the stability of the oxide layer formed on CPTi (and, consequently, its high corrosion resistance) and its relatively higher ductility (i.e., the ability to be cold worked) compared to Ti-6Al-4V has led to its use in porous coatings (e.g., fiber metal) of TJA components. Generally, Ti-6Al-4V (ASTM F136) is used for joint replacement components because

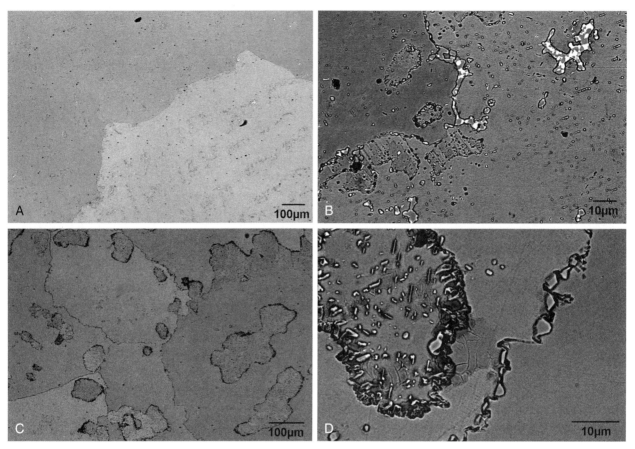

FIGURE 11-5 Backscatter-mode scanning electron micrographs of the microstructure of cast CoCrMo alloys. Alloy samples were taken from two TKA femoral components from two different manufacturers. The alloy shown in **(A)** has a grain size of several millimeters. In **(B)** the same alloy is shown at a higher magnification. Large mixed hard phases can be observed within the grain and along the grain boundaries. These hard phases consist of a lighter phase rich in Mo and Si (intermetallic phase), and a darker phase rich in Cr and carbon (carbides). Additionally, a dispersion of very fine globular hard phases can be observed throughout the grains. The other alloy in **(C)** exhibits a slightly smaller grain size of several hundreds of micrometers. **D:** Within grains, distinct areas can be observed that are rich in fine hard phases. These hard phases can be globular or elongated in shape. (Courtesy of Deborah J. Hall, Rush University Medical Center, Chicago, IL.)

of its superior mechanical properties in comparison to CPTi (**Table 11-2**). The Ti-6Al-4V alloy (also known as *Ti-6-4*) is composed of grains of two phases: an HCP phase and a BCC phase referred to as the *alpha-* and *beta-phases*, respectively (**Fig. 11-3**). Al (5.5% to 6.5% by weight) stabilizes the HCP phase, and V (3.5% to 4.5% by weight) stabilizes the BCC phase. The microstructure and mechanical properties of this alloy are highly dependent on the thermomechanical processing treatments. The Ti-6Al-4V alloy microstructure is generally composed of a fine-grained HCP phase with a sparse distribution of the BCC phase. If the material is cooled too slowly, the BCC phase becomes more prominent and lowers the strength and corrosion resistance of the alloy.

Ti alloys are particularly good implant materials because of their high corrosion resistance compared with stainless steel and Co-Cr-Mo alloys. A passive oxide film (primarily of TiO_2) protects Ti-6Al-4V and CPTi. This stable and adherent passive oxide film protects Ti alloys from pitting corrosion, intergranular corrosion, and crevice corrosion attack and in large part is responsible for the excellent biocompatibility of Ti alloys. Generally,

the strength of Ti-6Al-4V exceeds that of stainless steel, with a flexural rigidity roughly half of stainless steel and Co-Cr-Mo alloys. The torsional and the axial stiffness (moduli) of Ti alloys are therefore closer to bone and theoretically provide less stress shielding than do Co alloys and stainless steel. This attribute, along with excellent biocompatibility and corrosion resistance, is primarily responsible for the popularity of Ti alloys in fracture fixation devices (plates, screws), spinal fixation devices, and total hip replacement femoral components. However, Ti alloys are notch sensitive. This reduces the effective strength of a component by increasing the material's susceptibility to crack initiation and propagation through the component. This requires close attention to the design geometry and the fabrication of Ti alloy components. As would be expected in such a deformation sensitive material, finishing of Ti alloy implants is conducted using heat treatment or hot forging and not cold working similarly to Co alloys. Perhaps the greatest drawback to Ti alloys is their relative poor wear behavior when compared to Co-Cr-Mo alloys (**Table 11-3**). Generally a material's "hardness" (resistance to indentation) correlates with resistance to wear; however, this is not a direct correlation or always true. Ti-6Al-4V alloy is an example of a material that can be approximately 15% softer than Co-Cr-Mo alloys, yet when used in bearing applications, results in significantly more than 15% greater wear than Co-Cr-Mo when used in orthopedic applications (e.g., TKA or THA femoral heads). Thus, Ti alloys are seldom used as materials in which resistance to wear is the primary concern.[1-4,7]

Other Titanium Alloys

One new group of Ti alloys proposed for orthopedic applications are the so-called beta-Ti alloys, which contain metal alloying elements that stabilize the beta (BCC)-phase. One such alloy contains >10% Mo, a known beta-stabilizer. These beta-Ti alloys promise increased fatigue strength and 20% reduction in the elastic modulus, which is closer to bone, minimizing the potential for stress shielding. However, recent implant retrieval studies have shown an increase of catastrophic failures of femoral stems made of beta-Ti alloys, which need to be further investigated.[23,24]

Other attempts at improving traditional Ti-6Al-4V alloys seek to improve biocompatibility and mechanical properties by the substitution of V (a relatively toxic metal) with other less toxic metals. Two such Ti alloys include Ti5Al25Fe and Ti6Al7Nb. These alloys have higher fatigue strength and a lower modulus compared to Ti-6-4, thus enhancing bone to implant load transfer (**Table 11-3**).

Other Ti alloys are being developed for specific applications, such as TiTa30, which has been found to possess the same thermal coefficient of expansion as alumina (a ceramic currently used as femoral and head components) and can be bonded to the ceramic without induction of cracks within the metal. The combination of metal bonded to ceramic has the advantages of high fatigue resistance and high wear resistance. This couple is currently used in dental applications.

"Nitinol" is a Ni–Ti alloy that has "shape memory" properties and appears promising for orthopedic applications. After these alloys are preformed into specific shapes, they can be manipulated into new shapes at temperatures below their transition temperature. Then when heated to temperatures above their transition temperature (15°C to 75°C), they revert to their original shape. Biocompatibility concerns regarding nitinols are centered on the Ni composition (55%) of these alloys. Despite this high amount of a relatively toxic metal, these "memory alloys" may allow implant shape changes *in situ*, thereby expanding the capabilities of current implants.

OTHER ALLOYS AND SURFACE COATINGS

The quest for new metal alloys with improved biocompatibility and mechanical properties is ongoing. The use of Ti alloys, Co-Cr-Mo alloys, or stainless steels in a specific application generally involves tradeoffs of one desirable property for another. New alloys seek improved material properties to overcome or minimize necessary tradeoffs. "New" alloys are usually slight variations of the three categories of implant metals previously described, which are already approved for use as implant materials.

Zirconium (Zr) and tantalum (Ta) are characterized as refractory metals (others include Mo and W) because of their relative chemical stability (passive oxide layer) and high melting points. Zr and Ta alloys are currently in use and may be gaining popularity as orthopedic metals. Because of the surface layer stability, Zr and Ta (like Ti) are highly corrosion resistant. Corrosion resistance generally correlates with biocompatibility (although not always), because more stable metal alloys tend to be less chemically active and less participatory in biologic reactions. Additionally, these refractory metals generally possess high levels of hardness (12 GPa) and wear resistance (approximately tenfold that of Co and Ti alloys, using abrasion testing), which makes them well suited for bearing surface applications. The thickness of the surface oxide layer (approximately 5 μm) and ability to extend ceramic-like material properties (i.e., hardness) into the material through techniques such as oxygen enrichment has resulted in the production of TJA components using these alloys (e.g., oxidized zirconium TKA femoral components [Smith and Nephew, Largo, FL]). As difficulties associated with forming and machining these metals are overcome, the use of these materials is expected to grow. A common way refractory metals can be manufactured is through the process of hot isostatic pressure using alloying elements, such as copper, to catalyze the binding of the refractory powder into a solid component. Removing binding metals that remain within components as grain boundary impurities is problematic, however, and remains as a technical barrier to the use of these alloys as implant materials.[2-4,6,15]

CLINICAL CONCERNS REGARDING METAL IMPLANT DEGRADATION

Metal generated from implant material degradation is released into surrounding tissues. Although this metal may stay bound to local tissues, there is an increasing recognition that released metal products bind to specific proteins and are transported to remote organs. Elements used in modern orthopedic implant alloys (Ti, Al, V, Co, Cr, and Ni) are potentially toxic through (1) metabolic alterations, (2) alterations in host–parasite interactions, (3) immunologic interactions of metal moieties by virtue of their ability to act as haptens (specific immunologic activation) or antichemotactic agents (nonspecific immunologic suppression), and (4) chemical carcinogenesis.

Co, Cr, V, and possibly Ni are essential trace metals in that they are required for normal homeostasis. In excessive amounts, however, Co has been reported to lead to polycythemia, hypothyroidism, cardiomyopathy, and carcinogenesis; Cr can lead to nephropathy, hypersensitivity, and carcinogenesis; Ni can lead to eczematous dermatitis, hypersensitivity, and carcinogenesis; and V can lead to cardiac and renal dysfunction and has been associated with hypertension and manic-depressive psychosis.

Other nonessential metallic elements can also be toxic. Ti has been associated with pulmonary disease in patients with occupational exposure and with platelet suppression in animal models. Al has been associated with renal failure, anemia, osteomalacia, and neurologic dysfunction, possibly including Alzheimer disease. All these aforementioned toxicities generally apply to soluble forms of these elements or particulate aerosols and may not apply to the chemical species that result from prosthetic implant degradation. Therefore, it is important to note that despite the potential toxicologic possibilities, the association of metal release from orthopedic implants with any metabolic, bacteriologic, immunologic, or carcinogenic toxicity remains speculative: Cause and effect have not been well established in humans with TJAs.[25]

Metal Ion Release

There has always been concern regarding the release of chemically active metal ions from implants into surrounding tissues and the bloodstream. Normal human serum levels of prominent implant metals are approximately 1 to 10 ng per mL Al, 0.15 ng per mL Cr, <0.01 ng per mL V, 0.1 to 0.2 ng per mL Co, and <4.1 ng per mL Ti. After TJA, levels of circulating metal have been shown to increase (**Table 11-4**).

The values in this table show that after successful primary total joint replacement, there are measurable elevations in serum and urine Co, Cr, and Ti. Transient elevations of urine and serum Ni have been noted immediately after surgery. However, urine and serum Al and V concentrations have not been found to be greatly elevated in patients with TJA (**Table 11-4**).

Metal ion levels within serum and urine of TJA patients are affected by a variety of factors. For example, mechanically assisted crevice corrosion in patients with modular femoral THA stems has been associated with elevations in serum Co and urine Cr. It had been previously assumed that extensively porous, coated, cementless stems would give rise to higher serum and urine Cr concentrations owing to the larger surface area available for passive dissolution. However, recent studies suggest that disseminated Cr may predominantly come from fretting corrosion of the modular head–neck junction. Postmortem analyses of tissue obtained from subjects with total joint replacement components have indicated that significant increases in Ti, Al, V, Co, and Cr concentrations occur in such tissues as the heart, liver, kidney, spleen, bone marrow, and lymphatic tissue (**Table 11-4**).

In vitro investigations indicate that specific metals in ionic form within the ranges of metal concentrations reported to exist in periprosthetic tissue can affect the functionality of a variety of periimplant cells such as fibroblasts, osteoclasts, macrophages, and lymphocytes. Generally, the most toxic metal ions are Ni, Fe, Cu, Mn, and V, whereas others, such as Na, Cr, Mg, Mo, Al, Ta, and Co, demonstrate relatively less cellular reactivity *in vitro*. Different metals act through different cellular mechanisms to induce distinct responses. However, the form(s) of metal released from TJAs that result in adverse cellular response remain incompletely characterized. The bioreactivity of metal ions *in vitro* (e.g., in culture medium with 10% serum) may differ from *in vivo* conditions of essentially 100% serum, in which relatively inert compounds (e.g., metal oxides) or complexes, or both (e.g., metal–albumin), may more readily form and abrogate or exaggerate the toxic effects of metals such as Ni, Mn, and V. There is mounting evidence that adverse local and remote tissue responses associated with metal particles may be due in part to soluble forms of specific metal degradation products.[26-30]

Metal Particle Distribution

Generally, metal particles found disseminated beyond the periprosthetic tissue are submicron in size. Although variables influencing accumulation of wear debris in remote organs are not clearly identified, numerous case reports document the presence of metallic, ceramic, or polymeric wear debris from hip and knee prostheses in regional and pelvic lymph nodes. Postmortem studies have demonstrated that dissemination of wear particles to the liver, spleen, or abdominal lymph nodes is a common occurrence in patients who have a total hip or knee replacement. These studies also revealed metallic and polyethylene (PE) wear particles in the para-aortic lymph nodes of approximately 90% of patients with a joint replacement prosthesis. Metallic wear particles alone were present in the para-aortic lymph nodes of approximately 70% of patients with a hip or knee replacement. Of these, approximately 40% were reported to have particles disseminated to the liver or spleen. Most disseminated metallic particles have been reported to be less than 1 μm in size, but the range of particle sizes is material dependent. Particles of CPTi and Ti-Al-V alloy may range from 0.1 μm to as large as 50 μm in the lymph nodes and as large as 10 μm in the liver and spleen. In contrast, particles of Co–Cr and stainless steel alloys rarely exceed 3 μm. The response to metallic (and polymeric) debris in lymph nodes includes immune activation of macrophages and associated production of inflammatory cytokines. Metallic and PE wear particles in the liver or spleen are more prevalent in patients who have had a previously failed reconstruction when compared to patients with primary hip or knee arthroplasties.[29,31-35]

TABLE 11-4   Approximate Concentrations of Metal in Human Body Fluids and in Human Tissue With and Without Total Joint Replacements (9,17,19,20,26)

		Ti	Al	V	Co	Cr	Mo	Ni
Human body fluids (×10⁻³ mM)								
Serum	Normal	0.06	0.08	<0.02	0.003	0.001	*	0.007
	TJA	0.09	0.09	0.03	0.007	0.006	*	<0.16
	TJA-F	0.17	0.08	0.03	*	0.004	*	*
Urine	Normal	<0.04	0.24	0.01	*	0.001	*	*
	TJA	0.07	0.24	<0.01	*	0.009	*	*
Synovial fluid	Normal	0.27	4.0	0.10	0.085	0.058	0.219	0.086
	TJA	11.5	24	1.2	10	7.4	0.604	0.55
Joint capsule	Normal	15.0	35	2.4	0.42	2.6	0.177	69
	TJA	32.0	76	5.6	20	12.5	1.13	40
	TJA-F	399	47	29	14	64	4.65	100
Whole blood	Normal	0.35	0.48	0.12	0.002	0.058	0.009	0.078
	TJA	1.4	8.1	0.45	0.33	2.1	0.104	0.50
Human tissue (µg/g) (roughly equivalent to 0.10-0.01 mM)								
Skeletal muscle	Normal	*	*	*	<12	<12	*	*
	TJA	*	*	*	160	570	*	*
Liver	Normal	100	890	14	120	<14	*	*
	TJA	560	680	22	15,200	1130	*	*
Lung	Normal	710	9830	26	*	*	*	*
	TJA	980	8740	23	*	*	*	*
Spleen	Normal	70	800	<9	30	10	*	*
	TJA	1280	1070	12	1600	180	*	*
Pseudocapsule	Normal	<65	120	<9	50	150	*	*
	TJA	39,400	460	121	5490	3820	*	*
Kidney	Normal	*	*	*	30	<40	*	*
	TJA	*	*	*	60	<40	*	*
Lymphatic	Normal	*	*	*	10	690	*	*
Tissue	TJA	*	*	*	390	690	*	*
Heart	Normal	*	*	*	30	30	*	*
	TJA	*	*	*	280	90	*	*

*, data not available; Al, aluminum; Co, cobalt; Cr, chromium; Mo, molybdenum; Ni, nickel; Ti, titanium; TJA, total joint arthroplasty; V, vanadium.
Note: Normal, subjects without any metallic prosthesis (not including dental); TJA, subjects with well-functioning total joint arthroplasty; TJA-F, subjects with a poorly functioning total joint arthroplasty (needing surgical revision).

Metal Hypersensitivity Responses

Released metal can activate the immune system by forming complexes with native proteins. These metal–protein complexes somehow trigger an immune response. Metals accepted as sensitizers include Be, Ni, Co, and Cr, whereas occasional responses have been reported to Ta, Ti, and V. Ni is the most common metal sensitizer in humans followed by Co and Cr. Cross-sensitivity reactions between metals are also common. Metal hypersensitivity is a well-established phenomenon affecting approximately 10% to 15% of the population. Dermal contact and ingestion of metals have been reported to cause cell-mediated type IV delayed-type immune reactions, which most typically manifest as hives, eczema, redness, and itching. The incidence of metal sensitivity among patients with TJA implants is approximately 25% (roughly twice as high as that of the general population), and the average incidence of metal sensitivity among patients with a "failed" implant (in need of revision surgery) is approximately 50% to 60%.

The temporal and physical evidence associated with reactions of severe dermatitis, urticaria, or vasculitis, or all, to the implantation of orthopedic devices leaves little doubt that the phenomenon of metal-induced hypersensitivity does occur in some cases, currently accepted to be <1% of patients. *In vivo*, these metal hyperreactivity reactions may be associated with the presence of metallosis (darkened tissue staining), excessive periprosthetic fibrosis, or necrosis, or all. However, it is currently unknown whether metal sensitivity exists as a complication in only a few susceptible patients or is a more subtle and common phenomenon, which over time plays an important role in implant function. The degree to which a precondition of metal hypersensitivity may elicit an overaggressive immune response in a patient receiving an implant remains unknown.[36-38]

Metal-Induced Carcinogenesis

The carcinogenic potential of the metals used in TJA remains an area of concern. The carcinogenic potential of orthopedic implant materials has been documented in animal studies. Rat sarcomas were noted to correlate with high serum Co, Cr, or Ni content released from metal implants. Recent studies of human TJA populations have found no significant increase in leukemia or lymphoma in patients with implants, although these studies did not include large proportions of subjects with a metal-on-metal prostheses. Whether metal release from orthopedic implants is carcinogenic remains conjectural, because causality has not been established in human subjects. However, compared to the number of devices implanted on a yearly basis (>700,000), the incidence of cancer at the site of implantation is rare. Continued surveillance and longer-term epidemiologic studies are required to fully address these issues.[39-43]

STATUS OF METALS IN TKA

Most total knee arthroplasties today rely on a femoral component made from cast CoCrMo alloy articulating against a PE tibial liner. Tibial components are usually made from Ti6Al4V alloy or CoCrMo alloy. The clinical success of the CoCrMo-PE bearing couple is most evident in the rising number of TKAs performed per year and the increasing average implant life time.[44,45] The marked reduction of the PE wear rate over the last years has been mainly achieved by improvements of the ultrahigh-molecular-weight PE itself (sterilization in a nitrogen atmosphere, controlled cross-linking, and most recently vitamin-E doping). The femoral components may exhibit different grain sizes (hundreds of micrometers up to several millimeters), and hard phase type (carbide or intermetallic phases), size, and distribution depending on

the solidification sequence and subsequent heat treatment chosen by different manufacturers. So far, there has been no evidence that the microstructure of the CoCrMo alloy has a noticeable impact on the bearing performance or PE wear. Adverse local tissue reactions to corrosion products generated from CoCrMo alloy in THAs has raised concerns for the potential occurrence of similar problems in TKAs.[9,10] So far, there are only few isolated reports of corrosion in TKRs. Mostly corrosion has been found on modular components of revision stems.[46] It appears that corrosion damage is most noticeable on CoCrMo alloy stems compared to Ti alloy. However, there are currently no studies linking corrosion of TKA femoral or tibial components to adverse tissue reactions of any kind or implant failure in general. Despite the lack of evidence for clinical necessity, alternative materials for the femoral component are either already available (e.g., zirconia coatings) or may enter the market more broadly soon (e.g., ceramics). Although such alternative implants may eliminate the risk of corrosion, one has to consider potential downsides (e.g., fracture risk, costs) that need to be weighed against the benefits. Thus, the clinical performance of these implants needs to be carefully monitored. Judged by the great clinical performance of CoCrMo alloy in TKA, it is yet unclear if a more corrosion resistant alternative is needed and may come with unforseen risks.[44,47,48]

CONCLUSION

Ti alloys, Co alloys, and stainless steels remain the three dominant metal alloys used in orthopedics and particularly in TJA. Zr and Ta alloys have been recently introduced for TJA applications, although the use of such devices remains limited. Differences between the mechanical properties of these metals have resulted in specialized roles for each in TJA. Ti alloys are the most inert (with the highest corrosion resistance) of the popular alloys (excluding Zr and Ta alloys) and are widely considered to possess superior tissue compatibility under static conditions. However, due to their lower hardness compared to Co alloys, Ti alloys generally serve as load-bearing plates, screws, stems, and other applications without bearing surface articulation (e.g., femoral heads). Co alloys, although less resistant to electrochemical corrosion than Ti, possess the greatest wear resistance of the traditional orthopedic alloys and are the dominant materials used for applications such as TKA and THA femoral heads. Stainless steels are the most ductile of the three alloy categories and maintain mechanical property integrity after large deformations. Thus, they remain popular as cabling materials used to secure bone grafts and fractures.

This chapter has focused on the mechanical properties of metals used in TJA. The local and systemic biologic effects of long-term use of metal alloys remain largely uncharacterized. However, it is important to note that when evaluating the biocompatibility (or the ability of a material to demonstrate host and material response appropriate to its intended application) of a particular metal component, the results do not necessarily apply to all implants made of the same material. Reasons for poor implant performance can be attributed to many factors, which include manufacturing, mechanical design, and surgical errors, as well as inappropriate choice of material for a given application. Wise material selection cannot compensate for poor implant design or surgical error. It must be emphasized that there is no universal "best" material for all implant applications (in contrast to the claims touted by manufacturers' marketing departments). Terminology describing biologic performance such as "biocompatible" must be qualified with the type of application. For example, an appropriate statement might be "Co-Cr-Mo alloys are more biocompatible as bearing surfaces in TJA than Ti alloys, because higher hardness leads to less wear and particle-induced inflammation." Ultimately, the most prudent choice of a biomaterial (whether ceramic, polymer, or metal alloy) for a particular application depends on careful evaluation of which specific properties of available materials best satisfy the *in situ* demands and design characteristics of a particular implant component.

REFERENCES

1. Black J. *Orthopaedic Biomaterials in Research and Practice*. New York: Churchill Livingstone; 1988.
2. Black J. *Biomaterials*. New York: Marcel Dekker Inc; 1992.
3. Black J. *Prosthetic Materials*. New York: VCH Publishers; 1996.
4. Park J. *Biomaterials Science and Engineering*. US: Springer; 1984. Available at:https://www.springer.com/us/book/9781461297109. Accessed February 27, 2019.
5. Silver FH, Christiansen DL. *Biomaterials Science and Biocompatibility*. New York: Springer-Verlag; 1999. Available at:https://www.springer.com/us/book/9780387987118. Accessed March 4, 2019.
6. Breme J, Biehl V. Metallic biomaterials. In: Black J, Hastings G, eds. *Handbook of Biomaterial Properties*. London: Chapman and Hall; 2001:135-214.
7. Brunski M. Metals. In: Ratner B, Hoffman A, Schoen F, eds. *Biomaterials Science*. New York: Academic Press; 1996:37-50.
8. Laffargue P, Fialdes P, Frayssinet P, Rtaimate M, Hildebrand HF, Marchandise X. Adsorption and release of insulin-like growth factor-I on porous tricalcium phosphate implant. *J Biomed Mater Res*. 2000;49:415-421.
9. Cooper HJ, Urban RM, Wixson RI, Meneghini RM, Jacobs JJ. Adverse local tissue reactions arising from corrosion at the neck-body junction in a dual taper stem with a CoCr modular neck. *J Bone Jt Surg*. 2013;95:865-872.
10. Hall DJ, Pourzal R, Della Valle CJ, Galante JO, Jacobs JJ, Urban RM. Corrosion of modular junctions in femoral and acetabular components for hip arthroplasty and its local and systemic effects. In: Greenwald A, Kurtz S, Lemons J, Mihalko W, eds. *Modularity and Tapers in Total Joint Replacement Devices*. West Conshohocken, PA: ASTM International: 2015;410-427.
11. Gilbert JL, Buckley CA, Jacobs JJ. In vivo corrosion of modular hip prosthesis components in mixed and similar metal combinations. The effect of crevice, stress, motion, and alloy coupling. *J Biomed Mater Res*. 1993;27:1533-1544.
12. Hall DJ, Pourzal R, Lundberg HJ, Mathew MT, Jacobs JJ, Urban RM. Mechanical, chemical and biological damage modes within head-neck tapers of CoCrMo and Ti6Al4V contemporary hip replacements: damage modes in THR modular junctions. *J Biomed Mater Res B Appl Biomater*. 2018;106:1672-1685.
13. Gilbert JL, Mali S, Urban RM, Silverton CD, Jacobs JJ. In vivo oxide-induced stress corrosion cracking of Ti-6Al-4V in a neck-stem modular taper: emergent behavior in a new mechanism of in vivo corrosion. *J Biomed Mater Res B Appl Biomater*. 2011;100:584-594.
14. Jacobs JJ, Gilbert JL, Urban RM. Corrosion of metallic implants. *Total Revision Hip Arthroplasty*. 1994;2:279-319.
15. Jacobs JJ, Gilbert JL, Urban RM. Corrosion of metal orthopaedic implants. *J Bone Joint Surg Am*. 1998;80:268-282.
16. Pourbaix M. Electrochemical corrosion of metallic biomaterials. *Biomaterials*. 1984;5:122-134.
17. Liao Y, Pourzal R, Stemmer P, et al. New insights into hard phases of CoCrMo metal-on-metal hip replacements. *J Mech Behav Biomed Mater*. 2012;12:39-49.
18. Stemmer P, Pourzal R, Liao Y, et al. Microstructure of retrievals made from standard cast HC-CoCrMo alloys. In: Kurtz SM, Greenwald AS, Mihalko WH, Lemons JE, eds. *Metal-on-Metal Total Hip Replacement Devices*. West Conshohocken, PA: ASTM International; 2013:251-267.
19. Black J, Oppenheimer P, Morris DM, Peduto AM, Clark CC. Release of corrosion products by F-75 cobalt base alloy in the rat. III: effects of a carbon surface coating. *J Biomed Mater Res*. 1987;21:1213-1230.
20. Collier JP, Mayor MB, Williams IR, Surprenant VA, Surprenant HP, Currier BH. The tradeoffs associated with modular hip prostheses. *Clin Orthop Relat Res*. 1995;311:91-101.
21. Gilbert JL, Buckley CA, Jacobs JJ, Bertin KC, Zernich MR. Intergranular corrosion-fatigue failure of cobalt-alloy femoral stems. A failure analysis of two implants. *J Bone Joint Surg Am*. 1994;76:110-115.
22. McKellop HA, Sarmiento A, Brien W, Park SH. Interface corrosion of a modular head total hip prosthesis. *J Arthroplasty*. 1992;7:291-294.
23. Martin AJ, Jenkins DR, Van Citters DW. Role of corrosion in taper failure and head disassociation in total hip arthroplasty of a single design. *J Orthop Res*. 2018;36(11):2996-3003.
24. Morlock MM, Dickinson EC, Günther K-P, Bünte D, Polster V. Head taper corrosion causing head bottoming out and consecutive gross stem taper failure in total hip arthroplasty. *J Arthroplast*. 2018;33(11):3581-3590. Available at:https://linkinghub.elsevier.com/retrieve/pii/S0883540318306600. Accessed September 16, 2018.
25. Michel R, Nolte M, Reich M, Löer F. Systemic effects of implanted prostheses made of cobalt-chromium alloys. *Arch Orthop Trauma Surg*. 1991;110:61-74.
26. Dorr LD, Bloebaum R, Emmanual J, Meldrum R. Histologic, biochemical, and ion analysis of tissue and fluids retrieved during total hip arthroplasty. *Clin Orthop Relat Res*. 1990;(261):82-95.
27. Jacobs JJ, Silverton C, Hallab NJ, et al. Metal release and excretion from cementless titanium alloy total knee replacements. *Clin Orthop Relat Res*. 1999;(358):173-180.
28. Jacobs JJ, Skipor AK, Patterson LM, et al. Metal release in patients who have had a primary total hip arthroplasty. A prospective, controlled, longitudinal study. *J Bone Joint Surg Am*. 1998;80:1447-1458.
29. Stulberg BN, Merritt K, Bauer TW. Metallic wear debris in metal-backed patellar failure. *J Appl Biomater*. 1994;5:9-16.
30. Sunderman FW, Hopfer SM, Swift T, et al. Cobalt, chromium, and nickel concentrations in body fluids of patients with porous-coated knee or hip prostheses. *J Orthop Res*. 1989;7:307-315.
31. Jacobs null. Shanbhag null, glant null, black null, galante null. Wear debris in total joint replacements. *J Am Acad Orthop Surg*. 1994;2:212-220.
32. Jacobs JJ, Urban RM, Gilbert JL, et al. Local and distant products from modularity. *Clin Orthop Relat Res*. 1995;319:94-105.
33. Jasty M, Goetz DD, Bragdon CR, et al. Wear of polyethylene acetabular components in total hip arthroplasty. An analysis of one hundred and twenty-eight components retrieved at autopsy or revision operations. *J Bone Joint Surg Am*. 1997;79:349-358.

34. Urban RM, Jacobs JJ, Gilbert JL, Galante JO. Migration of corrosion products from modular hip prostheses. Particle microanalysis and histopathological findings. *J Bone Joint Surg Am.* 1994;76:1345-1359.

35. Urban RM, Jacobs JJ, Tomlinson MJ, Gavrilovic J, Black J, Peoc'h M. Dissemination of wear particles to the liver, spleen, and abdominal lymph nodes of patients with hip or knee replacement. *J Bone Joint Surg Am.* 2000;82:457-476.

36. Caicedo MS, Solver E, Coleman L, Jacobs JJ, Hallab NJ. Females with unexplained joint pain following total joint arthroplasty exhibit a higher rate and severity of hypersensitivity to implant metals compared with males: implications of sex-based bioreactivity differences. *J Bone Joint Surg Am.* 2017;99:621-628.

37. Hallab N, Merritt K, Jacobs JJ. Metal sensitivity in patients with orthopaedic implants. *J Bone Joint Surg Am.* 2001;83-A:428-436.

38. Merritt K, Brown SA. Metal sensitivity reactions to orthopedic implants. *Int J Dermatol.* 1981;20:89-94.

39. Gillespie WJ, Frampton CM, Henderson RJ, Ryan PM. The incidence of cancer following total hip replacement. *J Bone Joint Surg Br.* 1988;70:539-542.

40. Jacobs JJ, Urban RM, Wall J, Black J, Reid JD, Veneman L. Unusual foreign-body reaction to a failed total knee replacement: simulation of a sarcoma clinically and a sarcoid histologically. A case report. *J Bone Joint Surg Am.* 1995;77:444-451.

41. Mathiesen EB, Ahlbom A, Bermann G, Lindgren JU. Total hip replacement and cancer. A cohort study. *J Bone Joint Surg Br.* 1995;77:345-350.

42. Sinibaldi K, Rosen H, Liu SK, DeAngelis M. Tumors associated with metallic implants in animals. *Clin Orthop Relat Res.* 1976;(118):257-266.

43. Sunderman FW. Carcinogenicity of metal alloys in orthopedic prostheses: clinical and experimental studies. *Fundam Appl Toxicol.* 1989;13:205-216.

44. American Joint Replacement Registry. *Fourth AJRR Annual Report on Hip and Knee Arthroplasty Data.* 2017. http://www.ajrr.net/publications-data/annual-reports. Accessed March 4, 2019.

45. Kurtz S, Ong K, Lau E, Mowat F, Halpern M. Projections of primary and revision hip and knee arthroplasty in the United States from 2005 to 2030. *J Bone Joint Surg Am.* 2007;89:780-785.

46. Martin AJ, Seagers KA, Van Citters DW. Assessment of corrosion, fretting, and material loss of retrieved modular total knee arthroplasties. *J Arthroplasty.* 2017;32:2279-2284.

47. Vertullo CJ, Lewis PL, Graves S, Kelly L, Lorimer M, Myers P. Twelve-year outcomes of an oxinium total knee replacement compared with the same cobalt-chromium design: an analysis of 17,577 prostheses from the Australian Orthopaedic Association National Joint Replacement Registry. *J Bone Joint Surg Am.* 2017;99:275-283.

48. Xiang S, Zhao Y, Li Z, Feng B, Weng X. Clinical outcomes of ceramic femoral prosthesis in total knee arthroplasty: a systematic review. *J Orthop Surg Res.* 2019;14:57.

chapter 12

Polyethylene in Total Knee Arthroplasty

Pakdee Rojanasopondist, BA | Orhun Muratoglu, PhD

Ultrahigh-molecular-weight polyethylene (UHMWPE or polyethylene) is the material of choice as for the fabrication of tibial knee inserts and patellae components used in total knee arthroplasty. Owing to the relatively wide range of articular geometries, kinematics, and loading conditions, the analysis of the material properties and clinical performance of polyethylene in knee arthroplasty is more complex than in hip arthroplasty. The challenge in producing polyethylene for a prosthetic knee is to optimize the interplay of the basic material properties to allow a practically unlimited number of loading cycles without material failure—with the generation of a minimum of biologically active particles—for that specific design.

MEDICAL GRADE POLYETHYLENE

Ethylene is a gaseous hydrocarbon composed of two carbon atoms and four hydrogen atoms, C_2H_4. Polyethylene is a long-chain polymer of ethylene molecules in which all of the carbon atoms are linked, each of them holding its two hydrogen atoms[1] (**Fig. 12-1**). The mechanical properties of UHMWPE are strongly related to its chemical structure, molecular weight, crystalline organization, and thermal history.[2]

UHMWPE microstructure is a two-phase viscoplastic solid consisting of crystalline domains embedded within an amorphous matrix[2,3] (**Fig. 12-2**). Connecting the crystalline domains are bridging tie molecules.[3] UHMWPE is defined as polyethylene with an average molecular weight of more than 3 million g per mol.[2] The UHMWPE currently used in orthopedic applications has a molecular weight of 3 to 6 million g per mol, a melting point of 125°C–145°C, and a density of 0.930 to 0.945 g per

mL.[2,4] UHMWPE has been miscalled *high-density polyethylene* in the orthopedic literature, and it is important to distinguish between the two. *High-density polyethylene* is defined as polyethylene with a density greater than 0.940 g per mL and a molecular weight below 200,000 g per mol.[2] UHMWPE has a lower density than high-density polyethylene and has a much higher molecular weight, higher impact strength and toughness, and better wear characteristics under abrasive conditions.[3,4]

The nomenclature for UHMWPE resins has evolved. The current nomenclature is outlined in **Table 12-1**.[2] Ticona (Summit, NJ) is the sole supplier of medical grade UHMWPE resins to orthopedic manufacturers.

Ticona, previously Hoechst Celanese Corporation, produces GUR resins. GUR is an acronym as follows: The first letter represented the Hoechst nomenclature for polyethylene resins; in this case, G corresponds to "granular." The second letter represents the molecular weight in the old Hoechst system, with the higher letters equivalent to very high molecular weights; conveniently, U was selected for use with UHMWPE. The third letter, R, stands for Ruhrchemie AG (Oberhausen, Germany), the plant (which was partially owned by Hoechst) where this product was first produced.

For Ticona resins, the first digit of the grade was used to describe the loose bulk density of the resin; however, in 1998, the nomenclature was consolidated with the first digit uniformly "1." The second digit indicates the absence ("0") or presence ("1") of calcium stearate in

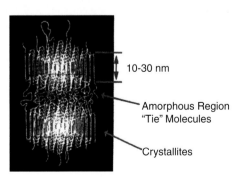

FIGURE 12-2 Molecular structure of ultrahigh-molecular-weight polyethylene. (From Spector M, Bellare A. Implant materials: metals, polyethylene, polymethylmethacrylate. In: Pellicci PM, Tria AJ Jr, Garvin KL, eds. *OKU-2—Hip and Knee Reconstruction.* Rosemont, IL: American Academy of Orthopedic Surgeons; 2000, with permission.)

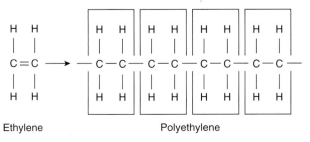

Ethylene   Polyethylene

FIGURE 12-1 Linear chemical structure of polyethylene.

TABLE 12-1 **Nomenclature of Medical Grades of Ultrahigh-Molecular-Weight Polyethylene. Note That GUR 1020 and GUR 1050 Are the Only Ones Currently in Clinical Use**

Resin Designation	Actual Producer	Previous Designation	Previous Producer
GUR 1150	Ticona (Summit, NJ)	GUR 4150	Hoechst
GUR 1050	Ticona (Summit, NJ)	GUR 4050	Hoechst
GUR 1120	Ticona (Summit, NJ)	GUR 4120	Hoechst
GUR 1020	Ticona (Summit, NJ)	GUR 4020	Hoechst
1900	Basell (Wilmington, DE)	–	Hercules–Himont–Montell
1900H	Basell (Wilmington, DE)	–	Hercules–Himont–Montell

the resin. Calcium stearate is an additive in the manufacturing process of many polyethylene resins, which acts as a corrosion inhibitor,[2,5] whitening agent,[4] and lubricant to facilitate the extrusion process.[2,5,6] The third digit is related to the average molecular weight of the resin; the number "2" is used for resins that have an average molecular weight of 3.5 millions g per mol, whereas the number "5" is used for resins with an average molecular weight between 5.5 and 6.0 million g per mol. The fourth digit is an internal code designation. The biggest difference between GUR resins is in impact strength and abrasion resistance. GUR 1020 and 1120 have higher levels of impact strength, whereas GUR 1050 and 1150 have higher abrasion resistance. The most commonly supplied UHMWPEs to orthopedic manufacturers in the United States are GUR 1050 and GUR 1020.[2]

In general, UHMWPE resin powders consist of numerous fused, spheroidal UHMWPE particles with a fine network of submicron-sized fibrils that interconnect the microscopic spheroids. Ticona resins have a mean particle size of approximately 140 μm.[2] Physical properties of Ticona resins are outlined in **Table 12-2**.

There are two methods to produce orthopedic devices with UHMWPE (**Fig. 12-3**). The first method is machining of components from stock polyethylene material. Stock material is available as cylindrical ram-extruded bars or large molded sheets, from which the implant is machined into its final shape.[2-4]

To produce ram-extruded bars, polyethylene powder is introduced into a cylinder that contains a reciprocating ram extruder. The powder is then compacted and heated at temperatures between 180°C and 200°C to become consolidated. Extruded bars are available in many diameters and lengths. The most commonly used are 2.0, 2.5, and 3 inch wide and 5 and 10 feet long.

To produce molded sheets, polyethylene powder is placed in a mold, usually with a size of 4 × 8 feet. Once in the mold, the powder is cold pressed under pressures between 5 and 10 megapascal (MPa) to reduce the amount of air trapped. The compressed powder is then heated at approximately 200°C until the powder is completely

TABLE 12-2 **Physical Properties of Ticona and Himont Resins**

Resin	Average Molecular Weight (10⁶ g/mol)[a]	Density (g/mL)[b]	Tensile Modulus (MPa)[b]	Yield Stress (MPa)[b]	Impact Strength (kJ/m²)[b]	Particle Size (μm)[a]	Calcium stearate[a]
GUR 1150	5.5-6.0	0.93	680[c]	≥17[c]	≥130[d]	140	Yes
GUR 1050	5.5-6.0	0.93	680[c]	≥17[c]	≥130[d]	140	No
GUR 1120	3.5	0.93	720[c]	≥17[c]	≥210[d]	140	Yes
GUR 1020	3.5	0.93	720[c]	≥17[c]	≥210[d]	140	No
1900	4.4-4.9	0.93	750[e]	19[f]	65[g]	300	No
1900H	>4.95	0.93	750[e]	19[f]	65[g]	300	No

MPa, megapascal. Note that the GUR 1020 and GUR 1050 are the only polyethylene resins currently in clinical use.

[a]Adapted from Kurtz SM, Muratoglu OK, Evans M, et al. Advances in the processing, sterilization, and crosslinking of ultrahigh molecular weight polyethylene for total joint arthroplasty. *Biomaterials*. 1999;20:1659-1688.

[b]Data from Ticona product data sheet and Basell product data sheet.

[c]International Standards Organization (ISO) 527 test method.

[d]ISO DIS 11542 test method.

[e]American Society for Testing and Materials (ASTM) D 790B test method.

[f]ASTM D 638 test method.

[g]Montell P 116 test method.

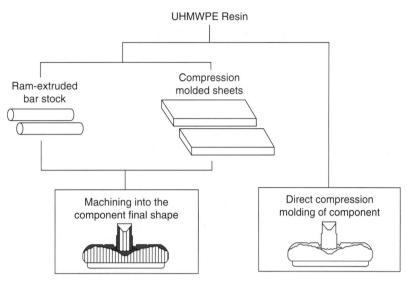

FIGURE 12-3 Manufacturing process of surgical implants from ultrahigh-molecular-weight polyethylene (UHMWPE). In components made by direct compression molding, the obtained surface finish is smooth and without machining marks.

fused. After that, the mold is cooled under approximately 7 to 10 MPa.[7] Most common molded sheet thicknesses are 60 mm, 2.25, 2.50, and 3.0 inch.

Although any type of resin can be used with either ram extrusion or compression molding, GUR 1050 is more commonly used for ram extrusion, whereas GUR 1020 is more commonly used for compression molding.[2]

Polyethylene components can also be made by direct compression molding. In this process, the manufacturer effectively converts the resin powder into the final component by placing it into a mold for the finished component, which is compressed and heated.[4] The obtained surface finish is smooth and without machining marks. Typically the direct compression molded parts are molded to a near net shape, where the final articular surface is formed during molding and the back side of the component is machined after molding.

Long-term performance of TKA implants can be compromised by adhesive/abrasive wear of the articular surface and the backside surface of the UHMWPE tibial insert as well as by articular surface wear of the patellar component. More importantly, pitting and delamination wear damage on the articular surface of the tibial insert and patellar components can adversely affect outcomes and, in catastrophic cases, lead to a revision surgery. There are many factors that may affect adhesive/abrasive wear and delamination damage of UHMWPE components such as articular surface geometry, metal backing, motion patterns, sterilization methods, level of crosslinking, and oxidative stability.

ARTICULAR SURFACE GEOMETRY

The geometry of an articulation can be generally described as a convex surface on a concave surface. In total knee replacement (TKR), the degree of conformity between tibial and femoral articulating surfaces can be described as the ratio of the radius of curvature of the tibial component (R_2) to the radius of curvature of the femoral component (R_1): R_2/R_1. Such an analysis can be done for the sagittal and coronal geometries. As the ratio approaches 1, the articular conformity increases. Thus, the most conforming articulation would have matched radii and a ratio of 1 (ie, a total hip replacement [THR] or a flat-on-flat surface). Because the sagittal radius of curvature of a femoral component may not be constant over the entire sagittal profile, conformity may vary throughout knee range of motion.[8] Constraint—the restriction of motion—is an independent result from increased conformity: A flat-on-flat articulation is completely conforming and has no constraint to motion, whereas a dished articulation of matched radii is completely conforming, yet motion is constrained to one plane.[8]

Condylar designs with conforming tibiofemoral articulations have large contact areas and lower contact stresses[9-11] but may not allow physiologic translational and rotational movements. Relatively flat tibial articulations can accommodate such motions but have smaller contact areas and higher contact stresses.[12-16]

Polyethylene contact stresses are a function of the load, the contact area, and component thickness.[17] The maximum contact stress on tibial components increases as the polyethylene thickness decreases.[16,18] The location of the maximum shear stress has implications for wear when conventional UHMWPE is used, owing to the fact that shear stresses are associated with propagation of subsurface cracks when the fatigue crack propagation resistance of UHMWPE is compromised by oxidation. In this regard, conformity is an important factor. In contrast to THRs in which the components are highly conforming and the maximum shear stress is at the surface, in TKRs, the maximum shear stress is located between 1 and 2 mm beneath the surface.[18] Unfortunately, this is also the location of maximum oxidation and the so-called white band, which develops in certain components after gamma radiation in air or in inert gas or after radiation cross-linking. The maximum stresses, occurring in the weakest zone of these components, cause subsurface fatigue, leading to aggressive delamination, high wear rates, and clinical failure.

METAL BACKING

Metal backing of the tibial component was introduced to improve the load distribution at the bone–implant interface, reducing the stress in the supporting bone.[18,19] Given sufficient polyethylene thickness, there is no apparent detrimental effect on the wear of the primary articulating surface as a result of metal backing.

The polyethylene insert–metal tibial base interface is, however, a potential additional source of wear debris (**Fig. 12-4**). Analysis of motion between the polyethylene tibial insert and metal baseplate of nine modular total knee implant designs, including five snap-fit (Miller-Galante II, Press-Fit Condylar, Duracon, Genesis, Ortholoc) and four tongue and groove designs (anatomic modular knee, IB II, Axiom, Maxim), showed that in every implant the polyethylene insert–metal base interface was subject to micromotion. No significant differences were observed in the motion allowed by each one of those mechanisms.[20] Because a significant correlation between severe wear on the back surface of polyethylene inserts and tibial osteolysis has been established,[21,22] locking mechanisms that minimize relative motion are desirable.

MOTION PATTERN

Polyethylene wear is a function of the motion pattern. In wear tests that use a linear motion path, such as a reciprocating pin on disc, the rate of polyethylene wear for a given set of test conditions is 10 to 100 times lower than that of wear tests that have crossing motion paths, such as in a hip simulator.[23] In theory, a total knee with simple linear motion pattern(s) would exhibit very low wear.

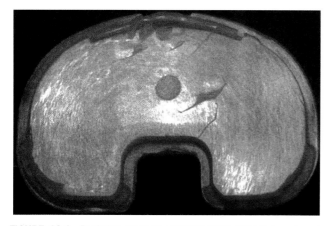

FIGURE 12-4 Backside wear on modular tibial polyethylene insert. Large gouges and gross deformation are due to implant extraction. Note, however, the diffuse burnishing and small scratches from relative motion against the metallic baseplate.

Yet, *in vivo* cine-fluoroscopic studies of clinically well-functioning total knees have demonstrated more complex motions that include variable degrees of rolling, sliding, and rotation on the same surface. In contrast to normal knees, the kinematics of posterior cruciate-retaining total knees is characterized by anterior femoral translation or "skidding" of between 3 and 9 mm.[24,25] Posterior cruciate-substituting knee systems demonstrate more posterior femoral rollback with flexion, although some anterior femoral translation can occur.[24] Additionally, low-conformity, cruciate-retaining designs can demonstrate paradoxic rotation or negative screw home around a lateral axis.[25] Condylar lift-off is a frequent occurrence in cruciate-retaining and cruciate-substituting designs. These motion patterns result in high polyethylene stresses and material failure, such as pitting and delamination.[26,27]

WEAR PARTICLES

The number, shape, and size of polyethylene wear particles are multifactorial: They are a function of the modes and mechanisms of wear that produce them, the stresses on the bearing surface, the motions, and the polyethylene molecular orientation. Most of the polyethylene wear particles produced in a prosthetic joint are micron to submicron in size and are produced in mode 1 in very large quantities by well-functioning joints.[28] Techniques have been developed to isolate and analyze wear particles generated *in vivo* by retrieving them from periprosthetic tissues.[28-34] The concentration of debris particles from prosthetic joints is directly correlated to the duration of implantation[35] and can extend into the billions per gram of tissue.[30-32,36]

Significant differences in polyethylene wear particles from THRs and TKRs have been found. THRs release a relatively high number of submicron polyethylene particles and relatively few particles several microns in dimension, whereas TKRs release a broader range of particles that include some very large flakes measuring hundreds of microns across but relatively fewer submicron particles.[37-39] Although some studies reported up to 71% submicron particles in TKR cases, compared to 85% in THR cases,[39] others have reported only 36% of submicron particles in such cases.[40] The overall average area of particles from total knees has been reported to be approximately twice that of total hips, owing to large flake-shaped particles, relatively common in knee specimens, measuring several microns in length and width.[39]

Such differences in polyethylene particles from TKRs and THRs can be explained by differences in the articulating surfaces, stresses, and motion patterns between them. Increased contact stresses resulting from a decreased conformity, as occurs in TKRs, can exceed the yield strength of polyethylene.[12,18,41] Furthermore, in a TKR with relative low conformity, the motion pattern can include rolling, sliding, and rotation on the same surface; rotation with anteroposterior sliding has been associated with high wear.[27] The combination of these factors results in differences in the balances of the wear mechanisms in THRs and TKRs. In THR, the predominant wear mechanisms appear to involve microadhesion and microabrasion with the generation of many polyethylene particles less than 1 µm in length. The resultant wear damage is predominately burnishing and scratching.[28] In contrast, pitting and subsurface delamination have been commonly identified as wear damages in TKRs because the wear mechanisms involve a greater amount of abrasion and fatigue. These mechanisms result in visually striking surface damage seen on some retrieved polyethylene tibial bearings.[42,43]

STERILIZATION METHODS

Clinical and laboratory research have revealed that sterilization methods can dramatically affect the *in vivo* performance of a polyethylene component. UHMWPE components for total joint arthroplasty can be sterilized using gamma irradiation, gas plasma, or ethylene oxide (EtO). Gamma irradiation in an air environment was the industry standard since the early 1970s until about the mid-1990s, using doses between 2.5 and 4.0 megarads (Mrad), most commonly between 3.0 and 3.5 Mrad.

In addition to sterilization, gamma radiation breaks covalent bonds in the polyethylene molecule. This produces free radicals—unpaired electrons from the broken covalent bonds—that can combine with oxygen (if present) during the irradiation process, during shelf-storage, and *in vivo*. Oxidation of the polyethylene molecule is a chemical reaction that results in chain scission (fragmentation and shortening of the large polymer chains) and introduction of oxygen moieties into the polymer molecules.[4] Such oxidation lowers the molecular weight of the polymer (which reduces its toughness), increases the density through increased crystallization, and results in a reduction in fracture strength, increase in modulus, and a decrease in elongation to break.[44-47]

Peak levels of oxidation typically occur approximately 0.5 to 2.0 mm below the surface of a polyethylene component, forming the so-called white bands seen on microtomed sections of components sterilized by gamma radiation (**Fig. 12-5**).[46] As the degree of oxidation increases, so does the occurrence of fatigue cracking and delamination, as is observed in retrieved tibial components (**Fig. 12-6**).[12,47-50] Why the peak level of oxidation is subsurfaced remains a topic of debate.

Oxygen can diffuse into the components during shelf-storage and *in vivo*. Components with less than 1 year from the time of sterilization to the time of implantation exhibit lower *in vivo* oxidation and better *in vivo*

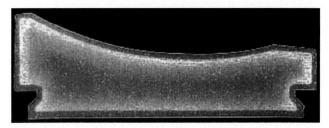

FIGURE 12-5 Microtome section of a polyethylene tibial component sterilized by gamma radiation. Peak levels of oxidation occur approximately 0.5 to 2.0 mm below the articular surface, forming the so-called white band. (Photo courtesy of Dr. John P Collier.)

performance than components with a longer so-called shelf-life before implantation.[51] A survival analysis performed on 108 TKRs sterilized by gamma irradiation in air showed that after 5 years of implantation, tibial-bearing surfaces that had shelf-lives of less than 4 years had a 100% survival rate, whereas those that had shelf-lives of 4 to 8 years and 8 to 11 years had survival rates of 88.6% and 79.2%, respectively.[52] In laboratory wear tests, polyethylene that had been gamma irradiated in air and aged exhibited a higher wear rate than nonirradiated material.[53] However, polyethylene components that have been irradiated in air and tested within months exhibit lower wear rates than identical components that have not been irradiated, owing to a favorable amount of *cross-linking* compared to the amount of oxidation.

Irradiation can produce a beneficial effect on polyethylene wear properties as a result of cross-linking. Cross-linking occurs when free radicals, located on the amorphous regions of polyethylene molecules, react to form a covalent bond between adjacent polyethylene molecules. Cross-linking can be accomplished using peroxide chemistry, variable dose ionizing radiation, or electron beam irradiation.

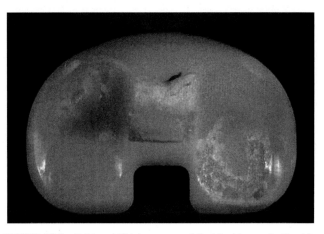

FIGURE 12-6 Retrieved tibial component that had been sterilized by gamma radiation in air with subsequent shelf-storage for 9 months. Note the gross material failure secondary to subsurface fatigue. This affects the tibiofemoral articulation.

It is believed that cross-linking of the polyethylene molecules resists intermolecular mobility, making it more resistant to deformation and wear in the plane perpendicular to the primary molecular axis. This has been demonstrated to dramatically reduce wear from crossing path motion, as it occurs in an acetabular cup.[54,55] Cross-linking has a detrimental effect on some fundamental material properties, including yield strength, ultimate tensile strength, and elongation to break.[54] The decrease in these properties is proportional to the degree of cross-linking.

Wear simulator studies indicate that with optimal cross-linking, adhesive wear rate of acetabular cups can be reduced by more than 95%.[56] Similarly, there is a marked reduction in adhesive wear rate of tibial knee inserts with increasing cross-link density.[57,58] The type of wear that occurs in total knees is different and more variable than wear in total hips. All total hip bearings are spherical and, consequently, have consistently high conformity and relatively uniform stresses in the polyethylene. In TKR, there are variable articular geometries that affect polyethylene stresses and motion patterns, both of which influence the type and amount of wear. Sources of variability include the design of the total knee prosthesis, as this affects the degree of conformity of the articulation over the range of motion. Surgical technique influences the loads and motion patterns through variability in coronal, sagittal, and axial alignment; ligament laxity and balance; and relative component position (to the other components and to the extensor mechanism). Mechanism that dominates wear in total hips is adhesive in nature and results in micron-sized particulate debris while in total knees, while there is adhesive wear, the dominant mechanism of wear is oxidation-induced delamination.

Gamma irradiation *in air* has been abandoned as a sterilization method in mid-1990s. Currently, two methods of sterilization are in use: gas sterilization (gas plasma and EtO) and gamma irradiation using inert environments (without air). Gas sterilization methods avoid the potential for high levels of oxidation, no free radicals are created, and there is no opportunity to produce cross-linking. Gamma irradiation in an oxygen-free environment still provides the benefits of cross-linking to the polyethylene but prevents oxidation and its deleterious effects during shelf-storage; however, once the components are exposed to lipids in the synovial fluid, cyclic load *in vivo* oxidation is unavoidable.[59-61]

EtO is a known sterilizing agent that acts by altering the DNA structure in bacteria, spores, and viruses. Sterilization is accomplished by diffusion of EtO into the near-surface regions.[2] The standard EtO sterilization process begins with a preconditioning period (at 46°C and 65% relative humidity) for 18 hours, followed by a 5-hour exposure to 100% EtO gas at 46°C and 0.04 MPa. An 18-hour forced air aeration period at the same temperature is required to allow diffusion of EtO out of UHMWPE.[62]

Gas plasma is a surface sterilization method in which plasma, an ionized body of gas (ie, peracetic acid, hydrogen peroxide), sterilizes surfaces by oxidizing biologic organisms.[48,63] Gas plasma sterilization is accomplished under dry, low-pressure, low-temperature conditions.[48] The sterilization cycle with gas plasma takes between 1.2 and 4.0 hours, at temperatures lower than 50°C.[2]

Components that have been sterilized by nonionizing methods, such as EtO or gas plasma, have no free radicals, thus there is no potential for oxidation either on the shelf or in the body. Ionizing radiation creates free radicals. Retrieval studies of total knee components revealed that components sterilized by EtO do not have a subsurface white band, and none of the components had delamination or cracking. In contrast, cracking (19%) and delamination (14%) were present in components sterilized by gamma irradiation in air.[46] Tibial components sterilized by gamma irradiation in air had nearly twice the average wear rate of those sterilized with EtO.[64]

Components that are irradiated in an oxygen-free environment (such as in nitrogen) and stored in an oxygen-free environment (such as in a vacuum, barrier package) have been shown to have improved oxidative stability during shelf-storage when compared to components that have been gamma-sterilized in air. Studies have shown that barrier packaging is highly successful at slowing oxidation in gamma-inert-sterilized components during shelf-storage for up to 5 years.[65,66] Due to the fact that the bearings are not already oxidized at the time of implantation, gamma-inert sterilization has been shown to improve the short-term survival of conventional polyethylene components.[67] Despite these short-term benefits, however, gamma-inert sterilization has not decreased the rate of *in vivo* oxidation or the incidence of long-term fatigue damage. Once implanted, gamma-inert-sterilized bearings have been shown to undergo an *in vivo* oxidation mechanism that mirrors its gamma-in-air-sterilized predecessor, in which residual free radicals in the polyethylene component react with the dissolved oxygen present in body fluids.[66] This oxidation reaction may also be accelerated by exposure of the polyethylene component to cyclic loading and synovial fluid lipids, which have both been shown to initiate oxidation in UHMWPE components independent of residual free radicals.[59-61] Long-term retrieval studies have found that gamma-inert-sterilized components demonstrate a trend of oxidation that exponentially increases with time and is projected to reach critical oxidation levels, above which catastrophic fatigue damage is increasingly likely to occur, after 11 to 14 years of *in vivo* service.[65-67] Therefore, gamma-inert sterilization is an improvement over gamma-in-air sterilization, but the technique has not yet solved the problem of *in vivo* oxidation.

CROSS-LINKING METHODS

Following an irradiation cross-linking step, the first generation of highly cross-linked UHMWPEs all featured a thermal processing step to stabilize the residual, radiation-induced free radicals. One approach to improving the oxidative stability of UHMWPE following irradiation is a below-melt-temperature annealing process. Annealing was theorized to help quench the free radicals that remain in HXPE following irradiation while also preserving the material's ultimate tensile strength and yield strength, which have been found to deteriorate if the material is completely remelted. The first commercially available highly cross-linked and annealed UHMWPE material was Crossfire (Stryker Orthopaedics; Mahwah, NJ), which is machined from extruded rod bar stock that has been 75-kGy gamma irradiated and annealed at 130°C. The material is then terminally gamma-sterilized with a dose of 30 kGy (resulting in a total dose of 105 kGy) and packaged in nitrogen gas.[68] Crossfire was clinically introduced for use in THA in 1998 but was never made available for TKA applications due to initial concerns raised by Wang et al,[69] who reported that patellar components fabricated from the material were reported to fracture through its support pegs during testing. These findings were also compounded by concerns about the detectable levels of free radicals that remained within the Crossfire material after annealing that could contribute to *in vivo* oxidation.[70,71] Subsequent retrieval analyses of failed Crossfire components would eventually confirm these concerns by discovering and correlating severe levels of oxidation, after less than 5 years of *in vivo* service, to observed delamination and fatigue damage within explanted acetabular components.[72,73] Crossfire acetabular liners are no longer in clinical use.

An alternative approach to quenching free radicals in first-generation highly cross-linked UHMWPEs is heating the material to a temperature above its crystalline melt point (approximately 150°C). Postirradiation remelting has been found to reduce free radical concentrations to undetectable levels, as measured by electron spin resonance, but at the cost of decreased mechanical properties due to a decrease in the material's crystallinity.[74] Although highly cross-linked and remelted UHMWPE was quickly adopted for use in THA, its use in TKA applications was initially delayed because of concerns about the material's reduced fracture toughness and resistance to fatigue crack propagation, as compared to conventional polyethylene.[75,76] Despite these concerns, early *in vitro* mechanical and wear simulator testing yielded positive results and the first commercially

available highly cross-linked and remelted UHMWPE tibial insert, Durasul (Zimmer; Warsaw, IN), became available in 2001.[57,58,77] Over the next several years, additional highly cross-linked and remelted UHMWPE tibial inserts were commercially introduced including Prolong (Zimmer; Warsaw, IN) in 2002, XLK (DePuy Synthes; Warsaw, IN) in 2005, and XLPE (Smith & Nephew; Memphis, TN) in 2008 (**Table 12-3**).

Early reports on the clinical performance of highly cross-linked and remelted tibial inserts are few and have all been generally positive. Several prospective and retrospective studies, with mean follow-up ranging from 2 to 6 years, have reported that patient-reported outcomes and radiographic evaluation of TKAs with Durasul,[78] Prolong,[79-81] and XLK[82] tibial inserts were not significantly different from TKAs with conventional, gamma-inert-sterilized tibial inserts. Currently, there are no clinical results available for the use of XLPE in TKA. Additionally, no difference has been found between the performance of highly cross-linked and remelted cruciate-retaining and posterior-stabilized tibial insert designs, and no published study has reported any instance of a highly cross-linked and remelted tibial insert having been revised due to excessive wear or catastrophic mechanical failure, such as the fracture of the tibial post in a posterior-stabilized knee, in the short- to mid-term follow-up period.[78-83] Due to the relatively short follow-up of all published clinical reports of highly cross-linked and remelted UHMWPE tibial components, additional follow-up will be needed in order to accurately assess if HXPE is not only as safe as its conventional, gamm-inert-sterilized predecessor, but also if it offers any additional clinical benefit to the patient in exchange for its increased cost.[81] Despite the lack of long-term clinical studies, registry findings, as we will discuss below, have indicated that highly cross-linked tibial inserts perform well and have a lower cumulative percent revision rate of 5.0%, compared to the 7.9% for non–cross-linked inserts, at 15 years after surgery.[84]

Echoing the early- to mid-term clinical results of highly cross-linked and remelted tibial inserts, early retrieval studies of explanted components manufactured from the same material have also had generally positive findings. Multiple retrieval studies have analyzed the surface damage and oxidation of several different first-generation highly cross-linked and remelted tibial inserts including

TABLE 12-3 Commercially Available First-Generation Highly Cross-linked Ultrahigh-Molecular-Weight Polyethylene (UHMWPE) Used in Total Knee Arthroplasty

Polyethylene Trade Name	Manufacturer	Available Since	Type of UHMWPE Resin	Irradiation Method	Irradiation Dose	Thermal Processing	Sterilization Method
Durasul	Zimmer	2001	GUR 1050	Electron beam	95 kGy	Remelted	Ethylene oxide
Prolong	Zimmer	2002	GUR1050	Electron beam	65 kGy	Remelted	Gas plasma
XLK	DePuy	2005	GUR 1020	Gamma	50 kGy	Remelted	Gas plasma
XLPE	Smith & Nephew	2008	GUR 1020	Gamma	75 kGy	Remelted	Ethylene oxide

Durasul,[85-88] Prolong,[87,89-94] XLK,[87,88,90,92-94] and HXPE[92-94] after short-term *in vivo* service. One of the first retrieval studies to study surface damage of highly cross-linked tibial inserts was conducted by Muratoglu et al and compared 8 Durasul and 71 conventional, gamma-inert-sterilized components that were mostly *in vivo* for under a year.[86] This study found that the only significant difference in damage between the two types of polyethylene inserts was in the elimination of machine marks in conventional inserts but not in the highly cross-linked inserts and suggested that highly cross-linked and remelted polyethylene has improved resistance to adhesive wear than its conventional polyethylene counterpart.[86] The findings of Muratoglu et al. are consistent with subsequent surface damage analyses of early remelted retrievals, which have all found no significant difference in either the type or severity of surface damage between highly cross-linked and remelted inserts and their conventional polyethylene counterparts. For both material types, the reported surface damage was primarily classified as burnishing, pitting, scratching, and abrasion; tabulated damage scores were comparable; and no studies reported any cracking, delamination, or signs of mechanical failure in any retrieved components.[89,91,92,94]

In addition to examining surface damage, several retrieval studies analyzed the oxidation of explanted highly cross-linked and remelted tibial inserts. These studies reported the surprising finding that remelted tibial inserts that have been *in vivo* for up to 3 to 4 years have detectable oxidation, with mean ketone peak height ratios, a measure of oxidation, ranging from 0.09 to 0.2.[85,87-91,93,94] Several studies have also reported that oxidation in remelted tibial inserts was positively correlated to the component's *in vivo* time prior to removal,[87-91] that measured oxidation was higher in loaded articular surfaces as compared to the unloaded bulk of the component,[89,93,94] and that increased oxidation was correlated with decreased cross-link density.[90,93] Furthermore, several studies reported that a portion of remelted tibial inserts, ranging from 16% to 45%, had subsurface oxidation peak at retrieval, mirroring the oxidation profiles found in conventional, gamma-inert-sterilized components.[87,88] It should be noted, however, that all reported oxidation levels of remelted tibial inserts were well below the critical oxidation threshold at which the mechanical properties of UHWMPE begin to deteriorate, a ketone peak height ratio >1.2, and that additional retrieval studies derived from components that have been *in vivo* for longer than 34 years are still needed to evaluate if the early oxidation trends observed in remelted tibial retrievals will match those of conventional gamma-inert-sterilized tibial inserts.[65]

The finding that retrieved remelted tibial inserts had measurable oxidation stood in stark contrast to the initial theory that remelted tibial inserts would undergo little to no *in vivo* oxidation given the absence of any measurable

free radicals after the remelting process[71,74] and any measured oxidative changes in remelted inserts that have been shelf-aged for 8 to 9 years.[87] These findings helped to not only spur additional research that demonstrated that synovial fluid lipids, such as squalene, and cyclic loading could both initiate the formation of new free radicals and facilitate *in vivo* oxidation,[59-61,95] but also encouraged the development of a second-generation highly cross-linked tibial inserts that would have improved oxidative stability (**Table 12-4**).

One proposed manufacturing method that could improve the oxidative stability of highly cross-linked tibial inserts was sequential annealing. By cycling a low-dose irradiation cross-linking step with a below-melt-temperature annealing process, it was theorized that low-dose irradiation steps would leave cross-links far enough apart that there would be sufficient mobility for free radicals to be more completely quenched during the annealing process.[96,97] Research suggested that this sequential cross-linking and annealing process would produce a material with an ideal balance of wear resistance (due to the high level of cross-linking), oxidative stability (due to the very low number of residual free radicals after the sequential annealing process), and mechanical properties (due to the lack of a remelting step).[96,97] The first commercially available highly cross-linked and sequentially annealed polyethylene was X3 (Stryker Orthopaedics, Mahwah, NJ), which is machined from GUR 1020 UHMWPE that has undergone three cycles of 30-kGy gamma irradiation followed by annealing at 130°C and then terminally gas plasma sterilized. X3 was approved for use in both THA and TKA applications in 2005.

Clinical studies on the *in vivo* performance of X3 tibial inserts are limited and have generally presented positive early- to mid-term results. The earliest study presenting clinical results of X3 tibial inserts was from Harwin et al,[98] who reported on the short-term follow-up of a cohort of 668 consecutive TKAs. This study reported excellent clinical and radiographic outcomes and no failures related to bearing complications. These results were supported by the findings of another study by Meneghini et al,[99] who presented the results of a prospective, single-surgeon series of 114 consecutive primary, posterior-stabilized TKAs (50 conventional, gamma-inert-sterilized and 64 X3 tibial inserts). Of the 103 knees (90%) with a mean 5-year follow-up, this study reported that patients with an X3 insert had significantly higher Knee Society Score (KSS) function scores and SF-36 physical function scores than patients who received a conventional insert and that there was no difference in the Lower Extremity Activity Scale (LEAS) between the two groups. Additionally, there was no radiographic osteolysis and no mechanical failures related to the tibial insert reported. In a separate, multicenter study that included the cohort originally reported on by Meneghini et al, similar clinical and

TABLE 12-4 Commercially Available Second-Generation Highly Cross-linked Ultrahigh-Molecular-Weight Polyethylene (UHMWPE) Used in Total Knee Arthroplasty

Polyethylene Trade Name	Manufacturer	Available Since	Type of UHMWPE Resin	Irradiation Method	Irradiation Dose	Free-Radical Stabilization Method	Sterilization Method
X3	Stryker	2005	GUR1020	Gamma	90 kGy over three steps	Annealed at 130°C after each irradiation	Gas plasma
E-Poly/E1	ZimmerBiomet	2007	GUR1020	Gamma	100 kGy	Vitamin E, diffused	Gamma
Vivacit-E	ZimmerBiomet	2013	GUR1020	Electron beam	>150 kGy	Vitamin E, blended[b]	Ethylene oxide
E+	DJO Surgical	2011	GUR 1020	Gamma	150 kGy	Vitamin E, blended	Gas plasma
E-CiMa	Corin	2010	GUR1020	Gamma	120 **kGy**	Vitamin E, blended[a]	Ethylene oxide
iPoly XE	Conformis	2017	GUR 1020	Gamma	100 kGy	Vitamin E, blended[a]	Gas plasma
Vitamys	Mathys	2009	GUR1020	Gamma	70-100 kGy	Vitamin E, blended	Gas plasma
AOX	DePuy	2012	GUR 1020	Gamma	75-80 kGy	Covernox	Gamma

[a]Material is mechanically annealed at 130°C to a compression ratio of 2.0 and subsequently annealed at 130°C to recover most of the deformation.
[b]Material is warm-irradiated at 120°C.

radiographic results were reported for a cohort of 307 primary, posterior-stabilized TKAs (168 conventional, gamma-inert-sterilized, 139 X3 tibial inserts).[100] Of the 224 TKAs (77%) that returned for a 4 to 5-year follow-up, patients with a X3 tibial insert had a higher KSS function and LEAS score than patients with a conventional tibial insert. No difference was reported between the two groups in active range of motion or in mean SF-6D scores, and no radiographic osteolysis or polyethylene insert failures were reported.

In contrast to early clinical results, retrieval studies analyzing the surface damage and oxidation of explanted sequentially annealed X3 tibial inserts are more mixed. Although some early-term retrieval studies have reported that the damage scores and primary damage modes (burnishing, pitting, and scratching) of X3 tibial inserts are not significantly different from a cohort of remelted tibial inserts,[92] other studies have reported more serious observed damage. In addition to findings of burnishing, pitting, and scratching within their respective cohort of X3 retrievals, Reinitz et al[101] reported 1 case of cracking and 7 cases of subsurface whitening, Kop et al[102] reported 4 cases of delamination and 2 cases of subsurface whitening, and MacDonald et al[103] reported 5 cases of delamination and/or subsurface whitening and 6 cases of posterior fracture. Subsurface whitening has been previously used as an indicator of oxidation in gamma-inert-sterilized components and is likely indicative of oxidation in X3 retrievals as well.[87,101] Given that many of these studies examined X3 retrievals that had been *in vivo* for an average of only 1 to 3 years, these findings are disturbing and significantly question the long-term performance of X3.

In addition to having more severe surface damage in some instances, several retrieval studies have reported that X3 also demonstrated high levels of oxidation after an average of less than 3 years *in vivo*. One early-term

retrieval study reported that a group of 27 X3 inserts had a significantly higher oxidation rate (0.16 ± 0.07/year) than a comparable group of 28 Prolong (0.07 ± 0.007/year) and 32 XLK (0.02 ± 0.02/year) components.[88] Similarly, Liu et al[93] reported that peak oxidation levels were higher for 17 retrieved X3 inserts, 0.66 (95% confidence interval (CI), 0.52-0.81), than a group of remelted tibial inserts, 0.40 (95% CI, 0.34-0.47), which consisted of 13 Prolong, 7 XLPE, and 3 XLP retrievals. These findings are in line with the findings of Reinitz et al,[101] who reported that the oxidation trend measured from a group of 74 X3 tibial inserts was significantly greater than that of historical gamma-sterilized tibial bearings and those of Kop et al,[102] who reported high levels of oxidation that ranged from 0.1 to 7.2 in a cohort of 8 retrieved X3 inserts (5 of which exhibited a ketone peak greater than 1.2, the critical oxidation threshold at which the mechanical properties of UHMWPE begin to deteriorate). In contrast to these previous studies, MacDonald et al[103] reported that the mean oxidation index measured for a group of 345 retrieved X3 inserts, 0.48 ± 0.56, was not significantly different from that of 111 matched, gamma-inert-sterilized inserts, 0.45 ± 0.67. Although the range of reported oxidation values of retrieved X3 tibial inserts may widely vary within this cohort of short-term explant studies, continued vigilance is critical as several studies reported that *in vivo* time was found to be correlated with oxidation, decreasing cross-link density, and a decrease in work to failure as measured using a small punch test.[88,90,101-103] Measured X3 *in vivo* oxidation may also be compounded by oxidation that occurred during shelf-aging because X3 not only has residual free radicals after annealing, but it is also packaged in gas-permeable packaging, which allows the component to come into contact with oxygen until it is implanted.[88] Additional retrieval analyses from components that have been *in vivo* for longer than an average of 1 to 3 years will be needed in order to determine if the concerning levels of oxidation that some studies have reported will translate into catastrophic fatigue damage within the mid- to long-term follow-up period.

An alternate method for improving the oxidative stability of highly cross-linked tibial inserts is the addition of an antioxidant into the UHMWPE. The addition of an antioxidant to highly cross-linked UHMWPE is theorized to not only quench the residual free radicals that remain after irradiation cross-linking and eliminate the need for a postirradiation remelting step but also provide active protection against oxidation that may be initiated by synovial fluid lipids or by cyclic loading during *in vivo* service.[59-61] Currently, the two most common antioxidants being added to UHMWPE for use in TJA applications are Vitamin E (α-tocopherol), normally found as a naturally occurring free radical scavenger in cell membranes, and pentaerythritol tetrakis(3-[3,5-ditertiary butyl-4-hydroxy phenyl]propionate) or PBHP, a hindered phenol antioxidant that has been trademarked by DePuy Synthes as Covernox.

In the case of Vitamin E, the two primary methods of incorporation into UHMWPE are through either postirradiation diffusion or through preconsolidation blending. In postirradiation diffusion, polyethylene resin is first consolidated into bar stock, cross-linked with an initial irradiation dose of approximately 100 kGy, and then immersed in Vitamin E at an elevated temperature below the polyethylene's melting point.[104-106] Then, to ensure that the Vitamin E is uniformly distributed across the polyethylene, the material undergoes a homogenization step where it is heated at an elevated temperature, typically around 130°C.[105-108] Following homogenization, the component is machined into its final shape and terminally gamma-sterilized with a dose of approximately 25 to 40 kGy.[105,106,108] Postirradiation diffusion has the benefit of ensuring that the presence of Vitamin E does not reduce cross-linking of UHMWPE and allows for higher concentrations of Vitamin E to be used, but it has the drawbacks of requiring a lengthy homogenization step that increases manufacturing time and having an uneven Vitamin E concentration throughout the final component.[105,106,108,109] Currently, the only commercially available highly cross-linked, Vitamin E–diffused polyethylene is E1 (ZimmerBiomet; Warsaw, IN), which was first approved for use in THA in 2007 and then for use in TKA in 2008. Although there have been multiple published reports summarizing excellent clinical and radiographic outcomes of several prospective studies of E1 acetabular liners in THA[110-118] for up to 5 years, there is only one clinical study tracking the use of E1 tibial inserts that has reported encouraging 3-year results with high patient-reported outcome measure (PROM) scores as well as low rates of complications and osteolytic potential.[119]

In preconsolidation blending, on the other hand, virgin polyethylene resin is first mixed with Vitamin E to the desired concentration and then subsequently radiation cross-linked, machined into its final form, and sterilized via gas plasma or ethylene oxide.[120-122] Preconsolidation blending has the benefit of allowing for greater control over the final Vitamin E concentration and results in a more uniform antioxidant concentration across the component, but the presence of Vitamin E also hinders the cross-linking of Vitamin E during the irradiation process.[120,123] There are currently three different manufacturing methods for producing blended Vitamin E tibial inserts. The first method involves consolidation of Vitamin E–blended UHMWPE resin, irradiation cross-linking with a total dose of approximately 100 kGy to 150 kGy at room temperature, and terminal sterilization via gas plasma or ethylene oxide. Commercially available tibial inserts produced using this first method include E+ (DJO Surgical; Vista, CA) and Vitamys (Mathys; Bettlach, Switzerland). The second method involves consolidating Vitamin E–blended UHMWPE resin, irradiation cross-linking with a dose of approximately 100 kGy, mechanical annealing by deformation at 130°C to a compression ratio of 2.0, annealing at 130°C to recover most of the deformation, and terminal sterilization via gas plasma or ethylene oxide. Mechanical annealing has been found to increase the crystallinity of the material from 60% to 66%, as opposed to decreasing it to 53% after remelting, and to decrease the concentration of free radicals by 99%.[121] Commercially available tibial inserts produced using this second method include iPoly XE (Conformis; Burlington, MA) and E-CiMa (Corin; Cirencester, United Kingdom). The third method involves consolidating Vitamin E–blended UHMWPE resin, irradiation cross-linking at an elevated temperature of 120°C, and terminal sterilization via ethylene oxide. Irradiation cross-linking of Vitamin E–blended UHMWPE has been shown to not only increase the cross-linking efficiency of the material and preserve the amount of active Vitamin E in the polymer but also provide the added benefit of increasing the amount of Vitamin E that becomes grafted onto the polyethylene.[124] Grafting has been theorized to improve the long-term stability of the implant by decreasing the extent of potential Vitamin E elution from the polyethylene during *in vivo* service. Currently, the only commercially available tibial insert produced using this third method is Vivacit-E (ZimmerBiomet; Warsaw, IN). There are several clinical studies that have described positive outcomes for highly cross-linked, Vitamin E–blended polyethylene for use in THA,[125-127] demonstrating high PROM scores and no polyethylene-related complications for up to 5 years after surgery, but none have yet been published on the outcomes of Vitamin E–blended tibial inserts.

In the case of Covernox, the antioxidant is blended with GUR 1020 to a concentration of 0.075%, consolidated, machined into tibial inserts, enclosed in vacuum barrier packaging, and terminally gamma-irradiated to achieve a final dose of 75 to 80 kGy. The only commercially available highly cross-linked tibial insert with Covernox is AOX (DePuy Synthes; Warsaw, IN). Currently, there are no published studies on the clinical outcomes of AOX tibial inserts.

Although there are very few clinical studies for highly cross-linked, antioxidant-stabilized tibial inserts, several retrieval reports have provided positive short-term results. One retrieval study analyzing 11 acetabular liners and 4 tibial inserts manufactured from Vitamin E–diffused polyethylene (E1), with *in vivo* times ranging from 2 days to 36.6 months, found that all retrieved components retained visible machining marks (indicating excellent early-term wear resistance), had little to no measurable oxidation, had material properties that were not significantly different from never-implanted controls, and had free radical signals that significantly decayed with *in vivo* duration.[128] The early oxidative stability of E1 was also confirmed in another study that examined the *ex vivo* stability of 9 Vitamin E–diffused (E1) acetabular liners and tibial inserts, 6 sequentially annealed (X3) acetabular liners and tibial inserts, 6 remelted (Longevity; ZimmerBiomet; Warsaw, IN) acetabular liners, and 6 remelted (Prolong) tibial inserts.[129] After accelerated aging (70°C with 5 atm of pure oxygen for 2 weeks), this study found that Vitamin E–diffused components had substantially lower oxidation levels before and after accelerated aging when compared to its highly cross-linked and remelted or sequentially annealed counterparts, confirming the antioxidant potential of Vitamin E.[129] Lastly, two early retrieval studies that compared a cohort of retrieved, antioxidant-stabilized tibial inserts (E1, Vitacit-E, and AOX), to either a cohort of conventional, gamma-inert-sterilized and remelted (HXL) tibial inserts or a cohort of only remelted tibial inserts (XLK, Prolong, and XLPE), found no difference in oxidation, cross-link density, or types and severity of damage to the articular surface between the groups.[94,130] Given these early retrieval studies, highly cross-linked, antioxidant-stabilized tibial inserts appear to be as wear resistant and oxidatively stable as their earlier predecessors. Longer-term retrieval clinical studies and retrieval analyses are still needed to confirm if the addition of antioxidants will improve long-term survival and decrease the incidence of catastrophic polyethylene failure secondary to severe oxidation.

In addition to clinical and retrieval studies, national registry reports can also provide important information on the overall performance of new, polyethylene technologies across a wide array of surgeons, practice settings, and patient populations. One national orthopedic registry that currently provides summary implant data is the Australian Orthopaedic Association National Joint Replacement Registry (AOANJRR). According to the 2018 Annual Report, the AOANJRR contained data for a total of 588,012 primary TKA cases.[84] Beginning in 2014, XLPE tibial inserts (irradiated with a dosage ≥50-kGy) are now more frequently used in TKA than their non–cross-linked counterparts, and, as of 2017, 61.0% of TKAs performed in Australia used highly cross-linked tibial inserts.

Furthermore, the 2018 Annual Report has found that TKAs performed with highly cross-linked polyethylene had a significantly lower cumulative percent revision rate of 5.0% at 15 years as compared to the 7.9% for non–cross-linked components. Adjusting for age and gender, the hazard ratio (HR) for revision for non–cross-linked versus highly cross-linked inserts in TKA was reported to be 1.73 (1.60-1.88) for any time greater than 3.5 years after surgery and was found to achieve statistical significance ($P < .001$). The main reason cited for this difference is the lower cumulative incidence for loosening in highly cross-linked cases, 0.8% at 15 years, compared to that of non–cross-linked cases, 2.0% at 15 years. The difference in revision rates between highly cross-linked and non–cross-linked TKA cases can especially be seen in patients younger than 65 years, who have a cumulative percent revision rate of 7.2% for highly cross-linked and 12.1% for non–cross-linked inserts at 15 years. In patients above the age of 65, the cumulative percent revision rate was 3.5% for highly cross-linked and 5.6% for non–cross-linked inserts at 15 years. When analyzed on an implant system level, those with a statistically significant HR for highly cross-linked versus non–highly cross-linked tibial inserts include Nexgen CR/Nexgen (Prolong), HR = 0.54 (0.38- 0.76) for greater than 4 years; Natural Knee II/Natural Knee II (Durasul), HR = 0.13 (0.08- 0.21) for greater than 5.5 years; Legion Oxinium PS/Genesis II (HXPE), HR = 0.68 (0.54- 0.85) for the entire period; and Triathlon PS/Triathlon (X3), HR = 0.78 (0.63- 0.96) for the entire period.

In the case of antioxidant-stabilized inserts, the AOANJRR only contains a total number of 16,828 prostheses with this bearing a short follow-up of 5 years. However, with the early data that have been collected, the 2018 Annual Report has found that there is no difference between the revision rates of highly cross-linked, 2.8% (2.7-2.9), and antioxidant-stabilized inserts, 2.7 (2.1-3.5) at 5 years. Adjusting for age and gender, the calculated HR for revision for antioxidant-stabilized versus highly cross-linked inserts was reported to be 0.89 (0.77-1.04) for the entire period and was found to not achieve statistical significance ($P = .133$).

Lastly, in a registry study using data collected as part of the Kaiser Permanente Total Joint Replacement Registry, a regional registry system, Paxton et al[131] analyzed a cohort of 77,084 TKAs performed between April 2001 and December 2011 in order to examine if highly cross-linked tibial inserts had a lower revision rate than conventional polyethylene inserts for patients with a cobalt-chrome femoral component. Within this cohort of patients, the cumulative incidence of revision was found to be 2.7% for conventional inserts and 3.1% for highly cross-linked inserts at 5-year follow-up. The adjusted risks of all-cause, aseptic, and septic revision were also found to not differ between the two material types. Additional analyses studying the risk of revision between XLK (DePuy) versus conventional polyethylene and for Prolong (Zimmer) versus conventional polyethylene also found no difference between the two material types in cumulative incidence of revision or in the risk of all-cause, aseptic, and septic revision.

CONCLUSION

Today, highly cross-linked UHMWPEs are the standard of care in total hip patients with 100% conversion from conventional polyethylene of a decade ago.[132] In total knees, over 70% of the components are highly cross-linked and the remaining are conventional UHMWPEs that are gamma-sterilized in an inert environment.[132] Despite previous concerns about the safety of highly cross-linked polyethylene in TKA applications, there is now definitive evidence from national registries like the AOANJRR that has demonstrated that the material is not only safe but also an improvement over conventional polyethylene. As described in the 2018 Annual Report of the AOANJRR, TKAs performed with highly cross-linked polyethylene had a significantly lower cumulative percent revision rate (5.0%) than its non–cross-linked counterparty (7.9%) at 15 years after surgery primarily due to a reduced cumulative incidence of loosening (0.8% for highly cross-linked versus 2.0% for non–cross-linked polyethylene at 15 years).[84] In the case of antioxidant-stabilized tibial inserts, early results are similarly promising and have shown no difference between the cumulative revision rates of highly cross-linked (2.8%) and antioxidant-stabilized (2.7%) inserts at 5 years.[84]

In conclusion, UHMWPE has shown satisfactory performance as a primary bearing surface in total knee arthroplasty. In the absence of material degradation secondary to oxidation, UHMWPE has demonstrated excellent wear resistance and clinical survivorship even in low-conformity designs. New polyethylene technologies including highly cross-linked and antioxidant-stabilized tibial inserts have demonstrated promising early- to mid-term results, but additional long-term follow-up is still needed in order to confirm the improved wear resistance and oxidative stability of these new bearing materials.

ACKNOWLEDGMENTS

The authors would like to acknowledge Mauricio Silva, MD, Thomas P. Schmalzried, MD, and Harvey S. Stein, PE, for their significant contributions to the original version of this chapter, which appeared in the previous edition of this textbook.

REFERENCES

1. Plastics and Polyolefins. In: *Petrothene Polyolefins: A Processing Guide*. 3rd ed. New York: National Distillers and Chemical Corporation; 1965:612.
2. Kurtz SM, Muratoglu OK, Evans M, Edidin AA. Advances in the processing, sterilization, and crosslinking of ultra-high molecular weight polyethylene for total joint arthroplasty. *Biomaterials*. 1999;20:1659-1688.
3. Ayers DC. Polyethylene wear and osteolysis following total knee replacement. *Instr Course Lect*. 1997;46:205-213.
4. Li S, Burstein AH. Ultra-high molecular weight polyethylene. The material and its use in total joint implants. *J Bone Joint Surg Am*. 1994;76:1080-1090.
5. Willie BM, Gingell DT, Bloebaum RD, Hofmann AA. Possible explanation for the white band artifact seen in clinically retrieved polyethylene tibial components. *J Biomed Mater Res*. 2000;52:558-566.
6. Tanner MG, Whiteside LA, White SE. Effect of polyethylene quality on wear in total knee arthroplasty. *Clin Orthop Relat Res*. 1995;317:83-88.
7. Sutula L, Collier JP, Wrona M. The role of polyethylene quality on wear. In: Callaghan JJ, Dennis D, Paprosky W, eds. *Orthopaedic Knowledge Update: Hip and Knee Reconstruction*. Rosemont: American Academy of Orthopaedic Surgeons; 1995:35-41.
8. Schmalzried TP, Callaghan JJ. Wear in total hip and knee replacements. *J Bone Joint Surg Am*. 1999;81:115-136.
9. Colizza WA, Insall JN, Scuderi GR. The posterior stabilized total knee prosthesis. Assessment of polyethylene damage and osteolysis after a ten-year-minimum follow-up. *J Bone Joint Surg Am*. 1995;77:1713-1720.
10. Huk OL, Bansal M, Betts F, et al. Polyethylene and metal debris generated by non-articulating surfaces of modular acetabular components. *J Bone Joint Surg Br*. 1994;76:568-574.
11. Kuster MS, Horz S, Spalinger E, Stachowiak GW, Gächter A. The effects of conformity and load in total knee replacement. *Clin Orthop Relat Res*. 2000;375:302-312.
12. Collier JP, Mayor MB, McNamara JL, Surprenant VA, Jensen RE. Analysis of the failure of 122 polyethylene inserts from uncemented tibial knee components. *Clin Orthop Relat Res*. 1991;273:232-242.
13. Goodfellow J, O'Connor J. The mechanics of the knee and prosthesis design. *J Bone Joint Surg Br*. 1978;60-B:358-369.
14. Goodfellow J. Knee prostheses—one step forward, two steps back. *J Bone Joint Surg Br*. 1992;74:1-2.
15. Heim C, Postak P, Greenwald A. Factors influencing the longevity of UHMWPE tibial components. In: Pritchard D, ed. *Instr. Course Lect.*, Rosemont, IL: American Academy of Orthopaedic Surgeons; 1996:303-312.
16. Bartel DL, Rawlinson JJ, Burstein AH, Ranawat CS, Flynn WF. Stresses in polyethylene components of contemporary total knee replacements. *Clin Orthop Relat Res*. 1995;317:76-82.
17. Barbour PSM, Barton DC, Fisher J. The influence of contact stress on the wear of UHMWPE for total replacement hip prostheses. *Wear*. 1995;181-183:250-257. doi:10.1016/0043-1648(95)90031-4.
18. Bartel DL, Bicknell VL, Wright TM. The effect of conformity, thickness, and material on stresses in ultra-high molecular weight components for total joint replacement. *J Bone Joint Surg Am*. 1986;68:1041-1051.
19. Lewis JL, Askew MJ, Jaycox DP. A comparative evaluation of tibial component designs of total knee prostheses. *J Bone Joint Surg Am*. 1982;64:129-135.
20. Parks NL, Engh GA, Topoleski LD, Emperado J. The Coventry Award. Modular tibial insert micromotion. A concern with contemporary knee implants. *Clin Orthop Relat Res*. 1998;356:10-15.
21. Ezzet KA, Garcia R, Barrack RL. Effect of component fixation method on osteolysis in total knee arthroplasty. *Clin Orthop Relat Res*. 1995;321:86-91.

22. Wasielewski RC, Parks N, Williams I, Surprenant H, Collier JP, Engh G. Tibial insert undersurface as a contributing source of polyethylene wear debris. *Clin Orthop Relat Res.* 1997;345:53-59.

23. McKellop H, Clarke I, Markolf K, Amstutz H. Friction and wear properties of polymer, metal, and ceramic prosthetic joint materials evaluated on a multichannel screening device. *J Biomed Mater Res.* 1981;15:619-653. doi:10.1002/jbm.820150503.

24. Dennis DA, Komistek RD, Colwell CE, et al. In vivo anteroposterior femorotibial translation of total knee arthroplasty: a multicenter analysis. *Clin Orthop Relat Res.* 1998;356:47-57.

25. Stiehl JB, Komistek RD, Dennis DA. Detrimental kinematics of a flat on flat total condylar knee arthroplasty. *Clin Orthop Relat Res.* 1999;365:139-148.

26. Wasielewski RC, Galante JO, Leighty RM, Natarajan RN, Rosenberg AG. Wear patterns on retrieved polyethylene tibial inserts and their relationship to technical considerations during total knee arthroplasty. *Clin Orthop Relat Res.* 1994;299:31-43.

27. Blunn GW, Walker PS, Joshi A, Hardinge K. The dominance of cyclic sliding in producing wear in total knee replacements. *Clin Orthop Relat Res.* 1991;273:253-260.

28. McKellop HA, Campbell P, Park SH, et al. The origin of submicron polyethylene wear debris in total hip arthroplasty. *Clin Orthop Relat Res.* 1995;311:3-20.

29. Campbell P, Ma S, Yeom B, McKellop H, Schmalzried TP, Amstutz HC. Isolation of predominantly submicron-sized UHMWPE wear particles from periprosthetic tissues. *J Biomed Mater Res.* 1995;29:127-131. doi:10.1002/jbm.820290118.

30. Hirakawa K, Bauer TW, Stulberg BN, Wilde AH. Comparison and quantitation of wear debris of failed total hip and total knee arthroplasty. *J Biomed Mater Res.* 1996;31:257-263. doi:10.1002/(SICI)1097-4636(199606)31:2<257::AID-JBM13>3.0.CO;2-I.

31. Maloney WJ, Smith RL, Schmalzried TP, Chiba J, Huene D, Rubash H. Isolation and characterization of wear particles generated in patients who have had failure of a hip arthroplasty without cement. *J Bone Joint Surg Am.* 1995;77:1301-1310.

32. Margevicius KJ, Bauer TW, McMahon JT, Brown SA, Merritt K. Isolation and characterization of debris in membranes around total joint prostheses. *J Bone Joint Surg Am.* 1994;76:1664-1675.

33. Schmalzried TP, Jasty M, Harris WH. Periprosthetic bone loss in total hip arthroplasty. Polyethylene wear debris and the concept of the effective joint space. *J Bone Joint Surg Am.* 1992;74:849-863.

34. Shanbhag AS, Jacobs JJ, Glant TT, Gilbert JL, Black J, Galante JO. Composition and morphology of wear debris in failed uncemented total hip replacement. *J Bone Joint Surg Br.* 1994;76:60-67.

35. Hirakawa K, Bauer TW, Stulberg BN, Wilde AH, Borden LS. Characterization of debris adjacent to failed knee implants of 3 different designs. *Clin Orthop Relat Res.* 1996;331:151-158.

36. Tipper JL, Ingham E, Hailey JL, et al. Quantitative analysis of polyethylene wear debris, wear rate and head damage in retrieved Charnley hip prostheses. *J Mater Sci Mater Med.* 2000;11:117-124.

37. Schmalzried TP, Jasty M, Rosenberg A, Harris WH. Polyethylene wear debris and tissue reactions in knee as compared to hip replacement prostheses. *J Appl Biomater.* 1994;5:185-190. doi:10.1002/jab.770050302.

38. Schmalzried TP, Campbell P. Isolation and characterization of debris in membranes around total joint prostheses. *J Bone Joint Surg Am.* 1995;77:1625-1626.

39. Schmalzried TP, Campbell P, Schmitt AK, Brown IC, Amstutz HC. Shapes and dimensional characteristics of polyethylene wear particles generated in vivo by total knee replacements compared to total hip replacements. *J Biomed Mater Res.* 1997;38:203-210.

40. Shanbhag AS, Bailey HO, Hwang DS, Cha CW, Eror NG, Rubash HE. Quantitative analysis of ultrahigh molecular weight polyethylene (UHMWPE) wear debris associated with total knee replacements. *J Biomed Mater Res.* 2000;53:100-110.

41. Hood RW, Wright TM, Burstein AH. Retrieval analysis of total knee prostheses: a method and its application to 48 total condylar prostheses. *J Biomed Mater Res.* 1983;17:829-842. doi:10.1002/jbm.820170510.

42. Landy MM, Walker PS. Wear of ultra-high-molecular-weight polyethylene components of 90 retrieved knee prostheses. *J Arthroplasty.* 1988;3 suppl:S73-S85.

43. Wright TM, Bartel DL. The problem of surface damage in polyethylene total knee components. *Clin Orthop Relat Res.* 1986;205:67-74.

44. McKellop HA, Shen FW, Campbell P, Ota T. Effect of molecular weight, calcium stearate, and sterilization methods on the wear of ultra high molecular weight polyethylene acetabular cups in a hip joint simulator. *J Orthop Res.* 1999;17:329-339. doi:10.1002/jor.1100170306.

45. Rose RM, Crugnola A, Ries M, Cimino WR, Paul I, Radin EL. On the origins of high in vivo wear rates in polyethylene components of total joint prostheses. *Clin Orthop Relat Res.* 1979;145:277-286.

46. Sutula LC, Collier JP, Saum KA, et al. The Otto Aufranc Award. Impact of gamma sterilization on clinical performance of polyethylene in the hip. *Clin Orthop Relat Res.* 1995;319:28-40.

47. Collier JP, Sperling DK, Currier JH, Sutula LC, Saum KA, Mayor MB. Impact of gamma sterilization on clinical performance of polyethylene in the knee. *J Arthroplasty.* 1996;11:377-389.

48. Collier JP, Sutula LC, Currier BH, et al. Overview of polyethylene as a bearing material: comparison of sterilization methods. *Clin Orthop Relat Res.* 1996;333:76-86.

49. Bell CJ, Walker PS, Abeysundera MR, Simmons JM, King PM, Blunn GW. Effect of oxidation on delamination of ultrahigh-molecular-weight polyethylene tibial components. *J Arthroplasty.* 1998;13:280-290.

50. Williams IR, Mayor MB, Collier JP. The impact of sterilization method on wear in knee arthroplasty. *Clin Orthop Relat Res.* 1998;356:170-180.

51. Currier BH, Currier JH, Collier JP, Mayor MB, Scott RD. Shelf life and in vivo duration. Impacts on performance of tibial bearings. *Clin Orthop Relat Res.* 1997;342:111-122.

52. Bohl JR, Bohl WR, Postak PD, Greenwald AS. The Coventry Award. The effects of shelf life on clinical outcome for gamma sterilized polyethylene tibial components. *Clin Orthop Relat Res.* 1999;367:28-38.

53. Fisher J, Chan KL, Hailey JL, Shaw D, Stone M. Preliminary study of the effect of aging following irradiation on the wear of ultrahigh-molecular-weight polyethylene. *J Arthroplasty.* 1995;10:689-692.

54. McKellop H, Shen FW, Lu B, Campbell P, Salovey R. Development of an extremely wear-resistant ultra high molecular weight polyethylene for total hip replacements. *J Orthop Res.* 1999;17:157-167. doi:10.1002/jor.1100170203.

55. Baker DA, Hastings RS, Pruitt L. Study of fatigue resistance of chemical and radiation crosslinked medical grade ultrahigh molecular weight polyethylene. *J Biomed Mater Res.* 1999;46:573-581.

56. Muratoglu OK, Bragdon CR, O'Connor D, et al. Larger diameter femoral heads used in conjunction with a highly cross-linked ultra-high molecular weight polyethylene: a new concept. *J Arthroplasty.* 2001;16:24-30. doi:10.1054/arth.2001.28376.

57. Muratoglu OK, Bragdon CR, O'Connor DO, Perinchief RS, Jasty M, Harris WH. Aggressive wear testing of a cross-linked polyethylene in total knee arthroplasty. *Clin Orthop Relat Res.* 2002;404:89-95.

58. Muratoglu OK, Bragdon CR, Jasty M, O'Connor DO, Von Knoch RS, Harris WH. Knee-simulator testing of conventional and cross-linked polyethylene tibial inserts. *J Arthroplasty.* 2004;19:887-897. doi:10.1016/j.arth.2004.03.019.

59. Muratoglu OK, Wannomae KK, Rowell SL, Micheli BR, Malchau H. Ex vivo stability loss of irradiated and melted ultra-high molecular weight polyethylene. *J Bone Joint Surg Am.* 2010;92:2809-2816. doi:10.2106/JBJS.I.01017.

60. Oral E, Ghali BW, Neils A, Muratoglu OK. A new mechanism of oxidation in ultrahigh molecular weight polyethylene caused by squalene absorption. *J Biomed Mater Res B Appl Biomater.* 2012;100:742-751. doi:10.1002/jbm.b.32507.

61. Medel F, Kurtz S, MacDonald D, Pascual FJ, Puértolas JA. Does cyclic stress play a role in highly crosslinked polyethylene oxidation? *Clin Orthop Relat Res.* 2015;473:1022-1029. doi:10.1007/s11999-015-4153-9.

62. Ries MD, Weaver K, Beals N. Safety and efficacy of ethylene oxide sterilized polyethylene in total knee arthroplasty. *Clin Orthop Relat Res.* 1996;331:159-163.

63. Bruck SD, Mueller EP. Radiation sterilization of polymeric implant materials. *J Biomed Mater Res.* 1988;22:133-144. doi:10.1002/jbm.820221306.

64. White SE, Paxson RD, Tanner MG, Whiteside LA. Effects of sterilization on wear in total knee arthroplasty. *Clin Orthop Relat Res.* 1996;331:164-171.

65. Berry DJ, Currier BH, Mayor MB, Collier JP. Gamma-irradiation sterilization in an inert environment a partial solution. *Clin Orthop Relat Res.* 2012;470:1805-1813. doi:10.1007/s11999-011-2150-1.

66. Currier BH, Currier JH, Mayor MB, Lyford KA, Van Citters DW, Collier JP. In vivo oxidation of gamma-barrier-sterilized ultra-high-molecular-weight polyethylene bearings. *J Arthroplasty.* 2007;22:721-731. doi:10.1016/j.arth.2006.07.006.

67. Medel FJ, Kurtz SM, Hozack WJ, et al. Gamma inert sterilization: a solution to polyethylene oxidation? *J Bone Joint Surg.* 2009;91:839-849. doi:10.2106/JBJS.H.00538.

68. Kurtz SM, Manley M, Wang A, Taylor S, Dumbleton J. Comparison of the properties of annealed crosslinked (Crossfire) and conventional polyethylene as hip bearing materials. *Bull Hosp Joint Dis.* 2006;61:17-26.

69. Wang A, Manley M, Serekian P. Wear and structural fatigue simulation of crosslinked ultra-high molecular weight polyethylene for hip and knee bearing applications. *J ASTM Int (JAI).* 2004;1:11593. doi:10.1520/JAI11593.

70. Ries MD, Pruitt L. Effect of cross-linking on the microstructure and mechanical properties of ultra-high molecular weight polyethylene. *Clin Orthop Relat Res.* 2005;440:149-156.

71. Collier JP, Currier BH, Kennedy FE, et al. Comparison of crosslinked polyethylene materials for orthopaedic applications. *Clin Orthop Relat Res.* 2003;414:289-304. doi:10.1097/01.blo.0000073343.50837.03.

72. Wannomae KK, Bhattacharyya S, Freiberg A, Estok D, Harris WH, Muratoglu O. In vivo oxidation of retrieved cross-linked ultra-high-molecular-weight polyethylene acetabular components with residual free radicals. *J Arthroplasty.* 2006;21:1005-1011. doi:10.1016/j.arth.2005.07.019.

73. Currier BH, Currier JH, Mayor MB, Lyford KA, Collier JP, Van Citters DW. Evaluation of oxidation and fatigue damage of retrieved crossfire polyethylene acetabular cups. *J Bone Joint Surg Am.* 2007;89:2023-2029. doi:10.2106/JBJS.F.00336.

74. Muratoglu OK, Bragdon CR, O'Connor DO, Jasty M, Harris WH. A novel method of cross-linking ultra-high-molecular-weight polyethylene to improve wear, reduce oxidation, and retain mechanical properties. Recipient of the 1999 HAP Paul Award. *J Arthroplasty.* 2001;16:149-160. doi:10.1054/arth.2001.20540.

75. Ries MD. Highly cross-linked polyethylene: the debate is over—in opposition. *J Arthroplasty.* 2005;20:59-62.

76. Wright TM. Polyethylene in knee arthroplasty: what is the future? *Clin Orthop Relat Res.* 2005;440:141-148.

77. Jasty M, Rubash HE, Muratoglu O. Highly cross-linked polyethylene: the debate is over—in the affirmative. *J Arthroplasty.* 2005;20:55-58.

78. Hodrick JT, Severson EP, McAlister DS, Dahl B, Hofmann AA. Highly crosslinked polyethylene is safe for use in total knee arthroplasty. *Clin Orthop Relat Res.* 2008;466:2806-2812. doi:10.1007/s11999-008-0472-4.

79. Minoda Y, Aihara M, Sakawa A, et al. Comparison between highly cross-linked and conventional polyethylene in total knee arthroplasty. *Knee.* 2009;16:348-351. doi:10.1016/j.knee.2009.01.005.

80. Kim YH, Park JW. Comparison of highly cross-linked and conventional polyethylene in posterior cruciate-substituting total knee arthroplasty in the same patients. *J Bone Joint Surg Am Vol.* 2014;96:1807-1813. doi:10.2106/JBJS.M.01605.

81. Lachiewicz PF, Soileau ES. Is there a benefit to highly crosslinked polyethylene in posterior-stabilized total knee arthroplasty? A randomized trial. *Clin Orthop Relat Res.* 2016;474:88-95. doi:10.1007/s11999-015-4241-x.

82. Kindsfater KA, Pomeroy D, Clark CR, Gruen TA, Murphy J, Himden S. In vivo performance of moderately crosslinked, thermally treated polyethylene in a prospective randomized controlled primary total knee arthroplasty trial. *J Arthroplasty.* 2015;30:1333-1338. doi:10.1016/j.arth.2015.02.041.

83. Long WJ, Levi GS, Scuderi GR. Highly cross-linked polyethylene in posterior stabilized total knee arthroplasty: early results. *Orthop Clin North Am.* 2012;43:e35-e38. doi:10.1016/j.ocl.2012.07.005.

84. AOANJRR. *Hip, Knee & Shoulder Arthroplasty – Annual Report 2018*; 2018.

85. Willie BM, Foot LJ, Prall MW, Bloebaum RD. Examining the influence of short-term implantation on oxidative degradation in retrieved highly crosslinked polyethylene tibial components. *J Biomed Mater Res.* 2008;85:385-397. doi:10.1002/jbm.b.30957.

86. Muratoglu OK, Ruberti J, Melotti S, Spiegelberg SH, Greenbaum ES, Harris WH. Optical analysis of surface changes on early retrievals of highly cross-linked and conventional polyethylene tibial inserts. *J Arthroplasty.* 2003;18:42-47.

87. Currier BH, Van Citters DW, Currier JH, Collier JP. In vivo oxidation in remelted highly cross-linked retrievals. *J Bone Joint Surg.* 2010;92:2409-2418. doi:10.2106/JBJS.I.01006.

88. Currier BH, Van Citters DW, Currier JH, Carlson EM, Tibbo ME, Collier JP. In vivo oxidation in retrieved highly crosslinked tibial inserts. *J Biomed Mater Res.* 2013;101B:441-448. doi:10.1002/jbm.b.32805.

89. MacDonald DW, Higgs G, Parvizi J, et al. Oxidative properties and surface damage mechanisms of remelted highly crosslinked polyethylenes in total knee arthroplasty. *Int Orthop.* 2013;37:611-615. doi:10.1007/s00264-013-1796-6.

90. Reinitz SD, Currier BH, Levine RA, Van Citters DW. Crosslink density, oxidation and chain scission in retrieved, highly crosslinked UHMWPE tibial bearings. *Biomaterials.* 2014;35:4436-4440. doi:10.1016/j.biomaterials.2014.02.019.

91. Currier BH, Currier JH, Franklin KJ, Mayor MB, Reinitz SD, Van Citters DW. Comparison of wear and oxidation in retrieved conventional and highly cross-linked UHMWPE tibial inserts. *J Arthroplasty.* 2015;30:2349-2353. doi:10.1016/j.arth.2015.06.014.

92. Liu T, Esposito C, Elpers M, Wright T. Surface damage is not reduced with highly crosslinked polyethylene tibial inserts at short-term. *Clin Orthop Relat Res.* 2016;474:107-116. doi:10.1007/s11999-015-4344-4.

93. Liu T, Esposito CI, Burket JC, Wright TM. Crosslink density is reduced and oxidation is increased in retrieved highly crosslinked polyethylene TKA tibial inserts. *Clin Orthop Relat Res.* 2017;475:128-136. doi:10.1007/s11999-016-4820-5.

94. Ponzio DY, Weitzler L, DeMeireles A, Esposito CI, Wright TM, Padgett DE. Antioxidant-stabilized highly crosslinked polyethylene in total knee arthroplasty: a retrieval analysis. *Bone Joint J.* 2018;100B:1330-1335. doi:10.1302/0301-620X.100B10.BJJ-2018-0061.R2.

95. Oral E, Fung M, Rowell SL, Muratoglu OK. In-vitro oxidation model for UHMWPE incorporating synovial fluid lipids. *J Orthop Res.* 2018;36(7):1833-1839. doi:10.1002/jor.23848.

96. Wang A, Yau SS, Essner A, Herrera L, Manley M, Dumbleton J. A highly crosslinked UHMWPE for CR and PS total knee arthroplasties. *J Arthroplasty.* 2008;23:559-566. doi:10.1016/j.arth.2007.05.007.

97. Kester MA, Herrera L, Wang A, Essner A. Knee bearing technology. Where is technology taking us? *J Arthroplasty.* 2007;22:16-20. doi:10.1016/j.arth.2007.05.012.

98. Harwin SF, Greene KA, Hitt K. Early experience with a new total knee implant: maximizing range of motion and function with gender-specific sizing. *Surg Technol Int.* 2007;16:199-205.

99. Meneghini RM, Lovro LR, Smits SA, Ireland PH. Highly cross-linked versus conventional polyethylene in posterior-stabilized total knee arthroplasty at a mean 5-year follow-up. *J Arthroplasty*. 2015;30:1736-1739. doi:10.1016/j.arth.2015.05.009.

100. Meneghini RM, Ireland PH, Bhowmik-Stoker M. Multicenter study of highly cross-linked vs conventional polyethylene in total knee arthroplasty. *J Arthroplasty*. 2016;31:809-814. doi:10.1016/j.arth.2015.10.034.

101. Reinitz SD, Currier BH, Van Citters DW, Levine RA, Collier JP. Oxidation and other property changes of retrieved sequentially annealed UHMWPE acetabular and tibial bearings. *J Biomed Mater Res*. 2015;103:578-586. doi:10.1002/jbm.b.33240.

102. Kop AM, Pabbruwe MB, Keogh C, Swarts E. Oxidation of second generation sequentially irradiated and annealed highly cross-linked X3™ polyethylene tibial bearings. *J Arthroplasty*. 2015;30:1842-1846. doi:10.1016/j.arth.2015.04.027.

103. MacDonald DW, Higgs GB, Chen AF, Malkani AL, Mont MA, Kurtz SM. Oxidation, damage mechanisms, and reasons for revision of sequentially annealed highly crosslinked polyethylene in total knee arthroplasty. *J Arthroplasty*. 2018;33:1235-1241. doi:10.1016/j.arth.2017.09.036.

104. Oral E, Wannomae KK, Hawkins N, Harris WH, Muratoglu OK. α-Tocopherol-doped irradiated UHMWPE for high fatigue resistance and low wear. *Biomaterials*. 2004;25:5515-5522. doi:10.1016/j.biomaterials.2003.12.048.

105. Oral E, Christensen SD, Malhi AS, Wannomae KK, Muratoglu OK. Wear resistance and mechanical properties of highly cross-linked, ultrahigh–molecular weight polyethylene doped with vitamin E. *J Arthroplasty*. 2006;21:580-591. doi:10.1016/j.arth.2005.07.009.

106. Haider H, Weisenburger JN, Kurtz SM, et al. Does vitamin E-stabilized ultrahigh-molecular-weight polyethylene address concerns of cross-linked polyethylene in total knee arthroplasty? *J Arthroplasty*. 2012;27:461-469. doi:10.1016/j.arth.2011.03.024.

107. Oral E, Wannomae KK, Rowell SL, Muratoglu OK. Diffusion of vitamin E in ultra-high molecular weight polyethylene. *Biomaterials*. 2007;28:5225-5237. doi:10.1016/j.biomaterials.2007.08.025.

108. Oral E, Malhi AS, Wannomae KK, Muratoglu OK. Highly cross-linked ultrahigh molecular weight polyethylene with improved fatigue resistance for total joint arthroplasty. Recipient of the 2006 hap Paul award. *J Arthroplasty*. 2008;23:1037-1044. doi:10.1016/j.arth.2007.09.027.

109. Rowell SL, Oral E, Muratoglu OK. Comparative oxidative stability of α-tocopherol blended and diffused UHMWPEs at 3 years of real-time aging. *J Orthop Res*. 2011;29:773-780. doi:10.1002/jor.21288.

110. Shareghi B, Johanson P-E, Kärrholm J. Femoral head penetration of vitamin E-infused highly cross-linked polyethylene liners. *J Bone Joint Surg Am Vol*. 2015;97:1366-1371. doi:10.2106/JBJS.N.00595.

111. Shareghi B, Johanson PE, Kärrholm J. Wear of vitamin E-infused highly cross-linked polyethylene at five years. *J Bone Joint Surg Am Vol*. 2017;99:1447-1452. doi:10.2106/JBJS.16.00691.

112. Sillesen NH, Greene ME, Nebergall AK, et al. Three year RSA evaluation of vitamin E diffused highly cross-linked polyethylene liners and cup stability. *J Arthroplasty*. 2015;30:1260-1264. doi:10.1016/j.arth.2015.02.018.

113. Nebergall AK, Greene ME, Laursen MB, Nielsen PT, Malchau H, Troelsen A. Vitamin E diffused highly cross-linked polyethylene in total hip arthroplasty at five years. *Bone Joint J*. 2017;99-B:577-584. doi:10.1302/0301-620X.99B5.37521.

114. Nebergall AK, Troelsen A, Rubash HE, Malchau H, Rolfson O, Greene ME. Five-year experience of vitamin E-diffused highly cross-linked polyethylene wear in total hip arthroplasty assessed by radiostereometric analysis. *J Arthroplasty*. 2016;31:1251-1255. doi:10.1016/j.arth.2015.12.023.

115. Salemyr M, Muren O, Ahl T, et al. Vitamin-E diffused highly cross-linked polyethylene liner compared to standard liners in total hip arthroplasty. A randomized, controlled trial. *Int Orthop*. 2015;39:1499-1505. doi:10.1007/s00264-015-2680-3.

116. Lindalen E, Nordsletten L, Høvik Ø, Röhrl SM. E-vitamin infused highly cross-linked polyethylene: RSA results from a randomised controlled trial using 32 mm and 36 mm ceramic heads. *Hip Int*. 2015;25:50-55. doi:10.5301/hipint.5000195.

117. Galea VP, Connelly JW, Shareghi B, et al. Evaluation of in vivo wear of vitamin E-diffused highly crosslinked polyethylene at five years. *Bone Joint J*. 2018;100–B:1592-1599. doi:10.1302/0301-620X.100B12.BJJ-2018-0371.R1.

118. Sillesen NH, Greene ME, Nebergall AK, et al. 3-year follow-up of a long-term registry-based multicentre study on vitamin E diffused polyethylene in total hip replacement. *HIP Int*. 2016;26:97-103. doi:10.5301/hipint.5000297.

119. Nielsen CS, Connelly J, Galea V, Huddleston J, Malchau H, Troelsen A. Safe performance of E-vitamin infused polyethylene in TKA at 3-year follow-up evaluated in a prospective, multicenter study. *European Federation of National Associations of Orthopaedics and Traumatology*. Barcelona, Spain 2018. Available at https://www.efort.org/barcelona2018/scientific-content/advanced-scientific-programme/details/?id={E786F68E-140-40C0-8D8C-8FB5B8CBBE8B}.

120. Oral E, Greenbaum ES, Malhi AS, Harris WH, Muratoglu OK. Characterization of irradiated blends of α-tocopherol and UHMWPE. *Biomaterials*. 2005;26:6657-6663. doi:10.1016/j.biomaterials.2005.04.026.

121. Oral E, Neils AL, Wannomae KK, Muratoglu OK. Novel active stabilization technology in highly crosslinked UHMWPEs for superior stability. *Radiat Phys Chem*. 2014;105:6-11. doi:10.1016/j.radphyschem.2014.05.017.

122. Wernle JD, Mimnaugh KD, Rufner AS, Popoola OO, Argenson JN, Kelly M. Grafted Vitamin-E UHMWPE may increase the durability of posterior stabilized and constrained condylar total knee replacements. *J Biomed Mater Res*. 2017;105:1789-1798. doi:10.1002/jbm.b.33710.

123. Oral E, Godleski Beckos C, Malhi AS, Muratoglu OK. The effects of high dose irradiation on the cross-linking of vitamin E-blended ultrahigh molecular weight polyethylene. *Biomaterials*. 2008;29:3557-3560. doi:10.1016/j.biomaterials.2008.05.004.

124. Oral E, Neils AL, Rowell SL, Lozynsky AJ, Muratoglu OK. Increasing irradiation temperature maximizes vitamin e grafting and wear resistance of ultrahigh molecular weight polyethylene. *J Biomed Mater Res*. 2013;101 B:436-440. doi:10.1002/jbm.b.32807.

125. Scemama C, Anract P, Dumaine V, Babinet A, Courpied JP, Hamadouche M. Does vitamin E-blended polyethylene reduce wear in primary total hip arthroplasty: a blinded randomised clinical trial. *Int Orthop*. 2017;41:1113-1118. doi:10.1007/s00264-016-3320-2.

126. Rochcongar G, Buia G, Bourroux E, Dunet J, Chapus V, Hulet C. Creep and wear in vitamin E-infused highly cross-linked polyethylene cups for total hip arthroplasty: a prospective randomized controlled trial. *J Bone Joint Surg Am*. 2018;100:107-114. doi:10.2106/JBJS.16.01379.

127. Wyatt M, Weidner J, Pfluger D, Beck M. The RM pressfit vitamys: 5-year swiss experience of the first 100 cups. *HIP Int*. 2017;27:368-372. doi:10.5301/hipint.5000469.

128. Rowell SL, Muratoglu OK. Investigation of surgically retrieved, vitamin E-stabilized, crosslinked UHMWPE implants after short-term in vivo service. *J Biomed Mater Res*. 2016;104:1132-1140. doi:10.1002/jbm.b.33465.

129. Rowell SL, Reyes CR, Malchau H, Muratoglu OK. In vivo oxidative stability changes of highly cross-linked polyethylene bearings: an ex vivo investigation. *J Arthroplasty*. 2015;30:1828-1834. doi:10.1016/j.arth.2015.05.006.

130. Currier BH, Currier JH, Holdcroft LA, Van Citters DW. Effectiveness of anti-oxidant polyethylene: what early retrievals can tell us. *J Biomed Mater Res*. 2017;106(1):353-359. doi:10.1002/jbm.b.33840.

131. Paxton EW, Inacio MCS, Kurtz S, Love R, Cafri G, Namba RS. Is there a difference in total knee arthroplasty risk of revision in highly crosslinked versus conventional polyethylene? *Clin Orthop Relat Res*. 2015;473:999-1008. doi:10.1007/s11999-014-4046-3.

132. AJRR. *American Joint Replacement Registry - Annual Report 2018*; 2018.

chapter 13

Damage of Implant Surfaces in Total Knee Arthroplasty

Ebru Oral, PhD | Markus A. Wimmer, PhD | Orhun Muratoglu, PhD

INTRODUCTION

Contemporary total knee arthroplasty (TKA) uses metallic, ceramicized, and polymeric materials to reconstruct the knee joint. The femoral component is, in general, manufactured from alloys of cobalt-chrome. The femoral component articulates against a tibial insert made of ultrahigh-molecular-weight polyethylene (UHMWPE)—in this chapter, UHMWPE and polyethylene terminology is used interchangeably and refers to the same polymer (i.e., UHMWPE). The tibial insert is typically metal-backed by titanium base alloy. If used, the patellar components are also fabricated from UHMWPE. These polyethylene components form the primary articulations present in the total knee (i.e., tibiofemoral and patellofemoral), and it is at these articulations where most damage is initiated. When the damage is extensive, the performance of the joint deteriorates and eventually leads to revision surgery.

The primary damage mode active at tibiofemoral and patellofemoral articulations is the wear of the polyethylene component. Articular wear is a highly complex process encompassing several different wear mechanisms. The wear mechanisms describe the mechanical, physical, and chemical interaction of the articulating elements in the joint. The two most active wear mechanisms in total knee replacement (TKR) are delamination and adhesive wear. Delamination occurs by the generation of subsurface cracks and their propagation to the surface, leading to the removal of large (more than 0.5 mm) pieces of polyethylene wear debris in the form of flakes (**Figs. 13-1 to 13-3**). This mechanism has been typically facilitated by the embrittlement (e.g., through oxidation) of polyethylene. Adhesive wear is initiated by the orientation and strain hardening of the polymer and the formation of microjunctions between the articulating bodies. During mechanical action, these microjunctions are torn off and fragments become small particles, usually on the order of a few micrometers or less in size. Abrasion is another wear mechanism that is typically observed in knee joints. Here, hard asperities on the femoral component and hard third body particles, such as bone chips or bone cement particles, generate wear debris by cutting and removing the softer polyethylene articular surface.

Besides wear, creep and plastic deformation also contribute to the damage seen on the polyethylene surface. Creep, which is the flow of the polymeric material under continued stress in loaded regions, leads to permanent deformation. This deformation is a function of time, the majority of which accumulates during approximately the first 2 years of *in vivo* use, at which time it reaches a steady state.

Among the earlier-described damage modes, delamination was recognized as the primary precursor of most device failures. Once initiated, delamination rapidly led to the loss of geometric conformity at articulation, disrupted the intended load distribution in the joint, and eventually led to implant failure in the form of tibial insert disengagement and fracture of polyethylene component. Thanks to improvements in UHMWPE processing techniques, sterilization, and packaging procedures in the last two decades, oxidation and oxidative embrittlement have been minimized and this wear mechanism is much less prominent. While late failure due to osteolysis and adhesive–abrasive wear was the most prevalent reason of failure in the late 1990s, this is no longer the case (**Table 13-1**).[1,2] According to the 2018 report of the American Joint Replacement Registry,[3] the two major reasons for TKR failure are now mechanical complications (23.7%) and aseptic loosening (21%). Wear of the articulating surface is listed in fifth place (2.2%).

Bone resorption secondary to particulate debris is at least still partially responsible for aseptic loosening, especially in the later stages.[4,5] Bone resorption or periprosthetic osteolysis is initiated by osteoclasts, which are stimulated by inflammatory mediators that are produced through the macrophage response to wear debris. Particularly submicron size wear debris (less than 1 µm) is thought to be easily phagocytosed by the macrophages. The progressive growth of inflammatory/granulomatous tissue and the increased bone resorption at the bone–implant interface eventually lead to loosening of the implant. Under certain circumstances, the amount of bone loss after TKR has been great, leading to component loosening or fracture.[6] Unfortunately, revision surgery in these cases is made particularly difficult, often necessitating the use of special augments to the components and bone grafts.[7]

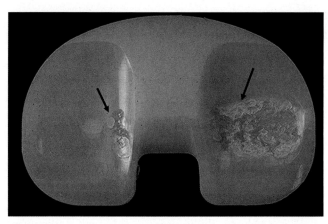

FIGURE 13-1   An example of delamination on the articular surface of a surgically retrieved polyethylene tibial insert. The delaminations (*arrows*) are well-accepted to have a strong correlation with oxidation-induced embrittlement secondary to gamma sterilization.

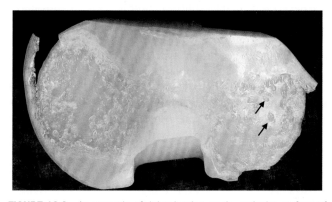

FIGURE 13-2   An example of delamination on the articular surface of a surgically retrieved polyethylene tibial insert. This explant also exhibited a yellow discoloration, due most likely to the penetration of synovial fluid into the cracks. Note that this implant shows pitting (*arrows*) on the new surface formed by delamination.

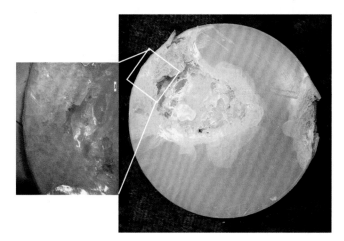

FIGURE 13-3   An example of delamination on the articular surface of a surgically retrieved polyethylene patellar component. Delamination, mostly on the lateral facet of the dome, is evident. There are also radial cracks apparent around the periphery of the explant. The inset is a high-magnification photograph of the highlighted superior-lateral region showing numerous cracks.

Delamination, adhesive–abrasive wear, creep, and plastic deformation contribute to the formation of the scar on articular surfaces of the polyethylene components. Unlike total hip replacement, in which the *in vivo* wear rate of polyethylene is well-quantified through various methods, the true rate at which the TKR damage modes proceed *in vivo* has only been recently quantified. It is impossible to quantify *in vivo* wear radiographically, mainly because of the complex geometry of the knee implants. The information on polyethylene damage in TKR available as of 2019 is largely based on the analysis of retrievals, which are inherently a selection of failures and do not necessarily represent the uncomplicated *in vivo* behavior. Yet, these explants are telling in determining the factors that can accelerate damage mechanisms. This chapter concentrates on the factors that affect the damage modes and the *in vivo* performance of the total knee. First, the historic design changes directed for the reduction of *in vivo* damage of tibial inserts and patellar components are outlined. The basic structure of polyethylene, mechanisms of *in vivo* damage, and factors that affect these damage modes are reviewed. Last, newly emerging technology of antioxidant stabilization of cross-linked polyethylene, modification of articular surfaces, and other technologies for use in the total knee are presented.

TIBIAL INSERTS

Total knee designs in the 1950s and 1960s were predominantly hinged devices such as the Guepar prosthesis.[8,9] These knees, by design, had a high degree of constraint between the tibial and femoral components, which led to high bone–cement interface shear stresses and, subsequently, a very high incidence of early failure secondary to aseptic loosening and infection.[9] To remedy this situation, resurfacing arthroplasty was introduced for the knee in the early 1970s by Gunston[10] with the polycentric knee. This design resurfaced the distal femur and proximal tibia with metallic and polyethylene runners, respectively. Among the downfalls of the polycentric knee were the failure to address the patellofemoral joint and a lack of instrumentation to allow reproducible implant insertion. The introduction of the total condylar design by Insall and associates in the mid-1970s revolutionized TKA.[11] This design was the predecessor of modern designs, as it allowed resurfacing of all three compartments of the knee, provided instrumentation for more reproducible insertion, and accommodated the collateral ligaments about the knee as no previous design had done. Subsequent to the total condylar design, knees fell into one of the two categories: posterior cruciate retaining or posterior cruciate substituting. The posterior cruciate–substituting designs substituted for the posterior cruciate ligament with a polyethylene post on the tibial component that articulated with a cam on the femoral component. This divergence in philosophy was fueled by controversy

TABLE 13-1	Historical and Current Ranking of Top Reasons for Revision			
	Sharkey et al, 2002[1]		Sharkey et al, 2014[2]	
Reason for Revision	Ranking (Early)	Ranking (Late)	Ranking (Early)	Ranking (Late)
UHMWPE	4	1	4	4
Loosening	3	2	2	1
Instability	2	3	3	3
Infection	1	4	1	2

regarding the function of the posterior cruciate ligament with respect to knee kinematics and anteroposterior stability after TKR. Both designs are still used and both have equally good long-term results to date. The advances in surgical technique, instrumentation, and component design (posterior stabilized and cruciate retaining) have made the operation more reproducible and markedly reduced the incidence of aseptic loosening.

Further advances in the total knee designs accompanied the use of modularity. Initially, tibial components were either all-polyethylene, or the polyethylene tibial surface was directly compression molded onto a tibial base plate.[12] Both types of tibial components were fixed using bone cement. Modularity allowed the surgeon to exchange the polyethylene tibial insert at revision surgery instead of revising the tibial metal plate in the event that the tibial component was well-fixed and aligned. Furthermore, the use of modular trial inserts and spacer blocks has allowed the refinement of accurate joint line placement and flexion–extension gap balancing. Today, the use of modular components is widespread and polyethylene inserts are made through a variety of methods that are discussed later (see Ultrahigh-Molecular-Weight Polyethylene).

PATELLAR COMPONENTS

In the early total knee designs, resurfacing of the patella was not common.[13,14] The long-term benefits of patellar resurfacing are still controversial. Although some surgeons always resurface the patella, some never perform resurfacing, and some resurface based on clinical or intraoperative findings.[15,16] The incidence of postoperative anterior knee pain is believed to be lower with the resurfacing of the patella.[17,18] In a 2018 systematic review and subsequent meta-analysis, the postoperative Knee Society (pain) score was significantly higher in the patellar resurfacing compared with the nonresurfacing group (OR 1.52, P = .004). Also, the percentage for reoperation is lower for the patellar resurfacing group (1% vs. 7%).[19]

Patellar complications are a source of poor outcome and require revision surgery after TKA.[20-23] Excessive wear, fracture, and maltracking of the patellar components have been associated with such complications[24-28] and have

been related to the surgical alignment and design.[29] Berger et al[30] have shown the importance of surgical alignment with a study of the ramifications of femoral rotation on patellar tracking. The combined internal rotation of the tibial and femoral components, judged from computed tomography scan measurements, correlated directly with the severity of patellofemoral complication in a group of 30 patients, suggesting that rotational malalignment may be the most important cause of patellofemoral complications. Among the design aspects that stimulate patellar complications are the polyethylene thickness, the nature of the backing (cement versus metal), and the articular surface geometry.[31-33] Furthermore, femoral design has been shown to affect the function of the patellofemoral joint. A femoral design with a trochlear groove that extends proximally to engage the patella in full extension, a deepened trochlear groove, and a gradual anterior to distal transition are desirable to optimize patellofemoral function after TKA.

ULTRAHIGH-MOLECULAR-WEIGHT POLYETHYLENE

UHMWPE is the material of choice for the fabrication of tibial inserts and patellar components and is used in all arthroplasties on the tibial side of the articulation regardless of the choice of counterface material on the femoral side. UHMWPE is synthesized by the polymerization of ethylene (CH_2=CH_2) gas leading to the formation of long-chain molecules with the chemical formula of $(-C_2H_4-)n$, where n is the degree of polymerization. As the degree of polymerization increases, so does the molecular weight of the polymer. The nomenclature of UHMWPE has changed considerably in the past five decades beginning in the early 60s as a form of HDPE[34] and it became possible to produce even higher-molecular-weight polyethylenes.

Today, UHMWPE is defined by ASTM D 4020 as a linear polyethylene with an average molecular weight of greater than 3.1 million g/mol[35] and greater than 1 million g/mol by ISO 11542. The first use of UHMWPE in orthopedics was in 1962 with Charnley,[36] who used the RCH 1000 resin—a grade of polyethylene available at the time—for his original acetabular components.

The available surgical grades of UHMWPE resins today are GUR1020 and GUR1050 (Celanese, Houston, TX) and have molecular weights of about 3.5 and 6 million g/mol, respectively.[37] Today, there is also a version of GUR1020 supplied premixed with 1000 ppm of vitamin E (GUR1020E). Until the disassembly of their production line in 2002, two other resins, 1900 and 1900H, which had a molecular weight in the range of 2 to 4 million g/mol, were supplied by Hercules Powder Company and Montell Polyolefins (Wilmington, DE, USA). The primary difference between the currently available resins is their molecular weight, which can affect their mechanical properties and adhesive–abrasive wear resistance. The Himont 1900 resin, although it exhibited the lowest mechanical properties among the three resins, also found widespread use in TKR devices primarily for its low incidence of delamination when consolidated through direct compression molding. The clinical comparison of the same implant made with the Himont 1900 resin and another resin such as the GUR4150 in MG-I and MG-II prostheses showed more delamination and oxidative damage with the latter resins[38] and suggested that resin type, consolidation method, or a combination of the two was effective in decreasing the oxidation potential. Muratoglu et al showed that oxidation is the highest at flake boundaries, in which calcium stearate contained in GUR4150 accumulated during consolidation.[39,40] Calcium stearate was added to GUR 4150 resin to protect the consolidation equipment from corrosion. It also acted as a lubricant and a release agent. While the Himont 1900 resin is no longer in production, the currently available GUR UHMWPEs do not contain calcium stearate anymore to avoid associated complications.

At the nanometer scale, UHMWPE is a semi-crystalline polymer with its crystalline domains embedded within an amorphous matrix. At room temperature, UHMWPE molecules pack themselves in a long-range order, forming crystalline lamellae, typically 10 to 50 nm in thickness and 10 to 50 μm in length (**Fig. 13-4**). There is a wide distribution of lamellar sizes within the polymer with the surrounding amorphous phase consisting of randomly oriented and entangled polymer chains traversed by tie molecules which interconnect lamellae and provide resistance to mechanical deformation.

After synthesis, UHMWPE is in the form of fine white powder resin particles which go through a consolidation process for the long polymer chains at the granule boundaries to diffuse effectively into the neighboring granules and fuse the polymer into stock forms. Consolidation into a stock material is done using ram extrusion, slab molding, or direct compression molding methods (**Fig. 13-5**). For the early designs of tibial inserts, for example, the MG-I and Insall-Burstein I (IB-I), the UHMWPE powder was directly molded into the metal base plate. Today, with the popularity of modular designs, the tibial inserts and patellar components

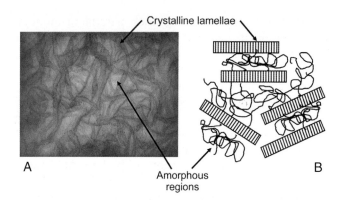

FIGURE 13-4 A transmission electron micrograph (**A**) and a schematic (**B**) of ultrahigh-molecular-weight polyethylene show the lamellae embedded in an amorphous matrix. The long-chain polyethylene molecules assume a random orientation in the amorphous regions. In the crystalline lamellae, the molecules are oriented in a long-range order.

are mostly manufactured by machining a ram-extruded or slab compression–molded stock material or by direct compression molding of the near-net or final shape.

The mechanical and wear properties of UHMWPE may be significantly affected by the manufacturing processes, such as the temperature and pressure cycles during molding and as such these processes are proprietary. The mechanical properties of UHMWPE are strongly related to the crystalline content and structure and the amount of interaction between its crystalline and amorphous phases. For example, the mechanical properties of consolidated UHMWPE vary as a function of the cooling rate during consolidation,[41] which affects the crystallization kinetics and may lead to lower crystallinity at higher cooling rates. Final implant shapes are further fashioned

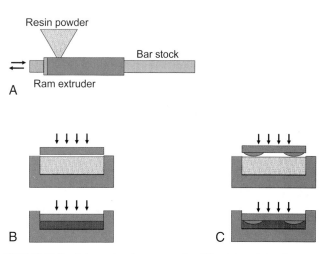

FIGURE 13-5 Schematic of ram extrusion (**A**), slab molding (**B**), and direction compression molding of ultrahigh-molecular-weight polyethylene powder (**C**). During ram extrusion, resin powder is consolidated to form bar stock. During slab molding, the mold is filled with resin powder and consolidated under high pressure and high temperature. Direct compression molding allows the consolidation of resin powder into the final geometry of the tibial insert. In the case of ram extrusion and slab molding, the consolidated stock is machined to fabricate tibial inserts and patellar components.

by either extensive machining stock material or minimal machining of the near-net shaped components obtained from direct compression molding. The final process in implant manufacture is sterilization. While gamma irradiation is the most common method of sterilization, ethylene oxide (EtO) and gas plasma sterilization are also used. Radiation processes including gamma irradiation produce long-lived free radicals in UHMWPE, the reactions of which with oxygen are a major factor in the long-term oxidation and degradation of the implant. One of the improvements in the technologies used in total knee implants in the last two decades has been radiation cross-linking of the UHMWPE-bearing surface to improve wear resistance.[42] We will discuss these processes and associated treatments to reduce oxidation in detail in further sections. Today, EtO and gas plasma sterilization, which do not introduce long-lived free radicals in UHMWPE, are also used in combination with radiation cross-linked materials to avoid increasing their oxidation potential (**Table 13-2**).

DAMAGE ON ARTICULATING AND NONARTICULATING SURFACES

During the activities of daily living, the articular surfaces of polyethylene components accumulate a scar. On tibial inserts, the scar is commonly localized to the articular condylar surfaces. Occasionally, damage may occur elsewhere, such as the tibial eminence. The scarring of the eminence may be induced by medial-lateral translation or, more typically, by a malrotated tibial component.[43] Rotation of the femoral component after progressive damage on the articular surface of the tibial insert is another mechanism that has been discussed in the literature.[44]

Another location where polyethylene surface damage occurs is the undersurface of tibial inserts. This damage is primarily a consequence of micromotion between the insert and baseplate, which produces small particles through adhesive wear, and has been commonly called "backside wear." It is estimated to contribute as much as 30% to the total wear volume in TKR.[45] In addition, the screw holes present on the tibial baseplate are often imprinted on the undersurface because of the effect of creep deformation of the polyethylene tibial insert into these openings.

The tibial post-cam articulation of posterior-stabilized (PS) designs has also been shown to contribute to the generation of particles. Puloski[46] reported on 23 retrieved PS tibial inserts of four different manufacturers (nine different designs), which had been implanted for a mean duration of 36 months, and performed quantitative and qualitative analysis of wear. About 30% exhibited severe damage with gross loss of polyethylene. Although the wear was primarily posterior at the post-cam articulation, damage of the medial, lateral, and anterior surfaces of the post was observed. Factors such as cam-post mechanics

and geometry may influence the wear at this articulation. On occasion, gross wear and even fracture of the post have also been observed.[46,47] Post fracture is a rare event and may be accelerated by the oxidative embrittlement of polyethylene.

WEAR MECHANISMS

There are several mechanisms of wear underlying the formation and progress of the scar on the polyethylene tibial and patellar components. The four main mechanisms are surface fatigue, adhesion, abrasion, and tribochemical reactions as defined by ASTM standard G40-05 and reported in the orthopedic literature.[45,48]

Surface fatigue results from repeated stress cycles in the subsurface of a material, during repeated sliding or rolling over the same wear track. The application of load through the femoral component on the tibial insert leads to compressive stresses immediately under the contact area and tensile stresses outside the contact.[49,50] The peak of the shear stresses occurs approximately 1 mm below the surface (**Fig. 13-6A**). Because of the rolling-sliding motion of the femoral component, the contact region of the polyethylene is subjected to a fluctuating stress environment (**Fig. 13-6B**), leading to crack initiation in the material. The formed microcracks can grow below the surface, and when they reach the surface cause detachments of large flaky particles, also known as delamination (**Figs. 13-3 to 13-3**). Delamination differs from other wear types as it is not a gradual release of material, but rather accumulated damage followed by surface destruction that leads to device failure *in vivo*. Pitting is also a fatigue-related phenomenon and is the outcome of the coalescence of shallow cracks or cracks initiated from the surface. Yet, this mode of damage mostly occurs on the articular surfaces without substantial material loss. In the absence of surface delamination, the adhesive–abrasive mechanisms prevail as the dominant wear processes in total knees.

Adhesion occurs when there is local bonding between asperities of both articulating surfaces under pressure. During relative motion, these microjunctions are torn off and fragments may form particles or are being transferred to the counterbody. Lubricant chemistry and film thickness between the two surfaces are important factors allowing the asperities to come into contact and bond. The rate of adhesive wear depends strongly on the relative motion of the metallic counterface against the polyethylene articular surface.[51-53] For example, cross-shear increases wear by an order of magnitude by shifting from a unidirectional, reciprocating wear path to a rectangular, bidirectional wear path when it is rubbed against an implant surface finish cobalt-chrome disc in the presence of bovine serum.[54] The unidirectional motion used in this pin-on-disc (POD) experiment is thought to orient and strain-harden the surface of polyethylene, resulting in low

TABLE 13-2   Current Alternatives of Medium to Highly Crosslinked Virgin (No Antioxidant) Polyethylenes in Total Knee Replacements

Trade Name	Manufacturer (Location)	Radiation Temperature (°C)	Radiation Dose (kGy[a])	Radiation Type	Postirradiation Treatment	Sterilization Method	Total Radiation Dose Level (kGy[a])
Prolong	Zimmer Biomet (Warsaw, IN)	~125	65	E-beam	Melted at 150°C	GP	65
ArCom XL	Zimmer Biomet (Warsaw, IN)	N/A	~50		Mechanical deformation	EtO	~50
Durasul	Zimmer Biomet (Warsaw, IN)	~120-125	95	E-beam	Melted at 150°C	EtO	95
X3	Stryker (Mahwah, NJ)	N/A	~90	Gamma	Sequentially annealed (~130°C) after each 30 kGy	GP	~90
XLK	Depuy Synthes (Warsaw, IN)	N/A	~50	Gamma	Melted at 155°C	GP	~50
XLPE	Smith & Nephew (Memphis, TN)	N/A	~75	Gamma	Melted at 147°C	EtO	~75

EtO, ethylene oxide; GP, gas plasma.
[a]10 kilograys (kGy) = 1 Mrad.

wear. On the other hand, with the rectangular, bidirectional motion, the surface strain hardens (strengthens) in the rubbing direction and weakens in the transverse direction. The metallic counterface encounters a weaker surface during changes in the direction of motion, leading to high wear. The microscopic analysis of the wear surfaces of

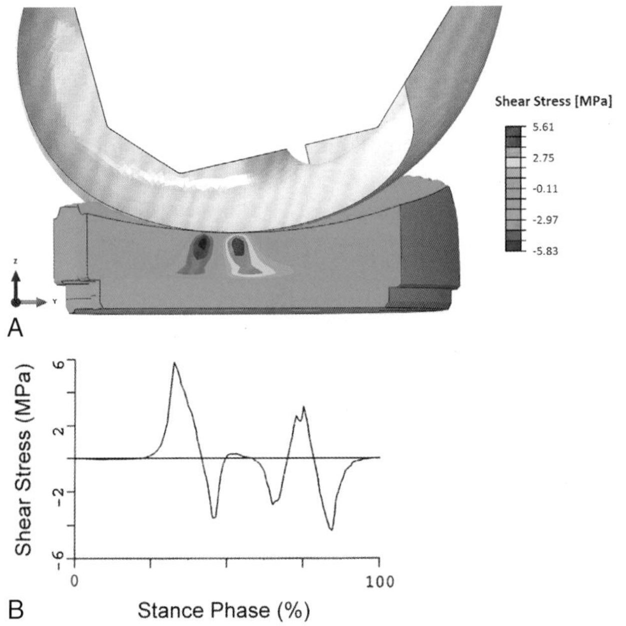

FIGURE 13-6   **A:** Shear stress contours shown cross section in a polyethylene implant. Note the maxima below the surface (FEM model from Mell et al[299]). **B:** Shear stress over time during stance phase of walking. Note the cyclic character of the stress pattern when viewed at a single location.

surgically retrieved tibial inserts has shown striated wear patterns with ripples oriented perpendicular and parallel to the primary direction of anterior–posterior motion.[55] These striations (**Fig. 13-7**) represent amorphous and crystalline regions of polyethylene[56] and develop during adhesive-type wear of polyethylene in the total knee.

Abrasion defines the action of hard counterface asperities or hard debris (so-called "third bodies") ploughing the softer material. Both hard asperities and third-body particles cause the release of polyethylene from the articular surfaces. Submechanisms include microcutting, microploughing, and microfatigue and are dependent on the material properties and sharpness of the asperities and/or third bodies. Third-body wear is common in TKR and can be generated by the fragmentation of bone cement used for fixation, bone chips, or metal debris from failure of metal-backed patellar components. Wasielewski reported on 55 tibial inserts retrieved at the time of revision surgery and found that 25% had severe insert damage related to third-body debris consisting of cement or metallic particles.[57] Third body can penetrate the articulation and accelerate the wear process, mainly in the form of material removal through extensive scratching of the polyethylene articular surfaces. With hard third-body particles, such as the barium sulfate additive in bone cement, scratching of the femoral counterface can occur, increasing the surface roughness. This in turn increases polyethylene wear.

Tribochemical reactions occur when surfaces in mechanical contact are activated due to friction and react with the interfacial medium, which results in the alternating formation and removal of chemical reaction products

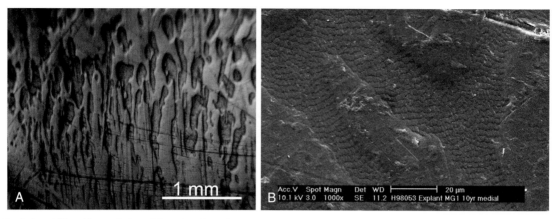

FIGURE 13-7   Striated ("lace") morphology **(A)** and surface ripples **(B)** on the articular surface of a surgically retrieved polyethylene tibial insert. These features are the likely precursors to adhesive–abrasive wear on tibial inserts.

at the surfaces. Whether this mechanism has any significance in TKR is currently unknown.

Adhesive and abrasive wear has been implicated in the generation of submicron polyethylene debris, capable of initiating adverse tissue reactions and periprosthetic osteolysis *in vivo*. The following section discusses the clinical observations on wear debris found in periprosthetic tissue and osteolysis in TKA.

WEAR APPEARANCE AND VOLUMETRIC MATERIAL LOSS

Unlike total hip replacement, in which the *in vivo* wear rate of polyethylene has been known through various methods, the true rate of TKR has only been established in the past few years based on retrieved UHMWPE components. There are no reliable radiographic methods developed for the quantification of *in vivo* wear, mainly because of the complex geometry of the knee implants.

Wear appearance, which describes the visible changes of surface texture, composition, or shape as a consequence

of wear, has been used as a surrogate for cumulative damage in many research studies. "Wear features," "wear patterns," or "wear damage" has been used synonymously in the literature. Originally developed by Hood et al,[58] the methodology has been cited over 350 times and applied to multiple retrieval studies. Polishing, burnishing, scratching, pitting, delamination, striation, abrasion, embedded debris, and surface deformation are typical wear features on retrieved polyethylene tibial inserts (**Fig. 13-8**). While the appearance of damage holds clues regarding the identification of the acting wear mechanism, damage patterns are only moderate predictors for material loss (except for delamination) as recently demonstrated in a study by Knowlton et al.[59]

The burnished feature occurs due to an adhesive wear mechanism that tears and pulls off fibrils during sliding of the femoral condoyle on the tibial insert. Scratches have linear features on the articulating surface, often due to the presence of third-body particles that act abrasively. Pitting is a common wear feature characterized by mostly round, small holes (<1 mm) at the surface.

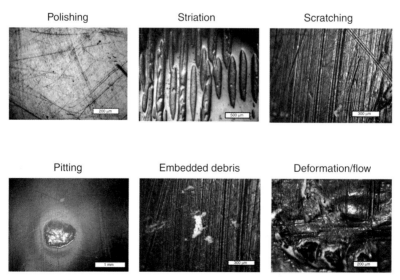

FIGURE 13-8   Various damage modes seen on the tibial polyethylene surface.

Pits can either be caused by local surface fatigue and ejection of material or by plastic deformation when third bodies (e.g., cement particles) are indented into the surface. Delamination is the most extreme wear feature and caused by surface fatigue as described above. It frequently occurred on components that were sterilized in air, accelerating oxidation and causing embrittlement of UHMWPE.[60]

Striations are a unique and frequent wear pattern that typically occurs within the first year after implantation of retrieved polyethylene inserts. The width of a single striation is about 70 to 100 μm and the darker elevations are separated from the brighter regions that form troughs in between.[55] Interestingly, it was recently found that striations accounted for the second highest material loss after delamination.[61] While little is known about the actual mechanism that causes striations, a recent FTIR microscopy study by Rad et al[56] suggests that striations are an arrangement of crystalline and amorphous regions. Other damage features that are reported in the literature are "abrasion," which is a rough and tufted region that can be visualized on the articulating surface of the tibial inserts, and "embedded debris," characterized by color or texture differences that suggest embedded particles in the polyethylene surface.[62] Deformation, which is a permanent change of the surface geometry due to plastic flow or creep, is also often mentioned. Obviously, this type of damage does not correspond to wear since no material is lost.[60]

The appearance of the scar observed on surgically retrieved patellar components is similar to those observed on tibial inserts. They generally develop on the lateral facet and the dome of the patellar component. Cameron[63] reported this type of scarring in 11 surgically revised Freeman-Swanson and Tricon (Smith & Nephew, Memphis, TN) knees. Scarring of the lateral facet of the patellar component is presumably induced by lateral loading of the patellar surface and excessive lateral subluxation or tilt, or both, of the patella during flexion, often associated with internal rotation of the femoral and tibial component.

Volumetric loss of material has been difficult to measure in TKR for various reasons. First, the loss of material is relatively subtle when delaminated components are excluded. Pourzal et al[64] found up to 60% less wear in total knees when compared to total hip components made out the same polyethylene. Next, the volumetric loss is easily confounded by plastic deformation/creep. Third, the geometry of TKR is complex, and tolerances are not always tight. Therefore, techniques had to be developed that allowed measurements from reconstructed surfaces, in an attempt to estimate the original surface.[65] Such methods also allowed differentiating wear from conformational changes due to plastic deformation and creep. Other studies approximated wear by linear thickness measurements or

stereoradiography. A summary of measurements that can be found in the literature is given in **Table 13-3**. It should be noted that some of the studies listed (e.g., CMM autonomous reconstructions) do not account for backside wear.

OSTEOLYSIS IN TOTAL KNEE REPLACEMENTS

Wear particles can trigger osteolysis in total joint arthroplasty.[5] This is true for both hip and knee joints, and the appearance of tissues surrounding prosthetic devices that have failed aseptically is similar between total knees and hips. In fact, Goodman et al[66] reported that these tissues are similar regarding cellular profile, structure, chemokine/cytokine signaling, and enzymatic profiles.

Compared with total hip, total knee patients exhibit a reduced rate of osteolysis, which is thought to be a consequence of fewer particles due to a smaller wear volume, but also the larger and more elongated polyethylene wear particles produced in the total knee.[67-69] Shanbhag et al performed an analysis of particulate wear debris retrieved from interfacial membranes around 18 failed total knees.[69] The mean particle size was 1.7 ± 0.7 μm, and this increase in size may contribute to a decrease in the biologic activity of particles. Still, 30% of the particles were less than 1 μm in size. We know now that a high proportion of the small particles is generated by backside wear.[45,70] With backside wear, the debris can find access to the periprosthetic interface through screw holes. Peters et al[71] showed the development of lytic lesions around screw–bone interfaces induced by polyethylene and metallic debris from modular interfaces.

Ultimately, particle size and total volumetric material loss of the polyethylene liner are dependent on implant design.[72] In addition, the particle load experienced by the tissue is in part a function of the joint space available, which makes the distribution of wear products less dense around knee arthroplasty when compared to hip arthroplasty. As a result, knee replacements demonstrate a lower number of particles per unit of surface compared to hip replacements even in the case where particle size and worn off material volume are identical. Therefore, osteolysis has been less frequent in TKR.

FACTORS AFFECTING DAMAGE AND SOLUTIONS TO MINIMIZE WEAR

The damage observed in tibial and patellar components is multifactorial and contributing factors will be discussed in detail below. Various damage mechanisms may require various solutions, and some may contradict each other. For example, to avoid *surface fatigue*, a large contact area with high conformity is needed. However, *adhesion* is reduced when the contact area is

TABLE 13-3	**Volumetric Wear of Tibial Components**				
	Study	**Knee Design (Type)**	**Assessment**	**Avg. Volume Loss [μL/y or /Mc]**	**No. of Studied Retrievals**
In vivo	Kop et al[289]	APG, LCS (MB, FB)	CMM	85	7
				77	10
	Atwood et al[290]	LCS (MB)	Thickness-based	54	100
	Engh et al[291]	Sigma RP, LCS, PFC Sigma (MB, FB CR/PS)	Micro-CT	43 ± 25	12
				74 ± 49	12
	Benjamin et al[292]	AMK (FB CR)	laser scan	794	33
	Lavernia et al[293]	PCA (FB-CR)	Thickness-based	32 ± 43	28 (PM)
	Gill et al[294]	AGC (FB-CR)	RSA	100	6
	Pourzal et al[139]	MGII (FB-CR)	CMM/autonomous reconstruction	18 ± 13 (no delamination)	17 (PM)
	Rad et al[137]	NexGen (FB-CR)	CMM/autonomous reconstruction	13.8 ± 2.0	83
	Knowlton[77]	NexGen (FB-CR/PS)	CMM/autonomous reconstruction	10.3 ± 6.5 (CR)	19 (PM)
				11.1 ± 4.2 (PS)	25 (PM)
In vitro	Muratoglu et al[42]	NKII (FB-CR)	CMM	8.3 ± 0.8	
			Gravimetric	8.8 ± 1.5	
	Schwenke et al[295]	MGII (FB-CR)	Gravimetric	22.4 (load control)−9.8 (display control)	
	Teeter et al[296]	Genesis II (FB-CR)	Micro-CT	24.7	
	Laurent et al[297]	NexGen (FB-CR)	Gravimetric	15.4 ± 1.2	
	Popoola et al[298]	NexGen (FB-CR)	Gravimetric	15.4 ± 3	

CR, cruciate-retaining; FB, fixed bearing; MB, mobile bearing; PM, postmortem; PS, posterior-stabilized.

minimized. Thus, an optimum between both should be chosen to balance these requirements.[73] The present section discusses factors that affect polyethylene wear and damage in detail.

Kinematics and Design

The kinematic conditions are determined based on the design, such as the retention or substitution of the posterior cruciate ligament, and conformity of the tibiofemoral articulation. In general, cruciate-retaining (CR) designs have less conforming tibiofemoral articulations than their posterior stabilized counterparts. This, in theory, allows the ligaments about the knee to exert their effect on the kinematics. In a video-fluoroscopy study comparing PS to CR knees, Dennis et al found a paradoxic anterior femoral translation with knee flexion in the CR design.[74] The posterior stabilized knees consistently exhibited posterior femoral rollback. In a similar study, Banks et al[75] studied the differences in the kinematics of CR and cruciate-sacrificing total knee designs and found that axial rotation and condylar translations decreased with the post-cam substitution of the posterior cruciate ligament. These design-related differences in tibiofemoral conformity and kinematics may be related to the distinct differences in wear behavior in CR and PS total knees described by

Hirakawa et al,[76] who showed smaller scars and reduced apparent wear with PS TKA. However, in a recent study by Knowlton,[77] who compared the wear of CR and PS knees of the same manufacturer and design family (Nexgen, Zimmer Inc.), no volumetric wear differences were found. Both groups were comprised of postmortem retrievals (19 vs. 25, respectively), which were on average 9 years *in situ*. The wear rates were 11.9 ± 5.0 mm³/y and 11.1 ± 4.2 mm³/y for the CR and PS design, respectively (wear on post of PS design not considered). There was also no statistically significant difference regarding creep and plastic deformation, although the CR design displayed a higher amount on average (70 vs. 32 mm³).

The state of kinematics determines the wear path that the femoral component follows on the articular surface of polyethylene. In the knee, the sliding motion, which is induced by the flexion–extension (typically 50 to 90°) and anteroposterior translation (typically 5 to 20 mm), produces unidirectional motion on articulating surfaces of the tibial insert. When superimposed on the sliding motion, any level of tibial rotation generates multidirectional motion. Unidirectional motion produces very little wear, whereas multidirectional motion is what causes an increase in wear rates.[54] Schwenke and Wimmer[78] experimentally determined the relationship between cross-shear motion and UHMWPE wear using a cobalt-chromium wheel that articulated in a gliding–rolling fashion on a flat polyethylene plateau. They found that it takes 6.4 times more work to remove a unit wear volume in the direction of principal motion (i.e., anteroposteriorly) than 90° perpendicular to it. This explains findings of Kawanabe et al,[79] Wang et al,[80] and Muratoglu et al[81] who showed that the wear rate of polyethylene tibial inserts increases with increasing extent of internal–external rotation of the tibia on *in vitro* knee simulators. Specifically, the study by Kawanabe et al[79] demonstrated that the addition of a ±5-degree tibial rotation increased the wear rate from 1.7 mg per million cycles to 10.6 mg per million cycles on a cruciate retaining design (AGC Biomet). Wang's study[80] showed a decrease in the rate of weight loss from 14.4 mm^3 per million cycles with a 13.5-degree internal–external rotation to 3.9 mm^3 per million cycles with no rotation of the tibia. Muratoglu's study[81] showed that the gravimetric weight loss of conventional polyethylene in a flat-on-flat design TKR (Natural-Knee II) increases from 0.4 to 23.0 mg per million cycles, with an increase of tibial rotation range from 5 to 14°. Excessive tibial rotation can also lead to damage on the intercondylar eminence further contributing to weight loss. Another kinematic consideration that has been discussed in the past is the potential separation of the femoral component from the tibial insert during articulation. Dennis et al[82] have fluoroscopically measured the occurrence and the degree of femoral liftoff with posterior-stabilizing and CR knees. The femoral condylar liftoff on one side of the tibial insert could lead to an edge loading condition on the opposite side. If the mechanical properties of the polyethylene tibial insert have degraded owing to oxidative embrittlement, liftoff could conceivably accelerate surface fatigue and lead to rapid delamination of the component.

Although the tibiofemoral kinematics substantially affects the adhesive wear behavior of tibial inserts, patellofemoral kinematics, such as the tracking, and patellar rotation and tilt influence the damage accumulation on the patellar components. The improved understanding of patellofemoral kinematics has led to alterations in surgical technique to improve patellofemoral tracking. These include obtaining proper rotation of the femoral components, slight lateral placement of the femoral component, and medial placement of the patellar component.[83] In a recent simulator study[84] that was performed under a malaligned conditions, it demonstrated that a constant 5° external rotation applied to the patella button can result in delamination if the polyethylene has undergone embrittlement due to oxidation. However, many of the observed patellar complications could be attributed to the design of the patellofemoral articulation. Design modifications with respect to the patellofemoral joint have decreased the incidence of patellofemoral complications. Berger reported on a series of 172 MG-I and 109 MG-II cemented total knees with a mean follow-up of 11 years. The MG-I and MG-II are similar in terms of the tibiofemoral articulation; however, the MG-II has

a more anatomic sagittal contour of the femoral sulcus, resulting in a decreased anterior radius of curvature of the patellofemoral articulation. In addition, the patellofemoral articulation was made more congruent, and an all-polyethylene patella was used instead of a metal-backed patellar component to decrease the stresses in the polyethylene. In this series, the MG-I group had a 9% prevalence of patellofemoral complications compared to 0% in the MG-II group.[85] In a similar series, Theiss and associates studied a group of 301 cemented primary total knees, 148 with the MG-I and 153 PFC prostheses followed for a minimum of 2 years postoperatively.[86] The patellofemoral complication rate was 10% for the MG-I group compared to 0.7% for the PFC group. From these studies it is apparent that patellofemoral complications are sensitive to design issues as well as rotational alignment of the femoral component. An anatomic sagittal contour of the femoral prosthesis, a congruent trochlear groove with a cemented all-polyethylene patellar component, and proper rotational alignment markedly reduced the prevalence of patellofemoral complications after TKA.

Oxidation

Oxidation and oxidative degradation constituted the most pervasive problem in total joint knee arthroplasty for several decades.[87,88] Historically, the polyethylene used in total knees was sterilized using gamma irradiation in air with a typical dose of 25 to 40 kilograys (kGy). These implants had high wear, high rates of degradation, and high rates of revision.[89] In 1995, gamma sterilization in air of UHMWPE implants was abandoned and implants started being sterilized while packaged in inert gas.[90] Gamma sterilization in air led to marked oxidative changes in polyethylene, which resulted in the significant degradation of its mechanical properties. This degradation was characteristically manifested in the form of a reduction in strength and ductility and an increase in modulus.[91-94] In the mid-1990s, these sterilization-induced changes in polyethylene were shown to strongly correlate with delamination, subsurface cracking, and pitting of tibial inserts.[89,95-97] Today, all gamma sterilization of polyethylene implants is carried out in an inert environment, such as nitrogen, argon, or vacuum. The oxidation rate observed in these implants has been much lower under shelf-storage than those sterilized in air; however, the oxidation rate *in vivo* still is measurable and progressive.[98,99]

Concerning gas sterilization methods, a study reported by Williams et al[95] demonstrated that, after ethylene oxide sterilization, UHMWPE-bearing surfaces showed no cracking or delamination, even after 15 years of *in vivo* use. Although very few implants are only processed by gas sterilization due to the general low wear resistance in nonirradiated surfaces,[300] gas sterilization as a terminal process is considered, especially in cases where radiation can be detrimental to the performance of the implanted material. The understanding of oxidation and oxidation potential in UHMWPE used for joint implants has been based largely on radiation-induced free radicals. During ionizing irradiation of UHMWPE (for sterilization as well as for cross-linking which will be discussed later), free radicals are formed, the most prevalent of which are the carbon free radicals resulting from the breakage of the C-H bonds.[100-103] Most of these free radicals recombine in the amorphous portion of the polymer,[104] resulting in cross-linking. The remaining free radicals are trapped in the crystalline lamellae.[105,106] Oxygen reacts with the primary free radicals to form peroxy free radicals.[103,107-110] These peroxy radicals abstract a hydrogen atom from other polyethylene chains, creating primary free radicals, which can then react with oxygen to further this cascade.[111,112] The reactions of polyethylene free radicals with oxygen and the decay of the formed hydroperoxides eventually result not only in carbonyl-containing species, which are defined as "oxidation" in UHMWPE, but also in chain scission, lowering the molecular weight of the material and degrading its material properties.[113] Oxidation is determined by spectroscopic techniques measuring carbonyl moieties on UHMWPE formed as hydroperoxides decay.[114]

Accelerated aging methods are used to evaluate the oxidative resistance of UHMWPEs *in vitro*. These commonly incorporate thermooxidative aging at high temperatures (70°C to 120°C) and high oxygen pressures (up to 5 atm. of oxygen) (ASTM 2102). While these methods do not simulate the oxidation profile as a function of depth as observed in retrievals, they can simulate clinically observed oxidation levels in UHMWPE with detectable residual free radicals. Recently, the unexpected levels of oxidation observed in irradiated and melted retrievals on the shelf after being implanted, even for very short periods of time,[115] suggested the possibility that exposure to synovial fluid lipids may be involved in initiating oxidation in UHMWPE. In light of this finding, new methods are developed to incorporate the influence of synovial lipids in accelerated aging methods.[116,117]

The overall mechanical degradation of UHMWPE is often determined through its mechanical strength or toughness as a function of oxidation. While *in vitro* studies often use the ultimate tensile strength or fatigue crack propagation resistance as indicators,[118] retrievals have limited amount of material, only amenable to "small punch testing" as an indicator of toughness.[119,120] For example, the fatigue strength of UHMWPE is often measured by measuring resistance to the propagation of a crack formed under fatigue stress (ASTM E-647, Section A1). Using this method, a stress factor range at crack inception, ΔK_i, is calculated with values ranging from 1.6 to 2.0 MPam$^{1/2}$ for consolidated UHMWPE without further processing. The fatigue strength of gamma-in-air-sterilized UHMWPE is significantly decreased from 1.29 to 0.18 MPam$^{1/2}$ upon oxidation via accelerated aging.[121]

While the rate of degradation in the mechanical properties of UHMWPEs have not been quantified widely *in vivo*, the overall impact toughness of oxidized conventional retrievals, measured by small punch testing, was shown to decrease.[122] It is also known that oxidation exacerbates fatigue-induced wear mechanisms such as delamination and can deteriorate implant performance without a catastrophic failure.

Although rare, complete *in vivo* fracture of the tibial insert can also result from extreme oxidation-induced embrittlement.[20,123] Other types of fracture-related failures include shearing of the pegs used in fixing all-polyethylene patellae,[124] which may be induced by a combination of plastic deformation and fatigue of the peg base and could also be accelerated by oxidative embrittlement.

Our understanding of oxidation resistance has long been centered on limiting the reactions of the residual free radicals with oxygen over the long term. The decrease in the oxidation rate of gamma-sterilized implants packaged in inert gas during irradiation and shelf-storage has been attributed to the decrease in the rates of reaction between polyethylene free radicals and oxygen. Another approach to limiting the reactions of the residual free radicals is eliminating them or decreasing them to undetectable levels before implantation, which will be discussed later in the section entitled "Technologies to reduce bearing surface damage."

Mechanical Stress: Conformity and Polyethylene Thickness

Many knee designs that were developed in the 70s and 80s focused either on maximizing surface area to reduce polyethylene stresses or on preserving the anatomical features of the joint. The latter provided not only less contact area but also less constraint and thus more freedom for secondary motions.[9] Total knees with highly conforming articulating surfaces have been shown to result in low stress state in polyethylene components[50] and are expected to exhibit higher delamination resistance *in vivo*. Conformity is defined as the ratio of the radius of curvature of the femoral component (R_1) to that of the tibial polyethylene component (R_2) and may be described in the sagittal or coronal plane. As the ratio of R_1 to R_2 approaches 1, the tibiofemoral conformity increases. In order to determine whether conformity is a predictor for polyethylene damage, Wimmer et al[125] performed a retrieval study of two implant designs with high and low conformity. The polyethylene inserts were made from the same UHMWPE resin and shared the identical processing history. Contrary to expectations, the more congruent contact did not mitigate fatigue-related wear mechanisms.[126] It was found that the conforming inserts were associated with higher delamination and pitting scores but lower polishing scores, even after adjusting for confounding variables including insert thickness and implantation duration. These findings were similar to those of Blunn et al[127] but not in agreement with those of Collier et al[128] and Willie et al[129] In a follow-up study, with a newer implant design, Knowlton and Wimmer[77] looked to the actual material volumes that were removed from the inserts due to wear, and the two designs showed identical material loss. Today, designs with high and low conformity are used in clinical practice. And although the choice of one over the other remains controversial, clinical results appear equivocal.[130]

Polyethylene thickness is another driver of stresses in polyethylene. Bartel and associates, in their classic paper from 1986, found that contact stresses remain unchanged above a critical polyethylene thickness (approximately 8 mm), below which the contact stresses increase exponentially.[50] They also pointed out that UHMWPE contact stresses are far more sensitive to tibiofemoral conformity in the coronal plane compared to the sagittal plane. Their finding was corroborated by many early retrieval studies that identified polyethylene thickness as a major factor in surface fatigue. In newer retrieval studies, for example, the one by Wimmer et al,[125] insert thickness no longer had an effect on surface damage, suggesting the minimum thickness of modern inserts (here 8 mm) is sufficient to mitigate the stress-rising effect of the underlying metal tray.

With patellar components, the contact stresses generated at the patellofemoral articulation have been reported to be several times higher than the compressive yield strength of UHMWPE[31,32,131]; this is true especially during deep knee bending or stair descent. Increased congruity between the patellar component and femoral groove has been shown to reduce the contact stresses in the patellar components and reduce polyethylene damage *in vivo*.[31,132] Similar to the tibial inserts, especially with rigid back support, such as with metal-backed patellae, contact stresses in polyethylene become more significant with decreasing polyethylene thickness (typically, less than 3 to 4 mm). Therefore, patellar buttons are typically directly cemented onto the bone, if replaced.[133]

Modularity and Backside Wear

The use of modularity in the fixed-bearing total knee designs allows the potential for micromotion between the components, such as the polyethylene insert and tibial base plate.[134,135] Depending on the locking mechanism and the congruity of the interface,[136] the extent of micromotion can be large enough to generate backside wear, increase the particle burden, and increase the potential for osteolysis. Parks et al[134] quantified the anteroposterior and mediolateral micromotion to be on the order of 0.2 to 1.0 mm and 0.1 to 0.5 mm, respectively, in nine different total knee designs using an extensometer placed across the interface between the tibial insert and the tibial base plate under a load of 100 N. The study by

Wasielewski et al[57] on autopsy and surgically retrieved polyethylene tibial inserts from cementless total knee arthroplasties showed a significant association between backside wear and radiographic evidence of osteolysis. Mikulak et al reported similar results in a retrieval analysis of PS tibial inserts.[47] Crowninshield et al[45] reported a linear wear rate of 4.1 μm/y of the backside, which was deemed moderate. In fact, this reflects about 10% of the topside wear[137]; however, the contact area on the backside is large and, thus, the removed volume can be considerable. In a wear simulation study that tested with actual patient waveforms during gait found that backside wear can be as high as 20% of total wear.[138] Therefore, modularity with minimal micromotion is desirable and is still an important issue for improving contemporary total knee design. Modularity allows determining the polyethylene insert thickness after the fixation of the tray and the ease of insert exchange during revision surgery and in the treatment of infection.

Clinical Variables

Several clinical variables could increase the load distribution across the polyethylene components, leading to accelerated damage in the form of delamination, adhesive wear, or even fracture. Among the pertinent clinical factors are malalignment of the components, ligamentous balancing, or varus–valgus alignment of the knee.

In a retrieval association study by Pourzal et al[139] who studied wear of 59 polyethylene inserts of a cruciate retaining knee design, several patient factors correlated with wear. Wear on the articular surface (topside) was quantitatively determined using a coordinate measuring machine, and backside wear was assessed qualitatively by scoring surface damage. Articular wear increased significantly with younger age and male sex. Also, patient weight and height were factors that correlated positively with wear rate; however, backside damage was not affected by these variables. Males typically require larger implant sizes, which could partially explain the higher wear rate due to a larger wear area. They are also more active[140] and display different physical activity patterns[141] than females. The effect of younger age on wear is likely related to higher patient activity as well: younger joint arthroplasty subjects execute more steps per day.[142]

Gait is another patient specific variable that has been implicated with wear. In a study by Harman et al,[143] six patients (eight knees) underwent posterior cruciate ligament-retaining TKA. All patients participated in fluoroscopic analysis during treadmill gait after arthroplasty, and articular contact was measured. After retrieval of the implants at autopsy or revision, a significant correlation between wear scar features and articular contact location measured fluoroscopically during the activity was found. Knowlton and Wimmer[59] investigated the polyethylene inserts of 17 patients with available bilateral inserts. The medial and lateral articular surfaces of tibial components exhibited higher wear symmetry contralaterally within a patient than across patients. This finding supports the notion that gait pattern affects wear.

Among implant positioning variables, joint line elevation and tibial slope were highly significant factors that contributed to polyethylene wear on both top- and backside of the cruciate retaining knee implant.[139] A similar association between implant wear and joint line elevation has been recently reported for PS polyethylene inserts.[144] These findings are corroborated by finite element analysis,[145] in which the effect of nine component alignments was studied. Among those parameters with the most effect on wear, the transverse plane rotation angle of femoral condyle and tibial insert, as well as tibial slope were identified. It is speculated that an increasing tibial slope can result in larger anterior–posterior translations of the knee joint during gait. This would lead to larger wear scars.[146]

Malalignment has been implicated as a critical factor in the failure of TKA.[147] Restoring the mechanical axis of the lower extremity so that a line from the center of the femoral head to the center of the ankle joint passes through the center of the knee is the single most important factor under the surgeon's control to avoid mechanical complications. A tibiofemoral angle of 6 ± 3° is generally considered to be acceptable after a TKA,[148,149] although patient factors, such as stature or concomitant hip and femoral or tibial deformity, may alter the standard recommendations. At this angle, the mechanical axis of the lower extremity passes close to the center of the knee and results in uniform medial and lateral load distribution at the knee.

Another general form of malalignment is associated with the varus knee. In such cases, the mechanical axis of the knee may shift medially and cause lateral liftoff. This can increase the load on the medial plateau of the tibial insert and cause increased creep and premature wear.[57,150,151] Mastuda, in a report on 20 total knees with a mean follow-up of 87 months, found that the coronal alignment had changed secondary to polyethylene wear.[127] The polyethylene wear rate correlated with the initial postoperative alignment, which was varus in 17 of the 20 knees.

An additional factor that could adversely affect the wear of polyethylene-bearing surfaces in the total knee is the ligamentous balancing in flexion. Improper ligament balancing is related to excessive wear, complications in patellofemoral tracking, and inferior clinical results.[20,152,153] In flexion, the proper balance depends on the rotation of the femoral component relative to the tibial resection.[153] Rotational malalignment of the femoral component leads to a trapezoidal flexion gap and uneven loading of the tibial condyles, which could accelerate the wear of polyethylene counterface.

In terms of the patellofemoral articulation, surgical rotational malalignment of the femoral component can cause patellofemoral maltracking.[29,154-156] Such conditions could result in increased contact stresses, plastic deformation processes, and acceleration of the wear. Medial placement of the patellar component and external rotation of the femoral component have been shown to improve patellar tracking in terms of a reduced postoperative patellar tilt and lateral subluxation. Berger et al have demonstrated the use of the surgical epicondylar axis in establishing femoral component rotation.[157] Tibial component rotation is equally important for optimal patellofemoral tracking. The tibial tubercle is almost always present, even in complex revision cases, and serves as the landmark for tibial component rotation. The tibial component should be centered over the medial aspect of the tubercle, in most cases, to provide optimal rotation. The combined (tibial plus femoral) component rotation has been shown to correlate directly with the severity of patellofemoral complications.[30] Rhoads et al[155] showed that postoperative patellar tilt, rotation, and mediolateral translation increased when the femoral component was placed at a 10° internal rotation. Similar to the surgical malalignment, complications with patellar tracking could also arise from increased tibiofemoral conformity that is known to reduce the rotational motion of the femur with respect to the tibia during flexion.[25] A recent *in vivo* determination of the angular rotations of the patellar component in the sagittal plane showed that patellar tilt increases as a function of tibiofemoral flexion.[158] At higher tilt angles, the contact area is smaller, increasing the contact stresses and plastic deformation of the patellar component.

TECHNOLOGIES TO REDUCE BEARING SURFACE DAMAGE

Highly Cross-Linked UHMWPEs and Thermal Treatment

While infection and component loosening are the most common reasons for revision in total knees,[85,159-162] historically the primary concern for long-term device performance in TKR has been the mechanical failures initiated by excessive polyethylene damage through surface wear in the form of adhesive–abrasive wear and/or delamination. While the prevalence of adhesive/abrasive wear is thought to be less in total knees than in hips due to the more unidirectional articular motion in knees,[53,78] improvement in wear resistance of tibial knee inserts through enhancement of material properties was still the focus of changes to improve device performance *in vivo* in TKR over the last two decades. Delamination wear, on the other hand, is caused by fatigue cracking initiated in the subsurface region of the implants, where the maximum stresses occur.[163] Since oxidative embrittlement was a major factor in the progress of delamination, improvement in delamination resistance of polyethylene could be mainly achieved by reducing the oxidation potential in the long term. This section will discuss the evolution of highly cross-linked UHMWPEs to improve wear resistance in combination with early thermal treatment for the reduction and elimination of free radicals and oxidation potential.

Wear resistance of UHMWPE has been increased by radiation cross-linking of UHMWPE using doses higher than the typical sterilization dose of 25 to 40 kGy. There are several methods used in cross-linked UHMWPEs without antioxidants to eliminate and reduce the concentration of free radicals after radiation cross-linking (**Table 13-2**). The first is postirradiation melting, which allowed the melting and disordering of the crystalline regions and the escape and recombination of the free radicals trapped within these regions. Then, implants fabricated from this type of material were sterilized using nonradiation methods such as gas plasma or ethylene oxide sterilization. The second postirradiation thermal method to address the residual free radicals is annealing below the melting point of the polymer. This method results in a decrease in the free radicals of the irradiated polymer. This is because the crystal melting range of the polydisperse polyethylene crystals is between 100°C and about 150°C with the peak melting temperature at 137°C. Thus, about 10% of the free radicals remain after annealing at 130°C.[164,165] Another method is the mechanical deformation of the cross-linked material at a temperature below the melting point to enhance the recombination of residual free radicals via increased mobility in the crystal regions.[166] This method decreases the residual free radicals in irradiated UHMWPE compared to thermal annealing only; it also results in structural and mechanical anisotropy due to directional alignment of the polymer chains during deformation.[167]

The development of laboratory pin-on-disk wear testers[54,168] and joint simulators[169-174] to simulate the crossing, multidirectional motion of articular joint surfaces commensurate with the development of cross-linked UHMWPEs showed that wear resistance was correlated with increasing radiation dose with significant improvements around 100 kGy.[175,176] While it is difficult to compare data between *in vitro* simulator studies due to variations in the type of kinematics and knee design used as well as serum conditions, various studies have shown a reduction of 65% to 90% in knee wear compared to conventional, gamma-sterilized UHMWPEs.[42,177-180] Wang et al[181] used gamma irradiation to cross-link polyethylene with subsequent annealing at 50°C. In this study, flexion motion was limited to 22°, providing a wear rate of approximately 20 mm³ per million cycles in the control inserts that had been sterilized with ethylene oxide gas. The cross-linked inserts exhibited no change in wear rate between 25 and 50 kGy of radiation dose. At 75 kGy, the wear rate decreased by 40% and at 100 kGy by 50%. The study by Schmidig et al[182] also showed a reduction in adhesive–abrasive wear rate of UHMWPE tibial knee inserts after a 100-kGy irradiation from a gamma source with subsequent annealing at 135°C, leaving behind some residual free radicals. That study was carried out on a force-driven knee simulator and showed a wear rate of approximately 12 mg per million cycles with conventional inserts, which had been sterilized with 30 kGy of gamma irradiation. The wear rate of the cross-linked inserts (100 kGy) was 1.3 mg per million cycles. In the previously noted studies, neither of the tibial inserts was subjected to accelerated aging; therefore, the effect of the respective cross-linking methods used on delamination resistance of polyethylene was not revealed.

Knee simulator studies[183,184] had observed delamination *in vitro* using shelf-aged, gamma-sterilized polyethylene. Currier et al[184] also observed that the extent of subsurface damage increased with the severity of the subsurface oxidation. Preconditioning of knee inserts by accelerated aging to simulate 3 to 7 years of shelf aging for gamma-in-air-sterilized UHMWPEs resulted in clinically relevant pitting, delamination, and subsurface cracking using knee simulators.[184,185] Combining accelerated aging preconditioning of highly cross-linked tibial inserts,[186] a polyethylene that was crosslinked to a dose level of 95 kGy at an elevated temperature (125°C) using electron beam irradiation with subsequent melt annealing showed delamination resistance on the articular surfaces after 10 million cycles of simulated gait compared to aged conventional polyethylene inserts showing delamination in less than 5 million cycles.

Axial or rotational malalignment contributes to implant failure by increasing the stress on the bearing materials[163] and by compromising the ligamentous balance. Failure risk can be reduced by design features such as a medial eminence and anterior flare,[187] but the decrease in the fatigue strength of UHMWPE with increasing radiation dose and postirradiation melting remained a concern,[188] especially considering adverse conditions such as undesired cam-post impingement in PS designs. There are compressive and shear forces on UHMWPE during articulation, and there may be residual tensile stresses that arise from accumulated stress during repeated load cycles.[189] The reversal of stress direction causes fatigue cracks to initiate causing delamination.[50,126] The fatigue crack propagation resistance of cross-linked UHMWPEs is decreased with increasing radiation dose and also further if the materials are postirradiation melted due to a decrease in crystallinity.[190] The radiation dose of many knee components was maintained lower than the radiation doses used for optimum wear resistance due to concerns about this decrease (**Table 13-2**). *In vitro*, even under adverse conditions of malignment, there was no evidence of increased risk of damage for highly cross-linked UHMWPEs compared to conventional UHMWPEs.

The performance of highly cross-linked UHMWPEs has been satisfactory for the first decade of use despite some unexpected observation of oxidation.[191,192] Compared to conventional, gamma-sterilized UHMWPE and first-generation irradiated annealed UHMWPE,[193] which showed significantly high levels of oxidation at 5 years implantation, the oxidation observed in irradiated and melted UHMWPEs in the same early follow-up period is low.[194,195] The rate of oxidation of sequentially irradiated and annealed cross-linked UHMWPE is faster than in irradiated and melted UHMWPE and higher in total knee implants,[196] but the clinical effects of this oxidation, if any, are not yet clear.

In total hips, where radiographic methods to monitor *in vivo* implant migration and wear are more available and accurate than in knees, the use of highly cross-linked UHMWPEs has resulted in an 87% decrease in the incidence of periprosthetic osteolysis in the first decade of their use.[197] Most of the information of highly cross-linked total knee implants is still based on retrieval analyses due to the lack of adequate clinical studies. In addition, the small scale of the existing studies does not enable differentiation between the different types of cross-linked UHMWPEs. At short-term follow-up (up to 3 years), the performance of highly cross-linked UHMWPEs is largely comparable to conventional UHMWPE.[191,198-200] Evaluation of the incidence of osteolysis has also been limited for knees. One retrospective series of 200 surgeries performed by a single surgeon (100 irradiated and melted highly cross-linked, 100 conventional) with a minimum follow-up of 5.8 years (mean 6.3 years) showed reduction in radiolucency in the highly cross-linked (irradiated and melted) cohort when compared to conventional, gamma-sterilized UHMWPE.[201] Another study with a minimum follow-up of 2 years showed no revisions and no osteolysis for both irradiated/melted and conventional UHMWPEs.[202] Regarding concerns about fatigue resistance, in a prospective cohort of 114 knees comparing highly cross-linked, annealed UHMWPE and conventional UHMWPE with a mean follow-up of 5 years utilizing a PS knee design, there were no complications regarding polyethylene wear or failure.[203] There was a report of five post fractures (0.5%) using a highly cross-linked and melted UHMWPE (Prolong, high-flexion) in a series of 955 consecutive cases.[204] All patients with polyethylene fracture had flexion above 120°, which was hypothesized to be a contributing factor by the authors. In a randomized, control study comparing less cross-linked and highly cross-linked UHMWPEs in a bilateral setting in 183 patients (366 knees), there was 100% survival at a mean follow-up of 5.8 years using the same design (Gender Flex). Further follow-up is required to fully understand the benefits and risks of using highly cross-linked UHMWPEs in TKR as well as to enable understanding differences between formulations.

Antioxidant Stabilization of Cross-Linked UHMWPEs

Antioxidants are used routinely in commercial manufacturing processes for polyolefins and polyethylenes,[205] but antioxidants as additives in UHMWPE joint implants have only been used since 2007. This is mainly because previous additives such as carbon fibers or process by-products such as calcium stearate have led to undesirable consequences.[206,207] However, extensive *in vitro* testing of the clinically relevant mechanical, tribological, and biological consequences of incorporating the antioxidant vitamin E into radiation cross-linked UHMWPE[121,208-217] led the way to the development of UHMWPE implants containing antioxidants. Since 2007, several joint implants manufactured from vitamin E–containing UHMWPE (E1, Biomet, Warsaw, IN; E+, DJO Global, Vista, CA; E-CiMa, Corin, UK; Vivacit-E, Zimmer, Warsaw, IN; E-Syntial, Mako Surgical, Ft Lauderdale, FL) and one containing a synthetic phenolic antioxidant (AOX, Depuy, Warsaw, IN) have been introduced into the clinic (**Table 13-4**).

Vitamin E is the most abundant and effective chain-breaking (phenolic) antioxidant present in the human body.[218] The physiological role of vitamin E is to react with free radicals in cell membranes and protect polyunsaturated fatty acids from degradation due to oxidation.[219] Oxidation of polyunsaturated fatty acids results in active free radicals. The antioxidant activity of vitamin E (RRR-α-tocopherol *in vivo*) is due to hydrogen donation from the phenolic OH group on the chroman ring to a free radical on the oxidized lipid chain. Hydrogen abstraction results in a tocopheryl free radical, which can combine with another free radical. Therefore, tocopherol can theoretically prevent two peroxy free radicals from attacking other fatty acid chains and producing more free radicals.[220-222] Therefore, the cascading nature of oxidation is stopped, and oxidative damage can be prevented. The oxidation cascade in irradiated polyethylene can therefore be hindered in the presence of vitamin E through a similar mechanism.

Antioxidants can be incorporated into UHMWPE either by diffusion into consolidated stock forms[121] or by blending with UHMWPE powder followed by consolidation and processing together.[223,224] The free radical scavenging ability of vitamin E enables its antioxidant activity, but it also hinders cross-linking of UHMWPE if it is present during radiation.[225,226] Diffusing vitamin E into solid form, previously radiation cross-linked UHMWPE prevents this complication. It is possible to diffuse vitamin E in pure form[210] or by dissolving it in a solvent or by the aid of a supercritical fluid into UHMWPE.[227]

TABLE 13-4   Current Applications of Highly Crosslinked Polyethylenes in Total Knee Replacements

TRADE Name	Manufacturer (Location)	Vitamin E Content (%)	Radiation Dose (kGy[a])	Radiation Type	Thermal Treatment	Sterilization Method	Total radiation Dose Level (kGy)
E1	Zimmer Biomet (Warsaw, IN)	~0.7	100	E-beam	Postdiffusion annealing	Gamma irradiation	~125
VivacitE	Zimmer Biomet (Warsaw, IN)	>0.2	>100	E-beam	Elevated temperature irradiation	E-beam irradiation	>100
AOX	Depuy Synthes (Warsaw, IN)	0.075	75-80	Gamma	N/A	Gamma irradiation	~75
E-Plus	DJO Surgical	0.1	Unknown	Gamma	N/A	Gamma irradiation	
E-CiMa	Corin Ltd	0.1	120 kGy	Gamma	Mechanical deformation followed by annealing	EtO	120

EtO, ethylene oxide.
[a]10 kilograys (kGy) = 1 Mrad.

Previous studies showed that melting the crystalline regions of the polymer after cross-linking prevented efficient recrystallization upon recooling and thus decreased the mechanical strength of the cross-linked polymer.[190] During diffusion, the process temperature was limited to below the melting point of the cross-linked polymer, which is about 137°C to 140°C. A two-step method was developed in which the first step comprised doping the radiation cross-linked UHMWPE in pure vitamin E to obtain a high surface concentration in a relatively short amount of time and the second step comprised homogenization of the high surface concentration into the component at a high temperature without vitamin E.[210] This way, an approximately 0.7 wt% vitamin E was obtained uniformly throughout the implant components.[228]

The implants machined out of the vitamin E–diffused UHMWPE are terminally sterilized using gamma irradiation. While this terminal step does not add any significant cross-linking to the material, there is some amount of vitamin E grafted onto the polymer.[229] Thus, terminal gamma irradiation may immobilize part of the antioxidant in the polymer, preventing against the loss of oxidation resistance in the long term.[230]

In simulator studies using both hip and knee implants, the wear rate of this highly cross-linked, vitamin E–diffused, and terminally sterilized UHMWPE was 70% to 90% less than conventional, gamma-sterilized UHMWPE[208,211,215,217] and was similar to that of clinically successful highly cross-linked UHMWPEs.[231,232] Their mechanical and fatigue strength was improved compared to the previous generation of irradiated and melted UHMWPE due to the elimination of postirradiation melting for oxidation resistance.[121]

A "real-time" aging study, where the irradiated, vitamin E–diffused, and terminally gamma-sterilized UHMWPE was placed in water at 40°C for 3 years, showed small amounts of surface oxidation and no changes in the mechanical properties.[213] This environment was comparable in oxygen concentration to the synovial fluid and also in temperature to an articulating joint. The small amount of surface oxidation was attributed to the oxidation reactions during radiation cross-linking before vitamin E was introduced into the polymer. The fast decay of the residual free radicals[209] and the lack of accumulation of hydroperoxides corroborated that vitamin E has hindered oxidative reactions in irradiated UHMWPE despite the presence of detectable free radicals.

Blending of the UHMWPE resin powder with vitamin E before further processing provides an easy alternative to the time-dependent diffusion of vitamin E into cross-linked UHMWPE. In fact, due to demand from the orthopedic device companies and stock consolidators, the manufacturer of the medical grade UHMWPE resin (Celanese) has been providing a vitamin E–blended powder at 0.1 wt%. Using this method, the polymer powder is blended with the antioxidant; the blend is consolidated into solid form products and preforms (slightly oversized versions of implants for processing) and further cross-linked by radiation at the desired dose. Initial studies investigating the feasibility of this method focused on improving the oxidation resistance of conventional, gamma-sterilized UHMWPE.[223,233] However, the success of high-dose cross-linking in terms of decreasing wear and osteolysis in UHMWPE implants has prompted the use of this method in highly cross-linked UHMWPEs.

Because vitamin E is a free radical scavenger and prevents cross-linking in UHMWPE when present during irradiation,[225,226] the vitamin E concentration in the blend as well as the radiation dose had to be modified to achieve high cross-link density. If the cross-link density and the commensurate wear rate of a 100-kGy irradiated, virgin UHMWPE without additives is the benchmark, the vitamin E concentration in the blend is limited to 0.3 wt% because cross-linking is saturated above this concentration.[226] In addition, even when a lower vitamin E concentration is used, such as 0.1 wt%, the radiation dose has to be increased compared to that used with a virgin UHMWPE to achieve the desired cross-link density.

The grafting of vitamin E onto the polymer is more extensive in vitamin E–blended UHMWPE because the terminal radiation dose to which vitamin E is exposed to is higher than the sterilization dose.[234] Also, the grafted amount increases with decreasing vitamin E concentration[235] such that for low vitamin E concentrations in the blend, such as 0.1 or 0.2 wt%, almost all of the vitamin E is immobilized and protected against migration.

For blended UHMWPEs, it has been shown *in vitro* that even trace amounts of the antioxidant in the polymer can increase the oxidation resistance of irradiated UHMWPE.[236] The clinical benefit of this increased oxidation resistance is not yet clear. Vitamin E–blended UHMWPE formulations have been in clinical use only in the last several years; therefore, there is little information yet on their clinical performance. There is also a synthetic antioxidant-stabilized, blended, and radiation cross-linked UHMWPE (AOX; **Table 13-4**). This material uses a 0.075 wt% concentration of the antioxidant (COVERNOX; medical grade pentaerythritol tetrakis[3-(3,5-di-tert-butyl-4-hydroxyphenyl) propionate][237] with a terminal gamma cross-linking/sterilization dose of 75 to 80 kGy.[238,239]

Since radiation-induced free radicals trapped in UHMWPE are a strong cause of oxidation in joint implants, their reduction or elimination from vitamin E–containing UHMWPEs can also increase the oxidation resistance of the polymer by preserving the antioxidant for long-term *in vivo* use. The mechanical deformation of irradiated UHMWPE followed by annealing below the melting point has been shown to eliminate detectable residual free radicals in virgin UHMWPE without antioxidants.[240,241] Mechanical deformation can induce anisotropic changes in UHMWPE where the mechanical strength in a preferred direction can be higher due to orientation[167]; however, the annealing step after deformation allows dimensional recovery and isotropic properties in the final implants.[242] A vitamin E–blended, radiation cross-linked, and mechanically deformed UHMWPE is expected to have high oxidative resistance by two mechanisms: incorporation of vitamin E and decrease in the free radical burden by deformation.[243] Since this material is not melted after irradiation, it is also expected to have mechanical properties comparable to irradiated but not melted, highly cross-linked UHMWPEs.

Another method by which the free radicals in radiation cross-linked, vitamin E–blended UHMWPE can be decreased is irradiation at elevated temperatures.[243] Increasing irradiation temperature, especially close to the melting point, not only enables free radical elimination

at the same time as cross-linking but also increases cross-link efficiency compared to irradiation at ambient temperature.[234] This method is only compatible with electron beam irradiation as accurate control of dose; dose rate and using a higher temperature during irradiation are only possible with this method. In addition to increased cross-link efficiency and commensurate lower wear rates, the grafting efficiency of vitamin E into UHMWPE is also higher. The implication is that slightly higher vitamin E concentrations can be used with lower radiation doses to obtain good wear resistance and improved oxidation resistance.

There are now a variety of antioxidant-stabilized UHMWPEs available for use in TKR (**Table 13-4**). Antioxidant-stabilized UHMWPEs have been available in total knees since 2008; thus, clinical follow-up information is scarce. In a retrieval study of 25 tibial inserts with implantation life of up to 3 years, Currier et al[244] studied the oxidation observed in antioxidant-stabilized UHMWPEs including different types of vitamin E–containing materials (E1, and Vivacit-E, Zimmer Biomet, Warsaw, IN) as well as synthetic hindered phenol-containing material (AOX, Depuy Synthes, Warsaw, IN). They showed that the antioxidants were effective in reducing oxidation levels compared to highly cross-linked UHMWPEs without antioxidants for the study period. Another study of 19 retrievals studying all three materials with implantation period up to 3.5 years, Ponzio et al[245] observed no clinical difference between the antioxidant materials and cross-linked and remelted UHMWPEs without antioxidants; however, they noted that the surface damage modes included burnishing more frequently and pitting and scratching more frequently.

Since the use of antioxidant-stabilized UHMWPEs has now become widespread especially in total hip arthroplasty, there are a number of investigations into their possible effects on the osteolytic potential of UHMWPE particles containing antioxidants.[214,246-251] These *in vitro* and preclinical studies indicate generally that the osteolytic potential of cross-linked UHMWPE particles containing antioxidants is low. Further, the antioxidants may decrease the osteolytic potential of UHMWPE particles and may have a favorable role to play in reducing oxidative processes in bone metabolism. However, a clear evaluation of these proposed effects can only be possible with clinical studies.

Surface Grafting of UHMWPE Using 2-Methacryloxyethyl Phosphorylcholine

One of the innate characteristics of articular cartilage is its superior lubricity. The dynamics between the osmotic pressure provided by the water in the cartilaginous network and the release of some of the free water from the network under load is partly responsible for the great wear and load-bearing properties of cartilage.[252] In contrast, the wear of UHMWPE is governed by surface-on-surface contact with little load sharing from a lubrication layer on the surface. Recently, a surface coating of UHMWPE comprising a phospholipid has been proposed to create a hydrophilic layer on the surface of UHMWPE, which can swell in water or synovial fluid and can create a fluid lubrication layer similar to cartilage under load.[253]

The incorporation and binding of 2-methacryloxyethyl phosphorylcholine (MPC) with the UHMWPE on the surface is enabled through a UV-mediated reaction.[254,255] In addition to the possible effects of wear reduction of the surface, MPC grafting was shown to reduce biological reactions *in vitro*[255] and was initially designed with the intention of reducing the osteolytic potential of polyethylene wear particles.[253] This method results in a roughly 100 nm-thick layer of the phospholipid on the surface, which could be detected by a cross-sectional transmission electron microscope image. In addition, contact angle measurements showed that the resulting surface was predominantly hydrophilic (water contact angle 'theta' <20°) in contrast to the native UHMWPE surface, which is very hydrophobic (theta ~70°).

Despite the nanometer-level thickness of the surface layer, the coated surfaces were reported to have lower wear in a hip simulator study compared to the base material, which was 75-kGy irradiated virgin (no antioxidant) UHMWPE that had been annealed at 130°C, presumably to decrease the concentration of free radicals.[256]

The main concern with any coating in this load-bearing application is its shear and scratch resistance due to the presence of high stresses and third-body particulate in the clinical environment. The wear of coated acetabular liners did not change over 5 million cycles (MC) in a routine knee simulator test in clean serum, suggesting longevity of the bearing under routine conditions.[257] MPC grafting of a 0.1 wt% vitamin E–containing, cross-linked UHMWPE has also been reported using a similar method.[258] The Japanese implant manufacturer Kyocera Medical introduced acetabular liners made out of this coated material for total hip arthroplasty applications in 2011 (Aquala) in Japan and this technology is currently under review with the FDA for use in hips. In knees, a vitamin E–stabilized UHMWPE (E-MAX; **Table 13-3**) without MPC grafting is available at this time from this company.

Ceramic and Ceramicized Femoral Components

One of the technologies introduced in knee implants in the last decade is a ceramicized surface for articulation against UHMWPE (Oxinium, Smith & Nephew, Memphis, TN).[259] The metallic alloy is made of zirconium and niobium followed by oxidation of the surface.[260,261] It was developed with the hypothesis of reducing

UHMWPE wear and damage caused by the roughening of the CoCrMo surfaces and also with the benefit of providing the ductility of metal in the bulk and hardness of ceramic on the surface for improved wear resistance.[261]

In a number of *in vitro* knee simulation studies, this oxidized zirconium surface showed better wear rates and resulted in general in less damage on the UHMWPE surfaces when compared to CoCrMo alternatives.[262,263]

In a retrieval study of 11 PS knee implants matched with oxidized zirconium femoral components, the UHMWPE surfaces showed less damage compared to a matched set articulating against CoCrMo.[264] In a community registry of nearly 3000 "premium" TKAs including mobile bearings, oxidized zirconium, and cross-linked polyethylene surfaces and high-flexion designs, there was no difference in revision rate at 7 to 8 years when compared to "traditional" TKAs.[265] In a large total joint replacement registry (Kaiser Permanente) of over 67,000 TKAs, zirconium oxide surfaces coupled with cross-linked polyethylenes had similar all-cause revision rates and risk of revision compared to "traditional" CoCr surfaces articulating against conventional polyethylene in the early period up to 4.9 years.[266] In the longest clinical cohort to date, the Australian Registry reported 12-year outcomes comparing the same knee design with Oxinium and CoCr surfaces for over 17,000 patients and about 6000 Oxinium knees[267]; although the hazard ratio was not found to be higher, the overall revision rate was higher with the Oxinium cohort (7.7% vs. 4.8%).

In addition to oxidized zirconium, there are alternatively coated components including titanium nitride coatings, which were developed to increase the abrasion resistance of metallic surfaces, especially in mobile-bearing components[268] (for example, ACS, Implantcast; Persona, Zimmer Biomet; Foundation, DJO Surgical) which have become available in the last few years. The follow-up has been reported in small cohorts up to 92 months with acceptable results and no unexpected complications.[269-273] Zirconium nitride (ZrN) coatings are available (Vega Knee, Aesculap) and silicon nitride (SiN) coatings are also available in other implants in the spine and hip and being considered in TKR.[274]

Other Technologies

Polyetheretherketone-Bearing Surfaces

Poly(aryl-ether-ether-ketone) (PEEK) is a high temperature, injection moldable, semi-crystalline polymeric material evaluated for and used in various medical applications including widespread use as spinal cages. Starting in the late 1990s when oxidative degradation and wear of gamma-in-air-sterilized UHMWPE resulted in severe damage to joint implants, carbon fiber–reinforced PEEK composite materials (CFR-PEEK) have also been evaluated as candidate-bearing materials for joint replacement.[275-277] For a review of the grades, processing, structure–property relationship, and history of PEEK materials in medical devices, we refer the reader to Ref. [275].

The elastic modulus of neat PEEK is close to that of UHMWPE, but it can be substantially increased by reinforcement with carbon fibers.[278] CFR-PEEK was originally developed for its increased elastic modulus in efforts to match the mechanical stiffness of bone and in the evaluation of PEEK as an alternative to metallic implants such as femoral stems and fixation plates.[278] The wear rate of CFR-PEEK was comparable to that of metallic or ceramic surfaces articulating against conventional UHMWPE in laboratory wear studies.[279] In studies looking at cylinder-on-flat or low conforming total knee articulation designs, the wear of PEEK as an alternative to UHMWPE was high.[276,280]

Although metal or ceramic-on-PEEK couples have shown good wear resistance *in vitro*, the increased wear resistance of UHMWPE by radiation cross-linking redirected the focus on finding a more wear-resistant couple using a new material in the articulation. In addition, the historic failure of carbon-reinforced polyethylene (Poly II,[206]) and the catastrophic clinical complications seen with metal-on-metal articulations proposed to increase the wear resistance of total hip replacements[281-285] may have contributed to decreased interest in PEEK materials as a replacement for UHMWPE.

Recently, there has been growing interest in looking at PEEK materials as an alternative to cobalt-chrome to replace the femoral component in TKA[286-288] due to the possibility of matching the mechanical stiffness of natural bone, the ease of manufacturing and its potential in decreasing adverse tissue reactions caused by metal ions. There is an active clinical trial (NCT03224689) in its recruitment stage to evaluate the safety and performance of a PEEK-OPTIMA (Invibio, Conshohocken, PA) femoral component in a total knee design (Freedom Total Knee, MAXX Orthopedics).

CONCLUSIONS AND FUTURE OUTLOOK

The last two decades have brought significant improvements to total knee implants to decrease bearing surface damage, particularly in the processing methods of the UHMWPE-bearing surface. The combination of radiation cross-linking and antioxidant stabilization is promising in decreasing adhesive/abrasive wear and oxidative damage, including delamination. In the light of these material improvements, the old debate of implant conformity versus implant constraint can be settled. As shown in this book chapter and other recent reviews, dished and flat tibial inserts work equally well in terms of surface damage when the original (as manufactured) polyethylene quality is maintained. Further reduction in surface wear can be achieved by optimizing implants and surgical procedures for the various activities of daily life, not just gait. This has been difficult in the past because wear testing was limited to *in vitro* experiments. However, more

recently, more and more in silico programs are predicting polyethylene wear rates with surprising accuracy. This will allow the investigation of several tens of variables in the time it took to conduct a single experiment on the simulator.

The future may also hold changes in femoral component material. While cobalt-chromium alloy has been shown good wear characteristics against abrasion, its corrosion resistance under tribological stress is currently debated. It will be exciting to see in the coming years if the ongoing evaluation of PEEK as a metal-free candidate for the femoral condyles articulating against improved polyethylenes can reduce adverse local tissue reactions linked to metal ion release.

REFERENCES

1. Sharkey PF, Hozack WJ, Rothman RH, Shastri S, Jacoby SM. Insall Award paper. Why are total knee arthroplasties failing today? *Clin Orthop Relat Res*. 2002;404:7-13.
2. Sharkey PF, Lichstein PM, Shen C, Tokarski AT, Parvizi J. Why are total knee arthroplasties failing today–has anything changed after 10 years? *J Arthroplasty*. 2014;29(9):1774-1778.
3. AJRR. *Annual Report on Hip and Knee Arthroplasty Data*. Rosemont, Illinois; 2018.
4. Gallo J, Goodman SB, Konttinen YT, Wimmer MA, Holinka M. Osteolysis around total knee arthroplasty: a review of pathogenetic mechanisms. *Acta Biomater*. 2013;9(9):8046-8058.
5. Jacobs JJ, Roebuck KA, Archibeck M, Hallab NJ, Glant TT. Osteolysis: basic science. *Clin Orthop Relat Res*. 2001;393:71-77.
6. Robinson EJ, Mulliken BD, Bourne RB, Rorabeck CH, Alvarez C. Catastrophic osteolysis in total knee replacement – a report of 17 cases. *Clin Orthop Relat Res*. 1995;(321):98-105.
7. Rorabeck CH, Smith PN. Results of revision total knee arthroplasty in the face of significant bone deficiency. *Orthop Clin N Am*. 1998;29(2):361-371.
8. Deburge A, Guepar. Guepar hinge prosthesis: complications and results with two years' follow-up. *Clin Orthop Relat Res*. 1976;(120):47-53.
9. Robinson RP. The early innovators of today's resurfacing condylar knees. *J Arthroplasty*. 2005;20(1):2-26.
10. Gunston FH. Polycentric knee arthroplasty. Prosthetic simulation of normal knee movement. *J Bone Joint Surg Br*. 1971;53(2):272-277.
11. Insall J, Ranawat CS, Scott WN, Walker P. Total condylar knee replacement: preliminary report. *Clin Orthop Relat Res*. 1976;(120):149-154.
12. Insall JN, Lachiewicz PF, Burstein AH. The posterior stabilized condylar prosthesis: a modification of the total condylar design. Two to four-year clinical experience. *J Bone Joint Surg Am Vol*. 1982;64(9):1317-1323.
13. Insall JN, Ranawat CS, Aglietti P, Shine J. A comparison of four models of total knee-replacement prostheses. *J Bone Joint Surg Am Vol*. 1976;58(6):754-765.
14. Scott RD. Prosthetic replacement of the patellofemoral joint. *Orthop Clin N Am*. 1979;10(1):129-137.
15. Bourne RB, Rorabeck CH, Vaz M, Kramer J, Hardie R, Robertson D. Resurfacing versus not resurfacing the patella during total knee replacement. *Clin Orthop Relat Res*. 1995;(321):156-161.
16. Stulberg SD, Stulberg BN, Hamati Y, Tsao A. Failure mechanisms of metal-backed patellar components. *Clin Orthop Relat Res*. 1988;(236):88-105.
17. Kajino A, Yoshino S, Kameyama S, Kohda M, Nagashima S. Comparison of the results of bilateral total knee arthroplasty with and without patellar replacement for rheumatoid arthritis – a follow-up note. *J Bone Joint Surg Am Vol*. 1997;79A(4):570-574.

18. Barrack RL, Wolfe MW, Waldman DA, Milicic M, Bertot AJ, Myers L. Resurfacing of the patella in total knee arthroplasty – a prospective, randomized, double-blind study. *J Bone Joint Surg Am Vol.* 1997;79A(8):1121-1131.

19. Longo UG, Ciuffreda M, Mannering N, D'Andrea V, Cimmino M, Denaro V. Patellar resurfacing in total knee arthroplasty: systematic review and meta-analysis. *J Arthroplasty.* 2018;33(2):620-632.

20. Cameron HU, Hunter GA. Failure in total knee arthroplasty: mechanisms, revisions, and results. *Clin Orthop Relat Res.* 1982;(170):141-146.

21. Laskin RS. Management of the patella during revision total knee replacement arthroplasty. *Orthop Clin N Am.* 1998;29(2):355-360.

22. Rand JA. Patellar resurfacing in total knee arthroplasty. *Clin Orthop Relat Res.* 1990;(260):110-117.

23. Brick GW, Scott RD. The patellofemoral component of total knee arthroplasty. *Clin Orthop Relat Res.* 1988;(231):163-178.

24. Doolittle KH II, Turner RH. Patellofemoral problems following total knee arthroplasty. *Orthop Rev.* 1988;17(7):696-702.

25. Grace JN, Rand JA. Patellar instability after total knee arthroplasty. *Clin Orthop Relat Res.* 1988;(237):184-189.

26. Hofmann GO, Hagena FW. Pathomechanics of the femoropatellar joint following total knee arthroplasty. *Clin Orthop Relat Res.* 1987;(224):251-259.

27. Ritter MA, Pierce MJ, Zhou H, Meding JB, Faris PM, Keating EM. Patellar complications (total knee arthroplasty) – Effect of lateral release and thickness. *Clin Orthop Relat Res.* 1999;(367):149-157.

28. Harwin SF. Patellofemoral complications in symmetrical total knee arthroplasty. *J Arthroplast.* 1998;13(7):753-762.

29. Lewonowski K, Dorr LD, McPherson EJ, Huber G, Wan Z. Medialization of the patella in total knee arthroplasty. *J Arthroplast.* 1997;12(2):161-167.

30. Berger RA, Crossett LS, Jacobs JJ, Rubash HE. Malrotation causing patellofemoral complications after total knee arthroplasty. *Clin Orthop Relat Res.* 1998;(356):144-153.

31. Collier JP, McNamara JL, Surprenant VA, Jensen RE, Surprenant HP. All-polyethylene patellar components are not the answer. *Clin Orthop Relat Res.* 1991(273):198-203.

32. Hsu HP, Walker PS. Wear and deformation of patellar components in total knee arthroplasty. *Clin Orthop Relat Res.* 1989;(246):260-265.

33. Cameron HU, Jung YB. Noncemented, porous ingrowth knee prosthesis - the 3-year to 8-year results. *Can J Surg.* 1993;36(6):560-564.

34. Kurtz S. A primer on UHMWPE. In: Kurtz S, ed. *UHMWPE Biomaterials Handbook*: New York: Elsevier; 2009.

35. Coughlan J, Hug D. Ultrahigh molecular weight polyethylene. In: Mark HF, Bikales NM, Overberger CG, Menges G, eds. *Encyclopedia of Polymer Science and Engineering*. New York: John Wiley & Sons; 1986.

36. Charnley J. *Low Friction Arthroplasty of the Hip*. London: Springer-Verlag; 1979.

37. Kurtz S. From ethylene gas to UHMWPE component: the process of producing orthopaedic implants. In: Kurtz S, ed. *UHMWPE Biomaterials Handbook*: New York: Elsevier; 2009:7-19.

38. Won CH, Rohatgi S, Kraay MJ, Goldberg VM, Rimnac CM. Effect of resin type and manufacturing method on wear of polyethylene tibial components. *Clin Orthop Relat Res.* 2000;(376):161-171.

39. Muratoglu OK, Jasty M, Harris WH. *High resolution synchrotron infra-red microscopy of the structure of fusion defects in UHMWPE*. In: *23rd Annual Meeting of Society for Biomaterials*. New Orleans, LA: Society for Biomaterials; 1997.

40. Kurtz SM, Muratoglu OK, Evans M, Edidin AA. Advances in the processing, sterilization, and crosslinking of ultra- high molecular weight polyethylene for total joint arthroplasty. *Biomaterials.* 1999;20(18):1659-1688.

41. Truss R, Han KS, Wallace JF, Geil PH. Cold compaction molding and sintering of UHMWPE. *J Appl Polym Sci.* 1981;26:79-88.

42. Muratoglu OK, Bragdon CR, Jasty M, O'Connor DO, VonKnoch RS, Harris WH. Knee-simulator testing of conventional and cross-linked polyethylene tibial inserts. *J Arthroplasty.* 2004;19(7):887-897.

43. Wasielewski RC, Galante JO, Leighty RM, Natarajan RN, Rosenberg AG. Wear patterns on retrieved polyethylene tibial inserts and their relationship to technical considerations during total knee arthroplasty. *Clin Orthop Relat Res.* 1994;(299):31-43.

44. Cadambi A, Engh GA, Dwyer KA, Vinh TN. Osteolysis of the distal femur after total knee arthroplasty. *J Arthroplast.* 1994;9(6):579-594.

45. Crowninshield RD, Wimmer MA, Jacobs JJ, Rosenberg AG. Clinical performance of contemporary tibial polyethylene components. *J Arthroplasty.* 2006;21(5):754-761.

46. Puloski SK, McCalden RW, MacDonald SJ, Rorabeck CH, Bourne RB. Tibial post wear in posterior stabilized total knee arthroplasty. An unrecognized source of polyethylene debris. *J Bone Joint Surg Am Vol.* 2001;83-A(3):390-397.

47. Mikulak SA, Mahoney OM, delaRosa MA, Schmalzried TP. Loosening and osteolysis with the press-fit condylar posterior-cruciate-substituting total knee replacement. *J Bone Joint Surg Am Vol.* 2001;83-A(3):398-403.

48. McKellop HA. The lexicon of polyethylene wear in artificial joints. *Biomaterials.* 2007;28(34):5049-5057.

49. Bartel DL, Rawlinson JJ, Burstein AH, Ranawat CS, Flynn WF. Stresses in polyethylene components of contemporary total knee replacements. *Clin Orthop Relat Res.* 1995;(317):76-82.

50. Bartel DL, Bicknell VL, Wright TM. The effect of conformity, thickness, and material on stresses in ultra-high molecular weight components for total joint replacement. *J Bone Joint Surg Am Vol.* 1986;68(7):1041-1051.

51. Pooley CM, Tabor D. Friction and molecular structure: the behavior of some thermoplastics. *Proc R Soc Lond.* 1972;329A:251-274.

52. Bragdon CR, O'Connor DO, Lowenstein JD, Jasty M, Syniuta WD. The importance of multidirectional motion on the wear of polyethylene. *Proc Instn Mech Engrs.* 1995;210:157-165.

53. Wang A. A unified theory of wear for ultra-high molecular weight polyethylene in multi-directional sliding. *Wear.* 2001;248:38-47.

54. Bragdon CR, O'Connor DO, Lowenstein JD, Jasty M, Biggs SA, Harris WH. A new pin-on-disk wear testing method for simulating wear of polyethylene on cobalt-chrome alloy in total hip arthroplasty. *J Arthroplasty.* 2001;16(5):658-665.

55. Wimmer MA, Andriacchi TP, Natarajan RN, et al. A striated pattern of wear in ultrahigh-molecular-weight polyethylene components of miller-galante total knee arthroplasty. *J Arthroplast.* 1998;13(1):8-16.

56. Rad EM. *Volumetric Wear Assessment and Characterization of Striated Pattern of Retrieved UHMWPE Tibial Inserts.* Northwestern: The University of Illinois at Chicago (UIC); 2015.

57. Wasielewski RC, Galante JO, Leighty RM, Natarajan RN, Rosenberg AG. Wear patterns on retrieved polyethylene tibial inserts and their relationship to technical considerations during total knee arthroplasty. *Clin Orthop Relat Res.* 1994;299:31-43.

58. Hood RW, Wright TM, Burstein AH. Retrieval analysis of total knee prostheses: a method and its application to 48 total condylar prostheses. *J Biomed Mater Res.* 1983;17(5):829-842.

59. Knowlton CB, Wimmer MA. *Design-dependent wear scar symmetry on polyethylene inserts in bilateral total knee replacements.* In: *Transactions of the Annual Meeting of the Orthopaedic Research Society (ORS).* Austin, Texas; 2019.

60. Galetz MC, Glatzel U. Molecular deformation mechanisms in UHMWPE during tribological loading in artificial joints. *Tribol Lett.* 2010;38(1):1-13.

61. Knowlton CB, Bhutani P, Wimmer MA. Relationship of surface damage appearance and volumetric wear in retrieved TKR polyethylene liners. *J Biomed Mater Res B Appl Biomater.* 2017;105(7):2053-2059.

62. Harman MK, DesJardins J, Benson L, Banks SA, LaBerge M, Hodge WA. Comparison of polyethylene tibial insert damage from in vivo function and in vitro wear simulation. *J Orthop Res.* 2009;27(4):540-548.

63. Cameron HU. Patellar wear patients in total knee replacements. *Acta Orthop Belg.* 1991;57(2):144-146.

64. Pourzal R, Knowlton CB, Hall DJ, Laurent MP, Urban RM, Wimmer MA. How does wear rate compare in well-functioning total hip and knee replacements? A postmortem polyethylene liner study. *Clin Orthop Relat Res.* 2016;474(8):1867-1875.

65. Knowlton CB, Wimmer MA. An autonomous mathematical reconstruction to effectively measure volume loss on retrieved polyethylene tibial inserts. *J Biomed Mater Res B Appl Biomater.* 2013;101(3):449-457.

66. Goodman SB, Huie P, Song Y, et al. Cellular profile and cytokine production at prosthetic interfaces. Study of tissues retrieved from revised hip and knee replacements. *J Bone Joint Surg Br.* 1998;80(3):531-539.

67. Campbell P, Ma S, Yeom B, McKellop H, Schmalzried TP, Amstutz HC. Isolation of predominantly submicron-sized UHMWPE wear particles from periprosthetic tissues. *J Biomed Mater Res.* 1995;29(1):127-131.

68. Schmalzried TP, Campbell P, Schmitt AK, Brown IC, Amstutz HC. Shapes and dimensional characteristics of polyethylene wear particles generated in vivo by total knee replacements compared to total hip replacements. *J Biomed Mater Res.* 1997;38(3):203-210.

69. Shanbhag AS, Bailey HO, Hwang DS, Cha CW, Eror NG, Rubash HE. Quantitative analysis of ultrahigh molecular weight polyethylene (UHMWPE) wear debris associated with total knee replacements. *J Biomed Mater Res.* 2000;53(1):100-110.

70. Galvin AL, Jennings LM, Tipper JL, Ingham E, Fisher J. Wear and creep of highly crosslinked polyethylene against cobalt chrome and ceramic femoral heads. *Proc Inst Mech Eng H.* 2010;224(10):1175-1183.

71. Peters PC Jr, Engh GA, Dwyer KA, Vinh TN. Osteolysis after total knee arthroplasty without cement. *J Bone Joint Surg Am Vol.* 1992;74(6):864-876.

72. Utzschneider S, Paulus A, Datz JC, et al. Influence of design and bearing material on polyethylene wear particle generation in total knee replacement. *Acta Biomater.* 2009;5(7):2495-2502.

73. Haider H, Joel NW, Beau SK. *For lower wear of total knee replacements, is higher or lower contact area better?.* In: *Transactions of the Annual Meeting of the American Academy of Orthopaedic Surgeons (AAOS).* New Orleans, LA; 2018.

74. Dennis DA, Komistek RD, Colwell CE. In vivo anteroposterior femorotibial translation of total knee arthroplasty: a multicenter analysis. *Clin Orthop Relat Res.* 1998;(356):47-57.

75. Banks BA, Markovich GD, Hodge WA. In vivo kinematics of cruciate-retaining and -substituting knee arthroplasties. *J Arthroplasty.* 1997;12(3):297-304.

76. Hirakawa K, Bauer TW, Yamaguchi M, Stulberg BN, Wilde AH. Relationship between wear debris particles and polyethylene surface damage in primary total knee arthroplasty. *J Arthroplast.* 1999;14(2):165-171.

77. Knowlton CB. *A Gait-dependent Model of Wear from Retrieved Polyethylene Components of TKR.* Chicago: The University of Illinois at Chicago (UIC); 2019.

78. Schwenke T, Wimmer M. Cross-shear in metal-on-polyethylene articulation of orthopaedic implants and its relationship to wear. *Wear.* 2013;301(1-2):727-734.

79. Kawanabe K, Clarke IC, Tamura J, et al. Effects of A-P translation and rotation on the wear of UHMWPE in a total knee joint simulator. *J Biomed Mater Res.* 2001;54(3):400-406.

80. Wang A, Sun DC, Stark C, Dumbleton JH. Wear mechanisms of UHMWPE in total joint replacements. *Wear.* 1995;181-183:241-249.

81. Muratoglu OK, Bragdon CR, O'Connor DO, Jasty M, Harris WH. A highly crosslinked, melted UHMWPE: expanded potential for total joint arthroplasty. In: Rieker C, Oberholzer S, Wyss U, eds. *World Tribology Forum in Arthroplasty.* Bern: Hans Huber; 2001:245-262.

82. Dennis DA, Komistek RD, Walker SA, Cheal EJ, Stiehl JB. Femoral condylar lift-off in vivo in total knee arthroplasty. *J Bone Joint Surg Br.* 2001;83(1):33-39.

83. Miller MC, Berger RA, Petrella AJ, Karmas A, Rubash HE. Optimizing femoral component rotation in total knee arthroplasty. *Clin Orthop Relat Res.* 2001;392:38-45.

84. Maiti R, Cowie RM, Fisher J, Jennings LM. The influence of malalignment and ageing following sterilisation by gamma irradiation in an inert atmosphere on the wear of ultra-high-molecular-weight polyethylene in patellofemoral replacements. *Proc Inst Mech Eng H.* 2017;231(7):634-642.

85. Berger RA, Rosenberg AG, Barden RM, Sheinkop MB, Jacobs JJ, Galante JO. Long-term followup of the Miller-Galante total knee replacement. *Clin Orthop Relat Res.* 2001;388:58-67.

86. Theiss SM, Kitziger KJ, Lotke PS, Lotke PA. Component design affecting patellofemoral complications after total knee arthroplasty. *Clin Orthop Relat Res.* 1996;(326):183-187.

87. Premnath V, Harris WH, Jasty M, Merrill EW. Gamma sterilization of UHMWPE articular implants: an analysis of the oxidation problem. *Biomaterials.* 1996;17:1741-1753.

88. Kurtz S. In vivo oxidation of UHMWPE. In: Kurtz S, ed. *UHMWPE Biomaterials Handbook.* New York: Academic Press; 2009:325-340.

89. Collier JP, Sperling DK, Currier JH, Sutula LC, Saum KA, Mayor MB. Impact of gamma sterilization on clinical performance of polyethylene in the knee. *J. Arthroplasty.* 1996;11(4):377-389.

90. Kurtz S. Packaging and sterilization of UHMWPE. In: Kurtz S, ed. *UHMWPE Biomaterials Handbook.* London: Elsevier; 2009:21-30.

91. Roe RJ, Grood ES, Shastri R, Gosselin CA, Noyes FR. Effect of radiation sterilization and aging on ultrahigh molecular weight polyethylene. *J Biomed Mater Res.* 1981;15(2):209-230.

92. Rose RM, Goldfarb EV, Ellis E, Crugnola AN. Radiation sterilization and the wear rate of polyethylene. *J Orthop Res.* 1984;2(4):393-400.

93. Eyerer P, Ke YC. Property changes of UHMW polyethylene hip cup endoprostheses during implantation. *J Biomed Mater Res.* 1984;18(9):1137-1151.

94. Eyerer P, Kurth M, McKellup HA, Mittlmeier T. Characterization of UHMWPE hip cups run on joint simulators. *J Biomed Mater Res.* 1987;21(3):275-291.

95. Williams IR, Mayor MB, Collier JP. The impact of sterilization method on wear in knee arthroplasty. *Clin Orthop Relat Res.* 1998;356:170-180.

96. White SE, Paxson RD, Tanner MG, Whiteside LA. Effects of sterilization on wear in total knee arthroplasty. *Clin Orthop Relat Res.* 1996;(331):164-171.

97. Sutula LC, Collier JP, Saum KA, et al. Impact of gamma sterilization on clinical performance of polyethylene in the hip. *Clin Orthop.* 1995;319:28-40.

98. Currier BH, Mayor MB, Lyford KA, Van Citters DW, Collier JP. In vivo oxidation of γ-barrier-sterilized ultra-high-molecular-weight polyethylene bearing. *J Arthroplasty.* 2007;22:721-731.

99. Berry D, Currier BH, Mayor MB, Collier JP. Gamma-irradiation sterilization in an inert environment – a partial solution. *Clin Ortop Relat Res.* 2012;470:1805-1813.

100. Libby D, Ormerod M, Charlesby A. Electron spin resonance spectra of some polymers irradiated at 77-degrees-K. *Polymer.* 1960;1:212-218.

101. Charlesby A, Libby D, Ormerod M. Radiation damage in polyethylene as studied by electron spin resonance. *Proceedings of the Royal Society (London).* 1961;A262(130):207.

102. Ohnishi S, Sugimoto S, Nitta I. Temperature dependence of the ESR spectrum of polyethylene. *J Chem Phys.* 1962;37:1283-1288.

103. Carlsson D, Chmela S, Lacoste J. On the structures and yields of the first peroxyl radicals in γ-irradiated polyolefins. *Macromolecules.* 1990;23:4934-4938.

104. Dole M. Free radicals in irradiated polyethylene. In: Dole M, ed. *The Radiation Chemistry of Macromolecules.* New York: Academic Press; 1972:335-348.

105. Keller A, Ungar G. Radiation effects and crystallinity in polyethylene. *J Phys Chem.* 1983;22(1/2):155-181.

106. Bhateja S, Duerst RW, Aus EB, Andrews EH. Free radicals trapped in polyethylene crystals. *J Macromol Sci Phys.* 1995;B34 (3):263-272.

107. Kuzuya M, Kondo S, Sugito M, Yamashiro T. Peroxy radical formation from plasma-induced surface free radicals of polyethylene as studied by electron spin resonance. *Macromolecules.* 1998;31:3230-3234.

108. Seguchi T, Tamura N. Mechanism of decay of alkyl radicals in irradiated polyethylene on exposure to air as studied by electron spin resonance. *J Phys Chem.* 1973;77(1):40-44.

109. Carlsson D, Dobbin C, Wiles D. Direct observations of macroperoxyl radical propagation and termination by electron spin resonance and infrared spectroscopies. *Macromolecules.* 1985;18:2092-2094.

110. Ohnishi S, Sugimoto S, Nitta I. Electron spin resonance study of radiation oxidation of polymers. IIIA. Results for polyethylene and some general remarks. *J Polym Sci A Polym Chem.* 1963;1:605-623.

111. Rabek J, Ranby B. Photochemical oxidation reactions of synthetic polymers. In: Kinell P, Ranby B, eds. *ESR Applications to Polymer Research.* Stockholm: Almqvist-Wiksell Forlag AB; 1973.

112. Al-Malaika S. Autoxidation. In: Scott G, ed. *Atmospheric Oxidation and Antioxidants.* Amsterdam: Elsevier Science Publishers B.V.; 1993:45-82.

113. Costa L, Luda MP, Trossarelli L. Ultra-high molecular weight polyethylene: I. Mechano-oxidative degradation. *Polym Degrad Stab.* 1997;55:329-338.

114. Carlsson DJ, Brousseau R, Can Z, Wiles DM. Polyolefin oxidation: quantification of alcohol and hydroperoxide products by nitric oxide reactions. *Polym Degrad Stab.* 1987;17:303-318.

115. Muratoglu O, Wannomae KK, Rowell SL, Micheli BR, Malchau H. Ex vivo stability loss of irradiated and melted UHMWPE. *J Bone Joint Surg Am.* 2010;92:2809-2816.

116. Oral E, Ghali BW, Neils A, Muratoglu OK. A new mechanism of oxidation in UHMWPE caused by squalene absorption. *J Biomed Mater Res.* 2012;100B:742-751.

117. Oral E, Fung M, Rowell SL, Muratoglu OK. An oxidation model for UHMWPE incorporating synovial fluid lipids. *J Orthop Res.* 2018;36(7):1833-1839.

118. Spiegelberg S. Characterization of physical, chemical and mechanical properties of UHMWPE. In: Kurtz S, ed. *UHMWPE Biomaterials Handbook*: London: Elsevier; 2009:365-368.

119. Kurtz SM, Foulds JR, Jewett CW, Srivastav S, Edidin AA. Validation of a small punch testing technique to characterize the mechanical behaviour of ultra-high-molecular-weight polyethylene. *Biomaterials.* 1997;18:1-5.

120. Villarraga ML, Kurtz SM, Herr MP, Edidin AA. Multiaxial fatigue behavior of conventional and highly crosslinked UHMWPE during cyclic small punch testing. *J Biomed Mater Res.* 2003;66A:298-309.

121. Oral E, Wannomae KK, Hawkins N, Harris WH, Muratoglu OK. α-Tocopherol doped irradiated UHMWPE for high fatigue resistance and low wear. *Biomaterials.* 2004;25(24):5515-5522.

122. Kurtz S, Hozack W, Marcolongo M, Turner J, Rimnac C, Edidin A. Degradation of mechanical properties of UHMWPE acetabular liners following long-term implantation. *J Arthroplast.* 2003;18(7 suppl 1):68-78.

123. Weightman B, Isherwood DP, Swanson SA. The fracture of ultra-high molecular weight polyethylene in the human body. *J Biomed Mater Res.* 1979;13(4):669-672.

124. Francke EI, Lachiewicz PF. Failure of a cemented all-polyethylene patellar component of a Press-Fit Condylar total knee arthroplasty. *J Arthroplast.* 2000;15(2):234-237.

125. Wimmer MA, Laurent MP, Haman JD, Jacobs JJ, Galante JO. Surface damage versus tibial polyethylene insert conformity: a retrieval study. *Clin Orthop Relat Res.* 2012;470(7):1814-1825.

126. Bartel DL, Rawlinson JJ, Burstein AH, Ranawat CS, Flynn WF. Stresses in polyethylene components of contemporary total knee replacements. *Clin Orthop Relat Res.* 1995;317:76-82.

127. Blunn GW, Joshi AB, Minns RJ, et al. Wear in retrieved condylar knee arthroplasties. A comparison of wear in different designs of 280 retrieved condylar knee prostheses. *J Arthroplasty.* 1997;12(3):281-290.

128. Collier JP, Mayor MB, McNamara JL, Surprenant VA, Jensen RE. Analysis of the failure of 122 polyethylene inserts from uncemented tibial knee components. *Clin Orthop Relat Res.* 1991;273:232-242.

129. Willie BM, Foot LJ, Prall MW, Bloebaum RD. Surface damage analysis of retrieved highly crosslinked polyethylene tibial components after short-term implantation. *J Biomed Mater Res B Appl Biomater.* 2008;85(1):114-124.

130. Beaupre LA, Sharifi B, Johnston DWC. A randomized clinical trial comparing posterior cruciate-stabilizing vs posterior cruciate-retaining prostheses in primary total knee arthroplasty: 10-year follow-up. *J Arthroplasty.* 2017;32(3):818-823.

131. Takeuchi T, Lathi VK, Khan AM, Hayes WC. Patellofemoral contact pressures exceed the compressive yield strength of UHMWPE in total knee arthroplasties. *J Arthroplast.* 1995;10(3):363-368.

132. Pappas MJ, Buechel FF. The patellofemoral joint - its function and influence IN patellar replacement design [review]. *J Orthop Rheumatol JOR.* 1994;7(2):75-80.

133. Russell RD, Huo MH, Jones RE. Avoiding patellar complications in total knee replacement. *Bone Joint Lett J.* 2014;96-B(11 suppl A):84-86.

134. Parks NL, Engh GA, Topoleski LD, Emperado J. The Coventry Award. Modular tibial insert micromotion. A concern with contemporary knee implants. *Clin Orthop Relat Res.* 1998;(356):10-15.

135. Wasielewski RC, Parks N, Williams I, Surprenant H, Collier JP, Engh G. Tibial insert undersurface as a contributing source of polyethylene wear debris. *Clin Orthop Relat Res.* 1997;(345):53-59.

136. Wasielewski RC. The causes of insert backside wear in total knee arthroplasty. *Clin Orthop Relat Res.* 2002;404:232-246.

137. Rad EM, Michel PL, Christopher BK, Hannah JL. Linear penetration as a surrogate measure for volumetric wear in TKR tibial inserts. In: Mihalko WM, Lemons JE, Greenwald AS, Kurtz SM, eds. *Beyond the Implant Retrieval Analysis Methods for Implant Surveillance.* West Conshohocken, PA: ASTM International; 2018.

138. Ngai V, Uth T, Kunze J, Wimmer MA. *Backside wear of tibial polyethylene components is affected by gait.* In: *Transactions of the Annual Meeting of the Orthopaedic Research Society (ORS).* Long Beach, CA; 2011.

139. Pourzal R, Cip J, Rad EM, Laurent MP, Jacobs JJ, Wimmer MA. *Joint line elevation is associated with increased polyethylene wear in cruciate retaining total knee replacements.* In: *Transactions of the Annual Meeting of the Orthopaedic Research Society (ORS).* Orlando, Florida; 2016.

140. Azevedo MR, Araújo CL, Reichert FF, Siqueira FV, daSilva MC, Hallal PC. Gender differences in leisure-time physical activity. *Int J Public Health.* 2007;52(1):8-15.

141. Moschny A, Platen P, Klaassen-Mielke R, Trampisch U, Hinrichs T. Physical activity patterns in older men and women in Germany: a cross-sectional study. *BMC Public Health.* 2011;13(11):559.

142. Naal FD, Impellizzeri FM. How active are patients undergoing total joint arthroplasty?: a systematic review. *Clin Orthop Relat Res.* 2010;468(7):1891-1904.

143. Harman MK, Banks SA, Andrew HW. Polyethylene damage and knee kinematics after kinematics during stair-stepping. *Clin Orthop Rel Res*. 2001;392:383-393.

144. Pang HN, Bin Abd Razak HR, Jamieson P, Teeter MG, Naudie DDR, MacDonald SJ. Factors affecting wear of constrained polyethylene tibial inserts in total knee arthroplasty. *J Arthroplasty*. 2016;31(6):1340-1345.

145. Mell SP, Wimmer MA, Jacobs JJ, Lundberg HJ. *Total knee replacement wear is most sensitive to transverse plane alignment-a parametric finite element study*. In *Transactions of the Annual Meeting of the Orthopaedic Research Society (ORS)*. Austin, Texas; 2019.

146. Marouane H, Shirazi-Adl A, Hashemi J. Quantification of the role of tibial posterior slope in knee joint mechanics and ACL force in simulated gait. *J Biomech*. 2015;48(10):1899-1905.

147. Lotke PA, Ecker ML. Influence of positioning of prosthesis in total knee replacement. *J Bone Joint Surg Am Vol*. 1977;59(1):77-79.

148. Dorr LD, Boiardo RA. Technical considerations in total knee arthroplasty. *Clin Orthop Relat Res*. 1986;(205):5-11.

149. Insall J. Total knee replacement. In: Insall J, ed. *Surgery of the Knee*. New York: Churchill Livingstone; 1984:587-696.

150. Shaw JA. Angled bearing inserts in total knee arthroplasty. A brief technical note. *J Arthroplast*. 1992;7(2):211-216.

151. Matsuda S, Hiromasa M, Ryuji N, et al. Changes in knee alignment after total knee arthroplasty. *J Arthroplast*. 1999;14(5):566-570.

152. Laskin RS. Flexion space configuration in total knee arthroplasty. *J Arthroplast*. 1995;10(5):657-660.

153. Fehring TK. Rotational malalignment of the femoral component in total knee arthroplasty. *Clin Orthop Relat Res*. 2000;(380):72-79.

154. Singerman R, Pagan HD, Peyser AB, Goldberg VM. Effect of femoral component rotation and patellar design on patellar forces. *Clin Orthop Relat Res*. 1997;(334):345-353.

155. Rhoads DD, Noble PC, Reuben JD, Mahoney OM, Tullos HS. The effect of femoral component position on patellar tracking after total knee arthroplasty. *Clin Orthop Relat Res*. 1990;(260):43-51.

156. Walker PS. Biomechanics of the patella in total knee replacement. *Knee Surg Sport Traumatol Arthrosc*. 2001;9(suppl 1):S3-S7.

157. Berger RA, Rubash HE, Seel MJ, Thompson WH, Crossett LS. Determining the rotational alignment of the femoral component in total knee arthroplasty using the epicondylar axis. *Clin Orthop Relat Res*. 1993;(286):40-47.

158. Komistek RD, Dennis DA, Mabe JA, Walker SA. An in vivo determination of patellofemoral contact positions. *Clin Biomech*. 2000;15(1):29-36.

159. Bozic K, Kurtz SM, Lau E, et al. The epidemiology of revision total knee arthroplasty in the United States. *Clin Ortho Rel Res*. 2010;468:45-51.

160. Colizza WA, Insall JN, Scuderi GR. The posterior stabilized total knee prosthesis. Assessment of polyethylene damage and osteolysis after a ten-year-minimum follow-up. [see comments.]. *J Bone Joint Surg*. 1995;77(11):1713-1720.

161. Diduch DR, Insall JN, Scott WN, Scuderi GR, Font-Rodriguez D. Total knee replacement in young, active patients. Long-term follow-up and functional outcome. *J Bone Joint Surg Am Vol*. 1997;79(4):575-582.

162. Berzins A, Jacobs JJ, Berger R, et al. Surface damage in machined ram-extruded and net-shape molded retrieved polyethylene tibial inserts of total knee replacements. *J Bone Joint Surg*. 2002;84A(9):1534-1540.

163. D'Lima D, Chen P, Colwell C Jr. Polyethylene contact stresses, articular congruity and knee alignment. *Clin Orthop Relat Res*. 2001;392:232-238.

164. Dumbleton J, D'Antonio JA, Manley MT, Capello WN, Wang A. The basis for a second-generation highly cross-linked UHMWPE. *Clin Ortho Rel Res*. 2006;453:265-271.

165. Wang A, Zeng H, Yau SS, et al. Wear, oxidation and mechanical properties of a sequentially irradiated and annealed UHMWPE in total joint replacement. *J Phys D Appl Phys*. 2006;39:3213-3219.

166. Oral E, Neils A, Wannomae K, Muratoglu O. Novel active stabilization technology in highly cross-linked UHMWPEs for superior stability. *Radiat Phys Chem*. 2014;105:6-11.

167. Kurtz SM, Mazzucco D, Rimnac CM, Schroeder D. Anisotropy and oxidative resistance of highly crosslinked UHMWPE after deformation processing by solid-state ram extrusion. *Biomaterials*. 2006;27(1):24-34.

168. Cooper J, Dowson D, Fisher J. Macroscopic and microscopic wear mechanisms in UHMWPE. *Wear*. 1993;162-164:378-384.

169. Scales J, Kelly P, Goddard D. Friction torque studies of total joint replacements. The use of a simulator. *Ann Rheum Dis*. 1969;28(5 suppl):30-35.

170. Saikko V, Paavolainen P, Kleimola M, Stätis P. A five-station hip joint simulator for wear rate studies. *Proc Inst Mech Eng H*. 1992;206:195-200.

171. Ramamurti B, Muratoglu O, Bragdon C, O'Connor D. How realistically do contemporary hip joint simulators reproduce physiologic gait motion. *Trans of the ORS, Atlanta*. 1996:457.

172. Shaw JA, Murray DG. Knee joint simulator. *Clin Orthop*. 1973;94:15-23.

173. Burgess IC, Kolar M, Cunningham JL, Unsworth A. Development of a six station knee wear simulator and preliminary wear results. *Proc Inst Mech Eng H J Eng Med*. 1997;211(1):37-47.

174. Walker P, Blunn GW, Broome DR. A knee simulating machine for performance evaluation of total knee replacements. *J Biomech*. 1997;30(1):83-89.

175. Muratoglu OK, Bragdon CR, O'Connor DO, et al. Unified wear model for highly crosslinked ultra-high molecular weight polyethylenes (UHMWPE). *Biomaterials*. 1999;20(16):1463-1470.

176. McKellop H, Shen FW, Lu B, Campbell P, Salovey R. Development of an extremely wear resistant ultra-high molecular weight polyethylene for total hip replacements. *J Orthop Res*. 1999;17(2):157-167.

177. Muratoglu OK, Bragdon CR, O'Connor DO, Perinchief RS, Jasty M, Harris WH. Aggressive wear testing of a cross-linked polyethylene in total knee arthroplasty. *Clin Orthop*. 2002;404:89-95.

178. McEwen H, Barnett PI, Bell CJ, et al. The influence of design, materials and kinematics on the in vitro wear of total knee replacements. *J Biomech*. 2005;38:357-365.

179. Wang A, Yau SS, Essner A, Herrera L, Manley M, Dumbleton J. A highly crosslinked UHMWPE for CR and PS total knee arthroplasties. *J Arthroplast*. 2008;23(4):559-566.

180. Hermida J, Fischler A, Colwell CW Jr, D'Lima DD. The effect of oxidative aging on the wear performance of highly crosslinked polyethylene knee inserts under conditions of severe malalignment. *J Orthop Res*. 2008;26(12):1585-1590.

181. Wang A, Polineni VK, Essner A, Sun DC, Stark C, Dumbleton JH. *Effect of radiation dosage on the wear of stabilized UHMWPE evaluated by kip and knee joint simulators*. In: *Trans 23rd Soc Biomater*. San Fransisco, CA; 1997.

182. Schmidig G, Essner A, Wang A. *Knee simulator wear of cross-linked UHMWPE*. In: *46th Annual Meeting, ORS*. Orlando, Florida; 2000.

183. Deluzio KJ, O'Connor DO, Bragdon CR, Rubash HE, Jasty M. *Development of an in vitro delamination model in a knee simulator with physiological load and motion*. In: *46th Annual Meeting of the Orthopaedic Research Society*. Rosemont, Illinois; 2000.

184. Currier JH, Duda JL, Sperling DK, Collier JP, Currier BH, Kennedy FE. In vitro simulation of contact fatigue damage found in ultra-high molecular weight polyethylene components of knee prostheses. *Proc Inst Mech Eng H J Eng Med*. 1998;212(4):293-302.

185. Hastings RS, Huston DE, Reber EW, DiMaio WG. *Knee wear testing of a radiation crosslinked and remelted UHMWPE*. In: *1999 Society for Biomaterials 25th Annual Meeting Transactions*. Providence, RI; 1999.

186. Muratoglu OK, Bragdon CR, O'Connor DO, et al. *Markedly improved adhesive wear and delamination resistance of a highly cross-linked UHMWPE for use in total knee arthroplasty*. In: *47th Annual Meeting of Orthopedic Research Society*. San Francisco; 2001.

187. Collier M, Engh CA Jr, Hatten KM, Ginn SD, Sheils TM, Engh GA. Radiographic assessment of the thickness lost from polyethylene tibial inserts that had been sterilized differently. *J Bone Joint Surg.* 2008;90A(7):1543-1552.

188. Rodriguez J. Crosslinked polyethylene in total knee arthroplasty. In opposition. *J Arthroplasty.* 2008;23(7 suppl 1):31-34.

189. Sathasivam S, Walker P. Computer model to predict subsurface damage in tibial inserts of total knees. *J Orthop Res.* 1998;16:564-571.

190. Oral E, Malhi A, Muratoglu O. Mechanisms of decrease in fatigue crack propagation resistance in irradiated and melted UHMWPE. *Biomaterials.* 2006;27:917-925.

191. Currier B, Currier JH, Franklin KJ, Mayor MB, Reinitz SD, Van Citters DW. Comparison of wear and oxidation in retrieved conventional and highly cross-linked UHMWPE tibial inserts. *J Arthroplast.* 2015;30(12):2349-2353.

192. Reinitz S, Currier BH, Levine RA, Van Citters DW. Crosslink density, oxidation and chain scission in retrieved, highly cross-linked UHMWPE tibial bearings. *Biomaterials.* 2014;35:4436-4440.

193. Currier BH, Currier JH, Mayor MB, Lyford KA, Collier JP, Van Citters DW. Evaluation of oxidation and fatigue damage of retrieved Crossfire polyethylene acetabular cups. *J Bone Joint Surg.* 2007;89A:2023-2029.

194. Currier B, Van Citters DW, Currier JH, Collier JP. In vivo oxidation in remelted highly crosslinked retrievals. *J Bone Joint Surg.* 2010;92A:2409-2418.

195. Currier B, Van Citters DW, Currier JH, Carlson EM, Tibbo ME, Collier JP. In vivo oxidation in retrieved highly crosslinked tibial inserts. *J Biomed Mater Res.* 2013;101B:441-448.

196. Reinitz SD, Franklin KJ, Gray LT, Dansu HJ, Currier BH, Van Citters DW. *Comparison of the in vivo perfomance of two highly crosslinked UHMWPE materials in the hip and knee.* In: *Annual Meeting of the Orthopaedic Research Society.* San Francisco, CA; 2012.

197. Kurtz S, Gawel H, Patel J. History and systematic review of wear and osteolysis outcomes for first-generation highly crosslinked polyethylene. *Clin Orthop Relat Res.* 2011;469:2262-2277.

198. Paulus A, Matthias W, Volkmar J, Sandra U. Conventional and highly crosslinked polyethylene in total knee arthroplasty - a design-independent wear investigation. *Lubricants.* 2017;5(25):5030025.

199. Boyer B, Bordini B, Caputo D, Neri T, Stea S, Toni A. Is crosslinked polyethylene an improvement over conventional UHMWPE in total knee arthroplasty?. *J Arthroplast.* 2018;33:908-914.

200. Kindsfater K, Pomeroy D, Clark CR, Gruen TA, Murphy J, Himden S. In vivo performance of moderately crosslinked, thermally treated polyethylene in a prospective, randomized controlled primary total knee arthroplasty trial. *J Arthroplast.* 2015;30:1333-1338.

201. Hodrick J, Severson EP, McAlister DS, Dahl B, Hofmann AA. Highly crosslinked polyethylene is safe for use in total knee arthroplasty. *Clin Orthop Relat Res.* 2008;466:2806-2812.

202. Minoda Y, Masaharu A, Akira S, et al. Comparison between highly crosslinked and conventional polyethylene in total knee arthroplasty. *Knee.* 2009;16(5):348-351.

203. Meneghini R, Lovro LR, Smits SA, Ireland PH. Highly crosslinked versus conventional polyethylene in posterior-stabilized total knee arthroplasty at a mean 5-year follow-up. *J Arthroplast.* 2015;30:1736-1739.

204. Diamond O, Howard L, Masri B. Five cases of tibial post fracture in posterior stabilized total knee arthroplasty using Prolong highly cross-linked polyethylene. *The Knee.* 2018;25:657-662.

205. Pritchard G. Plastics additives: an A-Z reference. In: Brewis D, Briggs D, ed. *Polymer Science and Technology.* Bristol, UK: Springer Science and Business Media B.V.; 1998:633.

206. Wright TM, Astion DJ, Bansal M, et al. Failure of carbon fiber-reinforced polyethylene total knee-replacement components. *J Bone and Joint Surg.* 1988;70-A:926-932.

207. Willie BM, Shea JE, Bloebaum RD, Hofmann AA. Elemental and morphological identification of third-body particulate and calcium stearate inclusions in polyethylene components. *J Biomed Mater Res.* 2000;53(2):137-142.

208. Oral E, Christensen SD, Malhi AS, Wannomae KK, Muratoglu OK. Wear resistance and mechanical properties of highly crosslinked UHMWPE doped with vitamin E. *J Arthroplasty.* 2006;21(4):580-591.

209. Oral E, Rowell S, Muratoglu O. The effect of alpha-tocopherol on the oxidation and free radical decay in irradiated UHMWPE. *Biomaterials.* 2006;27:5580-5587.

210. Oral E, Keith KW, Shannon LR, Orhun KM. Diffusion of vitamin E in ultra-high molecular weight polyethylene. *Biomaterials.* 2007;28(35):5225-5237.

211. Wannomae KK, Micheli BR, Lozynsky AJ, Malhi AS, Oral E, Muratoglu OK. *Vitamin E-stabilized, irradiated UHMWPE for cruciate-retaining knees.* In: *Transactions, 53rd Annual Meeting of the Orthopaedic Research Society.* San Diego, CA; 2007.

212. Oral E, Malhi AS, Wannomae KK, Muratoglu OK. Highly cross-linked UHMWPE with improved fatigue resistance for total joint arthroplasty. *J Arthroplast.* 2008;23(7):1037-1044.

213. Rowell S, Oral E, Muratoglu O. Comparative oxidative stability of alpha-tocopherol blended and diffused UHMWPEs at 3 years of real-time aging. *J Orthop Res.* 2009;29:773-780.

214. Jarrett B, Cofske J, Rosenberg AE, Oral E, Muratoglu O, Malchau H. In vivo biological response to vitamin E and vitamin E-doped polyethylene. *J Bone Joint Surg.* 2010;92(13):2672-2681.

215. Haider H, Weisenburger JN, Kurtz SM, et al. Does vitamin E-stabilized UHMWPE address concerns of cross-linked polyethylene in total knee arthroplasty. *J Arthroplasty.* 2012;27(3):461-469.

216. Wannomae K, Christensen SD, Micheli BR, Rowell SL, Schroeder DW, Muratoglu OK. Delamination and adhesive wear behavior of alpha-tocopherol-stabilized irradiated UHMWPE. *J Arthroplast.* 2010;25(4):635-643.

217. Micheli B, Wannomae KK, Lozynsky AJ, Christensen SD, Muratoglu OK. Knee simulator wear of vitamin E-stabilized irradiated UHMWPE. *J Arthroplast.* 2012;27(1):95-104.

218. Packer L. Protective role of vitamin E in biological systems. *Am J Clin Nutr.* 1991;53-1050S-1055S.

219. Packer L, Kagan VE. Vitamin E: the antioxidant harvesting center of membranes and lipoproteins. In: Packer L, Fuchs J, eds. *Vitamin E in Health and Disease.* New York: Marcel Dekker, Inc.; 1993:179-192.

220. Burton G, Ingold K. Autoxidation of biological molecules. 1. The antioxidant activity of vitamin E and related chain-breaking phenolic antioxidants in vitro. *J Am Chem Soc.* 1981;103:6472-6477.

221. Burton GW, Traber MG. Vitamin E: antioxidant activity, biokinetics, and bioavailability. *Annu Rev Nutr.* 1990;10:357-382.

222. Kamal-Eldin A, Appelqvist L. The chemistry and antioxidant properties of tocopherols and tocotrienols. *Lipids.* 1996;31(7):671-701.

223. Wolf C, Krivec T, Blassnig J, Lederer K, Schneider W. Examination of the suitability of α-tocopherol as a stabilizer for ultra-high molecular weight polyethylene used for articulating surfaces in joint endoprostheses. *J Mater Sci Mater Med.* 2002;13:185-189.

224. Oral E, Evan SG, Arnaz SM, William HH, Orhun KM. Characterization of irradiated blends of alpha-tocopherol and UHMWPE. *Biomaterials.* 2005;26(33):6657-6663.

225. Parth M, Aust N, Lederer K. Studies on the effect of electron beam radiation on the molecular structure of ultra-high molecular weight polyethylene under the influence of alpha-tocopherol with respect to its application in medical implants. *J Mater Sci Mater Med.* 2002;13(10):917-921.

226. Oral E, Godleski BC, Malhi AS, Muratoglu OK. The effects of high dose irradiation on the cross-linking of vitamin E-blended UHMWPE. *Biomaterials.* 2008;29:3557-3560.

227. Wolf C, Maninger J, Lederer K, Frühwirth-Smounig H, Gamse T, Marr R. Stabilisation of crosslinked ultra-high molecular weight polyethylene (UHMW-PE)-acetabular components with alpha-tocopherol. *J Mater Sci Mater Med.* 2006;17:1323-1331.

228. Rowell S, Oral E, Muratoglu O. *Three-year real-time aging of vitamin E-diffused, radiation cross-linked UHMWPE.* In: *Transactions of the 55th Annual Meeting of the Orthopaedic Research Society.* Las Vegas, NV; 2009.

229. Oral E, Neils AL, Rowell SL, Muratoglu OK. *Trace amounts of grafted vitamin E protect UHMWPE against squalene-initiated oxidation.* In: *Annual Meeting of the Orthopaedic Society.* Long Beach, CA; 2011.

230. Oral E, Rowell S, Muratoglu O. *Oxidation resistance of Vitamin E-doped, irradiated UHMWPE for total joints following forceful extraction of vitamin E.* In: *Transactions, 52nd Annual Meeting of the Orthopaedic Research Society.* Chicago, IL; 2006.

231. Saikko V, Calonius O, Keranen J. Wear of conventional and cross-linked ultra-high-molecular-weight polyethylene acetabular cups aganist polished and roughened CoCr femoral heads in a biaxial hip simulator. *Biomed Mater Red (Appl Biomater).* 2002;63:848-853.

232. Muratoglu OK, Burroughs BR, Bragdon CR, Christensen S, Lozynsky A, Harris WH. Knee simulator wear of polyethylene tibias articulating against explanted rough femoral components. *Clin Orthop Relat Res.* 2004;(428):108-113.

233. Bracco P, Valentina B, Marco Z, MariaPaola L, Costa L. Stabilisation of ultra-high molecular weight polyethylene with vitamin E. *Polym Degrad Stab.* 2007;92:2155-2162.

234. Oral E, Andrew N, Shannon R, Andrew JL, Orhun M. Increasing irradiation temperature maximizes vitamin E grafting and wear resistance of UHMWPE. *J Biomed Mater Res B Appl Biomater.* 2013;101B(3):436-440.

235. Neils A, Oral E, Muratoglu O. *The initial concentration of vitamin E in irradiated UHMWPE affects vitamin E grafting.* In: *59th Annual Meeting of the Orthopaedic Research Society.* San Antonio, TX; 2013.

236. Kurtz S, Dumbleton J, Siskey RS, Wang A, Manley M. Trace concentrations of vitamin E protect radiation crosslinked UHMWPE from oxidative degradation. *J Biomed Mater Res.* 2008;90A:549-563.

237. Narayan V. Spectroscopic and chromatographic quantification of an antioxidant-stabilized UHMWPE. *Clin Orthop Relat Res.* 2015;473:952-959.

238. King R, Narayan VS, Ernsberger C, Hanes M. *Characterization of gamma-irradiated UHMWPE stabilized with a hindered-phenol antioxidant.* In: *Transactions of the 55th Annual Meeting of the Orthopaedic Research Society.* Las Vegas, NV; 2009.

239. Narayan V, Ernsberger C, King R. *Pin-on-disk wear studies of antioxidant stabilized UHMWPE materials.* In: *Transactions of the 55th Annual Meeting of the Orthopaedic Research Society.* Las Vegas, NV; 2009.

240. Muratoglu OK, Oral E, Burroughs BR, et al. *Two second generation crosslinked UHMWPEs show improved mechanical properties and fatigue strength.* In: *Transactions, 51st Annual Meeting of the Orthopaedic Research Society.* Washington, DC; 2005.

241. Malhi AS, Wannomae KK, Christensen SD, Godleski CG, Muratoglu OK. *A novel processing methodology for improvement of mechanical properties in highly cross-linked UHMWPE.* In: *Transactions, 52nd Annual Meeting of the Orthopaedic Research Society.* Chicago, IL; 2006.

242. Wannomae KK, Micheli BR, Lozynsky AJ, Muratoglu OK. *A new method of stabilizing irradiated UHMWPE using vitamin E and mechanical annealing.* In: *Transactions of the 56th Annual Meeting of the Orthopaedic Research Society.* New Orleans, NV; 2010.

243. Oral E, Andrew N, Keith KW, Orhun M. Novel active stabilization technology in highly cross-linked UHMWPEs for superior stability. Radiation Physics and Chemistry. 2014;105:6-11.

244. Currier B, Currier JH, Holdcroft LA, Van Citters DW. Effectiveness of anti-oxidant polyethylene: what early retrievals can tell us. *J Biomed Mater Res.* 2018;106B:353-359.

245. Ponzio D, Weitzler L, deMeireles A, Esposito CI, Wright TM, Padgett DE. Antioxidant-stabilized highly crosslinked polyethylene in total knee arthroplasty. *Bone Joint J.* 2018;100B: 1330-1335.

246. Chen Y, Hallab NJ, Liao YS, Narayan V, Schwarz EM, Xie C. Antioxidant impregnated ultra-high molecular weight polyethylene wear debris particles display increased bone remodeling and a superior osteogenic:osteolytic profile vs. Conventional UHMWPE particles in a murine calvaria model. *J Orthop Res.* 2016;34:845-851.

247. Massaccesi L, Ragone V, Papini N, Goi G, CorsiRomanelli MM, Galliera E. Effects of vitamin E-stabilized UHMWPE on oxidative stress response and osteoimmunological response in human osteoblast. *Front Endocrinol.* 2019;10:203.

248. Teramura S, Russell S, Ingham E, et al. *Reduced biological response to wear particles from UHMWPE containing vitamin E.* In: *Transactions of the 55th Annual Meeting of the Orthopaedic Research Society.* Las Vegas, NV; 2009.

249. Bladen C, Teramura S, Russell SL, et al. Analysis of wear, wear particles, and reduced inflammatory potential of vitamin E ultrahigh-molecular-weight polyethylene for use in total joint replacement. *J Biomed Mater Res.* 2013;101B:458-466.

250. Bichara D, Malchau E, Sillesen NH, Cakmak S, Nielsen GP, Muratoglu OK. Vitamin E-diffused highly cross-linked UHMWPE particles induce less osteolysis compared to highly cross-linked virgin UHMWPE particles in vivo. *J Arthroplast.* 2014;29(suppl 2):232-237.

251. Green J, Hallab NJ, Liao YS, Narayan V, Schwarz EM, Xie C. Anti-oxidation treatment of ultra high molecular weight polyethylene components to decrease periprosthetic osteolysis: evaluation of osteolytic and osteogenic properties of wear debris particles in a murine calvaria model. *Curr Rheumatol Rep.* 2013;15:325.

252. Mankin HJ, Mow VC, Buckwalter JA. Articular cartilage structure, composition and function. In: Buckwalter JA, Einhorn T, Simon S, eds. *Orthopaedic Basic Science: The Biology and Biomechanics of the Musculoskeletal System.* Rosemont, IL: American Academy of Orthopaedic Surgeons; 2000:443-470.

253. Moro T, Takatori Y, Ishihara K, et al. Surface grafting of artificial joints with a biocompatible polymer for preventing periprosthetic osteolysis. *Nat Mater.* 2004;3(11):829-836.

254. Kyomoto M, Moro T, Miyaji F, et al. Effect of 2-methacryloyloxyethyl phosphorylcholine concentration on photo-induced graft polymerization of polyethylene in reducing the wear of orthopaedic bearing surface. *J Biomed Mater Res.* 2008;86A:439-447.

255. Ishihara K, Aragaki R, Ueda T, Watenabe A, Nakabayashi N. Reduced thrombogenicity of polymers having phospholipid polar groups. *J Biomed Mater Res.* 1990;24:1069-1077.

256. Moro T, Kawaguchi H, Ishihara K, et al. Wear resistance of artificial hip joints with poly(2-methacryloyloxyethyl phosphorylcholine) grafted polyethylene: comparisons with the effect of polyethylene crosslinking and ceramic femoral heads. *Biomaterials.* 2009;30:2995-3001.

257. Moro T, Takatori Y, Kyomoto M. Surface grafting of biocompatible phospholipid polymer MPC provides wear resistance of tibial polyethylene insert in artificial knee joints. *Osteoarthr Cartil.* 2010;18:1174-1182.

258. Kyomoto M, Shobuike T, Moro T, et al. Prevention of bacterial adhesion and biofilm formation on a vitamin E-blended, cross-linked polyethylene surface with a poly(2 methacryloyloxyethyl phosphorylcholine) layer. *Acta Biomater.* 2015;24:24-34.

259. Laskin R. An oxidized Zr ceramic surfaced femoral component for total knee arthroplasty. *Clin Orthop Relat Res.* 2003;416:191-196.

260. Benezra V, Mangin S, Treska M, Spector M, Hunter G, Hobbs LW. *Microstructural investigation of the oxide scale on Zr-2.5Nb and its interface with the alloy substrate.* In: *Materials Research Society Symposium: Biomedical Materials-Drug Delivery, Implants and Tissue Engineering.* Boston: Materials Research Society; 1999.

261. Hobbs L, Valarie Benezra R, Stephan M, Meri T, Gordon H. Oxidation microstructures and interfaces in the oxidized zirconium knee. *Int J Ceram Technol.* 2005;2(3):221-246.

262. Tsukomoto R, Chen S, Asano T, et al. Improved wear performance with crosslinked UHMWPE and zirconia implants in knee simulation. *Acta Orthopaedica.* 2006;77(3):505-511.

263. Innocenti M, Roberto C, Christian C, Fabrizio M, Marco V. The 5-year results of an oxidized zirconium femoral component for TKA. *Clin Orthop Relat Res.* 2010;468:1258-1263.

264. Heyse T, Chen DX, Kelly N, Boettner F, Wright TM, Haas SB. Matched-pair total knee arthroplasty retrieval analysis: oxidized zirconium vs. CoCrMo. *Knee.* 2016;18:448-452.

265. Gioe T, Sharma A, Tatman P, Mehle S. Do "premium" joint implants add value? *Clin Orthop Relat Res.* 2011;469:48-54.

266. Inacio M, Cafri G, Paxton EW, Kurtz SM, Namba RS. Alternative bearings in total knee arthroplasty: risk of early revision compared to traditional bearings. *Acta Orthopaedica.* 2013;84(2):145-152.

267. Vertullo C, Lewis PL, Graves S, Kelly L, Lorimer M, Myers P. Twelve-year outcomes of an Oxinium total knee replacement compared with the same cobalt-chromium design. *J Bone Joint Surg.* 2017;99:275-283.

268. vanHove R, Sierevelt IN, van Royen BJ, Nolte PA. Titanium-nitride coating of orthopaedic implants: a review of the literature. *BioMed Res Int.* 2015;2015:485975.

269. Mohammed A, Metcalfe A, Woodnutt D. Medium term outcome of Titanium Nitride, mobile bearing total knee Replacement. *Acta Orthop Belg.* 2014;80(2):269-275.

270. von Hove R, Brohet RM, van Royen BJ, Nolte PA. No clinical benefit of titanium nitride coating in cementless mobile-bearing total knee arthroplasty. *Knee Surg Sport Traumatol Arthrosc.* 2015;23:1833-1840.

271. Thienpont E. Titanium niobium nitride knee implants are not inferior to chrome cobalt components for primary total knee arthroplasty. *Achives of Orthopaedic and Trauma Surgery.* 2015;135:1749-1754.

272. Park C, Kang SG, Bae DK, Song SJ. Mid-term clinical and radiological results do not differ between fixedandmobile-bearing total knee arthroplasty using titanium-nitride-coated posterior-stabilized prostheses: a prospective randomized controlled trial. *Knee Surg Sport Traumatol Arthrosc.* 2019;27:1165-1173.

273. Breugem S, Linnartz J, Sierevelt I, Bruijn JD, Driessen MJM. Evaluation of 1031 primary titanium nitride coated mobile bearing total knee arthroplasties in an orthopedic clinic. *World J Orthop.* 2017;8(12):922-928.

274. Bal B, Rahaman M. Orthopaedic applications of silicon nitride ceramics. *Acta Biomater.* 2012;8:2889-2898.

275. Kurtz S, Devine J. PEEK biomaterials in trauma, orthopaedic, and spinal implants. *Biomaterials.* 2007;28:4845-4869.

276. Wang A, Lin R, Stark C, Dumbleton JH. Suitability and limitations of carbon fiber reinforced PEEK composites as bearing surfaces for total joint replacements. *Wear.* 1999;225-229:724-727.

277. Geringer J, Tatkiewicz W, Rouchouse G. Wear behavior of PAEK, poly(aryl-ether-ketone) under physiological conditions, outlooks for performing these materials in the field of hip prosthesis. *Wear.* 2011;271(11-12):2793-2803.

278. Skinner H. Composite technology for total hip arthroplasty. *Clin Orthop Relat Res.* 1988;(235):224-236.

279. Scholes S, Unsworth A. Wear studies on the likely performance of CFR-PEEK-CoCrMo for use as artificial joint bearing. *J Mater Sci Mater Med.* 2009;20(1):163-170.

280. Brockett C, Silvia C, John F, Jennings LM. PEEK and CFR-PEEK as alternative bearing materials to UHMWPE in a fixed bearing total knee replacement: an experimental wear study. *Wear.* 2017;374-375:86-91.

281. Willert H, Buchhorn GH, Fayyazi A, et al. Metal-on-metal bearings and hypersensitivity in patients with artificial hip joints. *J Bone Joint Surg.* 2005;87A(1):28-36.

282. Jacobs J, Hallab N. Loosening and osteolysis associated with metal-on-metal bearings-A local effect of metal hypersensitivity. *J Bone Joint Surg.* 2006;88(6):1171-1172.

283. Pandit H, Glyn-Jones S, McLardy-Smith P, et al. Pseudotumors associated with metal-on-metal hip resurfacings. *J Bone Joint Surg.* 2008;90B(7):847-851.

284. Medical Device Alert MDA/2010/033. Medicines and Healthcare products Regulatory Agency (MHRA), London, UK. 2010. Available at http://www.jisrf.org/pdfs/mediacl-device-alert.pdf.

285. Haddad F, Thakrar RR, Hart AJ, et al. Metal-on-metal bearings. *J Bone and Joint Surg Br.* 2011;93B:572-579.

286. Du Z, Zhu Z, Yue B, Li Z, Wang Y. Feasibility ans safety of a cemented PEEK-on-PE knee replacement in a goat model: a preliminary study. *Artif Organs.* 2018;42(8):E204-E214.

287. Meng X, Du Z, Wang Y. Characteristics of wear particles and wear behavior of retrieved PEEK-on-HXLPE total knee implants: a preliminary study. *RSC Adv.* 2018;8:30330.

288. Cowie R, Briscoe A, Fisher J, Jennings LM. PEEK-OPTIMATM as an alternative to cobalt chrome in the femoral component of total knee replacement: a preliminary study. *Proc Inst Mech Eng H J Eng Med.* 2016;230(11):1008-1015.

289. Kop AM, Swarts E. Quantification of polyethylene degradation in mobile bearing knees: a retrieval analysis of the Anterior-Posterior-Glide (APG) and Rotating Platform (RP) Low Contact Stress (LCS) knee. *Acta Orthop.* 2007;78(3):364-370.

290. Atwood S, Currier JH, Mayor MB, Collier JP, Van Citters DW, Kennedy FE. Clinical wear measurement on low contact stress rotating platform knee bearings. *J Arthroplast.* 2008;23(3):431-440.

291. Engh CA Jr, Zimmerman RL, Hopper RH Jr, Engh GA. Can microcomputed tomography measure retrieved polyethylene wear? Comparing fixed-bearing and rotating-platform knees. *Clin Orthop Relat Res.* 2013;471(1):86-93.

292. Benjamin J, Szivek J, Dersam G, Persselin S, Johnson R. Linear and volumetric wear of tibial inserts in posterior cruciate-retaining knee arthroplasties. *Clin Orthop Relat Res.* 2001;392:131-138.

293. Lavernia CJ, Sierra RJ, Hungerford DS, Krackow K. Activity level and wear in total knee arthroplasty: a study of autopsy retrieved specimens. *J Arthroplasty.* 2001;16(4):446-453.

294. Gill HS, Waite JC, Short A, Kellett CF, Price AJ, Murray DW. In vivo measurement of volumetric wear of a total knee replacement. *Knee.* 2006;13(4):312-317.

295. Schwenke T, Orozco D, Schneider E, Wimmer MA. Differences in wear between load and displacement control tested total knee replacements. *Wear.* 2009;267(5-8):757-762.

296. Teeter MG, Parikh A, Taylor M, Sprague J, Naudie DD. Wear and creep behavior of total knee implants undergoing wear testing. *J Arthroplasty.* 2015;30(1):130-134.

297. Laurent MP, Yao JQ, Bhambri S, et al. *High cycle wear of highly crosslinked UHMWPE tibial articular surfaces evaluated in a knee wear simulator.* In: *Transactions of the 48th Annual Meeting of the Orthopaedic Research Society (ORS).* Dallas, Texas, USA; 2002.

298. Popoola OO, Yao JQ, Johnson TS, Blanchard CR. Wear, delamination, and fatigue resistance of melt-annealed highly crosslinked UHMWPE cruciate-retaining knee inserts under activities of daily living. *J Orthop Res.* 2010;28(9):1120-1126.

299. Mell SP, Wimmer MA, Lundberg HJ. The choice of the femoral center of rotation affects material loss in total knee replacement wear testing - A parametric finite element study of ISO 14243-3. *J Biomech.* 2019;88:104-112.

300. Davis ET, Pagkalos J, Kopjar B. Polyethylene manufacturing characteristics have a major effect on the risk of revision surgery of cementless and hybrid total hip arthroplasties. *Bone Joint J.* 2020;102B(1):90-101.

chapter 14

Implant Fixation

Mick P. Kelly, MD | Brett R. Levine, MD, MS | Joshua J. Jacobs, MD | Dale Rick Sumner, PhD

INTRODUCTION

Total knee arthroplasty (TKA) relying on cement fixation remains the gold standard approach with proven long-term results.[1-4] However, due to an increasing number of procedures performed in a younger, more active patient population combined with advancements in biomaterials, there is renewed interest in cementless TKA.[5,6] Benefits of cementless fixation include potential for increased longevity, elimination of cement third-body wear, and perhaps decreased operative time. The purpose of this chapter is to describe the basic science of cemented and cementless fixation, with an emphasis on osseointegration in TKA. A thorough understanding of this topic is critical because it allows the surgeon to predict, recognize, and avoid common mechanisms of failure.

CEMENTED FIXATION

Basic Science of Polymethylmethacrylate

Bone cement comes in several different varieties that are typically supplied in a two-component system, a polymethylmethacrylate (PMMA) powder copolymer and a liquid methylmethacrylate monomer. Within the powder, there is typically an initiator (benzoyl peroxide), a radioopacifier (barium sulfate,[7] zirconium dioxide), possibly a coloring agent and/or an antibiotic. The liquid portion typically contains a stabilizer for the monomer (hydroquinone) and an accelerator (N,N-dimethyl para-toluidine, DMPT). Once the two components are mixed, the cement follows four stages as it sets up for use and will ultimately serve as a grout in aiding fixation of TKA components. The four phases are mixing, waiting, working, and hardening, and these may vary in length based upon the bone cement, local environment, and mixing process.[8]

There are numerous properties of bone cement that must be understood to evaluate all of the options currently available as well as to assure that it is utilized appropriately. One of the most commonly discussed properties of PMMA is viscosity, or the resistance to flow of a liquid, which can vary greatly based on the mixing method, molecular weight, liquid to powder ratio, and the addition of other materials to the cement (copolymers, antibiotics, etc.). High-viscosity cement typically has a shorter waiting phase and a longer working phase, which would seemingly be ideal for implanting TKA components.[8] However, there are some reports and concerns that these "thicker" cement options may not penetrate into the cancellous bone as well, leading to the potential for higher failure rates.[8-10] With modern cement techniques, it does not appear that these potential concerns have come to fruition in clinical practice with high-viscosity cement. Recently, Kelly et al confirmed this enthusiasm in regards to high-viscosity cement as its utilization has increased from 46% to 61.3% from 2012 to 2017,[11] even though survivorship studies are still needed prior to encouraging greater adoption of high-viscosity cements. Despite the less-than-ideal mixing conditions with low-viscosity cement, there have been reports with greater success than with high-viscosity cement.[11] An additional difference associated with cement viscosity includes the thermal energy produced during mixing and curing of the cement. High-viscosity cements tend to cure faster producing greater peak temperatures, while low-viscosity cements have lower heat release that lasts a longer time.[8] In the end, there is no consensus and both appear to work well if the appropriate steps are taken during the cementation process during a TKA.

During the cementation process, it is critical for cement to penetrate into the cancellous bone. The deeper and more complete the interdigitation is at the cement–bone interface, the greater the overall strength of the construct. To aid in this process, cement can be injected into the bone using a cement gun or finger packed using manual pressure. Both are successful techniques if the bony surface is cleaned and dried in preparation for receiving a cemented implant. Pulsatile lavage, drying the bone, and drilling into sclerotic areas of bone can aid in cement penetration and are encouraged prior to applying cement to the surface of the cancellous bone.[12,13] Typically, cement is quite strong in compression but is not as durable under shear forces, yet these properties can be greatly influenced by voids and deficiencies in the cement mantle. Therefore, meticulous cement preparation and mixing are critical and can intimately affect cement properties.

Mixing of cement can be performed by hand or under a vacuum preparation. The latter has been associated with decreased porosity and increased tensile strength.[8] Other concerns with hand mixing have been reports of higher mortality and pulmonary embolism rates.[8,14] Much of this data are based on case series in total hip arthroplasty but still remains a consideration in preparation for TKA. As mentioned previously, compounds can be added to PMMA as opacifying agents. Barium sulfate is often utilized in this regard, yet increasing concentrations can lead to a reduction in shear strength and polymerization temperatures, with possible further decreases in fatigue, compressive, and transverse bending strengths.[15,16] Alternatively, smaller size particles may aid in osteoblast adhesion as well as have a positive effect on fatigue strength.[8] Modern cement preparations in the United States often involve Simplex (Stryker, Mahwah, NJ) or Palacos (Heraeus Medical LLC, Yardley, PA) formulations with other options from alternative vendors being available. Classically, Simplex is an example of a low-viscosity cement and Palacos is a high-viscosity preparation. Some of the specific properties of these two commonly used cements include opacifier—zirconium dioxide for Palacos and barium sulfate for Simplex; higher-molecular-weight polymer for Palacos versus lower for Simplex; sterilizing method—ethylene oxide for Palacos and Gamma radiation for Simplex; initial bending strength 87 versus 72 MPa and residual strength after cycling, 17.8 versus 14.2 MPa, both favoring Palacos over Simplex.[17]

The final potential advantage of utilizing bone cement in TKA is the ability to deliver local antibiotics within the cement. This remains a relatively controversial topic as there is no definitive data to support the routine use of antibiotic-laden bone cement in primary TKA. In selecting an ideal antibiotic, it has to be heat stable, water soluble, bactericidal (against the bacteria of choice), and have minimal effect on the mechanical strength of the cement. Balancing cost (antibiotic bone cement can be up to three times that of plain cement) versus efficacy is an important concern regarding adding antibiotics routinely to the bone cement in primary TKA. The Norwegian and Swedish registries have shown a reduced risk of periprosthetic infection when antibiotics are preloaded into the cement during total hip procedures.[18,19] These early results have been favorable but must be weighed against the risks of compromised mechanical strength, drug-resistant bacteria, and hypersensitivity reactions.[20,21] Alternatively, Hinarejos et al reported on 2948 cemented TKAs with 1465 receiving PMMA without antibiotics and 1483 with erythromycin- and colistin-loaded cement. The study was a prospective randomized trial in which they found no difference in deep (1.4% vs. 1.35%) or superficial (1.2% vs. 1.8%) infection rates with the control group compared to the antibiotic–PMMA cohort.[22] Bohm et al. reported from the Canadian Joint Registry that 2-year revision rates were similar for those receiving antibiotic-loaded bone cement compared to those without antibiotics.[23] This included over 36,000 cases, and the revision rate for infection was similar between the groups at this short-term follow-up. Despite the potential advantage of adding antibiotics, there has been a trend of decreasing utilization in the American Joint Registry ranging from 44.2% to 34.5% from 2012 to 2017.[11] Some of the commonly used antibiotics for mixing with PMMA include vancomycin, gentamicin, tobramycin, ciprofloxacin, and voriconazole for fungal infections.

In regards to outcomes, cemented TKA remains the current gold standard. There are some recent studies that suggest equivalence between modern cementless versus cemented TKA. However, in general, the literature in the past has shown superior results with cemented implants as evidenced by the Swedish Registry reporting a 1.6× higher risk of revision if the tibial component is cementless.[24-26] In general, cemented components show smaller migration distances and rates compared to uncemented tibial implants. Cemented implants are typically cheaper, more forgiving during insertion, and can be used for all patients requiring TKA.

CEMENTLESS FIXATION

Biology of Cementless Fixation

Cementless fixation involves a connection between newly formed bone tissue and the implant's surface in contrast to cemented fixation, in which the polymer interdigitates with the surrounding trabecular bone to provide the bond between the host skeleton and the implant. An underlying assumption of the present chapter is that establishment and maintenance of a secure bony connection between the host skeleton and implant are prerequisites for long-term success. The theoretical advantage of cementless fixation is that the body relies on a self-repairing system of bone remodeling to maintain a mechanically competent interface, whereas with a cemented interface the mechanical properties of the polymer, if not the bone as well, would be expected to deteriorate with time.

Most of the initial studies of bone ingrowth in porous-coated implants indicated that bone ingrowth was a rare occurrence.[27,28] However, other studies which include a significant number of implants retrieved at autopsy from patients who had well-functioning implants indicate that bone ingrowth occurs more reliably than originally thought.[29,30] Even so, the topographic "coverage" by bone ingrowth typically involves less than one-third of the bone-contacting implant surface.[29-31] Despite this limited amount of osseous fixation, studies have shown comparable mechanical stability of TKA implants fixed by bone ingrowth and cement[32,33] and no differences in medium- to long-term survivorship based on revision for all causes in cemented versus cementless TKA in randomized controlled trials.[34] A meta-analysis of 15 studies which included 5 randomized controlled trials and 10 other studies found better survivorship and less aseptic loosening with cemented implants; although if the analyses were restricted to the randomized controlled trials, there were no significant differences between cemented and cementless TKA with respect to survivorship or aseptic loosening.[35]

From a mechanical standpoint, the load at the fixation interface could exceed the strength of the connecting bone tissue, in which case, one would expect fixation failure. This can occur if the area of fixation is insufficient, in which case interface stresses can exceed the capacity of newly formed bone to support the implant. Thus, implant designs need to accommodate this factor by providing broad enough areas of fixation. On the biologic side, it would seem advantageous to have surgical techniques and, perhaps, biologically active agents to ensure broad areas of bone ingrowth/apposition. Data suggest that most, if not all, cases of late aseptic loosening actually represent failure to obtain fixation initially.[36,37] Thus, the early mechanical and biologic events in cementless fixation are of critical importance.

The surgically induced trauma created at the time of implantation provides the context in which cementless fixation occurs.[38] The skeleton mounts a response leading to woven bone formation after hematoma formation and mesenchymal tissue development (**Fig. 14-1**). In this process of intramembranous bone regeneration, lamellar bone eventually forms on the spicules of woven bone and the hematopoietic marrow is reestablished. Under the correct conditions, this biologic response can result in the development of a mechanically competent connection between the implant's surface and host bone (**Fig. 14-2**).

After surgically induced intramembranous bone regeneration in sites where bone is not normally found (i.e., the diaphysis of a long bone), the newly formed bone will be completely resorbed and replaced by marrow unless an implant is present to provide a mechanical reason for the new bone to persist. In the context of knee arthroplasty, where the implants are placed in a trabecular bone bed, one would expect long-term persistence and functional adaptation of the newly formed bone tissue because fixation to the host skeleton imparts a mechanical function to the new tissue. Therefore, the distribution or amount of bone ingrowth would be expected to change over time and reflect areas of stress transfer from the implant to the host skeleton. Adaptation of the bone in periprosthetic regions has been identified in the context of knee replacement and is suspected to reflect changes in the local mechanical environment.[39-41]

The osteogenic potential of the implantation site would seem to be an important factor in cementless fixation. For instance, osteogenesis after skeletal trauma would be inhibited in the absence of appropriate stem cells. These cells are thought to reside in the marrow, especially in the region near the endosteum.[42-44] Although skeletal stem cells can be isolated from multiple anatomic locations, including bone marrow, periosteum, skeletal muscle, fat, and umbilical cord blood,[45] the general consensus is that only cells recruited locally serve as bone cell progenitors during bone repair.[46] If the local source-only concept for bone repair is correct, then decreased availability of stem cells is likely after aseptic loosening of cemented

implants, where the marrow spaces are filled by granuloma rather than normal marrow tissue, and may account for decreased bone formation in models of revision arthroplasty.[47,48] The issue of compromised osteogenic potential of stem cells as a function of aging is controversial.[49-55] Currently, there is limited clear-cut evidence of decreased osteogenesis in response to skeletal trauma in the aged skeleton.[56] However, diminished mechanical fixation related to osteopenia may pose problems.[57]

Studies of implant fixation and fracture healing indicate that many factors can inhibit bone regeneration. Perhaps of most concern are adjuvant treatments that are sometimes administered to patients receiving cementless joint replacements, especially for prevention of heterotopic ossification. For instance, it has been shown that the bisphosphonate disodium ethane-1-hydroxy-1, 1-diphosphonate,[58] indomethacin,[59,60] and certain doses of radiation[61,62] inhibit implant fixation. In addition, the anticoagulant warfarin has been shown to inhibit fixation strength.[63] In general, any factor that inhibits fracture healing should be assumed to have a similar effect on implant fixation unless otherwise demonstrated.

Various materials (e.g., bone graft substitutes), modalities (e.g., electrical stimulation), and implant surface modifications have been investigated for their ability to enhance cementless implant fixation. Treatment of interface gaps that exist at the time of surgery with autogenous bone or calcium phosphate bone graft substitute can enhance cementless fixation.[64,65] Additionally, certain growth factors such as recombinant transforming growth factor-β, bone morphogenetic protein-2, bone morphogenetic protein-7 (also known as *osteogenic protein-1*), and parathyroid hormone have been known for many years from preclinical models to enhance fixation,[66-68] but this strategy has not found its way to the clinic except for some occasional case reports. There is a vast literature on how treatment of implant surfaces can be manipulated to enhance implant fixation.[69] Broadly speaking, the approaches can be categorized as methods to affect surface topography from porous coatings at the millimeter scale to subtractive treatments (polishing, blasting, acid etching, oxidation) or additive processes (calcium phosphate coating, ion deposition) or surface chemistry manipulations (calcium phosphate surfaces, bioactive glasses, oxidized surfaces, and surfaces functionalized with peptides or proteins) at micrometer and nanometer scales. In addition, silver is being investigated as a surface treatment with antibacterial properties.[70] The most common of these, from a clinical point of view, is the use of calcium phosphate coatings, where a number of studies of the tibial component in TKA have reported beneficial findings.[69]

In the context of particle-induced osteolysis, a recent systematic review has shown that both anticatabolic and anabolic strategies can improve fixation in animal models.[65] While bisphosphonates are often delivered

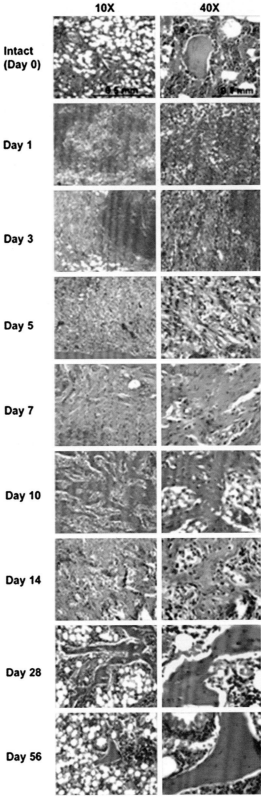

FIGURE 14-1   Time course of the histologic appearance in the rat following marrow ablation, which is a model of the biological response to the preparation of the implant site for joint replacement. This series of photomicrographs shows the progression from the intact marrow (day 0) which is typically populated by adipocytes and hematopoietic cells with some trabecular bone elements present. Day 1 post ablation is characterized by scattered polymorphonuclear cells in a forming blood clot. Day 3 shows infiltration of cells into the clot. Day 5 shows formation of fibrovascular structure with small vessels and an immature collagenous network. Days 7 and 10 show developing woven bone trabeculae. Day 14 is characterized by further development of the trabecular bone. Days 28 and 56 show maturation of the trabecular structure and reconstitution of the hematopoietic tissue. (From Wise JK, et al. Temporal gene expression profiling during rat femoral marrow ablation-induced intramembranous bone regeneration. *PLoS One*. 2010;5(10):e12987. doi:10.1371/journal.pone.0012987.)

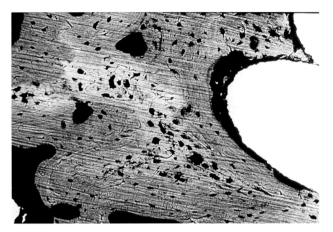

FIGURE 14-2 Backscatter scanning electron micrograph depicting bone ingrowth into a porous-coated joint replacement implant retrieved at autopsy. The subject was a 38-year-old male and the implant had been in place for 4 months. The implant had a porous surface made from titanium fiber metal. Note the presence of bone within the pores, with only occasional direct contact with the titanium wires. Thus, the basis of implant fixation by bone ingrowth into a porous surface is usually ascribed to mechanical interlock of bone and coating rather than direct bone–implant contact. The fiber metal wires were 0.25 mm thick.

locally, these and other anticatabolic agents as well as several anabolic agents can be administered systemically.[65,71] In particular, bisphosphonates and some other anticatabolic agents as well as intermittent parathyroid hormone administration and sclerostin antibody have been shown to block the development of particle-induced osteolysis.

STANDARD CONCEPTS IN ACHIEVING OSSEOINTEGRATION

Most cementless joint replacement implants in the United States involve the use of porous-coated surfaces, grit blasting, and/or plasma spray technology. In addition, a number of novel means of preparing implant surfaces are now under investigation, and some of these are likely to reach clinical practice in the future. Despite these options for cementless fixation, many of the basic concepts learned during the past 5 decades of research into the use of porous coatings remain relevant. The conditions for osseointegration include the following:

- Close contact between the implant surface and host bone
- Minimal relative motion at the bone–implant interface
- The presence of appropriate implant surface characteristics
- A bony bed with osteogenic potential

A number of studies have shown that gaps as small as 0.5 mm can inhibit bone ingrowth.[72] This is a matter of concern because gaps between the implant and host bone of 1 to 2 mm are routinely created in total knee replacement,[73] and even larger gaps occasionally occur, especially in the context of revision surgery.[74,75] Cutting

errors from saw toggle and motion of cutting guides are seen in traditional jig-based TKA.[73] Robotic arm–assisted TKA reduces cutting error in cadaveric specimens,[76] which in theory increases the likelihood of osseointegration by decreasing the distance between implant surface and host bone, but this has never been shown in clinical studies. Robotic surgery that uses an irrigated burr may also reduce heat necrosis of bone associated with a traditional saw blade cutting technique.

"Excessive" motion is universally accepted to be inhibitory to bone ingrowth, but the precise definition of "excessive" remains elusive. For example, implants in which a connection between the host skeleton and bone within the porous coating is maintained permit bone ingrowth with initial interface motions of 20 μm.[77] However, in the same study with initial motions of 40 μm or more, the connection with the host skeleton was subsequently lost or was never formed in the first place, even though bone tissue was observed within the porous coating. Another study demonstrated bony ingrowth with minimal motion of 28 μm, while motion >150 μm produced fibrous ingrowth.[78]

There has been considerable interest in how tibial component design in total knee replacement can be altered to minimize the initial motion between the implant and host bone. Screws were initially used for increased stability, but retrieval studies have shown that screw tracts or holes can serve as a conduit for particulate debris to gain access to the interface,[29] leading to osteolysis. This paradox underscores the complexity of implant design—generally, there truly is no perfect solution, only a series of compromises. The goal is to obtain ingrowth at the tibial baseplate and not on the screws or fixation pegs. A recent biomechanical study demonstrated less liftoff and rocking with a circumferential porous titanium undersurface tibial baseplate with a central keel and fixation pegs compared to a porous tantalum baseplate with dual-hex peg fixation,[79] but the optimal design is still unknown.

One of the most exciting recent advancements in cementless fixation is the design of new highly porous metals. Surface characteristics have been well studied in terms of the pore geometry of porous coatings, where a previous dogma stated the pores must be interconnecting and between 100 and 400 μm in size. New highly porous metals offer desirable characteristics for ingrowth. Porous tantalum, for example, has pore geometry up to 650 μm along with higher coefficient of friction and lower modulus of elasticity than previous porous-coated implants. In canine models, both porous tantalum and highly porous titanium demonstrated greater ingrowth and higher interference shear strength when compared to previous porous implants.[80,81] In addition, a retrieval study of failed hip and knee arthroplasty implants showed increased depth of ingrowth in porous tantalum compared to traditional porous metal designs.[82]

Surface coating with calcium phosphate treatments, especially plasma-sprayed hydroxyapatite, has been the subject of extensive investigation and growing clinical usage.[83] The ability of these coatings to enhance fixation, even under "ideal" conditions of implantation, has been recognized for some time.[84] This type of surface treatment appears to have beneficial effects even in the presence of interface motion. For instance, studies of impaired fixation because of interface motion have shown that a hydroxyapatite coating of the porous surface appears to permit bone ingrowth/ongrowth in the presence of 150 μm of interface motion, an amount of motion that normally does not permit bone ingrowth/ongrowth. As there are wide variations in the qualitative aspects of these coatings, a key development will be an improved understanding of the biologic effects and clinical correlates.[83] In addition, a clinical trial has shown that hydroxyapatite-treated porous-coated components and cemented components were equally stable and showed less migration at 1 to 2 years than porous-coated tibial components of the same design.[85]

As a consequence of the increased metal surface area of porous-coated or surface-structured cementless components and the fact that metal surfaces directly interact with the surrounding tissue without an intervening layer of bone cement, there has historically been concerns that cementless total joint replacement components are associated with a greater risk of systemic dissemination of metal debris and potentially a greater risk of adverse systemic effects. While comparative studies of metal release in cement versus cementless total knee replacements are limited, one study of cementless titanium alloy total knee replacements demonstrated statistically significant elevations in serum titanium only when there was a failed metal-backed patella or a carbon-fiber-reinforced polyethylene articulating surface, the latter implying accelerated femoral component wear. In comparison to patients without implants, there were no statistically significant elevations in serum titanium in patients with well-functioning cementless total knee replacements using conventional polyethylene.[86]

Furthermore, in a head to head comparison of metal release in patients with cemented versus cementless total hip replacements, passive dissolution from extensively coated cobalt-alloy stems was not found to be a dominant mode of metal release. Rather, metal release from metal/metal modular junctions was the likely dominant source of metal release.[87,88] Taken together, the available evidence suggests that it is unlikely that cementless total knee replacements, per se, are associated with a higher risk of systemic transport of metal debris or a higher risk of metal-induced systemic effects than cemented total knee replacements. However, wear through of a metal-backed patellar component, which is most commonly used in cementless TKA, can be associated with very high levels of serum titanium.[86,89]

IMPLANT CONSIDERATIONS: LEARNING FROM OUR MISTAKES

Past failures of cementless TKA have been linked to design failures and led many surgeons to abandon cementless fixation. Modern implant design has tried to account for these errors, but at the present time, there are no cementless knee implants with a proven long-term track record.

Tibial fixation is challenging using cementless techniques due to relatively poor bone stock, single-plane fixation compared to multiplanar fixation in the femur, and complex loading patterns on the tibial baseplate that may cause liftoff and/or micromotion that inhibits osseointegration. An early series of 108 uncemented porous-coated anatomic knee prostheses demonstrated 19% failure rate at average of 64 months of follow-up, and all failures were related to failure of osseointegration of the tibial component.[90] In an effort to improve initial stability and prevent liftoff, newer designs included screw augmentation. However, this led to the unanticipated observation of screw tract osteolysis as particulate debris gained access to the implant interface. In a series of 131 consecutive cementless total knee arthroplasties with a mean follow-up of 11 years, tibial components had 8% rate of aseptic loosening and 12% rate of osteolytic lesions, all occurring around screws or screw holes.[91] Improving locking mechanisms and improved polyethylene wear resistance will most likely reduce screw tract osteolysis by decreasing the polyethylene debris associated with backside and articular surface wear. The current goal for tibial baseplate design is to feature circumferential porous coating that achieves osseointegration at the baseplate rather than screw or peg fixation in order to achieve enough stability to prevent micromotion. Good long-term clinical data with any design are not available at this time.

Failure of metal-backed patella designs is well documented in the literature with patellar revision rate as high as 48% in a study with 11-year follow-up.[91] Failure mechanisms in that cohort were loosening and catastrophic polyethylene wear. Currently controversy remains regarding the best method of patella resurfacing in cementless fixation. Issues with cementless femoral fixation have included stress shielding of the anterior cortex due to fixation around the pegs, as well as fatigue fracture of the femoral component at thin regions.[92,93]

REVISION ARTHROPLASTY: ACHIEVING OSSEOINTEGRATION IN SETTING OF BONE LOSS

The revision environment appears to represent a severe challenge for cementless fixation because of the increased likelihood of interface gaps, motion, and, probably, an inherently diminished osteogenic capacity. This diminished osteogenic capacity is due to the replacement of normal medullary contents by granulation tissue. These observations were noted in an experimental total hip arthroplasty study[47] and may well apply to the knee. Although there is clinical as well as experimental evidence that the bony bed in revision surgery still retains some osteogenic potential, it is apparent that revision surgery presents the greatest challenge for bone ingrowth fixation and the greatest need for the development of means to enhance bone regeneration.

Highly porous metal cone augments are an attractive option to address large tibial and femoral metaphyseal bone defects. These augments take advantage of the mechanical properties of highly porous metals which provide stability yet allow for biologic integration. The cones provide modular defect reconstruction as they come in variable sizes and can be used across manufacturer's implant systems. Cement is typically used between the cone and implant, but the stem extension in the tibia or femur can be cemented or cementless. Metaphyseal titanium-tapered sleeves are a similar broach-only option that links the titanium sleeve to the implant through a modular taper. These new biomaterials increase the potential for biologic ingrowth with host bone and may lead to long-term success. The results from using porous tantalum metaphyseal cones for revision TKA with severe tibial bone loss at intermediate follow-up of 5 to 9 years suggest greater than 95% revision-free survival of the tibial component.[94] However, long-term clinical outcomes to demonstrate success are not available.

CONCLUSION

In conclusion, cemented TKA involves interdigitation of PMMA cement that serves as a grout between the implant and host bone. While cemented TKA remains the gold standard technique, cementless TKA is an attractive alternative because a biological fixation interface may have increased longevity. However, cementless fixation relies on a few important principles: close contact between the implant surface and host bone, minimal relative motion at the bone–implant interface, the presence of appropriate implant surface characteristics, and a bony bed with osteogenic potential.

ACKNOWLEDGMENTS

Some of the authors have been supported by NIH Grants R01AR066562 and R21AR075130. The content is solely the responsibility of the authors and does not necessarily represent the official views of the National Institutes of Health.

REFERENCES

1. Sartawi M, Zurakowski D, Rosenberg A. Implant survivorship and complication rates after total knee arthroplasty with a third-generation cemented system: 15-year follow-up. *Am J Orthop (Belle Mead NJ)*. 2018;47(3). doi:10.12788/ajo.2018.0018.

2. Ritter MA, Keating EM, Sueyoshi T, Davis KE, Barrington JW, Emerson RH. Twenty-five-years and greater, results after nonmodular cemented total knee arthroplasty. *J Arthroplasty*. 2016;31(10):2199-2202.

3. Patil S, McCauley JC, Pulido P, Colwell CW Jr. How do knee implants perform past the second decade? Nineteen- to 25-year followup of the Press-fit Condylar design TKA. *Clin Orthop Relat Res*. 2015;473(1):135-140.

4. Huizinga MR, Brouwer RW, Bisschop R, van der Veen HC, van den Akker-Scheek I, van Raay JJ. Long-term follow-up of anatomic graduated component total knee arthroplasty: a 15- to 20-year survival analysis. *J Arthroplasty*. 2012;27(6):1190-1195.

5. Gwam CU, George NE, Etcheson JI, Rosas S, Plate JF, Delanois RE. Cementless versus cemented fixation in total knee arthroplasty: usage, costs, and complications during the inpatient period. *J Knee Surg*. 2019;32(11):1081-1087.

6. Cohen RG, Sherman NC, James SL. Early clinical outcomes of a new cementless total knee arthroplasty design. *Orthopedics*. 2018;41(6):e765-e771.

7. Lai PL, Chen LH, Chen WJ, Chu IM. Chemical and physical properties of bone cement for vertebroplasty. *Biomed J*. 2013;36(4):162-167.

8. Saleh KJ, El Othmani MM, Tzeng TH, Mihalko WM, Chambers MC, Grupp TM. Acrylic bone cement in total joint arthroplasty: a review. *J Orthop Res*. 2016;34(5):737-744.

9. Kopec M, Milbrandt JC, Kohut N, Kern B, Allan DG. Effect of bone cement viscosity and set time on mantle area in total knee arthroplasty. *Am J Orthop (Belle Mead NJ)*. 2009;38(10):519-522.

10. Kopinski JE, Aggarwal A, Nunley RM, Barrack RL, Nam D. Failure at the tibial cement-implant interface with the use of high-viscosity cement in total knee arthroplasty. *J Arthroplasty*. 2016;31(11):2579-2582.

11. Kelly MP, Illgen RL, Chen AF, Nam D. Trends in the use of high-viscosity cement in patients undergoing primary total knee arthroplasty in the United States. *J Arthroplasty*. 2018;33(11):3460-3464.

12. Schlegel UJ, Bishop NE, Puschel K, Morlock MM, Nagel K. Comparison of different cement application techniques for tibial component fixation in TKA. *Int Orthop*. 2015;39(1):47-54.

13. Norton MR, Eyres KS. Irrigation and suction technique to ensure reliable cement penetration for total knee arthroplasty. *J Arthroplasty*. 2000;15(4):468-474.

14. Hazelwood KJ, O'Rourke M, Stamos VP, McMillan RD, Beigler D, Robb WJ III. Case series report: early cement-implant interface fixation failure in total knee replacement. *Knee*. 2015;22(5):424-428.

15. Combs SP, Greenwald AS. The effects of barium sulfate on the polymerization temperature and shear strength of surgical simplex P. *Clin Orthop Relat Res*. 1979;(145):287-291.

16. Haas SS, Brauer GM, Dickson G. A characterization of polymethylmethacrylate bone cement. *J Bone Joint Surg Am*. 1975;57(3):380-391.

17. Kuhn K-D. *Bone Cements: Up-to-Date Comparison of Physical and Chemical Properties of Commercial Materials*. 1st ed. Berlin, New York: Springer; 2000.

18. Espehaug B, Engesaeter LB, Vollset SE, Havelin LI, Langeland N. Antibiotic prophylaxis in total hip arthroplasty. Review of 10,905 primary cemented total hip replacements reported to the Norwegian arthroplasty register, 1987 to 1995. *J Bone Joint Surg Br Vol*. 1997;79(4):590-595.

19. Malchau H, Herberts P, Ahnfelt L. Prognosis of total hip replacement in Sweden. Follow-up of 92,675 operations performed 1978-1990. *Acta Orthop Scand*. 1993;64(5):497-506.

20. Illingworth KD, Mihalko WM, Parvizi J, et al. How to minimize infection and thereby maximize patient outcomes in total joint arthroplasty: a multicenter approach: AAOS exhibit selection. *J Bone Joint Surg Am Vol*. 2013;95(8):e50.

21. Chiu FY, Chen CM, Lin CF, Lo WH. Cefuroxime-impregnated cement in primary total knee arthroplasty: a prospective, randomized study of three hundred and forty knees. *J Bone Joint Surg Am Vol*. 2002;84-A(5):759-762.

22. Hinarejos P, Guirro P, Leal J, et al. The use of erythromycin and colistin-loaded cement in total knee arthroplasty does not reduce the incidence of infection: a prospective randomized study in 3000 knees. *J Bone Joint Surg Am.* 2013;95(9):769-774.

23. Bohm E, Zhu N, Gu J, et al. Does adding antibiotics to cement reduce the need for early revision in total knee arthroplasty? *Clin Orthop Relat Res.* 2013;472(1):162-168.

24. Karachalios T, Komnos G, Amprazis V, Antoniou I, Athanaselis SA. 9-Year outcome study comparing cancellous titanium-coated cementless to cemented tibial components of the advance medial-pivot knee arthroplasty. *J Arthroplasty.* 2018;33(12):3672-3677.

25. Robertsson O, Ranstam J, Sundberg M, W-Dhal A, Lidgren L. The Swedish knee arthroplasty register: a review. *Bone Joint Res.* 2014;3(7):217-222.

26. Zhou K, Yu H, Li J, Wang H, Zhou Z, Pei F. No difference in implant survivorship and clinical outcomes between full-cementless and full-cemented fixation in primary total knee arthroplasty: a systematic review and meta-analysis. *Int J Surg.* 2018;53:312-319.

27. Ranawat CS, Johanson NA, Rimnac CM, Wright TM, Schwartz RE. Retrieval analysis of porous-coated components for total knee arthroplasty. A report of two cases. *Clin Orthop Relat Res.* 1986;(209):244-248.

28. Cook SD, Scheller AD, Anderson RC, Haddad RJ Jr. Histologic and microradiographic analysis of a revised porous-coated anatomic (PCA) patellar component. A case report. *Clin Orthop Relat Res.* 1986;(202):147-151.

29. Sumner DR, Kienapfel H, Jacobs JJ, Urban RM, Turner TM, Galante JO. Bone ingrowth and wear debris in well-fixed cementless porous-coated tibial components removed from patients. *J Arthroplasty.* 1995;10(2):157-167.

30. Bloebaum RD, Bachus KN, Jensen JW, Hofmann AA. Postmortem analysis of consecutively retrieved asymmetric porous-coated tibial components. *J Arthroplasty.* 1997;12(8):920-929.

31. Hanzlik JA, Day JS, Rimnac CM, Kurtz SM. Is there a difference in bone ingrowth in modular versus monoblock porous tantalum tibial trays? *J Arthroplasty.* 2015;30(6):1073-1078.

32. Matsuda S, Tanner MG, White SE, Whiteside LA. Evaluation of tibial component fixation in specimens retrieved at autopsy. *Clin Orthop Relat Res.* 1999;(363):249-257.

33. Nilsson KG, Karrholm J, Linder L. Femoral component migration in total knee arthroplasty: randomized study comparing cemented and uncemented fixation of the Miller-Galante I design. *J Orthop Res.* 1995;13(3):347-356.

34. Prudhon JL, Verdier R. Cemented or cementless total knee arthroplasty? – comparative results of 200 cases at a minimum follow-up of 11 years. *Sicot J.* 2017;3:70.

35. Gandhi R, Tsvetkov D, Davey JR, Mahomed NN. Survival and clinical function of cemented and uncemented prostheses in total knee replacement: a meta-analysis. *J Bone Joint Surg Br.* 2009;91(7):889-895.

36. Ryd L, Albrektsson BE, Carlsson L, et al. Roentgen stereophotogrammetric analysis as a predictor of mechanical loosening of knee prostheses. *J Bone Joint Surg Br.* 1995;77(3):377-383.

37. Pijls BG, Plevier JWM, Nelissen R. RSA migration of total knee replacements. *Acta Orthop.* 2018;89(3):320-328.

38. Moran MM, Sena K, McNulty MA, Sumner DR, Virdi AS. Intramembranous bone regeneration and implant placement using mechanical femoral marrow ablation: rodent models. *Bonekey Rep.* 2016;5:837.

39. Regner LR, Carlsson LV, Karrholm JN, Hansson TH, Herberts PG, Swanpalmer J. Bone mineral and migratory patterns in uncemented total knee arthroplasties: a randomized 5-year follow-up study of 38 knees. *Acta Orthop Scand.* 1999;70(6):603-608.

40. Petersen MM, Olsen C, Lauritzen JB, Lund B. Changes in bone mineral density of the distal femur following uncemented total knee arthroplasty. *J Arthroplasty.* 1995;10(1):7-11.

41. Jaroma A, Soininvaara T, Kroger H. Periprosthetic tibial bone mineral density changes after total knee arthroplasty. *Acta Orthop.* 2016;87(3):268-273.

42. Ohgushi H, Caplan AI. Stem cell technology and bioceramics: from cell to gene engineering. *J Biomed Mater Res.* 1999;48(6):913-927.

43. Bruder SP, Kurth AA, Shea M, Hayes WC, Jaiswal N, Kadiyala S. Bone regeneration by implantation of purified, culture-expanded human mesenchymal stem cells. *J Orthop Res.* 1998;16(2):155-162.

44. Prockop DJ. Marrow stromal cells as stem cells for nonhematopoietic tissues. *Science.* 1997;276(5309):71-74.

45. Walmsley GG, Ransom RC, Zielins ER, et al. Stem cells in bone regeneration. *Stem Cell Rev.* 2016;12(5):524-529.

46. Worthley DL, Churchill M, Compton JT, et al. Gremlin 1 identifies a skeletal stem cell with bone, cartilage, and reticular stromal potential. *Cell.* 2015;160(1-2):269-284.

47. Turner TM, Urban RM, Sumner DR, Galante JO. Revision, without cement, of aseptically loose, cemented total hip prostheses. Quantitative comparison of the effects of four types of medullary treatment on bone ingrowth in a canine model. *J Bone Joint Surg Am.* 1993;75(6):845-862.

48. Soballe K, Mouzin OR, Kidder LA, Overgaard S, Bechtold JE. The effects of hydroxyapatite coating and bone allograft on fixation of loaded experimental primary and revision implants. *Acta Orthop Scand.* 2003;74(3):239-247.

49. D'Ippolito G, Schiller PC, Ricordi C, Roos BA, Howard GA. Age-related osteogenic potential of mesenchymal stromal stem cells from human vertebral bone marrow. *J Bone Miner Res.* 1999;14(7):1115-1122.

50. Bergman RJ, Gazit D, Kahn AJ, Gruber H, McDougall S, Hahn TJ. Age-related changes in osteogenic stem cells in mice. *J Bone Miner Res.* 1996;11(5):568-577.

51. Oreffo RO, Bennett A, Carr AJ, Triffitt JT. Patients with primary osteoarthritis show no change with ageing in the number of osteogenic precursors. *Scand J Rheumatol.* 1998;27(6):415-424.

52. Oreffo RO, Bord S, Triffitt JT. Skeletal progenitor cells and ageing human populations. *Clin Sci (Lond).* 1998;94(5):549-555.

53. Stenderup K, Justesen J, Eriksen EF, Rattan SI, Kassem M. Number and proliferative capacity of osteogenic stem cells are maintained during aging and in patients with osteoporosis. *J Bone Miner Res.* 2001;16(6):1120-1129.

54. Muschler GF, Nitto H, Boehm CA, Easley KA. Age- and gender-related changes in the cellularity of human bone marrow and the prevalence of osteoblastic progenitors. *J Orthop Res.* 2001;19(1):117-125.

55. Gao X, Lu A, Tang Y, et al. Influences of donor and host age on human muscle-derived stem cell-mediated bone regeneration. *Stem Cell Res Ther.* 2018;9(1):316.

56. Sumner DR, Turner TM, Cohen M, et al. Aging does not lessen the effectiveness of TGFbeta2-enhanced bone regeneration. *J Bone Miner Res.* 2003;18(4):730-736.

57. Lane JM, Cornell CN, Healey JH. Osteoporosis: the structural and reparative consequences for the skeleton. *Instr Course Lect.* 1987;36:71-83.

58. Rivero DP, Skipor AK, Singh M, Urban RM, Galante JO. Effect of disodium etidronate (EHDP) on bone ingrowth in a porous material. *Clin Orthop Relat Res* 1987;(215):279-286.

59. Keller JC, Trancik TM, Young FA, St Mary E. Effects of indomethacin on bone ingrowth. *J Orthop Res.* 1989;7(1):28-34.

60. Cook SD, Barrack RL, Dalton JE, Thomas KA, Brown TD. Effects of indomethacin on biologic fixation of porous-coated titanium implants. *J Arthroplasty.* 1995;10(3):351-358.

61. Sumner DR, Turner TM, Pierson RH, et al. Effects of radiation on fixation of non-cemented porous-coated implants in a canine model. *J Bone Joint Surg Am.* 1990;72(10):1527-1533.

62. Chin HC, Frassica FJ, Markel MD, Frassica DA, Sim FH, Chao EY. The effects of therapeutic doses of irradiation on experimental bone graft incorporation over a porous-coated segmental defect endoprosthesis. *Clin Orthop Relat Res* 1993;(289):254-266.

63. Callahan BC, Lisecki EJ, Banks RE, Dalton JE, Cook SD, Wolff JD. The effect of warfarin on the attachment of bone to hydroxyapatite-coated and uncoated porous implants. *J Bone Joint Surg Am.* 1995;77(2):225-230.

64. Kienapfel H, Sumner DR, Turner TM, Urban RM, Galante JO. Efficacy of autograft and freeze-dried allograft to enhance fixation of porous coated implants in the presence of interface gaps. *J Orthop Res.* 1992;10(3):423-433.

65. Moran MM, Wilson BM, Ross RD, Virdi AS, Sumner DR. Arthrotomy-based preclinical models of particle-induced osteolysis: a systematic review. *J Orthop Res.* 2017;35(12):2595-2605.

66. Sumner DR, Turner TM, Purchio AF, Gombotz WR, Urban RM, Galante JO. Enhancement of bone ingrowth by transforming growth factor-beta. *J Bone Joint Surg Am.* 1995;77(8):1135-1147.

67. Cook SD, Barrack RL, Shimmin A, Morgan D, Carvajal JP. The use of osteogenic protein-1 in reconstructive surgery of the hip. *J Arthroplasty.* 2001;16(8 suppl 1):88-94.

68. Skripitz R, Aspenberg P. Implant fixation enhanced by intermittent treatment with parathyroid hormone. *J Bone Joint Surg Br.* 2001;83(3):437-440.

69. Sumner D, Virdi A. *Materials in Hip Surgery: Bioactive Coatings for Implant Fixation.* New York, NY: Elsevier; 2013.

70. Gallo J, Panacek A, Prucek R, et al. Silver nanocoating technology in the prevention of prosthetic joint infection. *Materials (Basel).* 2016;9(5). pii: E337.

71. Ross RD, Hamilton JL, Wilson BM, Sumner DR, Virdi AS. Pharmacologic augmentation of implant fixation in osteopenic bone. *Curr Osteoporos Rep.* 2014;12(1):55-64.

72. Dalton JE, Cook SD, Thomas KA, Kay JF. The effect of operative fit and hydroxyapatite coating on the mechanical and biological response to porous implants. *J Bone Joint Surg Am.* 1995;77(1):97-110.

73. Otani T, Whiteside LA, White SE. Cutting errors in preparation of femoral components in total knee arthroplasty. *J Arthroplasty.* 1993;8(5):503-510.

74. Whiteside LA. Correction of ligament and bone defects in total arthroplasty of the severely valgus knee. *Clin Orthop Relat Res.* 1993;(288):234-245.

75. Whiteside LA. Cementless revision total knee arthroplasty. *Clin Orthop Relat Res.* 1993;(286):160-167.

76. Hampp EL, Chughtai M, Scholl LY, et al. Robotic-arm assisted total knee arthroplasty demonstrated greater accuracy and precision to plan compared with manual techniques. *J Knee Surg.* 2019;32(3):239-250.

77. Bragdon CR, Burke D, Lowenstein JD, et al. Differences in stiffness of the interface between a cementless porous implant and cancellous bone in vivo in dogs due to varying amounts of implant motion. *J Arthroplasty.* 1996;11(8):945-951.

78. Pilliar RM, Lee JM, Maniatopoulos C. Observations on the effect of movement on bone ingrowth into porous-surfaced implants. *Clin Orthop Relat Res.* 1986;(208):108-113.

79. Bhimji S, Meneghini RM. Micromotion of cementless tibial baseplates: keels with adjuvant pegs offer more stability than pegs alone. *J Arthroplasty.* 2014;29(7):1503-1506.

80. Bobyn JD, Stackpool GJ, Hacking SA, Tanzer M, Krygier JJ. Characteristics of bone ingrowth and interface mechanics of a new porous tantalum biomaterial. *J Bone Joint Surg Br.* 1999;81(5):907-914.

81. Frenkel SR, Jaffe WL, Dimaano F, Iesaka K, Hua T. Bone response to a novel highly porous surface in a canine implantable chamber. *J Biomed Mater Res B Appl Biomater.* 2004;71(2):387-391.

82. Hanzlik JA, Day JS. Bone ingrowth in well-fixed retrieved porous tantalum implants. *J Arthroplasty.* 2013;28(6):922-927.

83. Sun L, Berndt CC, Gross KA, Kucuk A. Material fundamentals and clinical performance of plasma-sprayed hydroxyapatite coatings: a review. *J Biomed Mater Res.* 2001;58(5):570-592.

84. Thomas KA, Kay JF, Cook SD, Jarcho M. The effect of surface macrotexture and hydroxylapatite coating on the mechanical strengths and histologic profiles of titanium implant materials. *J Biomed Mater Res.* 1987;21(12):1395-1414.

85. Onsten I, Nordqvist A, Carlsson AS, Besjakov J, Shott S. Hydroxyapatite augmentation of the porous coating improves fixation of tibial components. A randomised RSA study in 116 patients. *J Bone Joint Surg Br.* 1998;80(3):417-425.

86. Jacobs JJ, Silverton C, Hallab NJ, et al. Metal release and excretion from cementless titanium alloy total knee replacements. *Clin Orthop Relat Res.* 1999;(358):173-180.

87. Jacobs JJ, Skipor AK, Patterson LM, et al. Metal release in patients who have had a primary total hip arthroplasty. A prospective, controlled, longitudinal study. *J Bone Joint Surg Am.* 1998;80(10):1447-1458.

88. Levine BR, Hsu AR, Skipor AK, et al. Ten-year outcome of serum metal ion levels after primary total hip arthroplasty: a concise follow-up of a previous report. *J Bone Joint Surg Am.* 2013;95(6):512-518.

89. Leopold SS, Berger RA, Patterson L, Skipor AK, Urban RM, Jacobs JJ. Serum titanium level for diagnosis of a failed, metal-backed patellar component. *J Arthroplasty.* 2000;15(7):938-943.

90. Moran CG, Pinder IM, Lees TA, Midwinter MJ. Survivorship analysis of the uncemented porous-coated anatomic knee replacement. *J Bone Joint Surg Am.* 1991;73(6):848-857.

91. Berger RA, Lyon JH, Jacobs JJ, et al. Problems with cementless total knee arthroplasty at 11 years followup. *Clin Orthop Relat Res.* 2001;(392):196-207.

92. Whiteside LA, Fosco DR, Brooks JG Jr. Fracture of the femoral component in cementless total knee arthroplasty. *Clin Orthop Relat Res.* 1993;(286):71-77.

93. Campbell MD, Duffy GP, Trousdale RT. Femoral component failure in hybrid total knee arthroplasty. *Clin Orthop Relat Res.* 1998;(356):58-65.

94. Kamath AF, Lewallen DG, Hanssen AD. Porous tantalum metaphyseal cones for severe tibial bone loss in revision knee arthroplasty: a five to nine-year follow-up. *J Bone Joint Surg Am.* 2015;97(3):216-223.

Clinical Science

SECTION 3

JAMES I. HUDDLESTON III

chapter 15

Examination of the Knee Before and After Total Knee Replacement

Raj K. Sinha, MD, PhD

INTRODUCTION

This purpose of this chapter is to discuss the examination of the knee as it pertains specifically to total knee arthroplasty (TKA), rather than to be an exhaustive treatise on knee examination relevant to other surgical procedures. Although the examination of the soon-to-be-replaced knee is relatively streamlined, almost every pertinent finding has an important impact on planning and executing the knee replacement. Similarly, after knee replacement, particularly in an unhappy patient, examination is as important as imaging and other tests to help determine the etiology of an unsuccessful replacement. In the case of the happy knee replacement patient, of course, examination and imaging are usually both satisfactory!

EXAMINATION OF THE KNEE BEFORE KNEE REPLACEMENT

Inspection and Observation

Skin

As knee replacement will require a surgical incision, integrity of the skin is critical for a successful outcome. The skin at the surgical site should be healthy, without lesions, with excellent flexibility, vascularity, and turgor. In the case of inflammatory conditions such as psoriatic arthritis, all rashes should be optimized prior to surgery. The author employs the assistance of a rheumatologist or dermatologist to achieve this. When recent trauma has occurred, all ecchymosis and induration should be allowed to heal prior to surgery. Similarly, conditions such as prepatellar bursitis may affect the decision to proceed with TKA. For example, the prepatellar bursa may be so tense that the overlying skin appears compromised. The concern arises that healing may be delayed after surgery, thus unnecessarily raising the risk of infection in TKA. In such cases, the author has performed a bursa excision, in effect as a sham incision, to confirm that healing will proceed normally. Likewise, if vascularity is thought to be compromised, performing a sham incision is a reasonable approach before proceeding with knee replacement.[1] The use of transcutaneous pO_2 to assess vascularity has shown to be of some value, as areas of lower oxygen tension may demonstrate delayed healing.[2] Thin skin, especially in the

obese and elderly, is prone to persistent wound drainage and may require special closure techniques[3] (**Fig. 15-1A**). Of course, knee replacement should never be undertaken in the face of surgical site cellulitis or other infections.

A common situation encountered in TKA patients is previous surgical incisions. Prior arthroscopy, open meniscectomy and repair of fractures about the knee are quite frequent prior to TKA. The location of these incisions should be noted, particularly whether they will affect the TKA incision. In general, the most recent or most lateral incision should be utilized[4] (**Fig. 15-1B**), as the lateral side of the skin tends to be more hypoxic after surgery. Similarly, the longitudinal TKA incision should cross more transverse incisions as perpendicular as possible. Oblique incisions can frequently be extended proximally and distally, still allow excellent joint exposure, and result in a more cosmetically pleasing scar (**Fig. 15-1C and D**). Fortunately, in the last several decades, as TKA became a more reliable salvage solution after trauma, midline skin incisions have become more popular for fracture fixation, resulting in fewer issues for the arthroplasty surgeon. In cases of multiple incisions, with excessively scarred and immobile skin, pre-TKA tissue expanders can be utilized.[4] In conclusion, the condition of the skin is of paramount importance to an eventual successful outcome.

Gait

Evaluation of the patient's gait will demonstrate varus or valgus thrust, varus or valgus joint alignment, hip/spine/foot/ankle issues, and muscle strength. Dynamic thrust during gait is predictive of asymmetric joint loading and cartilage wear,[5] and the demonstration of a thrust helps to confirm the presence of advanced joint degeneration (**Fig. 15-2A to C**). Similarly, the degree of static varus or valgus alignment is reflective of degree of cartilage and/or bone loss. In terms of relevance to TKA surgery, thrust may indicate ligamentous laxity, whose presence may determine implant choice or adjustment in reconstruction technique. Thus, the presence of dynamic or static thrust necessitates a thorough examination of knee ligament functionality. Abnormal gait may also reveal hip/spine/foot/ankle pathology. Prior to proceeding with TKA, it is important to determine whether issues with other ipsilateral or contralateral joints may affect technique or

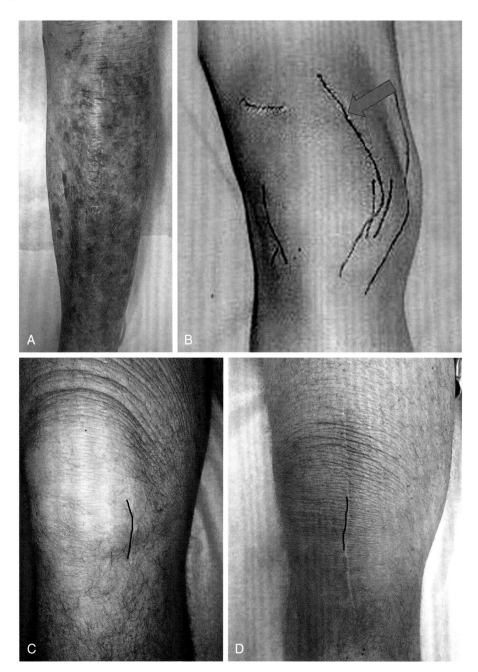

FIGURE 15-1   A: Thin skin, concerning for delayed postoperative healing or slough from postoperative swelling. **B:** Example of a knee with previous multiple incisions. In this case, the incision marked with the arrow would be most favorable for total knee arthroplasty (TKA). **C** and **D:** Example of a TKA performed incorporating a previous surgical scar. Preoperative (**C**—scar marked by line). 1 y postoperative (**D**).

postoperative rehab. For example, when severe hip joint osteoarthritis is present, total hip arthroplasty should be performed before TKA. Abnormal muscle strength may manifest in an abnormal gait pattern and should be addressed when considering TKA. A weak quadriceps will result in a forward lurch and may be indicative of an underlying neuromuscular condition or myopathy, both of which would affect rehabilitation after TKA. Thus, evaluation of gait will help the arthroplasty surgeon customize the knee reconstruction and possibly adjust the treatment plan to avoid a complication and optimize the outcome.

Deformity

INTRA-ARTICULAR

Within the joint, varus or valgus deformity can occur from cartilage loss, bone loss, malunions, ligamentous laxity, or some combination of all. Each of these parameters will affect the surgical reconstruction. For example, bone loss may necessitate the use of stems or wedges to create the proper joint line position and angle. Similarly, collateral ligament incompetence may require a more constrained polyethylene insert or even a hinged arthroplasty. Combined with imaging, physical examination will assist in planning the reconstruction.

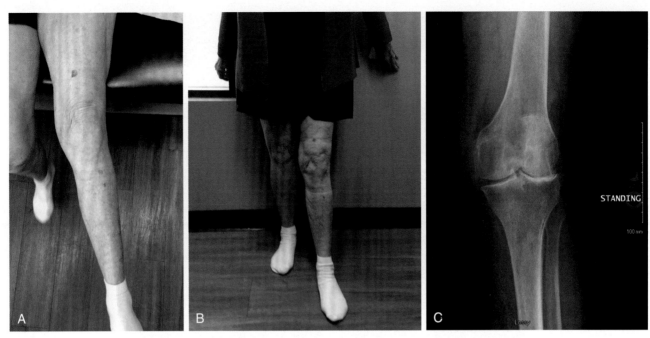

STANDING

100 mm

FIGURE 15-2 **A:** Example of valgus deformity. **B:** Same patient standing and taking a forward step. Note the increase in valgus alignment or valgus thrust. **C:** Corresponding X-ray with weight-bearing. Note lateral collapse with medial opening, suggestive of possible loss of medial collateral ligament integrity.

EXTRA-ARTICULAR

Deformity in the femur or tibia, from a congenital condition or prior trauma, will also affect the TKA reconstruction. Old fractures or excessive bowing of bones may compromise the use of intramedullary instruments for alignment. Malunions leading to leg length inequality may require shoe lifts to aid in rehabilitation and walking post reconstruction. With modern tools such as surgical robots, prenavigated instruments, customized patient-specific implants, and intraoperative surgical navigation, the surgeon should be able to successfully lessen the overall effect of extra-articular deformity on the surgery itself. However, consideration of the deformity will aid in postoperative recovery.

Palpation

RELEVANT BONY LANDMARKS

All the bony landmarks of the knee joint should be palpated during the examination. This includes compressing the patella in extension to assess for hypermobility and retinacular asymmetry (**Fig. 15-3A** and **B**). At 30° of flexion, the patellar facets contact the femoral trochlea. Compression at this flexion angle will indicate abnormal patellar tilt or maltracking, if present, as well as degree of pain (**Fig. 15-3C** and **D**). Tilt and tracking may affect patellar component position or the decision to perform a lateral retinacular release during surgery. The absence of pain may open the consideration for unicompartmental arthroplasty or leaving the patella unresurfaced during TKA in the proper clinical setting. On the femur, both condyles and epicondyles and the menisci should be examined. Condylar tenderness may suggest bone

marrow edema. Epicondylar tenderness may suggest collateral ligament injury. Meniscal integrity is not important to TKA since the menisci will be excised. However, meniscal injury may contribute to some other mechanical instability. The fibular head should also be palpated to assess the lateral collateral insertion as well as whether the peroneal nerve may be entrapped or tethered. The medial tibial plateau should be palpated to assess the medial collateral ligament (MCL) insertion and pes anserine bursa. Pes tenderness may indicate a combination of weak quadriceps and tight hamstrings. Palpation of the lateral plateau, including Gerdy's tubercle, will assess the iliotibial band (ITB) insertion. The ITB, along with the collateral ligaments, imparts stability to the joint in full extension, both before and after TKA.

Ligament Integrity and Stress Testing

ANTERIOR CRUCIATE LIGAMENT

Until recently, the anterior cruciate ligament (ACL) was sacrificed in all TKA surgeries. The recent introduction of ACL–posterior cruciate ligament (PCL) retaining TKA designs has been met with marginal success.[6] At the current time, ACL integrity is essentially irrelevant to TKA, although ACL dysfunction may contribute to posterior medial bony erosion.

POSTERIOR CRUCIATE LIGAMENT

TKA designs that retain the PCL (CR-TKA) remain popular in North America. If the surgeon is planning a CR-TKA, then obviously the PCL must be intact and functional for the TKA to be stable. The PCL can be assessed with a "posterior" Lachman's test and with a

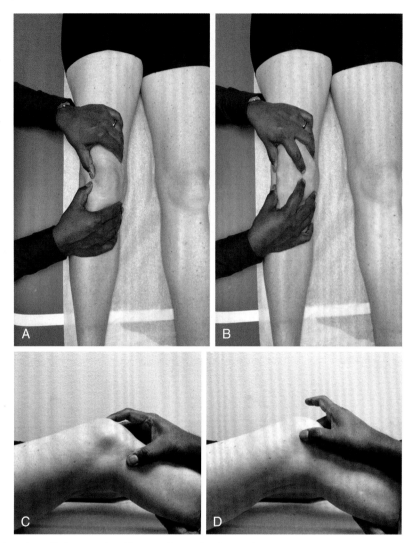

FIGURE 15-3   **A:** Examination of patella in extension. The examiner's thumbs push the patella medially to check for lateral retinacular tightness. **B:** Examination of patella in extension. The examiner's forefingers push the patella laterally to check for medial tightness. **C** and **D:** Examination of patella at 30° flexion demonstrating lateral tilt (C) and lack of movement medially (D).

posterior drawer test (**Fig. 15-4A** and **B**, respectively). In the former, with the patient supine, the knee is flexed to 30° and a posterior force is applied to the tibia. In the posterior drawer test, with the patient supine, the knee is flexed to 90°, and a posterior force is applied to the tibia. In both tests, there will be a firm end point if the PCL is intact.

MEDIAL COLLATERAL LIGAMENT

In all primary TKA designs, the MCL is critical for medial-sided stability. The MCL should be assessed at full extension and at 30° of flexion (**Fig. 15-5A** and **B**). In both positions, a valgus stress is applied to the tibia while the femur is held stably. At full extension, both the posterior capsule and MCL contribute to medial side stability and resistance to valgus stress. At 30°, the posterior capsule relaxes, and only the MCL acts as a restraint to valgus force. If there is no medial opening at 30° with valgus force, then the MCL is likely contracted or tethered

by osteophytes. This information will help the surgeon determine how aggressively to release the medial side during surgery. (It should be noted that in a fixed varus deformity, the five attachments of the semimembranosus tendon frequently contribute to the varus contracture and deformity and may have to be released during surgery.) If the knee corrects to a neutral position only, then the MCL is intact and is not contracted or tethered. In addition, bony integrity on the lateral side is also preserved. Thus, the medial release required should likely be minimal at the time of surgery. If the medial side opens with no clear-cut end point, then the MCL is likely incompetent or there is severe lateral bony compromise. Not only will release be unnecessary, but also increased implant constraint or bony augmentation may be necessary.

Lateral Side

The lateral side of the knee, normally, has much greater motion from anterior to posterior throughout the range

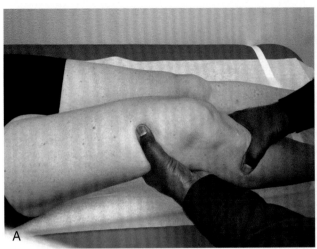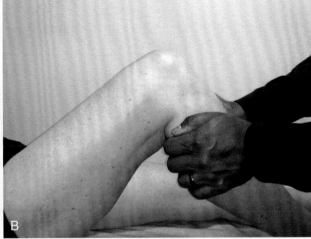

FIGURE 15-4　**A:** Posterior Lachman's test. With the knee flexed to 30°, the thigh is grasped with one hand. With the opposite hand, the examiner grasps the tibia and pushes it posteriorly. There should be a firm end point. **B:** Posterior drawer test. With the knee flexed to 90°, the tibia is manually directed posteriorly. A firm end point should be encountered.

of motion (ROM). In addition, the tibia externally rotates relative to the femur as the knee moves from flexion to extension, via the "screw-home" mechanism. As a result, the kinematics of the lateral side of the joint are more complex. The ITB inserts at Gerdy's tubercle. The lateral collateral ligament (LCL) extends from the lateral femoral epicondyle to the fibular head. The biceps femoris tendon inserts on the fibula head, proximal lateral tibia, and Gerdy's tubercle. At full extension, the ITB, LCL, and posterior capsule serve to resist varus stress. As flexion progresses, especially past 30°, and as the posterior capsule relaxes, the biceps femoris tendon joins the other

structures in providing lateral side stability. In addition, the arcuate complex contributes to posterolateral rotatory stability.

How does this lateral side complexity affect TKA? Prior to surgery, examination of the lateral side should consist of varus stress applied at full extension and 30° of flexion (**Fig. 15-6A and B**). At 90° of flexion, the varus stress should be applied in a "Figure 4" orientation. It is important to determine the degree of normal laxity and functional integrity of these structures. This information can be applied to the TKA reconstruction in a few ways. Since the lateral side has more anterior–posterior

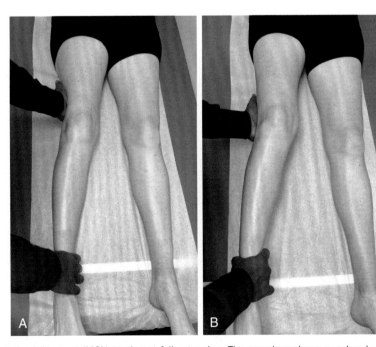

FIGURE 15-5　**A:** Medial collateral ligament (MCL) testing at full extension. The examiner places one hand on the lateral thigh. The other hand grasps the tibia and stresses it laterally. With an intact MCL (or in a varus knee with medial OA), there should be minimal medial-sided opening. **B:** MCL testing at 30° of flexion—note how valgus stress reveals laxity in the MCL. This may be physiologic or pathologic, depending upon degree of medial OA.

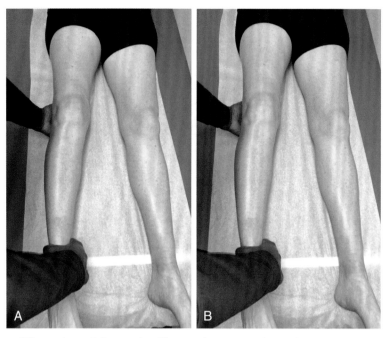

FIGURE 15-6   **A:** Lateral side stability testing at full extension. The examiner grasps the medial thigh with one hand and grasps the tibia with the other. A varus force is applied. **B:** Lateral side stability testing at 30° flexion. Note the increased varus angulation compared to full extension.

(A-P) translational rollback, even when replaced, advance knowledge of the patient's "normal" lateral side laxity will help the surgeon determine how much laxity to accept at surgery. Also, in an arthritic valgus knee, the degree of tightness or laxity will help determine how much release is needed on the lateral side to achieve flexion extension balance and mid-flexion stability. An example is provided in **Fig. 15-7A** and **B**.

Posterior Capsule

The posterior capsule of the knee is tight in extension and relaxes as the knee flexes. When testing varus–valgus stability, the examiner can be fooled if testing in full extension or slight hyperextension, as the tightened posterior capsule gives a false sense of knee stability. To examine the posterior capsule's integrity, the knee should be flexed to 90°. A-P translation should be measured. With the tibia

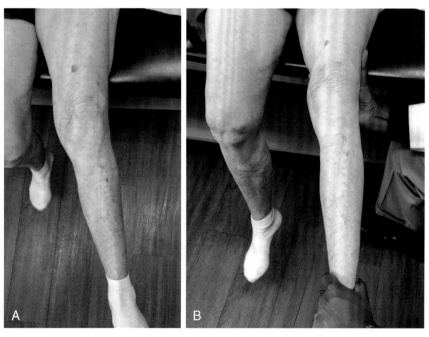

FIGURE 15-7   **A:** An arthritic valgus knee. When the patient actively extends the knee, note the valgus deformity. **B:** Varus stress applied to the knee corrects the knee to a neutral alignment, suggesting that the lateral collateral ligament and other lateral side structures are intact and functional.

externally rotated, an intact posteromedial capsule tightens and A-P translation decreases. The converse is true of the posterolateral capsule when the tibia is internally rotated. Posterior capsular tightness plays a role in TKA rotatory stability in flexion, especially in designs with minimal constraint. More importantly, if the posterior capsule is stretched out, the knee will come into recurvatum when extension is assessed. In TKA, recurvatum can be difficult to correct and therefore should not be missed during the examination.

Range of Motion

ROM should be tested both actively and passively (**Fig. 15-8A** and **B**). With the patient supine, the examiner should bring the knee to full extension and move it into full flexion. Active flexion and extension should also be addressed supine. If there is a residual flexion contracture, the etiology may be weak quadriceps/tight hamstrings, significant patellofemoral osteophyte, large anterior tibial osteophyte, or significant posterior femoral condyle osteophyte. The muscle imbalance may need to be corrected prior to surgery, whereas the osteophytes will need to be completely resected during TKA. If there is a restriction in flexion, this may be indicative of a short or scarred patellar tendon, significant patellofemoral arthrosis causing pain, or contracted capsule and collateral ligaments. Most of this can be addressed during surgery, although preoperative restriction of flexion frequently persists after TKA.

With the patient in a seated position, active ROM should be tested. Lack of full extension can be either due to a residual flexion contracture or some extensor mechanism pathology. Depending upon the pathology, it may need to be addressed prior to surgery or may be corrected during surgery. Regaining full extension after TKA

is critical to patient function and satisfaction; therefore, understanding its degree and etiology is imperative.

When considering ROM, the surgeon should also consider patellar mechanics. Tracking can be affected by muscle strength, Q-angle, trochlear dysplasia, sulcus angle, and tibial tubercle-trochlear groove/patellar ligament (TT-TG/PL) ratio.[7] In surgery, this knowledge can be applied to determine composite thickness of the patella and implant, implant position, joint line position, and need for lateral release.

Motor Testing

Quadriceps strength must be evaluated prior to undertaking TKA. A minimum grade of 3/5 is required for TKA, with a grade less than 3/5 widely considered an absolute contraindication. Similarly, hamstring strength should be at least 3/5 prior to surgery. Quadriceps atrophy and its effect on patellar mechanics should be assessed. In some cases, the patient will benefit from preoperative physical therapy.

Nonjoint Examination

PULSES

Distal pulses should be assessed to ensure there is no compromise of blood flow to the lower limb. Injury to the popliteal artery during TKA fortunately is rare. However, even minor injury can become problematic in a patient with already compromised circulation. Preoperative vascular consultation should be considered.

LYMPHEDEMA

Preexisting lymphedema frequently will be worsened after TKA surgery. Similarly, patients with poor tissue turgor in the calf are prone to postoperative swelling. In these patients, postoperative compression stockings may be considered.

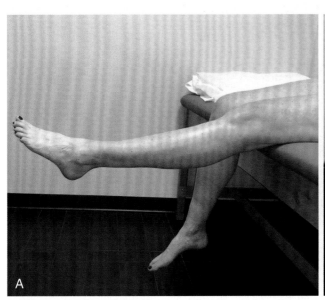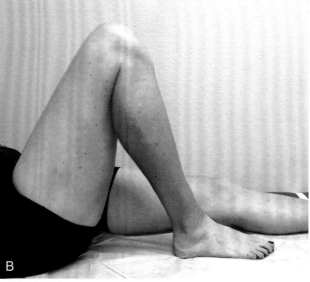

FIGURE 15-8   A: Active and passive extension should also be assessed by the examiner and differences between the two noted. **B:** Active flexion. Passive flexion should also be determined.

NEUROLOGIC EXAMINATION

The peroneal nerve can be injured during TKA, especially in patients with concomitant flexion contracture and valgus deformity. Therefore, documentation of distal neurologic function is good practice. In cases at high risk of neurologic injury, intraoperative neurologic monitoring may be considered.

EXAMINATION OF THE KNEE AFTER KNEE REPLACEMENT

Introduction

Normal Examination of the Postoperative TKA (Fig. 15-9A to E)

Hallmarks of the well-functioning TKA include full active and passive extension, active flexion to a minimum of 110°, passive flexion to 120°, symmetric ligamentous stability at full extension and 30° of flexion, minimal A-P translation at 90° of flexion, well-healed incision, minimal bony tenderness, and proper tracking of the patella, among others. A patch of lateral numbness is not uncommon due to transection of the infrapatellar branch of the saphenous nerve by the distal aspect of the incision.

Immediate Postoperative Findings of Concern

In the short term after surgery, some degree of lower extremity swelling is normal. Likewise, minimal eschar formation and discoloration of the incision line is normal (**Fig. 15-10**). However, wound issues should be aggressively evaluated and managed, lest a minor problem evolves into a deep periprosthetic infection. **Fig. 15-11** depicts a patient with poor skin who developed a skin tear from the surgical drape. The proximity to the wound raises concern for extension into the joint. Therefore, referral to the wound care service was made to ensure unremarkable healing.

Other short-term issues include slow recovery of ROM and effusion. **Fig. 15-12A** and **B** demonstrates a patient 1 month after surgery, with painful effusion and associated lack of full passive and active extension. Aspiration may be considered, although small effusions will usually resolve within 3 months. In this case, aspiration removed 40 cc of bloody joint fluid. Continued physical therapy, with special emphasis on regaining extension, was ordered. Static progressive bracing may also be considered if the patient is struggling.[8] Regaining extension is frequently more important functionally than regaining flexion.

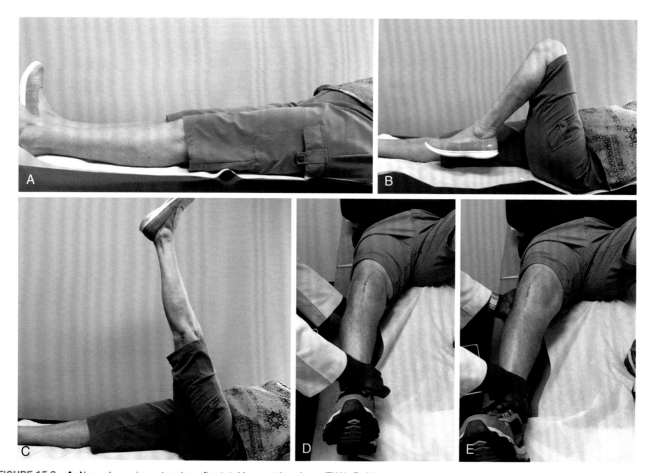

FIGURE 15-9 **A:** Normal passive extension after total knee arthroplasty (TKA). **B:** Normal active flexion after TKA. **C:** Normal active extension after TKA demonstrating no extensor lag. **D:** Varus stress and extension after TKA, demonstrating minimal lateral opening. **E:** Valgus stress applied to TKA demonstrating no medial-sided opening or laxity.

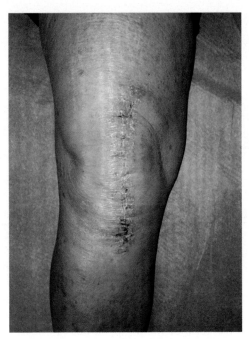

FIGURE 15-10   Appearance of knee two weeks postoperatively. Note minimal eschar and discoloration, both within normal limits.

Examination Findings in the Painful TKA

In most TKA cases, patients and surgeons are generally pleased with the results. A vexing situation for both surgeon and patient is the TKA with residual pain and stiffness. Radiographs frequently appear satisfactory, yet the patient is dissatisfied with the outcome. This situation is commonly referred to as a knee that "looks good, feels bad." The algorithmic workup for these TKAs has been discussed[9] and also elsewhere in this volume. This section will address the physical examination findings associated with the more common etiologies of the mysteriously painful TKA.

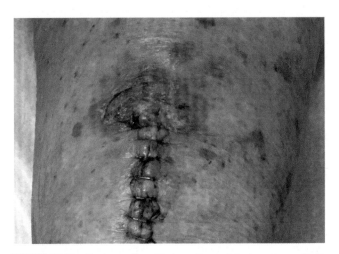

FIGURE 15-11   Postoperative skin tear. Even at 2 wk postoperatively, there has been no epithelialization. Referral to the wound care service was made to accelerate healing.

Rule Out Infection

The mysteriously painful knee, in the author's opinion, is infected until otherwise disproven. Definitive physical examination criteria for infection include purulent drainage and sinus tract formation[10] (**Fig. 15-13**). In the absence of these definitive criteria, other examination findings that should raise the suspicion for infection include erythema, induration, and stiffness. The diagnosis of infection can be confirmed by coupling physical examination findings with specific laboratory tests.[11]

Is It the Knee Prosthesis?

Causes of knee pain that are not directly due to the prosthesis but that can be diagnosed by physical examination include the following.

Hip Osteoarthritis

Internal and external rotation in extension and at 90° of flexion will be diminished with hip osteoarthritis. Similarly, extension and or flexion may also be limited. The ipsilateral knee may have a residual flexion contracture due to the hip's inability to extend fully. The patient will commonly complain of generalized anterior knee pain.

Spinal Pathology

Radicular tests (straight leg raising and sitting root test) should be performed to assess the spine as a possible source of referred pain to an otherwise well-functioning TKA. Examination of the knee is usually unremarkable, though the patient may complain of burning or aching anterior pain, often with distal radiation.

Complex Regional Pain Syndrome

Thankfully rare, complex regional pain syndrome (CRPS) should be suspected when the patient complains of burning pain worsened by tight clothing or bedsheets and deep aching worsened by motion or cold. The examiner should look for periarticular swelling rather than a joint effusion, discolored cyanotic skin, sensitivity to light touch, and cool skin.

Quadriceps Tendinitis

The patient will complain of anterior knee pain and palpation of the quadriceps tendon will elicit pain. Also, resisted extension will be painful.

Patellar Tendinitis

The patient will complain of anterior knee pain and palpation of the patellar tendon will elicit pain. Also, resisted extension will be painful.

Pes Anserine Bursitis

Palpation of the medial tibial plateau will elicit pain. There may also be localized swelling at the hamstring insertion.

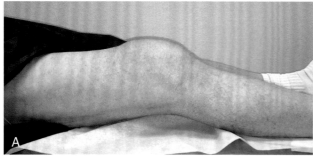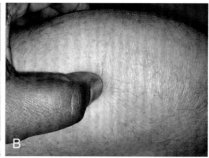

FIGURE 15-12   **A:** Flexion contracture 4 wk after surgery. **B:** Postoperative effusion. Note ballotable fluid under examiner's thumb.

Iliotibial Band Tendinitis

Tenderness with palpation of Gerdy's tubercle is suggestive of ITB tendinitis or tightness. There may also be localized swelling and pain may be worsened with varus stress.

There are several causes of pain after TKA that can be directly related to the prosthesis, and physical examination is extremely useful to elicit many of these conditions.

Overhang

Tenderness at the medial or lateral joint line should raise the suspicion for medial or lateral component overhang. As little as 3 mm of overhang can cause pain and restrict ROM.[12]

Patellar Impingement

At 30° of flexion, tenderness of the lateral patellar facet may be indicative of patellar tilt/maltracking or exposed lateral patellar bone.

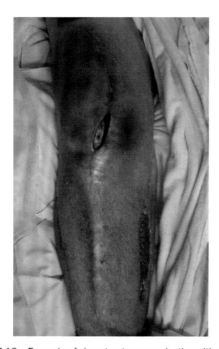

FIGURE 15-13   Example of sinus tract communicating with a total knee arthroplasty (TKA), pathognomonic for deep periprosthetic infection.

Limited ROM

Poor passive extension usually points to a tight posterior capsule or tight extension gap. Poor active extension (with normal passive extension) may occur with extensor mechanism injury or quadriceps weakness. Poor active flexion may result from poor pain control during physical therapy, a tight PCL, or overstuffing of the anterior compartment. When both poor flexion and extension are present, infection should be suspected, as well as oversized components, malalignment of components, ligamentous instability, or CRPS. Oversized components will overhang and impinge upon the capsule and collateral ligaments. The subsequent pain will cause the patient to avoid positions that worsen the pain, resulting in soft-tissue contracture. Similarly, malalignment will cause soft-tissue pain with the same cascade of events as oversizing.

Ligamentous Instability

Surgeons vary upon how much laxity to accept in a TKA. Some will accept up to 5 mm in full extension,[13] whereas others allow only 1 to 2 mm. When the patient is asymptomatic, more laxity can be accepted then when the patient is symptomatic. At 30° of flexion, typically there will be slightly more laxity with varus and valgus stress. However, greater than 5 mm more laxity then exists at full extension points to mid-flexion instability. This can be caused by overresecting the distal femur or improperly balancing the flexion and extension gaps. A-P instability suggests an incompetent PCL (**Fig. 15-14**) or an overly large flexion space. Recurvatum results from either a too loose extension gap or incompetent posterior capsule. Occasionally, with associated trauma, a collateral ligament can be ruptured (**Fig. 15-15**).

CONCLUSION

Preoperative examination of the knee in most cases should be straightforward. Nevertheless, thorough consideration of pertinent physical findings will allow the surgeon to execute TKA successfully in most cases. Similarly, several immediate postoperative findings will highlight potential

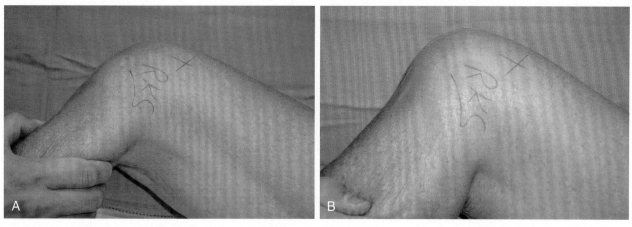

FIGURE 15-14   A: Anterior drawer demonstrating anterior translation in a CR-total knee arthroplasty (TKA). **B:** Posterior drawer showing increasing translation without firm end point, confirming incompetent posterior cruciate ligament after TKA.

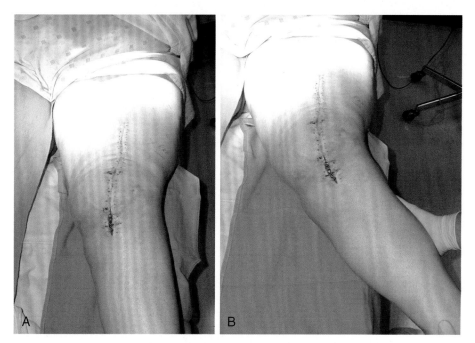

FIGURE 15-15   A: Six weeks postoperative. Patient fell and sustained medial collateral ligament (MCL) rupture. Neutral alignment of the leg with no stress applied. **B:** With valgus stress applied, the limb goes into significant valgus with no medial end point, confirming incompetence of the MCL. Revision to constrained total knee arthroplasty was required.

impending problems. When revision surgery is contemplated, accurate physical examination may point to the etiology of the initial failure and thus what to avoid during the revision.

REFERENCES

1. Sanna M, Sanna C, Caputo F, Piu G, Salvi M. Surgical approaches in total knee arthroplasty. *Joints*. 2013;1(2):34-44. Published online 2013 Oct 24.
2. Aso K, Ikeuchi M, Izumi M, Kato T, Tani T. Transcutaneous oxygen tension in the anterior skin of the knee after minimal incision total knee arthroplasty. *Knee*. 2012;19(5):576-579. Epub 2011 Nov 12.
3. Patel VP, Walsh M, Sehgal B, Preston C, DeWal H, Di Cesare PE. Factors associated with prolonged wound drainage after primary total hip and knee arthroplasty. *J Bone Joint Surg Am*. 2007;89(1):33-38.
4. Vince KG, Abdeen A. Wound problems in total knee arthroplasty. *Clin Orthop Relat Res*. 2006;452:88-90.
5. Sharma L, Chang AH, Jackson RD, et al. Varus thrust and incident and progressive knee osteoarthritis. *Arthritis Rheumatol*. 2017;69(11):2136-2143.
6. Christensen JC, Brothers J, Stoddard GJ, et al. Higher frequency of reoperation with a new bicruciate-retaining total knee arthroplasty. *Clin Orthop Relat Res*. 2017;475(1):62-69. doi: 10.1007/s11999-016-4812-5.
7. Hevesi M, Heidenreich MJ, Camp CL, et al. The recurrent instability of the patella (RIP) score: a statistically based model for prediction of long-term recurrence risk after first-time dislocation. *Arthroscopy*. 2019;35(2):537-543.
8. Sodhi N, Yao B, Khlopas A, et al. A case for the brace: a critical, comprehensive, and up-to-date review of static progressive stretch, dynamic, and turnbuckle braces for the management of elbow, knee, and shoulder pathology. *Surg Technol Int*. 2017;31:303-318.

9. Vince KG. The problem total knee replacement: systematic, comprehensive and efficient evaluation. *Bone Joint J*. 2014;96-B(11 suppl A):105-111.

10. Parvizi J. AAOS Workgroup consensus statement.

11. Gehrke T, Alijanipour P, Parvizi J. The management of an infected total knee arthroplasty. *Bone Joint J*. 2015;97-B(10 suppl A):20–9.

12. Mahoney OM, Kinsey T. Overhang of the femoral component in total knee arthroplasty: risk factors and clinical consequences. *J Bone Joint Surg Am*. 2010;92(5):1115-1121.

13. Babazadeh S, Stoney JD, Lim K, Choong PFM. The relevance of ligament balancing in total knee arthroplasty: how important is it? A systematic review of the literature. *Orthop Rev*. 2009;1(2):e26.

chapter 16

Imaging of the Native and Prosthetic Knee

Alissa J. Burge, MD | Hollis G. Potter, MD

INTRODUCTION

Determination of an appropriate imaging algorithm for evaluation of the knee depends on a number of factors. A variety of imaging modalities are available, each of which complements the others in terms of which tissues are best evaluated. Considerations when selecting an imaging modality include clinical and surgical history, as well as the suspected pathology and types of tissue that may be involved.

CONVENTIONAL RADIOGRAPHS

Standard Views

Radiographs are commonly the first imaging modality obtained for evaluation of the knee, being relatively easily obtained, and providing global assessment of the osseous anatomy, and to an extent, the soft-tissue structures. Standard examinations typically include weight-bearing anteroposterior (AP) and lateral views, with additional views added as warranted by the clinical concern. Routine AP views may demonstrate evidence of osteoarthritis, such as joint space narrowing and marginal osteophytes, while lateral views, which are typically obtained non–weight-bearing in 30° of flexion, allow evaluation of the anterior structures such as the extensor mechanism and suprapatellar region. Tangential views of the patellofemoral compartment are often included in the routine radiographic examination of the knees, allowing demonstration of patellofemoral alignment and joint space narrowing.[1]

Additional Views

Posteroanterior (PA) flexion views of the knee may be obtained for more sensitive evaluation of the posterior aspect of the femorotibial compartments and are useful for demonstrating chondral loss preferentially affecting the posterior aspect of the joint (**Fig. 16-1**).[1]

The tunnel view is obtained supine with the knee in flexion and the beam directed inferiorly perpendicular to the tibia, in order to best demonstrate the intercondylar notch. This view is useful for detecting pathology within the notch, such as loose bodies, tibial spine avulsions, and osteochondral lesions along the inner aspects of the condyles.[1]

The cross table lateral view is obtained with the patient supine and the leg extended; this view is often obtained in the patient who have suffered acute trauma and are unable to bear weight and may demonstrate a fat-fluid level within the suprapatellar region, indicative of lipohemarthrosis in the setting of an intra-articular fracture.[1]

COMPUTED TOMOGRAPHY

Computed tomography (CT) has been supplanted by magnetic resonance imaging (MRI) for many indications in evaluation of the knee; however, CT remains the gold standard evaluation of mineralized bone and fine details of osseous anatomy. CT also provides an alternative cross-sectional modality for evaluation of patients with contraindications to MRI, such as those with pacemakers or severe claustrophobia.

Routine CT evaluation of the knee is generally performed with the patient in the supine position and the knee extended, with the field of view extending from the supracondylar region of the femur through the proximal tibia utilizing submillimeter axial slices and reformats constructed in three planes. Reformatted images may also be constructed at unique obliquities in order to optimally demonstrate pathology, and 3D reformats are useful for a more global depiction of the knee. CT arthrography may be performed following intra-articular injection of iodinated contrast and air, in order to assess for soft-tissue pathology in patients unable to undergo MRI.[2]

One of the most common indications for CT evaluation of the knee is preoperative assessment of fracture morphology. CT provides accurate characterization of the degree of comminution, areas of cortical and articular surface displacement, and small ossific fragments within the joint space. CT is also useful for preoperative templating of custom arthroplasty implants, in which the implant is specifically tailored to the patient's individual anatomy.[3,4] In patients with painful total knee arthroplasty (TKA), modification of scan parameters allows reduction of metal artifact and improved visualization of the tissues surrounding the implant.[5] CT may demonstrate areas of osseous resorption, as may be seen in the setting of polymeric wear or mechanical

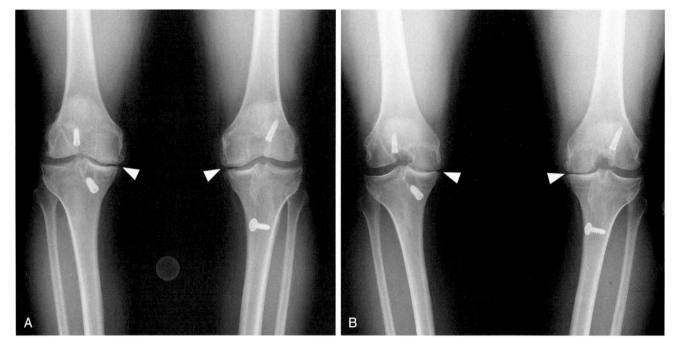

FIGURE 16-1 Anteroposterior **(A)** radiograph of the bilateral knees in a patient status post prior bilateral anterior cruciate ligament reconstructions demonstrates preferential medial femorotibial compartment joint space narrowing (white arrowheads) bilaterally. Posteroanterior flexion radiograph **(B)** in the same patient demonstrates accentuation of joint space narrowing (white arrowheads), indicating that chondral loss is most severe posteriorly.

component loosening. CT arthrography may demonstrate meniscal tears and chondral defects in native knees, as well as areas of synovial scarring in patients following TKA (**Fig. 16-2**).

NUCLEAR SCINTIGRAPHY

Much like CT, nuclear scintigraphy has largely been supplanted by MRI for most indications in the knee; however, nuclear imaging may be useful in patients with

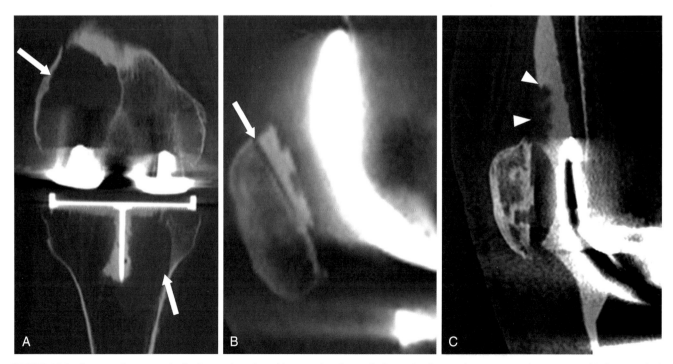

FIGURE 16-2 Computed tomography in the setting of total knee arthroplasty. **A:** Coronal reformat demonstrates large areas of bulky osteolysis (white arrows) along both the femoral and tibial components. **B:** Sagittal reformat demonstrates fibrous membrane formation (white arrow) along the patellar component, seen to extend along the entirety of the component upon review of all images, consistent with component loosening. **C:** Sagittal reconstruction of a CT arthrogram demonstrates scar nodule (white arrowheads) along the superior aspect of the patella, in keeping with patellar clunk.

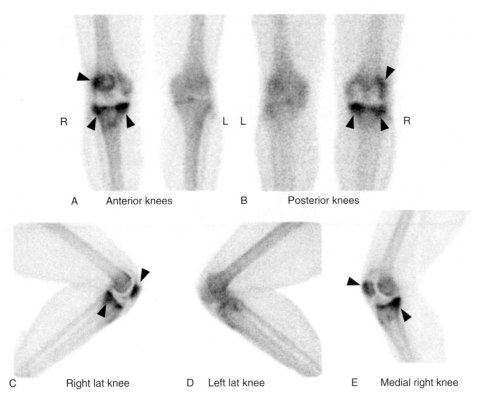

FIGURE 16-3 Bone scan of the bilateral knees in a 55-year-old man status post right total knee arthroplasty demonstrates areas of increased radiotracer uptake (black arrowheads) along the tibial and patellar components, compatible with osseous resorption and possible component loosening. **A:** Anterior knees, **B:** Posterior knees, **C:** Right lat knee, **D:** Left lat knee, **E:** Medial right knee.

contraindications to MRI, as well as for evaluation of suspected malignancy. Bone scans utilizing technetium-labeled bisphosphonate compounds detect areas of increased osteoblastic activity and therefore are useful in evaluation of conditions involving greater than normal osseous remodeling, such as fractures and stress reactions, neoplasm, and arthroplasty loosening (**Fig. 16-3**).[6,7] Other radiotracers are utilized for various specialized indications; for example, gallium and indium scans are useful in the setting of suspected infection. While highly sensitive, nuclear studies are generally of lower resolution than other modalities and are therefore generally less specific. Utilizing nuclear imaging in conjunction with other modalities may be useful in increasing the diagnostic specificities of these scans.

Following initial placement of TKA components, periprosthetic uptake of radiotracer may persist for approximately 1 year.[8] During this time period in particular, scanning utilizing a combination of radiotracers may yield improved diagnostic accuracy over scans utilizing a single tracer. These scans may be a useful data point in identifying implant loosening. Additionally, in patients with suspected infection, a combination leukocyte and sulfur colloid marrow scan provides increased specificity over either scan alone, as infection will manifest as increased uptake on the leukocyte scan without a concurrent increase in uptake of sulfur colloid, which accumulates in areas of altered marrow distribution; this combined technique results in accuracy of approximately

90% for diagnosis of infection.[9-11] It is important to point out that while these scans alone do not confirm periprosthetic joint infection, they may be one of multiple data points needed to confirm this diagnosis.

ULTRASOUND

Basic Principles

In addition to providing high-resolution images of the more superficial structures about the knee, ultrasound provides the additional benefits of potential dynamic evaluation and the performance of image-guided procedures. Evaluation of musculoskeletal structures is typically best performed with a linear array transducer of medium to high frequency, depending on the size and depth of the structure of interest.

Diagnostic Imaging

The more superficial tendons and ligaments about the knee are easily visualized with ultrasound.[12] Normal tendons and ligaments appear overall hyperechoic, with longitudinally oriented fibers resulting in a fibrillar internal architecture which is clearly visible on ultrasound. Tendinosis manifests as areas of hypoechogenicity, enlargement, and loss of normal fibrillar architecture; however, care must be taken to maintain the probe at an orientation perpendicular to the structure being interrogated, in order to

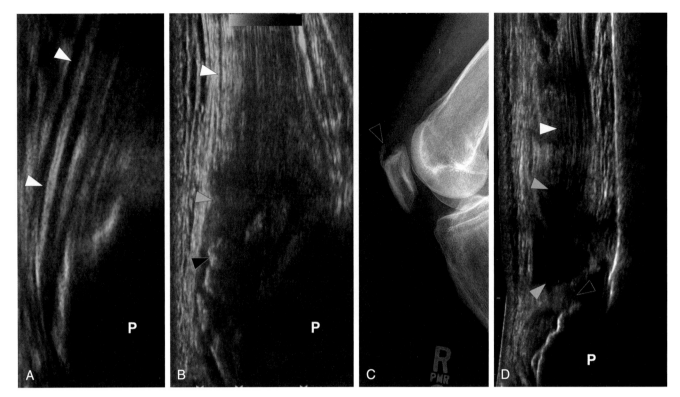

FIGURE 16-4 Ultrasound of the extensor mechanism. **A:** Longitudinal image demonstrates normal quadriceps tendon (white arrowheads) with hyperechoic fibers and striated appearance; P = patella. **B:** Longitudinal image demonstrates distal quadriceps tendinosis (gray arrowhead), with enthesopathic spur (black arrowhead, also visible on radiograph, **C**); note more normal appearing tendon proximally (white arrowhead). **D:** Longitudinal image demonstrates distal quadriceps tear yielding fluid-filled gap (gray arrowheads), with degenerated stump of torn tendon fibers (black arrowhead) at the superior patellar pole; the more proximal quadriceps tendon (white arrowhead) is somewhat tendinotic but otherwise intact.

avoid mistaking the effects of anisotropy for pathology. Frank tears appear as disruption of normal fibers with intervening fluid, often superimposed upon degeneration (Fig. 16-4).[13,14]

Synovial expansion is also often easily appreciated on ultrasound, particularly in the suprapatellar region. Doppler imaging may detect areas of hyperemia within inflamed synovium. Popliteal cysts in arthritic knees are a common cause of posterior knee discomfort and are easily visualized on ultrasound. In patients with TKA, ultrasound is particularly useful in assessment of patellar clunk, in which a nodule of scarred synovium along the patellofemoral articulation results in mechanical symptoms during range of motion. Dynamic evaluation allows visualization of the motion of the scar nodule during flexion and extension, offering confirmation that the scar is the cause of the patients' symptoms.[15]

Neurovascular structures are well-appreciated sonographically, provided they are relatively superficially positioned. Doppler evaluation of the popliteal vein is commonly performed to assess for deep venous thrombosis. Arterial abnormalities such as stenosis and pseudoaneurysm are also easily appreciated, and Doppler interrogation can provide waveform assessment for evaluation of vascular flow, potentially providing evidence of abnormalities both at and remote from the site of interrogation.[16] Many of the major nerves about the knee are superficially positioned and therefore quite amenable to sonographic evaluation.[17] Focal lesions such as neuromas and peripheral nerve sheath tumors are easily visualized. Areas of scar entrapment of extrinsic compression may also be identified. Nerves, much like tendons, are typically hyperechoic with internal longitudinal fascicular architecture; neuritis may manifest as fascicular swelling and hypoechogenicity, while injury may manifest as fascicular disruption.[18]

Ultrasound-Guided Intervention

Ultrasound is particularly well-suited for image-guided interventions.[19] While knee joint aspirations and steroid injections may be performed blindly, imaging guidance is often useful in patients with difficult anatomy. More complex procedures about the knee generally benefit from imaging guidance. Popliteal cyst aspirations are performed quite commonly under ultrasound, which allows visualization of cyst size and the degree of loculation, and confirmation of cyst collapse (Fig. 16-5). Perineural injections may be performed both as a treatment for neuropathic pain, as well as for anesthesia prior to surgical intervention.[17,20] Calcium hydroxyapatite deposition, while less common than in the shoulder, may occur in the knee and is amenable to ultrasound-guided lavage. Ultrasound injection of platelet rich

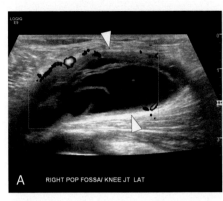
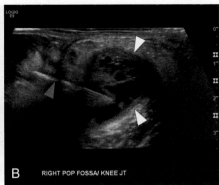
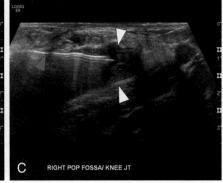

FIGURE 16-5 Ultrasound-guided popliteal cyst aspiration in a 48-year-old woman presenting with posterior pain. **A:** Initial preprocedural image demonstrates multilocular popliteal cyst (white arrowheads); note the lack of internal vascular flow on this power Doppler image. **B:** Image as the aspiration is in progress demonstrates the needle (gray arrowhead) within the cyst (white arrowheads), which is decreased in size. **C:** Image obtained prior to removing the needle (gray arrowhead) demonstrates complete aspiration of the fluid with collapse of the cyst, though the cyst walls (white arrowheads) remain visible.

plasma (PRP) may be used as a treatment for tendinosis and tears, particularly those involving the extensor tendons.

BASIC PRINCIPLES OF MAGNETIC RESONANCE IMAGING

Magnetic resonance imaging (MRI) provides excellent soft-tissue contrast as well as sensitivity for marrow changes and has therefore supplanted many traditional imaging techniques for evaluation of soft tissue and marrow within the knee.

Magnetic resonance imaging exploits the ability of spinning atomic species possessing an odd number of nucleons to induce a local magnetic field. 1H, containing a single proton, is the isotope upon which the vast majority of clinical MR imaging is based, due to its pervasiveness within biological tissues. Upon application of an external magnetic field, Bo, the normally randomly oriented hydrogen nuclei align their spins parallel to the long axis of the field, yielding a net magnetic vector, Mz, along the longitudinal axis of the field. While spinning, these nuclei simultaneously precess about the axis of the external magnetic field with a motion like that of a gyroscope, at a specific frequency which is determined by the field strength of Bo. When protons are aligned with Bo, this precessional motion is not synchronized among individual nuclei, therefore while a net magnetization vector is created in the longitudinal direction, no net magnetization vector is generated in the transverse plane. Through application of a brief radiofrequency pulse oriented at 90° to the longitudinal axis of the main magnetic field, the protons are raised to a higher energy state in which they are rotating in the transverse plane about the axis of the main magnetic field in a synchronized fashion, referred to as the state of being "in phase" with one another. This synchronicity results in the generation of a net transverse magnetization vector, Mxy, which allows transmission of the MR signal via the induction of magnetic flux within the receiver coil; the rotation of the nuclei in the transverse plane induces an alternating current within the receiver coil, which is subsequently subjected to series of digital manipulations in order to eventually form an image. Upon termination of the 90° RF pulse, the transverse magnetization vector decays via two simultaneous but independent processes: recovery of magnetization in the longitudinal axis (spin lattice, or T1, relaxation) and dephasing of rotation in the transverse plane (spin–spin, or T2, decay). These processes form the basis of MR tissue contrast, as the time required for each process depends upon the biochemical environment of each individual proton, thereby determining its signal characteristics on images generated by a given pulse sequence.[21]

Deliberate modification of pulse sequence acquisition parameters produces different types of soft-tissue contrast within the generated images, a concept referred to as image weighting. The main acquisition parameters contributing to image weighting are the interval between RF pulses (time to repetition, TR) and the interval from RF pulse to the sampled signal, or echo (time to echo, TE). Pulse sequences commonly employed for musculoskeletal MR imaging typically yield T1-weighted, T2-weighted, and proton density (PD)-weighted images and are obtained utilizing specific combinations of long and short TRs and TEs. Fat-suppressed, fluid-sensitive images allow sensitive detection of mobile water and are generally a part of routine clinical imaging algorithms. Knowledge of the expected signal characteristics and appearance of normal anatomic structures upon differently weighted images is key in image interpretation, facilitating recognition of pathology.[21]

The choice of optimal MR imaging sequences for a given algorithm depends on the body part and tissues being imaged. For orthopedic imaging, proton density (PD)-weighted fast spin echo (FSE) sequences provide excellent contrast between musculoskeletal tissues, allowing delineation of the major tissue types within the knee. The addition of fat-suppressed fluid-sensitive images

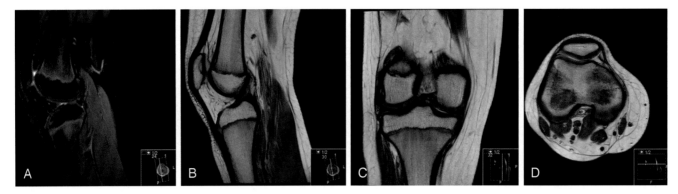

FIGURE 16-6   Routine clinical MRI of the knee. **A:** Sagittal inversion recovery (IR). **B:** Sagittal proton density (PD)–weighted fast spin echo (FSE). **C:** Coronal PD FSE. **D:** Axial PD FSE.

allows detection of fluid and edema. These sequences constitute the foundation of the majority of clinical imaging studies of the knee performed at the authors' institution, though additional sequences may be added on a per case basis (**Fig. 16-6**). For example, gradient echo images allow more sensitive detection of hemorrhagic products and are therefore commonly added for evaluation of patients with known or suspected pigmented villonodular synovitis (**Fig. 16-7**).[22] Imaging of the knee is typically performed with the patient in a supine position, utilizing a dedicated extremity coil.

MENISCI

Normal Meniscal Anatomy and Imaging

Normal meniscal tissue appears uniformly hypointense on all conventional MR pulse sequences, due to its being composed of highly ordered fibrocartilage, resulting in short relaxation times. Menisci are typically best visualized on coronal and sagittal images, with the anterior and posterior horns well seen on sagittal images, and the body segments best seen on coronal images (**Fig. 16-8**). The medial meniscus is larger than the lateral and has a more open C shape, with the posterior horn being generally larger than the anterior horn, while the lateral meniscus has a more circular configuration, and the horns are more uniform in size. The transverse meniscal ligament, which joins the anterior horns of both menisci, is also well seen on sagittal images, as are the meniscofemoral ligaments of Wrisberg and Humphrey, which extend from the medial femoral condyle to the posterior horn of the lateral meniscus.[23,24]

Meniscal Pathology

Meniscal degeneration results in decreased organization of collagen fibers and increases in mobile water content,

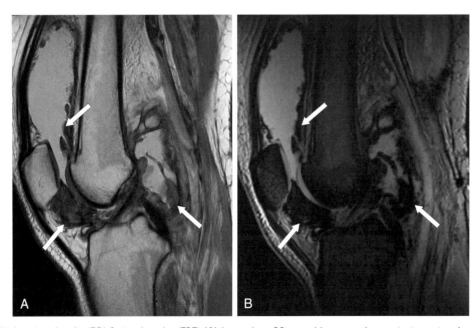

FIGURE 16-7   Sagittal proton density (PD) fast spin echo (FSE) **(A)** image in a 22-year-old woman demonstrates extensive proliferative synovitis (white arrows) consistent with her known history of pigmented villonodular synovitis. Sagittal gradient echo (GRE) **(B)** image demonstrates prominent blooming in the regions of synovial proliferation (white arrows) related to hemosiderin deposition.

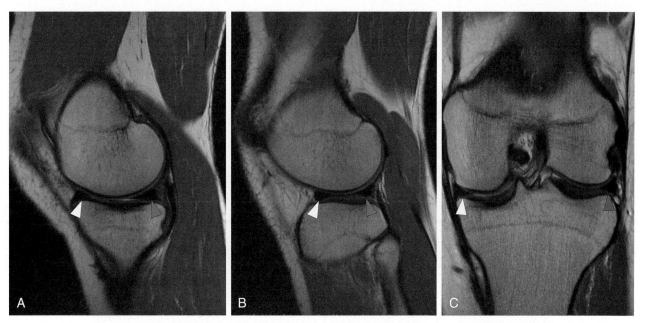

FIGURE 16-8 MRI of the normal menisci. **A:** Sagittal proton density (PD) fast spin echo (FSE) image demonstrates normal anterior (white arrowhead) and posterior (gray arrowhead) horns of the medial meniscus. **B:** Sagittal PD FSE image demonstrates normal anterior (white arrowhead) and posterior (gray arrowhead) horns of the lateral meniscus. **C:** Coronal PD FSE–weighted image demonstrates normal body segments of the medial (white arrowhead) and lateral (gray arrowhead) menisci.

resulting in increased signal relative to normal meniscal tissue. The presence of a frank meniscal tear is indicated by linear signal hyperintensity traversing the substance of the meniscus and contacting an articular surface, and/or changes in meniscal morphology. Meniscal tears are classified by their orientation with regard to the substance of the meniscus.

Horizontal tears, which are commonly degenerative, extend in an oblique but predominantly horizontal course across the substance of the meniscus (**Fig. 16-9**).

Vertical tears may be longitudinally or radially oriented. Longitudinal vertical tears commonly occur in the setting of acute trauma, such as pivot shirt injury, and are often amenable to repair, provided that they lie within the vascular periphery of the meniscus. Radial tears, if complete, disrupt the longitudinal fibers which provide hoop strength to the menisci, allowing for meniscal extrusion. A common location for radial tears is at the posterior horn root attachment junction; while these may be easily appreciated on coronal images, on sagittal images,

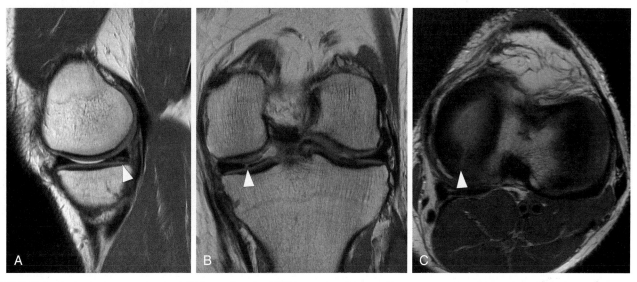

FIGURE 16-9 **A:** Sagittal proton density (PD) fast spin echo (FSE) image in a 60-year-old man presenting with medial pain demonstrates horizontal tear (white arrowhead) of the medial meniscal posterior horn. **B:** Coronal PD FSE image demonstrates superimposed radial component (white arrowhead) of the tear, which was not well-appreciated on sagittal images. **C:** Axial proton density image demonstrates the location and orientation of the radial component (white arrowhead) of the tear.

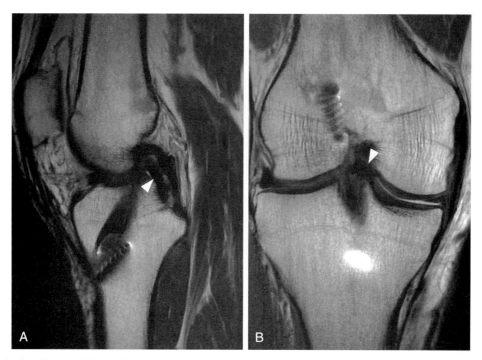

FIGURE 16-10 Bucket handle tear of the medial meniscus in a 29-year-old man presenting with locking. **A:** Sagittal proton density (PD) fast spin echo (FSE) image demonstrates the classic "double PCL" sign, in which the bucket handle fragment (white arrowhead), which is flipped centrally into the intercondylar notch, parallels and mimics the posterior cruciate ligament (gray arrowhead). **B:** Coronal PD FSE image demonstrates the bucket handle fragment within the intercondylar notch (white arrowhead). PCL, posterior cruciate ligament.

they may be subtle, appearing as "ghosting" on a single sagittal image, and sometimes not appearing on sagittal images at all, due to their orientation (**Fig. 16-9**). They may be evident on axial images, but again, this will largely depend on whether an axial image traverses the substance of the menisci.[23,24]

Bucket handle tears are longitudinally oriented vertical tears which allow the torn portion of the meniscus to displace, typically centrally, resulting in a "bucket handle" fragment of meniscal tissue which commonly results in mechanical symptoms. A "double PCL" sign is common on sagittal images, with the displaced bucket handle fragment paralleling the posterior cruciate ligament (PCL) (**Fig. 16-10**). The location of the vertical cleavage plane relative to the vascular periphery of the meniscus is important in terms of the potential for repair, as is the health of the nondisplaced meniscal remnant and bucket handle fragment, in terms of degeneration and additional areas of tearing.[23,24]

Flap tears are often obliquely oriented and may be subtle, with the flap largely visible only in a single plane (**Fig. 16-11**). Areas of abnormal meniscal truncation may provide a clue that there is a tear, allowing the radiologist to carefully scrutinize the images for a displaced flap.[23,24]

Meniscocapsular separation may occur in the setting of acute trauma, such as pivot shift injury. The posterior medial meniscocapsular junction and lateral fascicular attachments are well visualized on sagittal images. Laterally, injury manifests as fascicular hyperintensity and thickening and/or disruption. Medially, injury

manifests as signal hyperintensity, with a complete separation appearing as a fluid signal cleft along the meniscocapsular junction.[23]

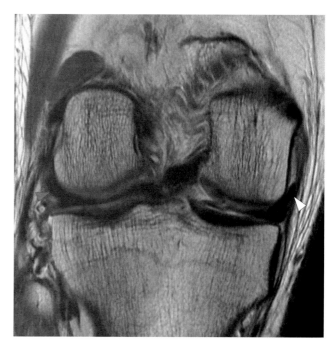

FIGURE 16-11 Coronal proton density (PD) fast spin echo (FSE) image in a 53-year-old man presenting with medial pain demonstrates flap tear of the medial meniscal body segment yielding flap (white arrowhead) which is flipped superiorly within the medial gutter. Note that on the lateral side, the popliteus tendon (gray arrowhead) may result in a similar appearance, a common potential pitfall.

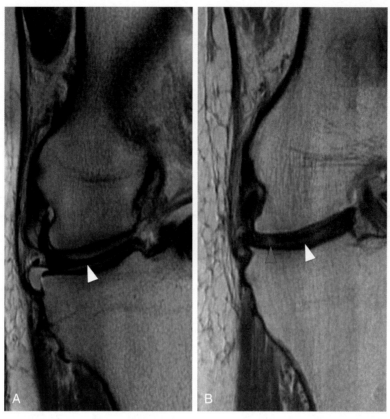

FIGURE 16-12   Discoid lateral menisci. **A:** Coronal proton density (PD) fast spin echo (FSE) image in a 54-year-old woman presenting with mechanical symptoms demonstrates discoid meniscus (white arrowhead) which is otherwise normal, without tear. **B:** Coronal PD FSE image in a 45-year-old woman presenting with lateral pain and mechanical symptoms demonstrates discoid meniscus (white arrowhead) with superimposed tear (gray arrowhead).

Discoid menisci are anatomic variants, more common laterally, resulting in meniscal tissue extending across the central and inner aspects of the compartment rather than being confined to the periphery (**Fig. 16-12**). This extra tissue is typically clearly visible on sagittal and coronal images, but is often markedly degenerated, to the point that it may not be easily recognizable as meniscal tissue.[23]

LIGAMENTS

Anterior Cruciate Ligament

The anterior cruciate ligament (ACL) is composed of parallel collagen fibers which are normally uniformly hypointense on clinical imaging sequences; these are typically interspersed with bands of fat, resulting in a striated appearance on non–fat-suppressed images (**Fig. 16-13**). The ACL has two distinct fiber bundles; the anteromedial bundle is slightly larger and is more taut in flexion, while the posterolateral bundle is more taut in extension.[25]

While complete ACL disruption is often evident clinically, MRI can provide valuable information in the setting of equivocal injury as well as in the assessment for concomitant injuries which may also warrant surgical intervention. In the acute setting, ACL tear appears as disruption of the normal ligament fibers, which typically appear hyperintense

and thickened due to the interstitial load experienced prior to rupture (**Fig. 16-14**). Rupture is commonly the result of pivot shift injury, which typically also results in transchondral impaction injuries over the anterior lateral femoral condyle and posterior lateral plateau. These will appear as focal areas of subchondral marrow edema on fluid-sensitive, fat-suppressed images, commonly with focal subchondral depression and overlying chondral abnormality.[26]

Partial ACL tears are often more difficult to diagnose on MRI than complete tears, as the injury tends to have a more subtle appearance. Partial tears generally manifest as hyperintensity and thickening of fibers, which may be accompanied by changes in ligament morphology such as attenuation and a somewhat wavy or concave appearance. The characteristic pivot shift contusions commonly seen in the setting of complete ACL rupture tend to be absent.[27]

In the chronic setting, persistent complete ligament disruption often results in horizontal lie of the torn ligament, which generally appears hypointense following scar remodeling (**Fig. 16-14**).[25] Torn ligament fibers may also be resorbed, resulting in absence of the ligament. Chronic ACL deficiency may allow anterior translation of the tibia, particularly within the lateral femorotibial compartment, with associated displacement/degeneration of the lateral meniscal posterior horn and preferential

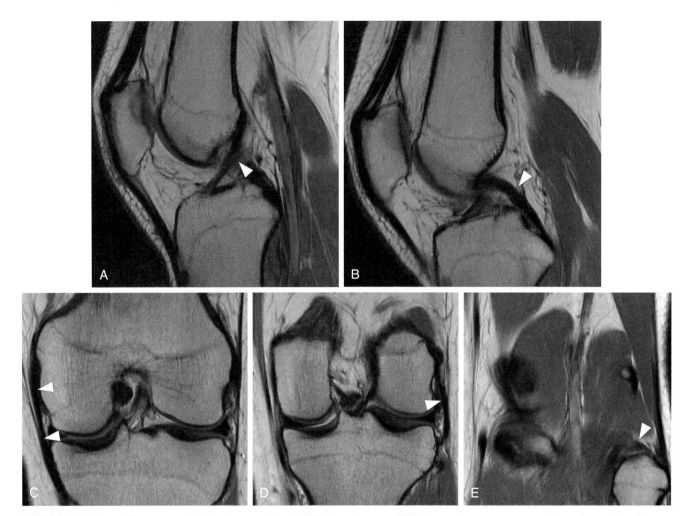

FIGURE 16-13 Normal ligaments. **A:** Sagittal proton density (PD) fast spin echo (FSE) image demonstrates normal anterior cruciate ligament (white arrowhead). **B:** Sagittal PD FSE image demonstrates normal posterior cruciate ligament (white arrowhead). **C:** Coronal PD FSE image demonstrates normal medial collateral ligament (white arrowheads). **D:** Coronal PD FSE image demonstrates normal fibular collateral ligament (white arrowhead). **E:** Coronal PD FSE image demonstrates normal popliteofibular ligament (white arrowhead).

wear of the subjacent articular cartilage.[28] Deficiency of the ACL may also allow recurrent pivot shift; therefore, the presence of pivot shift contusions does not necessarily indicate an acute ACL disruption.

A variety of associated injuries have been observed in conjunction with ACL tears sustained in the setting of pivot shift injury. In addition to the aforementioned lateral compartment transchondral impaction injuries, an additional area of impaction is often observed over the posterior aspect of the medial tibial plateau, thought to be related to contrecoup injury. Meniscal injury is not uncommon and often involved the meniscal periphery and/or meniscocapsular junction. Injury of the medial collateral ligament (MCL) and posterolateral corner (PCL) may also be observed and may warrant surgical intervention if severe.[29]

ACL ganglion, or mucinous degeneration, results in hyperintensity and thickening of ligament fibers and may be misinterpreted as acute injury (**Fig. 16-15**). The cysts are often visible insinuating along the ligament fibers and about the synovial reflections of the ligament and also often extend intraosseously along the tibial and femoral attachments.[26]

Posterior Cruciate Ligament

Tear of the PCL is encountered less commonly than injury to the ACL. The mechanism of PCL tear is often a hyperextension injury and therefore associated anterior contusions may be observed. Unlike the ACL, the PCL is typically uniformly hypointense of clinical imaging sequences and lacks the intrasubstance fat which gives the ACL a striated appearance. PCL tears often appear as hyperintensity and thickening of fibers, with a somewhat frayed appearance rather than a well-defined tear site, and can therefore often be challenging to characterize on imaging (**Fig. 16-16**).[26,30]

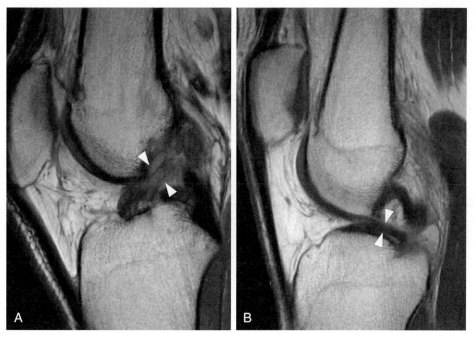

FIGURE 16-14 Anterior cruciate ligament tears. **A:** Sagittal proton density (PD) fast spin echo (FSE) image in a 25-year-old man following a skiing injury demonstrates acute anterior cruciate ligament tear (white arrowheads); note that while the ligament is torn and the fibers are hyperintense and thickened, the ligament retains its typical oblique orientation. **B:** Sagittal PD FSE image in a 32-year-old man with a history of remote soccer injury demonstrates chronic anterior cruciate ligament tear (white arrowheads), with characteristic horizontal lie of the ligament, which is hypointense due to scar remodeling.

Medial Collateral Ligament

Isolated tears of the MCL often result from a pure valgus load and are therefore often seen in conjunction with lateral-sided contusions. The MCL has both deep and superficial fibers; the deep fibers are comprised of meniscofemoral and meniscotibial ligaments and are the more commonly injured component in the setting of partial thickness tears (**Fig. 16-17**).[26,31]

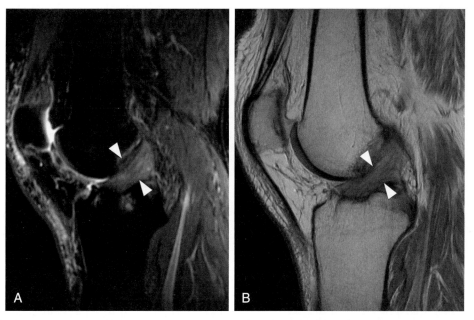

FIGURE 16-15 Sagittal inversion recovery (IR) **(A)** and proton density (PD) fast spin echo (FSE) **(B)** images in a 74-year-old man with chronic knee pain demonstrate pronounced hyperintensity and thickening of anterior cruciate ligament fibers (white arrowheads), related to intrasubstance ganglion formation, with intraosseous extension of ganglion visible along the tibial attachment.

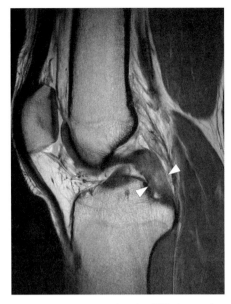

FIGURE 16-16 Sagittal proton density (PD) fast spin echo (FSE) image in a 33-year-old man presenting with pain following a basketball injury demonstrates acute tear of the posterior cruciate ligament (white arrowheads).

Fibular Collateral Ligament and Posterolateral Corner

A number of important ligaments and tendons are visible along the lateral aspect of the knee. The most anterior of these is the iliotibial band, which is not commonly torn, but which may result in a friction syndrome at the level of the lateral epicondyle or lateral tibial plateau. The fibular

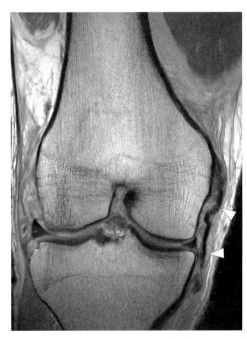

FIGURE 16-17 Coronal proton density (PD) fast spin echo (FSE) image in a 33-year-old man presenting with pain and instability following a football injury demonstrates complete disruption of the medial collateral ligament (white arrowheads).

collateral ligament inserts upon the fibular tip as a conjoined attachment with the biceps femoris tendon. The popliteus can be traced from its tendon attachment along the lateral condyle, extending inferiorly and medially across the posterior aspect of the knee, with the popliteofibular ligament extending as a fan-shaped structure from the fibular tip to the muscle tendon junction of the popliteus.[32-34]

PCL injury may occur in the setting of ACL tear and is of particular clinical import in that missed PLC injury is a known cause of anterior cruciate ligament reconstruction (ACLR) failure; therefore a high-grade injury to the PLC may warrant surgical intervention in a patient with ACL injury (**Fig. 16-18**).[32-34]

Knee Dislocation

Knee dislocation generally occurs in the setting of severe trauma and often results in multiligament disruption as well as concurrent neurovascular injury. MRI is useful in determining the degree and extent of soft-tissue injury, including ligament and tendon disruption, meniscal injury, and articular surface disruption.[29] Peripheral nerve injury also may be evident as changes in fascicular signal and morphology. Vascular injury may be evident clinically, in which case emergent surgical intervention is warranted; however, in a patient without obvious severe vascular injury, MR angiography may be utilized in order to assess for damage to the popliteal artery and branches. Time-resolved contrast-enhanced gradient images can provide accurate evaluation of the popliteal vessels in both the arterial and venous phases. A single MR examination can therefore provide a comprehensive assessment of the extent of damage in patients with these types of injuries.

Extensor Mechanism

Disorders of the extensor mechanism are a common cause of anterior knee pain. Patellar maltracking can result from anatomic abnormalities which disrupt the balance of stabilizing forces about the patella, resulting in abnormal tracking during range of motion. Predisposing factors may include trochlear dysplasia, patella alta, and excessive lateralization of the tibial tubercle, all of which may be characterized on MRI. Maltracking can lead to a variety of problems, including pain, lateral patellar dislocation, and osteoarthritis. Additionally, maltracking often results in impingement of the infrapatellar fat pad, with characteristic soft-tissue edema often visible along the superolateral aspect of the fat pad on fat-suppressed fluid-sensitive images.[35-37] The medial retinacular structures, and medial patellofemoral ligament (MPFL) in particular, are a primary restraint to lateral patellar displacement and are often injured in the setting of lateral patellar dislocation. MPFL insufficiency may contribute to recurrent lateral patellar dislocation, warranting surgical ligament reconstruction.[38]

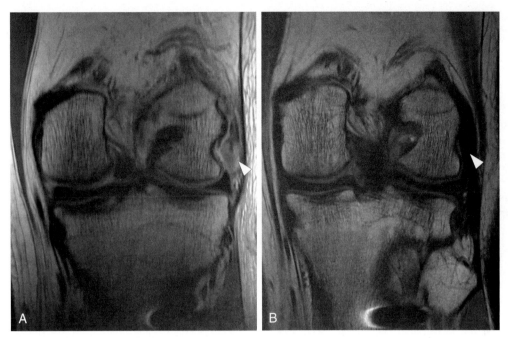

FIGURE 16-18   Posterolateral corner injury in a 40-year-old man following a skiing injury. **A:** Coronal proton density (PD) fast spin echo (FSE) image demonstrates acute avulsion of the fibular collateral ligament and popliteus tendon (white arrowhead) proximally. **B:** Coronal PD FSE image obtained 8 months following the initial injury demonstrates interval scar remodeling (white arrowhead) of the previously visible tear.

Extensor tendinosis is relatively common and may predispose to frank tendon rupture. In older patients, degeneration and tear of the quadriceps are not uncommon. The normal quadriceps tendon is largely hypointense, though may appear somewhat striated along its patellar insertion. Tendinosis results in hyperintensity and thickening of fibers. In the setting of a complete rupture, the torn tendon fibers will often retract, yielding a fluid-filled gap (**Fig. 16-19**). Accurate characterization of the degree of tear, extent of retraction, and overall health of the tendon tissue is valuable in aiding potential surgical planning.[39]

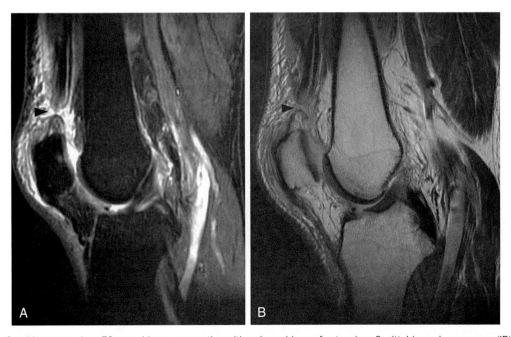

FIGURE 16-19   Quadriceps tear in a 70-year-old man presenting with pain and loss of extension. Sagittal inversion recovery (IR) **(A)** and proton density (PD) fast spin echo (FSE) **(B)** images demonstrate acute rupture of the distal quadriceps tendon yielding a small fluid-filled gap (black arrowheads).

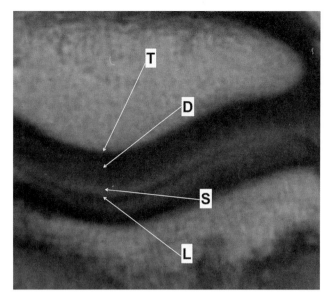

FIGURE 16-20 Magnified axial proton density (PD) fast spin echo (FSE) image of the patellofemoral articulation demonstrates normal chondral stratification over the patella. D, deep (radial) layer; L, lamina splendens; S, superficial (transitional) layer; T, tidemark.

ARTICULAR CARTILAGE

MRI allows direct visualization of the articular cartilage, with optimal sequencing allowing detection of early degeneration manifesting as changes in expected signal, in addition to detection of frank chondral defects. The signal characteristics of normal articular cartilage are dependent on the pulse sequence being utilized; sequencing for orthopedic imaging should provide adequate contrast between fibrocartilage, articular cartilage, subchondral bone, and synovial fluid. High-field, high-resolution proton density–weighted FSE sequences provide excellent depiction of normal chondral stratification with good tissue contrast

providing a clear delineation between adjacent subchondral bone and menisci and afford additional contrast with adjacent synovial fluid due to the effects of magnetization transfer.[40]

Normal hyaline articular cartilage is organized in layers, with the collagen orientation and proteoglycan content varying predictably within each layer relative to the others (**Fig. 16-20**). The deepest layer, called the tidemark, is a thin layer of cartilage which is mineralized, which therefore blends with the subchondral plate. The next layer, the radial zone, consists of highly organized parallel collagen fibers; this high degree of organization facilitated rapid energy transfer and results in short relaxation values. The next layer, called the transitional zone, consists of collagen fibers organized in arcades; energy transfer within this layer is less rapid relative to the deep layer and therefore relaxation values are longer. The most superficial layer of articular cartilage is the lamina splendens; this is a very thin layer of horizontally oriented collagen fibers organized perpendicular to one another; therefore, this layer also appears relatively hypointense due to shorter relaxation times. The earliest changes in cartilage undergoing degeneration include disorganization of collagen fibers, depletion of proteoglycan, and increases in water content. On clinical MR imaging sequences, these changes typically manifest as changes in expected signal, with degenerating cartilage becoming more hyperintense due to prolonged relaxation times, and losing its expected normal stratified appearance. Later changes include loss of chondral substance, including focal defects and well as more diffuse thinning (**Fig. 16-21**). Once arthrosis progresses to an advanced stage, full-thickness chondral defects with associated subchondral changes such as cysts and edema may be observed, as well as osseous remodeling resulting in sclerosis and osteophytes.[40]

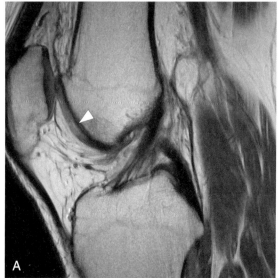
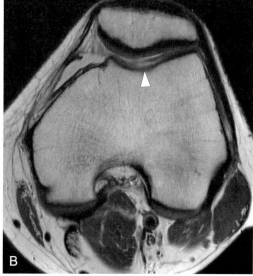

FIGURE 16-21 Sagittal (**A**) and axial (**B**) proton density (PD) fast spin echo (FSE) images in a 55-year-old woman presenting with anterior pain demonstrate an area of chondral delamination and flap formation over the central trochlea (white arrowheads).

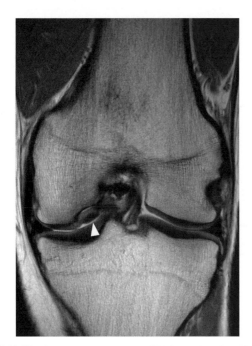

FIGURE 16-22   Coronal proton density (PD) fast spin echo (FSE) image in a 14-year-old boy presenting with medial pain demonstrates osteochondral lesion of the medial femoral condyle, with unstable in-situ osteochondral fragment (white arrowhead) which has flipped such that the articular cartilage is directed toward the underlying osseous bed. Also note that the signal within the osseous portion of the fragment is uniformly hypointense, suggesting devitalization.

Osteochondral lesions are well-evaluated on MRI, which may be useful in terms of determining whether a particular lesion may warrant surgical intervention. Lesions deemed likely to be unstable on imaging are less likely to heal spontaneously without intervention. Signs of lesion instability include a frank fluid interface and cystic change along the junction of the lesion and underlying osseous bed, as well as well-corticated sclerotic margins about the osseous portion of the fragment and along the osseous bed. Frank displacement is also an obvious sign of lesion instability (**Fig. 16-22**).[41-43]

Peripheral Nerves

MRI is capable of accurate evaluation of the major peripheral nerves at the knee, which may suffer traumatic and iatrogenic injury, as well as entrapment and inflammation, and neurogenic neoplastic lesions. Peripheral nerve MRI is often technically more challenging than routine knee MRI, due to the small cross-sectional diameter, extensive length, and complex course of many peripheral nerves. Optimal sequencing for evaluation of peripheral nerves must allow detailed evaluation of nerve signal and morphology; therefore, sequences should be obtained at high resolution and at an obliquity oriented to the axis of the nerve of interest. Neurogenic pain is often vague and potentially remote from the causative lesion, and therefore localization of lesions on imaging may be challenging. Patterns of associated muscle denervation may provide clues as to the nerve involved and the level of the causative lesion (**Fig. 16-23**).[18,44]

POSTOPERATIVE MRI

Postoperative Meniscus

Evaluation of the postoperative meniscus is often challenging. Knowledge of if and what type of surgery was performed is generally valuable in aiding in the interpretation of meniscal findings on imaging. Knowledge of

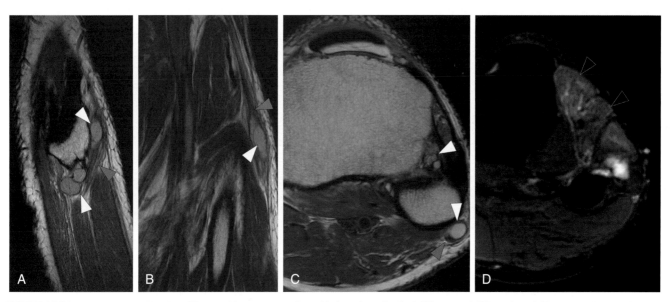

FIGURE 16-23   Peroneal ganglion in a 63-year-old man presenting with foot drop. Sagittal (**A**), coronal (**B**), and axial (**C**) proton density (PD) fast spin echo (FSE) images demonstrate multilocular ganglion (white arrowheads) along the course of the peroneal nerve (gray arrowheads), with associated denervation of the anterior compartment musculature on inversion recovery (IR) images (**D**, black arrowheads).

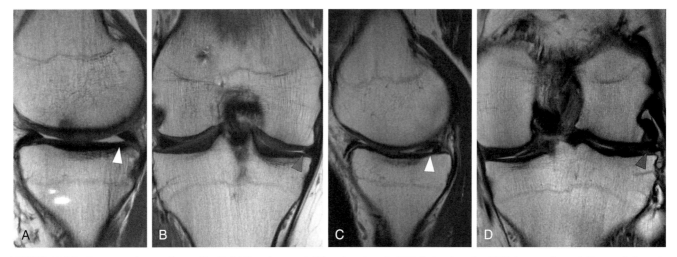

FIGURE 16-24   Postoperative meniscus. Sagittal **(A)** and coronal **(B)** proton density (PD) fast spin echo (FSE) images through the medial meniscus in a 50-year-old man status post partial meniscectomy demonstrate attenuation and blunting of the posterior horn (white arrowhead) and body segment (gray arrowhead), a normal appearance following partial meniscectomy. Sagittal **(C)** and coronal **(D)** PD FSE in a 64-year-old man following prior partial medial meniscectomy demonstrate a retear involving the posterior horn (white arrowhead) and body segment (gray arrowhead).

the expected postoperative appearance of the menisci is important in preventing expected postsurgical changes from being misinterpreted as pathology.

Partial meniscectomy is performed commonly in the setting of meniscal tears not amenable to surgical repair, typically degenerative horizontal cleavage tears. The postoperative meniscal remnant is typically diminished in size and blunted along the free edge, which should appear smooth and regular (Fig. 16-24). Signs of retear include fluid signal intensity clefts, displaced flaps, and frank fragmentation.[45,46]

Following meniscal repair, linear signal hyperintensity often persists along the repair site, an expected postoperative finding which does not indicate a retear unless the hyperintensity is of frank fluid intensity.[45,46]

Meniscal transplantation may be performed utilizing allograft tissue to replace a meniscus that is beyond repair in a patient without arthrosis advanced enough to warrant an arthroplasty. Characteristic fixation points will often be visible at the meniscal attachments; these tend to differ based on whether the transplant is lateral or medial, due to the differing morphology of the two menisci. Medial meniscal allografts typically possess two separate fixation points, while lateral allografts are commonly fixed utilizing a single block of donor bone for both root attachments, due to their closer proximity to one another (**Fig. 16-25**).

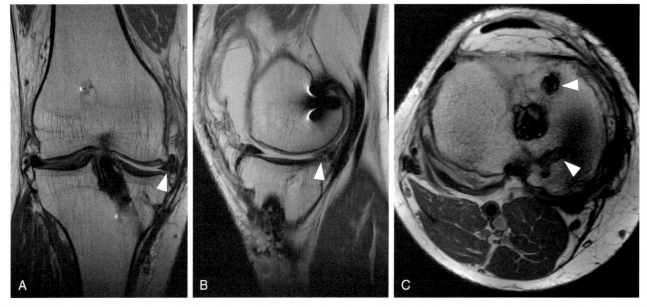

FIGURE 16-25   Medial meniscal transplant in a 40-year-old man returning with persistent pain. Coronal **(A)** and sagittal **(B)** proton density (PD) fast spin echo (FSE) images in a patient status post prior medial meniscal transplant demonstrate degeneration of the transplant meniscus with extrusion of the posterior horn and body segments (white arrowheads). Axial PD FSE image **(C)** demonstrates the typical fixation of a medial meniscal transplant with two separate fixation points along the anterior and posterior attachments (white arrowheads).

MRI allows evaluation of allograft degeneration, tear, and extrusion, as well as the degree and extent of chondral wear prior to and following surgery.[47]

Ligament Reconstruction

Evaluation of ligament reconstruction, and ACL reconstruction in particular, is a common indication for postoperative knee MRI. ACL grafts have been shown to undergo a predictable process of maturation over the first year post reconstruction. In the immediate postoperative period, graft fibers are typically uniformly hyperintense. Over the first few months following surgery, the graft undergoes a process of ligamentization, in which remodeling and vascularization occur, causing the graft to appear relatively hyperintense. Following this process, the graft typically decreases in signal, ultimately becoming hypointense once more, typically around 6 months to 1 year following surgery (**Fig. 16-26**).[48-50]

The orientation of an ACL graft is typically best assessed in the sagittal and coronal planes. On sagittal images, the graft should parallel the roof of the intercondylar notch. Excessive anterior positioning may result in impingement of the graft along the roof of the intercondylar notch, while too vertical a graft orientation may result in graft laxity. Scar may form around the synovial reflections of the graft, which may occasionally manifest as a cyclops lesion, a focal scar nodule along the anterior aspect of the graft distally, which can result in decreased range of motion with loss of terminal extension.[48-50]

Acute retear of an ACL graft generally results in imaging findings similar to those observed in a tear of the native ACL—hyperintensity and thickening of the graft with disruption of fibers and associated secondary findings. Lateral contusions indicative of acute pivot shift may be seen not only in the setting of graft retear but also in the setting of graft laxity, in which case the graft fibers are often completely normal appearing due to the fact that they are not experiencing load (**Fig. 16-27**). Chronic graft failure, like chronic insufficiency of the native ACL, can result in anterior tibial translation (**Fig. 16-28**).[48-51]

As in the native ACL, ganglion may be observed within the substance of the graft, often with intraosseous extension. In the setting of ACLR, this may result in widening of the osseous tunnels and may compromise the fixation, potentially necessitating revision.[49]

Repair of the Articular Surfaces

Evaluation following chondral or osteochondral repair is becoming a more common indication for knee MRI. A variety of techniques are available for repair of chondral and osteochondral lesions, and familiarity with their expected appearances is therefore valuable. Patients with unstable osteochondral lesions amenable to repair often undergo pinning of the unstable osteochondral fragment to fix it within the osseous bed. Microfracture involves abrading the subchondral bone in order to stimulate bleeding and formation of repair tissue. This tissue is typically fibrocartilaginous and therefore is expected to be lower in signal than normal hyaline cartilage and to lack normal chondral stratification. A variety of osteochondral grafts are available for repairing focal defects. These include autologous grafts, which are harvested from the patient, allografts, which are harvested from cadaveric donors, and synthetic grafts, engineered to behave similar to native articular cartilage and bone. Autologous grafts and allografts, because they are comprised of harvested native tissue, typically have the expected appearance of normal bone and hyaline articular cartilage, while synthetic grafts often possess a characteristic biphasic appearance. Allografts are commonly utilized for larger defects, due to the limited area available for harvest of native autograft tissue. Cell-based repair techniques are also available, utilizing either the patient's own chondrocytes, cultured following harvest, or cultured donor chondrocytes (**Fig. 16-29**).[50,52-57]

Various specialized MR imaging techniques are available for more advanced assessment of articular cartilage. Parametric mapping sequences can be utilized for detection of early chondral matrix depletion prior to changes becoming evident on routine clinical imaging sequences. These quantitative sequences include T2 mapping, which is sensitive to changes in collagen orientation and mobile water content, as well as T1rho, which detects early proteoglycan depletion (**Fig. 16-29**). Delayed gadolinium-enhanced MRI of cartilage (DGEMRIC) involves the

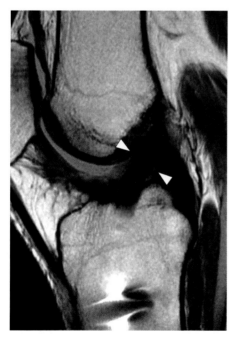

FIGURE 16-26 Sagittal proton density (PD) fast spin echo (FSE) image in a 43-year-old man status post remote anterior cruciate ligament (ACL) reconstruction demonstrates normal appearance of the graft, with mild scar along the synovial reflections of the graft (white arrowheads), but without focal nodule or globalized arthrofibrosis.

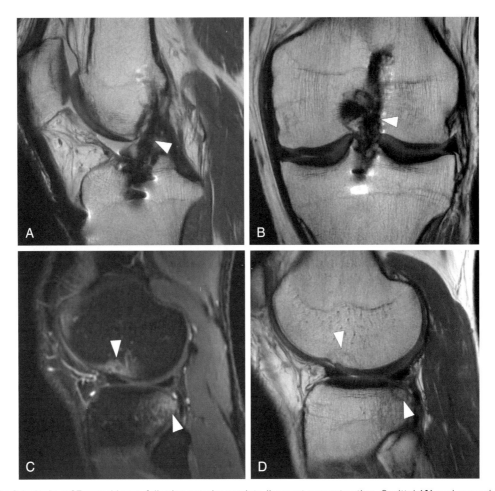

FIGURE 16-27 Graft laxity in a 37-year-old man following anterior cruciate ligament reconstruction. Sagittal **(A)** and coronal **(B)** proton density (PD) fast spin echo (FSE) images demonstrate intact graft (white arrowheads) with normal signal characteristics; however, the graft is somewhat vertical in orientation. Sagittal inversion recovery (IR) **(C)** and PD FSE **(D)** images through lateral femorotibial compartment in the same patient demonstrate acute transchondral impaction injuries (white arrowheads) indicative of recent pivot shift, related to laxity of the anterior cruciate ligament (ACL) graft.

administration of intravenous gadolinium in order to detect proteoglycan depletion. Sodium MRI can also detect changes in proteoglycan content but requires the use of dedicated hardware.[58-65]

Subchondroplasty is a relatively recent technique developed for treatment of painful subchondral lesions such as subchondral insufficiency fractures. The technique is minimally invasive and involves the injection of calcium phosphate into the site of the lesion in order to treat the cause of pain. On imaging, the injected material appears hypointense on routine clinical pulse sequences, replacing the normal fatty marrow on non–fat-suppressed sequences (**Fig. 16-30**).[66]

KNEE ARTHROPLASTY

Knee arthroplasty continues to increase in prevalence as an effective treatment for osteoarthritis; however, MR imaging of arthroplasty has often been avoided in the past due to the challenges inherent when imaging about metal. Because periprosthetic pathology is a common cause of

pain and implant failure, accurate imaging assessment of the various types of osseous and soft-tissue pathology is valuable in evaluation of patients with pain in the setting of arthroplasty.

Deliberate manipulation of MR imaging parameters may be applied to routine clinical pulse sequences in order to minimize the amount of artifact generated by a particular metallic implant. These parameter manipulations include widening the receiver bandwidth in order to increase the strength of the readout gradient, increasing the number of excitations (NEX), increasing the spatial resolution by decreasing the voxel size, and orienting the frequency encoding direction along long axis of the implant. Additionally, as the severity of artifact is proportional to field strength, implants should not be imaged at very high field strength, with 1.5 T preferable to 3.0 T. Frequency-selective fat-suppression techniques should be avoided in favor of more robust techniques, such as inversion recovery. Additionally, specialized sequences designed specifically for suppression of metal artifact are available, with two of the more common being

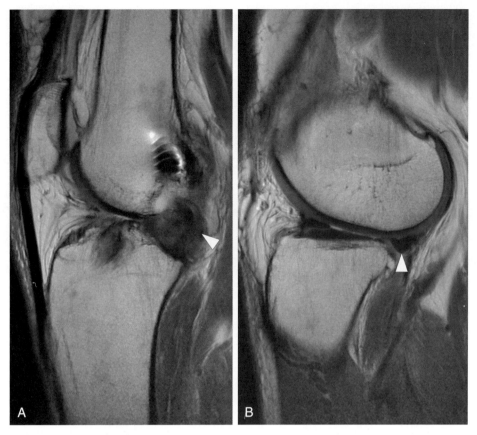

FIGURE 16-28   Failed graft in a 64-year-old woman with history of remote anterior cruciate ligament (ACL) reconstruction. **A:** Sagittal proton density (PD) fast spin echo (FSE) image demonstrates complete disruption of the ACL graft with secondary deformity of the somewhat remodeled posterior cruciate ligament (PCL) (white arrowhead) and amorphous scar within the intercondylar notch. **B:** Sagittal PD FSE obtained through the lateral compartment demonstrates associated anterior translation of the tibia relate to the femur, with posterior displacement of the lateral meniscal posterior horn (white arrowhead).

multiacquisition variable resonance image combination (MAVRIC) and slice encoding metal artifact correction (SEMAC).[67-73]

Pain in patients with TKA may be related to a variety of causes. Periprosthetic fractures may occur intraoperatively or may occur postoperatively in the setting of stress or trauma (**Fig. 16-31**). Displaced fractures are easily diagnosed on radiographs, while nondisplaced or incomplete fractures may warrant cross-sectional imaging. MRI is particularly useful in this scenario, given its sensitivity for marrow edema.[74,75]

Component alignment may contribute to early implant failure due to altered biomechanics and accelerated wear. Component rotational analysis requires cross-sectional imaging and may be performed on either CT or MRI. Relevant measurements include the relationship of the femoral component to the tibial component, the tibial component to the tibial tubercle, and the femoral component to the epicondylar axis of the distal femur (**Fig. 16-32**).[74,76]

Joint infection is a particularly serious complication in patients with TKA, as it often requires prolonged treatment and staged revisions for cure. On MRI, joint infection typically manifests as a pronounced inflammatory synovitis, with the synovium commonly possessing a hyperintense, thickened, and lamellated appearance which is highly specific for infection (**Fig. 16-33**). Additional signs of infection include marked soft-tissue edema, lymphadenopathy, and soft-tissue fluid collections and sinus tracts.[11,77,78] At most institutions, MRI is not used routinely to diagnose periprosthetic joint infection.

Mechanical component loosening is a common cause of implant failure. On MRI, mechanical loosening is confirmed by observation of a thin but circumferential rim of osseous resorption along the interface of the implant or bone cement; this type of resorption is termed fibrous membrane formation and corresponds to a synovialized space lined by a fibrous interface on histopathology (**Fig. 16-34**).[74,78,79]

Osteolysis is another common cause of implant loosening and results from particulate debris shed by the tibial polyethylene insert as the component wears over time. On MRI, polymeric synovitis classically contains isointense debris and often has areas frond-like synovial proliferation. Osteolysis is commonly observed in the setting of polymeric wear; if contrast to the aforementioned fibrous membrane formation, polymeric osteolysis tends to be bulky and lobular rather than thin and

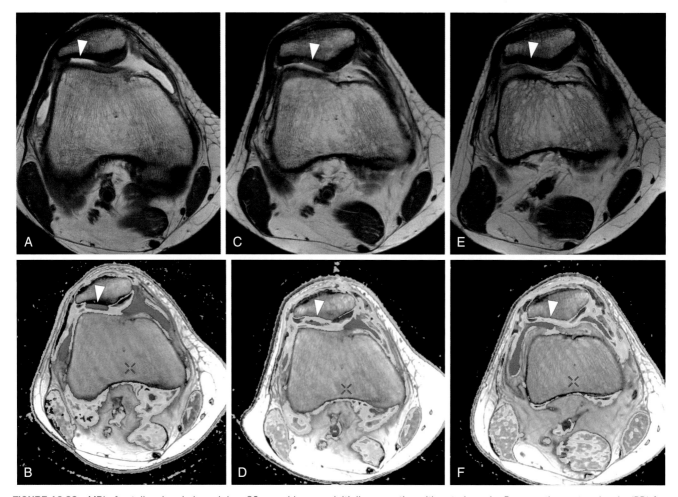

FIGURE 16-29 MRI of patellar chondral repair in a 30-year-old woman initially presenting with anterior pain. Preoperative proton density (PD) fast spin echo (FSE) **(A)** and T2 mapping **(B)** images demonstrate a focal full-thickness chondral defect over the lateral patellar facet (white arrowheads). Subsequent PD FSE images **(C)** following repair of the initial defect utilizing juvenile minced chondrocytes demonstrate good fill of the repair site (white arrowhead) with somewhat hyperintense repair tissue; corresponding prolongation of relaxation times is present on concomitant T2 mapping **(D**, white arrowhead). PD FSE images **(E)** obtained 12 months following repair demonstrate persistent good fill (white arrowhead) with decreased relative hyperintensity of repair tissue indicative of ongoing graft maturation and corresponding decrease in relaxation times on T2 mapping **(F**, white arrowhead).

linear (**Fig. 16-35**). Most polymeric osteolysis appears isointense with a well-marginated sclerotic rim but less commonly the osteolysis may be cystic.[74,78-80]

Fracture of the implant components is rare, and when it does occur, it most commonly affects the polyethylene post (**Fig. 16-36**). Familiarity with the appearance of different polyethylene components is valuable in this scenario, so as not to mistake the lack of polyethylene post in a cruciate sparing implant for a post fracture. In the setting of a post fracture, the fractured portion of the component is often displaced, and care should be taken to locate the fragment so that it can be retrieved at the time of revision.

Patellar clunk is a complication unique to knee arthroplasty and involves the formation of a prominent scar nodule in the peripatellar region, classically along the superior aspect of the articulation (**Fig. 16-37**). The nodule enters the intercondylar notch during flexion and catches on the box of the femoral component during extension, causing mechanical symptoms including a painful, palpable "clunk." This nodule is easily visualized on MRI, though dynamic ultrasound is particularly useful in order to demonstrate the nodule catching at the time the patient is experiencing their typical symptoms.[74,78,81]

Recurrent hemarthrosis may occur in the setting of TKA, causing recurrent episodes of pain and swelling. MR angiography may be helpful in determining the cause of the patient's bleeding and may allow localization of a target vessel for potential embolization (**Fig. 16-38**). While discovering a focal lesion such as a pseudoaneurysm is rare, oftentimes synovial blush indicative of synovitis and inflammation can be localized to the distribution of a specific genicular artery, when may subsequently be embolized in order to control the bleeding.[82,83]

Unicompartmental knee arthroplasty may be utilized for treatment of isolated unicompartmental knee osteoarthritis. These implants may suffer from the same complications as total knee implants, though in addition,

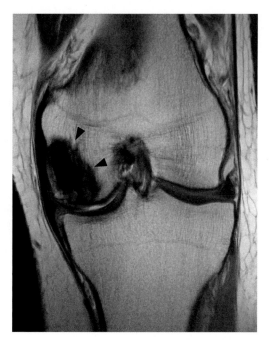

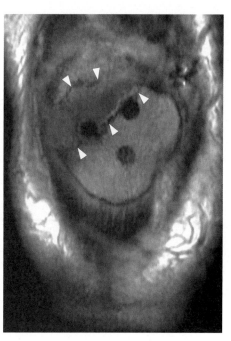

FIGURE 16-30 Coronal proton density (PD) fast spin echo (FSE) image in a 70-year-old woman with history of subchondral insufficiency fracture treated with subchondroplasty demonstrates large hypointense region (black arrowheads) within the medial femoral condyle, contacting the articular surface.

FIGURE 16-31 Coronal proton density (PD) fast spin echo (FSE) image through the patella in a 71-year-old man status post total knee arthroplasty presenting with chronic anterior pain demonstrates obliquely oriented distracted fracture line (white arrowheads) extending along the two superior most pegs.

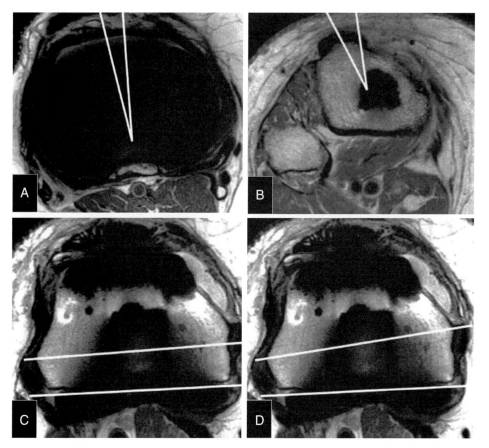

FIGURE 16-32 Axial proton density (PD) fast spin echo (FSE) images demonstrate measurement of rotation of the tibial component relative to the femoral component **(A)**, the tibial component relative to the tibial tubercle **(B)**, the femoral component relative to the surgical transepicondylar axis **(C)**, and the femoral component relative to the clinical transepicondylar axis **(D)**.

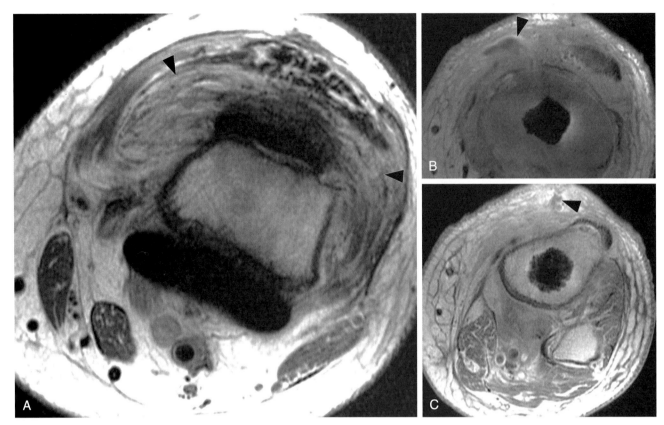

FIGURE 16-33 Joint infection following total knee arthroplasty (TKA) in a 64-year-old man presenting with pain and swelling. Multiple-axial FSE images in a patient status post total knee arthroplasty demonstrate severe inflammatory synovitis (**A**, black arrowheads) with a lamellated appearance, consistent with infection, as well as soft-tissue fluid collection extending to the underlying bone (**B**, black arrowhead) which also communicates with the skin surface via a sinus tract (**C**, black arrowhead).

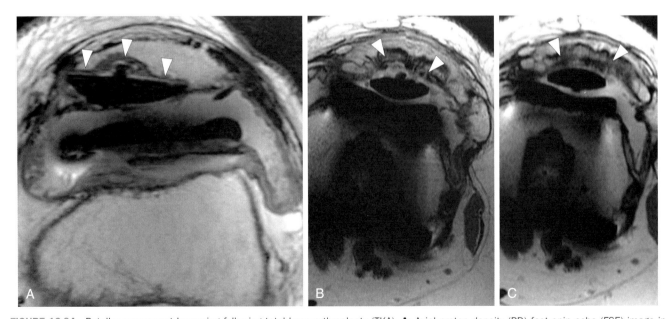

FIGURE 16-34 Patellar component loosening following total knee arthroplasty (TKA). **A:** Axial proton density (PD) fast spin echo (FSE) image in a 66-year-old woman status post TKA demonstrates extensive fibrous membrane formation (white arrowheads) along the patellar component, the extent of which is consistent with loosening. Axial PD FSE image **(B)** in a 56-year-old woman status post TKA demonstrates more bulky osseous resorption along the patellar component, with frank fluid interposed between the component and bone; upon follow-up imaging **(C)**, the patellar component is noted to have flipped such that the articular surface is facing the patella.

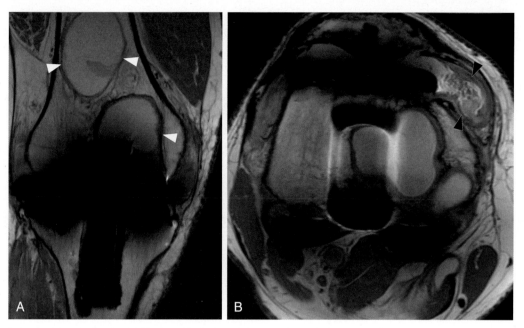

FIGURE 16-35   Polymeric wear following total knee arthroplasty (TKA) in a 69 year-old man presenting with pain and swelling. Coronal proton density (PD) fast spin echo (FSE) **(A)** demonstrates well circumscribed foci of largely cystic osseous resorption (white arrowheads), consistent with osteolysis, as well as synovitis with intermediate signal intensity debris (black arrowheads) on axial images **(B)**, consistent with polymeric wear.

patients with unicompartmental knee arthroplasty may also develop pain related to pathology within their remaining native compartments, such as meniscal tears and progressive osteoarthritis. The most common modes of implant failure in these patients are aseptic loosening and unexplained pain likely related to early fixation failure; therefore careful scrutiny of the bone–implant interface is warranted in these patients.[84]

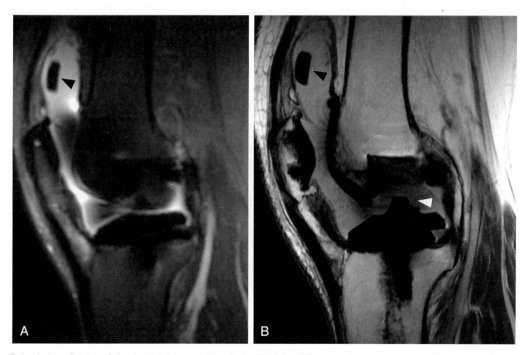

FIGURE 16-36   Polyethylene fracture following total knee arthroplasty (TKA) in a 59-year-old man presenting with acute mechanical symptoms and instability. Sagittal multiacquisition variable resonance image combination (MAVRIC) inversion recovery (IR) **(A)** and sagittal proton density (PD) fast spin echo (FSE) **(B)** demonstrate fracture of the polyethylene post (white arrow), with displacement of the fragment (black arrows) into the suprapatellar region.

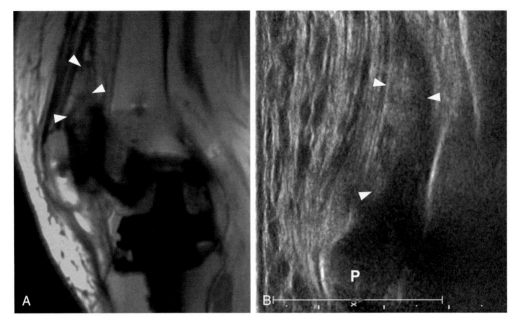

FIGURE 16-37 Patellar clunk in a 62-year-old man status post total knee arthroplasty (TKA). **A:** Sagittal proton density (PD) fast spin echo (FSE) image demonstrates scar nodule (white arrowheads) along the suprapatellar region, in keeping with patellar clunk. **B:** Subsequent dynamic ultrasound demonstrated impingement of the nodule (white arrowheads) during range of motion (P = patella).

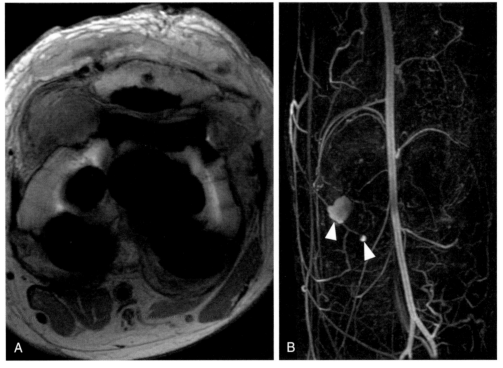

FIGURE 16-38 Hemarthrosis in a 43-year-old man status post recent total knee arthroplasty (TKA). **A:** Axial proton density (PD) fast spin echo (FSE) image demonstrates complex synovitis consistent with hemarthrosis. **B:** Time-resolved contrast-enhanced MR angiographic image demonstrates two early filling foci (white arrowheads) along the medial aspect of the knee, consistent with pseudoaneurysms.

CONCLUSION

Diagnostic imaging is a dynamic field, with rapid technological advances allowing evolution of imaging techniques in order to better demonstrate the multitude of conditions which may be present in patients presenting with a painful knee. The various imaging modalities each possess unique strengths and weaknesses and because of this tend to complement one another. Ultimately, the selection of the most appropriate imaging algorithm requires consideration of the patient's clinical and surgical history and should be tailored to provide optimum assessment of the patient's suspected pathology. Collaboration between radiologists and treating physicians is essential to avoid unnecessary testing, especially in cases where a rare diagnosis may be in question.

REFERENCES

1. Pavlov HBM, Giesa M, Seager K, White E. *Orthopaedist's Guide to Plain Film Imaging*. New York: Thieme Medical Publishers; 1999.
2. Ghelman B. Meniscal tears of the knee: evaluation by high-resolution CT combined with arthrography. *Radiology*. 1985;157(1):23-27. doi:10.1148/radiology.157.1.3839928.
3. An VV, Sivakumar BS, Phan K, Levy YD, Bruce WJ. Accuracy of MRI-based vs. CT-based patient-specific instrumentation in total knee arthroplasty: a meta-analysis. *J Orthop Sci*. 2017;22(1):116-120. doi:10.1016/j.jos.2016.10.007.
4. Wu XD, Xiang BY, Schotanus MGM, Liu ZH, Chen Y, Huang W. CT- versus MRI-based patient-specific instrumentation for total knee arthroplasty: a systematic review and meta-analysis. *Surgeon*. 2017;15(6):336-348. doi:10.1016/j.surge.2017.06.002.
5. Khodarahmi I, Fishman EK, Fritz J. Dedicated CT and MRI techniques for the evaluation of the postoperative knee. *Semin Musculoskelet Radiol*. 2018;22(4):444-456. doi:10.1055/s-0038-1653955.
6. Palmer ELSJ, Strauss HW. *Bone Imaging. Practical Nuclear Medicine*. Philadelphia: WB Saunders; 1992:121-183.
7. van der Bruggen W, Hirschmann MT, Strobel K, et al. SPECT/CT in the postoperative painful knee. *Semin Nucl Med*. 2018;48(5):439-453. doi:10.1053/j.semnuclmed.2018.05.003.
8. Duus BR, Boeckstyns M, Kjaer L, Stadeager C. Radionuclide scanning after total knee replacement: correlation with pain and radiolucent lines. A prospective study. *Investig Radiol*. 1987;22(11):891-894.
9. Ahmad SS, Shaker A, Saffarini M, Chen AF, Hirschmann MT, Kohl S. Accuracy of diagnostic tests for prosthetic joint infection: a systematic review. *Knee Surg Sports Traumatol Arthrosc*. 2016;24(10):3064-3074. doi:10.1007/s00167-016-4230-y.
10. Love C, Marwin SE, Tomas MB, et al. Diagnosing infection in the failed joint replacement: a comparison of coincidence detection 18F-FDG and 111In-labeled leukocyte/99mTc-sulfur colloid marrow imaging. *J Nucl Med*. 2004;45(11):1864-1871.
11. Taljanovic MS, Gimber LH, Omar IM, et al. Imaging of postoperative infection at the knee joint. *Semin Musculoskelet Radiol*. 2018;22(4):464-480. doi:10.1055/s-0038-1667119.
12. Peltea A, Berghea F, Gudu T, Ionescu R. Knee ultrasound from research to real practice: a systematic literature review of adult knee ultrasound assessment feasibility studies. *Med Ultrason*. 2016;18(4):457-462. doi:10.11152/mu-873.
13. Alves TI, Girish G, Kalume Brigido M, Jacobson JA. US of the knee: scanning techniques, pitfalls, and pathologic conditions. *Radiographics*. 2016;36(6):1759-1775. doi:10.1148/rg.2016160019.
14. Jacobson JA, Ruangchaijatuporn T, Khoury V, Magerkurth O. Ultrasound of the knee: common pathology excluding extensor mechanism. *Semin Musculoskelet Radiol*. 2017;21(2):102-112. doi:10.1055/s-0037-1599204.
15. Geannette C, Miller T, Saboeiro G, Parks M. Sonographic evaluation of patellar clunk syndrome following total knee arthroplasty. *J Clin Ultrasound*. 2017;45(2):105-107. doi:10.1002/jcu.22389.
16. Kraay MJ, Goldberg VM, Herbener TE. Vascular ultrasonography for deep venous thrombosis after total knee arthroplasty. *Clin Orthop Relat Res*. 1993;(286):18-26.
17. Nwawka OK, Miller TT. Ultrasound-guided peripheral nerve injection techniques. *AJR Am J Roentgenol*. 2016;207(3):507-516. doi:10.2214/AJR.16.16378.
18. Morag Y, Yang LJ. Imaging nerve pathology of the knee: magnetic resonance imaging and ultrasound. *Semin Musculoskelet Radiol*. 2017;21(2):122-136. doi:10.1055/s-0037-1599206.
19. Lueders DR, Smith J, Sellon JL. Ultrasound-guided knee procedures. *Phys Med Rehabil Clin N Am*. 2016;27(3):631-648. doi:10.1016/j.pmr.2016.04.010.
20. Nwawka OK, Miller TT, Jawetz ST, Saboeiro GR. Ultrasound-guided perineural injection for nerve blockade: does a single-sided injection produce circumferential nerve coverage? *J Clin Ultrasound*. 2016;44(8):465-469. doi:10.1002/jcu.22364.
21. Huda W. *Review of Radiologic Physics*. 4th ed. Philadelphia: Wolters Kluwer; 2016.
22. Friedman T, Chen T, Chang A. MRI diagnosis of recurrent pigmented villonodular synovitis following total joint arthroplasty. *HSS J*. 2013;9(1):100-105. doi:10.1007/s11420-012-9283-y.
23. Blake MH, Lattermann C, Johnson DL. MRI and arthroscopic evaluation of meniscal injuries. *Sport Med Arthrosc Rev*. 2017;25(4):219-226. doi:10.1097/JSA.0000000000000168.
24. Bolog NV, Andreisek G. Reporting knee meniscal tears: technical aspects, typical pitfalls and how to avoid them. *Insights Imaging*. 2016;7(3):385-398. doi:10.1007/s13244-016-0472-y.
25. Ruzbarsky JJ, Konin G, Mehta N, Marx RG. MRI arthroscopy correlations: ligaments of the knee. *Sport Med Arthrosc Rev*. 2017;25(4):210-218. doi:10.1097/JSA.0000000000000167.
26. Naraghi AM, White LM. Imaging of athletic injuries of knee ligaments and menisci: sports imaging series. *Radiology*. 2016;281(1):23-40. doi:10.1148/radiol.2016152320.
27. Phelan N, Rowland P, Galvin R, O'Byrne JM. A systematic review and meta-analysis of the diagnostic accuracy of MRI for suspected ACL and meniscal tears of the knee. *Knee Surg Sports Traumatol Arthrosc*. 2016;24(5):1525-1539. doi:10.1007/s00167-015-3861-8.
28. Keizer MNJ, Otten E. Passive anterior tibia translation in anterior cruciate ligament-injured, anterior cruciate ligament-reconstructed and healthy knees: a systematic review. *Musculoskelet Surg*. 2019;103(2):121-130. doi:10.1007/s12306-018-0572-6.
29. Hansford BG, Yablon CM. Multiligamentous injury of the knee: MRI diagnosis and injury patterns. *Semin Musculoskelet Radiol*. 2017;21(2):63-74. doi:10.1055/s-0037-1599208.
30. Badri A, Gonzalez-Lomas G, Jazrawi L. Clinical and radiologic evaluation of the posterior cruciate ligament-injured knee. *Curr Rev Musculoskelet Med*. 2018;11(3):515-520. doi:10.1007/s12178-018-9505-0.
31. Gimber LH, Hardy JC, Melville DM, Scalcione LR, Rowan A, Taljanovic MS. Normal magnetic resonance imaging anatomy of the capsular ligamentous supporting structures of the knee. *Can Assoc Radiol J*. 2016;67(4):356-367. doi:10.1016/j.carj.2015.11.004.
32. Porrino J, Sharp JW, Ashimolowo T, Dunham G. An update and comprehensive review of the posterolateral corner of the knee. *Radiol Clin N Am*. 2018;56(6):935-951. doi:10.1016/j.rcl.2018.06.006.
33. Vasilevska Nikodinovska V, Gimber LH, Hardy JC, Taljanovic MS. The collateral ligaments and posterolateral corner: what radiologists should know. *Semin Musculoskelet Radiol*. 2016;20(1):52-64. doi:10.1055/s-0036-1579677.
34. Grawe B, Schroeder AJ, Kakazu R, Messer MS. Lateral collateral ligament injury about the knee: anatomy, evaluation, and management. *J Am Acad Orthop Surg*. 2018;26(6):e120-e127. doi:10.5435/JAAOS-D-16-00028.
35. Jarraya M, Diaz LE, Roemer FW, Arndt WF, Goud AR, Guermazi A. MRI findings consistent with peripatellar fat pad impingement: how much related to patellofemoral maltracking? *Magn Reson Med Sci*. 2018;17(3):195-202. doi:10.2463/mrms.rev.2017-0063.
36. Lapegue F, Sans N, Brun C, et al. Imaging of traumatic injury and impingement of anterior knee fat. *Diagn Interv Imaging*. 2016;97(7-8):789-807. doi:10.1016/j.diii.2016.02.012.
37. Liu YW, Skalski MR, Patel DB, White EA, Tomasian A, Matcuk GR Jr. The anterior knee: normal variants, common pathologies, and diagnostic pitfalls on MRI. *Skelet Radiol*. 2018;47(8):1069-1086. doi:10.1007/s00256-018-2928-2.
38. Trinh TQ, Ferrel JR, Bentley JC, Steensen RN. The anatomy of the medial patellofemoral ligament. *Orthopedics*. 2017;40(4):e583–e588. doi:10.3928/01477447-20170223-03.

39. McMahon CJ, Ramappa A, Lee K. The extensor mechanism: imaging and intervention. *Semin Musculoskelet Radiol*. 2017;21(2):89-101. doi:10.1055/s-0037-1599207.

40. Potter HGF. L.F.F. Articular cartilage. In: Stoller D, ed. *Magnetic Resonance Imaging in Orthopaedics and Sports Medicine*. 1st ed. Baltimore: Lippincott Williams & Wilkins; 2007:1099-1130.

41. De Smet AA, Ilahi OA, Graf BK. Untreated osteochondritis dissecans of the femoral condyles: prediction of patient outcome using radiographic and MR findings. *Skelet Radiol*. 1997;26(8):463-467.

42. Gorbachova T, Melenevsky Y, Cohen M, Cerniglia BW. Osteochondral lesions of the knee: differentiating the most common entities at MRI. *Radiographics*. 2018;38(5):1478-1495. doi:10.1148/rg.2018180044.

43. Kocher MS, Tucker R, Ganley TJ, Flynn JM. Management of osteochondritis dissecans of the knee: current concepts review. *Am J Sports Med*. 2006;34(7):1181-1191. doi:10.1177/0363546506290127.

44. Burge AJ, Gold SL, Kuong S, Potter HG. High-resolution magnetic resonance imaging of the lower extremity nerves. *Neuroimaging Clin N Am*. 2014;24(1):151-170. doi:10.1016/j.nic.2013.03.027.

45. Chapin R. Imaging of the postoperative meniscus. *Radiol Clin N Am*. 2018;56(6):953-964. doi:10.1016/j.rcl.2018.06.007.

46. Cordle AC, Williams DD, Andrews CL. The postoperative meniscus: anatomical, operative, and imaging considerations. *Semin Musculoskelet Radiol*. 2018;22(4):398-412. doi:10.1055/s-0038-1661345.

47. Lee H, Lee SY, Na YG, et al. Surgical techniques and radiological findings of meniscus allograft transplantation. *Eur J Radiol*. 2016;85(8):1351-1365. doi:10.1016/j.ejrad.2016.05.006.

48. Tsifountoudis I, Karantanas AH. Current concepts on MRI evaluation of postoperative knee ligaments. *Semin Musculoskelet Radiol*. 2016;20(1):74-90. doi:10.1055/s-0036-1579676.

49. Viala P, Marchand P, Lecouvet F, Cyteval C, Beregi JP, Larbi A. Imaging of the postoperative knee. *Diagn Interv Radiol*. 2016;97(7-8):823-837. doi:10.1016/j.diii.2016.02.008.

50. Walz DM. Postoperative imaging of the knee: meniscus, cartilage, and ligaments. *Radiol Clin N Am*. 2016;54(5):931-950. doi:10.1016/j.rcl.2016.04.011.

51. Amano K, Li Q, Ma CB. Functional knee assessment with advanced imaging. *Curr Rev Musculoskelet Med*. 2016;9(2):123-129. doi:10.1007/s12178-016-9340-0.

52. Grawe B, Burge A, Nguyen J, et al. Cartilage regeneration in full-thickness patellar chondral defects treated with particulated juvenile articular allograft cartilage: an MRI analysis. *Cartilage*. 2017;8(4):374-383. doi:10.1177/1947603517710308.

53. Malempati C, Jacobs CA, Lattermann C. The early osteoarthritic knee: implications for cartilage repair. *Clin Sports Med*. 2017;36(3):587-596. doi:10.1016/j.csm.2017.02.011.

54. Wang T, Belkin NS, Burge AJ, et al. Patellofemoral cartilage lesions treated with particulated juvenile allograft cartilage: a prospective study with minimum 2-year clinical and magnetic resonance imaging outcomes. *Arthroscopy*. 2018;34(5):1498-1505. doi:10.1016/j.arthro.2017.11.021.

55. Wang T, Wang DX, Burge AJ, et al. Clinical and MRI outcomes of fresh osteochondral allograft transplantation after failed cartilage repair surgery in the knee. *J Bone Joint Surg Am Vol*. 2018;100(22):1949-1959. doi:10.2106/JBJS.17.01418.

56. Wuennemann F, Rehnitz C, Weber MA. Imaging of the knee following repair of focal articular cartilage lesions. *Semin Musculoskelet Radiol*. 2018;22(4):377-385. doi:10.1055/s-0038-1667301.

57. Zouzias IC, Bugbee WD. Osteochondral allograft transplantation in the knee. *Sport Med Arthrosc Rev*. 2016;24(2):79-84. doi:10.1097/JSA.0000000000000109.

58. Argentieri EC, Burge AJ, Potter HG. Magnetic resonance imaging of articular cartilage within the knee. *J Knee Surg*. 2018;31(2):155-165. doi:10.1055/s-0037-1620233.

59. Boesen M, Ellegaard K, Henriksen M, et al. Osteoarthritis year in review 2016: imaging. *Osteoarthr Cartil*. 2017;25(2):216-226. doi:10.1016/j.joca.2016.12.009.

60. Chang EY, Ma Y, Du J. MR parametric mapping as a biomarker of early joint degeneration. *Sports Health*. 2016;8(5):405-411. doi:10.1177/1941738116661975.

61. Eagle S, Potter HG, Koff MF. Morphologic and quantitative magnetic resonance imaging of knee articular cartilage for the assessment of post-traumatic osteoarthritis. *J Orthop Res*. 2017;35(3):412-423. doi:10.1002/jor.23345.

62. Hafezi-Nejad N, Demehri S, Guermazi A, Carrino JA. Osteoarthritis year in review 2017: updates on imaging advancements. *Osteoarthr Cartil*. 2018;26(3):341-349. doi:10.1016/j.joca.2018.01.007.

63. Lansdown DA, Wang K, Cotter E, Davey A, Cole BJ. Relationship between quantitative MRI biomarkers and patient-reported outcome measures after cartilage repair surgery: a systematic review. *Orthop J Sports Med*. 2018;6(4):2325967118765448. doi:10.1177/2325967118765448.

64. Link TM, Neumann J, Li X. Prestructural cartilage assessment using MRI. *J Magn Reson Imaging*. 2017;45(4):949-965. doi:10.1002/jmri.25554.

65. Nacey NC, Geeslin MG, Miller GW, Pierce JL. Magnetic resonance imaging of the knee: an overview and update of conventional and state of the art imaging. *J Magn Reson Imaging*. 2017;45(5):1257-1275. doi:10.1002/jmri.25620.

66. Agten CA, Kaplan DJ, Jazrawi LM, Burke CJ. Subchondroplasty: what the radiologist needs to know. *AJR Am J Roentgenol*. 2016;207(6):1257-1262. doi:10.2214/AJR.16.16521.

67. Chang EY, Bae WC, Chung CB. Imaging the knee in the setting of metal hardware. *Magn Reson Imag Clin N Am*. 2014;22(4):765-786. doi:10.1016/j.mric.2014.07.009.

68. Chen CA, Chen W, Goodman SB, et al. New MR imaging methods for metallic implants in the knee: artifact correction and clinical impact. *J Magn Reson Imaging*. 2011;33(5):1121-1127. doi:10.1002/jmri.22534.

69. Gupta A, Subhas N, Primak AN, Nittka M, Liu K. Metal artifact reduction: standard and advanced magnetic resonance and computed tomography techniques. *Radiol Clin N Am*. 2015;53(3):531-547. doi:10.1016/j.rcl.2014.12.005.

70. Hayter CL, Koff MF, Shah P, Koch KM, Miller TT, Potter HG. MRI after arthroplasty: comparison of MAVRIC and conventional fast spin-echo techniques. *AJR Am J Roentgenol*. 2011;197(3):W405-W411. doi:10.2214/AJR.11.6659.

71. Koch KM, Hargreaves BA, Pauly KB, Chen W, Gold GE, King KF. Magnetic resonance imaging near metal implants. *J Magn Reson Imaging*. 2010;32(4):773-787. doi:10.1002/jmri.22313.

72. Liebl H, Heilmeier U, Lee S, et al. In vitro assessment of knee MRI in the presence of metal implants comparing MAVRIC-SL and conventional fast spin echo sequences at 1.5 and 3 T field strength. *J Magn Reson Imaging*. 2015;41(5):1291-1299. doi:10.1002/jmri.24668.

73. Lu W, Pauly KB, Gold GE, Pauly JM, Hargreaves BA. SEMAC: slice encoding for metal artifact correction in MRI. *Magn Reson Med*. 2009;62(1):66-76. doi:10.1002/mrm.21967.

74. Fritz J, Lurie B, Potter HG. MR imaging of knee arthroplasty implants. *Radiographics*. 2015;35(5):1483-1501. doi:10.1148/rg.2015140216.

75. McDowell M, Park A, Gerlinger TL. The painful total knee arthroplasty. *Orthop Clin N Am*. 2016;47(2):317-326. doi:10.1016/j.ocl.2015.09.008.

76. De Valk EJ, Noorduyn JC, Mutsaerts EL. How to assess femoral and tibial component rotation after total knee arthroplasty with computed tomography: a systematic review. *Knee Surg Sports Traumatol Arthrosc*. 2016;24(11):3517-3528. doi:10.1007/s00167-016-4325-5.

77. Plodkowski AJ, Hayter CL, Miller TT, Nguyen JT, Potter HG. Lamellated hyperintense synovitis: potential MR imaging sign of an infected knee arthroplasty. *Radiology*. 2013;266(1):256-260. doi:10.1148/radiol.12120042.

78. Sneag DB, Bogner EA, Potter HG. Magnetic resonance imaging evaluation of the painful total knee arthroplasty. *Semin Musculoskelet Radiol*. 2015;19(1):40-48. doi:10.1055/s-0034-1396766.

79. Potter HG, Foo LF. Magnetic resonance imaging of joint arthroplasty. *Orthop Clin N Am.* 2006;37(3):361-373, vi-vii. doi:10.1016/j.ocl.2006.03.003.

80. Li AE, Johnson CC, Sneag DB, et al. Frondlike synovitis on MRI and correlation with polyethylene surface damage of total knee arthroplasty. *AJR Am J Roentgenol.* 2017;209(4):W231-W237. doi:10.2214/AJR.16.17443.

81. Heyse TJ, Chong le R, Davis J, Haas SB, Figgie MP, Potter HG. MRI diagnosis of patellar clunk syndrome following total knee arthroplasty. *HSS J.* 2012;8(2):92-95. doi:10.1007/s11420-011-9258-4.

82. Daniels SP, Sneag DB, Berkowitz JL, Trost D, Endo Y. Pseudoaneurysm after total knee arthroplasty: imaging findings in 7 patients. *Skelet Radiol.* 2019;48(5):699-706. doi:10.1007/s00256-018-3084-4.

83. Rodriguez-Merchan EC, Jimenez-Yuste V, Gomez-Cardero P, Rodriguez T. Severe postoperative haemarthrosis following a total knee replacement in a haemophiliac patient caused by a pseudo-aneurysm: early treatment with arterial embolization. *Haemophilia.* 2014;20(1):e86-e89. doi:10.1111/hae.12286.

84. Kleeblad LJ, Zuiderbaan HA, Burge AJ, Amirtharaj MJ, Potter HG, Pearle AD. MRI findings at the bone-component interface in symptomatic unicompartmental knee arthroplasty and the relationship to radiographic findings. *HSS J.* 2018;14(3):286-293. doi:10.1007/s11420-018-9629-1.

chapter 17

Knee Rating Scales for Clinical Outcome

David C. Ayers, MD | Patricia D. Franklin, MD, MPH, MBA | Matthew E. Deren, MD

KNEE RATING SCALES FOR CLINICAL OUTCOME

The evaluation of orthopedic surgical treatments dates back to Ernest Amory Codman in the early 20th century at Massachusetts General Hospital. Traditionally, measures of success after surgery were based on physical examination and radiographic parameters. Since the 1980s, outcome assessment after orthopedic surgery has focused increasingly on the patient's perspective. While this evolution toward the incorporation of patient-based measures is appropriate, traditional measures of outcome, including physical examination, imaging studies, and measures of knee laxity, are complimentary and should not be viewed as unnecessary.

Knee surgery is generally performed for symptoms and disability. Pain is the most common symptom for which surgery is performed. Disability varies among patients who undergo knee surgery and depends to a large extent on the individual. Disability for an elite athlete may involve inability to perform at their desired level of competition. For an elderly individual with knee arthrosis, disability may involve difficulties with activities of daily living (ADLs) or walking.

The objective of treatment must be taken into account when selecting a measure with which to evaluate an orthopedic procedure or treatment. If an inappropriate outcome is used to evaluate the result of anterior cruciate ligament (ACL) reconstruction or total knee arthroplasty (TKA), incorrect treatment decisions may be made for future patients. It is therefore critical to use measures of clinical outcome that are of importance to the patients who are evaluated, while also being relevant to the surgeon.

This chapter discusses measures of clinical outcome that may be used to evaluate different treatments for patients with disorders of the knee. The measurement properties of reliability, validity, and responsiveness are reviewed. Last, general health status measures, joint- and condition-specific instruments, and measures of activity level are reviewed.

Reliability, Validity, and Responsiveness

A measure of any kind is only useful if it is reproducible (reliable) and accurate (valid). In the assessment of health status, measures must also be able to detect improvement or worsening (termed *responsiveness* or *sensitivity to change*). This section is devoted to the concepts of reliability, validity, and responsiveness.

Reliability

An instrument is reliable if it is measuring something in a reproducible fashion.[1] *Reliability* is also known as *reproducibility*, because repeated administrations of the same questionnaire to stable patients should produce more or less the same results.[2]

There are two schools of thought with respect to the measurement of reliability for health status instruments. The first is test–retest reliability, which involves having patients who are in a stable state respond to the questionnaire at two points in time. The time period must not be too short, because the subject will remember their prior responses. As well, the time period must not be too prolonged, which will allow for the possibility of clinical change. In general, a time period ranging from 2 days to 2 weeks is used.

Measures of agreement, such as the intraclass correlation coefficient[3] or the limits of agreement statistic,[4-6] or both, are typically used to compare the scores.[7] The intraclass correlation coefficient is an index of concordance for dimensional measurements ranging between 0 and 1, where 0.75 or more is adequate for patients enrolled in a clinical trial.[8] This statistic is important to differentiate from measures of correlation, such as the Spearman or Pearson correlation coefficients, which do not measure agreement. These statistics may indicate excellent correlation in situations in which agreement is poor, and, therefore, they should not be used for studies of reliability. For example, if the first measure is twice as high as the second measure for all subjects in a study of reliability, the correlation would be perfect but the agreement would be poor.

The limit of agreement statistic is a descriptive measure of reproducibility. This value is the mean difference between the two tests ±2 standard deviations.[5] Ninety-five percent of the differences between the two test administrations will lie within this interval,[5] providing the investigator with an estimate of the precision of the measure.

Internal consistency is another method for measuring the reliability of rating scales. This concept was borrowed by clinicians from the field of psychometrics. The latter discipline involves the measurement of psychologic phenomena (e.g., depression or anxiety) or educational achievement.[9]

The concepts evaluated by psychometric scales are difficult to define or may involve learning or both. In these situations, it would not be possible to have the patients complete the questionnaire on two separate occasions, owing to recall or learning effects. The calculation of internal consistency involves a measurement of the inter-correlation of the responses to the questions on a single administration. The statistic generally used to describe internal consistency is termed *Cronbach alpha,* which ranges from 0 to 1, with 1 indicating perfect reliability.[10] Cronbach alpha has been used to evaluate the reliability of rating scales in orthopedic surgery[11]; however, it is questionable whether the principles of psychometric theory apply to the measurement of symptoms and disability. In practice, orthopedic scales that measure a wide variety of clinical phenomena have also been demonstrated to have high internal consistency.[12]

Validity

An instrument is valid if it measures what it is intended to measure. There are several types of validity that are reviewed briefly below.

The simplest way of validating a rating scale is to provide evidence that its results match a gold standard.[13] This is known as *criterion validity,* although it is generally not possible for instruments that measure quality of life. In such situations, we must rely on face validity, content validity, and construct validity.

Face validity is present when an expert clinician reviews the questions in the scale and believes that they appear to measure the concept in question. This form of validity is rather simple; however, it is important nevertheless.

Content validity is a more formal application of face validity. Content validity measures whether the scale includes representative samples of the concept that the investigator is attempting to measure. For example, if a rating scale was measuring quality of life, the content of the scale should include measures of physical, mental, and social health to provide adequate content validity.

Construct validity determines whether the questionnaire behaves in relation to other measures as would be expected. This requires several hypotheses about how the results of the questionnaires should correlate (positively or negatively) with other related or unrelated measures and in testing these hypotheses.

Responsiveness

Orthopedic surgeons generally use rating scales to measure improvement in health-related quality of life after treatment. An instrument that is not able to measure improvement in a patient who has been treated successfully would not be useful for clinical research or evaluation. Therefore, the characteristic of responsiveness is critical for the practical application of a rating scale.

There are many statistics that are available to determine responsiveness.[14,15] The standardized response mean (observed change/standard deviation of change) is most commonly used in orthopedic research.[16-18] This statistic incorporates the response variance, allowing statistical testing of the response means.[19]

Generic and Specific Measures

Specific measures may pertain to a certain pathologic entity (disease-specific), condition (condition-specific), or anatomic location (joint-specific). These measures focus not only on specific aspects of the condition (or anatomic location), but complaints are also usually attributed to the disorder (or anatomic location).[13,20,21] For example, a joint-specific instrument for the knee may ask patients if they have difficulty dressing because of their knee problem.

Generic tools have a broader perspective, including emotional, social, mental, and physical health, and do not restrict attribution to a particular disorder.[13,21] The advantage of generic health status instruments compared with specific instruments is that they allow comparisons across conditions and treatments. The disadvantage of these tools is that they may not be responsive to clinically important change, because a change in an isolated problem may not be reflected in the score of this more global measure.[13,21-23] The advantage of disease- or joint-specific measures is that they are generally more responsive to change in the specific phenomenon of interest, and they are more relevant to patients.

The most commonly used generic health status instrument is the Short Form 36 (SF-36). It is a 36-item questionnaire that measures general health.[24-26] Its use has been encouraged in conjunction with knee-specific instruments for studies of ACL-injured patients[27] and is commonly used in studies of TKA to describe the patients' overall status.[21] A physical component scale (PCS) and a mental component scale (MCS) can be derived from the SF-36, SF-12, VR-12, or PROMIS global. The PCS provides a summary score of the patients' physical function. The MCS provides a summary score of the patients' emotional function and accurately measures a patients' emotional health. The MCS is an excellent screening tool for a patients' emotional fitness for surgery. For example, a patient that has subclinical depression with trait anxiety disorder will have a MCS score less than 45.

KNEE RATING SCALES FOR ATHLETIC PATIENTS

There are many rating scales available to measure outcome in athletic patients with disorders of the knee. What defines an athletic individual may not always be clear. The activity level of the patient is an important prognostic variable, because active patients place greater demands on their knees than sedentary individuals and have different expectations of the results of treatment. Activity level is not always directly related to symptoms and disabilities and should be measured separately. This topic is discussed at the end of the chapter. A review of eight commonly used rating scales for athletic patients with disorders of the knee is presented.

The modified Lysholm scale[28] is an eight-item questionnaire that was originally designed to evaluate patients after knee ligament surgery.[29] It is scored on a 100-point scale, with 25 points attributed to knee stability; 25 to pain; 15 to locking; 10 each to swelling and stair climbing; and 5 each to limp, use of a support, and squatting.[28] Although this scale was developed without patient input, it has been used extensively for clinical research studies.[27,30-32] It has been demonstrated to have adequate test–retest reliability and good construct validity.[29,33]

The first version of the Cincinnati Knee Rating System was published in 1983 with additional modifications that were developed for occupational activities, athletic activities, symptoms and functional limitations with sports, and daily activities.[34,35] There are 11 components in the Cincinnati Knee Rating System. In addition to measuring symptoms and disability, there are sections of this rating system that measure physical examination, laxity of the knee based on instrumented testing, and radiographic evidence of degenerative joint disease.[36] This instrument is reliable, valid, and responsive to clinical change.[33,36]

The American Academy of Orthopaedic Surgeons Sports Knee Rating Scale[37] was included in the Musculoskeletal Outcomes Data Evaluation and Management System for athletic patients with disorders of the knee. There are five parts and 23 questions in this instrument: a core section, including stiffness, swelling, pain, and function (seven questions); a locking or catching on activity section (four questions); a giving way on activity section (four questions); a current activity limitations due to the knee section (four questions); and a pain on activity due to the knee section (four questions).

The five subscales are independent and are meant to be reported separately. As well, this scale has the response "cannot do for other reasons" for many questions. The scoring manual states that an item should be "dropped" if the patient selects that response, which may be interpreted as "scored as missing." These factors may lead to practical difficulties when using this questionnaire.[33] Despite these concerns, the measurement properties of this instrument were found to be satisfactory when the five subscales were combined and the mean was calculated.[33]

The Activities of Daily Living Scale of the Knee Outcome Survey was published with an evaluation of its reliability, validity, and responsiveness.[11] It was developed based on a review of relevant instruments and clinician input. This scale is designed for patients with disorders of the knee ranging from ACL injury to arthrosis. It includes 17 multiple-choice questions divided into two sections:

one for symptoms (7 questions) and one for functional disability (10 questions). This instrument was found to have slightly higher correlations with the Lysholm, Cincinnati, and American Academy of Orthopaedic Surgeons scales, as well as other measures of disability, indicating excellent construct validity.[33] It was also found to be slightly more sensitive to clinical improvement (responsive) than the three other scales in a group of athletic patients.[33] The questions that make up this tool are presented in Appendix A.

The single assessment numeric evaluation was devised to evaluate college-aged patients after ACL reconstruction.[38] The single assessment numeric evaluation asks the patient how they would rate their knee, from 0 to 100, with 100 being normal. This score was found to correlate well with the Lysholm scale in this patient population.[38] The advantage of this single question is its simplicity and the ease with which it can be administered. One potential pitfall is that a single, relatively broad question may be interpreted differently by patients with different disorders and varying levels of symptoms and disability. In the setting of a very homogeneous cohort, such as college-aged patients recovering from a specific procedure (such as ACL reconstruction), the range of pathology is relatively narrow and the instrument correlates well with a standard measure of knee function. The applicability of this tool to patients with a variety of diagnoses is unknown.

The Knee Injury and Osteoarthritis Outcome Score (KOOS) was developed with input from patients who underwent remote meniscal surgery.[39] The reliability, validity, and responsiveness were determined to be satisfactory in a cohort of 21 patients who underwent ACL reconstruction.[39] Five separate scores are calculated for pain, symptoms, ADLs, sport and recreation function, and knee-related quality of life. Of particular interest, the Western Ontario and McMaster Universities Osteoarthritis Index, discussed in greater detail later, is included in the KOOS, and its score can be determined from the KOOS.

The quality-of-life outcome measure for chronic ACL deficiency was developed by Mohtadi.[40] This instrument was developed by surveying ACL-deficient patients, primary care sports medicine physicians, orthopedic surgeons, athletic therapists, and physical therapists. The scale comprises 31 visual analog questions regarding symptoms and physical complaints, work-related concerns, recreational activities and sport participation, lifestyle, and social and emotional health status relating to the knee. This rating scale was found to be valid and responsive for patients with ACL insufficiency.[40] It is very specific to ACL deficiency and, therefore, would not be applicable to other disorders of the knee.

The International Knee Documentation Committee developed a rating scale for seven "objective" parameters relating to the knee.[41] These included effusion, motion, ligament laxity, crepitus, harvest site pathology, X-ray findings, and one-leg hop test. Patients were graded as normal, nearly normal, abnormal, or severely abnormal on each of these. The lowest grade for a given group determines the final patient grade.

More recently, the International Knee Documentation Committee has developed a questionnaire relating to "subjective" factors. These include symptoms, sports activities, and ability to function, including stairs, squatting, running, and jumping. It is currently available on the American Orthopaedic Society for Sports Medicine website at http://www.sportsmed.org/Research/Default.htm. At the time of this writing, the reliability, validity, and responsiveness testing have been completed.[42-44]

KNEE RATING SCALES FOR PATIENTS WITH DEGENERATIVE DISORDERS OF THE KNEE

There are several knee rating scales available for patients with arthrosis of the knee. These rating scales were generally designed to evaluate patients with a greater level of disability than the scales reviewed in Knee Rating Scales for Athletic Patients. The three scales discussed below are commonly used to evaluate patients after TKA.

A commonly used instrument for patients with knee arthrosis is the Western Ontario and McMaster Universities Osteoarthritis Index.[45-47] This scale involves 24 questions: 5 relating to pain, 2 relating to stiffness, and 17 relating to difficulty with ADLs. This scale has been found to be responsive and valid for patients with arthrosis.[21,48,49] The Western Ontario and McMaster Universities Osteoarthritis Index has been translated into many languages, and these versions have been validated as well.[45,50,51]

The index of severity for knee disease[52] was initially developed for nonsteroidal antiinflammatory drug trials. This questionnaire involves five questions related to pain, one question related to the maximum distance the patient can walk, and four questions relating to ADLs. This scale was initially intended to be interviewer administered, although a questionnaire format has subsequently been validated as well.[49]

Part of the Musculoskeletal Outcomes Data Evaluation and Management System package includes a knee core-rating scale. This section, which includes seven questions, is recommended for use in patients with osteoarthritis of the knee. The questions relate to knee stiffness; knee swelling; use of a support to get around, putting on socks; and pain with walking, stairs, and lying in the bed at night. This core scale is included in the American Academy of Orthopaedic Surgeons Sports Knee Rating Scale as one of the five subscores. This instrument has been shown to be reliable and valid.[53]

The Oxford Knee Score was developed by using patient input to select the most relevant items.[54] The developers of this tool interviewed multiple groups of 20 patients who were attending an outpatient clinic for consideration of TKA to determine which questions should be included. After each group of 20 patients tested, they modified the responses and retested the items. The questionnaire is comprised of 12 multiple-choice questions, each with five responses. It was tested in a prospective group of 117 patients undergoing TKA and was demonstrated to be reliable, valid, and responsive.[50,54]

In 1989, the Knee Society Clinical Rating System was developed as a simple objective scoring system to rate the function of the knee and the patient following TKA (Appendix B[55]). While this scoring system was a popular method of tracking and reporting outcomes after TKA, there were ambiguities and deficiencies that challenged its utility and validity in our contemporary patients, who have expectations, demands, and functional requirements that are different from earlier generations. Realizing the need for a new and improved validated knee scoring system, the Knee Society developed and published the new Knee Society Knee Scoring System (**Fig. 17-1**) in 2012.[56,57] This new scoring system is both surgeon- and patient-derived. The objective knee score completed by the surgeon includes a visual analog score for pain walking on level surfaces and on stairs, along with assessment of alignment, ligament stability, and range of motion. Patients record their overall satisfaction, expectations, and functional activities that include standard ADLs and patient-specific activities. This new validated score provides sufficient flexibility and depth to capture the diverse lifestyles and activities of our current TKA patients. It is broadly applicable across gender, age, activity level, and implant type.

The new Knee Society Knee Scoring System is a highly responsive outcome measurement tool that may be applied in both the clinical and research setting. However, in the routine clinical setting, the administration and scoring of outcome tools are resource intensive, especially with the length and complexity of the forms and amount of data collected. Patient responsiveness decreases with long forms and results in incomplete forms, unanswered questions, and limited data collection. Knowing that surgeons are increasingly being held accountable for tracking their surgical outcomes, as payors tie reimbursement to quality, cost, and outcome metrics, the Knee Society created a shorten version of their knee scoring system.[58] The Knee Society Knee Score Patient Short Form (**Fig. 17-2**) is a practical, reliable, responsive, and validated patient-reporting tool for assessing both patient function and satisfaction following TKA. The SF provides a brief measure for the three functional domains of the long form and can be used for monitoring patients in research studies or clinical practice. The long form of the Knee Society Knee Scoring System is recommended for research studies and as a more sensitive measurement of the outcomes of individual patients.

KNEE SOCIETY SCORE: SHORT FORM

DEMOGRAPHIC INFORMATION

1 - Sex
○ Male
○ Female

Enter dates as:
mm/dd/yyyy

2 - Date of birth
☐☐ / ☐☐ / ☐☐☐☐

3 - Height (ft' in")
☐ ☐☐

Weight (lbs.)
☐☐☐

4 - Today's date
☐☐ / ☐☐ / ☐☐☐☐

5 - Surgically treated knee
○ Left   ○ Right

*If both knees please use a different form for each one

6 - Race
○ American Indian or Alaska Native
○ Native Hawaiian or other Pacific Islander
○ Asian
○ Black
○ White
○ Other

7 - Ethnicity
○ Not Hispanic
○ Hispanic

SYMPTOMS

8 - Pain with level walking
○ 0   ○ 1   ○ 2   ○ 3   ○ 4   ○ 5   ○ 6   ○ 7   ○ 8   ○ 9   ○ 10
none   **severe**

9 - Pain with stairs or inclines
○ 0   ○ 1   ○ 2   ○ 3   ○ 4   ○ 5   ○ 6   ○ 7   ○ 8   ○ 9   ○ 10
none   **severe**

10 - Does this knee feel "normal" to you?
○ Always   ○ Sometimes   ○ Never

PATIENT SATISFACTION

11 - Currently, how satisfied are you with your knee function while performing light household activities?
○ very satisfied   ○ satisfied   ○ neutral   ○ dissatisfied   ○ very dissatisfied

FUNCTIONAL ACTIVITIES

12 - For how long can you walk (with or without aid) before stopping due to knee discomfort?
○ cannot walk   ○ 0-5 minutes   ○ 6-15 minutes
○ 16-30 minutes   ○ 31-60 minutes   ○ more than an hour

FIGURE 17-1   The new knee society knee scoring system. (Copyright © by The Knee Society. All rights reserved. Reproduced with permission.)

STANDARD ACTIVITIES

How much does your knee bother you during each of the following activities?	no bother 5	slight 4	moderate 3	severe 2	very severe 1	cannot do (because of knee) 0	I never do this
13 - Walking on an uneven surface	○	○	○	○	○	○	○
14 - Climbing up or decending a flight of stairs	○	○	○	○	○	○	○
15 - Getting up from a low couch or a chair without arms	○	○	○	○	○	○	○
16 - Running	○	○	○	○	○	○	○

DISCRETIONARY KNEE ACTIVITIES

Many people consider the following activities important. Of these activities, which one is the most important to you?

(please do not write in additional activities)

☐ Swimming   ☐ Weight-lifting

☐ Golfing (18 holes)   ☐ Leg Extensions

☐ Road Cycling (>30mins)   ☐ Stair-Climber

☐ Gardening   ☐ Stationary Biking / Spinning

☐ Bowling   ☐ Leg Press

☐ Racquet Sports (Tennis, Racquetball, etc.)   ☐ Jogging

☐ Distance Walking   ☐ Eliptical Trainer

☐ Dancing / Ballet   ☐ Aerobic Exercises

☐ Stretching Exercises (stretching out your muscles)

How much does your knee bother you during the activity checked above?

no bother 5	slight 4	moderate 3	severe 2	very severe 1	cannot do (because of knee) 0
○	○	○	○	○	○

FIGURE 17-2   The knee society knee score patient short form. (Copyright © by The Knee Society. All rights reserved. Reproduced with permission.)

Most recently, the Knee Injury and Osteoarthritis Outcome Score for Joint Replacement (KOOS, JR) was developed to create an abbreviated version of the KOOS which was relevant for patients undergoing total knee replacement (TKR).[59] This was internally validated in 2291 patients identified through a hospital registry, as well as externally validated using a national database, Function and Outcomes Research for Comparative Effectiveness in Total Joint Replacement (FORCE-TJR). This seven-question form was created with the intent of serving as a shorter version of an outcome score with questions relevant to osteoarthritis patients, particularly including pain which was absent from the KOOS-PS, a shorter form aimed at a more athletic population.[60] The KOOS JR was developed to reproduce the KOOS score with fewer questions. It unfortunately does not provide subscores in pain, function, and quality of life which are very useful when evaluating patients after TKR.

MEASURES OF ACTIVITY LEVEL FOR PATIENTS WITH DISORDERS OF THE KNEE

Patients' activity levels are related to prognosis in the sports medicine population, because people who are very active have different expectations and demands than those who are relatively sedentary.[31,61] A measure of activity is important for studies evaluating such individuals because the frequency and intensity of sports participation vary widely among these patients.[62] For example, a study describing a new surgical technique for a knee disorder should document the patients' activity level to ensure that the results can be applied to the appropriate patient population. For studies comparing two groups of patients, it is important for the activity levels of the two groups to be similar to avoid a biased comparison.[63]

In a systematic literature review,[63] five activity-level rating scales that are potentially applicable to outcome studies in sports medicine were identified.[28,64-67] There were inherent problems with each of the available instruments, which led to the construction of a new rating scale for this purpose.[63] This activity rating scale consists of four questions relating to the frequency with which the patient runs, cuts, pivots, and decelerates. It has been demonstrated to be reliable and valid.[63] This scale is recommended in addition to a knee outcome instrument for the evaluation of athletic patients with disorders of the knee.

As health care within the United States moves to a value-based system, payers and physicians alike have placed more emphasis on the value of care delivered. One method of measuring the quality of care is by using patient-reported outcome measures (PROMs[68]). PROMs have been instituted for the bundled payment system in the Centers of Medicare and Medicaid Services Comprehensive Care for Joint Replacement, which matches outcomes with reimbursement for hospitals.[69] It is important, though, that outcome be risk-adjusted to allow for fair comparisons between both hospitals and individual surgeons.[70] Without risk adjustment, those performing complex surgeries and having more medically complex patients would likely have inferior publicly reported outcomes due to a higher risk profile and subsequent lower reimbursement, in actuality a penalty for taking on increased complexity. The use of PROMs will only increase as they become more integrated into medical practice and assist further in shared medical decision-making with patients. The 42-item KOOS is a joint-specific, validated, knee PRO assessments used commonly in research. The KOOS is translated into multiple languages and are available free of charge to clinicians and researchers.[71] In 2010, when the FORCE-TJR registry was established, no single disease-specific PRO had emerged as the most common tool for use in US clinical practice. FORCE-TJR adopted the KOOS because the assessments include items to calculate key domains that are meaningful to patients and clinicians, namely: Pain, Activities of Daily Living, Quality of Life, Sport Activities, and Symptoms. Today, the pain and joint function (ADL) scores are used widely to assess knee disease severity and, after surgery, the impact of arthroplasty surgery. For example, CMS's Comprehensive Care for Joint Replacement bundled payment program accepts the KOOS as an outcome measure to meet quality incentives.

While easy access and broadly translated formats are benefits of the KOOS, the surveys' lengths are a barrier to adoption in busy orthopedic clinics. To address the need for a brief PRO that would retain the legacy subscores, Agency for Healthcare Research and Quality (AHRQ)-funded psychometric researchers use the FORCE-TJR national database to develop brief, joint-specific assessments that retain the ability to calculate the pain, ADL, and quality-of-life subscores. The KOOS-12 emerged. This brief PRO uses 12 of the original KOOS survey items to generate pain, ADL, and quality-of-life subscores that are comparable with the full survey's scores.[72-74] In addition, a comprehensive summary, or joint impact, score can be calculated. Yet, the KOOS-12 lower respondent burden by more than 70%. These brief surveys are also available on the public website1 for use in clinic and research. Full descriptions of the psychometric properties are published for user reference.

In conclusion, there are multiple outcome scores available in 2019. After years of discussions with all stakeholders in our professional community, it was agreed upon that a balance must be struck to ease responder burden yet maintain collection of essential data elements and maintain the ability to investigate the essential subscores in pain and function. Essential to this balance was inclusion of both general health as well as joint-specific surveys. For patients with knee osteoarthritis, this list includes either VR-12, SF-12, or PROMIS-10 global as well as the KOOS-12. In the future, we expect increased utilization of these instruments as process measures as well for determining appropriateness for surgery. A KOOS threshold of 58 has been established, over which patients are not likely to obtain a clinically meaningful improvement in function following TKA.[75] Given the intent of their designers, it is unlikely that the surgical community will ever embrace their use as performance measures, despite the desires of some stakeholders.

REFERENCES

1. Streiner DL, Norman GR. *Health Measurement Scales: A Practical Guide to Their Development and Use*. Oxford: Oxford University Press; 1989.
2. Guyatt GH, Bombardier C, Tugwell PX. Measuring disease-specific quality of life in clinical trials. *Can Med Assoc J*. 1986;134(8):889-895.
3. Bartko JJ. The intraclass correlation coefficient as a measure of reliability. *Psychol Rep*. 1966;19(1):3-11.
4. Bland JM, Altman DG. Comparing methods of measurement: why plotting difference against standard method is misleading. *Lancet*. 1995;346(8982):1085-1087.
5. Bland JM, Altman DG. A note on the use of the intraclass correlation coefficient in the evaluation of agreement between two methods of measurement. *Comput Biol Med*. 1990;20(5):337-340.
6. Bland JM, Altman DG. Statistical methods for assessing agreement between two methods of clinical measurement. *Lancet*. 1986;1(8476):307-310.
7. Deyo RA, Diehr P, Patrick DL. Reproducibility and responsiveness of health status measures. Statistics and strategies for evaluation. *Control Clin Trials*. 1991;12(4 suppl):142S-158S.
8. Rosner B. *Fundamentals of Biostatistics*. Toronto: Duxbury Press; 1995.
9. Wright JO, Feinstein AR. A comparative contrast of clinimetric and psychometric methods for constructing indexes and rating scales. *J Clin Epidemiol*. 1992;45(11):1201-1218.
10. Nunnally JC, Bernstein IH. *Psychometric Theory*. New York: McGraw-Hill; 1994.
11. Irrgang JJ, Snyder-Mackler L, Wainer RS, et al. Development of a patient-reported measure of function of the knee. *J Bone Joint Surg Am*. 1998;80(8):1132-1145.
12. Marx RG, Bombardier C, Hogg-Johnson S, et al. Clinimetric and psychometric strategies for development of a health measurement scale. *J Clin Epidemiol*. 1999;52(2):105-111.
13. Guyatt GH, Feeny DH, Patrick DL. Measuring health-related quality of life. *Ann Intern Med*. 1993;118(8):622-629.
14. Beaton DE, Hogg-Johnson S, Bombardier C. Evaluating changes in health status: reliability and responsiveness of five generic health status measures in workers with musculoskeletal disorders. *J Clin Epidemiol*. 1997;50(1):79-93.
15. Wright JG, Young NL. A comparison of different indices of responsiveness. *J Clin Epidemiol*. 1997;50(3):239-246.
16. Kirkley A, Griffin S, McLintock H, et al. The development and evaluation of a disease-specific quality of life measurement tool for shoulder instability. The Western Ontario Shoulder Instability Index (WOSI). *Am J Sports Med*. 1998;26(6):764-772.
17. L'Insalata JC, Warren RF, Cohen SB, et al. A self-administered questionnaire for assessment of symptoms and function of the shoulder. *J Bone Joint Surg Am*. 1997;79(5):738-748.
18. Martin DP, Engelberg R, Agel J, Swiontkowski MF. Comparison of the musculoskeletal function assessment questionnaire with the Short Form-36, the Western Ontario and McMaster Universities Osteoarthritis Index, and the sickness impact profile health-status measures. *J Bone Joint Surg Am*. 1997;79(9):1323-1335.
19. Liang MH, Fossel AH, Larson MG. Comparisons of five health status instruments for orthopedic evaluation. *Med Care*. 1990;28(7):632-642.
20. Bergner M, Rothman ML. Health status measures: an overview and guide for selection. *Annu Rev Public Health*. 1987;8:191-210.
21. Bombardier C, Melfi CA, Paul J, et al. Comparison of a generic and a disease-specific measure of pain and physical function after knee replacement surgery. *Med Care*. 1995;33(4 suppl):AS131-AS144.
22. MacKenzie CR, Charlson ME, DiGioia D, et al. Can the Sickness Impact Profile measure change? An example of scale assessment. *J Chronic Dis*. 1986;39(6):429-438.
23. MacKenzie CR, Charlson ME, DiGioia D, et al. A patient-specific measure of change in maximal function. *Arch Intern Med*. 1986;146(7):1325-1329.
24. McHorney CA, Ware JE Jr, Raczek AE. The MOS 36-Item Short-Form Health Survey (SF-36): II. Psychometric and clinical tests of validity in measuring physical and mental health constructs. *Med Care*. 1993;31(3):247-263.
25. McHorney CA, Ware JE Jr, Rogers W, et al. The validity and relative precision of MOS short- and long-form health status scales and Dartmouth COOP charts. Results from the Medical Outcomes Study. *Med Care*. 1992;30(5 suppl):MS253-MS265.
26. Ware JEJ, Snow KK, Kosinski M, et al. *SF-36 Health Survey Manual and Interpretation Guide*. Boston: The Health Institute; 1993.
27. Shapiro ET, Richmond JC, Rockett SE, et al. The use of a generic, patient-based health assessment (SF-36) for evaluation of patients with anterior cruciate ligament injuries. *Am J Sports Med*. 1996;24(2):196-200.
28. Tegner Y, Lysholm J. Rating systems in the evaluation of knee ligament injuries. *Clin Orthop Relat Res*. 1985;198:43-49.
29. Lysholm J, Gillquist J. Evaluation of knee ligament surgery results with special emphasis on use of a scoring scale. *Am J Sports Med*. 1982;10(3):150-154.
30. Gauffin H, Pettersson G, Tegner Y, et al. Function testing in patients with old rupture of the anterior cruciate ligament. *Int J Sports Med*. 1990;11(1):73-77.
31. Odensten M, Hamberg P, Nordin M, et al. Surgical or conservative treatment of the acutely torn anterior cruciate ligament. A randomized study with short-term follow-up observations. *Clin Orthop Relat Res*. 1985;198:87-93.
32. Roberts TS, Drez D Jr, McCarthy W, et al. Anterior cruciate ligament reconstruction using freeze-dried, ethylene oxide-sterilized, bone-patellar tendon-bone allografts. Two year results in thirty-six patients [published erratum appears in Am J Sports Med 1991;19(3):272]. *Am J Sports Med*. 1991;19(1):35-41.
33. Marx RG, Jones EC, Allen AA, et al. Reliability, validity and responsiveness of four knee outcome scales for athletic patients. *J Bone Joint Surg Am*. 2001;83-A(10):1459-1469.
34. Noyes FR, Matthews DS, Mooar PA, et al. The symptomatic anterior cruciate-deficient knee. Part II: the results of rehabilitation, activity modification, and counseling on functional disability. *J Bone Joint Surg Am*. 1983;65(2):163-174.
35. Noyes FR, Mooar PA, Matthews DS, et al. The symptomatic anterior cruciate-deficient knee. Part I: the long-term functional disability in athletically active individuals. *J Bone Joint Surg Am*. 1983;65(2):154-162.
36. Barber-Westin SD, Noyes FR, McCloskey JW. Rigorous statistical reliability, validity, and responsiveness testing of the Cincinnati knee rating system in 350 subjects with uninjured, injured, or anterior cruciate ligament-reconstructed knees. *Am J Sports Med*. 1999;27(4):402-416.

37. Academy of Orthopaedic Surgeons. *Scoring Algorithms for the Lower Limb Outcomes Data Collection Instrument Version 2.0.* Rosemont: Academy of Orthopaedic Surgeons; 1998.
38. Williams GN, Taylor DC, Gangel TJ, et al. Comparison of the single assessment numeric evaluation method and the Lysholm score. *Clin Orthop Relat Res.* 2000;373:184-192.
39. Roos EM, Roos HP, Lohmander LS, et al. Knee injury and osteoarthritis outcome score (KOOS)—development of a self-administered outcome measure. *J Orthop Sports Phys Ther.* 1998;28(2):88-96.
40. Mohtadi N. Development and validation of the quality of life outcome measure (questionnaire) for chronic anterior cruciate ligament deficiency. *Am J Sports Med.* 1998;26(3):350-359.
41. Hefti F, Muller W. Heutiger stand der evaluation von kniebandlasionen; das neue IKDC-knie-evaluationsblatt. *Der Orthopäde.* 1993;22:351-362.
42. Irrgang J. *ACL outcomes.* In: *Paper Presented at International Society of Arthroscopy, Knee Surgery and Orthopaedic Sports Medicine.* Montreux, Switzerland; 2001.
43. Irrgang JJ, Anderson AF, Boland AL, et al. Development and validation of the International knee documentation committee subjective knee form. *Am J Sports Med.* 2001;29:600-613.
44. Irrgang JJ, Anderson AF, Boland AL, et al. *Responsiveness of the IKDC subjective knee form.* In: *Paper Presented at Final Program of the Annual Meeting of the American Orthopaedic Society for Sports Medicine (AOSSM).* Orlando, FL; 2002.
45. Bellamy N. Outcome measurement in osteoarthritis clinical trials. *J Rheumatol Suppl.* 1995;43:49-51.
46. Bellamy N, Buchanan WW, Goldsmith CH, et al. Validation study of WOMAC: a health status instrument for measuring clinically important patient relevant outcomes to antirheumatic drug therapy in patients with osteoarthritis of the hip or knee. *J Rheumatol.* 1988;15(12):1833-1840.
47. Bellamy N, Sothem RB, Campbell J. Rhythmic variations in pain perception in osteoarthritis of the knee. *J Rheumatol.* 1990;17(3):364-372.
48. Kirkley A, Webster-Bogaert S, Litchfield R, et al. The effect of bracing on varus gonarthrosis. *J Bone Joint Surg Am.* 1999;81(4):539-548.
49. Theiler R, Sangha O, Schaeren S, et al. Superior responsiveness of the pain and function sections of the Western Ontario and McMaster Universities Osteoarthritis Index (WOMAC) as compared to the Lequesne-Algofunctional Index in patients with osteoarthritis of the lower extremities. *Osteoarthritis Cartilage.* 1999;7:515-519.
50. Dunbar MJ, Robertsson O, Ryd L, et al. Translation and validation of the Oxford-12 item knee score for use in Sweden. *Acta Orthop Scand.* 2000;71(3):268-274.
51. Wigler I, Neumann L, Yaron M. Validation study of a Hebrew version of WOMAC in patients with osteoarthritis of the knee. *Clin Rheumatol.* 1999;18(5):402-405.
52. Lequesne MG, Mery C, Samson M, et al. Indexes of severity for osteoarthritis of the hip and knee; validation—value in comparison with other assessment tests. *Scand J Rheumatol Suppl.* 1987;65:85-89.
53. Hunsaker FG, Cioffi DA, Amadio PC, et al. The American Academy of Orthopaedic Surgeons outcomes instruments: normative values from the general population. *J Bone Joint Surg Am.* 2002;84-A:208-215.
54. Dawson J, Fitzpatrick R, Murray D, et al. Questionnaire on the perceptions of patients about total knee replacement. *J Bone Joint Surg Br.* 1998;80(1):63-69.
55. Insall J, Dorr L, Scott R, et al. Rational of the knee society clinical rating system. *Clin Orthop Relat Res.* 1989;248:13-14.
56. Scuderi G, Bourne R, Noble P, et al. The new knee society knee rating system. *Clin Orthop Relat Res.* 2012;470:3-19.
57. Scuderi G, Sikorskii A, Bourne R, et al. The knee society short form reduces respondent burden in the assessment of patient-reported outcomes. *Clin Orthop Relat Res.* 2015;474:134-142.
58. Noble P, Scuderi G, Brekke A, et al. Development of a new knee society scoring system. *Clin Orthop Relat Res.* 2012;470(1):20-32.
59. Lyman S, Lee Y, Franklin P, et al. Validation of the KOOS, JR: a short-form knee arthroplasty outcomes survey. *Clin Orthop Relat Res.* 2016;474(6):1461-1471.
60. Perruccio A, Lohmander S, Canizares M, et al. The development of a short measure of physical function for knee OA KOOS-Physical Function Short form (KOOS-PS) – an OARSI/OMERACT initiative. *Osteoarthritis Cartilage.* 2008;16(5):542-550.
61. Barber SD, Noyes FR, Mangine RE, et al. Quantitative assessment of functional limitations in normal and anterior cruciate ligament-deficient knees. *Clin Orthop Relat Res.* 1990;255:204-214.
62. Armitage P, Berry G. *Statistical Methods in Medical Research.* London: Blackwell Science; 1994.
63. Marx RG, Stump TJ, Jones EC, et al. Development and evaluation of an activity rating scale for disorders of the knee. *Am J Sports Med.* 2001;29(2):213-218.
64. Daniel DM, Stone ML, Dobson BE, et al. Fate of the ACL-injured patient. A prospective outcome study. *Am J Sports Med.* 1994;22(5):632-644.
65. Noyes FR, Barber SD, Mooar LA. A rationale for assessing sports activity levels and limitations in knee disorders. *Clin Orthop Relat Res.* 1989;246:238-249.
66. Seto JL, Orofino AS, Morrissey MC, et al. Assessment of quadriceps/hamstring strength, knee ligament stability, functional and sports activity levels five years after anterior cruciate ligament reconstruction. *Am J Sports Med.* 1988;16(2):170-180.
67. Straub T, Hunter RE. Acute anterior cruciate ligament repair. *Clin Orthop Relat Res.* 1988;227:238-250.
68. Ayers D. Implementation of patient-reported outcome measures in total knee arthroplasty. *J Am Acad Orthop Surg.* 2017;25(suppl 1):S48-S50.
69. Center for Medicaid and Medicare Innovation (CMMI). *Comprehensive Care for Joint Replacement Model.* Washington, DC: Center for Medicare and Medicaid Services; 2015.
70. Ayers D, Fehring T, Odum S, et al. Using joint registry data from FORCE-TJR to improve the accuracy of risk-adjustment prediction models for thirty-day readmission after total hip replacement and total knee replacement. *J Bone Joint Surg Am.* 2015;97(8):668-671.
71. Knee Injury and Osteoarthritis Outcome Score (KOOS), English version LK1.0. http://koos.nu. Accessed May 23, 2019.
72. Gandek B, Roos E, Franklin P, et al. Item selection for 12-item short forms of the knee injury and osteoarthritis outcome score (KOOS-12) and hip disability and osteoarthritis outcome score (HOOS-12). *Osteoarthritis Cartilage.* 2019;27(5):746-753.
73. Gandek B, Roos E, Franklin P, et al. A 12-item short form of the Hip disability and Osteoarthritis Outcome Score (HOOS-12): tests of reliability, validity, and responsiveness. *Osteoarthritis Cartilage.* 2019;27(5):754-761.
74. Gandek B, Roos E, Franklin P, et al. A 12-item short form of the Knee injury and Osteoarthritis Outcome Score (KOOS-12): tests of reliability, validity, and responsiveness. *Osteoarthritis Cartilage.* 2019;27(5):762-770.
75. Berliner J, Brodke D, Chan V, et al. Can preoperative patient-reported outcome measures be sued to predict meaningful improvement in function after TKA? Clin Orthop Relat Res. 2017;475(1):149-157.

appendix a

Activities of Daily Living Scale of the Knee Outcome Survey

KNEE OUTCOME SURVEY

Instructions:

Please mark ONLY the response that best describes the symptoms and limitations that you have experienced because of your knee while performing each of these usual daily activities over the last 1 to 2 days.

To What Degree do the Following Affect Your Daily Activity Level? (Please Fill in ONLY ONE BUBBLE PER ROW)	Never Have It	Have It, But It Does Not Affect My Daily Activity	It Affects My Activity Slightly	It Affects My Activity Moderately	It Affects My Activity Severely	It Prevents Me From Performing All Daily Activities
1. **Pain in your knee**	○	○	○	○	○	○
2. **Grinding or grating of your knee**	○	○	○	○	○	○
3. **Stiffness in your knee**	○	○	○	○	○	○
4. **Swelling in your knee**	○	○	○	○	○	○
5. **Slipping of your knee**	○	○	○	○	○	○
6. **Buckling of your knee**	○	○	○	○	○	○
7. **Weakness or lack of strength of your leg**	○	○	○	○	○	○

Please fill in ONLY ONE BUBBLE for each question.

8. **How does your knee affect your ability to walk?**
   - ○ My knee does not affect my ability to walk.
   - ○ I have pain in my knee when walking, but it does not affect my ability to walk.
   - ○ My knee prevents me from walking more than 1 mile.
   - ○ My knee prevents me from walking more than ½ mile.
   - ○ My knee prevents me from walking more than 1 block.
   - ○ My knee prevents me from walking.

9. **Because of your knee, do you walk with crutches or a cane?**
   - ○ I can walk without crutches or a cane.
   - ○ My knee causes me to walk with 1 crutch or a cane.
   - ○ My knee causes me to walk with 2 crutches.
   - ○ Because of my knee, I cannot walk even with crutches.

10. **Does your knee cause you to limp when you walk?**
    - ○ I can walk without a limp.
    - ○ Sometimes my knee causes me to walk with a limp.
    - ○ Because of my knee, I cannot walk without a limp.

Please fill in ONLY ONE BUBBLE for each question.

11. How does your knee affect your ability to go UP stairs?

○ My knee does not affect my ability to go up stairs.

○ I have pain in my knee when going up stairs, but it does not limit my ability to go up stairs.

○ I am able to go up stairs normally, but I need to rely on use of a railing.

○ I am able to go up stairs one step at a time with use of a railing.

○ I have to use crutches or a cane to go up stairs.

○ I cannot go up stairs.

13. How does your knee affect your ability to stand?

○ My knee does not affect my ability to stand. I can stand for unlimited amounts of time.

○ I have pain in my knee when standing, but it does not limit my ability to stand.

○ Because of my knee, I cannot stand for more than 1 h.

○ Because of my knee, I cannot stand for more than ½ h.

○ Because of my knee, I cannot stand for more than 10 min.

○ I cannot stand because of my knee.

15. How does your knee affect your ability to squat?

○ My knee does not affect my ability to squat. I can squat all the way down.

○ I have pain when squatting, but I can still squat all the way down.

○ I cannot squat more than ¾ of the way down.

○ I cannot squat more than ½ of the way down.

○ I cannot squat more than ¼ of the way down.

○ I cannot squat at all.

17. How does your knee affect your ability to rise from a chair?

○ My knee does not affect my ability to rise from a chair.

○ Because of my knee, I can only rise from a chair if I use my hands and arms to assist.

12. How does your knee affect your ability to go DOWN stairs?

○ My knee does not affect my ability to go down stairs.

○ I have pain in my knee when going down stairs, but it does not limit my ability to go down stairs.

○ I am able to go down stairs normally, but I need to rely on use of a railing.

○ I am able to go down stairs one step at a time with use of a railing.

○ I have to use crutches or a cane to go down stairs.

○ I cannot go down stairs.

14. How does your knee affect your ability to kneel on the front of your knee?

○ My knee does not affect my ability to kneel on the front of my knee. I can kneel for unlimited amounts of time.

○ I have pain when kneeling on the front of my knee, but it does not limit my ability to kneel.

○ I cannot kneel on the front of my knee for more than 1 hour.

○ I cannot kneel on the front of my knee for more than ½ hour.

○ I cannot kneel on the front of my knee for more than 10 minutes.

○ I cannot kneel on the front of my knee.

16. How does your knee affect your ability to sit with your knee bent?

○ My knee does not affect my ability to sit with my knee bent. I can sit for unlimited amounts of time.

○ I have pain when sitting with my knee bent, but it does not limit my ability to sit.

○ I cannot sit with my knee bent for more than 1 h.

○ I cannot sit with my knee bent for more than ½ h.

○ I cannot sit with my knee bent for more than 10 min.

○ I cannot sit with my knee bent.

○ I have pain when rising from the seated position, but it does not affect my ability to rise from the seated position.

○ Because of my knee, I cannot rise from a chair.

appendix b

The Knee Society Score[56]

DEMOGRAPHIC INFORMATION   (To be completed by patient)

1. Today's date

☐☐ / ☐☐ / ☐☐☐☐

Enter dates as:
mm/dd/yyyy

2. Date of birth

☐☐ / ☐☐ / ☐☐☐☐

3. Height (ft' in")

☐ ☐☐

4. Weight (lbs.)

☐☐☐

5. Sex

○ Male   ○ Female

6. Side of this (surgically treated) knee

○ Left   ○ Right

If both knees have been operated on,
please use a different form for each knee

7. Ethnicity

○ Native Hawaiian or other Pacific Islander   ○ American Indian or Alaska Native   ○ Hispanic or Latino

○ Arab or Middle Eastern   ○ African American or Black   ○ Asian   ○ White

8. Please indicate date and surgeon for your knee replacement operation

Date

☐☐ / ☐☐ / ☐☐☐☐

Name of Surgeon

☐☐☐☐☐☐☐

Enter dates as:
mm/dd/yyyy

9. Was this a primary or revision knee replacement?

○ Primary   ○ Revision

To be completed by surgeon

10. Charnley Functional Classification   **(Use Code Below)** ☐

A Unilateral Knee Arthritis

B1 Unilateral TKA, opposite knee arthritic

B2 Bilateral TKA

C1 TKR, but remote arthritis affecting ambulation

C2 TKR, but medical condition affecting ambulation

C3 Unilateral or Bilateral TKA with Unilateral or Bilateral THR

OBJECTIVE KNEE INDICATORS   (To be completed by surgeon)

ALIGNMENT

1. Alignment: measured on AP standing Xray (Anatomic Alignment)   **25 point max**

> Neutral: 2-10 degrees valgus   (25 pts)
> Varus: < 2 degrees valgus   (-10 pts)
> Valgus: > 10 degrees valgus   (-10 pts)

INSTABILITY

2. Medial / Lateral Instability: measured in full extension   **15 point max**

> None   (15 pts)
> Little or < 5 mm   (10 pts)
> Moderate or 5 mm   (5 pts)
> Severe or > 5 mm   (0 pts)

3. Anterior / Posterior Instability: measured at 90 degrees   **10 point max**

> None   (10 pts)
> Moderate < 5 mm   (5 pts)
> Severe > 5 mm   (0 pts)

JOINT MOTION

4. Range of motion (1 point for each 5 degrees)

Deductions

Flexion Contracture   **Minus Points**
1-5 degrees   (-2 pts)
6-10 degrees   (-5 pts)
11-15 degrees   (-10 pts)
> 15 degrees   (-15 pts)

Extensor Lag   **Minus Points**
<10 degrees   (-5 pts)
10-20 degrees   (-10 pts)
> 20 degrees   (-15 pts)

SYMPTOMS   **(To be completed by patient)**

1. Pain with level walking   **(10 - Score)**

0	1	2	3	4	5	6	7	8	9	10

none   severe

2. Pain with stairs or inclines   **(10 - Score)**

0	1	2	3	4	5	6	7	8	9	10

none   severe

3. Does this knee feel "normal" to you?   **(5 points)**

○ Always (5 pts)   ○ Sometimes (3 pts)   ○ Never (0 pts)

Maximum total points (25 points)

PATIENT SATISFACTION

1. Currently, how satisfied are you with the pain level of your knee while sitting?   **(8 points)**

○ Very Satisfied   ○ Satisfied   ○ Neutral   ○ Dissatisfied   ○ Very Dissatisfied
(8 pts)   (6 pts)   (4 pts)   (2 pts)   (0 pts)

2. Currently, how satisfied are you with the pain level of your knee while lying in bed?   **(8 points)**

○ Very Satisfied   ○ Satisfied   ○ Neutral   ○ Dissatisfied   ○ Very Dissatisfied
(8 pts)   (6 pts)   (4 pts)   (2 pts)   (0 pts)

3. Currently, how satisfied are you with your knee function while getting out of bed?   **(8 points)**

○ Very Satisfied   ○ Satisfied   ○ Neutral   ○ Dissatisfied   ○ Very Dissatisfied
(8 pts)   (6 pts)   (4 pts)   (2 pts)   (0 pts)

4. Currently, how satisfied are you with your knee function while performing light household duties?   **(8 points)**

○ Very Satisfied   ○ Satisfied   ○ Neutral   ○ Dissatisfied   ○ Very Dissatisfied
(8 pts)   (6 pts)   (4 pts)   (2 pts)   (0 pts)

5. Currently, how satisfied are you with your knee function while performing leisure recreational activities?   **(8 points)**

○ Very Satisfied   ○ Satisfied   ○ Neutral   ○ Dissatisfied   ○ Very Dissatisfied
(8 pts)   (6 pts)   (4 pts)   (2 pts)   (0 pts)

Maximum total points (40 points)

PATIENT EXPECTATION   (To be completed by patient)

Compared to what you expected before your knee replacement:

1. My expectations for pain relief were...   **(5 points)**

○ Too High- 'I'm a lot worse than I thought' (1 pt)

○ Too High- 'I'm somewhat worse than I thought' (2 pts)

○ Just Right- 'My expectations were met' (3 pts)

○ Too Low- 'I'm somewhat better than I thought' (4 pts)

○ Too Low- 'I'm a lot better than I thought' (5 pts)

2. My expectations for being able to do my normal activities of daily living were...   **(5 points)**

○ Too High- 'I'm a lot worse than I thought' (1 pt)

○ Too High- 'I'm somewhat worse than I thought' (2 pts)

○ Just Right- 'My expectations were met' (3 pts)

○ Too Low- 'I'm somewhat better than I thought' (4 pts)

○ Too Low- 'I'm a lot better than I thought' (5 pts)

3. My expectations for being able to do my leisure, recreational or sports activities were...   **(5 points)**

○ Too High- 'I'm a lot worse than I thought' (1 pt)

○ Too High- 'I'm somewhat worse than I thought' (2 pts)

○ Just Right- 'My expectations were met' (3 pts)

○ Too Low- 'I'm somewhat better than I thought' (4 pts)

○ Too Low- 'I'm a lot better than I thought' (5 pts)

Maximum total points (15 points)

FUNCTIONAL ACTIVITIES   (To be completed by patient)

WALKING AND STANDING (30 points)

1. Can you walk without any aids (such as a cane, crutches or wheelchair)?   **(0 points)**

○ Yes   ○ No

2. If no, which of the following aid(s) do you use?   **(-10 points)**

○ wheelchair (-10 pts)   ○ walker (-8 pts)   ○ crutches (-8 pts)   ○ two canes (-6 pts)

○ one crutch (-4 pts)   ○ one cane (-4 pts)   ○ knee sleeve / brace (-2 pts)

○ other

3. Do you use these aid(s) because of your knees?   **(0 points)**

○ Yes   ○ No

4. For how long can you stand (with or without aid) before sitting due to knee discomfort?   **(15 points)**

○ cannot stand (0 pts)   ○ 0-5 minutes (3 pts)   ○ 6-15 minutes (6 pts)

○ 16-30 minutes (9 pts)   ○ 31-60 minutes (12 pts)   ○ more than an hour (15 pts)

5. For how long can you walk (with or without aid) before stopping due to knee discomfort?   **(15 points)**

○ cannot walk (0 pts)   ○ 0-5 minutes (3 pts)   ○ 6-15 minutes (6 pts)

○ 16-30 minutes (9 pts)   ○ 31-60 minutes (12 pts)   ○ more than an hour (15 pts)

Maximum points (30 points)

STANDARD ACTIVITIES (30 points)

How much does your knee bother you during each of the following activities?	no bother 5	slight 4	moderate 3	severe 2	very severe 1	cannot do (because of knee) 0	I never do this	
1. Walking on an uneven surface	○	○	○	○	○	○	○	
2. Turning or pivoting on your leg	○	○	○	○	○	○	○	
3. Climbing up or down a flight of stairs	○	○	○	○	○	○	○	
4. Getting up from a low couch or a chair without arms	○	○	○	○	○	○	○	
5. Getting into or out of a car	○	○	○	○	○	○	○	
6. Moving laterally (stepping to the side)	○	○	○	○	○	○	○	

Maximum points (30 points)

ADVANCED ACTIVITIES (25 points)

	no bother 5	slight 4	moderate 3	severe 2	very severe 1	cannot do (because of knee) 0	I never do this	
1. Climbing a ladder or step stool	○	○	○	○	○	○	○	
2. Carrying a shopping bag for a block	○	○	○	○	○	○	○	
3. Squatting	○	○	○	○	○	○	○	
4. Kneeling	○	○	○	○	○	○	○	
5. Running	○	○	○	○	○	○	○	

Maximum points (25 points)

DISCRETIONARY KNEE ACTIVITIES (15 points)

Please check 3 of the activities below that you consider *most important* to you.
(Please do not write in a additional activities)

Recreational Activities

☐ Swimming
☐ Golfing (18 holes)
☐ Road Cycling (>30mins)
☐ Gardening
☐ Bowling
☐ Racquet Sports (Tennis, Racquetball, etc.)
☐ Distance Walking
☐ Dancing / Ballet
☐ Stretching Exercises (stretching out your muscles)

Workout and Gym Activities

☐ Weight-lifting
☐ Leg Extensions
☐ Stair-Climber
☐ Stationary Biking / Spinning
☐ Leg Press
☐ Jogging
☐ Elliptical Trainer
☐ Aerobic Exercises

Please copy all 3 checked activities into the empty boxes below.

How much does your knee bother you during each of these activities?

Activity (Please write the 3 activites from list above)	no bother 5	slight 4	moderate 3	severe 2	very severe 1	cannot do (because of knee) 0	
1.	○	○	○	○	○	○	
2.	○	○	○	○	○	○	
3.	○	○	○	○	○	○	
						Maximum points (15 points)	

Maximum total points (100 points) ☐

Patellofemoral Disorders

ROBERT L. BARRACK

chapter 18

Etiology of Anterior Knee Pain in the Adult

Ronak M. Patel, MD | Robert H. Brophy, MD

Patellar pain, also known as *anterior knee pain*, *patellofemoral syndrome*, or even *chondromalacia*, refers to a number of conditions. The differential diagnosis of anterior knee pain can be divided into conditions extrinsic or intrinsic to the patellofemoral joint. Some of these conditions are readily apparent on the physical examination, whereas the diagnosis of others requires varying degrees of sophistication interpreting the history, physical examination, and imaging.

BACKGROUND

During the last 100 years, patellar instability has received greater attention from the orthopedic community than patellar pain. In 1959, Cotta counted more than 100 patellar realignment operations in the literature.[1] These were all designed to address instability (see Chapter 19). The causes of instability are indeed more obvious; they tend to be more mechanical in nature than pain-producing conditions, and consequently they give the appearance of being more amenable to a surgical solution. There are numerous structural and anatomic factors leading to mechanical instability such as ligamentous laxity and/or incompetence, muscle imbalance, patella alta, trochlear and femoral condyle dysplasia, and an increased tibial tubercle to trochlear groove distance. Surgical options to address these factors are described which include but are not limited to medial patellofemoral ligament (MPFL) repair and reconstruction, lateral release, tibial tubercle osteotomy, and trochleoplasty.

A misleading breakthrough occurred in 1928, when Aleman identified areas of softening and blistering on the patellar cartilage. He termed these "chondromalacia," from the Greek words for "cartilage" and "softening," and he understandably attributed patellar pain to these lesions.[2] However, this premise was not borne out. With the exception of deep, bone-exposing lesions, chondral lesions about the patella are not currently believed to correlate well with the presence or absence of pain. Therefore, the term "chondromalacia" in association with patellar pain is unfortunate, and its use should be discouraged, if not abandoned.[3]

"Patellar pain" is not a monolithic entity but rather a constellation of conditions subsequently discussed in this chapter. When tending to a patient, it behooves the physician to identify the condition by name rather than treat a nonspecific "patellofemoral syndrome."

ANATOMY

The extensor mechanism consists of the four quadriceps muscles (rectus femoris, vastus intermedius, vastus lateralis, and vastus medialis), the patella, the femoral trochlea, and the tibial tuberosity. But all structures from the pelvis down can indirectly be responsible for patellar pain.[4,5] The anterior knee fat pad, synovium, and capsule have some of the most sensitive afferent nerve fibers while, interestingly, patellar cartilage has nearly no pain response.[6] The lower portion of the vastus medialis is called the *vastus medialis obliquus* (VMO) and may have its own nerve supply.[7] It normally reaches at least as far down as the junction of the proximal and middle thirds of the patella, and its fibers normally lie at an angle of 50° to 65° from the long axis of the femur.[8] The lateral border of the trochlea is more prominent than its medial counterpart.

The patella features articular cartilage that is the thickest in the human body (up to 7 mm thick near the center of the patella), a testament to the stresses imposed on it. The cartilage is also peculiar in that it does not follow the contour of its bony bed. Thus, the apex of the articular cartilage can be either medial or lateral to the bony apex of the patella.[9] This anatomic quirk can be important when one assesses the congruence (fit) of the patellofemoral joint. The patellar cartilage is more permeable and more compressible than its trochlear counterpart.[10,11] This is postulated to explain the higher prevalence of chondrosis on the patella compared to the trochlea. The patellar cartilage offers many facets, the two most obvious being medial and lateral. However, approximately one-half of the time the median ridge separating these facets veers medially over the distal half of the patella.[12]

The resultant vector of the quadriceps muscles is not colinear with the patellar tendon. The two form an angle the complement of which is called the *Q angle* (see Physical Examination).

BIOMECHANICS

The patella is a complex lever that diminishes the effort required of the extensor mechanism by transmitting tensile forces of the quad tendon to the patellar tendon.[13] The patella descends 7 cm caudally by full flexion and has full patellofemoral contact at 45° of flexion. With increasing knee flexion, the patellofemoral joint reactive forces increase substantially.[14] Conversely, the absence of a patella causes the quadriceps to work harder during knee extension and during the heel-strike phase of gait.[15] The patella lies above the femoral trochlear groove ("trochlea") when the knee is fully extended, and it engages the trochlea in the first 10° to 20° of knee flexion. It is very slightly lateralized at full extension and is rapidly centered over the patella as the knee flexes.[13]

HISTORY

The clinician must inquire about the nature of the pain and its specific location; about factors that aggravate and quiet the pain; about the presence of skin sensitivity, numbness, tingling, or burning; about the presence or absence of swelling or redness; and about the factors that seem to have brought about the symptoms.[3,16,17] Pain typically occurs insidiously, but any history of an injury or prior surgery must be elicited. While difficult to sometimes elicit, overuse is a common theme in anterior knee pain. They should be asked about new activities or a recent increase in activities. Patients typically describe a vague anterior or retropatellar pain, but certain forms of patellar malalignment such as tilt and lateral displacement can cause medial or even popliteal pain.[18] Having the patient fill out a pain diagram to specifically localize the area of the pain is helpful.[19] Ask the patient what positions, movements, and activities make the pain worse, such as squatting, kneeling, sitting, stairs, running, etc. to understand the position of patellofemoral contact inciting pain.[17] A complaint of crepitus, locking, or catching may suggest a structural issue such as instability, osteochondral defect, or arthritis.

Burning, unrelenting pain should raise the suspicion of a radiculopathy or a complex regional pain syndrome–like condition. The onset of symptoms after an unusually stressful activity suggests overuse or even a stress fracture. A fall directly onto the knee may have caused a neuroma-like condition. Recurrent swelling may reflect a synovitis. The history must also inquire about other etiologies such as back, hip, or infectious etiologies of knee pain. Pain at night or rest should raise suspicion about a tumor.

PHYSICAL EXAMINATION

The physical examination begins with the patient standing. Limb alignment is evaluated as the examiner looks for signs of genu varum or valgum, or patellar squinting, whereby the patellae point inward (see "Miserable Malalignment" in this chapter and Fig. 19.1 in Chapter 19). As the patient walks, the feet are checked for pes planovalgus or cavovarus deformities. While standing, the patient's hip external rotator muscles should be evaluated.[17] As the patient does a single-legged squat, the presence of valgus collapse at the knee or internal rotation at

the hip should be observed. Weak external rotator muscles cause functional internal rotation at the hip which can lead to lateral patellar tracking and patellofemoral pain. Anterior knee pain with dynamic tests such as a deep squat or duck walk is another finding consistent with patellofemoral pathology.

One can check for joint laxity which is most commonly done using Beighton's criteria.[20] Does the patient stand with the knees in recurvatum? Can the thumb be pushed down far enough to touch the forearm? The patient is asked to sit at the edge of the table and to extend the knee. Sudden lateral to medial relocation of the patella as the knee nears extension is called the *J sign*. The knee is examined for any obvious skin discolorations or incisions, effusion, or deformity.

The Q angle assesses the patella's tendency to displace laterally when the quadriceps contract. It is subtended by two imaginary lines, one spanning the thigh from the anterior superior iliac spine to the center of the patella and a second going from the center of the patella to the tibial tuberosity. Historically, angles of less than 15° are normal, those more than 20° are abnormal, and those in the 15° to 20° range were judged on a case-by-case basis. However, the Q angle does not reliably predict diagnosis, treatment, or outcomes of the patellofemoral-related pain.[21] Its clinical utility remains in question.

The peripatellar tissues are palpated, including over the quadriceps and patellar tendons, patella, lateral and medial retinaculum, and iliotibial band (ITB). The patient is asked to tense his or her quadriceps muscles. The VMO and quadriceps muscle is examined for bulk and tone.

The patella proper is first examined by gently palpating its medial and lateral borders. An imaginary line between these two landmarks should be parallel to the floor when the limb is in neutral rotation. When one side is lower (more posterior) than its counterpart, the patella is said to be tilted.[22,23] In a patient with no history of previous surgery, tilt is always lateral—that is, the lateral side is down. Tilt is said to be reducible when the lateral border can be readily lifted out of its abnormal position. The examiner displaces the patella medially and laterally. Some patellae display abnormal amounts of play, and this can be quantified by quadrants of translation. The examiner's fingers are curled around the medial and lateral borders of the patella as the facets (and intervening soft tissues) are palpated for tenderness (**Fig. 18-1**).[23-25] Downward pressure is applied to the patella as the knee is put through a range of motion. If instability is suspected (see Chapter 19), a laterally directed force is applied to the patella as the knee extends from a flexed position. If the patient experiences pain or suddenly becomes apprehensive as the knee approaches extension, a positive apprehension sign is said to be present. The examiner can place their palm on the patella while the patient actively ranges the knee to feel for crepitus. The presence of crepitus near or at full

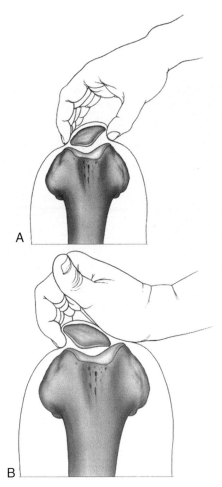

FIGURE 18-1   A and **B:** The patellar "facets" and intervening soft tissues are gently squeezed. This maneuver is normally painless.

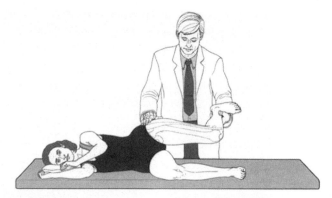

FIGURE 18-2   The Ober test assesses the tightness of the iliotibial band. With the hip extended to neutral and the knee flexed 90°, the knee should drop down to the examining table.

extension suggests a distal patellar chondral lesion, while crepitus at other flexion angles suggests a more proximal lesion.[17] The presence of a synovial plica should be considered, but this may be difficult given the lack of specific physical exam findings[26] (see Plica). There may be palpable and painful soft tissue band over the medial femoral condyle. Provocative maneuvers may elicit pain and/or a click with the knee ranged from extension to flexion. The popliteal space is examined, and if any mass is suspected, the patient is examined prone. The subject can now be placed in the lateral decubitus position, and the Ober test is performed to assess the tightness of the ITB (**Fig. 18-2**).

The remainder of the knee examination is carried out to look for nonpatellar sources of knee pain. The hip and back should be evaluated as well as potential sources of referred knee pain.

IMAGING

Plain X-Rays

Imaging confirms and refines the diagnosis suggested by the history and the physical examination; it does not supplant them. For the large majority of patients the radiographic examination begins and ends with plain x-rays.[3] A standing anteroposterior (AP) and even a standing tunnel (also known as the "schuss" view, Rosenberg view, standing flexion view) are taken to evaluate the femorotibial joint. The lateral and Merchant ("axial," "sunrise") views are most pertinent to the patella.

The lateral x-ray is taken with the knee at 30° of flexion and in such a way as to obtain near overlap of the posterior femoral condyles (**Fig. 18-3**).[27,28] Patellar height, patellar tilt, and trochlear dysplasia are thus assessed. *Patellar height* is defined as the position of the patella relative to the trochlear groove and to the tibia. A patella that is too high is called "alta," and one that is too low is called "infera" or "baja." Parameters used to calculate patellar height include the Insall-Salvati and Blackburne-Peel ratios, both of which normally equal approximately 1 (see Fig. 19.11 in Chapter 19).[29] The Insall-Salvati ratio is adversely affected by unusual shapes of the patella.[30] The Blackburne-Peel ratio has been shown to be more reliable and have less interobserver variability.[31] On the lateral radiograph the ventral aspect of the normal patella reveals two lines, the condensations of the bony median ridge and the lateral border of the patella. As the patella tilts, these lines become confluent and the patella becomes more globular in appearance (**Fig. 18-3**B).[3,27] Note that tilt varies with the degree of knee flexion, often becoming less pronounced as the knee flexes (in patients with malalignment). When seen on a lateral radiograph, the trochlea appears as a white line that normally remains parallel to the outline of the lateral femoral condyle (**Fig. 18-4**). Intersection of these two lines therefore signifies an absence of trochlear depth—that is, the bony aspect of the trochlea is flat. The trochlea is said to be dysplastic. This radiographic sign has been called the "crossing sign" and the "lateral trochlear sign."[32,33] The cartilage may actually be convex. The more distal the intersection of the lines, the more extensive the dysplasia.

The axial radiograph provides information on the medial-lateral position, tilt, and shape of the patella, and it provides a snapshot of the trochlear sulcus. Axial views obtained in the earlier degrees of flexion show the more

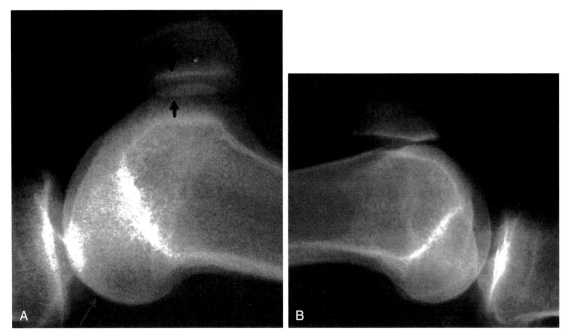

FIGURE 18-3 **A:** On an optimal lateral x-ray, the posterior condyles are superimposed. The ventral surface of the patella features two parallel lines that are clearly separate (*arrows*). These represent the bony median ridge and the lateral border of the patella. **B:** As the patella tilts laterally, the two lines become confluent.

proximal portion of the trochlea (where trochlear dysplasias begin), whereas views taken in deeper degrees of flexion reveal the more distal trochlea. Moreover, in the typical patient with patellar subluxation, lateral displacement of the patella is most apparent in the early degrees

of flexion, the patella reducing itself into the sulcus as the knee flexes. Axial views should therefore be obtained with the knee as close to extension as possible with 30° being a reasonable goal. By and large, this requires a simple leg rest placed at the end of the x-ray table as described by

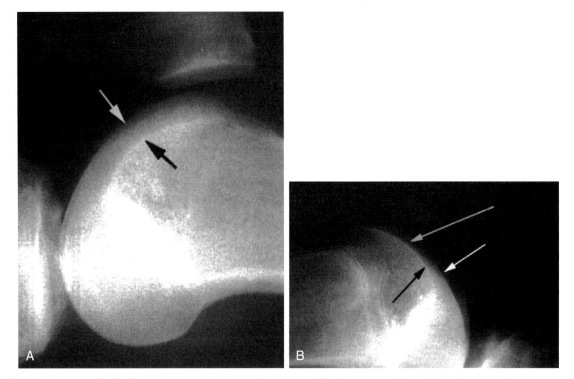

FIGURE 18-4 The crossing sign. **A:** The white lines, representing the trochlea (*black arrow*) and the subchondral bone of the lateral femoral condyle (*white arrow*), are normally parallel. The distance between the two is a measure of trochlear depth. **B:** Intersection and blending of the two lines indicate an absence of depth over the distance that they overlap. The more distal the point of intersection, the more extensive the dysplasia (*white arrow*, lateral femoral condyle; *gray arrow*, blending of the two lines—crossing sign; *black arrow*, trochlea).

Merchant et al.[34] Without such a leg rest, axial views are taken with the knee flexed 60° and are nearly useless for the purposes listed here. Note that if the knee appears in the middle of the x-ray film, one can deduce that the knee was flexed more than 45° when the x-ray was taken. If, on the contrary, the trochlea just barely appears over the bottom of the film, the knee was flexed closer to 30°. On a 30° axial view, the normal trochlear sulcus angle is approximately 140°. An angle of more than 145° signifies trochlear dysplasia.[35]

If trochlear dysplasia is present only at the proximal-most portion of the trochlea, it may not be detected on the best of axial views but may instead be appreciated on a good lateral view.

Merchant et al described a congruence angle to judge the medial-lateral position of the patella.[34] A normal angle is negative, whereas a positive value indicates lateral displacement. The congruence angle is relatively independent of leg rotation. When the axial view is obtained with the patient's leg in neutral rotation, tilt can be assessed relative to any horizontal line drawn on the film. Angles of less than 5° are normal, whereas tilt angles of more than 10° are frankly abnormal (see Fig. 19.10 in Chapter 19).[36] Many other parameters of tilt and displacement appear in the literature.[37]

Magnetic Resonance Imaging

Magnetic resonance imaging (MRI) is rarely required in the setting of patellofemoral pain and should not be a substitute for adequate x-ray films. In the preoperative patient, an MRI can help delineate chondral lesions and even differentiate between trochlear and/or patellar lesions.[38] If tumors, fractures, or osteochondritis dissecans are insufficiently delineated on x-rays, MRI can provide finer detail.

On routine MRI, the patella is centered over the femur. Lateral displacement, although not necessarily symptomatic, is abnormal.[39] As with the physical and roentgenographic examination, tilt is abnormal. The angle formed by the plane of the posterior femoral condyles and the slope of the lateral (bony) facet should be *more than* 7°.[40] Alternatively, the angle formed by the plane of the posterior femoral condyles and a line connecting the medial and lateral borders of the patella should be *less than* 10°.

Nuclear Imaging

A technetium bone scan reveals the metabolic activity of bone.[41] Studies have suggested patellofemoral pain may be related to increased bone metabolic activity.[42] While helpful to confirm metabolic activity in patients with pain, this imaging modality is not specific to elucidate the exact pathology. One can expect this activity to be increased in cases of overuse, stress fractures, tumors, infections, osteochondritis dissecans, and possibly even in

the malaligned (tilted) patella. A negative bone scan may not completely rule out an etiology but raises the possibility of psychosocial causes or malingering.

DIFFERENTIAL DIAGNOSIS

Soft Tissue

Overuse

Overuse is one of the most common sources of anterior knee pain, and except in a military or institutional setting, it rarely brings the patient to the doctor.[43,44] X-rays are unremarkable, as is the physical examination. The pain is self-limited. Treatment consists of rest, activity modification, analgesics, the application of heat and/or cold, and the gradual resumption of regular activities. A bone scan can be expected to be positive about the patella. The main condition from which it must be distinguished is a stress fracture (see Stress Fracture).

Adolescent Anterior Knee Pain

Adolescents can develop anterior knee pain for no apparent reason. There are no focal lesions, no malalignment, and no distant pathology referring pain to the knee. The pain is treated symptomatically, and assurance can be given that the condition is likely to be self-limited.

Tightness of the Iliotibial Band

It has long been appreciated that tightness of the hamstrings or quadriceps can cause anterior knee pain. Performing the Ober test will reveal that a number of patients also suffer from tightness of the ITB. Thus, a stretching program may need to include the ITB.

Tendinitis

The quadriceps and patellar tendons are prone to tendinitis especially when the quadriceps and hamstring muscles are not flexible.[45] On physical examination, tenderness is elicited over the tendon or at the inferior pole of the patella. Tendinitis is treated nonoperatively unless focal degeneration is noted on an MRI, in which case the diseased tissue may need to be excised.[46-48] Calcification can occur at the origin of the patellar tendon (Sinding-Larsen–Johansson condition), giving it a swordfish appearance that is different from that of a patella with long, nonarticulating inferior poles. Patellar tendinitis may be correlated with the position of the patella in the sagittal plane.[49,50]

Bursitis

The prepatellar and pes anserine bursas are the most commonly affected bursae in the knee. Bursitis is typically caused by trauma, infections, or most commonly repetitive use. Prepatellar bursitis is commonly seen in individuals who kneel often, including plumbers, carpenters, gardeners, housekeepers, and wrestlers.[51] Pes anserine bursitis is more common in athletes, especially middle- to older-aged females who run.[52] The diagnosis is typically made clinically based on history and careful examination. Treatment should initially focus on conservative measures. Steroid injections into the pes bursa may serve as a diagnostic and therapeutic purpose prior to pursuing bursectomy for refractory cases. Studies evaluating the role of injection for pes bursitis are limited and often confounded with knee osteoarthritis.

Plica Syndrome

Plicae are embryologic tissue remnants of synovium that are most commonly located mediopatellar, infrapatellar, and suprapatellar. They are thought to become symptomatic with overuse as they become thickened and this is referred to as plica syndrome. A suprapatellar plica may become thickened and contracted to potentially alter patellar tracking. Pain can be differentiated from a meniscal tear as tenderness is typically suprapatellar or above the joint line on the condyle. Hamstring tightness is also associated, and the hamstring-popliteal angle should be examined. Appropriate therapy should focus on isometric quad strengthening and hamstring stretching. Conservative treatments include rest, anti-inflammatories, physical therapy, and steroid injections[53] and tend to be successful in younger patients with shorter duration of symptoms, whereas surgical treatment may be needed for older patients with longer duration of symptoms and blunt or twisting type of trauma.[54] Arthroscopic resection of the plica is the mainstay of surgical treatment and tends to have a favorable outcome in those with an accurate diagnosis.[55,56] Resection of the plica is preferred over division to prevent scar reformation and recurrent symptoms. Excision can be accomplished with the use of a shaver, electrocautery, and/or scissors.

Hoffa Disease

Fat pad impingement syndrome, or Hoffa disease, is a less common etiology of anterior knee pain. The anterior suprapatellar, posterior suprapatellar, and infrapatellar fat pads are the most commonly symptomatic. The fat pad, capsule, and synovium are highly innervated and implicated as sources of intra-articular pain.[6] Diagnosis can be a challenge considering other more common causes of pain, but typically MRI can be helpful.[57] Conservative management takes precedence when this diagnosis is suspected and a diagnostic/therapeutic localized injection can help. In rare cases, arthroscopic fat pad excision may be considered.

Bone, Joint, and Cartilage

Bipartite Patella

A linear lucency can appear on the AP radiograph of a patella. The lucency is differentiated from a fracture by its smooth borders and by its commonly bilateral nature. It is classically present at the superolateral aspect of the patella but can run vertically from pole to pole. The

Saupe classification remains the most commonly used. The bipartite patella is usually an asymptomatic condition, but trauma can lead to pain, presumably because of motion between the fragments. Internal fixation can be required, and if malalignment is present, a lateral retinacular release can be contemplated.[5,58-60]

Stress Fracture

Relatively few cases of stress fracture of the patella have been reported. The fracture is usually transverse but can be longitudinal. It remains open to discussion whether these heal readily or not. Plain x-rays can remain normal for an extended period of time, an MRI or bone scan being required to make the diagnosis. The limited literature suggests that recognition and immobilization of the condition within a few weeks of onset lead to an uneventful healing, whereas delays in recognition increase the need for operative intervention.[61,62]

Osteochondritis Dissecans

More commonly found in the tibiofemoral compartments, osteochondritis dissecans can also be found in the patella and the trochlea, where the prognosis is less favorable. Other than being potentially separated from the surrounding cartilage, the articular cartilage has a normal appearance.[63-65]

Dorsal Defect

A dorsal defect is a benign osteochondral lesion featuring classically a "hole in the bone" appearance on the AP radiograph that must be differentiated from a Brodie abscess. It is readily differentiated from osteochondritis dissecans by the fibrillations of the articular cartilage.[66]

"Miserable Malalignment"

"Miserable malalignment" is the colloquial name given to complex torsional variations in limb alignment from the hip down to the ankle. When the patient is examined standing, the patella can point inward ("squinting") or outward ("grasshopper patella") (see Fig. 19.1 in Chapter 19). The hip is usually excessively anteverted, distal femoral torsion can be internal or external, external torsion of the upper tibia is a common finding (with a concomitant increase in the Q angle because of the lateralized tibial tuberosity), the tibia displays varus bowing, and external tibial torsion can be present at the ankle.[4] Such limb morphology can be associated with anterior knee pain. Clearly, the patella is an innocent bystander in this complex malalignment. Imaging will often reveal a horizontal patella overlying a rotated distal femur. Fortunately, pain can often be controlled with activity modification, stretching, and strengthening exercises. For the patient requiring surgery, so-called small procedures such as a lateral retinacular release are not usually successful. On the other hand, the requisite derotational procedures are substantial, but results have been favorable.[67,68]

Patella Malalignment

Outside of overuse and simple tendinitis, patella malalignment is arguably the greatest source of persistent knee pain in patients between the ages of 20 and 50.[3,17] Ironically, its very existence as a clinical entity remains a subject of dispute. Patella malalignment is a translational or rotational deviation of the patella relative to any axis. This theoretically includes patella alta and infers as well as abnormal Q angles. In practice, however, the term refers to patellar tilt, a condition where one side of the patella lies posterior to the other. In the nonoperated patient the lateral side is always the posterior one, and this is called "lateral tilt." Ficat in France and Merchant in the United States introduced this concept in the 1970s.

Patellar malalignment appears to be related to a number of factors that appear in varying degrees. These include constitutional laxity, paradoxical tightness of the ITB and of the lateral retinaculum, abnormal positioning and firing of the VMO, anatomic variations of the trochlea, patella alta, and a lateralized tibial tuberosity (elevated Q angle). The pain is presumed to result from excessive pressure on the subchondral bone of the overloaded lateral side of the patella. However, tilt itself does not completely account for the onset of pain, as evidenced by the observation that not every patient with malalignment is symptomatic. Pain appears to be related to multiple parameters with variable clinical expression, and many of these parameters have yet to be identified.

Blunt trauma to the front of the knee and overuse are two of the many potential triggering mechanisms. Nerve abnormalities have been noted in the lateral retinaculum, but it is not clear whether these are always present. As with tightness of the lateral retinaculum, it is also unclear whether the nerve abnormalities are the cause or the result of the condition.

The key features on the physical examination are a tilted patella that cannot readily be righted and tenderness about the lateral facet when the examiner's fingers are curled under the patella (**Fig. 18-1**).[22,25] This maneuver also compresses the soft tissues between the skin and the patella, and part of the pain may emanate from these tissues. The VMO is commonly barely visible or palpable. Its insertion onto the medial retinaculum is too proximal, its fibers are more vertical than normal, and the timing of its contractions are not well synchronized with the surrounding muscle groups.[5] The last two factors cannot be appreciated on routine examination.

During radiographic examination, tilt can often be appreciated on the Merchant view, especially if the x-rays are obtained with the leg in neutral rotation and the lower border of the cassette is maintained parallel to the floor. With the knee flexed 30°, tilt should be no greater than 10° relative to the horizontal.[36]

The large majority of patients with patella malalignment can be effectively treated with a nonoperative approach. This includes a traditional program of

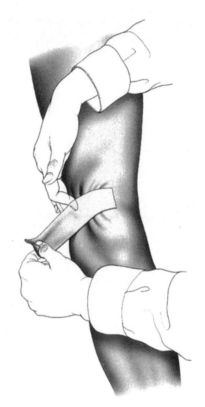

FIGURE 18-5 Patellar taping is an accepted, although controversial, part of physical therapy.

hamstring and quadriceps stretches, VMO strengthening, antiinflammatory medications, bracing, and activity modification. Newer concepts include taping (**Fig. 18-5**), ITB stretching, orthotics for select patients, and muscle coordination.[69]

For the rare patient requiring surgery, a balance must be struck between the obligation to address all the pathoanatomy and the need to perform the smallest possible procedure. The surgeon's goal is to create a centered, untilted, normally tracking patella without increasing the stresses on any chondral lesion.

Procedures to choose from include the isolated lateral retinacular release,[70] the medial plication,[71] the VMO advancement (these are called *proximal realignment procedures*),[72] tibial tuberosity transfers (*distal realignment procedures*),[73] patellofemoral replacements (**Fig. 18-6**),[74-76] patellectomy,[77] cartilage grafting,[78] and trochleoplasties.[79] The indications for these procedures remain controversial, and the reader is referred to dedicated publications on the subject.[3,17]

In performing a *lateral retinacular release*, the surgeon divides the lateral retinaculum beginning at approximately the superior pole of the patella. The procedure can be carried to the joint line or to the tibial tuberosity; it can be performed arthroscopically or via an open procedure; it can be performed in an outward direction from inside the knee or inward beginning in the subcutaneous tissues; and it can performed by way of a sharp instrument,

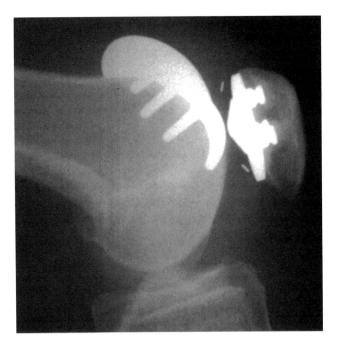

FIGURE 18-6   Lateral view of a patellofemoral replacement.

cautery, or a laser. The relative ease of the procedure led to great initial enthusiasm since then tempered by hematomas and inconsistent results.[70,80,81]

Medial plication and *advancement of the VMO* address the deficiencies of the medial soft tissues. The former can be carried out by way of an initial arthrotomy and subsequent pants-over-the-vest suturing or by arthroscopic plication. The combination of the lateral release and the medial arthrotomy provides a measure of denervation that may contribute to pain relief.[82]

Tibial Tuberosity Transfers

The *Elmslie–Trillat procedure* (called "Roux" in parts of Europe) transfers the tuberosity medially without any anterior or posterior displacement (see Fig. 19.27 in Chapter 19). It effectively diminishes the Q angle. The operation can lead to recurvatum in subjects whose tibial apophysis has not fused, can induce a "Charlie Chaplin" gait in patients who are very loose-jointed and who tend to walk with their legs in external rotation, and is of limited value when a subject's trochlea is very dysplastic. The Maquet operation anteriorizes the tibial tuberosity with the intent of decreasing patellofemoral stresses.[83,84] The diminution of stresses is more pronounced over the distal patella relative to the proximal patella, and the clinical benefits remain subject to debate.[85] An 8- to 10-cm incision minimized skin complications. It is an operation of decreasing popularity. The anteromedialization (*AMZ*, *Fulkerson*) operation combines the Elmslie–Trillat and the Maquet by slanting the cut of the tibial tuberosity, thus providing an element of medialization and of anteriorization.[3,86] It would appear to be most effective in the presence of distolateral patellar lesions and least efficacious when arthritic lesions are present throughout the patella

or involve the trochlea. The tibial tuberosity can also be transferred distally in cases of patella alta.[87] However, care must be taken also not to transfer the patella medially and posteriorly, in which case the surgeon would be performing a Hauser procedure. Although the Hauser operation was popular for many decades as a treatment for the unstable patella, the overtightening induced by the three-plane transfer led to long-term arthritis.[88]

Patellectomy

A favorite in times when the patella was thought to be a useless appendage, a *patellectomy* is truly an operation of last resort.[77] It represents a resection arthroplasty of an important joint. Uncomplicated patellar pain is no longer an indication for this procedure, but the presence of a severely comminuted patella or incurable osteomyelitis is. To minimize weakness of the extensor mechanism, some form of plication is required of the extensor mechanism about the knee.

Tumors

The patella is not a common site for tumors, but a number of benign and malignant neoplasms have been reported.[89,90]

Infection

Osteomyelitis in adults is relatively uncommon, and this is particularly true of the patella. If other signs and symptoms of infection are present, however, or if the host is particularly immunocompromised, the diagnosis should be considered. A patellectomy is an option in severe or intractable cases.

Rheumatologic Conditions

Rheumatologic conditions can cause pain and arthritis solely about the patellofemoral joint early in their course.

Nerve

Neuroma

Patients with tender areas over the retinaculum have histologic evidence of neuromatous degeneration.[91] Prior surgery or blunt trauma can also lead to sensitive areas of the anterior knee. Gentle scratching of the skin with a thumbnail or squeezing of the skin is painful. Neuroma-like conditions will not appear on any imaging study, but an MRI can help distinguish this from a bone bruise. Relief is obtained with subcutaneous injection of an anesthetic. Refractory cases can be treated with neuroma excision once the diagnosis is confirmed.[92]

Complex Regional Pain Syndrome

Complex regional pain syndrome (the current term for *reflex sympathetic dystrophy*) leads to persistent pain in the absence of obvious pathology or to pain out of proportion to existing pathology. It is caused by abnormal activity of the sympathetic fibers. It is beyond the control of the patient ("reflex") and in its worst form leads to atrophy and dysfunction ("dystrophy") about the knee. Radiographs may show patchy osteoporosis, and in its active stage, a nuclear scan is positive. The diagnosis is made after meeting four clinical criteria based upon well-established guidelines.[93] These include (1) pain disproportionate to an inciting event, (2) at least one symptom in last three categories including sensory, vasomotor, sudomotor/edema, and motor/trophic, (3) at least one sign (exam finding) in at least two of the categories above, and (4) no other diagnosis that fits the patient's signs and symptoms. Sensory symptoms include hyperesthesia or allodynia and signs such as hyperalgesia and allodynia to pinprick and light touch. Vasomotor symptoms include temperature changes and/or skin color and signs such as measurable temperature differences and skin color asymmetry. Sudomotor/edema signs and symptoms include edema and abnormal or asymmetric sweating patterns. Motor/trophic signs and symptoms include decreased motion, motor weakness, or trophic changes in hair, nails, and skin. Sympathetic blocks can be diagnostic and therapeutic.

Lateral Retinacular Neuroma and Fibrosis

Examination of the lateral retinaculum has revealed neural injury and fibrosis in patients with malalignment.[94,95] Whether this is the cause or the result of the malalignment has not been determined. A number of soft tissues about the knee including the lateral retinaculum may feature an overabundance of substance P.[96,97]

Venous Congestion

Some investigators have noted increased pressure within the patella of patients with anterior knee pain, and drilling of the patella has been reported to be successful.[98] The authors describe a minimally invasive technique to measuring intrapatellar pressure. An intraosseous pressure greater than 25 mmHg in the patella is considered abnormal.[99,100] Patients were indicated for surgery if raising the pressure with a 1 to 2 mL saline solution reproduced anterior knee pain. Of those treated with extra-articular drilling and decompression, 90% had prolonged relief at more than 3 years postoperatively.[101] Studies reporting on this approach have not commented on malalignment, and it is possible that venous congestion and tilt coexist. Moreover, drill holes and arthrotomies may have similar effects on venous congestion.

Other

Referred Pain (Hip, Spine)

Hip and spine pathology can refer pain to the knee in the absence of pain about the hip or spine. Careful examination of the spine and hip should be performed and imaging obtained when appropriate. When the diagnosis is unclear, a fluoroscopically guided injection in the hip joint or spine (epidural, nerve root, facet) can be diagnostic and/or therapeutic. Patients should be asked to keep a pain diary describing the timing and extent of any symptom relief.

CONCLUSION

Anterior knee pain has multiple etiologies. Rather than attribute this pain to the nonspecific and confusing "chondromalacia" the clinician must identify which of the above conditions is responsible for the pain and treat the patient accordingly.

REFERENCES

1. Cotta H. Zur Therapie der habituellen Patellarluxation. *Arch Orthop Unfall-Chir.* 1959;51:265-271.
2. Aleman O. Chondromalacia posttraumatica patellae. *Acta Chir Scand.* 1928;63:149-190.
3. Grelsamer RP. Patellar malalignment. *J Bone Joint Surg Am.* 2000;82-A:1639-1650.
4. Turner MS. The association between tibial torsion and knee joint pathology. *Clin Orthop Relat Res.* 1994;302:47-51.
5. Grelsamer RP, McConnell J. *The Patella: A Team Approach.* Gaithersburg, Maryland: Aspen Publishers; 1998.
6. Dye SF, Vaupel GL, Dye CC. Conscious neurosensory mapping of the internal structures of the human knee without intraarticular anesthesia. *Am J Sports Med.* 1998;26:773-777.
7. Günal I, Araç S, Sahinoğlu K, Birvar K. The innervation of vastus medialis obliquus. *J Bone Joint Surg Br.* 1992;74:624.
8. Raimondo RA, Ahmad CS, Blankevoort L, April EW, Grelsamer RP, Henry JH. Patellar stabilization: a quantitative evaluation of the vastus medialis obliquus muscle. *Orthopedics.* 1998;21:791-795.
9. Stäubli HU, Dürrenmatt U, Porcellini B, Rauschning W. Anatomy and surface geometry of the patellofemoral joint in the axial plane. *J Bone Joint Surg Br.* 1999;81:452-458.
10. Froimson MI, Ratcliffe A, Gardner TR, Mow VC. Differences in patellofemoral joint cartilage material properties and their significance to the etiology of cartilage surface fibrillation. *Osteoarthr Cartil.* 1997;5:377-386.
11. Herberhold C, Faber S, Stammberger T, et al. In situ measurement of articular cartilage deformation in intact femoropatellar joints under static loading. *J Biomech.* 1999;32:1287-1295.
12. Kwak SD, Colman WW, Ateshian GA, Grelsamer RP, Henry JH, Mow VC. Anatomy of the human patellofemoral joint articular cartilage: surface curvature analysis. *J Orthop Res.* 1997;15:468-472.
13. Grelsamer RP, Weinstein CH. Applied biomechanics of the patella. *Clin Orthop Relat Res.* 2001;389:9-14.
14. Hungerford DS, Barry M. Biomechanics of the patellofemoral joint. *Clin Orthop Relat Res.* 1979;144:9-15.
15. Sutton FS, Thompson CH, Lipke J, Kettelkamp DB. The effect of patellectomy on knee function. *J Bone Joint Surg Am.* 1976;58:537-540.
16. Post WR. Clinical evaluation of patients with patellofemoral disorders. *Arthroscopy.* 1999;15:841-851.
17. Fulkerson JP. Diagnosis and treatment of patients with patellofemoral pain. *Am J Sports Med.* 2002;30:447-456.
18. Karlson S. Chondromalacia patellae. *Acta Orthop Scand.* 1940;83:347.
19. Post WR, Fulkerson J. Knee pain diagrams: correlation with physical examination findings in patients with anterior knee pain. *Arthroscopy.* 1994;10:618-623.

20. Beighton P, Horan F. Orthopaedic aspects of the Ehlers-Danlos syndrome. *J Bone Joint Surg Br.* 1969;51:444-453.
21. Post WR. Current concepts clinical evaluation of patients with patellofemoral disorders. *Arthrosc J Arthrosc Relat Surg.* 1999;15:841-851.
22. Kolowich PA, Paulos LE, Rosenberg TD, Farnsworth S. Lateral release of the patella: indications and contraindications. *Am J Sports Med.* 1990;18:359-365.
23. Atkin DM, Fithian DC, Marangi KS, Stone ML, Dobson BE, Mendelsohn C. Characteristics of patients with primary acute lateral patellar dislocation and their recovery within the first 6 months of injury. *Am J Sports Med.* 2000;28:472-479.
24. Insall J, Falvo KA, Wise DW. Chondromalacia Patellae. A prospective study. *J Bone Joint Surg Am.* 1976;58:1-8.
25. Dehaven KE, Dolan WA, Mayer PJ. Chondromalacia patellae in athletes. *Am J Sports Med.* 1979;7:5-11.
26. Schindler OS. 'The Sneaky Plica' revisited: morphology, pathophysiology and treatment of synovial plicae of the knee. *Knee Surg Sport Traumatol Arthrosc.* 2014;22:247-262.
27. Malghem J, Maldague B. Patellofemoral joint: 30 degrees axial radiograph with lateral rotation of the leg. *Radiology.* 1989;170:566-567.
28. Malghem J, Maldague B. Depth insufficiency of the proximal trochlear groove on lateral radiographs of the knee: relation to patellar dislocation. *Radiology.* 1989;170:507-510.
29. Grelsamer RP, Meadows S. The modified Insall-Salvati ratio for assessment of patellar height. *Clin Orthop Relat Res.* 1992;282:170-176.
30. Grelsamer RP, Proctor CS, Bazos AN. Evaluation of patellar shape in the sagittal plane. *Am J Sports Med.* 1994;22:61-66.
31. Seil R, Müller B, Georg T, Kohn D, Rupp S. Reliability and interobserver variability in radiological patellar height ratios. *Knee Surg Sport Traumatol Arthrosc.* 2000;8:231-236.
32. Dejour H, Walch G, Neyret P, Adeleine P. Dysplasia of the femoral trochlea. *Rev Chir Orthop Reparatrice Appar Mot.* 1990;76:45-54.
33. Grelsamer RP, Tedder JL. The lateral trochlear sign. Femoral trochlear dysplasia as seen on a lateral view roentgenograph. *Clin Orthop Relat Res.* 1992;281:159-162.
34. Merchant AC, Mercer RL, Jacobsen RH, Cool RC. Roentgenographic analysis of patellofemoral congruence. *J Bone Joint Surg.* 1974;56:1391-1396.
35. Dejour H, Walch G, Nove-Josserand L, Guier C. Factors of patellar instability: an anatomic radiographic study. *Knee Surg Sport Traumatol Arthrosc.* 1994;2:19-26.
36. Grelsamer RP, Bazos AN, Proctor CS. Radiographic analysis of patellar tilt. *J Bone Joint Surg Br.* 1993;75:822-824.
37. McNally EG. Imaging assessment of anterior knee pain and patellar maltracking. *Skeletal Radiol.* 2001;30:484-495.
38. Harris JD, Brophy RH, Jia G, et al. Sensitivity of magnetic resonance imaging for detection of patellofemoral articular cartilage defects. *Arthroscopy.* 2012;28:1728-1737.
39. Grelsamer RP, Newton PM, Staron RB. The medial-lateral position of the patella on routine magnetic resonance imaging: when is normal not normal? *Arthroscopy.* 1998;14:23-28.
40. Schutzer SF, Ramsby GR, Fulkerson JP. The evaluation of patellofemoral pain using computerized tomography. A preliminary study. *Clin Orthop Relat Res.* 1986;204:286-293.
41. Dye SF, Chew MH. The use of scintigraphy to detect increased osseous metabolic activity about the knee. *Instr Course Lect.* 1994;43:453-469.
42. Draper CE, Fredericson M, Gold GE, et al. Patients with patellofemoral pain exhibit elevated bone metabolic activity at the patellofemoral joint. *J Orthop Res.* 2012;30:209-213.
43. Thomeé R, Renström P, Karlsson J, Grimby G. Patellofemoral pain syndrome in young women. I. A clinical analysis of alignment, pain parameters, common symptoms and functional activity level. *Scand J Med Sci Sports.* 1995;5:237-244.
44. Fairbank JC, Pynsent PB, van Poortvliet JA, Phillips H. Mechanical factors in the incidence of knee pain in adolescents and young adults. *J Bone Joint Surg Br.* 1984;66:685-693.
45. Witvrouw E, Bellemans J, Lysens R, Danneels L, Cambier D. Intrinsic risk factors for the development of patellar tendinitis in an athletic population. *Am J Sports Med.* 2001;29:190-195.
46. Popp JE, Yu JS, Kaeding CC. Recalcitrant patellar tendinitis. *Am J Sports Med.* 1997;25:218-222.
47. Griffiths GP, Selesnick FH. Operative treatment and arthroscopic findings in chronic patellar tendinitis. *Arthroscopy.* 1998;14:836-839.
48. Shalaby M, Almekinders LC. Patellar tendinitis: the significance of magnetic resonance imaging findings. *Am J Sports Med.* 1999;27:345-349.
49. Schmid MR, Hodler J, Cathrein P, Duewell S, Jacob HA, Romero J. Is impingement the cause of Jumper's knee? Dynamic and static magnetic resonance imaging of patellar tendinitis in an open-configuration system. *Am J Sports Med.* 2002;30:388-395.
50. Tyler TF, Hershman EB, Nicholas SJ, Berg JH, McHugh MP. Evidence of abnormal anteroposterior patellar tilt in patients with patellar tendinitis with use of a new radiographic measurement. *Am J Sports Med.* 2002;30:396-401.
51. Hong E, Kraft MC. Evaluating anterior knee pain. *Med. Clin. North Am.* 2014;98:697-717.
52. Alvarez-Nemegyei J, Canoso JJ. Evidence-based soft tissue rheumatology IV. *J Clin Rheumatol.* 2004;10:205-206.
53. Amatuzzi MM, Fazzi A, Varella MH. Pathologic synovial plica of the knee. Results of conservative treatment. *Am J Sports Med.* 1990;18:466-469.
54. Hardaker WT, Whipple TL, Bassett FH. Diagnosis and treatment of the plica syndrome of the knee. *J Bone Joint Surg Am.* 1980;62:221-225.
55. Dorchak JD, Barrack RL, Kneisl JS, Alexander AH. Arthroscopic treatment of symptomatic synovial plica of the knee. *Am J Sports Med.* 1991;19:503-507.
56. Gerrard AD, Charalambous CP. Arthroscopic excision of medial knee plica: a meta-analysis of outcomes. *Knee Surg Relat Res.* 2018;30:356-363.
57. Jacobson JA, Lenchik L, Ruhoy MK, Schweitzer ME, Resnick D. MR imaging of the infrapatellar fat pad of Hoffa. *Radiographics.* 1997;17:675-691.
58. Ogata K. Painful bipartite patella. A new approach to operative treatment. *J Bone Joint Surg Am.* 1994;76:573-578.
59. Fulkerson J. *Disorders of the Patellofemoral Joint.* Baltimore, Maryland: Williams & Wilkins; 1996.
60. Adachi N, Ochi M, Yamaguchi H, Uchio Y, Kuriwaka M. Vastus lateralis release for painful bipartite patella. *Arthroscopy.* 2002;18:404-411.
61. Brogle PJ, Eswar S, Denton JR. Propagation of a patellar stress fracture in a basketball player. *Am J Orthop.* 1997;26:782-784.
62. Orava S, Taimela S, Kvist M, Karpakka J, Hulkko A, Kujala U. Diagnosis and treatment of stress fracture of the patella in athletes. *Knee Surg Sports Traumatol Arthrosc.* 1996;4:206-211.
63. Smith JB. Osteochondritis dissecans of the trochlea of the femur. *Arthroscopy.* 1990;6:11-17.
64. Bruns J, Luessenhop S, Lehmann L. Etiological aspects in osteochondritis dissecans patellae. *Knee Surg Sport Traumatol Arthrosc.* 1999;7:356-359.
65. Peters TA, McLean ID. Osteochondritis dissecans of the patellofemoral joint. *Am J Sports Med.* 2000;28:63-67.
66. Smith JS, McLean ID. Letter to the Editor. *Am J Sports Med.* 2001;29:112-113.
67. Delgado ED, Schoenecker PL, Rich MM, Capelli AM. Treatment of severe torsional malalignment syndrome. *J Pediatr Orthop.* 1996;16:484-488.
68. Bruce WD, Stevens PM. Surgical correction of miserable malalignment syndrome. *J Pediatr Orthop.* 2004;24:392-396.

69. Crossley K, Bennell K, Green S, McConnell J. A systematic review of physical interventions for patellofemoral pain syndrome. *Clin J Sport Med.* 2001;11:103-110.

70. O'Neill DB. Open lateral retinacular lengthening compared with arthroscopic release. A prospective, randomized outcome study. *J Bone Joint Surg Am.* 1997;79:1759-1769.

71. Hughston JC, Walsh WM. Proximal and distal reconstruction of the extensor mechanism for patellar subluxation. *Clin Orthop Relat Res.* 1979;144:36-42.

72. Madigan R, Wissinger HA, Donaldson WF. Preliminary experience with a method of quadricepsplasty in recurrent subluxation of the patella. *J Bone Joint Surg Am.* 1975;57:600-607.

73. Cox JS. Evaluation of the Roux-Elmslie-Trillat procedure for knee extensor realignment. *Am J Sports Med.* 1982;10:303-310.

74. Cartier P, Sanouiller JL, Grelsamer R. Patellofemoral arthroplasty. 2-12-year follow-up study. *J Arthroplasty.* 1990;5:49-55.

75. Argenson JN, Guillaume JM, Aubaniac JM. Is there a place for patellofemoral arthroplasty? *Clin Orthop Relat Res.* 1995;321:162-167.

76. Arnbjörnsson AH, Ryd L. The use of isolated patellar prostheses in Sweden 1977-1986. *Int Orthop.* 1998;22:141-144.

77. Ziran BH, Goodfellow DB, Deluca LS, Heiple KG. Knee function after patellectomy and cruciform repair of the extensor mechanism. *Clin Orthop Relat Res.* 1994;302:138-146.

78. O'Driscoll SW. The healing and regeneration of articular cartilage. *J Bone Joint Surg Am.* 1998;80:1795-1812.

79. Masse Y. Trochleoplasty. Restoration of the intercondylar groove in subluxations and dislocations of the patella. *Rev Chir Orthop Reparatrice Appar Mot.* 1978;64:3-17.

80. Flandry F, Hughston JC. Complications of extensor mechanism surgery for patellar malalignment. *Am J Orthop.* 1995;24:534-543.

81. Schneider T, Fink B, Abel R, Jerosch J, Schulitz KP. Hemarthrosis as a major complication after arthroscopic subcutaneous lateral retinacular release: a prospective study. *Am J Knee Surg.* 1998;11:95-100.

82. Dellon AL, Mont MA, Mullick T, Hungerford DS. Partial denervation for persistent neuroma pain around the knee. *Clin Orthop Relat Res.* 1996;329:216-222.

83. Maquet P. Advancement of the tibial tuberosity. *Clin Orthop Relat Res.* 1976;115:225-230.

84. Ferguson AB. Elevation of the insertion of the patellar ligament for patellofemoral pain. *J Bone Joint Surg Am.* 1982;64:766-771.

85. Ferrandez L, Usabiaga J, Yubero J, Sagarra J, de No L. An experimental study of the redistribution of patellofemoral pressures by the anterior displacement of the anterior tuberosity of the tibia. *Clin Orthop Relat Res.* 1989;238:183-189.

86. Fulkerson JP, Becker GJ, Meaney JA, Miranda M, Folcik MA. Anteromedial tibial tubercle transfer without bone graft. *Am J Sports Med.* 1990;18:490-497.

87. AL-Sayyad MJ, Cameron JC. Functional outcome after tibial tubercle transfer for the painful patella alta. *Clin Orthop Relat Res.* 2002;396:152-162.

88. Crosby EB, Insall J. Recurrent dislocation of the patella. Relation of treatment to osteoarthritis. *J Bone Joint Surg Am.* 1976;58:9-13.

89. Ferguson PC, Griffin AM, Bell RS. Primary patellar tumors. *Clin Orthop Relat Res.* 1997;336:199-204.

90. Chaudhary D, Bhatia N, Ahmed A, et al. Unicameral bone cyst of the patella. *Orthopedics.* 2000;23:1285-1286.

91. Fulkerson JP, Tennant R, Jaivin JS, Grunnet M. Histologic evidence of retinacular nerve injury associated with patellofemoral malalignment. *Clin Orthop Relat Res.* 1985;197:196-205.

92. Kasim N, Fulkerson JP. Resection of clinically localized segments of painful retinaculum in the treatment of selected patients with anterior knee pain. *Am J Sports Med.* 2000;28:811-814.

93. Harden RN, Oaklander AL, Burton AW et al. Complex regional pain syndrome: practical diagnostic and treatment guidelines, 4th edition. *Pain Med.* 2013;14:180-229 .

94. Fulkerson JP, Gossling HR. Anatomy of the knee joint lateral retinaculum. *Clin Orthop Relat Res.* 1980;153:183-188.

95. Sanchis-Alfonso V, Rosello-Sastre E, Martinez-Sanjuan V. Pathogenesis of anterior knee pain syndrome and functional patellofemoral instability in the active young. *Am J Knee Surg.* 1999;12:29-40.

96. Wojtys EM, Beaman DN, Glover RA, Janda D. Innervation of the human knee joint by substance-P fibers. *Arthroscopy.* 1990;6:254-263.

97. Witoński D, Wągrowska-Danielewicz M. Distribution of substance-P nerve fibers in the knee joint in patients with anterior knee pain syndrome. *Knee Surg Sport Traumatol Arthrosc.* 1999;7:177-183.

98. Schneider U, Breusch SJ, Thomsen M, Wenz W, Graf J, Niethard FU. A new concept in the treatment of anterior knee pain: patellar hypertension syndrome. *Orthopedics.* 2000;23:581-586.

99. Schneider U, Graf J, Thomsen M, Wenz W, Niethard F. Das Hypertensionssyndrom der Patella - Nomenklatur, Diagnostik und Therapie. *Z Orthop Ihre Grenzgeb.* 2008;135:70-75.

100. Graf J, Christophers R, Schneider U, Niethard F. Chondromalacia patellae und intraossärer Druck. *Z Orthop Ihre Grenzgeb.* 2008;130:495-500.

101. Miltner O, Siebert CH, Schneider U, Niethard FU, Graf J. Patellar hypertension syndrome in adolescence: a three-year follow up. *Arch Orthop Trauma Surg.* 2003;123:455-459.

chapter 19

Patellar Instability

Paul M. Inclan, MD | Matthew J. Matava, MD

INTRODUCTION

In the ambulatory setting, up to one-fourth of all ortho-pedic office visits pertain to pathology involving the patellofemoral joint.[1] Though the differential diag-nosis for such pathology is broad, the vast majority of patellofemoral complaints can be subclassified into three general conditions: patellofemoral pain syndrome, patellofemoral arthritis, and patellofemoral instability, although some overlap may occur. For example, patients with patellofemoral instability often have associated acute articular cartilage defects, which may progress to focal or diffuse osteoarthritis over time. All three conditions result from a complex interplay of pathologic processes related to patellar maltracking, increased patellofemoral joint loading, and altered somatosensory processes.[2]

Patellofemoral pain syndrome is one of the most com-mon causes of knee pain in the United States with a prev-alence cited between 15% and 45% in young adults.[3,4] Often insidious in onset, and associated with overuse, this condition typically results in diffuse anterior knee pain most commonly in young, active individuals—especially females. This condition is not due to structural damage to the patellofemoral articulation but rather to func-tional muscle weakness of the core and lower extrem-ity. Therefore, patellofemoral pain syndrome is usually amenable to nonoperative management including phys-ical therapy with an emphasis on "closed-chain" quad-riceps and core muscle strengthening,[5,6] nonsteroidal anti-inflammatory drugs (NSAIDs),[7] and activity modifi-cation with avoidance of prolonged bent-knee activities and "open-chain" knee extension.

At the other end of the spectrum is *patellofemoral arthritis*. This condition results in focal or diffuse degener-ation of the patellar and/or trochlear articular surface(s), typically in middle-aged and older adults.[8] This condition is manifested as peripatellar pain exacerbated by activities that increase loading of the patellofemoral joint such as climbing stairs, rising from a seated position, or kneeling. Though nonoperative management remains the main-stay of treatment for isolated patellofemoral arthritis, a variety of operative procedures to realign, reconstruct, or replace the articulating surfaces are available based on patient age and activity, severity of arthritis, and associ-ated anatomical factors.

Both patellofemoral pain syndrome and patellofemo-ral arthritis exhibit pathomechanics and clinical features that overlap with the third, distinct clinical entity of *patellofemoral instability*. This condition is defined as either a single or recurrent episode(s) of patellar sublux-ation (partial pathological movement of the patella out of the trochlear groove with retention of some articular contact) or dislocation (complete movement of the patella out of the trochlear groove without retention of articular contact).[9] The vast majority of cases involve lateral patel-lar instability, with medial instability most commonly due to iatrogenic causes following surgical procedures intended to address lateral instability such as an exces-sive lateral retinacular release, detachment of the vastus lateralis, and/or an overly tightened medial patellofemo-ral ligament (MPFL) repair/reconstruction.[10] True medial patellar instability is extremely rare without a known inci-dence. Underlying hyperlaxity, trochlear dysplasia, and a deficient vastus lateralis musculature may play a role in patients medial instability with or without prior surgery.

With an annual incidence of 23.2 per 100,000 person-years,[11] a first-time patellar dislocation is a frequently encountered orthopedic complaint. Moreover, the ado-lescent population may experience an annual incidence nearly seven times that of the general population,[11] typi-cally while engaging in athletic activites.[12] Unfortunately, affected individuals have an approximately 25% risk of recurrent instability up to 5 years following the initial event.[13] This risk is higher in younger patients, females, and individuals with underlying anatomic predisposition such as patella alta, patellar and/or trochlear dysplasia, genu valgum, and lateral patellar maltracking[13] (discussed below). In addition to the risk of recurrent instability, almost half of all affected individuals will eventually develop patellofemoral arthritis,[14] likely secondary to either the initial traumatic insult or from repetitive patellar dislocation/relocation episodes. Therefore, patellar insta-bility affects young, active individuals, many of whom will experience some form of continued patellofemoral symptoms during their lifetime, either because of recur-rent instability or from articular cartilage damage.

ANATOMY AND BIOMECHANICS OF THE PATELLOFEMORAL JOINT

The patella represents the largest sesamoid bone in the body. Enveloped in the retinacular layer of the quadri-ceps tendon, it articulates with the trochlear groove of the distal femur and possesses the thickest articular cartilage of any joint (up to 6 mm).[15] The patella is typically described as containing two major facets—a long, shallow lateral facet and a short, steep medial facet—mirroring the anatomy of the trochlear groove. The anatomic symmetry between the patella and trochlea is evidence of the developmental codependence of these two structures, as abnormal articulation of the patella within the trochlea is theorized to yield a shallow trochlear groove with possible predisposition to patellar instability.[16] In addition to the two major facets, a far medial, or "odd," facet is often described, as are multiple subdivisions of the primary lateral and medial facets, based upon transverse ridges of the articular surface.[17]

Functionally, the patella serves as a vital link in the extensor mechanism by increasing the moment arm of the quadriceps tendon and providing a mechanical advantage to knee extension.[18] Not surprisingly, loss of the patella from partial or complete patellectomy results in decreased quadriceps force and knee extension weakness.[19] In addition to serving as a knee extensor, a portion of the quadriceps muscle—the vastus medialis obliquus (VMO)—is occasionally described as a "dynamic" stabilizer of the patella.[20] Originating from the intermuscular septum and adductor magnus approximately 3.3 cm proximal to the adductor tubercle,[21] the oblique orientation of this muscle allows for a medially directed force during contraction, providing dynamic stabilization of the patella against lateral translation. However, biomechanical evidence indicates that the actual contribution of the VMO to patellar stability may be minimal,[22] as isolated activation and strengthening of this structure for therapeutic purposes has proven difficult.[23]

At early degrees of flexion, the MPFL represents the most important stabilizer of the patella, responsible for 50% to 60% of resistance to lateral patellar translation.[21,22] Originating between the medial femoral epicondyle and adductor tubercle,[24] this trapezoidal-shaped "static" soft-tissue stabilizer receives decussating contributions from the proximal medial collateral ligament (MCL)[25] and is contained in layer II of the medial soft tissues, deep to the pes anserinus at the level of the superficial MCL.[25,26] The MPFL inserts over a 2.5 cm expansion on both the proximal one-half of the patella and the distal portion of the quadriceps tendon.[27] This ligament is variable in diameter, and may contribute as little as 23% of the stabilizing force against lateral patellar translation in select individuals.[21] The other soft-tissue stabilizers of the medial knee are of lesser importance during early flexion, with the medial patellomeniscal ligament (MPML) providing 22% and medial patellotibial ligament (MPTL) providing 5% of the resistance against lateral patellar translation in extension.[21] Both aforementioned structures provide increasing contributions to patellar stability with increasing knee flexion but provide the majority of soft-tissue restraint only after the patella has engaged in

the trochlear groove. In almost all cases of patellar dislocation, these medial soft-tissue stabilizers are at least partially disrupted in the form of an acute tear or attenuation from chronic instability resulting in a ligament that is intact but functionally incompetent.

Once the patella engages in the trochlear groove at approximately 30° of flexion, the bony configuration of the patellofemoral joint, rather than the soft-tissue stabilizers, becomes the primary restraint to lateral patellar translation. The lateral wall of the trochlea is more prominent anteriorly than its medial counterpart. The more posteriorly directed vector of the quadriceps tendon augments this bony stability during progressive knee flexion, which increases contact between the patella and lateral trochlear facet.[28,29]

Anatomic predispositions to instability primarily result in alteration of the normal biomechanics of the patellofemoral joint. Patella alta doubles the risk of recurrent patellar dislocation,[30] as higher degrees of flexion are required for the patella to engage the trochlear groove. As such, the medial soft-tissue restraints must resist the posterolateral pull of the quadriceps during knee flexion without the buttressing effect provided by the lateral femoral condyle placing these medial soft tissues at higher risk for failure. Similarly, in the case of a hypoplastic lateral femoral condyle, the buttressing effect of the trochlear groove is not available—even with progressive flexion—resulting in less resistance against lateral patellar translation[31,32] and higher risk of dislocation. Complex torsional abnormalities throughout the lower extremity, resulting in increased femoral neck anteversion, internal femoral rotation, and external tibial torsion, increase the risk of instability through a clinical variant known as "miserable malalignment syndrome" (**Fig. 19-1**).

CLASSIFICATION OF PATELLAR INSTABILITY

Numerous classification systems[9,33,34] have been proposed to aid in the understanding and treatment of patellar instability, as the condition represents a heterogenous collection of clinical entities (especially in the pediatric population). However, our approach to the classification of patellar instability is most similar to that described by Parikh and Lykissas[9] and is based primarily on the chronicity of the condition and degree of trauma.

Acute patellar dislocation describes an index dislocation event in a patient with no prior episodes of patellar instability and warrants further subdivision based on mechanism: *traumatic or atraumatic*. In the traumatic setting, individuals with no discernible anatomic predisposition to instability and good quadriceps tone experience a blow to the medial patella resulting in a lateral dislocation. This dislocation event is often accompanied by a traumatic hemarthrosis and osteochondral fracture, with a presentation not dissimilar to an acute anterior cruciate ligament (ACL) rupture.[35]

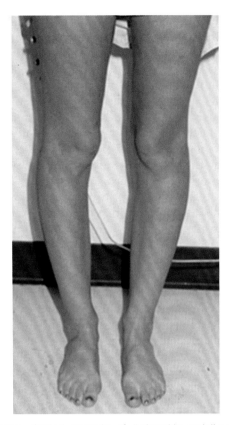

FIGURE 19-1 Clinical example of "miserable malalignment syndrome". (From Parikh SN. *Patellar Instability: Management Principles and Operative Techniques*. Philadelphia: Wolters Kluwer; 2020.)

The risk of subsequent osteochondral injury is inversely related to the degree of generalized ligamentous laxity. The medial soft-tissue restraints from the patella are at least partially disrupted either in their mid-substance or from their patellar or femoral insertions.[36] However, an avulsion fracture of the MPFL's patellar insertion may also occur.[37] Hiemstra and colleagues compare the STAID (Strong, Traumatic, Anatomy normal, Instability, and Dislocation) variant of acute traumatic patellar dislocation to the TUBS (Traumatic, Unilateral, Bankart lesion, and Surgery) variant of shoulder instability.[34] In contrast, an individual may also present with a first-time patellar dislocation without any identifiable trauma. These individuals report dislocation after turning, pivoting, or twisting. These *atraumatic dislocations* are less likely to be associated with a large hemarthrosis or osteochondral fracture and more likely to occur secondary to an underlying anatomic predisposition.[38] Hiemstra and colleagues summarize this as the WARPS (Weak, Atraumatic, Risky anatomy, Pain, and Subluxation) variant.[34] Importantly, these general descriptions provide merely a conceptual framework for patellar instability since actual clinical scenarios may not fit perfectly into one particular construct. For example, a patient suffering a traumatic dislocation may also possess an anatomic predisposition.

After presentation for acute patellar instability—either traumatic or atraumatic—subsequent subluxation and dislocation events are best classified as *recurrent patellar instability*.[9] Numerous risk factors exist for the progression from a single acute instability event to recurrent patellar instability. Young (<14 years), skeletally immature patients with both patella alta and trochlear dysplasia demonstrate a significant (88%) chance of recurrent instability.[30] The distinction between acute and recurrent instability is significant, as the current standard of care for a first-time dislocation is nonoperative treatment in the absence of significant structural damage (discussed below); whereas, recurrent instability is an indication for operative management.[39]

In less frequent cases, individuals may experience dislocation–relocation events with each flexion–extension cycle during ambulation. Such continuous dislocation–relocation is referred to as *habitual patellar instability* and is typically less painful than acute and recurrent episodes of instability.[40] Lateral patellar dislocation is required for knee flexion resulting from tight lateral soft tissues and a shortened extensor mechanism. This repetitive low-energy trauma results in severe chondral damage in young adulthood.[41] In the pediatric population, *congenital patellar dislocation* occurs *in utero* and results in a flexion contracture of the knee at birth.[42] Finally, patellar dislocation occurring during the early stages of ambulation is referred to as *developmental patellar dislocation*. These latter two subtypes are very uncommon and are rarely encountered in the routine clinical setting, particularly in adults.

HISTORY AND PHYSICAL EXAMINATION

History

As with all patient encounters, a thorough history is the initial step in patient evaluation. As discussed above, an understanding of the mechanism of injury and the activity at the time of dislocation is helpful in reaching a diagnosis. Further history should detail if a traumatic force was applied to the patella, whether the patella spontaneously reduced or required manual reduction, and if subsequent episodes occurred after the initial dislocation event. A history of giving-way, catching, clicking, or locking sensations occurring after the dislocation event is also informative, as osteochondral fractures commonly occur with patellar dislocation that results in loose bodies within the joint.[43] Moreover, instability of the tibiofemoral joint during twisting, pivoting, or landing may indicate ACL, meniscal, or collateral ligament injury, rather than isolated patellofemoral injury. Instability that occurs with only mild trauma suggests a greater degree of anatomic abnormalities, which increase the chance for recurrence. Additionally, since patellar instability affects young active patients, participation in sports and overall activity level prior to the dislocation should be determined. Assessment of past surgical history may indicate prior attempts at stabilization. A family history of patellar instability may predict both recurrent ipsilateral and future contralateral instability.[44]

Physical Examination

Our approach to the physical examination begins with general inspection of gait with an emphasis on dynamic lower limb alignment and the degree of foot pronation. The patient is examined in the standing position. With the feet pointing forward, the patellae should point straight ahead. A patella facing inward ("squinting patella") or outward ("grasshopper patella") may indicate significant underlying variation in torsional limb malalignment. Increased recurvatum in the sagittal plane should also be noted.

With the patient supine, general inspection of lower limb alignment will show generalized limb alignment, such as genu valgum (**Fig. 19-2**), and may reveal quadriceps atrophy in long-standing cases of instability. Although the patella tracks along an essentially straight line, the extensor mechanism forms an angle when viewed in the coronal plane. This is the quadriceps angle, commonly referred to as the *Q-angle*. This angle comprises a line connecting the anterior superior iliac spine to the center of the patella approximating the vector of the quadriceps musculature. The angle is completed by a line connecting the center of the patella to the tibial tuberosity. The existence of the Q-angle accounts for the tendency of the patella to displace laterally when the quadriceps muscles contract creating a

"bowstring" effect, analogous to a lax rope straightening when rendered taut. The Q-angle is directly related to the patella's tendency to displace laterally. Q-angle values greater than 20° are considered abnormal, though there may be variation in this angle based on whether the patient is sitting, standing, or supine. In general, the concept of the Q-angle must be questioned, given its variability and risk for false-negative measurements. For example, a patient with a patella that is "perched" on the lateral trochlea due to marked genu valgum or soft-tissue imbalance that is on the verge of dislocating will have a low Q-angle falsely suggesting a low risk of instability.

Systematic palpation of the tibiofemoral and patellofemoral joints will likely reveal an effusion and diffuse tenderness indicative of nonspecific structural damage to the knee. However, the majority of patients with patellar instability have tenderness over the medial femoral condyle at the attachment of the MPFL and, less commonly, at the medial patellar border.[45] Tightness of the lateral retinaculum can be determined by palpation of the space between the lateral patellar border and trochlea. Normally, the lateral patellar facet can be elevated from the lateral trochlea parallel to the transepicondylar axis with the knee in full extension (**Fig. 19-3**). A tight lateral retinaculum prevents this passive rotation and may be a predisposing factor to lateral patellar instability. Patients with generalized laxity rarely have tightness of the lateral retinaculum.

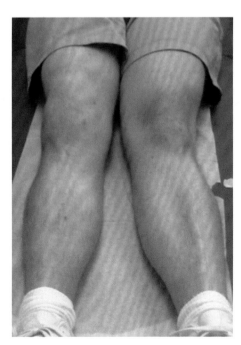

FIGURE 19-2 Patient demonstrating bilateral genu valgum.

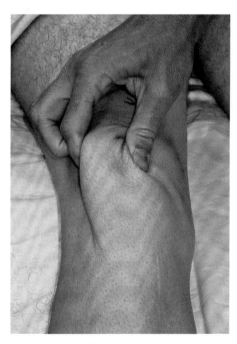

FIGURE 19-3 Tightness of the lateral retinaculum can be determined by the ability to elevate the lateral patellar facet away from the lateral trochlea. Normally, the lateral facet should be elevated to at least parallel to the transepicondylar axis with the knee in full extension. (From Johnson D, Amendola NA, Barber F. *Operative Arthroscopy.* Philadelphia: Wolters Kluwer; 2015.)

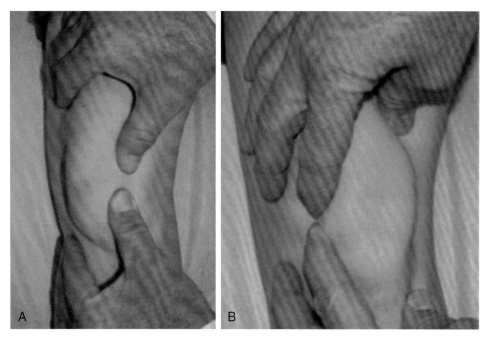

FIGURE 19-4 Medial and lateral patellar translation tested with the knee at 20° of flexion and divided into longitudinal quadrants. Normal medial translation is one quadrant and lateral translation is two quadrants. **A:** Medial and **B:** Lateral.

Active and passive knee range of motion should be measured with evaluation of patellar tracking and the presence of retropatellar crepitus throughout the arc of motion. Crepitus is accentuated with active knee extension because of the elevated compressive force rendered by quadriceps contraction. The degree of flexion associated with the onset of crepitus can provide information regarding the location of any patellar cartilage defect since patellar contact with the trochlea progresses from distal to proximal as the knee moves from extension into flexion. Patellar tracking is usually symmetrical and within the trochlear groove; however, an abrupt lateral jump ("J-sign") as the knee approaches full extension is indicative of lateral patellar subluxation.

Patellar translation in the coronal plane is quantified by dividing the patella into longitudinal quadrants, then placing a laterally and medially directed force on the patella at 20° of flexion to determine the amount of passive patellar translation (**Fig. 19-4**). It is important that this measurement be made in slight flexion in order to engage the patella in the trochlear groove and assess true ligamentous laxity. Normally, the patella cannot be translated more than two quadrants laterally and one quadrant medially. Increased passive lateral patellar translation is associated with patellar instability. A soft end point with lateral patellar translation may indicate either disruption or attenuation of the medial soft-tissue restraints. If the patient actively fires the quadriceps in an attempt to resist lateral patellar translation or endorses a sensation of anxiety due to impending subluxation, they are exhibiting a positive "apprehension sign." Some authors advocate applying this lateral force on the patella throughout a full arc of flexion and extension ("moving patellar apprehension test"), which yields a high degree of sensitivity and specificity for patellar instability.[46]

All patients with patellar instability should be assessed for generalized ligamentous laxity utilizing the Beighton criteria.[47] A score of 4 or more on this 9-point scale indicates generalized laxity, with females typically exhibiting higher scores than males.[48]

Tests for meniscal pathology (i.e., McMurray test, Thessaly test, and pain with hyperflexion), ACL insufficiency (e.g., Lachman, anterior drawer, and pivot shift tests), injury to the MCL and lateral collateral ligament (valgus and varus stress testing at 0° and 30° of flexion, respectively), and posterolateral corner injury (i.e., dial, reverse pivot shift, and extension-recurvatum tests) should be performed in all patients following an acute injury.

The examination concludes with determination of passive hip range of motion in both the supine and prone positions. With the patient prone, increased anteversion may be a predisposing factor for patellar instability (**Fig. 19-5**).

RADIOGRAPHIC EVALUATION

Plain Radiographs

A thorough radiographic assessment of the entire lower extremity is imperative in the comprehensive evaluation of patients with patellar instability. We routinely obtain four views of the knee: anteroposterior, 45°

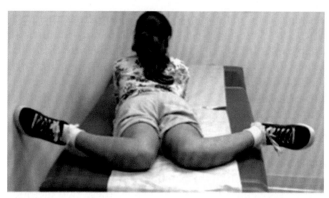

FIGURE 19-5 Prone patient demonstrating excessive femoral anteversion.

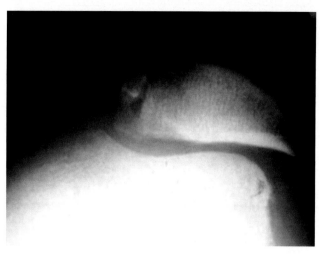

FIGURE 19-7 Axial (Merchant) X-ray demonstrating an avulsed bony fragment attached to the medial patellofemoral ligament.

flexion weight-bearing (Rosenberg), axial (Merchant), and 30° lateral. Fracture fragments from the lateral femoral condyle or medial patellar facet may be appreciated (**Fig. 19-6**). However, small pieces of bone where the MPFL was avulsed off the medial patellar border are typically *not* loose within the joint and do not require removal (**Fig. 19-7**). Degenerative changes of the patellofemoral cartilage may also be seen with long-standing instability (**Fig. 19-8**). Patellar position, in reference to the trochlea on the Merchant view (with contralateral comparison), may show asymmetrical lateral patellar translation or tilt (**Fig. 19-9**). The depth of the trochlear groove can be quantified through measurement of the sulcus angle (normal: 137° ± 6°),[49] with a shallow trochlea associated with both instability and trochlear dysplasia.[50] Additionally, subluxation can be quantified with the congruence angle (normal: −8°± 6°),[49] with a more positive congruence angle representing increasing lateral patellar subluxation (**Fig. 19-10**). Finally, the degree of patellar tilt is determined through the lateral patellofemoral angle, with excessive patellar tilt (defined as >5°)[51] potentially indicating a tight lateral retinaculum.

Patellar "height" is quantified with a 30° lateral radiograph. It is important that this measurement be made with the knee in a standardized degree of flexion. The anterior-most extent of the roof of the intercondylar fossa (Blumensaat line) should be at or just above the same level as the inferior pole of the patella. Numerous ratios (Insall–Salvati,[52] Caton–Deschamps,[53] and Blackburne–Peel[54]) have been developed for more objective quantification of patellar height (**Fig. 19-11**). The Insall–Salvati method divides the patellar tendon

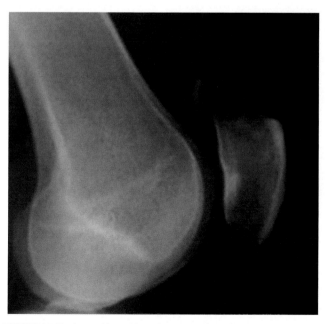

FIGURE 19-6 Lateral knee X-ray demonstrating a loose osteochondral body in the suprapatellar pouch.

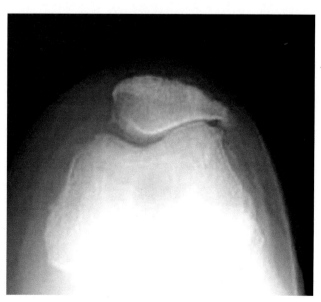

FIGURE 19-8 Axial (Merchant) X-ray demonstrating degenerative arthritis of the patellofemoral articulation seen with long-standing patellar instability.

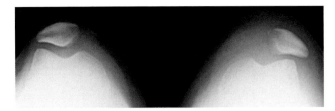

FIGURE 19-9 Bilateral axial (Merchant) X-ray showing asymmetric left lateral patellar subluxation.

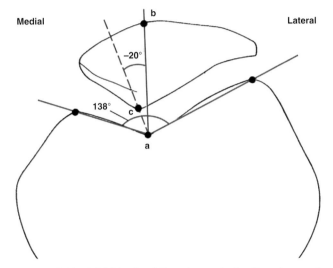

FIGURE 19-10 Axial (Merchant) X-ray demonstrating the sulcus angle (solid lines) and congruence angle (dashed lines). (From Miller MD, Dempsey IJ. *Making the Diagnosis in Orthopedics: A Video-Enhanced Guide to Identifying Musculoskeletal Disorders*. Philadelphia: Wolters Kluwer; 2020.)

length by the maximum patellar length from the superior to the inferior pole. This measurement requires an approximation of the tendon insertion into the tibial tubercle, which may introduce inconsistency into the measurement, especially in pediatric patients. Moreover, this ratio also remains unchanged during a tubercle osteotomy as neither patellar tendon nor patellar length change, potentially limiting its utility in the postoperative setting. The Caton–Deschamps and Blackburne–Peel methods utilize the length of the *articular surface* of the patella in relation to the patellar tendon length, with normal ratios being 0.8 to 1.2. As such, these two methods represent the most useful measurements for patella alta or baja, with the Blackburne–Peel ratio being the most consistently reproducible.[55] Patella alta can also be identified by the patella–plateau angle. This angle is formed by a line parallel to the tibial plateau and a line from the posterior tibial plateau to the most distal articulating surface of the patella. A normal angle is 25° with 90% of measurements between 20° and 30° (**Fig. 19-12**).[56]

The lateral radiograph can also be used to assess the trochlea for evidence of trochlear dysplasia, though the surgeon must take care to ensure perfect overlap of the medial and lateral femoral condyles. The most common classification for trochlear dysplasia is that of Dejour.[57] Type I dysplasia describes a shallow trochlear groove and is defined by the presence of the trochlear groove crossing the radiographic outline of the femoral condyles ("crossing sign") (**Fig. 19-13**). Type II dysplasia features a flat trochlea and a bony prominence at the proximal extent of the trochlea ("supratrochlear spur") (**Fig. 19-13**). Hypoplasia of the medial femoral condyle and a convex lateral femoral condyle defines type III

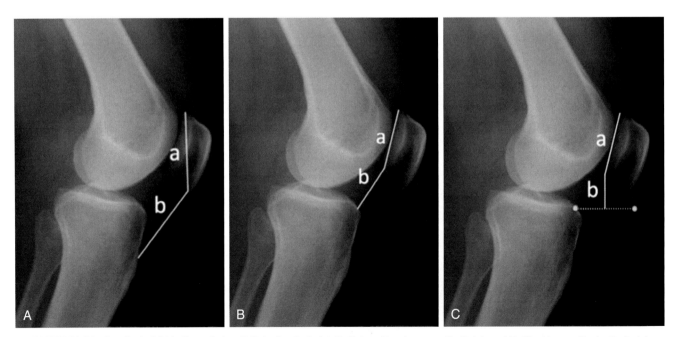

FIGURE 19-11 Patellar height indices. **A:** Insall–Salvati ratio (b/a), **B:** Caton–Deschamps ratio (b/a), and **C:** Blackburne–Peel ratio (b/a).

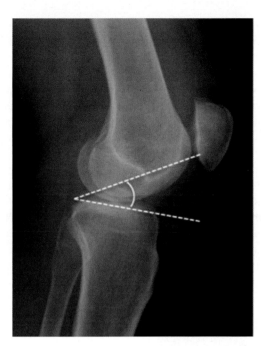

FIGURE 19-12 Lateral knee X-ray showing the plateau–patella angle used to measure patellar "height."

dysplasia, with the hypoplastic medial femoral condyle evident on the lateral radiographs as a "double contour sign." Type IV dysplasia is defined by a hypoplastic medial femoral condyle in the presence of a bony "cliff," "supratrochlear spur," and a "double contour sign."[29,57]

Finally, lower extremity alignment can be formally quantified with a long-cassette radiograph from the hip to ankle if excessive genu valgum or varum is suspected

based on the physical examination. The "mechanical axis" is the straight line from the center of the femoral head to the center of the tibial plafond. It should pass through the center of the knee between the tibial spines. The "femorotibial angle" is the angle formed by a line through the center of the intramedullary canals of the femur and of the tibia. Normal values are 178° in males and 174° in females.[58]

Computed Tomography

Computed tomography (CT) provides three-dimensional detail of potential injuries following patellar instability while also allowing for further understanding of trochlear dysplasia.[57] Sequential CT imaging in progressive knee flexion provides information regarding dynamic patellar tracking using static images in progressive degrees of flexion (**Fig. 19-14**). One distinct advantage of this imaging modality is the ability to calculate the tibial tubercle to trochlear groove (TT–TG) distance. This is defined as the distance from the apex of the tibial tubercle to the deepest portion of the trochlear groove on superimposed axial CT sections. This distance quantifies the lateral displacement of the tibial tubercle relative to the trochlear groove, with a distance more than 20 mm significantly increasing a patient's risk for

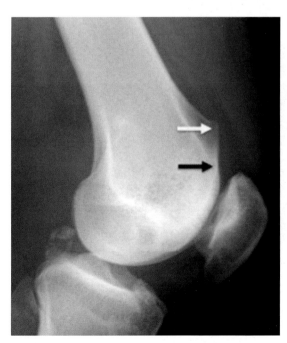

FIGURE 19-13 Radiographic evidence of trochlear dysplasia on lateral knee X-ray: "crossing sign" (black arrow) and "supratrochlear spur" (white arrow).

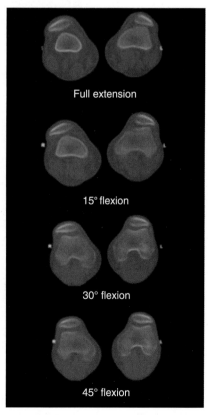

Full extension

15° flexion

30° flexion

45° flexion

FIGURE 19-14 Axial computed tomography of the left and right patellofemoral joints in progressive degrees of knee flexion demonstrating lateral patellar subluxation as a function of knee flexion.

recurrent instability (OR = 2.1).[13] A higher TT–TG distance has usually been used to indicate the need for a tibial tubercle ("distal") realignment.[59] However, this value should not be used as a rigid threshold when formulating a treatment plan as there is some variability in this measurement depending on the imaging modality (i.e., MRI)[60] and degree of knee flexion.[61] In general, CT imaging is used primarily in those patients with significant trochlear dysplasia or osteochondral fractures that may require fixation.

Magnetic Resonance Imaging

Magnetic resonance imaging (MRI) is most helpful to determine the integrity of the medial soft-tissue restraints and patellofemoral articular surfaces, the presence of loose bodies, and any concurrent meniscal or ligamentous injuries. It may also provide information regarding bony anatomy, such as trochlear geometry and the TT–TG distance (**Fig. 19-15**). MRI after acute lateral patellar dislocation shows complete or partial MPFL rupture in approximately 50% of cases,[36] with ruptures most often occurring at the femoral insertion site or mid-substance in adults (**Fig. 19-16**).[62] In the pediatric population, injury to the MPFL is most likely to occur through an avulsion of the patellar insertion, with femoral-sided avulsion fractures remaining more common than mid-substance rupture.[63,64] Additionally, 70% of MRIs demonstrate a chondral injury to the medial patellar facet and 15% show an intra-articular loose body following a lateral patellar dislocation (**Fig. 19-17**).[36] Beyond defining the degree of injury resulting from patellar dislocation, concurrent meniscal tears (11%) and MCL injuries (11%) are often identified, which may assist in planning surgical staging,

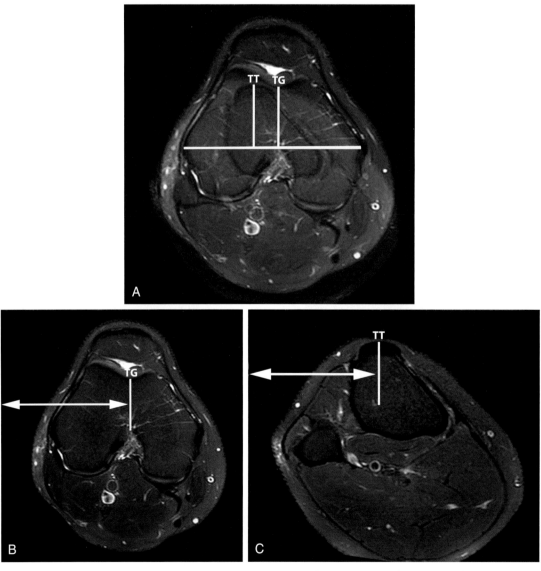

FIGURE 19-15   Axial MRI images showing the steps to calculate the tibial tubercle–trochlear groove (TT–TG) distance. **A:** Superimposed axial MRI images of the tibial tubercle (TT) and trochlear groove (TG). The distance between the two lines represents the TT-TG distance. **B:** Axial MRI image showing the sulcus of the TG. **C:** Axial MRI image showing the apex of the TT. (From Chew FS. *Musculoskeletal Imaging: The Essentials*. Philadelphia: Wolters Kluwer; 2019.)

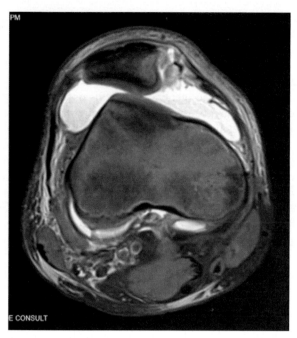

FIGURE 19-16 Axial MRI image showing avulsion of the medial patellofemoral ligament.

pre- and postoperative rehabilitation, and weight-bearing status. Given the variability of soft-tissue injury and bony anatomy, absence of ionizing radiation, and high occurrence of associated injuries, MRI is preferred over CT imaging for the majority of patients with patellar instability.[62] MRI is indicated in those patients with a tense effusion, an osteochondral loose body noted on plain radiographs, and undergoing surgical intervention.

TREATMENT OF PATELLAR INSTABILITY

Nonoperative Treatment

In the case of patellar subluxation, the patella repositions itself in the trochlea without assistance. Supportive care suffices in the acute setting. A dislocated patella, on the other hand, requires a reduction maneuver (**Fig. 19-18**). As the knee is slowly extended to the maximal extent (hyperextension is often possible in patients prone to dislocation), the patella is allowed to regain its normal position with manual manipulation occasionally required.

In the absence of a significant osteochondral fracture or loose body, nonoperative management is the standard of care for a first-time patellar dislocation in the majority of patients. Despite the increased risk of recurrent instability associated with younger patients, conservative management is indicated for first-time dislocations in the young athletic population as well.[65] This recommendation is due primarily to the essentially equivalent functional outcomes in both operative and nonoperative patient cohorts.[44,66-68] In addition, patients treated nonoperatively may actually have less pain and higher quality of life than those treated with surgical stabilization.[39,67] In the general population, stabilization of first-time dislocations does reduce the risk of recurrent instability by approximately 50%. However, primary stabilization has been associated with a sixfold increase in patellofemoral arthritis and no significant increase in quality of life.[69]

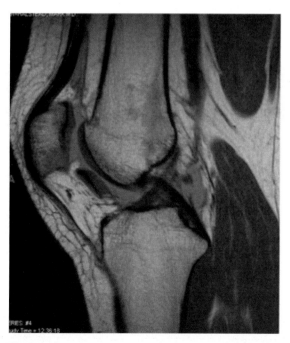

FIGURE 19-17 Sagittal T1-weighted MRI image demonstrating a chondral loose body between the patella and trochlea anterior to the intercondylar notch.

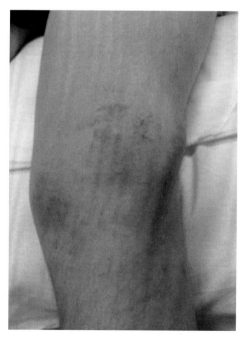

FIGURE 19-18 Patellar dislocation of left knee.

Nonoperative management may begin with arthrocentesis of a tense hemarthrosis to improve patient comfort. We place most patients in a knee immobilizer or hinged knee brace locked in extension for 7 to 10 days to allow the disrupted soft tissues to heal.[67] Flexion is avoided to protect the patella from the posterolateral pull of the quadriceps muscle. Intermittent icing, NSAIDs, joint compression, and elevation are initiated to reduce the inflammatory response. Quadriceps isometric strengthening exercises (i.e., straight leg raises) are also encouraged at this time. Weight-bearing as tolerated with the knee in extension is allowed since the patellofemoral articulation bears little weight in full extension.

After the first 7 to 10 days, the patient is placed in a patellar-stabilizing brace, and a gradual increase in range of motion is allowed. "Closed-chain" quadriceps strengthening (i.e., lunges, leg press, etc.) is initiated with avoidance of "open-chain" (i.e., knee extension) exercises which place increased sheer stress on the patellar articular surface.[70] Stationary cycling, treadmill ambulation, and core conditioning are introduced. Following the return of lower extremity strength and mobility, sports-specific functional drills are allowed. Return to full athletic activity is permitted when the patient is symptom free, exhibits full range of motion, and has 85% to 90% of contralateral lower extremity strength on isokinetic testing.

Operative Management

Surgical stabilization is most commonly indicated in patients with multiple instability episodes unresponsive to nonoperative treatment or a single instability event with concurrent articular cartilage injury resulting in a cartilaginous loose body or large osteochondral fragment. Recurrent instability is typically addressed surgically, as individuals with a second dislocation face a sevenfold increase in further instability episodes when compared to individuals with a single dislocation.[12]

There are three general surgical options used to address patellar instability—either alone or in combination—that repair/reconstruct the damaged ligamentous restraints and/or alter the anatomic relationship between the patella and trochlea. In the United States, "proximal realignment" is the mainstay of surgical treatment and involves repair, rebalancing, or reconstruction of the proximal ligamentous restraints in an attempt to statically guide the patella into the trochlear groove during knee flexion. "Distal realignment" refers to an osteotomy of the tibial tubercle with medialization of the patellar tendon insertion to provide a more congruent patellar articulation within the trochlear groove. Finally, "femoral trochleoplasty" involves altering the shape of the trochlea to either increase trochlear depth or augment the lateral trochlear buttress that contributes to lateral patellar stability. As each surgical technique attempts to address a distinct anatomic factor involved with patellar instability, the ideal procedure(s) selected depend on the particular structures that are damaged and/or pathologic anatomy responsible for the instability.[71]

A diagnostic arthroscopy is performed prior to all reconstructive procedures listed below. Arthroscopy provides the surgeon the ability to evaluate the patellar and trochlear surfaces, remove any loose cartilaginous bodies, repair displaced osteochondral fractures, perform a lateral retinacular release (discussed below), and treat any concurrent meniscal injuries (**Fig. 19-19**).

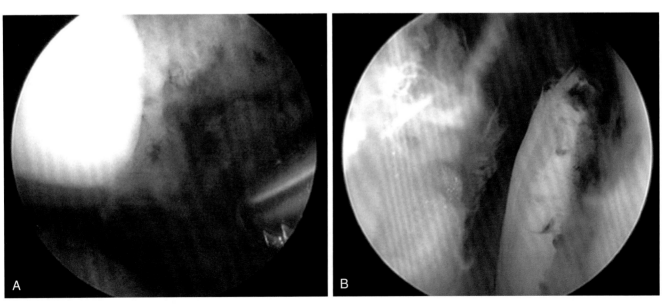

FIGURE 19-19   **A:** Arthroscopic view showing an articular defect of the medial patellar facet. **B:** corresponding loose body in the medial gutter.

Lateral Retinacular Release

A lateral retinacular release ("lateral release") is performed in those patients with excessive tightness of the lateral retinaculum as evidenced by an inability to manually elevate the lateral patellar facet past a position parallel to the transepicondylar axis in the axial plane. A lateral release should never be performed in isolation to address patellar instability or in patients with generalized ligamentous laxity. Rather, it should be used selectively as one component of the overall surgical treatment plan in those patients with excessive lateral retinacular tightness.

A lateral release is typically performed arthroscopically using electrocautery with care not to burn the overlying skin. A curved Mayo scissors is used to create a subcutaneous space lateral to the lateral retinaculum from the anterolateral to superolateral arthroscopic portal. The arthroscope is placed in the anteromedial portal viewing laterally. The fluid outflow portal is closed in order to allow the joint to distend, which causes the patella to rise away from the femur improving visualization. The electrocautery is used to make a linear incision through the synovium and lateral retinaculum from the superolateral portal to the anterolateral portal (**Fig. 19-20**). Care should be taken to avoid the superolateral geniculate artery. In addition to avoiding skin perforation with the electrocautery, care should be taken not to incise the vastus lateralis in order to prevent iatrogenic *medial* patellar subluxation. Following the release, the patella can usually be elevated 20° to 30°, though the lateral soft tissues will tighten over time. Concurrent procedures (discussed below) are then performed, as necessary.

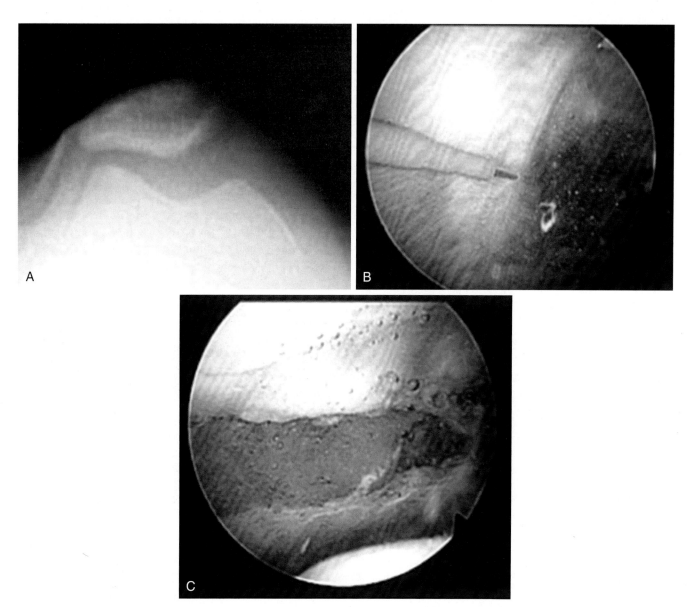

FIGURE 19-20   A: Axial (Merchant) X-ray showing lateral patellar tilt. **B:** Arthroscopic electrocautery incising the lateral retinaculum. **C:** Incised lateral retinaculum following the "lateral release."

Medial Patellofemoral Ligament Repair

Repair of the MPFL is often possible in patients who sustained a single dislocation event with avulsion/tear of the MPFL, which is otherwise robust (**Fig. 19-21**). The specific surgical approach depends on the location of the tear. Avulsions from either the femoral or patellar insertions are repaired with suture anchors through a 2 to 3 cm incision to secure the avulsed ligament to its anatomic origin. For mid-substance ruptures, a braided, nonabsorbable suture can be utilized for side-to-side repair. However, a mid-substance repair is less reliable than repair of a bony avulsion due to the enhanced biology of ligament-to-bone healing. Primary repair of the ligament has been shown to be equivalent to reconstruction in a small series of patients[72]; however, a larger meta-analysis of larger patient series indicates that an MPFL repair is inferior to reconstruction in preventing recurrent instability.[72] As such, we favor MPFL reconstruction over repair in most cases.

Medial Patellofemoral Ligament Reconstruction

Medial patellofemoral ligament reconstruction is the procedure of choice in cases where the MPFL has been attenuated due to chronic instability or when repair of a mid-substance rupture is not feasible. Isolated MPFL reconstruction has been shown to not only limit recurrent instability but also allow return to sports and other activities.[73] Given such favorable outcomes, MPFL reconstruction is the primary procedure for management of patellar instability either alone or in conjunction with other procedures.[39,71]

Successful reconstruction begins with appropriate graft selection with both autograft and allograft options available. Unlike ACL reconstruction, use of autograft tissue has not demonstrated clear superiority to allografts for MPFL reconstruction, though patient-reported outcomes do seem to favor autograft techniques.[74] We typically utilize the gracilis or semitendinosus autograft, which necessitates a small 2 to 3 cm incision just medial to the tibial tubercle. Either an open- or closed-ended tendon stripper is used for tendon harvest. Total tendon length is typically 20 to 24 cm, depending on patient size.[75] The gracilis tendon is adequate in most patients, but the semitendinosus should be considered in petite females whose gracilis may be too thin. Excess muscle should be stripped off the tendon prior to implantation (**Fig. 19-22**). Care should be taken to protect the superficial MCL and saphenous nerve during autograft harvest (**Fig. 19-23**). Allografts may be preferred in cases of hyperlaxity (as determined by the Beighton score), given the theoretical predisposition to graft attenuation in this patient population.

Appropriate graft placement is essential for optimal outcome, as graft malposition may lead to either recurrent instability from graft laxity, or loss of knee flexion, and pain from excessive graft tightness.[76] The MPFL's femoral origin is located in the sulcus between the adductor tubercle and medial epicondyle. Originally described in 2007 by Schöttle and colleagues, "Schöttle point" is a radiographic landmark representing the center of the MPFL's femoral origin located 1 mm anterior to the distal extension of the posterior femoral cortex 2.5 mm distal to the posterior origin of the medial femoral condyle, and proximal to the level of the posterior point of Blumensaat line on a lateral radiograph with

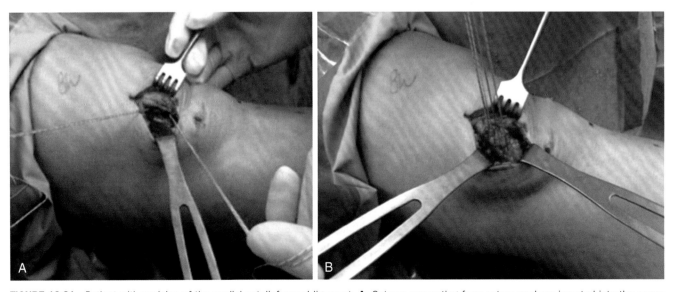

FIGURE 19-21 Patient with avulsion of the medial patellofemoral ligament. **A:** Sutures emanating from suture anchors inserted into the nonarticulating surface of the medial patellar border. **B:** Sutures imbricated through the torn medial retinaculum and medial patellofemoral ligament.

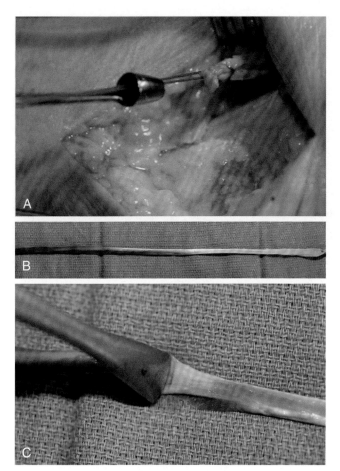

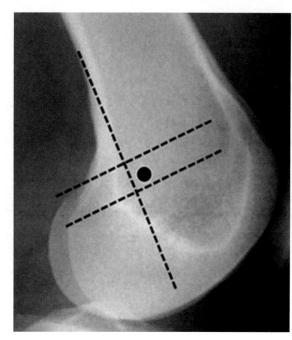

FIGURE 19-24 Schöttle point (black circle) seen on a lateral knee X-ray marking the center of the femoral attachment of the medial patellofemoral ligament.

FIGURE 19-22 Harvest and preparation of a gracilis autograft used for medial patellofemoral ligament reconstruction. **A:** A closed-ended tendon stripper used for graft harvest. **B:** The harvested tendon. **C:** Use of a Cobb elevator to remove all muscle from the gracilis tendon.

both posterior condyles projected in the same plane (**Fig. 19-24**).[24] We strongly recommend the use of fluoroscopic visualization to locate Schöttle point rather than relying solely on manual identification of the MPFL's origin to reduce the risk of error. A graft that is placed too proximally on the femur will prohibit full flexion and/or eventually fail. A graft placed too distally will result in ligament incompetence. A suture is used to check isometry throughout knee flexion between the medial patellar border and Schöttle point, as well as to estimate graft length.

Regardless of graft choice, we prefer a double-limb reconstruction to match the trapezoidal configuration of the native MPFL. The graft is folded in half to determine its diameter, though most grafts fit easily through a 5 to 7 mm drill sleeve or sizing guide to match the diameter of the femoral tunnel. Nonabsorbable #2 passing sutures are sewn into the free ends of the graft. Once Schöttle point is identified fluoroscopically, a Beath pin is drilled across the distal femur. This pin is overdrilled with the appropriately sized cannulated drill to a depth of 3 cm to prevent the graft from "bottoming out" in the femoral tunnel. The ends of the graft may be attached directly to the patella with two double-loaded 3.0 mm suture anchors and the looped end passed through the femoral tunnel (**Fig. 19-25**). Alternatively, the center of the graft may be attached to the nonarticular surface of the medial patellar border over the proximal 2.5 cm of the patella with similar anchors and the free ends of the graft docked into the femoral tunnel.[74] As a rule, we avoid large drill holes in the patella (especially those that

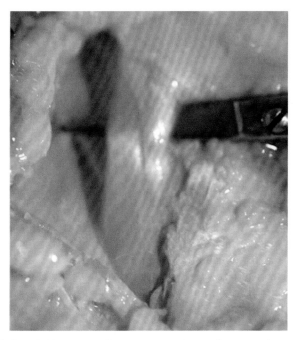

FIGURE 19-23 Fibers of the medial collateral ligament often mistaken for one of the hamstring tendons.

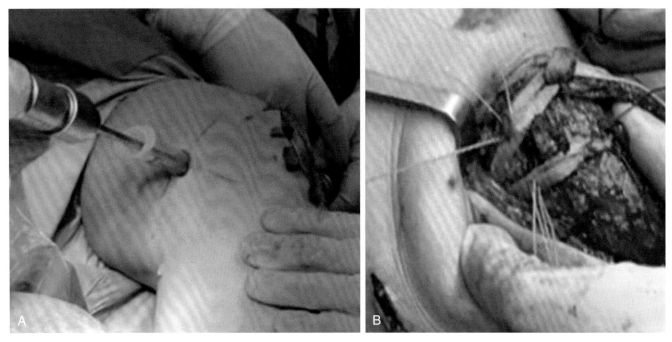

FIGURE 19-25   Reconstruction of the medial patellofemoral ligament. **A:** Drilling the femoral tunnel at Schöttle point. **B:** A double-limbed construct.

span the entire width of the bone) to reduce the risk for a postoperative patellar fracture. The graft is passed under layer II of the medial soft-tissue structures prior to final fixation. #2 passing sutures attached to the graft (free ends or looped end) are passed across the distal femur with the Beath pin, and the graft is docked into the femoral tunnel. Femoral graft fixation is accomplished with

either a bioabsorbable screw or suture button anchored external to the lateral femoral cortex (**Fig. 19-26**). The graft should be tensioned with the knee in 30° to 45° of knee flexion with the patella centered in the trochlear groove and minimal tension placed on the #2 sutures. The knee is then taken through a full range of motion to ensure normal patellar tracking and stability of the reconstruction. The sutures may be tied over a small polypropylene button external to the lateral femoral cortex for supplemental fixation.

Postoperatively, the patient is maintained in a hinged knee brace locked in full extension for 2 weeks. Physical therapy is initiated to address inflammation, regain knee motion and quadriceps strength, and ultimately, return the patient to their preinstability level of activity (**Table 19-1**). These general recommendations apply to both an MPFL repair and reconstruction.

Further complexity is added in the setting of an open distal femoral physis in skeletally immature patients, as the anatomic origin of the MPFL is an average of 3 mm distal to the distal femoral physis, though there is variability to this anatomic relationship.[77] Moreover, placement of the graft is determined relative to the femoral landmarks, which will change with continued growth. Interference screws should be avoided or used cautiously in skeletally immature patients due to the close proximity of the femoral drill hole to the distal femoral physis. Nevertheless, anatomic MPFL reconstruction remains a relatively safe and effective surgical option in skeletally immature patients.[78]

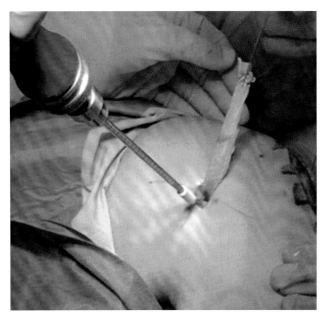

FIGURE 19-26   Femoral fixation of a medial patellofemoral ligament graft with a cannulated bioabsorbable screw.

TABLE 19-1 Postoperative Rehabilitation Following Medial Patellofemoral Ligament Reconstruction or Repair

Phase I: (0-1 mo)

Range of motion (passive)

Week 2: 0°-70°

Week 3: 0°-90°

Week 6: 0°-120°

Week 8: 0°-135°

Range of motion (active)

Week 2: Active extension allowed, active flexion as tolerated

Weight-bearing with brace locked in extension

0-2 wk: Toe-touch weight-bearing

2 wk: 25% body weight with increase of 25% per week

6-8 wk: Full weight-bearing

Modalities

Cryotherapy

Electrical stimulation to quadriceps

Exercises

Quadriceps, hamstring, gluteal isometrics

Ankle pumps

Four-way hip range of motion

Phase II: (1-3 mo)

Range of motion

At least 120°

Weight-bearing

Full with crutches, progress off crutches as tolerated

Emphasis on normal gait pattern

Modalities

Cryotherapy

Electrical stimulation to quadriceps as indicated

Exercises

Double-leg balance and coordination activities

Stationary bike at 8 wk

Upper body circuit training or ergometer

Strengthening

Isometric multiangle quadriceps sets

Closed-chain short arc strengthening in accordance with weight-bearing

Week 12: Isometric strength testing at 60° with quadriceps strength within 25% of contralateral limb

Phase III: >3 mo

Range of motion

Full

Weight-bearing

Full

Modalities

Cryotherapy

Exercises

Begin plyometrics

Stationary bike with progressive lowering of seat and increasing resistance

Light jogging

Swimming with flutter kick or stairmaster

Strengthening

Single-leg press

Single-leg balance board and proprioception exercises

Hip and core strengthening

Return to sports: 4-6 mo

Dynamic neuromuscular control exercises beginning with low-velocity single-plane progressing to higher velocity multiplane

Sport-specific functional progression

Isokinetic strength testing within 10% to 15% of contralateral limb

Tibial Tubercle Osteotomy

Though proximal realignment options restore the major soft-tissue restraints of the patella, distal realignment procedures address patellar instability by rectifying patellofemoral malalignment. In the setting of excessive lateralization of the extensor mechanism (i.e., elevated TT–TG distance, genu valgum, external tibial torsion[59,79]), a tibial tubercle osteotomy (TTO) serves to medialize the tibial tubercle to reduce the lateralizing force on the patella with active knee extension.

An Elmslie–Trillat osteotomy is the procedure of choice to medialize the patella in order to improve the articular congruence within the trochlea. This osteotomy is made parallel to the coronal plane so that there is pure medialization without anteriorization of the tubercle. A 4 to 6 cm incision is made just lateral to the tibial tubercle. The fascial attachment of the anterior compartment musculature is released with electrocautery leaving a small fascial sleeve at the tibial tubercle. The patellar tendon insertion is identified and an osteotomy is made in the axial plane with a 0.5″ straight osteotome just proximal to the patellar tendon insertion. A 3.2 mm drill is used

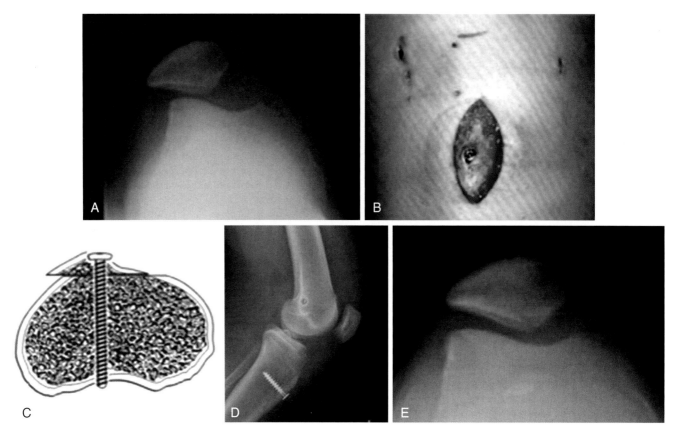

FIGURE 19-27 Elmslie–Trillat osteotomy. **A:** Axial (Merchant) X-ray showing lateral patellar tilt and subluxation. **B:** Incision used for final fixation of the transferred tibial tubercle. **C:** Figure showing medial translation of the osteotomized tibial tubercle. **D:** Lateral knee X-ray following a combined Elmslie–Trillat osteotomy and medial patellofemoral ligament reconstruction. **E:** Axial (Merchant) X-ray in the same patient following a combined Elmslie–Trillat osteotomy and medial patellofemoral ligament reconstruction.

to make sequential drill holes at a depth of 8 to 10 mm over a distance of 6 cm tapered anteriorly. These drill holes are connected with a curved 1″ osteotome in the coronal plane. The periosteum is incised medially, just enough to allow the osteotomized fragment to be rotated (not translated) medially 8 to 10 mm to normalize the TT–TG distance (assuming a value >20 mm). The knee should be passively taken through a full range of motion to monitor patellar tracking in order to avoid excessive medialization. Good bone-to-bone contact is imperative to allow healing. A single low-profile unicortical or bicortical screw is used for fixation (**Fig. 19-27**). We favor a unicortical low-profile screw as this avoids the neurovascular risks of drilling posterior to the tibia with avoidance of skin irritation from a round-headed screw. Bone wax is applied to the exposed cancellous surface of the proximal tibia, and a prophylactic fasciotomy is performed along the anterior compartment musculature; this facilitates reapproximation of the anterior compartment fascia to the tibial tubercle. In patients undergoing both a proximal MPFL reconstruction and TTO, the hamstring graft is harvested prior to the osteotomy. The osteotomy is performed prior to the proximal surgical exposure and insertion of the MPFL graft.

In patients with chondrosis of the lateral and/or distal patellar surface, *anteromedialization* of the tibial tubercle, as described by Fulkerson,[80] can be performed to unload the lateral and distal patellar facet, while also stabilizing the patella within the trochlear groove. This requires a triplane osteotomy in either a freehand fashion or with use of a cutting guide. The osteotomy is typically performed over a length of 10 cm at a 45° angle to the coronal plane, though this can be modified depending on the desired amount of anteriorization. A more "shallow" osteotomy results primarily in medialization, while a "steeper" osteotomy results in more anteriorization of the tubercle. Unlike an Elmslie–Trillat osteotomy, the Fulkerson osteotomy is fixed with two bicortical screws due to the larger bony fragment created. Closure is analogous to that for the Elmslie–Trillat osteotomy (**Fig. 19-28**).

Distal realignment provides clinically acceptable results with recurrent dislocation rates of less than 10% in the few studies available.[81] However, translation of the tubercle places the overlying skin at risk for infection or dehiscence, while the osteotomy site creates a risk for delayed union and nonunion. These risks are highest when the tibial tubercle is completely detached from

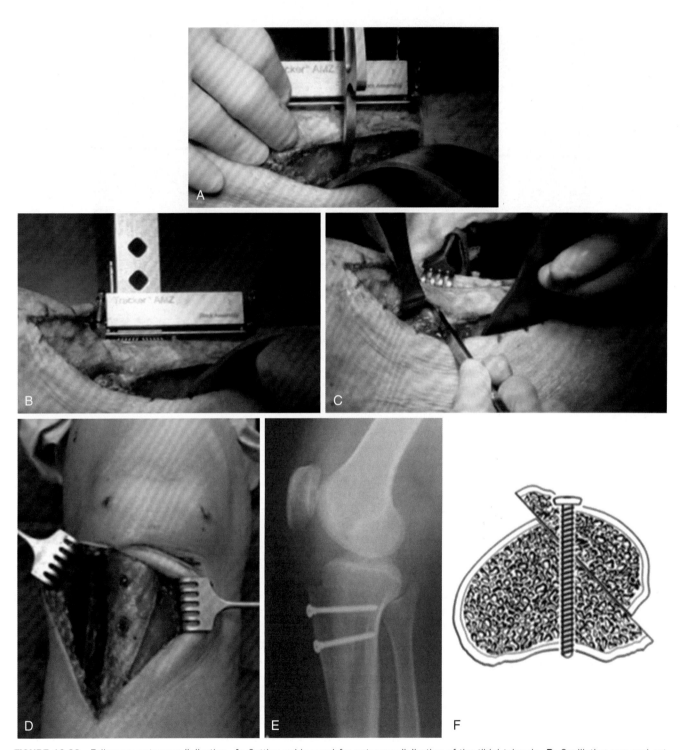

FIGURE 19-28 Fulkerson anteromedialization. **A:** Cutting guide used for anteromedialization of the tibial tubercle. **B:** Oscillating saw and cutting guide. **C:** Curved 1″ osteotome used to complete the osteotomy. **D:** Fixation of the transferred tibial tubercle using two bicortical screws. **E:** Postoperative lateral knee X-ray. **F:** Figure showing anterior and medial translation of the osteotomized tibial tubercle

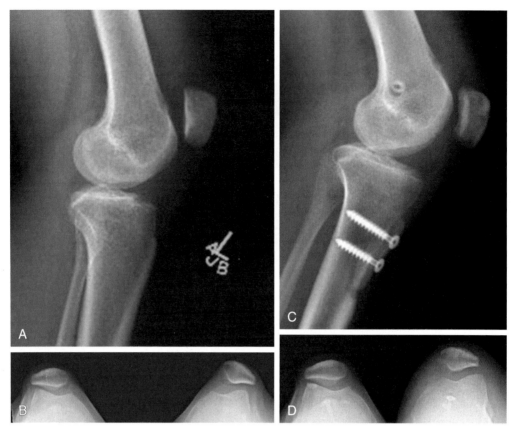

FIGURE 19-29   A: Lateral knee X-ray demonstrating patella alta. **B:** Axial (Merchant) X-ray showing asymmetrical lateral patellar subluxation of the left patella. **C:** Lateral knee X-ray showing combined distalization of the tibial tubercle and medial patellofemoral ligament reconstruction. **D:** Postoperative axial (Merchant) X-ray showing symmetrical realignment of the left patella.

the tibial shaft and in patients who smoke, use corticosteroids, or are overly aggressive in performing active knee extension during rehabilitation.[82] Regardless, a TTO is considered the accepted approach to addressing patellar instability in the setting of a TT–TG distance greater than 20 mm and often in patients with trochlear dysplasia.

For patients with patella alta, distalization of the tibial tubercle translates the patella closer to the tibiofemoral joint line. This causes the patella to engage the trochlear groove earlier in knee flexion allowing further support of the soft-tissue ligamentous stabilizers by the trochlear buttress. In this procedure, the medial and lateral retinaculum are released to allow distal mobilization of the tubercle. A rectangular osteotomy of the tibial tubercle is performed using a saw or osteotome (our preference to prevent thermal necrosis). The osteotomized tubercle is then pulled distally enough to reestablish a normal Caton–Deschamps or Blackburne–Peel ratio quantified by intraoperative fluoroscopy with the knee at 30°. The tubercle is provisionally held with two 0.62 mm Kirschner wires. A recipient trough is created in the proximal tibia to accommodate the distalized tubercle so as to maximize bone-to-bone contact. Two unicortical or bicortical screws are used for final fixation. Closure is similar to that of the other osteotomies. Proximal repair or reconstruction of the MPFL is then performed, as necessary (**Fig. 19-29**). Patients who smoke are strongly advised to discontinue tobacco use prior to a TTO of any type in order to enhance healing. Blood, urine, and salivary levels of cotinine (active metabolite of nicotine) can be monitored to confirm cessation of tobacco use in noncompliant patients at risk for delayed bone healing.

Postoperative rehabilitation following a TTO is more restrictive than the rehabilitation following an MPFL repair or reconstruction. Patients are maintained in a hinged knee brace with progressive increase in motion based on clinical symptoms and radiographic evidence of healing. Weight-bearing and quadriceps strengthening are advanced commensurate with tenderness at the osteotomy site and degree of radiographic healing (**Table 19-2**).

TABLE 19-2 **Postoperative Rehabilitation Following a Tibial Tubercle Osteotomy**

Phase I: (0-1 mo)

Range of motion (passive)

Week 2: 0°-70°

Week 3: 0°-90°

Week 6: 0°-120°

Week 8: 0°-135°

Range of motion (active)

No active extension allowed, active flexion as tolerated

Weight-bearing with brace locked in extension

Toe-touch weight-bearing only with brace locked in full extension

Modalities

Cryotherapy

Electrical stimulation to quadriceps

Exercises

Quadriceps, hamstring, gluteal isometrics

Ankle pumps

Four-way hip range of motion

Phase II: (1-3 mo)

Range of motion

At least 120°

Weight-bearing

Weeks 4-6: Toe-touch weight-bearing with brace locked in extension

Weeks 6-8: Weight bear as tolerated with brace locked in extension

Weeks 8-12: Emphasis on normal gait pattern

Modalities

Cryotherapy

Electrical stimulation to quadriceps as indicated

Exercises

Double-leg balance and coordination activities

Stationary bike at 8 wk

Upper body circuit training or ergometer

Strengthening

Isometric multiangle quadriceps sets

Closed-chain short arc strengthening in accordance with weight-bearing

Week 12: Isometric strength testing at 60° with quadriceps strength within 25% of contralateral limb

Phase III: >3 mo

Range of motion

Full

Weight-bearing

Full

Modalities

Cryotherapy

Exercises

Begin plyometrics

Stationary bike with progressive lowering of seat and increasing resistance

Light jogging

Swimming with flutter kick or stairmaster

Strengthening

Single-leg press

Single-leg balance board and proprioception exercises

Hip and core strengthening

Return to sports: 4-6 mo

Dynamic neuromuscular control exercises beginning with low-velocity single-plane progressing to higher velocity multiplane

Sport-specific functional progression

Isokinetic strength testing within 10% to 15% of contralateral limb

Femoral Trochleoplasty

In the setting of recurrent instability associated with a dysplastic trochlear groove, a femoral trochleoplasty attempts to restore the normal trochlear architecture. This is typically done by removing a triangular-shaped segment of subchondral bone under the central trochlear cartilage with a high-speed burr. The trochlear cartilage is then fractured in a "greenstick" fashion to depress the central articular surface. Alternatively, the lateral trochlea can be elevated up to 10 mm and supported with a structural graft under the elevated articular surface (Albee osteotomy) (**Fig. 19-30**). These techniques have been performed to deepen the trochlear groove with a high-level of success in Europe[83] with minimal complications (**Fig. 19-31**).[84] However, trochlear osteotomies are not widely utilized in the United States where the emphasis has been placed on addressing MPFL insufficiency and patellofemoral malalignment.

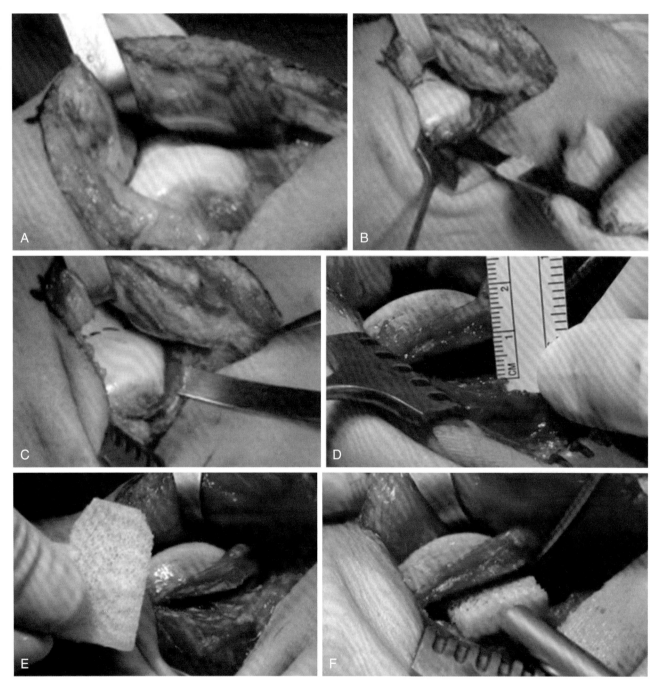

FIGURE 19-30 **A:** Arthrotomy of a patient with trochlear dysplasia. **B:** Osteotomy of the nonarticulating surface of the lateral trochlea. **C:** Osteotomy of the superolateral aspect of the trochlea. Note the dashed line indicating the deepest point of the trochlea. **D:** Measurement of the amount of elevation following the osteotomy. **E:** Allograft bone wedge used to support the elevated lateral trochlea. **F:** Implantation of the allograft wedge.

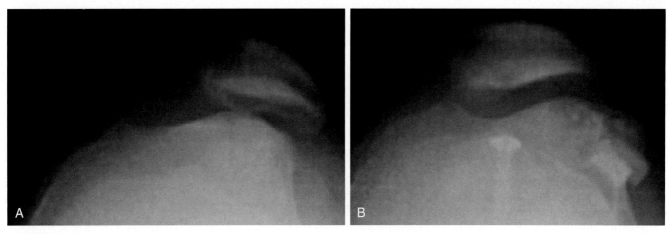

FIGURE 19-31 **A:** Axial (Merchant) X-ray of a patient with trochlear dysplasia. **B:** Postoperative axial X-ray of the same patient following an Albee osteotomy with elevation of the lateral trochlea.

CONCLUSION

Patellofemoral instability represents a spectrum of either a singular or recurrent episode(s) of patellar subluxation or dislocation. Instability results from either acute failure or chronic attenuation of the static soft-tissue restraints and/or pathologic biomechanics resulting from malalignment of the patellofemoral joint. Management of a first-time dislocation is typically nonoperative, with surgery reserved for acute, displaced osteochondral fractures or recurrent instability. Isolated or combined MPFL reconstruction, lateral retinacular release, TTO, and, occasionally, femoral trochleoplasty all represent surgical options for management of patellar instability. Ultimately, the patient's age, history, anatomy, physical examination, imaging, and activity goals all contribute to formulating the ideal treatment plan to address the instability and improve function.

REFERENCES

1. Devereaux MD, Lachmann SM. Patello-femoral arthralgia in athletes attending a Sports Injury Clinic. *Br J Sports Med.* 1984;18(1):18-21.
2. Powers CM, Witvrouw E, Davis IS, Crossley KM. Evidence-based framework for a pathomechanical model of patellofemoral pain. 2017 patellofemoral pain consensus statement from the 4th International Patellofemoral Pain Research Retreat, Manchester, UK: part 3. *Br J Sports Med.* 2017;51(24):1713-1723.
3. Crossley KM, Stefanik JJ, Selfe J, et al. Patellofemoral pain consensus statement from the 4th International Patellofemoral Pain Research Retreat, Manchester. Part 1: terminology, definitions, clinical examination, natural history, patellofemoral osteoarthritis and patient-reported outcome measures. *Br J Sports Med.* 2016;50:839-843.
4. Roush JR, Curtis Bay R. Prevalence of anterior knee pain in 18-35 year-old females. *Int J Sports Phys Ther.* 2012;7:396-401.
5. Baldon Rde M, Serrao FV, Scattone Silva R, Piva SR. Effects of functional stabilization training on pain, function, and lower extremity biomechanics in women with patellofemoral pain: a randomized clinical trial. *J Orthop Sports Phys Ther.* 2014;44(4):240-a248.
6. Crossley K, Bennell K, Green S, Cowan S, McConnell J. Physical therapy for patellofemoral pain: a randomized, double-blinded, placebo-controlled trial. *Am J Sports Med.* 2002;30(6):857-865.
7. Heintjes E, Berger MY, Bierma-Zeinstra SM, Bernsen RM, Verhaar JA, Koes BW. Pharmacotherapy for patellofemoral pain syndrome. *Cochrane Database Syst Rev.* 2004;3:CD003470.
8. McAlindon TE, Snow S, Cooper C, Dieppe PA. Radiographic patterns of osteoarthritis of the knee joint in the community: the importance of the patellofemoral joint. *Ann Rheum Dis.* 1992;51(7):844-849.
9. Parikh SN, Lykissas MG. Classification of lateral patellar instability in children and adolescents. *Orthop Clin North Am.* 2016;47(1):145-152.
10. Sanchis-Alfonso V, Merchant AC. Iatrogenic medial patellar instability: an avoidable injury. *Arthroscopy.* 2015;31(8):1628-1632.
11. Sanders TL, Pareek A, Hewett TE, Stuart MJ, Dahm DL, Krych AJ. Incidence of first-time lateral patellar dislocation: a 21-year population-based study. *Sports Health.* 2018;10(2):146-151.
12. Fithian DC, Paxton EW, Stone ML, et al. Epidemiology and natural history of acute patellar dislocation. *Am J Sports Med.* 2004;32(5):1114-1121.
13. Christensen TC, Sanders TL, Pareek A, Mohan R, Dahm DL, Krych AJ. Risk factors and time to recurrent ipsilateral and contralateral patellar dislocations. *Am J Sports Med.* 2017;45(9):2105-2110.
14. Sanders TL, Pareek A, Johnson NR, Stuart MJ, Dahm DL, Krych AJ. Patellofemoral arthritis after lateral patellar dislocation: a matched population-based analysis. *Am J Sports Med.* 2017;45(5):1012-1017.
15. Sherman SL, Plackis AC, Nuelle CW. Patellofemoral anatomy and biomechanics. *Clin Sports Med.* 2014;33(3):389-401.
16. Kaymaz B, Atay OA, Ergen FB, et al. Development of the femoral trochlear groove in rabbits with patellar malposition. *Knee Surg Sports Traumatol Arthrosc.* 2013;21(8):1841-1848.
17. Kwak SD, Colman WW, Ateshian GA, Grelsamer RP, Henry JH, Mow VC. Anatomy of the human patellofemoral joint articular cartilage: surface curvature analysis. *J Orthop Res.* 1997;15(3):468-472.
18. Kaufer H. Patellar biomechanics. *Clin Orthop Relat Res.* 1979;144:51-54.
19. Saltzman CL, Goulet JA, McClellan RT, Schneider LA, Matthews LS. Results of treatment of displaced patellar fractures by partial patellectomy. *J Bone Joint Surg Am.* 1990;72(9):1279-1285.
20. Ries Z, Bollier M. Patellofemoral instability in active adolescents. *J Knee Surg.* 2015;28(4):265-277.
21. Conlan T, Garth WP Jr, Lemons JE. Evaluation of the medial soft-tissue restraints of the extensor mechanism of the knee. *J Bone Joint Surg Am.* 1993;75(5):682-693.
22. Philippot R, Boyer B, Testa R, Farizon F, Moyen B. The role of the medial ligamentous structures on patellar tracking during knee flexion. *Knee Surg Sports Traumatol Arthrosc.* 2012;20(2):331-336.

23. Smith TO, Bowyer D, Dixon J, Stephenson R, Chester R, Donell ST. Can vastus medialis oblique be preferentially activated? A systematic review of electromyographic studies. *Physiother Theory Pract.* 2009;25(2):69-98.

24. Schottle PB, Schmeling A, Rosenstiel N, Weiler A. Radiographic landmarks for femoral tunnel placement in medial patellofemoral ligament reconstruction. *Am J Sports Med.* 2007;35(5):801-804.

25. Baldwin JL. The anatomy of the medial patellofemoral ligament. *Am J Sports Med.* 2009;37(12):2355-2361.

26. Tanaka MJ. The anatomy of the medial patellofemoral complex. *Sports Med Arthrosc Rev.* 2017;25(2):e8-e11.

27. Tanaka MJ. Variability in the patellar attachment of the medial patellofemoral ligament. *Arthroscopy.* 2016;32(8):1667-1670.

28. Amis AA. Current concepts on anatomy and biomechanics of patellar stability. *Sports Med Arthrosc Rev.* 2007;15(2):48-56.

29. LaPrade RF, Cram TR, James EW, Rasmussen MT. Trochlear dysplasia and the role of trochleoplasty. *Clin Sports Med.* 2014;33(3):531-545.

30. Jaquith BP, Parikh SN. Predictors of recurrent patellar instability in children and adolescents after first-time dislocation. *J Pediatr Orthop.* 2017;37(7):484-490.

31. Bollier M, Fulkerson JP. The role of trochlear dysplasia in patellofemoral instability. *J Am Acad Orthop Surg.* 2011;19(1):8-16.

32. Van Haver A, De Roo K, De Beule M, et al. The effect of trochlear dysplasia on patellofemoral biomechanics: a cadaveric study with simulated trochlear deformities. *Am J Sports Med.* 2015;43(6):1354-1361.

33. Frosch KH, Schmeling A. A new classification system of patellar instability and patellar maltracking. *Arch Orthop Trauma Surg.* 2016;136(4):485-497.

34. Hiemstra LA, Kerslake S, Lafave M, Heard SM, Buchko GM. Introduction of a classification system for patients with patellofemoral instability (WARPS and STAID). *Knee Surg Sports Traumatol Arthrosc.* 2014;22(11):2776-2782.

35. Harilainen A, Myllynen P, Antila H, Seitsalo S. The significance of arthroscopy and examination under anaesthesia in the diagnosis of fresh injury haemarthrosis of the knee joint. *Injury.* 1988;19(1):21-24.

36. Elias DA, White LM, Fithian DC. Acute lateral patellar dislocation at MR imaging: injury patterns of medial patellar soft-tissue restraints and osteochondral injuries of the inferomedial patella. *Radiology.* 2002;225(3):736-743.

37. Sillanpaa PJ, Salonen E, Pihlajamaki H, Maenpaa HM. Medial patellofemoral ligament avulsion injury at the patella: classification and clinical outcome. *Knee Surg Sports Traumatol Arthrosc.* 2014;22(10):2414-2418.

38. Stefancin JJ, Parker RD. First-time traumatic patellar dislocation: a systematic review. *Clin Orthop Relat Res.* 2007;455:93-101.

39. Liu JN, Steinhaus ME, Kalbian IL, et al. Patellar instability management: a survey of the International Patellofemoral Study Group. *Am J Sports Med.* 2018;46(13):3299-3306.

40. Batra S, Arora S. Habitual dislocation of patella: a review. *J Clin Orthop Trauma.* 2014;5(4):245-251.

41. Shen HC, Chao KH, Huang GS, Pan RY, Lee CH. Combined proximal and distal realignment procedures to treat the habitual dislocation of the patella in adults. *Am J Sports Med.* 2007;35(12):2101-2108.

42. Wada A, Fujii T, Takamura K, Yanagida H, Surijamorn P. Congenital dislocation of the patella. *J Child Orthop.* 2008;2(2):119-123.

43. Lee BJ, Christino MA, Daniels AH, Hulstyn MJ, Eberson CP. Adolescent patellar osteochondral fracture following patellar dislocation. *Knee Surg Sports Traumatol Arthrosc.* 2013;21(8):1856-1861.

44. Palmu S, Kallio PE, Donell ST, Helenius I, Nietosvaara Y. Acute patellar dislocation in children and adolescents: a randomized clinical trial. *J Bone Joint Surg Am.* 2008;90(3):463-470.

45. Ahmad CS, Brown GD, Shubin Stein BE. The docking technique for medial patellofemoral ligament reconstruction: surgical technique and clinical outcome. *Am J Sports Med.* 2009;37(10):2021-2027.

46. Ahmad CS, McCarthy M, Gomez JA, Shubin Stein BE. The moving patellar apprehension test for lateral patellar instability. *Am J Sports Med.* 2009;37(4):791-796.

47. Juul-Kristensen B, Rogind H, Jensen DV, Remvig L. Inter-examiner reproducibility of tests and criteria for generalized joint hypermobility and benign joint hypermobility syndrome. *Rheumatology.* 2007;46(12):1835-1841.

48. Singh H, McKay M, Baldwin J, et al. Beighton scores and cut-offs across the lifespan: cross-sectional study of an Australian population. *Rheumatology.* 2017;56(11):1857-1864.

49. Aglietti P, Insall JN, Cerulli G. Patellar pain and incongruence. I: measurements of incongruence. *Clin Orthop Relat Res.* 1983;176:217-224.

50. Davies AP, Costa ML, Shepstone L, Glasgow MM, Donell S. The sulcus angle and malalignment of the extensor mechanism of the knee. *J Bone Joint Surg Br.* 2000;82(8):1162-1166.

51. Grelsamer RP, Bazos AN, Proctor CS. Radiographic analysis of patellar tilt. *J Bone Joint Surg Br.* 1993;75(5):822-824.

52. Insall J, Salvati E. Patella position in the normal knee joint. *Radiology.* 1971;101(1):101-104.

53. Caton J, Deschamps G, Chambat P, Lerat JL, Dejour H. Patella infera. Apropos of 128 cases. *Rev Chir Orthop Reparatrice Appar Mot.* 1982;68(5):317-325.

54. Blackburne JS, Peel TE. A new method of measuring patellar height. *J Bone Joint Surg Br.* 1977;59(2):241-242.

55. Berg EE, Mason SL, Lucas MJ. Patellar height ratios: a comparison of four measurement methods. *Am J Sports Med.* 1996;24(2):218-221.

56. Portner O, Pakzad H. The evaluation of patellar height: a simple method. *J Bone Joint Surg Am.* 2011;93(1):73-80.

57. Dejour H, Walch G, Nove-Josserand L, Guier C. Factors of patellar instability: an anatomic radiographic study. *Knee Surg Sports Traumatol Arthrosc.* 1994;2(1):19-26.

58. Luo CF. Reference axes for reconstruction of the knee. *Knee.* 2004;11(4):251-257.

59. Duchman K, Bollier M. Distal realignment: indications, technique, and results. *Clin Sports Med.* 2014;33(3):517-530.

60. Camp CL, Stuart MJ, Krych AJ, et al. CT and MRI measurements of tibial tubercle-trochlear groove distances are not equivalent in patients with patellar instability. *Am J Sports Med.* 2013;41(8):1835-1840.

61. Camathias C, Pagenstert G, Stutz U, Barg A, Muller-Gerbl M, Nowakowski AM. The effect of knee flexion and rotation on the tibial tuberosity-trochlear groove distance. *Knee Surg Sports Traumatol Arthrosc.* 2016;24(9):2811-2817.

62. Weber-Spickschen TS, Spang J, Kohn L, Imhoff AB, Schottle PB. The relationship between trochlear dysplasia and medial patellofemoral ligament rupture location after patellar dislocation: an MRI evaluation. *Knee.* 2011;18(3):185-188.

63. Felus J, Kowalczyk B. Age-related differences in medial patellofemoral ligament injury patterns in traumatic patellar dislocation: case series of 50 surgically treated children and adolescents. *Am J Sports Med.* 2012;40(10):2357-2364.

64. Zheng L, Shi H, Feng Y, Sun BS, Ding HY, Zhang GY. Injury patterns of medial patellofemoral ligament and correlation analysis with articular cartilage lesions of the lateral femoral condyle after acute lateral patellar dislocation in children and adolescents: an MRI evaluation. *Injury.* 2015;46(6):1137-1144.

65. Cruz AI Jr, Richmond CG, Tompkins MA, Heyer A, Shea KG, Beck JJ. What's new in pediatric sports conditions of the knee? *J Pediatr Orthop.* 2018;38(2):e66-e72.

66. Apostolovic M, Vukomanovic B, Slavkovic N, et al. Acute patellar dislocation in adolescents: operative versus nonoperative treatment. *Int Orthop.* 2011;35(10):1483-1487.

67. Askenberger M, Bengtsson Mostrom E, Ekstrom W, et al. Operative repair of medial patellofemoral ligament injury versus knee brace in children with an acute first-time traumatic patellar dislocation: a randomized controlled trial. *Am J Sports Med.* 2018;46(10):2328-2340.

68. Vavken P, Wimmer MD, Camathias C, Quidde J, Valderrabano V, Pagenstert G. Treating patella instability in skeletally immature patients. *Arthroscopy*. 2013;29(8):1410-1422.

69. Smith TO, Song F, Donell ST, Hing CB. Operative versus non-operative management of patellar dislocation. A meta-analysis. *Knee Surg Sports Traumatol Arthrosc*. 2011;19(6):988-998.

70. McConnell J. Rehabilitation and nonoperative treatment of patellar instability. *Sports Med Arthrosc Rev*. 2007;15(2):95-104.

71. Weber AE, Nathani A, Dines JS, et al. An algorithmic approach to the management of recurrent lateral patellar dislocation. *J Bone Joint Surg Am*. 2016;98(5):417-427.

72. Dragoo JL, Nguyen M, Gatewood CT, Taunton JD, Young S. Medial patellofemoral ligament repair versus reconstruction for recurrent patellar instability: two-year results of an algorithm-based approach. *Orthop J Sports Med*. 2017;5(3):2325967116689465.

73. Schneider DK, Grawe B, Magnussen RA, et al. Outcomes after isolated medial patellofemoral ligament reconstruction for the treatment of recurrent lateral patellar dislocations: a systematic review and meta-analysis. *Am J Sports Med*. 2016;44(11):2993-3005.

74. Weinberger JM, Fabricant PD, Taylor SA, Mei JY, Jones KJ. Influence of graft source and configuration on revision rate and patient-reported outcomes after MPFL reconstruction: a systematic review and meta-analysis. *Knee Surg Sports Traumatol Arthrosc*. 2017;25(8):2511-2519.

75. Pichler W, Tesch NP, Schwantzer G, et al. Differences in length and cross-section of semitendinosus and gracilis tendons and their effect on anterior cruciate ligament reconstruction: a cadaver study. *J Bone Joint Surg Br*. 2008;90(4):516-519.

76. Sanchis-Alfonso V, Montesinos-Berry E, Ramirez-Fuentes C, Leal-Blanquet J, Gelber PE, Monllau JC. Failed medial patellofemoral ligament reconstruction: causes and surgical strategies. *World J Orthop*. 2017;8(2):115-129.

77. Shea KG, Martinson WD, Cannamela PC, et al. Variation in the medial patellofemoral ligament origin in the skeletally immature knee: an anatomic study. *Am J Sports Med*. 2018;46(2):363-369.

78. Nelitz M, Dreyhaupt J, Reichel H, Woelfle J, Lippacher S. Anatomic reconstruction of the medial patellofemoral ligament in children and adolescents with open growth plates: surgical technique and clinical outcome. *Am J Sports Med*. 2013;41(1):58-63.

79. Grawe B, Stein BE. Tibial tubercle osteotomy: indication and techniques. *J Knee Surg*. 2015;28(4):279-284.

80. Fulkerson JP. Anteromedialization of the tibial tuberosity for patellofemoral malalignment. *Clin Orthop Relat Res*. 1983;177:176-181.

81. Longo UG, Rizzello G, Ciuffreda M, et al. Elmslie-Trillat, Maquet, Fulkerson, Roux Goldthwait, and other distal realignment procedures for the management of patellar dislocation: systematic review and quantitative synthesis of the literature. *Arthroscopy*. 2016;32(5):929-943.

82. Payne J, Rimmke N, Schmitt LC, Flanigan DC, Magnussen RA. The incidence of complications of tibial tubercle osteotomy: a systematic review. *Arthroscopy*. 2015;31(9):1819-1825.

83. Longo UG, Vincenzo C, Mannering N, et al. Trochleoplasty techniques provide good clinical results in patients with trochlear dysplasia. *Knee Surg Sports Traumatol Arthrosc*. 2018;26(9):2640-2658.

84. van Sambeeck JDP, van de Groes SAW, Verdonschot N, Hannink G. Trochleoplasty procedures show complication rates similar to other patellar-stabilizing procedures. *Knee Surg Sports Traumatol Arthrosc*. 2018;26(9):2841-2857.

chapter 20

Cartilage Repair in the Patellofemoral Joint

Tom Minas, MD, MS | Takahiro Ogura, MD

INTRODUCTION

Anterior knee pain often occurs secondary to multifactorial causes including an abnormal quadriceps angle, valgus malalignment, patella alta, trochlea dysplasia, and others which can result in patellofemoral malalignment or maltracking and possible instability and pain. When treating articular cartilage lesions, the surgeon must uncover background factors as the causation of the articular lesions that must be addressed at the time of cartilage repair in order to obtain successful outcomes. This was noted by Brittberg et al[1] when patella autologous chondrocyte implantation (ACI) had initial poor outcomes; only 2/7 (29%) of patella had good/excellent outcomes in the initial series improving to 11/14 (79%) with realignment when maltracking was corrected.[2]

The goal of this chapter is to provide the orthopedic surgeon with practical and comprehensive management guidelines for unipolar and bipolar cartilage lesions in the patellofemoral (PF) joint. All cartilage repair procedures have shown worse outcomes in the PF joint than in the tibiofemoral (TF) joint. This is likely due to the complex anatomy and biomechanical environment of the PF joint. Special consideration is necessary for PF cartilage restoration; assessing the lesion size and location, the technique chosen should mirror good clinical outcomes in this compartment, and most importantly uncovering the correct background causation factors for the articular injury in order to obtain a successful outcome. Other considerations in the PF joint accounting for a slower and more prolonged recovery include the cartilage thickness (anywhere from 5 to 7 mm in the patella and trochlea thickness as compared to 2-3 mm in the weight-bearing condyles). In addition, the PF joint is loaded in shear as opposed to compression in the TF joint, which is less favorable for cellular repair and maturation of regenerating tissue.

NONSURGICAL TREATMENT

Nonsurgical treatment for cartilage lesions in the PF joints includes physical therapy, nonsteroidal anti-inflammatory medications, injection therapies including intra-articular corticosteroid, hyaluronic acid viscosupplementation, platelet-rich plasma, and stem cells (marrow/fat derived).

Physical therapy should focus on reducing pain and swelling. This can be improved by starting proximal to distal in the kinetic chain. Core strength; hip stabilization to prevent "dynamic valgus," working on external hip rotators; stretching of the ITB, quadriceps, and hamstrings; and improving the balance between vastus medialis and vastus lateralis. These maneuvers may decrease the loading of the PF joint. Quadriceps strength should be improved via closed chain strengthening and short arc quadriceps, avoiding loading the knee via open-chain resisted quadriceps strengthening between 40° and 70° where contact forces are maximal. Squatting and kneeling which impose relatively high stress on the PF joints should be avoided. The role for bracing or taping is unclear. Nonsurgical treatment should be attempted for at least 3 to 6 months before considering surgical treatment as most patients will experience pain relief, which may delay the need for surgery altogether. In senior author's practice for referred patients who have failed previous treatment, approximately 10% succeed with nonsurgical treatment after chondroplasty and physical therapy.

SURGICAL TREATMENT

Chondroplasty

Chondroplasty, or débridement, is the most commonly performed cartilage procedure. This technique is invasive and is performed arthroscopically. It consists of debriding the unstable cartilage tissue to a stable rim. In general, the indication for this procedure includes small (1-2 cm²) contained chondral lesions. Reports of the outcomes after chondroplasty in the PF joints are limited. Postoperative physical therapy is important for a good outcome. Recently, Anderson et al[3] reported good clinical outcomes with 2-year follow-up in patients who underwent mechanical chondroplasty in isolation in the cohort of patients, in which approximately half of those had chondral lesions in the PF joints. However, long-term outcomes still remain unclear.

Bone Marrow Stimulation

This procedure includes débridement of chondral lesions with removal of the calcified layer of cartilage tissue to enhance repair integration to the subchondral bone and penetration into the subchondral bone to release bone marrow elements to the defect surface. This allows stem cells and growth factors to form a "super clot" and stimulate cartilage repair via a cell-based repair. In general, the indication for this procedure has included an acute (<3-6 months post injury) small chondral and contained lesion (<2-3 cm^2). Bipolar lesions and uncontained lesions are contraindications to this procedure. Strict adhesion to the principle of the technique is necessary for a favorable outcome as well as a strict postoperative protocol of touch weight-bearing for 6 weeks and the use of continuous passive motion. Kreuz et al noted the decline of clinical outcomes after 2 years for chondral lesions treated with microfracture.[4] This is likely due to the nature of the repair tissue consisting of collagen type I instead of collagen type II. They also evaluated the outcomes after microfracture based on the compartment treated: PF versus TF. They demonstrated unfavorable results for the PF joints compared to TF joints.[4] The best results occurred when the patient was less than 40 years old, when surgery was performed within 12 months of the injury, and the body mass index was less than 30 kg/mm^2. In addition, although technically simple to perform, microfracture may require a mini arthrotomy to access the patella, and as the results for the patella are unpredictable one must always consider a subsequent salvage procedure such as ACI.[5,6] Unfortunately, following microfracture, ACI has been shown to have an increased failure rate. Microfracture can in fact "burn bridges" for future treatments.

Osteochondral Autograft Transplantation

Osteochondral autograft transplantation (OAT) is generally indicated for a lesion area of approximately 2 to 4 cm^2. This technique involves harvesting 10- to 15-mm-deep autologous osteochondral plugs from the femoral condyle and/or trochlea and transplanting them into the cartilage defect (**Fig. 20-1**). The defect is filled with harvested hyaline cartilage and the underlying subchondral bone as an "osteochondral unit." However, OAT takes from "Peter to pay Paul" and consequently may result in donor tissue morbidity. The osteochondral donor plugs should be harvested from the margins of the distal lateral and medial trochlea or intercondylar notch and stay out of the load-bearing portion of the PF joint. Further concerns include the unmatched shape or incongruous shape of the host and donor cartilage surfaces in addition to the limitation of defect size for relatively small lesions. Realistically lesions of 1.5 to 2 cm^2 are what most surgeons utilize as a cutoff for not causing donor site problems. The surgical technique requires a precise graft fit and making a smooth articular surface for the PF joint for a satisfactory outcome. The unique anatomy of the patella and trochlea specifically impose

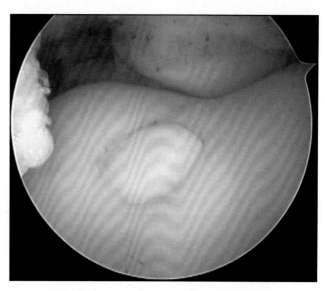

FIGURE 20-1 Autologous osteochondral plug for cartilage lesion in the trochlea.

surgical difficulties in matching the articular geometry of the donor to the patella or the trochlea. In addition, the articular thickness of the cartilage from the femoral surfaces is only 2 to 3 mm, whereas the patella thickness is 5 to 7 mm. In matching the surface topography, the donor plug is usually surrounded by articular cartilage and not subchondral bone and is therefore prone to resorption and collapse over time.

The outcomes of OAT in the PF joints are inconsistent. Hangody et al reported 79% good to excellent results in patients with chondral lesions in the PF joints, and 92% in the femoral condyle.[7] On the other hand, most others found almost a universal failure of OAT in the patella.[8] Bentley recommended universal abandonment of the technique in the patella because of the abysmal results when compared to ACI.[8] A recent study with a larger sample size by Astur and colleagues demonstrated OAT for patellar defects had better outcomes at 2 years for lesions smaller than 2.5 cm^2.[9] The inconsistency in outcomes may be explained by the fact that the results are likely dependent on the exacting surgical technique required, the importance of grafting perpendicular, and flush to the adjacent cartilage in order for satisfactory results in the PF joints.[10]

Autologous Chondrocyte Implantation/MACI

The FDA approved the use of ACI for the treatment of large cartilage defects of the femoral condyles and trochlea in 1997. Despite its "off-label" use, several studies have reported good and excellent clinical outcomes in patients who have undergone ACI for unipolar patellar and bipolar-patella and trochlea defects.[11-14] MACI (matrix autologous chondrocyte implantation), a third-generation cartilage repair technique using autologous chondrocytes, was recently approved by the FDA in December 2016

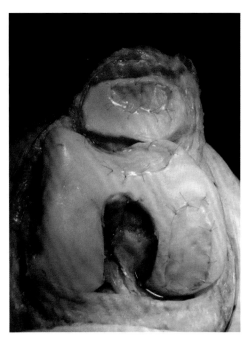

FIGURE 20-2 MACI for multiple cartilage lesions including PF joints.

(**Fig. 20-2**). Matrix-induced autologous chondrocyte implantation (MACI) are cultured in a three dimensional membrane. Its labeling was specific to all surfaces of the knee, and not just the femoral surfaces based on recent studies demonstrating improved clinical outcomes in the patella trochlea and bipolar lesions as noted above. The advantage of ACI/MACI includes the treatment of large defects (>3-4 cm²) easily matching the complex contour of the patella and trochlear articular surfaces.

ACI is a two-stage procedure. The initial surgery includes an arthroscopic evaluation of the joint and determination of the defect characteristics that may be suitable for ACI/MACI. If the defect(s) are well contained and are ICRS grade 3 or 4 in depth, a cartilage biopsy of approximately 200 to 300 mg of articular cartilage from a non–weight-bearing area, usually the superior intercondylar notch or a peripheral margin of the trochlea, is harvested. The tissue is then digested so that the chondrocytes may be freed, cultured, and then cryopreserved. After insurance approval for transplantation, they are then thawed and recultured for definitive implantation. Secondary surgery is then performed for implantation with arthrotomy. First-generation ACI uses the periosteum that was harvested from the proximal tibia or distal femur. A second-generation ACI uses a type I/III bilayer collagen membrane, derived from porcine peritoneum and skin instead of autologous periosteum. The use of a type I/III bilayer collagen membrane was off-label and used with an informed consent. The periosteum or collagen membrane was placed on the cartilage defect and secured with multiple absorbable sutures. In some uncontained defects, small wires are used to drill holes in adjacent bone and sutures are passed through these holes to

anchor the membrane. The suture line is waterproofed with fibrin glue and autologous cultured chondrocytes are then injected underneath the membrane.

When reviewing recent studies in the PF joint, one study stands out. In a multicenter study of 110 patients with cartilage defects in the patella treated with ACI, 92% of the patients stated that they would undergo the procedure again, 83% rated their clinical outcomes as good or excellent and improved at a mean of 7.5 years postoperatively.[11]

In another multicenter ACI study of 40 patients with cartilage defects in the trochlea, Mandelbaum et al reported improved functional outcomes at a mean follow-up at 59 months.[15] Our recent study evaluating bipolar, patella–trochlea defects, with an average of 9 years follow-up, showed comparable results to unipolar results (survival rate of 83% and 79% at 5 and 10 years, respectively). In addition, when defects were treated with unloading osteotomy as the primary surgery, the 10 year survivorship was 93%.[16] Subchondral bone abnormalities in the PF joint including cystic lesions, sclerotic bone, bone marrow edema, etc. were treated at same surgery using the ACI "sandwich" technique,[17,18] which may require autologous bone grafting. Excellent results after ACI sandwich technique has been reported in the cohorts of cartilage lesions in the TF and PF joints.[18]

Osteochondral Allograft Transplantation

The use of fresh osteochondral allograft (OCA) transplantation increased after the FDA imposed stricter guidelines for the procurement and storage of allograft tissues, which decreased the risk of disease transmission. In general, the indication of this procedure includes large full-thickness cartilage lesions with abnormal subchondral bone, traumatic osteochondral injuries, osteochondritis dissecans, avascular necrosis, articular injuries with subchondral cysts/stiffened subchondral bone/intralesional osteophytes after failed marrow stimulation procedures, or uncontained chondral defects with bone loss—usually posttraumatic (**Fig. 20-3**). OCA has the advantage of being a single-stage procedure and having the ability to treat large osteochondral lesions with mature, layered, viable tissue while avoiding potential donor site morbidity compared with OAT. Several studies have reported OCA failure rate to be higher in the PF joint than in the TF joint. In a recent systematic review, Assenmacher et al[19] reported failure rates of 50% for OCA after a mean follow-up of 12.3 years in the PF joints while 24% in the TF joints. On the other hand, a different recent systematic review (including five different high-volume centers) showed survival rates in the PF joints of 87.9% and 77.2% at 5 and 10 years, respectively.[20] Technically as with the OAT technique (but more so as the defects are larger),

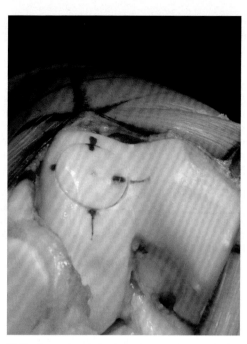

FIGURE 20-3 Osteochondral allograft transplantation for cartilage lesions in the trochlea.

matching the morphology is more challenging than for the femoral condyles. Precise matching of the congruity with perpendicular placement to the adjacent cartilage is critical for excellent outcomes and is based on surgeon skill to obtain good clinical outcomes. Inferior results were reported with bipolar lesions. Mizayan et al reported that comparable results to unipolar trochlea or patella grafts were comparable to grafts of the femoral condyles with an average follow-up of 33.2 months.[21] As good as fresh matched OCA results are in the short term when technically performed well, the long-term results tend to fail over time by creeping substitution of the bone and collapse of the allograft.[22,23]

Particulated Cartilage Procedures

The use of particulated or minced cartilage techniques are increasing in the United States because they are easy to perform and are less expensive than ACI. The indication includes focal full-thickness chondral defects between 1 and 6 cm². The particulated juvenile cartilage allograft is from fresh tissue donors and implanted in the defect and secured with the fibrin glue (**Fig. 20-4**). Several studies have reported good clinical outcomes over a short-term follow-up.[24-27] In addition, Farr et al reported that the repaired tissue are a mixture of hyaline and fibrocartilage with a dominance of type II collagen at 2 years postoperatively.[27] Long-term results are expected to hopefully confirm these good outcomes.

Disadvantages of these procedures are similar to fresh osteochondral allograft including the risk of transmission of infectious diseases, tissue rejection, and allograft availability.

Postoperative Rehabilitation

Postoperatively, we recommend the use of continuous passive motion for 6 to 8 hours every day. Patellar mobilizations in full extension—proximal–distal and medial–lateral—are implemented on the day of surgery to diminish the risk of Hoffa fat pad fibrosis. Partial weight-bearing in an extension locked brace is allowed with gradual progression to full weight-bearing by 6 to 8 weeks. Return to pivoting sports is not recommended until 12 to 18 months after surgery. The postoperative recovery protocol should be individually adjusted according to concurrent procedures, degree of graft maturation, and previous activity level.

Summary

The treatment of cartilage lesions in the PF joint is challenging despite having various procedures currently

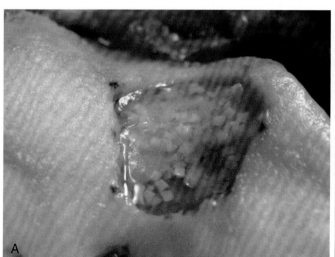
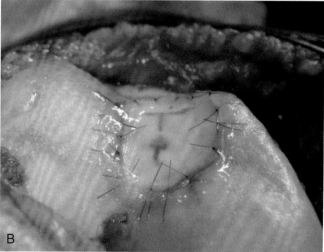

FIGURE 20-4 Particulated juvenile cartilage allograft for cartilage lesions in the trochlea. **A:** Standard technique, **B:** authors' preferred technique to maintain particulated allograft in defect during repair process due to shear forces in PF joint.

available. In any procedure, a careful assessment is necessary to uncover the background factors that must be addressed prior to or at the time of the cartilage repair procedure in order to have a successful outcome. Meticulous surgical technique is required to obtain a good outcome in addition to a compliant patient and good postoperative rehabilitation.

A thorough discussion between the patient and surgeon before surgery is crucial in order to match expectations to a realistic outcome to obtain a satisfied patient.

REFERENCES

1. Brittberg M, Lindahl A, Nilsson A, Ohlsson C, Isaksson O, Peterson L. Treatment of deep cartilage defects in the knee with autologous chondrocyte transplantation. *N Engl J Med.* 1994;331(14):889-895.
2. Peterson L, Minas T, Brittberg M, Nilsson A, Sjogren-Jansson E, Lindahl A. Two- to 9-year outcome after autologous chondrocyte transplantation of the knee. *Clin Orthop Relat Res.* 2000;374:212-234.
3. Anderson DE, Rose MB, Wille AJ, Wiedrick J, Crawford DC. Arthroscopic mechanical chondroplasty of the knee is beneficial for treatment of focal cartilage lesions in the absence of concurrent pathology. *Orthop J Sports Med.* 2017;5(5):2325967117707213.
4. Kreuz PC, Steinwachs MR, Erggelet C, et al. Results after microfracture of full-thickness chondral defects in different compartments in the knee. *Osteoarthr Cartil.* 2006;14(11):1119-1125.
5. Minas T, Gomoll AH, Rosenberger R, Royce RO, Bryant T. Increased failure rate of autologous chondrocyte implantation after previous treatment with marrow stimulation techniques. *Am J Sports Med.* 2009;37(5):902-908.
6. Pestka JM, Bode G, Salzmann G, Sudkamp NP, Niemeyer P. Clinical outcome of autologous chondrocyte implantation for failed microfracture treatment of full-thickness cartilage defects of the knee joint. *Am J Sports Med.* 2012;40(2):325-331.
7. Hangody L, Fules P. Autologous osteochondral mosaicplasty for the treatment of full-thickness defects of weight-bearing joints: ten years of experimental and clinical experience. *J Bone Joint Surg Am.* 2003;85-A(suppl 2):25-32.
8. Bentley G, Biant LC, Carrington RW, et al. A prospective, randomised comparison of autologous chondrocyte implantation versus mosaicplasty for osteochondral defects in the knee. *J Bone Joint Surg Br.* 2003;85(2):223-230.
9. Astur DC, Arliani GG, Binz M, et al. Autologous osteochondral transplantation for treating patellar chondral injuries: evaluation, treatment, and outcomes of a two-year follow-up study. *J Bone Joint Surg Am.* 2014;96(10):816-823.
10. Yabumoto H, Nakagawa Y, Mukai S, Saji T. Osteochondral autograft transplantation for isolated patellofemoral osteoarthritis. *Knee.* 2017;24(6):1498-1503.
11. Gomoll AH, Gillogly SD, Cole BJ, et al. Autologous chondrocyte implantation in the patella: a multicenter experience. *Am J Sports Med.* 2014;42(5):1074-1081.
12. von Keudell A, Han R, Bryant T, Minas T. Autologous chondrocyte implantation to isolated patella cartilage defects. *Cartilage.* 2017;8(2):146-154.
13. Minas T, Bryant T. The role of autologous chondrocyte implantation in the patellofemoral joint. *Clin Orthop Relat Res.* 2005;436:30-39.
14. Farr J. Autologous chondrocyte implantation improves patellofemoral cartilage treatment outcomes. *Clin Orthop Relat Res.* 2007;463:187-194.
15. Mandelbaum B, Browne JE, Fu F, et al. Treatment outcomes of autologous chondrocyte implantation for full-thickness articular cartilage defects of the trochlea. *Am J Sports Med.* 2007;35(6):915-921.
16. Ogura T, Bryant T, Merkely G, Minas T. Autologous chondrocyte implantation for bipolar chondral lesions in the patellofemoral compartment: clinical outcomes at a mean 9 years' follow-up. *Am J Sports Med.* 2019;47(4):837-846.
17. von Keudell A, Gomoll AH, Bryant T, Minas T. Spontaneous osteonecrosis of the knee treated with autologous chondrocyte implantation, autologous bone-grafting, and osteotomy: a report of two cases with follow-up of seven and nine years. *J Bone Joint Surg Am.* 2011;93(24):e149.
18. Minas T, Ogura T, Headrick J, Bryant T. Autologous chondrocyte implantation "sandwich" technique compared with autologous bone grafting for deep osteochondral lesions in the knee. *Am J Sports Med.* 2018;46(2):322-332.
19. Assenmacher AT, Pareek A, Reardon PJ, Macalena JA, Stuart MJ, Krych AJ. Long-term outcomes after osteochondral allograft: a systematic review at long-term follow-up of 12.3 years. *Arthroscopy.* 2016;32(10):2160-2168.
20. Chahla J, Sweet MC, Okoroha KR, et al. Osteochondral allograft transplantation in the patellofemoral joint: a systematic review. *Am J Sports Med.* 2019;47(12):3009-3018.
21. Mirzayan R, Charles MD, Batech M, Suh BD, DeWitt D. Bipolar osteochondral allograft transplantation of the patella and trochlea. *Cartilage.* 2018:1947603518796124. Epub 2018/09/04.
22. Gross AE, Shasha N, Aubin P. Long-term followup of the use of fresh osteochondral allografts for posttraumatic knee defects. *Clin Orthop Relat Res.* 2005;435:79-87.
23. Oakeshott RD, Farine I, Pritzker KP, Langer F, Gross AE. A clinical and histologic analysis of failed fresh osteochondral allografts. *Clin Orthop Relat Res.* 1988;233:283-294.
24. Tompkins M, Hamann JC, Diduch DR, et al. Preliminary results of a novel single-stage cartilage restoration technique: particulated juvenile articular cartilage allograft for chondral defects of the patella. *Arthroscopy.* 2013;29(10):1661-1670.
25. Bonner KF, Daner W, Yao JQ. 2-year postoperative evaluation of a patient with a symptomatic full-thickness patellar cartilage defect repaired with particulated juvenile cartilage tissue. *J Knee Surg.* 2010;23(2):109-114.
26. Buckwalter JA, Bowman GN, Albright JP, Wolf BR, Bollier M. Clinical outcomes of patellar chondral lesions treated with juvenile particulated cartilage allografts. *Iowa Orthop J.* 2014;34:44-49.
27. Farr J, Tabet SK, Margerrison E, Cole BJ. Clinical, radiographic, and histological outcomes after cartilage repair with particulated juvenile articular cartilage: a 2-year prospective study. *Am J Sports Med.* 2014;42(6):1417-1425.

chapter 21

Patellofemoral Arthroplasty

Joseph A. Karam, MD | Jess H. Lonner, MD

INTRODUCTION

While degenerative changes of the patellofemoral joint exist in at least half of patients with knee osteoarthritis, isolated patellofemoral osteoarthritis is not rare, and a recent meta-analysis revealed radiographic evidence of patellofemoral osteoarthritis in 17% of healthy individuals and 20% of patients presenting knee pain.[1,2] Risk factors include trauma, female gender, advanced age, increased body mass index (BMI), quadriceps and abductor weakness, as well as local anatomic factors such as trochlear dysplasia and valgus alignment of the lower extremity.[3,4] These patients may have significant impact on their quality of life, although it should be most profound with regard to activities that load the anterior knee and less impactful when patients are standing upright and walking on level surfaces.[5,6] Various nonsurgical and surgical options have been described for the management of patellofemoral arthritis.[7] Patellofemoral arthroplasty (PFA) is an effective treatment for isolated arthritis of the patellofemoral joint, especially after failure of reasonable nonoperative treatments. Total knee arthroplasty (TKA) was regarded as the standard and reproducible treatment for these patients in the past; however, it significantly alters knee kinematics and would sacrifice the otherwise-healthy tibiofemoral compartments.[8] Additionally, given that 50% of PFA candidates are 50 years old or younger,[9] TKA may be undesirable for many patients with isolated patellofemoral arthritis, particularly in light of recent data showing improved function after PFA compared to TKA performed for isolated patellofemoral arthritis.[10-12] Thus, PFA has gained greater interest as understanding of selection criteria has evolved and designs have improved.[9,13,14]

INDICATIONS AND CONTRAINDICATIONS

Perhaps the most critical factor determining the success of PFA remains appropriate patient selection. Indications for PFA include patients with isolated patellofemoral arthritis (or Outerbridge grade IV lateral patellar facet and/or lateral trochlear chondromalacia) due to primary osteoarthritis, posttraumatic arthritis, or secondary to trochlear dysplasia, patellar maltracking/subluxation, and/or patellar instability. Pain should be shown to be inadequately responsive to nonoperative treatment measures, which may include physical therapy, weight loss, nonsteroidal anti-inflammatory medication, activity modification, injections, or bracing.

On the other hand, this procedure should not be offered to individuals with pain on the medial or lateral aspects of the knee or evidence of arthritis or grade III-IV chondromalacia in the tibiofemoral compartments, as well as patients with inflammatory arthritis, chondrocalcinosis, fixed flexion contracture more than 10°, or uncorrected patellofemoral or tibiofemoral malalignment, as these suggest more diffuse pathology which cannot be adequately managed by isolated PFA.[15] While mild to moderate patellar maltracking or patellar tilt is easily addressed at the time of PFA with lateral retinacular release or recession and appropriate positioning of the trochlear and patellar components, severe patellofemoral malalignment or rotational deformity, noted on clinical examination and confirmed with imaging, is a relative contraindication if not correctable prior to, or simultaneous with, PFA. Patella baja, patellar tendon scarring, and quadriceps weakness are other reported relative contraindications to PFA.[4] Of note, PFA may be used in conjunction with a unicompartmental knee arthroplasty (so-called bicompartmental knee arthroplasty) in patients with medial or lateral tibiofemoral degenerative disease.[16,17] Additionally, focal femoral condylar cartilaginous lesions noted on preoperative magnetic resonance imaging (MRI) or at the time of PFA can be effectively addressed with combined PFA and osteochondral grafting.[18]

Intuitively, due to the increased patellofemoral stresses associated with increased weight, obese patients are thought to be at increased risk of failure after PFA, but more of an issue, is that obese patients are more likely to have subtle or overt tibiofemoral disease which can compromise the results of PFA. Indeed, this has been confirmed by previous studies, demonstrating that obese patients (BMI >30 kg/m^2) are at higher risk for revision for a variety of reasons.[19,20] However, to date, there is no accepted BMI cutoff for PFA. Similarly, there is currently no consensus regarding optimal age for patients undergoing PFA, though authors have generally advocated for a younger patient population (30-60 years old).[21,22] In one series, 50% of patients undergoing PFA were age 50 years or younger. Nonetheless, excellent outcomes are achievable even in octogenarians with isolated patellofemoral arthritis.[9] We would not typically recommend PFA for patients in their 20s.

TABLE 21-1   Indications and Contraindications for Patellofemoral Arthroplasty

Indications	Contraindications	Relative Contraindications
• Advanced primary isolated patellofemoral osteoarthritis • Posttraumatic patellofemoral osteoarthritis • Patellofemoral osteoarthritis secondary to patellar maltracking (with or without trochlear dysplasia) • Mild patellar subluxation or tilt • Outerbridge grade IV chondromalacia of lateral patellar facet and/or lateral trochlea • Retropatellar/peripatellar pain worsened by descending stairs, kneeling, squatting	• Tibiofemoral osteoarthritis or Outerbridge grade III-IV tibiofemoral chondromalacia • Inflammatory arthritis or chondrocalcinosis • Knee instability • Limb malalignment (valgus >8°, varus >5°) • Flexion contracture • Uncorrectable patellar malalignment	• BMI >40 • Isolated Outerbridge grade IV chondromalacia of medial patellar facet and/or medial trochlea • Preoperative opioid dependence • Disproportionate pain • Equivalent anterior pain walking on level ground as descending stairs, kneeling, or squatting • Age <30 years • Tibiofemoral tenderness on examination

Additional contraindications include active infection, complex regional pain syndrome, disproportionate pain, and narcotic dependence to manage patellofemoral pain. Patients who require opioid medications for patellofemoral osteoarthritis are generally considered poor candidates for PFA, and all attempts should be made to wean them from these medications prior to pursuing surgery. Last, previous studies have shown that coexisting psychological distress or psychiatric disease may be associated with poorer outcomes and/or poorer satisfaction postoperatively.[9] Accordingly, it is important for the practitioner to determine the mental status of patients prior to proceeding with PFA and set appropriate and realistic expectations for patients. Indications and contraindications are further summarized in **Table 21-1**.

PREOPERATIVE EVALUATION

Preoperative evaluation includes a thorough history and physical examination. The history usually reveals anterior (retropatellar or peripatellar) knee pain which is exacerbated during activities that particularly stress the patellofemoral joint such as descending stairs, kneeling, squatting, sitting for a prolonged period of time, or going from a sitting to a standing position. There should be little if any pain when walking on level ground. There may be a history of patellar trauma, dislocation, or patellar instability. Nonoperative treatment measures and prior procedures should be documented.

Physical examination is focused on the assessment of the patellofemoral joint as well as more global evaluation of the knee and lower extremity to exclude other pathology. Active patellar tracking is assessed with the limb dangling over the edge of the examination table. Typically, patellofemoral crepitus is felt and/or heard. Patellar maltracking may be observed with lateral deviation of the patella as the knee approaches full extension (J sign), indicating muscular imbalance or rotational deformity. For patients who have high Q angles, a tibial tubercle realignment procedure (anteromedialization) may be considered before, or at the same time as, PFA. Assessment for hypermobility, patella alta, and baja is

also useful. Provocative testing should include elicitation of tenderness with palpation around the patella, apprehension with attempted lateral subluxation, pain and crepitus with patellar compression, and recreation of patellofemoral crepitus and retropatellar knee pain with range of motion and squatting.

The examiner should also look for other causes of anterior knee pain such as patellar tendonitis, pes anserinus bursitis, synovitis, complex regional pain syndrome, referred pain from the hip or the lumbar spine...etc. Tenderness to palpation at the joint line medially or laterally should also be evaluated and would contraindicate PFA even in the absence of tibiofemoral arthritis on radiographic imaging.

Preoperative imaging includes four views of the knees (weight-bearing anteroposterior, weight-bearing mid-flexion posteroanterior, lateral, and sunrise views). These should identify the presence of patellofemoral degenerative changes and the absence of tibiofemoral arthritis, though small osteophytes and mild squaring of the femoral condyles may be acceptable in the context of normal tibiofemoral joint spaces and lack of clinical symptoms. Patellar tilt, subluxation, and patellar congruence are evaluated on the sunrise view. Patellar height should also be assessed on the lateral X-ray. If significant lower limb angular deformity is suspected, full-length standing plain films should be obtained.

MRI is routinely obtained when evaluating a patient being considered for PFA. While it is naturally used to confirm the findings of patellofemoral joint degeneration (chondral thinning, bony edema), equally important is its role in excluding the presence of substantial tibiofemoral compartment pathology such as meniscal injury, chondromalacia/arthritis, or subchondral edema. The presence of more substantial tibiofemoral chondral disease or edema would exclude isolated PFA, although consideration may be given to bicompartmental knee arthroplasty, combined PFA and chondral grafting, or TKA in these circumstances. Previous arthroscopy photographs or video, if available, may be especially valuable in documenting the extent of patellofemoral joint disease as well as the absence of disease elsewhere.

IMPLANT DESIGN

Implant design in PFA has witnessed significant progress over the years. Initial prostheses in the 1950s consisted of patellar resurfacing with vitallium implants, leaving the native trochlea untouched.[23] Later implants in the 1970s addressed the femoral trochlea and constituted first-generation PFA prostheses. These implants have an "inlay" design, whereby the trochlear implant only replaces the articular cartilage and sits flush with the surrounding cartilage.[14,21,24] These implants follow the alignment of the native trochlea—typically internally rotated 10° relative to the AP axis of the femur—which is the primary reason for high rates of secondary surgery and revision of inlay-style trochlear designs, mostly related to abnormal patellofemoral tracking and instability.[25-27]

Recognizing the etiology of failures with inlay-style trochlear designs, second-generation prostheses—considered an "onlay" trochlear design—were developed to be positioned flush with the anterior femoral cortical surface and perpendicular to the anteroposterior axis (Whiteside axis) of the femur.[14,21,24] The ability to rotationally position the trochlear implant independently of the native anterior trochlear anatomy has substantially improved patellofemoral tracking, reduced the need for secondary surgeries or revisions, and optimized functional outcomes and durability.[13,14] Several additional design features have contributed to the improvements in patellar tracking, including a less constrained trochlear groove, an anatomic radius of curvature, greater proximal extension, improved congruence, and asymmetric designs.[13]

SURGICAL TECHNIQUE

Nuances of the surgical technique will vary with surgeon preference and based on particulars of specific implant designs and instrumentation. Nonetheless, general principles described here can optimize outcomes. A dynamic leg holder can aid in placement of the knee in flexion. Alternatively, two static positioners can be secured to the table to stabilize knee flexion in roughly 20° and 60°. Initial exposure is obtained with standard medial parapatellar arthrotomy (**Fig. 21-1**). A midvastus or subvastus approach can also be utilized, and some authors alternatively prefer a lateral approach.[28] The exposure should be adequate to allow for ample exposure and placement of the femoral cutting guide. Care should be taken not to damage or incise the medial meniscus, intermeniscal ligament, femoral condyle articular cartilage, or the anterior cruciate ligament during the exposure (**Fig. 21-2**). The joint is inspected to ensure that isolated PFA is appropriate.

The patella is subluxated laterally, and osteophytes are resected from the patella and from the trochlea. Proper exposure is ensured proximally, including resection of synovium on the anterior femur extending 1.5 to 2 cm from the proximal edge of the trochlear surface,

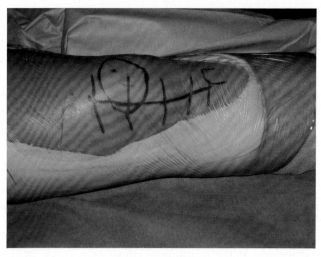

FIGURE 21-1 An incision is marked for a medial parapatellar, midvastus, or subvastus approach. (Reproduced from Lonner JH. Patellofemoral arthroplasty. In: Lotke PA, Lonner JH, eds. Master Techniques in Orthopedic Surgery: Knee Arthroplasty. 3rd ed. Philadelphia, PA: Lippincott Williams & Wilkins; 2008.)

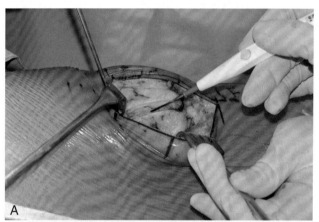

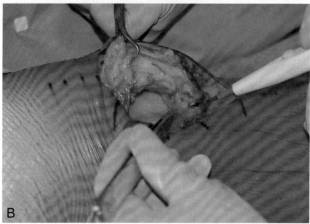

FIGURE 21-2 **A:** The arthrotomy is made taking care not to damage or incise the medial meniscus, intermeniscal ligament, femoral condyle articular cartilage, or the anterior cruciate ligament. **B:** The infrapatellar fat pad may be partially excised to facilitate exposure without damaging the menisci or intermeniscal ligament. (Reproduced from Lonner JH. Patellofemoral arthroplasty. In: Lotke PA, Lonner JH, eds. Master Techniques in Orthopedic Surgery: Knee Arthroplasty. 3rd ed. Philadelphia, PA: Lippincott Williams & Wilkins; 2008.)

to adequately visualize the anterior distal femur. With the knee in mid-flexion, the anterior femoral trochlea is prepared with a femoral cutting guide. The guide is rotated so that the anterior femoral resection is made perpendicular to the AP axis of the femur and positioned vertically to make the resection flush with the lateral anterior femoral cortex, creating the so-called "grand piano sign" (**Fig. 21-3**). The cut should avoid femoral notching on the one hand and anteriorization (anterior offset) on the other. This is step one in optimizing patellar tracking.

Sizing the femoral component is also critical. The trochlear implant should not extend entirely to the periphery of the femur. Instead, a few millimeters of resected bone should be left "uncovered" by the implant, particularly at the transitional edges, or corners, of the implant (where it bends into the intercondylar region of the femur distally), to reduce the tendency of the surrounding capsular and retinacular tissue from rubbing on the implant as the knee moves through flexion and

extension. Additionally, the distal portion of the component should not extend into the intercondylar notch, as this could then impinge on the anterior cruciate ligament in extension. The cartilage in the gap between the distal "tongue" of the implant and the notch can either be preserved or it can be removed, as typically, at this degree of knee flexion, the central portion of the patellar prosthesis is not contacting the central/distal trochlear surface. A notchplasty, with excision of notch osteophytes, is performed if needed. Once a properly sized implant trial is selected, the intercondylar bone and articular cartilage are prepared to accept the trial trochlear prosthesis, so that the edges of the distal tongue of the implant are flush with, or recessed 1 to 2 mm relative to, the adjacent condylar cartilage surfaces. In our case, we prefer a milling guide, which is most effective at preparing this region; other systems require more of a freehand technique (**Fig. 21-4**). The trochlear trial component is impacted into place.

The patella is then prepared, either with a freehand technique or instrumented, based on surgeon preference. Just proximal to the patella, the synovium on the undersurface of the quadriceps tendon should be excised. The key tenets to optimal patellar resurfacing should be followed. First, the resection should be parallel to the anterior patellar cortex. Second, the composite patellar thickness (residual bone and prosthesis) should be similar to the native patellar thickness. This may not always be feasible, given that substantial patellar wear and dysplasia often leave the native patella very thin. In these cases, even using the thinnest patellar component available may require slight patellar stuffing in order to avoid resecting the patella to a thickness of less than 12 mm. Of course, ideally, the remnant patella

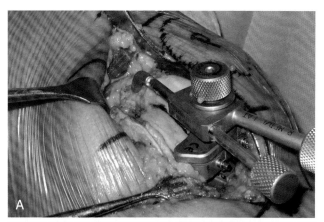

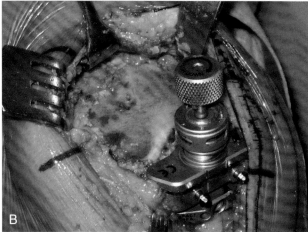

FIGURE 21-3 **A:** The femoral trochlear cutting guide is rotated so that the anterior femoral resection is made perpendicular to the anteroposterior axis of the femur and positioned vertically to make the resection flush with the lateral anterior femoral cortex. **B:** A "grand piano" sign is seen after completing the cut with the oscillating saw. (Reproduced from Lonner JH. Patellofemoral arthroplasty. In: Lotke PA, Lonner JH, eds. Master Techniques in Orthopedic Surgery: Knee Arthroplasty. 3rd ed. Philadelphia, PA: Lippincott Williams & Wilkins; 2008.)

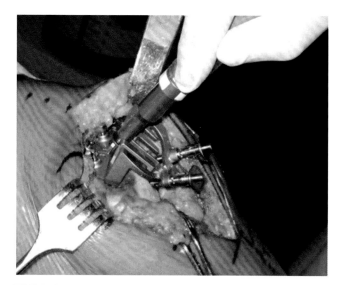

FIGURE 21-4 A milling guide is placed for preparation of the intercondylar bone and articular cartilage with a burr. (Reproduced from Lonner JH. Patellofemoral arthroplasty. In: Lotke PA, Lonner JH, eds. Master Techniques in Orthopedic Surgery: Knee Arthroplasty. 3rd ed. Philadelphia, PA: Lippincott Williams & Wilkins; 2008.)

should be 14 to 15 mm thick when possible. Third, the patellar button should be placed as medial as possible on the patella to optimize patellar tracking. Fourth, the portion of the lateral patella that is not covered by the patellar button should be excised to slacken the lateral retinaculum and remove a potential source of bony impingement (**Fig. 21-5**). Finally, patellar tracking should be assessed (**Fig. 21-6**). If there is slight patellar tilt or subluxation, first confirm appropriate implant position and sizing and make adjustments if needed. Then recess the retinacular attachment from the lateral patellar facet or perform a lateral retinacular release. If there is still maltracking (which is uncommon with the described method of surface preparation), antero-medialization of the tibial tubercle is performed if the Q angle is increased (greater than 20°) or soft-tissue proximal realignment is undertaken if it is not. Once positioning and tracking are deemed to be satisfactory, the surfaces are irrigated, dried, and the final components cemented into place.

POSTOPERATIVE COMPLICATIONS

While early postoperative complications can occur after PFA, like unicompartmental knee arthroplasty, the risk of complications such as thromboembolic disease, infection, mortality, neurovascular injury, fracture,...etc. is far less common than after TKA.[29-31]

Patellar maltracking, catching, and subluxation are common in the immediate postoperative period after "inlay-style" PFA and account for the majority of failures of this procedure, requiring secondary or revision surgery. Early patellar instability has been reported to occur in 7% to 36% of patients after inlay PFA.[13,32-35] Registry data have shown a dramatically increased incidence of early revisions with contemporary inlay compared to onlay-style implants due to patellar instability. The dichotomy in outcomes between inlay and onlay designs is highlighted in the Australian National Joint Registry, which shows that the 5-year cumulative revision rate was over 20% for inlay prostheses and under 10% for onlay

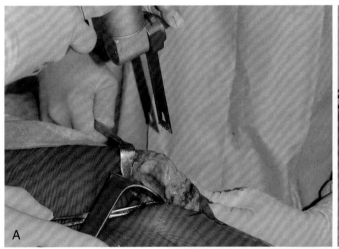
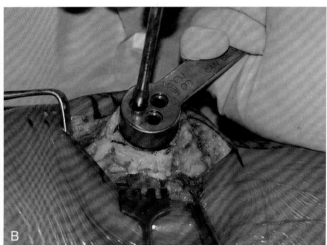
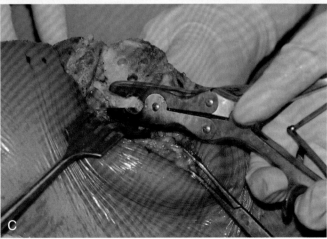

FIGURE 21-5   A: The patellar cut can be done using freehand technique with an oscillating saw as shown or using a guide. The cut can be performed with or without everting the patella. **B:** The patella is sized and the lug holes are drilled, taking care to medialize the position of the patellar component on the patella. **C:** Patellar bone lateral to the implant is excised to slacken the lateral retinaculum and avoid a potential source of bony impingement. (Reproduced from Lonner JH. Patellofemoral arthroplasty. In: Lotke PA, Lonner JH, eds. Master Techniques in Orthopedic Surgery: Knee Arthroplasty. 3rd ed. Philadelphia, PA: Lippincott Williams & Wilkins; 2008.)

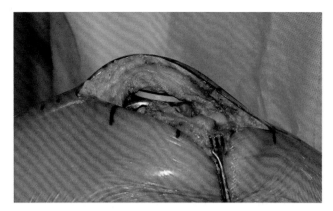

FIGURE 21-6 Patellar tracking is assessed with trial components in place. (Reproduced from Lonner JH. Patellofemoral arthroplasty. In: Lotke PA, Lonner JH, eds. Master Techniques in Orthopedic Surgery: Knee Arthroplasty. 3rd ed. Philadelphia, PA: Lippincott Williams & Wilkins; 2008.)

designs.[25] The most likely explanation for this has to do with trochlear component morphology and positioning relative to the femoral AP axis.

On the other hand, patellar instability with onlay trochlear designs has been shown to be less than 1% in most contemporary series.[9,36,37] Furthermore, an inlay trochlear component compromised by patellar maltracking can be revised to an onlay component with successful resolution of those patellar tracking problems.[38]

Arthritis progression is the most common cause of late failures after PFA. Van der List et al performed a recent systematic review of 36 cohort studies and 3 registry studies and found that the most common failure modes were progression of arthritis (38%), pain (16%), aseptic loosening (14%), and patellar maltracking (10%).[39] The causes of failure were significantly different between the early postoperative period (5 years from the index PFA) and the late postoperative period (more than 5 years from index PFA). When looking at early failures, the reasons were pain (31%), progression of arthritis (24%), and patellar maltracking (14%). Causes for late failure were found to be arthritis progression (46%), aseptic loosening (18%), pain (8%), and patellar maltracking (7%). Less common causes for failure included wear (responsible for 4% of all failures), infection, stiffness, and periprosthetic fracture. The risk of patellar fracture after PFA was reported to be 9% by King et al, who treated all of their cases nonoperatively.[40] A recent meta-analysis of 28 studies compared complications after PFA and TKA performed for isolated patellofemoral arthritis. The authors found an eightfold higher likelihood of reoperation and revision for PFA compared to TKA. However, when comparing second-generation onlay prostheses only, no significant differences in reoperation, revision, pain, or mechanical complications were found, indicating a significant effect of implant design and rotational positioning of the trochlear component. On subgroup analysis, first-generation inlay-style prostheses had over four times

higher rates of significant complications than second-generation onlay prostheses, likely biasing the overall results. These data indicate that modern onlay-style PFA and TKA likely have similar rates of complications in this patient population.[26]

FUNCTIONAL OUTCOMES AND SURVIVORSHIP

Functional outcomes, satisfaction, and implant durability after PFA have been shown to be dependent on a variety of factors including disease pattern, implant design, and patient characteristics, including etiology of patellofemoral arthritis, body habitus, and baseline mental health. Indeed, using the strict selection criteria and surgical technique outlined above, Kazarian et al found significant improvements in the mean knee range of motion and Knee Society knee and function scores at an average 4.9 years of follow-up after PFA with a modern onlay-style design.[9] Less than 4% of patients required revision arthroplasty, all for progressive tibiofemoral arthritis and none for patellar maltracking. No components were loose or worn at most recent follow-up. Despite these improvements, while patients with high mental health scores were satisfied and had their expectations met, those with poor mental health scores tended to be dissatisfied with their outcomes and their expectations were not met, suggesting that patient mental health may be a valid selection criteria for PFA.[9] Others have found that trochlear dysplasia is protective of revision due to progressive tibiofemoral osteoarthritis, whereas obesity and prior patellofemoral procedures increase the likelihood of failures.[19,20,41,42]

Comparing PFA to TKA performed for isolated patellofemoral arthritis, Dahm et al found lower postoperative morbidity and significantly higher activity scores after PFA at a mean 2.5-year follow-up.[10] Odgaard et al reported their results from a randomized controlled trial examining this issue.[11] Patients with isolated patellofemoral osteoarthritis were identified by clinical and radiographic assessment and randomized to receive either an onlay PFA or TKA. The patients and clinical evaluators were blinded (for the first year), and various patient outcome measures were collected at regular follow-up visits up to 2 years postoperatively. The authors found significantly improved clinical outcomes in the PFA patients at 2 years (Short Form-36 bodily pain, Knee Injury and Osteoarthritis Outcome Score (KOOS) symptoms, and Oxford Knee Score). No patient reported outcome favored conventional TKA at 2 years, but KOOS scores and knee range of motion were significantly more improved in the PFA group compared to the TKA group. Overall, there was not a statistically significant difference between PFA and TKA in regard to risk of revision, though the authors reported that one patient had PFA revision and one patient had conversion to TKA.[11]

While outcomes of onlay-style trochlear components have been optimized compared to inlay-style designs, failures primarily from tibiofemoral wear or unexplainable soft-tissue pain will predictably occur. Multiple centers have reported their outcomes after various onlay-type PFAs over the years with varying results. Metcalfe et al recently reported long-term outcomes with the Avon onlay prosthesis (Stryker Inc), using the United Kingdom National Joint Registry.[43] They included 483 PFAs in 368 patients with up to 18 years of follow-up. They found a 21.7% revision rate, more than half due to progression of osteoarthritis in the other knee compartments. Overall, the implant survival was 77.3% at 10 years and 67.4% at 15 years. The authors found that survivorship improved through the course of the study period, with a 9-year survivorship of 91.8% for cases performed in the latter 9 years. Middleton et al also reported a large independent-center study evaluating the same implant.[44] They included 103 PFAs in 85 patients with a mean follow-up of 5.6 years. They found a survivorship of 89% at 5 years and 86% at 10 years. Van der List et al recently conducted a meta-analysis looking at the outcomes and survivorship of PFA.[45] They included 60 studies (57 cohort studies and 3 registry studies), most being level III and level IV studies. The survivorship was found to be 91.7%, 83.3%, 74.9%, and 66.6% at 5, 10, 15, and 20 years, respectively, keeping in mind that the long-term studies mostly reported on the first-generation prostheses. They identified a revision rate of 9.4% among 9619 PFAs yielding a yearly revision rate of about 2% per year. In regard to functional outcomes, good to excellent results were reported in 87% to 92% of cases at short-term follow-up of 5 years, and the mean Knee Society Score was 87.5%. At long-term follow-up of 15 to 20 years, 79% to 82% of patients still reported good to excellent results. Long-term failures are primarily due to progressive tibiofemoral arthritis rather than loosening or wear of the patellofemoral components. Argenson et al found that patients with primary patellofemoral osteoarthritis have the greatest risk of developing tibiofemoral osteoarthritis, whereas the risk is lower in those who developed patellofemoral arthritis secondary to patellofemoral dysplasia/subluxation or trauma.[41,46]

While many regard conversion of PFA to TKA as a straightforward procedure similar to a primary TKA, Hutt et al compared patients undergoing conversion of PFA to TKA to a matched cohort of patients undergoing primary TKA and found that functional outcome scores were reduced in the conversion cohort.[47] Additionally, Lonner et al found that at a mean follow-up of 3.1 years after revision PFA to TKA using primary TKA components (without stems, augments, or bone grafting) for progressive tibiofemoral osteoarthritis, patellar instability, or both, there was significant improvement in Knee Society clinical and function scores ($P < .001$) and no clinical or radiographic evidence of patellofemoral maltracking,

loosening, or wear.[48] Parratte et al compared their series of PFA conversions to TKA to a matched control group of primary TKAs and found no significant difference in operative time, blood loss, or postoperative range of motion.[49] They did, however, identify higher functional outcome scores and decreased complications in the primary TKA group. Very recently, Lewis et al analyzed this matter based on the Australian Orthopaedic Association Joint Replacement Registry and looking at the risk of revision.[50] They included 482 PFAs revised to TKA among a total of 3251 PFAs in the registry. The risk of revision after conversion of PFA to TKA was found to be significantly higher than the risk of revision after primary TKA (hazard ratio of 2.39) and lower than the risk of revision after revision TKA (hazard ratio of 0.60). The risk of revision after conversion of PFA was not affected by the use of cruciate-retaining or cruciate-substituting implants or by revising the patellar component at the time of conversion to TKA.[50]

CONCLUSION

PFA, with newer generation onlay-style implants, represents a reliable surgical treatment for patients with isolated patellofemoral disease. This represents a less invasive procedure than TKA, with significant functional improvement and preservation of normal cartilage and soft tissues, which is especially critical in the younger patients. Patient selection is of utmost importance, and proper implant alignment and surgical technique help reduce the risk of mechanical complications from patellar instability that plagues inlay-style components. Unlike inlay trochlear components, using onlay-style trochlear implants has equivalent complications and reoperation rates compared to TKA. Given the typically younger demographic of patients with isolated patellofemoral arthritis, PFA with an onlay design should be considered as an alternative to TKA.

REFERENCES

1. Davies AP, Vince AS, Shepstone L, Donell ST, Glasgow MM. The radiologic prevalence of patellofemoral osteoarthritis. *Clin Orthop Relat Res.* 2002;402:206-212.
2. Hart HF, Stefanik JJ, Wyndow N, Machotka Z, Crossley KM. The prevalence of radiographic and MRI-defined patellofemoral osteoarthritis and structural pathology: a systematic review and meta-analysis. *Br J Sports Med.* 2017;51(16):1195-1208. doi:10.1136/bjsports-2017-097515.
3. Mills K, Hunter DJ. Patellofemoral joint osteoarthritis: an individualised pathomechanical approach to management. *Best Pract Res Clin Rheumatol.* 2014;28(1):73-91. doi:10.1016/j.berh.2014.01.006.
4. Pisanu G, Rosso F, Bertolo C, et al. Patellofemoral arthroplasty: Current Concepts and review of the literature. *Joints.* 2017;5(4):237-245. doi:10.1055/s-0037-1606618.
5. Coburn SL, Barton CJ, Filbay SR, Hart HF, Rathleff MS, Crossley KM. Quality of life in individuals with patellofemoral pain: a systematic review including meta-analysis. *Phys Ther Sport.* 2018;33:96-108. doi:10.1016/j.ptsp.2018.06.006.

6. Hart HF, Filbay SR, Coburn S, Charlton JM, Sritharan P, Crossley KM. Is quality of life reduced in people with patellofemoral osteoarthritis and does it improve with treatment? A systematic review, meta-analysis and regression. *Disabil Rehabil*. 2018;10:1-15. doi:10.1080/09638288.2018.1482504.

7. Mosier BA, Arendt EA, Dahm DL, Dejour D, Gomoll AH. Management of patellofemoral arthritis: from cartilage restoration to arthroplasty. *Instr Course Lect*. 2017;66:531-542.

8. Parvizi J, Stuart MJ, Pagnano MW, Hanssen AD. Total knee arthroplasty in patients with isolated patellofemoral arthritis. *Clin Orthop Relat Res*. 2001;392:147-152.

9. Kazarian GS, Tarity TD, Hansen EN, Cai J, Lonner JH. Significant functional improvement at 2 years after isolated patellofemoral arthroplasty with an onlay trochlear implant, but low mental health scores predispose to dissatisfaction. *J Arthroplasty*. 2016;31(2):389-394. doi:10.1016/j.arth.2015.08.033.

10. Dahm DL, Al-Rayashi W, Dajani K, Shah JP, Levy BA, Stuart MJ. Patellofemoral arthroplasty versus total knee arthroplasty in patients with isolated patellofemoral osteoarthritis. *Am J Orthop*. 2010;39(10):487-491.

11. Odgaard A, Madsen F, Kristensen PW, Kappel A, Fabrin J. The Mark Coventry Award: patellofemoral arthroplasty results in better range of movement and early patient-reported outcomes than TKA. *Clin Orthop Relat Res*. 2018;476(1):87-100. doi:10.1007/s11999.0000000000000017.

12. Shubin Stein BE, Brady JM, Grawe B, et al. Return to activities after patellofemoral arthroplasty. *Am J Orthop*. 2017;46(6):E353-E357.

13. Lonner JH. Patellofemoral arthroplasty: pros, cons, and design considerations. *Clin Orthop Relat Res*. 2004;428:158-165.

14. Lonner JH, Bloomfield MR. The clinical outcome of patellofemoral arthroplasty. *Orthop Clin North Am*. 2013;44(3):271-280. doi:10.1016/j.ocl.2013.03.002.

15. Leadbetter WB, Seyler TM, Ragland PS, Mont MA. Indications, contraindications, and pitfalls of patellofemoral arthroplasty. *J Bone Joint Surg Am*. 2006;88 suppl 4:122-137. doi:10.2106/JBJS.F.00856.

16. Biazzo A, Silvestrini F, Manzotti A, Confalonieri N. Bicompartmental (uni plus patellofemoral) versus total knee arthroplasty: a match-paired study. *Musculoskelet Surg*. 2018;103(1):63-68. doi:10.1007/s12306-018-0540-1.

17. Kooner S, Johal H, Clark M. Bicompartmental knee arthroplasty vs total knee arthroplasty for the treatment of medial compartment and patellofemoral osteoarthritis. *Arthroplasty Today*. 2017;3(4):309-314. doi:10.1016/j.artd.2017.02.006.

18. Lonner JH, Mehta S, Booth RE. Ipsilateral patellofemoral arthroplasty and autogenous osteochondral femoral condylar transplantation. *J Arthroplasty*. 2007;22(8):1130-1136. doi:10.1016/j.arth.2005.08.012.

19. Dahm DL, Kalisvaart MM, Stuart MJ, Slettedahl SW. Patellofemoral arthroplasty: outcomes and factors associated with early progression of tibiofemoral arthritis. *Knee Surg Sports Traumatol Arthrosc*. 2014;22(10):2554-2559. doi:10.1007/s00167-014-3202-3.

20. Liow MHL, Goh GS-H, Tay DK-J, Chia S-L, Lo N-N, Yeo S-J. Obesity and the absence of trochlear dysplasia increase the risk of revision in patellofemoral arthroplasty. *Knee*. 2016;23(2):331-337. doi:10.1016/j.knee.2015.05.009.

21. Lonner JH. Patellofemoral arthroplasty. *J Am Acad Orthop Surg*. 2007;15(8):495-506.

22. Lonner JH. Patellofemoral arthroplasty. *Orthopedics*. 2010;33(9):653. doi:10.3928/01477447-20100722-39.

23. McKeever DC. Patellar prosthesis. 1955. *Clin Orthop Relat Res*. 2002;404:3-6.

24. Lonner JH. Patellofemoral arthroplasty: the impact of design on outcomes. *Orthop Clin North Am*. 2008;39(3):347-354. doi:10.1016/j.ocl.2008.02.002.

25. Australian Orthopaedic Association National Joint Replacement Registry (AOANJRR). Hip, Knee & Shoulder Arthroplasty: 2018 Annual Report. Adelaide: AOA. 2018. Available at https://aoanjrr.sahmri.com/annual-reports-2018. Accessed April 6, 2019.

26. Dy CJ, Franco N, Ma Y, Mazumdar M, McCarthy MM, Gonzalez Della Valle A. Complications after patello-femoral versus total knee replacement in the treatment of isolated patellofemoral osteoarthritis. A meta-analysis. *Knee Surg Sports Traumatol Arthrosc*. 2012;20(11):2174-2190. doi:10.1007/s00167-011-1677-8.

27. Kamath AF, Slattery TR, Levack AE, Wu CH, Kneeland JB, Lonner JH. Trochlear inclination angles in normal and dysplastic knees. *J Arthroplasty*. 2013;28(2):214-219. doi:10.1016/j.arth.2012.04.017.

28. Imhoff AB, Feucht MJ, Bartsch E, Cotic M, Pogorzelski J. High patient satisfaction with significant improvement in knee function and pain relief after mid-term follow-up in patients with isolated patellofemoral inlay arthroplasty. *Knee Surg Sports Traumatol Arthrosc*. 2018;27(7):2251-2258. doi:10.1007/s00167-018-5173-2.

29. Levack A, Kamath AF, Lonner JH. Incidence of symptomatic thromboembolic disease after patellofemoral arthroplasty. *Am J Orthop*. 2012;41(10):456-460.

30. Longenecker AS, Kazarian GS, Boyer GP, Lonner JH. Radiographic imaging in the postanesthesia care unit is unnecessary after partial knee arthroplasty. *J Arthroplasty*. 2017;32(5):1431-1433. doi:10.1016/j.arth.2016.11.033.

31. Shaner JL, Karim AR, Casper DS, Ball CJ, Padegimas EM, Lonner JH. Routine postoperative Laboratory tests are unnecessary after partial knee arthroplasty. *J Arthroplasty*. 2016;31(12):2764-2767. doi:10.1016/j.arth.2016.05.052.

32. Blazina ME, Fox JM, Del Pizzo W, Broukhim B, Ivey FM. Patellofemoral replacement. *Clin Orthop Relat Res*. 1979;144:98-102.

33. Charalambous CP, Abiddin Z, Mills SP, Rogers S, Sutton P, Parkinson R. The low contact stress patellofemoral replacement: high early failure rate. *J Bone Joint Surg Br*. 2011;93(4):484-489. doi:10.1302/0301-620X.93B4.25899.

34. Krajca-Radcliffe JB, Coker TP. Patellofemoral arthroplasty. A 2- to 18-year followup study. *Clin Orthop Relat Res*. 1996;330:143-151.

35. de Winter WE, Feith R, van Loon CJ. The Richards type II patellofemoral arthroplasty: 26 cases followed for 1-20 years. *Acta Orthop Scand*. 2001;72(5):487-490. doi:10.1080/000164701753532826.

36. Ackroyd CE, Newman JH, Evans R, Eldridge JDJ, Joslin CC. The Avon patellofemoral arthroplasty: five-year survivorship and functional results. *J Bone Joint Surg Br*. 2007;89(3):310-315. doi:10.1302/0301-620X.89B3.18062.

37. Mont MA, Johnson AJ, Naziri Q, Kolisek FR, Leadbetter WB. Patellofemoral arthroplasty: 7-year mean follow-up. *J Arthroplasty*. 2012;27(3):358-361. doi:10.1016/j.arth.2011.07.010.

38. Hendrix MRG, Ackroyd CE, Lonner JH. Revision patellofemoral arthroplasty: three- to seven-year follow-up. *J Arthroplasty*. 2008;23(7):977-983. doi:10.1016/j.arth.2007.10.019.

39. van der List JP, Chawla H, Villa JC, Pearle AD. Why do patellofemoral arthroplasties fail today? A systematic review. *Knee*. 2017;24(1):2-8. doi:10.1016/j.knee.2015.11.002.

40. King AH, Engasser WM, Sousa PL, Arendt EA, Dahm DL. Patellar fracture following patellofemoral arthroplasty. *J Arthroplasty*. 2015;30(7):1203-1206. doi:10.1016/j.arth.2015.02.007.

41. Argenson JN, Guillaume JM, Aubaniac JM. Is there a place for patellofemoral arthroplasty? *Clin Orthop Relat Res*. 1995;321:162-167.

42. Willekens P, Victor J, Verbruggen D, Vande Kerckhove M, Van Der Straeten C. Outcome of patellofemoral arthroplasty, determinants for success. *Acta Orthop Belg*. 2015;81(4):759-767.

43. Metcalfe AJ, Ahearn N, Hassaballa MA, et al. The Avon patellofemoral joint arthroplasty. *Bone Joint J*. 2018;100-B(9):1162-1167. doi:10.1302/0301-620X.100B9.BJJ-2018-0174.R1.

44. Middleton SWF, Toms AD, Schranz PJ, Mandalia VI. Mid-term survivorship and clinical outcomes of the Avon patellofemoral joint replacement. *Knee*. 2018;25(2):323-328. doi:10.1016/j.knee.2018.01.007.

45. van der List JP, Chawla H, Zuiderbaan HA, Pearle AD. Survivorship and functional outcomes of patellofemoral arthroplasty: a systematic review. *Knee Surg Sports Traumatol Arthrosc.* 2017;25(8):2622-2631. doi:10.1007/s00167-015-3878-z.

46. Argenson J-NA, Flecher X, Parratte S, Aubaniac J-M. Patellofemoral arthroplasty: an update. *Clin Orthop Relat Res.* 2005;440:50-53.

47. Hutt J, Dodd M, Bourke H, Bell J. Outcomes of total knee replacement after patellofemoral arthroplasty. *J Knee Surg.* 2013;26(4):219-223. doi:10.1055/s-0032-1329233.

48. Lonner JH, Jasko JG, Booth RE. Revision of a failed patellofemoral arthroplasty to a total knee arthroplasty. *J Bone Joint Surg Am.* 2006;88(11):2337-2342. doi:10.2106/JBJS.F.00282.

49. Parratte S, Lunebourg A, Ollivier M, Abdel MP, Argenson J-NA. Are revisions of patellofemoral arthroplasties more like primary or revision TKAs. *Clin Orthop Relat Res.* 2015;473(1):213-219. doi:10.1007/s11999-014-3756-x.

50. Lewis PL, Graves SE, Cuthbert A, Parker D, Myers P. What is the risk of repeat revision when patellofemoral replacement is revised to TKA? An analysis of 482 cases from a Large National Arthroplasty Registry. *Clin Orthop Relat Res.* 2018;477(6):1402-1410. doi:10.1097/CORR.0000000000000541.

Alternatives to Arthroplasty for Knee Arthritis

BRETT R. LEVINE

chapter 22

Oral and Topical Agents and Injectables

Kathleen Weber, MD, MS | Shannon Powers, DO

INTRODUCTION

Osteoarthritis, the most prevalent form of arthritis, is a common cause of joint pain, functional loss, and disability. As the population ages, it is anticipated that the cost, care, and treatment of these individuals will exponentially increase. The treatment of those affected with osteoarthritis should consist of an individualized comprehensive management program that includes education about the disease, its degenerative process, and appropriate available conservative and surgical treatment options. The ultimate goal of conservative management is to improve function, reduce pain, and limit disease progression.

Conservative management (**Fig. 22-1**) includes maintaining or achieving a proper body weight and incorporating an exercise program comprised of stretching, strengthening, and aerobic fitness. When appropriate, the use of modalities, bracing, and activity modification should be considered. Pharmacological treatment is utilized when these measures are becoming less effective or patients' pain warrants their use. Pharmacological treatments include oral and topical medications and intra-articular injections. A variety of intra-articular injections are currently being utilized in osteoarthritis treatment including corticosteroids, hyaluronic acid, and biologics such as platelet-rich plasma (PRP) and stem cells.[1]

The optimal conservative management includes an individualized combination of nonpharmacological and pharmacological treatment(s) as well as potentially natural products (tumeric, glucosamine, etc.). This chapter will focus on the pharmacological and biologic treatments used in the management of osteoarthritis.

ORAL MEDICATIONS

Acetaminophen

When nonpharmacological interventions are failing or do not provide adequate pain control, initiating oral medications, such as acetaminophen, is typically a first-line therapy for symptom relief (i.e., pain, stiffness, swelling) related to knee osteoarthritis.[2] The American College of Rheumatology (ACR) and the Osteoarthritis Research Society International (OARSI) guidelines for nonsurgical management of knee osteoarthritis recommend the use of acetaminophen for those patients who have failed

nonpharmacologic treatment, have no relevant comorbidities, or have no contraindications to use.[3,4] One should consider short-term use of acetaminophen due to the potential for adverse events, such as elevated liver enzymes, hepatotoxicity, and organ failure.[5] If acetaminophen is not providing adequate pain relief, other oral agents should be considered.

Nonsteroidal Anti-inflammatory Drugs

Nonsteroidal anti-inflammatory drugs (NSAIDs) have been used for treatment of osteoarthritis for several decades. They are recommended for the management of knee osteoarthritis after use of acetaminophen and nonpharmacologic interventions have failed. NSAIDs function to reduce inflammation and pain by reversibly inhibiting cyclooxygenase (COX), the enzyme involved in the pathway of prostaglandin synthesis.[6] NSAIDs can be categorized into nonselective and COX-2 selective. Nonselective NSAIDs inhibit both COX-1 and COX-2, whereas COX-2 selective NSAIDs inhibit only COX-2.[2,6] Examples of nonselective NSAIDs include ibuprofen, naproxen, indomethacin, and diclofenac; COX-2 selective NSAIDs often include the suffix "-coxib" such as celecoxib and rofecoxib.

It is generally agreed upon by many organizations that NSAIDs are an appropriate treatment for knee osteoarthritis as they provide both analgesic effects and decrease inflammation.[2-4,7] However, when treating elderly patients, providers should consider initiating a topical NSAID due to the higher potential for adverse events in this age group.[4,8]

NSAIDs have the potential to cause side effects related to the gastrointestinal (GI), renal, and cardiovascular (CV) systems. In pertaining to the gastrointestinal system, patients taking NSAIDs can have an increased risk of gastritis, abdominal pain, ulcers, GI bleeding, and liver toxicity.[2,9,10] Patients may complain of dyspepsia, burning sensation, gastric reflux or they can be asymptomatic and present with hematemesis or hematochezia.[8,9,11-13] The gastric lining contains COX-1, and therefore nonselective NSAID therapy can have higher potential for adverse GI events in comparison to COX-2 selective NSAIDs.[10] In addition to age, risk factors for potential GI-related adverse events include use of anticoagulation, prior gastric ulcer, concurrent use of corticosteroids and/

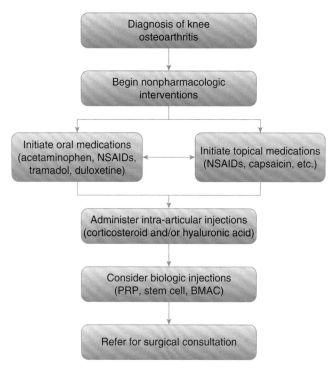

FIGURE 22-1 Approach to treatment of knee osteoarthritis.

or aspirin.[10,13] Concomitant use of a proton pump inhibitor should be considered in patients with comorbidities to reduce the risk of an adverse event.[3,4,10] COX-2 selective NSAIDs when first brought to market showed great promise in reducing GI complications while providing pain relief.[8,10,14-17] High rates of cardiovascular events (myocardial infarction, cerebrovascular events, and death) were noted and subsequently two of the COX-2 selective medications were withdrawn from the market.[8,10,18,19] The FDA has extended the potential for CV events to include all NSAIDs including both selective and nonselective NSAIDs.[10,20,21] The risk and benefits of NSAID use should be weighed when prescribing these medications especially in patients who have or suspected to have cardiovascular disease.[8,10,21] In those patients with comorbidities alternative therapeutic modalities should be considered.[3,10] Furthermore, NSAID therapy should be avoided in patients with known renal disease or who are at risk of renal toxicity.[4,6] When administered in appropriate doses and durations, NSAID utilization remains a first-line therapy for management of knee osteoarthritis.

Other Oral Medications

There are numerous oral medications that have been marketed and are indicated for the treatment of pain associated with knee osteoarthritis including duloxetine, tramadol, and other oral opioids. Duloxetine, a serotonin-norepinephrine reuptake inhibitor (SNRI), has demonstrated clinical benefit in treatment of chronic pain, including chronic knee osteoarthritis.[3,22] SNRI, as a class of medications, has the

potential for numerous drug interactions and an extensive list of common and serious adverse reactions. Common side effects can include fatigue, nausea, constipation, dizziness, and dry mouth, while more serious include seizures, hypertensive crisis, and suicidality.[3,23-25] Duloxetine can be considered for therapy in patients who fail to respond to other oral medications (such as acetaminophen and NSAIDs) or in those patients who have contraindications to use of these medications.

Tramadol, a nontraditional opioid, has therapeutic indications for symptom management in knee OA. Studies have reported similar therapeutic responses as oral NSAIDs, including reduction of joint stiffness and pain.[2,4,7,26] Although tramadol and other opioids may be considered in patients who failed or have contraindication to use of other first-line oral agents, many organizations do not make recommendations for or against the use of opioid agents for analgesia.[3,4,7] This is based on limited data to recommend for or against opioid use. Additionally these medications have a potential for side effects, abuse, and addiction.[27] The modern opioid epidemic in the United States has led to a push to discourage the use of these medications to treat osteoarthritis. Furthermore, preoperative utilization of opioids can be associated with poor outcomes and a greater chance for increased and sustained use of these drugs in the long-term.

TOPICAL TREATMENTS

Topical NSAIDs

Topical NSAIDs have therapeutic indications for the treatment of knee osteoarthritis.[3,4,7,28-31] Multiple studies have documented improvement in pain relief with use of topical NSAIDs compared to placebo[29,32] and noted similar benefits in relation to oral NSAIDs.[3,27,30] There is significantly less systemic absorption of topical NSAIDs compared to oral NSAIDs, with serum levels being less than 5% those of the oral route.[29,33,34] While there is an increased risk of dermatological side effects such as skin reactions, there is a decreased risk of GI adverse effects with use of these medications.[3,27,30,35] As a result of the potential reduction in GI side effects, topical NSAIDs are sometimes preferred to oral NSAIDs, especially in the geriatric population.[4,28] In conclusion, topical NSAIDs are a beneficial treatment choice for nonoperative knee osteoarthritis.

Topical Salicylates and Topical Capsaicin

Other topical agents exist for treatment of knee osteoarthritis, including topical salicylates and topical capsaicin. Unlike topical NSAIDs that are generally agreed upon as efficacious therapy for knee osteoarthritis, the evidence to support or not support the other topical treatments is less clear. This is partly due to the limited number of studies comparing these agents to placebo and/or other generally accepted therapies. When compared to placebo, topical salicylates have not demonstrated significant therapeutic benefit for treatment of knee osteoarthritis.[27,29,36] The literature has been riddled with mixed reviews suggesting that topical salicylates may have increased adverse events compared to placebo,[29,36] while other authors report there is no significant increase in adverse events.[37]

The OARSI guidelines recommend topical capsaicin as an appropriate treatment of knee osteoarthritis without comorbidities[3,38,39]; however, the ACR guidelines recommend against its use for the management of knee osteoarthritis.[4] Other publications support the use of topical capsaicin, but report that it is less effective than both topical and oral NSAIDs.[29] Capsaicin is reported to have the potential for increased adverse effects compared to placebo.[3,27] As a result, some providers turn to topical capsaicin for therapy only if comorbidities exist with use of alternative interventions.

CORTICOSTEROID INJECTIONS

Pharmacology and Mechanism of Action

Corticosteroid injections (CSIs) have been widely used as a mainstay treatment of knee osteoarthritis for several decades.[40] Hollander et al. documented the anti-inflammatory effect CSIs had on inflammatory/rheumatoid arthritis in 1951.[41] Despite the long-standing use of CSIs, the exact mechanism in which these intra-articular injections alleviate symptoms is not fully known. However, it is suggested that use of CSIs results in a reduction of inflammatory processes at the site of administration by interacting with cytokines typically recruited for the immune response.[40,42,43]

Several formulations of injectable corticosteroids exist. These are separated into two categories, water-soluble (nonparticulate) and water insoluble (particulate). Soluble corticosteroids are nonester preparations and these do not form microcrystals in water. These have a quicker onset but shorter duration of action. Sodium phosphate formulations are included in this category; examples include betamethasone sodium phosphate and dexamethasone. Insoluble corticosteroids are ester preparations and these form microcrystals in water. These have a slower onset but longer duration of action because these preparations remain in the synovial fluid longer. Acetate formulations are included in this category; examples include betamethasone acetate, methylprednisolone, and triamcinolone. Insoluble injections tend to have a lower potency and therefore require a higher dose to reach similar response compared to soluble injections.[40,43,44] According to the American College of Rheumatology, the preferred injectable corticosteroids are methylprednisolone acetate, triamcinolone hexacetonide, and triamcinolone acetonide.[42,45] Refer to **Table 22-1** for a list of common corticosteroid preparations.

Triamcinolone acetonide extended release (ER) is a new corticosteroid formulation. The steroid is packaged within a biodegradable bead, which allows the steroid

TABLE 22-1	**Common Corticosteroid Preparations Used for Intra-Articular Injections**
Water soluble	Betamethasone sodium phosphate
	Dexamethasone
Water insoluble	Betamethasone acetate
	Methylprednisolone
	Prednisone
	Triamcinolone

to remain in the joint for an extended period of time in comparison to immediate release injectable corticosteroids.[46,47] In 2019, Spitzer et al. conducted a study that demonstrated treatment with triamcinolone acetonide ER provided symptom relief without damage to cartilage with repeated injections.[46] While it has only been on the market for therapeutic use since 2017, the extended release injection shows promising results in its relatively early use in treatment of osteoarthritis.[48]

The duration of benefit from intra-articular CSIs is another topic of debate due to discrepancies in several studies in the literature. One meta-analysis reported significant efficacy in intra-articular CSIs at 3 to 4 weeks postinjection but not at 6 to 8 weeks postinjection compared to control.[49] In a different meta-analysis, patients were noted to have benefit from intervention lasting anywhere from 1 to 24 weeks in duration, although higher doses of steroid may be needed in order to have benefit from weeks 16 to 24.[42,50]

Indications

Intra-articular CSIs are often used when other oral and topical pharmacologic and nonpharmacologic modalities have failed to adequately provide symptom relief for knee osteoarthritis, including pain and stiffness.[42,51] CSIs can be used if there is a contraindication to oral and/or topical medications. CSIs are also used in the management of inflammatory arthritis, such as in rheumatoid arthritis, psoriatic arthritis, and gout/pseudogout.[42]

Local anesthetics, such as bupivacaine, lidocaine, and ropivacaine, are often used in combination with corticosteroid injections providing immediate short-term pain relief. There has been some literature to suggest that large amounts of local anesthetics have the potential to cause chondrolysis, with bupivacaine having a greater potential for toxicity.[43]

The American Academy of Orthopedic Surgeons (AAOS) released their updated guidelines in 2013 pertaining to treatment of knee osteoarthritis. According to these guidelines, the AAOS is "unable to recommend for or against" intra-articular CSIs for the treatment of knee osteoarthritis, with strength of recommendation rated to be "inconclusive."[7] Other organizations have released more definitive recommendations. OARSI recommends intra-articular CSIs to be "appropriate" for the treatment of knee osteoarthritis, resulting in short-term pain relief.[3] The ACR "conditionally recommends" the use of intra-articular CSIs when patients have an unsuccessful response from treatment with oral and topical pharmacologic interventions.[4]

Adverse Effects

Compared to the potential complications that are associated with surgical intervention, CSIs have been and continue to remain a relatively safe conservative therapeutic intervention for patients with knee osteoarthritis. That being said, there have been adverse side effects attributed to use of corticosteroids. The most common side effect is a postinjection flare, which has been documented to occur in anywhere from 2% to 25% of injection administrations.[40,43,52] This results in an acute pain crisis due to increased inflammation, typically occurring within hours of injection and can last up to 48 to 72 hours in duration.[53] It has been suggested that an aspiration to rule out infection should be considered if an intra-articular infection is suspected or if symptoms of postinjection flare persist longer than 24 hours,[40,43] Along with postinjection flare, postinjection pain is a commonly noted side effect.

The most concerning adverse event of intra-articular CSIs is septic arthritis due to the potential of high morbidity and mortality. However, studies have shown that the actual occurrence of postinjection septic arthritis is as low as 0.01% to 0.03%.[40,43,54] Additional complications that may occur include local tissue atrophy, skin hypopigmentation, and fat atrophy.[42,55] This can be due to improper placement of an intra-articular injection (not actually placed in the joint) or if the solution exits the joint space out along the pathway from the needle.[40,43] A concern that is frequently discussed is the thought that intra-articular CSIs could potentially lead to acceleration of cartilage loss and damage compared to placebo. Numerous studies have been performed with conflicting data. Several long-term studies and randomized control trials have been published indicating there were no significant negative effects to the knee anatomical structures or articular cartilage observed with long-term administration of intra-articular CSIs.[42,46,51] Furthermore, intervention with intra-articular CSIs had been noted to provide significant improvement in pain, nighttime symptoms, and joint stiffness.[51] In 2017, McAlindon et al. conducted a study comparing intra-articular CSIs in the knee joint to saline injections every 12 weeks for 2 years and reported greater cartilage volume loss in the intervention group compared to the control group.[56] It should be noted that the protocol of every 12-week injections is not typically done in practice and draws question to clinical relevance of the study conclusions.

Systemic adverse effects have also been documented. A commonly described effect is facial flushing, which can occur in up to 15% of recipients and is most commonly observed with administration of triamcinolone acetonide.[40,42,43,57] It is believed to result from a histamine-mediated response, and typically is self-limited resolving within 36 hours.[58] Hyperglycemia in diabetic patients is

another known effect from CSIs and can last 2 to 5 days in duration.[40,43,59] Diabetic patients should be counseled about this prior to administration of CSIs and it is not prudent to perform multiple injections in the same setting for such patients.

Contraindications

Intra-articular CSIs should be avoided or reconsidered in patients with absolute and/or relative contraindications. An absolute contraindication to intra-articular CSIs is evidence of an active septic arthritis or overlying superficial soft tissue infection.[40,42,43] A corticosteroid injection should be avoided in a systemic infection such as bacteremia. Patients with joint instability or an intra-articular fracture should not undergo an intra-articular CSI as this could worsen the underlying structure pathology and potentially delay healing.[40,43,60]

There is mixed literature to advise for or against performing intra-articular CSIs in patients on anticoagulation medications given the potential for hemarthrosis.[40,43,61] This is often left to the discretion of the provider, as is the decision on whether to hold anticoagulation prior to the procedure. A relative contraindication to a CSI is a recent intra-articular CSI in the same joint within the previous 6 weeks, or three injections within the previous year.[62] Juxta-articular osteoporosis is an additional contraindication for these procedures.[43] Refer to **Table 22-2** for a list of adverse events and contraindications associated with intra-articular CSIs.

HYALURONIC ACID INJECTIONS

Pharmacology and Mechanism of Action

A natural glycosaminoglycan polymer, hyaluronic acid (HA) is a key element of synovial fluid, which exists at a high molecular weight.[63,64] It functions to provide shock absorption, serves as a lubricant, protects cartilage, and has anti-inflammatory properties for joints.[65,66] Natural

TABLE 22-2 Adverse Events and Contraindications Associated With Intra-Articular Corticosteroid Injections

Adverse Events	Contraindications (Absolute and Relative)
Facial flushing	Absolute:
Hyperglycemia	Septic arthritis
Hypopigmentation	Superficial soft tissue infection
Hypothalamic–pituitary–adrenal axis suppression	Systemic infection
Local tissue atrophy	Relative:
Postinjection flare	Anticoagulation use
Postinjection pain	Osteoporosis
Septic arthritis	Recent CSI within past 6 wk
Tendon rupture	Recent CSI 3 injections within past 12 mo

HA within the joint decreases over time, and the intention of an intra-articular HA injection is to replenish the HA within synovial fluid and assist in production of new HA.[66]

Additionally, it can also provide pain relief and affect inflammatory mediator activity.[63,66]

Intra-articular HA injections exist in many different formulations. Molecular weight composition (high versus moderate versus low) varies between formulations.[67-69] Other differences include the source from which they are derived (biological versus avian), quantity/volume of injection, and frequency of injections needed ranging from one to five injections per series.[65,70,71] The efficacy between high- versus low-molecular-weight HA injections is frequently studied. Most literature supports the claim that high-molecular-weight HA injections provide better outcomes for treatment of knee osteoarthritis.[65,66,72] While biological and avian-derived HA injections have shown similar efficacy, biologically derived HA injections have demonstrated a better safety profile and have gained increasing popularity as a result.[65,70] There has yet to be a consensus as to which HA formulation is the best for use of knee osteoarthritis. Refer to **Tables 22-3** and **22-4** for a detailed composite of HA injections.

When compared to placebo, the efficacy of an intra-articular HA injection has statistically significant improvement in knee osteoarthritis pain and function.[73-75] The efficacy of intra-articular HA injections and intra-articular CSIs is often compared, as CSIs tend to have a quicker onset of symptom relief, but viscosupplementation injections have a longer duration of symptom relief.[63] Typically, there is better pain control in those receiving CSI during the first month after injection compared to those receiving HA injections.[63,73,75] However, at 4 to 26 weeks postinjection, administration of HA injections has been shown to be more beneficial than CSIs for symptom management.[73,75]

Indications

Viscosupplementation injections continue to be a popular treatment modality for knee osteoarthritis. They are often

TABLE 22-3 Single-Injection Viscosupplementation Injections

Name	Molecular Weight (kilodaltons)	Derivative (Avian vs. Biologic)
Durolane (Bioventus, Durham, NC)	N/A	Biologic
Gel-One (Zimmer Biomet, Warsaw, IN)	N/A	Avian
Monovisc (Anika Therapeutics, Bedford, MA)	1000-2900	Biologic
Synvisc-One (Genzyme Corporation, Cambridge, MA)	6000	Avian

TABLE 22-4 Multiple-Injection Series Viscosupplementation Injections

Name	Molecular Weight (kilodaltons)	Weekly Injections	Derivative (Avian vs. Biologic)
Euflexxa (Ferring Pharmaceuticals, Saint-Prex, Switzerland)	2400-3600	3	Biologic
Gelsyn-3 (Bioventus, Durham, NC)	1100	3	Biologic
Genvisc 850 (OrthogenRx, New Britain, PA)	620-1170 (average 850)	5	Biologic
Hyalgan (Fidia Pharma, Florham Park, NJ)	500-730	3-5	Avian
Orthovisc (Anika Therapeutics, Bedford, MA)	1000-2900	3	Biologic
Supartz (Bioventus, Durham, NC)	620-1170	3-5	Avian
Synvisc (Genzyme Corporation, Cambridge, MA)	6000	3	Avian
Visco-3 (Zimmer Biomet, Warsaw, IN)	620-1170	3	Avian

used for conservative management of knee osteoarthritis in terms of pain and function when initial treatment with oral and topical medications has failed to adequately provide relief or for patients with contraindications to these same medications, and have been demonstrated to have greater efficacy compared to placebo.[63,74,76] Intra-articular HAs can prolong the time before one requires a total knee replacement for knee osteoarthritis management,[63,77] with one study demonstrating this was delayed by 3.6 years for patients who received five or more intra-articular HA injection series.[78] This is important as some patients have coexisting conditions preventing them from being able to undergo surgery.

There continues to be on-going discussions about the use of intra-articular HA injections for treatment of knee osteoarthritis. This is in part due to differing opinions from consensus guidelines. In 2013, the AAOS stated they "cannot recommend using" HA injections for treatment of knee osteoarthritis, based on meta-analyses reporting that the treatment effects of intra-articular HAs did not meet the minimum clinically important improvement (MCII) threshold[7]; however, it did acknowledge HA injections provided "statistically significant treatment effects." The American Medical Society for Sports Medicine (AMSSM) argued against the AAOS recommendations and supported the use of viscosupplementation after conducting a network meta-analysis which showed patients receiving intra-articular HA had a better therapeutic response compared to those receiving intra-articular CSI or placebo.[75] The ACR also "conditionally supports" the use of viscosupplementation if a patient had an inadequate response to treatment with acetaminophen.[4] The European Society for Clinical and Economic Aspects of Osteoporosis and Osteoarthritis (ESCEO) task force also supports the use of intra-articular HA injections.[79] Because of varying conclusions among meta-analyses, the OARSI guidelines in 2014 have "uncertain" recommendations for use of intra-articular HA.[3]

Adverse Effects and Contraindications

Similar to those of intra-articular CSIs, some of the most common side effects due to intra-articular HA injections are often topical and include pain and postinjection flares due to an increase in inflammation.[63,65,80] These can last up to 48 to 72 hours, and an intra-articular aspiration should be considered if symptoms persist longer than 24 hours to exclude the possibility of septic arthritis or pseudogout. Joint stiffness and effusion are other common adverse events with viscosupplementation injections.[63,65] Urticaria, bleeding, rash, and erythema include some of the other local adverse events reported with these injections.[74] There is a higher frequency of side effects in intra-articular HA injections compared to intra-articular CSIs, which could be in part due to the repeated injections involved in administration of the injection series for various preparations.[63] Additional adverse events that can develop include pseudogout, septic arthritis, or an anaphylactoid reaction after receiving an HA injection.[67]

As is the case with any intervention, absolute and relative contraindications to use of viscosupplementation injections exist. Intra-articular HA injections share some of the same contraindications as was previously discussed with intra-articular CSIs. Septic arthritis is the most serious contraindication to intra-articular HA injections. Similarly, evidence of surrounding superficial soft tissue infection overlying the knee joint would because to postpone administration of an injection until the infection has resolved.[1] A prior adverse reaction to an intra-articular HA injection should be considered a relative contraindication to further treatment with this modality.

ORTHOBIOLOGICS

The utilization of biologics in orthopedics has significantly increased over the last few decades as has the published literature regarding biologic agents. It is anticipated that this trend will continue as both providers and patients strive for improved function and quality of life. An excellent understanding of the different types and formulation of biologics and current literature is necessary to provide the best possible outcomes. This section will provide you with the current information regarding biologics as it relates to the treatment of osteoarthritis.

Platelet-Rich Plasma

Platelets or thrombocytes are derived from bone marrow megakaryocytes. Normal platelet numbers range between 150,000 and 450,000 per microliter of blood.[81] The platelets function in coagulation and hemostasis but also function in regulating mechanisms involved in the healing process. Platelets contain numerous proteins including cytokines, messenger molecules, and growth factors. In fact, stored in the platelets' alpha and dense granules are more than 1500 active proteins.[82-84] The alpha granules contain numerous growth factors that are engaged in the normal healing response. These growth factors include platelet-derived growth factor (PDGF), transforming growth factor-beta 1 (TGF-β), epidermal growth factor (EGF), vascular endothelial growth factor (VEGF), insulin-like growth factor (IGF-1), and basic fibroblast growth factor (FGF).[83,85,86] When the granules release the growth factors, they enable recruitment of reparative cells to the injury site ultimately resulting in an increase in angiogenesis, cell proliferation, and tissue regeneration.[85-90]

Platelet-rich plasma (PRP) is autologous plasma with a higher number of platelets compared to the amount at baseline.[91] PRP is obtained by an initial blood draw. The autologous blood is then centrifuged resulting in a small volume of plasma containing a high concentration of platelets. The increased concentration of platelets yields greater numbers of growth factors and mediators. PRP has a proliferative effect on multiple cell types including fibroblasts, tenocytes, myocytes, osteoblasts, and chondrocytes.[89,92-95] Additionally, PRP may have a chondrocyte protective role by modifying and inhibiting the inflammatory response toward these cartilage cells.[96-99] The role that activated PRP plays in the treatment of knee OA likely stems from its ability to influence cellular proliferation, differentiation, angiogenesis, and tissue regeneration.

There are numerous available commercial systems used in the preparation of PRP. The quantity of blood needed to yield the end product of PRP will depend on the system used. Commercial systems' PRP formulations differ in the platelet count, leukocyte concentration, and the process of platelet activation. Mazzocca et al.[100] found when using the same commercial system that the PRP component concentrations varied significantly from person to person and this was also observed when blood samples were obtained at different times in the same subject. Others have corroborated these findings of varying concentrations.[100-102]

PRP is categorized by leukocyte concentration. PRP leukocyte concentrations are either leukocyte-rich PRP (LR-PRP) or leukocyte-poor PRP (LP-PRP) based on neutrophils concentrations above or below their normal baseline. The decision to use LR-PRP or LP-PRP may differ demanding on the target tissue. Braun and colleagues[103] found that LR-PRP, LP-PRP, RBC concentrate, and PPP (platelet-poor plasma) in a controlled laboratory setting had differing effects on human synovial cells. LP-PRP resulted in more anti-inflammatory cytokines opposed to LR-PRP and RBC concentrate that resulted in a significantly greater production of pro-inflammatory cytokines and more synovial cell death. The authors concluded that LP-PRP should be considered for intra-articular injections. Other investigators have also demonstrated improved outcomes in treating knee OA with LP-PRP.[104,105]

Platelet activation varies among the different PRP formulations. The activation of the platelets can be done chemically, for example, with thrombin or calcium chloride or PRP can be injected into the target site and endogenously activated through local tissue factors. Either technique, depending on the providers' platelet activation preference, results in the platelet degranulation and the release of mediators and growth factors.

Depending on the commercial PRP system used the protocol for the collection and preparation of the PRP will vary. In general, a specific whole-blood volume will be required to obtain the final platelet concentration. The whole blood is mixed with an anticoagulant factor and centrifuged. The blood is then centrifuged to separate the red blood cells (RBCs) from the PPP, and the concentrated platelets and leukocytes. Depending on the commercial system used will determine the leukocyte component resulting in either LR-PRP or LP-PRP. The concentrated platelet layer is separated out and the RBC and PPP layers are discarded (**Figs. 22-2** and **22-3**). Depending on the provider's platelet activation preference, the PRP is injected into the target treatment area.

PRP Use in Osteoarthritis

At the time of this publication, PRP injection use in the treatment of OA is considered off-label, as PRP is not currently FDA approved for injection therapy.

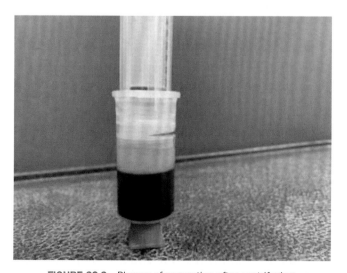

FIGURE 22-2 Phases of separation after centrifuging.

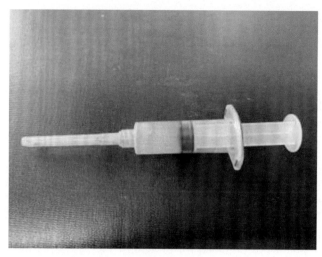

FIGURE 22-3 Syringe with platelet-rich plasma.

Studies involving PRP in the treatment of osteoarthritis have increased over the past decade. Most knee OA trials have looked to compare HA to PRP. Khoshbin and colleagues[106] published a quantitative systematic review of randomized controlled trials (RCTs) and prospective cohort studies evaluating the efficacy of PRP versus HA versus normal saline (NS) injections. The authors reported that Western Ontario and McMaster Universities Arthritis Index (WOMAC) and the International Knee Documentation Committee Scores (IKDC) at 6 months were significantly better or favored PRP-treated patients over HA and NS injections. A recent prospective RCT by Huang et al.[107] compared PRP, HA, and CS injections in the treatment of early knee OA. They reported that at 3 months all treatment groups had significant improvement in WOMAC scores. However, the PRP group had significant improvement at 6, 9, and 12 months compared to both the HA and CS groups. Others have reported WOMAC score improvements 12 months following PRP injections.[106,108,109]

Shen et al.[110] performed a systematic review of 14 RCTs with 1423 participants. PRP was compared to controls using a variety of treatments from HA, saline, ozone, and corticosteroid with follow-up ranging between 3 and 12 months. PRP injections were reported to significantly reduce total WOMAC scores and knee pain with concomitant improvement in physical function at 3, 6, and 12 months compared to controls. The authors also noted that there were no significant differences in the PRP group in adverse events compared to the other IA injections.

Studies show better efficacy with PRP, compared to HA in younger patients with low-grade knee osteoarthritis compared to individuals with more advanced OA.[108,111,112] In older patients with more advanced OA, PRP and HA injections shown similar efficacy.[111] It is important to note that not all studies comparing PRP to HA have found clinical improvement in subjects with knee OA, and this still remains a highly debated form of management by providers.[113,114]

Adverse Effects and Contraindications

Most PRP injection studies report adverse events related to the injections to be minimal and are limited to transient pain and swelling at the injection site.[114-116] Larger studies are needed to further determine immediate and long-term adverse events related to PRP injections.

Contraindications for PRP injections are similar to those of corticosteroid injections including cellulitis overlying the injection site, joint infection, or a septic illness. Other medical conditions that may affect the quality of PRP include platelet dysfunction and thrombocytopenia.

The most recent AAOS treatment of knee osteoarthritis guidelines published in 2013 stated that they were unable to recommend for or against PRP as a treatment of symptomatic knee osteoarthritis based on limited, low-level conflicting study results. They suggested that practitioners should be aware of new evidence and use clinical judgment when using PRP.[117]

The studies investigating the use of PRP in the treatment of osteoarthritis continue to grow in number. PRP appears to be a safe and promising treatment for osteoarthritis. The published literature lacks consistent methodology and PRP concentration reporting limiting the ability to compare studies. Future high-quality large clinical trials are needed to improve our understanding of the clinical application of PRP in the treatment of osteoarthritis.

Stem Cells

Mesenchymal stem cell (MSC) therapy has emerged as a promising treatment of osteoarthritis. MSCs have self-renewal ability and multilineage differentiation into specialized cell types including osteocytes, chondrocytes, myoblasts, and adipocytes.[118,119] It is not entirely clear how MSCs achieve their therapeutic effect on knee OA. Multiple processes are likely involved in symptom reduction and the regenerative process including the MSC's ability to stimulate endogenous cell repair and proliferate and regenerate both cartilage and subchondral bone.[120-122] In addition, MSCs have paracrine signaling capabilities that control inflammation and improve blood flow.[122-125] Ultimately it may be the anti-inflammatory effect that leads to a reduction in OA symptoms.

Embryonic stem cells can differentiate into numerous cell lineages making them the ideal cell source for regenerative medicine.[119] Ethical and regulatory factors limit embryonic stem cell use in humans.[119] There are other sources of MSCs that possess chondrogenic potential including bone marrow, adipose tissue, amniotic-derived from amniotic fluid, and umbilical cord.[119,122,126] MSCs derived from bone marrow aspirate (BMA) account for only 0.001% to 0.01% of cellular content of the bone marrow.[127] Depending on the pathology, determining the appropriate source for the MSCs to be utilized is important as the MSC source may affect the differentiation capabilities.[128]

Multiple trials have investigated MSC injections in the treatment of knee OA. Vega et al.[129] reported on a randomized, control trial with 30 subjects with knee OA pain refractory to conservative treatment. Half of the subjects received intra-articular allogeneic bone marrow MSCs, and the control group received a single dose of intra-articular HA. Clinical outcomes at 1 year found that the MSC treatment arm had significant improvement in quality-of-life outcomes versus the HA control group. Additionally, articular cartilage quality was evaluated by quantitative magnetic resonance imaging (MRI) T2 mapping showing in the MSC treated group cartilage quality improvement while there was a significant decrease in the poor cartilage area.

Orozco and colleagues[130] reported findings on their pilot study involving 12 patients with no controls. As with Vega, all subjects had refractory knee pain from OA. All subjects were treated with an intra-articular MSC injection. The subjects were found to have a rapid and progressive significant improvement in pain, function, and cartilage quality. 11 of 12 subjects by quantitative MRI T2 mapping revealed significant improvement in cartilage quality and a decrease in the area of poor cartilage. Wong et al.[131] reported similar clinical and MRI findings in subjects receiving MSC injections compared to controls. Kim et al.[132] performed BMAC injection with adipose tissue in subjects with degenerative OA, Kellgren-Lawrence (K-L) grade I-IV. Results showed all groups had significant improvement in pain and functional outcome scores, but K-L I-III had significant improvement over K-L IV. These findings suggest that these injections, although improvement in all OA groups was noted, may be more effective in earlier grade OA.

Cotter and colleagues[133] performed a critical review of the current clinical data regarding the utilization of bone marrow aspirate concentrate (BMAC) in the setting of focal cartilage defects of the knee. The authors reported after reviewing 1832 articles that BMAC demonstrated good clinical efficacy with favorable results in chondral defect repair either used as an isolated treatment or as an adjuvant treatment.

Adverse Events

Marenah et al.[134] published a systemic review evaluating the quality of regenerative medicine clinical research in the treatment of knee OA. They included adverse events in their review. A total of 35 studies out of the 152 identified met inclusion for review. A total of 3101 patients participated in the studies. They report that of the 35 studies, 31 studies (88.6%), reported their adverse events but some lacked precise descriptions of character and exact number of side effects. The reported events noted in this review included injection site pain, swelling, stiffness, warmth, and infection. Unfortunately, the review does not report the specific regenerative therapy used, making it hard to delineate if one type of regenerative therapy was more or less likely to have an associated adverse event. They reported that the adverse events findings were similar to reports from other types of intra-articular injections.[135-137]

Concerns have been expressed regarding the possibility of MSCs' neoplastic potential because of their enhancing angiogenesis and tumor proliferation capacity.[138] Yamasaki et al.[139] reported no observed tumors or infections after evaluating 10 years of preclinical and clinical study data from subjects that had autologous BMSC transplantation. Additionally, a systematic review published by Lalu and colleagues suggests that MSC therapy appears to be safe.[140]

Overall stem cell research tends to show improved functional outcomes and may have a positive effect on the articular cartilage. However, limitations exist in the present literature with clinical trials having relatively low subject numbers and lack high-level reproducible study methodology. In the future, large high-quality clinical trials are needed to determine the optimal source, timing, and frequency of stem cell injections while further determining the regenerative effect on the cartilage. Further diligence in monitoring and reporting adverse events will be necessary to assure safety.

CONCLUSION

It is important to have an excellent understanding of the pharmacological and biologics available for use in the treatment of osteoarthritis. The decision to use biologics for the treatment of osteoarthritis should be based on the current literature and individualized to specific patients' needs. The authors want to remind the reader that although orthobiologic research has made significant progress in recent years it is an evolving field and therefore encourage you to be diligent in keeping apprised of the current literature while making treatment recommendations. Ultimately osteoarthritis treatment should be individualized to allow for optimal function and pain control. Prudent use of the modalities mentioned can lead to successful management of knee OA symptoms with a relatively low adverse event profile, with the benefit of delaying further surgical needs.

REFERENCES

1. Ayhan E, Kesmezacar H, Akgun I. Intraarticular injections (corticosteroid, hyaluronic acid, platelet rich plasma) for the knee osteoarthritis. *World J Orthop.* 2014;5(3):351-361.
2. Jordan KM, Arden NK, Doherty M, et al. EULAR recommendations 2003: an evidence based approach to the management of knee osteoarthritis: report of a task force of the Standing Committee for International Clinical Studies Including Therapeutic Trials (ESCISIT). *Ann Rheum Dis.* 2003;62(12):1145-1155.
3. McAlindon TE, Bannuru RR, Sullivan MC, et al. OARSI guidelines for the non-surgical management of knee osteoarthritis. *Osteoarthr Cartil.* 2014;22(3):363-388.
4. Hochberg MC, Altman RD, April KT, et al. American College of Rheumatology 2012 recommendations for the use of nonpharmacologic and pharmacologic therapies in osteoarthritis of the hand, hip, and knee. *Arthritis Care Res.* 2012;64(4):465-474.
5. Craig DG, Bates CM, Davidson JS, Martin KG, Hayes PC, Simpson KJ. Staggered overdose pattern and delay to hospital presentation are associated with adverse outcomes following paracetamol-induced hepatotoxicity. *Br J Clin Pharmacol.* 2012;73(2):285-294.
6. Pepine CJ, Gurbel PA. Cardiovascular safety of NSAIDs: additional insights after PRECISION and point of view. *Clin Cardiol.* 2017;40(12):1352-1356.
7. Jevsevar DS, Brown GA, Jones DL, et al. The American Academy of Orthopaedic Surgeons evidence-based guideline on: treatment of osteoarthritis of the knee, 2nd edition. *J Bone Joint Surg Am.* 2013;95(20):1885-1886.
8. Sostres C, Gargallo CJ, Arroyo MT, Lanas A. Adverse effects of non-steroidal anti-inflammatory drugs (NSAIDs, aspirin and coxibs) on upper gastrointestinal tract. *Best Pract Res Clin Gastroenterol.* 2010;24(2):121-132.
9. Garg Y, Singh J, Sohal HS, Gore R, Kumar A. Comparison of clinical effectiveness and safety of newer nonsteroidal anti-inflammatory drugs in patients of osteoarthritis of knee joint: a randomized, prospective, open-label parallel-group study. *Indian J Pharmacol.* 2017;49(5):383-389.
10. Ong CK, Lirk P, Tan CH, Seymour RA. An evidence-based update on nonsteroidal anti-inflammatory drugs. *Clin Med Res.* 2007;5(1):19-34.
11. Laine L, Connors LG, Reicin A, et al. Serious lower gastrointestinal clinical events with nonselective NSAID or coxib use. *Gastroenterology.* 2003;124(2):288-292.
12. Rahme E, Barkun A, Nedjar H, Gaugris S, Watson D. Hospitalizations for upper and lower GI events associated with traditional NSAIDs and acetaminophen among the elderly in Quebec, Canada. *Am J Gastroenterol.* 2008;103(4):872-882.
13. Wolfe MM, Lichtenstein DR, Singh G. Gastrointestinal toxicity of nonsteroidal antiinflammatory drugs. *N Engl J Med.* 1999;340(24):1888-1899.
14. Singh G, Fort JG, Goldstein JL, et al. Celecoxib versus naproxen and diclofenac in osteoarthritis patients: SUCCESS-I Study. *Am J Med.* 2006;119(3):255-266.
15. Bombardier C, Laine L, Reicin A, et al. Comparison of upper gastrointestinal toxicity of rofecoxib and naproxen in patients with rheumatoid arthritis. VIGOR Study Group. *N Engl J Med.* 2000;343(21):1520-1528, 1522 p following 1528.
16. Schnitzer TJ, Burmester GR, Mysler E, et al. Comparison of lumiracoxib with naproxen and ibuprofen in the Therapeutic Arthritis Research and Gastrointestinal Event Trial (TARGET), reduction in ulcer complications: randomised controlled trial. *Lancet.* 2004;364(9435):665-674.
17. Silverstein FE, Faich G, Goldstein JL, et al. Gastrointestinal toxicity with celecoxib vs nonsteroidal anti-inflammatory drugs for osteoarthritis and rheumatoid arthritis: the CLASS study: a randomized controlled trial. Celecoxib Long-Term Arthritis Safety Study. *JAMA.* 2000;284(10):1247-1255.
18. Bresalier RS, Sandler RS, Quan H, et al. Cardiovascular events associated with rofecoxib in a colorectal adenoma chemoprevention trial. *N Engl J Med.* 2005;352(11):1092-1102.
19. Solomon SD, McMurray JJ, Pfeffer MA, et al. Cardiovascular risk associated with celecoxib in a clinical trial for colorectal adenoma prevention. *N Engl J Med.* 2005;352(11):1071-1080.
20. Kuehn BM. FDA panel: keep COX-2 drugs on market: black box for COX-2 labels, caution urged for all NSAIDs. *JAMA.* 2005;293(13):1571-1572.
21. Singh G, Wu O, Langhorne P, Madhok R. Risk of acute myocardial infarction with nonselective non-steroidal anti-inflammatory drugs: a meta-analysis. *Arthritis Res Ther.* 2006;8(5):R153.
22. Wang ZY, Shi SY, Li SJ, et al. Efficacy and safety of duloxetine on osteoarthritis knee pain: a meta-analysis of randomized controlled trials. *Pain Med.* 2015;16(7):1373-1385.
23. Brown JP, Boulay LJ. Clinical experience with duloxetine in the management of chronic musculoskeletal pain. A focus on osteoarthritis of the knee. *Ther Adv Musculoskelet Dis.* 2013;5(6):291-304.

24. Montgomery SA. Antidepressants and seizures: emphasis on newer agents and clinical implications. *Int J Clin Pract.* 2005;59(12):1435-1440.

25. Xue F, Strombom I, Turnbull B, Zhu S, Seeger J. Treatment with duloxetine in adults and the incidence of cardiovascular events. *J Clin Psychopharmacol.* 2012;32(1):23-30.

26. Beaulieu AD, Peloso PM, Haraoui B, et al. Once-daily, controlled-release tramadol and sustained-release diclofenac relieve chronic pain due to osteoarthritis: a randomized controlled trial. *Pain Res Manag.* 2008;13(2):103-110.

27. Chou R, McDonagh MS, Nakamoto E, Griffin J, eds. *Analgesics for Osteoarthritis: An Update of the 2006 Comparative Effectiveness Review.* Rockville, MD: Agency for Healthcare Research and Quality; 2011.

28. American Geriatrics Society Panel on Pharmacological Management of Persistent Pain in Older P. Pharmacological management of persistent pain in older persons. *J Am Geriatr Soc.* 2009;57(8):1331-1346.

29. Meng Z, Huang R. Topical treatment of degenerative knee osteoarthritis. *Am J Med Sci.* 2018;355(1):6-12.

30. Rannou F, Pelletier JP, Martel-Pelletier J. Efficacy and safety of topical NSAIDs in the management of osteoarthritis: evidence from real-life setting trials and surveys. *Semin Arthritis Rheum.* 2016;45(4 suppl):S18-S21.

31. Jorge LL, Feres CC, Teles VE. Topical preparations for pain relief: efficacy and patient adherence. *J Pain Res.* 2010;4:11-24.

32. Bruhlmann P, de Vathaire F, Dreiser RL, Michel BA. Short-term treatment with topical diclofenac epolamine plaster in patients with symptomatic knee osteoarthritis: pooled analysis of two randomised clinical studies. *Curr Med Res Opin.* 2006;22(12):2429-2438.

33. Klinge SA, Sawyer GA. Effectiveness and safety of topical versus oral nonsteroidal anti-inflammatory drugs: a comprehensive review. *Phys Sportsmed.* 2013;41(2):64-74.

34. McPherson ML, Cimino NM. Topical NSAID formulations. *Pain Med.* 2013;14(suppl 1):S35-S39.

35. Derry S, Conaghan P, Da Silva JA, Wiffen PJ, Moore RA. Topical NSAIDs for chronic musculoskeletal pain in adults. *Cochrane Database Syst Rev.* 2016;4:CD007400.

36. Shackel NA, Day RO, Kellett B, Brooks PM. Copper-salicylate gel for pain relief in osteoarthritis: a randomised controlled trial. *Med J Aust.* 1997;167(3):134-136.

37. Mason L, Moore RA, Edwards JE, McQuay HJ, Derry S, Wiffen PJ. Systematic review of efficacy of topical rubefacients containing salicylates for the treatment of acute and chronic pain. *BMJ.* 2004;328(7446):995.

38. Mason L, Moore RA, Derry S, Edwards JE, McQuay HJ. Systematic review of topical capsaicin for the treatment of chronic pain. *BMJ.* 2004;328(7446):991.

39. De Silva V, El-Metwally A, Ernst E, et al. Evidence for the efficacy of complementary and alternative medicines in the management of osteoarthritis: a systematic review. *Rheumatology.* 2011;50(5):911-920.

40. Freire V, Bureau NJ. Injectable corticosteroids: take precautions and use caution. *Semin Musculoskelet Radiol.* 2016;20(5):401-408.

41. Hollander JL, Brown EM Jr, Jessar RA, Brown CY. Hydrocortisone and cortisone injected into arthritic joints; comparative effects of and use of hydrocortisone as a local antiarthritic agent. *J Am Med Assoc.* 1951;147(17):1629-1635.

42. Cole BJ, Schumacher HR Jr. Injectable corticosteroids in modern practice. *J Am Acad Orthop Surg.* 2005;13(1):37-46.

43. MacMahon PJ, Eustace SJ, Kavanagh EC. Injectable corticosteroid and local anesthetic preparations: a review for radiologists. *Radiology.* 2009;252(3):647-661.

44. Benzon HT, Chew TL, McCarthy RJ, Benzon HA, Walega DR. Comparison of the particle sizes of different steroids and the effect of dilution: a review of the relative neurotoxicities of the steroids. *Anesthesiology.* 2007;106(2):331-338.

45. Centeno LM, Moore ME. Preferred intraarticular corticosteroids and associated practice: a survey of members of the American College of Rheumatology. *Arthritis Care Res.* 1994;7(3):151-155.

46. Spitzer AI, Richmond JC, Kraus VB, et al. Safety and efficacy of repeat administration of triamcinolone acetonide extended-release in osteoarthritis of the knee: a phase 3b, open-label study. *Rheumatol Ther.* 2019;6(1):109-124.

47. Bodick N, Lufkin J, Willwerth C, et al. An intra-articular, extended-release formulation of triamcinolone acetonide prolongs and amplifies analgesic effect in patients with osteoarthritis of the knee: a randomized clinical trial. *J Bone Joint Surg Am.* 2015;97(11):877-888.

48. Kaufman MB. Pharmaceutical approval update. *P&T.* 2017;42(12):733-755.

49. Godwin M, Dawes M. Intra-articular steroid injections for painful knees. Systematic review with meta-analysis. *Can Fam Physician.* 2004;50:241-248.

50. Arroll B, Goodyear-Smith F. Corticosteroid injections for osteoarthritis of the knee: meta-analysis. *BMJ.* 2004;328(7444):869.

51. Raynauld JP, Buckland-Wright C, Ward R, et al. Safety and efficacy of long-term intraarticular steroid injections in osteoarthritis of the knee: a randomized, double-blind, placebo-controlled trial. *Arthritis Rheum.* 2003;48(2):370-377.

52. Friedman DM, Moore ME. The efficacy of intraarticular steroids in osteoarthritis: a double-blind study. *J Rheumatol.* 1980;7(6):850-856.

53. Young P, Homlar KC. Extreme postinjection flare in response to intra-articular triamcinolone acetonide (Kenalog). *Am J Orthop (Belle Mead NJ).* 2016;45(3):E108-E111.

54. Gray RG, Tenenbaum J, Gottlieb NL. Local corticosteroid injection treatment in rheumatic disorders. *Semin Arthritis Rheum.* 1981;10(4):231-254.

55. Okere K, Jones MC. A case of skin hypopigmentation secondary to a corticosteroid injection. *South Med J.* 2006;99(12):1393-1394.

56. McAlindon TE, LaValley MP, Harvey WF, et al. Effect of intra-articular triamcinolone vs saline on knee cartilage volume and pain in patients with knee osteoarthritis: a randomized clinical trial. *JAMA.* 2017;317(19):1967-1975.

57. Pattrick M, Doherty M. Facial flushing after intra-articular injection of steroid. *Br Med J.* 1987;295(6610):1380.

58. Everett CR, Baskin MN, Speech D, Novoseletsky D, Patel R. Flushing as a side effect following lumbar transforaminal epidural steroid injection. *Pain Physician.* 2004;7(4):427-429.

59. Habib GS, Bashir M, Jabbour A. Increased blood glucose levels following intra-articular injection of methylprednisolone acetate in patients with controlled diabetes and symptomatic osteoarthritis of the knee. *Ann Rheum Dis.* 2008;67(12):1790-1791.

60. Pountos I, Georgouli T, Blokhuis TJ, Pape HC, Giannoudis PV. Pharmacological agents and impairment of fracture healing: what is the evidence? *Injury.* 2008;39(4):384-394.

61. Foremny GB, Pretell-Mazzini J, Jose J, Subhawong TK. Risk of bleeding associated with interventional musculoskeletal radiology procedures. A comprehensive review of the literature. *Skeletal Radiol.* 2015;44(5):619-627.

62. Ostergaard M, Halberg P. Intra-articular corticosteroids in arthritic disease: a guide to treatment. *BioDrugs.* 1998;9(2):95-103.

63. He WW, Kuang MJ, Zhao J, et al. Efficacy and safety of intraarticular hyaluronic acid and corticosteroid for knee osteoarthritis: a meta-analysis. *Int J Surg.* 2017;39:95-103.

64. Hisada N, Satsu H, Mori A, et al. Low-molecular-weight hyaluronan permeates through human intestinal Caco-2 cell monolayers via the paracellular pathway. *Biosci Biotechnol Biochem.* 2008;72(5):1111-1114.

65. Altman RD, Bedi A, Karlsson J, Sancheti P, Schemitsch E. Product differences in intra-articular hyaluronic acids for osteoarthritis of the knee. *Am J Sports Med.* 2016;44(8):2158-2165.

66. Moreland LW. Intra-articular hyaluronan (hyaluronic acid) and hylans for the treatment of osteoarthritis: mechanisms of action. *Arthritis Res Ther.* 2003;5(2):54-67.

67. Hamburger MI, Lakhanpal S, Mooar PA, Oster D. Intra-articular hyaluronans: a review of product-specific safety profiles. *Semin Arthritis Rheum.* 2003;32(5):296-309.

68. Goldberg VM, Buckwalter JA. Hyaluronans in the treatment of osteoarthritis of the knee: evidence for disease-modifying activity. *Osteoarthr Cartil.* 2005;13(3):216-224.

69. Colen S, van den Bekerom MP, Mulier M, Haverkamp D. Hyaluronic acid in the treatment of knee osteoarthritis: a systematic review and meta-analysis with emphasis on the efficacy of different products. *BioDrugs.* 2012;26(4):257-268.

70. Kirchner M, Marshall D. A double-blind randomized controlled trial comparing alternate forms of high molecular weight hyaluronan for the treatment of osteoarthritis of the knee. *Osteoarthr Cartil.* 2006;14(2):154-162.

71. Bowman S, Awad ME, Hamrick MW, et al. Recent advances in hyaluronic acid based therapy for osteoarthritis. 2018;7:6.

72. Altman RD, Manjoo A, Fierlinger A, Niazi F, Nicholls M. The mechanism of action for hyaluronic acid treatment in the osteoarthritic knee: a systematic review. *BMC Musculoskelet Disord.* 2015;16:321.

73. Campbell KA, Erickson BJ, Saltzman BM, et al. Is local viscosupplementation injection clinically superior to other therapies in the treatment of osteoarthritis of the knee: a systematic review of overlapping meta-analyses. *Arthroscopy.* 2015;31(10):2036-2045.e2014.

74. Navarro-Sarabia F, Coronel P, Collantes E, et al. A 40-month multicentre, randomised placebo-controlled study to assess the efficacy and carry-over effect of repeated intra-articular injections of hyaluronic acid in knee osteoarthritis: the AMELIA project. *Ann Rheum Dis.* 2011;70(11):1957-1962.

75. Trojian TH, Concoff AL, Joy SM, Hatzenbuehler JR, Saulsberry WJ, Coleman CI. AMSSM scientific statement concerning viscosupplementation injections for knee osteoarthritis: Importance for individual patient outcomes. *Clin J Sport Med.* 2016;26(1):1-11.

76. Bannuru RR, Vaysbrot EE, Sullivan MC, McAlindon TE. Relative efficacy of hyaluronic acid in comparison with NSAIDs for knee osteoarthritis: a systematic review and meta-analysis. *Semin Arthritis Rheum.* 2014;43(5):593-599.

77. Ong KL, Anderson AF, Niazi F, Fierlinger AL, Kurtz SM, Altman RD. Hyaluronic acid injections in medicare knee osteoarthritis patients are associated with longer time to knee arthroplasty. *J Arthroplasty.* 2016;31(8):1667-1673.

78. Altman R, Lim S, Steen RG, Dasa V. Hyaluronic acid injections are associated with delay of total knee replacement surgery in patients with knee osteoarthritis: evidence from a large U.S. health claims database. *PLoS One.* 2015;10(12):e0145776.

79. Bruyere O, Cooper C, Pelletier JP, et al. A consensus statement on the European Society for Clinical and Economic Aspects of Osteoporosis and Osteoarthritis (ESCEO) algorithm for the management of knee osteoarthritis-From evidence-based medicine to the real-life setting. *Semin Arthritis Rheum.* 2016;45(4 suppl):S3-S11.

80. Legre-Boyer V. Viscosupplementation: techniques, indications, results. *Orthop Traumatol Surg Res.* 2015;101(1 suppl):S101-S108.

81. Ross DW, Ayscue LH, Watson J, Bentley SA. Stability of hematologic parameters in healthy subjects. Intraindividual versus interindividual variation. *Am J Clin Pathol.* 1988;90(3):262-267.

82. Wu CC, Chen WH, Zao B, et al. Regenerative potentials of platelet-rich plasma enhanced by collagen in retrieving proinflammatory cytokine-inhibited chondrogenesis. *Biomaterials.* 2011;32(25):5847-5854.

83. Borrione P, Gianfrancesco AD, Pereira MT, Pigozzi F. Platelet-rich plasma in muscle healing. *Am J Phys Med Rehabil.* 2010;89(10):854-861.

84. Broggini N, Hofstetter W, Hunziker E, et al. The influence of PRP on early bone formation in membrane protected defects. A histological and histomorphometric study in the rabbit calvaria. *Clin Implant Dent Relat Res.* 2011;13(1):1-12.

85. Nurden AT. Platelets, inflammation and tissue regeneration. *Thromb Haemost.* 2011;105(suppl 1):S13-S33.

86. Nurden AT, Nurden P, Sanchez M, Andia I, Anitua E. Platelets and wound healing. *Front Biosci.* 2008;13:3532-3548.

87. Pufe T, Petersen WJ, Mentlein R, Tillmann BN. The role of vasculature and angiogenesis for the pathogenesis of degenerative tendons disease. *Scand J Med Sci Sports.* 2005;15(4):211-222.

88. Gawaz M, Vogel S. Platelets in tissue repair: control of apoptosis and interactions with regenerative cells. *Blood.* 2013;122(15):2550-2554.

89. Wang X, Qiu Y, Triffitt J, Carr A, Xia Z, Sabokbar A. Proliferation and differentiation of human tenocytes in response to platelet rich plasma: an in vitro and in vivo study. *J Orthop Res.* 2012;30(6):982-990.

90. Lynch SE, Nixon JC, Colvin RB, Antoniades HN. Role of platelet-derived growth factor in wound healing: synergistic effects with other growth factors. *Proc Natl Acad Sci U S A.* 1987;84(21):7696-7700.

91. Marx RE. Platelet-rich plasma (PRP): what is PRP and what is not PRP? *Implant Dent.* 2001;10(4):225-228.

92. Kasemkijwattana C, Menetrey J, Bosch P, et al. Use of growth factors to improve muscle healing after strain injury. *Clin Orthop Relat Res.* 2000(370):272-285.

93. Klein MB, Pham H, Yalamanchi N, Chang J. Flexor tendon wound healing in vitro: the effect of lactate on tendon cell proliferation and collagen production. *J Hand Surg Am.* 2001;26(5):847-854.

94. Akeda K, An HS, Okuma M, et al. Platelet-rich plasma stimulates porcine articular chondrocyte proliferation and matrix biosynthesis. *Osteoarthr Cartil.* 2006;14(12):1272-1280.

95. Graziani F, Ivanovski S, Cei S, Ducci F, Tonetti M, Gabriele M. The in vitro effect of different PRP concentrations on osteoblasts and fibroblasts. *Clin Oral Implants Res.* 2006;17(2):212-219.

96. LaPrade RF, Geeslin AG, Murray IR, et al. Biologic treatments for sports injuries II think tank-current concepts, future research, and barriers to advancement, Part 1: biologics overview, ligament injury, tendinopathy. *Am J Sports Med.* 2016;44(12):3270-3283.

97. Sun Y, Feng Y, Zhang CQ, Chen SB, Cheng XG. The regenerative effect of platelet-rich plasma on healing in large osteochondral defects. *Int Orthop.* 2010;34(4):589-597.

98. Sundman EA, Cole BJ, Fortier LA. Growth factor and catabolic cytokine concentrations are influenced by the cellular composition of platelet-rich plasma. *Am J Sports Med.* 2011;39(10):2135-2140.

99. Sundman EA, Cole BJ, Karas V, et al. The anti-inflammatory and matrix restorative mechanisms of platelet-rich plasma in osteoarthritis. *Am J Sports Med.* 2014;42(1):35-41.

100. Mazzocca AD, McCarthy MB, Chowaniec DM, et al. Platelet-rich plasma differs according to preparation method and human variability. *J Bone Joint Surg Am.* 2012;94(4):308-316.

101. Castillo TN, Pouliot MA, Kim HJ, Dragoo JL. Comparison of growth factor and platelet concentration from commercial platelet-rich plasma separation systems. *Am J Sports Med.* 2011;39(2):266-271.

102. Magalon J, Bausset O, Serratrice N, et al. Characterization and comparison of 5 platelet-rich plasma preparations in a single-donor model. *Arthroscopy.* 2014;30(5):629-638.

103. Braun HJ, Kim HJ, Chu CR, Dragoo JL. The effect of platelet-rich plasma formulations and blood products on human synoviocytes: implications for intra-articular injury and therapy. *Am J Sports Med.* 2014;42(5):1204-1210.

104. Riboh JC, Yanke AB, Cole BJ. Effect of leukocyte concentration on the efficacy of PRP in the treatment of knee OA: response. *Am J Sports Med.* 2016;44(11):NP66-NP67.

105. Buendia-Lopez D, Medina-Quiros M, Fernandez-Villacanas Marin MA. Clinical and radiographic comparison of a single LP-PRP injection, a single hyaluronic acid injection and daily NSAID administration with a 52-week follow-up: a randomized controlled trial. *J Orthop Traumatol.* 2018;19(1):3.

106. Khoshbin A, Leroux T, Wasserstein D, et al. The efficacy of platelet-rich plasma in the treatment of symptomatic knee osteoarthritis: a systematic review with quantitative synthesis. *Arthroscopy.* 2013;29(12):2037-2048.

107. Huang Y, Liu X, Xu X, Liu J. Intra-articular injections of platelet-rich plasma, hyaluronic acid or corticosteroids for knee osteoarthritis: a prospective randomized controlled study. *Der Orthopäde.* 2019;48(3):239-247.

108. Campbell KA, Saltzman BM, Mascarenhas R, et al. Does intra-articular platelet-rich plasma injection provide clinically superior outcomes compared with other therapies in the treatment of knee osteoarthritis? A systematic review of overlapping meta-analyses. *Arthroscopy.* 2015;31(11):2213-2221.

109. Raeissadat SA, Rayegani SM, Hassanabadi H, et al. Knee osteoarthritis injection choices: platelet- rich plasma (PRP) versus hyaluronic acid (A one-year randomized clinical trial). *Clin Med Insights Arthritis Musculoskelet Disord.* 2015;8:1-8.

110. Shen L, Yuan T, Chen S, Xie X, Zhang C. The temporal effect of platelet-rich plasma on pain and physical function in the treatment of knee osteoarthritis: systematic review and meta-analysis of randomized controlled trials. *J Orthop Surg Res.* 2017;12(1):16.

111. Kon E, Mandelbaum B, Buda R, et al. Platelet-rich plasma intra-articular injection versus hyaluronic acid viscosupplementation as treatments for cartilage pathology: from early degeneration to osteoarthritis. *Arthroscopy.* 2011;27(11):1490-1501.

112. Filardo G, Kon E, Buda R, et al. Platelet-rich plasma intra-articular knee injections for the treatment of degenerative cartilage lesions and osteoarthritis. *Knee Surg Sports Traumatol Arthrosc.* 2011;19(4):528-535.

113. Bennell KL, Hunter DJ, Paterson KL. Platelet-rich plasma for the management of hip and knee osteoarthritis. *Curr Rheumatol Rep.* 2017;19(5):24.

114. Filardo G, Di Matteo B, Di Martino A, et al. Platelet-rich plasma intra-articular knee injections show no superiority versus viscosupplementation: a randomized controlled trial. *Am J Sports Med.* 2015;43(7):1575-1582.

115. Sampson S, Reed M, Silvers H, Meng M, Mandelbaum B. Injection of platelet-rich plasma in patients with primary and secondary knee osteoarthritis: a pilot study. *Am J Phys Med Rehabil.* 2010;89(12):961-969.

116. Spakova T, Rosocha J, Lacko M, Harvanova D, Gharaibeh A. Treatment of knee joint osteoarthritis with autologous platelet-rich plasma in comparison with hyaluronic acid. *Am J Phys Med Rehabil.* 2012;91(5):411-417.

117. Jevsevar DS. Treatment of osteoarthritis of the knee: evidence-based guideline, 2nd edition. *J Am Acad Orthop Surg.* 2013;21(9):571-576.

118. Barry F, Murphy M. Mesenchymal stem cells in joint disease and repair. *Nat Rev Rheumatol.* 2013;9(10):584-594.

119. Wei X, Yang X, Han ZP, Qu FF, Shao L, Shi YF. Mesenchymal stem cells: a new trend for cell therapy. *Acta Pharmacol Sin.* 2013;34(6):747-754.

120. Hunziker EB, Rosenberg LC. Repair of partial-thickness defects in articular cartilage: cell recruitment from the synovial membrane. *J Bone Joint Surg Am.* 1996;78(5):721-733.

121. Caplan AI. Review: mesenchymal stem cells: cell-based reconstructive therapy in orthopedics. *Tissue Eng.* 2005;11(7-8):1198-1211.

122. Veronesi F, Giavaresi G, Tschon M, Borsari V, Nicoli Aldini N, Fini M. Clinical use of bone marrow, bone marrow concentrate, and expanded bone marrow mesenchymal stem cells in cartilage disease. *Stem Cells Dev.* 2013;22(2):181-192.

123. Chen FH, Tuan RS. Mesenchymal stem cells in arthritic diseases. *Arthritis Res Ther.* 2008;10(5):223.

124. Caplan AI. Adult mesenchymal stem cells for tissue engineering versus regenerative medicine. *J Cell Physiol.* 2007;213(2):341-347.

125. Caplan AI, Correa D. PDGF in bone formation and regeneration: new insights into a novel mechanism involving MSCs. *J Orthop Res.* 2011;29(12):1795-1803.

126. Antonucci I, Pantalone A, Tete S, et al. Amniotic fluid stem cells: a promising therapeutic resource for cell-based regenerative therapy. *Curr Pharm Des.* 2012;18(13):1846-1863.

127. Pittenger MF, Mackay AM, Beck SC, et al. Multilineage potential of adult human mesenchymal stem cells. *Science.* 1999;284(5411):143-147.

128. Mafi R, Hindocha S, Mafi P, Griffin M, Khan WS. Sources of adult mesenchymal stem cells applicable for musculoskeletal applications – a systematic review of the literature. *Open Orthop J.* 2011;5(suppl 2):242-248.

129. Vega A, Martin-Ferrero MA, Del Canto F, et al. Treatment of knee osteoarthritis with allogeneic bone marrow mesenchymal stem cells: a randomized controlled trial. *Transplantation.* 2015;99(8):1681-1690.

130. Orozco L, Munar A, Soler R, et al. Treatment of knee osteoarthritis with autologous mesenchymal stem cells: a pilot study. *Transplantation.* 2013;95(12):1535-1541.

131. Wong KL, Lee KB, Tai BC, Law P, Lee EH, Hui JH. Injectable cultured bone marrow-derived mesenchymal stem cells in varus knees with cartilage defects undergoing high tibial osteotomy: a prospective, randomized controlled clinical trial with 2 years' follow-up. *Arthroscopy.* 2013;29(12):2020-2028.

132. Kim JD, Lee GW, Jung GH, et al. Clinical outcome of autologous bone marrow aspirates concentrate (BMAC) injection in degenerative arthritis of the knee. *Eur J Orthop Surg Traumatol.* 2014;24(8):1505-1511.

133. Cotter EJ, Wang KC, Yanke AB, Chubinskaya S. Bone marrow aspirate concentrate for cartilage defects of the knee: from bench to bedside evidence. *Cartilage.* 2018;9(2):161-170.

134. Marenah M, Li J, Kumar A, Murrell W. Quality assurance and adverse event management in regenerative medicine for knee osteoarthritis: current concepts. *J Clin Orthop Trauma.* 2019;10(1):53-58.

135. Centeno CJ, Schultz JR, Cheever M, et al. Safety and complications reporting update on the re-implantation of culture-expanded mesenchymal stem cells using autologous platelet lysate technique. *Curr Stem Cell Res Ther.* 2011;6(4):368-378.

136. Centeno CJ, Bashir J. Safety and regulatory issues regarding stem cell therapies: one clinic's perspective. *PM R.* 2015; 7(4 suppl):S4-S7.

137. Peeters CM, Leijs MJ, Reijman M, van Osch GJ, Bos PK. Safety of intra-articular cell-therapy with culture-expanded stem cells in humans: a systematic literature review. *Osteoarthr Cartil.* 2013;21(10):1465-1473.

138. Suzuki K, Sun R, Origuchi M, et al. Mesenchymal stromal cells promote tumor growth through the enhancement of neovascularization. *Mol Med.* 2011;17(7-8):579-587.

139. Yamasaki S, Mera H, Itokazu M, Hashimoto Y, Wakitani S. Cartilage repair with autologous bone marrow mesenchymal stem cell transplantation: review of preclinical and clinical studies. *Cartilage.* 2014;5(4):196-202.

140. Lalu MM, McIntyre L, Pugliese C, et al. Safety of cell therapy with mesenchymal stromal cells (SafeCell): a systematic review and meta-analysis of clinical trials. *PLoS One.* 2012;7(10):e47559.

chapter 23

Physical Therapy and Bracing

Hassan Alosh, MD | P. Maxwell Courtney, MD | Roshan P. Shah, MD, JD

KNEE BRACING

The use of bracing in the management of knee osteoarthritis (OA) has been a widely adopted measure since the 1980s.[1-3] Since then, a vast range of knee braces have been promoted with the goal of restoring mechanical alignment of the arthritic joint and providing symptomatic relief.[4] To varying degrees, clinical and *in vitro* studies have attempted to determine the efficacy of knee bracing in unloading the arthritic compartment and providing clinical improvement.[5,6] The mixed data surrounding bracing in the management of OA have resulted in divergent practices, with a survey demonstrating 29% of physicians routinely prescribing unloader bracing and 32% rarely or never prescribing them.[7] It is estimated that in the United States, upwards of 125,000 knee braces are dispensed annually, with an estimated mean cost of $700 to $1000 per brace.[2] Based on total cost numbers, it is important to weigh the cost-to-benefit ratio when considering this treatment modality. Given the increased projected utilization and cost of bracing, it is important to understand the contemporary evidence surrounding this management option.

Indications and Design

Unicompartmental osteoarthritis in the absence of any significant sagittal joint contracture hypothetically allows an unloader knee brace to provide a counterforce and reduce the forces through the arthritic compartment.[7] The candidate for knee bracing is one with pain caused by mild to severe knee OA who is willing to tolerate an external brace. Most manufacturers recommend that coronal deformity not exceed 10°, and that patients with a flexion contracture of >10° may not be ideal candidates for bracing.[2] Coronal deformity does not need to necessarily correctable as there is evidence that bracing works by load sharing or limiting muscle contraction as opposed to altering the coronal angle.[8] Patients with ligamentous incompetence in the direction of the brace moment (e.g., medial collateral ligament instability for a valgus unloader brace) should be avoided, and patients with peripheral vascular disease or skin lesions should be assessed carefully to minimize the risk of complications.[9] Patellofemoral disease is not a contraindication to unloader bracing, though severe bicompartmental osteoarthritis may limit the benefit of this modality.[10] Timing and duration of brace use lacks consensus; mild OA may only benefit from bracing during high impact activities, while severe arthritis can benefit with a longer duration of bracing, e.g., during activities of daily living.[1]

Knee brace designs are fabricated in a range of configurations, with various degrees of angular moments generated and supportive struts utilized to provide a buttress against the arthritic knee deformity (**Fig. 23-1**). These braces apply mechanical leverage through the use of upright struts or bars, hinges, and cuffs. The factors that increase the brace leverage include the length of bars, the number of fixation points (with four points being superior to three for leverage), the fit of the brace, and the brace material properties.[11] Application points applied over subcutaneous bone, such as the anteromedial tibia, provides greater leverage than areas with larger amounts of soft-tissue coverage.

In the most common scenario, a valgus-producing force is utilized in medial compartment osteoarthritis using a three- or four-point bending moment, with the goal of relieving the arthritic medial compartment and shifting the mechanical axis laterally (**Fig. 23-2**). Designs can include a single or dual upright support, along a hinge mechanism that allows for knee motion. Hinge mechanisms can range from a basic mechanism permitting sagittal motion to polycentric designs aimed at providing more natural knee motion in greater than one plane.[12] A displacement mechanism for achieving angular correction is used in an unloading brace and can be accomplished by pads, straps, or a more elaborate mechanism for fine-tuning the degree of valgus moment created.

Radiographic Studies

Several prior investigations have assessed the magnitude of radiographic deformity correction with a valgus-producing brace. In one early study, 15 patients with unicompartmental OA were assessed with fluoroscopy to determine the degree of coronal alignment and condylar separation at heel strike while using a treadmill.[13] These subjects were then fitted with an unloader brace, and the fluoroscopic examination was repeated. The authors determined that the brace generated a small difference in the amount of mean condylar separation distance (1.2 mm) and mean condylar separation angle (2.2°), though there were three subjects that did not have any measurable difference in either parameter. A subsequent study proposed that if a medial unloader brace did indeed

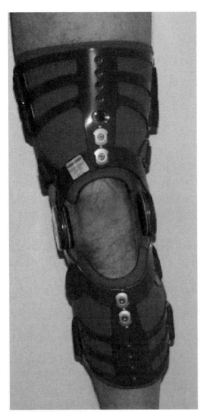

FIGURE 23-1 An example of a medial unloader brace, the MOS Genu brace. (Adapted from van Raaij TM, Reijman M, Brouwer RW, Bierma-Zeinstra SM, Verhaar JA. Medial knee osteoarthritis treated by insoles or braces: a randomized trial. *Clin Orthop Relat Res.* 2010;468(7):1926-1932.)

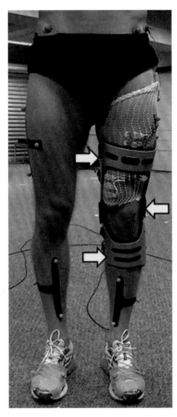

FIGURE 23-2 Direction of three-point bending moment in a valgus-producing unloader brace. (Adapted from Ebert JR, Hambly K, Joss B, Ackland TR, Donnelly CJ. Does an unloader brace reduce knee loading in normally aligned knees? *Clin Orthop Relat Res.* 2014;472(3):915-922.)

shift the mechanical axis laterally, a valgus-producing brace should increase that bone density of lateral compartment.[14] Utilizing dual-energy bone mineral density testing, they studied a series of patients with medial compartment osteoarthritis before and 3 months after wearing an unloader brace. There was a statistically significant increase in the lateral compartment bone density, whereas the lateral compartment in the unaffected contralateral limb did not show a significant increase in bone density.

Advances in dynamic three-dimensional imaging have allowed the ability to determine continuous changes in knee compartment space with an accuracy of submillimeter distances.[15] Previous studies were limited in their ability to determine changes in joint space in two planes at discrete point of the gait cycles (e.g., heel strike, stance, etc.). In a series of 10 patients with varus knee OA, Nagai and colleagues studied the medial compartment dynamic joint space (DJS) using continuous biplane radiography during gait with and without unloader bracing, in addition to determining changes in the ground reactive force (GRF) throughout the gait cycle.[16] The subjects had worn the unloader brace for 2 weeks prior to the radiographic study. Subjective improvement with the brace was determined with questionnaires. A small but statistically significant difference was found in medial compartment DJS

with brace use (0.3 mm, $P = .005$), though there was no difference in GRF. The patients also reported an improvement in pain with brace use.

Radiographic-based investigations have demonstrated modest though discernible radiographic effects of unloader bracing in the arthritic knee. Biomechanically, the postulated effect of unloader bracing on shifting the mechanical axis toward neutral alignment appears to have some supporting evidence, though its relevance clinically is debatable.

Gait Analysis Studies

Prior investigators have reasoned that if unloader bracing changes the static mechanical alignment of the limb, then an unloader brace should also improve the kinematics of gait in the arthritic knee. In addition to correcting the coronal deformity of the arthritic knee, the external coronal moment is an important contributor to force distribution across the knee.[2] This moment, or torque, is created when the foot contacts the ground during the stance phase of gait and the ground reaction force vector falls medial (varus knee) or lateral (valgus knee)[17] (**Fig. 23-3**). Also described as the knee adduction moment, this force is optimally counteracted with an unloader brace in addition to correction of the coronal deformity.[18]

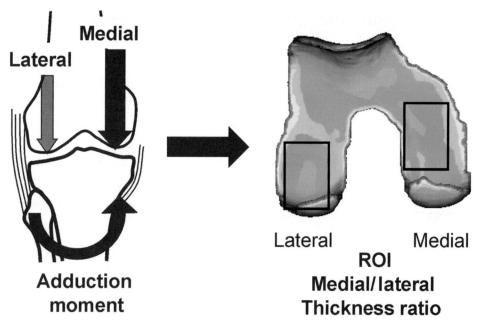

FIGURE 23-3   A depiction of the knee adductor moment. ROI, region of interest. (Adapted from Andriacchi TP, Koo S, Scanlan SF. Gait mechanics influence healthy cartilage morphology and osteoarthritis of the knee. *J Bone Joint Surg Am.* 2009;91(suppl 1):95-101.)

Small series have demonstrated changes in the varus moment created during gait with an unloader brace. In one investigation, five subjects with medial compartment osteoarthritis were fitted with a custom valgus-loading knee brace.[8] Three-dimensional analysis was coupled with force plate information to calculate the forces at the knee. The varus moment was found to be significantly reduced in the subjects during the early stance phase of gait when wearing an unloader brace. In another study using three-dimensional gait analysis, the authors attempted to quantify the decrease in the varus moment of 11 arthritic patients with and without an unloader brace. The authors determined that valgus bracing reduced the net moment around the knee by 13% and the medial compartment load of the knee by an average of 11%.[19]

More recently, Ramsey and colleagues coupled gait analysis studies with electromyography to determine the contribution of reduced muscle forces in the braced knee.[20] The authors hypothesized that rather than correcting the varus moment of the arthritic knee, unloader bracing mediated relief by stabilizing the joint and reducing muscle contractions and joint compression around the knee. The authors performed both gait analysis and dynamic EMG with the subjects wearing no brace, wearing the brace in neutral alignment, or wearing the brace in 4° of valgus (**Fig. 23-4**). When wearing the brace in neutral, patients experienced greater subjective knee stability and function than when wearing the brace in an unloader setting. Notably, the varus knee moments and muscle co-contraction were similar or improved when wearing a neutral brace in comparison to the brace in the valgus unloader mode, and the study concluded the benefits of bracing may emanate from a reduction in muscle contraction rather than a mechanical correction of the varus moment.

Schmalz and colleagues reported on the gait analysis of 16 patients who had worn an unloader brace for 4 weeks.[21] Beyond standard gait analysis, the authors also calculated the valgus moment created by the brace using a novel system that measured the deformation of the brace during the stance phase and measured the reaction force created by the brace. They determined that the brace reduced varus moment by approximately 10%, in addition to reducing the magnitude of gait asymmetry between the brace and contralateral leg while walking.

Clinical Data

Investigation into the clinical efficacy of unloader bracing has produced data suggesting improvements in knee pain and function. In a prospective cohort study assessing improvements in pain and function in patients with osteoarthritis, 18 subjects were evaluated for up to 1-year after initiating brace use.[22] The Cincinnati Knee Rating System and pain scale were used to analyze symptoms and functional limitation. In addition, subjects underwent gait analysis and were compared to control of nonarthritic patients matched for age and walking speed. Significant improvement in pain and clinical outcome scores was found 9 weeks after initiating brace use and continued up to 1-year. Before bracing, 78% had rated their knee condition as poor in comparison to 33% at 1-year follow-up. Of note, no significant differences were found in gait dynamics before and after brace use. The authors concluded that unloader bracing provides a significant improvement in pain scores, though there was not a discernible impact on gait dynamics.

Knee osteoarthritis outcome score

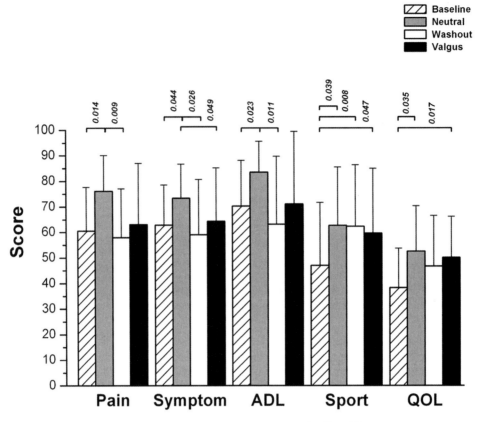

FIGURE 23-4 Clinical improvements with neutral knee bracing versus valgus unloader bracing in the arthritic knee. ADL, activity of daily living; QOL, quality of life. (Adapted from Ramsey DK, Briem K, Axe MJ, Snyder-Mackler L. A mechanical theory for the effectiveness of bracing for medial compartment osteoarthritis of the knee. *J Bone Joint Surg Am.* 2007;89(11):2398-2407.)

In a randomized clinical trial assessing clinical improvement with bracing, 119 patients with medial OA were randomized to a neoprene sleeve, and unloader brace, or a control group with no brace.[23] Clinical outcomes were assessed with Western Ontario and McMaster University Osteoarthritis (WOMAC) and McMaster-Toronto Arthritis Patient Preference Disability Questionnaire (MACTAR), and function was assessed with the use of a 6-minute walking and 30-second stair-climbing tests. At 6 months, there was a significant improvement in clinical outcome scores and function with both the neoprene sleeve and unloader brace cohorts. There was also a trend toward significance favoring the unloader brace in the WOMAC physical function scores relative to the neoprene sleeve.

Subsequent randomized trials have not demonstrated the same magnitude of clinical improvement with brace treatment. Brouwer and colleagues randomized 117 patients with unicompartmental osteoarthritis of the knee to conservative treatment consisting of medication and therapy with and without bracing.[24] The primary outcomes of interest were changes in pain severity and

knee function scores. They noted that while there were clinical improvements at 3 and 12 months in the bracing group, the improvements were of borderline statistical significance. Another trial comparing 91 patients randomized to either laterally wedged insoles or a valgus brace was assessed for pain scores and WOMAC outcomes measures.[24] The authors also utilized dynamic sensors throughout the gait cycle to determine any changes in the knee adduction moment or ground reaction force with the use of knee unloader bracing or lateral wedge shoe inserts (**Fig. 23-5**). The authors found no significant difference in WOMAC scores between the groups. Subsequently, in a secondary study, analysis demonstrated there was no significant change in the knee adduction moment or GRF with the use of an unloader brace.[25]

In a prospective study assessing improvement in activities of daily living, Larsen and colleagues followed a series of patients who had worn an unloader brace for 2 months.[26] They found that in patients with low to moderate osteoarthritis, there was an increase in activity while wearing the brace in addition to a

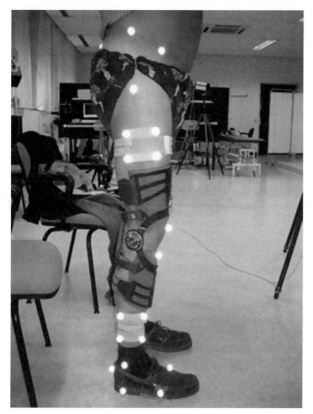

FIGURE 23-5 Dynamic sensors for the detection of ground reactive force and knee adduction moment with brace use. (Reproduced from Duivenvoorden T, van Raaij TM, Horemans HLD, et al. Do laterally wedged insoles or valgus braces unload the medial compartment of the knee in patients with osteoarthritis? *Clin Orthop Relat Res.* 2015;473(1):265-274.)

decrease in pain. The authors did not find a significant difference in the knee adduction moment while walking. Dessery et al reported on a series of 24 patients who wore three different types of custom knee brace: a valgus unloader brace, an unloader brace with external rotation function, and a functional knee brace used for ligament injuries.[27] The authors found that at 2 weeks, all subjects reported a decrease in pain. The valgus unloader brace was noted to reduce the velocity of gait, and patients all reported the bracing was cumbersome because of bulkiness. The authors concluded that all braces were similar in both pain relief and functional improvement.

Subsequent research has assessed the cost-efficacy of bracing in the long-term management of osteoarthritis. In a series of 63 patients who were fitted with a brace for medial osteoarthritis after having attempted medication and physical therapy (PT), the continued use of the brace was assessed at up to 8 years (mean 26 months).[28] The authors determined that at 4 months, the unloader brace was cost-effective in comparison to surgical management and demonstrated that for patients who tolerated the unloader brace for greater than 24 months, the chance of undergoing surgery was significantly reduced. The authors concluded that unloader bracing provides

a discernible difference in quality adjusted life years (QALY) and is a cost-effective management option after 4 months of use.

A meta-analysis of randomized trials evaluating clinical improvement with bracing reviewed pain and functional improvement with valgus unloader bracing.[29] The authors identified six randomized trials that met eligibility criteria. Complications and treatment adherence rates were also collected. The study determined that there was a statistically significant difference favoring valgus knee bracing in improving pain and function when wearing a brace. However, when compared to a control group that used a neutral orthosis that did function as an unloader brace, the effect size on pain was considerably reduced though remained statistically significant in favor of unloader bracing. The authors also reported that across studies, instructions for use were variable and compliance rates ranged from 45% to 100%. In addition, nearly 25% of patients reported minor complications as a consequence of brace use, including blistering, skin irritation, and swelling. Patients reported reasons for noncompliance including poor fit, brace slippage, or bulkiness of the bracing. A study specifically assessing compliance with brace use was conducted by Squyer and colleagues.[30] They administered a survey of 110 patients 12 to 40 months after being fitted with unloader bracing for unicompartmental OA. From those who responded, 28% reported regular brace utilization, defined as twice per week, 1 hour at a time, or more at 1-year follow-up. Patients reported a lack of relief, discomfort, and irritation as reason for discontinuing the brace. While clinical data suggest that brace wear provides symptomatic improvement and can be cost-effective, these investigations suggest that only a minority of patients continue bracing at 1-year.

While the majority of clinical studies investigating bracing demonstrate pain and clinical outcome score improvement, there is a paucity of high-quality randomized trials in this arena.[9] The American Academy of Orthopaedic Surgeons Clinical Practice Guidelines (Second edition) for the conservative management of osteoarthritis states "we are unable to recommend for or against the use of a valgus directing force brace for patients with symptomatic osteoarthritis of the knee."[31] This is due to only two high-quality randomized clinical trials investigating bracing, with conflicting data regarding the magnitude and duration of clinical efficacy of this management approach.[23,24]

Summary

Unloader bracing in the management of OA offers a noninvasive approach for alleviating pain and improving function in patients who wish to delay or defer surgical measures. The mechanism of effect may be due to unloading the arthritic compartment, though there is evidence to suggest that it may modulate its effect through limiting muscle contraction across the arthritic knee. Radiographic and gait analysis studies have demonstrated mixed results in the magnitude of deformity and varus moment correction with brace wear in the arthritic knee. Compliance issues and a lack of consensus on the indications for bracing have created divergent practices in the use of bracing for knee OA. The few existing high-quality randomized clinical trials assessing efficacy of bracing have demonstrated favorable improvements in pain and function, though more investigation is required to determine the magnitude and duration of treatment effect with this intervention.

REHABILITATION AND TOTAL KNEE ARTHROPLASTY

Osteoarthritis of the knee is the most common cause of chronic disability among older people in the United States. Common subjective complaints from patients include joint pain, decreased function, joint instability, muscle weakness, and fatigue. The onset of these symptoms is almost invariably insidious, with episodes of pain that may increase in frequency and duration. Patients with degenerative joint disease have demonstrated decreased quadriceps strength, impaired proprioception, decreased flexibility, and range-of-motion deficits. When loading stresses cannot be absorbed by the joints, surrounding weak muscles, opposing articular cartilages, and trabecular bone are disproportionately impacted. Quadriceps weakness has been reported by patients to be one of the most common and earliest symptoms of osteoarthritis. It is debated whether quadriceps weakness precedes the progression of osteoarthritis to knee pain or disability or both. The phenomenon of arthrogenous muscle inhibition has been attributed to abnormal afferent information from the diseased joint, which results in decreased motor output to the quadriceps muscles. Muscle function plays an important role in joint movement, stability, shock absorption, and proprioception. Impairment of neuromuscular mechanisms can induce the knee joint to abnormal loading, which may traumatize articular tissues.

When nonoperative treatment fails, patients consider electing for a total knee arthroplasty (TKA). Patients and surgeons often view postoperative rehabilitation as the lion's share of work during a TKA episode of care. The success of surgery in achieving optimal functional outcomes and patient satisfaction hinges on the postoperative course. Total knee replacement is somewhat unique. Very few other interventions in medicine require a fresh surgical wound to be stressed with immediate mobilization and stretching in order to have a successful outcome.

As already discussed, presurgical rehabilitation has great value in reducing pain and improving function. Nonetheless, many patients enter the surgical episode with a deconditioned, stiff, and painful knee. Therefore, postoperative rehabilitation must address the prior functional deficiencies of that knee in addition to the fresh surgical issues from knee replacement.

Preoperative Education

TKA rehabilitation in many ways begins before surgery. Mandatory preoperative education by a member of the surgical team or by a representative from the hospital has been shown to have value in arthroplasty outcomes for some variables, like discharge status and length of stay.[32] Although some studies have questioned the direct benefit of preoperative education, they have been widely adopted as part of Medicare bundle payment programs because of their understood successes. Patients who fully anticipate the required work of postoperative rehabilitation are most likely to actively engage in their recovery, strengthening, and achievement of functional milestones. In a systematic review, Louw et al found that there was also a limited benefit to controlling postoperative pain with the use of a preoperative education program.[33] Some personality types benefit more from preoperative education than others, though offering it to all patients is generally more feasible than assessing psychosocial qualities of all patients.[34]

Timing of Physical Therapy

With an increasing number of TKA cases moving to surgery centers and being discharged as ambulatory patients from the hospital, there is a change in the perception of the reliance on acute PT after surgery. Many surgery centers do not have access to trained therapists in the recovery room. Instead, nurses or mobility techs mobilize patients and begin the gait training, aid usage, and range of motion (ROM) exercises in a less structured and expedited manner in the recovery room. Following a short recovery period at home, these ambulatory patients may either receive at-home PT or begin outpatient therapy.

For traditional TKA admissions to the inpatient setting, there is good evidence that receiving therapy on the day of surgery is beneficial to functional outcomes and length of stay.[35] Studies showing a positive effect of same-day PT show improved function, reduced pain and opioid consumption, and reduced length of stay. Bohl et al, however, suggest that rapid mobilization may not have to happen on the same day of surgery. They found no significant difference in length of stay or patient satisfaction when comparing same-day PT versus on the morning after surgery.[36]

Goals of Acute Physical Therapy

While hospitals can differ in their functional milestones required prior to discharge from inpatient TKA, several principals are held in common. Therapists engage patients in a graduated activity program following surgery, teaching safe mobilization, with range-of-motion exercises, and neuromuscular training. Functional milestones for the TKA patient are as follows:

1. Independence in following prescribed exercise programs to enhance muscular control and optimize knee ROM
2. Successful transfer from supine to sit and from sit to stand (including entering and exiting bed, sitting, and standing from the toilet)
3. Ambulation of at least 100 ft with safe use of a walking aid
4. Negotiation of one flight of stairs

In the inpatient setting, these milestones can often be achieved after 2 days. The first day of PT involves baseline assessments, vital sign monitoring, assisted bed mobility, transfers from bed to chair, and short distance walking. Progression then occurs depending on the ability of the patient to incorporate the functional goals described above, including stairs, 100 ft ambulation, and navigating toilets.

Continuous passive motion, or CPM, has largely fallen out of favor in the United States. Reasons for its disappearance include cost, pain generation, no proven functional benefit, development of flexion contracture (machines do not do a great job with knee extension), and the risk of complications like peroneal palsy. Many studies have shown the lack of value of CPM, though there may be some reduction in manipulation rates and adverse events.[37]

Long-Term Goals of Physical Therapy

One of the drivers of satisfaction and function after TKA is the ability to obtain full knee extension. Therefore, early emphasis on achieving full extension is critical and often needs to address any preoperative hamstring tightness associated with flexion contractures. Longer term ROM is guided by our understanding of the functional ROM for activities of daily living. These include about 90° of flexion to successfully navigate stairs, 105° to stand from sitting, and 115° to squat. Conventional wisdom aims for 125° of motion. However, preoperative flexion is a strong determinant of ultimate postoperative flexion.

Flexion exercises become the second major focus of rehabilitation after TKA and can be achieved passively and actively after wound healing. Initially, while the wound is fresh, many surgeons will limit flexion to 100°. This also minimizes pain in the immediate perioperative period. Therapists have several mechanisms for pushing flexion, including passive stretch, use of bands, and specific postures to relax and stretch the quadriceps.

Quadriceps activation is another major component of recovery and is targeted with quad-sets and structured active exercises. Some have advocated for electrical stimulation, though the data are not overwhelmingly in favor or against its use.

Future Developments in Rehabilitation After Knee Arthroplasty

Total joint arthroplasty is moving to the ambulatory setting, as discussed. Medicare removed total knee from the inpatient-only list in 2018, which opens the door to the coverage of TKA done in hospital-connected surgery centers. As arthroplasty evolves from the traditional pathway of inpatient stay to ambulatory discharge home, technology will continue to develop to improve the rehabilitation process. These technologies include internet-based PT, phone and smart device apps, and wearable technologies. Klement et al found that a web-based, self-directed PT program showed promise for primary TKA patients discharged home.[38]

A first step was taken nationally when patients began to be discharged home instead of to inpatient facilities. Home-healthcare PT has been shown to be improved the early functional recovery after knee replacement in Medicare beneficiaries.[39] Christensen et al found, however, that immediately starting outpatient PT was superior and led to a more rapid recovery than first having home-health PT followed by outpatient PT.[40]

Ultimately with the fast-tracking of recovery and huge pressures on cost, it is conceivable that postoperative rehabilitation will become less of a focal and discrete cost during the episode of TKA. Online instructions and educated caregivers in the home may help patients rehabilitate, when combined with improved pain control measures and fewer medical stresses associated with modern TKA techniques.

ACKNOWLEDGMENTS

We would like to thank the authors from the last edition of this book for laying the groundwork for this chapter.

REFERENCES

1. Steadman JR, Briggs KK, Pomeroy SM, Wijdicks CA. Current state of unloading braces for knee osteoarthritis. *Knee Surg Sports Traumatol Arthrosc.* 2016;24(1):42-50.
2. Pollo FE, Jackson RW. Knee bracing for unicompartmental osteoarthritis. *J Am Acad Orthop Surg.* 2006;14(1):5-11.
3. Gravlee JR, Van Durme DJ. Braces and splints for musculoskeletal conditions. *Am Fam Physician.* 2007;75(3):342-348.
4. Rodriguez-Merchan EC, De La Corte-Rodriguez H. The role of orthoses in knee osteoarthritis. *Hosp Pract.* 2018;23:1-5.
5. Brand A, Klöpfer-Krämer I, Morgenstern M, et al. Effects of knee orthosis adjustment on biomechanical performance and clinical outcome in patients with medial knee osteoarthritis. *Prosthet Orthot Int.* 2017;41(6):587-594.
6. Chughtai M, Bhave A, Khan SZ, et al. Clinical outcomes of a pneumatic unloader brace for Kellgren-Lawrence Grades 3 to 4 osteoarthritis: a minimum 1-year follow-up study. *J Knee Surg.* 2016;29(8):634-638.
7. Beaudreuil J, Bendaya S, Faucher M, et al. Clinical practice guidelines for rest orthosis, knee sleeves, and unloading knee braces in knee osteoarthritis. *Joint Bone Spine.* 2009;76(6):629-636.
8. Self BP, Greenwald RM, Pflaster DS. A biomechanical analysis of a medial unloading brace for osteoarthritis in the knee. *Arthritis Care Res.* 2000;13(4):191-197.

9. Mistry DA, Chandratreya A, Lee PYF. An update on unloading knee braces in the treatment of unicompartmental knee osteoarthritis from the last 10 years: a literature review. *Surg J.* 2018;4(3):e110-e118.

10. Haladik JA, Vasileff WK, Peltz CD, Lock TR, Bey MJ. Bracing improves clinical outcomes but does not affect the medial knee joint space in osteoarthritic patients during gait. *Knee Surg Sports Traumatol Arthrosc.* 2014;22(11):2715-2720.

11. France EP, Paulos LE. Knee bracing. *J Am Acad Orthop Surg.* 1994;2(5):281-287.

12. Pollo FE. Bracing and heel wedging for unicompartmental osteoarthritis of the knee. *Am J Knee Surg.* 1998;11(1):47-50.

13. Komistek RD, Dennis DA, Northcut EJ, Wood A, Parker AW, Traina SM. An in vivo analysis of the effectiveness of the osteoarthritic knee brace during heel-strike of gait. *J Arthroplasty.* 1999;14(6):738-742.

14. Katsuragawa Y, Fukui N, Nakamura K. Change of bone mineral density with valgus knee bracing. *Int Orthop.* 1999;23(3):164-167.

15. Anderst WJ, Tashman S. A method to estimate in vivo dynamic articular surface interaction. *J Biomech.* 2003;36(9):1291-1299.

16. Nagai K, Yang S, Fu FH, Anderst W. Unloader knee brace increases medial compartment joint space during gait in knee osteoarthritis patients. *Knee Surg Sports Traumatol Arthrosc.* 2018;27(7):2354-2360.

17. Ebert JR, Hambly K, Joss B, Ackland TR, Donnelly CJ. Does an unloader brace reduce knee loading in normally aligned knees? *Clin Orthop Relat Res.* 2014;472(3):915-922.

18. Baliunas AJ, Hurwitz DE, Ryals AB, et al. Increased knee joint loads during walking are present in subjects with knee osteoarthritis. *Osteoarthr Cartil.* 2002;10(7):573-579.

19. Pollo FE, Otis JC, Backus SI, Warren RF, Wickiewicz TL. Reduction of medial compartment loads with valgus bracing of the osteoarthritic knee. *Am J Sports Med.* 2002;30(3):414-421.

20. Ramsey DK, Briem K, Axe MJ, Snyder-Mackler L. A mechanical theory for the effectiveness of bracing for medial compartment osteoarthritis of the knee. *J Bone Joint Surg Am.* 2007;89(11):2398-2407.

21. Schmalz T, Knopf E, Drewitz H, Blumentritt S. Analysis of biomechanical effectiveness of valgus-inducing knee brace for osteoarthritis of knee. *J Rehabil Res Dev.* 2010;47(5):419-429.

22. Hewett TE, Noyes FR, Barber-Westin SD, Heckmann TP. Decrease in knee joint pain and increase in function in patients with medial compartment arthrosis: a prospective analysis of valgus bracing. *Orthopedics.* 1998;21(2):131-138.

23. Kirkley A, Webster-Bogaert S, Litchfield R, et al. The effect of bracing on varus gonarthrosis. *J Bone Joint Surg Am.* 1999;81(4):539-548.

24. Brouwer RW, van Raaij TM, Verhaar JA, Coene LN, Bierma-Zeinstra SM. Brace treatment for osteoarthritis of the knee: a prospective randomized multi-centre trial. *Osteoarthr Cartil.* 2006;14(8):777-783.

25. Duivenvoorden T, van Raaij TM, Horemans HLD, et al. Do laterally wedged insoles or valgus braces unload the medial compartment of the knee in patients with osteoarthritis? *Clin Orthop Relat Res.* 2015;473(1):265-274.

26. Larsen BL, Jacofsky MC, Brown JA, Jacofsky DJ. Valgus bracing affords short-term treatment solution across walking and sit-to-stand activities. *J Arthroplasty.* 2013;28(5):792-797.

27. Dessery Y, Belzile EL, Turmel S, Corbeil P. Comparison of three knee braces in the treatment of medial knee osteoarthritis. *Knee.* 2014;21(6):1107-1114.

28. Lee PY, Winfield TG, Harris SR, Storey E, Chandratreya A. Unloading knee brace is a cost-effective method to bridge and delay surgery in unicompartmental knee arthritis. *BMJ Open Sport Exerc Med.* 2016;2(1):e000195.

29. Moyer RF, Birmingham TB, Bryant DM, Giffin JR, Marriott KA, Leitch KM. Valgus bracing for knee osteoarthritis: a meta-analysis of randomized trials. *Arthritis Care Res.* 2015;67(4):493-501.

30. Squyer E, Stamper DL, Hamilton DT, Sabin JA, Leopold SS. Unloader knee braces for osteoarthritis: do patients actually wear them? *Clin Orthop Relat Res.* 2013;471(6):1982-1991.

31. Brown GA. AAOS clinical practice guideline: treatment of osteoarthritis of the knee. Evidence-based guideline, 2nd edition. *J Am Acad Orthop Surg.* 2013;21(9):577-579.

32. Shah RP, Karas V, Berger RA. Rapid discharge and outpatient total joint arthroplasty introduce a burden of care to the surgeon. *J Arthroplasty.* 2019;34(7):1307-1311.

33. Louw A, Diener I, Butler DS, Puentedura EJ. Preoperative education addressing postoperative pain in total joint arthroplasty: review of content and educational delivery methods. *Physiother Theory Pract.* 2013;29(3):175-194.

34. McDonald S, Page MJ, Beringer K, Wasiak J, Sprowson A. Preoperative education for hip or knee replacement. *Cochrane Database Syst Rev.* 2014;(5):CD003526.

35. Yakkanti RR, Miller AJ, Smith LS, Feher AW, Mont MA, Malkani AL. Impact of early mobilization on length of stay after primary total knee arthroplasty. *Ann Transl Med.* 2019;7(4):69.

36. Bohl DD, Li J, Calkins TE, et al. Physical therapy on postoperative day zero following total knee arthroplasty: a randomized, controlled trial of 394 patients. *J Arthroplasty.* 2019;34(7 suppl):S173-S177.

37. Harvey LA, Brosseau L, Herbert RD. Continuous passive motion following total knee arthroplasty in people with arthritis. *Cochrane Database Syst Rev.* 2014;(2):CD004260.

38. Klement MR, Rondon AJ, McEntee RM, Greenky MR, Austin MS. Web-based, self-directed physical therapy after total knee arthroplasty is safe and effective for most, but not all, patients. *J Arthroplasty.* 2018;34(7 suppl):S178-S182.

39. Falvey JR, Bade MJ, Forster JE, et al. Home-health-care physical therapy improves early functional recovery of Medicare beneficiaries after total knee arthroplasty. *J Bone Joint Surg Am.* 2018;100(20):1728-1734.

40. Christensen JC, Paxton RJ, Baym C, et al. Benefits of direct patient discharge to outpatient physical therapy after total knee arthroplasty. *Disabil Rehabil.* 2019:1-7.

chapter 24

The Role of Arthroscopy in Treating Degenerative Joint Disease

Andrew D. Carbone, MD | Yair D. Kissin, MD, FAAOS | Michael A. Kelly, MD

INTRODUCTION

Degenerative joint disease of the knee is among the most common orthopedic conditions requiring treatment today. The breakdown of articular cartilage of the knee may present with symptomatic pain, swelling, and associated disability in both activities of daily living and recreation. The population at risk to develop osteoarthritis of the knee continues to grow rapidly with aging of the baby boomer generation, the obesity epidemic, and the increase in athletic injuries particularly among females during the past 2 decades.[1]

Unfortunately, as prevalent and disabling as knee arthritis is recognized to be, no specific medical or surgical remedy has effectively altered the natural history. Despite improvements in surgical procedures to repair or regenerate articular cartilage of the knee, these are largely focused on isolated cartilage lesions, rather than generalized degenerative changes of the knee. As in the past, the treatment strategies today continue to concentrate primarily on pain control and improvement in a patient's quality of life.

The pain associated with osteoarthritis of the knee is typically managed with nonsurgical treatments including activity modification, strengthening knee exercises, nonsteroidal anti-inflammatory medications, braces, and ambulatory aids. Much effort has been directed at intra-articular injections such as corticosteroids and a variety of hyaluronic acid derivatives.[2] Recently, biologic therapies such as platelet-rich plasma and bone marrow are receiving a great deal of attention with varied results.[3-6] Depending on severity and location, a variety of surgical options exist including femoral or tibial osteotomies, partial and total knee replacement. This chapter will focus on arthroscopic techniques designed to treat knee arthritis. Review of the published literature on these techniques over the past 2 decades has demonstrated more limited indications for arthroscopy for these patients. This has coincided with the success and durability of knee arthroplasty over the same time period.[7]

HISTORY OF ARTHROSCOPY IN KNEE OA

Surgical arthroscopy as a form of treatment for degenerative joint disease of the knee was first developed in the 1920s.[8] In the 1930s, Burman et al looked at 30 cases of patients treated with knee arthroscopy and found generally positive results.[9] Dr. Masaki Watanabe helped popularize the arthroscopic lavage in 1950s, perfecting the techniques of knee arthroscopy and also finding positive results when treating patients with knee OA.[10]

Bone marrow stimulation (BMS) has also been utilized in the treatment of OA. BMS was first devised in the 1950s as an open procedure and involves drilling through the damaged cartilaginous surface and into the subchondral bone to stimulate bleeding, clot formation, and migration of stem cells. While BMS has evolved into a variety of techniques utilized today for managing focal cartilage defects, they have not been successful in treating the diffuse nature of osteoarthritis of the knee.[11]

Without the long-term outcome data of total knee arthroplasty that we are privileged to have today,[7,12] many surgeons chose arthroscopy as treatment for knee OA, especially in younger patients. TKA was delayed for as long as possible, often at the expense of patients' continued pain and decreased function. Arthroscopic débridement was seen as a minimally invasive option, which would provide pain relief, albeit temporarily, in patients who would otherwise be TKA candidates. The goal was to delay the need for a TKA until patients were older and less active. Consequently, given the increasing rate of OA, along with the intention of minimizing surgical trauma to the knee, arthroscopy became widespread.

Initial studies supported the idea that arthroscopic débridement provided patients with significant pain relief.[13,14] Harwin found a 63% improvement in pain scores following surgical débridement, noting patients with more neutral mechanical axes had better results.[15] Fond reported similar results: 25 out of 36 patients at 5 years had satisfactory results and improved HSS scores, with flexion contractures >10° being a negative prognostic factor of outcome.[16]

However, these early studies were often small case series, which lacked robust control groups. In response to this, several large clinical trials were performed in the late 1990s and 2000s, which called into question the efficacy of arthroscopy. The most influential study on the subject was a large prospective, randomized controlled trial comparing sham surgery versus arthroscopic débridement and meniscectomy in 2002 by Moseley et al. This study, published in the *New England Journal of Medicine*, found no difference in terms of pain or function between sham surgery and the treatment group.[17] Likewise in 2006, a Cochrane review article found a "Gold level of evidence" against arthroscopic débridement in patients with knee OA.[18] A subsequent review by Barlow et al, a larger review than the Cochrane study, also found no indication for arthroscopy in OA. Though these studies, especially the Moseley study, were initially met with skepticism from the orthopedic community, they rightfully questioned orthopedists to evaluate the true indications for arthroscopy in knee OA patients.[19]

Following the release of the large controlled trials in the 2000s the indications for arthroscopy in patients with degenerative osteoarthritis of the knee decreased significantly. Improvements in radiography, as well as the more widespread availability of advanced imaging modalities including CT and MRI, have all but obviated the need for diagnostic arthroscopy to evaluate the extent of arthritis. In addition, large studies, including a well-known large randomized controlled trial from Finland, FIDELITY, have demonstrated no benefit of arthroscopic débridement in patients with either osteoarthritis or degenerative meniscus pathology, which had been one of the major indications.[20] Mechanical symptoms, once a fairly strong indication for arthroscopy, are no longer universally accepted following a recent review article which found no benefit from arthroscopy in this cohort either.[21] Indeed, a 2016 randomized controlled trial from a group in Norway, comparing physical therapy and arthroscopic meniscus débridement with physical therapy, found no difference in long-term outcome and noted that the physical therapy group trended toward improved thigh strength with no difference in pain scores or function.[22] Based on these data, along with other studies, the *British Medical Journal* recently released clinical practice guidelines strongly recommending against the use of arthroscopy for primary treatment of degenerative knee arthritis or degenerative meniscus tears.[23] Additionally, in a retrospective comparative study, Su et al demonstrated knee arthroscopy did not delay or decrease the knee for TKA, and did not provide pain relief past 2 years.[24] One

recent systemic review of 20 different studies found that knee arthroscopy did not obviate the need for TKA, and that the median time between knee arthroscopy and TKA was a mere 2 years.[25] These studies in conjunction with the publication of long-term outcomes data on the TKA demonstrating excellent results at 20 and even 30 years postoperatively gave surgeons confidence to indicate younger more active patients who had previously been seen as arthroscopy candidates, for TKA.[7,12]

Despite the literature against the use of arthroscopy in the arthritic knee, many surgeons felt these studies may have overreached in claiming that there was no place for arthroscopy in the treatment paradigm. None of these studies were specific for patients with new onset knee pain or patients with an acute change in their pain. Indeed, this group often was actively excluded in some of these studies.[26] A recent article by Lamplot and Brophy, which reviewed major studies from 1975 to 2015, found that despite the evidence against arthroscopy, given the lack of specificity and power for certain patient subgroups, there still existed a specific role for arthroscopic débridement in certain patients with mild OA and symptomatic tears.[27]

Often patients with stable, long-standing arthritis whose symptoms are controlled for an extended period may experience an acute change in their knee pain, both atraumatically and traumatically. MRIs in these patients may demonstrate flipped meniscus tears as seen in **Fig. 24-1**, which may become incarcerated between the femoral and tibial condyles and can cause severe pain, preventing knee extension. Similarly, loose bodies as seen in **Figs. 24-2** and **24-3** may cause locking of the knee and are another strong indication for arthroscopic débridement given their propensity to cause pain, mechanical symptoms as well as due to their potential to cause damage to the articular surface of the joint. Removal of these loose bodies has demonstrated reliable pain relief.[28] In patients with these pathologies who previously had relief of their knee pain with conservative measures, arthroscopic débridement may return them to their baseline level of pain and function.

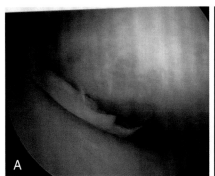 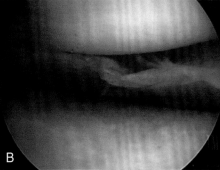 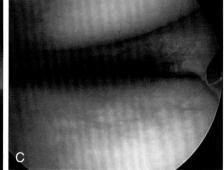

FIGURE 24-1   Flipped meniscus tears (**A** and **B**) are key contributors to mechanical knee symptoms such as locking and may benefit from débridement (**C**).

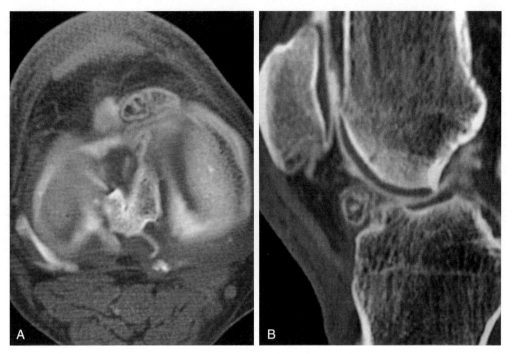

FIGURE 24-2   Axial **(A)** and sagittal **(B)** CT slices demonstrating a large intra-articular loose body in a patient with osteoarthritis.

CONTRAINDICATIONS

Presence of advanced degenerative changes in the knee is widely accepted as a major contraindication to arthroscopic débridement. To quantify the severity and extent of degenerative disease, surgeons often rely on the Kellgren-Lawrence grading system. This is a five-level radiographic grading system using weight-bearing radiographs, which ranges from grade 0 (no radiographic evidence of disease) to grade 4 (complete loss of joint space). Patients with advanced disease are categorized commonly as grade 3 and 4, while patients with more moderate disease are classified as having grades 1 and 2. Having worse than grade 2 is typically considered a contraindication to arthroscopy as these patients have been shown to have more rapid progression of arthritis following arthroscopic débridement than patients with grade 1 and 2.[25]

Studies suggest poor outcomes of arthroscopic débridement in patients with significant coronal plane angular deformity.[29] Valgus malalignment greater than 3° and varus greater than 5° may have poorer outcomes.[15,30,31] Younger patients with significant angular deformity may be candidates for osteotomy, while older patients may be indicated for arthroplasty.[31,32] Flexion contractures are also a contraindication to arthroscopy. Studies have shown patients with flexion contractures >10° have worse long-term outcomes following débridement.[16]

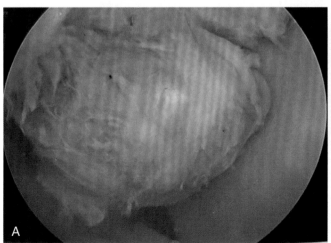
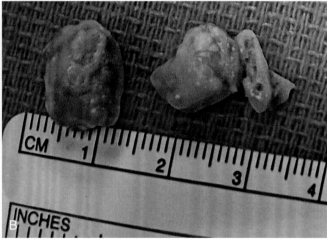

FIGURE 24-3   Intra-articular loose bodies seen arthroscopically **(A)** and grossly **(B)**.

Patients with inflammatory arthropathies are also contraindicated as often these patients have multicompartmental as well as polyarticular involvement. These patients should be referred to a rheumatologist for medical management of their disease. Today, far fewer patients with inflammatory arthritis require surgical procedures than in the past given the outstanding success of medical management of these patients.[33,34]

PREOPERATIVE ASSESSMENT

Thoroughly assessing the patient involves correlating symptoms, physical exam findings, and radiography. Information that is critical to obtain is the timing and onset of when and how symptoms began, as well as location of pain, radiation, and any exacerbating factors. Patients with previously mild or no symptoms not currently being treated for knee pain are more likely than those with chronic pain and advanced disease to experience pain relief following surgery. Other information to inquire about is the patient's usual activity level, history of prior injury to the knee, and whether the symptoms are related to a work injury. Patients will often describe mechanical symptoms such as locking or a sense of instability and/or buckling, which are important to note. Finally, any hip or back pain should be well documented.

On exam, initial focus should be on gait and alignment. Significant varus or valgus deformities should be noted. Localization of the patient's perceived pain through palpation should be performed. Patients noting diffuse tenderness on palpation in multiple compartments or patellofemoral tenderness should be excluded from consideration. The presence of a large knee effusion is sometimes indicative of an acute event and should be noted. Range of motion of the knee should be assessed along with any flexion contractures. Complete ligamentous exam should also be done, noting any laxity that is present. Evaluation of possible meniscus tears can be performed with rotatory maneuvers such as the McMurray test. A McMurray test is considered positive when the examiner apprentices a palpable or auditory click with rotation and extension of the knee. Finally, it is important to evaluate the ipsilateral hip and lumbar spine if indicated.

A proper radiographic evaluation of these patients is paramount to determining candidacy for arthroscopic treatment. This includes weight-bearing AP and lateral radiographs along with axial patellar views. Weight-bearing radiographs are much more sensitive at detecting OA and are preferred to non–weight-bearing images as can be demonstrated in **Fig. 24-4**. Additionally, Rosenberg views, which are posterior to anterior weight-bearing radiographs with the knee in 45° of flexion, are more sensitive for OA detection in the tibiofemoral compartments and should be obtained to assess for arthritis in the adjacent compartment, especially in patients with early or mild disease.[35] Full-length three joint films, as seen in **Fig. 24-5**, will allow for assessment of coronal plane deformity which may be otherwise difficult to detect from standard knee radiographs and are utilized on occasion.

Magnetic resonance imaging (MRI), though not indicated, is often obtained in OA patients prior to referral

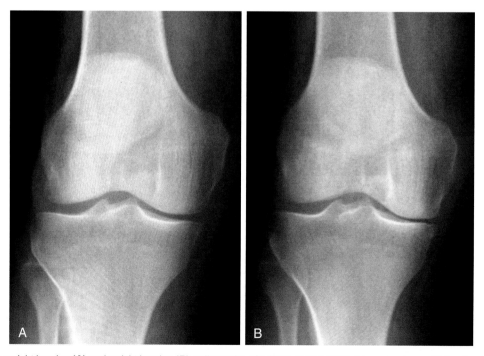

FIGURE 24-4 Non–weight-bearing **(A)** and weight-bearing **(B)** radiographs of a knee demonstrating increased sensitivity of weight-bearing images at detecting both joint space narrowing and varus malalignment.

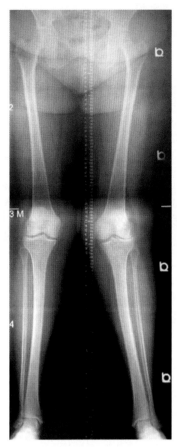

FIGURE 24-5 Full-length standing mechanical axis films allows for appreciation of significant coronal angular deformity.

to an orthopedic surgeon. These studies are frequently obtained in patients with mild disease and non–weight-bearing radiographs demonstrating Kellgren-Lawrence grade 0 or 1 changes. MRI provides much greater detail on the extent of disease in addition to detailed evaluation of surrounding soft-tissue structures. MRIs are sensitive at detecting meniscal tears, chondral lesions, and intra-articular loose bodies. Bone marrow edema, or bone marrow lesions (BMLs) as demonstrated in **Fig. 24-6**, are MRI findings which are commonly found following knee trauma. They are also found in patients with OA and have been spatially linked to the location of pain, as well as to persistence of knee pain in OA patients.[36]

In-office arthroscopy is a relatively new tool which offers a definitive, minimally invasive method to thoroughly examine all three compartments without subjecting patients to the risks of an operative procedure. This may be an ideal tool for patients with contraindications to MRI such as those with claustrophobia, metallic implants, pacemakers, etc.[37]

MANAGEMENT

Initial management of the OA patient should always begin conservatively, including weight control, NSAIDs, and physical therapy. The importance of these therapies cannot be understated. Weight loss has a tremendous impact on mechanical loading across the knee;

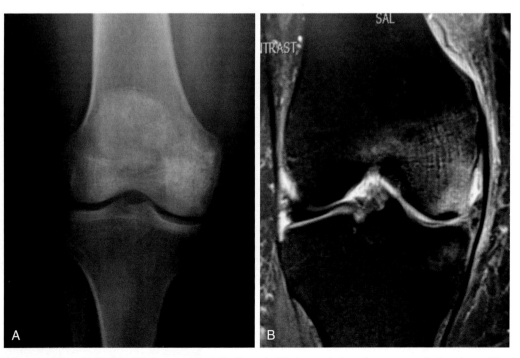

FIGURE 24-6 Radiograph **(A)** and MRI **(B)** of the same patient. Radiograph **(A)** demonstrates a bone marrow lesion along with associated meniscal and chondral pathology.

biomechanical studies have demonstrated that for every 1 kg of weight loss there is fourfold reduction in load across the knee.[38] These reductions in loading translate to significant pain reduction in a dose-dependent manner.[39] Additionally, in a study of patients with Kellgren-Lawrence grades 2 to 4, a significant number of patients with meniscus tears have good pain relief following a course of physical therapy.[26]

If no appreciable relief can be obtained following these therapies, a trial of intra-articular corticosteroid injections (CSI) may be considered. Patients with OA generally experience significant pain relief following CSI and can be managed with these injections intermittently.[40] Intra-articular viscosupplementation, although controversial, may also be effective early in the disease process.

Exhaustion of conservative treatments warrants discussion of operative management. Determination of appropriate surgical intervention depends on several considerations. The patient's age, acuity of symptoms, presence of mechanical symptoms, severity, location and extent of arthritic disease, presence of angular deformity, and knee ROM are all important considerations before proceeding with arthroscopic débridement. Most importantly, however, are the patient's goals and expectations, which should be discussed extensively prior to any planned surgical procedure. Surgical arthroscopy may be an appropriate option for a select number of patients. However, it is important for patients to have realistic expectations about their prognosis following surgery and it is critical that patients understand the limitations of arthroscopy.

AAOS strongly recommends against performing arthroscopy with lavage and/or débridement in patients with a primary diagnosis of symptomatic osteoarthritis of the knee in their Clinical Practice Guidelines for Treatment of Osteoarthritis of the Knee.[41] However, in patients with meniscal tears, they have found that there is inconclusive evidence and cannot recommend for or against use of arthroscopic surgery for these patients. The Appropriate Use Criteria Treatment guidelines for Non-Arthroplasty Treatment of Knee Osteoarthritis, an interactive guide to nonarthroplasty treatment options for patients with knee OA, were created by the AAOS based on evidence compiled for the clinical practice guidelines.[42] It provides evidence-based recommendations for or against various nonarthroplasty treatment options, both surgical and nonsurgical, for patients with knee OA based on different patient criteria, including pain limitation of function, ROM, ligamentous stability, arthritic pattern, amount of joint space, overall limb alignment, mechanical symptoms, and age. The AUC recommends the use of arthroscopic meniscectomy only in select conditions. Patients must be experiencing mechanical symptoms, and generally be relatively young or middle age with limited radiographic disease, and significant knee pain interfering with function.[43]

FUTURE TREATMENTS

New research has brought insight into the sources of pain in osteoarthritis, especially regarding BMLs. It is thought that these occur as a result of abnormal stresses across the joint and a reduced healing capacity of the bone. These injuries have been likened to nonhealing stress fractures of the subchondral bone and have been linked to persistent knee pain and pain location in patients with osteoarthritis.[36] In addition, these lesions are associated with more rapid progression of knee OA.[44] Compared to patients without a BML, patients with a MRI-observed BML were nearly nine times as likely to progress to TKA over a 3-year follow-up period.[45] One option which has been championed recently to resolve bone marrow edema and improve pain is the subchondroplasty. In this procedure, following an arthroscopic débridement, calcium phosphate bone substitute is injected into the compromised subchondral bone as demonstrated in **Fig. 24-7**. One study found clinically significant improvement in pain and function following this procedure in a recent retrospective series.[46] Another case series from Brazil found similar results.[47] Despite this, larger studies are needed to better assess the efficacy of the procedure, and indications are limited at this time.

AUTHOR PREFERRED INDICATIONS

We believe arthroscopic treatment of patients with knee OA may still have a limited role in select patients. However, patient selection is paramount to improving patient outcome and strict adherence to known

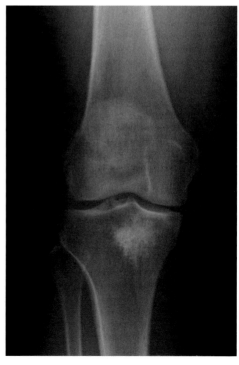

FIGURE 24-7 Radiograph of knee with mild osteoarthritis following subchondroplasty.

TABLE 24-1   **Contraindications to Knee Arthroscopy in Patients With Knee Osteoarthritis**
Contraindications to Arthroscopic Débridement
Baseline moderate to severe chronic knee pain
Kellgren-Lawrence grade III-IV
Angular deformity (varus >5°, valgus >3°)
Flexion contractures >10°
Inflammatory arthropathies

contraindications should be observed (**Table 24-1**). These include patients with mild disease, Kellgren-Lawrence grade 1 and 2, little no preinjury knee pain, and entrapped or flipped meniscus tears causing locking/catching. Arthroscopy can also be useful for the removal of intra-articular loose bodies, which are contributing to refractory pain and mechanical symptoms. MRI which demonstrates >2 mm of preserved joint space is favorable to more significant narrowing. Again, there should be adequate patient understanding that this procedure is a palliative procedure with a goal of providing pain relief and possibly delaying the need for a TKA.

AUTHOR'S PREFERRED TECHNIQUE

We prefer the use of general or short-acting spinal anesthesia although some surgeons utilize local anesthesia as well. Anterolateral diagnostic and anteromedial working portals are established and a generous lavage is performed. Partial meniscectomy is performed with a technique demonstrated in **Fig. 24-8**, where needed loose bodies, depending on their size, are managed with lavage or other appropriate techniques to remove them. Occasionally asymptomatic loose bodies can be present in the posterior compartments and may be left *in situ*. Conservative chondral shaving of articular lesions is performed and subchondral drilling such as microfracture is rarely recommended and indicated more for isolated defects. Loose particulate debris is irrigated out of the knee before removal of arthroscopic equipment and the patient is started on physical therapy in the days following surgery and advanced as tolerated.

SUMMARY

Arthroscopic treatment of degenerative joint disease of the knee remains a viable option in our treatment algorithm. Arthroscopic techniques provide marked reductions in morbidity and enhanced postoperative recovery in comparison to earlier open débridement procedures.

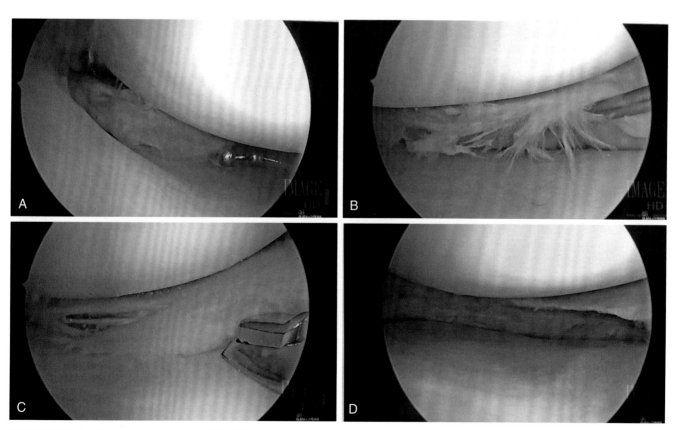

FIGURE 24-8 A radial meniscus tear (**A** and **B**). Following exposure (**C**), it is excised with an arthroscopic biter, to leave the patient with an intact rim of meniscus (**D**).

The frequency of these procedures has diminished in the past decade. They were often utilized in patients younger than 60 years with degenerative joint disease of the knee that was not responsive to nonoperative treatment. However, the durable results of TKA at 20- and 30-year follow-up and the erratic results of arthroscopy in relieving pain and restoring mobility have resulted in narrowed indication. Nonoperative treatment options have improved as well.

Indications for arthroscopic débridement are less clear today than contraindications, but this procedure is still beneficial in select patients. Surgical techniques have become more conservative with few if any indication of bone marrow stimulation procedures in patients with DJD. Careful preoperative discussion emphasizing the limited goals of arthroscopic débridement is critical to patient satisfaction.

REFERENCES

1. Srikanth VK, Fryer JL, Zhai G, Winzenberg TM, Hosmer D, Jones G. A meta-analysis of sex differences prevalence, incidence and severity of osteoarthritis. *Osteoarthr Cartil.* 2005;13(9):769-781.
2. Neustadt DH. Intra-articular injections for osteoarthritis of the knee. *Cleve Clin J Med.* 2006;73(10):897-911.
3. Meheux CJ, McCulloch PC, Lintner DM, Varner KE, Harris JD. Efficacy of intra-articular platelet-rich plasma injections in knee osteoarthritis: a systematic review. *Arthroscopy.* 2016;32(3):495-505. doi:10.1016/j.arthro.2015.08.005.
4. Kim J-D, Lee GW, Jung GH, et al. Clinical outcome of autologous bone marrow aspirates concentrate (BMAC) injection in degenerative arthritis of the knee. *Eur J Orthop Surg Traumatol.* 2014;24(8):1505-1511.
5. Jevsevar D, Donnelly P, Brown GA, Cummins DS. Viscosupplementation for osteoarthritis of the knee: a systematic review of the evidence. *J Bone Joint Surg Am.* 2015;97(24):2047-2060. Available at http://sk.sagepub.com/reference/globalhealth/n24.xml. Accessed January 20, 2019.
6. Shapiro SA, Kazmerchak SE, Heckman MG, Zubair AC, O'Connor MI. A prospective, single-blind, placebo-controlled trial of bone marrow aspirate concentrate for knee osteoarthritis. *Am J Sports Med.* 2017;45(1):82-90.
7. Long WJ, Bryce CD, Hollenbeak CS, Benner RW, Scott W. Total knee replacement in young, active patients: long-term follow-up and functional outcome. A concise follow-up of a previous report. *J Bone Joint Surg Am.* 2014;96(18):e159.
8. Kieser CW, Jackson RW. Eugen Bircher (1882–1956): the first knee surgeon to use diagnostic arthroscopy. *Arthroscopy.* 2003;19(7):771-776.
9. Burman M, Finkelstein H, Mayer L. Arthroscopy of the knee joint. *J Bone Joint Surg.* 1934;16(2):255-268.
10. Jackson RW. A history of arthroscopy. *Arthroscopy.* 2010;26(1):91-103. doi:10.1016/j.arthro.2009.10.005.
11. Bert JM. Arthroscopic treatment of degenerative arthritis of the knee. In: Scott WN, ed. *Insall & Scott Surgery of the Knee.* 5th ed. Philadelphia, PA: Elsevier; 2012:229-234. Available at http://www.crossref.org/deleted_DOI.html. Accessed November 25, 2018.
12. Diduch D, Insall J, Scott W, Scuderi G, Font-Rodriguez D. Total knee replacement in young, active patients: long-term follow-up and functional outcome. *J Bone Joint Surg.* 1997;79(4):575-582.
13. Ogilvie-Harris DJ, Fitsialos DP. Arthroscopic management of the degenerative knee. *Arthroscopy.* 1991;7(2):151-157.
14. Rand JA. Role of arthroscopy in osteoarthritis of the knee. *Arthroscopy.* 1991;7(4):358-363.
15. Harwin SF. Arthroscopic débridement for osteoarthritis of the knee: predictors of patient satisfaction. *Arthroscopy.* 1999;15(2):142-146. Available at http://linkinghub.elsevier.com/retrieve/pii/S0749806399000043. Accessed September 8, 2018.
16. Fond J, Rodin D, Ahmad S, Nirschl RP. Arthroscopic debridement for the treatment of osteoarthritis of the knee: 2- and 5-year results. *Arthroscopy.* 2002;18(8):829-834.
17. Moseley JB, O'Malley K, Pettersen N, et al. A controlled trial of arthroscopic surgery for osteoarthritis of the knee. *N Engl J Med.* 2002;347(2):81-88.
18. Wiroon L, Malinee L, Pisamai L, Chut S. Arthroscopic debridement for knee osteoarthritis. *Cochrane Database Syst Rev.* 2008;(1). Available at http://onlinelibrary.wiley.com/doi/10.1002/14651858.CD005118.pub2/abstract. Accessed September 8, 2018.
19. Ilahi OA. Selection bias results in misinterpretation of randomized controlled trials on arthroscopic treatment of patients with knee osteoarthritis. *Arthroscopy.* 2010;26(2):144-146.
20. Sihvonen R, Paavola M, Malmivaara A, et al. Arthroscopic partial meniscectomy versus sham surgery for a degenerative meniscal tear. *N Engl J Med.* 2013;369(26):2515-2524. doi:10.1056/NEJMoa1305189
21. Barlow T, Plant CE. Why we still perform arthroscopy in knee osteoarthritis: a multi-methods study. *BMC Musculoskelet Disord.* 2015;16(1):1-9. Available at https://bmcmusculoskeletdisord.biomedcentral.com/articles/10.1186/s12891-015-0537-y.
22. Kise NJ, Risberg MA, Stensrud S, Ranstam J, Engebretsen L, Roos EM. Exercise therapy versus arthroscopic partial meniscectomy for degenerative meniscal tear in middle aged patients: randomised controlled trial with two year follow-up. *Br J Sports Med.* 2016;50(23):1473-1480.
23. Siemieniuk R, Harris I, Agoritsas T, et al. Arthroscopic surgery for degenerative knee arthritis and meniscal tears: a clinical practice guideline. *BMJ.* 2017;357:1-8. doi:10.1136/bmj.j1982. Available at http://www.embase.com/search/results?subaction=viewrecord&from=export&id=L616112909%0A. Accessed January 10, 2019.
24. Su X, Li C, Liao W, et al. Comparison of arthroscopic and conservative treatments for knee osteoarthritis: a 5-year retrospective comparative study. *Arthroscopy.* 2018;34(3):652-659.
25. Winter AR, Collins JE, Katz JN. The likelihood of total knee arthroplasty following arthroscopic surgery for osteoarthritis: a systematic review. *BMC Musculoskelet Disord.* 2017;18(1):1-8.
26. Kirkley A, Birmingham T, Litchfield R, et al. A randomized trial of arthroscopic surgery for osteoarthritis of the knee. *N Engl J Med.* 2008;359(11):1097-1107. doi:10.1056/nejmoa0708333
27. Lamplot JD, Brophy RH. The role for arthroscopic partial meniscectomy in knees with degenerative changes: a systematic review. *Bone Joint J.* 2016;98-B(7):934-938. Available at https://www.ncbi.nlm.nih.gov/pubmed/27365471. Accessed January 15, 2019.
28. Samson L, Mazurkiewicz S, Treder M, Wisniewski P. Outcome in the arthroscopic treatment of synovial chondromatosis of the knee. *Ortop Traumatol Rehabil.* 2005;7(4):391-396. Available at https://www.ncbi.nlm.nih.gov/pubmed/17611458. Accessed January 26, 2019.
29. Fauno P, Nielsen AB. Arthroscopic partial meniscectomy: a long-term follow-up. *Arthroscopy.* 1992;8(3):345-349.
30. Tanamas S, Hanna FS, Cicuttini FM, Wluka AE, Berry P, Urquhart DM. Does knee malalignment increase the risk of development and progression of knee osteoarthritis? A systematic review. *Arthritis Care Res.* 2009;61(4):459-467.
31. Felson DT, Niu J, Gross KD, et al. Valgus malalignment is a risk factor for lateral knee osteoarthritis incidence and progression: findings from the Multicenter Osteoarthritis Study and the Osteoarthritis Initiative. *Arthritis Rheum.* 2013;65(2):355-362.
32. Huang T-L, Tseng KF, Chen WM, Lin RMH, Wu JJ, Chen TH. Preoperative tibiofemoral angle predicts survival of proximal tibia osteotomy. *Clin Orthop Relat Res.* 2005;432:188-195.

33. Shourt CA, Crowson CS, Gabriel SE, Matteson EL. Orthopedic surgery among patients with rheumatoid arthritis 1980-2007: a population-based study focused on surgery rates, sex, and mortality. *J Rheumatol.* 2012;39(3):481-485.

34. Momohara S, Inoue E, Ikari K, et al. Decrease in orthopaedic operations, including total joint replacements, in patients with rheumatoid arthritis between 2001 and 2007: data from Japanese outpatients in a single institute-based large observational cohort (IORRA). *Ann Rheum Dis.* 2010;69(1):312-313.

35. Duncan ST, Khazzam MS, Burnham JM, Spindler KP, Dunn WR, Wright RW. Sensitivity of standing radiographs to detect knee arthritis: a systematic review of Level I studies. *Arthroscopy.* 2015;31(2):321-328.

36. Felson DT, Chaisson CE, Hill CL, et al. The association of bone marrow lesions with pain in knee osteoarthritis. *Ann Intern Med.* 2001;134(7):541-549.

37. Gill TJ, Safran M, Mandelbaum B, Huber B, Gambardella R, Xerogeanes J. A prospective, blinded, multicenter clinical trial to compare the efficacy, accuracy, and safety of in-office diagnostic arthroscopy with magnetic resonance imaging and surgical diagnostic arthroscopy. *Arthroscopy.* 2018;34(8):2429-2435. doi:10.1016/j.arthro.2018.03.010.

38. Messier S, Gutekunst D, Davis C, DeVita P. Weight loss reduces knee-joint loads in overweight and obese older adults with knee osteoarthritis. *Arthritis Rheum.* 2005;52(7):2026-2032. Available at https://www.ncbi.nlm.nih.gov/pubmed/?term=Weight+loss+reduces+knee-joint+loads+in+overweight+and+obese+older+adults+with+knee+osteoarthritis. Accessed January 26, 2019.

39. Atukorala I, Makovey J, Lawler L, Messier S, Bennell K, Hunter D. Is there a dose-response relationship between weight loss and symptom improvement in persons with knee osteoarthritis? *Arthritis Care Res.* 2016;68(8):1106-1114. Available at https://www.ncbi.nlm.nih.gov/pubmed/?articles-search-by=subject&otool=mssmlib&holding=mssmlib&articles-scope=title-begins-with&term=Is+There+a+Dose-Response+Relationship+Between+Weight+Loss+and+Symptom-+Improvement+in+Persons+With+Knee+Osteoarthritis%3F. Accessed January 26, 2019.

40. Dieppe PA, Sathapatayavongs B, Jones HE, Bacon PA, Ring E. Intra-articular steroids in osteoarthritis. *Rheumatol Rehabil.* 1980;19(4):212-217. Available at http://ovidsp.ovid.com/ovidweb.cgi?T=JS&PAGE=reference&D=emed3&NEWS=N&AN=11232162. Accessed January 20, 2019.

41. Brown GA. AAOS clinical practice guideline: treatment of osteoarthritis of the knee: evidence-based guideline, 2nd edition. *J Am Acad Orthop Surg.* 2013;21(9):577-579. Available at http://www.ncbi.nlm.nih.gov/pubmed/23996989. Accessed December 12, 2018.

42. Riley LP. *AAOS Approves Appropriate Use Criteria (AUC) for Non-Arthroplasty Treatment of Osteoarthritis of the Knee.* 2013. Available at http://newsroom.aaos.org/media-resources/Press-releases/aaos-approves-appropriate-use-criteria-auc-for-non-arthroplasty-treatment-of-osteoarthritis-of-the-knee.tekprint. Accessed November 25, 2018.

43. AAOS. *Appropriate Use Criteria: Osteoarthritis of the Knee: Non-Arthroplasty Treatment.* 2013. Available at http://www.aaos.org/aucapp. Accessed November 25, 2018.

44. Felson DT, Mclaughlin S, Goggins J, et al. Bone marrow edema and its relation to progression of knee osteoarthritis. *Ann Intern Med.* 2003;139(5):330-337.

45. Scher C, Craig J, Nelson F. Bone marrow edema in the knee in osteoarthrosis and association with total knee arthroplasty within a three-year follow-up. *Skeletal Radiol.* 2008;37(7):609-617.

46. Cohen S, Sharkey P. Subchondroplasty for treating bone marrow lesions. *J Knee Surg.* 2016;29:555-563.

47. Bonadio MB, Giglio PN, Helito CP, Pécora JR, Camanho GL, Demange MK. Subchondroplasty for treating bone marrow lesions in the knee – initial experience. *Rev Bras Ortop.* 2017;52(3):325-330. Available at http://linkinghub.elsevier.com/retrieve/pii/S2255497117300496. Accessed November 25, 2018.

chapter 25

Cartilage Restoration Procedures of the Knee

Neal B. Naveen, BS I Taylor M. Southworth, BS I Alex Beletsky, BS I William M. Cregar, MD I Tracy M. Tauro, BS, BA I Kelechi R. Okoroha, MD I Toufic R. Jildeh, MD I Brian J. Cole, MD, MBA I Adam B. Yanke, MD, PhD

INTRODUCTION

Articular cartilage is a highly specialized unit of connective tissue that is paramount to the movement of joints by acting as a load-bearing structure and to minimize friction.[1,2] The articular cartilage overlies the subchondral bone and is a thin layer between 2 and 4 mm composed of chondrocytes and an extracellular matrix (ECM). It is divided into four layers, each with distinct morphology, biochemical composition, and biomechanical properties (from deep to superficial): The calcified cartilage layer (CCL), deep, transitional, and superficial zone.[3] The three cartilaginous zones range in collagen orientation and water composition, while the CCL is a thin layer that acts to offset the discontinuity in stiffness between the subchondral bone and cartilaginous layers, as well as securing the layers together.[1,4,5] Water is the largest component of the ECM, ranging from 65% in the deep zone of the osteochondral unit to almost 80% in the superficial zone, and serves to nourish the collagen network.[6,7]

The ECM is also composed of collagen fibers and proteoglycans, with a small component of other proteins and glycoproteins.[7] There are over eight different types of collagen fibers present in hyaline cartilage, with over 90% of the fibers being type II collagen.[8] The chondrocytes are of mesenchymal stem cell origin and are primarily responsible for the synthesis of the ECM. This complex framework of chondrocytes, macromolecules, and a collagen fibril mesh provides cartilage its tensile strength and unique structure.

Articular cartilage receives its nutritional supply and oxygen by diffusion through the surrounding synovial fluid and at times the subchondral bone.[9] Therefore, injuries to hyaline cartilage that do not penetrate the subchondral bone cannot produce an inflammatory response and thus have a low capacity for healing.[10,11] Full-thickness cartilage injuries do undergo some degree of regeneration by initiating a typical inflammatory response, which consists of hematoma formation, mitogenic chondrocyte activity, and vascular ingrowth.[12,13] Unfortunately, the fibrocartilage produced by this inflammatory response, as opposed to healthy hyaline cartilage, gradually deteriorates and leads to the progression of osteoarthritis (OA) due to its inferior biomechanical properties.[11,14-16]

Thus, due to its avascular and aneural nature, articular cartilage has poor intrinsic healing capacity and is often susceptible to injury and degeneration into chondral lesions.[6,17,18] Over time, the articular surface may become destabilized from the subchondral bone and resultant shear forces may wear away the resulting fragment in a process known as osteochondritis dissecans (OCD).[19] Some causes for chondral lesions may include repetitive microtrauma, genetic predisposition, or vascular ischemia.[20] Left unmanaged, these lesions can be debilitating for active patients and lead to the early onset of OA. One of the challenges of developing an adequate treatment for defects lies in the complex structure and function of healthy hyaline cartilage, as the entire osteochondral unit must be restored rather than just the articular surface.[11,12]

The prevalence of chondral defects is estimated at 15 to 30 per 100,000, the majority of which occur in the knee. Focal chondral defects have been reported in up to 89% of high-level athletes due to the repetitive load-bearing stresses that occur during activity.[21-24] However, these defects are not confined to solely athletes, as focal cartilage defects have been identified in over 60% of patients undergoing knee arthroscopies.[3,25,26] Nearly 80% of the cases involve the medial femoral condyle (MFC), 15% involve the lateral femoral condyle, and 5% involve the patellofemoral region.[27,28]

Patients may typically complain of catching, pain, crepitus, and effusion, which often prevent these patients from participating in their usual daily activities, and larger lesions have a significant risk of progressing to OA.[29] The challenge has been finding a process that restores the joint surface congruity, controls the patient's symptoms, is able to withstand the intra-articular forces of the knee over time, and prevents the progression of focal chondral injuries to end-stage OA. The treatment modality is largely contingent upon the stability of a lesion; patients having a short duration of symptoms and a stable lesion can be managed successfully with just a hiatus from sporting or high-impact activity. In the setting of an unstable lesion or failure of nonsurgical management, there are a number of treatment modalities that can be used to repair the lesion and can be classified as either palliative, reparative, restorative, or reconstructive procedures.

Palliative approaches may include loose body removal or débridement which may provide short-term symptom relief.[30-33] Reparative procedures may include microfracture/marrow stimulation or drilling, which stimulates the defect to be filled with fibrocartilage.[34] The resulting hyalinelike cartilage from restorative procedures such as autologous chondrocyte implantation (ACI) may provide better long-term durability than fibrocartilage due to its superior viscoelastic and force distribution properties.[34,35] Finally, reconstructive procedures place a preformed osteochondral unit directly into the defect area and include osteochondral allograft (OCA) or autograft. Each procedure comes with its own indications and contraindications—age, lesion characteristics, level of activity, and patient expectations are just a few factors that must be considered in order to choose the best treatment modality for a patient. The purpose of this chapter is to explore outcomes, discuss the general indications and contraindications, and postoperative management for each of these techniques.

More recently, the role of different techniques has been further defined with respect to lesion location, lesion size, and specific patient demands.[36] Although primary repair is preferred for any cartilage injury that is amenable to fixation in a natural position, microfracture is indicated in the case of moderate symptoms, small-to middle-sized lesions (i.e., <2-3 cm in size), and grade III/IV (modified Outerbridge classification) OA.[37,38] Microfracture represents an optimal treatment for femoral condyle lesions <2 to 3 cm in size in both low-demand patients but results can deteriorate in high-demand patients, patellofemoral lesions, or large (i.e., >2-3 cm) lesions.[36] Treatment decisions are more complex in patients with large femoral condyle lesions. OCA transplantation or ACI is the preferred treatment option in patients with high demands; however, in moderate demand patients, microfracture may be a reasonable alternative. Prior surgical treatment may also guide indications as patients with a history of failed microfracture treatment for the lesion in question may be best suited for a reconstructive option.[36] Lesion depth should also be considered, as deeper lesions often involve significant bone and are best treated with OCA[39] (**Fig. 25-1**).

OVERALL CARTILAGE INDICATIONS

General indications for cartilage treatment beyond débridement include full-thickness cartilage defects, unstable cartilage defects overlying subchondral bone, and unstable partial-thickness defects.[40] Concurrent angular deformity of the knee also needs to be addressed in these patients at the time of cartilage treatment.[41] Other important considerations include ligamentous insufficiency (i.e., anterior cruciate ligament [ACL], posterior cruciate ligament [PCL]) and meniscal deficiency, which may require concurrent treatment.[42,43] Partial

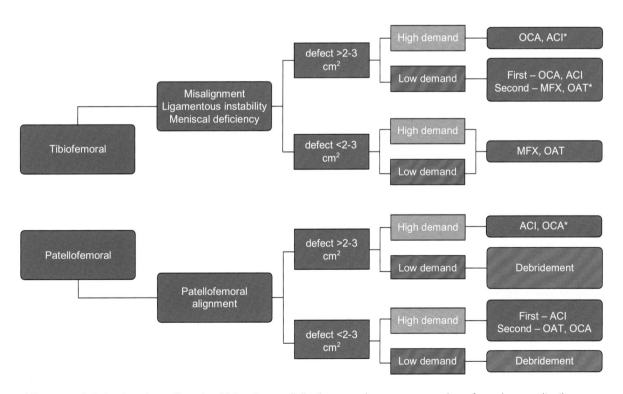

* Corresponds to treatment paradigms in which anteromedialization procedures are commonly performed concomitantly

FIGURE 25-1 Indications for cartilage treatment: an overview. ACI, autologous chondrocyte implantation; OCA, osteochondral allograft; MFX, Microfracture; OAT, osteochondral autograft.

meniscectomy is considered in patients with meniscal injury, although outcomes in those with severe chondral damage have demonstrated elevated rates of subsequent OA following meniscectomy.[44] Additionally, the role of anteromedialization procedures, particularly in the case of lateral patellofemoral lesions, is emerging.[36,45]

Contraindications for cartilage treatment include systemic diseases that may predispose to arthritis (i.e., posttraumatic, postinfectious), diseases altering the therapeutic release of marrow factors (i.e., systemic, immune-mediated disease), or primary cartilage diseases that may alter the functionality of the articular cartilage (i.e., polychondritis, OCD). Global degenerative osteoarthrosis, capsular contraction, synovitis, partial-thickness defects, or scarring of the anterior interval has previously been identified as contraindications.[46] Cartilage procedures should not be performed in patients unable to tolerate weight-bearing on the contralateral leg or unable to follow postoperative rehabilitation protocols.[46] When considering the defect location, overall alignment, defect size, and patient demands, one can understand the best treatment option available to the patient (**Fig. 25-1**).

MICROFRACTURE

Microfracture was originally designed as a surgical intervention for patients with posttraumatic cartilage lesions which progressed to full-thickness cartilage defects.[46] The procedure relies on an influx of marrow factors (i.e., mesenchymal stem cells, growth factors), formation of a fibrin clot, and subsequent remodeling into fibrocartilage.[47] Due to the advancement of more involved cartilage techniques (i.e., ACI, matrix-associated chondrocyte implantation [MACI]) as well as limited outcomes, microfracture has taken a lesser role in treatment of cartilage defects.[48,49] Due to its ease of implementation, microfracture has been utilized in settings that differ from large restorative or reconstructive options. Specifically, indications for correcting meniscal deficiency, alignment, and postoperative weight-bearing have not been as stringent as with other cartilage procedures. Current evidence suggests that optimal outcomes are seen in patients with lesions <2 to 3 cm^2, no prior cartilage surgery, and age <30 years old. Femoral condyle lesions also have better outcomes than the patella and other options should be considered in this region.

Technique

After general anesthesia allows for appropriate muscle relaxation, an examination under anesthesia is performed to confirm the absence of ligamentous laxity or possible mechanical symptoms suggestive of a possible meniscal injury. The patient is most commonly positioned supine. A posterior lesion can necessitate knee hyperflexion that should be accounted for prior to initiation of arthroscopy.

Diagnostic arthroscopy requires a standard three-portal system with an anteromedial, anterolateral, and optional proximal outflow portal. Tourniquet use is not required, and arthroscopic pump pressure is varied to optimize viewing. A complete diagnostic workup includes inspection of the suprapatellar pouch, gutters (i.e., medial, lateral), the intercondylar notch, and both the patellofemoral and tibiofemoral (i.e., medial, lateral compartment) joints. A graduated probe can be utilized to inspect tears of the inferior aspect of the meniscus. The intercondylar notch must be inspected to ensure ligamentous stability of the ACL and PCL. Unstable chondral lesions should be marginally debrided to create an appropriately stable chondral border, devoid of loose bodies. The final, clean, stable lesion should provide a perpendicular surface of healthy, viable cartilage to ensure appropriate clot creation and proliferation.[46,40] Chronic lesions can present a unique technical challenge due chronic cartilage degeneration, bony sclerosis, and subchondral thickening. In these scenarios, it becomes important to create a stable chondral surface with punctate bleeding uniformly over the cartilage surface to ensure appropriate propensity toward clot formation.[40] A degenerative knee may also warrant surgical release of the anterior interval via the intermeniscal interval, particularly if scarring is identified during the diagnostic portion of the procedure. Typically, if these procedures are necessary, the patient is poorly indicated for microfracture.

The microfracture is classically performed as the final intra-articular procedure of a case with the hopes of optimizing marrow release and fibrin clot formation.[40] Two important variations exist with respect to this instrumentation. Traditional methods utilize a microfracture awl to create perpendicular perforations in subchondral bone at depths of 2 to 4 mm.[40] More recent techniques utilizing microdrilling result in limiting bony compaction[50]; however, there are concerns of thermal necrosis[46] (**Fig. 25-2A and B**). Using the preferred instrumentation, subchondral bone is perforated beginning at the lesion periphery and ending with the central site of microfracture. Careful distances between perforations are approximated such that fracture across the subchondral bone plate is appropriately avoided (i.e., 2-4 mm).[36] Fat droplets are commonly visualized at the bony fracture site, and bony bleeding can be utilized to gauge appropriate depth of penetration. Intra-articular drains are generally avoided due to concerns of limiting efficient marrow factor release to propagating of a fibrin clot.[46] The fibrocartilage clot has previous been described by Cole and associates as a "superclot," due to the pluripotent nature of mesenchymal stem cells released from the marrow in the formation of fibrocartilage structure.[36] The microfracture can also be filled with micronized allogeneic cartilage which can help to act as a scaffold for the creation of hyalinelike cartilage. This allogeneic cartilage is typically mixed with platelet-rich plasma and applied in smaller defects and then sealed with a fibrin glue (**Fig. 25-2C and D**).[51]

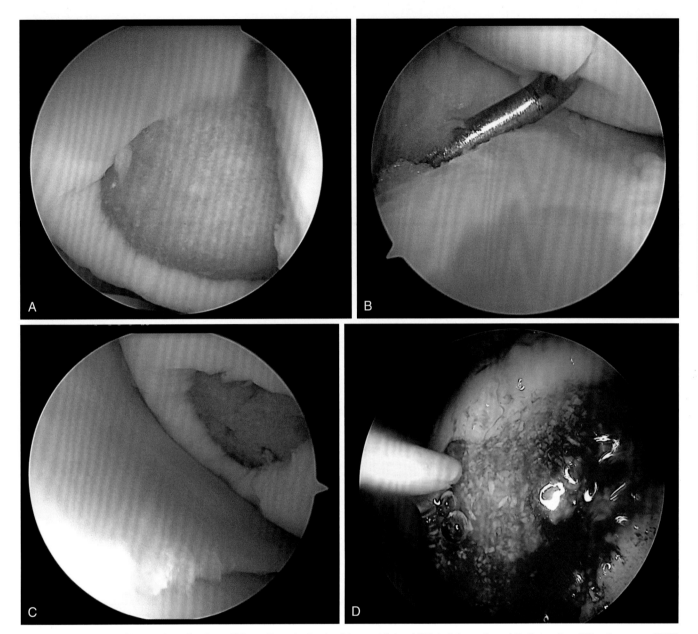

FIGURE 25-2   Microdrilling and application of biocartilage to the trochlea and lateral tibial plateau. **A** and **B:** Osteochondritis dissecans (OCD) lesion is debrided and the bone is microdrilled several times to release marrow elements. **C:** A mixture of platelet-rich plasma and allogeneic cartilage is applied to the site of the microfracture. **D:** A thin layer of fibrin glue is applied to the surface of the filled defect.

Outcomes

There are numerous results published in the literature detailing outcomes following microfracture with varying results.[52-58] **Table 25-1** summarizes the results of these previous studies.

Early investigations of microfracture generally demonstrated positive short-term outcomes.

Steadman and associated detailed clinical outcomes in 24 patients who underwent microfracture with a 24-month follow-up (61). Patients in their study were an average age of 38 years and injury date ranged from 1 day to 10 years. The author's reported that at 3 years postoperatively, 75% of patients (152 of 203) had less pain; 19% had unchanged pain; and 6% felt worse. Additionally,

the authors found negative predictors of postoperative outcomes to include preoperative joint space narrowing, age >30 years, chronicity of lesions, isolated defects, and non-CPM (continuous passive motion) use postoperatively. Outcomes in this study were not affected by lesion size, and survivability of the procedure demonstrated a small decline over 7 years (95% at 4 years, 92% at 7 years).

In 2000, Passler reported on subjective results on 162 of his patients who received microfracture (74). Seventy-eight percent of patients receiving a microfracture reported reduced pain, 18% reported no change, and 4% reported they were worse at a mean follow-up of 4.4 years (range, 3-6 years).

TABLE 25-1 Clinical and Functional Outcomes Following Microfracture

Study	Technique	Number of Patients	Outcome Measures	Results	Findings
Dzioba[55] (1-y follow-up)	Drilling	48	Pain	69% pain free; 31% had persistent pain and/or effusions	
Rodrigo et al[58]	Microfracture	77	Lesion appearance (second-look arthroscopy)	Better defect filling when CPM used postoperatively ($P = .003$)	Extent of filling did not correlate with functional outcome
Levy et al[53] (1-y follow-up)	Débridement of calcified cartilage layer only	15 soccer players	Brittberg scoring system	6 excellent; 9 good; 0 fair; 0 poor	High-demand population
Steadman et al[54] (5-y follow-up)	Microfracture		Subjective questionnaire, pain, ADLs, work, sports participation	Pain: 75% improved; 20% unchanged; 5% worse. ADLs and work: 67% improved; 20% unchanged; 13% worse. Sports: 65% improved	
Blevins et al[52]	Microfracture	38 "high-level" athletes and 140 recreational athletes	Subjective questionnaire: pain, swelling, giving way, locking. Lesion appearance (second-look arthroscopy)	All functional parameters were significantly improved in both groups after surgery. Grading of lesion improved in both groups ($P > .05$)	Numerous associated diagnoses and concomitant procedures
Passler[56] (3- to 6-y follow-up)	Microfracture	162	Subjective questionnaire: pain	78% improved; 18% unchanged; 4% worse	
Steadman et al[57] (3-y follow-up)	Microfracture	203	Subjective questionnaire: pain	75% improved; 19% unchanged; 6% worse	Negative predictors: Age >30 y Chronicity Isolated defect No CPM Size >300 mm² was not a negative predictor

ADL, activities of daily living; CPM, continuous passive motion.

Though early outcomes were encouraging, there is growing concern that these results may not be maintained. Mithoefer et al performed a systematic review of 3122 microfracture procedures with extended follow-up.[59] The author's reported a significant improvement in knee function postoperatively with a short-term clinical improvement rate of 75% to 100% at 24 months postoperatively. However, after 24 months, 47% to 80% of patients reported a subjective decline in functional outcomes. Other studies have corroborated the regression of positive outcomes at long-term follow-up.[60-62] More recently Solheim and colleagues reported on long-term (>15 years) outcomes following a randomized controlled trial comparing microfracture to mosaicplasty.[63] The author's found a significant improvement in all patients at 15-year follow-up. However, there was a clinically significant difference in Lysholm knee scores at all time

points postoperatively with mosaicplasty demonstrating more beneficial outcomes. Patient characteristics including greater BMI (>30 kg/m²), larger defects (>2.5 cm²), and higher physical activity level have been correlated with decreased outcomes following microfracture.[64-67] Kraeutler and associates performed a systematic review of three level 1 studies and two level 2 studies reporting 5-year outcomes following microfracture or ACI.[68] The authors found no difference in treatment failure at an average of 7 years postoperatively. Additionally, Lysholm score and Knee injury and Osteoarthritis Outcome Score (KOOS) were found to improve for both groups across studies, without a significant difference in improvement between the groups. In professional athletes including those in the National Basketball Association (NBA), there is a high rate of failure to return to sport (21%)[66,67]. In these high-level athletes, microfracture was correlated with decrease player efficiency, minutes per game, and points per game. It is evident that the induction of marrow stimulation to produce fibrocartilage does not recreate the natural structure and strength of hyaline articular cartilage. This renders the surface less durable and more prone to wearing out over time, especially when enduring high-impact activities. It should be noted that in more recent studies which have shown regression in outcomes with follow-up, the procedure was performed with an awl and impaction technique which has potential limitations in cartilage defect treatment. Current techniques of marrow stimulation utilize microdrilling which has been theorized to limit bony compaction and facilitate greater delivery of mesenchymal cells into the defect. Future studies should employ randomized controlled trials and prospective studies comparing long-term outcomes of newer generation microfracture techniques compared to alternative resurfacing techniques.

OSTEOCHONDRAL ALLOGRAFT/ AUTOGRAFT

Osteochondral allograft (OCA) implantation and osteochondral autograft transfer system (OATS) are procedures used to restore both the native bony and cartilaginous architecture at the site of the defect.[60,69] OCA can restore osseous, chondral, and mature hyaline cartilage components by matching the articular architecture with a donor allograft, whereas OATS involves harvesting bone and cartilage from a non–weight-bearing portion of the knee, such as the far proximal or far medial/lateral of the trochlea or the lateral intercondylar notch to the defect site, and transferring the tissue into the focal articular defect.[70,71] OCA is often regarded as a salvage procedure that should not be used as a first-line treatment due to the violation of the native subchondral architecture.[20]

These procedures can be used to either primarily repair large osteochondral lesions or as salvage procedures following a failed previous cartilage repair (such as failed microfracture or ACI). OCAs and OATS are particularly useful in restoring the anatomy of large full-thickness osteochondral defects and have the unique ability to be implemented in posttraumatic focal lesions, deep subchondral bone damage, or OCD.[72-74] Ideal candidates for this procedure are those with unipolar lesions of the patella, trochlea, or femoral condyle, high physical demands, neutral alignment, and low to normal BMI[36] (**Fig. 25-3A**).

OCA procedures are useful in lesions larger than 4 cm^2 and involves using a donor graft to match the patient's anatomy as closely as possible.[75,76] Osteochondral autograft transplantations (OATs) are useful in lesions <2.5 cm.[76] OAT procedures are limited to smaller lesions due to a limited supply of donor tissue and associated donor-site morbidity. These procedures are relatively contraindicated in patients with OA, avascular necrosis,

inflammatory arthropathies, BMI>30, or age older than 45 years,[39,77-80] and careful consideration must be made when considering surgical intervention within these demographics.

Osteochondral Allograft Technique

Dowel technique is the favored type of technique used for femoral OCA lesions.[81] The underlying principle when using this technique is conversion of the host cartilage defect to a cylindrical socket, which can be further filled with an osteochondral plug from an allograft. It involves driving a guidewire perpendicular to the curvature of the articular surface, which is centered over the sizing dowel (**Fig. 25-3B**). A reamer is used to remove the remaining articular cartilage and 3 to 4 mm of subchondral bone, not exceeding a depth of 8 to 10 mm. The guidewire is removed, and depth measurements are made at the four quadrants of the graft. The corresponding anatomic site is identified on the graft, and a graft harvesting site is used to procure the graft, perpendicular to the articular surface and matching the anatomic contours of the recipient site. Excess is trimmed with a saw, to ensure the graft is of appropriate depth (**Fig. 25-3C**). It is important to treat grafts with sustained pulsatile lavage prior to implantation to remove bone marrow elements that contribute to graft immunogenicity. Finally, the graft is press-fit by hand in a line-to-line manner, with special attention paid to the rotation. This graft can be gently tamped, and the joint is brought through a range of motion to fully seat the graft. If possible, impaction should be avoided to retain graft viability. It should be important to note that chondrocytes can be damaged during impaction, so the graft must be very carefully tamped flush with surrounding cartilage.[45,82] Typically, no other fixation is required; however, if needed, a bioabsorbable compression screw can be placed in the center of the graft[36] (**Fig. 25-3D**).

OAT Technique

Depending on the size of the defect, either one or multiple autologous osteochondral tissue plugs (i.e., "mosaicplasty") can be transferred from non–weight-bearing articular surfaces to the area of chondral defect.[76] Available donor sites include the medial or lateral femoral condyles proximal to the sulcus terminalis or the intercondylar notch.[76] The largest harvest size available for single-plug transfer is 1 cm^2 in diameter; however, multiple plugs can be harvested to treat larger lesions.[83] If doing so, multiple plugs can be harvested from the same side of the knee (i.e., medial–medial, lateral–lateral) by adjusting flexion/extension through a miniarthrotomy.[83] An all-arthroscopic technique is possible; however, lesion location, size, and surgeon preference/comfort dictate whether a formal arthrotomy is needed. Typically, condylar lesions are more easily accessed arthroscopically

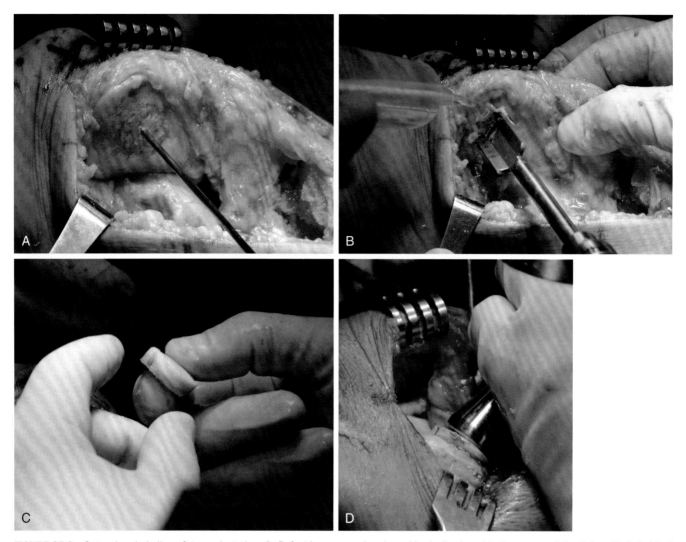

FIGURE 25-3 Osteochondral allograft transplantation. **A:** Defect is measured and a guidewire is placed in the center of the defect. **B:** Cylindrical socket in host tissue is created by reaming to a depth of 6 to 8 mm. **C:** Plug is harvested from the donor graft and trimmed to ensure congruity with recipient site. **D:** Graft is press-fit to be flush with the surrounding cartilage.

through satellite portals, whereas patellofemoral or tibial lesions are harder to access arthroscopically and may require a miniarthrotomy. We prefer to obtain donor plug(s) through a small lateral arthrotomy with implantation of the plug(s) arthroscopically if possible. Without performing these with any great frequency, the authors recommend surgeons perform this in an open fashion to obtain perpendicularity.

OATs begin with a diagnostic arthroscopy. The patient is positioned supine with the affected lower extremity placed in an ACL leg holder and the foot of the bed dropped such that the leg can be fully extended and hyperflexed to at least 120° with ease. The use of a leg positioner can aid in controlled placement of the limb and maintenance of limb position, especially if hyperflexion is required for access to the articular lesion. A well-padded, nonsterile tourniquet is placed on the thigh of the affected extremity. The contralateral leg is placed in a lithotomy-style well-leg holder ensuring that the common peroneal nerve is well padded. An examination under anesthesia

is carried out to document range of motion and ligamentous stability of both extremities for comparison. The affected leg is prepped and draped in a sterile fashion. A complete diagnostic arthroscopy is carried out using standard anteromedial and anterolateral portals. Attention is turned to the cartilage defect which is fully identified and classified. An arthroscopic probe is used to assess the boundaries and stability of the lesion. Any loose cartilage flaps are debrided, and the size of the defect is determined. Size-specific cannulas or measurement probes are used to determine the size of the lesion depending on the particular system being used. The surgeon can then plan the number and size of grafts needed. Satellite portals can be made with spinal needle localization to ensure that the articular defects can be accessed perpendicularly.

Once a plan for the size and number of harvest grafts is established, the donor site can be harvested. This can be done arthroscopically or through a miniarthrotomy (2-3 cm). We prefer to obtain donor osteochondral tissue through a small arthrotomy. A small incision is made at the superolateral aspect of the patella, and two retractors are positioned to expose the superolateral trochlea. There are many commercial systems available that differ slightly in the method of extraction and creation of a press-fit implant. Generally, a harvesting tube retractor is assembled based upon the size of the lesion, and the graft is procured by impacting perpendicular to the articular surface to a depth of about 12 to 15 mm and removing the intact plug.[36] It is important that the harvest graft is obtained at a perpendicular angle to the articular surface to aid in the creation of well-defined vertical walls such that the donor plug is a congruent fit.[11,18,84,85] The graft depth is measured and attention is turned to the recipient site.

The knee may need to be repositioned, and another satellite portal may need to be established in order to gain perpendicular access for drilling of the recipient site. An appropriately sized reamer is selected corresponding to the diameter of the harvest graft, and the recipient hole is impacted to a depth of 2 mm less than the length of the donor graft.[36] A motorized shaver or curettes are used to obtain a stable vertical margin, again aiding in graft congruency. If using multiple grafts, each recipient hole should be separated from each other by a 1 to 2 mm bridge.[86] The graft is then placed in the delivery tube and seated perpendicularly to the reamed recipient hole. Graft implantation is achieved by advancement with gentle taps of the impactor in a press-fit manner to avoid chondrocyte injury.[45,76,82,87] The final graft should be flushed with adjacent surrounding articular cartilage as a graft left proud can result in increased articular contact pressures.[88] The knee should be adequately cleared of all debris and incisions should be closed in a standard layered fashion.

OAT Outcomes

Overall, results of OATs in the literature are generally good; however, the major limitation hinges on the size of the articular cartilage defect along with donor-site morbidity. Braun et al demonstrated good clinical results at 5.5 years postoperatively with lesions >4 cm^2 with other literature reporting the successful use of osteochondral autograft in lesions as large as 8 cm^2. Despite this, treatment of lesions <2 cm^2 are associated with superior clinical outcomes.[74] A systematic review by Lynch et al demonstrated a high rate of return to sport as early as 6 months postoperatively with significant improvement in 607 patients and superior outcomes for patients with lesions <2 cm^2.[72] Pareek et al also published a systematic review in 2016 including 10 studies with a total of 610 patients and a mean follow-up of 10.2 years. They found significantly improved International Knee Documentation Committee (IKDC) and Lysholm scores in 72% of patients. However, there was a 19% reoperation rate.[74] Along the same lines, Riboh et al compared reoperation rates among OAT, microfracture, and second-generation ACI procedures. They found a slightly higher reoperation rate with OAT when compared to ACI, however, a lower

reoperation rate when compared with microfracture.[85] Hangody et al published one of the largest studies in 2010 describing 383 athletes who were treated with autograft osteochondral mosaicplasty with follow-up data averaging just below 10 years. They reported an overall good to excellent result in 91% of femoral condylar lesions with slightly inferior results seen in tibial lesions (86%) and patellofemoral lesions (74%).[89] Overall, OAT remains a viable option in a small subset of patients with small isolated articular lesions, neutral limb alignment, and normal BMI.[73,74] Despite this, donor-site morbidity remains a major drawback.

Osteochondral Allograft Outcomes

Osteochondral allograft (OCA) is primarily indicated for full-thickness osteochondral defects.[71] Overall, there is good evidence that the long-term success rates of OCA are very good, with subjective improvement in 75% of patients at 12.3 years postoperative and an overall 85% graft survival rate after 10 years.[73,74,90,91] OCA has also shown promising results in highly active individuals. Krych and colleagues reported an overall 80% return to sport rate in professional athletes with a 2.5-year mean follow-up.[92] Similarly, Cotter et al reported an 81.6% return to sport rate in patients self-identifying as athletes at an average of 14 months postoperatively.[93] Importantly, OCA can be a highly effective subsequent treatment after a prior failed cartilage intervention (i.e., microfracture, ACI, OAT). Gracitelli and colleagues reported an overall 10-year survival rate of 86% in patients undergoing OCA as a revision procedure following failed microfracture.[84] They also reported an overall 97% satisfaction rate among patients who underwent OCA following a failed prior cartilage procedure.[84] Finally, OCA can be an effective treatment method to address cartilage defects when used with concomitant procedures. Saltzman et al reported no difference in outcomes or survivorship among patients who underwent isolated meniscal allograft transplantation when compared to patients who underwent meniscus allograft transplantation (MAT) with OCA.[94]

AUTOLOGOUS CHONDROCYTE IMPLANTATION

For a patient who presents with a full-thickness, isolated defect larger than 2 cm^2 that may be deeper than 8 mm, techniques such as fragment removal, subchondral drilling, and microfracture may not suffice as the resulting fibrocartilage will be mechanically inferior to the hyaline cartilage.[8] For these deep defects necessitating the replacement of both the surface cartilage as well as subchondral bone, ACI can be used in order to create a hyalinelike cartilage layer and has been demonstrated to achieve excellent outcomes at over 5-year follow-up.[81,95-97] The procedure typically involves two stages, with chondrocytes first being harvested arthroscopically and culturing the cells in a chondroinductive matrix for at least 4 weeks before surgically reimplanting it in the lesion.[98]

Indications/Contraindications

ACI is indicated for symptomatic, full-thickness chondral lesions at least 2.5 to 3 cm² in patients who do not have a significant OA.[99] While most studies have reported an average defect size of less than 5 cm², ACI has been utilized for lesions as large as 10 cm².[100,101] Defects may be localized to the femoral condyles, trochlea, patella, or the tibial plateau. While ACI was traditionally viewed as a treatment for younger patients, efficacy of ACI has not shown inferior outcomes in patients older than 45 years.[102] ACI is generally not indicated as a treatment option for patients with BMI ≥ 35 kg/m² or advanced degenerative joint disease which is the most significant factor which must be taken into consideration.[99,103]

There are currently three different generations of ACI. The first-generation ACI involved injecting chondrocytes underneath a periosteal flap which was sown to the defect, while the periosteal flap was replaced with a collagen scaffold in second-generation ACI. These previous generations were replaced by the third-generation ACI or matrix-induced autologous chondrocyte implantation (MACI), in which the cultured cells are seeded onto a chondroinductive type I/III collagen gel scaffold, which is then implanted at the time of surgery. Some third-generation ACIs have recently employed a one-step approach by using allogenic fetal chondrocytes, thus reducing donor-site morbidity[104]; however, these are not approved for use in the United States at this time.

Surgical Approach/Initial Biopsy

An inferolateral portal incision is made, and a diagnostic arthroscopy is first performed in order to assess all articular surfaces, menisci, and possible loose bodies. Once damaged areas are debrided with a shaver and the defect is measured, 200 to 300 g of cartilage are obtained arthroscopically from the intercondylar notch and sent to a laboratory for expansion.[103] The tissue is enzymatically digested in order to release chondrocytes, and the cells are expanded with a chondroinductive matrix for at least 4 weeks in order to obtain a count between 15 and 20 million cells.

Implantation

A medial or lateral parapatellar arthrotomy is used to expose the corresponding chondral injury (**Fig. 25-4A**). These regions of damaged cartilage surrounding the chondral defect are then debrided vertically using a fresh No. 15 scalpel blade or a sharp ring curette through the cartilage down to the level of the subchondral bone plate, but not into, the subchondral lamina[103] (**Fig. 25-4 B**). The

result should be a vertically walled defect that will be able to better distribute forces at the lesion and act as a reservoir for the implanted cells.[97] Defect dimensions are then measured using a sterile ruler or tin foil to cut the precise size and shape of membrane necessary. Alternatively, a custom oval cutter may be used to debride the defect as well as prepare the appropriate size of membrane (**Fig. 25-4C**) to ensure a line-to-line fit and minimal handling of the tissue. Lastly, the scaffold is fixed with a minimal amount of fibrin glue and sown with 6-0 Vicryl, with the cell-seeded side facing the subchondral bone[103] (**Fig. 25-4D**). After the glue has cured, the knee is then brought into immediate range of motion to ensure that the implant is not grossly unstable. The arthrotomy is then closed in a layered fashion, and a soft sterile dressing is applied to the knee.

Sandwich Technique

The ACI sandwich technique, first developed by Jones and Peterson, involves autologous bone grafting in the subchondral bone and then placing the cells between two layers of collagen I/III.[105] After the defect is prepared by an 8 mm high-speed burr to reveal healthy appearing bone, a Kirschner wire is drilled at the base of the defect in multiple sites in order to enhance blood supply at the autologous bone graft site. Once the autologous bone chips are then placed in the prepared defect, fibrin glue is applied to the surface of the bone graft and the first collagen layer is on the layer of fibrin glue. Finally, the second collagen layer of cells is then sutured and glued to the surface, and cultured chondrocytes are injected between the two collagen membranes thus completing the ACI sandwich.

Outcomes

Results following MACI have been documented by numerous studies, achieving good clinical outcomes in patients, with varying results on return to activity and level of competition. At 5 years after MACI, Ebert et al reported a significant improvement in patient-reported outcomes, with 98% satisfaction with procedure's alleviation of knee pain and 89% of patients demonstrating good to excellent filling of the chondral defect on MRI.[106] In a prospective, randomized study of 91 patients comparing MACI to ACI, Bartlett et al found that both treatments resulted in improvements in the modified Cincinnati Knee score, International Cartilage Repair Society (ICRS) score, and visual analogue scale (VAS) score as well as showed hyalinelike cartilage with or without fibrocartilage at 1-year follow-up biopsy.[107] Ventura et al reported on 53 patients with isolated or multiple localized 2 to 10 cm² osteochondral lesions who underwent MACI at 2-year follow-up, finding significant improvement in patient-reported outcomes as well as complete integration with surrounding native cartilage on MRI in 88% of patients.[108]

Patients have also experienced a high rate of return to activities, with Niemeyer reporting a return to sport of 73.1%, although the duration of exercise and

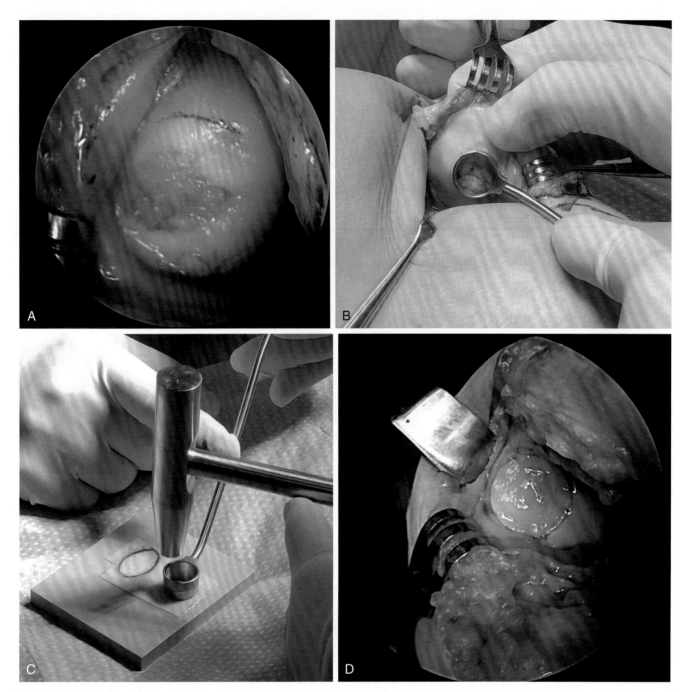

FIGURE 25-4 Matrix-induced autologous chondrocyte implantation of the patella and lateral femoral condyle. **A:** The lesion is identified and measured. **B:** A ring curette and sizer are used to debride and measure the appropriate area of the defects. **C:** A custom round cutter is used to maximize membrane congruity with the defect. **D:** Fibrin glue is placed to aid in implant fixation.

number of sessions per week significantly decreased after surgery.[109] Although only 31% of patients were able to return to their previous level of competition or work intensity, it was also found that level of activity was not correlated with defect location and size, thus showing promise for the use of ACI in the treatment of mid- to large-sized defects. Long-term outcomes for patients undergoing MACI have been documented by Zaffagnini et al, who reported 64.5% of athletes who were able to return to a competitive level at 10-year

follow-up. 58.1% returned to preinjury level of sport,[110] with previous surgeries being the most important factor in affecting return to prior level of play. Thus, while MACI can achieve good outcomes in patients, the level of high-demand activity in athletes may be more difficult to achieve, with high BMI, a degenerative etiology, and older age linked to a lower rate of return to sport.[110]

Numerous studies have compared the efficacies of marrow stimulation to those of MACI. Kon et al compared

ACI to microfracture and found a deterioration in clinical outcomes and sports activity in the microfracture group at 2- to 5-year follow-up, while they were maintained in the ACI group.[111] Although postoperative rehabilitation and recovery are traditionally slower in MACI than in microfracture, recent studies have shown equivalent, if not greater, functional outcomes and graft healing in patients undergoing an accelerated weight-bearing and rehabilitation regimen.[112,113]

Incidence of complications following MACI ranges between 0% and 6.3%, with one of the more common problems being graft hypertrophy.[107] Due to its low complication rates and significant improvements in patient-reported outcomes, MACI is an appealing option for patients with mid- to large-sized defects. While MACI has achieved encouraging results in patients at up to 10-year follow-up, it is not the definitive treatment for all cartilage lesions. An understanding of a patient's expectations and level of activity, along other preoperative factors, is crucial in determining whether ACI is a valid treatment option for those with large full-thickness symptomatic chondral injuries.

Concomitant Procedures

Multifactorial pathology such as ligamentous instability, meniscal injury, or malalignment is commonly found in patients with articular cartilage defects. Failure to correct any abnormalities can exacerbate existing cartilage defects and result in inferior outcomes following a cartilage restoration procedure.[42,114] Thus, it is imperative to perform a comprehensive physical examination and diagnostic imaging to identify combined pathology. Surgical correction should be performed at the time of the cartilage procedure in order to prevent any prolongation in rehabilitation, thus optimizing the biomechanics and stability of the environment following the cartilage repair.[115]

MENISCAL ALLOGRAFT TRANSPLANTATION

The meniscus plays a multifaceted role in the tibiofemoral joint, aiding in stability, load transmission, as well as proprioception. The presence of a healthy meniscus is crucial in the prevention of OA, with meniscectomies being linked to a four- to fivefold increased risk in the rate of OA and a 132-fold increased risk for a subsequent knee arthroplasty when compared to the contralateral knee.[116] Thus, in the setting of a symptomatic patient with a largely absent medial or lateral meniscus and cartilage pathology, treatment should be focused on restoring both deficiencies by performing a concomitant meniscal allograft transplant (MAT). One must be mindful of rehabilitation modification when performing a concomitant MAT, as tibial rotation must be avoided for 8 weeks postoperatively in order to protect the meniscus allograft.[117]

MALALIGNMENT (DFO/HTO) AND MALTRACKING (TTO)

In physiologic conditions, the knee is traditionally in 3° to 4° of varus, with the medial compartment bearing roughly 60% of the weight-bearing force.[118,119] Thus, any degree of varus malalignment can increase the load on the medial meniscus/MFC, with a valgus malalignment causing the converse.[115] Over time, this increased load may lead to meniscal and cartilage damage, increasing the risk for degenerative joint disease.[120,121] A standard weight-bearing radiograph series and long-leg alignment views are used to confirm malalignment. In patients undergoing an OCA and/or MAT, malalignment correction should be concomitantly performed if the mechanical axis crosses the knee in the same compartment of surgical intervention. General indications include patients younger than 60 years, normal ligamentous status, and unicompartmental OA. In the senior author's practice, malalignment of greater than 5° is an indication for surgical correction, in which a varus deformity is treated with a medial opening wedge high-tibial osteotomy, and a valgus malalignment is corrected with a lateral opening wedge distal femoral osteotomy.

Biomechanical data have shown the efficacy of osteotomies in decreasing peak pressures in the medial compartment of the knee, with the largest decrease in pressure occurring from neutral to 3° varus.[2] Bode et al helped to highlight the effect of malalignment of cartilage restoration procedures by comparing outcomes of patients with 1° to 5° of varus and concomitant articular cartilage defects. It was found that patients undergoing a combined HTO/ACI had significantly higher survival rates, lower reoperation rates, and superior clinical outcomes at 6-year follow-up, thus showing the importance of restoring normal biomechanical environment during a cartilage procedure.

CONCLUSION

With such a large population of today's athletes, chondral defects are an important pathology that should be diagnosed and addressed promptly. There are number of surgical and nonsurgical techniques that can be used for treating cartilage defects, and important factors that should be taken into consideration before choosing a treatment modality which include size and grade of the lesion, patient-specific demands, ligamentous stability, alignment, and location and stability of the lesion. While a stable lesion may be managed with simply a hiatus from activity or non–weight-bearing status, an unstable and large lesion may require a MACI, OCA, or OAT. Irrespective of the lesion, it is critical to combine the patient's expectations with findings from a comprehensive history and physical examination in order to determine the best course of management.

REFERENCES

1. Carballo CB, Nakagawa Y, Sekiya I, Rodeo SA. Basic science of articular cartilage. *Clin Sports Med.* 2017;36(3):413.

2. Van Thiel GS, Frank RM, Gupta A, et al. Biomechanical evaluation of a high tibial osteotomy with a meniscal transplant. *J Knee Surg.* 2011;24(1):45.

3. Curl WW, Krome J, Gordon ES, Rushing J, Smith BP, Poehling GG. Cartilage injuries: a review of 31,516 knee arthroscopies. *Arthroscopy.* 1997;13(4):456.

4. Norrdin RW, Kawcak CE, Capwell BA, McIlwraith CW. Calcified cartilage morphometry and its relation to subchondral bone remodeling in equine arthrosis. *Bone.* 1999;24(2):109.

5. Hwang J, Kyubwa EM, Bae WC, Bugbee WD, Masuda K, Sah RL. In vitro calcification of immature bovine articular cartilage: formation of a functional zone of calcified cartilage. *Cartilage.* 2010;1(4):287.

6. Mansour JM, Mow VC. The permeability of articular cartilage under compressive strain and at high pressures. *J Bone Joint Surg Am.* 1976;58(4):509.

7. Cohen NP, Foster RJ, Mow VC. Composition and dynamics of articular cartilage: structure, function, and maintaining healthy state. *J Orthop Sports Phys Ther.* 1998;28(4):203.

8. Baumann C, Hinkel BB, Bozynski CC, Farr J. *Articular Cartilage: Structure and Restoration.* New York, NY: Springer; 2019.

9. Danisovic L, Varga I, Polak S. Growth factors and chondrogenic differentiation of mesenchymal stem cells. *Tissue Cell.* 2012;44(2):69.

10. Brady MA, Waldman SD, Ethier CR. The application of multiple biophysical cues to engineer functional neocartilage for treatment of osteoarthritis. Part II: signal transduction. *Tissue Eng Part B Rev.* 2015;21(1):20.

11. Mankin HJ. Mitosis in articular cartilage of immature rabbits. A histologic, stathmokinetic (colchicine) and autoradiographic study. *Clin Orthop Relat Res.* 1964;34:170.

12. Buckwalter JA, Rosenberg LC, Hunziker EB. *Articular cartilage: composition, structure, response to injury, and methods of facilitating repair.* In: *Articular Cartilage and Knee Joint Function: Basic Science and Arthroscopy.* New York: Raven Press; 1990.

13. Miniaci A, Tytherleigh-Strong G. Fixation of unstable osteochondritis dissecans lesions of the knee using arthroscopic autogenous osteochondral grafting (mosaicplasty). *Arthroscopy.* 2007;23(8):845.

14. Pearle AD, Warren RF, Rodeo SA. Basic science of articular cartilage and osteoarthritis. *Clin Sports Med.* 2005;24(1):1.

15. Bhosale AM, Richardson JB. Articular cartilage: structure, injuries and review of management. *Br Med Bull.* 2008;87:77.

16. Lattermann C, Romine SE. Osteochondral allografts: state of the art. *Clin Sports Med.* 2009;28(2):285.

17. Bauer KL, Polousky JD. Management of osteochondritis dissecans lesions of the knee, elbow and ankle. *Clin Sports Med.* 2017;36(3):469.

18. Buckwalter JA, Mankin HJ. Articular cartilage: degeneration and osteoarthritis, repair, regeneration, and transplantation. *Instr Course Lect.* 1998;47:487.

19. Bekkers JE, Tsuchida AI, van Rijen MH, et al. Single-stage cell-based cartilage regeneration using a combination of chondrons and mesenchymal stromal cells: comparison with microfracture. *Am J Sports Med.* 2158;41(9):2013.

20. Aichroth P. Osteochondritis dissecans of the knee. A clinical survey. *J Bone Joint Surg Br.* 1971;53(3):440.

21. Flanigan DC, Harris JD, Trinh TQ, Siston RA, Brophy RH. Prevalence of chondral defects in athletes' knees: a systematic review. *Med Sci Sports Exerc.* 2010;42(10):1795.

22. Elleuch MH, Guermazi M, Mezghanni M, et al. Knee osteoarthritis in 50 former top-level soccer players: a comparative study. *Ann Readapt Med Phys.* 2008;51(3):174.

23. Roos H. Are there long-term sequelae from soccer?. *Clin Sports Med.* 1998;17(4):819.

24. Walczak BE, McCulloch PC, Kang RW, Zelazny A, Tedeschi F, Cole BJ. Abnormal findings on knee magnetic resonance imaging in asymptomatic NBA players. *J Knee Surg.* 2008;21(1):27.

25. Aroen A, Loken S, Heir S, et al. Articular cartilage lesions in 993 consecutive knee arthroscopies. *Am J Sports Med.* 2004;32(1):211.

26. Widuchowski W, Widuchowski J, Trzaska T. Articular cartilage defects: study of 25,124 knee arthroscopies. *Knee.* 2007;14(3):177.

27. Steinhagen J, Bruns J, Deuretzbacher G, Ruether W, Fuerst M, Niggemeyer O. Treatment of osteochondritis dissecans of the femoral condyle with autologous bone grafts and matrix-supported autologous chondrocytes. *Int Orthop.* 2010;34(6):819.

28. Prakash D, Learmonth D. Natural progression of osteo-chondral defect in the femoral condyle. *Knee.* 2002;9(1):7.

29. Felson DT, Lawrence RC, Dieppe PA, et al. Osteoarthritis: new insights. Part 1: the disease and its risk factors. *Ann Intern Med.* 2000;133(8):635.

30. Hubbard MJ. Articular debridement versus washout for degeneration of the medial femoral condyle. A five-year study. *J Bone Joint Surg Br.* 1996;78(2):217.

31. Livesley PJ, Doherty M, Needoff M, Moulton A. Arthroscopic lavage of osteoarthritic knees. *J Bone Joint Surg Br.* 1991;73(6):922.

32. Baumgaertner MR, Cannon WD Jr, Vittori JM, Schmidt ES, Maurer RC. Arthroscopic debridement of the arthritic knee. *Clin Orthop Relat Res.* 1990;253:197.

33. Gibson JN, White MD, Chapman VM, Strachan RK. Arthroscopic lavage and debridement for osteoarthritis of the knee. *J Bone Joint Surg Br.* 1992;74(4):534.

34. Frank RM, Cotter EJ, Nassar I, Cole B. Failure of bone marrow stimulation techniques. *Sports Med Arthrosc Rev.* 2017;25(1):2.

35. Peterson L, Minas T, Brittberg M, Nilsson A, Sjogren-Jansson E, Lindahl A. Two- to 9-year outcome after autologous chondrocyte transplantation of the knee. *Clin Orthop Relat Res.* 2000;374:212.

36. Cole BJ, Pascual-Garrido C, Grumet RC. Surgical management of articular cartilage defects in the knee. *J Bone Joint Surg Am.* 2009;91(7):1778.

37. Mithoefer K, Williams RJ III, Warren RF, et al. The microfracture technique for the treatment of articular cartilage lesions in the knee. A prospective cohort study. *J Bone Joint Surg Am.* 1911;87(9):2005.

38. Asik M, Ciftci F, Sen C, Erdil M, Atalar A. The microfracture technique for the treatment of full-thickness articular cartilage lesions of the knee: midterm results. *Arthroscopy.* 2008;24(11):1214.

39. Pisanu G, Cottino U, Rosso F, et al. Large osteochondral allografts of the knee: surgical technique and indications. *Joints.* 2018;6(1):42.

40. Steadman JR, Rodkey WG, Briggs KK. Microfracture: its history and experience of the developing surgeon. *Cartilage.* 2010;1(2):78.

41. Sterett WI, Steadman JR, Huang MJ, Matheny LM, Briggs KK. Chondral resurfacing and high tibial osteotomy in the varus knee: survivorship analysis. *Am J Sports Med.* 2010;38(7):1420.

42. Rue JP, Yanke AB, Busam ML, McNickle AG, Cole BJ. Prospective evaluation of concurrent meniscus transplantation and articular cartilage repair: minimum 2-year follow-up. *Am J Sports Med.* 2008;36(9):1770.

43. McCormick F, Harris JD, Abrams GD, et al. Survival and reoperation rates after meniscal allograft transplantation: analysis of failures for 172 consecutive transplants at a minimum 2-year follow-up. *Am J Sports Med.* 2014;42(4):892.

44. Maletius W, Messner K. The effect of partial meniscectomy on the long-term prognosis of knees with localized, severe chondral damage. A twelve- to fifteen-year followup. *Am J Sports Med.* 1996;24(3):258.

45. Brophy RH, Zeltser D, Wright RW, Flanigan D. Anterior cruciate ligament reconstruction and concomitant articular cartilage injury: incidence and treatment. *Arthroscopy.* 2010;26(1):112.

46. Steadman JR, Rodkey WG, Rodrigo JJ. Microfracture: surgical technique and rehabilitation to treat chondral defects. *Clin Orthop Relat Res.* 2001;391(suppl):S362.

47. Camp CL, Stuart MJ, Krych AJ. Current concepts of articular cartilage restoration techniques in the knee. *Sports Health.* 2014;6(3):265.

48. Brittberg M, Lindahl A, Nilsson A, Ohlsson C, Isaksson O, Peterson L. Treatment of deep cartilage defects in the knee with autologous chondrocyte transplantation. *N Engl J Med.* 1994;331(14):889.

49. Behrens P, Bitter T, Kurz B, Russlies M. Matrix-associated autologous chondrocyte transplantation/implantation (MACT/MACI)–5-year follow-up. *Knee.* 2006;13(3):194.

50. Chen H, Sun J, Hoemann CD, et al. Drilling and microfracture lead to different bone structure and necrosis during bone-marrow stimulation for cartilage repair. *J Orthop Res.* 2009;27(11):1432.

51. Hirahara AM, Mueller KW Jr. BioCartilage: a new biomaterial to treat chondral lesions. *Sports Med Arthrosc Rev.* 2015;23(3):143.

52. Blevins FT, Steadman JR, Rodrigo JJ, Silliman J. Treatment of articular cartilage defects in athletes: an analysis of functional outcome and lesion appearance. *Orthopedics.* 1998;21(7):761.

53. Levy AS, Lohnes J, Sculley S, LeCroy M, Garrett W. Chondral delamination of the knee in soccer players. *Am J Sports Med.* 1996;24(5):634.

54. Steadman JR, Rodkey WR, Briggs KK. *The Microfracture Technique.* Thorofare, NJ: SLACK; 2009.

55. Dzioba RB. The classification and treatment of acute articular cartilage lesions. *Arthroscopy.* 1988;4(2):72.

56. Passler HH. Microfracture for treatment of cartilage defects. *Zentralbl Chir.* 2000;125(6):500.

57. Steadman JR, Rodrigo JJ, Briggs KK, et al. *Debridement and microfracture ("pick technique") for full-thickness articular cartilage defects.* In: *Surgery of the Knee.* New York: Churchill Livingstone; 2000.

58. Rodrigo JJ, Steadman JR, Silliman JF, Fulstone HA. Improvement of full-thickness chondral defect healing in the human knee after debridement and microfracture using continuous passive motion. *Am J Knee Surg.* 1994;7:109.

59. Mithoefer K, Gill TJ, Cole BJ, Williams RJ, Mandelbaum BR. Clinical outcome and return to competition after microfracture in the athlete's knee: an evidence-based systematic review. *Cartilage.* 2010;1(2):113.

60. Gudas R, Kalesinskas RJ, Kimtys V, et al. A prospective randomized clinical study of mosaic osteochondral autologous transplantation versus microfracture for the treatment of osteochondral defects in the knee joint in young athletes. *Arthroscopy.* 2005;21(9):1066.

61. Gudas R, Gudaite A, Pocius A, et al. Ten-year follow-up of a prospective, randomized clinical study of mosaic osteochondral autologous transplantation versus microfracture for the treatment of osteochondral defects in the knee joint of athletes. *Am J Sports Med.* 2012;40(11):2499.

62. Harris JD, Walton DM, Erickson BJ, et al. Return to sport and performance after microfracture in the knees of National Basketball Association players. *Orthop J Sports Med.* 2013;1(6):1-4. doi: 10.1177/2325967113512759.

63. Solheim E, Hegna J, Strand T, Harlem T, Inderhaug E. Randomized study of long-term (15-17 years) outcome after microfracture versus mosaicplasty in knee articular cartilage defects. *Am J Sports Med.* 2018;46(4):826.

64. Mithoefer K, McAdams T, Williams RJ, Kreuz PC, Mandelbaum BR. Clinical efficacy of the microfracture technique for articular cartilage repair in the knee: an evidence-based systematic analysis. *Am J Sports Med.* 2009;37(10):2053.

65. Gobbi A, Nunag P, Malinowski K. Treatment of full thickness chondral lesions of the knee with microfracture in a group of athletes. *Knee Surg Sports Traumatol Arthrosc.* 2005;13(3):213.

66. Cerynik DL, Lewullis GE, Joves BC, Palmer MP, Tom JA. Outcomes of microfracture in professional basketball players. *Knee Surg Sports Traumatol Arthrosc.* 2009;17(9):1135.

67. Namdari S, Baldwin K, Anakwenze O, Park MJ, Huffman GR, Sennett BJ. Results and performance after microfracture in National Basketball Association athletes. *Am J Sports Med.* 2009;37(5):943.

68. Kraeutler MJ, Belk JW, Purcell JM, McCarty EC. Microfracture versus autologous chondrocyte implantation for articular cartilage lesions in the knee: a systematic review of 5-year outcomes. *Am J Sports Med.* 2018;46(4):995.

69. Bugbee WD, Convery FR. Osteochondral allograft transplantation. *Clin Sports Med.* 1999;18(1):67.

70. Magnussen RA, Carey JL, Spindler KP. Does operative fixation of an osteochondritis dissecans loose body result in healing and long-term maintenance of knee function? *Am J Sports Med.* 2009;37(4):754.

71. Oliver-Welsh L, Griffin JW, Meyer MA, Gitelis ME, Cole BJ. Deciding how best to treat cartilage defects. *Orthopedics.* 2016;39(6):343.

72. Lynch TS, Patel RM, Benedick A, Amin NH, Jones MH, Miniaci A. Systematic review of autogenous osteochondral transplant outcomes. *Arthroscopy.* 2015;31(4):746.

73. Assenmacher AT, Pareek A, Reardon PJ, Macalena JA, Stuart MJ, Krych AJ. Long-term outcomes after osteochondral allograft: a systematic review at long-term follow-up of 12.3 years. *Arthroscopy.* 2016;32(10):2160.

74. Pareek A, Reardon PJ, Macalena JA, et al. Osteochondral autograft transfer versus microfracture in the knee: a meta-analysis of prospective comparative studies at midterm. *Arthroscopy.* 2016;32(10):2118-2130.

75. Sherman SL, Garrity J, Bauer K, Cook J, Stannard J, Bugbee W. Fresh osteochondral allograft transplantation for the knee: current concepts. *J Am Acad Orthop Surg.* 2014;22(2):121.

76. Redondo ML, Naveen NB, Liu JN, Tauro TM, Southworth TM, Cole BJ. Preservation of knee articular cartilage. *Sports Med Arthrosc Rev.* 2018;26(4):e23.

77. Getgood A, Gelber J, Gortz S, De Young A, Bugbee W. Combined osteochondral allograft and meniscal allograft transplantation: a survivorship analysis. *Knee Surg Sports Traumatol Arthrosc.* 2015;23(4):946.

78. Chui K, Jeys L, Snow M. Knee salvage procedures: the indications, techniques and outcomes of large osteochondral allografts. *World J Orthop.* 2015;6(3):340.

79. Oakeshott RD, Farine I, Pritzker KP, Langer F, Gross AE. A clinical and histologic analysis of failed fresh osteochondral allografts. *Clin Orthop Relat Res.* 1988;233:283.

80. McCulloch PC, Kang RW, Sobhy MH, Hayden JK, Cole BJ. Prospective evaluation of prolonged fresh osteochondral allograft transplantation of the femoral condyle: minimum 2-year follow-up. *Am J Sports Med.* 2007;35(3):411.

81. Peterson L, Minas T, Brittberg M, Lindahl A. Treatment of osteochondritis dissecans of the knee with autologous chondrocyte transplantation: results at two to ten years. *J Bone Joint Surg Am.* 2003;85-A(suppl 2):17.

82. Pylawka TK, Wimmer M, Cole BJ, Virdi AS, Williams JM. Impaction affects cell viability in osteochondral tissues during transplantation. *J Knee Surg.* 2007;20(2):105.

83. Cole BJ, Sekiya JK. *Surgical Techniques of the Shoulder, Elbow, and Knee in Sports Medicine.* 2nd ed. Philadelphia, PA: Saunders; 2013.

84. Gracitelli GC, Meric G, Briggs DT, et al. Fresh osteochondral allografts in the knee: comparison of primary transplantation versus transplantation after failure of previous subchondral marrow stimulation. *Am J Sports Med.* 2015;43(4):885.

85. Riboh JC, Cvetanovich GL, Cole BJ, Yanke AB. Comparative efficacy of cartilage repair procedures in the knee: a network meta-analysis. *Knee Surg Sports Traumatol Arthrosc.* 2017;25(12):3786.

86. Day JB, Gillogly SD. Autologous chondrocyte implantation in the knee. In: Cole BJ, Sekiya JK, eds. *Surgical Techniques of the Shoulder, Elbow, and Knee in Sports Medicine*. Philadelphia: Saunders Elsevier; 2008:559.

87. Brophy RH, Wojahn RD, Lamplot JD. Cartilage restoration techniques for the patellofemoral joint. *J Am Acad Orthop Surg*. 2017;25(5):321.

88. Wu JZ, Herzog W, Hasler EM. Inadequate placement of osteochondral plugs may induce abnormal stress-strain distributions in articular cartilage –finite element simulations. *Med Eng Phys*. 2002;24(2):85.

89. Hangody L, Dobos J, Balo E, Panics G, Hangody LR, Berkes I. Clinical experiences with autologous osteochondral mosaicplasty in an athletic population: a 17-year prospective multicenter study. *Am J Sports Med*. 2010;38(6):1125.

90. Gross AE, Kim W, Las Heras F, Backstein D, Safir O, Pritzker KP. Fresh osteochondral allografts for posttraumatic knee defects: long-term followup. *Clin Orthop Relat Res*. 1863;466(8):2008.

91. Zouzias IC, Bugbee WD. Osteochondral allograft transplantation in the knee. *Sports Med Arthrosc Rev*. 2016;24(2):79.

92. Krych AJ, Pareek A, King AH, Johnson NR, Stuart MJ, Williams RJ III. Return to sport after the surgical management of articular cartilage lesions in the knee: a meta-analysis. *Knee Surg Sports Traumatol Arthrosc*. 2017;25(10):3186.

93. Cotter EJ, Frank RM, Wang KC, et al. Clinical outcomes of osteochondral allograft transplantation for secondary treatment of osteochondritis dissecans of the knee in skeletally mature patients. *Arthroscopy*. 2018;34(4):1105.

94. Saltzman BM, Meyer MA, Leroux TS, et al. The influence of full-thickness chondral defects on outcomes following meniscal allograft transplantation: a comparative study. *Arthroscopy*. 2018;34(2):519.

95. Hefti F, Beguiristain J, Krauspe R, et al. Osteochondritis dissecans: a multicenter study of the European Pediatric Orthopedic Society. *J Pediatr Orthop B*. 1999;8(4):231.

96. Harada YTN, Nakajima M, Ikeuchi K, Wakitani S. Effect of low loading and joint immobilization for spontaneous repair of osteochondral defect in the knees of weightless (tail suspension) rats. *J Orthop Sci*. 2005;10(5):508.

97. Dipaola JD, Nelson DW, Colville MR. Characterizing osteochondral lesions by magnetic resonance imaging. *Arthroscopy*. 1991;7(1):101.

98. Cruz AI Jr, Shea KG, Ganley TJ. Pediatric knee osteochondritis dissecans lesions. *Orthop Clin North Am*. 2016;47(4):763.

99. Niemeyer P, Albrecht D, Andereya S, et al. Autologous chondrocyte implantation (ACI) for cartilage defects of the knee: a guideline by the working group "Clinical Tissue Regeneration" of the German Society of Orthopaedics and Trauma (DGOU). *Knee*. 2016;23(3):426.

100. Ebert JR, Fallon M, Wood DJ, Janes GC. A prospective clinical and radiological evaluation at 5 years after arthroscopic matrix-induced autologous chondrocyte implantation. *Am J Sports Med*. 2017;45(1):59.

101. Foldager CB, Farr J, Gomoll AH. Patients scheduled for chondrocyte implantation treatment with MACI have larger defects than those enrolled in clinical trials. *Cartilage*. 2016;7(2):140.

102. Rosenberger RE, Gomoll AH, Bryant T, Minas T. Repair of large chondral defects of the knee with autologous chondrocyte implantation in patients 45 years or older. *Am J Sports Med*. 2008;36(12):2336.

103. Minas T, Ogura T, Bryant T. Autologous chondrocyte implantation. *JBJS Essent Surg Tech*. 2016;6(2):e24.

104. Brittberg M, Winalski CS. Evaluation of cartilage injuries and repair. *J Bone Joint Surg Am*. 2003;85-A(suppl 2):58.

105. Jones DG, Peterson L. Autologous chondrocyte implantation. *J Bone Joint Surg Am*. 2006;88(11):2502.

106. Ebert JR, Robertson WB, Woodhouse J, et al. Clinical and magnetic resonance imaging-based outcomes to 5 years after matrix-induced autologous chondrocyte implantation to address articular cartilage defects in the knee. *Am J Sports Med*. 2011;39(4):753.

107. Bartlett W, Skinner JA, Gooding CR, et al. Autologous chondrocyte implantation versus matrix-induced autologous chondrocyte implantation for osteochondral defects of the knee: a prospective, randomised study. *J Bone Joint Surg Br*. 2005;87(5):640.

108. Ventura A, Memeo A, Borgo E, Terzaghi C, Legnani C, Albisetti W. Repair of osteochondral lesions in the knee by chondrocyte implantation using the MACI(R) technique. *Knee Surg Sports Traumatol Arthrosc*. 2012;20(1):121.

109. Niemeyer P, Porichis S, Salzmann G, Sudkamp NP. What patients expect about autologous chondrocyte implantation (ACI) for treatment of cartilage defects at the knee joint. *Cartilage*. 2012;3(1):13.

110. Zaffagnini S, Vannini F, Di Martino A, et al. Low rate of return to pre-injury sport level in athletes after cartilage surgery: a 10-year follow-up study. *Knee Surg Sports Traumatol Arthrosc*. 2018;27(8):2502-2510.

111. Kon E, Gobbi A, Filardo G, Delcogliano M, Zaffagnini S, Marcacci M. Arthroscopic second-generation autologous chondrocyte implantation compared with microfracture for chondral lesions of the knee: prospective nonrandomized study at 5 years. *Am J Sports Med*. 2009;37(1):33.

112. Wondrasch B, Zak L, Welsch GH, Marlovits S. Effect of accelerated weightbearing after matrix-associated autologous chondrocyte implantation on the femoral condyle on radiographic and clinical outcome after 2 years: a prospective, randomized controlled pilot study. *Am J Sports Med*. 2009;37(suppl 1):88S.

113. Della Villa S, Kon E, Filardo G, et al. Does intensive rehabilitation permit early return to sport without compromising the clinical outcome after arthroscopic autologous chondrocyte implantation in highly competitive athletes? *Am J Sports Med*. 2010;38(1):68.

114. Harris JD, Cavo M, Brophy R, Siston R, Flanigan D. Biological knee reconstruction: a systematic review of combined meniscal allograft transplantation and cartilage repair or restoration. *Arthroscopy*. 2011;27(3):409.

115. Weber AE, Gitelis ME, McCarthy MA, Yanke AB, Cole BJ. Malalignment: a requirement for cartilage and organ restoration. *Sports Med Arthrosc Rev*. 2016;24(2):e14.

116. Fairbank TJ. Knee joint changes after meniscectomy. *J Bone Joint Surg Br*. 1948;30B(4):664.

117. Cotter EJ, Frank RM, Waterman BR, Wang KC, Redondo ML, Cole BJ. Meniscal allograft transplantation with concomitant osteochondral allograft transplantation. *Arthrosc Tech*. 2017;6(5):e1573.

118. Levine HB, Bosco JA III. Sagittal and coronal biomechanics of the knee: a rationale for corrective measures. *Bull NYU Hosp Jt Dis*. 2007;65(1):87.

119. Hsu RW, Himeno S, Coventry MB, Chao EY. Normal axial alignment of the lower extremity and load-bearing distribution at the knee. *Clin Orthop Relat Res*. 1990;255:215.

120. Sharma L, Song J, Felson DT, Cahue S, Shamiyeh E, Dunlop DD. The role of knee alignment in disease progression and functional decline in knee osteoarthritis. *J Am Med Assoc*. 2001;286(2):188.

121. Sharma L, Eckstein F, Song J, et al. Relationship of meniscal damage, meniscal extrusion, malalignment, and joint laxity to subsequent cartilage loss in osteoarthritic knees. *Arthritis Rheum*. 2008;58(6):1716.

chapter 26

Femoral and Tibial Osteotomy for the Degenerative Knee

Stephanie Swensen, MD | Niv Marom, MD | Scott A. Rodeo, MD

INTRODUCTION

Management of degenerative osteoarthritis of the knee in the young, active patient remains challenging. Accelerated cartilage degeneration in this patient population is often associated with increased medial or lateral knee compartment pressures due to lower extremity malalignment. Realignment osteotomies of the distal femur and proximal tibia function to offload the affected compartment and, therefore, function to prevent further cartilage degradation and improve pain.[1] Despite the increasing utilization of knee arthroplasty procedures, there remain limitations in the use of arthroplasty in a young patient population due to the risk of early revision rates and lower return to high-impact activities.[2,3] Osteotomies have garnered renewed attention in recent years as desirable alternatives to arthroplasty procedures due to the ability to preserve the native joint and potentially facilitate return to high-level activities and work.[4-7] Additionally, osteotomies about the knee may be combined with various ligament reconstructions and meniscus and cartilage procedures to improve the success of these surgeries.

The most commonly performed osteotomies for the degenerative knee include proximal tibial osteotomies ("high tibial osteotomy," HTO) for varus deformities and distal femoral osteotomies (DFOs) for valgus deformities. Advances in techniques and fixation devices have led to continued improvements in functional outcomes. The purpose of this chapter is to review the indications, preoperative planning strategies, and evolving surgical techniques for the various osteotomies utilized for treatment of the degenerative knee or realignment as part of cartilage repair/reconstruction.

PATIENT SELECTION

Appropriate patient selection is paramount for optimal outcomes following osteotomy procedures. Although the specific indications for femoral and tibial osteotomies differ, general patient characteristics are important to consider when performing a realignment osteotomy. The ideal patient is a relatively young (<60 years old), active, nonsmoking individual with localized knee pain. The patient must be capable of enduring the average 6-month recovery and adhering to a rehabilitation protocol. Commonly accepted contraindications for realignment osteotomy include inflammatory arthritis, severe tricompartmental osteoarthritis, multiplanar ligamentous instability, extreme deformity, and bone loss.[8,9] Anterior cruciate ligament (ACL) or posterior cruciate ligament (PCL) insufficiency is not considered to be a definite contraindication, as these ligaments deficiencies can be addressed concomitantly with the osteotomy.[10-12]

The role of obesity in patient selection for realignment osteotomy has been debated within the literature. Obesity is defined as 1.32 times ideal weight and as body mass index (BMI) greater than 30 kg/m². Multiple studies have demonstrated an association between obesity and poor outcomes following lower extremity realignment osteotomy.[13,14] Coventry et al[13] reported probability of survival after HTO of only 38% after 5 years and 19% after 10 years in obese patients, compared with 90 and 65% probabilities in patients with average weight, respectively. A recent study by Liska et al[15] demonstrated a significantly higher rate of nonunion in smokers and patients who underwent DFOs with BMI >30 kg/m². However, some authors argue that osteotomy is preferable to the high rate of complications in the obese patient population undergoing knee arthroplasty.[9,16]

The decision to perform a realignment osteotomy should be individualized. It is imperative that patients are counseled on their unique risks, and general health must be optimized.

History and Physical Examination

A thorough history and physical examination should be performed for all patients considered candidates for osteotomy surgery. The onset of pain is typically insidious in nature in cases of degenerative osteoarthritis. Prior traumatic knee injuries should be noted, as well as any previous surgeries. Coronal and sagittal malalignment are most commonly the result of meniscal, ligamentous, or cartilage injuries.[17] The patient should ideally be able to localize pain to a focal compartment of the knee. Diffuse knee pain should raise suspicion for arthritis involving multiple compartments. Additionally, any subjective sensation of instability may be due to chronic ligamentous injury. The patient should be assessed for current activity level and overall expectations for the proposed procedure.

Physical examination should begin with global inspection and careful evaluation of coronal, sagittal, and rotational alignment. Palpation of the joint lines may reveal tenderness in the affected compartment. A careful evaluation of knee range of motion is essential. Flexion contractures of greater than 15° and knee flexion of less than 90° are considered relative contraindications for osteotomy. Ligamentous examination is important in identifying cruciate ligament deficiency and varus or valgus laxity, assessing for any fixed deformity. Preoperative gait evaluation is crucial for identifying dynamic varus or valgus deformity. Several studies have found that HTO has the potential to modify gait mechanics and suggest overcorrection of the mechanical axis in patients with preoperative increased knee adduction moment and an associated lateral "thrust" during gait to improve outcomes.[18,19] A complete physical examination should include assessment of hip and spine pathologies that may contribute to knee pain, as well as an evaluation of the neurovascular status.

Imaging

Radiologic evaluation of the degenerative knee includes weight-bearing anterior–posterior, lateral, and patellar views of the knee. Posterior–anterior weight-bearing 45-degree flexion view (Rosenberg) is useful for identifying early osteoarthritis changes in the posterior part of the tibiofemoral compartment, as this view has been found to have a higher sensitivity for detecting early medial or lateral tibiofemoral compartment changes compared to standard anterior–posterior radiographs made in full extension.[20,21] The radiographs should be closely inspected for subtle joint space narrowing, osteophytes, and early changes in subchondral bone morphology and geometry of the joint surface. Careful evaluation of the lateral compartment when considering HTO to unload a degenerative medial compartment is important to ensure the best possible outcome following the procedure. Similarly, the medial compartment should be examined when planning for a varus-producing osteotomy to unload the valgus knee. The lateral radiographs are useful for examining tibial slope, particularly in cases of cruciate ligament deficiency.[12,22] Additionally, patellar height should be evaluated on the lateral radiograph, given the risk of patella baja following HTO procedures.[23-25] Lower extremity hip-to-ankle alignment radiographs are essential in the workup for measuring the mechanical axis of the limb and the degree of deformity for surgical planning.

Advanced imaging may be performed to identify concomitant intra-articular pathology and further delineate the status of the articular cartilage and menisci. MRI is a useful adjunct to plain radiographs for characterizing the progression of osteoarthritis by demonstrating subchondral bone edema, early changes in subchondral bone geometry and architecture, and the overlying articular cartilage. Computed tomography (CT) can be utilized to evaluate for rotational malalignment of the limb. However, these advanced imaging modalities are costly, and there is a significantly increased radiation risk associated with CT.

PREOPERATIVE PLANNING

Characterizing the nature of the deformity is critical for determining the optimal corrective osteotomy procedure for the degenerative knee. The surgeon must first determine the location, direction, and magnitude of the deformity. Knee alignment is analyzed by measuring the mechanical and anatomic axes of the lower extremity on standing alignment radiographs. The weight-bearing line of the knee is measured from a straight line drawn from the center of the femoral head to the center of the talus and crosses the tibial plateau at a point 48% to 62.5% of the distance from the medial proximal tibial edge in a normally aligned knee.[22,26] The deformity is determined based of the location of the center of the knee in relation to the weight-bearing line (**Fig. 26-1**).

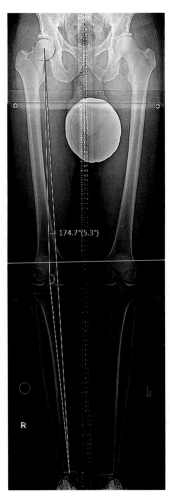

FIGURE 26-1 Standing alignment AP radiograph. Right leg mechanical limb axis falls within the medial compartment of the knee, which correlates with a varus deformity. Varus is measured 5.3°, based on mechanical axis of each bone separately.

The location of the osteotomy is traditionally determined to avoid joint line obliquity. Varus deformities with medial compartment wear are typically treated with an HTO, and valgus deformities are managed with DFOs to offload the lateral compartment. However, the decision as to the optimal location and type of osteotomy is ultimately based upon the individual patient's characteristics and degree of deformity. It is critically important to identify if the bony deformity is on the tibial versus femoral side, as this determines the site for the osteotomy. The mechanical lateral distal femoral angle and medial proximal tibial angle should be measured to more accurately identify the site of deformity (**Fig. 26-2**). For example, although a valgus deformity is felt to be usually associated with a degree of hypoplasia of the lateral femoral condyle and is thus typically corrected on the femoral side, Eberbach et al[27] measured coronal alignment on 420 standing long-leg radiographs of patients with valgus malalignment and found that 41% of valgus deformities were tibial based, 24% were femoral based, 27% were tibial and femoral based, and 9% were intra-articular/

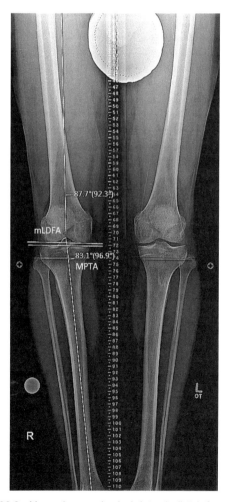

FIGURE 26-2 Measuring mechanical lateral distal femoral angle (mLDFA) and medial proximal tibial angle (MPTA) to determine the origin of deformity. In this case, MPTA is lower than the normal degree range (85 to 90), indicating tibial varus.

ligament based, suggesting that varus-producing osteotomy may need to be done on tibial side or as a double-level osteotomy in order to avoid an oblique joint line. Severe coronal deformities (greater than 10° to 15°) will often require combined tibial and femoral osteotomy to avoid joint line obliquity.[28] Schroter and colleagues[29] described the use of a double-level osteotomy in severe varus osteoarthritis (average 11°) and demonstrated good functional outcome with restoration of the joint line and improved angular measurements.

Opening wedge osteotomy is currently the preferred technique in the literature for both varus and valgus deformities. The opening wedge technique has the theoretical advantage of simplifying the procedure with a single bone cut, allowing for improved control over the degree of correction. The potential disadvantages include the risk of delayed union or nonunion. Closing wedge osteotomies have been suggested as a more favorable technique for patients with comorbidities that may increase the risk for nonunion, such as smoking and obesity.[22,30] Another proposed benefit of the closing wedge technique is the ability to bear weight earlier than opening wedge osteotomies; however, these differences are now less of a consideration with the development of newer implant devices that allow earlier weight-bearing with both techniques. Disadvantages of closing wedge osteotomies include bone loss and the technical challenge of the technique for achieving a precise angular correction.

HIGH TIBIAL OSTEOTOMIES

Indications

The primary indication for an HTO is symptomatic medial compartment osteoarthritis with varus deformity. The lateral closing wedge HTO was initially popularized by Coventry in the 1960s and demonstrates good long-term functional outcomes.[31,32] The medial opening wedge HTO has increased in acceptance over the past several decades and equally successful outcomes have been reported.[33-36] Additionally, the technique avoids the need to expose the lateral side of the leg and risks associated with peroneal nerve exposure, tibiofibular joint disruption, fibular osteotomy, and anterior compartment dissection. Medial opening wedge HTO does have the potential disadvantages of higher nonunion rates, patella baja, and risk of increasing tibial slope.[37] Dome-type tibial osteotomies are considered when a correction of greater than 10° to 15° is required, as this degree of correction is beyond the limits of the standard opening or closing wedge osteotomies. A coronal plane osteotomy can also be used, with the coronal plane bone cut oriented from the anterior-proximal aspect of the tibia to the posterior-distal tibia. This osteotomy starts just proximal to the tibial tubercle. Both varus and valgus correction can be done with this coronal plane cut. Concomitant fibular osteotomy is required to achieve the correction.

Degree of Correction

Deformity correction planning for tibial osteotomies is based on the lower extremity measurements on alignment radiographs and has evolved over recent years with the development of new technology. The overall goal is to shift the mechanical axis lateral to the center of the knee to unload the degenerative medial compartment. In general, a more modest correction is recommended for osteotomy that is performed in conjunction with concomitant cartilage repair or medial meniscus transplantation, as compared to osteotomy done in the setting of more advanced medial compartment arthritis.

Dugdale and colleauges[26] described a method of measuring the correction angle that can be utilized for both lateral closing wedge and medial opening wedge HTO techniques. This method involves identifying a reference point on the tibial plateau that is 62.5% from the medial cortex.[38] A line is then drawn from this point to the center of the femoral head, and a second line is drawn from this point to the center of the ankle. The intersection of these two lines is the angle of correction, also known as the alpha angle (**Fig. 26-3**). The correction angle is proportional to the measurement of the osteotomy distraction on the medial cortex of the tibia. Precise measurement of an angle is not easy to do intraoperatively, Rather, the height of the base of the opening or closing wedge can be measured. The height of the wedge is calculated as the tibial width at the level of the osteotomy multiplied by the tangent of the desired correction angle. As a rough guide, a 1-degree correction generally corresponds to approximately 1 mm distraction.

This calculation can be used for both opening wedge and closing wedge osteotomy.

Ligamentous instability is also taken into consideration when planning the correction angle. Varus ligamentous instability requires an additional 2° to 3° of correction to correct for the varus intra-articular deformity.[18] In the presence of anterior instability and ACL deficiency, the tibial slope can be decreased to restore alignment and potentially improve stability without ACL reconstruction.[39] Similarly, the tibial slope can be increased while performing HTO in the setting of PCL insufficiency to potentially decrease posterior instability. Alteration of tibial slope may also be considered during concomitant ACL or PCL reconstruction. Biomechanical studies demonstrate that increased posterior tibial slope results in higher forces on an ACL graft,[40] while PCL graft forces increased as tibial slope decreased (flattened).[41]

Numerous technological advances have led to the development of novel methods for preoperatively planning HTO correction. Preoperative computerized planning software programs using digital images have been recently developed. These programs have demonstrated excellent reliability and good consistency with real-size paper template methods.[42-44]

New methods have also been developed to intraoperatively assess the ability to achieve the preoperatively planned correction angle. Conventional methods of evaluating the angle of correction include using an alignment rod or cable and fluoroscopy to determine alignment. These methods have high variability and measurement error in addition to increasing radiation exposure with the multiple intraoperative fluoroscopy images necessary to evaluate the correction.[45-47] Kim and colleagues[48] evaluated the utility of three-dimensional (3D) printed models for opening wedge HTO procedures. The model based on preoperative CT allows for three-dimensional evaluation of the deformity and subsequent correction. The printed 3D osteotomy wedge can then be used as a guide intraoperatively to attain the desired correction angle. The authors found satisfactory results with the use of the 3D-printed model with accurate correction to the target point. In a similar manner, patient-specific cutting guides have also been proposed.[49] Computer-assisted navigation techniques have also been developed to improve

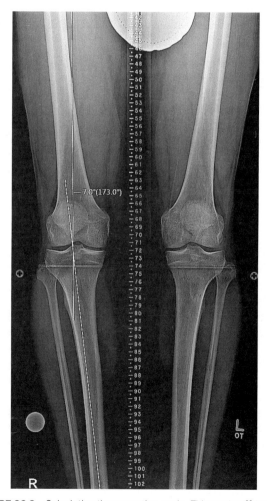

FIGURE 26-3 Calculating the correction angle. This method[26] involves identifying a reference point on the tibial plateau that is 62.5% from the medial cortex. A line is then drawn from this point to the center of the femoral head, and a second line is drawn from this point to the center of the ankle. The intersection of these two lines is the angle of correction, also known as the alpha angle.

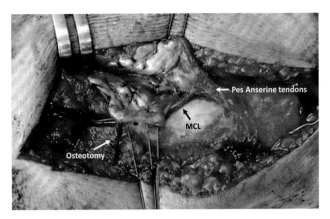

FIGURE 26-4 Pes anserine and medial collateral ligament (MCL) near osteotomy site.

accuracy, precision, and reliability of HTO.[47,50,51] A recent meta-analysis comparing navigated and conventional HTO for the treatment of the osteoarthritic varus knee demonstrated that navigated HTO resulted in more accuracy and precision of alignment correction. However, the authors noted that there was no difference in clinical outcomes between the two groups.[51]

Surgical Techniques

Medial Opening Wedge Osteotomy

Standard medial opening wedge osteotomies are performed through an approximately 5 cm longitudinal incision extending from 1 cm below the joint line to the medial border of the tibial tubercle. The sartorial fascia is divided; the pes tendons are identified and are then elevated as an L-shaped flap or retracted distally. The distal superficial medial collateral ligament (MCL) can either be subperiosteally elevated off the medial tibia or incised at the level of the osteotomy (**Fig. 26-4**). A biomechanical study demonstrated that medial opening wedge HTO maintains high medial compartment pressure after bony correction into valgus until there is complete release of the MCL.[52]

The posteromedial cortex of the tibia is dissected to the posterior tibiofibular joint, taking care to protect the neurovascular structures. Anteriorly, the patellar tendon is identified and protected with a retractor. Multiple novel jigs and guides have been developed to measure and cut the desired osteotomy angle once adequate exposure is obtained. Traditionally, the correction is templated with the placement of guidewires. The first guidewire is inserted from the anteromedial border of the tibia at the level of the proximal border of the tibial tubercle, aiming toward the fibular head. A second guidewire can be placed posterior to the first guidewire to determine the sagittal angle of the osteotomy cut. More superior placement of this guidewire will result in a decrease in the posterior tibial slope.

The osteotomy then begins on the anteromedial cortex at the level of the previously placed guidewires with a sagittal saw. Osteotomes are then used to advance the cut to a point 1 cm from the lateral tibial cortex. To minimize the risk of iatrogenic fracture, the tip of the osteotome should be 1.25 times further from the lateral tibial plateau than the distance to the lateral tibial cortex. Once the osteotomy is completed, a gentle valgus stress is applied to open the site. Stacked osteotomes or a calibrated wedge can be impacted into the osteotomy site to achieve the desired correction angle. The mechanical axis is then evaluated radiographically. The osteotomy is then fixed using a standard HTO plate and screws.

Lateral Closing Wedge Osteotomy

The lateral closing wedge osteotomy is a relatively simple procedure that requires more extensive dissection on the lateral aspect of the proximal tibia. An anterolateral incision is made over the proximal tibia, typically in an inverted L-shape with the horizontal limb just distal to the joint line. The anterior compartment musculature is subperiosteally elevated off the proximal lateral tibia. The patellar tendon is protected with a retractor anteriorly.

The proximal tibiofibular joint must be addressed with this osteotomy to prevent a tethering effect on the fibula. The options include disruption of the tibiofibular joint, osteotomy and resection of the fibular head, or osteotomy of the fibular shaft at any point distal to the osteotomy to allow shortening of the fibula. The common peroneal nerve is potentially at some risk with dissection around the proximal fibula. Maintenance of the knee in flexion allows the nerve to fall posteriorly and provides a degree of safety. Disruption of the proximal tibiofibular joint has the benefit of decreased risk of injuring the common peroneal nerve; however, the technique can result in superior migration of the fibula and subsequent lateral instability.[53] Osteotomy of the proximal fibular head or neck is often the preferred approach, and techniques with variable resection of the bone have been developed in an attempt to maintain the posterior cortex of the fibular head to protect the common peroneal nerve. Fibular shaft osteotomy has also been associated with multiple neurovascular complications, but the proximal 20 mm of the fibular shaft has been demonstrated to be a relatively safe zone.[54,55]

After the proximal tibiofibular joint has been addressed, the osteotomy is similarly templated with two guidewires. The first guidewire is placed parallel to the tibial articular surface approximately 2 to 2.5 mm below the joint line. The second guidewire is placed distal to the first guidewire at the measured correction angle. The guidewire is advanced obliquely to intersect with the first guidewire at the medial tibial cortex. The desired amount of bone is resected with a sagittal saw and then with osteotomes. A drill hole can be placed at the end of the osteotomy line on the medial tibial cortex to relax stresses at this point.[56] The wedge of the bone is then removed; the osteotomy is compressed with a valgus stress and then secured with a plate.

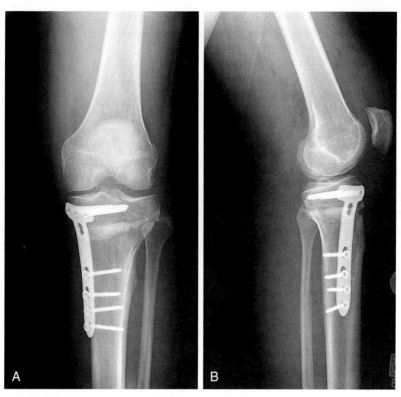

FIGURE 26-5   Anteroposterior **(A)** and lateral **(B)** postoperative radiographs after open wedge tibial osteotomy fixed with a locking plate.

Dome Osteotomy

The tibial dome osteotomy is typically reserved for larger deformity corrections (>20°). The procedure is technically challenging and may require an external fixator to stabilize the osteotomy. The osteotomy is performed in an inverted U-shaped bone cut and allows for correction at the center of the deformity.[57] The desired correction angle is marked with Steinman pins or specialized guides, and the osteotomy cut is begun with drill holes placed anterior to posterior. The cut is completed with osteotomes, taking care to protect the posterior neurovascular structures.[8,58]

The osteotomy is advantageous in cases of patellofemoral disease due to its ability to allow for anterior translation of the tubercle, thus maintaining patellar height. Additionally, leg length is preserved, and the alignment can be adjusted postoperatively. The osteotomy has the disadvantages of increased operative time due to complexity of the procedure and pin-site infections and other complications related to external fixation devices.

Fixation

Methods of stabilizing medial opening wedge and lateral closing wedge tibial osteotomies continue to evolve and are debated within the current literature. Historically, tibial osteotomies were stabilized with casting and no internal fixation. Casting is associated with complications of prolonged immobilization, such as increased joint stiffness and atrophy, further compounding the preexisting issues of the arthritic knee. Surgeons eventually moved away from casting in favor of devices that allow for early range of motion while maintaining corrected alignment.

Coventry and colleagues described the use of staples for fixation of lateral closing wedge HTO. This form of internal fixation should be supplemented with bracing to further stabilize the construct. Staples rely on the integrity of the medial hinge of the lateral closing wedge osteotomy.

Rigid internal fixation with plates and screws has become the preferred method of stabilization of both medial opening wedge and lateral closing wedge HTO (**Fig. 26-5**). With the exception of dome osteotomies, studies have demonstrated superiority of plates to external fixation devices for tibial osteotomy procedures.[59-61] Plate fixation maintains correction and permits early range of motion and partial weight-bearing.[62,63] Biomechanical studies have found that plates which contain a spacer have a significantly higher stiffness and reduced loss of osteotomy correction compared with conventional plates.[59]

Polyetheretherketone (PEEK) implants have recently been developed and are increasingly used for medial opening wedge HTO. These implants are lower profile and have a modulus of elasticity closer to the cortical bone.[64,65] Additionally, it is possible to drill through the PEEK material, allowing for easier concomitant ligamentous reconstruction and subsequent total knee arthroplasty (TKA). The implants are also radiolucent and do not produce artifact on MRI. Early reports suggested that the PEEK implants have limited ability to modify sagittal slope and have insufficient rigidity for maintaining large corrections.[64,66] However, a recent multicenter study comparing metal and PEEK implants for medial opening wedge HTO demonstrated that both implants were effective in obtaining and maintaining deformity correction with 88% overall arthroplasty-free survival at 5 years. Metal implants had a higher rate of hardware removal.[67]

Clinical Outcomes

Clinical outcomes for both medial opening wedge and lateral closing wedge HTO for varus deformity of the degenerative knee are good to excellent. Closing wedge HTO has a survivorship of 95% at 5 years and 60% at 15 years in patients younger than 50 years of age and with preoperative knee flexion greater than 120°.[33] Similarly, Hantes et al[68] found a 95% survival rate at 12 years following medial opening wedge HTO and no significant radiographic progression of osteoarthritis. Nerhus and colleagues[35] performed a prospective, randomized controlled trial comparing closing wedge and opening wedge HTO and reported no significant difference in clinical outcome scores between techniques. A 6-year follow-up randomized controlled trial comparing closing wedge and opening wedge HTO also found no difference in pain or functional outcome between the two groups. However, there was a higher complication rate in the opening wedge group (38% vs. 9%) and 22% of patients in the closing wedge group required conversion to a TKA within the 6-year period compared with 8% in the opening wedge group.[36] A study comparing radiologic outcomes of opening wedge and closing wedge HTO showed that posterior tibial slope and leg length changes were significantly different among the two techniques. The mean posterior slope was reduced by 2.5° in the closing wedge group and remained unchanged in the opening wedge group. The mean leg length was found to decrease by 5.7 mm in closing wedge HTO and increase 3.1 mm in opening wedge HTO.[69]

Unsuccessful outcome after HTO is often associated with inaccurate surgical planning and technique. Undercorrection of the weight-bearing line is associated with progression of medial compartment degeneration, while overcorrection may cause progressive wear in the lateral compartment.[6] A recent finite element model study suggested that correcting the weight-bearing axis to 55% of tibial width (1.7° to 1.9° of valgus) optimally distributes compartment pressures.[70]

Complications

Complication rates after HTO range from 2% to 55% in the literature and vary based on the approach.[71-74] Lateral closing wedge HTO is associated with peroneal nerve injury, anterior compartment syndrome, fibular osteotomy nonunion, lateral collateral ligament insufficiency,

and medial tibial cortex fractures. Complications of medial opening wedge HTO include hardware irritation (up to 40%), hardware failure, MCL injury, lateral cortex fracture, tibial plateau fracture, and nonunion.[75] Han et al[71] studied complications associated with medial opening wedge osteotomy using a locking plate. They noted that 30.6% of complications occurred intraoperatively and 40.3% of complications occurred within 3 months postoperatively. The most common complication in the study was nondisplaced lateral tibial hinge fracture (12%).

DISTAL FEMORAL OSTEOTOMIES

Indications

The primary indication for DFO is painful lateral compartment degenerative disease and valgus malalignment. Medial proximal tibial closing wedge osteotomies have been described as an option for valgus deformity correction.[32] However, tibial osteotomies should not be performed for larger deformities (greater than 12°) because they can result in tibiofemoral joint line obliquity.[32,76,77] Additionally, superolateral sloping of the tibiofemoral joint in the coronal plane cannot be corrected with tibial osteotomies. DFO has the ability to correct complex valgus deformity without compromising tibiofemoral joint stability.[76,78]

Degree of Correction

Similar to HTO for varus deformities, the degree of correction for valgus deformity is determined based on measurements obtained from lower extremity alignment films. The method initially described by Dugdale[26] is commonly used to determine the degree of correction. The weight-bearing line of the knee is measured to be approximately 48% to 50% of the width of the tibial plateau from the medial cortex. A line is drawn from the center of the femoral head to the planned weight-bearing line. A second line is then drawn from the center of the tibial plafond to the weight-bearing line. The correction angle is the angle at which the two lines intersect.

The ideal degree of correction has been debated within the literature. Unlike HTO, overcorrection of the deformity has traditionally been discouraged. Previous authors have recommended a goal of producing a 0° to 2° difference between the mechanical and anatomic axes.[9] However, recent biomechanical studies suggest that overcorrection may be more beneficial. In a cadaveric study, Quirno et al[79] demonstrated progressive unloading of the lateral compartment in full extension with increasing correction angle and recommended overcorrecting the osteotomy by 5° to restore near normal contact pressure in the lateral compartment. Wylie et al[80] examined the effect of DFO on tibiofemoral contact pressures from full extension through 75° of flexion. They demonstrated that DFO had the greatest unloading effect in the lateral compartment when the knee is in full extension, and the effect persisted through lower degrees of knee flexion.

Surgical Technique

Medial Closing Wedge Osteotomy

The medial closing wedge osteotomy was one of the earliest and most commonly utilized DFO techniques. The procedure affords the benefit of a reduced nonunion risk, and the medial location of the approach can be easily extended for subsequent TKA. However, the medial closing wedge technique requires two osteotomy cuts, thus increasing the technical complexity.

The first reported technique of medial closing wedge DFO was described by McDermott and colleagues.[76] The procedure is performed through an approximately 10 to 15 cm straight midline incision. A medial skin flap is developed, and the vastus medialis is retracted anteriorly to expose the medial femoral condyle. Care must be taken to subperiosteally dissect in this area to avoid injury to the femoral vessels in the adductor canal. A small arthrotomy is made just proximal to the adductor tubercle to visualize the intercondylar notch and joint line. A guidewire is then placed medial to lateral in the distal femur parallel and 1 cm proximal to the distal femoral articular surface with the knee flexed to 90°. A second guidewire is inserted approximately 2 cm proximal to the first guidewire to facilitate the entry of the blade plate chisel. A closing wedge osteotomy is made 1 cm proximal to the chisel. Converging pins are placed medial to lateral to mark the degree of the planned osteotomy. Once the two osteotomy cuts are performed with an oscillating saw, the 90-degree blade plate is applied along the medial femoral cortex to stabilize the correction.

Lateral Opening Wedge Osteotomy

Lateral opening wedge DFO has been increasingly performed due to the advantages of technical ease and improved intraoperative precision.[9,81,82] The technique also avoids risk of damage to the medial femoral neurovascular structures. Lateral plate fixation also has the mechanical advantage of acting as a tension band.[77]

The lateral opening wedge DFO is performed through a 10 to 15 cm longitudinal incision over the lateral aspect of the distal femur starting approximately two fingerbreadths below the lateral epicondyle and extending proximally. The iliotibial band is incised, and the vastus lateralis is dissected off the lateral intermuscular septum and retracted anteriorly. Contrary to the medial opening wedge DFO, an arthrotomy is not necessary for this procedure. Once the lateral cortex of the distal femur is exposed and the posterior neurovascular structures are protected, a guidewire is placed approximately three fingerbreadths above the lateral epicondyle, angled obliquely 20-degrees from proximal to distal toward the medial epicondyle. A second guidewire can be placed parallel to

the joint line for reference. The osteotomy is started with an oscillating saw, using the first guidewire as a template. Osteotomes are used to complete the osteotomy, preserving a 1 cm medial hinge. Placing gentle varus stress distracts the osteotomy site, taking care to preserve sagittal alignment. The mechanical axis correction is confirmed under fluoroscopy in the same manner as described for HTOs. A plate or external fixator is then applied.

Dome Osteotomy

The distal femoral dome osteotomy is performed in a similar manner to the proximal tibial dome osteotomy. Multiple techniques have been described within the literature, including both open and percutaneous techniques. The femoral cortex is perforated with drill holes, and a semicircular osteotomy is performed. The correction can be stabilized with a distal femoral plate, an external fixator, or a combination of retrograde nail and external fixation.[83-85] The dome osteotomy is useful for larger deformity corrections (up to 20°) and has the benefits of bony apposition and earlier weight-bearing.[83]

Fixation

Similar to the techniques for HTO, various fixation methods have been described for DFO. Options for fixation include casting, staples, plates, and external fixation. Mathews et al[86] evaluated the outcomes of medial closing wedge DFO with three different forms of fixation: plaster cast, staples supplemented with plaster cast, and rigid internal fixation with an AO blade plate. The authors noted that satisfactory results were obtained in patients who had lateral compartment grade I to III osteoarthritis, adequate correction of valgus deformity (anatomical axis within 2° of neutral), and rigid internal fixation to permit early postoperative mobilization.

External fixation allows for gradual correction of larger deformities with reduced soft-tissue damage. However, range of motion restriction and pin-site infections are potential downsides of external fixation. In a comparison of DFO stabilized with either external fixator or fixator-assisted plating, Seah et al[87] concluded that an accurate correction can be achieved with both techniques. Therefore, fixation choice should be individualized to each patient's deformity and characteristics.

In addition to the choice of fixation device, graft options for lateral opening wedge osteotomies are also an important consideration when planning for osteotomies around the knee. Puddu et al[9] suggested that gaps from smaller corrections may be left unfilled, but gaps larger than 7.5 mm should be grafted with autograft, allograft, or synthetic materials. Iliac crest bone graft remains the gold-standard graft material for DFOs. This graft option is desirable for its osteoconductive, osteoinductive, and osteogenic properties; however, it is associated with significant donor-site morbidity and pain. Numerous alternative grafts have been increasingly utilized, including various types of allograft bone graft and synthetic bone substitutes. The senior author routinely uses femoral head allograft bone for DFO with good outcomes. Autograft bone would be considered only in the setting of expected impaired bone healing, such as in a smoker or for revision osteotomy done for nonunion. Platelet-rich plasma and other biologic materials such as bone morphogenetic protein may also be considered to augment osteotomy gap healing.[88]

Clinical Outcomes

Overall, good to excellent outcomes have been reported for both medial closing wedge and lateral opening wedge osteotomies. Studies reporting on survivorship outcomes with both techniques have demonstrated the ability of DFO to delay the need for TKA in patients undergoing the procedure for degenerative joint disease.[89-92]

The majority of outcome studies in the literature have focused on medial closing wedge DFO. Multiple authors have reported good results with the McDermott technique of medial closing wedge DFO with a 90-degree blade plate.[76] Wang et al[93] demonstrated 83% satisfactory results and an 87% 10-year survival with this technique. Backstein[92] et al found a similar 10-year survivorship but noted a significant drop to 45% survival rate at 15 years. A more recent study by Kosashvili et al also showed satisfactory outcomes within the first 10 years but noted that conversion to TKA was expected to be required by 50% of patients at a mean of 15.6 years.[89] Good functional results have also been demonstrated with the use of a malleable semitubular plate[94] and angle-stable locking plate.[95]

Although there is less outcomes data regarding lateral closing wedge DFO techniques, the technique has been increasingly utilized with good results. Numerous authors have reported good to excellent outcomes with the T-shaped tooth plate designed by Puddu et al.[9] Dewilde et al[82] demonstrated significant improvement in knee functional outcome scores and 82% survival at 7-year follow-up using the Puddu plate and calcium phosphate cement to fill the osteotomy gap. Similar functional outcomes and 88% survival rate at 5-year follow-up have been reported using the Puddu plate and iliac crest bone grafting.[81,96] There was also noted to be no worsening of arthritic changes on subsequent radiographs, full incorporation of bone graft, and no hardware failure at 6.5-year follow-up with this technique.[96] Newer types of plate fixation for lateral opening wedge DFO have also demonstrated favorable functional outcomes with the benefit of earlier weight-bearing due to increased biomechanical stability.[30,91,97]

With the growing number of osteotomies performed in young patient populations, patient expectations and ability to return to work are of increasing importance.

Overall, patients have high expectations with regard to capacity to work, pain relief, and restoring knee function after DFO, HTO, and double-level osteotomy.[98] Grunwald et al[98] examined expectations of 264 patients undergoing osteotomies around the knee and found that expectations are high regarding all aspects of surgical outcome. A substantial proportion of the study population underestimated the natural course of osteoarthritis and possible need for conversion to TKA. Approximately 62% of patients expected that the surgery would prevent osteoarthritis and 32% expected that the osteotomy would prevent TKA. Therefore, it is important to preoperatively counsel patients on outcomes and survival rates. Despite some unrealistic expectations, recent studies demonstrate good return to work and high-level sports after DFO.[4,99] Hoorntje et al[99] demonstrated a 77% return to sport rate after DFO, with 71% of patients returning to sports within 6 months. The return to work rate was also high (91%) and 77% returned within 6 months.

Complications

Complication rates of DFO are fairly low within the literature and are similar to those reported for HTO. Common intraoperative complications for lateral opening wedge DFO include medial hinge fracture and osteotomy displacement, which may be remedied with a medial staple. Postoperative complication risks for lateral opening wedge DFO are nonunion and hardware irritation from the laterally placed plate under the iliotibial band. Medial closing wedge DFO has the intraoperative risk of damage to the neurovascular structures with medial dissection but less common risk of nonunion or need for postoperative hardware removal.

Ilizarov Technique

The Ilizarov technique involves placement of a specialized external fixator and frame which allows gradual distraction, translation, or rotation of the distal fragment following corticotomy. This technique may be used for complex, multiplanar corrections. This technique allows for a gradual correction over time and can be used for correction of either varus or valgus deformity.[100] Radiographic evaluation may be carried out to verify precise correction. Lengthening of the limb can be done in conjunction with correction of angular malalignment if needed. The downside is the risk of pin-site complications and the need for the patient to wear the frame for several months or more.

SUMMARY

Realignment osteotomies of the distal femur and proximal tibia are a powerful and effective tool. Whether used to improve patient's pain and decelerate cartilage degradation in the arthritic compartment or to protect and offload a compartment after a cartilage or meniscus surgery, realignment osteotomies have proven that when performed in the right indications with a well-executed surgery based on proper preoperative planning, they provide desirable results with low complication rates. Advances in techniques and fixation devices have led to improved and more accurate surgical procedure, lower complication rate, and superior functional outcomes.

REFERENCES

1. Parker DA, Beatty KT, Giuffre B, Scholes CJ, Coolican MR. Articular cartilage changes in patients with osteoarthritis after osteotomy. *Am J Sports Med.* 2011;39:1039-1045.
2. Witjes S, Gouttebarge V, Kuijer PP, van Geenen RC, Poolman RW, Kerkhoffs GM. Return to sports and physical activity after total and unicondylar knee arthroplasty: a systematic review and meta-analysis. *Sports Med.* 2016;46:269-292.
3. Schmalzried TP, Shepherd EF, Dorey FJ, et al. The John Charnley Award. Wear is a function of use, not time. *Clin Orthop Relat Res.* 2000;(381):36-46.
4. Hoorntje A, Witjes S, Kuijer P, et al. High rates of return to sports activities and work after osteotomies around the knee: a systematic review and meta-analysis. *Sports Med.* 2017;47:2219-2244.
5. Ekhtiari S, Haldane CE, de Sa D, Simunovic N, Musahl V, Ayeni OR. Return to work and sport following high tibial osteotomy: a systematic review. *J Bone Joint Surg Am.* 2016;98:1568-1577.
6. Bastard C, Mirouse G, Potage D, et al. Return to sports and quality of life after high tibial osteotomy in patients under 60 years of age. *Orthop Traumatol Surg Res.* 2017;103:1189-1191.
7. Voleti PB, Wu IT, Degen RM, Tetreault DM, Krych AJ, Williams RJ III: Successful return to sport following distal femoral varus osteotomy. *Cartilage.* 2019;10(1):19-25.
8. Preston CF, Fulkerson EW, Meislin R, Di Cesare PE. Osteotomy about the knee: applications, techniques, and results. *J Knee Surg.* 2005;18:258-272.
9. Puddu G, Cipolla M, Cerullo G, Franco V, Gianni E. Which osteotomy for a valgus knee?. *Int Orthop.* 2010;34:239-247.
10. Noyes FR, Barber SD, Simon R. High tibial osteotomy and ligament reconstruction in varus angulated, anterior cruciate ligament-deficient knees. A two- to seven-year follow-up study. *Am J Sports Med.* 1993;21:2-12.
11. Trojani C, Elhor H, Carles M, Boileau P. Anterior cruciate ligament reconstruction combined with valgus high tibial osteotomy allows return to sports. *Orthop Traumatol Surg Res.* 2014;100:209-212.
12. Herman BV, Giffin JR. High tibial osteotomy in the ACL-deficient knee with medial compartment osteoarthritis. *J Orthop Traumatol.* 2016;17:277-285.
13. Coventry MB, Ilstrup DM, Wallrichs SL. Proximal tibial osteotomy. A critical long-term study of eighty-seven cases. *J Bone Joint Surg Am.* 1993;75:196-201.
14. Bonasia DE, Dettoni F, Sito G, et al. Medial opening wedge high tibial osteotomy for medial compartment overload/arthritis in the varus knee: prognostic factors. *Am J Sports Med.* 2014;42:690-698.
15. Liska F, Haller B, Voss A, et al. Smoking and obesity influence the risk of nonunion in lateral opening wedge, closing wedge and torsional distal femoral osteotomies. *Knee Surg Sports Traumatol Arthrosc.* 2018;26:2551-2557.
16. Zusmanovich M, Kester BS, Schwarzkopf R. Postoperative complications of total joint arthroplasty in obese patients stratified by BMI. *J Arthroplasty.* 2018;33:856-864.
17. Sharma L, Song J, Felson DT, Cahue S, Shamiyeh E, Dunlop DD. The role of knee alignment in disease progression and functional decline in knee osteoarthritis. *J Am Med Assoc.* 2001;286:188-195.
18. Prodromos CC, Andriacchi TP, Galante JO. A relationship between gait and clinical changes following high tibial osteotomy. *J Bone Joint Surg Am.* 1985;67:1188-1194.
19. Lind M, McClelland J, Wittwer JE, Whitehead TS, Feller JA, Webster KE. Gait analysis of walking before and after medial opening wedge high tibial osteotomy. *Knee Surg Sports Traumatol Arthrosc.* 2013;21:74-81.
20. Rosenberg TD, Paulos LE, Parker RD, Coward DB, Scott SM. The forty-five-degree posteroanterior flexion weight-bearing radiograph of the knee. *J Bone Joint Surg Am.* 1988;70:1479-1483.
21. Duncan ST, Khazzam MS, Burnham JM, Spindler KP, Dunn WR, Wright RW. Sensitivity of standing radiographs to detect knee arthritis: a systematic review of Level I studies. *Arthroscopy.* 2015;31:321-328.
22. Uquillas C, Rossy W, Nathasingh CK, Strauss E, Jazrawi L, Gonzalez-Lomas G. Osteotomies about the knee: AAOS exhibit selection. *J Bone Joint Surg Am.* 2014;96:e199.
23. Phillips CL, Silver DA, Schranz PJ, Mandalia V. The measurement of patellar height: a review of the methods of imaging. *J Bone Joint Surg Br.* 2010;92:1045-1053.
24. El-Azab H, Glabgly P, Paul J, Imhoff AB, Hinterwimmer S. Patellar height and posterior tibial slope after open- and closed-wedge high tibial osteotomy: a radiological study on 100 patients. *Am J Sports Med.* 2010;38:323-329.
25. Bin SI, Kim HJ, Ahn HS, Rim DS, Lee DH. Changes in patellar height after opening wedge and closing wedge high tibial osteotomy: a meta-analysis. *Arthroscopy.* 2016;32:2393-2400.
26. Dugdale TW, Noyes FR, Styer D. Preoperative planning for high tibial osteotomy. The effect of lateral tibiofemoral separation and tibiofemoral length. *Clin Orthop Relat Res.* 1992;(274):248-264.
27. Eberbach H, Mehl J, Feucht MJ, Bode G, Sudkamp NP, Niemeyer P. Geometry of the valgus knee: contradicting the Dogma of a femoral-based deformity. *Am J Sports Med.* 2017;45:909-914.
28. Benjamin A. Double osteotomy for the painful knee in rheumatoid arthritis and osteoarthritis. *J Bone Joint Surg Br.* 1969;51:694-699.
29. Schroter S, Nakayama H, Yoshiya S, Stockle U, Ateschrang A, Gruhn J. Development of the double level osteotomy in severe varus osteoarthritis showed good outcome by preventing oblique joint line. *Arch Orthop Trauma Surg.* 2019;139(4):519-527.
30. Jacobi M, Wahl P, Bouaicha S, Jakob RP, Gautier E. Distal femoral varus osteotomy: problems associated with the lateral open-wedge technique. *Arch Orthop Trauma Surg.* 2011;131:725-728.
31. Coventry MB. Upper tibial osteotomy for gonarthrosis. The evolution of the operation in the last 18 years and long term results. *Orthop Clin North Am.* 1979;10:191-210.
32. Coventry MB. Proximal tibial varus osteotomy for osteoarthritis of the lateral compartment of the knee. *J Bone Joint Surg Am.* 1987;69:32-38.
33. Naudie D, Bourne RB, Rorabeck CH, Bourne TJ. The Insall Award. Survivorship of the high tibial valgus osteotomy. A 10- to -22-year followup study. *Clin Orthop Relat Res.* 1999;(367):18-27.
34. Ekeland A, Nerhus TK, Dimmen S, Thornes E, Heir S. Good functional results following high tibial opening-wedge osteotomy of knees with medial osteoarthritis: a prospective study with a mean of 8.3years of follow-up. *Knee.* 2017;24:380-389.
35. Nerhus TK, Ekeland A, Solberg G, Olsen BH, Madsen JE, Heir S. No difference in time-dependent improvement in functional outcome following closing wedge versus opening wedge high tibial osteotomy: a randomised controlled trial with two-year follow-up. *Bone Joint J.* 2017;99-B:1157-1166.
36. Duivenvoorden T, Brouwer RW, Baan A, et al. Comparison of closing-wedge and opening-wedge high tibial osteotomy for medial compartment osteoarthritis of the knee: a randomized controlled trial with a six-year follow-up. *J Bone Joint Surg Am.* 2014;96:1425-1432.

37. Smith TO, Sexton D, Mitchell P, Hing CB. Opening- or closing-wedged high tibial osteotomy: a meta-analysis of clinical and radiological outcomes. *Knee.* 2011;18:361-368.

38. Fujisawa Y, Masuhara K, Shiomi S. The effect of high tibial osteotomy on osteoarthritis of the knee. An arthroscopic study of 54 knee joints. *Orthop Clin North Am.* 1979;10:585-608.

39. Mehl J, Paul J, Feucht MJ, et al. ACL deficiency and varus osteoarthritis: high tibial osteotomy alone or combined with ACL reconstruction? *Arch Orthop Trauma Surg.* 2017;137:233-240.

40. Bernhardson AS, Aman ZS, Dornan GJ, et al. Tibial slope and its effect on force in anterior cruciate ligament grafts: anterior cruciate ligament force increases linearly as posterior tibial slope increases. *Am J Sports Med.* 2019;47:296-302.

41. Bernhardson AS, Aman ZS, DePhillipo NN, et al. Tibial slope and its effect on graft force in posterior cruciate ligament reconstructions. *Am J Sports Med.* 2019;47:1168-1174.

42. Specogna AV, Birmingham TB, DaSilva JJ, et al. Reliability of lower limb frontal plane alignment measurements using plain radiographs and digitized images. *J Knee Surg.* 2004;17:203-210.

43. Marx RG, Grimm P, Lillemoe KA, et al. Reliability of lower extremity alignment measurement using radiographs and PACS. *Knee Surg Sports Traumatol Arthrosc.* 2011;19:1693-1698.

44. Lee YS, Kim MK, Byun HW, Kim SB, Kim JG. Reliability of the imaging software in the preoperative planning of the open-wedge high tibial osteotomy. *Knee Surg Sports Traumatol Arthrosc.* 2015;23:846-851.

45. Iorio R, Pagnottelli M, Vadala A, et al. Open-wedge high tibial osteotomy: comparison between manual and computer-assisted techniques. *Knee Surg Sports Traumatol Arthrosc.* 2013;21:113-119.

46. Dahl MT. Preoperative planning in deformity correction and limb lengthening surgery. *Instr Course Lect.* 2000;49:503-509.

47. Hankemeier S, Hufner T, Wang G, et al. Navigated open-wedge high tibial osteotomy: advantages and disadvantages compared to the conventional technique in a cadaver study. *Knee Surg Sports Traumatol Arthrosc.* 2006;14:917-921.

48. Kim HJ, Park J, Park KH, et al. Evaluation of accuracy of a three-dimensional printed model in open-wedge high tibial osteotomy. *J Knee Surg.* 2019;32(9):841-846.

49. Munier M, Donnez M, Ollivier M, et al. Can three-dimensional patient-specific cutting guides be used to achieve optimal correction for high tibial osteotomy? Pilot study. *Orthop Traumatol Surg Res.* 2017;103:245-250.

50. Bae DK, Song SJ, Yoon KH. Closed-wedge high tibial osteotomy using computer-assisted surgery compared to the conventional technique. *J Bone Joint Surg Br.* 2009;91:1164-1171.

51. Wu ZP, Zhang P, Bai JZ, et al. Comparison of navigated and conventional high tibial osteotomy for the treatment of osteoarthritic knees with varus deformity: a meta-analysis. *Int J Surg.* 2018;55:211-219.

52. Agneskirchner JD, Hurschler C, Wrann CD, Lobenhoffer P. The effects of valgus medial opening wedge high tibial osteotomy on articular cartilage pressure of the knee: a biomechanical study. *Arthroscopy.* 2007;23:852-861.

53. Myrnerts R. Knee instability before and after high tibial osteotomy. *Acta Orthop Scand.* 1980;51:561-564.

54. Soejima O, Ogata K, Ishinishi T, Fukahori Y, Miyauchi R. Anatomic considerations of the peroneal nerve for division of the fibula during high tibial osteotomy. *Orthop Rev.* 1994;23:244-247.

55. Kirgis A, Albrecht S. Palsy of the deep peroneal nerve after proximal tibial osteotomy. An anatomical study. *J Bone Joint Surg Am.* 1992;74:1180-1185.

56. Kessler OC, Jacob HA, Romero J. Avoidance of medial cortical fracture in high tibial osteotomy: improved technique. *Clin Orthop Relat Res.* 2002;(395):180-185.

57. Paley D, Tetsworth K. Mechanical axis deviation of the lower limbs. Preoperative planning of multiapical frontal plane angular and bowing deformities of the femur and tibia. *Clin Orthop Relat Res.* 1992;(280):65-71.

58. Sundaram NA, Hallett JP, Sullivan MF. Dome osteotomy of the tibia for osteoarthritis of the knee. *J Bone Joint Surg Br.* 1986;68:782-786.

59. Spahn G, Muckley T, Kahl E, Hofmann GO. Biomechanical investigation of different internal fixations in medial opening-wedge high tibial osteotomy. *Clin Biomech.* 2006;21:272-278.

60. Zhim F, Laflamme GY, Viens H, Saidane K, Yahia L. Biomechanical stability of high tibial opening wedge osteotomy: internal fixation versus external fixation. *Clin Biomech.* 2005;20:871-876.

61. Kazimoglu C, Akdogan Y, Sener M, Kurtulmus A, Karapinar H, Uzun B. Which is the best fixation method for lateral cortex disruption in the medial open wedge high tibial osteotomy? A biomechanical study. *Knee.* 2008;15:305-308.

62. Insall JN, Joseph DM, Msika C. High tibial osteotomy for varus gonarthrosis. A long-term follow-up study. *J Bone Joint Surg Am.* 1984;66:1040-1048.

63. Billings A, Scott DF, Camargo MP, Hofmann AA. High tibial osteotomy with a calibrated osteotomy guide, rigid internal fixation, and early motion. Long-term follow-up. *J Bone Joint Surg Am.* 2000;82:70-79.

64. Getgood A, Collins B, Slynarski K, et al. Short-term safety and efficacy of a novel high tibial osteotomy system: a case controlled study. *Knee Surg Sports Traumatol Arthrosc.* 2013;21:260-269.

65. Heary RF, Parvathreddy N, Sampath S, Agarwal N. Elastic modulus in the selection of interbody implants. *J Spine Surg.* 2017;3:163-167.

66. Cotic M, Vogt S, Hinterwimmer S, et al. A matched-pair comparison of two different locking plates for valgus-producing medial open-wedge high tibial osteotomy: peek-carbon composite plate versus titanium plate. *Knee Surg Sports Traumatol Arthrosc.* 2015;23:2032-2040.

67. Hevesi M, Macalena JA, Wu IT, et al. High tibial osteotomy with modern PEEK implants is safe and leads to lower hardware removal rates when compared to conventional metal fixation: a multi-center comparison study. *Knee Surg Sports Traumatol Arthrosc.* 2019;27(4):1280-1290.

68. Hantes ME, Natsaridis P, Koutalos AA, Ono Y, Doxariotis N, Malizos KN. Satisfactory functional and radiological outcomes can be expected in young patients under 45 years old after open wedge high tibial osteotomy in a long-term follow-up. *Knee Surg Sports Traumatol Arthrosc.* 2018;26:3199-3205.

69. Nerhus TK, Ekeland A, Solberg G, Sivertsen EA, Madsen JE, Heir S. Radiological outcomes in a randomized trial comparing opening wedge and closing wedge techniques of high tibial osteotomy. *Knee Surg Sports Traumatol Arthrosc.* 2017;25:910-917.

70. Martay JL, Palmer AJ, Bangerter NK, et al. A preliminary modeling investigation into the safe correction zone for high tibial osteotomy. *Knee.* 2018;25:286-295.

71. Han SB, In Y, Oh KJ, Song KY, Yun ST, Jang KM. Complications associated with medial opening-wedge high tibial osteotomy using a locking plate: a multicenter study. *J Arthroplasty.* 2019;34(3):439-445.

72. Seo SS, Kim OG, Seo JH, Kim DH, Kim YG, Lee IS. Complications and short-term outcomes of medial opening wedge high tibial osteotomy using a locking plate for medial osteoarthritis of the knee. *Knee Surg Relat Res.* 2016;28:289-296.

73. Asik M, Sen C, Kilic B, Goksan SB, Ciftci F, Taser OF. High tibial osteotomy with Puddu plate for the treatment of varus gonarthrosis. *Knee Surg Sports Traumatol Arthrosc.* 2006;14:948-954.

74. Amendola A, Fowler PJ, Litchfield R, Kirkley S, Clatworthy M. Opening wedge high tibial osteotomy using a novel technique: early results and complications. *J Knee Surg.* 2004;17:164-169.

75. Woodacre T, Ricketts M, Evans JT, et al. Complications associated with opening wedge high tibial osteotomy–A review of the literature and of 15 years of experience. *Knee*. 2016;23:276-282.

76. McDermott AG, Finklestein JA, Farine I, Boynton EL, MacIntosh DL, Gross A. Distal femoral varus osteotomy for valgus deformity of the knee. *J Bone Joint Surg Am*. 1988;70:110-116.

77. Rosso F, Margheritini F. Distal femoral osteotomy. *Curr Rev Musculoskelet Med*. 2014;7:302-311.

78. Healy WL, Anglen JO, Wasilewski SA, Krackow KA. Distal femoral varus osteotomy. *J Bone Joint Surg Am*. 1988;70:102-109.

79. Quirno M, Campbell KA, Singh B, et al. Distal femoral varus osteotomy for unloading valgus knee malalignment: a biomechanical analysis. *Knee Surg Sports Traumatol Arthrosc*. 2017;25:863-868.

80. Wylie JD, Scheiderer B, Obopilwe E, et al. The effect of lateral opening wedge distal femoral varus osteotomy on tibiofemoral contact mechanics through knee flexion. *Am J Sports Med*. 2018;46:3237-3244.

81. Thein R, Bronak S, Thein R, Haviv B. Distal femoral osteotomy for valgus arthritic knees. *J Orthop Sci*. 2012;17:745-749.

82. Dewilde TR, Dauw J, Vandenneucker H, Bellemans J. Opening wedge distal femoral varus osteotomy using the Puddu plate and calcium phosphate bone cement. *Knee Surg Sports Traumatol Arthrosc*. 2013;21:249-254.

83. Luna-Pizarro D, Moreno-Delgado F, De la Fuente-Zuno JC, Meraz-Lares G. Distal femoral dome varus osteotomy: surgical technique with minimal dissection and external fixation. *Knee*. 2012;19:99-102.

84. El Ghazaly SA, El-Moatasem el HM. Femoral supracondylar focal dome osteotomy with plate fixation for acute correction of frontal plane knee deformity. *Strategies Trauma Limb Reconstr*. 2015;10:41-47.

85. Gugenheim JJ Jr, Brinker MR. Bone realignment with use of temporary external fixation for distal femoral valgus and varus deformities. *J Bone Joint Surg Am*. 2003;85-A:1229-1237.

86. Mathews J, Cobb AG, Richardson S, Bentley G. Distal femoral osteotomy for lateral compartment osteoarthritis of the knee. *Orthopedics*. 1998;21:437-440.

87. Seah KT, Shafi R, Fragomen AT, Rozbruch SR. Distal femoral osteotomy: is internal fixation better than external?. *Clin Orthop Relat Res*. 2011;469:2003-2011.

88. Koh YG, Kwon OR, Kim YS, Choi YJ. Comparative outcomes of open-wedge high tibial osteotomy with platelet-rich plasma alone or in combination with mesenchymal stem cell treatment: a prospective study. *Arthroscopy*. 2014;30:1453-1460.

89. Kosashvili Y, Safir O, Gross A, Morag G, Lakstein D, Backstein D. Distal femoral varus osteotomy for lateral osteoarthritis of the knee: a minimum ten-year follow-up. *Int Orthop*. 2010;34:249-254.

90. Zarrouk A, Bouzidi R, Karray B, Kammoun S, Mourali S, Kooli M. Distal femoral varus osteotomy outcome: is associated femoropatellar osteoarthritis consequential?. *Orthop Traumatol Surg Res*. 2010;96:632-636.

91. Saithna A, Kundra R, Getgood A, Spalding T. Opening wedge distal femoral varus osteotomy for lateral compartment osteoarthritis in the valgus knee. *Knee*. 2014;21:172-175.

92. Backstein D, Morag G, Hanna S, Safir O, Gross A. Long-term follow-up of distal femoral varus osteotomy of the knee. *J Arthroplasty*. 2007;22:2-6.

93. Wang JW, Hsu CC. Distal femoral varus osteotomy for osteoarthritis of the knee. *J Bone Joint Surg Am*. 2005;87:127-133.

94. Stahelin T, Hardegger F, Ward JC. Supracondylar osteotomy of the femur with use of compression. Osteosynthesis with a malleable implant. *J Bone Joint Surg Am*. 2000;82:712-722.

95. Forkel P, Achtnich A, Metzlaff S, Zantop T, Petersen W. Midterm results following medial closed wedge distal femoral osteotomy stabilized with a locking internal fixation device. *Knee Surg Sports Traumatol Arthrosc*. 2015;23:2061-2067.

96. Ekeland A, Nerhus TK, Dimmen S, Heir S. Good functional results of distal femoral opening-wedge osteotomy of knees with lateral osteoarthritis. *Knee Surg Sports Traumatol Arthrosc*. 2016;24:1702-1709.

97. Stoffel K, Stachowiak G, Kuster M. Open wedge high tibial osteotomy: biomechanical investigation of the modified Arthrex Osteotomy Plate (Puddu Plate) and the TomoFix Plate. *Clin Biomech*. 2004;19:944-950.

98. Grunwald L, Angele P, Schroter S, et al. Patients' expectations of osteotomies around the knee are high regarding activities of daily living. *Knee Surg Sports Traumatol Arthrosc*. 2019;27(9):3022-3031.

99. Hoorntje A, van Ginneken BT, Kuijer P, et al. Eight respectively nine out of ten patients return to sport and work after distal femoral osteotomy. *Knee Surg Sports Traumatol Arthrosc*. 2019;27(7):2345-2353.

100. Warner SJ, O'Connor DP, Brinker MR. Subtubercle osteotomy for medial compartment osteoarthritis of the knee using Ilizarov technique: survival analysis and clinical outcomes. *J Bone Joint Surg Am*. 2018;100:e1.

Primary Total Knee Arthroplasty

AARON G. ROSENBERG

BRETT R. LEVINE

HARRY E. RUBASH

HANY S. BEDAIR

chapter 27

Economics of Total Knee Arthroplasty

Jorge A. Padilla, MD | James E. Feng, MD, MS | Zlatan Cizmic, MD | Richard Iorio, MD

INTRODUCTION

Owing to its success in improving pain and functional status in patients afflicted with severe end-stage arthritis, total knee arthroplasty (TKA) is one of the most frequently performed surgical procedures in the United States. It is estimated that by 2030, the exponential growth for primary total joint arthroplasty (TJA) will rise to 4.05 million procedures per year, of which 3.48 million are expected to be TKA.[1-3] Several key factors have contributed to this rising demand, including the coming of age of the "baby boomer" population, the worsening obesity and metabolic syndrome epidemic, broadening of surgical indications to younger patients, and continued improvement in the standard of care.[1-5] However, as healthcare costs continue to increase at an unprecedented rate, cost containment is now at the forefront of discussion for patients, physicians, and payers alike. In 2016, $3.48 trillion US dollars (USD) was spent on healthcare, with over $9 billion dollars per annum attributed to TKA inpatient cost alone.[2,6-8]

In this chapter, we describe the economic burden associated with TKA including the cost of novel devices, in-hospital care, post-acute care, and the financial implications of technological advancements in the field. Furthermore, we will elaborate on the current era of innovative Alternative Payment Models (APM), which have been proven to improve cost-effectiveness for TKA.

COST OF TOTAL KNEE ARTHROPLASTY

In a 2015 study by the Blue Cross Blue Shield health insurance company, the average private insurer reimbursement for an elective primary TKA was estimated to be $34,124 per procedure.[9] However, in the same study, TKA reimbursements were found to vary significantly with geographic location despite similar outcomes in patient safety and care. In New York City, the average cost of an elective TKA was approximately $61,266 ranging from $56,945 to as high as $69,654 USD; meanwhile, the same procedure performed in the cities of Alabama reported an average cost of $16,096 ranging from as low as $11,317 to $20,984 USD.[9] These large discrepancies demonstrate the substantial inefficiencies in the current-day provision of TKA care.

Implant Costs

Implant costs have been proposed as the primary driver for increasing hospital charges following elective primary TKA, accounting for nearly 40% to 50% of the total costs per inpatient episode of care billed to Medicare.[9,10] Furthermore, implant prices have increased significantly, while substantive evidence demonstrating improved clinical or functional outcomes with newer, novel implants over previous generations remains equivocal.[11] As a result, select healthcare organizations have mandated value-based care initiatives, which have led to aggressive implant price restructuring. In 2011, New York University Langone Orthopedic Hospital (NYULOH) developed an implant cost-containment program.[12] A non-negotiable implant price ceiling was implemented, compelling vendors to compete for the hospital's market share. Eventually, all vendors decided to meet the implant price. Through this program, NYULOH reduced the average TKA implant cost, effectively decreasing the overall costs of TKA by 25.94%. After its first year, NYULOH saved $2 million through implant price negotiations for TJA alone. Similarly, an initiative at the Lahey Clinic demonstrated improved financial performance following the implementation of price negotiations with vendors. In their model, a single price per case purchasing program was developed. Vendors were required to provide all knee implants at one standard prenegotiated price for every TKA case irrespective of the implant being used during the cases.[13] The price was based on historical data on the use of implants at that institution. They successfully reduced the cost of knee implants by 23% at their institution.[13]

Fueled by the financial success of TKA, implant vendors have continued innovation while also producing an abundance of new medical device designs each year. However, as these new medical devices come to market at higher cost, questions have been raised concerning cost-efficacy and safety. The majority of these devices are often approved through the Food and Drug Administration's (FDA) 510(k) clearance process, a mandate passed by congress in 1976 as part of the FDA's Medical Device Amendments (MDA).[14] The 510(k) clearance process is a pragmatic approval

403

process for medical devices developed due to concerns for restricting continued medical innovation. This process allows for novel medical device approval based on claims of device similarity to preexisting medical devices on the market. Of even greater concern is the fact that the majority of the preexisting devices available on the market for comparison were also approved through a streamlined process for unregulated devices in 1976 as part of the MDA. As a result, there is a lack of supporting data for the durability, safety, and outcomes of these devices.[14,15] Studies supporting these existing devices may lack clinical trials altogether and in some cases, the preexisting device may also be approved through the 510(k) clearance process.[8,15] Due to the simplicity for acquiring approval of novel medical devices, approximately 35 TKA systems are approved by the FDA annually, further contributing to the financial burden of TKA.[8] However, as new medical devices continue to be brought to the market, there is a lack of scientific evidence that demonstrates conclusive clinical superiority over currently available devices.

With rising healthcare costs, it is critical to evaluate the value of medical device innovations in comparison to traditional devices that have existing evidence of safety and efficacy. Medical device innovations should be directed at solving unaddressed clinical challenges or should demonstrate improvements over previous iterations, such as improved range of motion, patient satisfaction, and survival for TKA implants.[16] Furthermore, introduction of these new medical devices can result in significant price variations between both new and old medical devices. Institutional cost-containment programs should therefore concentrate on maintaining negotiated prices when presented with new medical technologies, particularly when these new devices have yet to demonstrate evidence for clinical superiority over previous models, provide only theoretical clinical justification over the current standard of care, and have a currently unproven track record.

Navigation Cost

Modern day technological advancements have improved many aspects of medicine. In orthopedic surgery, the possibility of improving clinical and functional patient outcomes by reducing human error and improving surgical precision has been promising. Current innovative techniques center around the use of computer and robotic-assisted orthopedic surgery to improve precision, reproducibility, radiographic alignment, and implant positioning for TKA.[17-19] However, recent studies on the use of computer and robotic-assisted surgery fail to identify reproducible improvements in clinical or functional patient outcomes.[18-27] In addition, long-term clinical outcomes in orthopedic surgery and the economic implications secondary to these technological

innovations are yet to be clearly defined. The vast majority of existing literature has failed to demonstrate any substantial clinical advantage such as superior patient-reported outcomes, range of motion, survival, or revision rates attributed to the improvement in alignment achieved by the engagement of computer and robotic-assisted TKA.[18-27] Furthermore, concerns about the financial burdens secondary to increased surgical times, initial capital investment, and the additional training required with the use of the computer and robotic-assisted surgery have contributed to reservations about the use of these modern technological advancements as routine standard of care. One potential benefit of this technology is the possible use in learning curve improvement and surgeon education which may be used to provide immediate cutting precision and implant placement feedback.[21]

Computer-Assisted Navigation

Computer-assisted navigation systems exchange subjective decisions into precise, calculated, patient-specific surgical actions. Computer-assisted systems require less initial capital investment in comparison to robotic-assisted systems.[25] However, one study by Beringer et al described an additional expense with computer-assisted navigation ranging from $600 to $2000 per arthroplasty case.[28] Good clinical and functional outcomes following computer-assisted TKA have been reported.[18,19] Despite improving radiographic outcomes, it remains unclear whether computer-assisted navigation improves clinical outcomes or patient satisfaction in comparison to conventional methods.[25]

Robotic-Assisted Navigation

Robotic-assisted systems reportedly restore component alignment with greater accuracy than computer-assisted navigation; however, there is a paucity of evidence supporting improvement in clinical and functional outcomes.[25,29] Additionally, robotic technology requires a large initial capital investment for the robot, training, and software. There are currently four commonly used robotic platforms in the United States including Mako (Stryker, Mahwah, NJ), Navio (Smith and Nephew, London, UK), THINK (THINK Surgical Inc, Fremont, Ca), and OMNI (OMNIlife Science Inc., Raynham, MA). The initial cost for the robot is unique to each and therefore varies significantly. Capital investment for a robot ranges from $400,000 to $2.5 million.[30-32] For example, the Mako robotic system (Stryker, Mahwah, NJ) available for use in orthopedic surgery may cost upwards of $930,000 with an expected lifespan of merely 5 years.[31] There is also an additional inherent cost per year for the associated service contract bringing the total cost to an estimated $1.362 million. Furthermore, software licensing and annual maintenance for these robotic-assisted devices in general can range from $40,000 up to $250,000.[30-32] An additional variable expense inherent to robotic-assisted systems is attributed to disposable surgical kits. A study by Moschetti et al reported a $2743 increase in cost per surgical case for unicompartmental knee arthroplasty with the use of Mako.[31] Similarly, Belleman et al reported an additional $1360 per case for ancillaries required by the robot.[32] Many of the commonly used robotic-assisted systems require preoperative imaging to match anatomy during surgery, therefore further increasing expenditures, radiation exposure, and preoperative planning times and costs.[25] It is not yet clear whether the theoretical improvements in precision accomplished with the use of these robotic systems necessarily translate to objectively improved outcomes in TKA. Therefore, reservations persist in relation to the cost-effectiveness of these technological advancements.

ALTERNATIVE PAYMENT MODELS

In 2007, TKA was the procedure with the highest aggregate costs and was among the 10 procedures with the most rapidly increasing hospital inpatient cost in the United States.[33] From 2005 to 2011, the average hospital charges to Centers for Medicare and Medicaid Services (CMS) for TKA episodes of care increased by $15,419 from $36,756 to $52,175.[34] During that period the average reimbursement to hospitals from CMS reimbursements increased only $13,746 from $26,136 to $39,882, widening the deficit between hospital charges and CMS reimbursements from $10,620 to $12,293 per TKA. When adjusted for inflation, the growth in CMS reimbursement was 0.1%. Additionally, adverse events that may occur

during TKA or in the post-acute care period may further increase the average total cost up to $31,000.[35]

Traditionally fee for service and capitation models were the primary reimbursement models used for TKA, which incentivized quantity of service as opposed to the quality of care. In response to the rising demand of TKA and variability in healthcare outcomes, the CMS has ushered in an era of APM.[36] The Bundled Payments for Care Improvement (BPCI), Comprehensive Care for Joint Replacement (CJR), and BPCI Advanced are three of the most recent initiatives which strive to provide high quality of care and improved outcomes while simultaneously reducing the total cost of healthcare (**Table 27-1**). Early studies have been reassuring with reductions in healthcare expenditures following the implementation of these bundle payment models without negatively effecting quality. More importantly, changes, as the leading financier in the nation for US healthcare expenditures, modifications in reimbursements by the CMS reimbursement have the potential to judiciously change the economic landscape of healthcare.[37]

Bundled Payments for Care Improvement

The BPCI initiative was founded in 2013 by the Center for Medicare and Medicaid Innovation (CMMI), a program developed under the ACA.[38,39] BPCI was an early attempt to reduce the financial burden of healthcare, incentivize quality care improvement initiatives, and encourage coordination among healthcare providers.[36-42] Initially, the CMMI determined that BPCI was established as a 3-year experiment. Due to its success, CMS extended the initiative an additional 2 years. Under the BPCI initiative, healthcare organizations and CMS negotiate a fixed predetermined

TABLE 27-1 Alternative Payment Models

Model	Description	Conditions	Payment
BPCI Model 1	The episode of care includes the inpatient hospital setting only.	All MS-DRGs	Retrospective
BPCI Model 2	The episode of care includes the inpatient hospital setting and the post-acute care period. The post-acute care period may cover 30, 60, or 90 d following discharge and is to be determined by the healthcare organization.	48 MS-DRGs	Retrospective
BPCI Model 3	The episode of care covers the post-acute care setting only for 30, 60, or 90 d. Initiation of the episode follows discharge from an inpatient hospitalization.	48 MS-DRGs	Retrospective
BPCI Model 4	The episode of care includes the inpatient hospital setting only.	48 MS-DRGs	Prospective
CJR	The episode of care includes the inpatient hospital stay and the post-acute care setting for 90 d.	2 MS-DRGs	Retrospective
BPCI Advanced	The episode of care includes the inpatient hospital setting and the post-acute care period. The post-acute care period is a standard 90 d following discharge.	3 outpatient HCPCS and 29 inpatient MS-DRGs	Retrospective

BPCI, Bundled Payments for Care Improvement; CJR, Comprehensive Care for Joint Replacement; HCPCS, Healthcare Common Procedure Coding System; MS-DRGs, Medicare Severity-Diagnosis Related Groups.

"target" payment per episode of care. The target payment was derived from historical hospital reimbursements and discounted by 2% to 3%, essentially guaranteeing cost savings for CMS.[37] Healthcare institutions stood to benefit by delivering services at a lower cost than the target price, allowing them to reconcile the cost saving from CMS 30-days after an episode of care.[37,41-45] At the same time, these institutions became financially accountable for poor patient outcomes—the institution became financially responsible to repay the excess cost to CMS if the cost of all the services rendered during the episode of care exceeded the target price. Healthcare institutions became stakeholders in a patient's episode of care, whereby the success or failure of the patient was directly tied to their reimbursement.

To incentivize physicians in addition to healthcare institutions, CMS endorsed gainsharing. Institutions that achieve cost reductions greater than the determined target price can distribute their CMS reimbursements through gainsharing to providers involved in an episode of care. Substantial financial savings over time drive collaboration between providers to innovate and adhere to strategies that will provide further cost reduction which maintain or improve upon the current standard of care.

Depending on the model chosen, the episode of care may include a 72-hour preoperative period, acute inpatient hospital services, and/or a postoperative period of up to 90 days following surgery for unplanned readmissions (**Table 27-2**).[42,43,45] The specific inclusions and exclusions for each participant in a bundle must be clearly delineated and may include post-acute care services such as inpatient rehabilitation services, skilled nursing facilities, and inpatient and outpatient physician services. Furthermore, reimbursements may be paid to the hospital either prospectively or retrospectively depending on the model chosen by the hospital.

Institutions were allowed to pick from four models under the BPCI initiative. Payments were either retrospective or prospective and the episode of care is defined for each model as follows.[39] Model 1 is a retrospective

payment in which payments are made to healthcare organizations to cover the total episode of care in the acute inpatient hospital stay only. Under model 1 the episode of care includes all Medicare Severity-Diagnosis Related Groups (MS-DRGs). Model 2 is another retrospective form of payment where the episode of care consists of the inpatient stay and the post-acute care period for 48 specific MS-DRGs. The healthcare organizations may choose to define the post-acute care time frame as 30, 60, or 90 days following surgery. The minimum discounted price for plans that cover less than 90 days of the post-acute care period is 3%. Meanwhile the minimum discount for the 90-day post-acute care plan is established at 2%. Model 3 is another retrospective payment where the episode of care only covers the predetermined post-acute period (30, 60, or 90-day) for 48 specific MS-DRGs. Similarly, the minimum discount required by CMS varies from 2% to 3% depending on the post-acute care plan the healthcare organization decides upon. Model 4 is the only prospective payment model. The episode of care for model 4 is similar to model 1 in that it covers the acute inpatient hospital care setting. However, the episode of care under model 4 covers only 48 specific MS-DRGs. Model 2 is the most commonly designated by healthcare organizations for TJA including TKA.[37,41-49] Following the application of this initiative, providers must collaborate in order to achieve a common goal of cost reduction and healthcare quality control.

The fastest growing major Medicare spending category was post-acute care and therefore represented an opportunity for substantial reduction of healthcare expenditures.[50-52] Several elements of the post-acute care period have been targeted by BPCI participants' cost-containment programs, including but not limited to readmissions and discharge disposition. Post-acute care facility cost are a large portion of the total cost of care and has been cited at greater than 40% of the total cost for TKA.[16,46] One study by Dundon et al demonstrated a 20% cost reduction in TJA for their institution following the implementation of several cost-containment programs including risk factor optimization programs, improved care coordination, venous thromboembolism and infection protocols, and improved discharge disposition. The same authors reported that 88% of the total cost reduction for TJA was due to improving discharge disposition by reducing the use of post-acute inpatient care facilities.[40]

To reduce healthcare costs and maintain or improve quality, healthcare institutions implemented a variety of value-based care measures. Reducing the use of unnecessary and clinically insignificant routine testing along with decreasing the total length of stay in the inpatient setting following surgical intervention have been investigated as potential areas for reducing the cost per episode of care.[12,51,53-56] Additionally, by implementing an evidenced-based, multidisciplinary, standardized clinical pre- and postoperative pathway, the length of stay, readmission

TABLE 27-2	Episode of Care Coverage Per Model		
Model	**Outpatient Procedure**	**Acute Inpatient Hospital Stay**	**Post-Acute Care Services**[a]
BPCI Model 1		▓▓▓▓	
BPCI Model 2		▓▓▓▓▓▓▓▓▓▓▓	
BPCI Model 3			▓▓▓▓▓
BPCI Model 4		▓▓▓▓	
CJR		▓▓▓▓▓▓▓▓▓▓▓	
BPCI Advanced	▓▓▓▓▓▓▓▓▓▓▓▓▓		

BPCI, Bundled Payments for Care Improvement; CJR, Comprehensive Care for Joint Replacement.

[a]Post-acute care services for BPCI may be of either 30, 60, or 90-days duration. For CJR and BPCI Advanced, the duration is 90-days non-negotiable.

rate, and discharge to inpatient rehabilitation facilities have been successfully reduced, which have led to a total cost reduction per episode of care for both the hospital and CMS.[40,45,57] Several other studies have had similar cost saving results under BPCI.[12,51,55,56] Pain control following TKA is another factor which may affect the length of stay and should be taken into consideration. The adequate control of postoperative pain has been demonstrated to improve recovery time and reduce the length of stay following TKA.[58]

Post-acute care complications are frequently unpredictable and may result in readmission further increasing the financial burden. In 2004, the cost of readmissions to Medicare was approximately $17.4 billion.[59] The average financial burden of readmissions following primary TKA during the first 30 days postoperatively has been reported as greater than $13,000 per patient.[60] One such example has been in postoperative venous thromboembolic events (VTEs). A recent article by Luzzi and colleagues reported the most common complications following TKA were deep infection, myocardial infarction, and pulmonary embolism.[61] While aggressive preventative measures can be taken to prevent complications such as VTEs, they must be judiciously balanced against iatrogenic complications, such as the increased risk for bleeding and infection with aggressive anticoagulation.[53] As studies continue to evaluate the optimal protocol for VTE prophylaxis, current evidence-based guidelines have well-established that routine postoperative surveillance does not improve patient outcomes for suspected VTEs.[53]

Appropriate patient discharge has been another area of interest as the overutilization of inpatient facilities following TKA has been a significant contributor to increased episode of care costs.[50,52,59] Taken together, reducing readmissions through medical optimizations of comorbidities, appropriate patient selection, and discharge disposition have played a major role in the development of modern APM. In BPCI, the post-acute period includes readmissions ranging anywhere from 0 to 90 days following surgery. During this period, healthcare organizations do not receive additional reimbursements for services provided and are therefore incentivized to appropriately reduce unnecessary postoperative care services. Early results following the implementation of the BPCI initiative have demonstrated reduced readmission rates, discharge to post-acute care facilities, and overall cost to Medicare, while maintaining the same level of healthcare quality.[37,40-45,51,60]

Revision TKA in APM

In 2010, the average hospital cost of revision TKA was greater than $49,000 and similar to primary TKA varied greatly depending on the geographic region.[62] The annual financial burden to hospitals secondary to revision TKA was $2.9 billion in 2012 and is expected to exceed $13 billion by the year 2030.[62] Unlike primary TKA, the application of bundle payment models for revision TKA has been controversial.[44,63] The increased technical complexity of revision TKA cases, in addition to its heterogeneous and generally more comorbid patient population, further increases the cost per episode. Under the current payment model, a few outlier cases may have severe financial repercussions to smaller rural hospitals that do not have the financial resources to absorb these episodic costs.

Comprehensive Care for Joint Replacement

Building off of the success of BPCI model 2, CMS developed the CJR, a more bold 5-year TJA cost-containment program primarily focused on reducing the cost of the two most commonly billed inpatient procedures, MS-DRG 469 and 470.[64] The development of CJR aimed to increase hospital participation, improve quality of care, and reduce the total healthcare cost associated to TJA. In CJR, the episode of care is initiated at the time of admission and was completed at 90 days postoperatively.[38,64] Similar to BPCI, all costs incurred during the episode of care are reimbursed through the fee-for-service model at a 3% discounted price and reconciliation occurs at year's end.[64] However, the target price in CJR is also determined by comparing regional pricing based on Metropolitan Statistical Areas (MSA). As in BPCI, cost savings could be distributed among providers through gainsharing. Similarly, healthcare organizations bear the risk of financial loss if they fail to meet the target price.

Despite its similarities to BPCI model 2, CJR experienced substantial criticism due to several key differences. Upon its implementation, CJR became the first bundle payment program to enforce a mandatory enrollment for 802 hospitals that fell within 67 MSA.[64] Less than 1 year into its implementation, CMS annulled its mandatory regulation for participation in 33 of the MSA.[65] In addition, CJR also became the first APM to link payments to the collection of quality metrics; therefore, hospitals are incentivized to meet quality thresholds in order to reap the benefits of the cost savings.[66] Those who failed to meet quality thresholds would suffer financial losses. As a safeguard, CMS did not require hospitals to bear risk during its first performance year.[64] Beginning in performance year two, a stop loss limit of 5% protected hospitals from suffering severe financial losses. By the third year of the initiative, the stop loss increased to 10% and 20% for years four and five. Similarly, a stop gain limit of 5% was implemented for the first and second years, 10% in the third year, and 20% for fourth and fifth years. The extra cost savings achieved over the stop gain limit would be recovered by CMS. Physicians were not allowed to serve as episode initiators for CJR. Physician-led BPCI episodes were the most cost-effective for CMS.

BPCI Advanced

In 2018, the BPCI initiative concluded and CMS announced the launch of BPCI Advanced, a new bundle payment model.[67] This is a voluntary model which was created to build upon the success and experiences of the previous BPCI initiative. Similar to BPCI, the primary objective of BPCI Advanced is to reduce the financial burden to CMS and improve patient quality of care. Additionally, BPCI Advanced will continue to be a voluntary risk-sharing model and target prices for episodes of care will be set by CMS prior to commencement. Gainsharing will continue to serve as an incentive for healthcare organizations and providers to continue to improve healthcare efficiency and quality.

However, several differences exist between BPCI and BPCI Advanced. BPCI Advanced is comprised of solely a single model which is similar to model 2 of BPCI. Although the post-acute care period continues to form a portion of the entire episode of care, it will now be 90-day standard for every participant; therefore, healthcare organizations will not be allowed to choose a 30-day or 60-day plan. Furthermore, payments will now be linked to the quality of care provided. Initially, there will be seven quality measures during the first 2 years following implementation of BPCI Advanced and thereafter CMS may choose to modify or add additional measures. Under BPCI Advanced, CMS intends to improve quality of care and the use of evidenced-based care by linking payments with these quality control measures. Institutions that do not meet the quality criteria established will suffer financial losses by requiring institutions to repay up to 10% of their reimbursements. Conversely, healthcare organizations that meet the quality criteria will be reimbursed up to an additional 10%. Another major difference is that the clinical episode categories have been decreased and now comprise of 3 outpatient and 29 inpatient episodes only. Inpatient episodes will be identified by MS-DRGs, while outpatient episodes will be identified by Healthcare Common Procedure Coding System (HCPCS). Furthermore, the episode of care will begin the moment a patient is admitted to an acute care hospital for inpatient episodes or following the commencement of an outpatient procedure as opposed to BPCI model 2's 72 hour prior to admission rule. The episode is designed to terminate 90 days following the discharge from the inpatient hospital stay or 90 days after the outpatient procedure. Additional incentives have been applied to BPCI Advanced including a 20% stop loss protection. This deflates the financial burden which may otherwise have severe implications to smaller, rural participating hospitals. This new model will now qualify as an advanced APM; thus, CMS will provide eligible participants with an additional 5% incentive.

CONCLUSION

Healthcare costs continue to grow across the spectrum of medicine; TKA is no exception. CMS has responded with the implementation of APM, which has incentivized healthcare institutions and providers to engage in cost saving measures to reduce healthcare costs, while also making them financially accountable for the quality of care. In response, healthcare institutions have integrated new evidence-based care initiatives, which have effectively reduced costs and at this time have maintained the quality of care. Furthermore, while the medical device industry continues to market new and unproven innovative technologies, healthcare providers and institutions have emphasized the utilization of medical devices with proven track records that align with value-based care. Technologic innovation for TKA care delivery will need to prove value creation before widespread adoption will occur.

REFERENCES

1. Kurtz S, Ong K, Lau E, Mowat F, Halpern M. Projections of primary and revision hip and knee arthroplasty in the United States from 2005 to 2030. *J Bone Joint Surg Am.* 2007;89(4):780-785. doi:10.2106/JBJS.F.00222.
2. Kurtz SM, Ong KL, Lau E, Bozic KJ. Impact of the economic downturn on total joint replacement demand in the United States: updated projections to 2021. *J Bone Joint Surg Am.* 2014;96(8):624-630. doi:10.2106/JBJS.M.00285.
3. Inacio MCS, Graves SE, Pratt NL, Roughead EE, Nemes S. Increase in total joint arthroplasty projected from 2014 to 2046 in Australia: a conservative local model with international implications. *Clin Orthop Relat Res.* 2017;475(8):2130-2137. doi:10.1007/s11999-017-5377-7.
4. Sanders TL, Kremers HM, Schleck CD, Larson DR, Berry DJ. Subsequent total joint arthroplasty after primary total knee or hip arthroplasty. *J Bone Joint Surg.* 2017;99:396-401. doi:10.2106/JBJS.16.00499.
5. Maradit Kremers H, Larson DR, Crowson CS, et al. Prevalence of total hip and knee replacement in the United States. *J Bone Joint Surg Am.* 2015;97(17):1386-1397. doi:10.2106/JBJS.N.01141.
6. Healy WL, Rana AJ, Iorio R. Hospital economics of primary total knee arthroplasty at a teaching hospital. *Clin Orthop Relat Res.* 2011;469(1):87-94. doi:10.1007/s11999-010-1486-2.
7. 2016 National Health Expidenture Fact Sheet. Baltimore, MD; 2018.
8. Suter LG, Paltiel AD, Rome BN, et al. Placing a price on medical device Innovation: the example of total knee arthroplasty. *PLoS One.* 2013;8(5):e62709. doi:10.1371/journal.pone.0062709.
9. BlueShield B. A Study of Cost Variations For Knee and Hip Replacement Surgeries in the U.S. Blue Health Intelligence. 2015. Available at https://www.bcbs.com/the-health-of-america/reports/study-of-cost-variations-knee-and-hip-replacement-surgeries-the-us. Accessed May 7, 2018.
10. Healy W, Iorio R, Ko J, Appleby D, David L. Impact of cost reduction programs on short-term patient outcome and hospital cost of total knee arthroplasty. 2002;84(3):348-353.
11. Iorio R, Healy WL, Kirven FM, Patch DA, Pfeifer BA. Knee implant standardization: an implant selection and cost reduction program. *Am J Knee Surg.* 1998;11(2):73-79.
12. Bosco JA, Alvarado CM, Slover JD, Iorio R, Hutzler LH. Decreasing total joint implant costs and physician specific cost variation through negotiation. *J Arthroplasty.* 2014;29(4):678-680. doi:10.1016/j.arth.2013.09.016.

13. Healy WL, Iorio R, Lemos MJ, et al. Single price/case price purchasing in orthopaedic surgery: experience at the Lahey Clinic. *J Bone Joint Surg.* 2000;82(5):607-612. Available at http://ovidsp.ovid.com/ovidweb.cgi?T=JS&PAGE=reference&D=emed5&NEWS=N&AN=2000248538. Accessed December 1, 2017.

14. Health C for D and R. 510(k) Clearances. Available at https://www.fda.gov/medicaldevices/productsandmedicalprocedures/deviceapprovalsandclearances/510kclearances/. Accessed August 13, 2018.

15. Hines JZ, Lurie P, Yu E, Wolfe S. Left to their own devices: breakdowns in United States medical device premarket review. *PLoS Med.* 2010;7(7):e1000280. doi:10.1371/journal.pmed.1000280.

16. Braithwaite RS, Col NF, Wong JB. Estimating hip fracture morbidity, mortality and costs. *J Am Geriatr Soc.* 2003;51(3):364-370. doi:10.1046/j.1532-5415.2003.51110.x.

17. Keeney JA. Innovations in total knee arthroplasty: improved technical precision, but unclear clinical benefits. *Orthopedics.* 2016;39(4):217-220. doi:10.3928/01477447-20160628-03.

18. Liow MHL, Goh GSH, Pang HN, Tay DKJ, Lo NN, Yeo SJ. Computer-assisted stereotaxic navigation improves the accuracy of mechanical alignment and component positioning in total knee arthroplasty. *Arch Orthop Trauma Surg.* 2016;136(8):1173-1180. doi:10.1007/s00402-016-2483-z.

19. Goh GSH, Liow MHL, Lim WSR, Tay DKJ, Yeo SJ, Tan MH. Accelerometer-based navigation is as accurate as optical computer navigation in restoring the joint line and mechanical axis after total knee arthroplasty. A prospective matched study. *J Arthroplasty.* 2016;31(1):92-97. doi:10.1016/j.arth.2015.06.048.

20. Lee G-C. Take what you read with a grain of salt: commentary on an article by Richard N. de Steiger, MBBS, FRACS, FAOrthA, et al.: "Computer navigation for total knee arthroplasty reduces revision rate for patients less than sixty-five years of age". *J Bone Joint Surg Am.* 2015;97(8):e40. doi:10.2106/JBJS.O.00133.

21. Burnett RSJ, Barrack RL. Computer-assisted total knee arthroplasty is currently of no proven clinical benefit: a systematic review knee. *Clin Orthop Relat Res.* 2013;471(1):264-276. doi:10.1007/s11999-012-2528-8.

22. Gøthesen Ø, Espehaug B, Havelin LI, et al. Functional outcome and alignment in computer-assisted and conventionally operated total knee replacements a multicentre parallel-group randomised controlled trial. *Bone Joint J.* 2014;96:609-618.

23. Choong PF, Dowsey MM, Stoney JD. Does accurate anatomical alignment result in better function and quality of life? Comparing conventional and computer-assisted total knee arthroplasty. *J Arthroplasty.* 2009;24(4):560-569. doi:10.1016/j.arth.2008.02.018.

24. Cheng T, Zhang G, Zhang X. Imageless navigation system does not improve component rotational alignment in total knee arthroplasty. *J Surg Res.* 2011;171(2):590-600. doi:10.1016/j.jss.2010.05.006.

25. Wasterlain AS, Buza JA, Thakkar SC, Schwarzkopf R, Vigdorchik J. Navigation and robotics in total hip arthroplasty. *JBJS Rev.* 2017;5(3):1-8. doi:10.2106/JBJS.RVW.16.00046.

26. De Steiger RN, Liu YL, Graves SE. Computer navigation for total knee arthroplasty reduces revision rate for patients less than sixty-five years of age. *J Bone Joint Surg Am.* 2015;97(8):635-642. doi:10.2106/JBJS.M.01496.

27. Licini DJ, Meneghini RM. Modern abbreviated computer navigation of the femur reduces blood loss in total knee arthroplasty. *J Arthroplasty.* 2015;30(10):1729-1732. doi:10.1016/j.arth.2015.04.020.

28. Beringer DC, Patel JJ, Bozic KJ. An overview of economic issues in computer-assisted total joint arthroplasty. *Clin Orthop Relat Res.* 2007;463:26-30. doi:10.1097/BLO.0b013e318154addd.

29. Siddiqi A, Hardaker WM, Eachempati KK, Sheth NP. Advances in computer-aided technology for total knee arthroplasty. *Orthopedics.* 2017;40:338-352.

30. Tedesco G, Faggiano FC, Leo E, Derrico P, Ritrovato M. A comparative cost analysis of robotic-assisted surgery versus laparoscopic surgery and open surgery: the necessity of investing knowledgeably. *Surg Endosc.* 2016;30:5044-5051.

31. Moschetti WE, Konopka JF, Rubash HE, Genuario JW. Can robot-assisted unicompartmental knee arthroplasty be cost-effective? A Markov decision analysis. *J Arthroplasty.* 2016;31(4):759-765. doi:10.1016/j.arth.2015.10.018.

32. Bellemans J, Vandenneucker H, Vanlauwe J. Robot-assisted total knee arthroplasty. *Clin Orthop Relat Res.* 2007;464:111-116. doi:10.1097/BLO.0b013e318126c0c0.

33. Stranges E, Russo A, Friedman B. Procedures with the most rapidly increasing hospital costs, 2004-2007. *Value Heal.* 2010;13(3):A89. doi:10.1016/S1098-3015(10)72424-4.

34. Nwachukwu BU, McCormick F, Provencher MT, Roche M, Rubash HE. A comprehensive analysis of medicare trends in utilization and hospital economics for total knee and hip arthroplasty from 2005 to 2011. *J Arthroplasty.* 2015;30(1):15-18. doi:10.1016/j.arth.2014.08.025.

35. Culler SD, Jevsevar DS, Shea KG, McGuire KJ, Wright KK, Simon AW. The incremental hospital cost and length-of-stay associated with treating adverse events among medicare beneficiaries undergoing THA during fiscal year 2013. *J Arthroplasty.* 2016;31(1):42-48. doi:10.1016/j.arth.2015.07.037.

36. Skillman M, Cross-Barnet C, Singer RF, et al. Physician engagement strategies in care coordination: findings from the Centers for Medicare & Medicaid Services' Health Care Innovation Awards Program. *Health Serv Res.* 2017;52(1):291-312. doi:10.1111/1475-6773.12622.

37. Piccinin MA, Sayeed Z, Kozlowski R, Bobba V, Knesek D, Frush T. Bundle payment for musculoskeletal care: current evidence (Part 2). *Orthop Clin North Am.* 2018;49(2):147-156. doi:10.1016/j.ocl.2017.11.003.

38. CMS. About the CMS innovation center. Innov Cent. 2015:1-5. Available at http://innovation.cms.gov/About/index.html. Accessed December 1, 2017.

39. Services C for M and M. Centers for Medicare and Medicaid Services Bundled Payments for Care Improvement (BPCI) Initiative: General Information. Available at http://innovation.cms.gov/initiatives/bundled-payments/index.html. Accessed September 7, 2018.

40. Dundon JM, Bosco J, Slover J, Yu S, Sayeed Y, Iorio R. Improvement in total joint replacement quality metrics. *J Bone Joint Surg.* 2016;98(23):1949-1953. doi:10.2106/JBJS.16.00523.

41. Curtin BM, Russell RD, Odum SM. Bundled payments for care improvement: boom or bust? *J Arthroplasty.* 2017;32(10):2931-2934. doi:10.1016/j.arth.2017.05.011.

42. Greenwald AS, Bassano A, Wiggins S, et al. Alternative reimbursement models: bundled payment and beyond: AOA critical issues. *J Bone Joint Surg Am.* 2016;98(11):e45. doi:10.2106/JBJS.15.01174.

43. Froimson MI, Rana A, White RE, et al. Bundled payments for care improvement initiative: the next evolution of payment formulations. AAHKS bundled payment task force. *J Arthroplasty.* 2013;28(8):157-165. doi:10.1016/J.ARTH.2013.07.012.

44. Siddiqi A, White PB, Mistry JB, et al. Effect of bundled payments and health care reform as alternative payment models in total joint arthroplasty: a clinical review. *J Arthroplasty.* 2017;32(8):2590-2597. doi:10.1016/j.arth.2017.03.027.

45. Iorio R, Clair AJ, Inneh IA, Slover JD, Bosco JA, Zuckerman JD. Early results of medicare's bundled payment initiative for a 90-day total joint arthroplasty episode of care. *J Arthroplasty.* 2016;31(2):343-350. doi:10.1016/j.arth.2015.09.004.

46. Althausen PL, Mead L. Bundled payments for care improvement. *J Orthop Trauma.* 2016;30(12):S50-S53. doi:10.1097/BOT.0000000000000715.

47. Preston JS, Caccavale D, Smith A, Stull LE, Harwood DA, Kayiaros S. Bundled payments for care improvement in the private sector: a win for everyone. *J Arthroplasty.* 2018;33(8):2362-2367. doi:10.1016/j.arth.2018.03.007.

48. Anoushiravani AA, Iorio R. Alternative payment models: from bundled payments for care improvement and comprehensive care for joint replacement to the future? *Semin Arthroplasty.* 2016;27(3):151-162. doi:10.1053/j.sart.2016.10.002.

49. Iorio R. Strategies and tactics for successful implementation of bundled payments: bundled payment for care improvement at a large, urban, academic medical center. *J Arthroplasty.* 2015;30(3):349-350. doi:10.1016/j.arth.2014.12.031.

50. Chandra A, Dalton MA, Holmes J. Large increases in spending on postacute care in medicare point to the potential for cost savings in these settings. *Health Aff.* 2013;32(5):864-872. doi:10.1377/hlthaff.2012.1262.

51. Froemke CC, Wang L, DeHart ML, Williamson RK, Ko LM, Duwelius PJ. Standardizing care and improving quality under a bundled payment initiative for total joint arthroplasty. *J Arthroplasty.* 2015;30(10):1676-1682. doi:10.1016/j.arth.2015.04.028.

52. Whellan DJ, Ellis SJ, Kraus WE, et al. Large increases in spending on postacute care in Medicare point to the potential for cost savings in these settings. 2013;151(6):414-420. doi:10.1097/CCM.0b013e31823e986a.A.

53. Quick RC, Kwolek CJ, Minion DJ. Surveillance venous duplex is not clinically useful after total joint arthroplasty when effective deep venous thrombosis prophylaxis is used. *Ann Vasc Surg.* 2004;18(2):193-198.

54. Kocher MS, Erens G, Thornhill TS, Ready JE. Cost and effectiveness of routine pathological examination of operative specimens obtained during primary total hip and knee replacement in patients with osteoarthritis. *J Bone Joint Surg Am.* 2000;82(11):1531-1535.

55. Healy WL, Finn D. The hospital cost and the cost of the implant for total knee arthroplasty. A comparison between 1983 and 1991 for one hospital. *J Bone Joint Surg Am.* 1994;76:801-806. doi:10.1378/chest.13-2340.

56. Healy WL, Iorio R, Richards JA, Lucchesi C. Opportunities for control of hospital costs for total joint arthroplasty after initial cost containment. *J Arthroplasty.* 1998;13(5):504-507. doi:10.1016/S0883-5403(98)90048-1.

57. Healy WL, Ayers ME, Iorio R, Patch DA, Appleby D, Pfeifer BA. Impact of a clinical pathway and implant standardization on total hip arthroplasty: a clinical and economic study of short-term patient outcome. *J Arthroplasty.* 1998;13(3):266-276. doi:10.1016/S0883-5403(98)90171-1.

58. Duellman TJ, Gaffigan C, Milbrandt JC, Allan DG. Multi-modal, pre-emptive analgesia decreases the length of hospital stay following total joint arthroplasty. *Orthopedics.* 2009;32(3):167.

59. Mor V, Intrator O, Feng Z, Grabowski DC. The revolving door of rehospitalization from skilled nursing facilities. *Health Aff.* 2010;29(1):57-64. doi:10.1377/hlthaff.2009.0629.

60. Bosco JA, Karkenny AJ, Hutzler LH, Slover JD, Iorio R. Cost burden of 30-day readmissions following Medicare total hip and knee arthroplasty. *J Arthroplasty.* 2014;29(5):903-905. doi:10.1016/j.arth.2013.11.006.

61. Luzzi AJ, Fleischman AN, Matthews CN, Crizer MP, Wilsman J, Parvizi J. The "bundle busters": incidence and costs of postacute complications following total joint arthroplasty. *J Arthroplasty.* 2018;33(9):2734-2739. doi:10.1016/j.arth.2018.05.015.

62. Bhandari M, Smith J, Miller LE, Block JE. Clinical and economic burden of revision knee arthroplasty. *Clin Med Insights Arthritis Musculoskelet Disord.* 2012;5:89-94. doi:10.4137/CMAMD.S10859.

63. Courtney PM, Ashley BS, Hume EL, Kamath AF. Are bundled payments a viable reimbursement model for revision total joint arthroplasty? *Clin Orthop Relat Res.* 2016;474(12):2714-2721. doi:10.1007/s11999-016-4953-6.

64. Services C for M and M. Comprehensive Care for Joint Replacement Model | Center for Medicare and Medicaid Innovation. Available at https://innovation.cms.gov/initiatives/cjr. Accessed August 3, 2018.

65. Center for Medicare and Medicaid Services. CMS finalizes changes to the Comprehensive Care for Joint Replacement Model, cancels Episode Payment Models and Cardiac Rehabilitation Incentive Payment Model | CMS. Available at https://www.cms.gov/newsroom/press-releases/cms-finalizes-changes-comprehensive-care-joint-replacement-model-cancels-episode-payment-models-and. Accessed August 28, 2018.

66. Services C for M and M. Comprehensive Care for Joint Replacement Model | Center for Medicare & Medicaid Innovation Frequently asked questions. Available at https://innovation.cms.gov/initiatives/cjr. Accessed August 28, 2018.

67. Services C for M and M. BPCI Advanced. Available at https://innovation.cms.gov/initiatives/bpci-advanced. Accessed July 10, 2018.

chapter 28

Indications for Total Knee Arthroplasty

Alex J. Sadauskas, MD | Brett R. Levine, MD, MS

INTRODUCTION

Total knee arthroplasty (TKA) has been a mainstay for treating end-stage arthritic changes of the knee for decades and continues to grow in numbers worldwide. However, just because there have been improvements in polyethylene wear, success rates, and overall outcomes with TKA, it is only with stringent indications that such outstanding results can be achieved and improved upon. John Insall has written that, "It goes without saying that to warrant knee joint replacement, symptoms and disability must be severe. Patients who have had an unsatisfactory arthroplasty naturally gravitate to surgeons whose expertise lies in that area, and I have seen cases in which the selection of the original operation was questionable.[1]" Therefore, despite TKA being a revolutionary procedure for orthopedic surgeons and patients, it remains important to maintain appropriate and stringent indications and patient selection criteria. This becomes even more relevant in modern times, in which outpatient and short-stay knee arthroplasty may require a higher level of risk stratification and greater scrutiny of indications/optimization to attain the same degree of success.

Degenerative joint disease of the knee secondary to osteoarthritis is a common, costly, and disabling disease that impacts greater than 10% of individuals older than 60 years.[2] Osteoarthritis of the knee has been associated with worsening of quality-of-life (QoL) measures and has been associated with depressive symptoms when the pain is not adequately controlled.[2] While pain is a significant determining factor when indicating a patient for a knee arthroplasty, recently it has been shown that those reporting less pain and more advanced stages of radiographic osteoarthritis (Kellgren and Lawrence scores) had better functional and pain outcomes after TKA.[3] The concept of a clear clinical picture will resonate throughout this chapter, where there will be significant emphasis placed on indicating patients with a clinical, radiographical, and functional picture that corroborates the severity of disease in the knee. It is when these "moons align" that we stand the best chance for an optimal outcome with our patients.

Despite outstanding survivorship being reported at 20 years, there remains a dissatisfaction rate that has been reported to be as high as 17% to 41% after TKA.[4]

Being able to predict complications and satisfaction has been the focus of a tremendous amount of current research with several scoring systems being developed in the last decade. While some of these predictive scores have shown success, there is no widely accepted or validated scoring system that is being used to help indicate or contraindicate patients for TKA surgery at this time. Along with predictions tools, expectation management will be reviewed in light of indicating a good candidate for TKA. Expectation mismatch can occur on behalf of both the surgeon and the patient. It is important to align expectations adequately prior to surgery to avoid falling short of the perceived benefits of TKA and adding to the dissatisfied pool of patients.

With more than 700,000 TKAs being performed annually in the United States, it is important to follow a balanced algorithm to indicate patients for surgery as this burden is expected to increase to between 935,000 and 1.25 million by 2030.[5] Understanding predictive models, expectation management, and patient-related considerations as outlined in this chapter should afford a high rate of successful surgical outcomes. Identifying contraindications to TKA and optimizing patients may help fuel the concept of "cherry-growing" to replace that of the less well-received notion of "cherry-picking." In the end, it is imperative to maintain a team approach between the patient/family, orthopedic team, and primary care physicians so that appropriate indications for TKA are maintained and the limitations and risks of the procedure fully understood. Working together will allow us to achieve the greatest levels of success and open the door further for short-stay and outpatient indications for TKA.

DEFINING INDICATIONS

TKA is a unique procedure in orthopedic surgery since it is a completely elective surgery. This means the clinician must define the parameters for who may or may not be indicated for this optional (non–life-threatening conditions) operation. The literature has indicated that individuals' expectations play role in patient satisfaction postoperatively. In order to mitigate patient dissatisfaction, a clinician should have a general guideline in defining candidates for TKA. The primary indication for TKA is pain, with secondary factors being knee instability and decreasing range of motion or contracture development. The biggest issue with this is that pain is based wholly on a patient's perception; in other words, it is subjective and varies greatly from patient to patient. In order to try decrease this subjective nature in the surgical decision-making process, other parameters, such as severity of radiographic findings and response to nonoperative treatment modalities, have been found to supplement the complaint of pain.[6]

Radiographic imaging is an excellent surrogate to depict an objective level of arthritic changes occurring around the knee. Unfortunately, imaging alone cannot be used as an indication for TKA. The level of arthritic changes seen radiographically does not always correlate with clinical presentation, but imaging does provide confirmation for suspected arthritis if both examinations corroborate the diagnosis. In addition, patients with arthritic knee pain should undergo extensive nonoperative management before proceeding with surgical treatment. Any relief with nonoperative treatment would not only help verify the pain originating from the affected joint, but it would also provide temporary pain reduction while further treatment options are explored.

GOALS OF TOTAL KNEE ARTHROPLASTY

The goals of TKA are to relieve pain, restore function, and improve the patient's quality of life. To achieve these primary objectives, patients must undergo thorough evaluation to confirm the correction of arthritis will alleviate their discomfort. Patients should also have a clear understanding of all the risks and limitations associated with the surgery. While severe flexion contractures may show some relief with TKA, realistic expectations on postoperative range of motion should be understood. After TKA, knee function does improve by decreasing the pain associated with many movements. This permits activities of daily life to be performed relatively painlessly and improves the overall quality of life. It does not, however, restore the patient's knee back to a normal native knee, and this limitation has to be considered when discussing goals of the surgery with the patient. In fact, with setting goals, there are some good data on sporting activity recommendations post TKA that patients can be referred to both online and in the current literature.[7]

PATIENT SELECTION

Who Is a Candidate for Knee Arthroplasty

Individuals suffering from chronic knee pain, functional limitations, or a combination of the two are the best candidates to explore TKA as a potential treatment option. In general, individuals older than 60 years are better candidates due to lower postoperative expectations and diminished requirements for more intense activities. In addition, knee prostheses have a finite survivorship, so

younger individuals will likely require one if not two revision procedures from the daily "wear and tear" depending on how young they are at the time of surgery. TKA candidates must undergo a proper evaluation to make sure their medical history, physical examination, and radiographic findings are consistent, and the pain may be relieved and expectations met by TKA. Physicians should also be aware of any relative and absolute contraindications (see section below), so potential candidates could be appropriately excluded from TKA or better optimized to become a future surgical candidate.

When to Proceed with Knee Arthroplasty

Patients should proceed with TKA when they have met two criteria. First, they must be deemed appropriate candidates for the procedure. Second, they must have attempted and exhausted nonoperative treatment for the degenerative changes in their knee(s).[6]

Outpatient Patient Selection

Over the past 5 to 10 years, there has been a shift in focus on cost containment within our health care system. Among the biggest factors dictating the significant cost of TKAs are hospital length of stay and discharge to skilled facilities after surgery. In order to mitigate these costs, outpatient or "same-day" TKA became a popular trend among joint surgeons, taking place within hospitals and free-standing surgical centers. Though this new trend decreases the overall cost of the surgery, there are serious risks with TKA operations that must not be overlooked, and careful patient selection is necessary. There is no consensus at this time, but it is imperative that physicians adopt strong screening guidelines to select suitable patients for outpatient TKA procedures.

Currently, there lacks a significant amount of literature looking at outpatient, or less than 24-hour stay, TKA. One study by Sibia et al found that older, female patients with a history of atrial fibrillation or prior TKA on the contralateral side tended to stay in hospitals longer than their counterparts after TKA.[8] Furthermore, patients with American Society of Anesthesiologists score of 3 to 4 or patients who could not ambulate the day of the TKA demonstrated a longer recovery time compared to patients without these issues. Several other studies confirmed age, gender, presence of atrial fibrillation, and preoperative ambulation status correlated with increased length of stay after the procedure.[9-12] Contrary to this, an elevated body mass index (BMI) has surprisingly not been shown to increase the stay postoperatively.

Another study by Meneghini et al constructed an Outpatient Arthroplasty Risk Assessment (OARA) score to help identify individuals appropriate for outpatient total joint arthroplasty (TJA).[13] They utilized the expertise of a high-volume arthroplasty surgeon and a perioperative internist to risk stratify patients into low-moderate risk (score ≤ 59) and not appropriate for early discharge (score ≥ 60). Previously, the main classification systems used for TKA safety were ASA-PS (American Society of Anesthesiologists Physical Status Classification System) and CCI (Charlson Comorbidity Index). The former, ASA-PS, was a screening tool created by anesthesiologists to determine operative risk, but studies have shown great variability among physician-attributed scores compromising the effectiveness of the system.[14] The latter, CCI, has been effective in predicting 1-year patient mortality, but it does not specifically account for severity of symptoms. This causes the scale to lose much credibility for predicting candidates for outpatient TKA procedures.[15] The OARA score was specifically created for determining who can safely undergo outpatient or short-stay TKA. It takes in to consideration comorbidities relevant to TJA and has already been utilized successfully with over 2000 patients.[16] This updated study reported a 100% positive predictive value and 98.8% specificity for predicting patients that are candidates for outpatient surgery if there OARA score is between 0 and 79.

As more studies looking at outpatient patient selection criteria surface, guidelines for the selection process will continue being refined in order to balance all the risks and benefits of proceeding with an outpatient TKA.

Outcomes Prediction Tools

In order to cut health care costs, bundled payment and pay-for-performance models have become increasingly popular among orthopedic surgeons.[17-19] With such payment models, readmissions, reoperations, and discharge to skilled facilities are additional expenses, leading physicians to be more selective in choosing candidates for elective procedures, such as TKA. In order to prevent physicians and practices from taking the brunt of the financial burden, tools to anticipate the satisfaction in TKA patients postoperatively are essential. Since this economic shift in health care is relatively new, only a few of these outcome predictive tools exist. Additionally, it only seems rationale that if we can predict which patients will be the most satisfied and have the least complications one can work to optimize outcomes. Further, those at higher risk for complications or being dissatisfied can be counseled or optimized to educate them on how to improve their candidacy for surgery. After all, TKA should be a partnership between the physician and patient, with, both parties having to work on their end to achieve high levels of success.

The earliest TKA satisfaction predictive tool by Van Onsem et al consisted of a survey with 10 patient-answered questions.[20] This survey showed high sensitivity and positive predictive value internally, but two independent, external studies were unable to validate the predictiveness of the survey.[21,22] The discrepancies found

between studies exhibit the difficulty in finding an appropriate, outcome prediction tool. In addition, the survey by Van Onsem contained only nonmodifiable risk factors, which prevent any potential patient optimization. Kunze et al recently published an 11-question survey with eight of the questions consisting of modifiable risk factors.[23] This would allow for patient optimization before TKA if the patient did not meet the initial satisfactory threshold for the surgery. It is crucial that all factors be considered to further work on better prediction models so that we work to not limit the access to care but rather, increase the likelihood of a successful TKA outcome.

With patient satisfaction being paramount to medicine, outcome prediction tools should continue being studied and utilized preoperatively to help limit complications and achieve the best results possible for all TKA patients. It is also vital to understand that while patient-reported outcomes are an important measure, one has to consider the whole picture including radiographic follow-up as these may be predictive of failure even in a patient that is doing well score-wise.

Other Available Options

For certain patients, TKA may not be the best option. Patients with chronic pain, that may not be purely related to the knee joint itself, should consider going to a pain clinic for alternative options to treat their pain, since TKA may not resolve their symptoms. Patients with severe rheumatoid arthritis should consider rheumatologic treatment before proceeding with TKA. There also exist several alterative surgical procedures to TKA including osteotomy, unicompartmental arthroplasty, and arthrodesis. The procedures each have their own risks and benefits, which should be carefully weighed before to proceeding with any of these surgeries.

Osteotomy of the knee is appropriate in early degenerative joint disease in patients who have maintained full range of motion and good knee stability. The goal of this procedure is to redirect the weight-bearing portion of the joint from an area of degenerated cartilage to healthy, intact cartilage. Unicompartmental arthroplasty is appropriate for individuals with isolated medial or lateral arthritis without ligamentous instability, inflammatory arthritis, and minimal patellofemoral disease. Arthrodesis of the knee is rarely indicated (young, heavy laborer is the typical candidate) but remains an option for individuals with contraindications to TKA, such as active sepsis.

SETTING EXPECTATIONS

Surgeon Expectations

It is safe to say that in regards to TKA, surgeons have several expectations, but in the end, it boils down to, if I put the knee in correctly and it is well-fixed, then I would "expect" a successful outcome. Within these expectations are the inherent assumptions that patients will follow the physical therapy orders, work hard, wean off their pain medications, be compliant with venous thromboembolism (VTE) prophylaxis, follow-up at appropriate time intervals, and be invested in their own care and outcome. However, in the editor's spotlight by Dr Leopold, these assumptions are challenged as he posed the following question, "But is it possible that experienced surgeons have a no-better-than-chance likelihood of anticipating whether a patient undergoing one of the most common operations orthopedic surgeons perform—TKA—will improve enough to say the procedure is worthwhile?"[24] It was the study by Ghomrawi et al that spurred the asking of this question as their prospective study of eight high-volume orthopedic surgeons showed that for TKA, surgeon expectation scores were not accurate in predicting who would improve after surgery.[25] This is why it is critical that scoring systems are developed to help predict who will benefit from TKA so that surgeons are not just relying on a feeling or hunch that this patient is a good candidate for surgery and they will fulfill our ultimate expectations.

In this modern era of digital technology, it would seem that communication of a surgeon's expectations could occur via numerous modalities prior to surgery in order to make sure that the patient was clear on what was "expected" of them. It is also clear that surgeons are aware of this need as most have turned to total joint classes, handbooks, digital applications, establishing a coach, wearable devices, etc., to reach out to patients and try to set expectations.

With patient-reported outcomes being tied to reimbursement, there is an even greater push to make sure all parties are on the same page and meeting expectations. Making sure your expectations are clear to a patient will take time and communication, which is in direct contrast to the modern practice of being a high-volume surgeon. However, patients often want to please their doctor and show them that they are recovering well, so using tools that set goals and remind patients that they are ahead or behind can be quite valuable in furthering this relationship. Gautreau recently came up with a surgeon–patient communication checklist for TKA that may offer an alternative avenue for patients and doctors to set expectations and goals for one another that are clear and well contrived.[26] In the end, this will likely improve satisfaction and help with the reduction in dissatisfied patients (as this stands at ~20% currently).

Patient Expectations

While neither of the authors has had a TKA, it seems safe to say that reasonable patient expectations after TKA can be summarized as a reduction in knee pain, improved knee function, the ability to perform ADLs, restoration of disturbed sleep pattern, and the ability to return to some sporting activities. These are clearly attainable expectations but are by no stretch of the imagination the same as having no pain, restoring the ability to perform activities that they could do when they were younger but have not done in years, curing ailments in other locations, and being able to perform high-impact activities. If a patient was limited by spinal pathology or a remote condition from the knee, this will likely continue to limit them after a TKA and they should not anticipate returning to a higher level of function than this limiting factor. Additionally, there are no guarantees with surgery, and patients should understand their risk profile and the amount of work it will take to achieve their goals. If not there may be a failure to meet expectations and ultimately a dissatisfied patient. Another consideration is the timeframe for recovery as many are swayed by the fact that TKA is being performed as an outpatient, that this must be an easy and quick recovery. A recent study suggests that 1 year may be too short to be considered the final recovery and that physical and psychological support may be necessary to strive toward achieving a silent knee.[27]

Lützner et al reported on a prospective randomized controlled trial (RCT) including 103 patients at 5 years after surgery.[28] They found that a higher knee score and fulfillment of expectations were correlated with higher satisfaction. Therefore it is critical to establish realistic expectations for each individual patient along with the timeframe at which they can anticipate recovery. The authors tend to take a harder line on these expectations, painting a difficult and relatively painful road to recovery. This often leads to patients overestimating the recovery, rather than being surprised by what it takes to reach full strength. We would rather have the patient state that was easier than I expected, than say I didn't expect the recovery to be so hard. There is clearly a psychological nature to expectations, and it is important to incorporate this into your practice of indicating patients for surgery.

The last aspect of expectations includes the durability and longevity of TKA components. Patients should understand the importance of long-term follow-up and that a TKA will not last forever. The better they treat it (low-impact activity, maintaining a fit lifestyle, and regular follow-up), the longer it will likely last them. Modifying activities to keep them in the low-impact range can lead to excellent long-term survivorship. Abusing the knee by running, jumping, and high-impact activities will lead to a shorter lifespan of the replacement and revision surgery. While TKAs are currently expected to last 15 to 20 years, it is important after 10 years to make sure patients return for follow-up as wear may be relatively asymptomatic until it is "too late." The authors like to set the expectation for follow-up prior to the initial surgery, so it is clear that the patient will assume responsibility for their joint replacement and remember to take care of it over time. Putting this out on the table early helps the patient and surgeon determine if they are truly ready for a TKA or should other treatment options be explored.

PREOPERATIVE ASSESSMENT

It is important to remember, that every TKA candidate will present with a unique medical and orthopedic history, physical examination findings, and radiographic imaging results. Below represents some of the common complaints and findings found in a typical TKA candidate but is certainly not all encompassing. While not completely pathognomonic for end-stage knee degenerative changes, there are several commonalities found in TKA candidates. A recent consensus study from Germany came up with five core indication criteria for TKA[29]:

1. Intermittent or constant pain for a minimum of 3 to 6 months
2. Correlating knee radiographs that show structural damage (osteonecrosis or degenerative joint disease)
3. Failure of nonoperative measures (pharmacological and nonpharmacological) to provide relief after at least 3 to 6 months of trialing
4. Negative impact on the patient's quality of life for at least 3 to 6 months
5. Patient-reported impairment due to the knee pain/condition

History

The most common complaint in TKA-eligible individuals is worsening knee pain in the affected joint that has been impacting their quality of life. This pain should be further defined based on location, timing of symptoms, and specific aggravating factors. Usually the knee pain is fairly localized early on in the pathological process, but end-stage arthritic pain can elicit pain referred several centimeters superior and inferior to the actual knee. Complaints of anterior thigh, groin, or foot pain are all indications of pathologies that are likely separate from the knee and require a thorough adjacent joint assessment. Anterior thigh and groin pain point to potential hip pathologies, while radicular pain should be suspected with complaints of pain radiating down the leg below the knee. Often the patient notes worsening knee and stiffness pain during the day and with activity, but as the arthritis progresses, the pain can persist throughout the night and at rest. If the patient complains of sudden-onset knee pain that constantly hurts and responds minimally to nonoperative treatment or night pain, the physician should have some degree of suspicion for joint sepsis or a local tumor (bone or soft tissue).

If knee pain occurs mostly with activity, specific movements and functional disability caused by the pain should be determined. In addition, the physician should work with the patient to elicit the value in continuing these activities in the future, for example, continuing to ski black diamond runs, playing full court basketball games, etc. This can help determine the appropriate treatment path, as if the activities the patient wants to return to are not compatible with what a TKA will provide, this may limit their candidacy for the procedure. All other aggravating factors for the knee pain should be elicited as well as how much this impacts crucial activities important to that specific patient. Some important factors to inquire about are the ability to perform activities of daily life such as cleaning, driving, stair climbing, personal hygiene, and sleeping. After obtaining a good baseline understanding of what the ultimate activity goals are, the physician can determine how suitable TKA is at the time (refer to expectations section, above).

Previous operative treatment to the affected knee and any nonoperative intervention for the knee pain are critical components of the history to elucidate. Any prior operative treatment could alter the decision and approach used in TKA, so operative reports should be obtained if accessible. Additionally, prior surgical procedures may give information regarding the integrity and presence of the cruciate ligaments as well as degenerative findings in all compartments of the knee (may be important when deciding on anterior cruciate ligament (ACL)/ posterior cruciate ligament (PCL) retaining knees or unicompartmental knee arthroplasties [UKAs]). Nonoperative treatment can be broken into three different arenas: lifestyle management, pharmaceutical treatment, and interventional treatment. In lifestyle management, alterations in weight should be determined as this could alter the progression of the arthritic changes. Next, pharmaceutical treatment for pain or inflammation should be included in the history. Common pharmaceuticals include nonsteroidal anti-inflammatories and acetaminophen. Opioids should not be provided for the management of degenerative changes to the knee as this may make controlling postoperative pain more difficult.[30] AAOS clinical practice guidelines further recommend against opioid use since there is a lack of conclusive evidence exhibiting any benefits of opioids in the setting of knee osteoarthritis. Lastly, interventional treatment focused on prior physical therapy and knee injections should be elicited. The most recent injection, especially with corticosteroids, is important to determine since that could alter the scheduling of the TKA (potentially 6-week to 6-month delay).[25,26,31,32] Furthermore, if an appropriate response is not found after an injection, it may be prudent to investigate other sources of the patient's perceived knee pain. In general, all appropriate nonoperative measures should be attempted and determined to no longer be providing adequate pain relief and restoration of function before undergoing TKA.

The previous points have all mainly focused on the orthopedic history directly relating to the knee, but it is important not to have tunnel vision and dismiss pertinent medical history. Any adverse reactions to medications, specifically prophylactic antibiotics, are essential to determine to avoid potential surgical complications. Knowing any hereditary bleeding disorders or abnormal propensity toward clotting can further help prevent issues during and after the procedure. Comorbidities, such as diabetes, high BMI, and lower back pain, have lower outcome scores postoperatively and higher potential risks, so all comorbidities should be recorded at the initial patient visit.[33] In addition, inflammatory arthritis may need to be considered as a potential cause of the knee pathology if a relevant history is present. If the patient has an inflammatory arthropathy, all disease-modifying antirheumatic drugs (DMARDs), affected joints, systemic manifestations, as well as preoperative range of motion should be documented. Interestingly, Kobayashi et al determined that inflammatory arthritis patient satisfaction improves after TKA greater than those with osteoarthritis even though their functional activity remains lower overall.[34] Bleeding disorders, comorbidities, inflammatory arthritis, and DMARDs are important history points to cover for each TKA candidate, and there are numerous other confounding issues that should be explored on a case-by-case basis (see contraindications section below). The patient history gives invaluable information about the pathological process, but it is only the first of three prongs in determining whether or not the patient is an appropriate candidate for TKA.

Physical Examination

Physical examination should focus on overall gait, skin inspection, palpation of the joint, neurovascular status, range of motion, and ligamentous stability of the knee and adjacent joints.

An antalgic gait is common, and any excessive valgus or varus deformity should be noted particularly if leads to a medial or lateral thrust. Furthermore, a Trendelenburg gait can suggest the presence of hip pathology, which could be a source of referred pain to the knee. The foot should be assessed to look for excessive pronation or supination that can contribute to worsening standing alignment of the knee. Often the foot can accentuate a limb deformity at the knee and on occasion may need to be corrected prior to knee surgery. It is important to watch your patient ambulate, and this is often the first aspect of the physical examination you will notice as they stand up to move to introduce themselves. The act of standing up from the chair (or inability to do so) and how they initially move would be telling how limited the patient actually is.

Next, the skin around the knee should be inspected for any active lesions, prior incisions, or other abnormalities. Some lesions may even point to the cause of arthritis, as is the case with psoriatic arthritis. All active skin lesions around the knee should be closely monitored, since surgical intervention in the presence of such lesions is associated with high rate of postoperative infection.[35] Typically, standard arthroscopy portal scars can be ignored, yet open procedures about the knee must be respected and if possible to incorporate these scars (particularly if wide and associated with immobile skin) into the TKA incision.

If there are multiple incisions, try to use the lateral most incision to gain access to the knee joint.

Palpation of the joint should follow in order to determine where there is tenderness around the knee joint and will be used to assess consistency with other findings of the preliminary examinations. Though knee tenderness can occur diffusely throughout the joint in the setting of arthritis, specific areas of tenderness can help surgeons decide the appropriate surgical treatment. Most commonly, anterior knee and peripatellar pain can indicate the need for patellar resurfacing, since not all surgeons routinely perform this during TKA. Additionally, patella stability and apprehensive nature of lateral pressure on the patella should be assessed and noted. Once tenderness has been assessed, a neurovascular examination should begin with palpation of dorsalis pedis and posterior tibial pulses. Abnormal pulses could indicate vascular disease, which could limit tourniquet use during TKA, as well as a preoperative vascular consultation. Preoperative neurological deficits should be noted so that any incidental neurological damage occurring during the procedure could be clearly denoted.

Lastly, the range of motion and any ligamentous abnormalities should be evaluated. Range of motion is imperative to measure, since most times preoperative range of motion is predictive of postoperative range of motion.[36-38] Furthermore, any flexion contracture or extensor lag should be clearly measured and recorded, as should recurvatum (this may impact the procedure, i.e., performed and implants needed). Patients often have a misconception that they are guaranteed to regain lost motion after TKA, so the physician should attempt to clarify this fallacy preoperatively. The discussion should estimate ±10° range of motion from what they initially have in the office (more or less may depend on the intensity or lack thereof with postoperative physical therapy). After assessing the range of motion, ligamentous stability should be tested to confirm intact medial collateral ligament (MCL), lateral collateral ligament (LCL), PCL, and ACL, as well as any varus or valgus deformities that could be flexible and can be corrected preoperatively. It is important to note physical examination findings in correlation with the history provided and ultimately the radiographs that are obtained to make sure the pain and symptom pattern are consistent.

In addition to examining the knees, the physician should do an assessment of the back as well as the hips since pain can often be referred to the knee from these areas. Using the information from the patient history as well as the physical examination, the physician should move on to the third and final prong for determining the appropriate TKA candidate—radiographic analysis.

Radiograph Evaluation

Radiographic imaging is quintessential for confirming the arthritic etiology of the knee pain. It is important to note that some studies show little correlation between the severity of arthritic changes and initial clinical symptoms.[39] Due to this, imaging alone cannot be used as a reliable surgical candidacy determinant. However, the worse the degenerative disease is radiographically, the earlier the patient will typically feel better postoperatively.[40] Alternatively, if imaging shows no arthritic changes, a different diagnosis should be considered as TKA may not be indicated for such a patient.

The traditional radiographic views obtained for suspected knee arthritis include standing anteroposterior, Rosenberg (skier's view/flexed PA radiograph), lateral, and patellofemoral (Merchant or sunrise) views (**Fig. 28-1**).[41] The anteroposterior view must be standing to allow for observation of joint space narrowing under physiological conditions. An anteroposterior radiograph with the knee flexed exposes any joint space narrowing in the posterior aspect of the femur, which is difficult to observe on any other view. The lateral view shows any osteophytes or subchondral cysts at the posterior aspect of the affected knee. The patellofemoral view depicts any arthritic changes associated with the patella as well as patella tracking. This is important since some surgeons may opt out of patellar resurfacing if the patella is minimally affected. A full limb length radiograph can be utilized to determine mechanical axis deviations, other bony deformities, as well as a quick look at changes in the patient's hips and ankles. Bone

defects, quality, and abnormalities should be looked for as this could impact the surgical candidacy of the patient and/or the implants that may be required for the procedure.

After obtaining the appropriate views, the pathognomonic signs of arthritis are joint space narrowing, subchondral cysts, subchondral sclerosis, and the presence of osteophytes.[42] The Kellgren-Lawrence Classification System helped standardize the description of the osteoarthritis by creating a 0 to 4 grading scale. This scale allows clinicians to grade the knee in a simplified manner from 0 (no osteoarthritis present) to 4 (severe osteoarthritis present).[42] The K-L classification system was used as one of the scoring criteria in a recently published predictive outcome scale for patient satisfaction after TKA.[23] In general, radiographic evidence helps confirm the arthritic process, but it should not be used as the sole screening tool for the disease. A recent study by Alosh et al attempted to look at radiographic findings that were predictive of patient satisfaction and found that lateral compartment osteophytes and lateral patellar osteophytes were strongly associated with patient satisfaction.[43]

Patient history, physical examination findings, and radiographic analysis should all be used in conjugation to determine the TKA candidacy of each individual. Below will highlight conditions that warrant specific consideration when considering a patient a candidate for TKA with these concomitant findings on history, physical, or

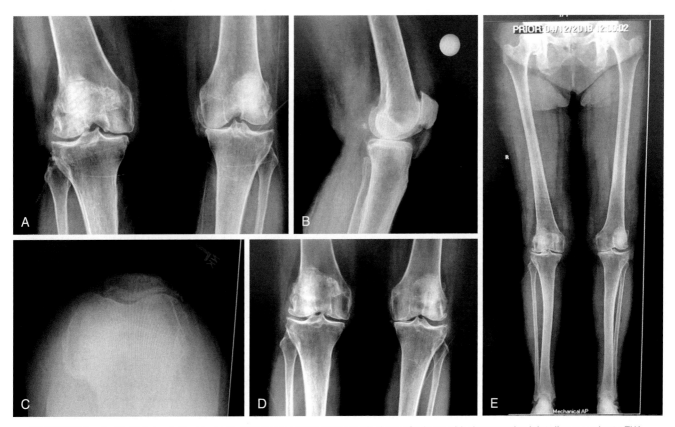

FIGURE 28-1   A: AP, **B:** lateral, **C:** skier's, **D:** Merchant, and **E:** limb length views of a knee with degenerative joint disease prior to TKA.

radiologic examination. This will be followed with contraindications for TKA as we again look for the clear picture of all aspects corroborating a patient's candidacy for the procedure.

SPECIFIC CONSIDERATIONS

When indicating patients for a primary TKA, there are several patient-related factors and conditions that can alter a patient's candidacy for the procedure and/or change some of the technical aspects in doing the surgery. The following is not an all-inclusive list of these considerations but is a good start, and all factors should be reviewed when contemplating TKA within these specific patient cohorts.

Age

Despite improving materials, pathways, and surgical techniques, it is important to consider a patient's age prior to TKA as implants will likely not last "forever," and with younger patients placing greater demands on the implants, there remains a question of how long and how much can they take. Charette et al recently reported a higher cumulative revision rate at 1 (3.4% vs. 1.8%), 2 (5.0% vs. 2.4%), and 5 (7.3% vs. 3.7%) years in patients younger than 55 years compared to those older than this age.[44] Another study by Karas and colleagues found a survivorship of 83.9% at 13 years for all-cause reoperations in patients between 45 and 54 years old.[45] In the 298 TKAs they reviewed, 20 died and 30 were lost to follow-up, leaving 248 knees. They found at an average of 13-year follow-up revisions occurred in, nine for tibial loosening, eight for deep infection, seven for polyethylene wear, and three for failed ingrowth of a cementless femoral component. Based on the fact that younger patients will likely need a revision in the future, and coupled with some of these early failure concerns, it is important to make the patient aware of these findings and risks prior to their TKA. The majority of cases are successful, yet these higher early to midterm failure rates are concerning. While younger age is not an absolute contraindication for TKA, it must be considered and discussed with the patient prior to surgery, as they may be likely signing up for one or two additional procedures in their lifetime.

At the other extreme, in the elderly, excellent results have been reported after TKA; however, these patients are typically not as healthy and require appropriate medical optimization and tight control of their comorbidities postoperatively. For the senior author (BL), it is not necessarily the number of the age but the whole package/physiologic age and concomitant comorbidities that have to be considered when indicating a patient for a TKA. Motivated elderly patients often outperform younger ones; and if carefully selected, octogenarians and nonagenarians can have successful results after TKA. Kodaira et al reported on 1003 TKAs in patients >80 years old at the

time of surgery and found no different in improvements in outcomes scores.[46] An increased length of stay, confusion, delayed wound healing, and acute heart failure occurred more frequently in their elderly cohort.

As such for younger patients, specific considerations include the possibility of using cementless technology for long-term implant fixation, assuring appropriate alignment is achieved, and using the least amount of constraint possible in an effort to improve the longevity of the TKA construct. Alternatively, for elderly patients, meticulous care of the soft tissues (be careful with adhesive dressings and skin tears), tight control and optimization of comorbidities, management of potentially "soft" bone, and the use of cemented implants can help achieve successful results even for patients in their 80s and 90s.

Body Mass Index

Obesity is a growing epidemic in the United States and is partially responsible for the increasing number of TKAs being performed annually. In fact ~37% of adults, or 1.12 billion people, are expected to be clinically obese by 2030, particularly among the developed countries in the world.[47] Clement and Deehan reported on 4740 TKAs and found that patients with increasing BMI class were noted to have an associated earlier age at the time of knee surgery.[48] Many overweight patients may be faced with the difficult task of trying to lose weight in the setting of a knee or knees that will not function to do higher level physical activity. A significant number of these patients revert to bariatric surgery to lose weight, which has controversial results with concerns for significant morbidity, malabsorption, and malnutrition after these operations. Further specifics for timing of such a procedure, also remains controversial and it is likely better for patients to work on weight loss without bariatric surgery. The senior author (BL) suggests a nutrition consult and referral for an exercise program for patients with a BMI over 40. Many of these patients, despite their weight in pounds, will be malnourished with suboptimal total protein and albumin levels. Ideally, a targeted weight loss program that is sustainable would be preferred to binge diets, with a goal to get below a BMI of 40 and closer to 35. Keeney et al reported that even losing a minimum of 20 pounds prior to TKA is associated with a shorter length of stay and decreased odds for discharge to nursing facility postoperatively.[49] Additionally, any associated medical comorbidities such as sleep apnea, peripheral vascular disease (PVD), lymphedema, and diabetes should be optimized preoperatively if they are present. It is important to take the whole clinical picture into consideration, and while not trying to restrict access to care, it is important that patients understand the significant added risk that obesity adds to their surgery. Unfortunately, restricting TJA from this population has not been successful in promoting weight loss and better incentives and programs are needed to optimize these patients.[50] This is a good opportunity to turn "cherry-picking" into "cherry growing" by getting the patient the help they need prior to an elective surgery.

Despite the concerns for performing TKA in morbidly and super morbidly obese patients, there are reports of improved outcomes after surgery and with meticulous techniques only slightly higher rates of complications. This led Hakim and colleagues to suggest that morbid obese patients are appropriate candidates for TKA and can still enjoy significant benefit from the surgery.[51] With many studies reporting excellent functional improvement in obese patients, there does seem to be a higher rate of periprosthetic infection in this cohort.[52] Other associated complications in obese TKA patients include higher readmission rates, delayed/poor wound healing, superficial and deep infections, MCL injury, and extensor mechanism injuries.[53] Patients of all obesity classes should have these risks discussed with them in the light of the potential benefit and opportunity for risk reduction with weight loss (**Table 28-1**). As such, special considerations for obese patients include meticulous surgery in regards to the adjacent ligaments of the knee and the skin/soft tissues. Longer incisions and extensile approaches for exposure are important so as to not have excessive retraction on the MCL and patellar tendon. Further considerations include adding short stems to the femur and or tibia, leaving the patella unresurfaced, and the possibility of using intramedullary guides to make cuts (as the tibia and ankle may be hard to palpate).

Diabetes Mellitus

Diabetics appear to have varying rates of complications after TKA, with many studies supporting higher rates of wound complications, deep infections, medical complications, and even need for manipulation under anesthesia.[54] It appears that immunomodulation occurs with elevated blood glucose impacting neutrophil and monocyte activity in the body. While many have tried to use a hemoglobin A1c cutoff as a marker for complication, Ryan et al found in their comparison study of 506 diabetics versus 900 nondiabetics that glycemic control markers were not predictive of an increased risk of periprosthetic joint infection (PJI) after TJA.[55] While an optimal hemoglobin A1c cutoff may be difficult to determine, a multicenter study reviewed 1004 TKAs determining a reasonable cutoff to work on optimization to be 7.7% (infection rate 0.8% vs. 5.4%, below and above this threshold, respectively).[56] Alternatively, fructosamine was recently reported to be a better predictor of adverse outcomes following TKA. Shohat et al reported an optimal cutoff of 293 µmol/L as patients above this level were 11.2 times more likely to develop PJI.[57] In fact they suggested that above this threshold should trigger a careful reevaluation of the risk to benefit ratio of TKA for the patient.

While infection rates and medical complications occur more frequently in diabetics, particularly with poor control of their daily blood sugars (blood sugar rates >180 on daily logs are concerning), it is equally concerning that there have been reports of lower functional scores and results. Cheuy et al found a negative relationship between the diagnosis of diabetes and the recovery paths for patients in the 4-m walk test, 30-second sit-to-stand test, and the timed up and go test.[58] Despite diabetic patients reporting high rates of satisfaction, Teo et al found poorer physical scores as compared to nondiabetics.[59] Decreased functional scores, higher infection rates, and a greater likelihood of medical complications necessitate close monitoring of diabetic patients and tight perioperative glycemic control. Special consideration for these patients include a wide exposure, so there is limited tension on the skin, endocrinology/medical consultation for

TABLE 28-1	Modified World Health Organization Classes of Obesity		
			Examples
BMI (kg/m²)	Classification	Height (inches)	Weight (Pounds)
<18.5	Underweight	65	100
18.5-24.9	Normal Weight	65	145
25-29.9	Overweight	65	175
30-34.9	Class I obesity	65	200
35-39.9	Class II obesity	65	225
≥40	Class III obesity	65	250
Modifications			
≥35	Severe obesity	65	225
≥40	Morbid obesity	65	250
≥50	Super obesity	65	305

glycemic control, utilization of antibiotic-impregnated bone cement, MSSA/MRSA nasal screening, and management and close monitoring of the postoperative wound (have a low threshold to limit range of motion to protect the wound).

Malnutrition

Malnutrition is a relatively underdiagnosed modifiable risk factor in many patients undergoing TKA that has been associated with increased risks of surgical site infection (SSI) and PJI.[60] Black et al found a 3.6% prevalence of malnutrition at single institution among 4047 TJA cases.[61] Their malnourished group had a greater length of stay (3.5 vs. 2.2 days), higher readmission rate (16% vs. 5%), a higher likelihood of discharge to a facility (30.8% vs. 14.7%), and a greater number of emergency room visits (30.8% vs. 9%), based on an optimal cutoff value for albumin levels of 3.94 g/dL. Screening for malnutrition often comes from routine preoperative labs with historically a cutoff for albumin being less than 3.5 g/dL. While the aforementioned study suggested a higher cutoff value, it is important to make this diagnosis preoperatively as altering the diet may have some benefit. Schroer et al found improved outcomes (decreased costs, reduced readmissions, and a shorter length of hospital stay) when a high-protein, anti-inflammatory diet was initiated in malnourished patients prior to surgery.[62] While not perfect, it is important to have some general thresholds of malnutrition to direct surgeons in educating patients that are working on preoperative optimization. It is suggested that an albumin <3.5 g/dL, prealbumin <15 mg/dL, and transferrin <200 mg/dL be used at this time to trigger the need for nutritional optimization and possible referral to a nutritionist in order to minimize post-TKA complications.[63] Special considerations for malnourished patients include pre- and postoperative diet modifications (i.e., replenishing vitamin and iron stores) as well as considering these patients higher risk with potential use of antibiotic-impregnated cement and maintaining meticulous handling of the soft tissues.

Osteonecrosis

Patients with osteonecrosis have varying degrees of presentation that often are related to the underlying etiology of the disease. The knee is the second most common joint affected by osteonecrosis behind the hip. Primary (spontaneous, older patients, isolated lesions) versus secondary osteonecrosis (younger patients, multifocal/systemic) carry different prognoses as the host is typically more compromised in the latter due to significant medical comorbidities associated with the pathogenesis and cause of the osteonecrosis. For example, primary, spontaneous, or postarthroscopy osteonecrosis is quite different than a patient with long-standing inflammatory arthritis and steroid-induced osteonecrosis. This would also hold true

for the plethora of systemic disorders that have the end result of osteonecrosis in the knee. Recently, Curtis et al reported on chronically immunosuppressed patients (often have secondary osteonecrosis), finding a higher risk for wound dehiscence, surgical site or organ infection, deep venous thrombosis, pneumonia, urinary tract infection, and sepsis.[64] These patients must not only be vetted carefully for medical concerns prior to surgery but also as to the extent of the osteonecrosis and depth of penetration into the femur and tibia (such factors may be associated with more complicated reconstructions). Much of the current literature focuses on isolated osteonecrotic lesions that are managed with arthroscopic procedures or UKA and is not as relevant to TKA patients. Additionally, there is some literature suggesting alternative options in treating osteonecrosis of the knee such as subchondral stem cell therapy that may be less risky and effective for young patients suffering from secondary osteonecrosis of the knee.[65]

In 1997, Mont and colleagues reported on 31 cementless TKAs in patients younger than 50 years with osteonecrosis of the femoral condyles and tibial plateaus. They found a 37% rate of aseptic loosening, 10% rate of PJI, and 44% successful outcomes in those with systemic lupus erythematosus.[66] Despite these disappointing results, Mont et al reported on 49 TKAs at a mean of 44 months follow-up that underwent a primary cementless TKA for osteonecrosis of the knee.[67] In this series, they found 97.9% aseptic implant survivorship and all-cause survivorship of 95.9%. They cautiously attributed the improved results to the new generation of cementless implants and are awaiting long-term data to validate the survivorship. Overall there remains conflicting data regarding TKA for osteonecrosis that often depends on the underlying etiology of the condition. Careful counseling and medical optimization are required in these patients. Further surgical considerations include meticulous handling and closure of the soft tissues as associated chronic conditions can weaken these tissues, cone or sleeve use for large osteonecrosis lesions, stem fixation for greater support at the joint line, and the use of antibiotic cement as this cohort may include high-risk patients.

Hemophilia

Hemophilia is a chronic condition that leads to an increased bleeding with subsequent frequent hemarthroses resulting in severe joint destruction, scarring, and pain. Additionally, transfusion-related complications such as viral transmission of hepatitis and/or HIV may further confound surgical intervention for knee pain in these patients. Historically, the combination of being HIV-positive and hemophilia was associated with a high rate of infection particularly with active disease and low CD4 counts.[68] Modern medicine has led to successful treatment of HIV to decrease viral loads with a concomitant reduction of infection rate in this group of patient as well. To maintain success in these patients requires close medical management of comorbidities and hematologic consultation before and after surgery to follow factor levels in the perioperative period. As TKA is an elective procedure, it is important to ascertain the patient's status regarding the presence of inhibitors, as this may be a contraindication for surgery.

Pain relief and patient satisfaction have been reported to be excellent for hemophilia patients treated with TKA. However, there are also significant rates of complications related to the underlying bleeding disorder as well as from other commonly associated conditions. A recent study reported on 43 TKAs (30 hemophilia patients), after a mean of 18 years of follow-up, there remained 21 TKAs (15 patients) that were assessed.[69] Thirty percent of the original cohort required revision surgery due to infection or aseptic loosening and the 20-year survivorship was reported to be 59% with revision for any reason as the end point. Despite this high rate of revision, the functional improvements were substantial as was patient satisfaction at long-term follow-up. Zingg et al reported on 43 TKAs in hemophilic patients in a 2012 study.[68] They found at a mean of 9.6 years follow-up that 94% of patient rated their result as good or excellent with 86% survivorship at 10 years with any component revision as the end point. Westberg et al described their results in 107 TKAs and a mean follow-up of 11.2 years.[70] Five- and ten-year survivorships were reported to be 92% and 88% for revision of any component as the end point. The overall infection rate was high at 6.5%, yet 93% reported a painless TKA at latest follow-up. Despite functional improvements and reduction in pain, the overall clinical outcomes for hemophilic patients remain inferior to TKA for osteoarthritis, with higher rates of complications (up to 31.5%) after surgery.[71] There have been some modern reports of computer-assisted and/or robotic-assisted TKAs in hemophilia patients with reasonable success.[72,73] Special surgical considerations include maintaining appropriate factor levels, possible use of an intra-articular drain, enhanced surgical exposure (quadriceps snip or tibial tubercle osteotomy) due to knee stiffness, use of revision style implants to help balance the knee and manage the poor bone quality, and use of antibiotic-impregnated bone cement.

Ipsilateral Hip Arthrodesis

Osteoarthritic changes of the knee may occur in up to 50% of those patients with an ipsilateral hip fusion.[74] In patients with a history of ipsilateral hip arthrodesis, it may be difficult to ascertain if their pain is primarily associated with the hip fusion or within the knee itself. Further, it can be quite a challenge to replace the knee in someone with a prior hip arthrodesis. Therefore, it may be worth considering managing the hip first with a fusion takedown and see if the knee pain persists or if the condition resolves without a TKA. It is controversial whether or not to proceed with the hip or knee first. Limited literature exists in this regard, with de la Hera et al reporting two successful cases of TKA after an ipsilateral hip arthrodesis.[75] While Garvin et al reported on nine TKAs that were performed below a hip arthrodesis with 78% good or excellent results, they did find a significant number of complications with seven knees being manipulated a total of 15 times, two nerve palsies and one infection.[76]

Koo and colleagues offered the following tips to replacing a knee in the setting of a hip arthrodesis, as they felt that positioning was critical to the success of the procedure: place a sandbag under the ipsilateral buttock (or can hang the leg off the side of the table) and rotate the table toward the operative knee.[77] Goodman et al reported tilting the table into increased Trendelenburg and episodically flexing the foot of table 90° facilitated making the bone cuts and the knee exposure.[78] They found successful results in two patients at a minimum of 2-year follow-up that had relative contraindications to proceed with arthrodesis takedown prior to the TKA. It is important to be aware that malpositioning of a fused hip can prohibit accurate positioning of a TKA, leading to compromised alignment and range of motion. Surgical considerations for these patients include assuring proper alignment of the hip fusion, adjusting the operating room table for exposure, consideration of hip fusion takedown prior to TKA, and extensive preoperative planning to include possibly robotics or navigation to direct bone cuts and implant placement.

Paget Disease ("Osteitis Deformans")

Paget disease of bone (PDB) is a chronic condition that affects 2% to 4% of the population older than 40 years and is hallmarked by an increase in osteoclastic bone resorption, followed by a secondary phase of osteoblast-mediated bone formation.[79] The exact etiology remains a mystery with some attributing the disease process to a viral infection in genetically predisposed hosts. The disease follows three distinct stages: osteolytic stage, mixed osteolytic/osteoblastic phase, and the osteoblastic/sclerotic phase.[80] The final process is a highly vascular bone that is mechanically weaker and more susceptible to fracture than normal adult bone. Osteoarthritis is typically found in approximately 10% to 12% of patients with PDB, and they can present with pain, temperature changes of the skin, or fractures. Treatment of PDB should be initiated, which includes the use of bisphosphonates and calcitonin, as this may, on occasion, alleviate the pain and obviate the need for surgery. Further, this medical treatment may decrease some of the complications associated with PDB in the perioperative timeframe, should surgery become necessary. The secondary degenerative changes of the knee should be initially managed with the same modalities as mentioned for typical osteoarthritis. When these treatments no longer provide relief, TKA may be performed with caution as the bone often is hypervascular with large cysts and sclerotic bone that can be challenging to deal with.

In a recent systematic review (includes all modern-day papers regarding PDB and TKA), Popat et al found four studies with a total of 54 TKAs at a mean follow-up of 7.5 years.[79] In this analysis, there were two cases of aseptic loosening, five cases of patellar tendon avulsion, and several challenging cases involving malalignment, bone loss, and soft-tissue contractures. Overall, they stressed the importance of preoperative planning to assess limb alignment/deformities, ability to utilize intramedullary guides, and plan for bony defects. Intraoperatively, a wide exposure is encouraged to take tension off of the patellar tendon; revision implants should be available to handle bone loss and ligamentous instability, and high-speed burrs may be required to manage dense and sclerotic bone. Additionally, a thorough blood management protocol should be followed with tranexamic acid and other blood salvage techniques being utilized. If care is taken, it is reasonable to anticipate an improvement in function and reduction in pain for patients with PDB following a primary TKA. Following these specific considerations for PDB and TKA, it is possible to maximize outcomes, appropriately indicate good candidates for surgery, and be prepared for any surprises that this comorbidity may pose during the procedure.

Posttraumatic Arthritis

Posttraumatic arthritis may stem from prior fractures, ligamentous injuries, and/or dislocation. The incidence of posttraumatic osteoarthritis ranges from 21% to 44% following fractures about the knee and may occur secondary to the injury itself, meniscal tears, malunion/malalignment, and ligamentous instability of the knee.[81] In such cases, there may be prior surgical incisions, hardware, and additional injuries that may affect the surgical technique and outcomes for TKA. Planning the appropriate surgical incision (utilize the lateral most scar and avoid parallel incisions), consideration of a plastic surgery consultation and staging hardware removal are potential hurdles to manage prior to considering TKA. When a previous surgical procedure has been performed, it is important to rule out infection and consider the soft-tissue trauma that is associated with the initial injury (**Fig. 28-2**).

In a recent institutional registry study, Khoshbin et al matched 5:1 osteoarthritic TKAs (375) to posttraumatic arthritis cases (75).[82] They found no demographic differences in their cohorts and that posttraumatic arthritis did not lead to higher revision rates or lower patient-reported outcomes. Two other studies have shown excellent survivorship of 88.6%[83] and 82%[84] for revision for any reason at 69 months and 15 years, respectively. This modern study is in contrast to prior publications that reported a higher risk of wound complications, longer operative times, increased blood loss, cellulitis, infection, higher revision rates, and lower outcome measures.[85-88] The recent turnaround in outcomes has been attributed to improving implant designs, meticulous soft-tissue handling, as well as the utilization of revision style implants. These improved techniques have led to there being no differences in prosthetic dislocation, bleeding complications, fractures, wear, osteolysis, neurovascular injury, or extensor mechanism rupture.[88] Overall if the specific considerations of having a detailed plan, appropriate management of the soft tissue, gaining wide exposure of the knee, and using revision style implants and constraint as needed, excellent survivorship can be obtained. However, it is important to counsel patients that there is clearly a high risk for needing a staged procedure for hardware removal and complications after TKA for posttraumatic arthritis despite the improved survivorship and patient-reported outcomes.

Neurologic Dysfunction

Neurologic dysfunction about the knee can have a dramatic impact on indications, surgical technique, and outcomes for TKA. When quadriceps function is severely affected, TKA may be contraindicated (further discussion below). Alternatively, neurologic diseases may also be associated with generalized hypotonia, ligamentous laxity, muscle spasm/rigidity, genu recurvatum, flexion contractures, excessive limb malalignment, and bony deformities. For many neurologic diseases, they are progressive and it is important to not only consider the patient's current condition but what things may look like in the future (i.e., Multiple sclerosis, Parkinson, Charcot Marie Tooth, etc.). Recent studies show that patient's with Parkinson disease have good functional results with only a minimal increase in hospital length of stay and in-hospital mortality. While the author's conclusion was that TKA is safe for this cohort and it is important to consider how future rigidity may impact outcomes later in life.[89] Ergin et al confirmed these successful results in their case-control study, showing similar outcomes compared to a general population after TKA at a little over 4-year mean follow-up.[90] While excellent results may be achieved in a significant number of cases, based on personal experience, rapidly progressive Parkinson disease is often associated with disabling rigidity and knee flexion contractures that can be quite severe after TKA.

Poliomyelitis is a highly infectious viral disease that impacts motor neurons to cause paralysis, muscle wasting, and hyporeflexia. While no longer commonly found in the United States, polio and postpolio syndrome impact a large number of children and adults worldwide. Prasad et al recently performed a systematic review of the literature and evaluated the data from six studies with 82 TKAs at an average of 5.5 years of follow-up.[91] They found a 7% revision rate at a mean of 6.2 years, and of the 36 knees that experienced preoperative recurvatum, there was a recurrence in 10 (28%) after TKA. While functional improvement may be achieved in these patients, it is important to assess the preoperative quadriceps muscle strength, as this appears to be an important prognostic factor (those that cannot hold the limb up against gravity should utilize constrained implants). These may be difficult patients to treat and complex surgeries to perform; therefore, it is important to plan these cases and be prepared for the worst. Joint line management is critical, as recurvatum (possible decreased distal femoral resection) or flexion contracture (increased distal femoral resection and posterior capsular release) may be severe and require technique alterations in those with a neurological disorder. Having component stems, augments, and hinged devices available is vital to achieving a successful outcome. Due to the progressive nature of these disorders, the authors typically suggest a higher level of constraint and consideration of some element of biologic fixation (cone or sleeve) to offset the added stress placed on the implants.

Workers' Compensation

When dealing with patients going through the workers' compensation (WC) program for a TKA, it is important to get a sense of the patient's motivation for surgery and make sure expectations are clear and fair. In and of itself, WC is not a contraindication for TKA despite these patients often having subjective findings that are much worse in nature than objective findings. Styron et al reported on patients returning to work after TKA and found the median time to return was 8.9 weeks, but the ability to return hinged more upon the person's

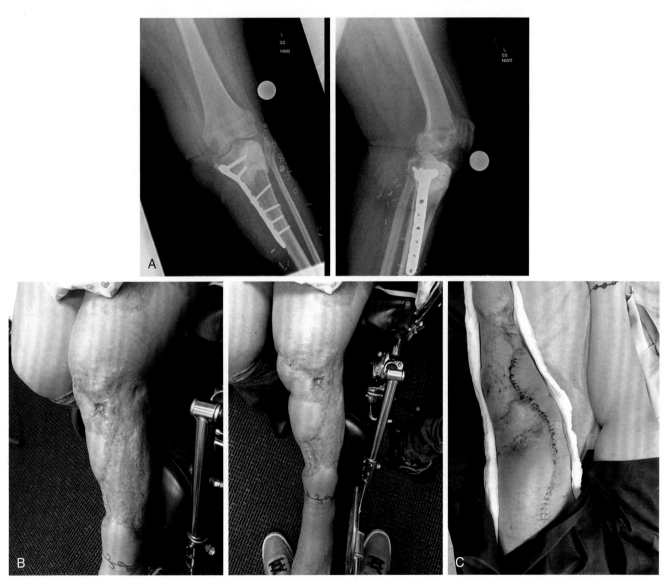

FIGURE 28-2 Posttraumatic degenerative joint disease **(A)** with a large soft-tissue injury **(B)** treated in a staged manner with plastic surgery **(C)**, hardware removal and a complex primary total knee arthroplasty with an extensor mechanism allograft **(D)**.

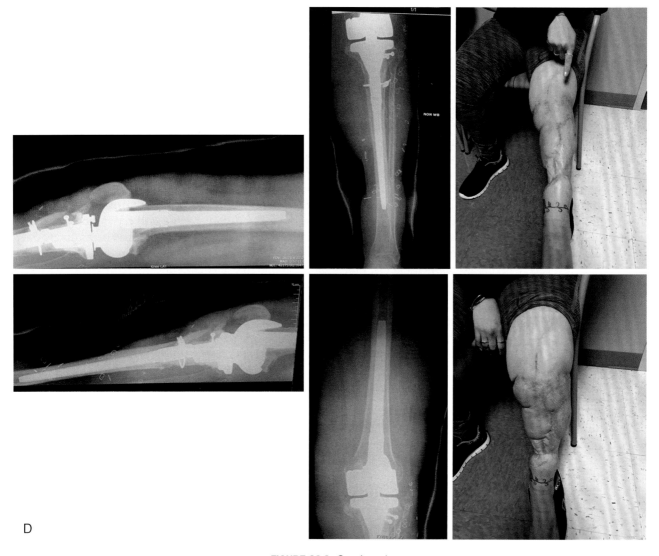

D

FIGURE 28-2 *Continued*

motivation rather than the physical demands of the job itself.[92] Clyde and colleagues reviewed WC patients and found that the average time to return to work was 16.4 weeks after a primary total joint with only 70.2% actually resuming their job.[93] This just highlights the concern for being able to predict a WC patient's motivation for the surgery and return to work. Additionally, other studies have shown inferior outcomes (higher pain scores, lower functional scores, and a decreased range of motion) for patients undergoing TKA through the WC pathway compared to those that followed the traditional route.[94-96] The authors suggest spending time with these patients prior to recommending TKA and make sure that there is a clear picture that surgery will benefit the patient and provide the functional outcome they are hoping to achieve. Additionally, early physical therapy and adequate pain management should be planned prior to surgery so that there is no confusion on the patient's and surgeon's expectations. Lastly, the authors would encourage that the treating physician not be part of the

causation determination for the claim, so as to remove that element of bias and conflict of interest for the surgeon and patient.

CONTRAINDICATIONS TO TOTAL KNEE ARTHROPLASTY

While it is important to know whom to indicate for TKA, it is equally important to recognize the absolute contraindications for surgery, as well. With aggressive preoperative patient optimization, navigation around many of the traditional relative contraindications for surgery is possible. These include morbid obesity (weight loss), remote local infection (two-stage primary procedures), tobacco use (smoking cessation program), malnutrition (nutrition consult), and neurologic dysfunction (constrained-type implants). As TKA is an elective procedure, it is critical to weigh the risks and benefits in these potentially more complicated cases. In general, it is best to look at the whole patient and what they stand to gain from the surgery versus what potentially could go wrong with intra- and postoperative complications. That being said, the following section represents suggested absolute contraindications to proceeding with a TKA.

Active Infection

In keeping with the concept of knee arthroplasty being an elective procedure, the authors would suggest delaying surgery in the setting of active sepsis, knee infection, or even a remote infection that could lead to future bacterial seeding of the bloodstream. A recent SSI risk score, developed by Everhart et al, includes lower extremity osteomyelitis, pyogenic arthritis, and history of staphylococcal septicemia as 6 points out of a 35-point scale for predicting SSI after primary TKA.[97] Intuitively, it makes sense that prior infection would increase the risk of a future infection as there may be some residual bacteria or it may serve as a marker to the hosts immune system or innate proclivity/susceptibility to infection. Jerry et al found a 7.7% risk of infection in patients with a history of prior sepsis or associated osteomyelitis.[98] More recently Lee and colleagues found a 5% recurrence of deep infection in treating 20 patients with septic arthritis or osteomyelitis about the knee.[99] They attributed their success to the utilization of antibiotic bone cement at the time of TKA as well as careful pre- and intraoperative evaluation.

While active sepsis may be relatively easy to diagnose, it is the more remote history of septic arthritis or osteomyelitis that is difficult to diagnose and manage. Preoperatively, the typical assessment may not lead to a definitive diagnosis with erythrocyte sedimentation rate (ESR), C-reactive protein (CRP), and knee aspiration results often being inconclusive. This was highlighted by Seo et al in their series of 62 patients with prior joint sepsis or osteomyelitis in which they followed a stringent algorithm (**Fig. 28-3**), yet still reported 9.7% infection rate with five out of six growing the same organism as their prior infection.[100] An independent risk factor for periprosthetic infection was the number of prior surgeries required to treat the native knee condition. In the setting of persistent infection or if it is inconclusive whether or not the remote infection was treated to completion, then a two-stage primary TKA is recommended. This involves a thorough débridement with removal of all of the native cartilage and bony resection in preparation for a future TKA. A spacer is placed, and the infection is treated appropriately, followed by reimplantation of TKA components during the second stage. Shaikh et al found no deep infections after this type of two-stage procedure in a series of 15 patients with a mean follow-up period of 4 years.[101] This two-stage approach for refractory infections has been supported by Nazarian and colleagues.[102] They reported no recurrence of infection in 14 patients at an average of 4.5-year follow-up, with an average of 3.1 months between stages of reconstruction. If the patient is not willing to undergo a two-stage procedure or accept the high risk of failure and/or repeat surgical intervention, then an arthrodesis may be a better option. In the end, prior infection is a concern for future complications as shown by Chalmers et al, who found that there is a threefold higher risk of prosthetic infection in patients with a prior hip or knee PJI and a subsequent primary TKA compared to match controls.[103] This compelling data lay emphasis on developing a detailed plan for managing any patients with a prior history of infection, pyogenic arthritis, or osteomyelitis about the knee (**Fig. 28-3**). This is further emphasized by Bedair et al that showed patients with a history of PJI were at higher risk of infection in another joint should they elect to undergo an additional TJA in the future.[104] In a matched controlled study, they found a ~11% infection rate versus zero in those with a prior TJA infection, with a second PJI occurring more frequently in females and in those with a history of a staphylococcal infection. Therefore, with any history of remote or joint infection, it is important to counsel patients on their risks and approach these elective cases with extreme caution.

Incompetent Extensor Mechanism

A primary TKA in the setting of an incompetent extensor mechanism will likely lead to persistent instability and dysfunction despite attempts at bracing the knee. Therefore, it is contraindicated to perform a TKA in a patient with an incompetent extensor mechanism, particularly if the primary etiology is neurologic in nature. When there has been a mechanical disruption of the extensor mechanism, then a grafting procedure (mesh, allograft, synthetic materials) with a primary TKA may be indicated (**Fig. 28-2**). Such procedures often require the use of revision style implants and are more difficult with a higher rate of complications. There remains minimal data on such grafting procedures for a primary TKA; however, there is ample data in reconstructing the extensor mechanism during revision surgery with a partial allograft, complete allograft, as well as synthetic mesh.[105-110]

Neuropathic Arthropathy

Neuropathic (Charcot) arthropathy is a chronic, progressive degenerative process resulting in collapse and destruction of weight-bearing joints due to the disruption of normal sensation leading to an insensate articulation.[111,112] Conditions commonly associated with this arthropathy include diabetes mellitus, neurosyphilis, and syringomyelia. Charcot-Marie-Tooth disease, multiple sclerosis, leprosy, amyloidosis, and congenital insensitivity to pain can lead to neuropathic arthropathy, which is categorized as a warm, swollen, and erythematous joint that is relatively painless. This is often associated with joint instability, but maintenance of a range of motion

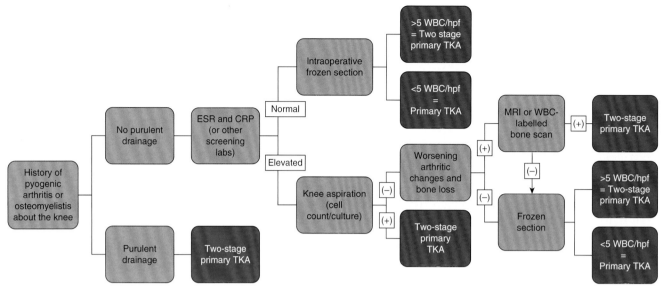

FIGURE 28-3   Algorithm for treating postpyogenic arthritis or osteomyelitis about the knee. CRP, C-reactive protein; ESR, erythrocyte sedimentation rate; TKA, total knee arthroplasty. (Adapted from Seo JG, Moon YW, Park SH, Han KY, Kim SM. Primary total knee arthroplasty in infection sequelae about the native knee. *J Arthroplasty.* 2014;29(12):2271-2275.)

that would not seem possible with the bony destruction was evidenced radiographically (**Fig. 28-4**). When a patient's presentation is suspicious for neuropathic arthropathy in the absence of an underlying diagnosis, a neurology consult should be obtained to identify the underlying etiology for the condition prior to considering surgery. Additionally, a Charcot knee can present much like septic arthritis, and preoperative lab and/or aspiration should be performed to rule this out. Historically, neuropathic arthropathy was considered an absolute contraindication for a TKA, yet with modern implants and techniques has become more controversial.

Patients with a neuropathic arthropathy of the knee should go through standard nonoperative management as well as considering bracing.[113] When this fails, a discussion regarding arthrodesis versus arthroplasty should be had to review potential risks and benefits of both procedures. Bone quality is often compromised and can lead to a significant challenge for both arthrodesis and primary TKA. With modern techniques and implants that are available, arthrodesis has been more relegated to a salvage procedure, and TKA has become more accepted as a treatment option for neuropathic arthropathy of the knee. A recent study by Tibbo et al reported on 37 TKAs for Charcot arthropathy with a 10-year survivorship of septic loosening of 88%.[112] By following a selective use of constraint and enhanced metaphyseal fixation, improved survivorship was found. However, they did find a high rate of complications (16%), revisions (16%), and reoperations (8%). Zeng et al found favorable outcomes in eight knees treated with constrained condylar or rotating hinge prostheses and autograft for large bone defects.[114] There have been numerous case reports related to a multitude of neuropathic arthopathy etiologies in the literature with varying levels of success.[113,115-118] Further, Bae et al

reported on 11 TKAs for neuropathic arthropathy due to neurosyphilis and found, at an average of 12.3-year follow-up, there were three complications and they suggest that this procedure is technically demanding and a rotating hinge prosthesis is strongly recommended.[119] If TKA is to be attempted in these cases, you must have numerous levels of constraint, stems, bone graft, cones/sleeves, and additional means of fixation such as cables, plates, and screws available to manage the expected bone loss, poor bone quality, and ligamentous instability. If revision principles are held, true successful outcomes can be achieved and in the future may remove this disease process from the contraindicated portion of the chapter.

Knee Arthrodesis

Conversion of a stable operative or spontaneous arthrodesis of the knee is quite controversial and has historically been considered a "no-brainer" contraindication to TKA. Concerns of muscle atrophy, poor range of motion, wound-healing complications, and ligamentous instability are among the common thoughts as to why most consider a stable arthrodesis a contraindication to primary TKA. A recent review paper attempted to answer the question of, what are the benefits and risks of TKA in arthrodesed knees?[120] The authors found that takedown of a fusion and TKA may increase functionality, but they were unsure if the increase in complications is worth the impact on pain or patient satisfaction. In a similar comprehensive literature search (10 studies included from 1998 to 2008), Jauregui et al reported on 98 surgically arthrodesed knees that underwent TKA.[121] The mean follow-up was 5 years, and they found an overall complication rate of 47%, with a 25% rate of revision surgery and an overall 11% failure rate. Despite this high complication

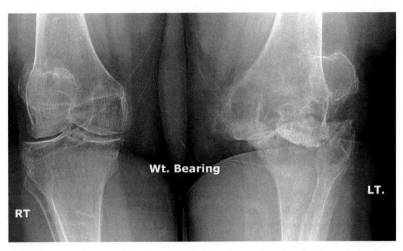

FIGURE 28-4 Neuropathic arthropathy due to long-standing uncontrolled diabetes. Despite significant bony destruction, the patient's pain was controlled with NSAIDs and her range of motion was from 10° to 105°.

rate, most patients remained happy with their outcome.[121] Lastly, Kernkamp and colleagues reviewed the literature to include six papers, with 123 TKAs and found 65% of the cases involved complications with the most frequent being skin necrosis (25%), arthrofibrosis (13%), infection (11%), revision (11%) and refusion, amputation, and death in <5% of all cases.[122] It is crucial to utilize revision techniques, respect the soft tissues (possible plastic surgery involvement), and counsel patients on the high risk of complications after converting a knee arthrodesis to a TKA. In the end with complication rates around 50% or higher, it may be prudent to advise patients against such a procedure as there is a near-equal likelihood of harm versus benefit.

Prohibitive Medical Comorbidities

As mentioned in prior sections of the chapter, comorbidities can impact the overall candidacy of a patient for an elective TKA. Modifiable risk factors should be assessed for all patients and, when possible, altered to give the patient the best chance for a successful outcome. Recently, several scoring systems have been introduced to aid in prediction of outcomes and patient satisfaction.[23,123,124] Machine learning and artificial intelligence are two new factors to prediction models and represent an exciting new means to gather data and interpret it in a rapid fashion to look at outcomes, function, and satisfaction after TKA.[125,126] These models are in their early phases, but significant advancements are anticipated over the next few years.

Many comorbidities can be optimized prior to considering surgery with a potential significant impact on outcomes and patient satisfaction. Examples include correction of malnutrition, weight loss for obesity, smoking cessation protocols, pain management plan to reduce preoperative opioid use, diabetes management (hemoglobin A1c or fructosamine monitoring), management of immune-compromising medications, hepatitis C

management/treatment, blood pressure and cholesterol control, and perioperative management of anticoagulation to name a few.[127-130] Further some conditions may require treatment but often are difficult to improve or optimize prior to surgery, making them potential contraindications to TKA surgery, such as lymphedema,[131] excessive reporting of allergies,[132] depression, fibromyalgia,[133] and neurologic disorders[134] (i.e., Parkinson). In this setting, if optimization cannot improve the risk profile and there is more chance of harm than benefit, it may be prudent to avoid any surgical interventions. Additionally, if functional improvement and pain relief may not be possible and the risk of morbidity and mortality are high, then TKA should not be recommended.

Peripheral Vascular Disease

Severe PVD can be a contraindication for TKA due to increased risks of delayed wound healing or catastrophic limb ischemia. Gronbeck et al found that the diagnosis of PVD was the most significant risk factor for medical complications and reoperations in a database review of 14,185 total joint arthroplasties (8934 of which were TKAs).[135] Abu Dakka and colleagues reviewed the literature finding very few studies related to PVD and TKA, yet they did suggest that patients with risk factors for PVD should be referred for a preoperative vascular assessment.[136] Additionally, if surgery is ultimately indicated, that use of a tourniquet should be avoided. While care should be taken with such patients, Walls et al recently reported a 7.5% rate of moderate PVD in 40 patients undergoing TKA.[137] They found that tourniquet use was okay in this cohort as long as the vasculature maintained an occlusion rate lower than 50%. In general, if there are diminished pulses or PVD is suspected, then an ankle-brachial-index examination should be ordered and if less than 0.9, a vascular consult is warranted.

In reviewing 4097 and 11,953 TKAs in two studies, Calligaro et al found a 0.17% incidence of acute limb-threatening ischemia that required urgent management.[138,139] They found that thrombectomy alone afforded poor results, and emergency bypass was generally necessary due to underlying chronic occlusive atherosclerotic disease in these patients. Further it appeared, intimal plaque disruption likely occurred with movements of the knee and/or tourniquet compression of the vessels. Some of the more common risk factors for PVD include asymmetric or weak distal pulses, calcified vasculature on preoperative radiographs, previous vascular surgery, or evidence of distal arterial insufficiency, and when identified on history and physical should trigger a consultation with a vascular surgeon.[140] While no longer considered an absolute contraindication, it is important to be diligent in making this diagnosis preoperatively and working with a vascular team to come up with a specific management plan on a case-by-case basis.

Unrealistic Patient Expectations

As discussed in earlier sections, patients and surgeons must share similar expectations for the anticipated outcome after a TKA. If there is a mismatch in what the two parties are "expecting" to occur, this may lead to unhappy patients, readmissions, and complications. Appropriate estimates of potential complications should be discussed as should any future restrictions in activity and the importance of long-term follow-up. It is paramount that the patient understands a TKA will treat the affected knee joint and is not going to make them feel like a teenager again. They must understand they will still be limited in postoperative function by the rest of their body, which may have its own level of dysfunction. If, at any point, the surgeon or the patient does not feel that the relationship is "working" or if there are concerns for the patients compliance and/or candidacy for TKA, a second opinion from another physician may be considered.

Deakin and colleagues reported on the expectations of 200 TKA patients using the Hospital for Special Surgery Knee Replacement Expectation Score.[141] They found at 6 weeks that 30% of expectations were fulfilled and that this increased to 48% at 1 year. The ability to provide pain relief and meet mobility expectations was the most predictive for postoperative patient satisfaction. Higher level activities, such as kneeling, squatting, paid work, and sexual function, were typically not fulfilled in this series. Expectations for return to high-impact sporting activities should be tempered and low-impact, sustainable, aerobic exercise plans should be encouraged. Ghomrawi and colleagues found that expectations that predicted patient dissatisfaction included the ability to kneel, leg straightening, and participation in recreational sports among 2279 TKAs.[142] This should be included in a thorough preoperative discussion as should the anticipation for hospital length of stay, discharge location, and length of postoperative recovery. It is important that these expectations are similar to assure that both physician and patient are on the same page for what will take place postoperatively.

CONCLUSION

Total knee replacement is a highly successful, elective procedure, when performed in the appropriately indicated patients. Coming to the decision for surgery and what makes an ideal patient is often a complex, multifaceted task. Effective communication is vital so that the patient and the surgeon form a team to provide the best opportunity for a successful outcome. Informed consent is a critical portion of the procedure and involves, setting expectations, detailing the potential risks and identifying the specific benefits of the individual prior to surgery. Modern-day advances have led to a push for outpatient TKA and patient selection for this type of procedure may follow a different set of rules compared to inpatient cases. Indicating a patient for surgery involves assuring the preoperative diagnosis is correct based on history, physical, and radiographic assessments and turning this into a plan that makes sure the patient will be compliant with postoperative protocols and restrictions. Special considerations and contraindications must be dealt with adequately to assure the highest level of success. In the end, as physicians, it is important that we do our part and work toward a goal of optimizing our patients and taking those that would benefit from a TKA but are not are a great candidate or even in the contraindicated category and striving to work with them to grow and optimize into that eventual ideal candidate for TKA. Those patients that know what they are getting into and are stringently indicated for TKA tend to be the most satisfied patients after surgery.

REFERENCES

1. Insall JN. *Indications and contraindications for total knee replacement*. In: *Surgery of the Knee*. Vol. 2. 2nd ed. London, England: Churchill Livingstone; 1993:719-722.
2. Tormalehto S, Aarnio E, Mononen ME, Arokoski JPA, Korhonen RK, Martikainen JA. Eight-year trajectories of changes in health-related quality of life in knee osteoarthritis: data from the Osteoarthritis Initiative (OAI). *PLoS One*. 2019;14(7):e0219902.
3. van de Water RB, Leichtenberg CS, Nelissen R, et al. Preoperative radiographic osteoarthritis severity modifies the effect of preoperative pain on pain/function after total knee arthroplasty: results at 1 and 2 years postoperatively. *J Bone Joint Surg Am*. 2019;101(10):879-887.
4. Robertsson O, Dunbar M, Pehrsson T, Knutson K, Lidgren L. Patient satisfaction after knee arthroplasty: a report on 27,372 knees operated on between 1981 and 1995 in Sweden. *Acta Orthop Scand*. 2000;71(3):262-267.
5. Sloan M, Premkumar A, Sheth NP. Projected volume of primary total joint arthroplasty in the U.S., 2014 to 2030. *J Bone Joint Surg Am*. 2018;100(17):1455-1460.
6. Manner PA, Tubb CC, Levine BR. AAOS appropriate use criteria: surgical management of osteoarthritis of the knee. *J Am Acad Orthop Surg*. 2018;26(9):e194-e197.

7. Klein GR, Levine BR, Hozack WJ, et al. Return to athletic activity after total hip arthroplasty. Consensus guidelines based on a survey of the Hip Society and American Association of Hip and Knee Surgeons. *J Arthroplasty.* 2007;22(2):171-175.

8. Sibia US, King PJ, MacDonald JH. Who is not a candidate for a 1-day hospital-based total knee arthroplasty? *J Arthroplasty.* 2017;32(1):16-19.

9. Husted H, Holm G, Jacobsen S. Predictors of length of stay and patient satisfaction after hip and knee replacement surgery: fast-track experience in 712 patients. *Acta Orthop.* 2008;79(2):168-173.

10. Aggarwal VK, Tischler EH, Post ZD, Kane I, Orozco FR, Ong A. Patients with atrial fibrillation undergoing total joint arthroplasty increase hospital burden. *J Bone Joint Surg Am.* 2013;95(17):1606-1611.

11. Smith TO, McCabe C, Lister S, Christie SP, Cross J. Rehabilitation implications during the development of the Norwich Enhanced Recovery Programme (NERP) for patients following total knee and total hip arthroplasty. *Orthop Traumatol Surg Res.* 2012;98(5):499-505.

12. Halawi MJ, Vovos TJ, Green CL, Wellman SS, Attarian DE, Bolognesi MP. Preoperative predictors of extended hospital length of stay following total knee arthroplasty. *J Arthroplasty.* 2015;30(3):361-364.

13. Meneghini RM, Ziemba-Davis M, Ishmael MK, Kuzma AL, Caccavallo P. Safe selection of outpatient joint arthroplasty patients with medical risk stratification: the "outpatient Arthroplasty risk assessment score". *J Arthroplasty.* 2017;32(8):2325-2331.

14. Fitz-Henry J. The ASA classification and peri-operative risk. *Ann R Coll Surg Engl.* 2011;93(3):185-187.

15. Charlson ME, Pompei P, Ales KL, MacKenzie CR. A new method of classifying prognostic comorbidity in longitudinal studies: development and validation. *J Chronic Dis.* 1987;40(5):373-383.

16. Ziemba-Davis M, Caccavallo P, Meneghini RM. Outpatient joint arthroplasty-patient selection: update on the outpatient arthroplasty risk assessment score. *J Arthroplasty.* 2019;34(7S):S40-S43.

17. Noble PC, Conditt MA, Cook KF, Mathis KB. The John Insall Award: patient expectations affect satisfaction with total knee arthroplasty. *Clin Orthop Relat Res.* 2006;452:35-43.

18. Barlow T, Dunbar M, Sprowson A, Parsons N, Griffin D. Development of an outcome prediction tool for patients considering a total knee replacement–the Knee Outcome Prediction Study (KOPS). *BMC Musculoskelet Disord.* 2014;15:451.

19. Belmont PJ Jr, Goodman GP, Hamilton W, Waterman BR, Bader JO, Schoenfeld AJ. Morbidity and mortality in the thirty-day period following total hip arthroplasty: risk factors and incidence. *J Arthroplasty.* 2014;29(10):2025-2030.

20. Van Onsem S, Van Der Straeten C, Arnout N, Deprez P, Van Damme G, Victor J. A new prediction model for patient satisfaction after total knee arthroplasty. *J Arthroplasty.* 2016;31(12):2660-2667.e2661.

21. Zabawa L, Li K, Chmell S. Patient dissatisfaction following total knee arthroplasty: external validation of a new prediction model. *Eur J Orthop Surg Traumatol.* 2019;29(4):861-867.

22. Calkins TE, Culvern C, Nahhas CR, et al. External validity of a new prediction model for patient satisfaction after total knee arthroplasty. *J Arthroplasty.* 2019;34(8):1677-1681.

23. Kunze KN, Akram F, Fuller BC, Zabawa L, Sporer SM, Levine BR. Internal validation of a predictive model for satisfaction after primary total knee arthroplasty. *J Arthroplasty.* 2019;34(4):663-670.

24. Leopold SS. Editor's spotlight/take 5: do surgeon expectations predict clinically important improvements in WOMAC scores after THA and TKA? *Clin Orthop Relat Res.* 2017;475(9):2146-2149.

25. Ghomrawi HMK, Mancuso CA, Dunning A, et al. Do surgeon expectations predict clinically important improvements in WOMAC scores after THA and TKA? *Clin Orthop Relat Res.* 2017;475(9):2150-2158.

26. Gautreau S, Gould ON, Aquino-Russell C, Forsythe ME. Developing a surgeon-patient communication checklist for total knee arthroplasty. *Musculoskelet Care.* 2019;17(1):91-96.

27. Skogo Nyvang J, Hedstrom M, Iversen MD, Andreassen Gleissman S. Striving for a silent knee: a qualitative study of patients' experiences with knee replacement surgery and their perceptions of fulfilled expectations. *Int J Qual Stud Health Well-Being.* 2019;14(1):1620551.

28. Lutzner C, Postler A, Beyer F, Kirschner S, Lutzner J. Fulfillment of expectations influence patient satisfaction 5 years after total knee arthroplasty. *Knee Surg Sports Traumatol Arthrosc.* 2019;27(7):2061-2070.

29. Schmitt J, Lange T, Gunther KP, et al. Indication criteria for total knee arthroplasty in patients with osteoarthritis - a multi-perspective consensus study. *Z Orthop Unfall.* 2017;155(5):539-548.

30. Kohn MD, Sassoon AA, Fernando ND. Classifications in brief: Kellgren-Lawrence classification of osteoarthritis. *Clin Orthop Relat Res.* 2016;474(8):1886-1893.

31. Bedard NA, Pugely AJ, Elkins JM, et al. The John N. Insall award: do intraarticular injections increase the risk of infection after TKA? *Clin Orthop Relat Res.* 2017;475(1):45-52.

32. Kokubun BA, Manista GC, Courtney PM, Kearns SM, Levine BR. Intra-articular knee injections before total knee arthroplasty: outcomes and complication rates. *J Arthroplasty.* 2017;32(6):1798-1802.

33. Loth FL, Giesinger JM, Giesinger K, et al. Impact of comorbidities on outcome after total hip arthroplasty. *J Arthroplasty.* 2017;32(9):2755-2761.

34. Kobayashi S, Niki Y, Harato K, Nagura T, Nakamura M, Matsumoto M. Rheumatoid arthritis patients achieve better satisfaction but lower functional activities as compared to osteoarthritis patients after total knee arthroplasty. *J Arthroplasty.* 2019;34(3):478-482.e471.

35. Stern SH, Insall JN, Windsor RE, Inglis AE, Dines DM. Total knee arthroplasty in patients with psoriasis. *Clin Orthop Relat Res.* 1989;248:108-110;discussion 111.

36. Anouchi YS, McShane M, Kelly F Jr, Elting J, Stiehl J. Range of motion in total knee replacement. *Clin Orthop Relat Res.* 1996;331:87-92.

37. Kawamura H, Bourne RB. Factors affecting range of flexion after total knee arthroplasty. *J Orthop Sci.* 2001;6(3):248-252.

38. Lizaur A, Marco L, Cebrian R. Preoperative factors influencing the range of movement after total knee arthroplasty for severe osteoarthritis. *J Bone Joint Surg Br.* 1997;79(4):626-629.

39. Claessens AA, Schouten JS, van den Ouweland FA, Valkenburg HA. Do clinical findings associate with radiographic osteoarthritis of the knee? *Ann Rheum Dis.* 1990;49(10):771-774.

40. Meding JB, Ritter MA, Faris PM, Keating EM, Harris W. Does the preoperative radiographic degree of osteoarthritis correlate to results in primary total knee arthroplasty? *J Arthroplasty.* 2001;16(1):13-16.

41. Bhatnagar S, Carey-Smith R, Darrah C, Bhatnagar P, Glasgow MM. Evidence-based practice in the utilization of knee radiographs–a survey of all members of the British Orthopaedic Association. *Int Orthop.* 2006;30(5):409-411.

42. Lespasio MJ, Piuzzi NS, Husni ME, Muschler GF, Guarino A, Mont MA. Knee osteoarthritis: a primer. *Perm J.* 2017;21:16-183.

43. Alosh H, Behery OA, Levine BR. Radiographic predictors of patient satisfaction following primary total knee arthroplasty. *Bull Hosp Joint Dis (2013).* 2018;76(2):105-111.

44. Charette RS, Sloan M, DeAngelis RD, Lee GC. Higher rate of early revision following primary total knee arthroplasty in patients under age 55: a cautionary tale. *J Arthroplasty.* 2019;34(12):2918-2924.

45. Karas V, Calkins TE, Bryan AJ, et al. Total knee arthroplasty in patients less than 50 years of age: results at a mean of 13 years. *J Arthroplasty.* 2019;34(10):2392-2397.

46. Kodaira S, Kikuchi T, Hakozaki M, Konno S. Total knee arthroplasty in Japanese patients aged 80 years or older. *Clin Interv Aging.* 2019;14:681-688.

47. Kelly T, Yang W, Chen CS, Reynolds K, He J. Global burden of obesity in 2005 and projections to 2030. *Int J Obes.* 2008;32(9):1431-1437.

48. Clement ND, Deehan DJ. Overweight and obese patients require total hip and total knee arthroplasty at a younger age. *J Orthop Res.* 2019. doi:10.1002/jor.24460.

49. Keeney BJ, Austin DC, Jevsevar DS. Preoperative weight loss for morbidly obese patients undergoing total knee arthroplasty: determining the necessary amount. *J Bone Joint Surg Am.* 2019;101(16):1440-1450.

50. Springer BD, Roberts KM, Bossi KL, Odum SM, Voellinger DC. What are the implications of withholding total joint arthroplasty in the morbidly obese? A prospective, observational study. *Bone Joint J.* 2019;101-B(7_suppl_C):28-32.

51. Hakim J, Volpin G, Amashah M, et al. Long-term outcome of total knee arthroplasty in patients with morbid obesity. *Int Orthop.* 2019. doi:10.1007/s00264-019-04378-y.

52. Chaudhry H, Ponnusamy K, Somerville L, McCalden RW, Marsh J, Vasarhelyi EM. Revision rates and functional outcomes among severely, morbidly, and super-obese patients following primary total knee arthroplasty: a systematic review and meta-analysis. *JBJS Rev.* 2019;7(7):e9.

53. Boyce L, Prasad A, Barrett M, et al. The outcomes of total knee arthroplasty in morbidly obese patients: a systematic review of the literature. *Arch Orthop Trauma Surg.* 2019;139(4):553-560.

54. Cartwright-Terry M, Cohen DR, Polydoros F, Davidson JS, Santini AJ. Manipulation under anaesthesia following total knee arthroplasty: predicting stiffness and outcome. *J Orthop Surg.* 2018;26(3):2309499018802971.

55. Ryan S, Dilallo M, McCoy K, Green C, Seyler T. Diabetes and total joint arthroplasty: infection risk may not be predictable by markers of glycemic control. *J Surg Orthop Adv.* 2019;28(2):127-131.

56. Tarabichi M, Shohat N, Kheir MM, et al. Determining the threshold for HbA1c as a predictor for adverse outcomes after total joint arthroplasty: a multicenter, retrospective study. *J Arthroplasty.* 2017;32(9S):S263–S267.e261.

57. Shohat N, Tarabichi M, Tan TL, et al. 2019 John Insall Award: fructosamine is a better glycaemic marker compared with glycated haemoglobin (HbA1C) in predicting adverse outcomes following total knee arthroplasty: a prospective multicentre study. *Bone Joint J.* 2019;101-B(7_suppl_C):3-9.

58. Cheuy VA, Loyd BJ, Hafner W, Kittelson AJ, Waugh D, Stevens-Lapsley JE. Influence of diabetes mellitus on the recovery trajectories of function, strength, and self-report measures after total knee arthroplasty. *Arthritis Care Res.* 2019;71(8):1059-1067.

59. Teo BJX, Chong HC, Yeo W, Tan AHC. The impact of diabetes on patient outcomes after total knee arthroplasty in an Asian population. *J Arthroplasty.* 2018;33(10):3186-3189.

60. Tsantes AG, Papadopoulos DV, Lytras T, et al. Association of malnutrition with periprosthetic joint and surgical site infections after total joint arthroplasty: a systematic review and meta-analysis. *J Hosp Infect.* 2019;103(1):69-77.

61. Black CS, Goltz DE, Ryan SP, et al. The role of malnutrition in ninety-day outcomes after total joint arthroplasty. *J Arthroplasty.* 2019;34(11):2594-2600.

62. Schroer WC, LeMarr AR, Mills K, Childress AL, Morton DJ, Reedy ME. 2019 Chitranjan S. Ranawat Award: elective joint arthroplasty outcomes improve in malnourished patients with nutritional intervention. A prospective population analysis demonstrates a modifiable risk factor. *Bone Joint J.* 2019;101-B(7_suppl_C):17-21.

63. Roche M, Law TY, Kurowicki J, et al. Albumin, prealbumin, and transferrin may be predictive of wound complications following total knee arthroplasty. *J Knee Surg.* 2018;31(10):946-951.

64. Curtis GL, Chughtai M, Khlopas A, et al. Perioperative outcomes and short-term complications following total knee arthroplasty in chronically, immunosuppressed patients. *Surg Technol Int.* 2018;32:263-269.

65. Hernigou P, Auregan JC, Dubory A, Flouzat-Lachaniette CH, Chevallier N, Rouard H. Subchondral stem cell therapy versus contralateral total knee arthroplasty for osteoarthritis following secondary osteonecrosis of the knee. *Int Orthop.* 2018;42(11):2563-2571.

66. Mont MA, Myers TH, Krackow KA, Hungerford DS. Total knee arthroplasty for corticosteroid associated avascular necrosis of the knee. *Clin Orthop Relat Res.* 1997;338:124-130.

67. Sultan AA, Khlopas A, Sodhi N, et al. Cementless total knee arthroplasty in knee osteonecrosis demonstrated excellent survivorship and outcomes at three-year minimum follow-up. *J Arthroplasty.* 2018;33(3):761-765.

68. Zingg PO, Fucentese SF, Lutz W, Brand B, Mamisch N, Koch PP. Haemophilic knee arthropathy: long-term outcome after total knee replacement. *Knee Surg Sports Traumatol Arthrosc.* 2012;20(12):2465-2470.

69. Ernstbrunner L, Hingsammer A, Catanzaro S, et al. Long-term results of total knee arthroplasty in haemophilic patients: an 18-year follow-up. *Knee Surg Sports Traumatol Arthrosc.* 2017;25(11):3431-3438.

70. Westberg M, Paus AC, Holme PA, Tjonnfjord GE. Haemophilic arthropathy: long-term outcomes in 107 primary total knee arthroplasties. *Knee.* 2014;21(1):147-150.

71. Moore MF, Tobase P, Allen DD. Meta-analysis: outcomes of total knee arthroplasty in the haemophilia population. *Haemophilia.* 2016;22(4):e275-e285.

72. Kim KI, Kim DK, Juh HS, Khurana S, Rhyu KH. Robot-assisted total knee arthroplasty in haemophilic arthropathy. *Haemophilia.* 2016;22(3):446-452.

73. Cho KY, Kim KI, Khurana S, Cho SW, Kang DG. Computer-navigated total knee arthroplasty in haemophilic arthropathy. *Haemophilia.* 2013;19(2):259-266.

74. Romness DW, Morrey BF. Total knee arthroplasty in patients with prior ipsilateral hip fusion. *J Arthroplasty.* 1992;7(1):63-70.

75. de la Hera B, Rubio-Quevedo R, Gomez-Garcia A, Gomez-Rice A. Total knee arthroplasty in patients with prior ipsilateral hip arthrodesis. *Eur J Orthop Surg Traumatol.* 2018;28(3):521-524.

76. Garvin KL, Pellicci PM, Windsor RE, Conrad EU, Insall JN, Salvati EA. Contralateral total hip arthroplasty or ipsilateral total knee arthroplasty in patients who have a long-standing fusion of the hip. *J Bone Joint Surg Am.* 1989;71(9):1355-1362.

77. Koo K, Pang KC, Wang W. Total knee arthroplasty in a patient with a fused ipsilateral hip. *J Orthop Surg Res.* 2015;10:127.

78. Goodman SB, Huddleston JI III, Hur D, Song SJ. Total knee arthroplasty in patients with ipsilateral fused hip: a technical note. *Clin Orthop Surg.* 2014;6(4):476-479.

79. Popat R, Tsitskaris K, Millington S, Dawson-Bowling S, Hanna SA. Total knee arthroplasty in patients with Paget's disease of bone: a systematic review. *World J Orthop.* 2018;9(10):229-234.

80. Lander PH, Hadjipavlou AG. A dynamic classification of Paget's disease. *J Bone Joint Surg Br.* 1986;68(3):431-438.

81. Srinivasan SS, Uthygarajan, Raj DG. Complex proximal malunited tibial plateau fracture treated primarily by total knee arthroplasty – a case report. *J Orthop Case Rep.* 2019;9(2):72-75.

82. Khoshbin A, Stavrakis A, Sharma A, et al. Patient-reported outcome measures of total knee arthroplasties for post-traumatic arthritis versus osteoarthritis: a short-term (5- to 10-year) retrospective matched cohort study. *J Arthroplasty.* 2019;34(5):872-876.e871.

83. Fuchs M, Effenberger B, Mardian S, et al. Mid-term survival of total knee arthroplasty in patients with posttraumatic osteoarthritis. *Acta Chir Orthop Traumatol Cech.* 2018;85(5):319-324.

84. Abdel MP, von Roth P, Cross WW, Berry DJ, Trousdale RT, Lewallen DG. Total knee arthroplasty in patients with a prior tibial plateau fracture: a long-term report at 15 years. *J Arthroplasty.* 2015;30(12):2170-2172.

85. Lonner JH, Pedlow FX, Siliski JM. Total knee arthroplasty for post-traumatic arthrosis. *J Arthroplasty.* 1999;14(8):969-975.

86. Lunebourg A, Parratte S, Gay A, Ollivier M, Garcia-Parra K, Argenson JN. Lower function, quality of life, and survival rate after total knee arthroplasty for posttraumatic arthritis than for primary arthritis. *Acta Orthop.* 2015;86(2):189-194.

87. Saleh KJ, Sherman P, Katkin P, et al. Total knee arthroplasty after open reduction and internal fixation of fractures of the tibial plateau: a minimum five-year follow-up study. *J Bone Joint Surg Am.* 2001;83(8):1144-1148.

88. Bala A, Penrose CT, Seyler TM, Mather RC III, Wellman SS, Bolognesi MP. Outcomes after total knee arthroplasty for post-traumatic arthritis. *Knee.* 2015;22(6):630-639.

89. Kleiner JE, Gil JA, Eltorai AEM, Rubin LE, Daniels AH. Matched cohort analysis of peri-operative outcomes following total knee arthroplasty in patients with and without Parkinson's disease. *Knee.* 2019;26(4):876-880.

90. Ergin ON, Karademir G, Sahin K, Meric E, Akgul T, Ozturk I. Functional outcomes of total knee arthroplasty in patients with Parkinson's disease: a case control study. *J Orthop Sci.* 2019. pii:S0949-2658(19)30184-8.

91. Prasad A, Donovan R, Ramachandran M, et al. Outcome of total knee arthroplasty in patients with poliomyelitis: a systematic review. *EFORT Open Rev.* 2018;3(6):358-362.

92. Styron JF, Barsoum WK, Smyth KA, Singer ME. Preoperative predictors of returning to work following primary total knee arthroplasty. *J Bone Joint Surg Am.* 2011;93(1):2-10.

93. Clyde CT, Goyal N, Matar WY, Witmer D, Restrepo C, Hozack WJ. Workers' Compensation patients after total joint arthroplasty: do they return to work? *J Arthroplasty.* 2013;28(6):883-887.

94. Mont MA, Mayerson JA, Krackow KA, Hungerford DS. Total knee arthroplasty in patients receiving Workers' Compensation. *J Bone Joint Surg Am.* 1998;80(9):1285-1290.

95. Saleh K, Nelson C, Kassim R, Yoon P, Haas S. Total knee arthroplasty in patients on workers' compensation: a matched cohort study with an average follow-up of 4.5 years. *J Arthroplasty.* 2004;19(3):310-312.

96. de Beer J, Petruccelli D, Gandhi R, Winemaker M. Primary total knee arthroplasty in patients receiving workers' compensation benefits. *Can J Surg.* 2005;48(2):100-105.

97. Everhart JS, Andridge RR, Scharschmidt TJ, Mayerson JL, Glassman AH, Lemeshow S. Development and validation of a preoperative surgical site infection risk score for primary or revision knee and hip arthroplasty. *J Bone Joint Surg Am.* 2016;98(18):1522-1532.

98. Jerry GJ Jr, Rand JA, Ilstrup D. Old sepsis prior to total knee arthroplasty. *Clin Orthop Relat Res.* 1988;236:135-140.

99. Lee GC, Pagnano MW, Hanssen AD. Total knee arthroplasty after prior bone or joint sepsis about the knee. *Clin Orthop Relat Res.* 2002;404:226-231.

100. Seo JG, Moon YW, Park SH, Han KY, Kim SM. Primary total knee arthroplasty in infection sequelae about the native knee. *J Arthroplasty.* 2014;29(12):2271-2275.

101. Shaikh AA, Ha CW, Park YG, Park YB. Two-stage approach to primary TKA in infected arthritic knees using intraoperatively molded articulating cement spacers. *Clin Orthop Relat Res.* 2014;472(7):2201-2207.

102. Nazarian DG, de Jesus D, McGuigan F, Booth RE Jr. A two-stage approach to primary knee arthroplasty in the infected arthritic knee. *J Arthroplasty.* 2003;18(7 suppl 1):16-21.

103. Chalmers BP, Weston JT, Osmon DR, Hanssen AD, Berry DJ, Abdel MP. Prior hip or knee prosthetic joint infection in another joint increases risk three-fold of prosthetic joint infection after primary total knee arthroplasty: a matched control study. *Bone Joint J.* 2019;101-B(7_suppl_C):91-97.

104. Bedair H, Goyal N, Dietz MJ, et al. A history of treated periprosthetic joint infection increases the risk of subsequent different site infection. *Clin Orthop Relat Res.* 2015;473(7):2300-2304.

105. Bateman DK, Preston JS, Kayiaros S, Tria AJ Jr. Synthetic mesh allograft reconstruction for extensor mechanism insufficiency after total knee arthroplasty. *Orthopedics.* 2019;42(4):e385-e390.

106. Browne JA, Hanssen AD. Reconstruction of patellar tendon disruption after total knee arthroplasty: results of a new technique utilizing synthetic mesh. *J Bone Joint Surg Am.* 2011;93(12):1137-1143.

107. Cottino U, Deledda D, Rosso F, Blonna D, Bonasia DE, Rossi R. Chronic knee extensor mechanism lesions in total knee arthroplasty: a literature review. *Joints.* 2016;4(3):159-164.

108. Deren ME, Pannu TS, Villa JM, Firtha M, Riesgo AM, Higuera CA. Meta-analysis comparing allograft to synthetic reconstruction for extensor mechanism disruption after total knee arthroplasty. *J Knee Surg.* 2019. doi:10.1055/s0039-1696656.

109. Lim CT, Amanatullah DF, Huddleston JI III, et al. Reconstruction of disrupted extensor mechanism after total knee arthroplasty. *J Arthroplasty.* 2017;32(10):3134-3140.

110. Wise BT, Erens G, Pour AE, Bradbury TL, Roberson JR. Long-term results of extensor mechanism reconstruction using Achilles tendon allograft after total knee arthroplasty. *Int Orthop.* 2018;42(10):2367-2373.

111. Delano PJ. The pathogenesis of Charcots joint. *Am J Roentgenol Radium Ther.* 1946;56(2):189-200.

112. Tibbo ME, Chalmers BP, Berry DJ, Pagnano MW, Lewallen DG, Abdel MP. Primary total knee arthroplasty in patients with neuropathic (Charcot) arthropathy: contemporary results. *J Arthroplasty.* 2018;33(9):2815-2820.

113. Patel A, Saini AK, Edmonds ME, Kavarthapu V. Diabetic neuropathic arthropathy of the knee: two case reports and a review of the literature. *Case Rep Orthop.* 2018;2018:9301496.

114. Zeng M, Xie J, Hu Y. Total knee arthroplasty in patients with Charcot joints. *Knee Surg Sports Traumatol Arthrosc.* 2016;24(8):2672-2677.

115. Goetti P, Gallusser N, Borens O. Bilateral diabetic knee neuroarthropathy in a forty-year-old patient. *Case Rep Orthop.* 2016;2016:3204813.

116. Sugitani K, Arai Y, Takamiya H, Minami G, Higuchi T, Kubo T. Total knee arthroplasty for neuropathic joint disease after severe bone destruction eroded the tibial tuberosity. *Orthopedics.* 2012;35(7):e1108-e1111.

117. Troyer J, Levine BR. Proximal tibia reconstruction with a porous tantalum cone in a patient with Charcot arthropathy. *Orthopedics.* 2009;32(5):358.

118. Yasin MN, Charalambous CP, Mills SP, Phaltankar PM, Nurron RW. Early failure of a knee replacement in a neuropathic joint. A case report. *Acta Orthop Belg.* 2011;77(1):132-136.

119. Bae DK, Song SJ, Yoon KH, Noh JH. Long-term outcome of total knee arthroplasty in Charcot joint: a 10- to 22-year follow-up. *J Arthroplasty.* 2009;24(8):1152-1156.

120. de Amesti M, Ortiz-Munoz L, Irarrazaval S. What are the benefits and risks of total arthroplasty in arthrodesed knees? *Medwave.* 2018;18(5):e7258.

121. Jauregui JJ, Buitrago CA, Pushilin SA, Browning BB, Mulchandani NB, Maheshwari AV. Conversion of a surgically arthrodesed knee to a total knee arthroplasty-is it worth it? A meta-analysis. *J Arthroplasty.* 2016;31(8):1736-1741.

122. Kernkamp WA, Verra WC, Pijls BG, Schoones JW, van der Linden HM, Nelissen RG. Conversion from knee arthrodesis to arthroplasty: systematic review. *Int Orthop.* 2016;40(10):2069-2074.

123. Twiggs JG, Wakelin EA, Fritsch BA, et al. Clinical and statistical validation of a probabilistic prediction tool of total knee arthroplasty outcome. *J Arthroplasty.* 2019;34(11):2624-2631.

124. Goltz DE, Ryan SP, Howell CB, Attarian D, Bolognesi MP, Seyler TM. A weighted index of Elixhauser comorbidities for predicting 90-day readmission after total joint arthroplasty. *J Arthroplasty.* 2019;34(5):857-864.

125. Harris AHS, Kuo AC, Weng Y, Trickey AW, Bowe T, Giori NJ. Can machine learning methods produce accurate and easy-to-use prediction models of 30-day complications and mortality after knee or hip arthroplasty? *Clin Orthop Relat Res.* 2019;477(2):452-460.

126. Huber M, Kurz C, Leidl R. Predicting patient-reported outcomes following hip and knee replacement surgery using supervised machine learning. *BMC Med Inform Decis Mak.* 2019;19(1):3.

127. Schwarzkopf R, Novikov D, Anoushiravani AA, et al. The preoperative management of Hepatitis C may improve the outcome after total knee arthroplasty. *Bone Joint J.* 2019;101-B(6):667-674.

128. Alamanda VK, Springer BD. The prevention of infection: 12 modifiable risk factors. *Bone Joint J.* 2019;101-B(1_suppl_A):3-9.

129. Bernstein DN, Liu TC, Winegar AL, et al. Evaluation of a preoperative optimization protocol for primary hip and knee arthroplasty patients. *J Arthroplasty.* 2018;33(12):3642-3648.

130. Roche M, Law TY, Kurowicki J, Rosas S, Rush AJ III. Effect of obesity on total knee arthroplasty costs and revision rate. *J Knee Surg.* 2018;31(1):38-42.

131. Shrader MW, Morrey BF. Insall Award paper. Primary TKA in patients with lymphedema. *Clin Orthop Relat Res.* 2003;416:22-26.

132. Otero JE, Graves CM, Gao Y, et al. Patient-reported allergies predict worse outcomes after hip and knee arthroplasty: results from a prospective cohort study. *J Arthroplasty.* 2016;31(12):2746-2749.

133. Sodhi N, Moore T, Vakharia RM, et al. Fibromyalgia increases the risk of surgical complications following total knee arthroplasty: a nationwide database study. *J Arthroplasty.* 2019;34(9):1953-1956.

134. Newman JM, Sodhi N, Wilhelm AB, et al. Parkinson's disease increases the risk of perioperative complications after total knee arthroplasty: a nationwide database study. *Knee Surg Sports Traumatol Arthrosc.* 2019;27(7):2189-2195.

135. Gronbeck C, Cote MP, Lieberman JR, Halawi MJ. Risk stratification in primary total joint arthroplasty: the current state of knowledge. *Arthroplast Today.* 2019;5(1):126-131.

136. Abu Dakka M, Badri H, Al-Khaffaf H. Total knee arthroplasty in patients with peripheral vascular disease. *Surgeon.* 2009;7(6):362-365.

137. Walls RJ, O'Malley J, O'Flanagan SJ, Kenny PJ, Leahy AL, Keogh P. Total knee replacement under tourniquet control: a prospective study of the peripheral arterial vasculature using colour-assisted duplex ultrasonography. *Surgeon.* 2015;13(6):303-307.

138. Calligaro KD, DeLaurentis DA, Booth RE, Rothman RH, Savarese RP, Dougherty MJ. Acute arterial thrombosis associated with total knee arthroplasty. *J Vasc Surg* 1994;20(6):927-930. discussion 930-922.

139. Calligaro KD, Dougherty MJ, Ryan S, Booth RE. Acute arterial complications associated with total hip and knee arthroplasty. *J Vasc Surg.* 2003;38(6):1170-1177.

140. Smith DE, McGraw RW, Taylor DC, Masri BA. Arterial complications and total knee arthroplasty. *J Am Acad Orthop Surg.* 2001;9(4):253-257.

141. Deakin AH, Smith MA, Wallace DT, Smith EJ, Sarungi M. Fulfilment of preoperative expectations and postoperative patient satisfaction after total knee replacement. A prospective analysis of 200 patients. *Knee.* 2019. pii:S0968-0160(18)30782-8.

142. Ghomrawi HMK, Lee LY, Nwachukwu BU, et al. Preoperative expectations associated with postoperative dissatisfaction after total knee arthroplasty: a cohort study. *J Am Acad Orthop Surg.* 2019. doi:10.5435/JAAOS-D-18-00785.

chapter 29

Preoperative Planning for Primary Total Knee Arthroplasty

Nathanael Heckmann, MD | Kevin Bigart, MD | Aaron G. Rosenberg, MD

INTRODUCTION

Modern total knee arthroplasty has revolutionized the treatment of degenerative diseases about the knee. Today, total knee arthroplasty offers both surgeons and patients a reliable treatment for these conditions. When total knee arthroplasty is compared to other medical and surgical interventions for common diseases, the cost of quality-adjusted life years associated with this procedure is unparalleled.[1-3]

The durability of modern total knee arthroplasty designs and component materials has led surgeons to broaden the indications for this procedure. Long-term follow-up of first-generation total condylar knee arthroplasty implants has shown survivorship of 77% to 91% at greater than 20-year follow-up.[4,5] With further improvements in operative techniques, instrumentation, and prosthetic design combined with a better understanding of the mechanisms of failure, long-term survivorship of total knee arthroplasty has improved. Newer knee designs have shown 20-year survivorship of 87% to 97% in some series.[6-8] Given the success of this procedure, surgeons have expanded the surgical indications, and a surgery once reserved for the elderly and low-demand patient is now being performed in younger, higher demand patients with increased frequency.[9]

Appropriate surgical indications are paramount to achieving successful outcomes. As the population continues to age, the number of patients with degenerative conditions of the knee will continue to increase. Furthermore, the recent increase in total knee arthroplasty procedures performed in patients 45 to 64 years old continues to change the overall population of patients undergoing this surgery. These demographic changes and broadened indications make an understanding of the limitations of total knee arthroplasty imperative for orthopedic surgeons, patients, and primary care physicians.

PATIENT SELECTION

With recent demographic changes and expanding indications, total knee arthroplasty has become one of the most common surgical procedures performed.[10] However, the increased utilization of total knee arthroplasty should be approached with appropriate caution as younger patients have been shown to have two- to fivefold greater revision rate with decreased long-term implant survival compared to older patients.[11-13] Despite these concerns, long-term improvements in pain and function can be achieved in young patients who undergo total knee arthroplasty.[14-16] However, any medical decision requires consideration of the risks and benefits of a given intervention, particularly surgical ones with rare but potentially catastrophic complications. Risk considerations should be weighed in light of the prospective benefits and limitations that a patient can experience following a total knee arthroplasty.

For total knee arthroplasty, any discussion about the appropriate indications for surgery mandates that the patient benefit from the intervention to warrant the specific risks involved. As with any surgery, determining whether or not a total knee arthroplasty is indicated or contraindicated involves the careful evaluation of the patient's complaints, pathology, and overall health status, as well as the weighing of multiple risk factors for adverse outcomes and prognostic factors associated with a successful surgery. Finally, these considerations should result in a judgment as to whether the final balance of risks and benefits is appropriate for the individual patient under consideration. This judgment should involve the patient, as an accurate assessment of the surgical benefit relies on realistic patient expectations and a thorough understanding of the limitations of total knee arthroplasty.

An important consideration in the performance of any elective surgical procedure is the relative risk of perioperative events that carry with them significant morbidity or mortality. Total knee arthroplasty as practiced before the risk of thromboembolic disease was well understood, carried with it a mortality risk from pulmonary embolism. Although the incidence of fatal pulmonary embolism has decreased, as have the rates of infection and other serious postsurgical morbidities, one must compare the potential long-term benefits of pain reduction and improved function with the short-term risks of death and other complications.

Risk and benefit analyses regarding total knee arthroplasty are dependent on several factors in addition to the underlying pathology, including patient age, activity level, and comorbid disease burden. These patient factors must be weighed in light of several assumptions before a surgeon can determine if a total knee arthroplasty is indicated for an individual patient. These assumptions include the finite durability of a total knee arthroplasty implant, the failure of nonsurgical treatment to alleviate pain, and the limitations to activity that are caused by a patient's degenerative knee disease. These three assumptions ought to inform any risk–benefit analysis when determining if total knee arthroplasty surgery is indicated.

The first assumption that a knee arthroplasty is a time-limited operation relies on an understanding of fixation longevity, material wear, and implant failure. While several previously referenced series demonstrate improved component survival in young and highly active patients, it is unreasonable to assume that young adults with a normal life span will reliably outlive a total knee implant in all instances. Thus, age becomes an important factor in the decision to proceed with total knee arthroplasty, particularly at extremely young ages, when the assumption that a total knee arthroplasty has a finite life span is thoughtfully considered. For this reason, ceteris paribus, older patients continue to be better candidates for total knee arthroplasty, as the likelihood that an implant will outlive the patient increases with age, obviating the need for revision surgery or potentially multiple subsequent surgical interventions. However, with improved surgical techniques, modern implant designs, and improved material properties, considerations about the time-limited nature of implants have led many surgeons to pursue knee arthroplasty in younger patients that were previously thought to be "out of bounds" based on age-related implant concerns. However, the pediatric and young adult patient clearly deserve an attempt at alternative treatments, such as osteotomy or cartilage restoration procedures, if such treatment will relieve symptoms sufficiently to postpone arthroplasty and not make subsequent treatment exceedingly complex.

Another assumption is that nonoperative treatment should be attempted before proceeding with arthroplasty. This may include the use of assistive devices for ambulation, weight loss, systemic or local medications, physiotherapy, bracing, and activity modification. A concerted effort at nonsurgical therapy may be more reasonable in the younger patient than in the elderly, in whom prolonged attempts are time consuming and rarely effective in relieving symptoms and improving function. These modalities should be attempted more aggressively in the younger patient than in the elderly. In some settings, the symptoms, physical findings, and radiographic changes are severe enough to warrant consideration of total knee arthroplasty even if the patient has had no prior nonoperative treatment. For example, in an elderly patient with progressively worsening localized knee pain and severe radiographic osteoarthritis (i.e., joint space obliteration, abundant marginal osteophytes, subchondral sclerosis or cystic changes, etc.), surgery may be indicated, given the futile likelihood that nonsurgical treatments will provide lasting relief. In most cases, however, particularly in

the younger individual, it may be wiser to demonstrate to the patient that conservative or nonsurgical treatment will not relieve symptoms or improve function before recommending more aggressive surgical treatment that has more substantial risk of complications.

The level of patient activity and symptom severity are other important factors to consider when determining whether arthroplasty is indicated. Although pain is the most common complaint before surgical intervention, in many cases, symptoms are activity related. If the patient's symptoms are clearly amenable to activity modification and if total knee arthroplasty is not an ideal option due to age, comorbidities, expectation mismatch, or other factors, the surgeon should opt for activity modification over operative intervention. If the individual has little or no symptoms with activity modification, then activity limitation may be a reasonable course of action. However, marked limitation in functional capacity may be an indication for joint arthroplasty in the elderly. Understanding the patient's requirements for performing activities of daily living is essential in this determination. A patient's ability to perform a job, do household tasks, and maintain personal hygiene can be used as measures of the effect of knee function on the patient's quality of life. Walking tolerance, defined as the length of time or distance one can walk without rest, can be an important benchmark in assessing the severity of disease and limitation of function. In general, if an elderly patient cannot perform activities of daily living despite nonoperative treatment, knee function has decreased to the point at which intervention is indicated. However, in a younger patient, surgery may be indicated following more moderate limitations in activity, provided the patient and surgeon have realistic expectations in terms of postoperative function, implant longevity, and postoperative complications.

In summary, total knee arthroplasty is often indicated in patients who have painful arthritic changes in the knee that limit or alter physical activity in a way that negatively affects their quality of life. However, the surgeon should bear in mind that the final determination of whether a knee arthroplasty is indicated for an individual should follow a risk–benefit analysis that takes into account a patient's age, comorbidities, functional limitation, and postsurgical expectations. This analysis should be followed by a shared patient–surgeon decision in which the surgeon bears the responsibility of ensuring that the patient has reasonable expectations following surgery, understands the limitation of a total knee arthroplasty, and is aware of the risks and benefits associated with the procedure and possible future procedures.

PATIENT EXPECTATIONS

The surgeon often encounters patients with unrealistic expectations for surgical intervention. These expectations must be tempered by the surgeon's experience and a thorough understanding of outcomes that can be obtained following total knee arthroplasty. A patient must understand that the goal of knee arthroplasty is to alleviate pain and improve function, not to restore the patient's knee to a prearthritic state. The patient must also understand that functional limitations may still exist after knee arthroplasty. Normal range of motion may not be restored after years of reduced motion and extensive flexion contracture. In some patients, range of motion may be less after surgery than before. These concepts should be discussed extensively with the patient prior to any surgical intervention as unmet expectations are associated with poor outcomes following total knee arthroplasty.[17]

Finally, it is important to discuss the responsibility patients must assume for their prosthetic knees. Patients must understand that this implant is a walking device designed to relieve pain and thus patients must be willing to modify their activity to prevent early mechanical failure. Although certain activities such as walking, swimming, and golf are compatible with a long-term successful outcome, higher impact sports such as long distance running may not be compatible with optimal implant longevity. By assuming responsibility for their actions, patients must realize that certain activities may result in diminished longevity of the knee and subsequent need for revision surgery. Along these same lines, before embarking on surgical intervention, the surgeon must be confident that a given patient is willing and able to comply with the necessary postoperative rehabilitation protocols compatible with a successful outcome.

PATIENT ASSESSMENT

Not unlike most orthopedic procedures, determining whether total knee arthroplasty is indicated for a given patient consists of obtaining a history that includes pain and disability, combined with corroborative physical examination and radiographic findings. These three facets of the patient evaluation should all confirm the presence of end-stage arthritis of the knee before the surgeon recommends a total knee arthroplasty. If any one of these evaluations fails to support this diagnosis, the surgeon should be alerted to the possibility of a mistaken diagnosis or the possibility that the patient's complaints will not be adequately addressed by this procedure.

History

The primary indication for total knee arthroplasty is recalcitrant pain in the knee caused by degenerative joint disease. Pain is the most reliably addressed symptom of knee arthritis after total knee arthroplasty is performed. The character and degree of pain is important to document, as is the presence of pain at night or at rest. If no other diagnosis is present, night or rest pain often heralds the final stage of knee osteoarthritis that may not

respond to nonoperative treatment. Inflammatory arthritis can also be associated with significant discomfort both at rest and at night. If the knee pain is associated with groin or anterior thigh pain, the clinician must be careful to evaluate the hip, as hip pathology may cause pain that is referred to the knee. Pain from knee osteoarthritis frequently extends below the knee, but pain down into the foot must be distinguished from radicular pain.

Pain associated with arthritis of the knee is typically related to activity, and the physician should establish the functional disability this has created. Specifically, the physician should determine how the patients' pain has affected their ability to perform their activities of daily living such as shopping, cleaning, and personal hygiene. These facets of the history are important to delineate, as pain is an individual experience that may hamper patients' ability to care for him- or herself and impact their lifestyle in uniquely individual ways. Patients who exhibit both severe pain and functional disability will derive the most benefit from total knee arthroplasty. It is also important to identify those patients with unrealistic expectations from total knee arthroplasty, such as those who only experience pain and disability in the context of intense physical exertion, in whom activity modification, rather than surgery, may be more appropriate.

The patient history should also include an assessment of prior nonoperative and operative treatments. A thorough trial of nonoperative treatment is appropriate for the majority of patients as previously discussed. Nonoperative treatment including activity modification, nonsteroidal anti-inflammatory medications, hyaluronate or corticosteroid injections, and the use of an assist device should all be considered and discussed with patients as potential forms of nonoperative management of knee arthritis. Failure of these modalities should be considered a good indication for surgery in the presence of corroborative physical examination and radiographic findings.

A prior history of operative treatment is also important to document, as various other operative treatments may influence the operative techniques used and compromise the final outcome of total knee arthroplasty. If possible, previous operative reports should be reviewed to confirm the surgical findings and treatment rendered.

The patient history should also include an assessment of the patient's general health including any medical problems. Appropriate preoperative medical consultation is imperative to identify medical comorbidities that can be optimized preoperatively or that may argue against elective surgery. A history of disease associated with an immunocompromised state (e.g., diabetes mellitus, renal failure, acquired immune deficiency syndrome, etc.) is also important to obtain, to more carefully counsel patients about the risks of periprosthetic joint infection. The history should also seek to identify other medical problems that may be associated with persistent bacteremia such as recurrent urinary tract infections in women, urinary outlet obstruction in men, or dental problems that can be addressed before operative intervention.

A thorough history should also include drug allergies and metal sensitivities. A notably small proportion of candidates for total knee arthroplasty who report a penicillin allergy actually have a true IgE-mediated reaction to cephalosporins.[18] However, given the potential severity of these types of reactions, the orthopedic surgeon should consider a preoperative skin testing with an allergist or a preoperative test dose, prior to the administration of a therapeutic dose of a preoperative first-generation cephalosporin. These considerations should be weighed with recent data suggesting patient who receive noncephalosporin antibiotics may be at increased risk of developing a postoperative periprosthetic joint infection.[19] Lastly, if a patient reports a history of metal sensitivity or metal allergies, the surgeon should consider sending the patient to an allergist for metal patch testing or ordering a lymphocyte transformation testing. In these patients, alternative implants that do not contain cobalt or chromium may be considered. However, one should note the lack of data supporting the use of preoperative allergy testing and alternative implants as a means to decrease complications in patients with metal allergies.

Physical Examination

Physical examination should begin with an assessment of gait. An antalgic gait is commonly encountered in patient with moderate to severe arthritis; however, the presence of a Trendelenburg gait should alert the physician to a problem with the ipsilateral hip joint or neuromuscular disease. A patient's gait is often illustrative of the amount of disability that they are encountering and helps the surgeon to determine if a given patient's arthritis warrants total knee arthroplasty. The alignment of the lower extremity is also noted to assist with preoperative planning of anticipated ligament releases if total knee arthroplasty is in fact indicated.

Inspection of the soft-tissue envelope is performed next. The location and age of prior incisions should be noted, as they may impact the surgical approach used in subsequent knee arthroplasty. If there is a question as to the suitability of the soft-tissue envelope for surgical intervention, a preoperative consultation with a plastic surgeon is recommended. The presence of cutaneous lesions is also important to note, because they may indicate the cause of arthritis (i.e., psoriatic arthritis) or may influence the decision to proceed with surgery, as surgery will need to be delayed for patients with active skin lesions until the soft-tissue envelope is intact to prevent an unacceptably high rate of infection.

A neurovascular examination including the palpation of dorsalis pedis and posterior tibial pulses follows. If they are not palpable, a vascular consultation may be warranted, and the avoidance of a tourniquet intraoperatively may be considered. The neurologic examination may alert the physician to the presence of preoperative neurologic deficits and may also identify a radiculopathy as the cause of the patient's pain. Other nonmusculoskeletal disease processes such as venous insufficiency, complex regional pain syndrome, and diabetic neuropathy can be identified with a thorough examination and should be noted as they may affect a patient's outcome.

Examination of the knee itself includes an assessment of range of motion, which is typically decreased. In addition, it is important to recognize that preoperative range of motion is often predictive of postoperative range of motion.[20] Some patients may seek total knee arthroplasty primarily to increase their range of motion, and the ability to improve their range of motion must be carefully discussed with the patient before surgery. Preoperative flexion contractures are also important to identify so that they can be appropriately addressed at the time of surgery. The knee is next palpated to determine areas of maximal tenderness. If the patient has pain in areas that do not correspond to the radiographic location of arthritis, other diagnoses should be examined. Ligamentous stability should be tested next, with care taken to examine the medial and lateral collateral ligaments, as well as the anterior and posterior cruciate ligaments. Lower extremity alignment should be noted and compared to the contralateral extremity. If any valgus or varus deformity is present, the ability to correct all or part of the deformity should be noted as should the ability to overcorrect the deformity.

The physical examination should include a thorough assessment of the lower back and hip to ensure that the pain experienced by the patient is not referred from a distant anatomic location. Lastly, the foot should also be evaluated as a pes planus deformity can accentuate a valgus deformity preoperatively and lead to valgus instability postoperatively. In cases in which the cause of the patient's pain is unclear, an intra-articular lidocaine injection can be used as a diagnostic test to confirm the pain is arising from the knee joint itself.

Radiographic Analysis

Radiographic confirmation of knee arthritis is important in the evaluation of the patient considered for total knee arthroplasty. Clinical symptoms, however, oftentimes do not correlate directly with the severity of radiographic findings. Specifically, the radiographic presence of severe arthritic changes in the absence of clinical symptoms or disability referable to the knee is clearly not an indication for total knee arthroplasty. Similarly, the absence of radiographic findings should alert the physician to an alternative diagnosis.

Radiographs obtained should include standing anteroposterior, lateral, and patellofemoral views. Standing radiographs are imperative to detect subtle joint space narrowing associated with loss of articular cartilage. A standing view with the knee flexed may further assist in identifying subtle joint space narrowing, particularly along the posterior femoral condyles. It is not uncommon for patients with minimal radiographic changes to undergo an extensive course of nonoperative treatment only for severe cartilaginous destruction to be found at the time of surgery. Thus, radiographs must always be interpreted in the context of clinical symptoms. Patellofemoral views are equally important as anteroposterior and lateral views alone can underestimate the degree of patellofemoral arthritis present. Full-length lower extremity mechanical axis views may provide the surgeon with additional information regarding the patient's coronal deformity. Lastly, if digital templating is performed, a calibrated radiographic marker should be used to increase accuracy.

CONTRAINDICATIONS AND ALTERNATIVES TO TOTAL KNEE ARTHROPLASTY

Contraindications

Although total knee arthroplasty is appropriate management for the majority of patients with a severely arthritic knee, the surgeon must be aware of alternate surgical therapies that may be more appropriate for certain patients. Alternative surgical options to total knee arthroplasty include osteotomy, unicompartmental arthroplasty, and arthrodesis. Osteotomy of the knee is reserved for patients with symptomatic unicompartmental arthritis who have a focal biomechanical derangement of the knee joint with an adjacent area of intact cartilage available for redirection into the weight-bearing portion of the joint. Osteotomy can be performed on either the tibial or femoral side of the joint. For these procedures, a congruous, stable knee with good range of motion is a prerequisite. These procedures are often used in younger patients with early degenerative arthritis that is limited to either the medial or lateral compartment. Unicompartmental arthroplasty is indicated for patients with unicompartmental tibiofemoral arthritis without significant deformity, concomitant patellofemoral disease, ligamentous instability, or inflammatory arthritis. Arthrodesis of the knee is infrequently indicated except for patients with a clear contraindication to total knee arthroplasty such as active sepsis.

Arthroscopy of the knee has a very limited role in the treatment of knee osteoarthritis and has been performed with decreasing frequency given its lack of efficacy.[21] However, patients with degenerative arthritis and mechanical symptoms may benefit from operative arthroscopy, but the surgeon should be aware that symptoms may worsen after surgery. Arthroscopic synovectomy may have a role in the treatment of patients with inflammatory arthritis of the knee before severe cartilaginous destruction has occurred; however, the long-term benefits of such intervention are currently unproven.[22]

SPECIFIC PATIENT-RELATED CONSIDERATIONS

Age

When a patient is considered for total knee arthroplasty, it is important to remember that arthroplasty has time-limited results. Although excellent results have been reported for younger, active patients undergoing total knee arthroplasty,[14-16,23] the necessity for revision and possibly multiple revision surgeries must be considered in patients with longer expected life spans, as previously discussed. Younger age should not be considered an absolute contraindication, as good results have been reported in adolescent patients with inflammatory arthropathies.[24]

Good results have also been reported in the very elderly, and likewise advanced age itself should not be considered a contraindication to total knee arthroplasty.[25-28] Functional improvements, however, may be less than those seen in more youthful patients. Medical comorbidities may be increased in this patient population, which make the risks of perioperative complications higher.

Weight

Many patients who have arthritis of the knee are obese,[29] and although weight loss prior to surgery may mitigate the risk of perioperative complication, this is often challenging for the patients to achieve. Obese patients are considered at risk for a higher rate of complications than nonobese controls.[30,31] Despite this, it has been reported that these patients can have satisfactory outcomes after total knee arthroplasty,[32-34] and obesity alone should not be considered as a contraindication to total knee arthroplasty. Even morbidly obese patients have been found to have adequate results, although functional outcomes are reported to be poorer for this subset of patients.[35,36] Perioperative complications, particularly wound healing issues, superficial infections, and medial collateral ligament avulsions, are reported more frequently than in nonobese comparative groups. Because of this, care with soft-tissue closure and operative technique is imperative in this population. Furthermore, obese patients must be counseled preoperatively on the specific problems of total knee arthroplasty that they may encounter.

Diabetes Mellitus

Patients with diabetes mellitus have been shown to have immune dysfunction secondary to abnormal neutrophil and monocyte activity that makes them predisposed to infection.[37] Clinical studies have shown that this patient population has a significantly higher rate of wound complications, deep prosthetic infection, and urinary tract infection after total knee arthroplasty.[38-40] Due to the increased risk of perioperative complications among these patients, a newfound interest has been placed on preoperative optimization of these patients. Tight glycemic control among diabetics, defined as an HbA1c ≤7%, may lower postoperative risk of infection. However, a high percentage of diabetic patients seeking elective total joint arthroplasty surgery may not be able to achieve this goal, while a HbA1c ≤8% was achieved by 98% of diabetic patients seeking total joint arthroplasty.[41] A multicenter review of 1645 patients undergoing total joint arthroplasty (1004 knees and 641 hips) reported an infection rate of 1.3%.[42] The authors found that patients with a HbA1c levels >7.7% had an infection rate of 5.4% compared to patients with a HbA1c levels <7.7% who had an infection rate of 0.8% and suggested that a HbA1c threshold of 7.7% be used for preoperative optimization. The addition of antibiotic bone cement and an extended duration of oral antibiotics may help decrease the risk of postoperative infection among patients with diabetes to levels close to those of nondiabetics.[43,44] However, these additional measures do not eliminate the need for preoperative optimization of glycemic control.

Osteonecrosis

Patients with osteonecrosis of the knee may have poor-quality bone that does not adequately support the prosthetic components leading to a higher rate of failure. It is important to keep in mind, however, that osteonecrosis of the knee is a heterogeneous disorder; idiopathic or spontaneous osteonecrosis of the knee occurs in older patients with more predictable outcomes, whereas younger patients with steroid-induced (secondary) osteonecrosis and diseases such as systemic lupus erythematosus have poorer outcomes. In the latter group, diseases such as lupus may make patients more susceptible to infection, perioperative medical complications, and poor functional outcomes. Although the results of total knee arthroplasty in this population may not be as predictable as patients with osteoarthritis, patients with severe joint involvement may not have other reasonable treatment options.

Mont et al reported on 31 knees in 21 patients with osteonecrosis of the knee younger than 50 years who had undergone total knee arthroplasty and were taking corticosteroids. The authors found only 55% of patients with good to excellent results with a 37% rate of aseptic loosening requiring revision at a mean of 8 years.[45] Similarly, Seldes et al. found a 16% rate of revision among 31 knees with three cases of aseptic loosening and two deep infections among patients with steroid-induced osteonecrosis after 5 years of follow-up.[46] In a later study by Mont et al, 48 knees treated with total knee arthroplasty for atraumatic osteonecrosis of the knee had a similarly disappointing rate of 71% clinically successful results at 9 years.[47] However, a follow-up study from Mont et al. found that 31 of 32 patients (97%) had successful outcomes at 4- to 12-year follow-up with cemented implants and stems when necrotic metaphyseal bone was present.[48]

Hemophilic Arthropathy

In patients affected with hemophilia, severe joint destruction and stiffness may occur. Specific problems encountered include poor bone quality and severe soft-tissue fibrosis, which leads to a high rate of complications, particularly an increased risk of infection compared to patients without hemophilia.[49-53] Hematologic consultation before and after surgery is essential to assist in the maintenance of factor levels in the perioperative period. The presence of antibodies directed against the deficient factors is a relative contraindication to total knee arthroplasty.

Figgie et al reported on 19 knees with an average follow-up of 9.5 years and found a 32% rate of fair and poor results.[49] Thomason et al. also reported poor results among 23 total knee arthroplasty procedures performed in 15 patients with hemophilic arthropathy.[52] At a mean of 7.5 years follow-up, 19 knees were rated as fair or poor with four infections (17%), all of which occurred in patients with human immunodeficiency virus infection. Norian et al reported on 53 total knee arthroplasties performed in 38 patients and reported a 13% infection rate at an average of 60 months.[51] In addition to the risk of infection, several studies have documented high rates of radiographic evidence of loosening[49,52] or complete failure from aseptic loosening.[53] Despite the problems encountered in this patient population, patient satisfaction is high with significant improvements in quality of life[54] and function[50] following total knee arthroplasty.

Ipsilateral Hip Fusion

Patients with a fusion of the hip may experience pain and arthrosis of the lumbar spine, ipsilateral knee, or contralateral hip. In general, it is advisable to perform a conversion arthroplasty of the hip before total knee arthroplasty, as patients may have significant pain relief in their knee after hip fusion takedown.[55-57] In addition, total knee arthroplasty with an ipsilateral hip fusion is technically challenging. Patients may have a frontal plane knee deformity if the ipsilateral hip is fused in excessive abduction or adduction, and ligamentous instability is common.[58]

Romness and Morrey reported on 16 knees in patients with an ipsilateral hip fusion; 12 patients had undergone total knee arthroplasty after conversion arthroplasty of the hip and 4 before such intervention.[59] At a mean of 5.5 years, 15 of 16 patients had no or minimal pain with no revisions reported in their cohort. Garvin et al. reported on nine knees that had undergone total knee arthroplasty with an ipsilateral hip fusion.[60] Although eight of the nine knees had good or excellent results at 7 years, all patients had at least one complication: seven knees required manipulation under anesthesia for poor range of motion, two experienced peroneal nerve palsies, and one patient developed a deep infection. Despite these complications, patients with an ipsilateral hip fusion can have good functional results even if they are unable to undergo a hip fusion takedown.

Paget Disease

Paget disease of bone is a disorder of abnormal bone remodeling with increased osteoclastic resorption followed by a secondary increase in reactive bone formation.[61] It is found in 3% to 4% of the population older than 50 years of age, although it is usually asymptomatic and often found incidentally on radiographs obtained for other reasons. The increased metabolic state leads to highly vascular bone that is weaker than normal which may compromise the success of a total knee arthroplasty.[61-63] Radiographic features include coarsened trabeculae with a blastic appearance with remodeling which may lead to bony enlargement and resultant deformity. The femur and tibia are frequently involved, and the disease process can cause severe deformity, pain, and degenerative joint disease of the hip and knee.

At times, it may be difficult to differentiate pain secondary to the disease process itself from pain in an adjacent joint secondary to arthritis. In these cases, an intra-articular injection of lidocaine into the knee may assist in differentiating the origin of pain. A sudden increase in pain may herald a pathologic fracture or the transformation of a Paget disease lesion into sarcoma, which should be ruled out before total knee arthroplasty is pursued. In these cases, radiographs may show cortical destruction and advanced imaging studies reveal an associated soft-tissue mass. Medical treatment before surgical intervention is recommended as it may decrease pain and thus obviate the need for surgery. In addition, if surgical intervention is indicated, medical management may decrease blood loss associated with operating on this highly vascular bone.

Clinical experience with total knee arthroplasty in patients with Paget disease is limited to several small series of patients.[63-67] These studies report difficulty in obtaining appropriate alignment secondary to deformity. Extramedullary alignment or navigation may be required for cases with extensive deformity. In addition, exposure may be challenging, with one series reporting partial patellar tendon avulsion in 3 of 21 cases (14%) due to difficulty mobilizing the patella during exposure.[66] Despite these technical challenges, good clinical and radiographic results are attainable, with little difference seen between these patients and matched osteoarthritic controls.

Posttraumatic Arthritis

Patients with posttraumatic arthritis of the knee may have previously undergone surgical intervention or have had severe soft-tissue injuries that may complicate total knee arthroplasty.[68] The location of previous incisions should be carefully noted, as should the overall condition of the soft-tissue envelope. These patients may also have severe deformity, bone loss, or associated ligamentous deficiencies that may need to be addressed at the time of surgery. Furthermore, the removal of internal fixation implants may both complicate the operative approach and mandate the use of stemmed components to span areas of potential weakness. If prior operative intervention has been carried out, the presence of an infection must also be considered.

Patients who sustain a tibial plateau fracture are over five times as likely to require a total knee arthroplasty compared to age- and sex-matched controls without a fracture.[69] As such, these patients are frequently encountered by the arthroplasty surgeon. Saleh et al. reported on 15 total knee arthroplasties performed after open reduction and internal fixation of a tibial plateau fracture.[70] Perioperative complications included four knees with poor wound healing which led to a deep infection in three cases, two patellar ligament ruptures, and three knees that required a manipulation under anesthesia for stiffness. At a mean of 6 years postoperatively, 12 of the 15 patients had good or excellent results. Given the high rate of infection observed, the authors recommended preoperative joint aspiration and the use of antibiotic-loaded cement. Weiss et al. reported on 62 total knee arthroplasties and reported marked improvement in function and pain relief.[71] However, these authors reported an intraoperative complication rate of 10% and a reoperation of 21%.

Neurologic Dysfunction

Neurologic diseases can affect the results of total knee arthroplasty. Patients with Parkinson disease may obtain good results following total knee arthroplasty; functional scores may be poorer in those with severe disease or disease that progresses in severity following surgery.[72-75] Poliomyelitis may similarly affect the results of total knee arthroplasty, particularly if significant knee instability or quadriceps weakness is present.[76-81] As the incidence of poliomyelitis continues to decrease, reports of patients with this disorder who undergo total knee arthroplasty are limited to small case series. These patients tend to have less pain relief and progressive deterioration in knee function following total knee arthroplasty. In summary, the presence of chronic neurologic diseases is associated with higher rates of complications and poorer functional outcomes following total knee arthroplasty.

Workers' Compensation

Patients receiving workers' compensation have been shown to have significantly poorer outcomes than matched subjects not receiving workers' compensation after total knee arthroplasty. Interestingly, whereas objective postoperative indicators such as range of motion and radiographic findings are similar to those in matched patients, subjective findings, particularly measures of pain, and overall outcomes are far worse. Although receipt of workers' compensation is not a contraindication to total knee arthroplasty, the surgeon should spend a substantial amount of time getting to know such patients preoperatively to build a strong relationship with them and to attempt to understand their motivations in seeking surgical intervention.

CONCLUSION

Surgical planning for total knee arthroplasty may range from simple to complex. However, it is the job of the surgeon to assess all of the relevant patient-related factors involved in the surgical planning including patient-specific risks and challenges of operative intervention. Clear communication with patients about perioperative risks, realistic outcomes, and postoperative limitation is paramount to a successful surgical outcome and patient satisfaction. Time spent communicating will reward the surgeon with patients who fully understand the goals of surgery, are better able to cooperate with their own recovery, and have a greater understanding of expected outcomes. In our experience, this tends to make for a happier patient population and a more satisfying surgical practice—perhaps the ultimate goals for the knee arthroplasty surgeon.

REFERENCES

1. Ethgen O, Bruyère O, Richy F, Dardennes C, Reginster J-Y. Health-related quality of life in total hip and total knee arthroplasty. A qualitative and systematic review of the literature. *J Bone Joint Surg Am*. 2004;86-A(5):963-974.
2. Konopka JF, Lee Y-Y, Su EP, McLawhorn AS. Quality-adjusted life years after hip and knee arthroplasty: health-related quality of life after 12,782 joint replacements. *JB JS Open Access*. 2018;3(3):e0007.
3. Dimitriou D, Antoniadis A, Flury A, Liebhauser M, Helmy N. Total hip arthroplasty improves the quality-adjusted life years in patients who exceeded the estimated life expectancy. *J Arthroplasty*. 2018;33(11):3484-3489.
4. Pavone V, Boettner F, Fickert S, Sculco TP. Total condylar knee arthroplasty: a long-term followup. *Clin Orthop Relat Res*. 2001;(388):18-25.
5. Rodriguez JA, Bhende H, Ranawat CS. Total condylar knee replacement: a 20-year followup study. *Clin Orthop Relat Res*. 2001;(388):10-17.
6. Ritter MA, Meneghini RM. Twenty-year survivorship of cementless anatomic graduated component total knee arthroplasty. *J Arthroplasty*. 2010;25(4):507-513.
7. Ritter MA. Twenty-year follow-up of the AGC total knee arthroplasty. *J Arthroplasty*. 2008;23(2):328.
8. Patil S, McCauley JC, Pulido P, Colwell CW Jr. How do knee implants perform past the second decade? Nineteen- to 25-year followup of the Press-fit Condylar design TKA. *Clin Orthop Relat Res*. 2015;473(1):135-140.
9. Kurtz SM, Lau E, Ong K, Zhao K, Kelly M, Bozic KJ. Future young patient demand for primary and revision joint replacement: national projections from 2010 to 2030. *Clin Orthop Relat Res*. 2009;467(10):2606-2612.

10. Losina E, Thornhill TS, Rome BN, Wright J, Katz JN. The dramatic increase in total knee replacement utilization rates in the United States cannot be fully explained by growth in population size and the obesity epidemic. *J Bone Joint Surg Am*. 2012;94(3):201-207.
11. Losina E, Katz JN. Total knee arthroplasty on the rise in younger patients: are we sure that past performance will guarantee future success?. *Arthritis Rheum*. 2012;64(2):339-341.
12. Paxton EW, Namba RS, Maletis GB, et al. A prospective study of 80,000 total joint and 5000 anterior cruciate ligament reconstruction procedures in a community-based registry in the United States. *J Bone Joint Surg Am*. 2010;92 suppl 2:117-132.
13. Meehan JP, Danielsen B, Kim SH, Jamali AA, White RH. Younger age is associated with a higher risk of early periprosthetic joint infection and aseptic mechanical failure after total knee arthroplasty. *J Bone Joint Surg Am*. 2014;96(7):529-535.
14. Long WJ, Bryce CD, Hollenbeak CS, Benner RW, Scott WN. Total knee replacement in young, active patients: long-term follow-up and functional outcome: a concise follow-up of a previous report. *J Bone Joint Surg Am*. 2014;96(18):e159.
15. Diduch DR, Insall JN, Scott WN, Scuderi GR, Font-Rodriguez D. Total knee replacement in young, active patients. Long-term follow-up and functional outcome. *J Bone Joint Surg Am*. 1997;79(4):575-582.
16. Lonner JH, Hershman S, Mont M, Lotke PA. Total knee arthroplasty in patients 40 years of age and younger with osteoarthritis. *Clin Orthop Relat Res*. 2000;(380):85-90.
17. Bourne RB, Chesworth BM, Davis AM, Mahomed NN, Charron KDJ. Patient satisfaction after total knee arthroplasty: who is satisfied and who is not?. *Clin Orthop Relat Res*. 2010;468(1):57-63.
18. Park MA, Koch CA, Klemawesch P, Joshi A, Li JT. Increased adverse drug reactions to cephalosporins in penicillin allergy patients with positive penicillin skin test. *Int Arch Allergy Immunol*. 2010;153(3):268-273. doi:10.1159/000314367. Epub 2010 May 19. PubMed PMID: 20484925.
19. Wyles CC, Hevesi M, Osmon DR, et al. 2019 John Charnley Award: increased risk of prosthetic joint infection following primary total knee and hip arthroplasty with the use of alternative antibiotics to cefazolin: the value of allergy testing for antibiotic prophylaxis. *Bone Joint J*. 2019;101-B(6 suppl B):9-15. doi:10.1302/0301-620X.101B6.BJJ-2018-1407.R1. PubMed PMID: 31146571.
20. Ritter MA, Harty LD, Davis KE, Meding JB, Berend ME. Predicting range of motion after total knee arthroplasty. Clustering, log-linear regression, and regression tree analysis. *J Bone Joint Surg Am*. 2003;85-A(7):1278-1285.
21. Moseley JB, O'Malley K, Petersen NJ, et al. A controlled trial of arthroscopic surgery for osteoarthritis of the knee. *N Engl J Med*. 2002;347(2):81-88.
22. Klug S, Wittmann G, Weseloh G. Arthroscopic synovectomy of the knee joint in early cases of rheumatoid arthritis: follow-up results of a multicenter study. *Arthroscopy*. 2000;16(3):262-267.
23. Mont MA, Sayeed SA, Osuji O, et al. Total knee arthroplasty in patients 40 years and younger. *J Knee Surg*. 2012;25(1):65-69.
24. Cage DJ, Granberry WM, Tullos HS. Long-term results of total arthroplasty in adolescents with debilitating polyarthropathy. *Clin Orthop Relat Res*. 1992;(283):156-162.
25. Belmar CJ, Barth P, Lonner JH, Lotke PA. Total knee arthroplasty in patients 90 years of age and older. *J Arthroplasty*. 1999;14(8):911-914.
26. Pagnano MW, McLamb LA, Trousdale RT. Total knee arthroplasty for patients 90 years of age and older. *Clin Orthop Relat Res*. 2004;(418):179-183.
27. Kuo F-C, Hsu C-H, Chen W-S, Wang J-W. Total knee arthroplasty in carefully selected patients aged 80 years or older. *J Orthop Surg Res*. 2014;9:61.
28. Hosick WB, Lotke PA, Baldwin A. Total knee arthroplasty in patients 80 years of age and older. *Clin Orthop Relat Res*. 1994;(299):77-80.

29. George J, Klika AK, Navale SM, Newman JM, Barsoum WK, Higuera CA. Obesity epidemic: is its impact on total joint arthroplasty underestimated? An analysis of national trends. *Clin Orthop Relat Res.* 2017;475(7):1798-1806.

30. Bozic KJ, Lau E, Ong K, et al. Risk factors for early revision after primary TKA in Medicare patients. *Clin Orthop Relat Res.* 2014;472(1):232-237.

31. Wagner ER, Kamath AF, Fruth K, Harmsen WS, Berry DJ. Effect of body mass index on reoperation and complications after total knee arthroplasty. *J Bone Joint Surg Am.* 2016;98(24):2052-2060.

32. Foran JRH, Mont MA, Etienne G, Jones LC, Hungerford DS. The outcome of total knee arthroplasty in obese patients. *J Bone Joint Surg Am.* 2004;86-A(8):1609-1615.

33. Lizaur-Utrilla A, Miralles-Muñoz FA, Sanz-Reig J, Collados-Maestre I. Cementless total knee arthroplasty in obese patients: a prospective matched study with follow-up of 5-10 years. *J Arthroplasty.* 2014;29(6):1192-1196.

34. Jackson MP, Sexton SA, Walter WL, Walter WK, Zicat BA. The impact of obesity on the mid-term outcome of cementless total knee replacement. *J Bone Joint Surg Br.* 2009;91(8):1044-1048.

35. Dewan A, Bertolusso R, Karastinos A, Conditt M, Noble PC, Parsley BS. Implant durability and knee function after total knee arthroplasty in the morbidly obese patient. *J Arthroplasty.* 2009;24(6 suppl):89-94, 94.e1-e3.

36. Winiarsky R, Barth P, Lotke P. Total knee arthroplasty in morbidly obese patients. *J Bone Joint Surg Am.* 1998;80(12):1770-1774.

37. Casqueiro J, Casqueiro J, Alves C. Infections in patients with diabetes mellitus: a review of pathogenesis. *Indian J Endocrinol Metab.* 2012;16 suppl 1:S27-S36.

38. Meding JB, Reddleman K, Keating ME, et al. Total knee replacement in patients with diabetes mellitus. *Clin Orthop Relat Res.* 2003;(416):208-216.

39. Iorio R, Williams KM, Marcantonio AJ, Specht LM, Tilzey JF, Healy WL. Diabetes mellitus, hemoglobin A1C, and the incidence of total joint arthroplasty infection. *J Arthroplasty.* 2012;27(5):726-729.e1.

40. Yang K, Yeo SJ, Lee BP, Lo NN. Total knee arthroplasty in diabetic patients: a study of 109 consecutive cases. *J Arthroplasty.* 2001;16(1):102-106.

41. Giori NJ, Ellerbe LS, Bowe T, Gupta S, Harris AHS. Many diabetic total joint arthroplasty candidates are unable to achieve a preoperative hemoglobin A1c goal of 7% or less. *J Bone Joint Surg Am.* 2014;96(6):500-504.

42. Tarabichi M, Shohat N, Kheir MM, et al. Determining the threshold for HbA1c as a predictor for adverse outcomes after total joint arthroplasty: a multicenter, retrospective study. *J Arthroplasty.* 2017;32(9S):S263-S267.e1.

43. Chiu FY, Lin CF, Chen CM, Lo WH, Chaung TY. Cefuroxime-impregnated cement at primary total knee arthroplasty in diabetes mellitus. A prospective, randomised study. *J Bone Joint Surg Br.* 2001;83(5):691-695.

44. Inabathula A, Dilley JE, Ziemba-Davis M, et al. Extended oral antibiotic prophylaxis in high-risk patients substantially reduces primary total hip and knee arthroplasty 90-day infection rate. *J Bone Joint Surg Am.* 2018;100(24):2103-2109.

45. Mont MA, Myers TH, Krackow KA, Hungerford DS. Total knee arthroplasty for corticosteroid associated avascular necrosis of the knee. *Clin Orthop Relat Res.* 1997;(338):124-130.

46. Seldes RM, Tan V, Duffy G, Rand JA, Lotke PA. Total knee arthroplasty for steroid-induced osteonecrosis. *J Arthroplasty.* 1999;14(5):533-537.

47. Mont MA, Baumgarten KM, Rifai A, Bluemke DA, Jones LC, Hungerford DS. Atraumatic osteonecrosis of the knee. *J Bone Joint Surg Am.* 2000;82(9):1279-1290.

48. Mont MA, Rifai A, Baumgarten KM, Sheldon M, Hungerford DS. Total knee arthroplasty for osteonecrosis. *J Bone Joint Surg Am.* 2002;84-A(4):599-603.

49. Figgie MP, Goldberg VM, Figgie HE III, Heiple KG, Sobel M. Total knee arthroplasty for the treatment of chronic hemophilic arthropathy. *Clin Orthop Relat Res.* 1989;(248):98-107.

50. Panotopoulos J, Ay C, Trieb K, Schuh R, Windhager R, Wanivenhaus HA. Outcome of total knee arthroplasty in hemophilic arthropathy. *J Arthroplasty.* 2014;29(4):749-752.

51. Norian JM, Ries MD, Karp S, Hambleton J. Total knee arthroplasty in hemophilic arthropathy. *J Bone Joint Surg Am.* 2002;84-A(7):1138-1141.

52. Thomason HC III, Wilson FC, Lachiewicz PF, Kelley SS. Knee arthroplasty in hemophilic arthropathy. *Clin Orthop Relat Res.* 1999;(360):169-173.

53. Westberg M, Paus AC, Holme PA, Tjønnfjord GE. Haemophilic arthropathy: long-term outcomes in 107 primary total knee arthroplasties. *Knee.* 2014;21(1):147-150.

54. Schick M, Stucki G, Rodriguez M, et al. Haemophilic; arthropathy: assessment of quality of life after total knee arthroplasty. *Clin Rheumatol.* 1999;18(6):468-472.

55. Kilgus DJ, Amstutz HC, Wolgin MA, Dorey FJ. Joint replacement for ankylosed hips. *J Bone Joint Surg Am.* 1990;72(1):45-54.

56. Hamadouche M, Kerboull L, Meunier A, Courpied JP, Kerboull M. Total hip arthroplasty for the treatment of ankylosed hips: a five to twenty-one-year follow-up study. *J Bone Joint Surg Am.* 2001;83-A(7):992-998.

57. Hardinge K, Murphy JC, Frenyo S. Conversion of hip fusion to Charnley low-friction arthroplasty. *Clin Orthop Relat Res.* 1986;(211):173-179.

58. Amstutz HC, Sakai DN. Total joint replacement for ankylosed hips. Indications, technique, and preliminary results. *J Bone Joint Surg Am.* 1975;57(5):619-625.

59. Romness DW, Morrey BF. Total knee arthroplasty in patients with prior ipsilateral hip fusion. *J Arthroplasty.* 1992;7(1):63-70.

60. Garvin KL, Pellicci PM, Windsor RE, Conrad EU, Insall JN, Salvati EA. Contralateral total hip arthroplasty or ipsilateral total knee arthroplasty in patients who have a long-standing fusion of the hip. *J Bone Joint Surg Am.* 1989;71(9):1355-1362.

61. Kaplan FS, Singer FR. Paget's disease of bone: pathophysiology, diagnosis, and management. *J Am Acad Orthop Surg.* 1995;3(6):336-344.

62. Merkow RL, Lane JM. Paget's disease of bone. *Orthop Clin North Am.* 1990;21(1):171-189.

63. Broberg MA, Cass JR. Total knee arthroplasty in Paget's disease of the knee. *J Arthroplasty.* 1986;1(2):139-142.

64. Gabel GT, Rand JA, Sim FH. Total knee arthroplasty for osteoarthrosis in patients who have Paget disease of bone at the knee. *J Bone Joint Surg Am.* 1991;73(5):739-744.

65. Schai PA, Scott RD, Younger AS. Total knee arthroplasty in Paget's disease: technical problems and results. *Orthopedics.* 1999;22(1):21-25.

66. Lee G-C, Sanchez-Sotelo J, Berry DJ. Total knee arthroplasty in patients with Paget's disease of bone at the knee. *J Arthroplasty.* 2005;20(6):689-693.

67. Popat R, Tsitskaris K, Millington S, Dawson-Bowling S, Hanna SA. Total knee arthroplasty in patients with Paget's disease of bone: a systematic review. *World J Orthop.* 2018;9(10):229-234.

68. Stevenson I, McMillan TE, Baliga S, Schemitsch EH. Primary and secondary total knee arthroplasty for tibial plateau fractures. *J Am Acad Orthop Surg.* 2018;26(11):386-395.

69. Wasserstein D, Henry P, Paterson JM, Kreder HJ, Jenkinson R. Risk of total knee arthroplasty after operatively treated tibial plateau fracture: a matched-population-based cohort study. *J Bone Joint Surg Am.* 2014;96(2):144-150.

70. Saleh KJ, Sherman P, Katkin P, et al. Total knee arthroplasty after open reduction and internal fixation of fractures of the tibial plateau: a minimum five-year follow-up study. *J Bone Joint Surg Am.* 2001;83-A(8):1144-1148.

71. Weiss NG, Parvizi J, Trousdale RT, Bryce RD, Lewallen DG. Total knee arthroplasty in patients with a prior fracture of the tibial plateau. *J Bone Joint Surg Am*. 2003;85-A(2):218-221.

72. Rondon AJ, Tan TL, Schlitt PK, Greenky MR, Phillips JL, Purtill JJ. Total joint arthroplasty in patients with Parkinson's disease: survivorship, outcomes, and reasons for failure. *J Arthroplasty*. 2018;33(4):1028-1032.

73. Mehta S, Vankleunen JP, Booth RE, Lotke PA, Lonner JH. Total knee arthroplasty in patients with Parkinson's disease: impact of early postoperative neurologic intervention. *Am J Orthop*. 2008;37(10):513-516.

74. Ashraf M, Priyavadhana S, Sambandam SN, Mounasamy V, Sharma OP. Total knee arthroplasty in patients with Parkinson's disease- A critical analysis of available evidence. *Open Orthop J*. 2017;11:1087-1093.

75. Duffy GP, Trousdale RT. Total knee arthroplasty in patients with Parkinson's disease. *J Arthroplasty*. 1996;11(8):899-904.

76. Giori NJ, Lewallen DG. Total knee arthroplasty in limbs affected by poliomyelitis. *J Bone Joint Surg Am*. 2002;84-A(7):1157-1161.

77. Jordan L, Kligman M, Sculco TP. Total knee arthroplasty in patients with poliomyelitis. *J Arthroplasty*. 2007;22(4):543-548.

78. Gan ZJ, Pang HN. Outcomes of total knee arthroplasty in patients with poliomyelitis. *J Arthroplasty*. 2016;31(11):2508-2513.

79. Tigani D, Fosco M, Amendola L, Boriani L. Total knee arthroplasty in patients with poliomyelitis. *Knee*. 2009;16(6):501-506.

80. Prasad A, Donovan R, Ramachandran M, et al. Outcome of total knee arthroplasty in patients with poliomyelitis: a systematic review. *EFORT Open Rev*. 2018;3(6):358-362.

81. Patterson BM, Insall JN. Surgical management of gonarthrosis in patients with poliomyelitis. *J Arthroplasty*. 1992;7 suppl:419-426.

chapter 30

Principles of Implantation—Flexion/Extension

Joseph A. Karam, MD | Jess H. Lonner, MD

INTRODUCTION

The main goals of total knee arthroplasty (TKA) are to alleviate pain and improve function, while restoring alignment, balance, and knee motion. Indeed, one of the most impactful technical factors to optimize the outcome of TKA is proper balancing of the soft tissues, in both the coronal plane (varus/valgus) as well as the sagittal plane (flexion and extension) gaps.[1,2] Creating equal rectangular gaps in flexion and in extension after bone resection and surface preparation ensures a stable knee throughout the range of motion, while providing full extension and maximal flexion.

Most arthritic knees will present with some modicum of underlying soft-tissue imbalance, often with a flexion contracture, which will need to be corrected at the time of surgery. A balanced knee is important in order to attain proper knee function, compatible with an active lifestyle, and to optimize the longevity of the prosthesis by avoiding uneven strain that could lead to early failure by implant loosening or wear of the polyethylene insert, even in the setting of suboptimal bone resections.[3] This chapter will focus on standard methods of flexion/extension gap balancing.

PREOPERATIVE EVALUATION

Proper preoperative planning vis-à-vis flexion–extension gap balancing begins during preoperative evaluation. The physical examination should note (and document) the preoperative knee range of motion, paying particular attention to the presence and magnitude of flexion contracture, extension lag or recurvatum deformity, and assessment of coronal and sagittal instability and coronal alignment. Standard imaging includes weightbearing anteroposterior, flexed posteroanterior, lateral, as well as sunrise radiographs. These are evaluated for coronal deformity, presence and size of osteophytes, loose bodies, tibial translation relative to the femur, and coronal alignment. Taken together, these assessments will help the surgeon plan resections and anticipate required soft-tissue releases and types of implants to be available.

INTRAOPERATIVE ASSESSMENT

Evaluation of flexion and extension gaps during surgery can be done with the use of spacer blocks, quantified ligament-tensioning devices or pressure sensors, laminar spreaders, or manual traction with visual evaluation. The goal is to have equally sized and balanced rectangular gaps (coronal balancing) in both full extension and 90° of flexion. Gap assessment by manual varus/valgus stress with trial implants in place after bony resection, and anterior/posterior drawer testing, is also performed. Scott and Chmell described the "pull-out lift-off test" (POLO test) for proper balancing of posterior cruciate ligament (PCL) tightness in cruciate retaining (CR) TKA with use of a stemless tibial component trial.[4] A positive pullout test reflects a loose flexion gap: the tibial trial can easily be pulled out and/or slid into place in 90° of flexion. Conversely, a tibial trial that lifts anteriorly off of the tibial bone surface with the knee in flexion reflects a PCL that is too tight (positive lift-off test). Alternatively, a femoral component that rolls back excessively also suggests a flexion gap that is too tight (**Fig. 30-1**). An everted patella should be reduced into place when assessing for a lift-off test because it may lead to a false-positive result due to an eccentric proximal pull of the patellar tendon on the tibia.

Proper intraoperative assessment of adequate coronal and sagittal balancing can also be aided with the use of a sensor-embedded tibial insert trial.[5] These devices can quantify contact pressures in the medial and lateral compartments both in extension and flexion positioning, identifying the maximal contact points in the medial and lateral compartments and assisting in guiding soft-tissue releases or bone resection adjustments (**Fig. 30-2**). Kinetic tracking can identify patterns of femoral rollback with passive flexion. In a knee with adequate sagittal balance, contact points will cluster in the central third of the bearing surface in 90° of flexion. In cases with a tight flexion gap, there will be posterior positioning of the contact points with increased loads and minimal excursion during posterior drawer testing. On the other hand, if a loose flexion gap is present, there will be increased excursion of the femoral contact points during posterior drawer testing and anterior translation of the femoral contact points.

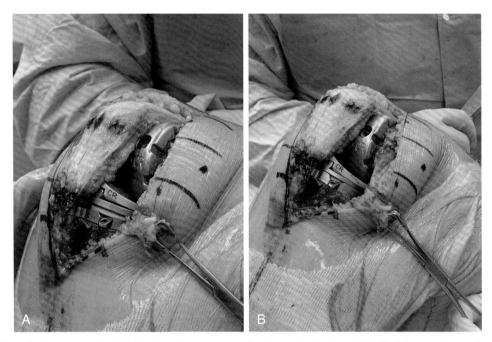

FIGURE 30-1   **A:** Tight flexion space with trials in place. There is excessive femoral rollback and lift off of the anterior portion of the tibial insert. **B:** After partial recession of the posterior cruciate ligament, the trial is appropriately seated and the femoral component is positioned perfectly relative to the tibial insert.

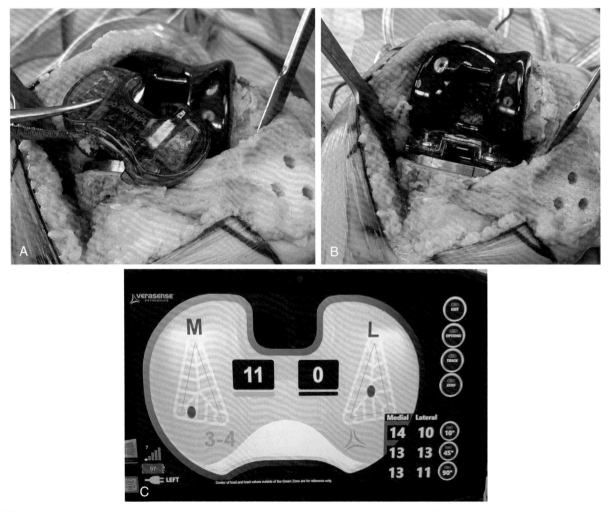

FIGURE 30-2   A sensor-embedded tibial insert trial can assist in gap balancing by detecting medial and lateral compartment pressures in extension, 90° flexion, and mid-flexion. **A:** A sensor-embedded tibial trial insert that matches the implant system and sizes is selected. **B:** The sensor-embedded trial is impacted into the metal tibial tray similarly to a standard plastic trial insert. **C:** The screen displays the amount of pressure and the point of maximal contact in both the medial and lateral compartments at different degrees of flexion. (Photos courtesy of George Branovacki, MD, Chicago, IL.)

This technology is used by some surgeons to objectively assess soft-tissue balancing instead of relying on subjective feel. Indeed, Elmallah et al demonstrated improved balancing with the use of an electronic sensor over manual balancing by an experienced arthroplasty surgeon.[6] Whether this translates to improved kinematics and functional outcomes has yet to be determined.

ACHIEVING A SAGITTALLY BALANCED KNEE

As previously stated, the target for a "balanced knee" is equal tightness medially and laterally throughout the range of motion. This is achieved by obtaining equal and rectangular gaps between the resected bone surfaces in extension (between the distal femoral cut and the tibial cut) and flexion (between the posterior femoral and the proximal tibial resection) (**Fig. 30-3**). Two techniques have been traditionally described to achieve a balanced knee: the measured resection technique and the gap balancing technique. In measured resection, the surgeon aims to remove equivalent bone and cartilage as will be replaced by the prosthesis, and the bone cuts are made in reference to anatomical landmarks. In the true gap balancing method, bone cuts are made based on soft-tissue tension as opposed to anatomical landmarks. The most important difference is the way femoral component rotation is determined. In measured resection, the femoral cutting block determining femoral component rotation is placed in reference to Whiteside line, the posterior condylar axis, and/or the transepicondylar axis. In gap balancing, the cutting guide is placed parallel to the tibial cut

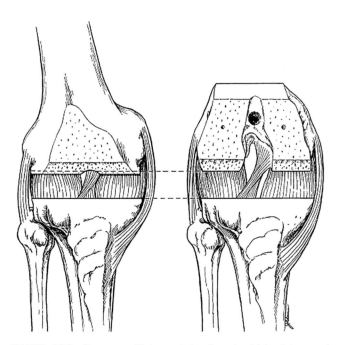

FIGURE 30-3 Proper sagittal gap balancing should lead to equal extension and flexion gaps. In this example, the flexion gap is tighter than the extension gap, requiring either additional posterior release or distal femoral resection to equalize gaps.

with use of a tensioning device or spacer block. In reality, whether acknowledging it or not, most surgeons use a combination of the two methods, although the sequences may vary. In any case, soft-tissue releases may still be necessary after bone cuts are made to ensure proper balancing. Indeed, a well-balanced knee is achieved through combined modification of bone cuts, soft-tissue releases, and/or component modification (sizing, augments, alignment, and rotation).

Matsumoto et al looked at 135 gap-balanced TKAs using navigation and compared them to 120 measured resection TKAs.[7] They found significantly higher sagittal gap imbalance in PCL-sacrificing/-substituting (PS) knees compared to CR knees, mostly consisting of an increased flexion gap, with both measured resection and gap balancing methods. CR knees were also found to have a significantly higher rate of achieving equalized rectangular gaps in both flexion and extension as compared to PS knees both with measured resection and gap balancing methods. Despite these differences, functional outcomes and range of motion at minimum 2-year follow-up were similar among all groups. Moon et al conducted a meta-analysis comparing soft-tissue balancing, femoral component rotation, and joint line change between gap balancing and measured resection methods.[8] They found no significant overall differences in flexion and extension gaps between the two techniques, although medial/lateral gaps in extension were found to be more balanced using gap balancing. The gap balancing method resulted in more external rotation of the femoral component and more joint line elevation compared to the measured resection technique. These changes had minimal clinical relevance, as they were typically in the 1 mm or 1° range. Another meta-analysis in 2017 found similar results, with no difference in flexion gap, extension gap, or flexion/extension differences between the two approaches and more joint line elevation when gap balancing.[9] However, the study found that patients who received TKA with the gap balancing technique had significantly higher functional scores 2 years postoperatively. On the contrary, a 5-year follow-up report of their randomized controlled trial by Babazadeh et al showed no difference in functional outcomes between measured resection and gap balancing techniques despite greater joint line elevation in the gap balancing group.[10] Of note, the joint line elevation was still well below 8 mm, which is the classically described threshold for either optimal or poor functional outcome after TKA with joint line elevation.[11]

THE INTERPLAY BETWEEN FLEXION AND EXTENSION GAPS: WHICH GAP TO BALANCE FIRST?

Depending on one's preference, the surgeon can choose to balance the extension gap first and then the flexion gap at 90° of flexion, or the flexion gap can be determined and balanced first. The extension gap is balanced first by many, because the bone cuts are often (but not always) made independent of the soft tissues. The distal femoral cut is typically made at a predetermined angle of valgus relative to the axis of the femur, although it may be individualized according to preoperative alignment measures or based on whether the planned tibial cut is made perpendicular to the mechanical axis or using a kinematic alignment method. Others may prefer to prepare the flexion gap first, arguing that it reduces the risk of joint line elevation; however, contemporary implant size intervals, appropriate femoral sizing, and maintenance of posterior condylar offset reduce this risk.[2,12]

MANAGING THE TIGHT EXTENSION GAP AND STEPWISE APPROACH TO FLEXION CONTRACTURES

Clinically, a tight extension gap will present as an inability to achieve full extension, leading to a flexion contracture. Persistent flexion contracture postoperatively can have detrimental effects on the outcome after TKA with increased pain, altered gait, decreased functional scores, increased energy expenditure during gait, and diminished quality of life.[13-15] Intraoperatively, a small flexion contracture is first addressed by resection of osteophytes from the posterior femoral condyles, which may tent the posterior capsule and may prevent terminal extension. They may also potentially lead to coronal asymmetry

if the posterior condylar osteophytes are unilateral or larger on one side of the knee than the other (**Fig. 30-4A**). Resection of the posterior femoral osteophytes has to be handled with care, in order to avoid excessive posterior condylar resection (which may compromise implant support) or inadvertent injury to the neurovascular bundle. Usually this is done with the knee in flexion and a laminar spreader between the tibia and the posterior femur. Pushing back on the posterior tibia (as if performing a posterior drawer test) can also optimize visualization of, and access to, posterior osteophytes and loose bodies. The osteophytes are removed with the use of a ¾″ curved osteotome (**Fig. 30-4B**).

In addition to affecting the extension gaps, posterior osteophytes can also affect flexion range by causing impingement on the posterior aspect of the tibial component in deep flexion. Indeed, Yau et al showed that residual posterior osteophytes after TKA were an independent risk factor for decreased flexion at 1 year after PS TKA, in addition to limited preoperative range of motion and overstuffing of the patellofemoral joint.[16] Sriphirom et al in a recent prospective study on patients undergoing computer-assisted TKA showed a significant increase in both flexion and extension gaps after removal of posterior osteophytes.[17] This further underlines the necessity to excise these osteophytes early on during the surgery in order to avoid unnecessary soft-tissue releases and excessive bony resection, especially if a gap balancing method is used and tension is assessed with the presence of these osteophytes.

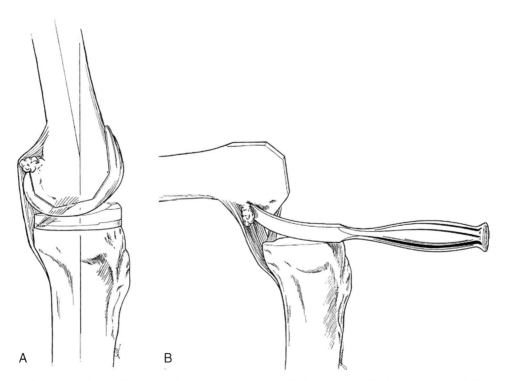

A   B

FIGURE 30-4   A: Posterior osteophytes can tent the posterior capsule and prevent full extension. **B:** Technique of removal of posterior osteophytes with the knee in flexion using a curved osteotome.

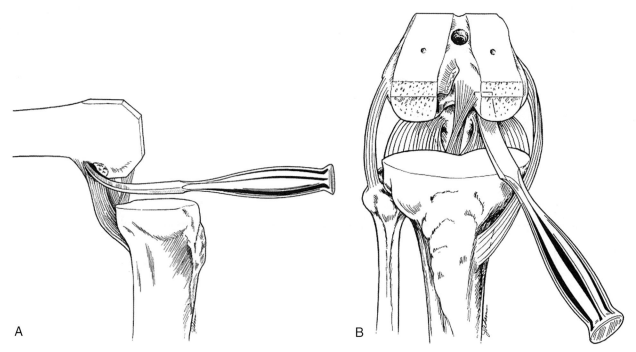

FIGURE 30-5 Technique of subperiosteal release of the posterior capsule off of the distal femur in cases of residual flexion contracture after resection of posterior osteophytes. **A:** Lateral view. **B:** Anterior view.

If flexion contracture persists after resection of posterior osteophytes and loose bodies in the posterior recess, the posterior capsule is released subperiosteally using a Cobb elevator from the posterior femur in a controlled fashion to avoid injury to the superior geniculate arteries or to the popliteal neurovascular bundle (**Fig. 30-5**). In severe concomitant varus deformity with flexion contracture, adequate medial release should be ensured before too aggressive of a posterior release. This should include the posteromedial capsule and the semimembranosus insertion and that should help decrease extension gap tightness. In revision cases, actual excision of scar tissue posteriorly may be necessary.

Finally, if a flexion contracture still persists despite appropriate release of the posterior soft tissues, additional resection of the distal femur can help achieve full extension of the knee. Bengs and Scott showed that an average of 9° of flexion contracture is corrected for every 2 mm of distal femoral bone resection.[18] Others found more limited correction, with 1.8° restoration for each 1 mm of distal femoral resection.[19] A more recent study using computer navigation revealed findings in between the two aforementioned studies with 3.5 mm of distal femoral resection required to correct a 10° flexion contracture.[20] In most severe flexion contractures, additional bone resection to the epicondylar attachments can be performed, but additional constraint will likely be needed to address the possibility of mid-flexion instability that may result from such dramatic joint line elevation. Kim et al looked at extension gain in patients with over 15° flexion contracture after each separate intervention on the soft-tissue tissues or osseous structures to address flexion

contracture.[21] They found an initial 5° gain after medial release, an additional 9° gain from standard bone cuts and soft-tissue releases including PCL release and posterior capsular release, and finally an additional 4.8° gain was noted after an extra 2 mm distal femoral resection, which was needed in patients who still had significant contracture despite standard soft-tissue releases and bone cuts.

To summarize, Lombardi's classification of flexion contractures into three grades based on the degree of deformity and algorithmic approach is a useful way to address this common problem in TKA (**Fig. 30-6**)[22]:
- Grade I (mild): less than 15° flexion contracture
- Grade II (moderate): 15°-30° flexion contracture
- Grade III (severe): more than 30° flexion contracture

Lombardi recommends a limit of 2 mm distal resection if using a CR knee design, as further resection significantly alters the kinematics of the PCL and would require switching to a PS implant. Grade II flexion contractures are not suitable for the use of CR knee designs, and grade III contractures require the use of constrained or hinged TKA due to difficulty in balancing flexion and extension gaps or mid-flexion instability. Severe grade III deformities may present with redundancy of the extensor mechanism, which may be addressed at the time of TKA with distal and lateral advancement of the vastus medialis obliquus (VMO). Postoperative rehabilitation protocols in these patients should focus on extension exercises, and a night extension splint may be beneficial in the early postoperative period to limit recurrent contracture.

On the opposite end of the spectrum, a minority of patients will present with preoperative knee recurvatum.

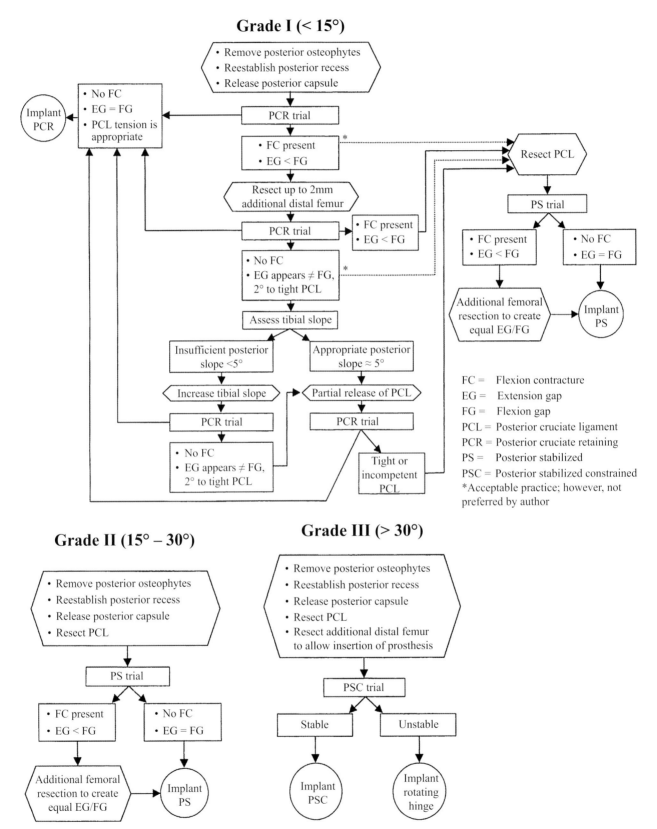

FIGURE 30-6 Lombardi's algorithmic approach for surgical management of grade I, grade II, and grade III flexion contractures during total knee arthroplasty.[22]

This is usually the result of a weak quadriceps with compensatory knee hyperextension during gait. In severe cases of recurvatum, neuropathic causes should be investigated. Correcting this deformity necessitates tightening up the extension gap, which can be accomplished by reducing the distal femoral resection and possibly using distal femoral augments in some severe cases. Complete correction of the recurvatum deformity may not be desired in patients with severe quadriceps weakness as this would deprive them from the ability to lock the knee during gait. A constrained or hinged knee construct may be necessary in these patients especially in the setting of neuromuscular disease such as poliomyelitis or tabes dorsalis.[23,24] Prasad et al performed a recent systematic review on TKA in patients with poliomyelitis.[25] Forty-four percent of patients had recurvatum deformity preoperatively, and quadriceps power was found to be an important prognostic factor for functional outcome of TKA. Despite a higher revision rate of 7%, functional improvement and outcomes in these patients are comparable to the general population.[25,26]

MANAGING THE FLEXION GAP

A tight flexion gap can result in increased joint reaction forces in flexion with limited range of motion and pain, as well as early posterior wear of the polyethylene insert. While managing the extension gap is relatively straightforward through release of posterior tissues and adjustment of the distal femoral resection, flexion gap management is more challenging with interplay of multiple factors and a different approach based on implant design, femoral implant thickness, intrinsic posterior offset, and PCL management (CR versus PS TKA). Indeed, Scott and Chmell recommended cutting the distal femur with 2 mm less than that to be replaced by the prosthesis when describing their technique for posterior CR TKA in order to avoid a situation where the flexion gap is tighter than the extension gap.[4] Likewise, due to the additional 2 mm of flexion gap laxity that results from PCL resection, some surgeons routinely resect two additional millimeters of distal femur to match the gaps when using PS or ultracongruent (UC) designs. Nonetheless, the need for these additional resections will vary from patient to patient and may be addressed by intrinsic system-specific implant modifications such as variable thicknesses in some PS designs between the extension and flexion surfaces. Therefore, knowing the geometric details of the components used in each case is important before reflexive resection of bone or release of soft tissues.

In et al sought to identify risk factors for flexion gap tightness in CR TKAs.[27] In their series, 21% of knees underwent PCL recession to address a tighter flexion gap. After looking into various demographic and preoperative factors, the only factor that was found to be significantly independently associated with flexion gap tightness after multivariate analysis was insufficient posterior tibial slope. Other factors such as lower extent of preoperative flexion contracture and the use of posterior referencing sizing technique were found to be significantly associated with a tight flexion gap in bivariate analysis but lost significance in the multivariate analysis model. Fujimoto et al also evaluated the role of multiple surgical factors in flexion/extension gap change and postoperative range of motion in patients undergoing CR TKA.[28] Multivariate analysis revealed that the posterior tibial slope and the medial/lateral balance in deep flexion had significant effect on gap change between full extension and deep flexion. In a more recent study, Hatayama et al evaluated risk factors for flexion gap tightness in CR TKA.[29] In their series, 30% of patients had to undergo PCL release due to flexion gap tightness. Univariate analysis showed multiple risk factors for PCL release: limited preoperative knee range of flexion, preoperative anterior cruciate ligament (ACL) disruption, decreased posterior femoral condylar offset, varus femorotibial alignment, higher preoperative posterior tibial slope angle, lower postoperative posterior tibial slope angle, as well as more pronounced decrease in tibial slope angle from preoperative to postoperative measurements. Of those risk factors, ACL disruption had the largest effect with patients, being four times more likely to undergo PCL release. Multivariate analysis showed that independent risk factors for PCL release were: varus alignment and decrease in the posterior tibial slope angle. When the decrease in posterior tibial slope exceeded 5°, the odds ratio for PCL release was 2.65. Okazaki et al aimed to quantify the effect of posterior tibial slope on the flexion gap and showed a 2 mm increase in the flexion gap for a 5° increase in the tibial slope in CR TKA.[30] They also looked at PS TKA designs and found a 1 mm increase in the flexion gap for 5° increase in the posterior tibial slope.

Addressing flexion gap tightness in CR knees includes releasing or recessing the PCL, increasing the posterior tibial slope or downsizing the femoral component. Three techniques have been described for release of the PCL[31]: sharp release of the PCL off of the medial femoral condyle, subperiosteal release of the PCL from the posterior proximal tibia, and finally removing a V-shaped piece of bone from the posterior proximal tibia that includes the distal insertion of the PCL (**Fig. 30-7**). In the latter case, the piece of bone still has capsular attachments posteriorly and heals in an elongated position. Clinically, it is not clear which method of flexion gap management is optimal. One cadaveric study recommended increasing the posterior tibial slope over recession of the PCL in knees that are tight in flexion, if the intention is to maintain a CR insert.[32] Using finite element analysis, another study also advocated for increasing the posterior tibial slope over recessing the PCL in a finite element study, mostly based on more significant alteration of knee kinematics after PCL recession and paradoxical

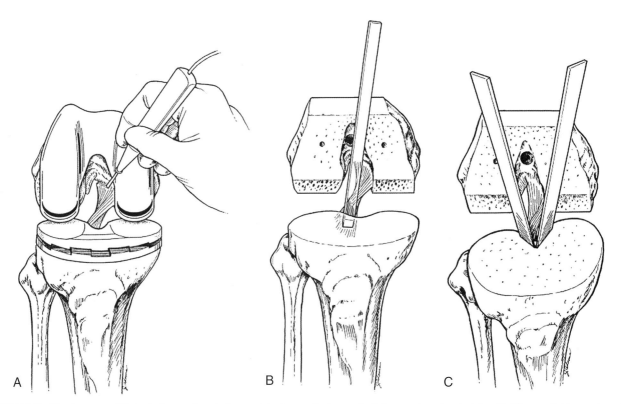

FIGURE 30-7   The three possible techniques of posterior cruciate ligament release: **A:** Release of proximal origin off of the medial femoral condyle. **B:** Release off of the posterior aspect of the proximal tibia. **C:** Release of the posterior cruciate ligament (PCL) distally with a V-shaped osteotomy of the proximal posterior tibia preserving posterior soft-tissue attachments.

anterior femoral rollback.[33] Whether there is an optimal extent or upper limit of posterior tibial slope in CR TKA is still not clear. Finally, downsizing the femoral component may be suboptimal unless the femoral component is overhanging medially and laterally at the selected size or if the interval between femoral sizes is only 2 to 3 mm. Larger intervals between sizes can otherwise have too great an impact on posterior femoral offset if downsizing.

Management of the flexion gap is quite different in PS TKA designs, where more relative laxity of the flexion gap is common. Mihalko and Krackow demonstrated a significant increase in the flexion gap size after resection of the PCL in cadaveric knees with a resected ACL (about 5 mm at rest and in excess of 6 mm under tension), with no change in the extension gap.[34] Kadoya et al found comparable results when using navigation to quantify their measurements in patients during TKA.[35] A similar 5 mm increase in the flexion gap was identified after PCL release, with less than a millimeter difference in the extension gap. The authors suggested using PCL release as a method to address flexion–extension gap imbalances where the flexion gap is tighter than the extension gap without having to resect more bone or change the prosthesis. These results were again reproduced by Park et al who further showed the repercussions of PCL resection on the change in navigation planning: the majority of patients required an increase in the femoral size (reducing

the posterior condylar resection and increasing the posterior condylar offset) and/or an increase in polyethylene size with appropriate management of the extension space.[36]

Based on these findings, Mihalko and Whiteside recommended a more proximal distal femoral cut when the PCL is to be sacrificed in order to compensate for the increased flexion gap, assuming equal thickness of the femoral component distally and posteriorly.[31,34] Alternatively, some PS femoral components have slightly greater posterior thickness than CR femoral components, so knowing these features is imperative. In knees with severe varus deformity, posteromedial release may lead to further opening of the flexion gap. Decreasing the slope of the tibial resection may help decrease excessive flexion gap laxity secondary to PCL sacrifice and decrease the risk of cam jump. As a reminder, posterior tibial slope in PS knees should not typically exceed 5° in most cases, anyway, in order to minimize the risk of cam-post impingement in extension.

ALGORITHMIC APPROACH FOR INTRAOPERATIVE SAGITTAL BALANCING

With all of the above taken into consideration, **Table 30-1** represents a guide to address the possible scenarios that may present intraoperatively while balancing flexion and extension gaps.

TABLE 30-1 Management of the Different Scenarios of Flexion/Extension Gap Imbalance

		Extension		
		Tight	**Balanced**	**Loose**
Flexion	**Tight**	Downsize tibial insert and/or resect more proximal tibia	• PCL recession or resection ± conversion to PS or UC TKA (in CR TKA) • Resect more posterior condyles and downsize femoral component • Increase tibial slope	Downsize femur and augment distally
	Balanced	• Release posterior capsule • Resect more distal femur • Incrementally decrease tibial slope toward zero degrees	Mission accomplished!	Augment distal femur
	Loose	• Upsize femoral component and augment posteriorly • Incrementally decrease tibial slope toward zero degrees • Resect more distal femur and use thicker insert	• Upsize femoral component and augment posteriorly • Resect more distal femur and use thicker insert	Use thicker polyethylene insert (± tibial augments)

CR, cruciate retaining; PCL, posterior cruciate ligament; PS, PCL-sacrificing/-substituting; TKA, total knee arthroplasty; UC, ultracongruent.

MID-FLEXION INSTABILITY: BALANCING THE FORGOTTEN GAP

Mid-flexion instability is an important but poorly defined and underdiagnosed cause of persistent pain after TKA. Patients present with pain, thought to be secondary to abnormal stresses on the soft-tissue envelope in mid-flexion from subtle instability, and often have recurrent effusions.[37] They may have difficulty with some activities of daily living such as negotiating stairs or standing up from a seated position, and they may have subtle instability. These patients will have a knee that is balanced and stable in full extension and in 90° of flexion, but some degree of instability can be appreciated in mid-flexion.

PS knee designs are at a higher risk of mid-flexion instability, particularly with joint line elevation, because the cam-post mechanism is not engaged during mid-flexion to supply additional stability that would have otherwise been provided by the PCL.[38] Indeed, Hino et al compared PS and CR knees using computer navigation and found significantly increased varus–valgus laxity in PS knees at 10° and 30° of flexion.[39] Joint laxity at full extension and 90° of flexion was not statistically different between the two designs.

Failure to achieve proper sagittal gap balancing and an elevated joint line to deal with a tight extension gap can contribute to mid-flexion instability. Minoda et al showed that patients who had a flexion gap looser than the extension gap prior to implantation demonstrated increased mid-flexion instability.[40] The authors recommended achieving a smaller flexion gap than the extension gap prior to implantation in order to minimize mid-flexion instability.

Martin and Whiteside showed in a cadaver study that positioning the femoral component more proximal and more anterior led to knee instability in flexion beyond 30°. They were among the first to draw the attention to the fact that despite balanced flexion and extension gaps, instability may still occur in mid-flexion if the joint line is significantly elevated.[41] Indeed joint line elevation is one of the most prominent etiologies of mid-flexion instability and can especially occur with overresection of the distal femur in patients with a severe flexion contracture or in those with very loose flexion gaps. The increased distal femoral resection and subsequent joint line elevation lead to decreased tension of the collateral ligaments in flexion and thus mid-flexion instability.[31,42] This was exemplified by Cross et al on cadaveric knee specimens where a 10° flexion contracture was created after standard bony resection using computer navigation and a measured resection technique.[43] While additional distal femoral resection helped decrease the flexion contracture deformity, it led to increased coronal imbalance in mid-flexion: an additional 2 mm distal femoral resection led to 4° medial–lateral laxity at 30° of flexion and an additional 4 mm distal femoral resection led to 6° of medial–lateral laxity at 30° of flexion. Some newer femoral implant designs with intermediate constraint have the potential of reducing mid-flexion instability and may be considered in cases where the joint line is elevated.

Maintaining the joint line is thus one of the most important technical factors to prevent mid-flexion instability. In addition to mid-flexion instability, an elevated joint line also alters PCL kinematics in CR knees and can lead to patella baja and impingement of the patella on the anterior edge of the tibial component with subsequent knee pain, increased wear and possibly patellar tendon erosion. Several anatomical landmarks have been described to ensure the joint line is at the proper level intraoperatively: the joint line should be at the level of the meniscal scar if present, 1 cm distal to the inferior patellar pole in full extension, 25 to 30 mm distal to the medial femoral epicondyle, 20 to 25 mm distal to the lateral femoral epicondyle, and 10 to 15 mm proximal to the tip of the fibular head. Nonetheless, given the importance of balancing the flexion and extension gaps, there will be times when compromising kinematics with suboptimal decisions will be necessary, such as increasing the extension space (elevating the joint line) by moving the femur more proximal or increasing the flexion space by reducing the posterior condylar offset (increasing posterior condylar resection).

CONCLUSION

In conclusion, restoring rectangular and equal flexion and extension gaps, while avoiding a significant shift in the joint line, is of paramount importance for a successful TKA. A simple understanding of the effect of the different soft-tissue releases, bony resections, and implant modifications can help address any given intraoperative scenario of sagittal and coronal imbalance. A stepwise approach is necessary when managing flexion contractures in order to avoid overresection of the distal femur and joint line elevation when possible. Implants with appropriate mid-level, mid-flexion constraint may be helpful. Proper balancing of the tight flexion gap in CR knees includes adjustment of the posterior tibial slope, recession of the PCL, and/or revision of the posterior condylar cut. In PS knee designs, a slightly more lax flexion gap may dictate a reduced posterior tibial slope and possibly a more generous distal femoral cut. In all cases, proper joint line restoration is desirable in order to avoid mid-flexion instability as well as other alterations in knee kinematics and biomechanics. In rare situations with substantial mismatch between flexion and extension gaps, especially in the revision setting, a constrained or hinged component should be considered in order to obtain a properly balanced and stable knee.

REFERENCES

1. Insall J, Scott WN, Ranawat CS. The total condylar knee prosthesis. A report of two hundred and twenty cases. *J Bone Joint Surg Am.* 1979;61(2):173-180.
2. Minoda Y, Sakawa A, Aihara M, Tada K, Kadoya Y, Kobayashi A. Flexion gap preparation opens the extension gap in posterior cruciate ligament-retaining TKA. *Knee Surg Sports Traumatol Arthrosc.* 2007;15(11):1321-1325. doi:10.1007/s00167-007-0394-9.
3. Parratte S, Pagnano MW, Trousdale RT, Berry DJ. Effect of postoperative mechanical axis alignment on the fifteen-year survival of modern, cemented total knee replacements. *J Bone Joint Surg Am.* 2010;92(12):2143-2149. doi:10.2106/JBJS.I.01398.
4. Scott RD, Chmell MJ. Balancing the posterior cruciate ligament during cruciate-retaining fixed and mobile-bearing total knee arthroplasty: description of the pull-out lift-off and slide-back tests. *J Arthroplasty.* 2008;23(4):605-608. doi:10.1016/j.arth.2007.11.018.
5. Roche M, Elson L, Anderson C. Dynamic soft tissue balancing in total knee arthroplasty. *Orthop Clin North Am.* 2014;45(2):157-165. doi:10.1016/j.ocl.2013.11.001.
6. Elmallah RK, Mistry JB, Cherian JJ, et al. Can we really "feel" a balanced total knee arthroplasty? *J Arthroplasty.* 2016;31(9 suppl):102-105. doi:10.1016/j.arth.2016.03.054.
7. Matsumoto T, Muratsu H, Kawakami Y, et al. Soft-tissue balancing in total knee arthroplasty: cruciate-retaining versus posterior-stabilised, and measured-resection versus gap technique. *Int Orthop.* 2014;38(3):531-537. doi:10.1007/s00264-013-2133-9.
8. Moon Y-W, Kim H-J, Ahn H-S, Park C-D, Lee D-H. Comparison of soft tissue balancing, femoral component rotation, and joint line change between the gap balancing and measured resection techniques in primary total knee arthroplasty: a meta-analysis. *Medicine.* 2016;95(39):e5006. doi:10.1097/MD.0000000000005006.
9. Huang T, Long Y, George D, Wang W. Meta-analysis of gap balancing versus measured resection techniques in total knee arthroplasty. *Bone Joint J.* 2017;99-B(2):151-158. doi:10.1302/0301-620X.99B2.BJJ-2016-0042.R2.
10. Babazadeh S, Dowsey MM, Vasimalla MG, Stoney JD, Choong PFM. Gap balancing sacrifices joint-line maintenance to improve gap symmetry: 5-year follow-up of a randomized controlled trial. *J Arthroplasty.* 2018;33(1):75-78. doi:10.1016/j.arth.2017.08.021.
11. Figgie HE, Goldberg VM, Heiple KG, Moller HS, Gordon NH. The influence of tibial-patellofemoral location on function of the knee in patients with the posterior stabilized condylar knee prosthesis. *J Bone Joint Surg Am.* 1986;68(7):1035-1040.
12. Sugama R, Kadoya Y, Kobayashi A, Takaoka K. Preparation of the flexion gap affects the extension gap in total knee arthroplasty. *J Arthroplasty.* 2005;20(5):602-607. doi:10.1016/j.arth.2003.12.085.
13. Goudie ST, Deakin AH, Ahmad A, Maheshwari R, Picard F. Flexion contracture following primary total knee arthroplasty: risk factors and outcomes. *Orthopedics.* 2011;34(12):e855-e859. doi:10.3928/01477447-20111021-18.
14. Koh IJ, Chang CB, Kang YG, Seong SC, Kim TK. Incidence, predictors, and effects of residual flexion contracture on clinical outcomes of total knee arthroplasty. *J Arthroplasty.* 2013;28(4):585-590. doi:10.1016/j.arth.2012.07.014.
15. Ritter MA, Lutgring JD, Davis KE, Berend ME, Pierson JL, Meneghini RM. The role of flexion contracture on outcomes in primary total knee arthroplasty. *J Arthroplasty.* 2007;22(8):1092-1096. doi:10.1016/j.arth.2006.11.009.
16. Yau WP, Chiu KY, Tang WM, Ng TP. Residual posterior femoral condyle osteophyte affects the flexion range after total knee replacement. *Int Orthop.* 2005;29(6):375-379. doi:10.1007/s00264-005-0010-x.
17. Sriphirom P, Siramanakul C, Chanopas B, Boonruksa S. Effects of posterior condylar osteophytes on gap balancing in computer-assisted total knee arthroplasty with posterior cruciate ligament sacrifice. *Eur J Orthop Surg Traumatol.* 2018;28(4):677-681. doi:10.1007/s00590-017-2118-2.
18. Bengs BC, Scott RD. The effect of distal femoral resection on passive knee extension in posterior cruciate ligament-retaining total knee arthroplasty. *J Arthroplasty.* 2006;21(2):161-166. doi:10.1016/j.arth.2005.06.008.
19. Smith CK, Chen JA, Howell SM, Hull ML. An in vivo study of the effect of distal femoral resection on passive knee extension. *J Arthroplasty.* 2010;25(7):1137-1142. doi:10.1016/j.arth.2009.05.030.
20. Liu DW, Reidy JF, Beller EM. The effect of distal femoral resection on fixed flexion deformity in total knee arthroplasty. *J Arthroplasty.* 2016;31(1):98-102. doi:10.1016/j.arth.2015.07.033.
21. Kim SH, Lim J-W, Jung H-J, Lee H-J. Influence of soft tissue balancing and distal femoral resection on flexion contracture in navigated total knee arthroplasty. *Knee Surg Sports Traumatol Arthrosc.* 2017;25(11):3501-3507. doi:10.1007/s00167-016-4269-9.
22. Lombardi AV. Soft tissue balancing of the knee - flexion. In: Callaghan JJ, Rosenberg AG, Rubash HE, Simonian PT, Wickiewicz TL, eds. *The Adult Knee.* 1st ed. Philadelphia, PA: Lippincott Williams & Wilkins; 2002.

23. Tigani D, Fosco M, Amendola L, Boriani L. Total knee arthroplasty in patients with poliomyelitis. *Knee*. 2009;16(6):501-506. doi:10.1016/j.knee.2009.04.004.

24. Jordan L, Kligman M, Sculco TP. Total knee arthroplasty in patients with poliomyelitis. *J Arthroplasty*. 2007;22(4):543-548. doi:10.1016/j.arth.2006.03.013.

25. Prasad A, Donovan R, Ramachandran M, et al. Outcome of total knee arthroplasty in patients with poliomyelitis: a systematic review. *EFORT Open Rev*. 2018;3(6):358-362. doi:10.1302/2058-5241.3.170028.

26. Gan Z-WJ, Pang HN. Outcomes of total knee arthroplasty in patients with poliomyelitis. *J Arthroplasty*. 2016;31(11):2508-2513. doi:10.1016/j.arth.2016.04.019.

27. In Y, Kim J-M, Woo Y-K, Choi N-Y, Sohn J-M, Koh H-S. Factors affecting flexion gap tightness in cruciate-retaining total knee arthroplasty. *J Arthroplasty*. 2009;24(2):317-321. doi:10.1016/j.arth.2007.10.022.

28. Fujimoto E, Sasashige Y, Masuda Y, et al. Significant effect of the posterior tibial slope and medial/lateral ligament balance on knee flexion in total knee arthroplasty. *Knee Surg Sports Traumatol Arthrosc*. 2013;21(12):2704-2712. doi:10.1007/s00167-012-2059-6.

29. Hatayama K, Terauchi M, Hashimoto S, Saito K, Higuchi H. Factors associated with posterior cruciate ligament tightness during cruciate-retaining total knee arthroplasty. *J Arthroplasty*. 2018;33(5):1389-1393. doi:10.1016/j.arth.2017.12.026.

30. Okazaki K, Tashiro Y, Mizu-uchi H, Hamai S, Doi T, Iwamoto Y. Influence of the posterior tibial slope on the flexion gap in total knee arthroplasty. *Knee*. 2014;21(4):806-809. doi:10.1016/j.knee.2014.02.019.

31. Mihalko WM, Saleh KJ, Krackow KA, Whiteside LA. Soft-tissue balancing during total knee arthroplasty in the varus knee. *J Am Acad Orthop Surg*. 2009;17(12):766-774.

32. Jojima H, Whiteside LA, Ogata K. Effect of tibial slope or posterior cruciate ligament release on knee kinematics. *Clin Orthop Relat Res*. 2004;426:194-198.

33. Zelle J, Heesterbeek PJC, De Waal Malefijt M, Verdonschot N. Numerical analysis of variations in posterior cruciate ligament properties and balancing techniques on total knee arthroplasty loading. *Med Eng Phys*. 2010;32(7):700-707. doi:10.1016/j.medengphy.2010.04.013.

34. Mihalko WM, Krackow KA. Posterior cruciate ligament effects on the flexion space in total knee arthroplasty. *Clin Orthop Relat Res*. 1999;360:243-250.

35. Kadoya Y, Kobayashi A, Komatsu T, Nakagawa S, Yamano Y. Effects of posterior cruciate ligament resection on the tibiofemoral joint gap. *Clin Orthop Relat Res*. 2001;391:210-217.

36. Park S-J, Seon J-K, Park J-K, Song E-K. Effect of PCL on flexion-extension gaps and femoral component decision in TKA. *Orthopedics*. 2009;32(10 suppl):22-25. doi:10.3928/01477447-20090915-54.

37. Park CN, White PB, Meftah M, Ranawat AS, Ranawat CS. Diagnostic algorithm for residual pain after total knee arthroplasty. *Orthopedics*. 2016;39(2):e246-e252. doi:10.3928/01477447-20160119-06.

38. Minoda Y, Nakagawa S, Sugama R, et al. Intraoperative assessment of midflexion laxity in total knee prosthesis. *Knee*. 2014;21(4):810-814. doi:10.1016/j.knee.2014.04.010.

39. Hino K, Ishimaru M, Iseki Y, Watanabe S, Onishi Y, Miura H. Mid-flexion laxity is greater after posterior-stabilised total knee replacement than with cruciate-retaining procedures: a computer navigation study. *Bone Joint J*. 2013;95-B(4):493-497. doi:10.1302/0301-620X.95B4.30664.

40. Minoda Y, Nakagawa S, Sugama R, Ikawa T, Noguchi T, Hirakawa M. Midflexion laxity after implantation was influenced by the joint gap balance before implantation in TKA. *J Arthroplasty*. 2015;30(5):762-765. doi:10.1016/j.arth.2014.11.011.

41. Martin JW, Whiteside LA. The influence of joint line position on knee stability after condylar knee arthroplasty. *Clin Orthop Relat Res*. 1990;259:146-156.

42. Parratte S, Pagnano MW. Instability after total knee arthroplasty. *J Bone Joint Surg Am*. 2008;90(1):184-194.

43. Cross MB, Nam D, Plaskos C, et al. Recutting the distal femur to increase maximal knee extension during TKA causes coronal plane laxity in mid-flexion. *Knee*. 2012;19(6):875-879. doi:10.1016/j.knee.2012.05.007.

chapter 31

Principles of Implantation: Measured Resection

Hiba K. Anis, MD | Trevor G. Murray, MD | Robert M. Molloy, MD

INTRODUCTION

In addition to pain relief, the goal of total knee arthroplasty (TKA) is to achieve joint stability and a balanced knee with improved function and range of motion. Malpositioned implants are currently the leading cause of failure and revision after TKA.[1] Implant survivorship was historically limited by polyethylene wear and osteolysis; however, for the contemporary TKA, instability and malalignment have been found to be the most common indications for revision.[1,2] The risk of instability is unsurprising given that many stabilizing structures are removed or damaged in the process of implant positioning.[2]

The success of a TKA is dependent on achieving balanced and symmetric flexion and extension gaps. Accurate bone resection and precise soft-tissue balancing determine proper femoral component alignment and rotation. Although patient satisfaction is seldom correlated with normal knee kinematics after TKA, there is an abundance of literature associating instability and malrotation to poor patient outcomes and early implant failures.[3-5] Specific clinical consequences of improper femoral rotation and alignment include anterior knee pain, patellofemoral instability, flexion gap instability, and arthrofibrosis, which in many cases necessitate revision. Measured resection and gap balancing are two different surgical techniques utilized by surgeons to achieve proper alignment and stability in TKA.

Currently, controversy exists regarding the optimal method of implantation.[5-7] The measured resection technique relies on anatomic landmarks to determine femoral component positioning. With this method, fixed bone resections are made prior to soft-tissue balancing. Conversely, the gap balancing technique addresses soft-tissue balancing first whereby ligamentous releases are typically performed before the femoral cuts. Proponents of both techniques argue one is more effective than the other at achieving alignment and correct femoral component rotation. In this chapter, we will discuss the measured resection technique along with its advantages, disadvantages, and review the current evidence on this approach.

SURGICAL TECHNIQUE

The measured resection technique was developed and introduced in the 1980s by Hungerford, Kenna, and Krackow.[8,9] In order to balance the knee throughout the entire range of motion, this technique emphasizes preservation of the preoperative joint line with accurate prosthetic alignment.[9] Since the joint line position is largely preserved, adequate posterior cruciate ligament (PCL) tension is maintained, and therefore cruciate retaining implants were initially associated with the measured resection technique. However, the principles of measured resection may be used with posterior stabilized implants as well and surgeons now use either implant design with this technique.[10]

With this approach, fixed bone resections are made based on patient anatomy and implant dimensions. Typically, surgeons begin with the distal femoral cut followed by femoral component sizing. Then, anterior and posterior femoral cuts along with the chamfer cuts are made followed by the proximal tibial cut. Finally, after trial component implantation, ligament balance is assessed and any imbalance or laxity corrected with appropriate soft-tissue releases. In order to achieve optimal femoral component positioning and rotation, three anatomic axes derived from bony landmarks are used to guide the bone resections.

Transepicondylar Axis

The transepicondylar axis (TEA) connects the lateral epicondylar prominence to the medial epicondylar ridge (clinical TEA) or the medial epicondylar sulcus (surgical TEA). These bony landmarks mark the origin of the collateral ligaments on the femur and are therefore useful in determining the neutral rotational orientation of the femoral component. The surgical TEA is perpendicular to the tibial mechanical axis at 90° of flexion and closely approximates the optimal flexion–extension axis of the knee.[11,12]

In measured resection, the femoral component is placed parallel to the surgical TEA, and several authors have found that this positioning results in ideal knee kinematics. Specifically, it improves patellofemoral tracking as demonstrated by Miller et al[13] who found that using the TEA as a rotational landmark resulted in the most normal patellar tracking and minimal patellofemoral shear forces. Additionally, Insall et al[14] found that in patients with femoral components placed parallel to the TEA, there was a reduced incidence of femoral condylar lift off and therefore a lower risk of eccentric polyethylene wear. Furthermore, using the TEA as a reference for femoral component positioning has also been shown to consistently achieve balanced and rectangular flexion gaps.[15]

Anteroposterior Axis

The anteroposterior (AP) axis, also known as the Whiteside line, connects the center of the trochlear sulcus anteriorly to the center of the intercondylar notch posteriorly. The AP axis is easily identified with the knee in flexion and is perpendicular to the surgical TEA in normal patient anatomy. With the measured resection technique, the goal is to establish femoral rotation perpendicular to the AP axis by placing the femoral component perpendicular to the AP axis. The AP axis has been found to be a reliable reference for establishing correct femoral rotational alignment and improved patellar tracking, particularly in the setting of a valgus knee or when the surgical TEA is difficult to identify.[16,17]

Posterior Condylar Axis

The posterior condylar axis (PCA) is the third landmark commonly used with measured resection and refers to a line connecting the posterior aspects of the lateral and medial femoral condyles. In relation to the PCA, the surgical TEA is approximately 3° to 4° externally rotated in a patient with normal anatomy. Therefore, externally rotating the femoral component 3° to 4° from the PCA allows for a symmetric, rectangular flexion gap.[18] This reference for femoral alignment is best used in patients with neutral or varus knees with little to no deformity.[7] It is important to note that the PCA should be used in conjunction with other anatomic references as studies have shown that due to the variability in patient anatomy, external rotation between the surgical TEA and the PCA can range between −1° and 10°.[16,19]

In summary, the measured resection technique entails positioning the femoral component parallel to the surgical TEA, perpendicular to the AP axis, and 3° to 4° externally rotated from the PCA in order to achieve optimal prosthetic alignment and rotation. Unlike in the gap balancing technique, proximal tibial resections are performed independent of the femoral resections. After these fixed bone resections are complete, joint stability and balance are assessed with trial implants throughout a complete range of motion and corrected accordingly with selective ligamentous releases.[20] The measured

resection technique often creates a flexion gap that is larger laterally; however, several authors have noted that some lateral laxity is inherent to the native knee joint and therefore many surgeons permit this residual lateral laxity.[9,21,22] Furthermore, Hungerford suggests that the lateral compartment is dynamically stabilized by several surrounding structures (popliteus, iliotibial tract, biceps femoris, and lateral head of the gastrocnemius) and in fact the slight increase in flexion gap allows for rotational freedom on the lateral side which mimics normal knee kinematics.[9]

ADVANTAGES

The principles of measured resection favor the preservation of normal knee kinematics and anatomy; major advantages of this technique are largely based on this concept. Studies comparing joint line elevation between measured resection and gap balancing techniques consistently demonstrate the former maintains a more physiologic joint line.[23,24] Joint line elevation has been associated with poor functional outcomes after TKA including impaired PCL function, midflexion instability, and reduced range of motion. A study on PCL biomechanics revealed that PCL strain increased with progressive joint line elevation at all flexion angles above 30° with statistically significant increases observed at elevations of 4 mm or more.[25] Martin and Whiteside studied the effect of joint line position on knee stability and found a 5 mm elevation led to a significant increase in midflexion laxity.[26] Additionally, a review of 100 TKA patients found that those with a joint line elevations of 5 mm or more had reduced range of motion and kneeling ability.[27]

As a result of a preserved joint line, the measured resection technique is also associated with enhanced patellar tracking. Elevation of the joint line has been correlated with impingement of the patella and increased patellofemoral contact force which may lead to postoperative pain as well as accelerated component wear.[28-30] As such, it has been suggested that measured resection should be considered in patients with preoperative shortening of the patella tendon or in cases of patella infera.[23]

Some authors have found that the measured resection technique offers more reliable and accurate implant positioning compared to gap balancing.[31-33] This may be explained by the use of multiple references as they provide multiple methods of assessing femoral component alignment and rotation. It has been found that surgeons who utilize the anatomic axes discussed earlier in conjunction with each other are more likely to achieve accurate femoral alignment and adequate rotational stability.[31] Since only fixed bone resections are performed according to patient anatomy, only bone that will be replaced by metal tends to be resected which may also facilitate accurate implant positioning.

DISADVANTAGES

The major criticism of this technique is that its dependence on anatomic references makes it vulnerable to errors due to misidentification of bony landmarks or anatomic variability between patients. Some authors have found that identifying the TEA can be difficult and imprecise.[34,35] Jerosch et al[35] examined interindividual reproducibility of the TEA on cadaveric specimens between eight experienced orthopedic surgeons and found that their marked reference points varied up to 22.3 mm for the medial epicondyle and up to 13.8 mm for the lateral epicondyle. Yau et al[36] compared the precision of rotational alignment between four alignment methods: TEA, 3° external rotation from the PCA, perpendicular to the AP axis, or flexion gap balancing. The authors found that the rates of rotational malalignment (errors of more than 5° from neutral alignment) were the highest when using the PCA (72%). The rates of rotational error were also higher with the AP axis (60%) and TEA (56%) methods when compared to the flexion gap balancing method (20%).

Asymmetric flexion and extension gaps are often reported with the measured resection technique.[24,33,37] The flexion and extension gaps are balanced with soft-tissue releases which may introduce asymmetry and laxity that is difficult to correct since the fixed bone resections cannot be modified.[38] Moon et al[33] conducted a meta-analysis and found that the mean difference in medial and lateral extension gaps was significantly greater with measured resection compared to gap balancing (−0.58 mm, 95% CI −1.01 to −0.15 mm; $P = .008$). Some authors suggest that implications of the resulting flexion gap asymmetry may include femoral condylar lift off and uneven polyethylene wear patterns.[6,37]

Advantages	Disadvantages
Joint line position is largely preserved[23]	Identification of landmarks may be difficult intraoperatively[34]
Midflexion stability[9,26]	Ligamentous release after trialing may result in gap asymmetry and laxity[33,38]
Optimal patellofemoral mechanics[28-30]	
Accurate implant positioning by referencing multiple anatomic landmarks[31]	

CLINICAL STUDIES

Measured resection and gap balancing techniques are two fundamentally different techniques used to achieve the same goal. Proponents and detractors of both methods have argued superiority of one method over the other based on a multitude of studies focused on the biomechanics of the knee. However, the vast majority of clinical studies have demonstrated that patient outcomes are comparable between the two.

Moon et al[33] conducted a meta-analysis of eight studies comparing knee biomechanics between measured resection and gap balancing in primary TKA. The authors found although there was no difference in flexion gap symmetries between the techniques, measured resection led to greater extension gap asymmetry. Gap balancing was associated with greater femoral component external rotation and joint line elevation. The authors concluded that although statistically significant, these differences were minimal (approximately 1 mm or 1°).

A randomized controlled trial by Babazadeh et al[24] compared both patient outcomes and knee kinematics in 103 patients over a 2-year period. The group found that there was no significant difference in femoral component rotation; however, gap balancing led to better gap symmetry whereas the measured resection technique was associated with a smaller change in joint line position. In this study, clinical outcomes and quality of life were assessed with the International Knee Society Score (IKSS) and short-form 12 (SF-12) questionnaires. At 2 years postoperatively, no difference in these clinical outcomes were observed between the two techniques.

Similarly, a recent review of 214 primary TKAs performed by a single surgeon found similar patient outcomes and excellent aseptic survivorship (98%) with both measured resection and gap balancing.[39] At a mean follow up of 3 years, patients in both groups had the same mean range of motion (123 versus 123°, $P = .990$) as well as similar Knee Society (KS) function scores (86 versus 85, $P = .829$) and KS pain scores (93 versus 92, $P = .425$).

SUMMARY

For the modern TKA, instability and malrotation are important etiologies of poor patient outcomes and implant failure. Although TKA is known to be a successful procedure, as many as one in five patients remains dissatisfied after surgery.[40] The measured resection technique has been used by surgeons worldwide for decades and is a valuable tool in achieving accurate femoral component alignment and rotational stability. However, as with many technical procedures, flaws exist with both measured resection and gap balancing. Ultimately, the selection of the most appropriate technique must be made by the surgeon based on a thorough understanding of what each method has to offer and its suitability to the individual patient.

In recent years, a hybrid technique has evolved which combines the strengths of both techniques in an effort to achieve optimal implant positioning in three planes as well as precise gap balancing. Although some small-scale clinical studies have compared outcomes between measured resection and gap balancing techniques, there is a lack of evidence on how hybrid techniques compare with these traditional approaches. Future research with large-scale studies is warranted to determine long-term outcomes in a sizable study population to effectively compare outcomes between measured resection, gap balancing, and hybrid techniques.

REFERENCES

1. Thiele K, Perka C, Matziolis G, Mayr HO, Sostheim M, Hube R. Current failure mechanisms after knee arthroplasty have changed: polyethylene wear is less common in revision surgery. *J Bone Joint Surg Am.* 2015;97:715-720. doi:10.2106/JBJS.M.01534.
2. Victor J. Optimising position and stability in total knee arthroplasty. *EFORT Open Rev.* 2017;2:215-220. doi:10.1302/2058-5241.2.170001.
3. Incavo SJ, Wild JJ, Coughlin KM, Beynnon BD. Early revision for component malrotation in total knee arthroplasty. *Clin Orthop Relat Res.* 2007;458:131-136. doi:10.1097/BLO.0b013e3180332d97.
4. Romero J, Stahelin T, Binkert C, Pfirrmann C, Hodler J, Kessler O. The clinical consequences of flexion gap asymmetry in total knee arthroplasty. *J Arthroplasty.* 2007;22:235-240. doi:10.1016/j.arth.2006.04.024.
5. Springer BD, Parratte S, Abdel MP. Measured resection versus gap balancing for total knee arthroplasty. *Clin Orthop Relat Res.* 2014;472:2016-2022. doi:10.1007/s11999-014-3524-y.
6. Dennis DA, Komistek RD, Kim RH, Sharma A. Gap balancing versus measured resection technique for total knee arthroplasty. *Clin Orthop Relat Res.* 2010;468:102-107. doi:10.1007/s11999-009-1112-3.
7. Daines BK, Dennis DA. Gap balancing vs. measured resection technique in total knee arthroplasty. *Clin Orthop Surg.* 2014;6:1-8. doi:10.4055/cios.2014.6.1.1.
8. Hungerford DS, Kenna RV, Krackow KA. The porous-coated anatomic total knee. *Orthop Clin North Am.* 1982;13:103-122.
9. Hungerford DS. Measured resection: a valuable tool in TKA. *Orthopedics.* 2008;31:941-942.
10. Sheth NP, Husain A, Nelson CL. Surgical techniques for total knee arthroplasty: measured resection, gap balancing, and hybrid. *J Am Acad Orthop Surg.* 2017;25:499-508. doi:10.5435/JAAOS-D-14-00320.
11. Churchill DL, Incavo SJ, Johnson CC, Beynnon BD. The transepicondylar axis approximates the optimal flexion axis of the knee. *Clin Orthop Relat Res.* 1998;356:111-118.
12. Aglietti P, Sensi L, Cuomo P, Ciardullo A. Rotational position of femoral and tibial components in TKA using the femoral transepicondylar axis. *Clin Orthop Relat Res.* 2008;466:2751-2755. doi:10.1007/s11999-008-0452-8.
13. Miller MC, Berger RA, Petrella AJ, Karmas A, Rubash HE. Optimizing femoral component rotation in total knee arthroplasty. *Clin Orthop Relat Res.* 2001;392:38-45.
14. Insall JN, Scuderi GR, Komistek RD, Math K, Dennis DA, Anderson DT. Correlation between condylar lift-off and femoral component alignment. *Clin Orthop Relat Res.* 2002;403:143-152.
15. Olcott CW, Scott RD. A comparison of 4 intraoperative methods to determine femoral component rotation during total knee arthroplasty. *J Arthroplasty.* 2000;15:22-26.
16. Whiteside LA, Arima J. The anteroposterior axis for femoral rotational alignment in valgus total knee arthroplasty. *Clin Orthop Relat Res.* 1995;321:168-172.
17. Arima J, Whiteside LA, McCarthy DS, White SE. Femoral rotational alignment, based on the anteroposterior axis, in total knee arthroplasty in a valgus knee. A technical note. *J Bone Joint Surg Am.* 1995;77:1331-1334.
18. Nagamine R, Miura H, Inoue Y, et al. Reliability of the anteroposterior axis and the posterior condylar axis for determining rotational alignment of the femoral component in total knee arthroplasty. *J Orthop Sci.* 1998;3:194-198.
19. Poilvache PL, Insall JN, Scuderi GR, Font-Rodriguez DE. Rotational landmarks and sizing of the distal femur in total knee arthroplasty. *Clin Orthop Relat Res.* 1996;331:35-46.
20. Whiteside LA. Soft tissue balancing: the knee. *J Arthroplasty.* 2002;17:23-27.
21. Tokuhara Y, Kadoya Y, Nakagawa S, Kobayashi A, Takaoka K. The flexion gap in normal knees. An MRI study. *J Bone Joint Surg Br.* 2004;86:1133-1136.
22. Sekiya H, Takatoku K, Takada H, Sasanuma H, Sugimoto N. Postoperative lateral ligamentous laxity diminishes with time after TKA in the varus knee. *Clin Orthop Relat Res.* 2009;467:1582-1586. doi:10.1007/s11999-008-0588-6.
23. Tigani D, Sabbioni G, Ben Ayad R, Filanti M, Rani N, Del Piccolo N. Comparison between two computer-assisted total knee arthroplasty: gap-balancing versus measured resection technique. *Knee Surg Sports Traumatol Arthrosc.* 2010;18:1304-1310. doi:10.1007/s00167-010-1124-2.
24. Babazadeh S, Dowsey MM, Stoney JD, Choong PFM. Gap balancing sacrifices joint-line maintenance to improve gap symmetry: a randomized controlled trial comparing gap balancing and measured resection. *J Arthroplasty.* 2014;29:950-954. doi:10.1016/j.arth.2013.09.036.
25. Emodi GJ, Callaghan JJ, Pedersen DR, Brown TD. Posterior cruciate ligament function following total knee arthroplasty: the effect of joint line elevation. *Iowa Orthop J.* 1999;19:82-92.
26. Martin JW, Whiteside LA. The influence of joint line position on knee stability after condylar knee arthroplasty. *Clin Orthop Relat Res.* 1990;259:146-156.
27. Hassaballa M, Gbejuade HO II, Porteous A, Murray IV JR. The effect of joint line restoration on kneeling ability after primary total knee replacement. *SA Orthop J.* 2012;11(3):79-83.
28. Partington PF, Sawhney J, Rorabeck CH, Barrack RL, Moore J. Joint line restoration after revision total knee arthroplasty. *Clin Orthop Relat Res.* 1999;367:165-171.
29. Konig C, Sharenkov A, Matziolis G, et al. Joint line elevation in revision TKA leads to increased patellofemoral contact forces. *J Orthop Res.* 2010;28:1-5. doi:10.1002/jor.20952.
30. Fornalski S, McGarry MH, Bui CNH, Kim WC, Lee TQ. Biomechanical effects of joint line elevation in total knee arthroplasty. *Clin Biomech.* 2012;27:824-829. doi:10.1016/j.clinbiomech.2012.05.009.
31. Hanada H, Whiteside LA, Steiger J, Dyer P, Naito M. Bone landmarks are more reliable than tensioned gaps in TKA component alignment. *Clin Orthop Relat Res.* 2007;462:137-142. doi:10.1097/BLO.0b013e3180dc92e7.
32. Luyckx T, Peeters T, Vandenneucker H, Victor J, Bellemans J. Is adapted measured resection superior to gap-balancing in determining femoral component rotation in total knee replacement? *J Bone Joint Surg Br.* 2012;94:1271-1276. doi:10.1302/0301-620X.94B9.28670.
33. Moon Y-W, Kim H-J, Ahn H-S, Park C-D, Lee D-H. Comparison of soft tissue balancing, femoral component rotation, and joint line change between the gap balancing and measured resection techniques in primary total knee arthroplasty: a meta-analysis. *Medicine (Baltimore)* 2016;95:e5006. doi:10.1097/MD.0000000000005006.
34. Katz MA, Beck TD, Silber JS, Seldes RM, Lotke PA. Determining femoral rotational alignment in total knee arthroplasty: reliability of techniques. *J Arthroplasty.* 2001;16:301-305.
35. Jerosch J, Peuker E, Philipps B, Filler T. Interindividual reproducibility in perioperative rotational alignment of femoral components in knee prosthetic surgery using the transepicondylar axis. *Knee Surg Sports Traumatol Arthrosc.* 2002;10:194-197. doi:10.1007/s00167-001-0271-x.
36. Yau WP, Chiu KY, Tang WM. How precise is the determination of rotational alignment of the femoral prosthesis in total knee arthroplasty: an in vivo study. *J Arthroplasty.* 2007;22:1042-1048. doi:10.1016/j.arth.2006.12.043.
37. Fehring TK. Rotational malalignment of the femoral component in total knee arthroplasty. *Clin Orthop Relat Res.* 2000;380:72-79.

38. Christensen CP, Stewart AH, Jacobs CA. Soft tissue releases affect the femoral component rotation necessary to create a balanced flexion gap during total knee arthroplasty. *J Arthroplasty.* 2013;28:1528-1532. doi:10.1016/j.arth.2013.01.008.

39. Churchill JL, Khlopas A, Sultan AA, Harwin SF, Mont MA. Gap-balancing versus measured resection technique in total knee arthroplasty: a comparison study. *J Knee Surg.* 2018;31:13-16. doi:10.1055/s-0037-1608820.

40. Noble PC, Conditt MA, Cook KF, Mathis KB. The John Insall Award: patient expectations affect satisfaction with total knee arthroplasty. *Clin Orthop Relat Res.* 2006;452:35-43. doi:10.1097/01.blo.0000238825.63648.1e.

chapter 32

Principles of Instrumentation and Component Alignment

Anthony P. Gualtieri, MD I Jonathan M. Vigdorchik, MD I Ran Schwarzkopf, MD, MSc

INTRODUCTION

Current instrumentation for total knee arthroplasty (TKA) facilitates the ability of the surgeon to make reproducible and accurate bone cuts that consistently restore the mechanical axis of the limb. Additionally, instruments may have the versatility to make adjustments that can accommodate for bone deficiency/deformity, ligament imbalance, and anatomic variations. This chapter focuses on the role and application of instruments in TKA.

NORMAL ANATOMY

There is great variation in native limb alignment. Individual differences in height, weight, and bone morphology affect the static knee alignment, and these differences are further affected by eccentric and asymmetric degenerative changes that are typically associated with the arthritic knee.

The mechanical axis of a knee normally aligned in the coronal plane is defined as a line drawn from the center of the femoral head passing through the center of the knee and ending in the center of the ankle joint. The *anatomic axis* refers to the intersection of a line down the axis of the femoral and tibial shafts (**Fig. 32-1**). On average, the anatomic axis of the knee is 5° to 7° of valgus. This angle represents a combination of the valgus alignment for the femoral condyles (a mean of ~7°) and the varus tilt of the tibial plateau (a mean of ~3°).[1]

The axis of rotation of the femur (flexion) also has a wide deviation, as the amount of the posterior condyles that falls below the transepicondylar axis can vary greatly. This is important if we make a transverse cut on the tibia and want to establish a rectangular space in flexion during TKA.

The flexion axis of rotation is complex but generally believed to transect the medial and lateral epicondyles at the origins of the collateral ligaments. It is transverse to the long axis of the tibia. At 90° of flexion, the medial condyle extends approximately 3 mm (1 to 6°) below (more posterior) the lateral condyles (**Fig. 32-2**).

BIOMECHANICS

In a limb with anatomic alignment of 7° of valgus, during normal gait, 60% to 70% of weight-bearing forces in stance phase pass through the medial compartment of the knee. Small changes in alignment can lead to substantial changes in load distribution in each of the compartments, which ultimately may predispose to the joint to developing osteoarthritis.[2-5] This may explain why there is often asymmetric chondral degeneration noted with progressive varus or valgus deformity in osteoarthritis.

Restoration of limb and component alignment during TKA normalizes the distribution of forces across the implant and enhances implant survival and performance. Lotke and Ecker[6] first established the overall importance of limb alignment and subsequent balance of soft tissues to optimize the results of total condylar knee replacement. Hsu et al[7] demonstrated that a 5-degree axial malalignment can change the load distribution up to 40%. These studies were corroborated by Ritter et al,[8] who showed that early failures occurred with tibial varus of more than 5°.

THEORIES OF AXIAL IMPLANT ALIGNMENT

The potential for errors of component implantation is great when we consider that the femoral and tibial components each have 6° of freedom in which they can be implanted: varus–valgus tilt, flexion–extension, proximal–distal position, internal–external rotation, anterior–posterior translation, and medial–lateral translation. The overall limb alignment and patella each has 3° of freedom. Combining all of the possibilities of implanting the components in relationship to one another, there exist more than 11,000 ways to get component alignment wrong. Fortunately, proper placement and alignment of components can be thought of as a range of satisfactory positions; however, implantation errors can be minimized by adhering to proven principles of TKA.

Restoring the mechanical limb alignment to neutral is a primary goal of TKA. There are three primary techniques for achieving alignment in TKA: mechanical alignment; anatomical alignment; and kinematic alignment. While mechanical and anatomical alignments were first proposed in the 1980s, kinematic alignment was only described in the mid 2000s. In order to make an informed decision on which technique to utilize, it is important to understand the philosophies that guide each surgical technique.

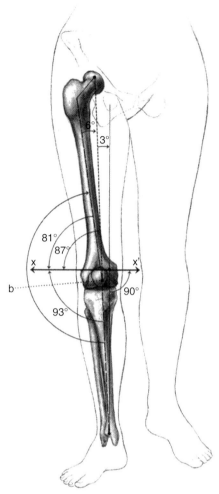

FIGURE 32-1   The reference axes for correct alignment are the anatomic axis along the shaft of the bone and the mechanical axis from the femoral head to the center of the ankle.

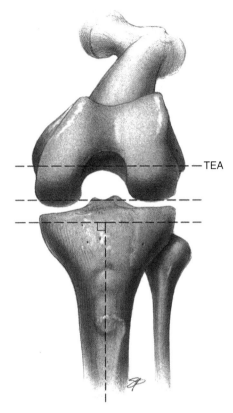

FIGURE 32-2   In flexion, the posterior medial condyle falls approximately 3° (3 mm) further below the transepicondylar axis (TEA) than the lateral posterior condyle. The medial tibial plateau is approximately 3° (3 mm) more distal than the lateral tibial plateau. If you make a transverse tibial osteotomy, to maintain a balanced rectangular flexion space, you will resect more bone from the medial posterior condyle.

Mechanical Alignment

The mechanical alignment for TKA was first described by John Insall in 1985.[9] The mechanical axis, as discussed previously, passes from the center of the femoral head to the center of the ankle joint. At the level of the knee, the mechanical axis typically passes just medial to the tibial spine.[10] Mechanical alignment depends on the distal femoral cut and the tibial cut, both being made perpendicular to their respective mechanical axes. This translates to a distal femoral cut of ~6° of valgus and a tibial cut of ~0° of varus/valgus.[9]

The philosophy behind this technique was based on Insall's belief that anatomically aligned knees were at risk for medial tibial plateau fixation failure due to the already established fact of increased forces across the medial aspect of the joint.[2-5,9] Insall pointed out that although the loading forces were even in the medial and lateral compartments during stance, these loading forces would be uneven during gait because of a laterally directed ground reaction force.[9,11]

Anatomical Alignment

The anatomic axis of the lower extremity is defined by the intramedullary (IM) canals of the femur and tibia. As described above, the anatomic and mechanical axes of the tibia match, while the anatomic axis of the femur is more valgus than the mechanical axis by an 8° to 9° angle.[1,10] Additionally, it is critical to remember that the normal knee joint is aligned at 2° to 3° of varus relative to the mechanical axis of the lower limb.[1] Therefore, the overall alignment of the lower extremity is a combined 5° to 7° of valgus.[1,10]

Hungerford and Krackow described the anatomical alignment technique for TKA in 1985.[12] The goal of anatomical alignment is to anatomically recreate the joint line. The tibia is cut at 2° to 3° of varus to the anatomical/mechanical axis of the tibia. The distal femoral cut is made at 8° to 9° of valgus, which is that same anatomical/mechanical difference mentioned previously. The overall alignment of the implanted components is therefore approximately 6° of valgus, which roughly matches the normal tibiofemoral angle of 5° to 7°.[12,13] This anatomic alignment technique purportedly improves the load distribution in the tibial component and improves patellar biomechanics by reducing lateral retinacular ligament stretching in knee flexion.[14,15]

Issues associated with the anatomical alignment technique include the difficulty of obtaining a tibial cut at 2° to 3° of varus and creating an oblique joint line. Consistently cutting the tibia at 2° to 3° requires a level of precision that may only be available through computer-assisted technologies. Creating an oblique joint line, rather than one parallel to the ground, has risks of higher chance of early failure.[8]

Kinematic Alignment

Kinematic alignment technique is the newest of the three techniques for TKA, first being performed in the mid-2000s. The notion of kinematic alignment for TKA is dependent on the work of Hollister and colleagues, who performed much of the original research on kinematics of the knee.[16] Additionally, much of the basic concepts of kinematic alignment hinges upon the technique of anatomical alignment, specifically the objective of reconstituting normal knee kinematics through resecting and replacing as little bone as possible.[12,17] Kinematic alignment is advocated as being patient-specific and ligament sparing.

Critical to the understanding of the kinematic alignment technique for TKA is the understanding of the three axes of movement in the knee. These three axes describe the movement of the patella and tibia in relation to the femur:

- The first and primary axis is a transverse axis that passes through the center of a circle fit to the articular surface of the femoral condyles from 10° to 160° of flexion. This is the axis about which the tibia flexes and extends.
- The second is a transverse axis that describes the motion of the patella as it flexes and extends around the distal femur. This axis is parallel, proximal, and anterior to the primary transverse axis.
- The third axis is longitudinal and centered in the tibia and is that about which the tibia internally and externally rotates around the distal femur. It is perpendicular to the first and second axes.

The main goal of kinematic alignment for TKA is to match the transverse axis of the femoral component to the primary transverse axis of the femur about which the tibia flexes and extends.[16,18] By aligning these axes and restoring the native tibial-femoral articular surfaces, the kinematic alignment method uses bony resection to maintain the native resting lengths of the collateral, retinacular, and posterior cruciate ligaments, thereby foregoing any need for ligamentous releases.[18]

Although the kinematic alignment technique proposes improved clinical outcomes through restoring native knee kinematics, there are some risks associated with this technique. It is a relatively new technique, so long-term survivorship data are sparse. Additionally, as mentioned previously, the varus tibial positioning inherent to this technique is a theoretical risk factor for earlier failure.[8]

MECHANICAL ALIGNMENT

Outcomes

The mechanical alignment technique has been the mainstay of TKA for decades. Mechanical alignment aims to align the hip–knee–ankle angle of the limb in neutral, thereby achieving a more balanced load distribution in the medial and lateral compartments. This classical approach has shown predictably good results and reliably high survivorship data.[19-23] A 2009 retrospective survivorship analysis of over 6000 TKAs showed that postoperative alignment was the chief predictor of failure and revision surgery, regardless of preoperative alignment. This study produced an "ideal" coronal alignment of 2.4° to 7.2° of valgus which was associated with the best overall survivorship.[22] An older study by Jefferey et al reported that when the mechanical axis fell in the medial 1/3 of the TKA, the rate of aseptic loosening was markedly lower than when the mechanical axis was further medial or lateral from this neutral position (3% vs. 24%).[23] Another prospective study on mechanical alignment using computer-assisted surgery found that patients with a postoperative alignment within 3° of a neutral axis had increased International Knee Society Score and Short-Form 12 Physical Scores at both 6 weeks and 12 months postoperatively.[24] In summary, these extensive data contribute to our knowledge that when performed well, the mechanical axis technique for TKA yields excellent results and survivorship.

Unfortunately, the method of mechanical axis alignment is associated with a persistent population of dissatisfied patients. A study of 1703 patients in Canada found that approximately 20% of patients were dissatisfied with their TKA.[25] These data were echoed by a US report of more than 10,000 patients, which showed 18.2% dissatisfaction.[26] Across numerous studies, these results have been reinforced, with 11% to 18% of patients remaining dissatisfied with their TKA.[27-34] The etiology for this dissatisfaction has been multifactorial, but possible causes could be alteration in limb alignment from natural valgus to a postoperative neutral position and collateral ligament tensioning changes.[35] Ultimately, it seems that while a large proportion of patients are satisfied after TKAs performed by the surgical technique of mechanical axis alignment, somewhere between one in every five to six patients are dissatisfied with their results.

Instrumentation

Classically, extramedullary and IM instruments have been used for the tibial and femoral osteotomies in the mechanical alignment technique. Both extramedullary and IM guides have been shown to be equally effective for the tibial osteotomy (**Fig. 32-3**).[36] For the femoral osteotomies, both extramedullary and IM guides have been utilized, although IM guides have been preferred due to studies

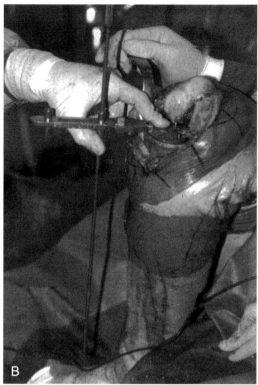

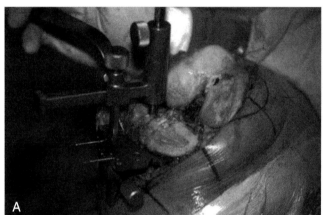

FIGURE 32-3   Intramedullary **(A)** or extramedullary **(B)** guides may be used to make a transverse osteotomy of the tibia.

showing improved relative accuracy.[3,37-43] Additionally, there are two important femoral osteotomies. The distal osteotomy, which relies on extramedullary or IM guides, sets axial alignment and the anterior–posterior osteotomies that determine rotational alignment, which will be discussed in a later section.

For the proximal tibial osteotomy, the extramedullary guide is placed parallel to the tibial crest in the coronal plane, with ability to adjust for a posterior slope. Extramedullary systems bypass any potential deformity of the tibial shaft, which can bias alignment. They also reduce the risk of fat embolism syndrome and allow for easy adjustment of alignment in all planes. Although this technique can be highly effective and accurate, Cates et al[37] reviewed alignment of the proximal tibial cut with the use of extramedullary guides and found a significant percentage of alignment errors. In morbidly obese patients, in whom external landmarks are obscure, these guides have a greater potential for error.

IM guides can also create reproducible osteotomies.[44,45] This technique is applicable for most knees, except when there is significant tibial deformity or obstruction of the tibial canal by previous fracture or hardware. IM instrumentation is placed through a drill hole in the tibial plateau. The pilot hole is often started at the junction of the insertion of the anterior cruciate ligament and the anterior horn of the lateral meniscus. Proximally, the drill hole should be wide enough so the guide is not biased at this level and marrow pressures can be released during rod insertion. It has been shown that a 12.7-mm drill hole

can reduce the risk of intraoperative oxygen desaturation when using an 8-mm alignment rod designed to allow venting of the canal.[46] It has also been shown that fluted and hollow rods significantly reduce IM pressures within the canal,[47] offering an explanation in the mechanism of reduced fat embolization.

Both IM and extramedullary guides have telescoping elements that are used to place a cutting block at the desired resection level (**Fig. 32-4**). The varus and valgus alignment is adjusted to parallel the mechanical axis of the tibia, and the posterior slope is "dialed in" by the cutting block to approximate the native posterior slope. The block is pinned at an appropriate resection level and

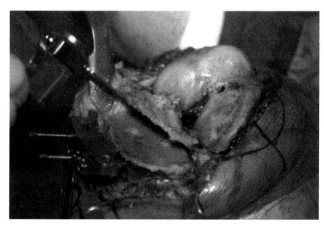

FIGURE 32-4   A tibial cutting block is fixed in place and used to guide the transverse tibial osteotomy.

the osteotomy is performed. A measuring guide (stylus) can be used to accurately determine the amount of bone to be resected, generally seeking to remove approximately 10 mm (depending on the implant and anatomy) of bone and cartilage from the less arthritic hemiplateau. Adjustments in placement of the stylus may be necessary in the presence of subchondral loss and abnormal contouring of the plateau.

For the distal femoral osteotomy, mechanical alignment technique dictates the osteotomy be aligned in 4° to 7° of valgus. IM and extramedullary guides are available for the distal femoral resection. However, most surgeons find that the IM devices are reproducible, easy, and applicable in the vast majority of cases (**Fig. 32-5**).[3,37-43] Cates et al[37] reviewed 200 consecutive TKAs in which IM femoral guides were used in 125 cases and extramedullary femoral guides in 75 cases. The distal femoral resection angle was outside the accepted range (4° to 10° of femoral valgus) in 28% of the extramedullary group and in only 14% of the IM group. Joint line orientation was also outside the normal range twice as frequently in the extramedullary alignment group. The authors suggested that IM guides improve the accuracy of distal femoral osteotomy. Teter et al[38] reviewed 201 TKAs in which IM

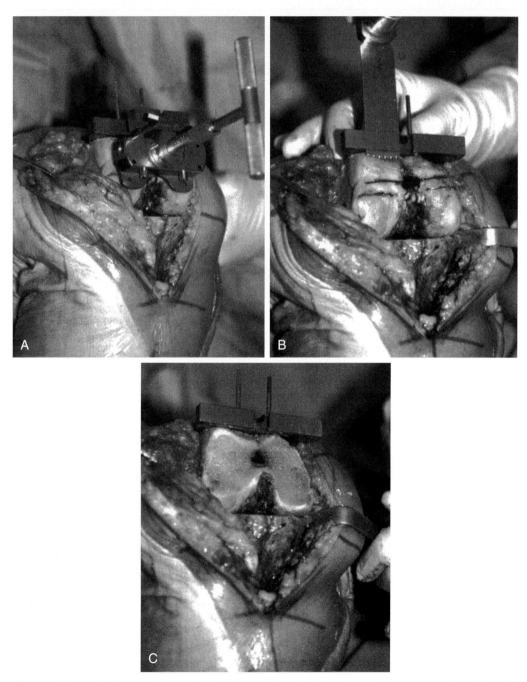

FIGURE 32-5   An intramedullary guide is set at 4°-6° of valgus and placed into the femur **(A)**. The rod is removed, and the osteotomy is taken in the distal femur **(B)**. The contour of the cut surface should approximate a "figure of eight" **(C)**.

femoral guides were used. Distal femoral alignment was considered inaccurate in only 8% of the x-rays. Risk factors for inaccurate alignment included capacious femoral canals and distal femoral bowing. Regardless of the technique, IM or extramedullary, attention to detail and confirmatory assessments are critical in minimizing alignment errors.

If opting to use an IM system, a drill hole is made in the femoral notch anterior to the origin of the posterior cruciate ligament, with the knee flexed. Standard full-length femoral radiographs can show the optimal placement of the drill hole to access the femoral canal. This position is usually slightly medial to the center of the apex of the intercondylar notch. Insertion of the IM guide too far medially leads to a relative varus cut; too far laterally leads to a valgus cut. The canal is overdrilled at the entry so as to not bias the IM guide, allowing the rod to engage diaphyseal bone. This also allows for the release of medullary contents and minimizes pressure within the canal.[46] Fluted rods placed in the canal have been shown to decrease IM pressures and possibly reduce the incidence of fat emboli syndrome.[46,47] Most jigs allow for adjustment of the valgus angle of the distal cut from 4° to 7°.

As a technical note, when seating the distal femoral cutting jig, an important note to remember is to ensure that the guide is seated medially and sitting just slightly off on the lateral condyle. If the guide is flush laterally, there is a risk of raising the joint line and therefore over-resecting the distal femur. It is also important to ensure that the distal femoral cutting is not placed in an extended or flexed position, as this will greatly impact the later positioning of the 4-in-1 cutting guide.

KINEMATIC ALIGNMENT

Outcomes

This consistent level of dissatisfaction, discussed in the previous section on outcomes of mechanical alignment, was partially responsible for the movement to adopt alternative alignment techniques. In addition, recent research has shown that there is a large variability in the "normal" parameters of individual's lower limb alignment; indeed, a large proportion of patients have a "constitutional varus" in their native knees.[35,48] Therefore, aiming for a neutral value on every patient, as with the mechanical axis technique, may alter some patients' natural alignment and kinematics. This dissatisfaction and evolving understanding of "normal" alignment has contributed to recent interest in the kinematic alignment technique for TKA.

A systemic review and metaanalysis of nine studies by Coutney et al[35] comparing kinematic alignment to mechanical alignment showed similar survivorship at 38 months and improved Knee Society Scores (KSS) in the kinematically aligned TKA group. A randomized control study of patients assigned to either patient-specific instruments with kinematic alignment or conventional instrumentation with mechanical alignment resulted in improved pain relief, restoration of function, and range of motion at 2-year follow-up.[49] A radiographic analysis of this group showed similar hip–knee–ankle angles between kinematic alignment with patient-specific guides and mechanical alignment with conventional guides, but increased femoral component valgus and tibial component varus in the kinematic alignment group.[50] Good results have also been demonstrated in a study performed utilizing the kinematic alignment technique with non–patient-specific, or conventional, instrumentation.[51]

Although these studies have demonstrated improved short-term results with kinematic alignment in comparison to mechanical alignment, not all of the literature about kinematic alignment has been so positive. Another randomized control trial of 95 patients was unable to replicate the results of Dossett et al.[49,50,52] This trial by Young et al showed no statistically significant difference in pain or function scores between kinematically and mechanically aligned knees at 2 years.[52] Additionally, it should be noted that long-term data regarding kinematically aligned TKA are lacking, due to its relatively recent introduction. Although a 6-year follow-up study of 219 knees showed 97.5% survivorship, there is no significant data regarding any longer-term results.[53] This is important due to the varus position into which the tibial component is placed during the kinematic alignment technique and the theoretical detriment this could have on implant longevity. As discussed previously, excess tibial component varus positioning is associated with a higher risk for early failure.[8] Additionally, the femoral component positioning during kinematically aligned TKA has been reported as being 2° more internally rotated than during mechanically aligned TKA.[52] This relative internal rotation poses a theoretical risk for patellofemoral maltracking, although patellofemoral issues have not yet been reported to be a statistically more significant issue with kinematic alignment than with mechanical alignment.[49-51,53-55] In conclusion, although short-term data regarding the outcomes for kinematic alignment seem promising, further long-term data are required.

Instrumentation

The key difference between the instrumentation utilized for mechanical alignment and that utilized for kinematic alignment is that the former is classically generic and the latter is typically patient-specific, or custom. The kinematic alignment technique aims to position implants so as to match the pre-arthritic anatomy of the individual, therefore the advantage of individualized instrumentation.[50,55,56] This technique utilizes the bone cuts to replace and resurface the native joint, with the ultimate goal of preserving natural knee anatomy.

As mentioned, most reports on kinematic alignment utilize patient-specific instrumentation to guide resection.[50,55,56] This necessitates preoperative advanced imaging with either computed tomography (CT) or MRI. Patient-specific instrumentation is associated with increased cost, due to the cost of manufacturing individualized guides, the need for advanced imaging, and increased preoperative planning time by the surgeon.[57,58] Proponents of kinematic alignment argue that patient-specific instrumentation may reduce operative time and improve implant alignment and therefore survivorship, and so while these guides may not be cost-effective, now they may be in the future.[57] There has been one report in the literature of kinematic alignment technique performed using generic, or conventional, instrumentation. This study by Howell et al utilized a cruciate-retaining fixed-bearing implant and reported excellent results in alignment and function, similar to those reported in studies utilizing patient-specific instrumentation. The surgical technique utilized by Howell in this paper is similar to that described in his paper describing kinematic alignment technique using patient-specific instrumentation.[51]

ROTATION

Femoral Component Rotation

External rotation of the femoral component is the key to creating a rectangular flexion gap and facilitating patella tracking.[59,60] Several methods are used to determine femoral component rotation. Each is effective but has some inherent errors (**Fig. 32-6**).

1. The transepicondylar axis—a line drawn between the medial and lateral epicondyles.[61] Some surgeons find this anatomy difficult to identify (**Fig. 32-2**).
2. The anterior–posterior line of Whiteside[62,63]—a line from the deepest portion of the trochlea to the center of the intercondylar notch. A line drawn perpendicular to this is considered to be an effective

degree of femoral component external rotation (**Fig. 32-6**). This technique relies on consistent trochlear anatomy, which can be distorted by patellofemoral and severe tibiofemoral osteoarthritis.[64]

3. Posterior condylar axis—a line drawn between the posterior surface of the medial and lateral condyles with a prefixed use of a 3-degree external rotation guide[65] (**Fig. 32-2**). With cartilage wear and bone defects of the posterior femoral condyles, this technique can be less reliable.[66]
4. Tensioned gap technique places a spreader to tension the flexion gap. Osteotomies are made to establish a rectangular gap in flexion with the tibial shaft axis.[67] This technique may be difficult when there is a substantial preexisting ligamentous imbalance. Errors in tibial resection can compromise femoral component rotation (**Fig. 32-7**).

These various techniques have had several advocates and detractors in the literature. Olcott and Scott[68] prospectively analyzed 100 TKAs and compared how these intraoperative femoral landmarks performed. Using the tensioning rectangular flexion space as the control, the transepicondylar axis most consistently created a balanced flexion gap when they compared the anteroposterior "line of Whiteside" and 3° of external rotation of the posterior condyles. Three degrees of external rotation performed least favorably, especially in preoperative valgus-aligned knees. Akagi et al[69] reported similar inaccuracies with the use of posterior condylar axis. They performed CT scans on 111 knees with symptomatic arthritis and evaluated the transepicondylar axes (clinical and surgical), the posterior condylar axis, and the anteroposterior axis. These values were then compared with the tibiofemoral and femoral valgus angles of the individual patients studied. The authors found that when tibiofemoral valgus exceeded 9°, the posterior femoral axis became increasingly unreliable. In 25% of the cases, the surgical transepicondylar axis could not be reconstructed due to

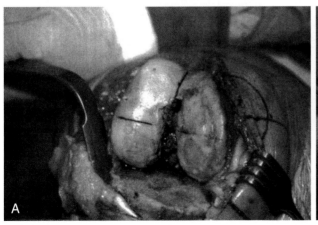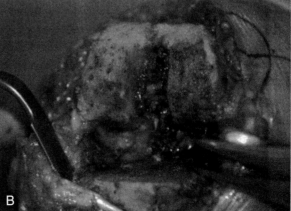

FIGURE 32-6 A knee with a transepicondylar axis and Whiteside's lines drawn on the distal femur **(A)**. After the posterior condylar osteotomy, the flexion gap should be rectangular under tension of a laminar spreader **(B)**.

Because of the vagaries and errors of any one technique, most surgeons will use several of these techniques in combination during each case to estimate femoral component rotation. We have found that for routine total knees, without too much deformity, we have relied more on the tension technique at 90° of flexion to confirm a rectangular flexion gap.

Another check for proper rotation is the "footprint" created by the anterior osteotomy ("grand piano sign"). It should look like a low and high bimodal curve (**Fig. 32-8**). If a reasonable contour is obtained, it can be a crude estimate of appropriate rotation.

Patellofemoral tracking is directly influenced by rotation of the femoral component.[59,71] External rotation of the femoral component brings the trochlea in closer proximity to the center of the patella. In addition, internal rotation leads to under-resection of the medial femoral condyle and a tight medial flexion gap. If this malrotation is not identified, unnecessary release of the medial structures may be performed. Problems with maltracking of the patella or a tight medial sleeve may be an indication of femoral component internal rotation. Excessive external rotation does not adversely affect patellofemoral tracking. However, it does create a trapezoidal flexion space and a flexion imbalance. Therefore, appropriate rotational alignment is essential for creating the perfect total knee.

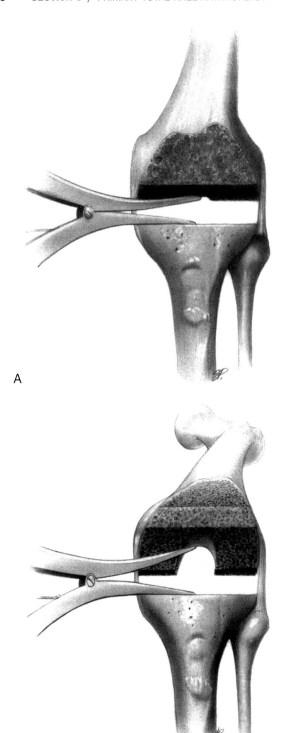

A

B

FIGURE 32-7 The tension technique makes a transverse tibial osteotomy first **(A)**, and the femoral osteotomy is determined with tension to make equal rectangular spaces in flexion and extension **(B)**.

medial epicondylar sulcus being unrecognized. In knees with greater valgus alignment, the authors believe the anteroposterior axis is more reliable. The authors advocate CT scans in severe valgus cases to help define femoral component rotation. Katz et al[70] showed that the tension technique was the most reliable and that estimating the transepicondylar axis had the greatest variation.

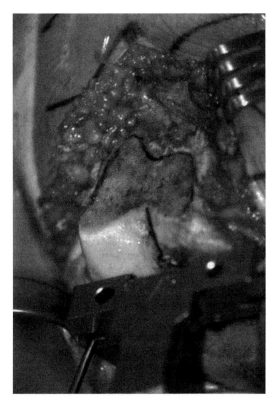

FIGURE 32-8 When the appropriate anterior osteotomy has been completed, the contours of the osteotomy should have a "bimodal" shape and enough area to receive the anterior flange of the femoral component.

Tibial Component Rotation

Tibial component rotation affects the kinematics of the femorotibial joint as well as patellar tracking, and therefore malrotation of the tibial component can contribute to poor outcomes following TKA. There is a wide range of literature focusing on the correct rotational alignment of the femoral component, but less so on the correct rotational alignment of the tibial component. This may be in part due to the difficulty in assessing the tibial component rotation. There are numerous proposed anatomical landmarks for tibial component rotation, including (1) the medial border of the tibial tuberosity, (2) the medial third of the tibial tuberosity, (3) the anterior tibial crest, (4) the medial border of the patellar tendon, (5) the middle of the posterior cruciate ligament, and (6) the second ray of the foot.[9,72-77]

Classically, the position of the tibial component was determined by centering its rotation with the border of the medial third and central third of the tibial tubercle, as advocated by Insall.[9] At least three studies, however, have suggested that this classic technique may cause excess tibial component external rotation.[75-77] Akagi et al utilized preoperative CT scans and identified the medial edge of the patellar tendon as a reliable and accurate anterior anatomic landmark.[76,77] Ikeuchi et al compared the anterior reference point obtained by ranging the knee with femoral and tibial components in place and reported that the best rotational orientation of the tibial component is close to the medial border of the attachment of the patellar tendon.[78]

Whichever technique is used, what is solidly established in the literature is the danger of excessive internal rotation of the tibial component. It has been reported that nearly 5% of TKA tibial components were significantly internally rotated on retrospective advanced imaging analysis.[79] This same study, by Nicoll and Rowley, also found that tibial component internal rotation greater than 9° was associated with pain and functional deficit after TKA.[79] A study by Barrack et al of more than 100 TKA patients at 5 years post-surgery found that patients with anterior knee pain had an average tibial component internal rotation of 6° and painless knees had an average external rotation of 0.4°.[80] Another study by Bedard et al on 34 TKAs complicated by stiffness that required surgical revision found 33 of 34 tibial components to be internally rotated at a mean of 13.7°.[81] All of these studies base their degree of rotation off of the tibial tubercle axis, which defines neutral as 18° of internal tibial component rotation in relation to the tibial tuberosity.[82]

On a technical note, there are some special situations that need unique consideration. In situations wherein there is extreme external rotation at the tibial tubercle, several of these techniques are impossible. For instance, externally rotating to the medial third of the tibial tubercle in a case with an extremely externally rotated tibial tubercle will shift the tibial component so much that it will not align underneath the femoral component. As another consideration, in PS implants, one must ensure that after setting the external rotation of the tibial component, the tibial post still aligns suitably with the femoral component's box.

PATELLAR ALIGNMENT

It is important to remember that the kinematics of the knee is characterized by the motions of not only the femur and tibia but also the patella.[83] The patella is a sesamoid bone within the tendon of the extensor mechanism that facilitates extension of the knee by increasing the efficiency of the quadriceps muscle.[84] The motion of the patella, both native and resurfaced, is complex and reinforced by extrinsic stabilizers, muscles, and soft tissue, as well as its intrinsic stability, determined by the retropatellar surface. When the quadriceps muscle is contracted, because of its oblique orientation in regard to the patella, it creates a line of pull with a laterally directed horizontal component. This angle between the quadriceps and the patellar tendon is often referred to as the Q angle, which is responsible for the tendency of the patella to shift laterally. In the native knee, this laterally directed force is offset by the more anteriorly prominent lateral femoral condyle and the more distally inserting muscle fibers of the vastus medialis.[83]

The asymmetric native retropatellar surface has a natural high point that is located more medial than lateral. Therefore, when using a dome patella, aligning the medial margin of the symmetric insert with the medial margin of the cut surface helps recreate this natural high point, but leaves more of the lateral retropatellar surface unresurfaced. An anatomic patellar implant has a shorter medial facet, which overcomes this shortcoming but necessitates correct rotational position to allow for correct alignment of the retropatellar high point within the trochlear groove.[85] Because the majority of patellar implants currently used are either dome-shaped or anatomic, the most commonly accepted position is superomedial relative to the center of the retropatellar surface, as this most closely emulates the location of the native retropatellar high point.[85]

Medialization of the patellar implant by 2 mm in cadaveric knees has been shown to reduce the peak lateral shear force by 10 to 15N, but a corresponding medial shear force was observed in knee flexion less than 25°.[86] This biomechanical study has been reflected in clinical data, with clinical series showing lateral retinacular release rates of 13% to 17% with patellar implant medialization compared to 46% to 48% with central placement.[87,88]

Further cadaveric study on patellar component medialization by Anglin et al has shown a significant reduction of patellofemoral contact forces above 60° of knee flexion associated with increasing medialization of the patellar implant. However, it was noticed that as the patella was more medialized it had a higher propensity to tilt laterally relative to the femur.[89] This tendency toward lateral tilt is thought to result from the medio-lateral moment created when the extensor mechanism, which is positioned centrally on the patella and acts posteriorly, becomes off-center from the implant after medialization.[85] To maximally reduce the patellofemoral contact force while minimizing the lateral patellar tilt, Anglin et al recommended medialization no greater than 2.5 mm.[89] Excessive medialization can also leave excessive exposed bone on the lateral patellar facet, a potential source of painful contact with the lateral femoral condyle.[90] Chamfering the lateral patellar rim has been advocated to reduce the risk of this bony impingement.[91]

NEW TECHNOLOGIES

Technology has advanced significantly since Theophilus Gluck performed one of the earliest recorded TKA procedures in the 1890s with an ivory implant.[92] In the most recent decades, advances in computer sciences have shepherded computer navigation and the current "robotic TKA" from fantasy to reality. This new technology is one of the most rapidly expanding tools being utilized, with trends from the Medicare database showing a steady increase over the last two decades.[93] TKA has had consistently excellent outcomes, and this newer technology seeks to improve on these already outstanding results to create a longer lasting, more kinematically natural knee.

Computer-assisted navigation systems have been utilized in TKA to improve accuracy in component positioning. As mentioned previously, malalignment can negatively affect patient-reported outcomes and implant survivorship[23,79]; computer-assisted TKA (CATKA) aims to eliminate these outlier errors. Several studies have utilized postoperative imaging to demonstrate the superiority of CATKA in accurate component positioning.[94-96] A randomized control trial by Matziolis et al found a much more precise and accurate range of implants' frontal and sagittal alignments with CATKA compared to conventional TKA.[94] These results were reproduced by Mizu-uchi et al, showing significantly improved component positioning with CATKA, especially in regard to rotational alignment.[95] Another prospective randomized control trial by Perlick et al found that CATKA was significantly more likely to result in a postoperative leg alignment within ±3° of neutral than conventional technique (92% vs. 72%).[96]

Outside of just improving component positioning on postoperative imaging, CATKA had demonstrated clinical benefits as well. At least two different studies have demonstrated significantly decreased blood loss with CATKA versus conventional technique.[97,98] This is most likely due to the lack of IM guide utilization in CATKA technique, reduces the risk of transfusion for the patient, and indicates CATKA may be a useful technique for whom blood products are not acceptable.[98] Additionally, CATKA has been associated with decreased embolic load

during and immediately after surgery. A study by Church et al utilized intraoperative transesophageal ECG to measure embolic load, finding significantly lower embolic scores with CATKA than conventional technique.[99] Another study on systemic emboli during and immediately after TKA showed a significant reduction in systemic emboli during TKA compared to conventional technique as measured by transcranial Doppler ultrasonography.[100] This reduction in embolic load has also been attributed to the lack of IM instrumentation during CATKA technique.[99,100] Additionally, a nationwide database study of over 100,000 TKA patients found that patients who underwent CATKA had a statistically significant lower rate of cardiac complications as well as nonsignificant trend toward shorter length of hospital stay and fewer postoperative hematomas.[101]

The advantages of CATKA in regard to component positioning, blood loss, emboli, and other clinical factors are well-established, but the benefits on functional outcome remain controversial. A study of almost 100 knees by Seon and Song showed better functional scores, pain, and range of motion at 1 year after CATKA compared to conventional technique.[102] Interestingly, in their small subcohort of bilateral patients who had had CATKA and conventional TKA, patients tended to prefer the side that had undergone CATKA compared to conventional. Another randomized prospective study by Hoffart et al of almost 200 knees found improved KSS scores at 5 years in the CATKA group compared to the conventional technique group.[103] On the other hand, other studies have failed to show significant functional outcome differences. A prospective study with a 10-year follow-up by Kim et al wherein patients underwent staged bilateral knee replacements, one side with CATKA and one with conventional technique, failed to show significant differences between the two techniques in terms of function, pain scores, activity scores, or survivorship.[104] This same research group replicated these results with the same protocol, finding no significant difference when looking at all outcomes at 12.3 years of follow-up.[105] Another retrospective study looking at more than 9000 cases of TKA in the New Zealand National Joint Registry found no differences in functional outcome or survivorship between cases performed via CATKA compared to conventional technique.[106]

In summation, the data regarding the positive impact of CATKA in several categories including radiographic alignment, blood loss, emboli, and cardiac events seem well-established; however, the impact of computer assistance on functional outcomes and survivorship in TKA is still a topic of much debate.

CONCLUSION

Alignment in total knee replacement has evolved over the last decade and better instrumentation has enabled the surgeon to perform total knee replacements with increasing consistency and reliability. The techniques outlined are the parameters we used to aid in the proper alignment and placement of femoral and tibial implants. Understanding the goals and principles of restoring limb alignment is essential in creating a well-balanced total knee replacement and will ultimately contribute to the success of the implant; contemporary instruments can aid in achieving these goals.

REFERENCES

1. Johnson F, Leitl S, Waugh W. The distribution of load across the knee. *J Bone Joint Surg Br.* 1992;62:346.
2. Harrington IJ. A bioengineering analysis of force actions at the knee in normal and pathologic gait. *Biomed Eng.* 1976;11:167.
3. Harrington IJ. Static and dynamic loading patterns in knee joints with deformities. *J Bone Joint Surg Am.* 1983;65:247-259.
4. Hsu RWW, Himeno S, Coventry MB. Normal axial alignment of the lower extremity and load-bearing distribution at the knee. *Clin Orthop Relat Res.* 1990;255:215-217.
5. Morrison JB. Bioengineering analysis of force actions transmitted by the knee joint. *Biomed Eng.* 1968;3:164.
6. Lotke PA, Ecker ML. Influence of positioning of prosthesis in total knee replacement. *J Bone Joint Surg Am.* 1977;59:77.
7. Hsu HP, Garg A, Walker PS, et al. Effect on knee component alignment on tibial load distribution with clinical correlation. *Clin Orthop Relat Res.* 1989;248:135.
8. Ritter MA, Faris PM, Keating EM, et al. Postoperative alignment of total knee replacement. Its effect on survival. *Clin Orthop Relat Res.* 1994;299:153-156.
9. Insall JN, Binazzi R, Soudry M, Mestriner LA. Total knee arthroplasty. *Clin Orthop Relat Res.* 1985;192:13-22.
10. Luo CF. Reference axes for reconstruction of the knee. *Knee.* 2004;11(4):251-257.
11. Cherian JJ, Kapadia BH, Banerjee S, Jauregui JJ, Issa K, Mont MA. Mechanical, anatomical, and kinematic axis in TKA: concepts and practical applications. *Curr Rev Musculoskelet Med.* 2014;7(2):89-95.
12. Hungerford DS, Krackow KA. Total joint arthroplasty of the knee. *Clin Orthop Relat Res.* 1985;192:23-33.
13. Johnson AJ, Harwin SF, Krackow KA, Mont MA. Alignment in total knee arthroplasty: where have we come from and where are we going? *Surg Technol Int.* 2011;21:183-188.
14. Klatt BA, Goyal N, Austin MS, Hozack WJ. Custom-fit total knee arthroplasty (OtisKnee) results in malalignment. *J Arthroplasty.* 2008;23(1):26-29.
15. Ghosh KM, Merican AM, Iranpour-boroujeni F, Deehan DJ, Amis AA. Length change patterns of the extensor retinaculum and the effect of total knee replacement. *J Orthop Res.* 2009;27(7):865-870.
16. Hollister AM, Jatana S, Singh AK, Sullivan WW, Lupichuk AG. The axes of rotation of the knee. *Clin Orthop Relat Res.* 1993;290:259-268.
17. Hungerford DS, Kenna RV, Krackow KA. The porous-coated anatomic total knee. *Orthop Clin North Am.* 1982;13(1):103-122.
18. Howell SM, Hull ML, Mahfouz MR. Kinematically aligned total knee arthroplasty. In: Scott WN, ed. *Surgery of the Knee.* 6th ed. Philadelphia, PA: Elsevier; 2018.
19. Aglietti P, Buzzi R. Posteriorly stabilised total-condylar knee replacement. Three to eight years' follow-up of 85 knees. *J Bone Joint Surg Br.* 1988;70(2):211-216.
20. Bargren JH, Blaha JD, Freeman MA. Alignment in total knee arthroplasty. Correlated biomechanical and clinical observations. *Clin Orthop Relat Res.* 1983;173:178-183.
21. Berend ME, Ritter MA, Meding JB, et al. Tibial component failure mechanisms in total knee arthroplasty. *Clin Orthop Relat Res.* 2004;428:26-34.
22. Fang DM, Ritter MA, Davis KE. Coronal alignment in total knee arthroplasty: just how important is it? *J Arthroplasty.* 2009;24(6 suppl):39-43.
23. Jeffery RS, Morris RW, Denham RA. Coronal alignment after total knee replacement. *J Bone Joint Surg Br.* 1991;73(5):709-714.1.
24. Choong PF, Dowsey MM, Stoney JD. Does accurate anatomical alignment result in better function and quality of life? Comparing conventional and computer-assisted total knee arthroplasty. *J Arthroplasty.* 2009;24(4):560-569.
25. Bourne RB, Chesworth BM, Davis AM, Mahomed NN, Charron KD. Patient satisfaction after total knee arthroplasty: who is satisfied and who is not? *Clin Orthop Relat Res.* 2010;468(1):57-63.
26. Baker PN, Van der meulen JH, Lewsey J, Gregg PJ. The role of pain and function in determining patient satisfaction after total knee replacement. Data from the National Joint Registry for England and Wales. *J Bone Joint Surg Br.* 2007;89(7):893-900.
27. Anderson JG, Wixson RL, Tsai D, Stulberg SD, Chang RW. Functional outcome and patient satisfaction in total knee patients over the age of 75. *J Arthroplasty.* 1996;11(7):831-840.
28. Chesworth BM, Mahomed NN, Bourne RB, Davis AM. Willingness to go through surgery again validated the WOMAC clinically important difference from THR/TKR surgery. *J Clin Epidemiol.* 2008;61(9):907-918.
29. Hawker G, Wright J, Coyte P, et al. Health-related quality of life after knee replacement. *J Bone Joint Surg Am.* 1998;80(2):163-173.
30. Heck DA, Robinson RL, Partridge CM, Lubitz RM, Freund DA. Patient outcomes after knee replacement. *Clin Orthop Relat Res.* 1998;356:93-110.
31. Noble PC, Conditt MA, Cook KF, Mathis KB. The John Insall Award: patient expectations affect satisfaction with total knee arthroplasty. *Clin Orthop Relat Res.* 2006;452:35-43.
32. Robertsson O, Dunbar M, Pehrsson T, Knutson K, Lidgren L. Patient satisfaction after knee arthroplasty: a report on 27,372 knees operated on between 1981 and 1995 in Sweden. *Acta Orthop Scand.* 2000;71(3):262-267.
33. Wylde V, Learmonth I, Potter A, Bettinson K, Lingard E. Patient-reported outcomes after fixed- versus mobile-bearing total knee replacement: a multi-centre randomised controlled trial using the Kinemax total knee replacement. *J Bone Joint Surg Br.* 2008;90(9):1172-1179.
34. Dunbar MJ, Robertsson O, Ryd L, Lidgren L. Appropriate questionnaires for knee arthroplasty. Results of a survey of 3600 patients from The Swedish Knee Arthroplasty Registry. *J Bone Joint Surg Br.* 2001;83(3):339-344.
35. Courtney PM, Lee GC. Early outcomes of kinematic alignment in primary total knee arthroplasty: a meta-analysis of the literature. *J Arthroplasty.* 2017;32(6):2028-2032.e1.
36. Dennis DA, Channer M, Susman MH, et al. Intramedullary versus extramedullary tibial alignment systems in total knee arthroplasty. *J Arthroplasty.* 1993;8:43.
37. Cates HE, Ritter MA, Keating EM, et al. Intramedullary versus extramedullary alignment systems in total knee replacement. *Clin Orthop Relat Res.* 1993;286:32-39.
38. Teter KE, Bregman D, Colwell CW Jr. The efficacy of intramedullary alignment in total knee replacement. *Clin Orthop Relat Res.* 1995;321:117-121.
39. Engh GA, Peterson M. Comparative experience with intramedullary and extramedullary alignment in total knee arthroplasty. *J Arthroplasty.* 1990;5:1.
40. Manning M, Elloy M, Johnson R. The accuracy of intramedullary alignment in total knee replacement. *J Bone Joint Surg Br.* 1988;70:852.
41. Ritter MA, Campbell ED. A model for easy location of the center of the femoral head during total knee arthroplasty. *J Arthroplasty.* 1988;3(suppl.):S59.
42. Siegel JL, Shall LM. Femoral instrumentation using the antero-superior iliac spine as a landmark in total knee arthroplasty. *J Arthroplasty.* 1991;6:317.

43. Tillett ED, Engh GA, Petersen T. A comparative study of extra-medullary and intramedullary alignment systems in total knee arthroplasty. *Clin Orthop Relat Res.* 1988;230:176.
44. Laskin RS, Turtel A. The use of an intramedullary tibial alignment guide in total knee replacement. *Am J Knee Surg.* 1989;2:123.
45. Simmons ED Jr, Sullivan JA, Rackemann S, et al. The accuracy of tibial intramedullary alignment devices in total knee arthroplasty. *J Arthroplasty.* 1991;6:45.
46. Fahmy NR, Chandler HP, Danylchuk K, et al. Blood-gas and circulatory changes during total knee replacement. Role of the intramedullary alignment rod. *J Bone Joint Surg Am.* 1990;72:19-26.
47. Gleitz M, Hopf T, Hess T. Experimental studies on the role of intramedullary alignment rods in the etiology of fat embolisms in knee endoprosthesis. *Z Orthop Ihre Grenzgeb* 1996;134:254-259.
48. Bellemans J, Colyn W, Vandenneucker H, Victor J. The Chitranjan Ranawat Award: is neutral mechanical alignment normal for all patients? The concept of constitutional varus. *Clin Orthop Relat Res.* 2012;470(1):45-53.
49. Dossett HG, Estrada NA, Swartz GJ, Lefevre GW, Kwasman BG. A randomised controlled trial of kinematically and mechanically aligned total knee replacements: two-year clinical results. *Bone Joint J.* 2014;96-B(7):907-913.
50. Dossett HG, Swartz GJ, Estrada NA, Lefevre GW, Kwasman BG. Kinematically versus mechanically aligned total knee arthroplasty. *Orthopedics.* 2012;35(2):e160-9.
51. Howell SM, Papadopoulos S, Kuznik KT, Hull ML. Accurate alignment and high function after kinematically aligned TKA performed with generic instruments. *Knee Surg Sports Traumatol Arthrosc.* 2013;21(10):2271-2280.
52. Young SW, Walker ML, Bayan A, Briant-evans T, Pavlou P, Farrington B. The Chitranjan S. Ranawat Award. No difference in 2-year functional outcomes using kinematic versus mechanical alignment in TKA: a randomized controlled clinical trial. *Clin Orthop Relat Res.* 2017;475(1):9-20.
53. Howell SM, Papadopoulos S, Kuznik K, Ghaly LR, Hull ML. Does varus alignment adversely affect implant survival and function six years after kinematically aligned total knee arthroplasty? *Int Orthop.* 2015;39(11):2117-2124.
54. Berger RA, Crossett LS, Jacobs JJ, Rubash HE. Malrotation causing patellofemoral complications after total knee arthroplasty. *Clin Orthop Relat Res.* 1998;356:144-153.
55. Howell SM, Howell SJ, Kuznik KT, Cohen J, Hull ML. Does a kinematically aligned total knee arthroplasty restore function without failure regardless of alignment category? *Clin Orthop Relat Res.* 2013;471(3):1000-1007.
56. Howell SM, Hull ML. Kinematically aligned TKA with MRI-based cutting guides. *Improving Accuracy in Knee Arthroplasty.* 1st ed. Jaypee Brothers Medical Publishing; 2012.
57. Nunley RM, Ellison BS, Ruh EL, et al. Are patient-specific cutting blocks cost-effective for total knee arthroplasty? *Clin Orthop Relat Res.* 2012;470(3):889-894.
58. Sassoon A, Nam D, Nunley R, Barrack R. Systematic review of patient-specific instrumentation in total knee arthroplasty: new but not improved. *Clin Orthop Relat Res.* 2015;473(1):151-158.
59. Anouchi YS, Whiteside LA, Kaiser AD. The effects of axial rotational alignment of the femoral component on instability and patellar tracking in total knee arthroplasty demonstrated on autopsy specimens. *Clin Orthop Relat Res.* 1993;287:170.
60. Rhoads DD, Noble PC, Reuben JD, et al. The effect of femoral component position on patellar tracking after total knee arthroplasty. *Clin Orthop Relat Res.* 1990;260:43.
61. Stiehl JB, Abbott BD. Morphology of the transepicondylar axis and its application in primary and revision total knee arthroplasty. *J Arthroplasty.* 1995;10:785-789.
62. Arima J, Whiteside LA, McCarthy DS, et al. Femoral rotational alignment, based on the anteroposterior axis in total knee arthroplasty in a valgus knee: a technical note. *J Bone Joint Surg Am.* 1995;77:1331-1334.
63. Whiteside LA, Arima J. The anteroposterior axis for femoral rotational alignment in valgus total knee arthroplasty. *Clin Orthop Relat Res.* 1995;321:168.
64. Poilvache PL, Insall JN, Scuderi GR, et al. Rotational landmarks and sizing of the distal femur in total knee arthroplasty. *Clin Orthop Relat Res.* 1996;331:35-46.
65. Berger RA, Rubash HE, Seel MJ, et al. Determining the rotational alignment of the femoral component in total knee arthroplasty using the epicondylar axis. *Clin Orthop Relat Res.* 1993;286:40-47.
66. Griffin FM, Insall NJ, Scuderi GR. The posterior condylar angle in osteoarthritis knees. *J Arthroplasty.* 1988;13:812.
67. Stiehl JB, Cherveny PM. Femoral rotational alignment using the tibial shaft axis in total knee arthroplasty. *Clin Orthop Relat Res.* 1996;331:47.
68. Olcott CW, Scott RD. A comparison of 4 intraoperative methods to determine femoral component rotation during total knee arthroplasty. *J Arthroplasty.* 2000;15:22-26.
69. Akagi M, Yamashita E, Nakagawa T, et al. Relationship between frontal knee alignment and reference axes in the distal femur. *Clin Orthop Relat Res.* 2001;388:147-156.
70. Katz MA, Beck TD, Silber JS, et al. Determining femoral rotational alignment in total knee arthroplasty: reliability of techniques. *J Arthroplasty.* 2001;16:301.
71. Berger RA, Crossett LS, Jacobs JJ, et al. Malrotation causing patellofemoral complications after total knee arthroplasty. *Clin Orthop Relat Res.* 1998;356:144.
72. Feczko PZ, Pijls BG, Van steijn MJ, Van rhijn LW, Arts JJ, Emans PJ. Tibial component rotation in total knee arthroplasty. *BMC Musculoskelet Disord.* 2016;17:87.
73. Merkow RL, Soudry M, Insall JN. Patellar dislocation following total knee replacement. *J Bone Joint Surg Am.* 1985;67:1321-1327.
74. Moreland JR. Mechanisms of failure in total knee arthroplasty. *Clin Orthop Relat Res.* 1988;226:49-64.
75. Yoshioka Y, Siu DW, Scudamore RA, Cooke TD. Tibial anatomy and functional axes. *J Orthop Res.* 1989;7:132-137.
76. Akagi M, Oh M, Nonaka T, Tsujimoto H, Asano T, Hamanishi C. An anteroposterior axis of the tibia for total knee arthroplasty. *Clin Orthop Relat Res.* 2004;420:213-219.
77. Akagi M, Mori S, Nishimura S, Nishimura A, Asano T, Hamanishi C. Variability of extraarticular tibial rotation references for total knee arthroplasty. *Clin Orthop Relat Res.* 2005;436:172-176.
78. Ikeuchi M, Yamanaka N, Okanoue Y, Ueta E, Tani T. Determining the rotational alignment of the tibial component at total knee replacement: a comparison of two techniques. *J Bone Joint Surg Br.* 2007;89(1):45-49.
79. Nicoll D, Rowley DI. Internal rotational error of the tibial component is a major cause of pain after total knee replacement. *J Bone Joint Surg Br.* 2010;92(9):1238-1244.
80. Barrack RL, Schrader T, Bertot AJ, Wolfe MW, Myers L. Component rotation and anterior knee pain after total knee arthroplasty. *Clin Orthop Relat Res.* 2001;392:46-55.
81. Bédard M, Vince KG, Redfern J, Collen SR. Internal rotation of the tibial component is frequent in stiff total knee arthroplasty. *Clin Orthop Relat Res.* 2011;469(8):2346-2355.
82. Gromov K, Korchi M, Thomsen MG, Husted H, Troelsen A. What is the optimal alignment of the tibial and femoral components in knee arthroplasty? *Acta Orthop.* 2014;85(5):480-487.
83. Steindler A. *Kinesiology of the Human Body Under Normal and Pathological Conditions.* Springfield, IL: Charles C Thomas; 1964.
84. Haxton H. The function of the patella and the effects of its excision. *Surg Gynecol Obstet.* 1945;80:389-395.
85. Schindler OS. Patellar resurfacing in total knee arthroplasty. In: Scott W, Diduch DR, Iorio R, eds. *Insall & Scott Surgery of the Knee.* 6th ed. Elsevier Inc; 2018:1585-1629.
86. D'Lima D, Chen PC, Kester MA, et al. Impact on patellofemoral design on patellofemoral forces and polyethylene stresses. *J Bone Joint Surg Am.* 2003;85:85-93.

87. Hofmann AA, Tkach TK, Evanich CJ, et al. Patellar component medialization in total knee arthroplasty. *J Arthroplasty.* 1997;12:155-160.

88. Lewonowski K, Dorr LD, McPherson EJ, et al. Medialization of the patella in total knee arthroplasty. *J Arthroplasty.* 1997;12:161-167.

89. Anglin C, Brimacombe JM, Wilson DR, et al. Biomechanical consequences of patellar component medialization in total knee arthroplasty. *J Arthoplasty.*2010;25:793-802.

90. Doerr TE, Eckhoff DG. Lateral patellar burnishing in total knee arthroplasty following medialization of the patellar button. *J Arthroplasty.* 1995;10:540-542.

91. Lonner JH. Lateral patellar chamfer in total knee arthroplasty. *Am J Orthop.* 2001;30:713-714.

92. Shiers LG. Arthroplasty of the knee; preliminary report of new method. *J Bone Joint Surg Br.* 1954;36-B(4):553-560.

93. Bala A, Penrose CT, Seyler TM, Mather RC, Wellman SS, Bolognesi MP. Computer-navigated total knee arthroplasty utilization. *J Knee Surg.* 2016;29(5):430-435.

94. Matziolis G, Krocker D, Weiss U, Tohtz S, Perka C. A prospective, randomized study of computer-assisted and conventional total knee arthroplasty. Three-dimensional evaluation of implant alignment and rotation. *J Bone Joint Surg Am.* 2007;89(2):236-243.

95. Mizu-uchi H, Matsuda S, Miura H, Okazaki K, Akasaki Y, Iwamoto Y. The evaluation of post-operative alignment in total knee replacement using a CT-based navigation system. *J Bone Joint Surg Br.* 2008;90(8):1025-1031.

96. Perlick L, Bäthis H, Tingart M, Perlick C, Grifka J. Navigation in total-knee arthroplasty: CT-based implantation compared with the conventional technique. *Acta Orthop Scand.* 2004;75(4):464-470.

97. Chauhan SK, Scott RG, Breidahl W, Beaver RJ. Computer-assisted knee arthroplasty versus a conventional jig-based technique. A randomised, prospective trial. *J Bone Joint Surg Br.* 2004;86(3):372-377.

98. Kalairajah Y, Simpson D, Cossey AJ, Verrall GM, Spriggins AJ. Blood loss after total knee replacement: effects of computer-assisted surgery. *J Bone Joint Surg Br.* 2005;87(11):1480-1482.

99. Church JS, Scadden JE, Gupta RR, Cokis C, Williams KA, Janes GC. Embolic phenomena during computer-assisted and conventional total knee replacement. *J Bone Joint Surg Br.* 2007;89(4):481-485.

100. Kalairajah Y, Cossey AJ, Verrall GM, Ludbrook G, Spriggins AJ. Are systemic emboli reduced in computer-assisted knee surgery? A prospective, randomised, clinical trial. *J Bone Joint Surg Br.* 2006;88(2):198-202.

101. Browne JA, Cook C, Hofmann AA, Bolognesi MP. Postoperative morbidity and mortality following total knee arthroplasty with computer navigation. *Knee.* 2010;17(2):152-156.

102. Seon JK, Song EK. Functional impact of navigation-assisted minimally invasive total knee arthroplasty. *Orthopedics.* 2005;28(10 suppl):s1251-s1254.

103. Hoffart HE, Langenstein E, Vasak N. A prospective study comparing the functional outcome of computer-assisted and conventional total knee replacement. *J Bone Joint Surg Br.* 2012;94(2):194-199.

104. Kim YH, Park JW, Kim JS. Computer-navigated versus conventional total knee arthroplasty a prospective randomized trial. *J Bone Joint Surg Am.* 2012;94(22):2017-2024.

105. Kim YH, Park JW, Kim JS. The clinical outcome of computer-navigated compared with conventional knee arthroplasty in the same patients: a prospective, randomized, double-blind, long-term study. *J Bone Joint Surg Am.* 2017;99(12):989-996.

106. Roberts TD, Clatworthy MG, Frampton CM, Young SW. Does computer assisted navigation improve functional outcomes and implant survivability after total knee arthroplasty? *J Arthroplasty.* 2015;30(9 suppl):59-63.

chapter 33

Patient Specific Instrumentation

Jessica Morton, MD | Ran Schwarzkopf, MD, MSc | Jonathan M. Vigdorchik, MD

BACKGROUND

Patient specific instrumentation (PSI) has undergone several iterations as technology has improved. Initially instruments were manufactured from three-dimensional imaging to accurately place pins for conventional cutting guides and preoperatively template the implant size. This has advanced to modern-day custom-engineered cutting guides through which bony resection can be performed as part of single-use disposable instrument trays. Unlike robotic or computer-navigated surgery, planning is performed preoperatively and no registration of bone position or computer system is necessary in the operating room.

The instruments are templated using three-dimensional imaging, computed tomography (CT) scan, or magnetic resonance imaging (MRI). Initially a three-dimensional model of the patient's anatomy is created; subsequently, using templating software, bone resections are templated and components are sized. Surgeons review and edit the proposed resection and sizing of implants with the company technician. Finally, after surgeon approval using three-dimensional printing and layered resin the custom guides are created and sterilized for use.

The driving forces behind the creation of PSI is to improve accuracy of bone resections, increase reproducibility, reduce blood loss, improve clinical outcomes, decrease operative time, and lower costs by decreasing intraoperative decision making and reducing the number of instrument trays, and turnover time.[1] Studies have demonstrated the reliability, safety, and accuracy of PSI; however, they have failed to show improved patient outcomes and cost-efficiency over conventional TKA instrumentation, and controversy around this topic continues.

ALIGNMENT

Approximately 15% to 25% of patients who undergo primary TKA are not satisfied with their outcome.[2-4] The source of that dissatisfaction remains debated, but deviations in mechanical alignment have been attributed as a potential source of this dissatisfaction.

While not in the scope of this chapter, there remains debate whether mechanical or kinematic alignment is the best method of component positioning.[5] We will briefly discuss both types of alignment as it is important in understanding the radiographic outcomes and proposed uses of PSI.

Kinematic Alignment

Kinematic alignment strives to restore an individual's alignment to its prearthritic state, using the kinematic axes of the knee. Kinematic alignment seeks to restore the native 3D alignment of the knee and three axes of normal knee motion. The specific goals of kinematic alignment are to restore native tibial-femoral articular surfaces, native knee and limb alignment, and native laxities.[5-7] This native alignment can vary significantly between individuals and is proposed as a source of postoperative dissatisfaction after TKA. Using three-dimensional imaging to model conditions prior to onset of arthritis, restore native anatomy, and custom generate cutting guides allows physicians using PSI to recreate a patient's kinematic alignment.

Mechanical Alignment

The mechanical axis of the lower extremity is the line drawn from the center of the femoral head to the center of the talus.[8,9] The mechanical alignment of the femur is about 3° of valgus, and the tibia is generally aligned with the mechanical alignment of the limb.[8] The postoperative restoration of limb mechanical axis within 3° of neutral has been an established predictor of success in TKA.[8,10-13] Implant malalignment has been reported as high as 20% to 40%,[14] and outliers, those greater than 3° from neutral, are at a higher risk of failure. Malalignment exceeding 3° of varus or valgus in the coronal plane increases aseptic loosening of implants, at a rate of 24% compared with a rate of 3% in patients within 3° of neutral mechanical axis. Malalignment can also lead to accelerated polyethylene wear and medial bone collapse.[9]

Establishing a patient's mechanical axis requires long-leg radiographs to accurately measure the hip–knee–ankle (HKA) angle, tibia mechanical axis (TMA), femoral mechanical axis (FMA). Although there are studies that demonstrate correlation between mechanical and anatomic axis, measured on short-leg radiographs, long-leg radiographs are the gold standard[15-17] (**Fig. 33-1**).

Hip–Knee–Ankle Angle

Despite extensive research and several meta-analyses on the topic there is no significant difference in outliers of greater than 3° from neutral mechanical axis in the hip–knee–ankle angle when comparing conventional instrumentation and PSI.[18-22]

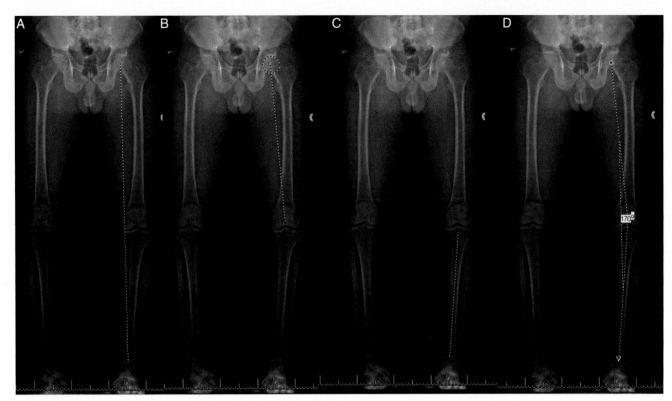

FIGURE 33-1   The mechanical axis **(A)**, femoral mechanical axis (FMA) **(B)**, tibial mechanical axis (TMA) **(C)**, and hip–knee–ankle angle (HKA) **(D)** in a patient undergoing preoperative evaluation. Mechanical axis of the knee is measured from the center of the femoral head to the center of the talus. In this patient the line passes medial to the center of the knee demonstrating a varus deformity **(A)**. FMA is defined as a line from the center of the femoral head to the center of the intercondylar notch **(B)**. TMA is defined as a line from the center of the tibia to the talus **(C)**. The HKA is defined as the angle between the TMA and the FMA **(D)**.

Coronal Alignment

Coronal alignment of the tibial and femoral components is key to component positioning and successful TKA. Multiple studies have reported on tibial component coronal alignment with mixed results. In metanalysis both Thienpont et al and Zhang et al found significantly increased risk of malalignment,[20,22] while Cavaignac et al. fond no significant difference.[18] Femoral component coronal alignment was slightly favored in metanalysis of PSI but infrequently reached statistical significance.[18–22]

Sagittal Alignment

Sagittal alignment remains more difficult to judge and is infrequently evaluated or reported. Flexion of the femoral component greater than 3° or sagittal alignment of the tibial component less than neutral, or tibial slope greater than 7° has been identified as a risk factor for failure.[23] Sagittal instability can occur secondary to this malalignment. While infrequently evaluated in the literature, a meta-analysis by Zhang et al found more tibial slope outliers when using PSI rather than conventional instrumentation[22] and Thienpont et al found a significantly higher probability of malalignment of the tibial component in the sagittal plane with use of PSI,

although neither of these studies reached statistical significance.[20,22] In a multicenter, randomized, clinical trial, Boonen et al reported a significant increase in outliers in the sagittal plane of the femoral component when using custom cutting guides.[24]

TEMPLATING AND PREOPERATIVE PLANNING

Preoperative planning for PSI is system dependent, but generally starts with three-dimensional imaging with or without long-leg radiographs to generate a working model of the knee. A proposed surgical plan with bone resection and implant sizing is provided to the surgeon who makes adjustments and returns the plan to the manufacturer. The cutting guides are then created offsite and sent to the surgeon for intraoperative use. **Figs. 33-2** and **33-3** demonstrate three-dimensional models of the knee with custom printed resection guides.

MANUFACTURER

There are several PSI total knee systems commercially available at this time, each with its accompanying template generation software and prosthetic options. Average lead time needed to generate cutting guides varies from

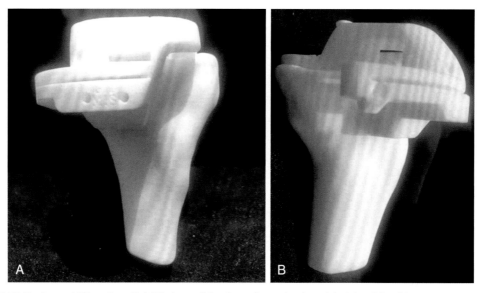

FIGURE 33-2   Coronal **(A)** and sagittal **(B)** views of the three-dimensional model of the tibia with custom cutting guide.

18 to 30 days.[25] **Table 33-1** lists some of the currently available PSI systems, preferred imaging modality, and average lead time in working days.

CT VERSUS MRI

The superior imaging modality for the creation of modeling and cutting guides remains debated. CT is less expensive with shorter imaging time, however does include the risk of increased radiation despite low-dose protocols. Radiation remains equivalent to a standard yearly background radiation dose or approximately 70 chest X-rays.[26] MRI does not utilize ionizing radiation; however, protocols often require the concurrent use of full-leg standing radiographs. MRI is a longer study and in most health systems more expensive. MRI has the advantage of providing additional information regarding soft tissue structures including ligaments and residual cartilage thickness which can influence guide fit and cut thickness.[20]

In animal models White et al found CT-generated bone models were superior to MRI-generated models with increased accuracy and bony landmark resolution.[26,27] However, using a similar sheep model Rathnayaka et al found no significant difference in 3D models generated with CT or MRI.[28] Ensini et al and Pfitzner et al performed randomized controlled trials in human patients demonstrating more outliers in the coronal plane with CT- versus MRI-generated templates.[29,30] Whereas Cenni et al and Schotanus et al found no significant difference between accuracy of MRI- and CT-generated PSI templates.[31,32] A meta-analysis by An et al supports MRI-generated PSI producing a lower proportion of mechanical axis outliers; however, there was no significant difference in the tibial or femoral component alignment in the coronal or sagittal plane.[33]

While superior imaging modality remains highly contested, what has shown to be significant in reducing intraoperative changes and accuracy of resection guides is surgeon review and alteration of the operative plan.

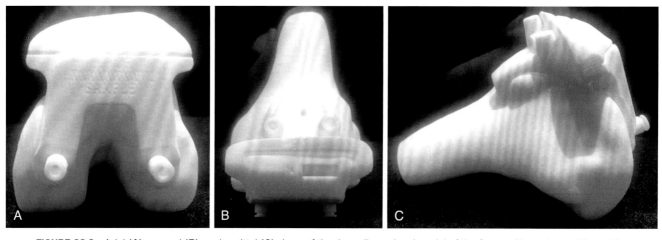

FIGURE 33-3   Axial **(A)**, coronal **(B)**, and sagittal **(C)** views of the three-dimensional model of the femur with custom cutting guide.

Company Name	System	CT vs MRI	Standing Long-Leg X-ray	Average Lead Time in Working Days
Biomet	Signature	CT or MRI	No	20
DuPuy-Synthes	Trumatch	CT	No	30
Medacta	MyKnee	CT or MRI	No	21
Smith and Nephew	Visionaire	MRI	Yes	28
Wright Medical	Prophecy	CT or MRI	Yes	20
Zimmer	PSI	MRI	No	18

TABLE 33-1   Listing of Several Companies, the Product Name of Available Patient Specific Instrumentation, Whether the System Is Based on CT- or MRI-Generated Images, Requirement for Long-Leg Radiographs, and Average Lead Time Necessary to Generate 3D Printed Guides

Surgeon-approved MRI and CT templates correctly predicted femoral size 93.9% of the time and tibial size 91.1%.[32] Surgeon-approved MRI-based templates had 95.5% and 93% accuracy in predicting implant size.[34] Technician templates without physician input were found to be less accurate and resulted in more intraoperative size changes.[32] Surgeon review and alteration of templates is necessary for accurate preoperative planning and prevention of intraoperative adjustments and abandonment.[35]

Intraoperative Adjustments and Abandonment

Surgeon involvement in templating and accurate recent three-dimensional imaging is key to preventing intraoperative adjustment and abandonment of PSI. Furthermore, like all techniques there is a learning curve associated with using PSI and surgeons have reported adjustments for surgeon preference. Stronach et al reported making "frequent intraoperative changes to the alignment and implant sizing" averaging 2.4 changes per knee and abandoned several PSI cases for traditional instruments secondary to poor tibial and femoral cutting guide fit.[36] More recent literature reports decreased to no crossover between PSI and traditional instrumentation and infrequent changes to implant sizing and alignment which may be secondary to better templating and increased guide stability.[24,37] Ultimately final component sizing and alignment is the responsibility of the surgeon and there should remain a low threshold to make adjustments or abandon PSI as necessary for ideal surgical outcomes.

CLINICAL OUTCOMES

At this time there have been no prospective studies demonstrating significantly improved outcomes after TKA with use of PSI over conventional instrumentation. In several studies PSI did not lead to advantages in early recovery at 2 days, 2 months, or 2 years.[38–40]

Abane et al performed a multicenter randomized trial of patients undergoing PSI compared to conventional TKA and found no differences in Oxford knee scores or Knee Society Scores.[38] Pietsch found no difference in Knee Society Score at 2, 6, and 12 weeks and no difference in attained knee flexion or postoperative swelling and pain.[41] Nam et al also found no difference in range of motion, Oxford knee scores, University of California Los Angeles activity score, and short form-12 health status questionnaire physical scores. Zhu et al found no significant differences in clinical outcomes at 6 or 24 months postoperatively.[42] Abdel et al found no significant difference in gait patterns during three-dimensional gait analysis in patients 3 months following knee replacement with PSI or conventional instruments.[39] However, in a meta-analysis by Thienpont et al postoperative Knee Society Scores favored the PSI group by a mean of 1.5 points but did not reach statistical significance ($P = .93$). Functional score also favored PSI with an increase of 4.3 points ($P = .003$) although they qualify these findings as preliminary as the majority of the studies in the meta-analysis could not be included in the evaluation.[20] At this time the literature does not support improved clinical outcomes with the use of PSI.

PERIOPERATIVE BLOOD LOSS

Intramedullary instrumentation is thought to be a source of significant perioperative and postoperative blood loss in TKA. By avoiding violation of the intramedullary canal and decreased surgical time, proponents of PSI believe it may reduce blood loss.[43] However, clinical studies have not consistently supported this claim.

Pietsch et al found a difference in intraoperative blood loss in TKA performed when a tourniquet was used only during cementing, but no significant difference in hemoglobin decrease or transfusion requirements postoperatively.[41] Boonen et al found intraoperative blood loss to be 100 mL less in the PSI group as compared to conventional TKA but again no significant difference in transfusion or hemoglobin decrease postoperatively.[24] Rathod et al found a trend toward decreased hemoglobin drop and lower transfusion rate but did not reach statistical significance.[44] Thienpont et al among others found no statistically significant difference in calculated blood loss, hemoglobin or hematocrit drop, or postoperative transfusion rate between PSI and conventional TKA.[37,38,43,45,46] In a meta-analysis Voleti et al also found no significant difference in intraoperative blood loss.[21]

Current data are unable to support significant differences in intraoperative or postoperative blood loss despite lack of violation of the medullary canal and slightly decreased operative times.

ECONOMIC EVALUATION

Operative Time

Patient specific guides, presurgical templating, and component sizing are proposed to decrease the number of intraoperative decisions surgeons need to do and therefore decrease operative time. Decreased trays and less time spent opening and organizing trays can also contribute to decreased case time and turnover time. Multiple studies have found slightly decreased surgical time when comparing PSI to conventional instrumentation.[24,37,45–47] Nunley et al found similar tourniquet time but decreased total in room time.[48] However, Hamilton et al and Voleti et al found that PSI cases do not decrease operative time compared to conventional TKA.[21,49] A recent meta-analysis by Thienpont et al of 3480 knees found decreased mean total operative time of 4.4 minutes ($P = .0002$) with no significant difference found in mean tourniquet time. Despite the trend toward decreased operative time with PSI, savings of several minutes in each case does not translate to an increase in the amount of cases an OR can perform in a day, and often does not translate to minute per minute savings of operative time as staff often remains in the OR during those minutes.

Cost Considerations

With decreased operative time, less instruments, and single-use trays, it is conceivable that PSI could offer institutional cost benefits. However, in the era of bundled payments these operative efficiency savings must be balanced against the cost of custom guides and three-dimensional imaging.

A significant decrease in the number of trays has been consistently reported in the literature. Ng et al reported a reduction in the number of trays from ten to five (50%), Watters et al reduced trays from six to one (83%), and Tibesku et al reported a reduction from six trays to two trays (67%), and a significant difference in OR turnaround time saving 20 minutes per case, and decreasing the number of surgical trays also decreases processing cost.[50-52] Barrack et al found time savings of 90 minutes for sterile processing and total cost savings of $30.96 per tray.[45] These time and cost savings may not be translatable to all hospital or surgical center systems.

In a prospective trial Renson et al found that PSI did significantly reduce the surgical time, OR time, and number of surgical trays required (55%).[53] However, decreasing operative trays and operative time may not decrease the overall cost to the healthcare system with three-dimensional imaging and cost of custom guide generation. Barrack et al found a net increase in cost of approximately $1775 per case due to the cost of preoperative imaging and the cost of the custom cutting guides[45]; this finding was coupled with no superiority of coronal alignment with PSI leading them to conclude PSI is of unproven value.

FUTURE DIRECTIONS

At this time data demonstrate alignment of components to the HKA axis is not superior when using PSI as compared to conventional instruments, nor does it provide superior clinical outcomes in the immediate to 2-year time frame. As briefly mentioned in kinematically aligned knees, three-dimensional modeling and individual anatomy play a larger role and custom guides may prove beneficial to surgeons attempting to provide kinematic alignment. At this time mid-term data of 5 year follow-up in 163 patients were recently published by Schoctanus et al demonstrating no significant clinical differences at mean of 5-year follow up. There were slightly increased revisions in the conventional group (one in the PSI group, three in the conventional group) which did not meet statistical significance.[54] Currently there are no studies with long-term data regarding PSI versus conventional TKA; however, further follow-up studies may show differences in long-term results.

From a financial standpoint implant cost and three-dimensional imaging may make PSI unfavorable in some healthcare settings. However, the application of PSI in a low-volume setting where instrumentation is not kept in house, or hospitals/surgery centers with decreased sterile processing on site where surgeons may be able to perform additional cases with PSI due to reduced number of trays and increased operative efficiency may prove to be financially beneficial. In the end total cost to the healthcare system is what must be assessed and balanced with long-term patient outcomes to determine if PSI is advantageous.

REFERENCES

1. Lee G-C. Patient-specific cutting blocks. *Bone Joint J.* 2016;98-B: 78-80. Available at http://www.ncbi.nlm.nih.gov/pubmed/26733647. Accessed December 27, 2018.
2. Baker PN, van der Meulen JH, Lewsey J, Gregg PJ. The role of pain and function in determining patient satisfaction after total knee replacement. Data from the National Joint Registry for England and Wales. *J Bone Joint Surg Br.* 2007;89:893-900. Available at http://online.boneandjoint.org.uk/doi/10.1302/0301-620X.89B7.19091. Accessed December 28, 2018.
3. Bourne RB, Chesworth BM, Davis AM, Mahomed NN, Charron KDJ. Patient satisfaction after total knee arthroplasty: who is satisfied and who is not? *Clin Orthop Relat Res.* 2010;468:57-63. Available at http://link.springer.com/10.1007/s11999-009-1119-9. Accessed December 28, 2018.

4. Choi Y-J, Ra HJ. Patient satisfaction after total knee arthroplasty. *Knee Surg Relat Res.* 2016;28:1-15. Available at http://www.ncbi.nlm.nih.gov/pubmed/26955608. Accessed December 28, 2018.

5. Dossett HG, Swartz GJ, Estrada NA, LeFevre GW, Kwasman BG. Kinematically versus mechanically aligned total knee arthroplasty. *Orthopedics.* 2012;35:e160-e169. Available at http://www.ncbi.nlm.nih.gov/pubmed/22310400. Accessed December 28, 2018.

6. Howell SM, Hodapp EE, Vernace JV, Hull ML, Meade TD. Are undesirable contact kinematics minimized after kinematically aligned total knee arthroplasty? An intersurgeon analysis of consecutive patients. *Knee Surg Sports Traumatol Arthrosc.* 2013;21:2281-2287. Available at http://link.springer.com/10.1007/s00167-012-2220-2. Accessed January 2, 2019.

7. Howell SM, Hull ML, Mahfouz MR. Kinematically aligned total knee arthroplasty. In: Scott WN, ed. *Insall & Scott Surgery of the Knee.* Philadelphia, PA: Elsevier; 2018:1784-1796.

8. Abdel MP, Oussedik S, Parratte S, Lustig S, Haddad FS. Coronal alignment in total knee replacement. *Bone Joint J.* 2014;96-B:857-862. Available at http://online.boneandjoint.org.uk/doi/10.1302/0301-620X.96B7.33946. Accessed November 20, 2018.

9. Jeffery RS, Morris RW, Denham RA. Coronal alignment after total knee replacement. *J Bone Joint Surg Br.* 1991;73:709-714. Available at http://www.ncbi.nlm.nih.gov/pubmed/1894655. Accessed December 28, 2018.

10. D'Lima DD, Chen PC, Colwell CW. Polyethylene contact stresses, articular congruity, and knee alignment. *Clin Orthop Relat Res.* 2001;(392):232-238. Available at http://www.ncbi.nlm.nih.gov/pubmed/11716388. Accessed January 6, 2019.

11. D'Lima DD, Hermida JC, Chen PC, Colwell CW. Polyethylene wear and variations in knee kinematics. *Clin Orthop Relat Res.* 2001;(392):124-130. Available at http://www.ncbi.nlm.nih.gov/pubmed/11716373. Accessed January 6, 2019.

12. Green GV, Berend KR, Berend ME, Glisson RR, Vail TP. The effects of varus tibial alignment on proximal tibial surface strain in total knee arthroplasty: the posteromedial hot spot. *J Arthroplasty.* 2002;17:1033-1039. Available at http://linkinghub.elsevier.com/retrieve/pii/S0883540302002607. Accessed January 6, 2019.

13. Werner FW, Ayers DC, Maletsky LP, Rullkoetter PJ. The effect of valgus/varus malalignment on load distribution in total knee replacements. *J Biomech.* 2005;38:349-355. Available at http://linkinghub.elsevier.com/retrieve/pii/S0021929004000958. Accessed January 6, 2019.

14. Hetaimish BM, Khan MM, Simunovic N, Al-Harbi HH, Bhandari M, Zalzal PK. Meta-analysis of navigation vs conventional total knee arthroplasty. *J Arthroplasty.* 2012;27:1177-1182. Available at https://linkinghub.elsevier.com/retrieve/pii/S088354031100708X. Accessed January 2, 2019.

15. Colebatch AN, Hart DJ, Zhai G, Williams FM, Spector TD, Arden NK. Effective measurement of knee alignment using AP knee radiographs. *Knee.* 2009;16:42-45. Available at https://linkinghub.elsevier.com/retrieve/pii/S0968016008001269. Accessed January 2, 2019.

16. Lombardi AV, Berend KR, Ng VY. Neutral mechanical alignment: a requirement for successful TKA: affirms. *Orthopedics.* 2011;34(9):e504-e506. Available at http://www.slackinc.com/doi/resolver.asp?doi=10.3928/01477447-20110714-40. Accessed January 2, 2019.

17. Moreland JR, Bassett LW, Hanker GJ. Radiographic analysis of the axial alignment of the lower extremity. *J Bone Joint Surg Am.* 1987;69:745-749. Available at http://www.ncbi.nlm.nih.gov/pubmed/3597474. Accessed January 2, 2019.

18. Cavaignac E, Pailhé R, Laumond G, et al. Evaluation of the accuracy of patient-specific cutting blocks for total knee arthroplasty: a meta-analysis. *Int Orthop.* 2015;39:1541-1552. Available at http://link.springer.com/10.1007/s00264-014-2549-x. Accessed November 20, 2018.

19. Jiang J, Kang X, Lin Q, et al. Accuracy of patient-specific instrumentation compared with conventional instrumentation in total knee arthroplasty. *Orthopedics.* 2015;38:e305-e313. Available at http://www.healio.com/doiresolver?doi=10.3928/01477447-20150402-59. Accessed November 20, 2018.

20. Thienpont E, Schwab P-E, Fennema P. Efficacy of patient-specific instruments in total knee arthroplasty. *J Bone Joint Surg.* 2017;99:521-530. Available at http://www.ncbi.nlm.nih.gov/pubmed/28291186. Accessed November 20, 2018.

21. Voleti PB, Hamula MJ, Baldwin KD, Lee G-C. Current data do not support routine use of patient-specific instrumentation in total knee arthroplasty. *J Arthroplasty.* 2014;29:1709-1712. Available at http://www.ncbi.nlm.nih.gov/pubmed/24961893. Accessed January 5, 2019.

22. Zhang Q, Chen J, Li H, et al. No evidence of superiority in reducing outliers of component alignment for patient-specific instrumentation for total knee arthroplasty: a systematic review. *Orthop Surg.* 2015;7:19-25. Available at http://doi.wiley.com/10.1111/os.12150. Accessed January 2, 2019.

23. Kim Y-H, Park J-W, Kim J-S, Park S-D. The relationship between the survival of total knee arthroplasty and postoperative coronal, sagittal and rotational alignment of knee prosthesis. *Int Orthop.* 2014;38:379-385. Available at http://link.springer.com/10.1007/s00264-013-2097-9. Accessed January 2, 2019.

24. Boonen B, Schotanus MGM, Kerens B, van der Weegen W, van Drumpt RAM, Kort NP. Intra-operative results and radiological outcome of conventional and patient-specific surgery in total knee arthroplasty: a multicentre, randomised controlled trial. *Knee Surg Sports Traumatol Arthrosc.* 2013;21:2206-2212. Available at http://link.springer.com/10.1007/s00167-013-2620-y. Accessed November 20, 2018.

25. Thienpont E, Bellemans J, Delport H, et al. Patient-specific instruments: industry's innovation with a surgeon's interest. *Knee Surg Sports Traumatol Arthrosc.* 2013;21:2227-2233. Available at http://link.springer.com/10.1007/s00167-013-2626-5. Accessed January 5, 2019.

26. Stirling P, Valsalan Mannambeth R, Soler A, Batta V, Malhotra RK, Kalairajah Y. Computerised tomography vs magnetic resonance imaging for modeling of patient-specific instrumentation in total knee arthroplasty. *World J Orthop.* 2015;6:290-297. Available at http://www.wjgnet.com/2218-5836/full/v6/i2/290.htm. Accessed January 6, 2019.

27. White D, Chelule KL, Seedhom BB. Accuracy of MRI vs CT imaging with particular reference to patient specific templates for total knee replacement surgery. *Int J Med Robot.* 2008;4:224-231. Available at http://doi.wiley.com/10.1002/rcs.201. Accessed January 2, 2019.

28. Rathnayaka K, Momot KI, Noser H, et al. Quantification of the accuracy of MRI generated 3D models of long bones compared to CT generated 3D models. *Med Eng Phys.* 2012;34:357-363. Available at https://linkinghub.elsevier.com/retrieve/pii/S1350453311001925. Accessed January 6, 2019.

29. Ensini A, Timoncini A, Cenni F, et al. Intra- and post-operative accuracy assessments of two different patient-specific instrumentation systems for total knee replacement. *Knee Surg Sports Traumatol Arthrosc.* 2014;22:621-629. Available at http://link.springer.com/10.1007/s00167-013-2667-9. Accessed January 6, 2019.

30. Pfitzner T, Abdel MP, von Roth P, Perka C, Hommel H. Small improvements in mechanical axis alignment achieved with MRI versus CT-based patient-specific instruments in TKA: a randomized clinical trial. *Clin Orthop Relat Res.* 2014;472:2913-2922. Available at http://www.ncbi.nlm.nih.gov/pubmed/25024031. Accessed January 6, 2019.

31. Cenni F, Timoncini A, Ensini A, et al. Three-dimensional implant position and orientation after total knee replacement performed with patient-specific instrumentation systems. *J Orthop Res.* 2014;32:331-337. Available at http://doi.wiley.com/10.1002/jor.22513. Accessed January 6, 2019.

32. Schotanus MGM, Schoenmakers DAL, Sollie R, Kort NP. Patient-specific instruments for total knee arthroplasty can accurately predict the component size as used peroperative. *Knee Surg Sports Traumatol Arthrosc.* 2017;25:3844-3848. Available at http://link.springer.com/10.1007/s00167-016-4345-1. Accessed January 2, 2019.

33. An VVG, Sivakumar BS, Phan K, Levy YD, Bruce WJM. Accuracy of MRI-based vs. CT-based patient-specific instrumentation in total knee arthroplasty: a meta-analysis. *J Orthop Sci.* 2017;22:116-120. Available at http://www.ncbi.nlm.nih.gov/pubmed/27823847. Accessed January 3, 2019.

34. Issa K, Rifai A, McGrath M, et al. Reliability of templating with patient-specific instrumentation in total knee arthroplasty. *J Knee Surg.* 2013;26:429-434. Available at http://www.thieme-connect.de/DOI/DOI?10.1055/s-0033-1343615. Accessed January 2, 2019.

35. Pietsch M, Djahani O, Hochegger M, Plattner F, Hofmann S. Patient-specific total knee arthroplasty: the importance of planning by the surgeon. *Knee Surg Sports Traumatol Arthrosc.* 2013;21:2220-2226. Available at http://link.springer.com/10.1007/s00167-013-2624-7. Accessed January 2, 2019.

36. Stronach BM, Pelt CE, Erickson J, Peters CL. Patient-specific total knee arthroplasty required frequent surgeon-directed changes. *Clin Orthop Relat Res.* 2013;471:169-174. Available at http://link.springer.com/10.1007/s11999-012-2573-3. Accessed January 3, 2019.

37. Ferrara F, Cipriani A, Magarelli N, et al. Implant positioning in TKA: comparison between conventional and patient-specific instrumentation. *Orthopedics.* 2015;38:e271-e280. Available at http://www.healio.com/doiresolver?doi=10.3928/01477447-20150402-54. Accessed January 6, 2019.

38. Abane L, Anract P, Boisgard S, Descamps S, Courpied JP, Hamadouche M. A comparison of patient-specific and conventional instrumentation for total knee arthroplasty. *Bone Joint J.* 2015;97-B:56-63. Available at http://online.boneandjoint.org.uk/doi/10.1302/0301-620X.97B1.34440. Accessed November 20, 2018.

39. Abdel MP, Parratte S, Blanc G, et al. No benefit of patient-specific instrumentation in TKA on functional and gait outcomes: a randomized clinical trial. *Clin Orthop Relat Res.* 2014;472:2468-2476. Available at http://link.springer.com/10.1007/s11999-014-3544-7. Accessed January 7, 2019.

40. Nam D, Park A, Stambough JB, Johnson SR, Nunley RM, Barrack RL. The Mark Coventry Award: custom cutting guides do not improve total knee arthroplasty clinical outcomes at 2 years followup. *Clin Orthop Relat Res.* 2016;474:40-46. Available at http://link.springer.com/10.1007/s11999-015-4216-y. Accessed January 7, 2019.

41. Pietsch M, Djahani O, Zweiger C, et al. Custom-fit minimally invasive total knee arthroplasty: effect on blood loss and early clinical outcomes. *Knee Surg Sports Traumatol Arthrosc.* 2013;21:2234-2240. Available at http://link.springer.com/10.1007/s00167-012-2284-z. Accessed January 6, 2019.

42. Zhu M, Chen JY, Chong HC, et al. Outcomes following total knee arthroplasty with CT-based patient-specific instrumentation. *Knee Surg Sports Traumatol Arthrosc.* 2017;25:2567-2572. Available at http://www.ncbi.nlm.nih.gov/pubmed/26410097. Accessed January 5, 2019.

43. Thienpont E, Grosu I, Paternostre F, Schwab P-E, Yombi JC. The use of patient-specific instruments does not reduce blood loss during minimally invasive total knee arthroplasty? *Knee Surg Sports Traumatol Arthrosc.* 2015;23:2055-2060. Available at http://link.springer.com/10.1007/s00167-014-2952-2. Accessed January 5, 2019.

44. Rathod PA, Deshmukh AJ, Cushner FD. Reducing blood loss in bilateral total knee arthroplasty with patient-specific instrumentation. *Orthop Clin North Am.* 2015;46:343-350, ix. Available at https://linkinghub.elsevier.com/retrieve/pii/S0030589815000309. Accessed January 6, 2019.

45. Barrack RL, Ruh EL, Williams BM, Ford AD, Foreman K, Nunley RM. Patient specific cutting blocks are currently of no proven value. *J Bone Joint Surg Br.* 2012;94-B:95-99. Available at http://www.ncbi.nlm.nih.gov/pubmed/23118393. Accessed December 27, 2018.

46. Chareancholvanich K, Narkbunnam R, Pornrattanamaneewong C. A prospective randomised controlled study of patient-specific cutting guides compared with conventional instrumentation in total knee replacement. *Bone Joint J.* 2013;95-B:354-359. Available at http://online.boneandjoint.org.uk/doi/10.1302/0301-620X.95B3.29903. Accessed November 20, 2018.

47. Bali K, Walker P, Bruce W. Custom-fit total knee arthroplasty: our initial experience in 32 knees. *J Arthroplasty.* 2012;27:1149-1154. Available at https://linkinghub.elsevier.com/retrieve/pii/S088354031100684X. Accessed January 5, 2019.

48. Nunley RM, Ellison BS, Ruh EL, et al. Are patient-specific cutting blocks cost-effective for total knee arthroplasty? *Clin Orthop Relat Res.* 2012;470:889-894. Available at http://link.springer.com/10.1007/s11999-011-2221-3. Accessed January 5, 2019.

49. Hamilton WG, Parks NL, Saxena A. Patient-specific instrumentation does not shorten surgical time: a prospective, randomized trial. *J Arthroplasty.* 2013;28:96-100. Available at https://linkinghub.elsevier.com/retrieve/pii/S0883540313004804. Accessed November 20, 2018.

50. Ng VY, DeClaire JH, Berend KR, Gulick BC, Lombardi AV. Improved accuracy of alignment with patient-specific positioning guides compared with manual instrumentation in TKA. *Clin Orthop Relat Res.* 2012;470:99-107. Available at http://link.springer.com/10.1007/s11999-011-1996-6. Accessed January 2, 2019.

51. Tibesku CO, Hofer P, Portegies W, Ruys CJM, Fennema P. Benefits of using customized instrumentation in total knee arthroplasty: results from an activity-based costing model. *Arch Orthop Trauma Surg.* 2013;133:405-411. Available at http://link.springer.com/10.1007/s00402-012-1667-4. Accessed January 7, 2019.

52. Watters TS, Mather RC, Browne JA, Berend KR, Lombardi AV, Bolognesi MP. Analysis of procedure-related costs and proposed benefits of using patient-specific approach in total knee arthroplasty. *J Surg Orthop Adv.* 2011;20:112-116. Available at http://www.ncbi.nlm.nih.gov/pubmed/21838072. Accessed January 7, 2019.

53. Renson L, Poilvache P, Van den Wyngaert H. Improved alignment and operating room efficiency with patient-specific instrumentation for TKA. *Knee.* 2014;21:1216-1220. Available at https://linkinghub.elsevier.com/retrieve/pii/S0968016014002270. Accessed January 7, 2019.

54. Schotanus MGM, Boonen B, van der Weegen W, et al. No difference in mid-term survival and clinical outcome between patient-specific and conventional instrumented total knee arthroplasty: a randomized controlled trial. *Knee Surg Sports Traumatol Arthrosc.* 2018;27(5):1463-1468. Available at http://www.ncbi.nlm.nih.gov/pubmed/29725747. Accessed January 17, 2019.

chapter 34

Computer Guidance

Hiba K. Anis, MD | Nipun Sodhi, MD | Joseph O. Ehiorobo, MD | Michael A. Mont, MD

INTRODUCTION

For the modern total knee arthroplasty (TKA), some of the common mechanisms of failure are malalignment and instability.[1,2] Poor positioning and malalignment often lead to prosthetic loosening and subsequent revision procedures, which in themselves are associated with higher risks for poorer outcomes. Computer guidance in arthroplasty was developed in the 1990s as a strategy to improve implant alignment and therefore improve long-term implant survivorship. Following several years of research, the first computer-navigated TKA was performed in 1997 by Saragaglia in France.[3] Computer guidance has since been used worldwide for TKA as well as for unicompartmental knee arthroplasty (UKA) and conversions to TKA.[4]

Computer assistance in knee arthroplasty can be classified as passive, semi-active, or active.[5-7] Computer navigation is a passive system in which intraoperative measurements are made by the system to guide implant positioning; however, the surgeon is in complete control of executing the surgical plan. In semi-active systems, although surgeons maintain control of the surgical tools, bone resections are restricted to within a three-dimensional (3D) space determined by the computer software. Active computer-assisted systems plan and execute surgical tasks without intervention of the surgeon. Although they are one of the earliest systems developed, there are no active systems currently approved by the Food and Drug Administration (FDA).

Comparisons between computer-assisted techniques and conventional instrumentation in knee arthroplasty have been well-documented at several institutions since the adoption of this new technology. Many historical and contemporary studies have reported the negative consequences of improper alignment on patient outcomes and implant longevity.[8-10] Computer-assisted arthroplasty aims to minimize the effects of surgeon-dependent variability on implant alignment by providing real-time surgical feedback to increase the precision of bone resections and implant positioning. Compared to conventional surgical techniques, computer-assisted TKAs have been shown to increase the accuracy of limb alignment to within 3° of neutral.[11-19] In an early prospective study comparing the two methods, Bäthis et al[16] found that neutral alignment was achieved in 78% of TKAs performed with conventional technique versus 96% with computer assistance.

Although computer-assisted surgeries currently account for a small percentage of knee arthroplasty procedures, there have been great advances in this field in a relatively short period of time. Given the rapid pace of technological evolution and the growing evidence of promising results, computer guidance has the potential to become a mainstay for knee arthroplasty. Therefore, it is important for orthopedic surgeons to understand the concepts underlying computer-assisted surgery and to assess its applicability to their practices. In this chapter, we will discuss the features of different types of computer guidance available for knee arthroplasty and will review the current literature on outcomes.

COMPUTER NAVIGATION SYSTEMS

While there are several available surgical applications, certain components are common to all computer-navigated TKA systems: computer platforms, tracking systems, and registration.[6,20] A computer platform interprets acquired data from the surgical field and integrates it with implant data and medical images. The resultant information is displayed in real time as a 3D image on a monitor for continuous monitoring throughout the procedure. Tracked instruments are placed either on patients' bones or on cutting block adaptors and are detected by a tracking system. Registration of these tracked instruments by the surgeon onto the computer system allows him/her to navigate the 3D anatomical model.

Computer navigation can be broadly categorized into image-based systems or imageless systems. With image-based navigation, preoperative computed tomography (CT) or intraoperative fluoroscopy can be used to reconstruct the 3D image of the surgical field for intraoperative referencing. Imageless computer-assisted surgery is currently the most widely used modality[5,6] and may involve optical or accelerometer-based navigation systems.

IMAGE-BASED COMPUTER NAVIGATION

Preoperative image-based computer navigation allows for detailed operative plans including patient-specific anatomic implant matching before surgery. These systems largely consist of two key components: (1) computer-generated models from preoperative scans and (2) intraoperative matching and registration.[21]

With image-based systems, sagittal and axial CT scans are used to create digital 3D models of the patient's anatomy preoperatively. Surgical planning software utilizes these models to obtain precise measurements of anatomical axes including the mechanical and transepicondylar axes as well as other key reference points. Implant sizes, implant positions, and bony resections for optimal alignment and implant contact are then calculated according to these measurements. These comprehensive virtual plans are presented for review by the surgeons preoperatively and therefore, in addition to the benefit of precise implant alignment, these modalities may also improve operating room efficiency by accurately predicting implant component sizes.

During surgery, the 3D models of the distal femur and tibia are typically displayed and are matched to the position and orientation of the patient's anatomy following a registration process. In order to make the bony resections determined in the preoperative plan, the system uses tracking technology to guide the placement of cutting jigs.

IMAGELESS COMPUTER NAVIGATION

Imageless computer navigation systems are more widely utilized compared to image-based systems for the simple reason that the former avoids the additional costs and radiation exposure associated with additional imaging. Instead of a preoperative scans, imageless systems intraoperatively construct 3D models of the surgical field based on the patients' osseous anatomy with both kinematic and surface registration processes. The intraoperative acquisition of information on patients' anatomy, including bone cysts, osteophytes, and bone density measurements, is then utilized and integrated into the surgical plan and execution.

Kinematic Registration

Accurate registration of anatomical axes and landmarks is critical for a dependable virtual bone map and ultimately for the restoration of neutral limb alignment. Kinematic registration is utilized to reference important anatomic landmarks that are not exposed and usually covered by surgical drapes during knee arthroplasty, namely the centers of the femoral head and the distal tibia which are required to identify the mechanical axes of the femur and tibia, respectively.[5]

Surgeons can register the center of the femoral head by stabilizing the pelvis and circumducting the femur around the hip joint. This passive, circular motion of the femur effectively creates the base of a cone and the apex of this cone closely approximately the center of the hip joint. Thus, the computer algorithm integrates dynamic reference points on the femur, tracked by an optical camera, and determines the location of the femoral head center by calculating the projected apex of the circular motion. The center of the distal tibia may be referenced with both kinematic and surface registration methods.[5] Multiple kinematic methods to reference the distal tibia have been described including one which estimates the center with passive movement of the ankle from dorsiflexion to plantarflexion and another treating the ankle as a ball-and-socket joint.[5,22-25]

Surface Registration

Surface registration involves the surgeon contacting dozens of points on the surface of the distal femur and proximal tibia with a calibrated probe. In order to limit the time spent matching reference points between the patient's bony surface and the virtual bone map, the reference areas are limited to small patches, or point clouds, on the bone. The computer system utilizes these reference points to identify the remaining landmarks required to establish anatomical axes.

Optical Navigation Systems

Optical and accelerometer-based systems are the two most commonly used imageless computer navigation systems in knee arthroplasty. The optical navigation system has been utilized since the inception of computer-assisted knee arthroplasty and serves as the link between the surgical field and the computer platform. Two or three charge-coupled device (CCD) cameras on a separate, standalone tower are placed approximately 2 meters from the surgical field and are used as sensors to detect markers that are attached to the femur and tibia rather than the bone itself. These markers also called as "rigid bodies" can be active or passive.[6,20] Active markers are light-emitting diodes, whereas passive markers are reflecting spheres both of which are detected by the camera. In passive systems, infrared flashes are sent from the camera system and reflected back by the spheres. Optical navigation systems allow a high degree of accuracy (100 measurements/second and an accuracy of <0.1 mm at 2 m)[20,26] and provide detailed intraoperative data which allow for the instantaneous calculations of flexion/extension gaps, coronal alignments, sagittal alignments, and implant sizes. Disadvantages of this system include the requirement of unobstructed line of sight between the trackers and CCD, which may force surgeons to adapt their techniques, and reduced accuracy with increasing distance between the camera and trackers.

Accelerometer-Based Systems

Unlike optical systems, the more recently developed accelerometer-based navigation systems do not require the placement of pins on the femur and tibia on which markers are mounted.[27] Instead, a handheld accelerometer device which displays alignment information is attached onto tibial and femoral resection instruments. Mechanical axes of the tibia and femur are determined with a combination of surface and kinematic registration. For example, to determine the femoral mechanical axis, the device is fixed to the distal anatomic location of the femoral mechanical axis and detects the center of the femoral head with kinematic registration through multiple passive movements of the femur by the surgeon.[28,29] This system does not require an unobstructed line of sight between the surgical field and a distant computer system, as it effectively places the navigation system within the surgical field. It is important to note that accelerometer-based systems can only guide distal femoral and proximal tibial resections and therefore conventional instrumentation is required for the remaining bone cuts, implant sizings, and rotational alignments.

ROBOTIC-ASSISTED KNEE ARTHROPLASTY

Robotic-assisted knee arthroplasty has been gaining attention in recent years due in part to the growing body of literature demonstrating its potential to improve the accuracy of implant positioning and therefore implant survivorship and patient outcomes.[30-34] Depending on the specific robotic-assisted knee system, either image-based or imageless navigation is utilized to determine the surgical plan. Unlike computer navigation systems, robotic-assisted surgery integrates predetermined, patient-specific plans with haptic feedback to allow for safe and accurate surgical execution.

Once the operative plan is determined and the robotic arm or surgical instrument is registered, the surgeon is able to burr or resect bone within a defined "safety zone." The surgeon receives haptic feedback which can be auditory, visual, or tactile, when the boundaries of this zone are approached. Thus, quantitative data from the operative plan are utilized to enforce haptic restraints in order to improve the accuracy of bone resections. Moreover, limiting the cutting tool to within an accurately determined 3D frame of reference may better protect the surrounding soft tissues and ligaments.

Robotic-assisted knee systems that utilize image-based navigation benefit from anatomic implant matching and positioning in the preoperative period. The compatibility of implant systems is dependent on whether a closed or open platform is utilized. For closed platforms, a specific manufacturer's implant can be used. With open platforms, different implant manufacturers and designs can be used; however, a degree of specificity and predictive value may be lost in such systems.[30]

CLINICAL OUTCOMES

Computer Navigation

Since its inception in the late 1990s, potential advantages of computer-assisted knee arthroplasty have been extensively investigated in a wide variety of clinical studies, reviews, and meta-analyses (**Table 34-1**). Computer navigation has been associated with better implant alignment in TKA compared to conventional techniques.[11-17] In a prospective cohort study of 80 TKA patients,[16] neutral alignment of the mechanical axis was achieved in 96% ($n = 77$) of the patients in the computer-assisted cohort and 78% ($n = 62$) in the conventional cohort, whereby neutral alignment was defined as ±3° of varus/valgus. Moreover, neutral coronal alignment of the femoral component was achieved in 92% ($n = 72$) of the patients in the computer-assisted cohort and 86% ($n = 69$) in the conventional cohort.

In a prospective study by McClelland et al,[35] radiographic and gait analyses were performed on 121 patients who underwent computer-assisted TKA ($n = 42$), conventional TKA ($n = 39$), or served as normal controls without knee surgery or pain ($n = 40$). Compared to the conventional group, the knee biomechanics of patients in the computer-assisted cohort more closely resembled that of a normal knee. Ideal mechanical axis alignment (180°) and the position of the weight-bearing line relative to the medial tibial border (50%) were significantly closer in the computer-assisted group (179° and 46%) compared to the conventional group (177° and 32%, $P < .01$ and $P = .01$, respectively). Upon gait analysis, it was found that patients in the computer-assisted group walked faster on average ($1.24 ± 0.02$ m/s) compared to the conventional group ($1.14 ± 0.02$ m/s, $P < .01$). After accounting for speed, patients in the conventional cohort had significantly less flexion during stance and swing compared to control patients with normal knees ($P < .01$); however, no significant differences were observed between the computer-assisted cohort and control.

Computer guidance is proposed to be a more accurate alternative to the medullary guides used in conventional knee arthroplasty, particularly in patients with bony deformities that make the identification of bony landmarks and measurements of cardinal axes more susceptible to error. Studies have shown that patients who have extra-articular deformity benefit from computer-assisted TKA with both optical and accelerometer-based navigation systems.[36-39] A study including patients with radiographic femoral extra-articular deformities undergoing TKA with computer-assisted navigation reported mean increases in Knee Society Scores (KSS) knee scores from 62 to 92 points ($P < .05$) and functional scores from 52 to 83 points ($P < .05$), as well as mean improvements in range of motion from 4° to 74° preoperatively to 0.6° to 98° at minimum 1-year follow-up.[36]

The use of intramedullary guides is avoided with computer assistance which potentially reduces the associated risk of fat embolism and excessive blood loss. Studies have reported reduced blood loss with the use of computer navigation in TKA.[40-42] McConnell et al[40] compared blood loss in 136 patients undergoing either computer-navigated TKA ($n = 68$) or conventional TKA ($n = 68$) with the use of intramedullary rods. Average total blood loss was 1,137 mL in the computer-navigated TKA cohort which was significantly less than the average blood loss of 1,362 mL in the conventional TKA group ($P = .016$). In

TABLE 34-1 **Clinical Studies Reporting Outcomes After Computer-Navigated Knee Arthroplasty and Conventional Knee Arthroplasty**

Study	Type of Navigation	Name of System	Outcomes	Results
Saragaglia et al (2001)[52]	Imageless, optical	OrthoPilot (Aesculap, Tuttlingen, Germany)	• Hip-knee-ankle (HKA) angle (goal 180°±3°) • Femoral angle from mechanical axis (90°) • Tibial angle from mechanical axis (90°)	$n = 25$ navigated; $n = 25$ conventional • HKA angle of 180 ± 3°: 84% navigated vs. 75% conventional • HKA angle: 179.0 ± 2.5° navigated vs. 181.2 ± 2.72° conventional ($P > .05$) • Femoral angle: 89.6 ± 1.6° navigated vs. 91.1 ± 2.1° conventional ($P = .048$) • Tibial angle: 89.5 ± 1.3° navigated vs. 90.2 ± 1.6° conventional ($P > .05$)
Jenny et al (2001)[22]	Imageless, optical	OrthoPilot (Aesculap, Tuttlingen, Germany)	• Mechanical femorotibial angle 177°-183° • Coronal orientation of femoral component 88-92° • Sagittal orientation of femoral component 88-92° • Coronal orientation of tibial component 88-92° • Sagittal orientation of tibial component 88-92° • Global implantation: all 5 criteria met	$n = 30$ navigated; $n = 30$ conventional • Mechanical femorotibial angle: 83% vs. 70% conventional ($P > .05$) • Coronal femoral alignment: 93% navigated vs. 83% conventional ($P > .05$) • Sagittal femoral alignment: 90% navigated vs. 63% conventional ($P > .05$) • Coronal tibial alignment: 93% navigated vs. 80% conventional ($P > .05$) • Sagittal tibial alignment: 83% navigated vs. 67% conventional ($P > .05$) • Optimal global implantation: 77% navigated vs. 27% conventional ($P < .001$)
Perlick et al (2004)[53]	Image-based, preoperative computed tomography (CT)	VectorVision CT-Based Knee 1.1 (BrainLAB, Munich, Germany)	• Limb axis alignment • Limb axis within 3° • Coronal femoral component alignment within 3° • Coronal tibial component alignment within 3°	$n = 50$ navigated; $n = 50$ conventional • Limb axis alignment: +0.4 ± 1.8° navigated vs. −1.2 ± 2.9° conventional ($P = .01$) • Limb axis within 3°: 92% navigated vs. 72% conventional • Femoral alignment: 96% navigated vs. 88% conventional • Tibial alignment: 96% navigated vs. 94% conventional
Bäthis et al (2004)[16]	Imageless, optical	VectorVision CT-free Knee (BrainLAB, Munich, Germany)	• Deviation from mechanical axis • Within 3° of mechanical axis	$n = 80$ computer-navigated; $n = 80$ conventional • Median (interquartile) deviation: 0° (−1 to +1°) navigated vs. 1° (−2 + 2°) ($P = .016$) • Within 3° of mechanical axis: 96% navigation vs. 78% conventional
Victor et al (2004)[54]	Image-based, intraoperative fluoroscopy	FluoroKnee (Smith & Nephew, Memphis, Tennessee, USA, and Medtronic SNT, Louisville, Colorado, USA)	• Coronal mechanical alignment within 2° • Coronal mechanical alignment • Lateral femur angle • Lateral tibia angle	$n = 50$ navigated; $n = 50$ conventional • Mechanical alignment: 100% navigated vs. 73.5% conventional • Alignment in the conventional group was more variable ($P < .0001$) • Mechanical alignment: −0.1 ± 2.1° navigated vs. −0.0 ± 1.2° conventional ($P > .05$) • Lateral femur angle: 2.4 ± 1.5° navigated vs. 2.9 ± 1.8° conventional ($P > .05$) • Lateral tibia angle: 3.4 ± 1.4° navigated vs. 2.9 ± 1.1° conventional ($P > .05$)

Study	Type	System	Parameters	Results
Mullaji et al (2007)[55]	Imageless, optical	Ci navigation system (BrainLab, Munich, Germany)	• Restoration of mechanical axis to ±1°, ±2°, and ±3° of neutral	$n = 282$ navigated; $n = 185$ conventional • Mechanical axis ±1°: 49% navigated vs. 30% conventional ($P = .0001$) • Mechanical axis ±2°: 79% navigated vs. 53% conventional ($P = .001$) • Mechanical axis ±3°: 91% navigated vs. 78% conventional ($P = .001$)
Martin et al (2007)[56]	Imageless, optical	CT-free VectorVision knee navigation system (BrainLAB, Munich, Germany)	• Alignment within 3° of mechanical axis • Posterior tibial slope within 3° of mechanical tibial axis • Lateral distal femoral component angle (LDFA) alignment within 3° • Medial proximal tibial angle (MPTA) alignment within 3°	$n = 100$ navigated; $n = 100$ conventional • Neutral mechanical axis: 92% navigated vs. 76% conventional ($P = .002$) • Posterior tibial slope within 3°: 98% navigated vs. 80% conventional ($P < .001$) • LDFA • LDFA within 3°: 95% navigated vs. 86% conventional ($P = .008$) • MPTA within 3°: 97% navigated vs. 85% conventional ($P = .003$)
Choong et al (2009)[12]	Imageless, optical	Ci System (Depuy, Leeds, UK)	• Alignment within 3° of mechanical axis • Femoral rotation aligned with epicondylar axis	$n = 57$ computer-navigated; $n = 52$ conventional • Neutral alignment: 88% navigated vs. 61% conventional ($P = .003$) • Neutral alignment in subgroup analysis of patients with body mass index ≥30: 93% navigated vs. 56% conventional ($P = .003$) • Median femoral rotation angles: 0.2° of internal rotation navigated vs. 0.6° external rotation conventional ($P = .061$)
Liow et al (2016)[57]	Imageless, accelerometer-based	iAssist (Zimmer Incorporated, Warsaw, Indiana, USA)	• Angle between mechanical axis of femur and mechanical axis of tibia (MA) • Angle between femoral component and mechanical axis of femur (CFA) • Angle between tibia base plate and mechanical axis of tibia (CTA) • Mechanical axis outliers (more than 3° varus/valgus from neutral)	$n = 92$ navigated; $n = 100$ conventional • MA: 1.9 ± 1.4° accelerometer vs. 2.8 ± 2.0° conventional ($P = .001$) • CFA: 1.6 ± 1.3° accelerometer vs. 2.1 ± 1.5° conventional ($P = .035$) • CTA: 1.6 ± 1.2° accelerometer vs. 2.1 ± 1.5° conventional ($P = .024$)
Goh et al (2016)[29]	Imageless: accelerometer-based versus optical	Accelerometer: iAssist (Zimmer Incorporated, Warsaw, Indiana, USA) Optical: Ci Mi TKR version 1.0 (BrainLAB/Depuy Orthopaedics Inc., Leeds, UK)	• Angle between mechanical axis of femur and mechanical axis of tibia (MA) • Angle between femoral component and mechanical axis of femur (CFA) • Angle between tibia base plate and mechanical axis of tibia (CTA) • Mechanical axis outliers (more than 3° varus/valgus from neutral)	$n = 38$ accelerometer-based, $n = 38$ optical • MA: 1.8 ± 1.3° accelerometer vs. 2.0 ± 1.5° optical ($P = .543$) • CFA: 1.3 ± 1.1° accelerometer vs. 1.9 ± 1.6° optical ($P = .074$) • CTA: 1.6 ± 1.3° accelerometer vs. 1.3 ± 1.0° optical ($P = .265$)

(Continued)

SECTION 6 / PRIMARY TOTAL KNEE ARTHROPLASTY

TABLE 34-1 Clinical Studies Reporting Outcomes After Computer-Navigated Knee Arthroplasty and Conventional Knee Arthroplasty—Continued

Study	Type of Navigation	Name of System	Outcomes	Results
McClelland et al (2017)[35]	Imageless, optical	Image Free BrainLAB Navigation System (BrainLAB, Munich, Germany)	• Mechanical axis • Weight-bearing line in relation to medial tibial border • Walking speed	$n = 40$ normal control; $n = 42$ navigated, $n = 39$ conventional • Mechanical axis: normal 180°, navigated 179°, conventional 177° ($P < .01$) • Weight-bearing line: normal 50%, navigated 46%, conventional 32%, ($P = .01$) • Walking speed: normal 1.27 ± 0.02 m/s, navigated 1.24 ± 0.02 m/s, conventional 1.14 ± 0.02 m/s ($P < .01$)
Gharaibeh et al (2017)[58]	Imageless, accelerometer-based	KneeAlign navigation system (OrthAlign, Aliso Viejo, California, USA)	• HKA angle within 3° of neutral • Femoral coronal angle (FCA) within 3° • Sagittal femoral angle (SFA) within 3° • Tibial coronal angle (TCA) within 3° • Tibial slope (TS) within 3°	$n = 89$ navigated; $n = 90$ conventional • Neutral HKA angle: 87% navigated vs. 82% conventional ($P = .54$) • Neutral FCA: 99% navigated vs. 94% conventional ($P = .21$) • Neutral SFA: 100% navigated vs. 98% conventional ($P = .50$) • Neutral TCA: 98% navigated vs. 99% conventional ($P = .62$) • Neutral TS: 98% navigated vs. 99% conventional ($P = .62$)
d'Amato et al (2019)[44]	Imageless, optical	Image-free knee navigation system (Stryker-Leibinger, Freiburg-im-Breisgau, Germany)	• 10-year implant failure rates • Limb mechanical axis deviation • 10-year Knee Society Score-Knee Score (KSS-K) • 10-year Knee Society Score-Function Score (KSS-F) • 10-year Knee Injury and Osteoarthritis Outcome Score (KOOS)	$n = 60$ navigated; $n = 60$ conventional • Implant failure: 4.2% navigated (aseptic loosening) vs. 6.4% conventional (aseptic loosening) ($P = .9$) • Mechanical axis deviation: $1.7 \pm 2.4°$ navigated vs. and $1.5 \pm 2.8°$ conventional ($P = .7$) • KSS-K: 85.9 ± 11.1 navigated vs. 85.0 ± 9.7 ($P = .42$) • KSS-F: 82.2 ± 19.3 navigated vs. 83.8 ± 18.0 ($P = .74$) • KOOS: 82.3 ± 14.3 navigated vs. 78.6 ± 14.4 conventional ($P = .12$)

(Continued)

TABLE 34.2   Clinical Studies Reporting Outcomes After Robotic-Assisted Knee Arthroplasty and Conventional Knee Arthroplasty

Study	Type of Surgery (UKA/TKA)	Name of System	Outcomes	Results
Cobb et al (2006)[59]	UKA	Acrobot System (The Acrobot Co. Ltd., London, UK)	• Coronal tibiofemoral angle within 2° • American Knee Society (AKS) score improvements at 18 wk • Western Ontario and McMaster Universities Osteoarthritis (WOMAC) score improvements at 18 wk	$n = 13$ robotic-assisted; $n = 15$ conventional • Tibiofemoral angle ±2°: 100% robotic vs. 40% ($P = .001$) • AKS score improvement: 65.21 ± 8.36 robotic vs. 32.5 ± 27.46 conventional ($P = .004$) • WOMAC pain: 8 ± 2 robotic vs. 6 ± 2 conventional ($P > .05$) • WOMAC stiffness: 3 ± 2 robotic vs. 2 ± 2 conventional ($P > .05$) • WOMAC function: 24 ± 10 robotic vs. 17 ± 11 conventional ($P > .05$)
Lonner et al (2010)[60]	UKA	Tactile Guidance System (MAKO Surgical, Fort Lauderdale, Florida, USA)	• Tibial slope error • Coronal tibial alignment error	$n = 31$ robotic-assisted; $n = 27$ conventional • Tibial slope error: 1.9° robotic vs. 3.1° conventional • Variance in tibial slope 2.6 times greater in conventional cohort ($P = .02$) • Coronal tibial alignment error: +0.2 ± 1.8° robotic vs. +2.7 ± 2.1° conventional ($P < .0001$)
MacCallum et al (2016)[61]	UKA	RIO Robotic Arm system (Stryker Orthopedics, Mahwah, New Jersey, and MAKO Surgical, Fort Lauderdale, Florida, USA)	• Tibial baseplate coronal alignment (goal 0°–3° varus) • Tibial slope in sagittal plane (goal 3°–9°)	$n = 87$ robotic-assisted; $n = 117$ conventional • Tibial baseplate alignment: 2.6 ± 1.5° robot vs. 3.9 ± 2.4° conventional ($P < .0001$) • Tibial slope: 2.4 ± 1.6° robot vs. 4.9 ± 2.8° conventional ($P < .0001$) • Robotic cohort had less variability and fewer outliers in coronal alignment ($P < .0001$) • Robotic cohort had less variability and fewer outliers in posterior slope ($P < .0001$)
Liow et al (2014)[49]	TKA	ROBODOC Surgical System with software version 4.3.6 (Curexo Technology Corp, Fremont, California, USA)	• Coronal plane mechanical axis • Coronal plane mechanical axis outliers (>3°) • Joint line deviation • Joint line deviation >5 mm • Anterior femoral notching • 6-mo extension • 6-mo flexion • 6-mo Oxford Knee Score • 6-mo Knee Society Score (KSS)	$n = 31$ robotic-assisted; $n = 29$ conventional • Mechanical axis: 1.3 ± 0.9° robotic vs. 1.8 ± 1.2° conventional ($P > .05$) • Mechanical axis outliers: 0% robotic vs. 19.4% conventional ($P = .049$) • Joint line deviation: 1.9 ± 1.1 mm robotic vs. 3.5 ± 2.8 conventional ($P = .010$) • Joint line deviation >5 mm: 3.2% robotic vs. 20.6% conventional ($P = .049$) • Anterior femoral notching: 0% robotic vs. 10.3% conventional ($P = .238$) • Extension: 5.3 ± 4.8° robotic vs. 4.5 ± 4.0° conventional ($P = .499$) • Flexion: 116.0 ± 17.8° robotic vs. 122.4 ± 10.7° conventional ($P = .112$) • Oxford knee scores: 18.8 ± 5.7 robotic vs. 19.6 ± 6.8 conventional ($P = .619$) • KSS scores: no significant differences in function or knee components ($P > .05$)

TABLE 34.2 Clinical Studies Reporting Outcomes After Robotic-Assisted Knee Arthroplasty and Conventional Knee Arthroplasty—Continued

Study	Type of Surgery (UKA/TKA)	Name of System	Outcomes	Results
Marchand et al (2018)[46]	TKA	Mako Robotic-Arm Assisted System (Stryker, Mahwah, New Jersey, USA)	• Post-bone cut medial versus lateral extension gap difference • Post-bone cut medial versus lateral flexion gap difference • Robot-predicted implant size	$n = 335$ robotic-assisted • Extension gap difference: 100% between −1 and 1 mm (mean, 0 mm) • Flexion gap difference: 99% between −2 and 2 mm (mean, 0 mm) • Robotic software predicted within 1 size of the tibial or femoral implant size used in 98% of knees
Marchand et al (2019)[31]	TKA	Mako Robotic-Arm Assisted System (Stryker, Mahwah, New Jersey, USA)	• 1-y WOMAC total scores • 1-y WOMAC function scores • 1-y WOMAC pain scores	$n = 14$ robotic-assisted; $n = 53$ conventional • Total scores: 6 ± 6 robotic vs. 9 ± 8 conventional ($P < .05$) • Function scores: 4 ± 4 robotic vs. 6 ± 5 conventional ($P < .05$) • Pain scores: 2 ± 3 robotic vs. 3 ± 4 conventional ($P > .05$) • Use of robotic-assisted surgery had a significant association with better total and function WOMAC scores ($P < .05$) on multivariate analysis
Batailler et al (2019)[62]	UKA	BlueBelt Navio robotic surgical system (Smith and Nephew, Pittsburgh, Pennsylvania, USA)	• Limb alignment lateral UKA outliers • Limb alignment medial UKA outliers • Tibial baseplate alignment outliers (±3°) • Tibial slope outliers (<82°) • Satisfaction rates • International Knee Society (IKS) scores • Conversion to TKA	$n = 80$ robotic-assisted; $n = 80$ conventional • Lateral UKA alignment outliers: 26% robotic vs. 61% conventional ($P = .018$) • Medial UKA alignment outliers: 16 vs. 32% conventional ($P = .038$) • Tibial baseplate outliers: 11% robotic vs. 35% conventional ($P < .001$) • Lateral UKA tibial slope outliers: 4.3% robotics vs. 17.4% conventional ($P > .05$) • Medial UKA tibial slope outliers ($P = .015$) • Satisfaction rates: 74% robotics vs. 79% conventional ($P > .05$) • IKS scores: knee and function scores not significantly different ($P > .05$) • Conversion rates: 5% robotic vs. 9% control ($P > .05$)
Figueroa et al (2019)[63]	TKA	iBlock/NanoBlock and APEX OMNIbotics system (OMNIlife Science, Raynham, Massachusetts, USA)	• Femoral coronal alignment (FCA) concordance with postoperative CT (±3°) • Femoral sagittal alignment (FSA) concordance (±3°) • Femoral rotational alignment (FRA, related to transepicondylar axis) concordance (±3°) • Tibial coronal alignment (TCA) concordance (±3°) • Tibial sagittal alignment (TSA) concordance (±3°) • HKA angle concordance (±3°)	$n = 173$ robotic-assisted • FCA ±3°: 98% • FSA ±3°: 100% • FRA ±3°: 94% • TCA ±3°: 99% • TSA ±3°:93% • HKA ±3°: 83%

CT, computed tomography; TKA, total knee arthroplasty; UKA, unicompartmental knee arthroplasty.

another study by Tabatabee et al,[42] the authors compared in-hospital complications between 787,809 conventional TKAs and 13,246 computer-assisted TKAs performed between 2005 and 2011 using a national database. Compared to the computer-assisted cohort, patients in the conventional cohort were at significantly increased risks for blood transfusions (odds ratio [OR] 1.15, 95% confidence interval [CI] 1.06–1.24, $P < .001$) and perioperative complications overall (OR 1.17, 95% CI 1.03–1.33, $P = .01$) after adjusting for several baseline variables including patient comorbidities. Interestingly, the study did not find significant differences in complication rates between image-based and imageless computer-assisted TKA (3.41% vs. 3.47%, $P = .34$).

Functional outcomes after computer-navigated TKA have also been assessed; however, the current evidence is inconclusive. Panjwani et al[43] conducted a meta-analysis of all prospective studies until 2018 which included 3060 knees, 1538 of which underwent computer-assisted TKA and 1522 of which underwent conventional TKA. Pooled mean KSS function scores ($P = .03$) and Western Ontario and McMaster Universities Osteoarthritis Index (WOMAC; $P < .001$) scores were significantly better with computer-assisted TKA at 5 to 8-year follow-up. In contrast, a 10-year follow-up study by d'Amato et al[44] reported that KSS scores, WOMAC scores, and Knee Injury and Osteoarthritis Outcome Scores (KOOS) were not significantly different between patients after computer-assisted ($n = 60$) and conventional TKA ($n = 60$, $P > .05$). Moreover, in a meta-analysis of 33 studies including 3423 patients, computer navigation was not reported to have a significant effect on functional outcomes.[18] However, findings from the same meta-analysis did reveal that computer navigation significantly reduced the risk of malalignment by >3° (risk ratio [RR] 0.79, 95% CI 0.71–0.87, $P < .001$) and by >2° (RR 0.76, 95% CI 0.71–0.82, $P < .001$) from the mechanical limb axis.

Robotic-Assisted Knee Arthroplasty

Promising results have also been demonstrated with robotic-assisted knee arthroplasty[17-19] (**Table 34-2**). Several clinical studies and randomized controlled trials have shown that robotic-assisted techniques improve the accuracy and precision of component positioning and thus lead to better limb alignment and implant survival after UKA and TKA.[30-34,45-50] A recent matched cohort analysis including 246 robotic-assisted UKAs and 492 conventional UKAs found that revision rates at 2 years postoperatively were significantly lower in the computer-assisted cohort (0.8% vs. 5.3%, $P = .002$).[47]

Results from a prospective randomized controlled trial of 100 TKA patients with 5-year follow-up demonstrated that robotic-assisted TKA reduced the number of mechanical axis outliers (defined as >3°) and minimized flexion–extension gap imbalances.[48] In a prospective cohort study of 330 robotic-assisted TKAs, Marchand et al[51] reported that postoperative neutral alignment (0° ± 3°) from the mechanical axis was achieved in all patients who had less than 7° of preoperative varus deformity. Moreover, most patients (64%) with severe varus deformities (>7°) and all patients with severe valgus deformities (>7°) also achieved neutral alignment postoperatively.

Heterogeneities in outcome scoring systems and follow-up periods limit the current evidence on the effect of robotic-assisted techniques on patient-reported outcomes. However, some studies have demonstrated that the benefits of accurate implant positioning with robotic-assisted techniques often translate to better functional outcomes. Early results from a multicenter study reported by Khlopas et al[32] found that of the 252 TKA patients who underwent surgery between 2016 and 2018 (150 robotic-assisted and 102 conventional), patients who underwent robotic-assisted TKA had equal or greater improvements in 9 out of 10 components of the KSS at 3 months postoperatively. In another prospective study, 1-year outcomes after 53 robotic-assisted TKAs were compared to those after 53 conventional TKAs, all of which were performed by a single high-volume surgeon.[31] Total WOMAC scores (6 ± 6 vs. 9 ± 8, $P < .05$) and physical function component scores (13 ± 5 vs. 14 ± 5, $P < .05$) were significantly better in the robotic-assisted cohort compared to the conventional cohort; these associations remained significant after adjusting for age, sex, and body mass index.

In summary, with many prosthetic manufacturers developing various forms of robotic platforms often using computer assistance, it is expected that these technologies will continue to increase in relation to standard conventional instrumentation for TKA.

REFERENCES

1. Thiele K, Perka C, Matziolis G, Mayr HO, Sostheim M, Hube R. Current failure mechanisms after knee arthroplasty have changed: polyethylene wear is less common in revision surgery. *J Bone Joint Surg Am*. 2015;97:715-720. doi:10.2106/JBJS.M.01534.
2. Victor J. Optimising position and stability in total knee arthroplasty. *EFORT Open Rev*. 2017;2:215-220. doi:10.1302/2058-5241.2.170001.
3. Saragaglia D, Rubens-Duval B, Gaillot J, Lateur G, Pailhe R. Total knee arthroplasties from the origin to navigation: history, rationale, indications. *Int Orthop*. 2019;43:597-604. doi:10.1007/s00264-018-3913-z.
4. Saragaglia D, Marques Da Silva B, Dijoux P, Cognault J, Gaillot J, Pailhe R. Computerised navigation of unicondylar knee prostheses: from primary implantation to revision to total knee arthroplasty. *Int Orthop*. 2017;41:293-299. doi:10.1007/s00264-016-3293-1.
5. Siston RA, Giori NJ, Goodman SB, Delp SL. Surgical navigation for total knee arthroplasty: a perspective. *J Biomech*. 2007;40:728-735. doi:10.1016/j.jbiomech.2007.01.006.
6. Bae DK, Song SJ. Computer assisted navigation in knee arthroplasty. *Clin Orthop Surg* 2011;3:259-267. doi:10.4055/cios.2011.3.4.259.
7. Picard F, Moody J, DiGioia A. Clinical classification of CAOS systems. *Comput Robot Assist Knee Hip Surg*. 2004:43-48.
8. Lotke PA, Ecker ML. Influence of positioning of prosthesis in total knee replacement. *J Bone Joint Surg Am*. 1977;59:77-79.

9. Tew M, Waugh W. Tibiofemoral alignment and the results of knee replacement. *J Bone Joint Surg Br.* 1985;67:551-556.

10. Ritter MA, Faris PM, Keating EM, Meding JB. Postoperative alignment of total knee replacement. Its effect on survival. *Clin Orthop Relat Res.* 1994;299:153-156.

11. Picard F, Deakin AH, Clarke JV, Dillon JM, Gregori A. Using navigation intraoperative measurements narrows range of outcomes in TKA. *Clin Orthop Relat Res.* 2007;463:50-57. doi:10.1097/BLO.0b013e3181468734.

12. Choong PF, Dowsey MM, Stoney JD. Does accurate anatomical alignment result in better function and quality of life? Comparing conventional and computer-assisted total knee arthroplasty. *J Arthroplasty.* 2009;24:560-569. doi:10.1016/j.arth.2008.02.018.

13. Fu Y, Wang M, Liu Y, Fu Q. Alignment outcomes in navigated total knee arthroplasty: a meta-analysis. *Knee Surg Sports Traumatol Arthrosc.* 2012;20:1075-1082. doi:10.1007/s00167-011-1695-6.

14. Hetaimish BM, Khan MM, Simunovic N, Al-Harbi HH, Bhandari M, Zalzal PK. Meta-analysis of navigation vs conventional total knee arthroplasty. *J Arthroplasty.* 2012;27:1177-1182. doi:10.1016/j.arth.2011.12.028.

15. Lee D-H, Park J-H, Song D-I, Padhy D, Jeong W-K, Han S-B. Accuracy of soft tissue balancing in TKA: comparison between navigation-assisted gap balancing and conventional measured resection. *Knee Surg Sports Traumatol Arthrosc.* 2010;18:381-387. doi:10.1007/s00167-009-0983-x.

16. Bathis H, Perlick L, Tingart M, Luring C, Zurakowski D, Grifka J. Alignment in total knee arthroplasty. A comparison of computer-assisted surgery with the conventional technique. *J Bone Joint Surg Br.* 2004;86:682-687.

17. van der List JP, Chawla H, Joskowicz L, Pearle AD. Current state of computer navigation and robotics in unicompartmental and total knee arthroplasty: a systematic review with meta-analysis. *Knee Surg Sports Traumatol Arthrosc.* 2016;24:3482-3495. doi:10.1007/s00167-016-4305-9.

18. Bauwens K, Matthes G, Wich M, et al. Navigated total knee replacement. A meta-analysis. *J Bone Joint Surg Am.* 2007;89:261-269. doi:10.2106/JBJS.F.00601.

19. Banerjee S, Cherian JJ, Elmallah RK, Jauregui JJ, Pierce TP, Mont MA. Robotic-assisted knee arthroplasty. *Expert Rev Med Devices.* 2015;12:727-735. doi:10.1586/17434440.2015.1086264.

20. Picard F, Deep K, Jenny JY. Current state of the art in total knee arthroplasty computer navigation. *Knee Surg Sports Traumatol Arthrosc.* 2016;24:3565-3574. doi:10.1007/s00167-016-4337-1.

21. Delp SL, Stulberg SD, Davies B, Picard F, Leitner F. Computer assisted knee replacement. *Clin Orthop Relat Res.* 1998;354:49-56. doi:10.1097/00003086-199809000-00007.

22. Jenny J-Y, Boeri C. Computer-assisted implantation of total knee prostheses: a case-control comparative study with classical instrumentation. *Comput Aided Surg.* 2001;6:217-220. doi:10.3109/10929080109146086.

23. Stulberg SD, Loan P, Sarin V. Computer-assisted navigation in total knee replacement: results of an initial experience in thirty-five patients. *J Bone Joint Surg Am.* 2002;84-A(suppl 2):90-98.

24. van den Bogert AJ, Smith GD, Nigg BM. In vivo determination of the anatomical axes of the ankle joint complex: an optimization approach. *J Biomech.* 1994;27:1477-1488.

25. Siston RA, Daub AC, Giori NJ, Goodman SB, Delp SL. Evaluation of methods that locate the center of the ankle for computer-assisted total knee arthroplasty. *Clin Orthop Relat Res.* 2005;439:129-135. doi:10.1097/01.blo.0000170873.88306.56.

26. Pitto RP, Graydon AJ, Bradley L, Malak SF, Walker CG, Anderson IA. Accuracy of a computer-assisted navigation system for total knee replacement. *J Bone Joint Surg Br.* 2006;88:601-605. doi:10.1302/0301-620X.88B5.17431.

27. Waddell BS, Carroll K, Jerabek S. Technology in arthroplasty: are we improving value? *Curr Rev Musculoskelet Med.* 2017;10:378-387. doi:10.1007/s12178-017-9415-6.

28. Scuderi GR, Fallaha M, Masse V, Lavigne P, Amiot L-P, Berthiaume M-J. Total knee arthroplasty with a novel navigation system within the surgical field. *Orthop Clin North Am.* 2014;45:167-173. doi:10.1016/j.ocl.2013.11.002.

29. Goh GS-H, Liow MHL, Lim WS-R, Tay DK-J, Yeo SJ, Tan MH. Accelerometer-based navigation is as accurate as optical computer navigation in restoring the joint line and mechanical axis after total knee arthroplasty: a prospective matched study. *J Arthroplasty.* 2016;31:92-97. doi:10.1016/j.arth.2015.06.048.

30. Jacofsky DJ, Allen M. Robotics in arthroplasty: a comprehensive review. *J Arthroplasty.* 2016;31:2353-2363. doi:10.1016/j.arth.2016.05.026.

31. Marchand RC, Sodhi N, Anis HK, et al. One-year patient outcomes for robotic-arm-assisted versus manual total knee arthroplasty. *J Knee Surg.* 2019;32(11):1063-1068. doi:10.1055/s-0039-1683977.

32. Khlopas A, Sodhi N, Hozack WJ, et al. Patient-reported functional and satisfaction outcomes after robotic-arm-assisted total knee arthroplasty: early results of a prospective multicenter investigation. *J Knee Surg.* 2019. doi:10.1055/s-0039-1684014.

33. Hampp EL, Chughtai M, Scholl LY, et al. Robotic-arm assisted total knee arthroplasty demonstrated greater accuracy and precision to plan compared with manual techniques. *J Knee Surg.* 2019;32:239-250. doi:10.1055/s-0038-1641729.

34. Khlopas A, Sodhi N, Sultan AA, Chughtai M, Molloy RM, Mont MA. Robotic arm–assisted total knee arthroplasty. *J Arthroplasty.* 2018;33:2002-2006. doi:10.1016/j.arth.2018.01.060.

35. McClelland JA, Webster KE, Ramteke AA, Feller JA. Total knee arthroplasty with computer-assisted navigation more closely replicates normal knee biomechanics than conventional surgery. *Knee.* 2017;24:651-656. doi:10.1016/j.knee.2016.12.009.

36. Bottros J, Klika AK, Lee HH, Polousky J, Barsoum WK. The use of navigation in total knee arthroplasty for patients with extra-articular deformity. *J Arthroplasty.* 2008;23:74-78. doi:10.1016/j.arth.2007.01.021.

37. Matassi F, Cozzi Lepri A, Innocenti M, Zanna L, Civinini R, Innocenti M. Total knee arthroplasty in patients with extra-articular deformity: restoration of mechanical alignment using accelerometer-based navigation system. *J Arthroplasty.* 2019;34:676-681. doi:10.1016/j.arth.2018.12.042.

38. Sculco PK, Kahlenberg CA, Fragomen AT, Rozbruch SR. Management of extra-articular deformity in the setting of total knee arthroplasty. *J Am Acad Orthop Surg.* 2019;27(18):e819-e830. doi:10.5435/JAAOS-D-18-00361.

39. Klein GR, Austin MS, Smith EB, Hozack WJ. Total knee arthroplasty using computer-assisted navigation in patients with deformities of the femur and tibia. *J Arthroplasty.* 2006;21:284-288. doi:10.1016/j.arth.2005.07.013.

40. McConnell J, Dillon J, Kinninmonth A, Sarungi M, Picard F. Blood loss following total knee replacement is reduced when using computer-assisted versus standard methods. *Acta Orthop Belg.* 2012;78:75-79.

41. Millar NL, Deakin AH, Millar LL, Kinninmonth AWG, Picard F. Blood loss following total knee replacement in the morbidly obese: effects of computer navigation. *Knee.* 2011;18:108-112. doi:10.1016/j.knee.2010.03.002.

42. Tabatabaee RM, Rasouli MR, Maltenfort MG, Fuino R, Restrepo C, Oliashirazi A. Computer-assisted total knee arthroplasty: is there a difference between image-based and imageless techniques? *J Arthroplasty.* 2018;33:1076-1081. doi:10.1016/j.arth.2017.11.030.

43. Panjwani TR, Mullaji A, Doshi K, Thakur H. Comparison of functional outcomes of computer-assisted vs conventional total knee arthroplasty: a systematic review and meta-analysis of high-quality, prospective studies. *J Arthroplasty.* 2019;34:586-593. doi:10.1016/j.arth.2018.11.028.

44. d'Amato M, Ensini A, Leardini A, Barbadoro P, Illuminati A, Belvedere C. Conventional versus computer-assisted surgery in

total knee arthroplasty: comparison at ten years follow-up. *Int Orthop.* 2019;43:1355-1363. doi:10.1007/s00264-018-4114-5.

45. Sodhi N, Khlopas A, Ehiorobo JO, et al. Robotic-assisted total knee arthroplasty in the presence of extra-articular deformity. *Surg Technol Int.* 2019;34:497-502.

46. Marchand RC, Sodhi N, Bhowmik-Stoker M, et al. Does the robotic arm and preoperative CT planning help with 3D intraoperative total knee arthroplasty planning? *J Knee Surg.* 2018;32(8):742-749. doi:10.1055/s-0038-1668122.

47. Cool CL, Needham KA, Khlopas A, Mont MA. Revision analysis of robotic arm-assisted and manual unicompartmental knee arthroplasty. *J Arthroplasty.* 2019;34:926-931. doi:10.1016/j.arth.2019.01.018.

48. Song E-K, Seon J-K, Yim J-H, Netravali NA, Bargar WL. Robotic-assisted TKA reduces postoperative alignment outliers and improves gap balance compared to conventional TKA. *Clin Orthop Relat Res.* 2013;471:118-126. doi:10.1007/s11999-012-2407-3.

49. Liow MHL, Xia Z, Wong MK, Tay KJ, Yeo SJ, Chin PL. Robot-assisted total knee arthroplasty accurately restores the joint line and mechanical axis. A prospective randomised study. *J Arthroplasty.* 2014;29:2373-2377. doi:10.1016/j.arth.2013.12.010.

50. Park SE, Lee CT. Comparison of robotic-assisted and conventional manual implantation of a primary total knee arthroplasty. *J Arthroplasty.* 2007;22:1054-1059. doi:10.1016/j.arth.2007.05.036.

51. Marchand RC, Sodhi N, Khlopas A, et al. Coronal correction for severe deformity using robotic-assisted total knee arthroplasty. *J Knee Surg.* 2018;31:2-5. doi:10.1055/s-0037-1608840.

52. Saragaglia D, Picard F, Chaussard C, Montbarbon E, Leitner F, Cinquin P. Computer-assisted knee arthroplasty: comparison with a conventional procedure. Results of 50 cases in a prospective randomized study. *Rev Chir Orthop Reparatrice Appar Mot.* 2001;87:18-28.

53. Perlick L, Bathis H, Tingart M, Perlick C, Grifka J. Navigation in total-knee arthroplasty: CT-based implantation compared with the conventional technique. *Acta Orthop Scand.* 2004;75:464-470.

54. Victor J, Hoste D. Image-based computer-assisted total knee arthroplasty leads to lower variability in coronal alignment. *Clin Orthop Relat Res.* 2004;428:131-139. doi:10.1097/01.blo.0000147710.69612.76.

55. Mullaji A, Kanna R, Marawar S, Kohli A, Sharma A. Comparison of limb and component alignment using computer-assisted navigation versus image intensifier-guided conventional total knee arthroplasty: a prospective, randomized, single-surgeon study of 467 knees. *J Arthroplasty.* 2007;22:953-959. doi:10.1016/j.arth.2007.04.030.

56. Martin A, Wohlgenannt O, Prenn M, Oelsch C, von Strempel A. Imageless navigation for TKA increases implantation accuracy. *Clin Orthop Relat Res.* 2007;460:178-184. doi:10.1097/BLO.0b013e31804ea45f.

57. Liow MHL, Goh GS-H, Pang H-N, Tay DKJ, Lo NN, Yeo SJ. Computer-assisted stereotaxic navigation improves the accuracy of mechanical alignment and component positioning in total knee arthroplasty. *Arch Orthop Trauma Surg.* 2016;136:1173-1180. doi:10.1007/s00402-016-2483-z.

58. Gharaibeh MA, Solayar GN, Harris IA, Chen DB, MacDessi SJ. Accelerometer-based, portable navigation (KneeAlign) vs conventional instrumentation for total knee arthroplasty: a prospective randomized comparative trial. *J Arthroplasty.* 2017;32:777-782. doi:10.1016/j.arth.2016.08.025.

59. Cobb J, Henckel J, Gomes P, et al. Hands-on robotic unicompartmental knee replacement: a prospective, randomised controlled study of the acrobot system. *J Bone Joint Surg Br.* 2006;88:188-197. doi:10.1302/0301-620X.88B2.17220.

60. Lonner JH, John TK, Conditt MA. Robotic arm-assisted UKA improves tibial component alignment: a pilot study. *Clin Orthop Relat Res.* 2010;468:141-146. doi:10.1007/s11999-009-0977-5.

61. MacCallum KP, Danoff JR, Geller JA. Tibial baseplate positioning in robotic-assisted and conventional unicompartmental knee arthroplasty. *Eur J Orthop Surg Traumatol.* 2016;26:93-98. doi:10.1007/s00590-015-1708-0.

62. Batailler C, White N, Ranaldi FM, Neyret P, Servien E, Lustig S. Improved implant position and lower revision rate with robotic-assisted unicompartmental knee arthroplasty. *Knee Surg Sports Traumatol Arthrosc.* 2019;27:1232-1240. doi:10.1007/s00167-018-5081-5.

63. Figueroa F, Wakelin E, Twiggs J, Fritsch B. Comparison between navigated reported position and postoperative computed tomography to evaluate accuracy in a robotic navigation system in total knee arthroplasty. *Knee.* 2019;26(4):869-875. doi:10.1016/j.knee.2019.05.004.

chapter 35

Robotic Applications for Total Knee Arthroplasty

Kenneth Gustke, MD

INTRODUCTION

Orthopedic surgeons continue to seek a better technique to perform total knee arthroplasty to match the greater perceived outcomes of total hip replacement surgery. There may be an element of inappropriate expectations for total knee arthroplasty.[1,2] Several series of revision knee arthroplasties report malalignment in 25% and instability in 20% to 25% of revisions.[3,4] Total knee imbalance with either too tight or loose soft tissues accounts for up to 54% of revisions in one series.[5] Gross component malalignment will lead to increased stress on the polyethylene, locking mechanism and supporting bone, thereby resulting in polyethylene wear and early loosening. Gross instability is easily perceived by patients necessitating early revision. Subtle instability and poor kinematics are more difficult to diagnose by both patients and surgeons. It can result in stiffness and perhaps may be the reason for the approximate 20% of unsatisfied patients who live with their arthroplasty.[2,6] Being able to consistently obtain an accurately aligned knee arthroplasty within acceptable alignment parameters that would not be expected to overstress the polyethylene and implant interfaces and obtain a perfectly balanced knee should result in the best short- and long-term outcomes.

Total knee arthroplasty performed with standard instruments has an inherent margin of error with implant and axial alignment. Even though many native knees are in constitutional varus or valgus,[7] most surgeons will aim for neutral mechanical alignment to minimize final alignment outliers outside of 3° of mechanical varus to 3° of mechanical valgus. Despite usual oblique joint lines in native knees, 90° angle proximal tibial cuts are usually performed because they are easier to make with conventional instruments. Unfortunately, following these techniques, axial alignment within 3° is obtained in only 70% to 80% of cases using standard instruments.[8,9] This lack of accuracy certainly prohibits consideration of following a constitutional, true kinematic, or hybrid kinematic alignment philosophy.[10-13] Standard total knee kits lack instruments to assist with soft tissue balancing. Soft tissue balancing is based on feel and visualization of gaps under applied varus and valgus stress. Subjective balance is less accurate and highly influenced by surgeon experience. Instrumented sensor trials can be helpful by providing quantitative information while balancing the soft tissues mainly through tissue releases may provide better short-term outcomes.[14-18] However, excellent long-term outcomes are predicated on both a perfectly balanced and aligned knee.

Computer navigation was developed to improve accuracy of implant alignment. Studies have shown a decrease in alignment outliers.[19-21] This technology may allow surgeons to consider constitutional or kinematic alignment of implants.[22] Computer navigation may aid with soft tissue balancing by showing gap equality and symmetry. However, most outcome studies of computer-navigated knee arthroplasty have not shown a difference in patient satisfaction, clinical function, and positioning of implants.[23,24] The Australian National Joint Registry has shown better survivorship of computer-navigated total knees in patients less than 65 years of age.[25] Younger patients would be expected to apply more stress on the polyethylene and component interfaces, thereby revealing a difference in survivorship which may not be noted in older, less demanding patients. Perhaps the use of sensor trials with computer-navigated knees, providing quantitative information on balance, may demonstrate improved short-term outcomes.

Patient-specific instrumentation (PSI) was also developed to assist with bone cuts to more accurately obtain implant alignment. Chosen alignment is based on the surgeon's preoperatively determined alignment parameters. Some alignment inaccuracy has been reported, particularly with the tibial cut.[26-28] Unfortunately, back-up instruments may still be needed if intraoperative changes are necessary.[29] One study demonstrated worse alignment with PSI than with computer navigation.[30] Typically, these systems do not include instruments to assist with soft tissue balancing. Use of custom-manufactured implants to match patient's anatomy inserted with PSI has been developed to theoretically reproduce better kinematics than with use of off-the-shelf implants. This may not be achievable without having anterior and posterior cruciate ligaments and in severe deformities. Callies et al have shown comparable results between kinematic aligned total knee arthroplasties and patient-specific instruments to mechanically aligned total knee arthroplasties with standard instruments.[31] However, they noted more outliers with poor outcomes in the PSI kinematic aligned group.

Robotic assistance for knee replacement can also accurately create bone cuts to align components in exactly the surgeon's desired position.[32-38] It is a unique technology because it can also allow individualized patient component alignment that can be adjusted preoperatively as well as intraoperatively. It also gives the surgeon the ability to modify alignment confidently within their desired parameters off the neutral mechanical axis in order to balance the knee and minimize soft tissue releases.

ROBOTIC ARM–ASSISTED TOTAL KNEE ARTHROPLASTY (MAKO—STRYKER ORTHOPEDICS)

General Overview

This system utilizes a saw that is attached to a robotic arm which places the saw cutting blade in the correct cutting plan (**Fig. 35-1**). This is a semi-active system that requires the surgeon to press the trigger to active the saw. The surgeon manipulates the robotic arm placing the saw tip close to the desired bone cut. Initial depression of the trigger will orient the saw tip in the exact plane and position to perform the bone cut. The tip of the saw operates only within haptic boundaries that are determined by the edges of the component positions (**Fig. 35-2**). Haptic boundaries significantly reduce the risk for soft tissue injury during bone resections.[39-41] Component position, size, and axial and rotational alignment are determined from preoperative planning of a 3D virtual model obtained from a computed tomography (CT) scan. The CT scan is performed under a protocol with scanning of just the hip, knee, and ankle. The radiation exposure is approximately 4.0 millisieverts (mSv), which is equivalent to 1/2 the dose of an abdominal CT, 1/4 the dose of a coronary angiogram,[42] or 1/13 of the occupational dose limit of 50 mSv.[43] Femoral and tibial infrared tracker arrays are inserted either inside or outside the incision depending on length of incision and surgeon's preference. The knee is surgically exposed. Various anatomic points and hip center are registered with probes to synchronize the patient's anatomy to the preoperative CT scan virtual model.

After removal of visualized osteophytes, varus and valgus stresses are applied to the knee in extension and flexion to demonstrate gaps and the soft tissue balance with the component aligned within the preoperative plan. A hybrid gap balancing/measured resection technique is used. The preoperative plan can be modified to change component position and alignment within the surgeon's acceptable parameters to facilitate better soft tissue balance and minimize soft tissue releases (**Fig. 35-3A and B**). Component realignment may be preferred to performing soft tissue releases due to the concern that soft tissue releases can be unpredictable and may stretch out postoperatively.[44,45] After all initial bone cuts are made and with trial components in place, varus and valgus stresses are

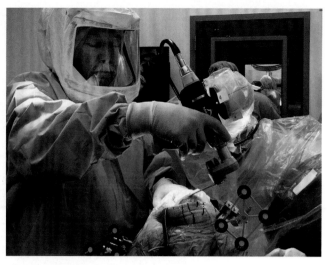

FIGURE 35-1 Robotic arm–directed placement of saw blade in appropriate cutting plane and position.

again applied in extension and flexion to visualize gaps and soft tissue balance. Alternatively, some of the bone cuts can be made and tensioner instruments used to show gap balance prior to trialing components. Further modification of component position and alignment can be considered and additional bone cuts are performed under haptic guidance to facilitate soft tissue balance. Generally tibial component modifications are performed if a change of balance is needed in both flexion and extension, and the femoral component alignment is adjusted if only extension rebalance is needed. Component alignment and position modifications are considered as long as they are still within the ranges acceptable to the surgeon. My final desired coronal alignment is between 2° of valgus and 3° of varus. Otherwise, soft tissue releases are performed to

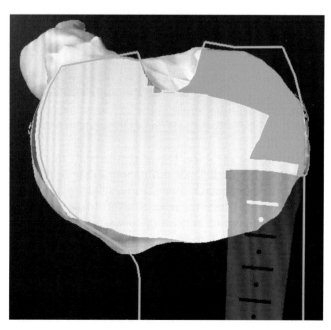

FIGURE 35-2 Saw tip cutting bone within haptic boundaries.

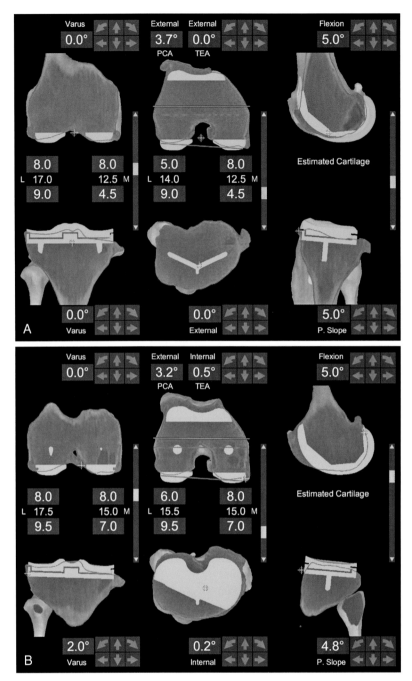

FIGURE 35-3 **A:** Initial preoperative plan with neutral coronal mechanical axial and tibial component alignments. **B:** Modified preoperative plan adding 2° of tibial component varus and subtracting a half degree of femoral external rotation.

further balance the knee. Use of sensor trials that show compartment load balance throughout range of motion, maximum load contact points, and tracking pattern can be used to also titrate the release of soft tissue and assist with determining the amount of component realignment needed[46] (**Fig. 35-4A** and **B**).

Indications

All patients with severe tricompartmental arthritis are candidates for this technique. The same robotic arm technology and setup can be utilized for unicompartmental,

patellofemoral, or bicompartmental arthroplasty when more isolated arthritis is present. The preoperative plan is modified depending on the type of arthroplasty desired.

Preoperative Planning

The surgeon's choice to use a posterior cruciate retaining or substituting knee design will change the haptic cutting boundaries around the posterior cruciate ligament. Also in substituting designs, the combined femoral flexion and tibial slope should not be greater

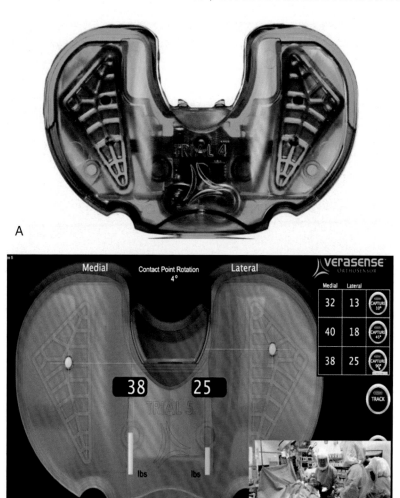

FIGURE 35-4   A: Sensor trial for Stryker Triathlon total knee system. **B:** Medial and lateral compartment pressure in near full extension, mid-flexion, and 90° of flexion. Location of maximum pressure contact points.

than 8° or the anterior edge of the tibial post could impingement against the femoral intercondylar notch in hyperextension.

The default plan will place the components in positions where they would be with traditional resections as if using conventional instruments and a neutral mechanical alignment (**Fig. 35-3A**). The tibial component is in a neutral mechanical axis with a 7 mm resection level of the least involved tibial condyle and 3° posterior slope for a cruciate retaining knee. The tibial component has 0° posterior slope for a posterior stabilized knee. Sizing is based on best tibial coverage without overhang. The femoral component is in a neutral mechanical vagus with an 8 mm distal femoral resection level from the least worn distal femoral condyle. The femoral component is flexed 3° to 5° to avoid anterior notching, placed 2 mm outside CT dimensions of the distal and mid-condyle on the less worn side to account for cartilage thickness, and rotated parallel to the transepicondylar line.

If an oblique joint line is desired, the tibial component can be changed to a few degrees of varus and femoral component to a few degrees of valgus. Also the femoral component rotation can be decreased. If the knee has a constitutional varus and a postoperative varus axial alignment is acceptable, it may be preferable in order to facilitate better soft tissue balance to place the tibial component in a few degrees of varus. My preferred postoperative coronal alignment range is 3° of mechanical varus to 2° of mechanical valgus, and 3° to 0° of tibial varus. Most tibial component coronal re-alignment is used for constitutional varus knees. If there is more than 5° of natural tibial slope and if the posterior cruciate ligament is to be retained, the tibial slope can be increased. If the knee has a constitutional valgus, the preoperative plan may be modified by adding increased femoral valgus and femoral external rotation. Also less bone resection is performed from the tibia and/or distal femur.

Patient Setup

The robot is placed on the side of the operated extremity at approximately the level of the hip. The

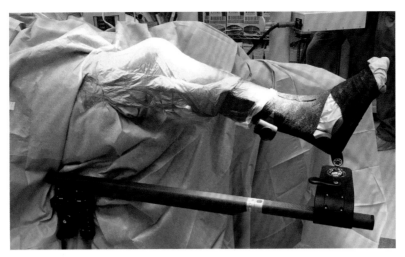

FIGURE 35-5 Stryker leg holder.

computer monitor and infrared camera are placed on the opposite side of the table. The operative leg can be draped free as with a typical total knee setup with or without a leg holder placed on the operating table. Alternatively, a specialized leg holder (Stryker Orthopedics) is attached to the distal end of the table on the side of the operated leg (**Fig. 35-5**). The lower third of the operating table is dropped down and the contralateral extremity is draped free and placed on a leg stirrup. This allows either the surgeon or assistant to stand between the lower extremities. Use of this specialized leg holder will also allow the use of self-retraining retractors (**Fig. 35-6**).

Surgical Exposure

The knee arthrotomy is performed per the surgeon's usual preferred technique. Osteophytes are not removed until after bone registration.

Tracker Array Placement

The femoral and tibial tracker arrays can be inserted either inside or outside the incision, depending on length of incision and surgeon's preference (**Fig. 35-6**). Two 3.2 mm pins arc drilled in place for each tracker array using the tibial or femoral stabilizers as guide. Bicortical stability is obtained. The stabilizers are kept in place to further stabilize the arrays. The intra-incisional femoral tracker pins are inserted at the metaphyseal/diaphyseal junction area at a 45° angle from anteromedial to posterolateral, parallel to the distal femoral joint surface. Extra-incisional femoral pins are placed in the distal diaphysis at a similar angle. The intra-incisional tibial tracker pins are inserted in the medial tibia metaphysis. The intra-incisional tibial pin placement may require modifying the saw handle placement for tibial bone cuts and pin removal before tibial stem preparation. The extra-incisional tibial pins are placed in tibial diaphysis just proximal to the mid tibia.

The clamps and arrays are attached to the pins, with the arrays angled slightly convergent. The knee is placed in extension and full flexion to verify that the arrays remain visible to the infrared camera.

Check point pins are inserted in the medial femoral and tibial metaphyses to be used to verify during the case that the tracker arrays have not moved.

Bone Registration

The center of femoral head rotation is registered by rotating the hip through increased circles. The blunt tip green probe is used to register the check points of the most medial and lateral aspects of the medial and lateral tibial malleoli, respectively. The blue probe is used to register the femur and tibia following the pattern noted on the monitor screen (**Fig. 35-7**). In areas of remaining cartilage, the sharp tip is placed through cartilage to bone. Registration accuracy is confirmed by placing the blue probe tip at large blue sphere locations.

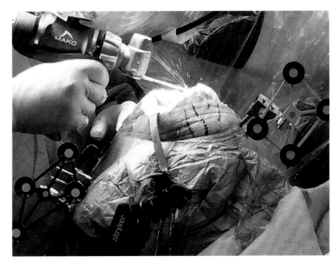

FIGURE 35-6 Self-retaining retractors in place attached to leg holder.

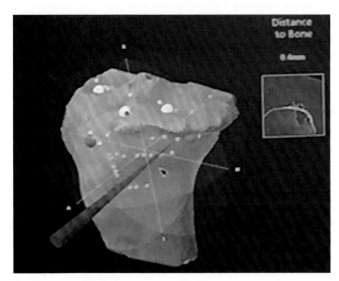

FIGURE 35-7 Bone registration points.

Pose Capture

The surgeon can eliminate this step, accept the component positions from preoperative planning, and proceed with bone cuts. However, use of an intraoperative gap balancing step is part of the power of using robotic assistance because it will assist in getting closer to ultimate soft tissue balance via component realignment and lessen the amount of soft tissue releases needed.

All exposed tibial and femoral osteophytes are removed. Varus and valgus stress is applied with the knee in 10° to 20° from full extension (**Fig. 35-8A**). The stressed medial and lateral gaps are recorded (**Fig. 35-8B**). Varus and valgus stress is applied at 90° of flexion. Accurate gaps may not be noted because resultant femoral rotation may make it difficult to maintain visualization of the tracker arrays. Alternatively, 1 mm increment spoons are inserted simultaneously to maximally distract the medial and lateral compartments. The flexion medial and lateral gaps are recorded. Ideally, the medial gaps should be equal in extension and flexion, with the lateral gaps equal to the medial gap in extension and 1 to 2 mm wider in flexion. If large osteophytes are still present medially on posterior femur or tibia, full distraction of the medial extension gap may not occur. In this situation, the extension gap medially is left 1 to 2 mm tighter than the medial flexion gap in anticipation of the medial extension gap increasing after these osteophytes are removed. Component position and alignment can be modified in the

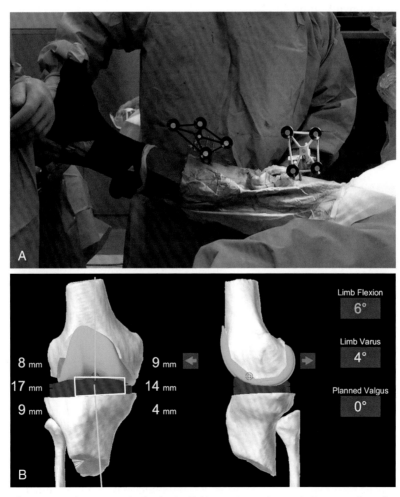

FIGURE 35-8 **A:** Application of varus or valgus stress to the knee. **B:** Varus stress demonstrates correction of medial gap in extension only to 14 mm and coronal alignment correction to 4° of mechanical varus.

preoperative plan to obtain the desired gap balance, as long as component and axial alignment is still within acceptable parameters. If the knee cannot be balanced by altering the component position within the preferred parameters, the need for soft tissue releases should be anticipated.

BONE CUTS PER MEASURED RESECTION TECHNIQUE

At this point the surgeon can proceed with a measured resection technique and make all the bone cuts or make a few bone cuts and utilize more gap balancing information before making the final bone cuts. A curved retractor is applied medially along the joint line to protect the medial collateral ligament. A curved retractor is placed along the lateral joint line during femoral cuts and a sharp tip retractor is placed over the anterolateral tibia to protect the patellar tendon especially during the tibial cut. All bone cuts are performed with the robotic-arm guiding the resection angles and the haptics limiting soft tissue injury. All remaining posterior osteophytes are removed. The posterior cruciate ligament is resected if the plan is for posterior stabilized components. Trial components are inserted and medial and lateral stressed gaps assessed near full extension and 90° of flexion while applying varus and valgus stress or by inserting 1 mm increment spoons. Use of an additional sensor tibial trial can be used to titrate soft tissue balance and assist with determining the amount of component realignment needed, but this is not a requisite component of robotic total knee arthroplasty.[46]

The knee can now be balanced with soft tissue releases only or by component repositioning. Alignment can be adjusted on the plan to balance the gaps medially in flexion and extension, and the lateral gap equal to the medial gap in extension and equal to or 2 mm wider in flexion. A tight posterior cruciate ligament can be managed with increasing tibial slope, a pie-crusting release and use of a cruciate substituting (CS) tibial liner, or resection and use of posterior-stabilized components. Component position and alignment changes are made as long as one's acceptable axial alignment parameters are maintained. The robotic arm is used to make new bone cuts following the haptic boundaries. The ability to do multiplanar bone recuts is unique to robotic assistance technology. Trial components are inserted again. If there is still imbalance present and component and axial alignment has been changed to the limits of the surgeon's acceptable parameters, soft tissue releases are then performed to balance the knee.

BONE CUTS PER TIBIAL CUT FIRST TECHNIQUE

The tibial cut is performed with robotic arm assistance. The tibial bone fragment is removed. This is easier to perform if the posterior cruciate ligament is excised. Posterior femoral osteophytes are removed. Laminar spreaders are

inserted in 90° of flexion to tension the flexion space. The patella should not be everted during this step. Ideally, the lateral flexion space should be equal to 1 to 2 mm looser than the medial flexion space. Femoral component rotation and/or tibial component alignment on the plan can be modified to obtain balance. Typical parameters for the acceptable range of femoral external rotation are between 3° of internal or external rotation from the transepicondylar line. Medial and lateral flexion gaps are recorded. Laminar spreaders are inserted with the knee near full extension to tension the extension space. The patella again should not be everted. Femoral component alignment and resection level are modified on the plan to equalize the medial flexion and extension gaps within the surgeon's acceptable component and axial alignment parameters. The remaining femoral bone cuts are made with robotic arm guidance. Trial components with or without a sensor tibial insert are inserted. If there is still imbalance to varus and valgus stress and maximum alignment changes have been made, soft tissue releases are performed. Usually these releases are minimal in comparison to releases that would have been needed if no component realignment was performed.

BONE CUTS PER TIBIAL CUT AND DISTAL FEMUR CUT FIRST TECHNIQUE

The tibial and distal femoral cuts are made with robotic arm assistance. The tibial bone fragment is removed in extension. Posterior femoral osteophytes are removed. There is a little more room to remove the tibial bone fragment and still retain the posterior cruciate ligament and remove posterior osteophytes with this technique. Laminar spreaders are inserted with the knee near full extension to tension the extension space. The patella should not be everted. If imbalance is present, the distal femoral or proximal tibial cut can be modified on the plan to equalize the extension gaps within the surgeon's acceptable component and axial alignment parameters. If there is still imbalance to varus and valgus stress and maximum alignment changes have been made, soft tissue releases are performed. Medial and lateral extension gaps are recorded. Laminar spreaders are inserted in 90° of flexion to tension the flexion space. The patella should not be everted. The medial flexion gap should be equal to the extension gap. Ideally, the lateral flexion space should be equal to 1 to 2 mm looser than the medial flexion space. Femoral component rotation and anteroposterior placement can be modified to obtain balance. The acceptable range of femoral external rotation is typically between 3° of internal or external rotation from the transepicondylar line. The remaining femoral cuts are made. Trial components are inserted with or without a sensor tibial insert. If there is still imbalance to varus and valgus stress and maximum alignment changes have been made, soft tissue releases are performed.

BONE CUTS PER FEMORAL CUTS FIRST TECHNIQUE

All femoral bone cuts are made based on modifications of the preoperative plan as a result of pose capture stressed gap information. Posterior tibial and femoral osteophytes are removed. Laminar spreaders are inserted with the knee near full extension to tension the extension space. The patella should not be everted. If imbalance is present, proximal tibial cut can be modified on the plan to equalize the extension gaps within the surgeon's acceptable component and axial alignment parameters. Medial and lateral extension gaps are recorded. Laminar spreaders are inserted in 90° of flexion to tension the flexion space. The patella should not be everted. The medial flexion gap should be equal to the medial extension gap. Ideally, the lateral flexion space should be equal to 1 to 2 mm looser than the medial flexion space. Tibial component slope can be adjusted on the plan to obtain balance. The tibial cut is made. Trial components with or without a sensor tibial insert are inserted. If there is still imbalance to varus and valgus stress and maximum alignment changes have been made, soft tissue releases are performed.

IMPLANTATION

The patellar bone resection and bone preparation for the femoral box, if posterior stabilized components are being used, is performed with standard instruments. Final components are implanted with or without cement. Final alignment and stressed medial and lateral extension and flexion gaps are recorded.

EARLY CLINICAL RESULTS

A review of the initial consecutive series of 100 robotic total knee replacements performed by the author using a semi-active haptic guided system demonstrated that the procedure is safe, reliable, and provides excellent clinical results.[47] Average follow-up was 1.54 years. Operative reports, 2, 6, 12 weeks, and yearly follow-up visit reports were reviewed and there were no inadvertent injuries to the medial collateral ligament, patellar tendon, or a neurovascular structure from the cutting tool. No cases were partially or completely aborted due to any issue. Review of outcome scores demonstrated an improvement in preoperative Knee Society Knee Scores and Knee Society Functional Scores of 44.7 and 50 to 98.1 and 87.8 at 1-year, 93.8 and 83.1 at 2-year, 98.5 and 87.7 at 3-years, and 99 and 85 at 4-year follow-up.

SUMMARY

Robotic arm assistance allows the surgeon to individualize and accurately align and place components to balance the patient's unique knee soft tissue envelope. As information is gathered about the patient's soft tissue balance, component position can be modified preoperatively using a CT-derived 3D virtual model, after initial arthrotomy and before any bone cuts are made, as well as intraoperatively after a few or all bone cuts are made. Femoral and tibial alignments achieved with robotic assistance are significantly more accurate than manual techniques.[32,35] The intraoperative alignment values are accurate when compared to postoperative radiographs,[48] so the surgeon can trust what effect component realignment will have on final alignment. Bone cuts with robotic arm assistance and haptic guidelines are safe and create less soft tissue damage than with standard instruments.[39-41] Preliminary data show a trend toward better function with knee balance performed with component realignment rather than with soft tissue balance alone.[49]

Clinical follow-up with this technology at this time is limited due to a short period of use. Compared to conventional total knee arthroplasty, one study has shown decreased pain, improved early function, and reduced hospital stay.[50] A 3-year review of the initial cases in the robotic arm total knee arthroplasty IDE study showed a Knee Society Knee Score of 98.8 and Knee Society Functional Score of 87.5.[51]

The capital cost of the robot and per case cost addition for CT scan, bone pins, and array pads is a hurdle for this technology to achieve universal acceptance as standard of care. However, economic models considering anticipated increased volume and improved outcomes with a decrease in manipulations and revisions will demonstrate surgical value.[52,53]

REFERENCES

1. Suda AJ, Seeger JB, Bitsch RG, et al. Are patients' expectations of hip and knee arthroplasty fulfilled? A prospective study of 130 patients. *Orthopedics*. 2010;33:76-80.
2. Bourne RB, Chesworth BM, Davis AM, et al. Patient satisfaction after total knee arthroplasty: who is satisfied and who is not? *Clin Orthop Relat Res*. 2010;468:57-63.
3. Fehring TK, Odum S, Griffin WL, et al. Early failures in total knee arthroplasty. *Clin Orthop Relat Res*. 2001;392:315-318.
4. Sharkey PF, Hozack WJ, Rothman RH, et al. Insall award paper: why are total knee arthroplasties failing today? *Clin Orthop Relat Res*. 2002;404:7-13.
5. Mulhall KJ, Ghomrawi HM, Scully S, et al. Current etiologies and modes of failure in total knee arthroplasty revision. *Clin Orthop Relat Res*. 2006;446:45-50.
6. Noble PC, Conditt MA, Cook KF, Mathis KB. The John Insall Award: patient expections affect satisfaction with total knee arthroplasty. *Clin Orthop Relat Res*. 2006;452:35.
7. Bellemens J, Colyn W, Vandenneucker H, Victor J. The Chitranjan Ranawat award: is neutral mechanical alignment normal for all patients? The concept of constitutional varus. *Clin Orthop Relat Res*. 2012;470:45-53.
8. Mahaluxmivala J, Bankes MJ, Nicolai P, et al. The effect of surgeon experience on component positioning in 673 press fit condylar posterior cruciate-sacrificing total knee arthroplasties. *J Arthroplasty*. 2001;16:635-640.
9. Petersen TL, Engh GA. Radiographic assessment of knee alignment after total knee arthroplasty. *J Arthroplasty*. 1988;3:67-72.
10. Delport H, Labey L, Innocenti B, et al. Restoration of constitutional alignment in TKA leads to more physiological strains in the collateral ligaments. *Knee Surg Sports Traumatol Arthrosc*. 2015;23:2159-2169.

11. Howell SM, Kuznik K, Hull ML, Siston RA. Results of an initial experience with custom-fit positioning total knee arthroplasty in a series of 48 patients. *Orthopedics*. 2008;31:857-863.
12. Almaawi AM, Hutt JRB, Masse V, et al. The impact of mechanical and restricted kinematic alignment on knee anatomy in total knee arthroplasty. *J Arthroplasty*. 2017;32:2133-2140.
13. Courtney PM, Lee G-C. Early outcomes of kinematic alignment in primary total knee arthroplasty: a meta-analysis of the literature. *J Arthroplasty*. 2017;32:2028-2032.
14. Gustke KA, Golladay GJ, Roche MW, et al. A new method for defining balance. Promising short-term clinical outcomes of sensor-guided TKA. *J Arthroplasty*. 2014;29:955-960.
15. Gustke K. Use of smart trials for soft-tissue balancing in total knee replacement surgery. *J Bone Joint Surg Br*. 2012;94(suppl A):147-150.
16. Gustke KA, Golladay GJ, Roche MW, et al. Primary TKA patients with quantifiably balanced soft-tissue achieve significant clinical gains sooner than unbalanced patients. *Adv Orthop*. 2014. doi:10.1155/2014/628695.
17. Gustke KA, Golladay GJ, Roche MW, et al. Increased satisfaction after total knee replacement using sensor-guided technology. *Bone Joint J*. 2014;96-B:1333-1338.
18. Krebs VE, Golladay MD, Gordon AC, et al. *Does a Balanced TKA Produce a More Forgotten Joint? Presented at the AAHKS Annual Meeting*. Dallas, Tx; 2017.
19. Hetaimish BM, Khan MM, Simunovic N, et al. Meta-analysis of navigation vs conventional total knee arthroplasty. *J Arthroplasty*. 2012;27:1177-1182.
20. Bolognesi M, Hofmann A. Computer navigation versus standard instrumentation for TKR. *Clin Orthop Relat Res*. 2005;440:162-169.
21. Haaker RG, Stockheim M, Kamp M, et al. Computer-assisted navigation increases precision of component placement in total knee arthroplasty. *Clin Orthop Relat Res*. 2005;433: 152-159.
22. Hutt JRB, LeBlanc MA, Masse V, et al. Kinematic TKA using navigation: surgical technique and initial results. *Orthop Traumatol Surg Res*. 2016;102:99-104.
23. Kim JH, Park JW, Kim JS. The clinical outcome of computer-navigated compared with conventional knee arthroplasty in the same patients: a prospective, randomized, double-blind, long-term study. *J Bone Joint Surg Am*. 2017;99:989-996.
24. Baumens K, Matthes G, Wich M, et al. Navigated total knee replacement. A meta-analysis. *J Bone Joint Surg*. 2007;89:261-269.
25. de Steiger RN, Liu YL, Graves SE. Computer navigation for total knee arthroplasty reduces revision rate for patients less than sixty-five years of age. *J Bone Joint Surg Am*. 2015;97:635-642.
26. Zambianchi F, Colombelli A, Digennaro V, et al. Assessment of patient-specific instrumentation precision through bone resection measurements. *Knee Surg Sports Traumatol Arthrosc*. 2017;25:2841-2848.
27. Stronach BM, Pelt CE, Erickson JA, Peters CL. Patient-specific instrumentation in total knee arthroplasty provides no improvement in component alignment. *J Arthroplasty*. 2014;29:1705-1708.
28. Victor J, Dujardin J, Vandenneucker H, et al. Patient-specific guides do not improve accuracy in total knee arthroplasty: a prospective randomized controlled trial. *Clin Orthop Relat Res*. 2014;472:263-271.
29. Stronach BM, Pelt CE, Erickson J, Peters CL. Patient-specific total knee arthroplasty required frequent surgeon-directed changes. *Clin Orthop Relat Res*. 2013;47:169-174.
30. Ollivier M, Tribot-Laspiere Q, Amzallag J, et al. Abnormal rate of intraoperative and postoperative implant positioning outliers using "MRI-based patient-specific" compared to "computer assisted" instrumentation in total knee replacement. *Knee Surg Sports Traumatol Arthrosc*. 2016;24:3441-3447.
31. Calliess T, Bauer K, Stukenborg-Colsman C, et al. PSI kinematic versus non-PSI mechanical alignment in total knee arthroplasty: a prospective, randomized study. *Knee Surg Sports Traumatol Arthrosc*. 2017;25:1743-1748.
32. Hampp EL, Chughtai M, Scholl LY, et al. Robotic-arm assisted total knee arthroplasty demonstrated greater accuracy and precision to plan compared with manual techniques. *J Knee Surg*. 2018;32(3):239-250. doi:10.1055/s-0038-1641729. [Epub ahead of print].
33. Urish KL, Conditt M, Roche M, Rubash HE. Robotic total knee arthroplasty: surgical assistant for a customized normal kinematic knee. *Orthopedics*. 2016;39:e822-827.
34. Sinha RK. Outcomes of robotic arm-assisted unicompartmental knee arthroplasty. *Am J Orthop*. 2009;38(2 suppl):20-22.
35. Citak M, Suero EM, Citak M, et al. Unicompartmental knee arthroplasty: is robotic technology more accurate than conventional technique? *Knee*. 2013;20:268-271.
36. Lonner JH, John TK, Conditt M. Robotic arm-assisted UKA improves tibial component alignment: a pilot study. *Clin Orthop Relat Res*. 2010;468:141-146.
37. Liow MH, Xia Z, Wong MK, Tay KJ, Yeo SJ, Chin PL. Robot-assisted total knee arthroplasty accurately restores the joint line and mechanical axis. A prospective randomized study. *J Arthroplasty*. 2014;29:2373-2377.
38. Bell SW, Anthony I, Jones B, MacLean A, Rowe R, Blyth M. Improved accuracy of component positioning with robotic-assisted unicompartmental knee arthroplasty: data from a prospective, randomized controlled study. *J Bone Joint Surg Am*. 2016;98: 627-635.
39. Conditt M, Gustke K, Coon T, et al. Intra-operative safety and early patient recovery in robotic arm assisted total knee arthroplasty. *Bone Joint J*. 2016;98-B(suppl.):49.
40. Khlopas A, Chughtai M, Hampp EL, et al. Robotic-arm assisted total knee arthroplasty demonstrated soft tissue protection. *Surg Technol Int*. 2017;30:441-446.
41. Kayani B, Konan S, Peitrzak JRT, Haddad FS. Iatrogenic bone and soft tissue trauma in robotic-arm assisted total knee arthroplasty compared with conventional jig-based total knee arthroplasty: a prospective cohort study and validation of a new classification system. *J Arthroplasty*. 2018;33:2496-2501.
42. Mettler FA, Jr, Huda W, Yoshizumi TT, Mahesh M. Effective doses in radiology and diagnostic nuclear medicine: a catalog. *Radiology*. 2008;248:254-263.
43. NRC Regulations Title 10, Code of Federal Regulations, Subpart C- Occupational Dose Limits, United States Nuclear Regulatory Commission.
44. Kwak DS, In Y, Kim TK, et al. The pie-crusting technique using a blade knife for medial collateral ligament release if unreliable in varus total knee arthroplasty. *Knee Surg Sports Traumatol Arthrosc*. 2016;24:188-194.
45. Meneghini RM, Daluga AT, Sturgis LA, Liebermann JR. Is the pie-crusting technique safe for MCL release in varus deformity correction in total knee arthroplasty? *J Arthroplasty*. 2013;28:1306-1309.
46. Gustke KA, Golladay GJ, Roche MW, et al. A targeted approach to ligament balancing using kinetic sensors. *J Arthroplasty*. 2017;32:2127-2132.
47. Gustke KA. *Robotic total knee arthroplasty with a semi-active haptic guided technique is safe and reliable. Presented at the International Society for Technology in Arthroplasty*. London, England; 2018.
48. Roche M, Law T, Vakharia R, et al. *Does intraoperative robotic arm assisted total knee arthroplasty alignment correlate with standing long leg postoperative alignment? Presented at the International Society of Technology in Arthroplasty Annual Meeting*. London, England; 2018.
49. Gustke KA. *Implant Realignment: an alternative to ligament release in TKR balancing. Presented at the International Society of Technology in Arthroplasty Annual Meeting*. London, England; 2018.

50. Kayani B, Konan S, Tahmassebi J, et al. Robotic-arm assisted total knee arthroplasty is associated with improved early functional recovery and reduced time to hospital discharge compared with conventional jig-based total knee arthroplasty. *Bone Joint J.* 2018;33:2496-2501.

51. Gustke KA. *Robotic total knee arthroplasty with a semi-active haptic guided technique is safe and reliable. Presented at the International Society of Technology in Arthroplasty Annual Meeting.* London, England; 2018.

52. Moschetti WE, Konopka JF, Rubash HE, Genuario JW. Can robotic-assisted unicompartmental knee arthroplasty be cost-effective? A Markov decision analysis. *J Arthroplasty.* 2016;31:759-765.

53. Jacofsky DJ, Allen M. Robotics in arthroplasty: a comprehensive review. *J Arthroplasty.* 2016;311:2353-2363.

chapter 36

A POSTERIOR CRUCIATE LIGAMENT RETENTION IN TOTAL KNEE REPLACEMENT

J. Joseph Gholson, MD I Brett R. Levine, MD, MS

Posterior cruciate ligament (PCL) retention in a well-balanced total knee arthroplasty (TKA) construct continues to be the standard by which other designs are compared. There is ongoing debate as to whether posterior cruciate–substituting or posterior cruciate–sacrificing designs provide improved kinematics and increased patient satisfaction. Proponents of PCL retention point to superior range of motion, strength, stability, and durability as reasons to spare the ligament in total knee replacement (TKR).[1] With similar enthusiasm, advocates of PCL substitution argue that resection eases exposure and correction of deformity, decreases polyethylene wear, and provides reliable sagittal plane stability.[2] Studies of both systems have demonstrated the long-term durability of PCL substitution and retention at 10 years (**Table 36A-1**), with many cohorts demonstrating 20-year survival of approximately 90%.[5-15] Furthermore, posterior cruciate retention in TKA allows for improved bone preservation, a smaller flexion gap secondary to maintaining the PCL, and the lowest long-term revision rates in registries for a multitude of implant designs. It is for these reasons that cruciate-retaining (CR) TKA continues to be a mainstay of TKA designs throughout the world. In this chapter, we review pertinent anatomy to CR TKA, discuss the kinematics of cruciate retention, address controversies in CR TKA, provide rationale for continued use of CR TKA over other designs, and describe our surgical technique for PCL-retaining TKA.

POSTERIOR CRUCIATE LIGAMENT ANATOMY

The PCL runs in a slightly oblique direction from the lateral aspect of the medial femoral condyle to the lateral aspect of the posterior intercondylar area of the tibia (**Fig. 36A-1**). The tibial insertion flares out for a distance of 2 cm below the articular surface. The broad, distal insertion makes PCL retention and balance during TKR feasible. Two anatomically inseparable bands comprise the PCL. A large anterolateral band tightens in flexion, and a smaller posteromedial band tightens in extension.[16] The anterior cruciate ligament (ACL) crosses in front of the PCL, running from the medial aspect of the lateral femoral condyle to the medial aspect of the anterior intercondylar area of the tibia. The synovium covers the anterior surface of the PCL and then fans out laterally onto the surface of the capsule.[17] Inflammatory arthritides such as rheumatoid

arthritis often spare the PCL because the synovium does not surround the ligament, making it an extrasynovial structure. In contrast, patients with rheumatoid arthritis often lack an ACL, as it is entirely surrounded by synovium.

KNEE KINEMATICS PERTAINING TO THE POSTERIOR CRUCIATE LIGAMENT

Bony contours provide little inherent stability to the knee. The lateral tibial plateau is convex in the sagittal and coronal planes. The medial tibial plateau is slightly larger than the lateral plateau and concave in both planes. Muscles, ligaments, and capsule combine to provide knee stability. Studies of sequential sectioning of the PCL reveal that in isolation the ligament has a limited role in providing varus/valgus and rotational stability.[18] The PCL plays a large role in preventing anterior/posterior translation of the tibia relative to the femur. Prosthetic designs must account for this stability through prosthetic geometry, a post-and-cam mechanism, or PCL retention.

A combination of rolling, sliding, and rotation occurs in normal knee motion. The synchrony of these motions depends on the articular contours of the tibia and femur, menisci, capsular structures, and an intact ACL/PCL in the nondiseased native knee. During the first 30° of knee flexion, motion occurs predominantly from rolling of the tibial and femoral surfaces relative to one another. As the knee further flexes, tightening of the PCL leads to sliding at the articular interface. This sliding, also referred to as *femoral rollback*, prevents impingement of the posterior surface of the tibia and femur during maximal flexion and allows flexion of approximately 140° in the nondiseased knee. The convex lateral tibial plateau allows more sliding than the more conforming, concave surface of the medial plateau. This creates an obligatory internal rotation of the tibia relative to the femur with knee flexion. Femoral rollback also lengthens the moment arm and improves the direction of pull of the quadriceps, which increases the strength of the quadriceps as the knee flexes.[19]

EVOLUTION OF THE CRUCIATE-RETAINING TOTAL KNEE REPLACEMENT

In the early 1970s, many different prosthetic knee designs were being used. Early hinge designs suffered many early and late complications, including infection

TABLE 36A-1 Long-Term Follow-Up to Cruciate-Retaining Total Knee Replacement

Study	Prosthesis	Manufacturer	No. of Patients/ Knees	Average Follow-Up (y)	Mean Age (y)	Osteoarthritis (%)	Rheumatoid Arthritis (%)	10-y Survivorship	Infection (%)	Radiographic Lucent Lines (%)	Instability (%)	Reoperation/ Revision Other than Infection (%)
Dennis et al[30]	Posterior cruciate condylar	Howmedica	35/42	11	62.8	50	50	N/A	0	75	2.3	4.7
Schai et al[31]	Press-Fit Condylar	Johnson & Johnson	122/155	10.5	68	62	33	90	1.2	Tibia 16 Femur 3 Patella 3	0	13.5
Berger et al[5]	Miller-Galante II	Zimmer	92/109	9	72	94.4	4.6	100	2.8	Tibia 13 Femur 11 Patella 1.4	0	1.8
Parker et al[6]	Miller-Galante I	Zimmer	67/67	12.8	66	100	0	90	6	N/A	0	52
Gill and Joshi[7]	Kinematic condylar	Howmedica	177/216	10.1	68	88	11	98.2	1	Femur 4.5 Tibia 8.3 Patella 4	0.5	3
Buechel et al[8]	Low contact stress (LCS) meniscal bearing	DePuy Orthopaedics	116/140	12.3	65	89	6.5	100	0.7	Femur 0 Tibia 6.6 Patella 0	0.7	5.7
Ritter et al[9]	Anatomic graduated components	Biomet	3054/4583	N/A	70.4	87	N/A	98	1.3	N/A	N/A	N/A
Sextro et al[10]	Kinematic condylar	Howmedica	118/168	15.7	65.2	64.9	31	96.5	1.2	N/A	0.6	7.7

N/A, not available.

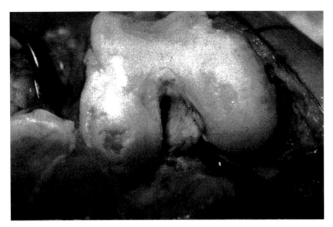

FIGURE 36A-1 Dissection of the posterior cruciate ligament during total knee replacement. Note the robust nature of the posterior cruciate ligament passing from the lateral aspect of the intercondylar notch to the posterior tibia.

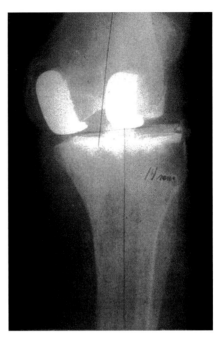

FIGURE 36A-2 Early resurfacing total knee replacement (Marmor) demonstrating lateral subluxation of the tibia on the femur.

and loosening, which made their routine use unacceptable. Early resurfacing knee replacements included the polycentric (1970), modular (1972), UCI (1972), McKeever (1960), Geometric (1971), and Duocondylar (1973). These surface replacement designs relied on intact native ligaments and capsule to provide knee stability. These prostheses consisted of medial and/or lateral polyethylene tibial components that were separate or connected by a small bar. Early techniques preserved both cruciate ligaments and made no provision for the patellofemoral joint. The conformity of the articulation of early TKAs varied based on the designer's philosophy. Less conforming articulations attempted to simulate normal knee rollback and motion (polycentric and Duocondylar). Other designs focused on stability and provided more congruent femoral and tibial articular surfaces (Geometric). Problems of tibial subsidence and loosening, patellofemoral pain, and lateral subluxation of the tibia on the femur complicated these early designs (**Fig. 36A-2**).[20-23]

Modern total knee designs reflect the lessons learned from the shortcomings of early resurfacing knee replacements. These include a one-piece metal condylar femoral component with a trochlear flange, a one-piece metal-backed or all-polyethylene tibial component, and resurfacing of the patella with an all-polyethylene component. From these early condylar designs emerged two schools of thought, namely, preservation or sacrifice of the PCL. The latter school, recognizing limited flexion in early cruciate-sacrificing designs and the advantage of femoral rollback and improved patellofemoral mechanics, evolved into cruciate substitution by the addition of a central polyethylene eminence on the tibial component. This eminence engaged in mid-flexion (60° to 80°) to achieve these goals.

Advocates of cruciate sacrifice/substitution developed the total condylar prosthesis in 1973 in response to their experience with the Duocondylar TKR (**Fig. 36A-3**).[24]

This design provided a femoral component with an anterior femoral flange and allowed patellar resurfacing. The tibial component was a one-piece all-polyethylene component that necessitated sacrifice of the PCL. The total condylar prosthesis proved durable and gave reliable results.[25,26] Limitations of this prosthesis related to range of motion and posterior subluxation of the tibia relative to the femur. To overcome these shortcomings, the posterior-stabilized (PS) total knee was introduced in 1978. These devices possess built-in posterior constraint and achieved femoral rollback by a post-and-cam mechanism. Numerous authors have subsequently reported excellent results with PS designs.[27]

Over the same time frame, advocates of CR designs of TKR grew as a result of the limitations these surgeons experienced with the Duocondylar, McKeever, Modular, and other early knee replacements.[20,28] One

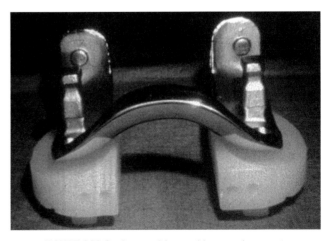

FIGURE 36A-3 Duocondylar total knee replacement.

example of an early PCL-retaining design, the Duo-Patellar, evolved from experience with the Duocondylar TKR. Implantation of the Duo-Patellar prosthesis at the Robert Breck Brigham Hospital began in 1974.[3] The femoral component provided an anterior flange to facilitate patellar tracking. The initial tibial component consisted of separate medial and lateral tibial pieces and allowed for ACL and PCL retention. The tibial contour changed from flat in the sagittal plane to a curved surface to increase articular constraint. The Duo-Patellar was redesigned in 1978 to a one-piece tibial component with a stem to better distribute weight-bearing forces (**Fig. 36A-4**).[4] This tibial component mandated sacrifice of the ACL but maintained a cutout for preservation of the PCL.

Over the next 7 years, gradual refinement of the femoral, tibial, and patellar components occurred and the Duo-Patellar evolved into Robert Breck Brigham Hospital and Kinematic total knee systems.[29] The goals of these prostheses were to increase range of motion, improve fixation of the tibial component, and maintain the overall excellent clinical results of the previous designs. The trochlear groove of the femoral component was deepened and aligned in 7° of valgus to improve patellar tracking. In 1980, the tibial component changed to a metal-backed design and reverted to a flattened surface in the sagittal plane to allow rollback. Femoral and tibial intramedullary stems were made available for situations of bone deficiency. Experience with the Kinematic total knee continued the clinical success of previous designs and taught valuable lessons on axial alignment, component position, and cementing technique.[23,30]

Advocates of cruciate retention remained concerned about a kinematic conflict if a conforming polyethylene surface directed motion antagonistic to the strong intact PCL. Moreover, cruciate tension was variable and difficult to match with tibiofemoral conformity. This concern led to the development of flat-on-flat cruciate-sparing designs. Unfortunately, these designs did not compensate for the abduction/adduction moments during gait and caused edge loading and polyethylene wear. Additionally, if the PCL was too tight, there was abnormal rollback and posterior polyethylene wear; if the PCL was too loose, random contact leading to abnormal shear stresses and even paradoxical roll forward occurred during flexion.

Recognizing the concerns of kinematic conflict and the problems of flat-on-flat designs, a new direction to cruciate retention was introduced. The Press-Fit Condylar (PFC) design incorporated different tibial contact patterns (posterior-lipped and curved) to accommodate for different cruciate tensions (**Fig. 36A-5**). Balancing the PCL by recession from either the tibia or femur allowed cruciate retention while accommodating sufficient conformity to allow low contact stress. In a series of patients from our institution who had posterior CR TKR with the PFC system, Schai et al found no tibial or femoral loosening at a minimum of 10-year follow-up.[31] Similarly, Buehler et al had 98.7% survivorship with posterior cruciate retention with the PFC system at 9-year follow-up.[32] The PFC modular cruciate-substituting design was introduced, thus coupling the PCL-retention and PCL-substituting philosophies. In 1996, the PFC Sigma design was introduced as a merged philosophy to allow smooth transition

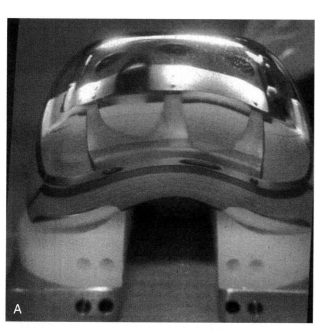
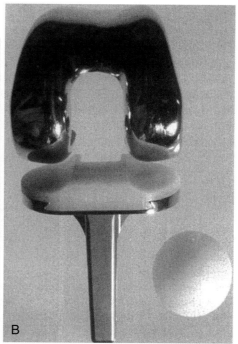

FIGURE 36A-4 **A:** Duo-Patellar total knee replacement. **B:** Design change with one-piece, stemmed tibial component.

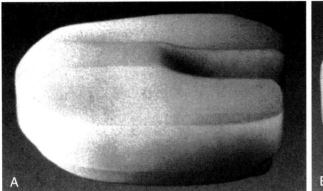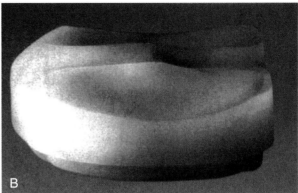

FIGURE 36A-5   A: Posterior-lipped polyethylene insert. **B:** Curved polyethylene insert.

between cruciate retention and substitution, expand revision capabilities, and eliminate gamma-radiated polyethylene sterilized in air. Since that time, multiple CR designs have incorporated a more conforming polyethylene with improved kinematics, range of motion, and excellent survivorship.

CURRENT CONTROVERSIES IN POSTERIOR CRUCIATE LIGAMENT–RETAINING AND POSTERIOR CRUCIATE LIGAMENT–SUBSTITUTING TOTAL KNEE REPLACEMENT

Rollback and Kinematics

Neither the cruciate-retaining nor cruciate-substituting knee can reproduce the kinematics of the normal knee. In fact, the unique aspects of the knee with the material properties of the articular cartilage, the cruciate ligaments, and the medial and lateral menisci confer very different properties than seen in metal-to-plastic condylar designs. Meniscal-bearing and rotating-platform knees attempt to more closely mimic normal knees but fall short of this goal. Most meniscal-bearing designs demonstrate paradoxical motion, whereas rotating-platform designs rotate about a fixed central axis rather than accomplishing the complex motion that occurs in the normal knee. It was originally believed that with proper conformity or mobile-bearing designs, normal kinematics could be achieved.

Recent fluoroscopic and gait laboratory data have contrasted with these early beliefs.[33-35] Fluoroscopic studies demonstrate that cruciate-retaining and cruciate-substituting designs fail to reproduce normal rollback. Strain-gauge studies also demonstrate the inability of TKR to reproduce normal ligament strain behavior.[36] As these studies would predict, clinical comparisons show little difference in range of motion achieved in either design.[37-41] Similarly, difference in quadriceps efficiency and stair-climbing ability also appears equivocal in cruciate-retaining and cruciate-substituting devices.[42,43] Excellent

clinical results and range of motion can be achieved with the use of recession to balance the PCL in conjunction with more conforming polyethylene inserts.[44-47]

At the present time, clinical and laboratory data fail to produce a clear advantage for PCL retention or substitution with regard to achieving femoral rollback or quadriceps function. Both designs produce predictable functional range of motion and clinical results.

Wear and Loosening

In the past, proponents of cruciate retention have argued that an intact PCL would decrease wear and loosening. The native PCL would theoretically act to absorb shear forces.[1] If this biologic structure for absorption was lost, the anterior–posterior shear forces would reroute through the metal–polyethylene and bone–cement interface, leading to a higher rate of wear and loosening.

Reports of excessive polyethylene wear in the literature focusing on CR designs contrast with this theoretical benefit of PCL retention.[48-50] Most of these cases of polyethylene failure, however, involve flat-on-flat articulations subject to edge loading and high contact stresses if the PCL is not properly balanced.[51,52] These failures also occurred at a time in the evolution of TKR in which thin tibial inserts with heat-pressed polyethylene were used.

More conforming articulations in conjunction with retention of the PCL have not had this high rate of wear.[30,53] Improved polyethylene and focus on balancing the PCL should minimize these wear failures in CR designs.[45,46] Polyethylene wear has not proved to be a major problem in cruciate-substituting designs in long-term follow-up.[27] Aseptic loosening is an uncommon phenomenon in cruciate-sacrificing, cruciate-sparing, and cruciate-substituting designs in long-term follow-up.[53-55]

Range of Motion

A number of studies have found conflicting results when comparing range of motion between CR and PS

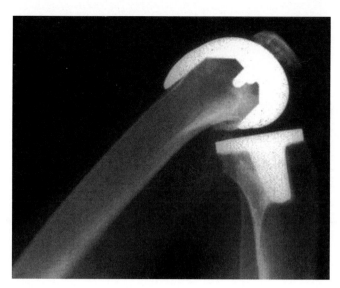

FIGURE 36A-6 This radiograph of a cruciate-retaining total knee replacement after posterior cruciate ligament recession demonstrates flexion.

knees, with some recent studies finding greater range of motion when a similar implant is used with a CR insert over a PS insert.[56] However, a recent meta-analysis and systematic review found slight improvement in range of motion with PS knees,[57,58] though the clinical significance of this small improvement is unclear. It is most likely that when the TKA designs are the same, and only the insert is varied between CR and PS, the range of motion is similar.[59-61] Regardless, both CR and PS designs have been found to have similarly excellent range of motion after well-performed and balanced TKA (**Fig. 36A-6**).

Proprioception

Retention of mechanoreceptors within the PCL has been used as an argument to retain the PCL. Theoretically this could improve knee proprioception and provide a more "normal-feeling" knee. Most authors agree that arthritic conditions lead to histologic changes within the ligament and significantly alter proprioception.[62,63] The hope that TKA could restore normal joint proprioception is unrealistic. Attempts to evaluate proprioception in knee arthroplasty patients reveal improvement in proprioception after implantation. These studies, however, do not indicate a clear advantage for cruciate-retaining or cruciate-substituting designs with regard to proprioception.[37,64,65]

Stability

Retention of the PCL provides anteroposterior stability for the knee. Less conforming polyethylene inserts used in conjunction with PCL retention require an intact PCL to provide this stability. Numerous authors report either flexion or extension instability if the PCL is not properly balanced or late rupture occurs.[66-69] This is a rare complication even in the rheumatoid patient.[70,71] Cruciate-substituting knee replacement relies on a post-and-cam mechanism to provide anterior and posterior stability. This design requires careful balancing of the flexion and extension gaps to prevent dislocation of the post. Moreover, cam engagement can lead to peg wear or back-sided wear in metal-backed tibial components.[72,73] Regardless of the design used for TKR, careful balancing of the soft tissues is required to avoid these pitfalls. Both cruciate-retaining and cruciate-substituting designs of TKR provide reliable stability in the sagittal plane if properly balanced.

AUTHORS' ARGUMENTS FOR POSTERIOR CRUCIATE LIGAMENT RETENTION

Balancing Flexion and Extension Gaps

Advocates of PCL substitution argue that resecting the PCL eases exposure and facilitates balancing the flexion and extension spaces.[74] In our experience, the PCL acts as a tether for the flexion space. If the PCL is resected, only the posterior capsule balances the flexion space. The posterior capsule is subject to late attenuation. Retaining the tether of the PCL eases balance of the flexion space and prevents attenuation of the posterior capsule and subsequent late instability or peg wear.

The broad, long medial collateral ligament running from the femur to the tibia tethers the medial side of the knee. In contrast, the lateral side of the knee is restrained by the less robust, round lateral collateral ligament running from the femur to the fibula. The PCL helps balance these disparate structures, serving as a checkrein to the lateral aspect of the medial compartment of the knee.

Bone Sparing

We submit that PCL retention is bone sparing, which eases management of the femur in the revision setting. Retaining the PCL allows one to retain the intercondylar bone. If the PCL is resected, the flexion gap increases. The surgeon must resect a commensurate increase in distal femur to balance this increased flexion gap. Thus, the amount of distal femur that must be resected in a PCL-retaining TKR is less than in a substituting design.

Patellar Clunk and Post Dislocation

The PCL provides anterior and posterior stability in CR designs. In contrast, a post-and-cam mechanism affords stability in this plane in cruciate-substituting TKR. This post may dislocate in the improperly balanced knee.[75,76]

The complication of patellar clunk is also associated with cruciate-substituting designs of TKR.[77] Although more recent designs limit these complications, the use of CR TKR avoids these problems altogether without adversely affecting patellar tracking. Recent reports of TKR with PCL retention have a very low rate of patellofemoral complications with a low incidence of lateral release.[5-7,9,10,32]

Ease of Management of Supracondylar Femur Fractures

Fractures of the distal femur above a TKR are an uncommon but difficult-to-treat complication.[78,79] With PCL-sparing TKR, it is easier to manage a supracondylar femur fracture. Intramedullary nailing of these fractures is possible without the closed box present in cruciate-substituting designs. Recent innovations with supracondylar rods, however, have eased this problem. Moreover, the lack of a box in the intercondylar notch provides a larger area for screw purchase when distal femoral periarticular plates are used for fracture fixation.

Avoidance of Peg Wear and Fracture

Recent studies have shown peg wear can be a problem in poorly balanced cruciate-substituting knees.[72,73] If the soft tissues are not balanced in flexion, the anterior translocation of the femur is stopped by the polyethylene eminence, leading to posterior peg wear. If the posterior capsule is not tightened, or if the tibial component is significantly sloped posteriorly, component hyperextension will occur, leading to anterior peg wear. Moreover, any rotational mismatch or increased rotation between the components due to soft-tissue balance can lead to rotational peg wear and fracture. Any of these constraining forces will also lead to back-sided wear when metal-backed tibial components are used.

Assessing differences in back-sided wear between cruciate-retaining and cruciate-substituting designs is difficult. Very few studies address the issue of back-sided wear, and confounding variables make comparisons of different systems impossible. In Schai and colleague's follow-up at 10 years with the PFC CR design, however, no osteolysis was noted.[31]

Survivorship

Recent studies of registry databases have demonstrated improved survivorship of CR implants over PS designs, particularly for CR on highly cross-linked polyethylene designs.[80] After controlling for patient and surgeon variables, a series out of the Australian Orthopaedic Association Registry found a 45% higher risk of revision when using a PS implant compared to a CR implant over a 13-year period.[81] Similarly, a study out of the Dutch

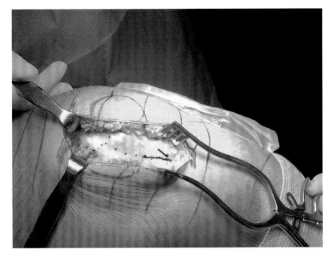

FIGURE 36A-7   Location of low-midvastus arthrotomy is marked.

Arthroplasty Registry found PS TKA patients were 1.5 times more likely to require a revision within 8 years of TKA compared to matched patients having CR TKA.[82] These studies support the use of CR TKA over PS TKA, with decreased constraint resulting in improved implant survival.

SURGICAL TECHNIQUE

Retaining the PCL does not pose a hindrance to operative exposure. A vertical midline incision is made, extending from the distal femur to just medial to the tibial tubercle, followed by a medial parapatellar incision in the capsule or a low midvastus incision (**Fig. 36A-7**). The knee is then flexed, the patella is subluxated, and the ACL and anterior horns of the menisci are resected. Next, a subperiosteal medial release of the proximal tibia using electrocautery or sharp dissection is directed beneath the medial collateral ligament at the joint line into the semimembranosus bursa (**Fig. 36A-8**). The medial dissection is tailored to the degree and type of deformity. A larger, more extensive dissection is performed for varus deformity, with minimal dissection performed for valgus deformity. This medial dissection combined with resection of any ACL remnant allows the proximal tibia to be externally rotated and subluxated anterior to the femur, aiding exposure and relaxation of the patellar tendon. Next, the posterior horns of the menisci are removed, and a PCL retractor facilitates displacing the tibia anteriorly. This sequence provides excellent exposure for the bony cuts whether the tibia or femur is initially prepared (**Fig. 36A-9**).

With PCL-retaining designs, it is not important whether the tibia or femur is cut first as long as measured resection with restoration of the native joint line is performed. For the tibial cut, a central reference point of the proximal tibia is marked at the junction of the medial one-third and lateral two-thirds of the tibial tubercle. Although

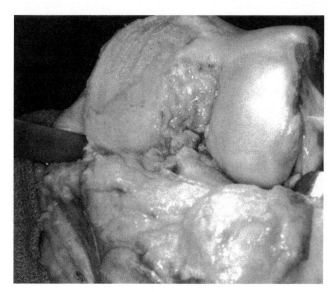

FIGURE 36A-8 An osteotome is passed beneath the medial collateral ligament and into the semimembranosus bursa for medial dissection.

optional, a triangular or square bony block is outlined with an osteotome anterior to the PCL to protect the ligament during tibial resection. The PCL inserts distally on the tibia so that proximal tibial resection is possible without injuring the ligament. The proximal cut is made to retain as much proximal tibia as possible, cutting to a depth equal to the anticipated thickness of the prosthetic tibial component with a few degrees of posterior slope in the sagittal plane. The largest tibial component without overhang is used.

An intramedullary guide is used for the femoral bony cut, typically in 5° to 7° of valgus. Valgus knees are cut in no more than 5° of femoral valgus. Care is taken to ensure the anterior femoral cortex is not notched. Cuts are again based on anatomic considerations, with every

attempt made to restore the joint line. The distal cut falls just distal to the PCL insertion on the lateral aspect of the medial femoral condyle. In the varus knee the distal cut will leave an intact bridge between the medial and lateral condylar resections. In contrast, the distal cut in the valgus knee usually leaves independent medial and lateral condylar resections due to the deficient lateral femoral condyle. Rotational alignment of the femoral component is based on a combination of the epicondylar axis, anteroposterior axis (Whiteside line), the posterior femoral condyles, and our previous tibial cut.[83,84] Great care must be taken in the valgus knee, as referencing from the deficient posterolateral femoral condyle will cause a relative internal rotation of the femoral component, adversely affecting patellar tracking.

Patellar thickness is assessed and the patella resurfaced with a thickness of polyethylene equivalent to the amount of bone resected. A patellar cutting guide or freehand technique may be used for this cut. The patellar cut should pass through the chondral–osseous junction both medially and laterally with complete resection of the medial and lateral facets. Proximally the cut passes just superficial to the quadriceps insertion and distally passes through the nose of the patella. No remnant cartilage should remain after adequate patellar resection.

With the trial components in place, a trial reduction is performed (**Fig. 36A-10**). The collateral ligaments should balance on both the medial and lateral sides through a full range of motion. Medial tightness is relieved by further subperiosteal dissection of the superficial medial collateral ligament when necessary. The iliotibial band is initially released with the knee in full extension in a piecrust fashion for lateral tightness. Although rarely necessary, further lateral release is achieved by

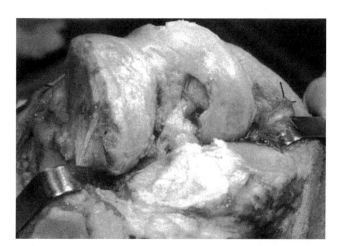

FIGURE 36A-9 Excellent exposure for bony cuts of the femoral and tibial surfaces with the posterior cruciate ligament intact is obtained after release of the patellofemoral ligaments, medial dissection, anterior cruciate ligament resection, and removal of remnant menisci.

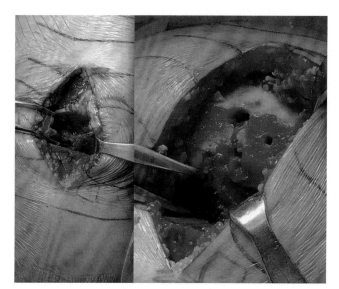

FIGURE 36A-10 Before trial reduction, laminar spreaders can be used to tension the medial and lateral soft tissues to assess balance in both flexion and extension.

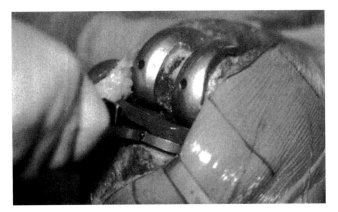

FIGURE 36A-11 Pullout/liftoff test. In 90° of flexion, the surgeon should not be able to pull out the tibial tray and there should be no liftoff of the anterior tibial tray.

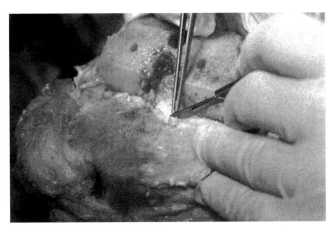

FIGURE 36A-12 An excessively tight posterior cruciate ligament is released from the posterior tibia.

subperiosteal dissection of the lateral structures from the epicondyle.

In many knees, the PCL will need to be recessed to accommodate a more conforming tibial polyethylene insert to increase contact area. Alternatively, some systems provide less conforming inserts suitable for low-demand patients, obviating the need for PCL recession. An initial release is achieved by peeling the PCL attachment off the retained tibial spine or removing the tibial spine at the level of the tibial cut. After this initial release, PCL tension is checked with the knee flexed 90°. In this position, the femoral component should articulate with the middle one-third of the polyethylene on the medial side of the knee. If the PCL is too tight and excessive rollback occurs, the posterior lip of the tibial insert riding on the posterior femoral condyle will cause the anterior aspect of the tibial tray to lift off the tibia as the knee is flexed.[85] To ensure that the PCL and flexion gap are tight enough, the surgeon should not be able to pull out the tibial tray with its handle in place at 90° of flexion (**Fig. 36A-11**).[86] The surgeon can also palpate the PCL with the components in place and the ligament should be compressible but not excessively taught and rigid.

If the PCL remains tight after the initial release, the ligament can be further released from the posterior aspect of the tibia (**Fig. 36A-12**).[1,47] Alternatively, the ligament may be released from the distal femoral attachment to selectively release tight bundles (usually the anterolateral bundle).[23] If liftoff continues in spite of these releases and the ligament is not too tight to palpation, impingement may occur between the posterior lip of the polyethylene insert and retained posterior femoral osteophytes (**Fig. 36A-13**). These osteophytes should be excised (**Fig. 36A-14**).

Patellar tracking is observed without the medial capsule sutured or clamped. As the knee flexes, the patella should remain within the trochlea without manual stabilization—"no touch technique."[23] Good contact between the medial facet of the patella and medial femoral condyle

should be maintained as the knee is flexed. If the patella dislocates, subluxates, or tilts laterally, a lateral release should be performed. This release is performed with the knee extended with slight valgus stress. The synovium and lateral retinaculum are incised in a longitudinal fashion from the joint line extending superiorly proximal to the patella. The lateral superior genicular vessels are identified at the inferior margin of the vastus lateralis and protected during the release.

After assessment of medial/lateral balance, PCL tension, and patellar tracking, all bony surfaces are irrigated with pulsatile lavage and dried. Cementing is performed in the sequence of tibia followed by the femur. The knee is then extended, with the final polyethylene insert in place. With the knee in extension for compression on the tibial and femoral components, the patellar component is cemented in place. A careful inspection for loose cement and debris is undertaken and the tourniquet released. After careful hemostasis and thorough irrigation, the knee is closed with the capsule, subcutaneous layers, and skin layers closed independently (**Fig. 36A-14**).

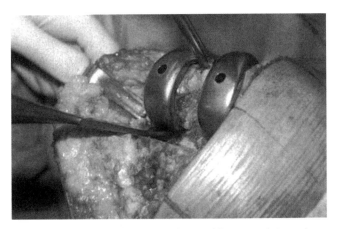

FIGURE 36A-13 Excision of posterior condylar osteophytes using a curved osteotome.

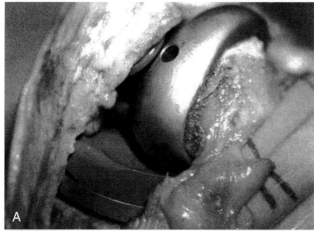

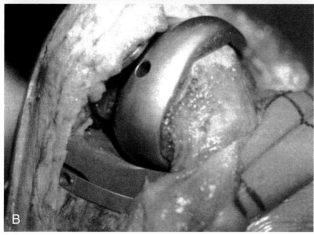

FIGURE 36A-14 A: Excessive femoral rollback and liftoff of the anterior tibial tray occur if the posterior cruciate ligament is too tight. **B:** After posterior cruciate ligament recession and removal of osteophytes, there is normal rollback and no anterior liftoff.

CONCLUSION

The published results of PCL-retaining and PCL-substituting TKR are identical. During the 1980s, PCL-retaining designs kept poor company with flat-on-flat tibial articulations, metal-backed patellae, indiscriminate uncemented fixation, and heat-pressed polyethylene.[4,47,58,87] These factors, combined with techniques that stressed bone cuts while ignoring important soft tissues, led to the misconception that PCL substitution was superior to PCL retention. Current techniques with proper soft-tissue balancing, PCL recession as necessary, and use of a curved polyethylene insert yield excellent long-term clinical results. The major benefits of PCL retention over other designs include improved bone preservation, a smaller flexion gap, and lower long-term revision rates.

ACKNOWLEDGMENTS

We would like to sincerely thank the authors of the previous edition of this chapter, Dr. Creg A. Carpenter and Dr. Thomas S. Thornhill, whose excellent original chapter from the first edition required only limited updating.

REFERENCES

1. Barnes CL, Sledge CB. Total knee arthroplasty with posterior cruciate ligament retention designs. In: Insall JN, Windsor RE, Scott WN, eds. *Surgery of the Knee.* 2nd ed. New York: Churchill Livingstone; 1993:815-827.
2. Freeman MAR, Railton GT. Should the posterior cruciate ligament be retained or resected in condylar nonmeniscal knee arthroplasty: the case for resection. *J Arthroplasty.* 1988;3:83.
3. Thomas WH. Duopatellar total knee arthroplasty. *Orthop Trans.* 1980;4:329.
4. Scott RD. Duopatellar total knee replacement: the Brigham experience. *Orthop Clin North Am.* 1982;13:89-102.
5. Berger RA, Rosenberg AG, Barden RM, et al. Long-term followup of the Miller-Galante total knee replacement. *Clin Orthop.* 2001;388:58-67.
6. Parker DA, Rorabeck CH, Boume RB. Long-term followup of cementless versus hybrid fixation for total knee arthroplasty. *Clin Orthop.* 2001;388:68-76.
7. Gill GS, Joshi AB. Long-term results of Kinematic Condylar knee replacement. *J Bone Joint Surg Br.* 2001;83:355-358.
8. Buechel FF Sr, Buechel FF Jr, Pappas MJ. Twenty year evaluation of meniscal bearing and rotating platform knee replacements. *Clin Orthop.* 2001;388:41-50.
9. Ritter MA, Berend ME, Meding JB, et al. Long term followup of anatomic graduated components posterior cruciate-retaining total knee replacement. *Clin Orthop.* 2001;388:51-57.
10. Sextro GS, Berry DJ, Rand JA. Total knee arthroplasty using cruciate retaining kinematic condylar prosthesis. *Clin Orthop.* 2001;388:33-40.
11. Laskin RS. The Genesis total knee prosthesis: a ten year followup study. *Clin Orthop.* 2001;388:95-102.
12. Pavone V, Boettner F, Fickert S, et al. Total condylar knee arthroplasty: a long term followup. *Clin Orthop.* 2001;388:18-25.
13. Callaghan JJ, Beckert MW, Hennessy DW, Goetz DD, Kelley SS. Durability of a cruciate-retaining TKA with modular tibial trays at 20 years. *Clin Orthop Relat Res.* 2013;471(1):109-117. doi:10.1007/s11999-012-2401-9.
14. Patil S, McCauley JC, Pulido P, Colwell CW. How do knee implants perform past the second decade? Nineteen- to 25-year followup of the press-fit condylar design TKA. *Clin Orthop Relat Res.* 2015;473(1):135-140. doi:10.1007/s11999-014-3792-6.
15. Ma H-M, Lu Y-C, Ho F-Y, Huang C-H. Long-term results of total condylar knee arthroplasty. *J Arthroplasty.* 2005;20(5):580-584. doi:10.1016/j.arth.2005.04.006.
16. Grigis FG, Marshall JL, Monajem ARS. The cruciate ligaments of the knee. *Clin Orthop.* 1975;106:216-231.
17. Williams PL, Warwick R, eds. *Gray's Anatomy.* 36th ed. Philadelphia: WB Saunders; 1980.
18. Gollehan DL, Torzilli PA, Warren RF. The role of the posterolateral and cruciate ligaments in the stability of the knee: a biomechanical study. *J Bone Joint Surg Am.* 1987;69:233-242.
19. Andriacchi TP, Galante JO. Retention of the posterior cruciate in total knee arthroplasty. *J Arthroplasty.* 1988;3(Suppl):S13-S19.
20. Ewald FC, Scott RD, Thomas WH, et al. The importance of intercondylar stability in knee arthroplasty: comparison of McKeever, modular and duocondylar types. *J Bone Joint Surg Am.* 1975;57:1033.
21. Gunston FH, MacKenzie RJ. Complications of polycentric knee arthroplasty. *Clin Orthop.* 1976;120:11.
22. Ilstrup DM, Coventry MB, Skolnick MD. A statistical evaluation of geometric total knee arthroplasties. *Clin Orthop.* 1976;120:27.
23. Scott RD, Volatile TB. Twelve years' experience with posterior cruciate retaining total knee arthroplasty. *Clin Orthop.* 1986;205:100-107.
24. Ranawat CS, Insall J, Shine J. Duocondylar knee arthroplasty: hospital for special surgery design. *Clin Orthop.* 1976;120:76.
25. Ranawat CS, Flynn WF, Saddler S, et al. Long-term results of the total condylar knee arthroplasty: a 15 year survivorship study. *Clin Orthop.* 1993;286:94-102.

26. Vince KG, Insall JN, Kelly MA. The total condylar prosthesis: 10- to 12-year results of a cemented knee replacement. *J Bone Joint Surg Br.* 1989;71:793-797.

27. Colizza WA, Insall JN, Scuderi GR. The posterior stabilized total knee prosthesis: assessment of polyethylene damage and osteolysis after a ten year-minimum follow-up. *J Bone Joint Surg Am.* 1995;77:1713-1720.

28. Sledge CB, Stern PJ, Thomas WH, et al. Two-year follow-up of the Duocondylar total knee replacement. *Orthop Trans.* 1978;2:193.

29. Ewald FC, Jacobs MA, Miegel RE, et al. Kinematic total knee replacement. *J Bone Joint Surg Am.* 1984;66:1032-1040.

30. Dennis DA, Clayton ML, O'Donnel S, et al. Posterior cruciate condylar total knee arthroplasty. *Clin Orthop.* 1992;281:168-176.

31. Schai PA, Thornhill TS, Scott RD. Total knee arthroplasty with the PFC system. *J Bone Joint Surg Br.* 1998;80:850-858.

32. Buehler KO, Venn-Watson E, D'Lima DD, et al. The press-fit condylar total knee system: 8- to 10-year results with posterior cruciate retaining design. *J Arthroplasty.* 2000;15:698-701.

33. Banks SA, Markovich GD, Hodge WA. In vivo kinematics of cruciate retaining and substituting knee arthroplasties. *J Arthroplasty.* 1997;12:297-304.

34. Dennis DA, Komistek RD, Colwell CE, et al. In vivo anteroposterior femorotibial translation of total knee arthroplasty: a multicenter analysis. *Clin Orthop.* 1998;356:47-57.

35. Stiehl JB, Komistek RD, Dennis DA, et al. Fluoroscopic analysis of kinematics after posterior cruciate-retaining knee arthroplasty. *J Bone Joint Surg Br.* 1995;77:884-889.

36. Incavo SJ, Johnson CC, Beynnon BD, et al. Posterior cruciate ligament strain biomechanics in total knee arthroplasty. *Clin Orthop.* 1994;309:88-93.

37. Becker MW, Insall JN, Fans PM. Bilateral total knee arthroplasty. *Clin Orthop.* 1991;271:122-124.

38. Dorr LD, Ochsner JL, Gronley J. Functional comparison of posterior cruciate-retained versus cruciate-sacrificed total knee arthroplasty. *Clin Orthop.* 1988;236:36-43.

39. Hirsch HS, Lotke PA, Morrison LD. The posterior cruciate ligament in total knee surgery. *Clin Orthop.* 1994;309:64-68.

40. Pereira DS, Jaffe FF, Ortiguera C. Posterior cruciate ligament sparing versus posterior cruciate ligament sacrificing arthroplasty. *J Arthroplasty.* 1998;13:138-144.

41. 41 Udomkiat P, Meng B, Dorr LD, et al. Functional comparison of posterior cruciate retention and substitution knee replacement. *Clin Orthop.* 2000;378:192-201.

42. Schoji H, Wolf A, Packard S, et al. Cruciate retained and excised total knee arthroplasty. *Clin Orthop.* 1994;305:218-222.

43. Wilson SA, McCann PD, Gotlin RS, et al. Comprehensive gait analysis in posterior-stabilized knee arthroplasty. *J Arthroplasty.* 1996;11:359-367.

44. Arima I, Whiteside LA, Martin JW, et al. Effect of partial release of the posterior cruciate ligament in total knee arthroplasty. *Clin Orthop.* 1998;353:194-202.

45. Ritter MA, Faris PM, Keating EM. Posterior cruciate ligament balancing during total knee arthroplasty. *J Arthroplasty.* 1988;3:323-326.

46. Scott RD, Thornhill TS. Posterior cruciate supplementing total knee replacement using conforming inserts and cruciate recession. *Clin Orthop.* 1994;309:146-149.

47. Worland RI, Jessup DE, Johnson J. Posterior cruciate recession in total knee arthroplasty. *J Arthroplasty.* 1997;12:70-73.

48. Landy MM, Walker PS. Wear of ultrahigh molecular weight polyethylene in cruciate ligament-retaining total knee arthroplasty: a case study. *J Arthroplasty.* 1993;8:439-446.

49. Stiehl JB, Komistek RD, Dennis DA. Detrimental kinematics of a flat on flat total condylar knee arthroplasty. *Clin Orthop.* 1999;365:139-148.

50. Swany MR, Scott RD. Posterior polyethylene wear in posterior cruciate ligament retaining total knee arthroplasty. *J Arthroplasty.* 1993;8:439-446.

51. Blunn GW, Walker PS, Joshi A, et al. The dominance of cyclic sliding in producing wear in total knee replacements. *Clin Orthop.* 1991;273:254-260.

52. Wright TM, Rimnac CM, Stulberg SD, et al. Wear of polyethylene in total joint replacement: observations from retrieved PCA knee implants. *Clin Orthop.* 1992;276:126-134.

53. Ritter MA, Herbst SA, Keating EM, et al. Long term survival analysis of a posterior cruciate retaining total condylar total knee arthroplasty. *Clin Orthop.* 1994;309:136-145.

54. Malkani AL, Rand JA, Bryan RS, et al. Total knee arthroplasty with the kinematic condylar prosthesis: a ten-year follow-up study. *J Bone Joint Surg Am.* 1995;77:423-431.

55. Rand JA, Ilstrup DM. Survivorship analysis of total knee arthroplasty: cumulative rates of survival of 9200 total knee arthroplasties. *J Bone Joint Surg Am.* 1991;73:397-409.

56. Kleinbert FA, Bryk E, Evangelista J, et al. Histologic comparison of posterior cruciate ligaments from arthritic and age-matched knee specimens. *J Arthroplasty.* 1996;11:726-731.

57. Koralewicz LM, Engh GA. Comparison of proprioception in arthritic and age-matched normal knees. *J Bone Joint Surg Am.* 2000;82:1582-1588.

58. Simmons S, Lephart S, Rubash HE, et al. Proprioception following total knee arthroplasty with and without the posterior cruciate ligament. *J Arthroplasty.* 1996;11:763-768.

59. Kolisek FR, McGrath MS, Marker DR, et al. Posterior-stabilized versus posterior cruciate ligament-retaining total knee arthroplasty. *Iowa Orthop J.* 2009;29:23-27. http://www.ncbi.nlm.nih.gov/pubmed/19742081. Accessed January 30, 2019.

60. Jiang C, Liu Z, Wang Y, Bian Y, Feng B, Weng X. Posterior cruciate ligament retention versus posterior stabilization for total knee arthroplasty: a meta-analysis. *PLoS One.* 2016;11(1):e0147865. doi:10.1371/journal.pone.0147865.

61. Longo UG, Ciuffreda M, Mannering N, et al. Outcomes of posterior-stabilized compared with cruciate-retaining total knee arthroplasty. *J Knee Surg.* 2018;31(04):321-340. doi:10.1055/s-0037-1603902.

62. Mayne A, Harshavardhan H, Johnston L, Wang W, Jariwala A. Cruciate Retaining compared with Posterior Stabilised Nexgen total knee arthroplasty: results at 10 years in a matched cohort. *Ann R Coll Surg Engl.* 2017;99(8):602-606. doi:10.1308/rcsann.2017.0086.

63. Sartawi M, Zurakowski D, Rosenberg A. Implant survivorship and complication rates after total knee arthroplasty with a third-generation cemented system: 15-year follow-up. *Am J Orthop.* 2018;47(3). doi:10.12788/ajo.2018.0018.

64. Serna-Berna R, Lizaur-Utrilla A, Vizcaya-Moreno MF, Miralles Muñoz FA, Gonzalez-Navarro B, Lopez-Prats FA. Cruciate-retaining vs posterior-stabilized primary total arthroplasty. Clinical outcome comparison with a minimum follow-up of 10 years. *J Arthroplasty.* 2018;33(8):2491-2495. doi:10.1016/j.arth.2018.02.094.

65. Warren PJ, Olanlokun TK, Cobb AG, et al. Proprioception after knee arthroplasty: the influence of prosthetic design. *Clin Orthop.* 1993;297:182-187.

66. Dejour D, Deschamps G, Garotta L, et al. Laxity in posterior cruciate sparing and posterior stabilized total knee prostheses. *Clin Orthop.* 1999;364:182-193.

67. Laskin RS, O'Flynn HM. Total knee replacement with posterior cruciate ligament retention in rheumatoid arthritis. *Clin Orthop.* 1997;345:24-28.

68. Matsuda S, Miura H, Nagamine R, et al. Knee stability in posterior cruciate ligament retaining total knee arthroplasty. *Clin Orthop.* 1999;366:169-173.

69. Pagnano MW, Hanssen AD, Lewallen DG, et al. Flexion instability after primary posterior cruciate retaining total knee arthroplasty. *Clin Orthop.* 1998;356:39-46.

70. Gill GS, Joshi AB. Long term results of retention of the posterior cruciate ligament in total knee replacements in rheumatoid arthritis. *J Bone Joint Surg Br.* 2001;83:510-512.

71. Schai PA, Scott RD, Thornhill TS. Total knee arthroplasty with posterior cruciate retention in patients with rheumatoid arthritis. *Clin Orthop*. 1999;367:96-106.

72. Mikulak SA, Mahoney OM, dela Rosa MA. Loosening and osteolysis with press fit condylar posterior cruciate substituting total knee replacement. *J Bone Joint Surg Am*. 2001;83:398-403.

73. Puloski SK, McCalden RW, MacDonald SI. Tibial post wear in posterior stabilized total knee arthroplasty. An unrecognized source of polyethylene debris. *J Bone Joint Surg Am*. 2001;83:390-397.

74. Laskin RS. Total knee replacement with posterior cruciate ligament retention in patients with a fixed varus deformity. *Clin Orthop*. 1996;331:29-34.

75. Lombardi AV, Mallory TH, Vaughn BK, et al. Dislocation following primary posterior stabilized total knee arthroplasty. *J Arthroplasty*. 1993;8:633-639.

76. Sharkey PF, Hozack WI, Booth RE, et al. Posterior dislocation of total knee arthroplasty. *Clin Orthop*. 1992;278:128-133.

77. Beight JL, Yao B, Hozack WI. The patellar "clunk" syndrome after posterior stabilized total *knee* arthroplasty. *Clin Orthop*. 1994;299:139-142.

78. Aaron RK, Scott RD. Supracondylar fracture of the femur after total knee arthroplasty. *Clin Orthop*. 1987;219:136-139.

79. Healy WL, Siliski JM, Incavo SJ. Operative treatment of distal femoral fractures proximal to total knee replacements. *J Bone Joint Surg Am*. 1993;75:27-34.

80. Berger RA, Rubash HE, Seel MI, et al. Determining the rotational alignment of the femoral component in total knee arthroplasty using the epicondylar axis. *Clin Orthop*. 1993;286:40-47.

81. Whiteside LA, Arima J. The anteroposterior axis for femoral rotational alignment in valgus total knee arthroplasty. *Clin Orthop*. 1995;321:168-172.

82. Chmell MI, Scott RD. Balancing the posterior cruciate ligament during cruciate-retaining total knee arthroplasty: description of the P.O.L.O. test. *J Orthop Tech*. 1996;4:12-15.

83. Vertullo CJ, de Steiger RN, Lewis PL, Lorimer M, Peng Y, Graves SE. The effect of prosthetic design and polyethylene type on the risk of revision for infection in total knee replacement. *J Bone Joint Surg*. 2018;100(23):2033-2040. doi:10.2106/JBJS.17.01639.

84. Vertullo CJ, Lewis PL, Lorimer M, Graves SE. The effect on long-term survivorship of surgeon preference for posterior-stabilized or minimally stabilized total knee replacement. *J Bone Joint Surg*. 2017;99(13):1129-1139. doi:10.2106/JBJS.16.01083.

85. Spekenbrink-Spooren A, Van Steenbergen LN, Denissen GAW, Swierstra BA, Poolman RW, Nelissen RGHH. Higher mid-term revision rates of posterior stabilized compared with cruciate retaining total knee arthroplasties: 133,841 cemented arthroplasties for osteoarthritis in The Netherlands in 2007-2016. *Acta Orthop*. 2018;89(6):640-645. doi:10.1080/17453674.2018.1518570.

86. Scott RD. Ligament releases. *Orthopedics*. 1994;17:883-885.

87. Bartel DL, Burstein AH, Toda MD, et al. The effect of conformity and plastic thickness on contact stresses in metal-backed plastic implants. *J Biomech Eng*. 1985;107:193.

B POSTERIOR STABILIZATION IN TOTAL KNEE ARTHROPLASTY

Giles R. Scuderi, MD, FACS | Douglas Vanderbrook, MD

HISTORICAL PERSPECTIVE

The present day posterior-stabilized (PS) total knee arthroplasty (TKA) design is the product of over six decades of innovation. During the late 1960s at Imperial College London Hospital, the Freeman Swanson prosthesis was designed which necessitated resection of both cruciate ligaments.[1] This design innovation occurred concurrently with the design of prosthesis such as the polycentric and geometric designs.[2] These designs proved to have a high incidence of early component loosening, breakage, subsidence, in addition to high incidence of early infections.[3] Early failures did not deter other innovators from proceeding and two distinct schools of thought emerged: the anatomical approach versus the functional approach.

The anatomical approach involved an implant that preserved one or both cruciate ligaments. The Duocondylar and subsequent Duo-Patellar implants were the first of their kind within the United States, developed at the Hospital for Special Surgery (HSS) by Peter Walker with contributions from John Insall. The Duo-Patellar design had excellent results at HSS, but the popularization of cruciate-retaining (CR) TKA would occur at the Robert Breck Brigham Hospital in Boston.[4,5]

The functional approach aimed at simplifying the biomechanics of the arthroplasty design by removing, and ultimately substituting, the cruciate ligaments. The first functional design was the total condylar prosthesis (TCP) developed in 1973 at HSS.[6] The total condylar design was successful; however, the lack of a femoral cam and tibial post mechanism in this early design led to anterior femoral translation on the tibia, which occasionally led to tibial component loosening and flexion instability. It is thought that these complications were the result of errors in surgical technique rather than implant design.[7] In addition, the early TCP design had limited flexion, averaging only 90°.[8] Insall and his colleagues redesigned the TCP and incorporated a high tibial post to prevent femoral translation in the TCP II design. The TCP II was implanted between 1976 and 77 and discontinued due to early tibial component loosening. In 1978 the Insall-Burstein (IB-I) prosthesis was introduced to address the issues experienced with the TC design.[9] The design changes included substituting the PCL with a tibial post and femoral cam mechanism along with a dished conforming articular surface. The femoral cam engaged the tibial post at approximately 70° of flexion and produced reliable femoral roll-back and facilitated

greater knee flexion, averaging 115°. While the original IB-I tibial monoblock design had an all-polyethylene tibial component, studies showed that metal-backed tibial components had a more uniform load dispersal and the original design was soon changed to incorporate a metal-backed tibial component.[10]

The IB-I had an excellent history of clinical performance and survivorship, with recent reports at 15- to 19-year follow-up showing survival of 92.4% when using revision as the end point (**Fig. 36B-1**).[11-14] The design was modified in 1988 and the IB-II, providing a modular tibial component (**Fig. 36B-2**) and the ability to add augments and stem extensions to the prosthesis, was introduced to the market. These modifications allowed the surgeon more flexibility in obtaining optimal knee alignment and stability while accommodating bone deficiencies. The IB-II design performed exceptionally well for over a decade before further advancements were made.

In the mid-1990s the Insall legacy of PS design continued with NexGen Legacy Posterior Stabilized (LPS) (Zimmer, Warsaw, IN) and subsequently the NexGen Legacy Posterior Stabilized Flex (LPS-flex) designs (Zimmer, Warsaw, IN). Major advancements in the LPS design included laterality with anatomic-specific femoral components with an enhanced lateral phalange and an elongated and deepened trochlear recess. These design modifications had the goal of improving patellofemoral kinematics and avoiding patellar clunk, which had been reported in the IB-II design. Elongation of the trochlear groove moved the femoral cam more posterior on the femoral component. This posterior position of the femoral cam mechanism had a beneficial effect on post/cam kinematics in that the cam continued to engage the post at 70° of flexion as it had with the predecessor IB-II prosthesis, but in the LPS implant the cam would ride down the tibial post, thus increasing jump distance and providing stability in flexion. Fuchs et al[15] reported a Knee Society Score of 96 in the LPS TKA at 2- to 6-year follow-up, and multiple survivorship studies report highly favorable outcomes with this design.

A desire by Insall to expand TKA to the Middle East and Asia, both cultures which require higher degrees of knee flexion for social and religious activities, led to the development of the LPS-flex total knee. Augmentation of the posterior femoral condyles allowed for greater clearance before impingement in deep knee flexion as well as enhanced posterior condylar geometry which provided

512

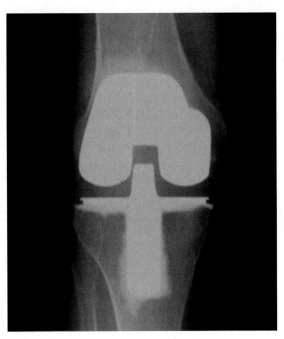

FIGURE 36B-1   AP radiograph of IB I prosthesis at 30 years.

greater contact surface area. Modifications made to the anterior lip of the tibial polyethylene articular surface permitted increased flexion without patellar tendon impingement. The LPS-flex was designed to obtain 140° to 150° of flexion compared with the 120° permitted by traditional PS implants. Later these implants were modified to include narrow versions to better accommodate anatomic differences between the genders. Since this time, numerous modifications from other vendors have expanded the implant inventory for higher flexion and gender-friendly designed femoral components.

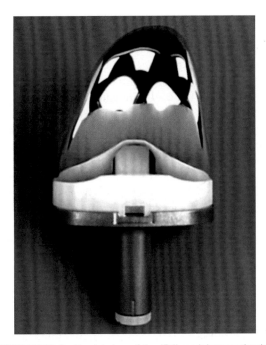

FIGURE 36B-2   Frontal view of the IB II modular prosthesis.

KINEMATICS

Retention of the posterior cruciate ligament (PCL) in CR designs was intended to preserve near-normal knee kinematics and facilitate femoral rollback. Literature, however, did not support this claim and suggested that the *in vivo* kinematics of the PCL-retaining knee are unpredictable. CR implants often led to paradoxical motion with anterior translation of the femur on the tibia, believed to be due in large part to incorrect PCL balancing.[16,17] Due to difficulty appropriately balancing the PCL as well as reports of late PCL failure and subsequent instability, implant design shifted to replacing, rather than retaining, the PCL. Biomechanical studies have shown PS designs to produce a femoral rollback more closely replicating that of the normal knee than the CR design.[16,18] This has further evolved into a relatively new category of ultracongruent or guided-rollback designs that sacrifice the PCL but do not substitute with the cam–post mechanism.

Specific Design Features

Post/Cam Mechanism

The IB-I was the first design to incorporate a tibial spine and femoral cam mechanism to facilitate femoral rollback and enhanced range of motion. This mechanism substitutes the function of the PCL and provides a mechanism for reliable femoral rollback. The tibial post engages the femoral cam at approximately 70° of flexion and allows for a controlled femoral rollback.[18] Fluoroscopic studies have shown PS femoral rollback to more closely represent that of a native knee than previous CR designs.[19,20] It bears noting that post–cam mechanisms are highly variable in design features and all PS knee designs do not function in the same way. Arnout et al[21] demonstrated large variations in the flexion angle at which the post and cam engage, maximal contact force, contact pressure, and contact area. They found that post–cam mechanisms that engage at lower flexion angles provide more normal rollback and tibial rotation.

The femoral cam of the IBPS initially engaged the lowest part of the tibial spine and as flexion increased the cam incrementally climbed the posterior tibial spine. This was not an issue when flexion was not expected to exceed 115° to 120°, but as patient demands for greater knee flexion increased the issue of stability in higher degrees of flexion arose. The sensitivity of the spine cam mechanism to instability became evident when the IB-I was changed to the IB-II. Following the initial introduction of the IB-II, there was a series of knee dislocations.[22] To address this problem, the tibial spine was moved 2 mm anterior and 2 mm higher. This design change improved the resistance of the femoral cam riding over the top of the tibial spine. Further modification of the spine cam mechanism occurred with later designs. In the mid 1990s Insall improved upon his IB-II design with the NexGen LPS prosthesis. The femoral cam was moved to a more posterior position, which had a beneficial effect of engaging the tibial post at 70° of flexion and riding down, rather than climbing up, the tibial spine. This feature increased the jump distance and produced increased stability with deep knee flexion.[23] Modern implants including the Smith & Nephew Genesis II as well as the Depuy Attune also utilize similar designs which rely upon implant surface geometry and soft-tissue balancing for stability through the first 60° of flexion, with cam–post engagement occurring at 60° to 75° of flexion. Additional advancements have been made in post geometry. For example, the patented "S-shape" of the Attune cam–post mechanism was developed to provide a large contact area as the cam engages the post and then smoothly translate the contact force distal down the spine as the knee moves into deeper flexion. In deeper degrees of flexion this design produces a compressive vector of force through the insert into the proximal tibia rather than a shear force that has the potential to ultimately lead to post wear and fracture.

Articular Conformity

A more conforming articular surface with a PS design is advantageous, since it increases the contact area and hence decreases polyethylene contact stress. This increased articular congruity evident in PS knees offers the advantage of lower shear forces that has been demonstrated in CR knees with paradoxical anterior femoral translation, with implications on polyethylene wear.[24]

Increased articular congruity also proves beneficial in the event of femoral condylar liftoff. Femoral condylar liftoff has been demonstrated via fluoroscopic motion analysis studies.[25,26] In the event of condylar liftoff, the conforming femoral–tibial articulation reduces the degree of tibial edge loading. In a prospective study of patients with bilateral paired posterior CR and PS TKAs performed by Lee et al,[26] they demonstrated condylar liftoff in 28% and 67% of knees, respectively. They postulated that the lack of PCL constraint in flexion contributes to this liftoff. Insall et al[27] examined the correlation between condylar liftoff and femoral component alignment in an LPS TKA, and reported that placement of the femoral component parallel to the transepicondylar axis could lessen the incidence of liftoff. Using computed tomography, it was determined that 69.2% of the subjects had a correlation between condylar liftoff and malalignment of the femoral component relative to the epicondylar axis. Therefore, it is thought that this phenomenon is multifactorial and variables such as ligament balance, component position, and static and dynamic limb alignment should be considered and the benefits of the PS design is advantageous.

High Flexion Designs

Consideration of patients' activities, lifestyle, and cultural practices drove innovation of high flexion designs and continue to be a factor that surgeons must consider. Activities that require high flexion include squatting,

sitting cross-legged, and kneeling with the knee fully flexed. These activities require up to 165° of flexion.[28] Additionally, everyday activities such as climbing stairs, sitting in a chair, and stepping in and out of a bathtub require between 90° and 135° of flexion.[29]

PS knees have consistently shown greater degrees of flexion attributed to unique implant design and surgical techniques intended to prevent impingement of the posterior tibial articulating surface and the posterior femoral metaphysis. High flexion is traditionally defined as greater than 125° of flexion after TKA. However, current high flexion implants are designed to accommodate 135° to 155° of flexion. Design modifications to the implant aimed at attaining deeper degrees of flexion include:

- Thickening and extension of the posterior condylar surface of the femoral component proximally (increases posterior femoral condylar offset and continued radius of curvature in an attempt to prevent posterior impingement).[30-32]
- An elongated trochlear groove is required as the contact region of the patella moves distally in deeper degrees of flexion in order to prevent the patella from being caught in the intercondylar box.[33]
- Recession of the anterior aspect of the tibial polyethylene (prevents patellar-polyethylene impingement in deep flexion).[33]
- Posterior placement of tibial post (cam engages the post earlier and allows for greater femoral rollback).[33]

In addition to implant design, a number of surgical considerations are important when attempting to maintain a high degree of knee flexion. Above all, soft-tissue balancing must remain of paramount importance to attain a stable and balanced articulation in both flexion and extension. Restoration of posterior condylar offset is critical for balance, and meticulous surgical technique cannot be understated. Additionally, attention must be paid to restoration of the posterior recess through removal of impinging posterior osteophytes.[31] Placement of appropriately sized and positioned components also impacts the final clinical outcome. Current contemporary designs with more anatomically shaped femoral and tibial components provide a more precise fit of the components without intraoperative compromise (**Fig. 36B-3**). Component malalignment must be avoided as deviation from optimal alignment has detrimental effects on patellar tracking, condylar liftoff, increased tibiofemoral wear, and an association with arthrofibrosis.[27,34] When preparing the patella, care must be taken to avoid overstuffing the patellofemoral joint. Reconstruction with too thick a patellar component or a femoral component with increased trochlear height have both been shown to limit flexion.[35,36]

Appropriate soft-tissue balancing and implant positioning allows for maintenance of preoperative joint line, which is vital to obtaining high flexion. Elevation of the joint line from a preoperative level creates a relative patella infera, which leads to early impingement and decreased motion.[37]

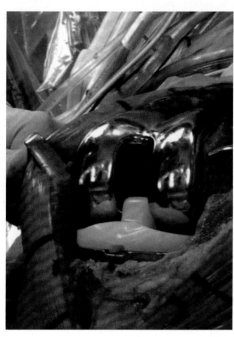

FIGURE 36B-3   Intraoperative view of the Persona PS prosthesis.

Several studies have demonstrated increased contact stress during deep knee flexion in some high flexion designs with the potential for adverse wear characteristics.[38,39] However, modern biomechanical research comparing PS high flexion designs with CR high flexion designs has demonstrated equivalent prosthetic load in deep flexion, though the amount of femoral rollback produced by the CR implants was inferior to that of PS implants.[40] This limited femoral rollback is likely due to inappropriate PCL balancing which may be a limitation when considering high flexion implants in a CR design.

INDICATIONS

Specific indications for PS TKA remain a topic of controversy. CR loyalists claim that correction of nearly all deformities except for severe flexion contractures can be addressed through PCL retention. With the more recent introduction of the ultracongruent polyethylene, characterized by an elevated anterior lip and a deeper trough, surgeons have expanded their use of CR implants on patients who previously may not have been candidates for PCL retention.[41,42] However, traditional indications for PCL substitution remain popular among arthroplasty surgeons.

First, severe flexion contracture is best treated with PCL substitution. Severe flexion contracture is an ill-defined term, but most comparative studies exclude patients from receiving CR implants with contractures greater than 15°.[43] PCL retention in cases of severe flexion contracture requires extensive release which may compromise function and predispose to early failure and/or attritional rupture. PS implants are more easily balanced in such cases.

PCL substitution is more appropriate in several additional preoperative conditions including inflammatory arthritis, postpatellectomy, periarticular osteotomy, and PCL deficiency.[44-48] Inflammatory arthritis, most commonly rheumatoid arthritis, is associated with extensive synovitis. It is this inflammatory synovitis that contributes to tissue laxity and ultimate ligament incompetence.[44] Reports exist of an increased incidence of late instability and recurvatum with CR knees in patients with rheumatoid arthritis.[45] Modern advances in antirheumatologic treatments have drastically decreased the severity of this disease process, but the pathologic condition does still exist and needs to be considered when TKA is indicated.[46]

In instances of previous patellectomy, most often performed following trauma and fracture, greater stress is placed on the PCL as a result of a disruption of knee kinematics.[47] In such patients the already compromised extensor mechanism is at risk of experiencing even greater quadriceps weakness should posterior subluxation of the tibia occur in cases of PCL attrition. However, recent data published out of the Mayo clinic has failed to demonstrate any statistically significant difference in postoperative complications or revisions between postpatellectomy patients treated with PS versus CR knees, thus challenging the long-held dogma that PS implants are needed in such cases.[48]

Patients with history of periarticular osteotomies or posttraumatic extra-articular deformity are often best served with a PS implant. The PS implant simplifies the process of soft-tissue balancing which often poses the greatest difficulty in angular deformity cases. Such cases often require augmentation, which may affect the position of the joint line which is crucial to maintain in order to optimize the extensor mechanism lever-arm.[49]

SURGICAL TECHNIQUE

The posterior substituting total knee technique is predicated upon a well-aligned prosthesis with coronal balance, equal flexion and extension gaps, and constant collateral ligament tension through the arc of motion. Soft-tissue balancing remains of paramount importance. Preoperative radiographic and physical examination will influence bone resections and soft-tissue releases. Unique features of the PS technique are PCL removal and femoral intercondylar bone resection to accommodate the femoral box. Care must be taken when performing femoral intercondylar bone resection as errant cuts, retractor placement, or knee manipulation may result in femoral condyle fractures. While femoral condyle fractures have been reported, especially in osteoporotic bone and in individuals with small femurs, this complication is usually an error in surgical technique. Alden and colleagues at the Mayo clinic reported a relative risk of distal femoral fracture in PS versus CR knees to be 4.74.[50] This was related to the aforementioned box resection, bone quality, patient gender, and technical placement of the femoral component either excessively lateral or medial thus leaving a narrow column of bone. However, the results of this database study must be considered in the context of inherent selection bias, as surgeons often elect to utilize a PS knee for complex cases due to ease of soft-tissue balancing.[51,52] Furthermore, advancements in implant designs are facilitating conservation of bone in femoral box resections.[53]

CLINICAL OUTCOMES

Posterior substituting total knees have an extensive history of exceptional patient satisfaction as well as long-term survivorship (**Table 36B-1**). At this time, greater than 15-year follow-up has been recorded for multiple prosthetic designs. Within the older patient population, cemented TKA has been shown to have excellent implant longevity and performance, but until recently little information existed on the clinical outcomes of the expanding population of young and active patients receiving TKA. Meftah et al[53] recently evaluated the long-term radiographic results, clinical outcomes, and quality of function with PS TKA in young and active patients, as defined by age less than 60 years and University of California Los Angeles (UCLA) activity score of 5 or greater. With a mean follow-up of 12.3 years they found no patients within their series underwent revision for osteolysis or loosening, the mean KSS was 93, and Kaplan–Meier survivorship was 98%. Furthermore, 68% of patients within the cohort were still participating in regular recreational activities at final follow-up. These results are consistent with previous literature by Diduch et al[62] in which a population of young and active patients aged 55 years or less at the time of primary PS TKA had an overall implant survivorship rate, with failure defined as revision of either the femoral or tibial components, of 94% at 18 years. Long et al[63] performed a follow-up study of this same patient population and found implant survivorship at 30 years without revision for any cause to be 70.1%.

TABLE 36B-1 Knee Society Score (KSS) and Survivorship Data for Various Contemporary Posterior-Stabilized Total Knee Arthroplasty Designs

	KSS (Mean)	Survivorship
LPS	96.0[15]	94.3% at 10 y[54]
Genesis II	93.2[55]	98.1% at 15 y[56]
Vanguard	92.0[57]	97.8% at 7 y[57]
Attune	89.4[58]	98.8 at 3 y[59]
PFC Sigma	90.7[58]	90.6% at 15 y[60]
Triathlon	89.5[61]	94.5% at 10 y[59]

PATIENT-REPORTED OUTCOME MEASURES

Patient-reported outcome measures (PROMs) are an increasingly important tool for documenting patient satisfaction and achievement of expectations. PROMs have consistently and overwhelmingly indicated that patients receiving PS total knees obtain superior flexion. Recent meta-analysis results have supported the improved range of motion in PS implants.[53]

Multiple meta-analyses and Cochrane reviews performed in recent years have assessed outcome measures including the Knee Society Score (KSS), Knee Society Functional Score (KSFS), Hospital for Special Surgery Score (HSS), and Western Ontario and McMaster Universities osteoarthritis index (WOMAC) when evaluating outcomes of PS knees.[64-66] The KSS is a widely used, validated outcome score, covering both objective and subjective variables with a focus on patient activity and satisfaction.[67] Several individual RCTs performed since 2012 have reported KSS for PS knees ranging from 83 to 93.5, each of which is within the excellent range of reported outcome.[68-71] In fact, Fuchs et al[15] published data on their first cohort of NexGen LPS prosthesis and reported improvements in KSS from a preoperative mean of 48 to a postoperative mean of 96 at a mean follow-up of 48 months. Likewise, Wang[72] in 2004 and Kim[73] in 2009 reported KSFS of 87 and 83.7, respectively. The HSS knee rating scale was an early score used to qualify the outcome of TKA and was developed to both evaluate a patient preoperatively, as well as to evaluate and monitor postoperative function. HSS knee scores for PS arthroplasty reported in the literature consistently exhibit scores in excess of 90, with a score ≥85 being considered excellent.[73-75] The WOMAC osteoarthritis index, developed by Bellamy et al,[76] is one of the most commonly used PROMs. The questionnaire covers three dimensions, pain, stiffness, and function, and has been tested for validity, reliability, feasibility, and responsiveness to change over time. Since 2001 five RCTs have utilized the WOMAC to evaluate outcomes after PS knee arthroplasty. These results demonstrate favorable outcomes with mean WOMAC scores ranging from 4.9 to 27.9.[43,70,73,75,77]

SURVIVORSHIP

Survivorship analysis provides a tool to predict the probability of implant success and an estimate of time to failure. PS implants have a long history of excellent survivorship. Long et al[63] reported on the Insall-Burstein prosthesis with a minimum 20-year follow-up (mean follow-up of 25.1 years). Data analysis revealed that survivorship, with failure defined as aseptic revision of the tibial or femoral components, was 82.5% at 30 years. The unmatched long-term survivorship associated with the IB PS condylar knee prosthesis has solidified this as the benchmark to which all modern and future prosthesis have and will be compared. Current contemporary PS designs are showing promising longevity (**Table 36B-1**).

Bozic et al[78] have reviewed their experience with the NexGen LPS. The 5- and 8-year survivorship for the NexGen LPS prosthesis were 100% and 94.6%, respectively. Only one knee in this cohort of 148 patients was revised for aseptic loosening. Likewise, Martin et al[79] recently reported long-term results of their experience with the Scorpio total knee system (Stryker, Mahwah NJ). They found all-cause survivorship at 10 years to be better than 96%.

Registry Data

The 2017 American Joint Replacement Registry fourth annual report indicated that approximately 50% of total knees performed from 2012 to 2016 were PS TKA. Over that same time period CR implants displayed a 5% decline in use, constituting approximately 35% of total knees in 2016.[80]

The Australian Orthopaedic Association National Joint Replacement Registry 2017 Annual Report reported on cumulative percent revision of primary TKA. PS primary TKA performed for osteoarthritis as the primary diagnosis exhibited a cumulative revision rate of 8.4% at 16 years (**Table 36B-2**). When the revision data were further compartmentalized into specific implant manufacturers, a large discrepancy in revision rate was found, implying that implant design may impact survivorship. For instance, the 10-year data on NexGen LPS and LPS Flex identified a 3.3% and 3.6% revision, respectively. This is in contrast to the 6.1% cumulative revision rate over the same time period.[59]

SPECIFIC COMPLICATIONS

Complications following TKA are fortunately rare; however, when occurring, they have the potential for catastrophic outcomes. Most risks can be minimized with proper surgical technique. For instance, infection risk has been proven to decrease with expeditious surgical time and minimizing room traffic. Appropriate soft-tissue balancing prevents instability and excessive polyethylene wear. Though many complications are universal to both PS and CR designs, there are several design-specific complications with PS TKA.

Tibial Post Wear

The tibial post is a unique feature of the PS knee design. The added articulation of the tibial post and the femoral cam introduces the potential for generation of particulate debris. This particulate debris can lead to osteolysis and ultimate component failure. In 1994 Scott and colleagues published wear analysis of retrieved PS knees in which evidence of tibial post wear was noted in all specimens, including those revised for infection.[81] The degree of wear and variability in wear patterns among different designs may be due to differences in cam–post mechanics, post location, and post geometry (**Fig. 36B-4**). In extreme cases the tibial post may fracture, which would indicate that the knee was grossly unstable and the tibial post had fatigued over time, ultimately resulting in a catastrophic failure.[82] Additionally, a femoral component placed in a flexed position risks anterior impingement upon the post which may also result in post wear and fracture even in an otherwise reasonably stable knee.

Component malrotation may result in post impingement throughout the range of motion.[83] Additionally, hyperextension of the knee can result in anterior

TABLE 36B-2 **Posterior-Stabilized Cumulative Percent Revision as Reported by the Australian Orthopaedic Association National Joint Replacement Registry**	
Posterior-Stabilized Total Knee Cumulative Revision Rate (Primary Diagnosis OA) N Total: 142,780 N Revision: 5786	
Duration	**Cumulative % Revision**
1 y	1.2
3 y	3.1
5 y	4.1
10 y	6.1
15 y	8.1
16 y	8.4

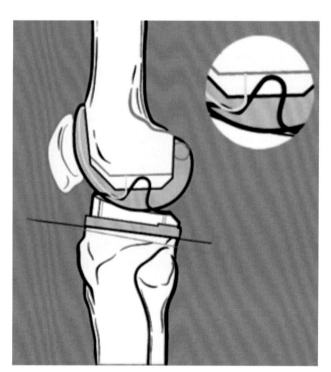

FIGURE 36B-4 Tibial post impingement may be the result of increased femoral component flexion or increased tibial posterior slope.

impingement of the femoral component on the tibial post. This may be a result of an undersized tibial polyethylene articulation, a femoral component placed in relative flexion, or a tibial resection with excessive posterior slope.[84,85]

Recent advances in polyethylene mechanical properties have improved wear characteristics.[86] A 2011 *in vitro* performance evaluation of wear, delamination, and tibial post durability was published comparing highly cross-linked polyethylene (HXPE) with conventional polyethylene. In this study, the use of HXPE in a PS TKA design resulted in a significant reduction in wear debris volume by 67% to 75% during knee simulator testing. In addition to reduced wear, only minor deformation was observed at the anterior surface of the tibial post of the HXPE components during wear testing, in contrast to the delamination and more severe deformation observed for conventional polyethylene components.[87] HXPE confers better wear performance compared to conventional polyethylene, but it comes with the drawback of reduced resistance to fatigue crack propagation.[88,89] These differences in mechanical properties contributed to the comparatively slow adoption of use in total knees relative to total hips. Although HXPE has performed reasonably well since its implementation, additional long-term retrieval studies are needed to draw more definitive conclusions.

Patellar Clunk

Patellar clunk is a design-related complication noted with PS knees originally described by Hozack et al[90] Patellar clunk is the result of a fibrous nodule that rarely forms at the junction of the quadriceps tendon and the superior pole of the patella. This nodule may become lodged within the femoral intercondylar box during flexion, and when the knee is extended, the nodule displaces back into the suprapatellar region at approximately 30° to 45° from full extension.[91] It is this displacement that results in a painful and audible "clunk." This complication was much more common with early PS designs, as high as 21% with the original IB design.[92] This was thought to be secondary to femoral trochlear geometry that had a short trochlea with a sharp transition into the intercondylar notch. Changes made in the sagittal geometry of the femoral component in the IB-II prosthesis reduced patellar clunk to between 3% and 8%.[93-95] A more recent study evaluating the incidence of patellar clunk in the third generation NexGen Legacy Posterior-Stabilized implant, with a more anatomic trochlear design, found no cases of this complication in 238 total knees.[96] It is believed that modifications made to modern implants including an elongated trochlear groove, side-specific implants, and a variety of available implant sizes have rendered this complication nearly historical.

Initial treatment of patellar clunk is physical therapy followed by arthroscopic débridement for recalcitrant and symptomatic cases. Arthroscopy has been found to successfully eliminate soft-tissue impingement associated with patellar clunk in over 70% of cases without recurrence.[97] Investigation into potential component malposition or loosening should be performed prior to surgical intervention to correctly identify the etiology of the clunk.

SUMMARY

Posterior-stabilized total knee arthroplasty has a long and storied history of success. Widely regarded for its outcome reproducibility and broad applicability across all deformities has contributed to its increasing use within the United States. Advancements made within the last two decades have further refined the design of posterior-stabilized implants. As registry data continue to gather implant information, including clinical outcomes and survivorship, the merits of posterior-stabilized TKA will be further acknowledged.

REFERENCES

1. Freeman MA, Samuelson KM, Levack B, de Alencar PG. Knee arthroplasty at the London Hospital. 1975-1984. *Clin Orthop Relat Res.* 1986;(205):12-20.
2. Mattingly PC, Bentley G, Cohen ML, Mowat AG. Preliminary experience with the geomedic total knee replacement. *Rheumatology.* 1977;16(4):241-247.
3. Goldberg VM, Henderson BT. The Freeman-Swanson ICLH total knee arthroplasty. Complications and problems. *J Bone Joint Surg Am.* 1980;62(8):1338-1344.
4. Ranawat CS, Shine JJ. Duo condylar total knee arthroplasty. *Clin Orthop Relat Red.* 1973;(94):185-195.
5. Scott RD. Duopatellar total knee replacement: the Brigham experience. *Orthop Clin North Am.* 1982;13(1):89-102.
6. Insall J, Ranawat CS, Scott WN, Walker P. Total condylar knee replacement: preliminary report. *Clin Orthop Relat Res.* 2001;(388):3-6.
7. Vince KG, Insall JN, Kelly MA. The total condylar prosthesis. 10- to 12-year results of a cemented knee replacement. *J Bone Joint Surg Br.* 1989;71(5):793-797.
8. Robinson RP. The early innovators of today's resurfacing condylar knees. *J Arthroplasty.* 2005;20(1 suppl 1):2-26.
9. Insall JN, Lachiewicz PF, Burstein AH. The posterior stabilized condylar prosthesis: a modification of the total condylar design. Two to four-year clinical experience. *J Bone Joint Surg Am.* 1982;64(9):1317-1323.
10. Bartel DL, Burstein AH, Santavicca EA, Insall JN. Performance of the tibial component in total knee replacement. *J Bone Joint Surg.* 1982;64(7):1026-1033.
11. Abdeen AR, Collen SB, Vince KG, Vince KG. Fifteen-year to 19-year follow-up of the Insall-Burstein-1 total knee arthroplasty. *J Arthroplasty.* 2010;25(2):173-178.
12. Colizza WA, Insall JN, Scuderi GR. The posterior stabilized total knee prosthesis: assessment of polyethylene damage and osteolysis after a ten-year-minimum follow-up. *J Bone Joint Surg Am.* 1995;77(11):1713-1720.
13. Scuderi GR, Insall JN. The posterior stabilized knee prosthesis. *Orthop Clin North Am.* 1989;20(1):71-78.
14. Scuderi GR, Insall JN, Windsor RE, Moran MC. Survivorship of cemented knee replacements. *J Bone Joint Surg Br.* 1989;71(5):798-803.
15. Fuchs R, Mills EL, Clarke HD, Scuderi GR, Scott WN, Insall JN. A third-generation, posterior-stabilized knee prosthesis. Early results after follow-up of 2 to 6 years. *J Arthroplasty.* 2006;21(6):821-825.

16. Dennis DA, Komistek RD, Colwell CE, et al. In vivo anteroposterior femorotibial translation of total knee arthroplasty: a multicenter analysis. *Clin Orthop Relat Res.* 1998;(356):47-57.

17. Komistek RD, Mahfouz MR, Bertin KC, Rosenberg A, Kennedy W. In vivo determination of total knee arthroplasty kinematics. A multicenter analysis of an asymmetrical posterior cruciate retaining total knee arthroplasty. *J Arthroplasty.* 2008;23(1):41-50.

18. Argenson JNA, Scuderi GR, Komistek RD, Scott WN, Kelly MA, Aubaniac JM. In vivo kinematic evaluation and design considerations related to high flexion in total knee arthroplasty. *J Biomech.* 2005;38(2):277-284.

19. Dennis DA, Komistek RD, Mahfouz MR, Haas BD, Stiehl JB. Conventry Award Paper: multicenter determination of in vivo kinematics after total knee arthroplasty. *Clin Orthop Relat Res.* 2003;(416):37-57.

20. Komistek RD, Dennis DA, Mahfouz M. In vivo fluoroscopic analysis of the normal human knee. *Clin Orthop Relat Res.* 2003;(410):69-81.

21. Arnout N, Vanlommel L, Vanlommel J, et al. Post-cam mechanics and tibiofemoral kinematics: a dynamic in vitro analysis of eight posterior-stabilized total knee designs. *Knee Surg Sport Traumatol Arthrosc.* 2015;23(11):3343-3353.

22. Lombardi AV, Mallory TH, Vaughn BK, et al. Dislocation following primary posterior-stabilized total knee arthroplasty. *J Arthroplasty.* 1993;8(6):633-639.

23. Scuderi GR, Scott WN, Tchejeyan GH. The Insall legacy in total knee arthroplasty. *Clin Orthop Relat Res.* 2001;(392):3-14.

24. Komistek R, Mahfouz M, Dennis D. *Biomechanics of the knee.* In: *Orthopedic Knowledge Update. Hip and Knee Reconstruction.* Rosemant, IL: American Academy of Orthopaedic Surgeons; 2006:17-29.

25. Dennis DA, Komistek RD, Walker SA, Cheal EJ, Stiehl JB. Femoral condylar lift-off in vivo in total knee arthroplasty. *J Bone Joint Surg Br.* 2001;83(1):33-39.

26. Lee SY, Matsui N, Kurosaka M, et al. A posterior-stabilized total knee arthroplasty shows condylar lift-off during deep knee bends. *Clin Orthop Relat Res.* 2005;(435):181-184.

27. Insall JN, Scuderi GR, Komistek RD, Math K, Dennis DA, Anderson DT. Correlation between condylar lift-off and femoral component alignment. *Clin Orthop Relat Res.* 2002;(403):143-152.

28. Mulholland SJ, Wyss UP. Activities of daily living in non-Western cultures: range of motion requirements for hip and knee joint implants. *Int J Rehabil Res.* 2001;24(3):191-198.

29. Rowe PJ, Myles CM, Walker C, Nutton R. Knee joint kinematics in gait and other functional activities measured using flexible electrogoniometry: how much knee motion is sufficient for normal daily life?. *Gait Posture.* 2000;12(2):143-155.

30. Li G, Most E, Sultan PG, et al. Knee kinematics with a high-flexion posterior stabilized total knee prosthesis: an in vitro robotic experimental investigation. *J Bone Joint Surg Am.* 2004;86(8):1721-1729.

31. Goldstein WM, Raab DJ, Gleason TF, Branson JJ, Berland K. Why posterior cruciate-retaining and substituting total knee replacements have similar ranges of motion: the importance of posterior condylar offset and cleanout of posterior condylar space. *J Bone Joint Surg Am.* 2006;88 suppl 4:182-188.

32. Massin P, Gournay A. Optimization of the posterior condylar offset, tibial slope, and condylar roll-back in total knee arthroplasty. *J Arthroplasty.* 2006;21(6):889-896.

33. Long WJ, Scuderi GR. High-flexion total knee arthroplasty. *J Arthroplasty.* 2008;23(7):6-10.

34. Boldt JG, Stiehl JB, Hodler J, Zanetti M, Munzinger U. Femoral component rotation and arthrofibrosis following mobile-bearing total knee arthroplasty. *Int Orthop.* 2006;30(5):420-425.

35. Kim AD, Shah VM, Scott RD. The effect of patellar thickness on intraoperative knee flexion and patellar tracking in patients with arthrofibrosis undergoing total knee arthroplasty. *J Arthroplasty.* 2016;31(5):1011-1015.

36. Mihalko W, Fishkin Z, Krakow K. Patellofemoral overstuff and its relationship to flexion after total knee arthroplasty. *Clin Orthop Relat Res.* 2006;449:283-287.

37. Figgie HE, Goldberg VM, Heiple KG, Moller HS, Gordon NH. The influence of tibial-patellofemoral location on function of the knee in patients with the posterior stabilized condylar knee prosthesis. *J Bone Joint Surg Am.* 1986;68(7):1035-1040.

38. Sharma A, Komistek RD, Scuderi GR, Cates HE. High-flexion TKA designs: what are their in vivo contact mechanics? *Clin Orthop Relat Res.* 2007;464:117-126.

39. Nagura T, Dyrby CO, Alexander EJ, Andriacchi TP. Mechanical loads at the knee joint during deep flexion. *J Orthop Res.* 2002;20(4):881-886.

40. Zelle J, Van der Zanden AC, De Waal Malefijt M, Verdonschot N. Biomechanical analysis of posterior cruciate ligament retaining high-flexion total knee arthroplasty. *Clin Biomech.* 2009;24(10):842-849.

41. Lützner J, Firmbach F-P, Lützner C, Dexel J, Kirschner S. Similar stability and range of motion between cruciate-retaining and cruciate-substituting ultracongruent insert total knee arthroplasty. *Knee Surg Sport Traumatol Arthrosc.* 2015;23(6):1638-1643.

42. Rajgopal A, Aggarwal K, Khurana A, Rao A, Vasdev A, Pandit H. Gait parameters and functional outcomes after total knee arthroplasty using persona knee system with cruciate retaining and ultracongruent knee inserts. *J Arthroplasty.* 2017;32(1):87-91.

43. Clark CR, Rorabeck CH, Macdonald S, Macdonald D, Swafford J, Cleland D. Posterior-stabilized and cruciate-retaining total knee replacement: a randomized study. *Clin Orthop Relat Res.* 2001;(392):208-212.

44. Hanyu T, Murasawa A, Tojo T. Survivorship analysis of total knee arthroplasty with the kinematic prosthesis in patients who have rheumatoid arthritis. *J Arthroplasty.* 1997;12(8):913-919.

45. Laskin RS, O'Flynn HM. The Insall Award. Total knee replacement with posterior cruciate ligament retention in rheumatoid arthritis. Problems and complications. *Clin Orthop Relat Res.* 1997;(345):24-28.

46. Pincus T, Sokka T, Kautiainen H. Patients seen for standard rheumatoid arthritis care have significantly better articular, radiographic, laboratory, and functional status in 2000 than in 1985. *Arthritis Rheum.* 2005;52(4):1009-1019.

47. Paletta GA Jr, Laskin RS. Total knee arthroplasty after a previous patellectomy. *J Bone Joint Surg Am.* 1995;77(11):1708-1712.

48. Haque OJ, Maradit Kremers H, Kremers WK, et al. Increased risk of postoperative complications after total knee arthroplasty in patients with previous patellectomy. *J Arthroplasty.* 2016;31(10):2278-2281.

49. Khakharia S, Scuderi GR. Restoration of the distal femur impacts patellar height in revision TKA. *Clin Orthop Relat Res.* 2012;470(1):205-210.

50. Alden KJ, Duncan WH, Trousdale RT, Pagnano MW, Haidukewych GJ. Intraoperative fracture during primary total knee arthroplasty. *Clin Orthop Relat Res.* 2010;468(1):90-95.

51. Scuderi G, Tria A. *The Knee: A Comprehensive Review.* 1st ed. New York: World Scientific; 2010.

52. Nett M, Roehrid G, Scuderi G, Scott W. *Posterior cruciate ligament substituting total knee arthroplasty.* In: *Insall & Scott Surgery of the Knee.* 5th ed. Philadelphia: Elsevier/Churchill Livingstone; 2012.

53. Meftah M, White PB, Ranawat AS, Ranawat CS. Long-term results of total knee arthroplasty in young and active patients with posterior stabilized design. *Knee.* 2016;23(2):318-321.

54. Mayne A, Harshavardhan HP, Johnston LR, Wang W, Jariwala A. Cruciate Retaining compared with Posterior Stabilised Nexgen total knee arthroplasty: results at 10 years in a matched cohort. *Ann R Coll Surg Engl.* 2017;99(8):602-606.

55. Jain NP, Lee SY, Morey VM, Chong S, Kang YG, Kim TK. Early clinical outcomes of a new posteriorly stabilized total knee arthroplasty prosthesis: comparisons with two established prostheses. *Knee Surg Relat Res.* 2017;29(3):180-188.

56. Victor J, Ghijselings S, Tajdar F, et al. Total knee arthroplasty at 15-17 years: does implant design affect outcome?. *Int Orthop.* 2014;38(2):235-241.
57. Schroer WC, Stormont DM, Pietrzak WS. Seven-year survivorship and functional outcomes of the high-flexion Vanguard complete knee system. *J Arthroplasty.* 2014;29(1):61-65.
58. Ranawat CS, White PB, West S, Ranawat AS. Clinical and radiographic results of Attune and PFC Sigma knee designs at 2-year follow-up: a prospective matched-pair analysis. *J Arthroplasty.* 2017;32(2):431-436.
59. Australian Orthopaedic Association. *Australian Orthopaedic Association National Joint Replacement Registry; Hip, Knee & Shoulder Arthroplasty: Annual Report 2017*; 2017.
60. Bistolfi A, Massazza G, Rosso F, et al. Cemented fixed-bearing PFC total knee arthroplasty: survival and failure analysis at 12-17 years. *J Orthop Traumatol.* 2011;12(3):131-136.
61. Palmer J, Sloan K, Clark G. Functional outcomes comparing Triathlon versus Duracon total knee arthroplasty: does the Triathlon outperform its predecessor? *Int Orthop.* 2014;38(7):1375-1378.
62. Diduch D, Insall J, Scott W, Scuderi G, Font-Rodriguez D. Total knee replacement in young, active patients: long-term follow-up and functional outcome. *J Bone Joint Surg.* 1997;79(4):575-582.
63. Long WJ, Bryce CD, Hollenbeak CS, Benner RW, Scott W. Total knee replacement in young, active patients: long-term follow-up and functional outcome: a concise follow-up of a previous report. *J Bone Joint Surg Am.* 2014;96(18):e159.
64. Bercik MJ, Joshi A, Parvizi J. Posterior cruciate-retaining versus posterior-stabilized total knee arthroplasty: a meta-analysis. *J Arthroplasty.* 2013;28(3):439-444.
65. Jiang C, Liu Z, Wang Y, Bian Y, Feng B, Weng X. Posterior cruciate ligament retention versus posterior stabilization for total knee arthroplasty: a meta-analysis. *PLoS One.* 2016;11(1):e0147865.
66. Verra WC, van den Boom LG, Jacobs W, Clement DJ, Wymenga AA, Nelissen RG. Retention versus sacrifice of the posterior cruciate ligament in total knee arthroplasty for treating osteoarthritis. *Cochrane Database Syst Rev.* 2013;(10):CD004803.
67. Scuderi GR, Sikorskii A, Bourne RB, Lonner JH, Benjamin JB, Noble PC. The knee society short form reduces respondent burden in the assessment of patient-reported outcomes. *Clin Orthop Relat Res.* 2016;474(1):134-142.
68. Yagishita K, Muneta T, Ju YJ, Morito T, Yamazaki J, Sekiya I. High-flex posterior cruciate-retaining vs posterior cruciate-substituting designs in simultaneous bilateral total knee arthroplasty. A prospective, randomized study. *J Arthroplasty.* 2012;27(3):368-374.
69. Matsumoto T, Muratsu H, Kubo S, Matsushita T, Kurosaka M, Kuroda R. Intraoperative soft tissue balance reflects minimum 5-year midterm outcomes in cruciate-retaining and posterior-stabilized total knee arthroplasty. *J Arthroplasty.* 2012;27(9):1723-1730.
70. van den Boom LGH, Halbertsma JPK, van Raaij JJ, Brouwer RW, Bulstra SK, van den Akker-Scheek I. No difference in gait between posterior cruciate retention and the posterior stabilized design after total knee arthroplasty. *Knee Surg Sport Traumatol Arthrosc.* 2014;22(12):3135-3141.
71. Vermesan D, Trocan I, Prejbeanu R, Poenaru DV, Haragus H, Gratian D. Reduced operating time but not blood loss with cruciate retaining total knee arthroplasty. *J Clin Med Res.* 2015;7(3):171-175.
72. Wang CJ, Wang JW, Chen HS. Anonymous. Comparing cruciate-retaining total knee arthroplasty and cruciate-substituting total knee arthroplasty: a prospective clinical study. *Chang Gung Med J.* 2004;27(8):578-585.
73. Kim YH, Choi Y, Kwon OR, Kim JS. Functional outcome and range of motion of high-flexion posterior cruciate-retaining and high-flexion posterior cruciate-substituting total knee prostheses: a prospective, randomized study. *J Bone Joint Surg Am.* 2009;91(4):753-760.
74. Catani F, Leardini A, Ensini A, et al. The stability of the cemented tibial component of total knee arthroplasty: posterior cruciate-retaining versus posterior-stabilized design. *J Arthroplasty.* 2004;19(6):775-782.
75. Seon JK, Park JK, Shin YJ, Seo HY, Lee KB, Song EK. Comparisons of kinematics and range of motion in high-flexion total knee arthroplasty: cruciate retaining vs. substituting designs. *Knee Surg Sport Traumatol Arthrosc.* 2011;19(12):2016-2022.
76. Bellamy N, Buchanan WW, Goldsmith CH, Campbell J, Stitt LW. Validation study of WOMAC. *J Rheumatol.* 1988;15(12):1833-1840.
77. Harato K, Bourne RB, Victor J, Snyder M, Hart J, Ries MD. Midterm comparison of posterior cruciate-retaining versus -substituting total knee arthroplasty using the Genesis II prosthesis. A multicenter prospective randomized clinical trial. *Knee.* 2008;15(3):217-221.
78. Bozic KJ, Kinder J, Menegini M, Zurakowski D, Rosenberg AG, Galante JO. Implant survivorship and complication rates after total knee arthroplasty with a third-generation cemented system: 5 to 8 years followup. *Clin Orthop Relat Res.* 2005;435:277.
79. Martin A, Quah C, Syme G, Lammin K, Segaren N, Pickering S. Long term survivorship following Scorpio total knee replacement. *Knee.* 2015;22(3):192-196.
80. Data A. First AJRR annual report on hip and knee arthroplasty. *AJRR.* 2014.
81. Scott RD, Thornhill TS. Posterior cruciate supplementing total knee replacement using conforming inserts and cruciate recession: effect on range of motion and radiolucent lines. *Clin Orthop Relat Res.* 1994;(309):146-149.
82. Clarke HD, Math KR, Scuderi GR. Polyethylene post failure in posterior stabilized total knee arthroplasty. *J Arthroplasty.* 2004;19(5):652-657.
83. Lombardi AV, Mallory TH, Fada RA, Adams JB, Kefauver CA. Fracture of the tibial spine of a Total Condylar III knee prosthesis secondary to malrotation of the femoral component. *Am J Knee Surg.* 2001;14(1):55-59.
84. Callaghan JJ, O'Rourke MR, Goetz DD, Schmalzried TP, Campbell PA, Johnston RC. Tibial post impingement in posterior-stabilized total knee arthroplasty. *Clin Orthop Relat Res.* 2002;(404):83-88.
85. Banks SA, Harman MK, Hodge WA. Mechanism of anterior impingement damage in total knee arthroplasty. *J Bone Joint Surg Am.* 2002;84-A(suppl 2):37-42.
86. Hodrick JT, Severson EP, McAlister DS, Dahl B, Hofmann AA. Highly crosslinked polyethylene is safe for use in total knee arthroplasty. *Clin Orthop Relat Res.* 2008;466(11):2806-2812.
87. Stoller AP, Johnson TS, Popoola OO, Humphrey SM, Blanchard CR. Highly crosslinked polyethylene in posterior-stabilized total knee arthroplasty: in vitro performance evaluation of wear, delamination, and tibial post durability. *J Arthroplasty.* 2011;26(3):483-491.
88. Diamond OJ, Howard L, Masri B. Five cases of tibial post fracture in posterior stabilized total knee arthroplasty using Prolong highly cross-linked polyethylene. *Knee.* 2018;25(4):657-662.
89. Paxton EW, Inacio MCS, Kurtz S, Love R, Cafri G, Namba RS. Is there a difference in total knee arthroplasty risk of revision in highly crosslinked versus conventional polyethylene?. *Clin Orthop Relat Res.* 2015;473(3):999-1008.
90. Hozack WJ, Rothman RH, Booth RE, et al. The patellar clunk syndrome. A complication of posterior stabilized total knee arthroplasty. *Clin Orthop.* 1989;241:203.
91. Beight JL, Yao B, Hozack WJ, Hearn SL, Booth RE. The patellar "clunk" syndrome after posterior stabilized total knee arthroplasty. *Clin Orthop Relat Res.* 1994;(299):139-142.
92. Aglietti P, Buzzi R, Gaudenzi A. Patellofemoral functional results and complications with the posterior stabilized total condylar knee prosthesis. *J Arthroplasty.* 1988;3(1):17-25.
93. Lucas TS, DeLuca PF, Nazarian DG, Bartolozzi AR, Booth RE. Arthroscopic treatment of patellar clunk. *Clin Orthop Relat Res.* 1999;(367):226-229.

94. Ip D, Wu WC, Tsang WL. Comparison of two total knee prostheses on the incidence of patella clunk syndrome. *Int Orthop.* 2002;26(1):48-51.

95. Maloney WJ, Schmidt R, Sculco TP. Femoral component design and patellar clunk syndrome. *Clin Orthop Relat Res.* 2003;410(410):199-202.

96. Clarke HD, Fuchs R, Scuderi GR, Mills EL, Scott WN, Insall JN. The influence of femoral component design in the elimination of patellar clunk in posterior-stabilized total knee arthroplasty. *J Arthroplasty.* 2006;21(2):167-171.

97. Diduch DR, Scuderi GR, Scott WN, et al. The efficacy of arthroscopy following total knee replacement. *Arthroscopy.* 1997;13:166.

C | MEDIAL PIVOT KNEE

Mark Oyer, MD | Ryan E. Harold, MD | Richard Nicolay, MD | Matthew D. Beal, MD

PERSONAL STATEMENT

There is a strong bias in this chapter favoring the medial pivot design for total knee arthroplasty. The senior author primarily uses a medial pivot knee for his current arthroplasty surgeries. We acknowledge that results presented in this chapter may be biased. We believe the biomechanical studies presented to be accurate and thank Dr. Freeman for his work on the subject.

INTRODUCTION

More than 700,000 total knee arthroplasties (TKAs) are performed in the United States yearly.[1] It is estimated that primary TKA will increase by 600% by the year 2030.[2] TKA has proven to decrease patient preoperative pain levels and increase preoperative function; however, rate of satisfaction stands at 82% to 89%, leaving orthopedic surgeons and researchers with room for improvement.[3-5] Today's patient expectations go beyond pain relief and activity of daily living as some patients require higher levels of activity to be satisfied.[6] From previous studies we know that reasonable postoperative radiographs and adequate range of motion do not guarantee satisfaction.[7] Many patients complain of instability. The hypothesis of "paradoxical motion" attempts to explain these symptoms. Paradoxical motion is described by the abnormal anterior movement of the femoral component on the tibial plateau, particularly in early flexion.[8] "Mid-flexion instability" may also lead to poor results and was described by Vince as a condition when a TKA is stable in full extension and flexion at 90° but unstable between the two positions.[9] Instability after TKA leads us to question if implant designs are replicating natural knee kinematics. The medial pivot knee was introduced in the early 1990s. It was designed to replicate normal tibiofemoral kinematics.[10] This chapter will discuss kinematics of the knee and how these biomechanics have influenced the medial pivot implant design. Potential complications, the surgical procedure, case review, and current literature will also be covered in this chapter.

KINEMATICS

Evolution of Knee Motion Measurements

Measuring the motion of the knee joint has proved to be a challenging endeavor. Our measurement tools have advanced over the years. Beginning measurement techniques focused on goniometers; however, this technique could only be applied to the static knee, was inaccurate, and had no varus/valgus measures.[11] In order to capture angular movement, goniometers were attached to pins driven into bones and combined with reflective markers.[12-15] These results were more reliable; however, ethical issues led to fewer subjects in studies. Angular motion has been successfully measured in cadavers using electromagnetic sensors fixed to bones about the knee.[16] Advancement in imaging modalities has allowed researchers to study the relative motion of the articular surface. Displacement during motion can now be imaged by cine-CT,[17] static CT combined with computerized image matching,[18] CT combined with fluoroscopy, X-rays combined with fluoroscopy,[19,20] or radiosteriometric analysis (RSA) plus CT.[21] To avoid radiation, MRI has been used; however, it has only been found to track static or quasi-static knee joint motion.[11] Today, 3D imaging and motion may be measured using three techniques: RSA in conjunction with CT or MRI; fluoroscopy in conjunction with CT, MRI, or radiographs; or MRI by itself.[11]

In order to make measurements of the knee in motion, a coordinate system had to be established. A coordinate system based on posterior femoral circles was proposed by McPherson et al in 2004.[21] This system places an origin at the center of the posterior spherical portion of the medial femoral condyle so that the origin of the axis system approximately coincides with the center of rotation of the knee.[11] Flexion facet centers (FFCs) were defined by Iwaki and Pinskerova as the center of the posterior articular surfaces of both femoral condyles in a sagittal view[22,23] (**Fig. 36C-1**). A transverse line through the femoral flexion facet centers (medial and lateral condyles) marks the first axis of McPherson's coordinate system. Iwaki and Pinskerova also described tibial flexion facets, which are the posterior border of the tibial articular surface.[22,23] The second axis of the coordinate system is perpendicular to the first and perpendicular to the tibial flexion facet. The second axis will penetrate the medial femoral flexion facet center and run distally to the posterior tibial cortex. The third axis in this coordinate system is 90° to both the first and second axes in the anteroposterior direction. It also penetrates the femoral flexion facet center. The proposed coordinate system allows for measurements of the FFCs relative to the articular surface of the tibia at varying degrees of flexion (**Fig. 36C-2**). Hill et al and Johal et al also displayed similar information with motion of the femoral condyle at their FFCs in each compartment (**Fig. 36C-3**).[24,25]

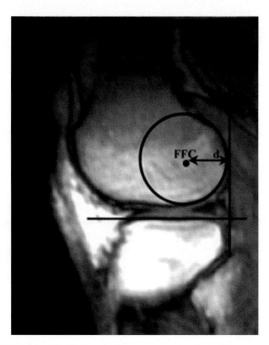

FIGURE 36C-1 Sagittal magnetic resonance imaging of the knee depicting flexion facet center (FFC) and distance ("d") from the FFC to the posterior border of the tibial plateau. (Reproduced with permission from Johal P, Williams A, Wragg P, Hunt D, Gedroyc W. Tibio-femoral movement in the living knee. A study of weight bearing and non-weight bearing knee kinematics using "interventional" MRI. *J Biomech*. 2005;38(2):269-276.)

Movement of Condyles

Many have studied the movement of the femoral condyles throughout knee range of motion. These studies depend upon tracking the movement of the individual femoral condyles by measuring the distances between the center of their posterior circular surfaces and the posterior border of the tibia.[11] The arc of active function is defined by some researchers as 10° to 30° of flexion to 110° to 120° of flexion.[11] The medial femoral condyle, during this arc, may be viewed as a sphere which rotates to produce a variable combination of flexion, longitudinal rotation (and minimal varus if liftoff occurs laterally). Translation in the anteroposterior direction in this arc of the medial femoral condyle is minimal and has been measured to be ±1.5 mm[25] (**Figs. 36C-2** and **36C-3**). The lateral femoral condyle also rotates, but in contrast to the medial side it tends to translate posteriorly about 15 mm by a mixture of rolling and sliding[18,25-27] (**Figs. 36C-2** and **36C-3**). As a result, during the arc of active function, the femur tends to externally rotate as the tibia internally rotates. This motion has been shown in the living non–weight-bearing knee.[24,25] In the living weight-bearing knee during a squat the general pattern of motion is again the same although backward movement of the lateral femoral condyle may occur earlier in flexion.[24,25]

Movement of Contact Area

Contact area of the tibiofemoral joint should not be confused with the movement of the condyles. In imaging studies "contact area" is defined as the point in the tibiofemoral joint where the subchondral plates of the tibia and femur are closest.[11] In 1990, O'Connor et al reviewed the subject of contact area and cadaveric studies and concluded that the areas moved posteriorly with flexion on both medially and laterally, but more so laterally[27] (see **Fig. 36C-4**). In a cadaveric MRI study, Pinskerova et al found contact area displacements both medially and laterally to be up to 8 mm from 0° to 30°, but at greater than 30° of flexion, found the medial contact area stationary and lateral contact area moving posteriorly up to 15 mm.[23] Dynamic studies, using fluoroscopy, of the contact areas in various activities, such as stairs and using a chair, were performed by Komistek et al and Kanisawa et al Both groups showed posterior motion of medial and lateral contact areas past the first 10° of flexion.[8,19] Komistek et al found only 2 mm of posteriorly shifted contact area in all activities but variably posterior shift from 4 to 14 mm depending on the activity performed.[8] Kanisawa et al found no medial contact area change from 0° to 60° but up to 4 mm of posterior movement from 60° to 80°. Laterally, Kanisawa found from 10° to 30° the contact area was shifted posteriorly 5 mm. Surprisingly, the lateral contact area moved anteriorly by 5 mm during 30° to 80° of flexion.[19] These results show the variability of contact area during knee range of motion and the differences between contact area and movement of the condyles. **Fig. 36C-4** displays the concept of minimal movement of the FFCs and posterior movement of the contact area during flexion.[28]

IMPLANT DESIGN

Rationale

Stability is a key principle in TKA. Coronal plane stability is generally provided by the collateral ligaments. Sagittal plane stability has been predicated on the retention of the PCL, retention of both the ACL and PCL, or resection of the cruciates with substitution of a cam and post mechanism.[29] Historically, the kinematics of the knee was thought of as a "cross-four-bar link" model.[27] In this model, the femur translates posteriorly on the tibia during flexion and anteriorly during extension. This phenomenon was termed "femoral rollback." Therefore, historically, tibial inserts had little conformity in order to avoid conflict to this theoretical motion. Dennis et al showed that femoral rollback may not actually occur in patients with TKAs. Patients in this study did not always display posterior femoral displacement during flexion; in fact, some displayed anterior displacement during flexion. This action was termed "paradoxical motion."[30] This idea, combined with relatively low TKA satisfaction rates, led researchers to question whether implant designs were providing sufficient anteroposterior stability. **Fig. 36C-5** displays what might happen during gait in a PCL-retaining TKA that does not provide sagittal stability. As the foot becomes flat and loads the knee, anterior translation of the femur or paradoxical motion may

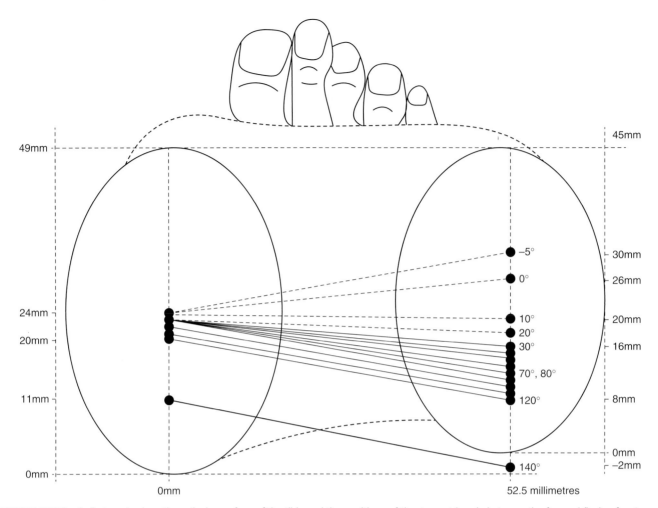

FIGURE 36C-2 A diagram to show the articular surface of the tibia and the positions of the geometric axis between the femoral flexion facet centers (FFCs) in various degrees of flexion. The points at the ends of the lines show the positions (in mm) of the FFCs medially and laterally relative to the ipsilateral posterior tibial cortex. (Reproduced with permission from Johal P, Williams A, Wragg P, Hunt D, Gedroyc W. Tibio-femoral movement in the living knee. A study of weight bearing and non-weight bearing knee kinematics using "interventional" MRI. *J Biomech*. 2005;38(2):269-276.)

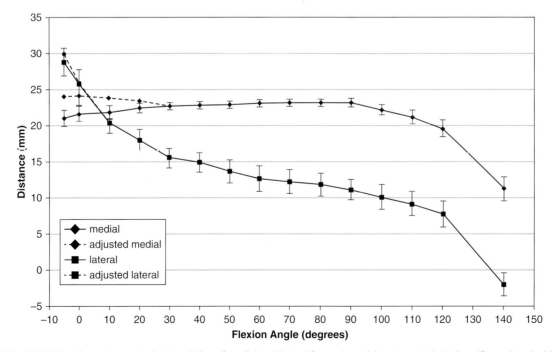

FIGURE 36C-3 Weight-bearing anteroposterior translation of medial and lateral femoral condyles at neutral rotation. (Reproduced with permission from Johal P, Williams A, Wragg P, Hunt D, Gedroyc W. Tibio-femoral movement in the living knee. A study of weight bearing and non-weight bearing knee kinematics using "interventional" MRI. *J Biomech*. 2005;38(2):269-276.)

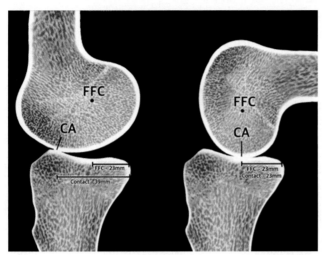

FIGURE 36C-4 Sagittal sections through the medial compartment at −5° and 90°. There is no movement of the femoral condyle (FFC; flexion facet centers) but the contact area (CA) moves posterior during flexion. (Values used from from Pinskerova V, Johal P, Nakagawa S, et al. Does the femur roll-back with flexion? *J Bone Joint Br.* 2004;86(6):925-931.)

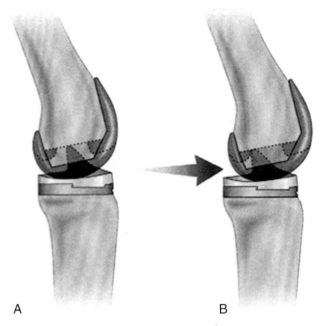

A   B

FIGURE 36C-6 **A:** At the time of load acceptance, a PCL-substituting prosthesis does not have cam and spine engagement. **B:** Forward motion of the femoral component can occur until the cam and spine engage. (Reproduced with permission from Blaha JD. The rationale for a total knee implant that confers anteroposterior stability throughout range of motion. *J Arthroplasty.* 2004;19(4 suppl 1):22-26.)

occur. The PCL is the only structure that can prevent this motion. However, in the normal knee, the PCL is not tight until at least 45° of flexion and therefore will not be able to prevent forward sliding.[29] Patients may change their gait patterns in order to prevent the femur from sliding anteriorly. They may limit knee flexion at load acceptance as well as lean forward to bring their center of mass forward and avoid a flexion moment. This gait is known

as a "quadriceps avoidance gait" because quadriceps contracture during stance phase is limited.[31] Patients may also walk slower, shorten stride length, and spend less time in stance phase to limit their paradoxical motion.[29]

Posterior cruciate substitution designs attempt to prevent paradoxical motion with a cam and post mechanism. Cam and post engagement often takes place between 20° and 65° of flexion. Therefore, forward sliding of the femur on the tibia can occur during early flexion of the load phase (**Fig. 36C-6**). The amount of forward sliding of the femur is dependent on the design of the cam and spine and, to a lesser degree, the position in which the component was implanted.[29]

In both CR and PS knees, paradoxical motion may occur. The instability in the anteroposterior plane may be part of the reason for unsatisfactory TKA. This theory along with the kinematic studies mentioned in this chapter led to the rationale for the medial pivot design. The medial ball and socket provides the anteroposterior stability to prevent paradoxical motion (**Fig. 36C-7**).[29]

Polyethylene

The design of the tibial insert separates the medial pivot knee from other implant designs such as the conventional posterior-stabilizing (PS) knee and the cruciate-retaining (CR) knee. Technically speaking, the medial pivot design is a PS knee due to its posterior lip on the medial concavity that provides constraint. However, unlike the

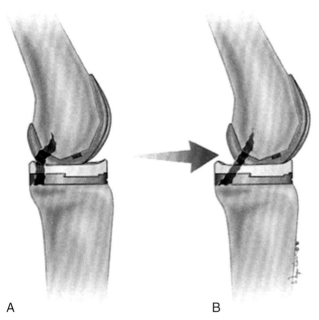

A   B

FIGURE 36C-5 **A:** A PCL-retaining prosthesis centered on the tibia just before load acceptance. **B:** At load acceptance, the lack of conformity between the femoral and tibial components allows the femur to slide forward in "paradoxical" motion. (Reproduced with permission from Blaha JD. The rationale for a total knee implant that confers anteroposterior stability throughout range of motion. *J Arthroplasty.* 2004;19(4 suppl 1):22-26.)

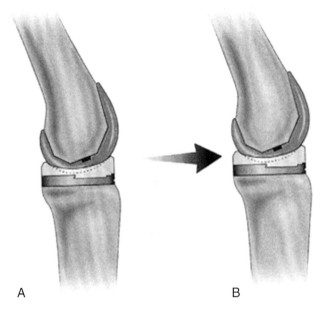

FIGURE 36C-7 The conformity of the medial ball-in-socket articulation prevents anterior slide of the femur on the tibia. (Reproduced with permission from Blaha JD. The rationale for a total knee implant that confers anteroposterior stability throughout range of motion. *J Arthroplasty.* 2004;19(4 suppl 1):22-26.)

conventional PS knee, there is no cam or post mechanism. Unlike the CR knee, the cruciates are sacrificed. The medial compartment of a medial pivot polyethylene consists of a concavity that allows for a ball-in-socket articulation with a stable point for the medial femoral condyle.[32] Besides the medial spherical concavity, the medial tibial insert also features anterior and posterior lips, which provide anteroposterior stability throughout range of motion (**Fig. 36C-8**). The tibial insert is asymmetrical as the lateral compartment has less conformity and allows for the lateral femoral condyle to roll slightly from anterior to posterior during flexion.

Femoral Component

The first medial pivot prosthesis designs contained a single radius of femoral curvature. This design is believed to enhance quadriceps power, especially in early flexion, by promoting early rollout of the femur.[33] Greater leverage for the extensor mechanism is maintained by preventing anterior sliding and shortening of the quadriceps lever/arm,[34] which may also improve patellofemoral mechanics by engaging the patella earlier in flexion. Newer femoral designs include a single radius of curvature on the medial side and a J-curve on the lateral side. J-curves are characterized by a decreasing radius from full extension to flexion.

Some companies have begun making CR and PS knees with medial congruent polyethylene inserts to help mimic what biomechanical studies have shown. Similar to a strictly medial pivot tibial insert, these medial congruent inserts have greater medial conformity via a concave medial compartment with an anterior lip. The lateral compartment is also similar in that lateral condyle is free to move in an arcuate path.[35] Tibial inserts that retain either CR or PS properties but include a medial concavity are typically known as "medial congruent" knees.

SURGICAL TECHNIQUE

The surgical technique for a medial pivot knee does not differ substantially from a conventional PS or CR knee. The approach to the knee is per the surgeon's preference. **Fig. 36C-9** shows a standard midline incision with a medial parapatellar approach. Tibial and femoral cuts are dependent on surgeon preference as well as the implant instrumentation. The medial pivot implant does not require the surgeon to change the way he or she cuts either the femur or tibia. One should note that when using a medial pivot system that sacrifices the cruciates, it is vital to completely sacrifice the PCL. **Fig. 36C-10**

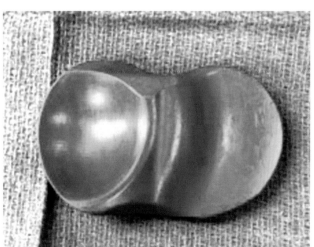
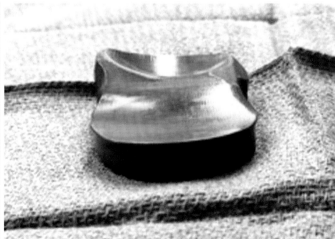

FIGURE 36C-8 A trial tibial polyethylene insert is shown. Note the medial sided concavity with anterior and posterior lips. The lateral side has less conformity but allows for lateral femoral condyle to slide posteriorly during flexion.

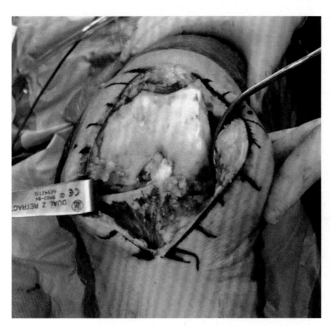

FIGURE 36C-9 View of the knee from a standard midline incision and medial parapatellar approach.

depicts the PCL completely denuded from the lateral femoral condyle. Leaving portions of the PCL attached will not allow the medial pivot knee to function as intended. PCL retention with a medial pivot system theoretically leaves the PCL to be an obstacle to lateral femoral posterior translation.[36] It should be noted that controversy exists as to whether the PCL should be sacrificed or retained. Bae et al reported there was no clinical difference in medial pivot knees when the PCL was sacrificed or retained. They did note that the PCL

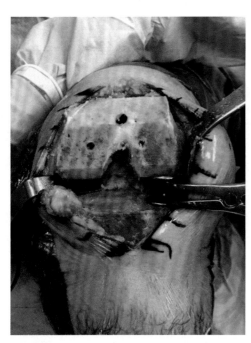

FIGURE 36C-10 Anterior view of the knee depicting importance of denuding posterior cruciate ligament from the lateral femoral condyle for a medial pivot implant.

may make appropriate tension difficult when evaluating flexion and extension gaps.[36] Placement of the tibial baseplate and femoral component are not specific to the medial pivot implant. Sizing of the polyethylene insert is similar to conventional PS and CR knees. The surgeon should be cognizant of the medial and lateral thickness of the system's polyethylene. Some systems have a polyethylene that is thicker medially, leaving the medial side of the knee tight. Soft-tissue releases on the medial side may be more extensive when using these implants. Balancing the knee in flexion, extension, and mid-flexion is vital.

When the trial is placed, the surgeon should be cognizant that the femoral component is pivoting on the medial side as the knee is taken from extension to flexion. Concurrently, the lateral femoral condyle should translate posteriorly. Discrepancies in this observation should lead the surgeon to question soft-tissue balancing or component positioning. **Fig. 36C-11** depicts the knee in extension and flexion. The medial side rotates as a ball and socket as the lateral side translates posteriorly during flexion. Easier visualization of these mechanics is seen in **Fig. 36C-12**.

CASES

The authors use standard anterior–posterior and lateral weight-bearing radiographs of the knee. There are currently no studies comparing varus versus valgus deformities being treated with a medial pivot knee. There are also no studies displaying the effects of the magnitude of deformity on the outcomes of a medial pivot TKA. Currently, the authors use a medial pivot knee despite the degree varus or valgus angulation as long as the knee is able to be balanced. If unable to be balanced, the next option would be a semiconstrained implant (which would also have a medial pivot polyethylene insert). **Fig. 36C-13** displays preoperative and postoperative radiographs of a varus knee. **Fig. 36C-14** displays preoperative and postoperative radiographs of a valgus knee.

RESULTS

Survivorship Studies

Clinical results of the medial pivot TKA are ongoing. Karachalios et al, in 2016, reported survival analysis of 284 consecutive TKAs with a mean follow-up of 13.4 years at 97.3%. Failures in their cohort included aseptic loosening, infection, and traumatic dislocation.[10] Fitch et al performed a systematic review and meta-analysis of the Advanced Medial Pivot (AMP) TKA (MicroPort Orthopaedics Inc., Arlington, Tennessee) from eight studies that included 1146 TKAs. Survivorship at 5 and 8 years postoperatively was 99.2% and 97.6%, respectively.[37] The National Joint registry of England, Wales, and Northern Ireland reported a survival rate of 96% at 10 years for 5985 AMP TKA.[38]

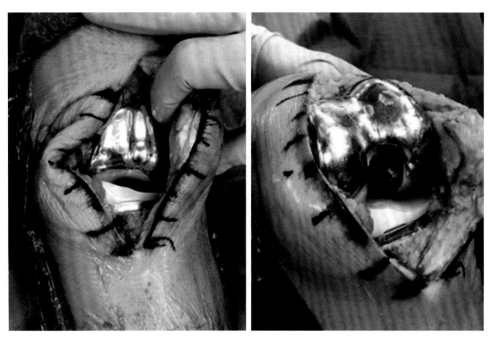

FIGURE 36C-11   Left: Knee in extension with medial pivot implant. Right: Knee in flexion showing the lateral rollback of the femoral condyle.

Survivorship data of medial pivotTKA, to this point, have proven to be equivalent to CR and PS TKAs. Further long-term survivorship studies and randomized controlled trials are still needed to draw further conclusions on the medial pivot TKA.

Comparison Studies

In 2017, Samy et al retrospectively compared a medial pivot TKA to a PS TKA in regard to patient-report outcomes (Forgotten Joint Score) and radiographic outcomes. No significant difference between range of motion or survivorship was found between the two groups at 1-year follow-up. Forgotten Joint Scores were significantly better in the medial pivot group; however, that group also had a significantly better preoperative range of motion.[39]

In 2011, Pritchett performed a randomized prospective study with 440 patients receiving staged bilateral TKAs with different types of implant designs on each extremity. Prostheses used were anterior–posterior cruciate-retaining (ACL/PCL), posterior cruciate-retaining (PCL), Medial Pivot (MP), posterior cruciate-substituting (PS), and mobile bearing (MB). Patients were asked which knee they preferred. When comparing ACL/PCL-retaining knee versus MP knees, there was no difference. Medial pivot knees were preferred over PCL, PS, and MB knees.

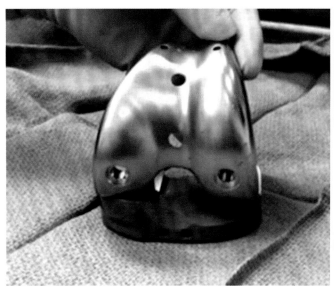
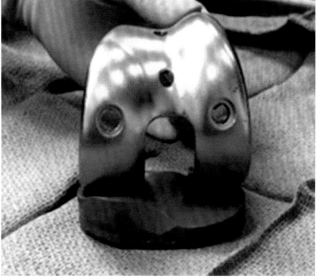

FIGURE 36C-12   Depiction of the lateral posterior translation as the knee moves from extension (left) to flexion (right).

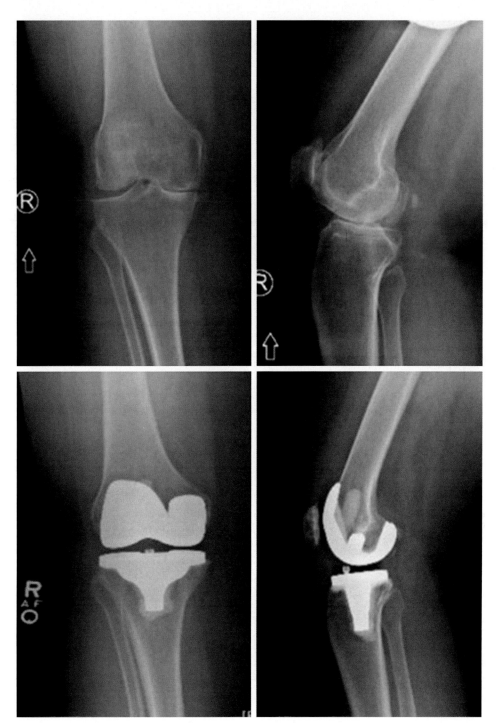

FIGURE 36C-13   Top: Anteroposterior and lateral radiographs of a varus knee. Bottom: Anteroposterior and lateral radiographs after a medial pivot design total knee arthroplasty.

Patients gave the following reasons for their preference for one knee design over the other: feels more normal; stronger on stairs; superior single-leg weight bearing; flexion stability; feels more stable overall; fewer clunks, pops, and clicks; and don't know.[33] It should also be noted there were no statistical differences in pain scores, Knee Society Scores, range of motion, function scores, or radiographic signs of loosening between groups. Mean follow-up was 6.8 years.

Benjamin et al compared the function of medial pivot and condylar knee designs in regard to patient outcomes and parameters of gait in 2018. They summarize that compared to a conventional PS knee, a medial pivot knee provides stability in the anteroposterior direction throughout the entirety of range of motion. However, they also summarize that when comparing gait analysis and clinical outcomes between a conventional single radius design and medial pivot design, there are no differences.[40]

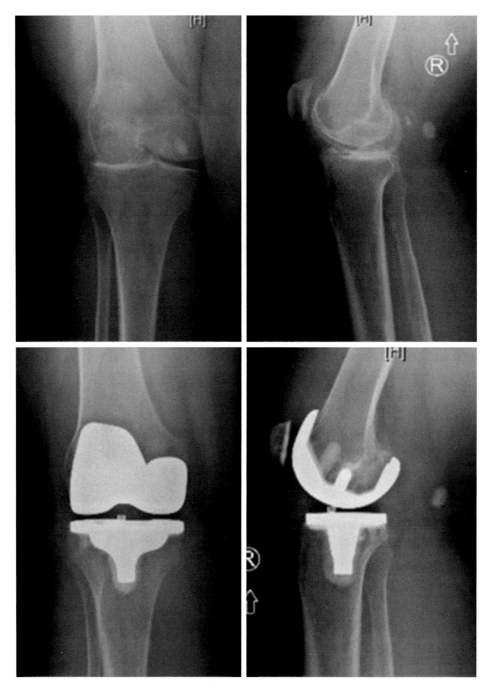

FIGURE 36C-14 Top: Anteroposterior and lateral radiographs of a valgus knee. Bottom: Anteroposterior and lateral radiographs after a medial pivot design total knee arthroplasty.

Radiographic Evaluation

In 2003, Schmidt et al reported that under fluoroscopic evaluation following a medial pivot TKA, the medial compartment does remain constrained as the lateral compartment does experience posterior translation (during the stance phase of gait).[8] It should be noted that the average posterior translation of the lateral femoral condyle in this study was less than 3 mm.

Warth et al looked at intraoperative medial pivot kinematic patterns using sensor-embedded tibial trials.

They compared patients who had a medial pivot pattern intraoperatively with those who did not have a medial pivot pattern. The authors concluded that only 40% of the TKAs performed, using a modern implant designed to replicate native knee motion, produced an intraoperative medial pivot kinematic pattern. At a minimum of 1-year follow-up, there were no differences in Knee Society objective, satisfaction, function, walking pain, stair pain, and University of California Los Angeles (UCLA) activity level.[41]

COMPLICATIONS

Theoretically, there is concern with a medial pivot knee system at the bone–implant interface. This theory lies in the concern for an increased transfer of stress due to the constraining effect of the convex hemispherical medial femoral condyle in a matching concavity on the medial polyethylene insert.[10] At this point, there are no data to support this theory. If this theory is proven true, one would expect to see changes in alignment and migration of components. Without a cam and post mechanism or retained cruciates, theories of dislocation exist. However, at this point, there are no such reported cases in the literature.

CONCLUSION

Studies of the native knee in the late 1990s and early 2000s concluded that throughout flexion the medial condyle experiences minimal anteroposterior motion, whereas the lateral condyle moves in a pivot motion around the medial condyle.[11,22,42] These attributes of native knee kinematics led the concept of a medially conforming ball-in-socket articulation known as a medial pivot knee. Survivorship studies have shown no differences between medial pivot designs compared to conventional PS and CR knee designs. Pritchett showed patients prefer a medial pivot or bicruciate design over a conventional PS, CR, and mobile-bearing knee.[33] However, radiographic studies have mixed results questioning whether the medial pivot design has a clinical or functional significance. As TKA satisfaction rates are relatively low compared to total hip arthroplasty, it is essential that surgeons and researchers continue to investigate designs, such as the medial pivot, to provide patients with the total knee that give them the highest satisfaction.

REFERENCES

1. Kurtz S, Mowat F, Ong K, Chan N, Lau E, Halpern M. Prevalence of primary and revision total hip and knee arthroplasty in the United States from 1990 through 2002. *J Bone Joint Surg Am Vol.* 2005;87(7):1487-1497.
2. Kurtz S, Ong K, Lau E, Mowat F, Halpern M. Projections of primary and revision hip and knee arthroplasty in the United States from 2005 to 2030. *J Bone Joint Surg Am Vol.* 2007;89(4):780-785.
3. Bourne RB, Chesworth BM, Davis AM, Mahomed NN, Charron KD. Patient satisfaction after total knee arthroplasty: who is satisfied and who is not? *Clin Orthop Relat Res.* 2010;468(1):57-63.
4. Chesworth BM, Mahomed NN, Bourne RB, Davis AM. Willingness to go through surgery again validated the WOMAC clinically important difference from THR/TKR surgery. *J Clin Epidemiol.* 2008;61(9):907-918.
5. Noble PC, Conditt MA, Cook KF, Mathis KB. The John Insall Award: patient expectations affect satisfaction with total knee arthroplasty. *Clin Orthop Relat Res.* 2006;452:35-43.
6. Nilsdotter AK, Toksvig-Larsen S, Roos EM. Knee arthroplasty: are patients' expectations fulfilled? A prospective study of pain and function in 102 patients with 5-year follow-up. *Acta Orthopaedica.* 2009;80(1):55-61.
7. Robertsson O, Dunbar M, Pehrsson T, Knutson K, Lidgren L. Patient satisfaction after knee arthroplasty: a report on 27,372 knees operated on between 1981 and 1995 in Sweden. *Acta Orthopaedica Scandinavica.* 2000;71(3):262-267.

8. Schmidt R, Komistek RD, Blaha JD, Penenberg BL, Maloney WJ. Fluoroscopic analyses of cruciate-retaining and medial pivot knee implants. *Clin Orthop Relat Res.* 2003;(410):139-147.
9. Vince K. Mid-flexion instability after total knee arthroplasty: woolly thinking or a real concern? *Bone Joint J.* 2016;98-B(1 suppl A):84-88.
10. Karachalios T, Varitimidis S, Bargiotas K, Hantes M, Roidis N, Malizos KN. An 11- to 15-year clinical outcome study of the Advance Medial Pivot total knee arthroplasty: pivot knee arthroplasty. *Bone Joint J.* 2016;98-B(8):1050-1055.
11. Freeman MA, Pinskerova V. The movement of the normal tibio-femoral joint. *J Biomech.* 2005;38(2):197-208.
12. Ishii Y, Terajima K, Terashima S, Koga Y. Three-dimensional kinematics of the human knee with intracortical pin fixation. *Clin Orthop Relat Res.* 1997;(343):144-150.
13. Lafortune MA, Cavanagh PR, Sommer HJ III, Kalenak A. Three-dimensional kinematics of the human knee during walking. *J Biomech.* 1992;25(4):347-357.
14. Levens AS, Inman VT, Blosser JA. Transverse rotation of the segments of the lower extremity in locomotion. *J Bone Joint Surg Am Vol.* 1948;30A(4):859-872.
15. Reinschmidt C, vdBA, Lundberg A, et al. Tibiofemoral and tibio-calcaneal motion during walking: external vs. skeletal markers. *Gait Posture.* 1997;(69):98-109.
16. Churchill DL, Incavo SJ, Johnson CC, Beynnon BD. The transepi-condylar axis approximates the optimal flexion axis of the knee. *Clin Orthop Relat Res.* 1998;(356):111-118.
17. Shapeero LG, Dye SF, Lipton MJ, Gould RG, Galvin EG, Genant HK. Functional dynamics of the knee joint by ultrafast, cine-CT. *Investig Radiol.* 1988;23(2):118-123.
18. Asano T, Akagi M, Tanaka K, Tamura J, Nakamura T. In vivo three-dimensional knee kinematics using a biplanar image-matching technique. *Clin Orthop Relat Res.* 2001;(388):157-166.
19. Kanisawa I, Banks AZ, Banks SA, Moriya H, Tsuchiya A. Weight-bearing knee kinematics in subjects with two types of anterior cruciate ligament reconstructions. *Knee Surg Sports Traumatol Arthrosc.* 2003;11(1):16-22.
20. Komistek RD, Dennis DA, Mahfouz M. In vivo fluoroscopic analysis of the normal human knee. *Clin Orthop Relat Res.* 2003;(410):69-81.
21. McPherson A, Karrholm J, Pinskerova V, Sosna A, Martelli S. Imaging knee position using MRI, RSA/CT and 3D digitisation. *J Biomech.* 2005;38(2):263-268.
22. Iwaki H, Pinskerova V, Freeman MA. Tibiofemoral movement 1: the shapes and relative movements of the femur and tibia in the unloaded cadaver knee. *J Bone Joint Surg Br.* 2000;82(8):1189-1195.
23. Pinskerova V, Iwaki H, Freeman MAR. The shapes and relative movemnts of the femur and tibia in the unloaded cadaveric knee: a study using MRI as an anatomical tool. In: Insall J, ed. *Surgery of the Knee.* 3rd ed. Philadelphia: Saunders; 2001.
24. Hill PF, Vedi V, Williams A, Iwaki H, Pinskerova V, Freeman MA. Tibiofemoral movement 2: the loaded and unloaded living knee studied by MRI. *J Bone Joint Surg Br.* 2000;82(8):1196-1198.
25. Johal P, Williams A, Wragg P, Hunt D, Gedroyc W. Tibio-femoral movement in the living knee. A study of weight bearing and non-weight bearing knee kinematics using "interventional" MRI. *J Biomech.* 2005;38(2):269-276.
26. Kurosawa H, Walker PS, Abe S, Garg A, Hunter T. Geometry and motion of the knee for implant and orthotic design. *J Biomech.* 1985;18(7):487-499.
27. O'Connor J, Shercliff T, Fitzpatrick D, Biden E, Goodfellow J. Mechanics of the knee. In: Daniel DM, Akeson WH, O'Connor JJ, eds. *Knee Ligaments: Structure, Function, Injury, and Repair.* New York: Raven Press; 1990:201-238, chap 11.
28. Pinskerova V, Johal P, Nakagawa S, et al. Does the femur roll-back with flexion?. *J Bone Joint Surg Br.* 2004;86(6):925-931.
29. Blaha JD. The rationale for a total knee implant that confers anteroposterior stability throughout range of motion. *J Arthroplasty.* 2004;19(4 suppl 1):22-26.

30. Dennis DA, Komistek RD, Mahfouz MR. In vivo fluoroscopic analysis of fixed-bearing total knee replacements. *Clin Orthop Relat Res.* 2003;(410):114-130.

31. Andriacchi TP. Functional analysis of pre and post-knee surgery: total knee arthroplasty and ACL reconstruction. *J Biomech Eng.* 1993;115(4B):575-581.

32. Risitano S, Karamian B, Indelli PF. Intraoperative load-sensing drives the level of constraint in primary total knee arthroplasty: surgical technique and review of the literature. *J Clin Orthop Trauma.* 2017;8(3):265-269.

33. Pritchett JW. Patients prefer a bicruciate-retaining or the medial pivot total knee prosthesis. *J Arthroplasty.* 2011;26(2):224-228.

34. D'Lima DD, Poole C, Chadha H, Hermida JC, Mahar A, Colwell CW Jr. Quadriceps moment arm and quadriceps forces after total knee arthroplasty. *Clin Orthop Relat Res.* 2001;(392):213-220.

35. Sabatini L, Risitano S, Parisi G, et al. Medial pivot in total knee arthroplasty: literature review and our first experience. *Clin Med Insights Arthritis Musculoskelet Disord.* 2018;11:1179544117751431.

36. Bae DK, Song SJ, Cho SD. Clinical outcome of total knee arthroplasty with medial pivot prosthesis a comparative study between the cruciate retaining and sacrificing. *J Arthroplasty.* 2011;26(5):693-698.

37. Fitch DA, Sedacki K, Yang Y. Mid- to long-term outcomes of a medial-pivot system for primary total knee replacement: a systematic review and meta-analysis. *Bone Joint Res.* 2014;3(10):297-304.

38. Vecchini E, Christodoulidis A, Magnan B, Ricci M, Regis D, Bartolozzi P. Clinical and radiologic outcomes of total knee arthroplasty using the Advance Medial Pivot prosthesis. A mean 7 years follow-up. *Knee.* 2012;19(6):851-855.

39. Samy DA, Wolfstadt JI, Vaidee I, Backstein DJ. A retrospective comparison of a medial pivot and posterior-stabilized total knee arthroplasty with respect to patient-reported and radiographic outcomes. *J Arthroplasty.* 2018;33(5):1379-1383.

40. Benjamin B, Pietrzak JRT, Tahmassebi J, Haddad FS. A functional comparison of medial pivot and condylar knee designs based on patient outcomes and parameters of gait. *Bone Joint J.* 2018;100-B(1 suppl A):76-82.

41. Warth LC, Ishmael MK, Deckard ER, Ziemba-Davis M, Meneghini RM. Do medial pivot kinematics correlate with patient-reported outcomes after total knee arthroplasty?. *J Arthroplasty.* 2017;32(8):2411-2416.

42. Moonot P, Mu S, Railton GT, Field RE, Banks SA. Tibiofemoral kinematic analysis of knee flexion for a medial pivot knee. *Knee Surg Sports Traumatol Arthrosc.* 2009;17(8):927-934.

D ULTRACONGRUENT TOTAL KNEE ARTHROPLASTY

Adolph V. Lombardi Jr, MD, FACS | Noah T. Mallory, Pre-medical Year-4

INTRODUCTION

Total knee arthroplasty (TKA) is a widely successful surgical procedure to help severe cases of arthritis in the knee.[1] TKA can attribute much of its success to its continuously evolving and refining the procedure and implants, with each advancement taking surgeons one step closer to restoring the stability and function of a healthy, anatomical knee. One of the many debated aspects of primary TKA is the retention or sacrifice of the posterior cruciate ligament (PCL).[2,3] Orthopedic surgeons are divided into camps over whether to choose: (1) the anatomic approach of always preserving one or both of the cruciate ligaments and using bicruciate-retaining or posterior cruciate-retaining (CR) implants, or (2) the functional approach of sacrificing and substituting for the cruciate ligaments with posterior-stabilized (PS) implants, or (3) to choose based on pathology. Although no clear answer is apparent, it is universally agreed that the best clinical results occur when the function of the PCL is retained or restored if it is resected.[4] Specifically, the implant must permit femoral rollback, prevent the femoral condyles from subluxing anteriorly, and restore the anteroposterior stability of the knee.[5-7] PS implants substitute for the PCL with a cam and post mechanism, but these bearings are not without complications, which include post dislocation and breakage,[5-8] patellar clunk syndrome and patellar crepitation,[5-7,9] intercondylar distal femoral fracture,[10] increased wear around the post, as well as noise from the contact of the cam and post.[6,9,11] The ultracongruent (UC) bearing was designed as an alternative to the PS bearing, substituting for the PCL but without the above-noted complications.

The UC bearing, sometimes known as anterior stabilized or condylar stabilized, is a deep-dished polyethylene insert with a large anterior buildup and a more conforming articular surface to prevent the condyles from subluxing anteriorly.[7] This large anterior buildup replaces the function of the post and thereby eliminates post-related complications. Because the UC is used with a CR femoral component, the need to resect bone from the intercondylar notch to accommodate a PS femoral is avoided and the procedure requires less time under tourniquet, which can be a factor in postoperative pain,[12,13] and makes the UC a bone-conserving alternative to the PS.[6,14,15] According to the most recent annual report of the American Joint Replacement Registry,[16] PS implants continue to be the most common device used for primary

TKA in the Unites States, but the use of UC bearings has increased steadily over time, from 1.1% in 2012 to 4.5% in 2018. For 2018, PS designs were utilized in 51.6% of primary TKA, followed by CR designs in 43.8%, and UC bearings, which, while starting to build momentum, are still relatively limited in use.

The UC is not solely a replacement for a PS bearing but also a noteworthy alternative to a standard CR implant as well.[7] One of the major difficulties in putting in a CR implant is balancing the soft tissues, but this becomes considerably easier when the PCL is resected.[5,7] The PCL can also rupture or become deficient in a knee with a standard CR bearing, rendering the patient unstable and in need of a revision, another complication not associated with the UC.[17]

INDICATIONS AND SURGICAL TECHNIQUE

PCL retention is heavily debated, and every surgeon takes a different stance regarding their preference and training; the use of the UC is no different.[18] Regardless of the condition of the PCL, some surgeons will resect it while others will try to balance it.[2,3,18] The view of the senior author is to spare whenever possible and put in the least amount of constraint that stabilizes the knee. Current TKA systems offer a continuum of constraint, from CR designs with variable degree of posterior slope, CR-lipped designs without posterior slope, to UC deep-dished anterior-stabilized bearings, to PS bearings, to mid-level PS bearings with a degree of varus/valgus constraint, to superstabilized constrained bearings, and ultimately to rotating hinges. The goal in both primary and revision TKA is to obtain balanced flexion/extension gaps.

The CR standard bearing in one particular system has 3° of posterior slope built into it (**Fig. 36D-1**). This allows the surgeon to cut the tibia at approximately 5° of posterior slope. With the additional 3° built into the insert and the tibia cut to 5°, the knee will have approximately 8° of posterior slope. This allows for satisfactory retention of the PCL and minimizes the need to balance the PCL. Therefore, when the PCL is intact, the medial and lateral collateral ligaments are intact and are balanced, and the flexion and extension gaps are balanced and equal, a CR standard bearing can be used. Upon completion of preparation of the distal femur and proximal tibial and balancing of the medial and lateral collaterals, there is occasionally a scenario where the flexion gap is slightly less than the extension gap. A way to treat this is to increase the posterior slope which will increase the flexion

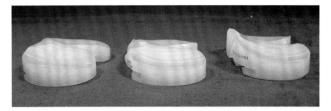

FIGURE 36D-1 Three bearing options for use with a cruciate-retaining femoral component are, from left to right, a standard cruciate-retaining that incorporates 3° of built-in posterior slope to facilitate ligamentous balancing, a cruciate-retaining–lipped bearing with no posterior slope that is approximately 2 mm thicker posteriorly, and an ultracongruent deep-dished bearing with an anterior build-up of polyethylene to afford stability. (Reproduced courtesy of Joint Implant Surgeons, Inc.)

gap. This allows the surgeon to appropriately balance the medial and collateral ligament. The extramedullary alignment jig is reapplied to the tibia and the tibial cut is refined with increased posterior slope, which increases the flexion space. With the trial components put back in place, an anteroposterior (AP) drawer test is performed. The knee should be stable in multiple degrees of flexion and articulating at the junction of the medial and posterior third. The knee should be balanced in extension when brought to full extension. The problem of knee with a tight flexion space and with a well-balanced extension space is solved by increasing the posterior slope and the surgeon may proceed with utilizing a standard CR bearing.

The indications for a CR-lipped bearing are an intact PCL, balanced medial and lateral collateral ligaments, and a flexion gap that is slightly greater than the extension gap. There is no posterior slope in a CR-lipped bearing (**Fig. 36D-1**). Therefore, the CR-lipped bearing is approximately 2 mm thicker posteriorly than the CR

standard bearing with 3° of posterior slope. The CR-lipped bearing can be used to the surgeon's advantage in a scenario where, with a 10 mm thick CR standard bearing placed, the AP drawer test reveals the knee to be loose in flexion. When the knee is brought to full extension, it is well balanced, it is stable, and it obtains full extension. The medial and lateral collateral ligaments are stable. When the knee is flexed, there is instability. The surgeon can certainly tighten the flexion gap by increasing the thickness of the bearing, going from a 10 mm to a 12 mm, but what effect will this have on extension? It should leave the knee with a slight flexion contracture. With a 12 mm bearing placed, testing in both flexion and extension reveals the knee to be springy in extension—it does not quite get full extension. When the knee is flexed it is balanced, is stable in flexion, and has a very satisfactory drawer test. This situation is where a CR-lipped bearing can provide a solution. The surgeon can place a 10 mm CR-lipped bearing, which will be approximately 2 mm thicker in flexion than the CR standard bearing that has 3° of posterior slope built in (**Fig. 36D-1**). When the CR-lipped bearing is inserted, it will tighten the flexion gap relative to the CR standard bearing and should balance our flexion/extension gap. The surgeon looks for full, stable extension with stable medial and lateral collateral ligaments. When the knee is brought to flexion, the AP drawer test will now be appropriate. The knee is balanced simply by placing a CR-lipped bearing.

When performing TKA with PCL-retaining designs, just as one balances the medial and lateral collateral ligaments, there is a need, occasionally, to balance the PCL. There are three techniques that can be utilized (**Fig. 36D-2**). One is releasing the PCL from the posterior aspect of

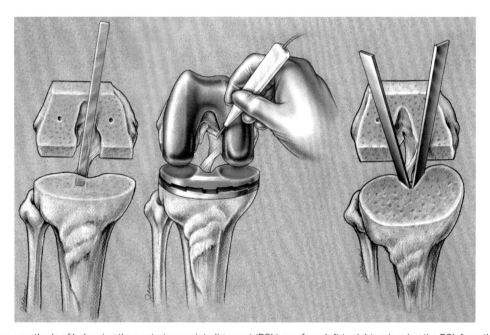

FIGURE 36D-2 Three methods of balancing the posterior cruciate ligament (PCL) are, from left to right, releasing the PCL from the posterior aspect of the tibia, performing a selective recession of fibers from their insertion on the distal femur, and performing a "V" osteotomy. (Reproduced courtesy of Joint Implant Surgeons, Inc.)

the tibia. Another is performing a femoral recession. And the final one is performing a "V" osteotomy.

For the femoral recession technique of balancing the PCL, with the knee flexed, the surgeon performs the AP drawer test and the knee appears tight in flexion. Is it tight because of the medial collateral ligament or because of the PCL? If the medial collateral appears satisfactory but the PCL is tight, the surgeon can selectively release fibers of the PCL from their insertion on the femur using electrocautery. This will allow us to balance the PCL just like we balance the medial collateral and the lateral collateral in this TKA. As fibers are selectively removed, the surgeon gently pushes on the tibia to see if appropriate balance has been obtained. The patella is now reduced and the knee is taken through a range of motion, first checking it in flexion, checking the AP drawer test, noting that indeed there is a good AP drawer test. The knee should feel balanced. The PCL is palpated and should appear to be satisfactory and more normal. The knee is then brought to extension and the varus/valgus stability is assessed. When brought back to flexion, appropriate drawer test verifies that knee is balanced. The PCL has been partially released and obtained a stable arthroplasty obtained.

To balance the PCL with an osteotomy of the insertion of the PCL on the tibia, the knee is tested in flexion with the trial components in place. The medial collateral ligament should appear satisfactory, but the PCL is tight when palpated. Performing the AP drawer test confirms that the PCL is tight. The knee is balanced in extension, tight in flexion secondary to a tight PCL. Therefore, the trial components are removed and the proximal tibia is exposed with appropriate retractors placed. The insertion of the PCL is outlined with methylene blue marker. The surgeon then takes a quarter inch osteotome and carefully performs a semilunar osteotomy of the insertion.

The osteotome is driven in approximately a centimeter to a centimeter and a half, and angled slightly posterior. The osteotomy is then completed with a broader osteotome and a mallet to displace the fragment. This will free the PCL insertion. Trial components are again placed. The stability of the knee is the assessed in flexion. By performing the osteotomy, the insertion autoregulates and the tension autoregulates. The AP drawer test will now be appropriate with an intact PCL that has been released to the appropriate tension for a good drawer test and good stability in flexion as well as extension. The knee is checked in multiple degrees of flexion as well as extension to be certain that it is balanced and stabilized, and the articulation is appropriate.

The indications for an UC anterior-stabilized bearing are similar to those for a PS bearing (**Fig. 36D-3**). There are many surgeons who, in light of the excellent results afforded by these bearings, prefer to always use either a UC or PS insert and avoid the necessity of ligamentous balancing required for a CR standard bearing, while other surgeons, including the senior author, reserve UC and PS bearings for situations where the required ligamentous balancing for a CR standard bearing cannot be achieved.[2,3] For surgeons who prefer to use selective constraint, the UC is indicated where the PCL is deficient but the medial and lateral collateral ligament are balanced and the flexion and extension gaps are equal.

The UC anterior-stabilized bearing is useful when instability in flexion is noted with the standard CR bearing; however, in extension the knee is well balanced and stable. When the knee is brought to flexion, the PCL is deficient. The surgeon can substitute for the deficient PCL in such a knee by using an UC bearing, while still using a CR femoral component and avoiding additional bony resection that would be required to switch to PS device.

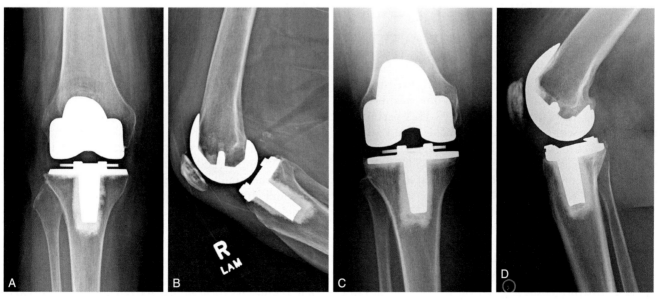

FIGURE 36D-3 Radiographic comparison of an ultracongruent implant (**A:** anteroposterior and **B:** lateral views) versus a posterior-stabilized device (**C:** anteroposterior and **D:** lateral views) for total knee arthroplasty. (Reproduced courtesy of Joint Implant Surgeons, Inc.)

An UC bearing is designed to provide stability by virtue of a long, broad anterior bumper. This enhanced polyethylene anteriorly will prevent posterior subluxation of the tibia when the knee is in flexion. When the UC trial bearing has been placed and the knee is brought to extension, it is stable in extension, both medially and laterally. In flexion the UC bearing provides resistance to posterior subluxation. The knee is balanced in flexion and extension. A high degree of flexion is obtainable with UC bearing and stability is provided by the anterior bumper. The trial bearing is exchanged for the definitive UC bearing, inserted, and assessed a final time for stability. It should be stable in both flexion and extension, with an appropriate AP drawer test, again noting resistance to posterior subluxation afforded by the anterior bumper of the UC bearing.

It is mandatory to balance the PCL in posterior CR TKA. This requires appropriate tibial resection with appropriate posterior slope. This also requires being facile with various techniques of PCL balance such as femoral recession or osteotomy of the insertion. Utilization of various degrees of constraint, including posterior CR standard bearings, posterior CR-lipped bearings, and UC anterior-stabilized bearings, may be required to address the full spectrum of instability and deformity encountered in primary TKA.

OUTCOMES

Extensive data and literature from randomized controlled trials, comparative cohort studies, meta-analyses, and systematic reviews support that there are excellent results with both posterior CR and PS TKA procedures.[19-25] However, many large registry studies report lower survival for PS TKA.[26-29] In a retrospective review of the Mayo Clinic registry that included 8117 TKA, with 5389 CR and 2728 PS performed between 1988 and 1998, survival at 15 years was 90% for CR compared with 77% for PS TKA ($P < .001$), and remained better for CR knees after adjusting for age, sex, and preoperative diagnosis and deformity.[26] In an international comparative evaluation from registries in six countries of 371,527 fixed-bearing TKA implanted from 2001 to 2010 for treatment of osteoarthritis, it was found that non-PS TKA performed better with or without patellar resurfacing than PS TKA, with the effect most pronounced in the first 2 years.[27] In a study encompassing 63,416 TKA and 138 high-volume surgeons from the Australian National Joint Replacement Registry, researchers examined the effect of surgeon preference for PS versus minimally stabilized TKA on long-term survivorship.[29] At 13 years there was a 45% higher risk of revision for patients of surgeons who preferred PS TKA compared with patients of surgeons who preferred minimally stabilized TKA. A recent study from the Dutch Arthroplasty Register of 8-year revision rates for 133,841 cemented, fixed-bearing primary CR and PS TKA performed from 2007 to 2016 found that PS knees

were 1.5 times (95% CI 1.4-1.6) more likely to be revised than CR knees.[28]

Several cohort studies have examined clinical outcomes using a range of UC TKA devices by different manufacturers with varying results (**Table 36D-1**). An early study by Sathappan et al reported 95% survival at 10 years in 77 patients (114 TKA) with UC implants.[30] With mean follow-up of 8.3 years, three patients (4 knees) were revised; two as a consequence of traumatic falls and one bilateral patient for polyethylene wear treated with bearing exchanges. Likewise, a recent study by Yoon and Yang reported 100% survival at 8.1 years in 233 patients with UC TKA in which a navigation-assisted gap-balancing technique was used.[1] A smaller study by Chavoix reported 100% survival at 5.6 years in 28 patients with a mobile-bearing design UC TKA device, which was comparable to his center's experience with a mobile-bearing PS TKA.[32] In contrast, other cohort studies have reported inferior results with UC devices.[4,12,34] In the largest study by Marion et al, in 121 TKA patients implanted with a UC insert made of conventional gamma-irradiated polyethylene, survival was only 88% ± 17% at 9 years with alarming incidence of osteolysis with aseptic loosening.[34] They concluded the device was inferior to PS TKA and discontinued its use. While the authors theorize that sheer stresses associated with the deep-dished design may increase backside wear and compromise fixation, the primary failure mechanism appears to be poor polyethylene quality rather than inferiority of the UC bearing concept. In two smaller studies involving intraoperative measurements of kinematics and stability, authors reported unsatisfactory findings associated with UC inserts.[4,12] Massin et al conducted intraoperative testing with navigation on 10 knees with UC inserts and concluded that posterior stabilization was imperfect.[12] Likewise, Akkawi et al treated 20 patients with UC TKA assisted by navigation and followed up at 6 months.[4] They observed that UC inserts failed to prevent anterior translation of the patella, thus causing inferior clinical scores.

Several published reports compare UC bearings with standard CR bearings in TKA (**Table 36D-2**). With the PCL resected, the UC high anterior buildup restores normal knee kinematics and provides comparable results to the CR.[5,6,36] Several studies support that functional outcomes and postoperative range of motion do not differ significantly between standard CR and UC implants,[6,15,39,40] and several report that the UC was better.[5,14,43] In the earliest published report of UC bearings, Scott and Thornhill compared patients undergoing CR TKA using a single TKA system with 50 having a flatter posterior-lipped insert (CR) and 50 having a sagittally curved, more conforming insert with retention but balancing of the PCL.[36] Range of motion and incidence of tibial radiolucencies were similar at 1 year, and the authors concluded that UC inserts form an attractive compromise between schools of cruciate preservation and cruciate substitution, maximizing advantages while minimizing disadvantages

TABLE 36D-1   Cohort Studies of Total Knee Arthroplasty Using Ultracongruent Bearings

Study	# UC-TKA	Device	Outcomes	Conclusions
Sathappan et al[30]	114	Osteonics Series 7000[1]	95% survivorship at 10 y	UC insert provides good to excellent mid-term results whether PCL is recessed or sacrificed
Chaidez-Rosales et al[31]	66	Consensus[2]	92% of patients were satisfied with procedure	UC is recommended as an alternative to prevent the possible complications that occur with PS
Massin et al[12]	10	Natural II[3]	At 1 y, 4 had persistent paradoxical displacement, 1 was revised to thicker poly for instability	UC partially stabilizes femoral condyles at flexion, but posterior stabilization was imperfect
Chavoix[32]	28	E-motion[4]	100% survival at 5.6 y; KSS functional and clinical were 68.1 ± 31.5 and 91.7 ± 7.2	UC prosthesis had promising outcomes, comparable to LCS (gold standard) historic control
Roh et al[33]	42[a] 43[b]	E-Motion[4]	UC with [a]preservation vs. [b]sacrifice of PCL. Preserving had more varus rotation at 90° and more anterior translation overall; 3 preserving vs. no sacrificed revised at ≥2 y	Preservation of PCL was not helpful for improving kinematics or clinical outcome in mobile-bearing UC TKA
Marion et al[34]	121	Wallaby I[5]	88% ± 17% survivorship at 9 y, concerning osteolysis	Wallaby I was inferior to PS, should no longer be used, and patients with device should be followed with CT; concerns with poor polyethylene quality
Ko et al[35]	76[a] 155[b]	[a]E-motion UC[4], [b]LCS-RP[6]	At 5 y, no differences in ROM, pain, clinical scores, or radiographic findings	Newer mobile-bearing UC could be considered with theoretical advantages and comparable outcomes to established LCS-RP
Akkawi et al[4]	20	Gemini-Light[7]	Patellar tendon angle and anterior translation increased significantly and correlated to lower clinical scores; ROM decreased	UC inserts did not prevent anterior translation, thus causing inferior clinical scores
Yoon and Yang[1]	233	Columbus[4]	100% survival at 8.1 y	Satisfactory short-term outcome aided by strict gap-balancing technique using offset-type force-controlled spreader system

[1]Osteonics, now Stryker, Mahwah, NJ; [2]Hayes Medical, now Consensus Orthopedics, El Dorado Hills, CA; [3]Zimmer Biomet, Warsaw, IN; [4]Aesculap, Tuttlingen, Germany; [5]Sulzer/Centerpulse, now Zimmer Biomet; [6]DePuy Synthes, Warsaw, IN; [7]Waldemar Link, Hamburg, Germany.

CT, computed tomography; KSS, Knee Society Score; LCS, low contact stress; PCL, posterior cruciate ligament; PS, posterior stabilized; RP, rotating platform; TKA, total knee arthroplasty; UC, ultracongruent.

and preserving bone. Likewise, a recent study by Song et al comparing 38 patients with CR and 38 with UC inserts in a single TKA system found similar clinical and functional outcomes and *in vivo* stability between groups at 3.7 years, and concluded that UC inserts are a good option when the PCL is damaged without the need for a bony intercondylar box cut required for a PS device.[6] Interestingly, Roh et al conducted a study using the same implant system as Song et al, but compared preservation versus sacrifice of the PCL when using UC inserts at a minimum follow-up of 2 years.[33] In 42 patients with PCL preservation versus 43 with PCL sacrifice, PCL-preserving knees had more varus rotation over 90° flexion, more anterior translation of the femur in all ranges of flexion than PCL-sacrificing knees, and more revisions—two for instability and one for PCL tightness, versus none revised

in the PCL-sacrificing group. The authors concluded that preserving the PCL was not helpful for improving kinematics and clinical outcomes in UC TKA. Hofmann et al compared 100 patients with primary and revision UC TKA to a matched group of 100 patients with CR TKA.[5] At 5 years mean follow-up, range of motion and clinical outcome scores were similar between groups, but there was a higher rate of revision for anteroposterior instability and PCL insufficiency in the CR group (5 of 100) compared with no revisions in the UC group. Similarly, Peters et al reported higher revision rates with CR versus UC TKA.[40] In their comparison of 228 patients with UC bearings and 240 with CR in a single TKA system with mean follow-up of 3.5 years, 3.1% of patients with UC TKA required revision versus 8.8% of CR TKA ($P = .03$), with six CR knees revised for instability versus no UC knees.

TABLE 36D-2   Comparative Studies of Total Knee Arthroplasty Using Ultracongruent Versus Standard Cruciate-Retaining (CR) or -Lipped Bearings

Study	# UC-TKA	# CR TKA	Devices	Outcomes	Conclusions
Scott and Thornhill[36]	50	50 CR-L	Press-Fit Condylar[1]	Same ROM preoperative and at 1 y in both groups, same frequency of tibial radiolucencies (4 each, nonprogressive)	Use of UC inserts offers an attractive compromise between schools of cruciate preservation and substitution, maximizing their advantages and minimizing disadvantages
Hofmann et al[5]	100	100	Natural Knee[2]	No UC revisions for instability vs. 5 CR; 98% vs. 92% survival at 5 y	Supports the UC insert as a viable alternative in primary and revision TKA
Uvehammer et al[37]	20	20	AMK[1]	At 2 y, no differences in RSA exam, clinical scores, and patient satisfaction; UC group had better sense of stability ($P = .04$); ΔHSS was 16 CR vs. 27 UC	Clinical outcome was similar in patients with CR or UC inserts
Daniilidis et al[38]	9	22	Genesis II[3]	UC had lower AP translation and nonphysiologic rollback; neither insert restored native knee kinematics	While UC reduces AP translation, centralization of contact pressure results in nonphysiological rollback
Argenson et al[39]	38 FB 199 MB	76 FB 63 MB	Variety of implants	10-y survivorship was 94% and 93% for UC FB and MB vs. 95% and 91% for CR FB and MB; KSS for UC was 87/89 and for CR was 73/75	10-year survival was >90% independent of design or mechanical stress level. No significant differences according to model
Peters et al[40]	228	240	Vanguard[2]	8.8% CR vs. 3.1% UC revised at 3.5 y; 88% CR vs. 97% UC survivorship at 5 y	UC had comparable clinical and radiographic outcomes with fewer revisions, making it an attractive option
Berend et al[14]	312 UC	1334 CR-S 803 CS-L	Vanguard[2]	At 2.3 y ΔROM was highest for UC (5.9°) vs. CR-S (3.1°) or CR-L (3.0°), and manipulation rate was lowest	Substitution for the PCL in the form of a PS design may not be necessary, even when the PCL is deficient
Mont et al[41]	32	139	Triathlon[5]	Survival was 100% for UC at 2.7 y and 99% for CR at 2.9 y with 1 revised for instability at 6 months	While the senior author typically uses the CR, the increased constraint of the UC occasionally is required to maintain stability
Lützner et al[15]	39	39	Columbus[4]	Intraoperative measurements in same knee before resections, with CR, then with PCL resection and UC, then UC outcomes at 1 y	Similar stability and ROM with CR and UC. UC inserts are a bone-preserving solution if PCL needs to be substituted
Emerson et al[42]		930 CR-S 228 CR-L	Vanguard[2]	At 3 y KSS was 92.4 for CR-S and 92.1 for CR-L, ROM arc was 2.1° to 116.2° for CR-S and 0.9° to 114.4° for CR-L	Clinical outcomes and survivorship were no different between insert groups
Song et al[6]	38	38	E-motion[4]	At 3.7 y similar KSS with 92.3 UC and 89.6 CR, ROM was 130.8° for UC and 128.7° for CR	UC had comparable functional outcomes and stability to CR, and is a good option when PCL is damaged without need for bony box cut
Rajgopal et al[43]	105	105	Persona[2]	No revisions at 2 y; modified KSS was 79.7 for UC vs. 72.8 for CR ($P < .001$)	UC had significantly better functional outcomes than CR, but no differences in gait parameters

[1]Johnson & Johnson, now DePuy Synthes, Warsaw, IN; [2]Zimmer Biomet, Warsaw, IN; [3]Smith and Nephew, Schenefeld, Germany; [4]Aesculap, Tuttlingen, Germany; [5]Stryker, Mahwah, NJ.

AMK, Anatomic Medullary Knee; AP, anteroposterior; CR, cruciate-retaining; CR-L, posterior cruciate-retaining lipped; CR-S, posterior cruciate-retaining standard; FB, fixed bearing; HSS, Hospital for Special Surgery score; KSS, Knee Society Score.; MB, mobile bearing; PCL, posterior cruciate ligament; ROM, range of motion; RSA, radiostereometric; TKA, total knee arthroplasty; UC, ultracongruent; Δ, improvement or change.

Knee Society Scores, radiographic results, frequency of nonsurgical complications, and frequency of manipulation under anesthesia were similar between groups. In a study from the current authors' center by Berend et al, using the same TKA system as the study by Peter et al, 312 patients with UC inserts were compared to 1334 with standard CR inserts and 803 with CR-lipped inserts.[14] At mean follow-up of 2.3 years, improvement in ROM was greatest in the UC group (5.9°) compared with 3.1° with standard CR and 3.0° with CR-lipped inserts, and the manipulation rate was lowest in the UC group, despite those patients having less preoperative ROM and greater tibiofemoral deformity and flexion contracture. In contrast to the findings of Hofmann et al and Peters et al in their series with longer follow-ups, no knees were revised for instability in any group. Mont et al reported on 32 knees in 29 patients with UC inserts and 139 knees in 124 patients with CR inserts in a single TKA system and observed similarly excellent clinical and functional outcomes.[41] Survival was 100% in the UC group at 2.7 years and 99% in the CR group at 2.9 years with one knee revised for instability at 6 months. The senior author in that study preferentially uses CR inserts but occasionally requires the UC to achieve stability. There are concerns that the increased conformity and constraint of the UC potentially could cause increased polyethylene wear. In a recent study by Rajgopal et al with 2-year follow-up comparing knees in 105 patients treated with simultaneous bilateral TKA using UC inserts on one side and CR inserts contralaterally, they reported that knees with UC inserts had statistically better Western Ontario and McMaster Universities Osteoarthritis Index scores, Modified Knee Society Score, and ROM than knees with CR inserts.[43] There were no revision surgeries in either group, and gait analysis measuring foot pressures and step length showed no differences between insert groups.

The decision between using a PS and a UC can be difficult considering they both serve the same function in replacing the PCL. Both inserts have benefits and drawbacks. The PS suffers from mechanical issues such as post dislocation or breakage,[5-8,11] patellar clunk syndrome,[5-7,9] intercondylar fracture,[10] and increased wear around the post,[6] all of which are not issues with UC designs. Several studies have directly compared UC and PS bearings (**Table 36D-3**). Laskin et al in 2000 reported on a prospective randomized clinical trial (RCT) that included 114 patients with UC inserts and 62 with PS inserts in the same TKA system.[44] At follow-up there were no differences between groups in ROM (both 116°), stair climbing ability, pain, or knee scores. They concluded that using UC inserts obviates the need to resect intercondylar femoral bone, thereby decreasing the potential for fracture and preserving bone. Parsley et al compared 88 patients with UC inserts to 121 patients with PS at 1-year follow-up.[46] While postoperative ROM was greater for PS patients at 119.9° than UC patients at 116.7° (P = .04), improvement from preoperative levels was similar (9.7°

PS vs. 11.5° UC; P = .46). Likewise, there were no differences in Knee Society Score, function score, or patient satisfaction between groups, and the authors concluded that there was no clear evidence proving superiority or need for posterior stabilization in PCL-sacrificing TKA. Machhindra et al prospectively collected data on 103 patients with UC inserts and 99 patients with PS inserts in the same mobile-bearing TKA system.[50] At 2 years follow-up they observed less postoperative ROM (126° vs. 131°) and improvement in ROM (−2° vs. 6°) in UC patients compared with PS patients, but found no other differences in functional outcomes, satisfaction, or incidence of adverse events. They concluded the mobile-bearing UC was a safe and viable alternative to the PS but with expectation of smaller postoperative ROM. In a prospective RCT reported by Kim et al of 45 UC patients and 45 PS patients with the same mobile-bearing TKA system as studied by Machhindra et al, at 3.3 years mean follow-up, the authors found no differences in ROM, clinical and functional scores, and radiographic results.[51] Intraoperative kinematic measurements with navigation showed differences in paradoxical anterior translation of the femur and paradoxical internal rotation of the femur between UC and PS knees; however, despite different kinematics, the equivalent clinical outcomes make the UC design an alternative to consider. In a prospective RCT by Lützner et al comparing 63 patients with UC inserts and 64 with PS inserts within a single TKA system, again intraoperative measurements with navigation showed kinematic differences between UC and PS inserts, but these seem to have no negative influence on short-term clinical outcomes.[54] There was no difference in ROM intraoperatively or at 1 year postoperative, Knee Society Scores were similar, and the Oxford knee score was better in the UC group. Additionally, operative time for UC TKA was 7 minutes faster. The authors conclude the UC seems to be a practical alternative to the established PS for substitution of the PCL.

Two studies have reported 5-year results of prospective RCTs comparing patients with UC and PS inserts with the same single TKA system. In a study by Sur et al with 22 UC patients and 22 PS patients, the authors observed no difference in functional outcomes and radiographic results, but found UC TKA had greater AP laxity (9.8 mm UC vs. 3.0 mm PS, P > .001) and greater posterior displacement (−9.5 mm UC vs. −1.7 mm PS, P < .001) on stress radiographs at latest follow-up.[7] The increase in AP laxity correlated to a lower Knee Society objective score for UC knees. The authors concluded that although midterm functional outcomes were similar, the UC could not restore AP stability with PCL sacrifice and therefore has no benefits with regard to knee stability after TKA. In the other RCT reported at 5 years follow-up and earlier at a minimum of 2 years, Scott et al studied 55 patients with UC inserts and 56 with PS inserts.[9,13] They observed essentially equivalent and excellent clinical scores and radiographic results between groups, with significantly

TABLE 36D-3 **Comparative Studies of Total Knee Arthroplasty Using Ultracongruent Bearings Versus Posterior-Stabilized Bearings**

Study	# UC-TKA	# PS TKA	Devices	Outcomes	Conclusions
Laskin et al[44]	114	62	Genesis II[1]	No difference in ROM (both 116°), stair climbing, pain, or knee scores (both 94)	Using UC obviates need to resect inter-condylar femoral bone, decreasing potential for fracture and preserving bone
Uvehammer et al[45]	25	22	AMK[2]	At 2 y, 1 patient in each group was revised; HSS scores were 88 UC and 90 PS; expectations met for 91% UC vs. 83% PS patients	The choice between the two designs can be left to preference of surgeon as long as PCL is resected
Parsley et al[46]	88	121	Apollo PS, Natural Knee-II UC[3]	At 1-year minimum follow-up postoperative ROM was slightly better with PS, but all other measures were similar	No clear evidence proving superiority and need for posterior stabilization in PCL-sacrificing TKA
Wajsfisz et al[47]	26	24 PS 22 PS-flex	SAL UC, NexGen PS[4]	Intraoperative flexion measurements before soft-tissue closure: UC 124°, PS 130°, PS flex 134°	Better intraoperative flexion with PS than UC. However, high-flexion PS was not superior to standard PS
Argenson et al[39]	38 FB 199 MB	216 FB 254 MB	Variety of implants	10-year survivorship was 94% and 93% for UC FB and MB vs. 90% and 94% for PS FB and MB; KSS for UC was 87/89 and for PS was 77/92	10-year survival was >90% independent of design or mechanical stress level. No significant differences according to model
Bignozzi et al[48]	30[a]	30[b] 30[c]	[a]Gemini UC[5], [b]FIRST PS[6], [c]HLS Noetos PS[7]	No difference in ROM, kinematics, clinical scores, or radiographic results at 2 y	With no clinical differences between cohorts, author cannot recommend one design over the other
Scott and Smith[13]	55	56	Triathlon[8]	At 3.8 y functional and radiographic outcomes were similar; UC had lower transfusion rate in males and tourniquet time overall	Results provide concrete support for UC as alternative to PS, with comparable outcomes, shorter tourniquet times, and trend toward decreased blood loss.
Sur et al[7]	22	22	Triathlon[8]	No difference in functional and radiographic outcomes at 5 y; however, UC had greater AP laxity than PS	UC could not restore posterior stability with sacrifice of the PCL
Appy Fedida et al[49]	35[a] 36[b]	43[a]	[a]Triathlon[8] (UC and PS); [b]BalanSys[9] (UC+)	At 2 y, sagittal laxity was similar for UC and UC+ but lower for PS ($P < .0001$); IKS was lower for UC+ than UC or PS ($P = .0007$)	Ideal sagittal laxity is unknown; however, greater laxity with UC raises concerns for long-term risk of complications (function and wear-related)
Machhindra et al[50]	103	99	E-motion[10]	At 2 y, functional outcomes and satisfaction were similar, but motion arc was smaller for UC than PS	MB-UC can be considered a safe and viable alternative to MB-PS, but with an expectation of less maximum flexion
Kim et al[51]	45	45	E-motion[10]	At 3.3 y, no differences in ROM, and clinical and radiographic outcomes	Despite different intraoperative kinematics, UC and PS had similar clinical outcomes. UC can be considered as an alternative to PS
Singh[52]	21	26	Natural Knee II UC[4], variety of PS types	After 3 mo, UC patients had greater postoperative flexion contracture and lower knee score	Asymmetric tibial base plates of UC device did not provide adequate bone coverage in Indian population; use was discontinued after just 21 cases

TABLE 36D-3 Comparative Studies of Total Knee Arthroplasty Using Ultracongruent Bearings Versus Posterior-Stabilized Bearings—Continued

Study	# UC-TKA	# PS TKA	Devices	Outcomes	Conclusions
Biyani et al[53]	43	39	Triathlon[8]	At 1 y, both UC and PS had equivalent function scores and satisfaction	UC is an adequate substitute for PS in patients undergoing TKA with PCL excision
Lützner et al[54]	63	64	Columbus[10]	No difference in ROM intraoperatively or at 1 y, or outcome scores at 1 y. PS had 5 mm less sagittal translation at 90° flexion and more posterior rollback. UC OR time was 7 min faster	For UC, reduced posterior femoral rollback had no deleterious effect on short-term clinical outcome. UC seems to be a practical alternative to PS for substitution of the PCL.
Fritsche et al[55]	40	40	Columbus[10]	Intraoperative kinematic measurement of 40 patients with UC then PS insert placed resulted in less AP stability and flexion with UC than PS	Surgeons should be aware of differences between UC and PS inserts when selecting one of these options to substitute for the PCL
Scott[9]	55	56	Triathlon[8]	At 5 y 21% of PS and 9% of UC patients had painless mechanical sensations (clicking, clunking, or popping; $P = .01$)	The UC provides excellent clinical, functional, and radiographic outcomes comparable to PS, with lower incidence of mechanical sensations

[1]Smith and Nephew, Andover, MA; [2]Johnson & Johnson, now DePuy Synthes, Warsaw, IN; [3]Sulzer, now Zimmer Biomet, Warsaw, IN; [4]Zimmer Biomet; [5]Waldemar Link, Hamburg, Germany; [6]Symbios SA, Switzerland; [7]Wright-Tornier, Montbonnet, France; [8]Stryker, Mahwah, NJ; [9]Mathys Ltd., Bettlach, Switzerland; [10]Aesculap, Tuttlingen, Germany.

AMK, Anatomic Medullary Knee; AP, anteroposterior; FB, fixed bearing; HSS, Hospital for Special Surgery score; KSS, Knee Society Score; MB, mobile bearing; OR, operating room; PCL, posterior cruciate ligament; PS, posterior-stabilized; ROM, range of motion; SAL, self-aligning mobile-bearing knee; TKA, total knee arthroplasty; UC, ultracongruent; UC+, ultracongruent with higher anterior edge.

fewer incidences of postoperative painless mechanical sensations in UC knees (9% vs. 21% PS, $P = .01$), such as clicking, clunking, or popping. In contrast to Sur et al, Scott et al concluded their results support the use of UC devices as an alternative to PS.

In summary, some studies show more AP laxity and posterior rollback in the UC when compared to the PS,[7,49,55,56] but despite this laxity, the two inserts show no significant difference in functional score, suggesting that the AP laxity may not be detrimental to the patient.[9,11,51,53,54,56,57] Bae et al, in a meta-analysis review of 13 studies comparing UC inserts (n = 757) and PS (n = 1040) inserts, concluded that PS inserts are preferable to UC based on more favorable intraoperative kinematics and stability in spite of reporting no significant differences in clinical outcomes between groups, including similar pain and function scores.[56] Several studies demonstrate that UC and PS inserts have no difference in range of motion.[44,48,51,54] UC devices eliminate disadvantages of cam-and-post PS designs that include risk of intercondylar fracture from the box cut, and an articulation that is a source of wear, post deformation, breakage or dislocation, and patellar clunk.[8,10,11] Finally, some studies suggest the operative procedure for UC TKA is more streamlined with shorter operative and tourniquet time, and reduced need for blood transfusions.[13,54] Overall, data suggest that both PS and UC implants are suitable for use with a deficient PCL, but the UC offers a bone-preserving procedure with no significant difference in clinical outcome.

REFERENCES

1. Yoon JR, Yang JH. Satisfactory short-term results of navigation-assisted gap-balancing total knee arthroplasty using ultracongruent insert. *J Arthroplasty.* 2018;33(3):723-728. doi:10.1016/j.arth.2017.09.049.
2. Lombardi AV Jr, Berend KR. Posterior cruciate ligament-retaining, posterior stabilized, and varus/valgus posterior stabilized constrained articulations in total knee arthroplasty. *Instr Course Lect.* 2006;55:419-427.
3. Lombardi AV Jr, Mallory TH, Fada RA, et al. An algorithm for the posterior cruciate ligament in total knee arthroplasty. *Clin Orthop Relat Res.* 2001;(392):75-87.
4. Akkawi I, Colle F, Bruni D, et al. Deep-dished highly congruent tibial insert in CR-TKA does not prevent patellar tendon angle increase and patellar anterior translation. *Knee Surg Sports Traumatol Arthrosc.* 2015;23(6):1622-1630.
5. Hofmann AA, Tkach TK, Evanich CJ, Camargo MP. Posterior stabilization in total knee arthroplasty with use of an ultracongruent polyethylene insert. *J Arthroplasty.* 2000;15(5):576-583.
6. Song EK, Lim HA, Joo SD, Kim SK, Lee KB, Seon JK. Total knee arthroplasty using ultra-congruent inserts can provide similar stability and function compared with cruciate-retaining total knee arthroplasty. *Knee Surg Sports Traumatol Arthrosc.* 2017;25(11):3530-3535. doi:10.1007/s00167-017-4553-3.
7. Sur YJ, Koh IJ, Park SW, Kim HJ, In Y. Condylar-stabilizing tibial inserts do not restore anteroposterior stability after total knee arthroplasty. *J Arthroplasty.* 2015;30(4):587-591.

8. Lombardi AV Jr, Mallory TH, Vaughn BK, et al. Dislocation following primary posterior-stabilized total knee arthroplasty. *J Arthroplasty.* 1993;8(6):633-639.

9. Scott DF. Prospective randomized comparison of posterior-stabilized versus condylar-stabilized total knee arthroplasty: final report of a five-year study. *J Arthroplasty.* 2018;33(5):1384-1388.

10. Lombardi AV Jr, Mallory TH, Waterman RA, Eberle RW. Intercondylar distal femoral fracture. An unreported complication of posterior-stabilized total knee arthroplasty. *J Arthroplasty.* 1995;10(5):643-650.

11. Meneghini RM, Stefl MD, Hodge WA, Banks SA. A cam-post mechanism is no longer necessary in modern primary total knee arthroplasty. *J Knee Surg.* 2019. 32(8):710-713. doi:10.1055/s-0039-1681030.

12. Massin P, Boyer P, Sabourin M. Less femorotibial rotation and AP translation in deep-dished total knee arthroplasty. An intraoperative kinematic study using navigation. *Knee Surg Sports Traumatol Arthrosc.* 2012;20(9):1714-1719.

13. Scott DF, Smith RR. A prospective, randomized comparison of posterior stabilized versus cruciate-substituting total knee arthroplasty: a preliminary report with minimum 2-year results. *J Arthroplasty.* 2014;29(9 suppl):179-181.

14. Berend KR, Lombardi AV Jr, Adams JB. Which total knee replacement implant should I pick? Correcting the pathology: the role of knee bearing designs. *Bone Joint J.* 2013;95-B(11 suppl A):129-132.

15. Lützner J, Firmbach FP, Lützner C, Dexel J, Kirschner S. Similar stability and range of motion between cruciate-retaining and cruciate-substituting ultracongruent insert total knee arthroplasty. *Knee Surg Sports Traumatol Arthrosc.* 2015;23(6):1638-1643. doi:10.1007/s00167-014-2892-x.

16. American Joint Replacement Registry 2019. *Sixth Annual Report on Hip and Knee Arthroplasty Data.* https://connect.ajrr.net/hubfs/Campaigns/All%20Annual%20Reports/AAOS_AJRR_2019_Annual_Report_FINAL.pdf.

17. Siebel T, Käfer W. In vitro investigation of knee joint kinematics following cruciate retaining versus cruciate sacrificing total knee arthroplasty. *Acta Orthop Belg.* 2003;69(5):433-440.

18. Lombardi AV Jr, Berend KR, Tria AJ Jr, et al. Choices, compromises, and controversies in total knee arthroplasty. *Instr Course Lect.* 2019;68:187-215.

19. Bercik MJ, Joshi A, Parvizi J. Posterior cruciate-retaining versus posterior-stabilized total knee arthroplasty: a meta-analysis. *J Arthroplasty.* 2013;28(3):439-444. doi:10.1016/j.arth.2012.08.008.

20. Jiang C, Liu Z, Wang Y, Bian Y, Feng B, Weng X.Posterior cruciate ligament retention versus posterior stabilization for total knee arthroplasty: a meta-analysis. *PLoS One.* 2016;11(1):e0147865. doi:10.1371/journal.pone.0147865.

21. Li N, Tan Y, Deng Y, Chen L. Posterior cruciate-retaining versus posterior stabilized total knee arthroplasty: a meta-analysis of randomized controlled trials. *Knee Surg Sports Traumatol Arthrosc.* 2014;22(3):556-564. doi:10.1007/s00167-012-2275-0.

22. Longo UG, Ciuffreda M, Mannering N, et al. Outcomes of posterior-stabilized compared with cruciate-retaining total knee arthroplasty. *J Knee Surg.* 2018;31(4):321-340. doi:10.1055/s-0037-1603902.

23. Migliorini F, Eschweiler J, Tingart M, Rath B. Posterior-stabilized versus cruciate-retained implants for total knee arthroplasty: a meta-analysis of clinical trials. *Eur J Orthop Surg Traumatol.* 2019;29(4):937-946. doi:10.1007/s00590-019-02370-1.

24. Verra WC, van den Boom LG, Jacobs W, Clement DJ, Wymenga AA, Nelissen RG. Retention versus sacrifice of the posterior cruciate ligament in total knee arthroplasty for treating osteoarthritis. *Cochrane Database Syst Rev.* 2013;(10):CD004803. doi:10.1002/14651858.CD004803.pub3.

25. Verra WC, Boom LG, Jacobs WC, Schoones JW, Wymenga AB, Nelissen RG. Similar outcome after retention or sacrifice of the posterior cruciate ligament in total knee arthroplasty. *Acta Orthop.* 2015;86(2):195-201. doi:10.3109/17453674.2014.973329.

26. Abdel MP, Morrey ME, Jensen MR, Morrey BF. Increased long-term survival of posterior cruciate-retaining versus posterior cruciate-stabilizing total knee replacements. *J Bone Joint Surg Am.* 2011;93(22):2072-2078. doi:10.2106/JBJS.J.01143.

27. Comfort T, Baste V, Froufe MA, et al. International comparative evaluation of fixed-bearing non-posterior-stabilized and posterior-stabilized total knee replacements. *J Bone Joint Surg Am.* 2014;96 suppl 1:65-72. doi:10.2106/JBJS.N.00462.

28. Spekenbrink-Spooren A, Van Steenbergen LN, Denissen GAW, Swierstra BA, Poolman RW, Nelissen RGHH. Higher mid-term revision rates of posterior stabilized compared with cruciate retaining total knee arthroplasties: 133,841 cemented arthroplasties for osteoarthritis in the Netherlands in 2007-2016. *Acta Orthop.* 2018;89(6):640-645. doi:10.1080/17453674.2018.1518570.

29. Vertullo CJ, Lewis PL, Lorimer M, Graves SE. The effect on long-term survivorship of surgeon preference for posterior-stabilized or minimally stabilized total knee replacement: an analysis of 63,416 prostheses from the Australian Orthopaedic Association National Joint Replacement Registry. *J Bone Joint Surg Am.* 2017;99(13):1129-1139. doi:10.2106/JBJS.16.01083.

30. Sathappan SS, Wasserman B, Jaffe WL, Bong M, Walsh M, Di Cesare PE. Midterm results of primary total knee arthroplasty using a dished polyethylene insert with a recessed or resected posterior cruciate ligament. *J Arthroplasty.* 2006;21(7):1012-1016.

31. Chaidez-Rosales PA, Briseño-Estrada CA, Aguilera-Zepeda JM, Ilizaliturri-Sánchez VM, Ruiz-Suárez M. Total knee arthroplasty with ultracongruent tibial insert. Two-year follow-up. *Acta Ortop Mex.* 2011;25(1):17-20.

32. Chavoix JB. Functionality and safety of an ultra-congruent rotating platform knee prosthesis at 5.6 years: more than 5- year follow-up of the e.motion ((®)) UC-TKA. *Open Orthop J.* 2013;7:152-157. doi:10.2174/1874325001307010152.

33. Roh YW, Jang J, Choi WC, et al. Preservation of the posterior cruciate ligament is not helpful in highly conforming mobile-bearing total knee arthroplasty: a randomized controlled study. *Knee Surg Sports Traumatol Arthrosc.* 2013;21(12):2850-2859. doi:10.1007/s00167-012-2265-2.

34. Marion B, Huten D, Boyer P, Jeanrot C, Massin P. Medium-term osteolysis with the Wallaby I® deep-dished total knee prosthesis. *Orthop Traumatol Surg Res.* 2014;100(4):403-408. doi:10.1016/j.otsr.2014.03.014.

35. Ko YB, Jang EC, Park SM, Kim SH, Kwak YH, Lee HJ. No difference in clinical and radiologic outcomes after total knee arthroplasty with a new ultra-congruent mobile bearing system and rotating platform mobile bearing systems after minimum 5-year follow-up. *J Arthroplasty.* 2015;30(3):379-383. doi:10.1016/j.arth.2014.09.025.

36. Scott RD, Thornhill TS. Posterior cruciate supplementing total knee replacement using conforming inserts and cruciate recession. Effect on range of motion and radiolucent lines. *Clin Orthop Relat Res.* 1994;(309):146-149.

37. Uvehammer J, Regnér L, Kärrholm J. Flat vs. concave tibial joint surface in total knee arthroplasty: randomized evaluation of 39 cases using radiostereometry. *Acta Orthop Scand.* 2001;72(3):257-265.

38. Daniilidis K, Skwara A, Vieth V, et al. Highly conforming polyethylene inlays reduce the in vivo variability of knee joint kinematics after total knee arthroplasty. *Knee.* 2012;19(4):260-265. doi:10.1016/j.knee.2011.04.001.

39. Argenson JN, Boisgard S, Parratte S, et al. Survival analysis of total knee arthroplasty at a minimum 10 years' follow-up: a multicenter French nationwide study including 846 cases. *Orthop Traumatol Surg Res.* 2013;99(4):385-390. doi:10.1016/j.otsr.2013.03.014.

40. Peters CL, Mulkey P, Erickson J, Anderson MB, Pelt CE. Comparison of total knee arthroplasty with highly congruent anterior-stabilized bearings versus a cruciate-retaining design. *Clin Orthop Relat Res.* 2014;472(1):175-180.

41. Mont MA, Costa CR, Naiziri Q, Johnson AJ. Comparison of 2 polyethylene inserts for a new cruciate-retaining total knee arthroplasty prosthesis. *Orthopedics.* 2013;36(1):33-35. doi:10.3928/01477447-20121217-04.

42. Emerson RH Jr, Barrington JW, Olugbode SA, Alnachoukati OK. A comparison of 2 tibial inserts of different constraint for cruciate-retaining primary total knee arthroplasty: an additional tool for balancing the posterior cruciate ligament. *J Arthroplasty.* 2016;31(2):425-428. doi:10.1016/j.arth.2015.09.032.

43. Rajgopal A, Aggarwal K, Khurana A, Rao A, Vasdev A, Pandit H. Gait parameters and functional outcomes after total knee arthroplasty using Persona knee system with cruciate retaining and ultracongruent knee inserts. *J Arthroplasty.* 2017;32(1):87-91. doi:10.1016/j.arth.2016.06.012.

44. Laskin RS, Maruyama Y, Villaneuva M, Bourne R. Deep-dish congruent tibial component use in total knee arthroplasty: a randomized prospective study. *Clin Orthop Relat Res.* 2000;(380):36-44.

45. Uvehammer J, Kärrholm J, Regnér L, Carlsson L, Herberts P. Concave versus posterior-stabilized tibial joint surface in total knee arthroplasty: randomized evaluation of 47 knees. *J Arthroplasty.* 2001;16(1):25-32.

46. Parsley BS, Conditt MA, Bertolusso R, Noble PC. Posterior cruciate ligament substitution is not essential for excellent postoperative outcomes in total knee arthroplasty. *J Arthroplasty.* 2006;21(6 suppl 2):127-131.

47. Wajsfisz A, Biau D, Boisrenoult P, Beaufils P. Comparative study of intraoperative knee flexion with three different TKR designs. *Orthop Traumatol Surg Res.* 2010;96(3):242-248. doi:10.1016/j.otsr.2009.12.006.

48. Bignozzi S, Zaffagnini S, Akkawi, et al. Three different cruciate-sacrificing TKA designs: minor intraoperative kinematic differences and negligible clinical differences. *Knee Surg Sports Traumatol Arthrosc.* 2014;22(12):3113-3120. doi:10.1007/s00167-014-3200-5.

49. Appy Fedida B, Krief E, Havet E, Massin P, Mertl P. Cruciate-sacrificing total knee arthroplasty and insert design: a radiologic study of sagittal laxity. *Orthop Traumatol Surg Res.* 2015;19. pii:S1877-0568(15):00276-5.

50. Machhindra MV, Kang JY, Kang YG, Chowdhry M, Kim TK. Functional outcomes of a new mobile-bearing ultra-congruent TKA system: comparison with the posterior stabilized system. *J Arthroplasty.* 2015;30(12):2137-2142. doi:10.1016/j.arth.2015.06.011.

51. Kim TW, Lee SM, Seong SC, Lee S, Jang J, Lee MC. Different intraoperative kinematics with comparable clinical outcomes of ultracongruent and posterior stabilized mobile-bearing total knee arthroplasty. *Knee Surg Sports Traumatol Arthrosc.* 2016;24(9):3036-3043. doi:10.1007/s00167-014-3489-0.

52. Singh AD. Retrospective study of asymmetric vs symmetric tibial plates and ultracongruent vs posterior stabilized inserts in Indian population: an Indian experience of Natural Knee II. *J Clin Orthop Trauma.* 2016;7(suppl 2):184-190. doi:10.1016/j.jcot.2016.07.005.

53. Biyani RK, Ziemba-Davis M, Ireland PH, Meneghini RM. Does an anterior-lipped tibial insert adequately substitute for a post-cam articulation in total knee arthroplasty. *Surg Technol Int.* 2017;30:341-345.

54. Lützner J, Beyer F, Dexel J, Fritzsche H, Lützner C, Kirschner S. No difference in range of motion between ultracongruent and posterior stabilized design in total knee arthroplasty: a randomized controlled trial. *Knee Surg Sports Traumatol Arthrosc.* 2017;25(11):3515-3521. doi:10.1007/s00167-016-4331-7.

55. Fritzsche H, Beyer F, Postler A, Lützner J. Different intraoperative kinematics, stability, and range of motion between cruciate-substituting ultracongruent and posterior-stabilized total knee arthroplasty. *Knee Surg Sports Traumatol Arthrosc.* 2018;26(5):1465-1470. doi:10.1007/s00167-017-4427-8.

56. Bae JH, Yoon JR, Sung JH, Shin YS. Posterior-stabilized inserts are preferable to cruciate-substituting ultracongruent inserts due to more favourable kinematics and stability. *Knee Surg Sports Traumatol Arthrosc.* 2018;26(11):3300-3310. doi:10.1007/s00167-018-4872-z.

57. Mazzucchelli L, Deledda D, Rosso F, et al. Cruciate retaining and cruciate substituting ultra-congruent insert. *Ann Transl Med.* 2016;4(1):2. doi:10.3978/j.issn.2305-5839.2015.12.52.

E MOBILE-BEARING KNEE REPLACEMENT

Humza S. Shaikh, MD | Malcolm E. Dombrowski, MD | Richard A. Wawrose, MD | Lawrence S. Crossett, MD

HISTORY AND DEVELOPMENT OF MOBILE BEARINGS

The need for mobile bearings in knee replacement developed after analysis of failed fixed-bearing knee replacements. Significant component loosening was seen in early fixed-hinge devices and congruent fixed-bearing nonhinged devices in less than 2 years of active use.[1,2] Incongruent knee replacements that were developed to avoid loosening problems were plagued with wear-related problems in less than 5 years.[3,4] Modular fixed-bearing polyethylene inserts were developed to allow intraoperative adjustment of component stability, but their locking mechanisms created a new source of wear debris that compounded the existing wear problems.[5]

It was established that congruity without mobility, and mobility without congruity, were flawed design concepts that caused premature loosening or excessive wear. Congruity with mobility has become the ideal stress and movement concept to minimize loosening and wear problems. That is to say, mobile bearings without locking mechanisms represent the most effective way to avoid the identified problems seen with fixed-bearing knee designs over the past three decades.

The kinematic tibiofemoral motion requirements dictate the use of spherical upper tibial bearing surfaces and a flat undersurface to accommodate the variety of movements in the most congruent way. The Oxford meniscal knee uses matching spherical surfaces for the femoral component and the upper meniscal-bearing surface and a flat surface to match a flat tibial component.[6]

This preferred geometry appears to work well as a medial unicompartmental replacement but has had dislocation problems in other applications.[6,7] These problems most likely are caused by a larger than normal single radius of curvature of the femoral component, which under the pull of the posterior cruciate ligament (PCL) in flexion moves the bearing too far posteriorly.

A design solution to the Oxford problem in the presence of cruciate ligaments is seen in the low contact stress (LCS) femoral component, which uses the same spherical surface of revolution in the medial–lateral plane but decreases the radius of curvature from extension to flexion, thus maintaining full-area contact on the upper meniscal-bearing surface from 0° to 45°, where walking loads are encountered, and maintaining at least spherical line contact at deeper flexion angles.[8] This surface geometry allows a more central femoral component position in flexion by reducing the PCL tension, which tends to pull the femur posteriorly when overstretched. Another design solution to prevent meniscal-bearing dislocation is the use of radial tracks on the LCS tibial components. These tracks allow axial rotation and controlled anteroposterior translation, which impedes direct dislocation by means of the cruciate bone bridge posteriorly and the patellar tendon anteriorly. When combined with stable flexion and extension gaps at surgery, the LCS meniscal bearings could be safely used when both cruciate ligaments are intact or if only the PCL is intact.

In the event of a nonfunctional or absent PCL, central stability with the ability to axially rotate is essential. Long-term survivorship studies have demonstrated that a centrally stabilized total condylar knee replacement is predicted to last for 15 years in more than 90% of cases when used in elderly patients with low loading demands.[9,10] These important studies prove that cruciate function is not essential for successful long-term fixation and function in low-demand situations.

Because wear increases as the loads and demands increase, it seems most appropriate to use the proven fixation and central stabilizing concepts of the total condylar device and provide a more wear-resistant and dislocation-resistant bearing surface to achieve better long-term survivorship and reduce wear-related failures. These concepts led to the development of a rotating-platform total knee device that uses the same spherical surface geometry as the meniscal bearings (**Fig. 36E-1**).

The patellofemoral design process, like the tibiofemoral design process, seeks to provide proper motion and maintain contact stresses below the ideal 5 megapascals (MPa) during walking, stair climbing, and deep-knee bending.[11] Button or nonrotating anatomic-type patellar replacements suffer from either point or line contact stresses or from overconstraint. High contact stress will cause early wear failure, whereas overconstraint will cause early loosening failure.[12] For these reasons, a rotating bearing patellar replacement was developed to maintain spherical area contact on the medial and lateral facets while congruently matching the surface of revolution of the deep sulcus femoral groove. Rotating bearing patellar replacement of the LCS design greatly improves on the contact stress seen in other design configurations.[11]

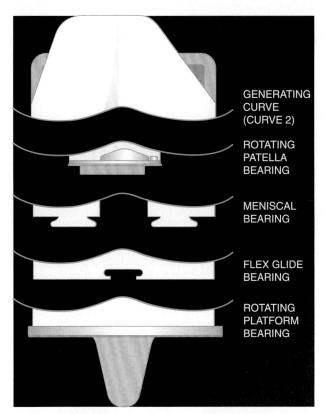

GENERATING
CURVE
(CURVE 2)

ROTATING
PATELLA
BEARING

MENISCAL
BEARING

FLEX GLIDE
BEARING

ROTATING
PLATFORM
BEARING

FIGURE 36E-1 LCS rotating-platform bearing design: spherical surface geometry matches meniscal-bearing designs + rotating bearing patella maintains spherical contact on the medial and lateral facets while congruently matching the surface of revolution of the deep sulcus femoral groove.

EVOLUTION OF THE NEW JERSEY LOW CONTACT STRESS MOBILE-BEARING KNEE

The first mobile-bearing application was seen in shoulder replacement in which two eccentrically placed spherical elements improved the range of motion over simple ball-and-socket systems. These "floating-socket" bearings were developed in 1974 and used clinically from 1975 to 1979, when less constrained

shoulder implants were developed.[13] Later, knee and ankle bearings were developed using similar concepts.[8]

The first complete systems approach to total knee replacement (TKR) using meniscal bearings, introduced in 1977, was the LCS Complete Knee System. At the time, the LCS system managed unicompartamental, bicompartamental, and tricompartamental disease by providing three options, the bicruciate-retaining, posterior-cruciate retaining, and the cruciate sacrificing rotating-platform design. Additionally, the first metal-backed, rotating bearing patellar replacement was developed in 1977 to provide mobility with congruity in patellofemoral articulation. This LCS Total Knee System, which initially received U.S. Food and Drug Administration Investigational Device Exemption (FDA-IDE) for clinical trials of cemented knees in 1980, and for uncemented knees in 1983, first came to market in 1985. Buechel and Pappas published the earliest clinical results of cemented LCS in 1986, reporting that 88.3% of the first 123 cemented knees had good to excellent outcomes at 2 to 7-year follow-up, with no reported mechanical failures or bearing dislocations.[14] The LCS remains the only knee system in the United States to have undergone formal FDA-IDE clinical trials in both cemented and uncemented applications before being released for general clinical use (**Fig. 36E-2**).

Early Results

While the majority of early LCS knee implants were posterior cruciate-retaining meniscal-bearing designs, early clinical results challenged their efficacy leading to a paradigm shift. In 2001, Buechel reported minimum 10-year follow-up results for 373 LCS prostheses. Survivorship for the posterior cruciate-retaining uncemented meniscal-bearing group was 83%, for the cemented cruciate sacrificing rotating-platform group was 97.7%, and for the uncemented cruciate sacrificing rotating-platform group was 98.3%. Thus, affirming what most had come to find

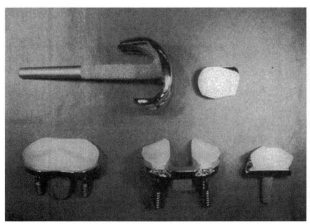
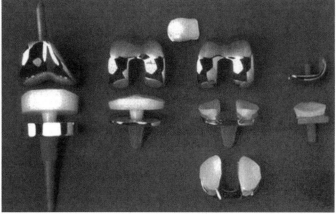

FIGURE 36E-2 History of mobile-bearing designs, from right to left: unicondylar / bicondylar, LCS RP, revision LCS RP.

over the years, that the rotating-platform prosthesis was not only an easier implant to utilize, but yielded superior survivorship than meniscal-bearing prosthesis.

BIOMECHANICAL CONSIDERATIONS

Component Surface Geometry

Surface congruence is essential to improve wear life in ultra-high-molecular-weight polyethylene bearings, especially in major repetitive load-bearing activities, such as walking, which generates loads of 2.5 times body weight, and stair climbing, which can generate loads of eight times body weight. Aside from direct compressive loading, however, the tibiofemoral bearings must be able to accommodate flexion of 155°, varus–valgus movements of 10°, axial rotation of 30°, and anteroposterior translation of 15 mm when the cruciate ligaments are retained. The patellofemoral articulation is also loaded mainly in

compression and needs to accommodate similar flexion to 155°, axial rotation of 6°, and the ability to tilt laterally and medially in the femoral groove without dislocating or rubbing on an edge.

The LCS knee was designed to accommodate for these parameters. Medical-grade polyethylene manufacturers recommend that contact stress ideally remain less than 5 MPa, and no greater than 10 MPa (**Fig. 36E-3A**). Maximizing the contact surface area between the femoral component and the polyethylene insert by maximizing conformity accomplishes this goal (**Fig. 36E-3B**). The unique geometry of the LCS knee maximizes conformity by matching the curvature of radii between femoral component and tibial insert, and femoral component with patellar insert. This conformity occurs between femur and tibia from 0° to 30° during gait, and between femur and patella from 0° to 110°. In the weight-bearing segment of the femoral component, segment 2, the anteroposterior radius of curvature equals the medial–lateral

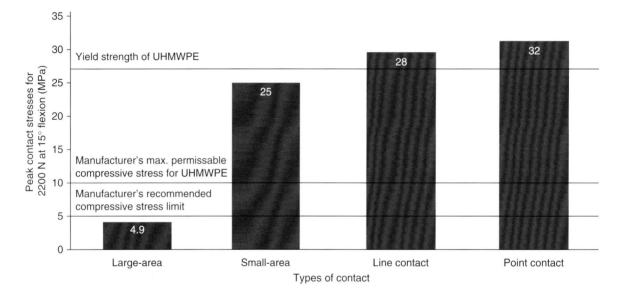

A

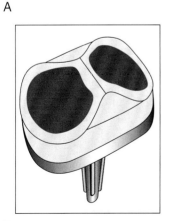 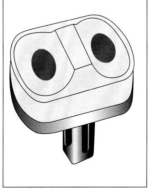 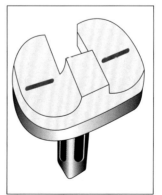 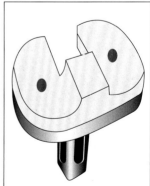

B

FIGURE 36E-3   A: Industry recommendations are to keep contact stress between femoral implant and polyethylene, ideally, less than 5 MPa, and no greater than 10 MPa. **B:** Maximizing the contact surface area between the femoral component and the polyethylene insert by maximizing conformity accomplishes this goal by reducing contact stress.

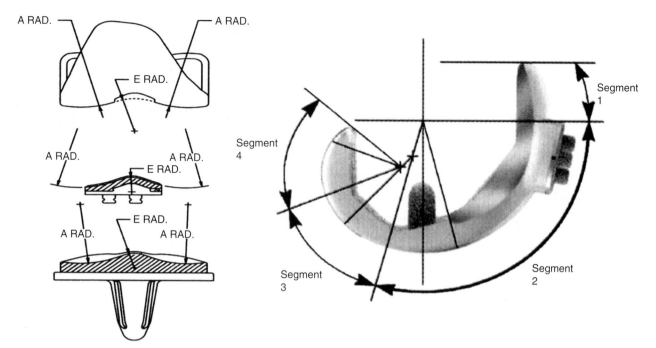

FIGURE 36E-4 Curvature of radii between femoral component and tibial insert, and femoral component with patellar insert is matched in LCS knee. This conformity occurs between femur and tibia from 0° to 30° during gait, and between femur and patella from 0° to 110°. In the weight-bearing segment of the femoral component, segment 2, the anteroposterior radius of curvature equals the medial–lateral radius.

radius (**Fig. 36E-4**). Therefore, during gait the contact area between the femoral and tibial components is a large sphere, 877 mm².

The importance of maximizing surface area to maximize conformity was elucidated by Kuster and Stachowiak, who examined the interplay between conformity and load.[15] A conformity ratio of 0.99 connotes fully conforming femoral and tibial components, while a ratio of 0 represents a femoral condyle and a flat tibial insert. Using finite element modeling, the authors found increasing conformity ratios has a greater effect on polyethylene stress than reducing loads. In their analysis, as expected, polyethylene stress was higher for a 1000 N load (standing) on a flat tibial insert than a 6000 N load (running) on a conforming insert. However, an increase in the conformity ratio from 0.95 to 0.99 had a greater effect on surface and shear stresses than a load increase of 3000 N. Thus, they posited that a high conformity ratio reduced tibial polyethylene insert delamination and accelerated wear more significantly than load restrictions due to activity modification in nonconforming total knee arthroplasty (TKA) designs. The LCS Total Knee System has a conformity ratio of 0.99 in gait.

Wear Properties

Recent advances have significantly improved the quality of polyethylene inserts. Gamma irradiation in a vacuum pouch has replaced gamma sterilization in air, and calcium stearate has been eliminated from polyethylene resins, both reducing the potential for polyethylene oxidation which is known to reduce polyethylene insert mechanical

properties. In spite of this, retrieval of component studies continue to demonstrate reductions in volumetric wear under high loads for LCS total knees in comparison to fixed-bearing prosthesis.[5,16-18] Similar retrieval analyses of meniscal bearings, rotating-platform bearings, and rotating patellar bearings demonstrated significantly less wear than with fixed bearings. Although mobile bearings allow reduced contact stress, they can be overloaded to failure by excessive weight, excessive activity, malalignment, or a combination of these factors. However, by their nature, spherically surfaced mobile bearings accommodate malalignment without overload more easily than fixed bearings. Whether the overall knee alignment is in neutral (5° valgus) or not, the spherical bearing surface always sees congruent contact with the femoral component as compared with a flat-on-flat bearing surface that becomes overloaded during normal condylar liftoff. By design, the rotating platform couples rotational forces between the femoral component and tibial polyethylene insert, and between the tibial insert and the tibial tray surface. In the LCS knee, rotation primarily occurs between the distal polyethylene surface and tibial tray, producing a unidirectional wear pattern. Similarly, rotation at the femoral component and polyethylene interface is largely during flexion–extension, again producing unidirectional wear. Thus, the LCS rotating-platform design reduces complex knee kinematics into predominately unidirectional motions (**Fig. 36E-5**). As various studies have shown, unidirectional motion reduces polyethylene wear rates, particularly with the newer, highly cross-linked polyethylene inserts[19,20] (**Fig. 36E-6**).

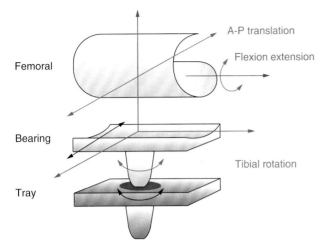

FIGURE 36E-5 The rotating platform decouples the femoral-bearing contact area and tibial-bearing mobility to reduce bone–prosthesis interface stressed as well as polyethylene stress.

In their biomechanical study, Wang et al analyzed the source of microscopic wear particles generated from modern polyethylene articular surfaces.[19] They found that the polyethylene chain reorganizes due to surface strain secondary to femoral component motion. When stressed, the molecular chain responds favorably when loaded on-axis, but unfavorably when loaded off-axis. Multidirectional joint simulators, mimicking fixed-bearing femoral component–tibial tray interaction, create complex, off-axis loads. They found that this multidirectional motion causes failure along three modes, in accordance with increasing degree of off-axis motion: tensile rupture, shear rupture, and transverse splitting. These mechanisms all produce fiber-like wear particles, with increased wear associated with large degrees

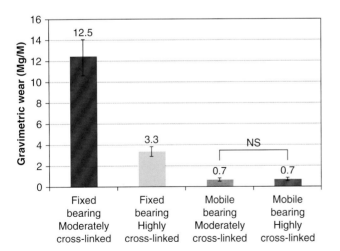

FIGURE 36E-6 Wear patterns for fixed versus mobile bearing, early moderately cross-linked versus newer highly cross-linked. Results show significant improvement in wear rate for fixed-bearing prosthesis when using highly cross-linked polyethylene inserts, but no significant change in wear rates between the two inserts between fixed- and mobile-bearing knees.

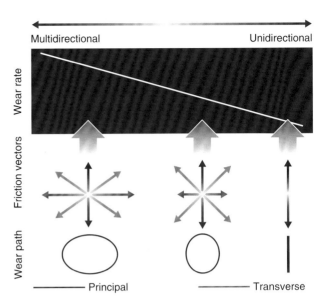

FIGURE 36E-7 Multidirectional wear patterns introduce friction vectors in various planes, increasing wear rates in the polyethylene insert. As motion is made more unidirectional, friction vectors align, minimizing the polyethylene wear rate.

of off-axis motion. Another biomechanical study by Marrs et al examined polyethylene wear rates, comparing unidirectional and multidirectional motion.[20] They similarly found that unidirectional motion reduces ultra-high-molecular-weight polyethylene wear (**Fig. 36E-7**). Numerous studies directly comparing the wear rates between fixed and mobile-bearing designs have corroborated these biomechanical findings. McEwen et al investigated polyethylene wear using various total knee prosthesis and stressing them in knee simulators, finding that rotating-platform mobile-bearing implants had reduced wear rates in comparison to fixed-bearing components.[21] Examination of wear patterns suggested improved wear characteristics in this prosthesis was due to redistribution of knee motion to two articulating interfaces with more linear motion at each interface.

FIXATION OF MOBILE BEARINGS

The use of methyl methacrylate bone cement was the initial adjunctive method of bony attachment for the first LCS unicompartmental meniscal-bearing device used in 1977 and for subsequent bicompartmental and tricompartmental devices.[14]

The tibial fixation surface of the LCS unicompartmental knee replacement has a flat tibial loading plate and a short-angled stem to resist tipping and shear loads. PCR LCS meniscal-bearing and LCS rotating-platform tibial components use a short, conical metaphyseal fixation stem centered in the proximal tibia. All femoral components use shallow cement-locking pockets and centralized femoral fixation pegs.

The rotating bearing patellar replacement uses cruciform fin geometry for fixation. This geometry reinforces the thin metal plate against torsional failure and reinforces the patellar remnant against fractures while engaging the patellar bone stock sufficiently to prevent loosening.

Uncemented fixation with sintered-bead cobalt-chromium-molybdenum porous coating on the cobalt-chromium-molybdenum substrate using the same articulating and fixation geometries was first used clinically in early 1981. Cruciate retaining and rotating-platform tibial components were developed with four screw holes and spherical seats. These implants used 6.5-mm cancellous bone screws to augment fixation.

Concerns over fretting corrosion, screw breakage, osteolysis, and potential neurovascular injuries from screw penetration led the developers away from screw fixation later in the same year. These early concerns are now complications that have been documented by several authors in other uncemented knee devices.[16,18,22]

Press-fit non–screw-fixed mobile-bearing knee replacements with porous coating have been in successful clinical use since 1981. Jordan et al, in their survivorship analysis on 473 uncemented cruciate-retaining meniscal-bearing implants, found that 3.6% were revised due to mechanical failure, 2.5% due to polyethylene failure, 1% due to ligamentous instability and subsequent tibial subluxation, and just 0.04% due to aseptic loosening. At 8 years from surgery, survivorship was 99% with failure due to mechanical loosening.[23] Longer-term 20-year rotating-platform studies have demonstrated a 99.4% overall fixation survivorship with these devices.

CLINICAL APPLICATION OF MOBILE BEARINGS

Unicompartmental Knee Replacement

Unicompartmental meniscal bearings are well adapted for knee replacement because they allow retention of both cruciate ligaments and allow the normal forward and backward translational movement of the femur on the tibia as well as axial rotation and varus–valgus movement with excellent congruity of the bearing surfaces. The Oxford meniscal-bearing unicompartmental device has had excellent success when used as a medial unicompartmental replacement but has functioned less consistently as a lateral compartment replacement because of significant dislocation problems.[6,7]

The uncemented LCS unicompartmental knee replacement was approved by the FDA Orthopaedic Advisory Panel in August 1991 and released for general use by the FDA in November 1992 after successful completion of an FDA-IDE clinical trial. Good or excellent results using a strict knee scoring scale were seen in 98.4%

of 122 patients followed up for 2 to 6 years (mean of 3.3 years).[24] One bearing fractured after trauma, and one tibial component loosened in a patient with posttraumatic osteoporotic bone deficiency. Progressive disease in the opposite knee compartment was an additional cause for revision. Such disorders represent current failure mechanisms for this device and are now considered contraindications. Long-term studies have shown that while severe lateral patellofemoral joint degeneration remains a contraindication to medial unicompartmental arthroplasty, less severe lateral PF and medial PF arthrosis of any severity do not affect survival or overall function of unicompartmental replacements at 15-year follow-up.[25]

Unicompartmental Oxford meniscal bearings showed a minimal wear rate of 0.02 mm per year, attesting to the concept of increased congruity decreases the wear rate[26] (**Fig. 36E-8**). Survivorship of the cemented device was 98% at 10 years in the developer's series[27] and 90% at 5 years in a National Swedish Arthroplasty study.[28] Bearing dislocation was the major problem leading to failure in both studies. Interestingly, low wear rates and favorable survivorship of these implants are often felt to be counterintuitive to the wear patterns anticipated with fixed, unicompartmental meniscal bearings. The Oxford, due to a single radius design, allows for normal AP translation and rotation. Such designs should be subject to the same multidirectional pattern seen in fixed-bearing knee designs. Thus, a healthy, functional anterior cruciate ligament is crucial to maintaining the desired wear patterns of the Oxford knee. Motion of the medial and lateral compartments is constrained such that apparent multidirectional wear is in fact repeated in a uniform arc along the polyethylene, thereby creating a unidirectional wear pattern.

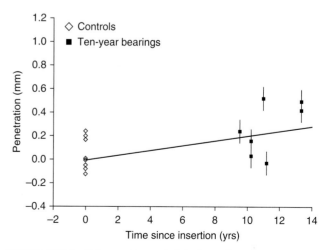

FIGURE 36E-8 Unicompartmental Oxford meniscal bearings show minimal wear rate, 0.02 mm per year.

Bicompartmental Knee Replacement

The articulating geometry of the femoral component is critical to the success or failure of the patellar component. A bispherical, continuous-surface-of-revolution femoral groove matching a bispherical congruently tracking patellar component will provide for a long service life for the patellar bearing. This same femoral groove can match the anatomic patellar geometry and can allow retention of the natural patella. No difference has been reported between bicompartmental (retention of natural patella) and tricompartmental (replaced patella) knee replacements, using the unique femoral groove of the LCS design, in a 10-year clinical series of 52 patients in whom one patella was replaced and the other patella was retained, as reported by Keblish et al[29]

Such predictability can allow patellar retention in patients such as farmers or laborers who require repetitive squatting loads that may increase patellar component wear. Additionally, patellar retention in conditions such as patella infera, patella alta, or hypoplasia can facilitate central tracking without fear of early knee replacement failure. Finally, those patients with previous patellectomies can undergo a patellar tendon bone grafting and enjoy a well-functioning bicompartmental replacement with improvement in both quadriceps leverage and tibiofemoral dislocation resistance.[30]

Rotating Bearing Patella Replacement

Failures of the rotating bearing patella have been rare and usually associated with displaced patellar fractures, malposition, subluxation, or excessive, repetitive hyperflexion loads.

The overall complications of rotating bearing patellar replacements that required revision surgery in 515 knees originally followed up for 6 months to 11 years (53) and now followed up for 8 to 19 years (mean of 12.5 years) were 5 of 515, or 0.97%. Wear-through of the bearing on the lateral facet and transverse bearing fractures have been the dominant mechanisms of mechanical failure. These have been associated with unrecognized poor-quality polyethylene and gamma radiation oxidation, which has also negatively affected the tibial bearings of the past two decades.

In their review of mobile-bearing patella components, Jordan L and Dowd J et al followed up 256 primary uncemented meniscal-bearing total knee arthroplasties with LCS metal-backed anatomic mobile patella.[31] At an average 11.5-year follow-up, no patellae were revised fixation failure due to dislocation or subluxation. Only one patellar implant in their series was revised due to polyethylene wear, and one functioning patellar implant was removed during revision TKA to facilitate range of motion and wound closure. At 12 years, the authors found 99.5% survivorship.

Similarly, Tarkin et al, in their long-term series of 70 LCS RP knees, found survivorship with respect to aseptic loosening was 97% at 17 years, with only 1 knee revision in that time for aseptic loosening.[32] However, overall survivorship was 76%, primarily due to failures of the metal-backed rotating patella. Compared to the high incidence of failure of metal-backed fixed-bearing patellae components, the anatomic rotating patella provides durable long-term results with a low incidence of complications.

SURVIVORSHIP

Few meta-analyses have sought to aggregate large national registries and systematic reviews to compare survivorship and functional outcomes between differing TKA prostheses. Carothers et al sought to compare the performance of LCS MB knees, LCS AP Glide knees, PFC Sigma Rotating Platform, and LCS RP knees, finding higher survivorship with the rotating-platform knees (PFC Sigma and LCS RP) than with the LCS MB knees.[33] With aggregate analysis including 3506 total knee arthroplasties, they found 15-year survivorship for rotating-platform designs versus meniscal-bearing implants was 96.4% vs. 86.5%.

More recently, Hopley, Crossett, and Chen reported on survivorship and function of LCS rotating-platform knees and compared RP results to fixed-bearing results over the same time period. Their analyses included 29 papers, including 4 level 1 randomized controlled trials, totaling 6437 LCS RP total knee arthroplasties done from 1980 to 2005.[34] The outcomes of their meta-analysis included Knee Society Scores (KSS) and cumulative revision rates (CRR). As comparison, they pooled survivorship data from two independent systematic reviews (the Agency for Healthcare, Research and Quality [AHRQ] and the Ontario Reviews) and the Swedish Knee Arthroplasty Registry, totaling over 100,000 implants, of which 94% were fixed-bearing or cemented designs.[35-37]

With regard to clinical outcomes (KSS), there was no significant difference in pre- and postoperative scores between the LCS RP studies and the fixed-bearing systematic reviews. Postoperative KSS from LCS RP studies were, on average, higher at 2 to 3 years and 7 to 10 years for knee scores, and higher at 2 to 3 years and 13 to 15 years for function scores, although none of these differences were significant at any time point.

With regard to survivorship, revision rates with the LCS RP knee implanted between 1981-1997 and 1988-2005 were lower (i.e., higher survivorship), on average, than the fixed-bearing cemented knees reported in the Swedish Knee Registry during those same time periods. The studies that reported survivorship for LCS RP knees at 15 years reported figures of 98.3%, 98%, 96.5%, 92.1%, and 76%. An additional two studies reported

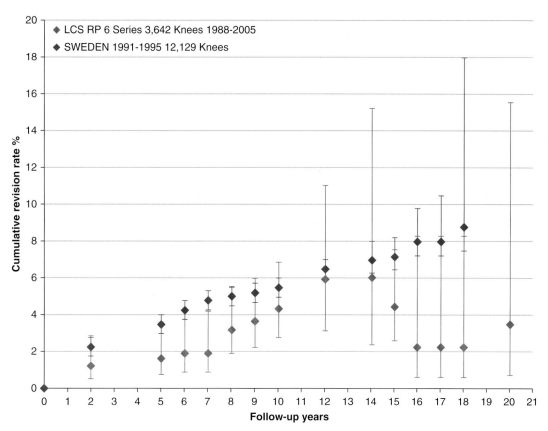

FIGURE 36E-9   Cumulative revision rate—LCS RP knees implanted in 1981 to 1997 and Swedish Registry Knees implanted in 1991 to 1995.

LCS RP survivorship at 18 years, of 98.3% and 96.5%. The longest reported survivorship with the LCS RP knee was 96.5% at 20 years.

These data suggest LCS RP implants are associated with equivalent clinical outcomes when compared to fixed-bearing knee prostheses. Additionally, pooled data for LCS RP implants show survivorship of 94% to 97% at 12 years, and 96% to 98% at 18 years. Survivorship data can be further sorted into two periods according to surgical date: 1981-1997 and 1998-2005. Though these intervals do not perfectly match Swedish Knee Registry–reported intervals, they were matched as closely as possible for analysis purposes. For imperfectly matched cohorts, LCS RP knee results were always compared to the more recent Swedish Registry results to provide a more rigorous comparison. Roughly, the pooled CRR of the LCS RP knee was lower on average than the CRR of the Swedish Knee Registry at all reporting times out to 9 and 12 years (**Figs. 36E-9** and **36E-10**). The survivorship in more contemporary studies (1988-2005) was substantially higher than older studies, a similar improvement to that reported in the Swedish Registry during a similar time frame. These data ultimately suggest a very high survivorship out to 20 years, with a very low incidence of wear-related revision in the second decade. The LCS RP knee has a comparable long-term

clinical outcome (KSS) to those reported in the recent AHRQ and Ontario systematic reviews of the TKA implants as a class.

POSTERIOR-STABILIZED LOW CONTACT STRESS MOBILE-BEARING KNEE

The design rationale for the posterior-stabilized LCS RP followed in-depth analyses of LCS RP kinematics. Dennis et al performed an *in vivo* kinematic study, examining multiple TKA designs, including the LCS.[38] They found that in gait, the LCS RP knee had the least variability in translation, predominantly due to its sagittal conformity which prevented anteroposterior movement. However, in deep knee bend, the decreased conformity resulted in, on average, a small anterior femoral translation. They also noted high variability in the amount of AP translation between subjects during deep knee bend. This paradoxical anterior translation was an obvious issue. During flexion, anterior slide of the femoral condyles caused early posterior femoral impingement as the posterior femoral cortex abutted the posterior lip of the conforming polyethylene insert. Dennis et al also found that in the posterior-stabilized designs, spine-cam engagement forces posterior femoral rollback in flexion, thereby limiting the extent to which the posterior femoral

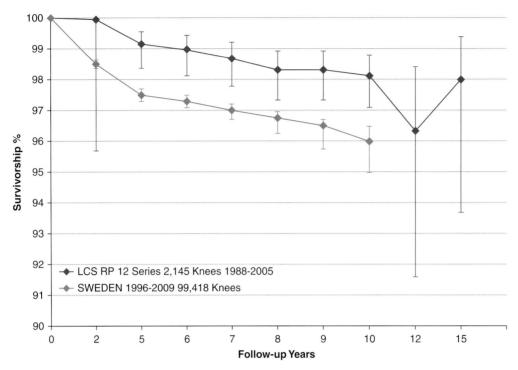

FIGURE 36E-10 Cumulative revision rate—LCS RP knees implanted in 1988 to 2005 and Swedish Registry Knees implanted in 1996 to 2009.

cortex abuts the polyethylene, increasing the amount of flexion possible with those implants. They noted that the femoral rollback forced by the PS design was the most predictable of flexion kinematics in the study. Indeed, the study confirmed that the LCS RP had lowest average *in vivo* range of motion, with 108° and 99° of passive and weight-bearing *in vivo* range of motion, compared to 139° and 135° for native knees, 127° and 113° for fixed-bearing posterior stabilized knees, and 121° and 100° for LCS MB knees.

Thus, the LCS RP PS design was born. Initially introduced in 2000, the first-generation LCS RP PS was halted due to issues of anterior impingement and hemarthrosis in early clinical trials, with early clinical data suggesting 8% to 10% hemarthrosis rate.[39] The large anterior lip of the highly conforming polyethylene was largely believed to be at fault for this complication.

In 2005, a second design the LCS RP PS knee was initiated (**Fig. 36E-11**). Goals of this design were predictable flexion kinematics, limited box resection, prevention of patellar crepitus and clunk, limited polyethylene wear, and providing adequate subluxation resistance. The design team sought to maintain every design feature and geometry of the LCS RP, while adding a post that mirrored the kinematics of the original posterior-stabilized implant, the Insall–Burstein PS prosthesis. The flexion kinematics were designed to limit femoral rollback, as excessive rollback was postulated to increase eccentric forces that could contribute to tray liftoff, especially for uncemented implants, as discussed below. Limited

box resection with an open box design was also of key importance, both to preserve native bone stock and prevent femoral condyle fracture, and to allow insertion of intramedullary nails for fixation of periprosthetic fractures. Box volume comparison studies by the design team found the first-generation LCS RP PS had a box volume of 10.3 mL, compared to the 17.0 mL volume of the IB-II femoral component. Finally, in an effort to reduce patellofemoral clunk, the trochlear groove was carried further anteriorly and distally. Coupling more favorable anterior flange geometry with an anatomic patella design and improved femoral rollback kinematics helped decrease patellofemoral tilt during knee flexion. Less of extension of the patella during flexion was thought to decrease the incidence of patellar clunk, making it less likely that the super pole of the patellar component would catch against the anterior aspect of the femoral box.[39]

The desired aspects of the second-generation LCS RP PS design have been confirmed in subsequent *in vivo* kinematic studies, which have documented that cam–post engagement occurs no earlier than 60° of knee flexion, and holds the femur in dwell position until 90°, after which the femoral component begins to roll back. Rollback was designed to be limited to prevent eccentric forces on the tibia and polyethylene, forces that contribute to liftoff, and aseptic loosening of the femoral and tibial components. For the LCS RP PS, rollback was limited to a maximum of 3 to 4 mm after 90° past the dwell point.

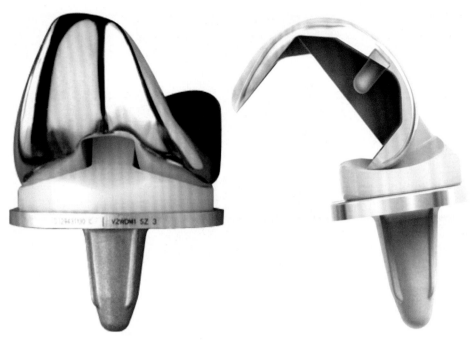

FIGURE 36E-11   LCS RP PS (posterior-stabilized) knee.

Stiehl at al. in 1999 had already confirmed that condylar liftoff during gait occurs in both cruciate-retaining and cruciate-sacrificing designs, suggesting that 85% of LCS RP implants demonstrate liftoff, 41% on medial plateau, 59% on lateral plateau.[40] However, given the medial–lateral conformity of the LCS articulation, this manifested as subluxation of the femoral component rather than rotational liftoff. Thus, the post of the LCS RP PS was developed with a unique design, such that the base of the post was slightly narrower than the top of the post, to accommodate for this translation of the femoral component. Because of the narrower nature of the post, a reinforcing rod was placed to support this post. Radiographically, a metal post should indicate to surgeons that PS design is being used, not a constrained design (**Fig. 36E-12**).

A small, in-house study conducted by the design surgeon confirmed improved outcomes with the LCS RP PS design. Evaluating the pre- and postoperative KSS and ROM scores for patients undergoing TKA with the LCS RP PS implant, the design surgeon found that, preoperative versus 12 months postoperatively, clinical score went from 40 to 86, functional score from 59 to 89, pain score from 15 to 45, stair score from 32 to 44, and range of motion increases from 109° to 120° (**Fig. 36E-13**).

Though long-term outcomes for the posterior-stabilized LCS RP are limited, recently nondesign surgeons have begun publishing their outcome data for the implant. Ulivi et al reported on 112 LCS RP PS knees, reporting 96.6% survivorship at 10 years postoperatively.[41] They reported a 0% incidence of spinout or radiographic osteolysis in their cohort. Maniar et al has reported the longest-term results thus far on 88 LCS RP PS knees followed up for

13 years.[42] They found that mean flexion improved from 107° to 127°. KSS knee score improved from 28 to 96, and function score improved from 53 to 78. There were no reported spinouts in their cohort, no radiographic evidence of osteolysis, nor any revisions, suggesting 100% implant survivorship.

Of note, spinout, which was a unique complication of the rotating-platform meniscal-bearing prosthesis, involved the femoral condyle subluxing anteriorly over the anterior edge of the polyethylene. With the posterior stabilized design, that phenomenon has been eliminated as found in the studies above.

REVISION TOTAL KNEE REPLACEMENT

If you believe in the concept of Low Contact Stress arthroplasty, does it not follow to apply these principles to the clinically compromised situation

Lawrence S. Crossett, MD

The benefits of rotating-platform implants in revision knee arthroplasty can be distilled to two factors: rotation and fixation.

Rotation

In the revision setting, rotation helps to minimize polyethylene wear, reduce loosening forces, and reduce post wear. Polyethylene wear accounts for 24.5% of failures in revision TKA. As discussed earlier in this chapter, multidirectional motion, as seen with fixed-bearing implants, accelerates polyethylene wear, while implants that promote unidirectional motion reduce polyethylene wear

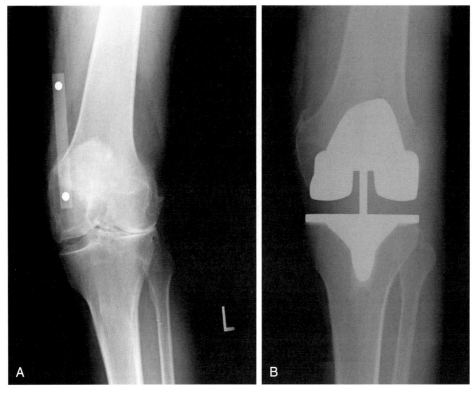

FIGURE 36E-12   Radiograph of LCS RP PS design with metal reinforcing rod in the post.

(**Fig. 36E-1**). Any effort to reduce polyethylene wear, and the potential for osteolysis, should play a central role in revision TKA. Second, aseptic loosening in knee replacement has the potential to cause massive bone loss and instability, making subsequent surgeries increasingly difficult. Tibial loosening accounts for 22% of failures in all revision

TKA. Mobile-bearing prosthesis can reduce torque at the proximal tibia by 68% to 73%, reducing rotatory forces at the bone–prosthetic interface, thereby minimizing these loosening forces.[43] Long-term studies have corroborated these findings. Callaghan et al, in their 15-year follow-up of cemented, rotating-platform knee, found no instance of

	Pre-Op Mean (SD)	3-Month Mean (SD)	6-Month Mean (SD)	12 Month Mean (SD)
Clinical Score (100 points possible)	40 (16)	82 (14)	86 (12)	86 (13)
Function Score (100 polnts possible)	59 (19)	78 (19)	85 (19)	89 (15)
Pain Score (50 points possible)	15 (10)	40 (12)	43 (10)	45 (9)
Stair Score (50 points possible)	32 (7)	38 (9)	41 (9)	44 (8)
ROM (degrees)	109 (18)	112 (13)	116 (12)	120(9)

FIGURE 36E-13   Results of in-house functional outcomes study of LCS RP PS design conducted by the design surgeon.

TC3 Fixed Bearing

TC3 Rotating Platform

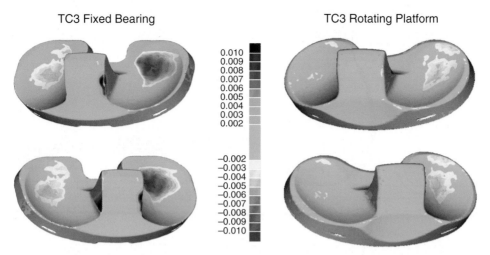

FIGURE 36E-14 Fixed-bearing revision polyethylene inserts show decreased thickness and greater wear at similar time points as rotating-platform revision inserts.

tibial loosening in 119 patients.[44] Similarly, Sorrels et al reported only one instance of tibial loosening in their cohort of 528 uncemented RP knees at 5 to 12 years follow-up.[45] Finally, post wear and impingement continue to be significant issues in the revision setting. Retrieval studies in knees being revised have found 100% of posts show some wear, with on average, 40% of the post exhibiting some wear.[46] They also noted that the posts with wider medial–lateral dimensions (i.e., constrained) showed additional wear. Orthopedic industry estimates that up to 80% of revision arthroplasty in the United States today is being done with constrained polyethylene inserts.[39] A native knee allows 16.5° and 5.7° of internal rotation during deep knee flexion and gait, respectively.[47] In comparison, constrained prosthesis at best allows 4.3° of rotation, while revision rotating-platform prosthesis, by design, allows rotation as required. Examination of wear similarly finds that fixed-bearing revision implants demonstrate greater polyethylene wear than their rotating-platform counterparts (**Fig. 36E-14**).

Fixation

Goals of fixation of the revision implant include filling of substantial bony defects, providing strong structural foundation, restoration of the joint line, and compressive loading of the bone. Tibial and metaphyseal sleeve designs are based on the proven S-ROM sleeve concept, which has a mobile-bearing hinge and has shown excellent midterm results.[48] The modular concept of the prosthesis sleeve device remains unique to the mobile-bearing arthroplasty family. In the development of the Attune fixed and mobile-bearing revision systems, the decision was made not to offer sleeve fixation on fixed-bearing implants, due to concerns that excessive rotational stresses would be transferred to the tibial and femoral components.[39]

The senior author of this chapter strongly believes that metaphyseal sleeves offer multiple advantages in revision arthroplasty. The first advantage is for the management of massive bone loss. Large tibiofemoral defects can be filled with titanium sleeves with porous ingrowth, fulfilling all of the goals of a revision implant. The second advantage is the increase in relative stability of the implant. As noted by Jean-Louis Briard in 2008, the failure of revision total knee arthroplasties is on the femoral side. In a healthy, native knee, the posterior femoral condyles control rotational stability at 90° flexion (**Fig. 36E-15A**). Mild posterior condylar defects create larger wedges, causing greater instability in flexion (**Fig. 36E-15B**). Meanwhile, complete posterior condylar defects result in a complete absence of control of the femoral torque at 90° flexion (**Fig. 36E-15C**). While stems contribute to varus/valgus stability in full extension, they add little to rotational stability (**Fig. 36E-15D and E**). A sleeve significantly improves rotational stability, controlling femoral torque at 90° flexion (**Fig. 36E-15F**). Finally, the third advantage for sleeves in revision arthroplasty is for uncemented long term fixation. Though long-term data are lacking, similar to uncemented fixation in total hip arthroplasty, the senior author agrees that bony ingrowth confers added stability and portends better long-term survival of the revision implant.

FUTURE DIRECTIONS OF MOBILE-BEARING KNEE REPLACEMENT

Industry trends suggest that the future of mobile-bearing TKA will involve a shift away from pure gap balancing. We have already come a long way from early LCS designs that had just three femoral component sizes (small, medium, large). The modern Attune TKA System offers 10 sizes, each varied by 3 mm increments. The senior author believes that the key to improving kinematics and

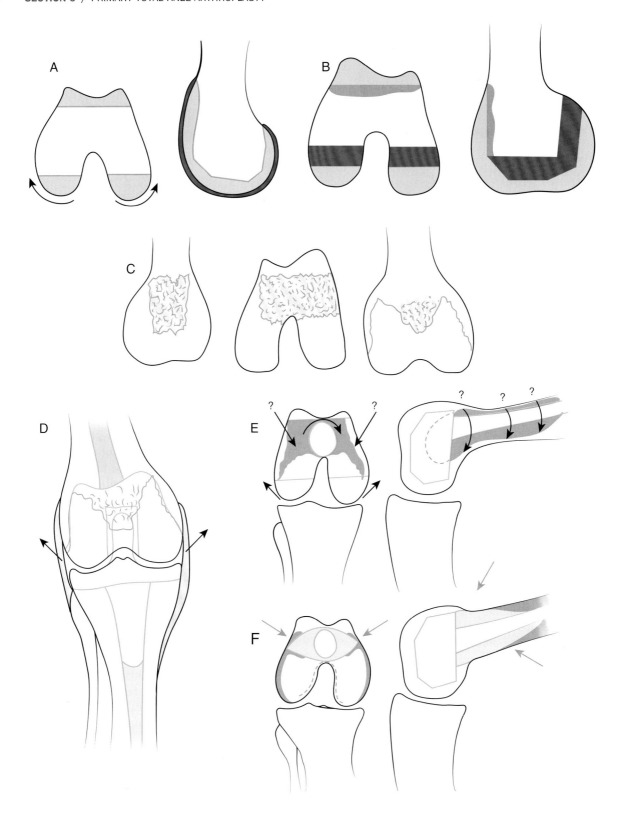

FIGURE 36E-15   A: posterior femoral condyles control rotational stability at 90° flexion. **B:** Mild posterior condylar defects create larger wedges, causing greater instability in flexion. **C:** Complete posterior condylar defects result in a complete absence of control of the femoral torque at 90° flexion. **D/E:** While stems contribute to varus/valgus stability in full extension, they add little to rotational stability. **F:** A sleeve significantly improves rotational stability, controlling femoral torque at 90° flexion.

eliminating midstance instability, following measured resection in extension, is the removal of **all** flexion deformity before going into flexion and continuing posterior femoral cuts. This includes a thorough posteromedial release, removing the large posteromedial osteophytes that contribute to capsular tenting and residual flexion deformity. By minimizing the extension gap and carefully manipulating the flexion gap, we hope to reliably and repeatably maximize isometry of the MCL in TKA.

REFERENCES

1. Rand JA, Chao EY, Stauffer RN. Kinematic rotating-hinge total knee arthroplasty. *J Bone Joint Surg Am.* 1987;69(4):489-497. PubMed PMID: 3571306.
2. Riley D, Woodyard JE. Long-term results of Geomedic total knee replacement. *J Bone Joint Surg Br.* 1985;67(4):548-550. PubMed PMID: 4030848.
3. Lewallen DG, Bryan RS, Peterson LF. Polycentric total knee arthroplasty. A ten-year follow-up study. *J Bone Joint Surg Am.* 1984;66(8):1211-1218. PubMed PMID: 6490696.
4. Collier JP, Mayor MB, McNamara JL, Surprenant VA, Jensen RE. Analysis of the failure of 122 polyethylene inserts from uncemented tibial knee components. *Clin Orthop Relat Res.* 1991;(273):232-242. PubMed PMID: 1959276.
5. Engh GA, Dwyer KA, Hanes CK. Polyethylene wear of metal-backed tibial components in total and unicompartmental knee prostheses. *J Bone Joint Surg Br.* 1992;74(1):9-17. PubMed PMID: 1732274.
6. Carr A, Keyes G, Miller R, O'Connor J, Goodfellow J. Medial unicompartmental arthroplasty. A survival study of the Oxford meniscal knee. *Clin Orthop Relat Res.* 1993;(295):205-213. PubMed PMID: 8403650.
7. Goodfellow JW, O'Connor J. Clinical results of the Oxford knee. Surface arthroplasty of the tibiofemoral joint with a meniscal bearing prosthesis. *Clin Orthop Relat Res.* 1986;(205):21-42. PubMed PMID: 3698380.
8. Buechel FF, Pappas MJ. New Jersey low contact stress knee replacement system. Ten-year evaluation of meniscal bearings. *Orthop Clin North Am.* 1989;20(2):147-177. PubMed PMID: 2922189.
9. Ranawat CS, Flynn WF Jr, Saddler S, Hansraj KK, Maynard MJ. Long-term results of the total condylar knee arthroplasty. A 15-year survivorship study. *Clin Orthop Relat Res.* 1993;(286):94-102. PubMed PMID: 8425373.
10. Scuderi GR, Insall JN, Windsor RE, Moran MC. Survivorship of cemented knee replacements. *J Bone Joint Surg Br.* 1989;71(5):798-803. PubMed PMID: 2584250.
11. Buechel FF, Pappas MJ, Makris G. Evaluation of contact stress in metal-backed patellar replacements. A predictor of survivorship. *Clin Orthop Relat Res.* 1991;(273):190-197. PubMed PMID: 1959271.
12. Wright TM, Rimnac CM, Stulberg SD, et al. Wear of polyethylene in total joint replacements. Observations from retrieved PCA knee implants. *Clin Orthop Relat Res.* 1992;(276):126-134. PubMed PMID: 1537143.
13. Buechel FF, Pappas MJ, DePalma AF. "Floating-socket" total shoulder replacement: anatomical, biomechanical, and surgical rationale. *J Biomed Mater Res.* 1978;12(1):89-114. doi:10.1002/jbm.820120109. PubMed PMID: 632319.
14. Buechel FF, Pappas MJ. The New Jersey Low-Contact-Stress Knee Replacement System: biomechanical rationale and review of the first 123 cemented cases. *Arch Orthop Trauma Surg.* 1986;105(4):197-204. PubMed PMID: 3753173.
15. Kuster MS, Stachowiak GW. Factors affecting polyethylene wear in total knee arthroplasty. *Orthopedics.* 2002;25(2 suppl):s235-s242. PubMed PMID: 11866159.
16. Collier JP, Mayor MB, Surprenant VA, Surprenant HP, Dauphinais LA, Jensen RE. The biomechanical problems of polyethylene as a bearing surface. *Clin Orthop Relat Res.* 1990;(261):107-113. PubMed PMID: 2245536.
17. Bohl JR, Bohl WR, Postak PD, Greenwald AS. The Coventry Award. The effects of shelf life on clinical outcome for gamma sterilized polyethylene tibial components. *Clin Orthop Relat Res.* 1999;(367):28-38. PubMed PMID: 10546595.
18. Peters PC Jr, Engh GA, Dwyer KA, Vinh TN. Osteolysis after total knee arthroplasty without cement. *J Bone Joint Surg Am.* 1992;74(6):864-876. PubMed PMID: 1634576.
19. Wang A, Stark C, Dumbleton JH. Mechanistic and morphological origins of ultra-high molecular weight polyethylene wear debris in total joint replacement prostheses. *Proc Inst Mech Eng H J Eng Med.* 1996;210(3):141-155. doi:10.1243/pime_proc_1996_210_407_02. PubMed PMID: 8885651.
20. Marrs H, Barton DC, Jones RA, Ward IM, Fisher J, Doyle C. Comparative wear under four different tribological conditions of acetylene enhanced cross-linked ultra high molecular weight polyethylene. *J Mater Sci Mater Med.* 1999;10(6):333-342. doi:10.1023/A:1026469522868.
21. McEwen HM, Barnett PI, Bell CJ, et al. The influence of design, materials and kinematics on the in vitro wear of total knee replacements. *J Biomech.* 2005;38(2):357-365. doi:10.1016/j.jbiomech.2004.02.015. PubMed PMID: 15598464.
22. Schatzker J, Horne JG, Sumner-Smith G. The effect of movement on the holding power of screws in bone. *Clin Orthop Relat Res.* 1975;(111):257-262. PubMed PMID: 1157420.
23. Jordan LR, Olivo JL, Voorhorst PE. Survivorship analysis of cementless meniscal bearing total knee arthroplasty. *Clin Orthop Relat Res.* 1997;(338):119-123. PubMed PMID: 9170372.
24. Buechel FF. A simplified evaluation system for the rating of knee function. *Orthop Rev.* 1982;11:5.
25. Hamilton TW, Pandit HG, Maurer DG, et al. Anterior knee pain and evidence of osteoarthritis of the patellofemoral joint should not be considered contraindications to mobile-bearing unicompartmental knee arthroplasty: a 15-year follow-up. *Bone Joint J.* 2017;99-B(5):632-639. doi:10.1302/0301-620x.99b5.Bjj-2016-0695.R2. PubMed PMID: 28455472.
26. Price AJ, Short A, Kellett C, et al. Ten-year in vivo wear measurement of a fully congruent mobile bearing unicompartmental knee arthroplasty. *J Bone Joint Surg Br.* 1005;87(11):1493-1497. doi:10.1302/0301-620x.87b11.16325. PubMed PMID: 16260665.
27. Murray DW, Goodfellow JW, O'Connor JJ. The Oxford medial unicompartmental arthroplasty: a ten-year survival study. *J Bone Joint Surg Br.* 1998;80(6):983-989. PubMed PMID: 9853489.
28. University L. *Swedish Knee Arthroplasty Registry.* 2018.
29. Keblish PA, Varma AK, Greenwald AS. Patellar resurfacing or retention in total knee arthroplasty. A prospective study of patients with bilateral replacements. *J Bone Joint Surg Br.* 1994;76(6):930-937. PubMed PMID: 7983122.
30. Buechel FF. Patellar tendon bone grafting for patellectomized patients having total knee arthroplasty. *Clin Orthop Relat Res.* 1991;(271):72-78. PubMed PMID: 1914316.
31. Jordan LR, Dowd JE, Olivo JL, Voorhorst PE. The clinical history of mobile-bearing patella components in total knee arthroplasty. *Orthopedics.* 2002;25(2 suppl):s247-s250. PubMed PMID: 11866161.
32. Tarkin IS, Bridgeman JT, Jardon OM, Garvin KL. Successful biologic fixation with mobile-bearing total knee arthroplasty. *J Arthroplasty.* 2005;20(4):481-486. doi:10.1016/j.arth.2004.09.026. PubMed PMID: 16124964.
33. Carothers JT, Kim RH, Dennis DA, Southworth C. Mobile-bearing total knee arthroplasty: a meta-analysis. *J Arthroplasty.* 2011;26(4):537-542. doi:10.1016/j.arth.2010.05.015. PubMed PMID: 20634039.
34. Hopley CD, Crossett LS, Chen AF. Long-term clinical outcomes and survivorship after total knee arthroplasty using a rotating platform knee prosthesis: a meta-analysis. *J Arthroplasty.* 2013;28(1):68-77.e1-3. doi:10.1016/j.arth.2012.04.026. PubMed PMID: 23006218.
35. The Swedish National Knee Arthroplasty Register Annual Report 2011. Department of Orthopedics University of Lund Annual. Available at http://www.knee.nko.se/. Accessed March 6, 2019.

36. Kane RSK, Wilt TJ, et al. *Total Knee Replacement. Evidence Report/Technology Assessment. Number 86. AHRQ Publication No. 04-E006-2.* Rockville, MD: Agency for Healthcare Research and Quality; 2003. http://www.ahrw.gov/downloads/pub/evidence/pdf/knee/knee.pdf.

37. The Medical Advisory Secretariat Ministry of Health and Long-Term Care Canada: Total Knee Replacement Health Technology Literature Review June 2005 [Internet].

38. Dennis DA, Komistek RD, Mahfouz MR, Haas BD, Stiehl JB. Multicenter determination of in vivo kinematics after total knee arthroplasty. *Clin Orthop Relat Res.* 2003;(416):37-57. doi:10.1097/01.blo.0000092986.12414.b5. PubMed PMID: 14646738.

39. Crossett L. *Personal Communication*; 2019.

40. Stiehl JB, Dennis DA, Komistek RD, Crane HS. In vivo determination of condylar lift-off and screw-home in a mobile-bearing total knee arthroplasty. *J Arthroplasty.* 1999;14(3):293-299. PubMed PMID: 10220182.

41. Ulivi M, Orlandini L, Meroni V, Consonni O, Sansone V. Survivorship at minimum 10-year follow-up of a rotating-platform, mobile-bearing, posterior-stabilised total knee arthroplasty. *Knee Surg Sports Traumatol Arthrosc.* 2015;23(6):1669-1675. doi:10.1007/s00167-014-3118-y. PubMed PMID: 24938395.

42. Maniar RN, Singhi T, Maniar PR, Kumar V. Ten- to 13-year results of mobile bearing posterior-stabilized rotating-platform knee implants, reported by nondesigner surgeon. *J Arthroplasty.* 2017;32(3):830-835. doi:10.1016/j.arth.2016.09.001. PubMed PMID: 27789096.

43. Bottlang M, Erne OK, Lacatusu E, Sommers MB, Kessler O. A mobile-bearing knee prosthesis can reduce strain at the proximal tibia. *Clin Orthop Relat Res.* 2006;447:105-111. doi:10.1097/01.blo.0000203463.27937.97. PubMed PMID: 16456313.

44. Callaghan JJ, O'Rourke MR, Iossi MF, et al. Cemented rotating-platform total knee replacement. A concise follow-up, at a minimum of fifteen years, of a previous report. *J Bone Joint Surg Am.* 1005;87(9):1995-1998. doi:10.2106/jbjs.D.03039. PubMed PMID: 16140814.

45. Sorrells RB, Voorhorst PE, Murphy JA, Bauschka MP, Greenwald AS. Uncemented rotating-platform total knee replacement: a five to twelve-year follow-up study. *J Bone Joint Surg Am.* 2004;86-A(10):2156-2162. PubMed PMID: 15466723.

46. Puloski SK, McCalden RW, MacDonald SJ, Rorabeck CH, Bourne RB. Tibial post wear in posterior stabilized total knee arthroplasty. An unrecognized source of polyethylene debris. *J Bone Joint Surg Am.* 2001;83-A(3):390-397. PubMed PMID: 11263643.

47. Dennis DA, Komistek RD, Mahfouz MR, Walker SA, Tucker A. A multicenter analysis of axial femorotibial rotation after total knee arthroplasty. *Clin Orthop Relat Res.* 2004;(428):180-189. PubMed PMID: 15534541.

48. Jones RE. Mobile bearings in revision total knee arthroplasty. *Instr Course Lect.* 2005;54:225-231. PubMed PMID: 15948450.

F BICRUCIATE RETAINING IN TOTAL KNEE ARTHROPLASTY

Christopher E. Pelt, MD, FAAOS

INTRODUCTION

While originally utilized for elderly, low-demand with good outcomes, the use of total knee arthroplasty (TKA) for younger and more active patients is becoming more common. In addition to patients with higher demands, longer life expectancy, and higher expectations, there also remains a significant percentage of patients with a level of dissatisfaction following TKA.[1-3] While many theories exist as to the reason for dissatisfaction following TKA, no one single reason has been identified. Ultimately patients with less significant arthritis, younger age, higher activity levels, higher demands, or higher expectations tend to fall into this dissatisfied category.[4,5] Surgeons, implant manufacturers, and other thoughtful professionals working toward improving outcomes have looked at implant design as a potential source of either dissatisfaction, or opportunity for improvement.

Historical discussions regarding implant designs that retain or eliminate the cruciate ligaments have discussed the PCL primarily. Cruciate-retaining (CR) and posterior-substituting (PS) TKA designs have been the mainstay in knee arthroplasty design for the past many decades, with data that continue to fail to demonstrate superiority of one design over the other.[6] Recent interest has developed regarding the potential for retention of both cruciates, including the anterior cruciate ligament (ACL), to potentially improve outcomes and address the issues of dissatisfaction.[7-10]

The ACL has rarely been discussed as a structure of importance in TKA. Recent studies have demonstrated that many patients undergoing routine TKA maintain an intact anterior cruciate ligament.[11] If retaining the anterior cruciate ligament during TKA had the potential to re-create more normal knee kinematics and create a knee that feels more natural, it is possible that the patient could be more satisfied with their TKA. Retention of native soft tissues for knee stability, as opposed to traditional reliance on stability from the implant, could additionally afford decreased mechanical wear of the implant. Decreased prosthetic constraint with more normal kinematics and perception in a bicruciate TKA could potentially help address issues of dissatisfaction and even implant survivorship, with appropriate implant technologies and materials.

With all of these theoretical benefits, it is important to understand the background and current understanding of bicruciate TKA.

HISTORY

While the concept of bicruciate-retaining (BCR) knee arthroplasty at first seems to be a novel concept, knee arthroplasty designs as early as the 1960s included implants that preserved both cruciate ligaments. Gunston Polycentric Knee was among the first to develop a BCR knee arthroplasty, with the goal of more naturally mimicking native knee kinematics.[12] The Polycentric Knee utilized independent cemented semicircular stainless-steel caps of the femoral condyles and independent polyethylene components on the medial and lateral tibia. Later designs, such as the Duocondylar and the Geomedic Knee, evolved toward a single femoral component to improve femoral preparation and continued to preserve the ACL,[13-15] though tibial preparation and implants, along with durable tibial fixation, remained problematic. While early survivorship looked promising in these earliest BCR TKA designs, possibly related to the decreased level of constraint, long-term results, like many of the early TKA designs, were not as good, with limitations in materials properties, implant design, and surgical techniques leading to loosening, polyethylene wear, osteolysis, patellofemoral problems, and poor postoperative motion.[16,17]

Over time, along with increasing and improving material properties of implants, additional bicruciate TKAs were designed and released to the market. Among the most successful of those included Cloutier bicruciate TKA (Hermes 2C).[18,19] While successful clinically, the implant was not widely accepted due to the complex ligament balancing and surgical technique.

The work on BCR TKA described by Pritchett using Townley Anatomic TKA and later the TKO bicruciate knee (BioPro, Port Huron, MI, USA) probably lead to the most recent enthusiasm in bicruciate TKAs.[20] With long-term survivorship reported at 23 years of 89% for all-cause revision, and 94% when eliminating polyethylene wear, which was the most common cause of failure in the early design, their results appear promising. However, his further publications that showed significant patient preferences of bicruciate knees compared to CR or PS knees offered perhaps the most compelling reasons to revisit bicruciate TKA as a potential opportunity to improve patient satisfaction following TKA.[20,21]

KINEMATICS

In order to understand the potential benefit of saving the ACL during TKA, it may be helpful to understand its function and the kinematics in the native and replaced knee. The native knee is a complex joint with multiple static and dynamic structures all working together to guide motion and provide stability. The cruciate ligaments provide both rotational as well as translational stability throughout the arc of motion. The ACL, with its two bundles, help to limit anterior tibial translation and guide knee rotation. The anteromedial bundle becomes tighter in flexion while the posterolateral bundle is taut in extension.[22] The screw home mechanism further aids stability in extension as the tibia externally rotates relative to the femur due to asymmetry between the femoral condyles and restraint from the taut ACL.[23] With flexion, femoral rollback occurs as the PCL tightens and drives the femoral condyles posteriorly on the tibia and internally rotates the tibia. In addition to improving flexion ability, the rollback further enhances the lever arm of the quadriceps muscle and patellar tracking.[24]

Beyond the guided motion afforded by the cruciates, the ACL also likely provides proprioceptive sensory feedback in the knee as it has been shown to contain mechanoreceptors.[25] In the setting of arthroplasty, work by Fuchs et al[26] compared proprioception between a BCR arthroplasty to healthy controls and concluded that a "total knee arthroplasty that retains all intraarticular ligaments achieves proprioceptive results comparable with healthy subjects." Advocates of BCR TKA have suggested that improved outcomes may be realized both due to the potential for more normal kinematics as well as a more natural feel of the artificial knee that results from the retained proprioception, which may be more similar to that seen in unicompartmental arthroplasty.[27]

In order to perform a BCR TKA, the presence of the ACL would seem to be an obvious requisite of the surgery. Common perception of knees undergoing TKA surgery is that an ACL is often absent. Contrary to this belief, however, Johnson et al[28] found the presence of an intact ACL in patients undergoing TKA in 78% of patients. Lachman exam under anesthesia had a poor sensitivity when used alone at 33%. MRI had 90% sensitivity when a reading of indeterminate was considered to be intact. Sagittal wear was also evaluated on a lateral radiograph, and anterior wear of the medial tibial plateau had an intact ACL and all patients with posterior medial tibial wear had an incompetent ACL. Prior to that, Sabouret et al[19] had concluded in their series that the presence of a functional ACL, even if degenerated or frayed, was adequate for the carrying out of BCR TKA.

Several studies have looked at the kinematics, gait, and motion of early BCR TKA designs. Andriacchi et al[29] performed gait analysis and showed abnormal gait that was more pronounced with stair ascent or descent than level walking, and was different based on total knee implant design, with more abnormality seen with increased constraint, and less seen with increased cruciate ligament preservation, including BCR designs. Using *in vivo* fluoroscopy to look at 16 BCR TKAs and 6 PS TKAs, Stiehl et al[30] showed BCR knees demonstrated more natural kinematic appearance with gradual femoral rollback and limited anterior–posterior translation in flexion. A later study of level-ground walking fluoroscopy in subjects with PS-and ACL-retaining TKA again concluded that an ACL-retaining knee experienced kinematic patterns more similar to the native knee, likely due to the retention of the ACL which limited anterior translation (an anterior contact point occurred in 67% of ACL-retaining TKA compared to 80% of PS knees) and increased axial rotation related to the preserved four-bar linkage.[31] Similarly, Moro-oka et al[32] performed fluoroscopic gait analysis of BCR versus PCL-retaining (CR) TKA and found that BCR TKAs exhibited more posterior translation of the lateral femoral condyle in maximum flexion and stair activity, more translation of both condyles in stance and swing phase and in midflexion, and concluded that BCR TKA maintained more features that mimic native knee kinematics than did CR TKA.

With the recent resurgence in interest in BCR TKA, along with two recent commercial introductions of BCR implants (Vanguard XP, Zimmer Biomet, Warsaw, IN and Smith and Nephew Journey II XR, Memphis, TN), additional studies have looked at the kinematics of these newer designs. Heyse et al[33] looked at seven cadaveric specimens pre- and postimplantation of one of the modern designs and found findings similar to those seen with fixed-bearing unicompartmental arthroplasty, in so much as the BCR TKA in the unloaded knee closely resembles native knee kinematics including preserving the rollback mechanism. They go on to suggest that the loss of tibial internal rotation and slight paradoxical AP motion of the medial femoral condyle with BCR TKA may be attributable to the loss of the conforming anatomy of menisci and tibial cartilage and replacement with a flatter polyethylene insert. Their group additionally looked at the influence of differential bearing thickness placed medially and laterally to more closely mimic native tibial varus as well as the impact of upsizing or downsizing the bearing thicknesses to over- or understuff the joint with limited impact of any of these changes, and again concluded that changes introduced to tibiofemoral kinematics by removal of the conforming meniscus and cartilage and replacement with a flat insert and femoral component are of more impact than different inlay sizes.[34] In another cadaveric study, Halewood et al[35] found that the AP laxity seen in BCR TKA was less than that seen with the traditional CR implant and more similar to that of the native knee prior to implantation. Wada et al,[36] in a cadaveric study with six specimens, looked at the use of a more constrained medial-sided bearing insert with a flat insert on the lateral side compared to a flat bearing insert on both the medial and lateral side, and found that creating a more medially constrained design recreated more natural knee kinematics, suggesting that perhaps there could be a role for some added conformity to the medial articular surface that may address the loss of the meniscus and articular congruity that was mentioned above. Similarly, Hamada et al[36] showed that the rotational kinematics seen with BCR TKA were retained with femoral component replacement and even meniscectomy, but were lost after resection and replacement of the tibial articular surface in their cadaveric experiment, and suggested that BCR TKA should be used to focus on enhanced anteroposterior stability as opposed to the rotational kinematics.

Among the few *in vivo* studies looking at the kinematics of a modern BCR TKA design, Simon et al[37] collected motion and EMG data on 12 subjects following BCR TKA and 15 following traditional CR TKA and found no significant differences in measures during level walking, but did show some beneficial differences during downhill activities in muscle activity, flexion moment, and knee flexion during heel strike. They concluded that BCR TKAs may offer some neuromuscular benefits for stabilizing the knee joint.

In summary, many studies of historical and even modern BCR TKA designs support the notion that BCR TKA may recreate more natural knee kinematics and preserve some proprioception. The kinematics of most BCR TKA studies show kinematics that more closely mimic those seen in unicompartmental arthroplasty, or even the native knee, than traditional PS or CR TKA designs. Certainly, these findings sound encouraging, but in order to consider BCR TKA more widely, these findings would need to be weighed against the increased surgical complexity and need to be supported by clinical outcomes.

CLINICAL OUTCOMES

The outcomes of the earlier designs of BCR TKA, described above, showed many promising features, including increased patient preference for a BCR TKA versus traditional TKA designs, improved proprioception, more natural kinematics, and good survivorship, particularly when excluding failures related to polyethylene wear. With failures seemingly related to shortfalls in materials properties, such as polyethylene wear and osteolysis, poor design with lack of consideration for the patellofemoral joint or enhanced tibial fixation, and challenging surgical techniques, modern implant manufacturers and surgeon designers felt that there could be an opportunity to improve upon the shortcomings of yesteryear.

Baumann et al[27] demonstrated promising results when looking at the Forgotten Joint Score and joint awareness,

when they showed modern BCR TKA outcomes that were similar to unicompartmental arthroplasty and better than seen in traditional PS TKA. To date, few other studies have been able to demonstrate superior patient-reported outcomes with the use of BCR TKA compared to traditional TKA designs.

Alnachoukati et al[10] at only 12 months follow-up looked at a series of 146 BCR TKAs and found high satisfaction and two revisions (1.4%) and one manipulation under anesthesia. Our own group had previously published our early results on the same implant using similar surgical technique on 66 of our first 78 BCR TKAs performed in the first year of our use of the novel implant with less favorable results.[9] At 12-month follow-up, we published 3/66 (5%) revisions and a higher number of radiolucent lines radiographically. Given these findings, our group later limited our ongoing use of the implant, but continued to follow up all of the patients we had performed BCR TKA in.

In our most recent review of our entire experience using a modern BCR TKA design at our center, currently in submission but yet unpublished, we looked at the entire cohort of 175 BCR TKAs performed at our institution between May 2013 and October 2015 to investigate if there was a potential improvement in these outcomes with longer-term follow-up or any impact on a learning curve explaining the early higher revision rates. Thirty-four knees (19%) missing 2-year follow-up were excluded. With follow-up time as either within the last 12 months or ended at the time of revision, mean follow-up was 3 years (range, 0.0434 to 4.9). Survivorship at 3-years was 88% (82% to 93%). Revisions were for: isolated tibial loosening (5/19), ACL impingement (3/19), pain (4/19), unknown reasons (3/19), femoral and tibial loosening (2/19), ACL deficiency (1/19), and arthrofibrosis (1/19). Using the NIH PROMIS system for evaluating patient-reported outcomes, the mean physical function computer adaptive test (PF CAT) T-score was 45 units (range, 23 to 63), which is similar to that seen in prior reviews of our traditional CR/CS TKA. There was no clustering of revisions in the early experience, nor any change in the rate of revision over time, suggesting no correlation of our revisions with a learning curve effect. With a revision-free survival of 88% at 3 years, with primary failure mechanisms of tibial loosening, ACL impingement, and pain and PROs that are not different than seen in traditional TKA, we are currently left to conclude that further refinement in implant design or surgical technique may be needed prior to widespread use of this, or similar implant designs.

COMPLICATIONS

Our experience, as well as that of others, has identified some unique failure patterns and challenges that are introduced when using BCR TKA compared to traditional TKA designs. Modern designs have added various design adaptations including cross-linked polyethylene to address the issues of polyethylene wear seen with preceding implants,[21] though the long-term outcomes of this change are unproven. Anterior cruciate ligament sacrifice certainly allows for wider exposure, ease of surgical technique, avoidance of intercondylar impingement as well as improved ability to correct deformity and contractures.[38] However, cruciate-sacrificing designs may trade the increased ease and reproducibility of surgical technique for loss of normal knee kinematics.[29-31]

Because restoration of the normal joint line is of importance to appropriately balance all four retained ligaments in the setting of BCR TKA, increased tibial bone resection is often required compared to PS and CR TKA. If not adequately resected, joint line elevation may occur. Altering the joint line (primarily joint line elevation or overstuffing) can lead to increased ACL tension in extension, and intraoperative and late ligament failure and bone island fractures have also been reported.[7,9,10] Furthermore, the ACL must be protected throughout the duration of the operation from iatrogenic injury, and often requires the use of additional cutting jigs, smaller saw blades, and protective guides. The central bone block at the ACL insertion determines tibial component rotation and becomes another possible step to introduce error into the surgical technique. Tibial fixation, with dominant modes of failure including tibial loosening, appears to be problematic.[9] There may be the potential for imperfect ligament balance and abnormal kinematics to occur in some patients, particularly if unique patient morphologies are not recreated with nonpersonalized surgical techniques. Tibial loosening may also be influenced by cement technique, which may be more difficult in the setting of reduced tibial exposure, or reduced tibial fixation, given the challenges of adding a central keel while preserving a central tibial bone block.[39] Clinical studies of the most recent modern BCR TKA design introduced (Smith and Nephew Journey II XR, Memphis, TN) are not yet available to tell if the addition of such a keel, among other modifications, may address these issues of tibial fixation. While attempting to couple the medial and lateral tibial resections and implant with a single baseplate design has been adopted by most modern BCR TKA designs, the connection between the medial and lateral tibial plateau is an area at risk for mechanical fatigue fracture of the tibial implant. Postoperative stiffening in patients suffering from preoperative stiffness has been described to be more common in BCR TKA than PS TKA.[40] Further, the cyclops lesion has been described as a source of mechanical impingement and stiffness following BCR TKA.[9,41]

SUMMARY

The demographics, demands, and expectations of patients undergoing TKA are changing and dissatisfaction continues to be an issue that implant designers hope to improve upon. With the belief that improved proprioception and

more natural kinematics could improve upon this issue, bicruciate TKA designs have seen a resurgence in interest. Despite the introduction of modern BCR TKA designs that aim to improve upon the shortcomings of previous implant materials properties and designs, several technical complexities unique to BCR TKA along with few studies showing significant differences in patient-reported outcomes between BCR and traditional TKA may ultimately limit the widespread adoption of this implant design during TKA.

REFERENCES

1. Robertsson O, Dunbar M, Pehrsson T, Knutson K, Lidgren L. Patient satisfaction after knee arthroplasty: a report on 27,372 knees operated on between 1981 and 1995 in Sweden. *Acta Orthopaedica Scandinavica.* 2000;71:262-267.
2. Scott CE, Howie CR, MacDonald D, Biant LC. Predicting dissatisfaction following total knee replacement: a prospective study of 1217 patients. *J Bone Joint Surg Br.* 2010;92:1253-1258.
3. Lutzner C, Kirschner S, Lutzner J. Patient activity after TKA depends on patient-specific parameters. *Clin Orthop Relat Res.* 2014;472:3933-3940.
4. Scott CE, Oliver WM, MacDonald D, Wade FA, Moran M, Breusch SJ. Predicting dissatisfaction following total knee arthroplasty in patients under 55 years of age. *Bone Joint J.* 2016;98-B:1625-1634.
5. Ghomrawi HMK, Lee LY, Nwachukwu BU, et al. Preoperative expectations associated with postoperative dissatisfaction after total knee arthroplasty: a cohort study. *J Am Acad Orthop Surg.* 2019. doi:10.5435/JAAOS-D-18-00785.
6. Serna-Berna R, Lizaur-Utrilla A, Vizcaya-Moreno MF, Miralles Munoz FA, Gonzalez-Navarro B, Lopez-Prats FA. Cruciate-retaining vs posterior-stabilized primary total arthroplasty. Clinical outcome comparison with a minimum follow-up of 10 years. *J Arthroplasty.* 2018;33:2491-2495.
7. Pagnano MW. The bi-cruciate retaining knee: a bridge too far - affirms. *Orthop Proc.* 2017;99-B(SUPP_7):86.
8. Lombardi AV. The bi-cruciate retaining knee: a bridge too far - opposes. *Orthop Proc.* 2017;99-B(SUPP_7):87.
9. Christensen JC, Brothers J, Stoddard GJ, et al. Higher frequency of reoperation with a new bicruciate-retaining total knee arthroplasty. *Clin Orthop Relat Res.* 2017;475:62-69.
10. Alnachoukati OK, Emerson RH, Diaz E, Ruchaud E, Ennin KA. Modern day bicruciate-retaining total knee arthroplasty: a short-term review of 146 knees. *J Arthroplasty.* 2018;33:2485-2490.
11. Cushner FD, La Rosa DF, Vigorita VJ, Scuderi GR, Scott WN, Insall JN. A quantitative histologic comparison: ACL degeneration in the osteoarthritic knee. *J Arthroplasty.* 2003;18:687-692.
12. Cracchiolo A III, Benson M, Finerman GA, Horacek K, Amstutz HC. A prospective comparative clinical analysis of the first-generation knee replacements: polycentric vs. geometric knee arthroplasty. *Clin Orthop Relat Res.* 1979;(145):37-46.
13. Goldie IF, Raner C, Cappelen-Smith J. The relationship between the position of a duocondylar knee-prosthesis (St. Georg) and the function of the knee. A clinical follow-up and radiographic study. *Arch Orthop Trauma Surg.* 1979;95:1-5.
14. Little EG. A static experimental stress analysis of a single plateau of the Geomedic knee joint using embedded strain gauges. *Eng Med.* 1985;14:69-74.
15. van Loon CJ, Hu HP, Van Horn JR, De Waal Malefijt MC. The Geomedic knee prosthesis. A long-term follow-up study. *Acta Orthop Belg.* 1993;59:40-44.
16. Lewallen DG, Bryan RS, Peterson LF. Polycentric total knee arthroplasty. A ten-year follow-up study. *J Bone Joint Surg Am Vol.* 1984;66:1211-1218.
17. Rand JA, Coventry MB. Ten-year evaluation of geometric total knee arthroplasty. *Clin Orthop Relat Res.* 1988;(232):168-173.

18. Cloutier JM. Results of total knee arthroplasty with a non-constrained prosthesis. *J Bone Joint Surg Am*. 1983;65:906-919.

19. Sabouret P, Lavoie F, Cloutier JM. Total knee replacement with retention of both cruciate ligaments: a 22-year follow-up study. *Bone Joint J*. 2013;95-B:917-922.

20. Pritchett JW. Bicruciate-retaining total knee replacement provides satisfactory function and implant survivorship at 23 years. *Clin Orthop Relat Res*. 2015;473:2327-2333.

21. Pritchett JW. Patients prefer a bicruciate-retaining or the medial pivot total knee prosthesis. *J Arthroplasty*. 2011;26:224-228.

22. Petersen W, Zantop T. Anatomy of the anterior cruciate ligament with regard to its two bundles. *Clin Orthop Relat Res*. 2007;454:35-47.

23. Bull AM, Kessler O, Alam M, Amis AA. Changes in knee kinematics reflect the articular geometry after arthroplasty. *Clin Orthop Relat Res*. 2008;466:2491-2499.

24. Pinskerova V, Johal P, Nakagawa S, et al. Does the femur roll-back with flexion?. *J Bone Joint Surg Br*. 2004;86:925-931.

25. Cabuk H, Kusku Cabuk F. Mechanoreceptors of the ligaments and tendons around the knee. *Clin Anat*. 2016;29:789-795.

26. Fuchs S, Tibesku CO, Genkinger M, Laass H, Rosenbaum D. Proprioception with bicondylar sledge prostheses retaining cruciate ligaments. *Clin Orthop Relat Res*. 2003;(406):148-154.

27. Baumann F, Bahadin O, Krutsch W, et al. Proprioception after bicruciate-retaining total knee arthroplasty is comparable to unicompartmental knee arthroplasty. *Knee Surg Sports Traumatol Arthrosc*. 2017;25:1697-1704.

28. Johnson AJ, Howell SM, Costa CR, Mont MA. The ACL in the arthritic knee: how often is it present and can preoperative tests predict its presence?. *Clin Orthop Relat Res*. 2013;471:181-188.

29. Andriacchi TP, Galante JO, Fermier RW. The influence of total knee-replacement design on walking and stair-climbing. *J Bone Joint Surg Am*. 1982;64:1328-1335.

30. Stiehl JB, Komistek RD, Cloutier JM, Dennis DA. The cruciate ligaments in total knee arthroplasty: a kinematic analysis of 2 total knee arthroplasties. *J Arthroplasty*. 2000;15:545-550.

31. Komistek RD, Allain J, Anderson DT, Dennis DA, Goutallier D. In vivo kinematics for subjects with and without an anterior cruciate ligament. *Clin Orthop Relat Res*. 2002;(404):315-325.

32. Moro-oka TA, Muenchinger M, Canciani JP, Banks SA. Comparing in vivo kinematics of anterior cruciate-retaining and posterior cruciate-retaining total knee arthroplasty. *Knee Surg Sports Traumatol Arthrosc*. 2007;15:93-99.

33. Heyse TJ, Slane J, Peersman G, et al. Kinematics of a bicruciate-retaining total knee arthroplasty. *Knee Surg Sports Traumatol Arthrosc*. 2017;25:1784-1791.

34. Peersman G, Slane J, Dirckx M, et al. The influence of polyethylene bearing thickness on the tibiofemoral kinematics of a bicruciate retaining total knee arthroplasty. *Knee*. 2017;24:751-760.

35. Halewood C, Traynor A, Bellemans J, Victor J, Amis AA. Anteroposterior laxity after bicruciate-retaining total knee arthroplasty is closer to the native knee than ACL-resecting TKA: a biomechanical cadaver study. *J Arthroplasty*. 2015;30:2315-2319.

36. Wada K, Hamada D, Takasago T, et al. The medial constrained insert restores native knee rotational kinematics after bicruciate-retaining total knee arthroplasty. *Knee Surg Sports Traumatol Arthrosc*. 2018;27(5):1621-1627.

37. Simon JC, Della Valle CJ, Wimmer MA. Level and downhill walking to assess implant functionality in bicruciate- and posterior cruciate-retaining total knee arthroplasty. *J Arthroplasty*. 2018;33:2884-2889.

38. Freeman MA, Insall JN, Besser W, Walker PS, Hallel T. Excision of the cruciate ligaments in total knee replacement. *Clin Orthop Relat Res*. 1977;(126):209-212.

39. Saxena V, Anari JB, Ruutiainen AT, Voleti PB, Stephenson JW, Lee GC. Tibial component considerations in bicruciate-retaining total knee arthroplasty: a 3D MRI evaluation of proximal tibial anatomy. *Knee*. 2016;23:593-599.

40. Lavoie F, Al-Shakfa F, Moore JR, Mychaltchouk L, Iguer K. Postoperative stiffening after bicruciate-retaining total knee arthroplasty. *J Knee Surg*. 2018;31:453-458.

41. Klaassen MA, Aikins JL. The cyclops lesion after bicruciate-retaining total knee replacement. *Arthroplast Today*. 2017;3:242-246.

chapter 37

Cement Fixation for Total Knee Arthroplasty

John B. Meding, MD

Historically, cement has been the preferred method of fixation among knee surgeons for total knee arthroplasty (TKA). Although some cementless TKA designs have provided excellent patient results with respect to function and survivorship,[1-6] cemented TKA continues to remain the standard by which the success of cementless fixation in TKA is judged.[1,7] On one hand, midterm results of cementless posterior-stabilized (PS) TKA have shown 8-year survivorship of 98%[5] to 99.5%.[1] In addition, longer-term results in cementless cruciate-retaining (CR) TKA have reported excellent survivorship[2-4,6] between 93% at 12 years[2] and 97% at 20 years.[4] On the other hand, numerous studies of cemented TKA, including a variety of modular, nonmodular, CR, and PS designs, have demonstrated excellent clinical and radiographic outcomes[8-18] between 98% at 10 years[12,14] and 94% at 25 years[17] with survivorship in some cases over 92% into the fourth decade.[17] Furthermore, registry data on 7174 TKAs noted a higher 5-year survival for cemented TKA (95.9%) versus cementless TKA (88.3%) with 2.2 times the risk of early failure with cementless fixation.[19] Finally, a meta-analysis of 15 studies comparing cemented and cementless fixation in TKA found the combined odds ratio for failure due to aseptic loosening was 4.2 for the cementless TKA between 2 and 11 years.[20] Thus, as cementless TKA has rarely been shown to be superior to cemented TKA,[21] careful consideration is needed when choosing cementless fixation over cemented fixation in TKA.

Relative indications for cemented TKA may include poor bone quality, cases where immediate rigid implant fixation in mandatory (multiple lower extremity joint arthritis or inflammatory arthropathy), and when the addition of antibiotics in the cement is desired. However, because concern may exist over the bone–cement interface deteriorating over time,[5] the so-called "biologic fixation"[5,22] of cementless TKA may be considered appealing, especially in the relatively younger, heavier, and potentially more active patient.[5]

It is axiomatic that obtaining rigid implant fixation at the time of cemented TKA is a primary goal for the surgeon and a fundamental prerequisite for long-term survivorship. Achieving implant stability while maintaining adequate bone stock is a key objective.[21] The surgical technique begins with an adequate exposure. This is required not only for proper bone cuts and osteophyte removal but also for bone preparation, cement pressurization, implantation of the prosthesis, and removal of cement excrescences. Commonly, the tibia is subluxed anterior to the femur, with or without eversion of the patella. Because optimal implant fixation requires 3 to 4 mm of cement penetration into bone,[23] sclerotic bone may be drilled at this time creating multiple fenestrations allowing the cement to penetrate into more cancellous bone (**Fig. 37-1A**). Blood and bone debris inhibit cement penetration and can decrease the shear strength at the bone–cement interface by 50%[24] (**Fig. 37-1B**). This interlock is the main factor in interface strength. Thus, the bone surfaces must be thoroughly cleaned with high-pressure, high-volume, jet lavage. Simple manual syringe irrigation has been shown to be inferior with respect to cement penetration into bone. Ritter et al. clearly demonstrated that proper bone preparation, jet lavage, suction drying, and cement pressurization (digital or cement gun) yielded less radiolucencies at the bone–cement interface and improved prosthetic survival at 5 years (98% vs. 82%) when compared to manual irrigation alone.[25] The bony surfaces are kept clean and dry with suction and/or sponges (**Fig. 37-1C**). Most surgeons recognize that bleeding is minimized with maximal knee flexion. Still, the use of a tourniquet at this point in the procedure remains controversial and is left to surgeon preference. Some authors suggest using a tourniquet to minimize bleeding.[21] However, Ejaz et al prospectively randomized 70 patients into a tourniquet and a nontourniquet group using radiostereometric analysis to evaluate implant motion. At 2 years there was no significant difference in tibial component migration between the two groups.[26] Generally, one cement mix allows sufficient time to apply cement to all three surfaces. (One or two 40-g bags are most commonly used based on prosthesis size and/or surgeon preference. In many cases, one bag of cement may be sufficient.) Digital compression is used with particular attention given to pressurizing cement into the posterior femoral condyles (**Fig. 37-1D**). After cement is applied directly to both femoral and tibial components, the implants are impacted into place, excess cement is removed, and the knee is brought out into full extension with a trial insert to enhance cement penetration (**Fig. 37-1E**). If indicated, the patella is similarly prepared, cemented, and clamped either first or last according to surgeon preference. Care is taken to avoid component malposition at this point, either flexion of the formal component or rotation of the tibial component. The knee is held in place until the cement has hardened. Checking knee range of motion and laxity while the cement is hardening should be avoided as these procedures may disturb the bone–cement and, especially, the cement–prosthesis interface. All cement excrescences are removed. Again, adequate visualization is needed to remove any excess cement from about the posterior aspect of the femoral condyles and, especially, the posterior and lateral corner of the tibial component (**Fig. 37-1F**). A generous amount of irrigation with the jet lavage is used to remove the residual particulate debris prior to placing the tibial insert if a modular design is used (**Fig. 37-1G**). Postoperative radiographs are obtained either in the recovery room or at early postoperative period or both. They serve not only as a baseline to monitor any implant migration or signs of loosening but also provide unbiased and objective feedback on the surgeon's cement technique (**Fig. 37-2A** and **B**).

Along with cement technique, implant design may also influence the durability, quality, and sheer strength of the bone–cement or cement–prosthesis interface.[27] Implants differ with respect to keel shape and length, surface roughness, and other modifications to improve cement penetration into bone and fixation of the prosthesis. Surgeons should carefully evaluate and be familiar with each manufacturer's recommended surgical protocol and cement technique based on the specific prosthetic design. For example, the decision to surface cement the tibial tray versus fully cementing the tray and keel, while somewhat controversial, may or may not influence tibial component fixation. While simply cementing the proximal tibial bone may seem beneficial in enhancing proximal loading, it may increase the likelihood of micromotion and subsequent loosening. Ryd et al suggested that surface cementing might lead to a compromised seal, allowing fluid to penetrate the cement–prosthesis interface resulting in inadequate fixation[28] (**Fig. 37-3A-C**).

Recently, in the United States, the use of high-viscosity cement (HVC) has increased among knee arthroplasty surgeons.[29] Presumably, this change is due to the appealing nature of the increased working time of HVC as compared to low-viscosity cement (LVC). Yet, as the intrusion depth of LVC into bone is almost double that of HVC at multiple pressures,[21] some authors have raised concern over the routine use of HVC with certain

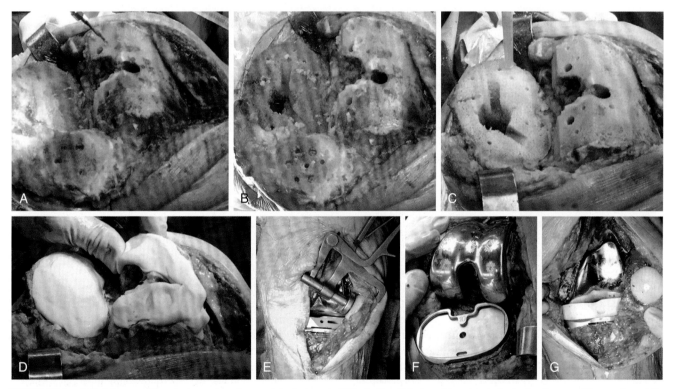

FIGURE 37-1 **A–G:** Intraoperative photographs of cement technique in TKA. **A:** The tibia is subluxed anterior to the femur, with eversion of the patella providing optimal exposure to all bony surfaces. Sclerotic bone may be drilled creating multiple fenestrations that allow cement to penetrate into the deeper cancellous bone. **B:** Blood, bone debris, and soft tissue will inhibit cement penetration and compromise the strength of the bone–cement interface. The bony surfaces must be thoroughly cleaned with high-pressure, high-volume, jet lavage. **C:** After all blood and bone debris are removed, the bony surfaces are kept clean and dry with suction or gauze sponges. **D:** Cement is pressurized either with a cement gun or digital pressure to the desired depth. Simply placing cement on the bony surfaces is insufficient. Special attention is given to pressurizing cement into the posterior femoral condyles. **E:** After the implants are impacted into place, excess cement is removed and the knee is brought out into full extension with a trial insert to enhance cement penetration. Avoid component malposition. The knee is held in place until the cement has hardened. **F:** All cement excrescences are removed. Adequate visualization is needed to remove any excess cement from about the posterior femoral condyles and the posterior tibial tray. **G:** If a modular tibial prosthesis is used, it is inserted only after irrigation with jet lavage to remove any residual particulate debris.

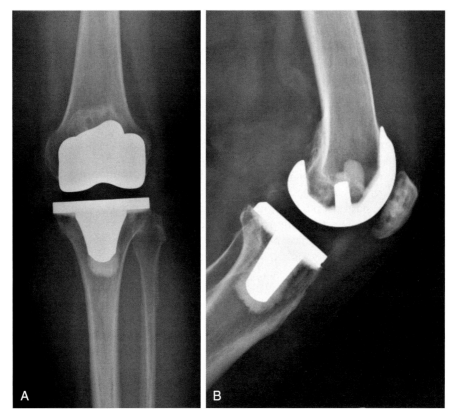

FIGURE 37-2 A–B: Postoperative anteroposterior (**A**) and lateral (**B**) radiographs. The quality of cement penetration is critically evaluated. Note cement penetration into posterior femoral condyles on lateral radiograph.

prostheses.[30] While the etiology of aseptic loosening in TKA is multifactorial, cement choice and cement technique are surgeon dependent. A practical understanding and appreciation of the working time and quality of cement penetration is needed for each type of cement that is used. Cement choice can influence fixation of the prosthesis. Even minor differences in fatigue strength, depth of penetration into bone, and cement porosity influence both the bone–cement and cement–prosthesis interface and can lead to early loosening of the implant.

The routine use of antibiotic-laden bone cement (ALBC) is controversial as well.[6,31] In the United States, ALBC is only FDA approved for the second stage of a reimplanted infected joint arthroplasty when the infection has been cured. Nevertheless, some surgeons routinely use ALBC as an adjunct to prophylaxis against deep periprosthetic infection, especially in patients with an increased risk of deep infection. While the most compelling evidence comes from total hip arthroplasty (THA) data, multiple studies have found ALBC to be at least as good as systemic antibiotics in preventing deep infection.[32-36] A review of the Norwegian hip registry found the lowest infection rate with the use of systemic antibiotics and ALBC.[34] Malchau et al., in a review of 92,675 THAs, noted a lower risk of infection with the use of operating room laminar airflow and ALBC with the lowest revision rates in hips where gentamicin ALBC was used.[36] In contradistinction, Tayton et al. actually

noted a relative increase risk of infection with ALBC in a review of 64,566 TKAs in the New Zealand Joint Registry.[37] A recent review[30] of seven controlled trials, comparing ALBC (8189 TKAs) and plain bone cement (26,475 TKAs), demonstrated no significant difference in the deep infection rate (1.1% vs. 0.9%, respectively). The authors concluded that ALBC in TKA might be an unnecessary cost to the healthcare system.[31] In contrast, Chiu et al. randomized 340 TKA patients to receive either cefuroxime bone cement or plain bone cement.[32] The authors reported a significant advantage of ALBC noting a 0% infection rate in the cefuroxime group and a 3.1% infection rate in the control group.

At the author's institution, 750 mg of cefuroxime is routinely added to each 40-g bag of cement prior to adding the liquid monomer (**Fig. 37-4**). Cefuroxime is prepared as a fine white powder and mixed well with the cement powder. It is thermally stable allowing satisfactory elution.[32] Up to 2 g of powder may be added to each 40-g bag of cement without adversely affecting the tensile or compressive strength of the bone cement.[32,38] ALBC is not used at our institution in patients with preexisting allergy concerns. Other potential and theoretical concerns with the routine use of ALBC include the development of antibiotic-resistant bacteria and antibiotic toxicity.[31] While it may be difficult to justify the routine use of ALBC in all TKA patients, selective use in high-risk patients may still be warranted.[39]

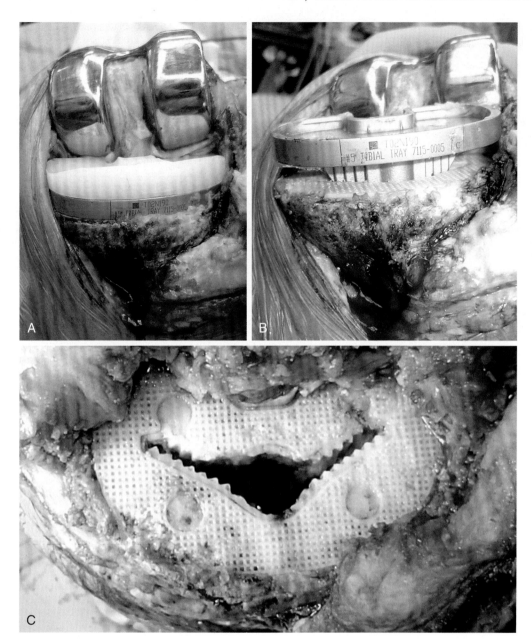

FIGURE 37-3 A–C: Intraoperative photograph during revision total knee arthroplasty (TKA) depicting surface cementing of the tibial component and subsequent loosening. **A:** After maximal knee flexion, the tibia is subluxed anterior. The gap between the bone cement and tibial component is easily visualized medially. **B:** Failure of cement to adhere to the undersurface of the tibial tray. The tibial component is easily removed. **C:** Surface cementing only with no cement in area of the keel. This allows for the possibility of fluid, fat, or blood to penetrate the cement–prosthesis interface resulting in inadequate fixation.

A number of authors have reported on the long-term success of cemented TKA with specific attention given to survivorship in terms of aseptic loosening. The total condylar TKA has been studied extensively. In particular, Gill et al[11] reported a 99% survival at 20 years, Ma et al,[40] a 92% survival at 20 years, Rodriguez et al,[18] a 94% at 20 years, and Pavone et al,[16] a 93% survival at 23 years. Buechel et al. followed 223 low-contact stress TKAs and noted a 98% survivorship at 20 years.[8] Ritter and colleagues[17] published the results of 5649 Anatomic Graduated Component (AGC) TKAs in a multicenter study and found a 94% survivorship at 25 years and a remarkable 92% survivorship of the prosthesis at 30 years. Similarly, Huizinga et al[41] in a 15- to 20-year follow-up study of 211 AGC TKAs noted only 12 of 211 (94%) knees revised for aseptic loosening of any component. McCalden et al[13] studied 469 Genesis II TKAs with a 15-year survival of 97.5%. In patients 55 years of age and younger, Diduch et al[10] reported a 94% survival of 114 cemented PS and CR TKAs at 18 years. Finally, published results of the Press-Fit Condylar (PFC) knee yielded a 10-year survival of 98% in 117 rotating platform PFC

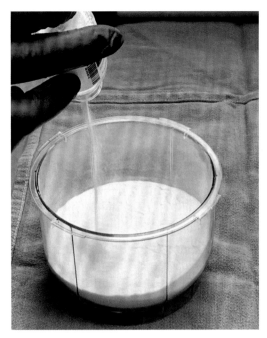

FIGURE 37-4 Photograph showing 750 mg of cefuroxime mixed with the dry cement powder prior to the adding the liquid monomer. This custom mixing may be done in lieu of using commercially available low-dose antibiotic-laden bone cement (ALBC).

TKAs,[14] a 15-year survival of 92% in 203 fixed-bearing PFC TKAs,[15] and a 20-year survival of 91% in 101 fixed-bearing PFC TKAs.[9]

The longevity of a cemented TKA depends on multiple patient, prosthesis, and surgeon factors. These include proper patient selection, appropriate choice of the prosthesis, and careful attention to surgical technique. Clearly, based on the overall success of cemented TKA and the proven durability of cement fixation, the routine use of cement as the fixation of choice in TKA appears well justified in most patients.

REFERENCES

1. Harwin SF, Patel NK, Chughtai M, et al. Outcomes of newer generation cementless total knee arthroplasty: beaded periapatite-coated vs highly porous titanium-coated implants. *J Arthroplasty.* 2017;32(7):2156-2160.
2. Hofmann AA, Evanich JD, Ferguson RP, Camargo MP. Ten- to 14-year clinical followup of the cementless natural knee system. *Clin Orthop Relat Res.* 2001(388):85-94.
3. Park JW, Kim YH. Simultaneous cemented and cementless total knee replacement in the same patients: a prospective comparison of long-term outcomes using an identical design of NexGen prosthesis. *J Bone Joint Surg Br.* 2011;93(11):1479-1486.
4. Ritter MA, Meneghini RM. Twenty-year survivorship of cementless anatomic graduated component total knee arthroplasty. *J Arthroplasty.* 2010;25(4):507-513.
5. Sultan AA, Khlopas A, Sodhi N, et al. Cementless total knee arthroplasty in knee osteonecrosis demonstrated excellent survivorship and outcomes at three-year minimum follow-up. *J Arthroplasty.* 2018;33(3):761-765.
6. Chiu FY, Chen CM, Lin CF, Lo WH. Cefuroxime-impregnated cement in primary total knee arthroplasty: a prospective, randomized study of three hundred and forty knees. *J Bone Joint Surg Am.* 2002;84-A(5):759-762.

7. Ranawat CS, Meftah M, Windsor EN, Ranawat AS. Cementless fixation in total knee arthroplasty: down the boulevard of broken dreams - affirms. *J Bone Joint Surg Br.* 2012;94(11 suppl A):82-84.
8. Buechel FF Sr, Buechel FF Jr, Pappas MJ, Dalessio J. Twenty-year evaluation of the New Jersey LCS rotating platform knee replacement. *J Knee Surg.* 2002;15(2):84-89.
9. Callaghan JJ, Beckert MW, Hennessy DW, Goetz DD, Kelley SS. Durability of a cruciate-retaining TKA with modular tibial trays at 20 years. *Clin Orthop Relat Res.* 2013;471(1):109-117.
10. Ejaz A, Laursen AC, Jakobsen T, Rasmussen S, Nielsen PT, Laursen MB. Absence of a tourniquet does not affect fixation of cemented TKA: a randomized RSA study of 70 patients. *J Arthroplasty.* 2015;30(12):2128-2132.
11. Gill GS, Joshi AB, Mills DM. Total condylar knee arthroplasty. 16- to 21-year results. *Clin Orthop Relat Res.* 1999(367):210-215.
12. Gudnason A, Hailer NP, A WD, Sundberg M, Robertsson O. All-polyethylene versus metal- backed tibial components-an analysis of 27,733 cruciate-retaining total knee replacements from the Swedish knee arthroplasty register. *J Bone Joint Surg Am.* 2014;96(12):994-999.
13. McCalden RW, Hart GP, MacDonald SJ, Naudie DD, Howard JH, Bourne RB. Clinical results and survivorship of the GENESIS II total knee arthroplasty at a minimum of 15 years. *J Arthroplasty.* 2017;32(7):2161-2166.
14. Meftah M, Ranawat AS, Ranawat CS. Ten-year follow-up of a rotating-platform, posterior-stabilized total knee arthroplasty. *J Bone Joint Surg Am.* 2012;94(5):426-432.
15. Oliver WM, Arthur CHC, Wood AM, Clayton RAE, Brenkel IJ, Walmsley P. Excellent survival and good outcomes at 15 years using the press-fit condylar sigma total knee arthroplasty. *J Arthroplasty.* 2018;33(8):2524-2529.
16. Pavone V, Boettner F, Fickert S, Sculco TP. Total condylar knee arthroplasty: a long-term followup. *Clin Orthop Relat Res.* 2001(388):18-25.
17. Ritter MA, Keating EM, Sueyoshi T, et al. After nonmodular cemented total knee arthroplasty. *J Arthroplasty.* 2016;31(10):2199-2202.
18. Rodriguez JA, Bhende H, Ranawat CS. Total condylar knee replacement: a 20-year followup study. *Clin Orthop Relat Res.* 2001(388):10-17.
19. Furnes O, Espehaug B, Lie SA, Vollset SE, Engesaeter LB, Havelin LI. Early failures among 7,174 primary total knee replacements: a follow-up study from the Norwegian Arthroplasty Register 1994-2000. *Acta Orthop Scand.* 2002;73(2):117-129.
20. Gandhi R, Tsvetkov D, Davey JR, Mahomed NN. Survival and clinical function of cemented and uncemented prostheses in total knee replacement: a meta-analysis. *J Bone Joint Surg Br.* 2009;91(7):889-895.
21. Cawley DT, Kelly N, McGarry JP, Shannon FJ. Cementing techniques for the tibial component in primary total knee replacement. *Bone Joint J.* 2013;95-B(3):295-300.
22. Bagsby DT, Issa K, Smith LS, et al. Cemented vs cementless total knee arthroplasty in morbidly obese patients. *J Arthroplasty.* 2016;31(8):1727-1731.
23. Walker PS, Soudry M, Ewald FC, McVickar H. Control of cement penetration in total knee arthroplasty. *Clin Orthop Relat Res.* 1984(185):155-164.
24. Bannister GC, Miles AW. The influence of cementing technique and blood on the strength of the bone-cement interface. *Eng Med.* 1988;17(3):131-133.
25. Ritter MA, Herbst SA, Keating EM, Faris PM. Radiolucency at the bone-cement interface in total knee replacement. The effects of bone-surface preparation and cement technique. *J Bone Joint Surg Am.* 1994;76(1):60-65.
26. Ejaz A, Laursen AC, Jakobsen T, Rasmussen S, Nielsen PT, Laursen MB. Absence of a tourniquet does not affect fixation of cemented TKA: a randomized RSA study of 70 patients. *J Arthroplasty.* 2015;30(12):2128-2132.

27. Crook PD, Owen JR, Hess SR, Al-Humadi SM, Wayne JS, Jiranek WA. Initial stability of cemented vs cementless tibial components under cyclic load. *J Arthroplasty*. 2017;32(8):2556-2562.

28. Ryd L, Hansson U, Blunn G, Lindstrand A, Toksvig-Larsen S. Failure of partial cementation to achieve implant stability and bone ingrowth: a long-term roentgen stereophotogrammetric study of tibial components. *J Orthop Res*. 1999;17(3):311-320.

29. Kelly MP, Illgen RL, Chen AF, Nam D. Trends in the use of high-viscosity cement in patients undergoing primary total knee arthroplasty in the United States. *J Arthroplasty*. 2018;33(11):3460-3464.

30. Kopinski JE, Aggarwal A, Nunley RM, Barrack RL, Nam D. Failure at the tibial cement-implant interface with the use of high-viscosity cement in total knee arthroplasty. *J Arthroplasty*. 2016;31(11):2579-2582.

31. King JD, Hamilton DH, Jacobs CA, Duncan ST. The hidden cost of commercial antibiotic-loaded bone cement: a systematic review of clinical results and cost implications following total knee arthroplasty. *J Arthroplasty*. 2018;33(12):3789-3792.

32. Chiu FY, Chen CM, Lin CF, Lo WH. Cefuroxime-impregnated cement in primary total knee arthroplasty: a prospective, randomized study of three hundred and forty knees. *J Bone Joint Surg Am*. 2002;84-A(5):759-762.

33. Cummins JS, Tomek IM, Kantor SR, Furnes O, Engesaeter LB, Finlayson SR. Cost-effectiveness of antibiotic-impregnated bone cement used in primary total hip arthroplasty. *J Bone Joint Surg Am*. 2009;91(3):634-641.

34. Engesaeter LB, Lie SA, Espehaug B, Furnes O, Vollset SE, Havelin LI. Antibiotic prophylaxis in total hip arthroplasty: effects of antibiotic prophylaxis systemically and in bone cement on the revision rate of 22,170 primary hip replacements followed 0-14 years in the Norwegian Arthroplasty Register. *Acta Orthop Scand*. 2003;74(6):644-651.

35. Espehaug B, Engesaeter LB, Vollset SE, Havelin LI, Langeland N. Antibiotic prophylaxis in total hip arthroplasty. Review of 10,905 primary cemented total hip replacements reported to the Norwegian arthroplasty register, 1987 to 1995. *J Bone Joint Surg Br*. 1997;79(4):590-595.

36. Malchau H, Herberts P, Ahnfelt L. Prognosis of total hip replacement in Sweden. Follow-up of 92,675 operations performed 1978-1990. *Acta Orthop Scand*. 1993;64(5):497-506.

37. Tayton ER, Frampton C, Hooper GJ, Young SW. The impact of patient and surgical factors on the rate of infection after primary total knee arthroplasty: an analysis of 64,566 joints from the New Zealand Joint Registry. *Bone Joint J*. 2016;98-B(3):334-340.

38. Meding JB, Reddleman K, Keating ME, et al. Total knee replacement in patients with diabetes mellitus. *Clin Orthop Relat Res*. 2003(416):208-216.

39. Gandhi R, Backstein D, Zywiel MG. Antibiotic-laden bone cement in primary and revision hip and knee arthroplasty. *J Am Acad Orthop Surg*. 2018;26(20):727-734.

40. Ma HM, Lu YC, Ho FY, Huang CH. Long-term results of total condylar knee arthroplasty. *J Arthroplasty*. 2005;20(5):580-584.

41. Huizinga MR, Brouwer RW, Bisschop R, van der Veen HC, van den Akker-Scheek I, van Raay JJ. Long-term follow-up of anatomic graduated component total knee arthroplasty: a 15- to 20-year survival analysis. *J Arthroplasty*. 2012;27(6):1190-1195.

chapter 38

Cementless Total Knee Arthroplasty

R. Michael Meneghini, MD | Lucian C. Warth, MD

INTRODUCTION

Initially popularized in the 1980s,[1,2] cementless fixation for total knee arthroplasty (TKA) has enjoyed variable rates of success over the last 3 decades. Historical registry data demonstrate a relatively small percentage of usage internationally for cementless fixation in TKA, with slightly higher failure rate consistently observed with uncemented fixation.[3] While arthroplasty surgeons have been relatively slow to embrace cementless fixation in TKA, interest has recently surged in large part due to the increasing incidence of TKAs performed in younger,[4] more active, and more demanding patients. Additionally, recent improvements in biomaterials and robust implant designs to enhance initial component stability and osseointegration, improved polyethylene, and a better understanding of the failure mechanisms of past designs portend a bright future for cementless fixation in TKA. While cemented fixation has a well-established track record and remains the gold standard,[5-11] aseptic loosening with fragmentation and debonding of the cement interface continues to be a major failure mechanism.[12-15] This is particularly concerning with TKA in young patients[16,17] with whom a more durable biological fixation method holds the promise of improved longevity. Moreover, improved operating room and procedural efficiency via eliminating cement cure time can yield improved operating room efficiency and translate directly into healthcare dollars saved.[18] It is documented that decreasing surgical procedure duration has a positive impact on postoperative infection rate, and this may be a potential advantage to cementless fixation in TKA.[19] Additionally, the longevity of a biologic ingrowth interface may yield decreased long-term revision burden in patients who would have outlived traditional cemented fixation, particularly in younger more active patients.

Despite potential advantages, improved materials, and advances in design, cementless fixation remains controversial. Past failures in the early cementless implant designs are well documented and are often directly attributable to various design flaws or inferior biomaterials.[20-24] Poor-quality polyethylene, inferior polyethylene locking mechanisms, tibial patch-porous coating,[25,26] tibial screw augmentation, fatigue fracture of the femoral component,[27] and patellar failures[28-30] have all contributed to poor outcomes. Despite these early failures, certain cementless TKA designs have yielded excellent long-term results on par with those of cemented TKA.[31-35] With the emergence of porous ingrowth metals and improved polyethylene, the current generation of modern cementless designs is an enticing option for fixation in TKA.

EARLY CEMENTLESS DESIGNS: LEARNING FROM HISTORICAL FAILURES

As with early generations of cementless total hip arthroplasty (THA), close clinical follow-up has identified several design-related failures associated with early cementless TKA systems. These unanticipated shortcomings of early designs underscore the significance of close clinical follow-up as new technologies and cementless TKA designs are introduced into the marketplace. The somewhat checkered history of cementless TKA has left us with a cache of knowledge which can be implemented to enhance future designs. In most systems, the femoral component has achieved reliable long-term fixation to bone in both in hybrid and cementless TKA constructs,[33,36] while the tibial and patellar components remained problematic in many series[25,26,28-30] and are considered the "Achilles heel" of successful uncemented TKA.

Successful fixation on the femoral side has not been problematic and is attributed to the inherent mechanical stability obtained with multiplanar press-fit. Although fixation was not an issue, some early-generation cementless femoral component designs demonstrated catastrophic failures due to fatigue fracture of the thin regions of the implant.[27,37] Additionally, designs with porous-coated femoral pegs have been shown to cause stress-shielding which can lead to loss of anterior femoral bone at revision surgery for cementless TKA systems. Early-generation femoral components, both cemented and cementless, were not designed to optimize patellar tracking[38,39] and likely contributed to polyethylene wear and metal-backed patellar component failure frequently observed in series of early designs.

Tibial component fixation and design in cementless TKA continues to be the main area of focus for optimizing performance and outcomes. Early designs achieved fixation with short pegs which did not attain adequate initial mechanical stability for osseointegration, instead allowing deleterious micromotion, liftoff, and subsidence. The addition of stems or screws to augment initial tibial component stability has been shown in biomechanical studies to minimize micromotion and prevent tray liftoff. While supplemental screw fixation can enhance initial stability, there has been reported failure of ingrowth and metaphyseal osteolytic lesions predominating around tibial screw tracks. Berger et al reported results in a series of 131 consecutive cementless Miller-Galante-1 (Zimmer, Warsaw, IN) with an ingrowth tibial interface and screw augmentation, finding 8% tibial aseptic loosening rate due to failure of ingrowth and a 12% incidence of osteolytic lesions around screw holes at a mean 11-year follow-up. The incidence of screw hole osteolysis is reported to be greater than 30% in some cementless tibial component designs and has been attributed to the screw holes acting as access channels for particulate debris to the proximal tibial metaphysis.

While screw holes provide access, the osteolytic process is likely multifactorial and tied to the polyethylene quality, polyethylene thickness, and integrity of the polyethylene locking mechanism. Hofmann et al reported no cases of screw track osteolysis in a series of 176 cementless Natural Knee prostheses (Zimmer, Warsaw, IN) at minimum 10-year clinical follow-up.[33] In the next iteration of this design, the Natural Knee II (Zimmer, Warsaw, IN) screw augmentation was found to be unnecessary by Ferguson et al.[40] This study evaluating 116 consecutive TKAs study demonstrated equivalent stability and ingrowth at average 67-month follow-up in cementless TKA both with and without screw fixation.[40]

Tibial baseplates that contain patch-porous coating and/or smooth metal tracks separating pads of porous coating on the undersurface of the tibial tray allow a path of minimal resistance for egress of particulate wear debris and the subsequent development of osteolysis in the proximal tibia.[25,26] Whiteside et al reported a high rate of osteolysis in the first-generation Ortholoc Modular tibial component (Wright Medical Technology, Arlington, TN), which contained such a configuration. When compared to the next-generation Ortholoc II tibial component (Wright Medical Technology, Arlington, TN) that utilized continuous porous coating, no cases of osteolysis in 675 cementless TKAs were identified. These clinical findings support that maintaining a circumferential and fully porous-coated cementless tibial tray is important to effectively seal off the tibial metaphysis from particulate debris and can prevent particulate egress and subsequent tibial lysis in cementless TKA tibial designs.

The most commonly reported complication in early cementless TKA designs was failure of cementless metal-backed patellar components.[20,24,41,42] Failure mechanisms included dissociation of the metal–polyethylene interface,[41] dissociation of the peg–baseplate junction due to lack of osseointegration of the baseplate,[24] and excessive polyethylene wear with subsequent metal–metal articulation,[42] proliferative synovitis, and pain. These complications were linked to both component design as well as errant surgical technique such as excessive femoral component internal rotation. Berger et al[20] reported a 48% failure rate requiring reoperation for failed Miller-Galante (Zimmer, Warsaw, IN) cementless patellar components with the two failure mechanisms being failure of ingrowth and excessive polyethylene wear and metallosis.

EARLY CEMENTLESS DESIGNS: SUCCESS STORIES

Despite the early design failures and complications reported with cementless TKA, there are a number of designs that have obtained successful long-term results similar to cemented TKA with 10-year survival rates greater than 95% (**Table 38-1**). Hofmann et al reported on the cruciate-retaining (CR) cementless Natural Knee system (Zimmer, Warsaw, IN) that utilized a tibial tray with a stem and screw augmentation and a countersunk metal-backed patella, reported 99.1%, 99.6%, and 95.1% 14-year survivorship for the femoral, tibial, and patellar components, respectively.[33] As with most cementless systems, the majority of failures were attributed patellar edge wear, and the authors attributed the excellent long-term results to the asymmetric tibial component, coating the bone surfaces with autograft bone slurry and a countersunk patella component.[33]

TABLE 38-1	Long-Term Follow-Up of Traditional Cementless TKA Designs				
Authors	**Patient Number**	**Knee System**	**Tibial Fixation**	**10-Year Survivorship**	**Comments**
Buechel et al[43]	309	LCS	Stem	97%	One tibial component aseptic loosening at 0.9 y
Hofmann et al[33]	176	Natural	Stem and screws	95.10%	No screw-associated osteolysis
Ritter et al[10]	73	AGC	Stem	98.60%	Two tibial component failures, 98.6% 20-y survivorship
Eriksen et al[45]	114	AGC	Stem	97%	84.4% 20-y survivorship
Watanabe et al[34]	54	Osteonics	Stem and screws	100%	
Whiteside[35]	163	Ortholoc	Stem and smooth pegs	94.10%	23% lost to follow-up

Whiteside reported the 10-year results of 163 CR Ortholoc I (Wright Medical Technology, Arlington, VA) cementless tibial and femoral components.[35] The tibial component had a fully porous-coated undersurface with a smooth central stem and smooth pegs, while the femoral component had porous coating on the distal surface; the anterior and posterior chamfers with a less rough and relatively smooth anterior and posterior condylar flanges to avoid transmitting axial forces to those bone regions. Considering loosening and infection as failure criteria, Whiteside reported a 97% at 10-year follow-up. However, 91 of the original 256 knees were lost to follow-up or had died prior to follow-up in this series.[35] Buechel et al reported the 20-year results of the Low Contact Stress (LCS, Depuy, Warsaw, IN) cementless CR meniscal bearing and rotating platform designs with a rotating-bearing cementless metal-backed patellar component.[43] Using revision for any mechanical reason, including bearing wear, survivorship of the cementless CR meniscal-bearing knee was 97% at 10-year and 83% at 16-year follow-up. Survivorship of the cementless rotating platform knee group was 98% at both 10- and 16-year follow-up. The tibial component was fully porous-coated and stabilized with a stem without screw augmentation. In the total 309 cementless tibial and femoral components, there was only one reported tibial component loosening and no femoral component loosening.[43] A report of 76 CR cementless Osteonics series 3000 (Osteonics, Allendale, NJ) total knee replacements documented a 100% survival rate at 10 years and 97% at 13 years.[34] The femoral and tibial components were both made of cobalt-chrome with cobalt-chrome beads on the undersurface, and the tibial components were stemmed and secured with supplemental screw fixation.[34]

The cementless Anatomic Graduated Component (AGC) knee system (Biomet, Warsaw, IN) has demonstrated excellent long-term results. The system consists of a CR, nonmodular tibial component with a porous-coated undersurface, and a grit-blasted central stem without screw fixation. In an update of a previously reported cohort,[44] a series of 73 cementless AGC total knee arthroplasties were reviewed at a minimum of 10 years by the original designer. The investigators discovered a 97% cumulative survivorship at 20 years, with only two cases of tibial component loosening at 1 and 9 years. There were 12 cases of metal-backed patellar failure and metallosis requiring revision.[32] Eriksen also reported on the Anatomic Graduated Component (AGC) knee system (Biomet, Warsaw, IN), finding an 84.4% all component survivorship at 20 years for this system, with the majority of failures being attributable to patellar component failures. An impressive 97.2% and 100% 20-year survival was found for the tibial and femoral components, respectively.[45]

It is clear that certain cementless TKA systems provide durable long-term results. The implant design features common in these successful systems include a tibial component that achieved initial implant stability with either a stem, supplemental screw fixation, or both. High-quality compression-molded polyethylene in a nonmodular design appears to avoid the problem of osteolysis, and utilizing either a countersunk or mobile-bearing patellar component yields satisfactory long-term results if patellar resurfacing is indicated.

MODERN CEMENTLESS TKA DESIGNS: IMPROVED BIOMATERIALS AND DESIGNS

Recently developed biomaterials including hydroxyapatite (HA), porous titanium, and porous tantalum and improved polyethylene have demonstrated enhanced fixation and improved wear characteristics, respectively. These biomaterials have achieved acceptance through clinical success in a wide variety of hip and knee arthroplasty applications, and it is hopeful that they will be translated to improve primary cementless TKA designs and outcomes.

Hydroxyapatite (HA) has emerged as excellent surface coating to facilitate osseointegration of prosthetic components. Soballe et al documented three times greater interface shear strength with implants coated with HA when compared to titanium alloy without HA.[46] Gejo et al examined a prospective cohort of patients that underwent CR TKA using the cementless NexGen (Zimmer, Warsaw, IN) knee system with either a titanium porous-coated tibial component and supplemental screw fixation or a HA-coated tibial tray without screws.[47] At 12-month follow-up of the 92 knees, the authors documented clear zones radiographically under 32% of the tibial components in the non-HA group, while the HA-coated tibial components demonstrated only a single clear zone underneath the medial aspect of one tibial tray. The authors suggest the HA provides additional interface strength and bone ingrowth that allows for tibial fixation without screws.[47]

Porous metals, most notably porous tantalum and more recently porous titanium, have emerged as biologically and mechanically friendly options which have a number of applications in knee replacement surgery. In addition to rapid bone ingrowth and increased interface strength,[48] porous tantalum provides improved material elasticity and an increased surface coefficient of friction. The coefficient of friction for porous tantalum on cancellous bone (0.88 to 0.98) is significantly greater than that previously reported for traditional porous-coated and sintered-bead materials (0.50 to 0.66).[49] Furthermore, the modulus of elasticity of porous tantalum is in between cortical and cancellous bone, significantly less than titanium and chromium cobalt materials. This elasticity of porous tantalum may create a more physiologic stress transfer to the periprosthetic bone, which may affect initial mechanical stability and adaptive bone response, while minimizing stress-shielding in the longer term.

Highly porous titanium has also been developed to improve fixation strength to bone through a more biologically friendly macro- and microstructure. A canine study was conducted to determine the fixation strength of traditional titanium beads (porosity 30% to 35%), cobalt-chrome beads (porosity 35% to 40%), and a newly developed highly porous titanium surface treatment that has a porosity of 65% to 70%.[50] The authors reported a far greater amount of bone ingrowth and mechanical strength with the highly porous titanium over the other two traditional porous surfaces.[50] Ultimately, the advantage of these newly developed biomaterials, such as porous metals, will likely improve cementless fixation and long-term patient outcomes in knee replacement through greater initial mechanical prosthesis fixation and more rapid osseointegration.

MODERN CEMENTLESS TKA: EARLY CLINICAL PERFORMANCE

While there are a number of modern designs utilizing porous metals currently available on the market, there is minimal literature evaluating short- and mid-term clinical outcomes of these implants. An exception is the cementless, monoblock porous Trabecular Metal tibial component (Zimmer Inc, Warsaw, IN) which has been shown to exhibit excellent initial mechanical stability with two hex pegs for fixation without screws and has emerged with encouraging early clinical outcomes (**Table 38-2**).[51-54]

In a randomized, controlled trial, Fernandez-Fairen compared 74 cementless TKAs utilizing the porous tantalum monoblock tibial component against 71 hybrid TKAs utilizing cemented tibial components.[51] Patients receiving the cementless tibiae had slightly improved Knee Society Scores (KSS) as well as WOMAC scores and were found to have no increased frequency of complications, reoperations, or tibial loosening at an average 5-year follow-up. Kamath et al reported on a series of 100 patients younger than 55 years who received a cementless TKA with the porous tantalum monoblock tibial component.[52] At a minimum 5-year follow-up in this cohort, there were no component-related failures, significant radiographic lucencies, osteolysis, or changes in component positioning. In a randomized clinical trial,

Pulido et al compared 106 cementless porous tantalum monoblock tibial components against 115 partially cemented porous tantalum monoblock tibial components and a 126 traditional modular cemented tibial components.[53] At minimum 2 years, survivorship with revision for all causes was not different among the groups, and the 5-year cumulative risk of aseptic loosening of the tibia was greater in the traditional cemented modular tibia group than in the uncemented cohort (3.1% vs. 0%). Unger reported average 4.5-year follow-up data on a cohort of 108 cementless TKAs with the Trabecular Metal monoblock tibial component noting no tibial revision and no progressive lucencies.[54]

These early successes are tempered by the findings of Meneghini and de Beaubien[55] in a study of 106 consecutive cementless TKAs utilizing porous tantalum monoblock tibial components. In this cohort, nine tibial failures occurred at a mean of 18 months postoperatively and were predominantly identified in tall, heavy, male patients. Although not statistically significant, the authors identified a trend toward the failure group having a greater postoperative varus tibiofemoral angle. Refinements in patient selection, implant design, and surgical technique remain to be made. The early success and acceptance of porous tantalum materials in primary knee replacement[56] has ushered in a new era of cementless TKA designs and strategies.

A successful modern cementless TKA system has emerged with excellent short-term results.[57,58] The system (Triathlon, Stryker; Mahwah, NJ) consists of a 3-D printed highly porous tibial component with a robust central keel and four peripheral pegs matched with a cobalt-chrome femoral component with a fixation surface of HA-coated beads. Substantiated with a robust biomechanical basis and validation of design,[59-61] the porous titanium implant has performed well in the short-term. Nam and coauthors reported on 66 cementless TKAs with this design and reported no failures at a mean of 1.4 years with similar outcomes to a matched cohort of 62 cemented TKAs of identical design.[58] Miller and coauthors reported on 200 cementless TKAs of this design (matched to 200 cemented TKAs of identical design) and at a mean of 2.4 years reported a single case of aseptic loosening of the tibial component.[57] While these early-term clinical results are promising and need to be followed into the longer term,

TABLE 38-2	**Short-Term Follow-Up of Modern Cementless TKA Designs**				
Authors	**Patient Number**	**Knee System**	**PS CR**	**Mean Follow-up**	**Tibial Component Survivorship**
Fernandez-Fairen et al[51]	74	NexGen (Zimmer)	CR	5 y	100.0%
Kamanth et al[52]	100	NexGen (Zimmer)	PS	5 y	100.0%
Meneghini et al[55]	106	NexGen (Zimmer)	PS	3.4 y	84.9%
Pulido et al[53]	106	NexGen (Zimmer)	PS	5 y	100.0%
Unger and Duggan[54]	108	NexGen (Zimmer)	CR	4.5 y	100.0%

they support that contemporary designs with premarket scientific and biomechanical study and development with modern biomaterials have excellent and promising results.

SURGICAL CONSIDERATIONS AND PREFERRED TECHNIQUE

When compared to cemented designs, cementless TKA is a more technically demanding procedure, with less room for error which can be compounded with each consecutive cut. Cemented fixation is forgiving and achieves maximal fixation strength immediately and can be used as a grout to accommodate bony defects, imperfect surgical cuts, and varying levels of bone porosity. With cementless TKA, optimal cut orientation, cut quality, ligament balance, and limb alignment can minimize micromotion from eccentric loading during knee motion and weight-bearing and will improve the biomechanical milieu of the joint, maximizing potential for osseointegration. This is considered an essential surgical principle inherent in the success of cementless TKA, and the performing surgeon should accept very little imperfection in achieving planar cuts and intimate bone–implant apposition.

Currently, there is little clinical evidence to guide patient selection and determine the optimal candidate for cementless TKA. However, it is the contention of the authors that bone quality and viability are essential for mechanical stability and subsequent osseointegration, and there is biomechanical evidence supporting this notion. Meneghini and coauthors reported decreased mechanical stability of uncemented tibial components in an osteoporotic bone model, compared to normal controls.[61] The authors further reported that utilizing a keeled design conferred enhanced stability in the osteoporotic model compared to a smaller two-peg-designed tibial component and that mechanical stability is dependent on implant design and host bone quality. It is therefore reasonable to reserve cementless fixation in TKA for patients with sufficient bone quality. However, objectively quantifying sufficient bone quality remains a challenge. The authors' current preference is to offer cementless TKA to those patients younger than 65 years who do not have radiographic osteopenia, clinical osteoporosis, or any medical condition that could potentially compromise bone quality such as nicotine addiction, long-term immunosuppression, or autoimmune arthropathy. However, this conservative approach has expanded with success of modern cementless designs to include healthy active individuals older than 65 years, who are more commonly male, and have robust radiodense bone quality radiographically. The final confirmation of sufficient bone quality occurs intraoperatively with a critical visual inspection of the cancellous and cortical bone along with confirmation of final implant stability with manual assessment.

The senior author does not alter the surgical approach whether utilizing cementless fixation, as optimal visualization is mandatory whether using cemented or cementless fixation in TKA. Our preferred surgical approach is the median parapatellar approach, and the incision should be adequate enough to provide excellent exposure to visualize the entire femoral and tibial and provide enough excursion to provide a clear path for execution of accurate planar saw cuts. The anterior fat pad is excised to enhance visualization, and a standard medial release to the mid-coronal plane is performed in all knees and titrated appropriately to gain adequate visualization and protection of the surrounding ligamentous structures. The author prefers posterior cruciate ligament (PCL)-retaining implant systems, where the majority of cementless TKA clinical data exist and the anterior cruciate ligament (ACL) is sacrificed.

Preparation of the femur begins with the distal femoral cut. The author's preference is to use computer navigation to make the distal femoral cut, and it has reported decreased blood loss in cemented and cementless TKA, which is further potentiated with the use of tranexamic acid.[62,63] Executing an accurate planar cut of the distal femur is of critical importance, as any error or irregularities will be magnified in the chamfer and condyle cuts due to the linked planar cuts through the four-in-one cutting guide. Therefore, the distal femoral cut must be performed with great attention to detail and accuracy to ensure a perfectly flat surface. Differential hardness of bone is frequently encountered, and the surgeon must be cognizant of this during all planar cuts, including the distal femur, as the saw blade may tend to skive as it encounters sclerotic bone on the medial or lateral femoral condyle with varus or valgus knees, respectively. This can be checked and confirmed by placing the flat surface of the distal femoral guide or edge of the saw blade on the distal femoral cut and ensuring no gaps or undulations exist. The four-in-one cutting block is applied to the distal femoral cut, and the authors' preference is to anchor this particular guide to bone with threaded pins for extra secure fixation and adherence to the distal femoral cut planar surface. Finally, ensure that when removing osteophytes, no irregularities or indentations are introduced onto the planar cut surfaces.

The tibia resection is prepared with the same attention to planar accuracy and awareness of differential bone hardness, particularly the medial tibial plateau in severe varus knees with medial osteoarthritis. The authors' preference is to replicate the native tibial slope (**Fig. 38-1A**) in order to maintain the isometric tension of the PCL and prevent excessive tightness in flexion, which may create anterior liftoff of the tibial component, particularly in large, tall, and heavy male patients.[55] The tibial resection depth is minimized with an aim to utilize the thinnest polyethylene when possible, as a deeper resection into the more soft metaphyseal bone has been reported to significantly increase the proximal tibial strain.[64] As with

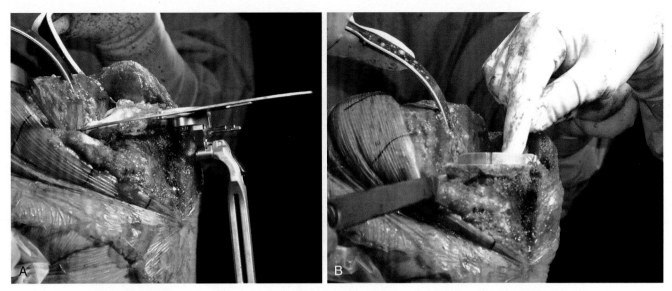

FIGURE 38-1 **A:** Using a flat guide to approximate the native tibial slope with the saw cut. **B:** The "four-corner" test to ensure a planar tibial cut with a flat surface.

the femoral cuts, the tibial cut must be perfectly planar, and the surgeon must be cognizant that the saw will tend to skive off the sclerotic bone on the side most affected by disease and dive more deeply into softer bone on the unaffected side. In order to confirm the planar accuracy and "flatness" of the tibial cut, the authors' employ the "four-corner test," popularized by Leo Whiteside, MD. The four-corner test is performed by placing a trial tibial baseplate on the cut tibial surface and attempting to rock it by pushing down on the four corners or quadrants (posterolateral, posteromedial, anterolateral, and anteromedial) of the trial baseplate (**Fig. 38-1B**). Any rocking will indicate that the surface is not perfectly flat and must be readdressed and potentially recut to ensure a perfectly flat surface. Once tibial and bone preparation is performed and gaps assessed for optimal balance, trial femoral and tibial implants are inserted, and the femoral trial is closely inspected to ensure intimate contact and interference fit of the trial to the planar cuts of the femur. This ensures that the final component will be seated properly and optimize contact of the ingrowth surface and ensure mechanical stability. Once the optimal tibial baseplate position and rotation are determined, the tibial keel is prepared with the appropriate broach. It is critical to ensure the broach is not allowed to deviate from its path within the guide, in order to maintain the optimal interference fit when the final implant is inserted. Most press-fit and cementless TKA systems employ an interference fit between the broach and final implant keel, which provides essential mechanical stability. Due to the mechanical challenge of maintaining mechanical stability of two flat planar surfaces (tibial baseplate and tibial cut surface), the authors are strong proponents of adjuvant fixation into the peripheral tibial bone, in addition to a robust tibial keel. The robust keel and peripheral fixation has been shown to optimize stability and minimize

micromotion compared to peripheral fixation alone.[59,60] The peripheral pegs are meticulously prepared to optimize interference fit, similarly to the keel and the trial tibial baseplate must be adequately secured during preparation to ensure optimal interference fit. Finally, the authors routinely prepare areas of sclerotic bone with small drill holes, which serves to stress-relax the bone to minimize fracture occurs during the tight interference impaction of the final implant.

An asymmetric tibial component (to maximize ingrowth surface area) with circumferential highly porous titanium baseplate undersurface and supplemental fixation with cruciform pegs is preferred by the senior author (**Fig. 38-2A**). An important surgical technique is to ensure that during impaction of the tibial component, the tibial baseplate and tibial bone surface are parallel and coplanar to ensure that the keel and adjuvant pegs are traversing the path prepared within the cancellous bone to optimize interference fit. Impacting the keel off-axis or at an oblique angle can disrupt the press-fit imparted by the carefully prepared path within the cancellous bone. The coplanar and parallel baseplate position should be monitored throughout impaction until the final resting position on the proximal tibial cut surface (**Fig. 38-B**). As a final step, the implant–bone interface should be inspected closely to ensure there are no gaps, which confirms a uniform and intimate contact of the highly porous undersurface of the tibial implant and viable host bone (**Fig. 38-C**).

Femoral component impaction requires similar scrutiny and critique to ensure clinical success. A press-fit cementless femoral component (**Fig. 38-A**) has the tendency to assume a relatively flexed position during impaction due to the initial contact of the longer anterior condyle on the anterior femoral bone with frictional resistance from porous metal. The frictional resistance then creates a tendency for the surgeon's hand to drop as a consequence,

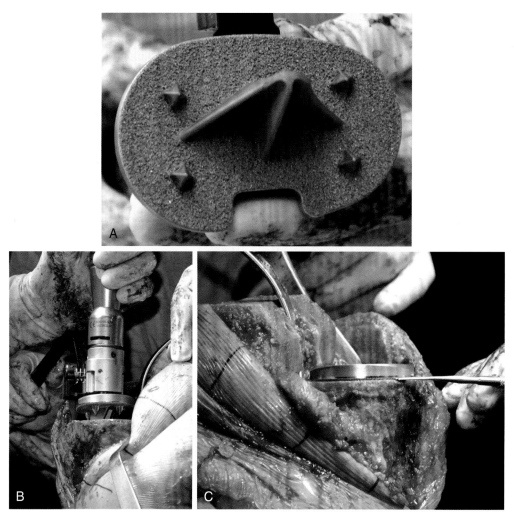

FIGURE 38-2 **A:** A modern contemporary asymmetric highly porous tibial baseplate (Empower 3D, DJO; Austin, TX) with a robust central keel and four peripheral cruciform pegs to enhance fixation. **B:** Impaction of the final tibial implant ensuring the tibial baseplate is coplanar to the cut tibial bone surface. **C:** Ensuring intimate tibial contact of the baseplate to host bone with a scalpel blade.

which could result in excessive gap between the anterior chamfer cut and implant, most notable anteriorly. This should be mitigated by using a captured femoral component inserter handle and maintaining a relatively extended position of the femur during impaction of the femoral component, resisting the tendency to flex the implant, and the femoral implant–bone interfaces should be closely inspected for excessive gaps (**Fig. 38-3B**). However, unlike the tibial implant, small gaps less than 1 mm are typically acceptable if isolated to select locations such as the anterior aspect of the anterior chamfer and may be filled with bone graft or slurry, although this is not typically needed (**Fig. 38-3C**). The intrinsic mechanical stability of the femoral implant due to the three-dimensional shape, distal lugs, and interference fit afforded between the anterior and posterior femoral condyles, along with the larger surface area of ingrowth material in contact with host bone provides a factor of safety for clinical success. While a perfectly intimate fit of the femoral component with the host bone is desired, as opposed to the tibial, minor gaps can be tolerated and do

not lead to clinical failure as long as mechanical stability of the implant is robust.

Viable options for addressing the patella in cementless TKA include nonresurfacing,[65] a cemented allpolyethylene component,[66] or a metal-backed cementless component. As described earlier, most metal-backed cementless components in traditional designs have had a poor track record and have been associated with early polyethylene failure and metallosis. Standard surgical techniques which have evolved to enhance patellar tracking should be used in all cases irrespective of how the patella is addressing intraoperatively. These include attention to appropriate femoral rotation, tibial rotation, medialization of the patellar component, lateralization of the tibial component, and soft-tissue release when necessary. If the surgeon considers resurfacing the patella with a cementless patella, particular attention should be paid to the implant design. Most modern designs incorporate modern tenets of maximizing high-quality polyethylene, highly porous metal ingrowth surface, and an optimized robust polyethylene–metal interface to minimize risk of

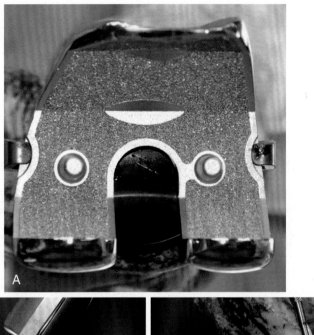

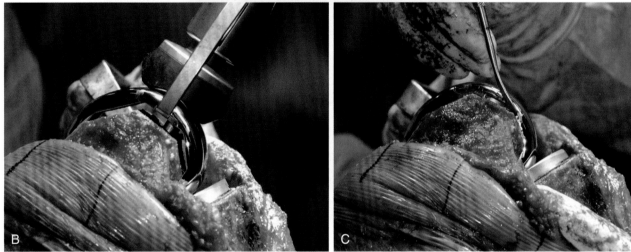

FIGURE 38-3   A: Cobalt-chrome femoral component with porous-coated fixation surface (3D Matrix, Empower 3D, DJO; Austin, TX). **B:** Impaction of the femoral component ensuring coplanar orientation of all five cuts via optimal orientation of femoral insertion handle. **C:** Intimate contact of femoral component against host bone.

dissociation. Further enhancing the modern cementless patellofemoral articulations are patella-friendly trochlear designs of modern femoral components.

In current practice, the senior author discusses all three patella options with the patient during preoperative counseling; however, a definitive choice is determined after intraoperative assessment for presence of arthritis and evaluation of patellar tracking when trialing components. If there is minimal to no arthritic change of the patella in a young patient and the patella tracks congruently without tilt intraoperatively, it is left unresurfaced, which has the advantage of preserving patellar bone stock in young patients typically younger than 65 years and is supported with data on selective patella resurfacing.[67] If there is moderate or significant arthritic change, the patella is resurfaced with a cemented component in older patients with less optimal bone quality as well as patients with borderline patellar tracking. If patellar tracking is excellent and

there is significant arthritic change of the patella, a metal-backed cementless component is selectively utilized in the younger patient typically younger than 65 years.

Clinical and Perioperative Considerations

Postoperative management of modern cementless TKA patients is nearly identical to those of cement fixation. Patients are allowed to be full weight-bearing and progress in their activity level as tolerated. It is the senior authors experience that cementless TKA patients have greater drain output; however, the use of tranexamic acid has been instrumental in minimizing this blood loss in uncemented fixation and is used routinely in all patients.[62,68,69]

Patients are seen in follow-up at regular intervals and radiographic evaluation performed with attention to visualizing the bone–implant interface (**Fig. 38-4A** and **B**). This requires diligence on the part of the technologist to

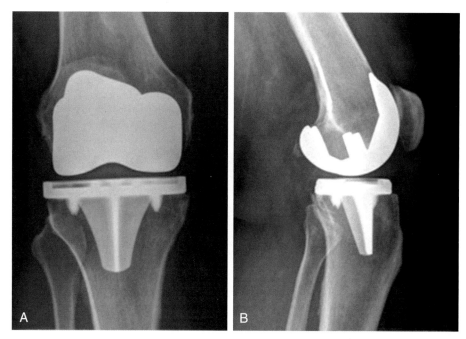

FIGURE 38-4   A: Anteroposterior radiograph of cementless TKA (Empower 3D, DJO; Austin, TX) with excellent osseointegration without radiolucencies. **B:** Lateral radiograph of cementless TKA (Empower 3D, DJO; Austin, TX) with excellent osseointegration without radiolucencies and approximation of the native tibial slope.

direct the X-ray beam perpendicular the implant, so that the prosthesis–bone interface is visualized in line with the planar cut. This methodology is well described in the updated Knee Society Radiographic Methodology.[70]

CONCLUSIONS

The long-term results of cementless TKA designs, combined with examination of early failure of some designs, support the notion that once osseointegration is achieved, fixation and the structural integrity of the bone–prosthesis interface are maintained into the long-term. Fixation will likely be enhanced and improved through newly developed biomaterials, such as highly porous tantalum and titanium. If osteolysis is prevented through improved-quality polyethylene and minimization of backside wear through modern tibial tray locking mechanisms and nonmodular tibial components, need for revision surgery should be minimal out past 20 years. The bone preserving nature of cementless total knee replacement, combined with abovementioned benefits, suggests that cementless TKA is likely the future of knee replacement, particularly in the young patient with an active lifestyle.

REFERENCES

1. Landon GC, Galante JO, Maley MM. Noncemented total knee arthroplasty. *Clin Orthop Relat Res.* 1986;205:49-57.
2. Laskin RS. Tricon-M uncemented total knee arthroplasty. A review of 96 knees followed for longer than 2 years. *J Arthroplasty.* 1988;3(1):27-38.
3. Ranawat CS, Meftah M, Windsor EN, Ranawat AS. Cementless fixation in total knee arthroplasty: down the boulevard of broken dreams - affirms. *J Bone Joint Surg Br.* 2012;94(11 suppl A):82-84.
4. Kurtz SM, Lau E, Ong K, Zhao K, Kelly M, Bozic KJ. Future young patient demand for primary and revision joint replacement: national projections from 2010 to 2030. *Clin Orthop Relat Res.* 2009;467(10):2606-2612.
5. Meneghini RM, Hanssen AD. Cementless fixation in total knee arthroplasty: past, present, and future. *J Knee Surg.* 2008;21(4):307-314.
6. Font-Rodriguez DE, Scuderi GR, Insall JN. Survivorship of cemented total knee arthroplasty. *Clin Orthop Relat Res.* 1997;345:79-86.
7. Berger RA, Rosenberg AG, Barden RM, Sheinkop MB, Jacobs JJ, Galante JO. Long-term followup of the Miller-Galante total knee replacement. *Clin Orthop Relat Res.* 2001;388:58-67.
8. Ranawat CS, Flynn WF Jr, Saddler S, Hansraj KK, Maynard MJ. Long-term results of the total condylar knee arthroplasty. A 15-year survivorship study. *Clin Orthop Relat Res.* 1993;286: 94-102.
9. Rasquinha VJ, Ranawat CS, Cervieri CL, Rodriguez JA. The press-fit condylar modular total knee system with a posterior cruciate-substituting design. A concise follow-up of a previous report. *J Bone Joint Surg Am.* 2006;88(5):1006-1010.
10. Ritter MA, Berend ME, Meding JB, Keating EM, Faris PM, Crites BM. Long-term followup of anatomic graduated components posterior cruciate-retaining total knee replacement. *Clin Orthop Relat Res.* 2001;388:51-57.
11. Rodriguez JA, Bhende H, Ranawat CS. Total condylar knee replacement: a 20-year followup study. *Clin Orthop Relat Res.* 2001;388:10-17.
12. Ducheyne P, Kagan A II, Lacey JA. Failure of total knee arthroplasty due to loosening and deformation of the tibial component. *J Bone Joint Surg Am.* 1978;60(3):384-391.
13. Faris PM, Ritter MA, Keating EM, Meding JB, Harty LD. The AGC all-polyethylene tibial component: a ten-year clinical evaluation. *J Bone Joint Surg Am.* 2003;85-A(3):489-493.
14. Lonner JH, Hershman S, Mont M, Lotke PA. Total knee arthroplasty in patients 40 years of age and younger with osteoarthritis. *Clin Orthop Relat Res.* 2000;380:85-90.
15. Moreland JR. Mechanisms of failure in total knee arthroplasty. *Clin Orthop Relat Res.* 1988;226:49-64.

16. McCalden RW, Robert CE, Howard JL, Naudie DD, McAuley JP, MacDonald SJ. Comparison of outcomes and survivorship between patients of different age groups following TKA. *J Arthroplasty.* 2013;28(8 suppl):83-86.

17. Meehan JP, Danielsen B, Kim SH, Jamali AA, White RH. Younger age is associated with a higher risk of early periprosthetic joint infection and aseptic mechanical failure after total knee arthroplasty. *J Bone Joint Surg Am.* 2014;96(7):529-535.

18. Dexter F, Weih LS, Gustafson RK, Stegura LF, Oldenkamp MJ, Wachtel RE. Observational study of operating room times for knee and hip replacement surgery at nine U.S. community hospitals. *Health Care Manag Sci.* 2006;9(4):325-339.

19. Pugely AJ, Martin CT, Gao Y, Schweizer ML, Callaghan JJ. The incidence of and risk factors for 30-day surgical site infections following primary and revision total joint arthroplasty. *J Arthroplasty.* 2015;30(9 suppl):47-50.

20. Berger RA, Lyon JH, Jacobs JJ, et al. Problems with cementless total knee arthroplasty at 11 years followup. *Clin Orthop Relat Res.* 2001;392:196-207.

21. Engh GA, Parks NL, Ammeen DJ. Tibial osteolysis in cementless total knee arthroplasty. A review of 25 cases treated with and without tibial component revision. *Clin Orthop Relat Res.* 1994;309:33-43.

22. Kim YH, Oh JH, Oh SH. Osteolysis around cementless porous-coated anatomic knee prostheses. *J Bone Joint Surg Br.* 1995;77(2):236-241.

23. Nafei A, Nielsen S, Kristensen O, Hvid I. The press-fit Kinemax knee arthroplasty. High failure rate of non-cemented implants. *J Bone Joint Surg Br.* 1992;74(2):243-246.

24. Rosenberg AG, Andriacchi TP, Barden R, Galante JO. Patellar component failure in cementless total knee arthroplasty. *Clin Orthop Relat Res.* 1988;236:106-114.

25. Ward WG, Johnston KS, Dorey FJ, Eckardt JJ. Extramedullary porous coating to prevent diaphyseal osteolysis and radiolucent lines around proximal tibial replacements. A preliminary report. *J Bone Joint Surg Am.* 1993;75(7):976-987.

26. Whiteside LA. Effect of porous-coating configuration on tibial osteolysis after total knee arthroplasty. *Clin Orthop Relat Res.* 1995;321:92-97.

27. Whiteside LA, Fosco DR, Brooks JG Jr. Fracture of the femoral component in cementless total knee arthroplasty. *Clin Orthop Relat Res.* 1993;286:71-77.

28. Andersen HN, Ernst C, Frandsen PA. Polyethylene failure of metal-backed patellar components. 111 AGC total knees followed for 7-22 months. *Acta Orthop Scand.* 1991;62(1):1-3.

29. Levi N, Kofoed H. Early failure of metal-backed patellar arthroplasty. *J Bone Joint Surg Br.* 1994;76(4):675.

30. Baech J, Kofoed H. Failure of metal-backed patellar arthroplasty. 47 AGC total knees followed for at least 1 year. *Acta Orthop Scand.* 1991;62(2):166-168.

31. Buechel FF Sr, Buechel FF Jr, Pappas MJ, Dalessio J. Twenty-year evaluation of the New Jersey LCS rotating platform knee replacement. *J Knee Surg.* 2002;15(2):84-89.

32. Ritter MA, Meneghini RM. Twenty-year survivorship of cementless anatomic graduated component total knee arthroplasty. *J Arthroplasty.* 2010;25(4):507-513.

33. Hofmann AA, Evanich JD, Ferguson RP, Camargo MP. Ten- to 14-year clinical followup of the cementless Natural Knee system. *Clin Orthop Relat Res.* 2001;388:85-94.

34. Watanabe H, Akizuki S, Takizawa T. Survival analysis of a cementless, cruciate-retaining total knee arthroplasty. Clinical and radiographic assessment 10 to 13 years after surgery. *J Bone Joint Surg Br.* 2004;86(6):824-829.

35. Whiteside LA. Cementless total knee replacement. Nine- to 11-year results and 10-year survivorship analysis. *Clin Orthop Relat Res.* 1994;309:185-192.

36. Illgen R, Tueting J, Enright T, Schreibman K, McBeath A, Heiner J. Hybrid total knee arthroplasty: a retrospective analysis of clinical and radiographic outcomes at average 10 years follow-up. *J Arthroplasty.* 2004;19(7 suppl 2):95-100.

37. Campbell MD, Duffy GP, Trousdale RT. Femoral component failure in hybrid total knee arthroplasty. *Clin Orthop Relat Res.* 1998;356:58-65.

38. Varadarajan KM, Rubash HE, Li G. Are current total knee arthroplasty implants designed to restore normal trochlear groove anatomy? *J Arthroplasty.* 2011;26(2):274-281.

39. D'Lima DD, Chen PC, Kester MA, Colwell CW Jr. Impact of patellofemoral design on patellofemoral forces and polyethylene stresses. *J Bone Joint Surg Am.* 2003;85-A(suppl 4):85-93.

40. Ferguson RP, Friederichs MG, Hofmann AA. Comparison of screw and screwless fixation in cementless total knee arthroplasty. *Orthopedics.* 2008;31(2):127.

41. Lombardi AV Jr, Engh GA, Volz RG, Albrigo JL, Brainard BJ. Fracture/dissociation of the polyethylene in metal-backed patellar components in total knee arthroplasty. *J Bone Joint Surg Am.* 1988;70(5):675-679.

42. Kraay MJ, Darr OJ, Salata MJ, Goldberg VM. Outcome of metal-backed cementless patellar components: the effect of implant design. *Clin Orthop Relat Res.* 2001;392:239-244.

43. Buechel FF Sr, Buechel FF Jr, Pappas MJ, D'Alessio J. Twenty-year evaluation of meniscal bearing and rotating platform knee replacements. *Clin Orthop Relat Res.* 2001;388:41-50.

44. Kavolus CH, Ritter MA, Keating EM, Faris PM. Survivorship of cementless total knee arthroplasty without tibial plateau screw fixation. *Clin Orthop Relat Res.* 1991;273:170-176.

45. Eriksen J, Christensen J, Solgaard S, Schrøder H. The cementless AGC 2000 knee prosthesis: 20-year results in a consecutive series. *Acta Orthop Belg.* 2009;75(2):225-233.

46. Soballe K, Toksvig-Larsen S, Gelineck J, et al. Migration of hydroxyapatite coated femoral prostheses. A Roentgen Stereophotogrammetric study. *J Bone Joint Surg Br.* 1993;75(5):681-687.

47. Gejo R, Akizuki S, Takizawa T. Fixation of the NexGen HA-TCP-coated cementless, screwless total knee arthroplasty: comparison with conventional cementless total knee arthroplasty of the same type. *J Arthroplasty.* 2002;17(4):449-456.

48. Bobyn JD, Stackpool GJ, Hacking SA, Tanzer M, Krygier JJ. Characteristics of bone ingrowth and interface mechanics of a new porous tantalum biomaterial. *J Bone Joint Surg Br.* 1999;81(5):907-914.

49. Dammak M, Shirazi-Adl A, Zukor DJ. Fixation response of two cementless tibial implants under static and fatigue compression loading. *Technol Health Care.* 2003;11(4):245-252.

50. Frenkel SR, Jaffe WL, Dimaano F, Iesaka K, Hua T. Bone response to a novel highly porous surface in a canine implantable chamber. *J Biomed Mater Res B Appl Biomater.* 2004;71(2):387-391.

51. Fernandez-Fairen M, Hernández-Vaquero D, Murcia A, Torres A, Llopis R. Trabecular metal in total knee arthroplasty associated with higher knee scores: a randomized controlled trial. *Clin Orthop Relat Res.* 2013;471(11):3543-3553.

52. Kamath AF, Lee GC, Sheth NP, Nelson CL, Garino JP, Israelite CL. Prospective results of uncemented tantalum monoblock tibia in total knee arthroplasty: minimum 5-year follow-up in patients younger than 55 years. *J Arthroplasty.* 2011;26(8):1390-1395.

53. Pulido L, Abdel MP, Lewallen DG, et al. The Mark Coventry Award: trabecular metal tibial components were durable and reliable in primary total knee arthroplasty. A randomized clinical trial. *Clin Orthop Relat Res.* 2015;473(1):34-42.

54. Unger AS, Duggan JP. Midterm results of a porous tantalum monoblock tibia component clinical and radiographic results of 108 knees. *J Arthroplasty.* 2011;26(6):855-860.

55. Meneghini RM, de Beaubien BC. Early failure of cementless porous tantalum monoblock tibial components. *J Arthroplasty.* 2013;28(9):1505-1508.

56. Levine B, Sporer S, Della Valle CJ, Jacobs JJ, Paprosky W. Porous tantalum in reconstructive surgery of the knee: a review. *J Knee Surg.* 2007;20(3):185-194.

57. Miller AJ, Stimac JD, Smith LS, Feher AW, Yakkanti MR, Malkani AL. Results of cemented vs cementless primary total knee arthroplasty using the same implant design. *J Arthroplasty*. 2018;33(4):1089-1093.

58. Nam D, Kopinski JE, Meyer Z, Rames RD, Nunley RM, Barrack RL. Perioperative and early postoperative comparison of a modern cemented and cementless total knee arthroplasty of the same design. *J Arthroplasty*. 2017;32(7):2151-2155.

59. Bhimji S, Meneghini RM. Micromotion of cementless tibial baseplates: keels with adjuvant pegs offer more stability than pegs alone. *J Arthroplasty*. 2014;29(7):1503-1506.

60. Bhimji S, Meneghini RM. Micromotion of cementless tibial baseplates under physiological loading conditions. *J Arthroplasty*. 2012;27(4):648-654.

61. Meneghini RM, Daluga A, Soliman M. Mechanical stability of cementless tibial components in normal and osteoporotic bone. *J Knee Surg*. 2011;24(3):191-196.

62. Fleischman M, Hood M Jr, Ziemba-Davis M, Meneghini RM. Tranexamic acid and computer-assisted surgery in cemented and cementless total knee arthroplasty: are the effects additive for blood conservation? *Surg Technol Int*. 2017;30:268-273.

63. Licini DJ, Meneghini RM. Modern abbreviated computer navigation of the femur reduces blood loss in total knee arthroplasty. *J Arthroplasty*. 2015;30(10):1729-1732.

64. Berend ME, Small SR, Ritter MA, Buckley CA. The effects of bone resection depth and malalignment on strain in the proximal tibia after total knee arthroplasty. *J Arthroplasty*. 2010;25(2):314-318.

65. Burnett RS, Boone JL, McCarthy KP, Rosenzweig S, Barrack RL. A prospective randomized clinical trial of patellar resurfacing and nonresurfacing in bilateral TKA. *Clin Orthop Relat Res*. 2007;464:65-72.

66. Johnson TC, Tatman PJ, Mehle S, Gioe TJ. Revision surgery for patellofemoral problems: should we always resurface? *Clin Orthop Relat Res*. 2012;470(1):211-219.

67. Roberts DW, Hayes TD, Tate CT, Lesko JP. Selective patellar resurfacing in total knee arthroplasty: a prospective, randomized, double-blind study. *J Arthroplasty*. 2015;30(2):216-222.

68. Mutsuzaki H, Ikeda K. Intra-articular injection of tranexamic acid via a drain plus drain-clamping to reduce blood loss in cementless total knee arthroplasty. *J Orthop Surg Res*. 2012;7:32.

69. Ishii Y, Noguchi H, Sato J, Tsuchiya C, Toyabe S. Effect of a single injection of tranexamic acid on blood loss after primary hybrid TKA. *Knee*. 2015;22(3):197-200.

70. Meneghini RM, Mont MA, Backstein DB, Bourne RB, Dennis DA, Scuderi GR. Development of a modern knee society radiographic evaluation system and methodology for total knee arthroplasty. *J Arthroplasty*. 2015;30(12);2311-2314.

Surgical Exposures in Total Knee Arthroplasty

Kenneth L. Urish, MD, PhD | Jason P. Zlotnicki, MD | Michael J. O'Malley, MD

INTRODUCTION

The surgical approach selected in total knee arthroplasty has significant implications for the surgeon and patient. The selection of an approach must consider patient characteristics including existing deformity, prior surgical incisions, and level of exposure required to correctly place components and protect the soft tissue. It should provide the surgeon a level of flexibility for intraoperative modification in the setting of unexpected complexity or complication. In this chapter, the technical considerations of each approach will be described, with attention to the advantages, disadvantages, and associated outcomes.

SKIN INCISION AND SOFT-TISSUE HANDLING

Surgical approach to the knee joint starts with an understanding of the anatomy of the anterior knee soft tissues (**Fig. 39-1**). The classic approach to the knee, in absence of wound or prior surgical scars, is centered on the anterior knee. The incision is placed over the patella at midline, extending in both proximal and distal direction to a total of approximately 10 cm in length, and terminating 1 cm medial to the tibial tubercle. An alternative is to make a medial parapatellar skin incision, with the goal of achieving less tension across the incision in flexion. No differences have been noted in clinical studies comparing these approaches.[1-3] In this region where soft-tissue coverage is limited, it is critical for the surgeon to preserve skin vascularity for effective wound healing. The operating surgeon must be familiar with the vascular anatomy of the knee and minimize superficial dissection as to not devascularize the superficial skin and soft tissue. Moreover, a thick subcutaneous flap must be maintained above the extensor mechanism to preserve blood supply and prevent necrosis.

The neurovascular network of the anterior knee skin and soft tissue originates from the saphenous and descending geniculate arteries on the medial aspect of the knee. Therefore through the classic midline incision, the lateral skin flap experiences a greater level of hypoxia during the surgery.[1,4,5] The anastomoses that feed the anterior

skin exist superficial to the deep fascia of the knee, and thus care should be taken to avoid superficial dissection that may put the overlying skin at risk for necrosis (**Fig. 39-2**). Likewise, the infrapatellar branch of the saphenous nerve is usually sacrificed with midline incision leading to lateral knee numbness. Though this is associated with no morbidity, the potential for lateral knee numbness after surgery should be disclosed with patients in the preoperative period.

An understanding of the medial-based neurovascular anatomy about the knee is important for all cases but critical for the creation of skin incisions in the patient with previous incisions. When selecting an area to place the incision, the surgeon must stay as lateral as possible to avoid devascularizing a large section of anterior soft tissue. It is also preferable to incorporate previous longitudinal skin incision and incise at right angles to previous horizonal incisions to better preserve skin perfusion and eliminate avascular skin bridges that lead to necrosis. Subcutaneous tissue flaps should be developed directly ventral to the extensor mechanism. This preserves the blood supply for the superficial flap carried through the subcutaneous tissue. A far lateral incision can be selected, and medial exposure can still be obtained because of the ability to lengthen the incision and develop large flexible flaps that provide that necessary exposure. Surgeons should be aware of large scars or soft-tissues defects that may be threatened by an anterior- or medial-based knee incision. Important characteristics include the age of the incision or scar, the circumstances, and history of difficulty with wound healing. In the setting of complex history with any of the above criteria, a plastic surgery consult should be considered preoperatively.

After skin incision and soft-tissue flap preparation, the extensor mechanism is clearly visualized (**Fig. 39-3**). All subsequent exposures described differ in their management of the extensor mechanism; however, the goal of any approach is to achieve adequate visualization for bone resection, component insertion, and soft-tissue balancing. The major anatomic landmarks and the different intervals that can be utilized for approach are described in **Fig. 39-3**.

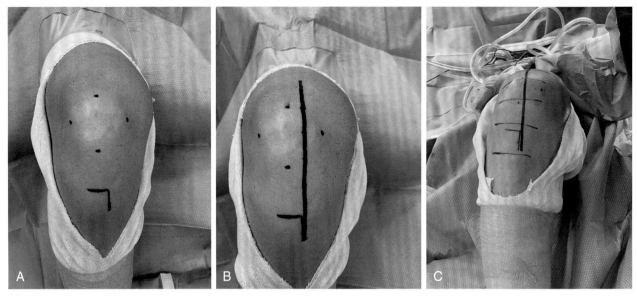

FIGURE 39-1   Anterior knee landmarks. **A:** Knowledge of anterior bone and soft-tissue landmarks about the knee promotes appropriate position of anterior midline incision. The border of the patella and tibial tubercle has been annotated. **B:** Author's preferred skin incision is placed relevant to the annotated landmarks. **C:** Orthogonal lines used to assist in accurate reapproximation of the skin during closure are then added. (Image Library, K. Urish, with permission.)

MEDIAL PARAPATELLAR APPROACH

Initially described by von Langenbeck in 1879, the medial parapatellar approach (i.e., median parapatellar or paramedian approach) offers an easily reproducible and extensile approach to the knee.[6] More recently popularized by Insall, the approach provides excellent exposure and can be modified when additional exposure or soft-tissue release is required (as discussed in the following difficult exposures section). The classic version of this approach splits the quadriceps tendon in the medial one-third and releases both the rectus femoris tendon and vastus medialis fibers from the patella. More recent modifications of this approach have medialized the quadriceps incision, leaving the majority of the quadriceps tendon intact and only removing the vastus medialis from its patellar insertion. Insall's modification describes dissection of the

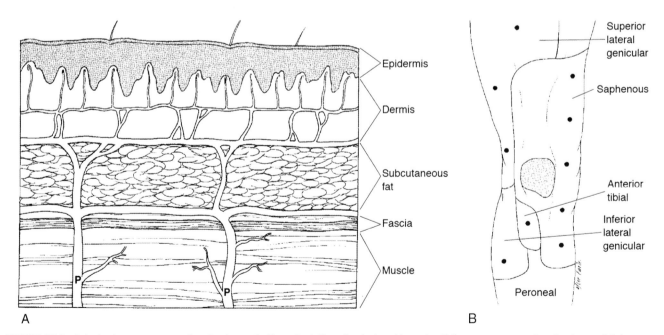

FIGURE 39-2   Anterior knee neurovascular structures. **A:** The orientation of anterior skin and soft-tissue neurovascular structures dictate proper soft-tissue handling. Microvascular anatomy of skin and subcutaneous tissue requires thick flaps to preserve blood flow to wound edges from deep perforator vessels (P). **B:** Due to medial-based circulation the lateral flap experiences more hypoxia (solid circles refer to position of deep perforators). The course of the infrapatellar branch of saphenous nerve explains post-op lateral skin numbness. (From Younger AS, Duncan CP, Masri BA. Surgical exposures in revision total knee arthroplasty. *J Am Acad Orthop Surg.* 1998;6:56, Figs 1A and B, with permission.)

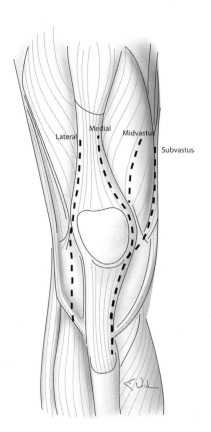

FIGURE 39-3 Extensor mechanism and relationship of approaches. The extensor mechanism includes the quadriceps muscle and tendon, patella, patellar tendon, and tibial tubercle among other soft-tissue structures. The different approaches to the knee vary in how they incise capsule to avoid or manipulate the extensor mechanism for exposure. (Image Library, K. Urish, with permission.)

extensor mechanism in a straight line over the anterior patella surface, continuing distal along the medial border of the patellar tendon.[6] From there, the quadriceps expansion is peeled from the anterior patellar surface with sharp dissection until the medial border of the patella is visualized. At this point, the synovium is then divided, the fat pad is split in the midline, and the patella is everted laterally. Closure can be performed in either flexion or extension, as randomized prospective trial has shown no effect on outcome based on knee position during closure.[7]

The authors of this chapter prefer the following step-by-step approach, utilizing different modifications as needed for a repeatable and extensile exposure to the knee (**Fig. 39-4**).

Surgical Technique

The patient is positioned supine on a standard operating table. Two L-bars affixed to the table are used to hold the foot, stabilizing the knee while in flexion during surgery. One is placed under the proximal calf and used to stabilize the leg in maximal flexion; the other is placed under the distal calf to hold the knee at 90° of flexion. Alternative devices can be used to allow the surgeon to select different levels of flexion that will be needed during the procedure.

The incision is made with the knee at 90° of flexion, tensioning the anterior skin, causing the skin edges to retract as the incision is made. The incision is made just medial to midline, starting roughly 5 cm (3 fingerbreadths) proximal to the superior pole of the patella, and extends distal to the inferomedial boarder of the tibial tubercle. This optimizes soft-tissue coverage on the distal extensor mechanism where it can sometimes be tenuous and translates the incision directly off a pressure point when kneeling. The incision is taken sharply down to the extensor mechanism. Full-thickness skin flaps are made to preserve superficial blood supply. The medial skin flap is reflected off the fascia to the medial boarder of the patella, and minimal lateral dissection is performed. Large skin flaps are avoided to prevent disruption of the anastomotic blood supply to the skin.

The medial parapatellar arthrotomy is started at the proximal quadriceps tendon, 1 to 2 mm lateral to the vastus medialis oblique insertion, and extends distal around the medial boarder of the patella. Care is taken to leave 3 to 5 mm of medial retinaculum on the patella to ensure adequate tissue for repair of the arthrotomy during closure. The arthrotomy is then continued distally to the medial edge of the tibial tubercle. The capsule and synovium are incised in line with the arthrotomy. The anterior horn of the medial meniscus is incised. The synovium and fat pad are released from under the patellar tendon to the level of the tibial tubercle. This aids in patellar mobility. If the patella remains difficult to evert, the surgeon can release the lateral patellofemoral ligament and should ensure the capsular folds in the suprapatellar pouch are incised. Once the patella is mobilized, the infrapatellar fat pad is debulked or excised based on surgeon preference. The author prefers to revert the patella and retract it laterally rather than evert the patella for the remainder of the operation. If additional mobility of the extensor mechanism is required for exposure, the proximal quadriceps split can be extended roughly 5 cm before risking denervation.

For a standard varus knee, the medial capsule and deep medial collateral ligament (MCL) are reflected subperiosteally as a triangular sleeve of tissue starting from the medial boarder of the tubercle and extending around the medial plateau to posterior medial corner. The release extends 5 to 10 mm below the medial joint line. Care is taken not to release further distal as the superficial MCL attaches 3 to 5 cm distal to the medial joint line. An additional suggestion for improving exposure is the removal of the tibial and femoral osteophytes early in the operation subsequently relaxing the capsule. If the patella is being resurfaced, performing the patella cut early in the exposure also helps with extensor mechanism mobilization. In this case, the surgeon should consider placing a shield over the patella to avoid damaging or fracturing the patella.

Closure of the arthrotomy can be accomplished based on surgeon preference with either absorbable or nonabsorbable sutures. Running barbed suture closures have gained favor recently as their use can decrease operative

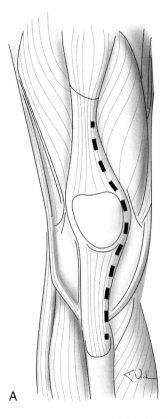
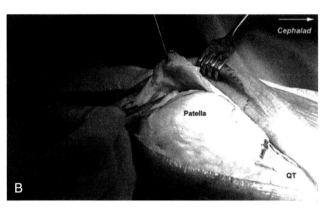

A   B

FIGURE 39-4   Median parapatellar approach. **A:** Author's preferred skin incision. **B:** After creation of thick soft-tissue flaps, quadriceps tendon and medial approach are marked out to facilitate creation of soft-tissue cuff that is easily approximated during closure. QT, quadriceps tendon. (A, Image Library, K. Urish, with permission. B and C, From Photo Library – Department of Orthopaedics (Adult Reconstruction), London Health Sciences Centre, London, Ontario, Canada, with permission.)

time without increase in complications.[8] The subcutaneous skin layer is closed with absorbable 2-0 monofilament. Surgeon preference, including subcuticular monocryl, staples, or coaptive film,[9] can be used for skin closure. Regardless of the specific technique to close, meticulous attention to hemostasis, gentle soft-tissue handling, and reapproximating the edges of each tissue plane is important in avoiding wound complications. Postoperatively, the patient is allowed to bend the knee as tolerated and does not have weight-bearing restrictions.

The advantages of this workhorse approach are the universal nature and reproducible ease for exposure in primary knee replacement. Purported disadvantages include removal of the vastus medialis from the remainder of the quadriceps and extensor mechanism, as well as disruption of the medial-based patellar vascularity.[10,11] Despite these theoretical disadvantages, no obvious clinical morbidity or inferiority has been demonstrated in clinical outcomes.

MIDVASTUS APPROACH

The midvastus approach has been well described by Engh and Parks.[12] It utilizes an interval in the midsubstance of the vastus medialis at the superomedial border of the patella. By using this interval, it avoids disruption of the

quadriceps tendon and vastus medialis insertion thereby maintains an intact extensor mechanism.

A standard anterior midline incision is created in flexion, and dissection is performed to fascia. The medial aspect of the patella and vastus medialis insertion should be adequately exposed with creation of the medial soft-tissue flap. The prepatellar bursa is reflexed medially off the anterior surface of the patella, while the dissection in the distal aspect of the incision is limited to skin and fat only. With the knee in a flexed position, the superomedial corner of the patella is identified and blunt dissection is performed full thickness through the vastus medialis parallel to muscle fibers approximately 4 cm proximal to the superomedial patella. The arthrotomy is then performed in this region, proximal to the patella and deep to the vastus split, and is carried through the retinaculum along the medial aspect of patella to 1 cm medial to the distal aspect of the tibial tubercle (**Fig. 39-5**). Care must be taken to preserve a cuff of soft tissue on the patella for closure. A subperiosteal release is then performed to the midcoronal plane while capsule, synovium, and bursa are reflected to the medial border of the tubercle. Necessary soft-tissue releases from the proximal tibia may now be performed. Note that, in order to fully evert the patella from this approach, the capsular folds of the suprapatellar pouch must also be released. With lateral patellofemoral

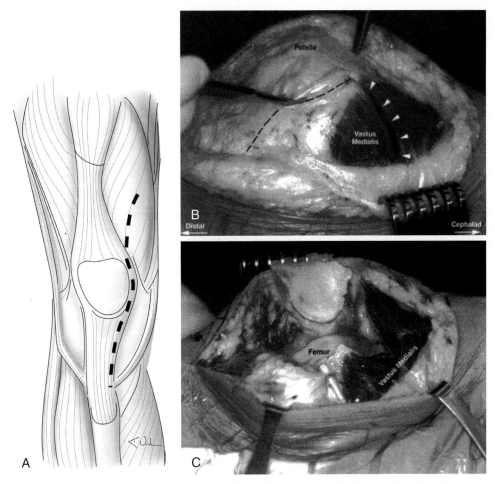

FIGURE 39-5 Midvastus approach. **A:** View of surgical interval during midvastus approach. Note relationship of extensor mechanism, medial border of patella, and vastus medialis obliquus. **B:** The interval is parallel to the vastus medialis muscle fibers (white arrow heads). **C:** The patella is everted after incision is carried into the retinaculum. (A, Image Library, K. Urish, with permission. B and C, From Engh GA, Parks NL. Surgical technique of the midvastus arthrotomy. *Clin Orthop Relat Res.* 1998;351:271, Figs. 2B and C, with permission.)

ligament release and fat pad excision, the joint capsule is reflected until the lateral plateau is clearly visualized, completing the approach. Closure of the arthrotomy and approach should be performed at 60° of flexion, starting at the intersection of the capsular and muscle-splitting region of the incision. The muscle split itself does not need to be sutured.[13]

Proponents of this approach contend the midvastus approach avoids disruption of the quadriceps tendon while providing excellent exposure. However, this approach should not be performed in obese patients, hypertrophic arthridities, knees that lack greater than 80° of flexion, and in the setting of previous high tibial osteotomies.[12] In addition, the surgeon must be aware of the maximal safe distance for proximal sharp dissection, 4.5 cm, which was demonstrated by Cooper et al.[14] In comparing the midvastus approach to the median parapatellar approach, the avoidance of the extensor mechanism demonstrates some early improvement in pain control and return of function. An early study from White et al showed postoperative improvement in pain at both 8 day and 6 week time points, with an improved time to achieve

straight leg raise. However, no differences were seen at 6-month follow-up between the midvastus and median.[15] From an intraoperative standpoint, fewer lateral releases were observed with the midvastus approach. Early pain control and return of quadriceps function were confirmed in a study by Dalury and Jiranek,[16] but refuted by Keating et al[17] who found no significant differences at early or late time point. Interestingly, Parentis et al showed the midvastus split to alter EMG findings suggestive of an underlying component of nerve injury to the vastus medialis. They also noted a decrease in the number of lateral releases and overall blood loss in the midvastus approach compared to medial parapatellar approach.[18] Despite these findings, no corresponding clinical deficits or outcome differences were noted in the study. A more recent meta-analysis performed by Liu et al combined 32 randomized controlled trials with a total of 2451 total knee arthroplasty cases to evaluate both the midvastus approach and subvastus approach to the median parapatellar. The midvastus approach demonstrated improved visual analog scale (VAS) pain scores and knee motion in the 1 to 2 week postoperative period but an overall increase in operative time. No significant differences were noted in long-term clinical outcome.[19] Overall, there is evidence of the theoretical benefit of sparing the extensor mechanism to decrease the early pain and aid in early recovery of knee motion and quadriceps function. However, this improvement does not persist at later time points and amounts to no significant clinical improvement at long-term follow-up.

SUBVASTUS APPROACH

The subvastus (or Southern approach) to the knee joint was first described in 1929 but has been more recently described and popularized by Hoffman et al.[20] Proponents of this approach state that it is a more anatomic approach, respecting the boundaries of the normal knee anatomy. In comparison to the medial parapatellar approach, the extensor mechanism is left undisrupted with preservation of the medial patellar blood supply. However, the subvastus approach has important contraindications to recognize for use and cannot be extended in cases of difficult exposure. These contraindications include revision arthroplasty, prior knee arthrotomy, previous high tibial osteotomy, and obese patients.[20,21] In these cases, proper exposure will be difficult to obtain because the arthrotomy cannot be extended, and there are limited options to further mobilize the extensor mechanism.

A standard anterior incision over the midline is performed with the knee in 90° of flexion. Dissection is performed to the superficial fascia. The superficial fascia is then incised in line with the skin incision and curving slightly medial at the level of the patella. This creates a plane that is then bluntly dissected to separate the fascia layer from the perimuscular fascia of the vastus medialis at the site of insertion. The inferior edge of the vastus is identified, and blunt dissection is continued as the surgeon lifts the muscle off the periosteum and intermuscular septum to a distance of approximately 10 cm proximal to the adductor tubercle. The insertion of the vastus medialis to the medial capsule must then be identified by placing the dissected muscle belly under tension. At this location, a transverse incision of the insertion is performed at the midpatellar level without disrupting the underlying synovium. The remainder of the vastus insertion remains attached to the patella and quadriceps tendon (**Fig. 39-6**). The extensor mechanism is then retracted in an anterolateral direction, while a curvilinear arthrotomy is performed from the suprapatellar pouch to the tibial tubercle underneath the tensioned muscle belly. The fat pad is incised along the medial edge, and soft-tissue releases are performed around the proximal tibia. With the knee in extension, the patella is then everted and dislocated laterally. The knee is then placed back into flexion slowly, while additional blunt dissection is performed to prevent excessive tension through the vastus

medialis and patellar insertion. Once instrumentation is complete, patellar tracking can be assessed. If a lateral release is required, it is performed in an outside-to-inside fashion with the knee in full flexion. This differs from the standard inside-to-outside direction as the lateral aspect of the dorsal portion of the extensor mechanism has limited exposure. Closure of the approach is then initiated with a suture at the apex of the curvilinear fascial incision and completed with interrupted close of both capsule and fascial layers.

The reported advantages of this approach focus on the "anatomic-nature" of the dissection and arthrotomy, with preservation of the extensor mechanism and patellar blood supply. Early studies comparing the subvastus approach with the median parapatellar demonstrated improved patellar tracking and a decreased need for lateral release.[22] In addition, multiple more recent analyses have reported a faster return of quadriceps function with decreased pain, improved motion, and outcome scores at early time points.[19,23-27] However, these same studies fail to demonstrate persistence of these findings or superiority to other approaches at later time points with the exception of one.[19] A most recent systematic review reiterates a faster return of straight leg raise postoperatively but highlights the inconsistency and variability in the findings of improved Knee Society Scores at both early and late time points.[28] A table has been provided for comparison (see **Table 39-1**).[24,26,29-41] Preservation of the extensor mechanism may possibly decrease pain and enhance function in the immediate postoperative period, but these benefits do not persist at later time points.

MEDIAL TRIVECTOR-RETAINING APPROACH

First described by Bramlett,[42] the medial trivector-retaining approach combines the extensile approach of the medial parapatellar and extensor mechanism preservation of the subvastus approach. The underlying principle is that the quadriceps muscle has medial, lateral, and superior vectors that contribute to the extensor mechanism. With an incision through the vastus medialis, the muscle never becomes detached from the quadriceps tendon and therefore a maximal amount of the medial vector is unaltered. In one clinical study, straight leg raise returned 2 days faster in the trivector-retaining approach, but no clinical significance was demonstrated.[43] Though quadriceps function may be improved with this approach in the immediate perioperative period, the long-term effect of dividing the muscle fibers has not been extensively studied or validated.

In this approach, a standard anterior midline incision is utilized with dissection performed to expose the extensor mechanism. Approximately 6 cm proximal to the patella, an incision and separation through the vastus medialis is performed approximately 10 to 15 mm medial to the

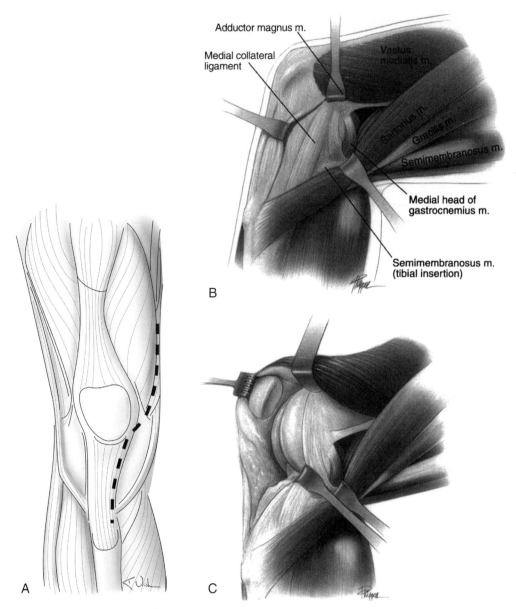

FIGURE 39-6 Subvastus approach. **A:** View of surgical interval during subvastus approach. **B** and **C:** Interval is carried to the inferior aspect of vastus medialis, with retraction of important anatomic structures and subvastus arthrotomy to expose joint space. (A, Image Library, K. Urish, with permission. B and C, From Scuderi G. Chapter 7. Removal of the femoral and tibial components for revision total knee arthroplasty. In: Insall N, Scott WN, eds. *Surgery of the Knee*. Vol 1. 3rd ed. Philadelphia: WB Saunders; 2000:195, Fig. 7.5, with permission.)

vastus medialis insertion to quadriceps tendon. This split is carried distal until approximately 1 cm medial to the patella and then is continued on to the tibial tubercle. Eversion of the patella and all subsequent soft-tissue release are performed as needed to achieve visualization of femur and tibia. Proponents claim a similar level of exposure comparable to the medial parapatellar, while preserving vastus medialis tendon contribution to the extensor mechanism. However, as previously highlighted, the long-term effect in terms of healing and innervation of the intermuscular incision has not been well studied. No long-term clinical superiority has been demonstrated with this approach.[43]

LATERAL PARAPATELLAR APPROACH

First described by Keblish,[44] the lateral parapatellar approach was developed as a counter to the medial-based approach in the treatment of valgus knee deformity. Proponents of the approach believe that a medial-based approach does not provide direct access to the tight lateral structures, exacerbates the need for external tibial rotation, and requires additional lateral release for patellar tracking and soft-tissue balancing in the valgus knee. Therefore, a lateral-based approach would theoretically provide better access to the lateral joint pathology while incorporating necessary lateral releases into the approach

TABLE 39-1 Comparison of Reported Outcomes Between the Subvastus and Medial Parapatellar Approach

Author	Year	N (SV)	N (MPP)	Knee Society Score at 6 wk			Knee Society Score at 1 y			Return of Straight Leg Raise (days)		
				SV Mean (SD)	MPP Mean (SD)	Significance	SV Mean (SD)	MPP Mean (SD)	Significance	SV Mean (SD)	MPP Mean (SD)	Significance
Bourke et al[24]	2012	36	40	127.7 (37.9)	125.9 (29.2)		153.1 (29.7)	162.7 (23)		1.9 (1.6)	2.8 (1.9)	*
Pan et al[35]	2010	35	33	173 (30.1)	158 (30.9)	*	181.6 (23.9)	178.5 (24.2)		1.9 (2.8)	4.2 (2.8)	*
Wegrzyn et al[40]	2013	18	18	162 (14)	152 (28)		NR	NR		NR	NR	
van Hemert et al[38]	2011	20	20	142 (20)	154 (20)		NR	NR		NR	NR	
Hart et al[31]	2006	40	40	158 (22.9)	138 (24.6)	*	NR	NR		NR	NR	
Varela-Egocheaga et al[39]	2010	50	50	131.8 (23.2)	111.6 (28.5)	*	181.6 (10.9)	172.7 (20.3)	*	NR	NR	
Koh et al[34]	2016	50	50	125 (22.9)	123 (24.6)		180 (36.9)	189 (36.9)		NR	NR	
Bridgman et al[30]	2009	108	107	95.6 (27.7)	98.5 (28.9)		129.1 (31)	125.8 (31.1)		NR	NR	
Tomek et al[37]	2014	62	65	122.3 (18.2)	124.4 (18.2)		NR	NR		NR	NR	
Dutka et al[26]	2011	97	83	104.4 (11.2)	92.9 (12.8)	*	137.4 (10.7)	135.4 (9.8)		NR	NR	
Weinhardt et al[41]	2004	26	26	NR	NR		NR	NR		8.3 (2.8)	12 (3.1)	*
Jung et al[33]	2009	21	19	NR	NR		NR	NR		0.5 (0.8)	2.2 (1.4)	*
Roysam and Oakley[36]	2001	46	43	NR	NR		NR	NR		3.2 (1.4)	5.8 (1.7)	*
Boerger et al[29]	2005	60	60	NR	NR		NR	NR		3.2 (1.3)	4.1 (1.5)	*
Jain et al[32]	2013	100	100	NR	NR		NR	NR		1.6 (1.4)	2.1 (1.7)	*

*Statistical significance achieved.

NR indicates outcome not reported in study.

MPP, medial parapatellar; SV, subvastus.

Adapted from Berstock JR, Murray JR, Whitehouse MR, Blom AW, Beswick AD. Medial subvastus versus the medial parapatellar approach for total knee replacement: A systematic review and meta-analysis of randomized controlled trials. *EFORT Open Rev.* 2018;3(3):78-84.

and arthrotomy.[44] It is important to understand that a lateral-based approach decreases medial side visualization, makes patellar eversion more difficult, and requires diligent soft-tissue management to prevent a large lateral defect upon closure.

An anterior midline incision is made over the knee along the vector of the Q-angle, ending approximately 1 to 2 cm lateral to the tibial tubercle (**Fig. 39-7**). Exposure of the extensor mechanism is achieved via dissection through fat and superficial fascia. Arthrotomy is then performed starting proximal along the lateral border of the quadriceps tendon, extending distal to a point that is 1 to 2 cm lateral to the tibial tubercle and through the medial edge of the Gerdy tubercle. The arthrotomy should terminate in the anterior compartment of the lower extremity, approximately 2 cm lateral to the tibial tubercle. The fat pad should be protected, such that it maintains a viable

blood supply and can be utilized for closure of soft-tissue gap. Per description by Keblish, sharp dissection under the patellar tendon will create a "graft" containing rim of lateral meniscus, fat pad, and intermeniscal ligament that can be mobilized and incorporated into the soft-tissue gap at the time of closure. This is performed by suturing the graft into the capsule proximally and the lateral aspect of the quadriceps and patellar tendons. It is important that the surgeon pays continuous attention to this gap during intraoperative dissection and soft-tissue balancing such that it remains manageable at the conclusion of the case. A recent study by Jiang et al describes the reduction of complications and the improvement of clinical outcome with this defect closure technique as described by Keblish and continuous attention to the lateral soft-tissue defect.[45]

The benefit of the lateral approach in the case of valgus deformity is the anatomic structures responsible for the

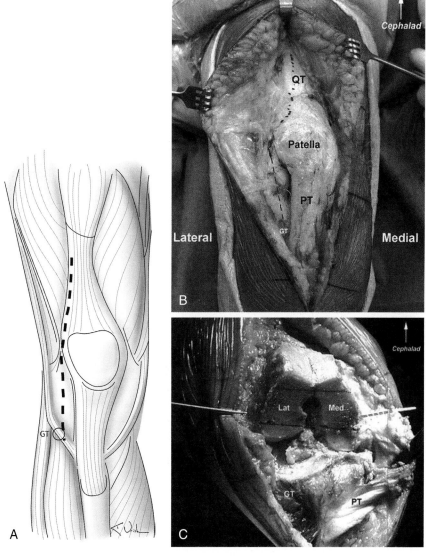

FIGURE 39-7 Lateral Parapatellar Approach. **A** and **B:** View of surgical interval during lateral parapatellar approach. **C:** Final view after mobilization of extensor mechanism to the medial side once distal femur cuts have been made. GT, gerdy's tubercle; PT, patella tendon; QT, quadriceps tendon. (A, Image Library, K. Urish, with permission. B and C, From Photo Library – Department of Orthopaedics (Adult Reconstruction), London Health Sciences Centre, London, Ontario, Canada, with permission.)

deformity are encountered during approach and may be released for correction of deformity. Per initial description, iliotibial (IT) band release should be performed 10 cm proximal to the joint line as part of the exposure if the coronal alignment is not correctable to neutral during arthroplasty. Furthermore, in cases of severe deformity (more than 40°), the release is performed by elevating Gerdy tubercle with a continuous sleeve of fascia. In this scenario, the lateral 50% of tibial tubercle is elevated with an osteotome (including tendon, tubercle, and anterior compartment fascia) to aid in eversion of patella during exposure.[44] Any osteophytes or adhesions that are contributing to deformity should be removed at this point, and an osteoperiosteal release can be performed on the femoral side.

Numerous modifications have since been described to the lateral parapatellar approach to address difficult exposure and deformity. Buechel describes three different releases to be performed based on the level of deformity, including IT band alone, IT band with collateral ligament and popliteus release, or a fibular head resection for severe fixed deformity.[46] If the tibia is translating forward and cannot be subluxed beneath the femur at the 90° position, a posterior cruciate ligament release should be performed. Fidian et al modified the lateral parapatellar approach via an extension of the quadriceps tendon incision 2 to 3 cm in the proximal direction beneath the fat and skin to release the contracted vastus lateralis from the extensor mechanism.[47] Closure of the arthrotomy is then performed at 75° of flexion under gentle tension to proximally advance the lateralis tendon. The authors of this modification claim that this avoids elevation of the tibial tubercle and improved patellofemoral mechanics.[47] Medial quadriceps snip[48] and tibial tubercle osteotomy[49] have also been described in combination with the lateral parapatellar approach to aid in exposure and visualization of the joint.

Studies have shown no significant clinical difference in medial versus lateral parapatellar approaches to the fixed valgus knee deformity. A recent study by Gunst et al prospectively analyzed 424 knees with a preoperative valgus deformity ranging from 3° to 10° (109 medial approach vs. 315 lateral approach).[50] No significant differences were noted in tourniquet time, complications, postoperative limb alignment, or clinical outcome scores. However, a tibial tubercle osteotomy was performed more frequently in the lateral approach (*P* < .05) noting the need for additional surgical dissection/preparation in the lateral approach to achieve adequate exposure.

DIFFICULT EXPOSURES: SPECIALIZED TECHNIQUES

In complex primary and revision scenarios, supplemental techniques may be required to establish adequate exposure. Identifying these patients reinforces the importance of preoperative planning to optimize outcomes and

minimize complications in arthroplasty surgery. Exposure of the knee can be challenging in severe varus and valgus deformities, significant patella baja, or with a significant contractures such as with arthrofibrosis. The challenge in these cases is the ability to safely remove arthroplasty components by mobilization of the extensor mechanism while avoiding tendon avulsion.

Exposure can be obtained using a hierarchical approach (**Fig. 39-8**). In the majority of cases, the medial parapatellar approach can establish the needed exposure by including more extensive releases. When this is inadequate, a quadriceps snip can be supplemented. This approach allows approximately 95% of knee revisions to be completed.[51] In rare cases, the extensor mechanism needs to be detached to establish exposure, typically either distally with a tibial tubercle osteotomy or proximally with a V-Y quadricepsplasty. Other alternative techniques could be substituted for these approaches. This primarily occurs with the stiff or arthrofibrotic knee with less than 90° of flexion.[5,52] The overall goal is optimizing exposure with the simplest technique to minimize complications.

When a quadriceps snip is insufficient to mobilize the extensor mechanism, the decision between a tibial tubercle osteotomy and V-Y quadricepsplasty is a balance between the advantages and disadvantages of each. The location of the patella can serve as a guide. In patella baja,

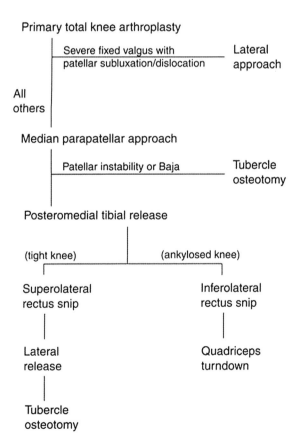

FIGURE 39-8 Algorithm to determine surgical approach to the knee in challenging scenarios. This can be anticipated when there is limited flexion less than 90°, patella baja, or severe varus or valgus deformity.

with the limitations of exposure distal, a tibial tubercle osteotomy will provide optimum exposure. When the patella is in a normal position, the limit to exposure is occurring proximally. In a severely ankylosed knee (less than 60° flexion), a V-Y quadricepsplasty will provide the exposure necessary to remove the proximal adhesions limiting motion, and the extensor mechanism can be lengthened to improve motion. The area of exposure needed can also serve as a guide. A tibial tubercle osteotomy is advantageous with the removal of a long-stemmed tibial component. If inadequate bone stock or distal soft-tissue coverage is an issue, a proximal approach should be used.

MODIFICATIONS TO THE MEDIAL PARAPATELLAR APPROACH IN CHALLENGING EXPOSURES

The standard medial parapatellar approach remains the primary tool in revision and complex arthroplasty cases. The addition of more extensive articular releases helps facilitate exposure and mobilization of the extensor mechanism. This is first executed by performing a radical and complete synovectomy to restore the synovial recesses over the femoral condyles. Debulking of hypertrophied capsular tissue and excision of the adhesions are made in each of the five main surfaces of the knee: the medial and lateral gutters, suprapatellar pouch, dorsal aspect of the extensor mechanism, and the posterior capsule once the polyethylene liner is removed. These adhesions limit the surgical exposure when the knee is brought into deep flexion.

A medial release of the capsule is performed. A sequential subperiosteal dissection of the medial retinaculum, deep MCL, and semimembranous insertion is completed. In a revision scenario, it is often necessary to extend this medial capsule release around the posterior corner of the medial tibial plateau. This increases visualization of the posterior capsule and ultimately allows subluxation of the tibia anterior to the femoral condyles.

The extensor mechanism is then mobilized. A pin can be placed in the medial third of the tibial tubercle to protect the patella tendon from avulsion. The pin should be directed toward the lateral plateau as to not interfere with placement of stemmed tibial components. The fibrous tissue along the dorsal aspect of the extensor mechanism is removed. It is especially important to define and release the space between the anterior tibia and patella tendon to mobilize the proximal patella tendon. These maneuvers increase the flexibility of the extensor mechanism. Limited partial lateral retinacular release may help facilitate displacement of the patella. External rotation of the tibia decreases tension on the extensor mechanism.[13,53] These combined maneuvers of total synovectomy, mobilization of the extensor mechanism, and rotation of the tibia permit flexion and improve exposure.

Finally, the posterior capsule is released and debrided. Posterior capsule débridement allows the tibia to be subluxed in relation to the femur to improve exposure of the posterior aspect of the implants for removal. Care should be taken to respect the posterior neurovascular structures. These maneuvers allow components to be removed in approximately 90% of knee revisions.[51]

QUADRICEPS SNIP OR RECTUS SNIP

When the initial standard approach of extensive intra-articular releases does not provide the needed exposure, the next maneuver is the quadriceps snip. The proximal quadriceps tendon is released diagonally. There are many advantages: It is a simple technique to execute, provides a large increase in exposure, not associated with extensor lag, and does not alter the postoperative rehabilitation protocol.[54] There are almost no disadvantages as there is no clinical difference in morbidity as compared to the standard medial parapatellar approach.[55]

The initial technique was described by Insall.[56] After the medial parapatellar release, a classic quadriceps snip is an extension of this approach. At the proximal portion of the arthrotomy, the apical portion of the quadriceps tendon is incised in a lateral obliques fashion to transect the rectus femoris tendon from the myotendinous junction (**Fig. 39-9**). This facilitates patella mobilization

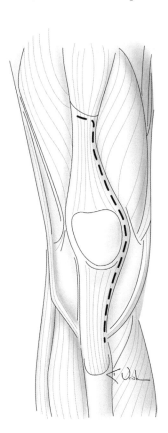

FIGURE 39-9 The quadriceps snip. After a standard medial parapatellar arthrotomy, the incision is extended laterally at the myotendinous junction of the quadriceps. (Image Library, K. Urish, with permission.)

distally and laterally. Insall developed this approach as an initial step to the V-Y patella turndown.[56] An alternative technique includes a standard medial parapatellar arthrotomy with a small perpendicular release of the tendon at the midpoint between the superior pole of the patella and myotendinous junction of the quadriceps. If a quadriceps snip does not develop the necessary exposure and extensor mechanism mobilization, it can be converted into any of the other more specialized exposure approaches.

A variation on the quadriceps snip has been termed the "wandering resident." A standard arthrotomy in a revision scenario follows the medial border of the quadriceps tendon. An alternative approach is to let the arthrotomy drift laterally as it is extended in the proximal direction. This detaches the quadriceps tendon in an oblique fashion from its insertion on the patella (**Fig. 39-10**). The technique is termed the "wandering resident" as it implies a lack of appreciation for the anatomy by an inexperienced junior resident.[57] The one clinical study of this approach included only 18 patients.[58] The rehabilitation course included ambulation with a knee brace locked in extension for 6 weeks while passive range of motion was allowed during this period. There are no apparent advantages of this approach over the

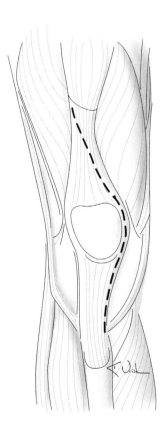

FIGURE 39-10 The "wandering resident." A medial arthrotomy is extended proximally in an oblique direction across the quadriceps tendon. This approach gives a similar result as a quadriceps snip but must be planned for initially and does not respect the anatomic borders. (Image Library, K. Urish, with permission.)

quadriceps snip while the quadriceps snip respects the anatomic structures of the extensor mechanism, and this technique does not.

TIBIAL TUBERCLE OSTEOTOMY

When a quadriceps snip does not provide the needed exposure, a popular next step to mobilize the extensor mechanism is the tibial tubercle osteotomy. Initially described by Dolin,[59] the technique was standardized by Whiteside with the first report of clinical outcomes.[60,61] It is useful in revision scenarios for removal of tibial-stemmed components. Initial reports were variable with concerns for higher rates of complications with nonunions, fractures, and wound issues.[62,63] Recent studies suggest that proper technique can minimize these complications.[62,64-67] An advantage of this technique allows adjustment of the osteotomy fragment medial or proximal to improve patella tracking, patellar height, motion, and quadriceps tension.[66-68] It has increased popularity in the scenario of periprosthetic joint infection where staged procedures will be performed.[69] Contraindications for this procedure include inadequate bone stock, osteoporosis, or comorbidities that would prevent osteotomy healing including tobacco use, diabetes, rheumatoid arthritis, and steroid use.[66]

The tibia tubercle osteotomy is a coronal osteotomy from the medial side. The most important aspects of the technique are to take a fragment of adequate thickness and length, to leave a lateral soft-tissue hinge intact, and to achieve stable fixation. To avoid postoperative fracture, the stemmed tibial component needs to bypass the osteotomy defect. The chevron osteotomy is typically 7 to 10 cm in length, along the medial and lateral edge of the patella tendon, and is beveled toward the anterior cortex distally. There must be sufficient bone of at least 1 to 1.5 cm between anterior tubercle and the deepest part of the osteotomy accounting for the cement mantle and tibia implant. Distally, the depth tapers to 5 mm. The proximal transverse osteotomy is made parallel to the joint line. When possible, a proximal bone bridge should be maintained to assist in preventing proximal migration of the osteotomy. An alternative technique is to include a chevron osteotomy with the apex at the midpoint of the osteotomy[66] (**Fig. 39-11**). Large osteotomes are used to elevate the fragment off the tibia while preserving the lateral soft-tissue envelope and distal periosteal sleeve intact, hinging the fragment laterally to evert the patella. Fixation can be accomplished with screws, wires, or both. If screws are used, two 6.5 mm cancellous screws are usually placed with offset entry points on the tubercle to avoid splitting the fragment and diverging away from the tibial component stem. If wires are used, three Luque wires or wires of comparable gauge are used, with the first through the fragment and the distal two around the fragment. The wires are angled distally from lateral to medial to tension the fragment

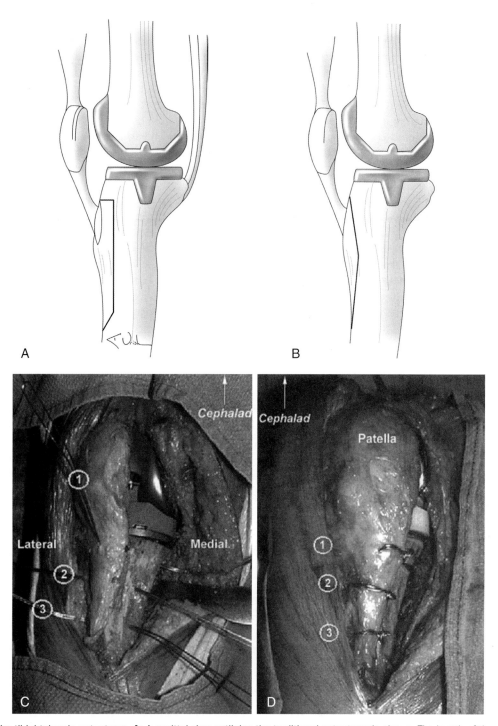

FIGURE 39-11   The tibial tubercle osteotomy. **A:** A sagittal view outlining the traditional osteotomy is shown. The length of the osteotomy should be 6-10 cm in length. A proximal bone bridge can prevent proximal migration of the osteotomy. **B:** An alternative shape of the chevron osteotomy is to place the apex at the midpoint of the tubercle. This facilitates exposure of the stem. **C:** The osteotomy is closed by passing three wires (or use of a cortical screw) and is then stabilized by compression of the cortical bone. The first wire is passed through the osteotomized fragment to prevent proximal migration. The more distal two wires (wire 2 and 3) are placed through lateral drill holes that are placed more proximally than the medial drill holes. This draws the osteotomy distally with compression. **D:** Stability of fixation is assessed by observing the wires while putting the knee through an arc of flexion–extension. (A and B, from Image Library of K. Urish. C and D, from Photo Library – Department of Orthopaedics, London Health Sciences Centre, London, Ontario, Canada, with permission.)

distally. A known complication with this technique is irritation of the fixation device, and so hardware should be placed as posterior and medial as possible to avoid prominence.[13,53,66,67]

For postoperative rehabilitation, weight-bearing is at the discretion of the surgeon, but initial weight-bearing is not contraindicated for the osteotomy itself. Range of motion is initially restricted to the maximum safe flexion observed during the intraoperative stress test of the osteotomy which is typically around 90°. At 1 month, range of motion can be gradually increased with discontinuation of the brace at 6 weeks. The author preference is to limit range of motion during the first 2 weeks of any major revision surgery to avoid tension across the incision and soft tissues and then start range of motion at 2 weeks from the flexion angle observed during the stress test. This can then progress every 2 weeks by 10° with discontinuation of brace at 6 weeks.

Biomechanical testing has demonstrated that screw fixation has superior strength over tension wires,[70,71] but clinically both fixation techniques have good outcomes. Recent reports have noted that fixation with bioabsorbable sutures (Vicryl 1.0) with the suture needle directly penetrating the cortex has comparable rates of union and osteotomy migration as compared to direct fixation techniques. This suggests that the surgeon has some latitude in fixation technique.[72]

A series of clinical studies have demonstrated reasonable outcomes with the tibia tubercle osteotomy and an ability to minimize complications (**Table 39-2**). The initial series of the current standardized technique from Whiteside reported a 100% union rate and a flexion range of more than 90°. Complications included extensor lag, patella tendon avulsions, and postoperative tibia fractures.[60] Multiple studies have supported the initial rate of union of the osteotomy. A series of retrospective studies have reported a near complete osseous union rate, postoperative knee range of motion greater than 90°, and improved functional patient-reported outcome scores. A variety of complications have been reported in these studies including extensor lag, osteotomy migration, delayed union, painful hardware, tibia fracture, and extensor mechanism disruption. More recent reports of complication rates range from 1% to 5%.[64,67-69,73-80] Earlier studies reported complications at 37%. The most common pitfall included extensor lag. Tibial osteotomy migration was also observed in up to 20% of patients but did not have an observed clinical effect on function or range of motion.[81] To avoid these pitfalls and the most serious complication of nonunion, the osteotomy fragment should be a minimum of 6 to 7 cm. Shorter osteotomies have been shown to have a higher rate of loss of fixation and extensor lag.[74,77]

V-Y QUADRICEPSPLASTY OR QUADRICEPS TURNDOWN

An alternative technique for mobilizing the extensor mechanism includes proximal detachment with the V-Y quadricepsplasty. This technique was initially popularized by Coonse and Adams as a v-type exposure for intra-articular fracture repair.[82] The approach was modified by Insall to allow an extensile exposure with a more limited tendinous incision.[56] Other modifications were made by Siliski et al to facilitate an easier conversion from a standard medial parapatellar approach and avoid the superior lateral geniculate artery.[83]

A quadricepsplasty is used as an alternative to a tibial tubercle osteotomy based on the advantages and disadvantages of each approach and the specific details of each unique revision scenario. It is most useful as compared to a tibial tubercle osteotomy in extremely stiff knees with less than 60° flexion where a lengthening of the extensor mechanism will be necessary or when a tibial tubercle osteotomy cannot be performed secondary to poor tibia bone stock or soft-tissue concerns distally. During repair and closure, the tendon can be lengthened in stiff knees to increase flexion. Disadvantages include risk of devascularization of the patella, extensor lag, and compared to the tibial tubercle osteotomy the biomechanical repair is weaker.[53] Also, it is difficult to use more than once in a scenario where repeat procedures may be required.[84]

A V-Y quadricesplasty is a proximal exposure to the knee. The exposure can be performed as a sequence with each step providing greater exposure (**Fig. 39-12**). A standard medial parapatellar arthrotomy is completed with revision modifications as discussed above. A V-Y turndown is completed by establishing appropriate lateral exposure of the extensor mechanism so that the quadriceps tendon and vastus lateralis can be easily distinguished. From the proximal extent of the quadriceps tendon, an oblique 45° cut is made to the lateral edge of the tendon at its border with the vastus lateralis. This is in contrast to a rectus snip that typically extends in a proximal direction. If sufficient exposure is obtained with this step, the vastus lateralis remains intact, the blood supply to the superior geniculate is not in danger, and a direct closure of the tendon can be completed. In the rare circumstance where exposure remains inadequate, the exposure can be continued distally across the vastus lateralis tendon and upper portion of the iliotibial tract. Completion of the V-Y turndown facilities access to the lateral gutter, allowing for release of dense adhesions and mobilization of the extensor mechanism.[13] A modification by Siliski et al. to preserve the superior geniculate artery includes extending the incision across the vastus lateralis insertion.[85] A formal lateral release can be included when necessary but increases the risk of injury to the superior lateral geniculate.[83]

Closure should be completed with an appropriate degree of tension. The goal is to complete the closure that permits 90° of flexion without an extensor lag. An intraoperative stress test of the repair is completed by allowing the knee to flex by gravity and observing the angle at which the repair comes under tension. Postoperative rehabilitation should limit flexion to the intraoperative stress point until the extensor lag is less than 15° or for 6 weeks to allow initial tendon healing. The tendon can be lengthened up to 2 cm by conversion of the "V" shaped incision to a "Y" shape, and lateral retinaculum can be left open as a lateral release.[84] Active extension should be avoided in this time frame.

TABLE 39-2 Comparison of Reported Outcomes and Complications Between Tibial Tubercle Osteotomy Clinical Studies

Author	Year	Type	Number in Study	Fixation Type	ROM Pre-op	ROM Post-op	Follow-Up (yrs)	KSS Preop	KSS PostOp	Total PostOp (N)	Fracture (N)	Nonunion (N)	Migration Proximal (N)	Extensor Lag (N)
Young et al[79]	2006	IV Retrospective	41	Wire	66	87	8.4	73	124	NR	NR	1	9	6
van den Broek et al[96]	2008	IV Retrospective	37	Screws	81	93	28.4	72	125	NR	NR	0	2	0
Tabutin et al[75]	2011	IV Retrospective	20	Screws	73	88	4.5	58	84	NR	NR	0	0	NR
Ries and Richman[64]	1996	IV Retrospective	29	Screws	83	101	1.5	NR	NR	NR	1	NR	1	0
Choi et al[69,80]	2012	IV Retrospective	13	Wire	60	94	4.6	39	78	NR	1	0	3	0
Chalidis and Reis[77]	2009	IV Retrospective	74	Screw/wire	60	95	4	NR	NR	NR	3	0	2	0
Mendes et al[68]	2004	IV Retrospective	67	Wire	101	107	2.5	56	86	NR	0	2	13	3
Hirschmann et al[97]	2012	II Prospective	76	Screws	112	118	2.1	50	93	NR	0	0	0	0
Choi et al[69,80]	2012	IV Retrospective	36	Wire	40	92	4.75	47	82	NR	2	1	5	0
Whiteside et al[61]	1995	IV Retrospective	136	Wire	NR	93.7	2	NR	NR	NR	2	0	0	2
Bruni et al[87]	2013	I Prospective	39	Wire	60	94	8	11	88	NR	0	0	NR	5
Sun et al[88]	2015	IV Retrospective	28	Screw		94.1	4	93.4	126	3	2	0	0	0
Barrack et al[73]	1998	IV Retrospective	15	Wire	73	81	1.5	77	117	NR	NR	NR	0	NR
Vandeputte et al[98]	2017	IV Retrospective	13	Screw/wire	NR	NR	2	30	75	NR	0	0	0	NR
Punwar et al[99]	2017	IV Retrospective	42	Screw	85	95	0.3-2	NR	NR	3		1	0	0
Segur et al[100]	2015	IV Retrospective	26	Wire	90	95	3.4	26	78	3	0	0	2	1
Biggi et al[67]	2018	IV Retrospective	79	Screw	78.7	90.5	7.4	40.7	75	11	0	0	0	1
Zonnenberg et al[72]	2014	IV Retrospective	23	Suture	87.9	95.3	1.25	NR	99.5	3	1	2	0	0

Postoperative extensor lag is reported as 0 if less than 5°.

Infection was excluded from being listed as major complication given the high rate of infection recurrence in PJI cohorts where TTO was used for revision exposure.

NR indicates outcome not reported in study.

Adapted from Bruni D, Iacono F, Sharma B, Zaffagnini S, Marcacci M. Tibial tubercle osteotomy or quadriceps snip in two-stage revision for prosthetic knee infection? A randomized prospective study. Clin Orthop Relat Res. 2013;471(4):1305-1318.

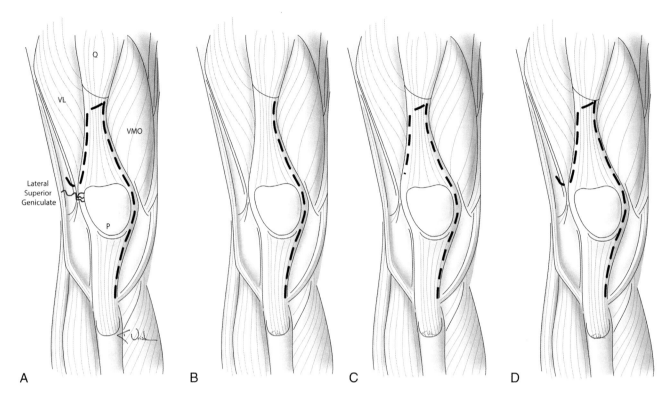

A   B   C   D

FIGURE 39-12 The V-Y quadricepsplasty. **A:** The overall outline of the arthrotomy modified by Siliski[83] and labeled anatomic structures are shown (VMO: vastus medialis oblique; Q: quadriceps; VL: vastus lateralis; P: patella). **B:** Standard medial parapatellar incision is performed. **C:** The arthrotomy is extended down the lateral border of the quadriceps tendon. **D:** If additional exposure is needed, lateral incision should stay curved around the vastus lateralis to avoid the lateral superior geniculate artery. Only as much of the lateral incision should be made to achieve the incision as necessary. A lateral release can be used distally in rare scenarios. (Image Library, K. Urish, with permission.)

COMPARISON OF REVISION APPROACHES

There have been minimal clinical studies comparing outcomes between different exposures in total knee arthroplasty revision. Results support little difference between a medial parapatellar approach and a rectus snip. Given the decreased technical challenge and lower complication rate, the medial parapatellar approach and the addition of a rectus snip, if needed, are used in the vast majority of revision scenarios. The tibial tubercle osteotomy and V-Y quadricepsplasty have recognized disadvantages, making them procedures to use only when necessary. There are a few alternative approaches that are discussed in the next section as there are limited clinical reports of their use and no direct comparisons to other approaches.

One of the first clinical studies to compare difficult exposure techniques was completed by Barrack and involved a retrospective series of 94 patients. The medial parapatellar incision and quadriceps snip had equivalent outcomes for all parameters. Tibial tubercle osteotomy and quadricepsplasty had equivalent outcomes that were significantly lower than the standard approach and rectus snip. Compared to the tibial tubercle osteotomy, the quadricepsplasty group had greater extensor lag but improved function with squatting and greater motion.[73] Other groups have observed that the extensor

lag commonly observed after a quadricepsplasty usually resolved by 6 months[83] and that active extension returns to near normal.[86]

Bruni et al completed a prospective randomized study on 81 patients between quadriceps snip and tibial tubercle osteotomy in two-stage periprosthetic knee infections. The tibial tubercle osteotomy group had improved patient-reported outcome score and comparable complication rate.[87] This is the only study that demonstrated the tibial tubercle osteotomy had a superior outcome. These results are supported by a recent retrospective review comparing quadriceps snip to tibial tubercle osteotomy. In the retrospective analysis of 48 patients, there were no differences in functional outcomes, range or motion, or complication rates.[88] A limitation is the lack of analysis to appreciate the power necessary to observe a clinical difference.

ALTERNATIVE TECHNIQUES

There are a series of alternative techniques to obtain exposure that have been reported. These techniques can be utilized using a similar concept of considering these approaches as either a distal or proximal release of the extensor mechanism similar to a tibial tubercle osteotomy or V-Y quadricepsplasty. There is a minimal amount of clinical studies available to evaluate their clinical utility and success as compared to the other more popular distal and proximal releases of the extensor mechanism.

A medial epicondylar osteotomy can be used for exposure in contractures associated with flexion or varus deformity. Popularized by Engh, it has been recommended in varus deformity and difficult exposures where good visualization of the posterior capsule is required such as capsular fibrosis, conversion of a knee arthrodesis, distal femur allograft reconstruction, and revision of a posterior dislocation of a cruciate-retaining arthroplasty.[13,57,89]

The procedure is performed through a standard revision medial arthrotomy. The epicondylar osteotomy is performed with the knee at 90° or at the maximum of flexion. The adductor tubercle and insertion of the adductor magnus tendon are identified by palpating the proximal medial femoral condyle. The osteotomy is demarcated by incising the synovium with electrocautery. A 1.5 inch osteotome is placed parallel to the long axis of the femur, lateral to the origin of the MCL. A fragment of bone is detached approximately 1 cm thick and 4 cm in diameter. The osteotome should exit above the adductor magnus tendon to ensure a full release of the medial structures. The osteotomy is hinged open in a posterior direction, and the tibia is externally rotated to provide direct visualization of the posterior capsule (**Fig. 39-13**). A release of the posterior capsule can be performed under direct visualization allowing the posterior recess of the knee to be restored if absent. The tibia will then fall behind the femur improving exposure. The epicondyle fragment

is repaired in 90° of flexion with heavy nonabsorbable suture. A cortical bridge should be left on the anterior portion of the femur to anchor the screws.[57,78]

An alternative method to the medial epicondyle osteotomy is the femoral peel. After a standard revision medial parapatellar exposure, there is a partial or complete subperiosteal dissection and release of the MCL where the distal femur is essentially skeletonized.[90,91] In knees with a normal soft-tissue envelope, stripping the capsular attachments and ligaments would result in instability. In knees with limited flexion secondary to a hypertrophied capsular envelope, stability is restored after reapproximation of the arthrotomy secondary to the inelastic mechanical properties of the capsular tissue.

The decision between an osteotomy and a femoral peel is dictated by the character of the capsular tissue. The medial epicondyle osteotomy can be completed with or without a dense hypertrophied capsule as it does not rely on a scarred, noncompliant soft-tissue envelope to provide stability. The femoral peel depends on hypertrophied tissue and should not be performed when normal compliant capsular tissue is present.

Reservation should be used with these approaches given the limited clinical studies. With the medical epicondyle osteotomy, one clinical study with 60 patients was completed to correct varus deformity in only primary knee arthroplasty. The authors noted improved Knee Society Scores and function but did not have a comparison control group. Bone union occurred in 54% of patients and fibrous union occurred in the remainder of

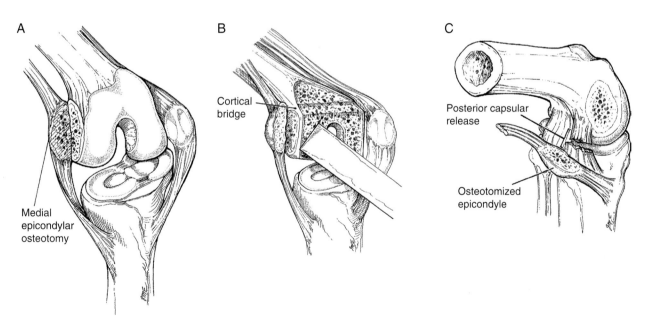

FIGURE 39-13 Medial epicondyle osteotomy. **A:** The osteotomized epicondyle with intact adductor magnus tendon and collateral ligaments is displaced to the medial femoral condyle. Exposure is enhanced by external rotation and varus angulation of the knee in a flexed position. **B:** A cortical bridge is established between the anterior femoral bone resection and the osteotomized medial femoral condyle. Sutures are passed beneath the bridge of cortical bone to anchor the repair of the epicondyle. **C:** The posteromedial capsule, including fibers of the posterior oblique ligament, is released with cautery to fully correct the varus deformity and flexion contracture of the knee. (From Engh GA. Medial epicondyle osteotomy: a technique used with primary and revision total knee arthroplasty to improve surgical exposure and correct varus deformity. *Inst Course Lect.* 1999;48:153-156, Figs 1 to 3 with permission.)

the group.[92] A separate study supported these results and demonstrated improved function, observed no instability in flexion or extension, and no difference in outcomes between bone and fibrous union.[93] In a cadaveric study, other groups have suggested that the osteotomy can leave the knee with less stability in flexion than a standard release of the MCL.[94] In the femoral peel technique, there has been one retrospective clinical study of 87 patients. The authors reported improved range or motion and an overall complication rate of 17%.[95]

A variation on the distal release of the extensor mechanism includes the "banana peel." Instead of a tibial tubercle osteotomy, the insertion of the patella tendon is removed as a periosteal sleeve from the tibia. A standard medial arthrotomy with a quadriceps snip is performed. The patella is then everted, and gentle force is used to peel the patella tendon off the tibial tubercle as a continuous sleeve. According to its initial description, electrocautery, sharp dissection, or a cobb is *not* used to create the sleeve. The peel must maintain continuity with the soft tissues laterally and distally. At closure, the arthrotomy is repaired with sutures alone. There is no special attention directed at reattaching the periosteal sleeve such as with suture anchors.[89] Similar to the femoral peel, the success of this approach may be based on the thickened, inelastic, and noncompliant fibrotic capsular tissue. This approach is not to be recommended when a normal soft-tissue envelope around the knee is present. Given the limited clinical evidence, discretion should be used with this technique. The one clinical study notes acceptable postoperative range of motion but has limited evidence to support postoperative quadriceps function or residual extensor lag.[89] In practice, use of this approach is probably underreported secondary to its unplanned utilization during revision cases while trying to increase exposure and inadvertently partially or completely peeling the extensor mechanism off the tibia tubercle.

CONCLUSION

The surgical exposure to perform total knee arthroplasty is a basic fundamental skill in orthopedic surgery. Attention to detail is essential from the initial skin incision to final closure to maximize exposure for correct placement of implants and avoid unnecessary morbidity. In primary total knee arthroplasty, the common methods have comparable outcomes. It is the authors' preference to use a medial parapatellar approach. In a revision, scenario, a more extensive parapatellar approach typically provides the necessary exposure. When this is inadequate, a rectus snip commonly allows appropriate visualization. Only in rare cases, are more specialized techniques needed. An important surgical axiom reinforces the importance of proper preoperative planning and surgical exposure—exposure begets confidence and confidence begets exposure (Raskin, Kevin. 2013).

REFERENCES

1. Johnson DP. Midline or parapatellar incision for knee arthroplasty. A comparative study of wound viability. *J Bone Joint Surg Br.* 1988;70(4):656-658.
2. Johnson DP, Houghton TA, Radford P. Anterior midline or medial parapatellar incision for arthroplasty of the knee. A comparative study. *J Bone Joint Surg Br.* 1986;68(5):812-814.
3. Langer K. On the anatomy and physiology of the skin: conclusions by Professor K. Langer. *Br J Plast Surg.* 1978;31(4):277-278.
4. Haertsch PA. The blood supply to the skin of the leg: a post-mortem investigation. *Br J Plast Surg.* 1981;34(4):470-477.
5. Younger AS, Duncan CP, Masri BA. Surgical exposures in revision total knee arthroplasty. *J Am Acad Orthop Surg.* 1998;6(1):55-64.
6. Insall J. A midline approach to the knee. *J Bone Joint Surg Am.* 1971;53(8):1584-1586.
7. Masri BA, Laskin RS, Windsor RE, Haas SB. Knee closure in total knee replacement: a randomized prospective trial. *Clin Orthop Relat Res.* 1996;331:81-86.
8. Krebs VE, Elmallah RK, Khlopas A. Wound closure techniques for total knee arthroplasty: an evidence-based review of the literature. *J Arthroplasty.* 2018;33(2):633-638.
9. Grottkau BE, Rebello G, Merlin G, Winograd JM. Coaptive film versus subcuticular suture: comparing skin closure time after posterior spinal instrumented fusion in pediatric patients with spinal deformity. *Spine.* 2010;35(23):2027-2029.
10. Bonutti PM, Miller BG, Cremens MJ. Intraosseous patellar blood supply after medial parapatellar arthrotomy. *Clin Orthop Relat Res.* 1998;352:202-214.
11. Kayler DE, Lyttle D. Surgical interruption of patellar blood supply by total knee arthroplasty. *Clin Orthop Relat Res.* 1988;229:221-227.
12. Engh GA, Parks NL. Surgical technique of the midvastus arthrotomy. *Clin Orthop Relat Res.* 1998;351:270-274.
13. Parker DA, Tsigaras H, Rorabeck CH. Surgical exposure for primary total knee arthroplasty. In: Callaghan JJ, et al. *The Adult Knee.* Vol. 2. 1st ed. New York: Wolters Kluwer; 2005.
14. Cooper RE Jr, Trinidad G, Buck WR. Midvastus approach in total knee arthroplasty: a description and a cadaveric study determining the distance of the popliteal artery from the patellar margin of the incision. *J Arthroplasty.* 1999;14(4):505-508.
15. White RE Jr, Allman JK, Trauger JA, Dales BH. Clinical comparison of the midvastus and medial parapatellar surgical approaches. *Clin Orthop Relat Res.* 1999;367:117-122.
16. Dalury DF, Jiranek WA. A comparison of the midvastus and paramedian approaches for total knee arthroplasty. *J Arthroplasty.* 1999;14(1):33-37.
17. Keating EM, Faris PM, Meding JB, Ritter MA. Comparison of the midvastus muscle-splitting approach with the median parapatellar approach in total knee arthroplasty. *J Arthroplasty.* 1999;14(1):29-32.
18. Parentis MA, Rumi MN, Deol GS, Kothari M, Parrish WM, Pellegrini VD Jr. A comparison of the vastus splitting and median parapatellar approaches in total knee arthroplasty. *Clin Orthop Relat Res.* 1999;367:107-116.
19. Liu HW, Gu WD, Xu NW, Sun JY. Surgical approaches in total knee arthroplasty: a meta-analysis comparing the midvastus and subvastus to the medial peripatellar approach. *J Arthroplasty.* 2014;29(12):2298-2304.
20. Hofmann AA, Plaster RL, Murdock LE. Subvastus (Southern) approach for primary total knee arthroplasty. *Clin Orthop Relat Res.* 1991;269:70-77.
21. Fauré BT, Benjamin JB, Lindsey B, Volz RG, Schutte D. Comparison of the subvastus and paramedian surgical approaches in bilateral knee arthroplasty. *J Arthroplasty.* 1993;8(5):511-516.
22. Matsueda M, Gustilo RB. Subvastus and medial parapatellar approaches in total knee arthroplasty. *Clin Orthop Relat Res.* 2000;371:161-168.

23. Bourke MG, Buttrum PJ, Fitzpatrick PL, Dalton PA, Jull GA, Russell TG. Systematic review of medial parapatellar and subvastus approaches in total knee arthroplasty. *J Arthroplasty.* 2010;25(5):728-734.

24. Bourke MG, Jull GA, Buttrum PJ, Fitzpatrick PL, Dalton PA, Russell TG, Comparing outcomes of medial parapatellar and subvastus approaches in total knee arthroplasty: a randomized controlled trial. *J Arthroplasty.* 2012;27(3):347-353.e1.

25. Curtin B, Yakkanti M, Malkani A. Postoperative pain and contracture following total knee arthroplasty comparing parapatellar and subvastus approaches. *J Arthroplasty.* 2014;29(1):33-36.

26. Dutka J, Skowronek M, Sosin P, Skowronek P. Subvastus and medial parapatellar approaches in TKA: comparison of functional results. *Orthopedics.* 2011;34(6):148.

27. Teng Y, Du W, Jiang J, et al. Subvastus versus medial parapatellar approach in total knee arthroplasty: meta-analysis. *Orthopedics.* 2012;35(12):e1722-e1731.

28. Berstock JR, Murray JR, Whitehouse MR, Blom AW, Beswick AD. Medial subvastus versus the medial parapatellar approach for total knee replacement: a systematic review and meta-analysis of randomized controlled trials. *EFORT Open Rev.* 2018;3(3):78-84.

29. Boerger TO, Aglietti P, Mondanelli N, Sensi L. Mini-subvastus versus medial parapatellar approach in total knee arthroplasty. *Clin Orthop Relat Res.* 2005;440:82-87.

30. Bridgman SA, Walley G, MacKenzie G, Clement D, Griffiths D, Maffulli N. Sub-vastus approach is more effective than a medial parapatellar approach in primary total knee arthroplasty: a randomized controlled trial. *Knee.* 2009;16(3):216-222.

31. Hart R, Janecek M, Cizmár I, Stipcák V, Kucera B, Filan P. Minimally invasive and navigated implantation for total knee arthroplasty: X-ray analysis and early clinical results. *Orthopäde.* 2006;35(5):552-557.

32. Jain S, Wasnik S, Mittal A, Hegde C. Outcome of subvastus approach in elderly nonobese patients undergoing bilateral simultaneous total knee arthroplasty: a randomized controlled study. *Indian J Orthop.* 2013;47(1):45-49.

33. Jung YB, Lee YS, Lee EY, Jung HJ, Nam CH. Comparison of the modified subvastus and medial parapatellar approaches in total knee arthroplasty. *Int Orthop.* 2009;33(2):419-423.

34. Koh IJ, Kim MW, Kim MS, Jang SW, Park DC, In Y. The patient's perception does not differ following subvastus and medial parapatellar approaches in total knee arthroplasty: a simultaneous bilateral randomized study. *J Arthroplasty.* 2016;31(1):112-117.

35. Pan WM, Li XG, Tang TS, Qian ZL, Zhang Q, Zhang CM. Mini-subvastus versus a standard approach in total knee arthroplasty: a prospective, randomized, controlled study. *J Int Med Res.* 2010;38(3):890-900.

36. Roysam GS, Oakley MJ. Subvastus approach for total knee arthroplasty: a prospective, randomized, and observer-blinded trial. *J Arthroplasty.* 2001;16(4):454-457.

37. Tomek IM, Kantor SR, Cori LA, et al. Early patient outcomes after primary total knee arthroplasty with quadriceps-sparing subvastus and medial parapatellar techniques: a randomized, double-blind clinical trial. *J Bone Joint Surg Am.* 2014;96(11):907-915.

38. van Hemert WL, Senden R, Grimm B, van der Linde MJ, Lataster A, Heyligers IC. Early functional outcome after subvastus or parapatellar approach in knee arthroplasty is comparable. *Knee Surg Sports Traumatol Arthrosc.* 2011;19(6):943-951.

39. Varela-Egocheaga JR, Suárez-Suárez MA, Fernández-Villán M, González-Sastre V, Varela-Gómez JR, Rodríguez-Merchán C. Minimally invasive subvastus approach: improving the results of total knee arthroplasty. A prospective, randomized trial. *Clin Orthop Relat Res.* 2010;468(5):1200-1208.

40. Wegrzyn J, Parratte S, Coleman-Wood K, Kaufman KR, Pagnano MW. The John Insall award: no benefit of minimally invasive TKA on gait and strength outcomes: a randomized controlled trial. *Clin Orthop Relat Res.* 2013;471(1):46-55.

41. Weinhardt C, Barisic M, Bergmann EG, Heller KD. Early results of subvastus versus medial parapatellar approach in primary total knee arthroplasty. *Arch Orthop Trauma Surg.* 2004;124(6):401-403.

42. Stern SH. Surgical exposures in total knee arthroplasty. In: Fu FH, Harner CD, Vince KG, eds. *Knee Surgery.* Vol 2. Baltimore: Williams & Wilkins; 1994:1289-1302.

43. Fisher DA, Trimble SM, Breedlove K. The medial trivector approach in total knee arthroplasty. *Orthopedics.* 1998;21(1):53-56.

44. Keblish PA. The lateral approach to the valgus knee. Surgical technique and analysis of 53 cases with over two-year follow-up evaluation. *Clin Orthop Relat Res.* 1991;271:52-62.

45. Jiang J, Fernandes JC. A lateral approach defect closure technique with deep fascia flap for valgus knee TKA. *J Orthop Surg Res.* 2015;10:173.

46. Buechel FF. A sequential three-step lateral release for correcting fixed valgus knee deformities during total knee arthroplasty. *Clin Orthop Relat Res.* 1990;260:170-175.

47. Fiddian NJ, Blakeway C, Kumar A. Replacement arthroplasty of the valgus knee. A modified lateral capsular approach with repositioning of vastus lateralis. *J Bone Joint Surg Br.* 1998;80(5):859-861.

48. Hendel D, Weisbort M. Modified lateral approach for knee arthroplasty in a fixed valgus knee–the medial quadriceps snip. *Acta Orthop Scand.* 2000;71(2):204-205.

49. Burki H, von Knoch M, Heiss C, Drobny T, Munzinger U. Lateral approach with osteotomy of the tibial tubercle in primary total knee arthroplasty. *Clin Orthop Relat Res.* 1999;362:156-161.

50. Gunst S, Villa V, Magnussen R, Servien E, Lustig S, Neyrest P. Equivalent results of medial and lateral parapatellar approach for total knee arthroplasty in mild valgus deformities. *Int Orthop.* 2016;40(5):945-951.

51. Della Valle CJ, Berger RA, Rosenberg AG. Surgical exposures in revision total knee arthroplasty. *Clin Orthop Relat Res.* 2006;446:59-68.

52. Masri BA, Campbell DG, Garbuz DS, Duncan CP. Seven specialized exposures for revision hip and knee replacement. *Orthop Clin North Am.* 1998;29(2):229-240.

53. Abdel MP, Della Valle CJ. The surgical approach for revision total knee arthroplasty. *Bone Joint J.* 2016;98-B(1 suppl A):113-115.

54. Barrack RL. Specialized surgical exposure for revision total knee: quadriceps snip and patellar turndown. *Instr Course Lect.* 1999;48:149-152.

55. Meek RM, Greidanus NV, McGraw RW, Masri BA. The extensile rectus snip exposure in revision of total knee arthroplasty. *J Bone Joint Surg Br.* 2003;85(8):1120-1122.

56. Garvin KL, Scuderi G, Insall JN. Evolution of the quadriceps snip. *Clin Orthop Relat Res.* 1995;321:131-137.

57. Engh GA. Exposure options for revision total knee arthroplasty. In: Bono JV, Scott RD, eds. *Revision Total Knee Arthroplasty.* Boston, MA: Springer; 2005.

58. Hendel D, Weisbort M, Garti A. "Wandering resident" surgical exposure for 1- or 2-stage revision arthroplasty in stiff aseptic and septic knee arthroplasty. *J Arthroplasty.* 2004;19(6):757-759.

59. Dolin MG. Osteotomy of the tibial tubercle in total knee replacement. A technical note. *J Bone Joint Surg Am.* 1983;65(5):704-706.

60. Whiteside LA, Ohl MD. Tibial tubercle osteotomy for exposure of the difficult total knee arthroplasty. *Clin Orthop Relat Res.* 1990;260:6-9.

61. Whiteside LA. Exposure in difficult total knee arthroplasty using tibial tubercle osteotomy. *Clin Orthop Relat Res.* 1995;321:32-35.

62. Masini MA, Stulberg SD. A new surgical technique for tibial tubercle transfer in total knee arthroplasty. *J Arthroplasty.* 1992;7(1):81-86.

63. Ritter MA, Carr K, Keating EM, Faris PM, Meding JB. Tibial shaft fracture following tibial tubercle osteotomy. *J Arthroplasty.* 1996;11(1):117-119.

64. Ries MD, Richman JA. Extended tibial tubercle osteotomy in total knee arthroplasty. *J Arthroplasty.* 1996;11(8):964-967.

65. Whiteside LA. Distal realignment of the patellar tendon to correct abnormal patellar tracking. *Clin Orthop Relat Res.* 1997;344:284-289.

66. DeHaan A, Shukla S, Anderson M, Ries M. Tibial tubercle osteotomy to aid exposure for revision total knee arthroplasty. *JBJS Essent Surg Tech.* 2016;6(3):e32.

67. Biggi S, Divano S, Tedino R, Capuzzo A, Tornago S, Camera A. Tibial tubercle osteotomy in total knee arthroplasty: midterm results experience of a monocentric study. *Joints.* 2018;6(2):95-99.

68. Mendes MW, Caldwell P, Jiranek WA. The results of tibial tubercle osteotomy for revision total knee arthroplasty. *J Arthroplasty.* 2004;19(2):167-174.

69. Choi HR, Kwon YM, Burke DW, Rubash HE, Malchau H. The outcome of sequential repeated tibial tubercle osteotomy performed in 2-stage revision arthroplasty for infected total knee arthroplasty. *J Arthroplasty.* 2012;27(8):1487-1491.

70. Davis K, Caldwell P, Wayne J, Jiranek WA. Mechanical comparison of fixation techniques for the tibial tubercle osteotomy. *Clin Orthop Relat Res.* 2000;380:241-249.

71. Caldwell PE, Bohlen BA, Owen JR, et al. Dynamic confirmation of fixation techniques of the tibial tubercle osteotomy. *Clin Orthop Relat Res.* 2004;424:173-179.

72. Zonnenberg CB, van den Bekerom MP, de Jong T, Nolte PA. Tibial tubercle osteotomy with absorbable suture fixation in revision total knee arthroplasty: a report of 23 cases. *Arch Orthop Trauma Surg.* 2014;134(5):667-672.

73. Barrack RL, Smith P, Munn B, Engh G, Rorabeck C. The Ranawat Award. Comparison of surgical approaches in total knee arthroplasty. *Clin Orthop Relat Res.* 1998;356:16-21.

74. Wolff AM, Hungerford DS, Krackow KA, Jacobs MA. Osteotomy of the tibial tubercle during total knee replacement. A report of twenty-six cases. *J Bone Joint Surg Am.* 1989;71(6):848-852.

75. Tabutin J, Morin-Salvo N, Torga-Spak R, Cambas P-M, Vogt F. Tibial tubercule osteotomy during medial approach to difficult knee arthroplasties. *Orthop Traumatol Surg Res.* 2011;97(3):276-286.

76. Piedade SR, Pinaroli A, Servien E, Neyret P. Tibial tubercle osteotomy in primary total knee arthroplasty: a safe procedure or not? *Knee.* 2008;15(6):439-446.

77. Chalidis BE, Ries MD. Does repeat tibial tubercle osteotomy or intramedullary extension affect the union rate in revision total knee arthroplasty? A retrospective study of 74 patients. *Acta Orthop.* 2009;80(4):426-431.

78. Chinzei N, Ishida K, Kuroda R, et al. Tibial tubercle osteotomy with screw fixation for total knee arthroplasty. *Orthopedics.* 2014;37(4):e367-e73.

79. Young CF, Bourne RB, Rorabeck CH. Tibial tubercle osteotomy in total knee arthroplasty surgery. *J Arthroplasty.* 2008;23(3):371-375.

80. Choi HR, Burke D, Malchau H, Kwon YM. Utility of tibial tubercle osteotomy in the setting of periprosthetic infection after total knee arthroplasty. *Int Orthop.* 2012;36(8):1609-1613.

81. Philips HC, Grant L, Berkowitz J. The prevention of chronic pain and disability: a preliminary investigation. *Behav Res Ther.* 1991;29(5):443-450.

82. Coonse K, Adams J. A new operative approach to the knee joint. *Surg Gynecol Obstet.* 1943;77:344-347.

83. Scott RD, Siliski JM. The use of a modified V-Y quadricepsplasty during total knee replacement to gain exposure and improve flexion in the ankylosed knee. *Orthopedics.* 1985;8(1):45-48.

84. Siliski JM, Austin KS. Extensile exposures of the knee. In: Siliski JM ed. *Traumatic Disorders of the Knee.* New York: Springer-Verlag; 1994.

85. Ritter MA, Campbell ED. Postoperative patellar complications with or without lateral release during total knee arthroplasty. *Clin Orthop Relat Res.* 1987;219:163-168.

86. Trousdale RT, Hanssen AD, Rand JA, Cahalan TD. V-Y quadricepsplasty in total knee arthroplasty. *Clin Orthop Relat Res.* 1993;286:48-55.

87. Bruni D, Iacono F, Sharma B, Zaffagnini S, Marcacci M. Tibial tubercle osteotomy or quadriceps snip in two-stage revision for prosthetic knee infection? A randomized prospective study. *Clin Orthop Relat Res.* 2013;471(4):1305-1318.

88. Sun Z, Patil A, Song EK, Kim HT, Seon JK. Comparison of quadriceps snip and tibial tubercle osteotomy in revision for infected total knee arthroplasty. *Int Orthop.* 2015;39(5):879-885.

89. Lahav A, Hofmann AA. The "banana peel" exposure method in revision total knee arthroplasty. *Am J Orthop.* 2007;36(10):526-529; discussion 529.

90. Huff TW, Russel E. Difficult exposures in total knee arthroplasty: the femoral peel. *Curr Orthop Pract.* 2008;19:272-275.

91. Windsor RE, Insall JN. Exposure in revision total knee arthroplasty: the femoral peel. *Tech Orthop.* 1988;3:1-4.

92. Engh GA, Ammeen D. Results of total knee arthroplasty with medial epicondylar osteotomy to correct varus deformity. *Clin Orthop Relat Res.* 1999;367:141-148.

93. Sim JA, Na YG, Go JY, Lee BK. Clinical and radiologic evaluation of medial epicondylar osteotomy for varus total knee arthroplasty. *Knee.* 2018;25(1):177-184.

94. Mihalko WM, Saeki K, Whiteside LA. Effect of medial epicondylar osteotomy on soft tissue balancing in total knee arthroplasty. *Orthopedics.* 2013;36(11):e1353-e1357.

95. Lavernia C, Contreras JS, Alcerro JC. The peel in total knee revision: exposure in the difficult knee. *Clin Orthop Relat Res.* 2011;469(1):146-153.

96. Van den Broek CM, van Hellemondt GG, Jacobs WC, Wymenga AB. Step-cut tibial tubercle osteotomy for access in revision total knee replacement. *Knee.* 2006;13:430-434.

97. Hirschmann MT, Hoffmann M, Krause R, Jenabzadeh R-A, Arnold MP, Friederich NF. Anterolateral approach with tibial tubercle osteotomy versus standard medial approach for primary total knee arthroplasty: does it matter? *BMC Musculoskelet Disord.* 2010;11:167.

98. Vandeputte FJ, Vandenneucker H. Proximalisation of the tibial tubercle gives a good outcome in patients undergoing revision total knee arthroplasty who have pseudo patella baja. *Bone Joint J.* 2017;99(7):912-916.

99. Punwar SA, Fick DP, Khan RJK. Tibial Tubercle Osteotomy in Revision Knee Arthroplasty. *J Arthroplasty.* 2017;32(3):903-907.

100. Segur JM, Vilchez-Cavazos F, Martinez-Pastor JC, Macule F, Suso S, Acosta-Olivo C. Tibial tubercle osteotomy in septic revision total knee arthroplasty. *Arch Orthop Trauma Surg.* 2014;134(9):1311-1315.

chapter 40

Unicompartmental Knee Arthroplasty

Axel Schmidt, MD | Matthieu Ollivier, MD, PhD | Jean-Noël A. Argenson, MD, PhD

INTRODUCTION

Surgical options for unicompartmental osteoarthritis of the tibiofemoral joint vary according to the stage of disease and patient characteristics. Options are arthroscopic débridement, high tibial or distal femoral osteotomies, unicompartmental arthroplasty (UKA), and total knee arthroplasty (TKA).

In this chapter dedicated to UKA, we will detail indications for UKA, the different implant designs, the technical procedures, modes of failures, and the outcomes of UKA.

INDICATIONS AND PATIENT SELECTION

Anteromedial Osteoarthritis

Anteromedial osteoarthritis (AMOA), the primary indication of medial UKA, is defined by a reduction of 75% of the tibiofemoral joint space, associated with condylar or tibial osteophytes or grade IV disease. Function of the knee is relatively normal with an intact anterior cruciate ligament (ACL), reducible varus deformity, both clinically and on valgus stress radiographs. The lateral compartment is nondegenerative with no pain on the lateral side of the knee, less than 25% loss of joint space on stress radiographs, and a normal aspect of the cartilage found intraoperatively.

Varus deformity >10° and >15° of flexion contracture are not considered as absolute contraindications, but they are classically associated with ACL deficiency, or not correctable on valgus stress. In those conditions, UKA cannot be recommended.

Avascular Osteonecrosis

Avascular osteonecrosis (AVN) is a common cause of knee pain both in elderly and younger populations. It is the second most common indication of medial UKA when medical treatment fails, in primary disease or following previous surgeries (arthroscopic débridement with drilling).

Diagnosis is based on radiographs and confirmed with MRI allowing locoregional extension map of the necrosis. UKA is possible only in isolated disease localized to the subchondral region of one compartment without extension to epiphyseal or metaphyseal bone. However, MRI can be misleading as to the severity of disease when extensive edema is evident, while adequate bone support needs still to be present for successful UKA.

As reported by Marmor et al,[1] UKA has been used with success in the treatment of spontaneous or idiopathic medial femoral condyle osteonecrosis with good results. Our own results have confirmed this indication with favorable outcomes at long-term follow-up.[2,3]

Obesity

High body mass index (BMI) was considered as a contraindication of UKA because fixed-bearing all-polyethylene implants have been shown to have poor survival in obese patients (**Fig. 40-1**).

Recent series on modern metal-backed designs, whether fixed or mobile bearing, have shown excellent survivorship in obese patients, equivalent to normal weight patients, associated with fewer reoperations, reduced deep infection risk, fewer perioperative complications, and better functional scores including range of motion after UKA comparable or even better than with TKA (**Fig. 40-2**).[4] UKA wear is more related to activity, rather than BMI.

In conclusion, obesity and increasing BMI are no longer considered as contraindications to a metal-backed UKA, as recently described in a new perspective on UKA indications by members of the Knee Society.[5]

Age

In patients with AMOA, age is no longer considered as a contraindication to UKA[6] because revision UKAs are not correlated to activity or age.

Young patients have a greater level of activity, including professional activities and sport. They also have a greater expectation for the surgery results to restore knee function. UKA could appear to be an attractive alternative in this age category, as a conservative "first" arthroplasty allowing a better knee function, reducing the rehabilitation time, and preserving sporting activity. Young patients should be educated on the risk of earlier degradation in intensive high-impact activity and the potential for future revision.

Patellofemoral Osteoarthritis

The status of the patellofemoral joint continues to be a source of debate concerning indications of UKA.

In cases of AMOA associated with full-thickness cartilage loss of the lateral trochlea and/or lateral facet of the

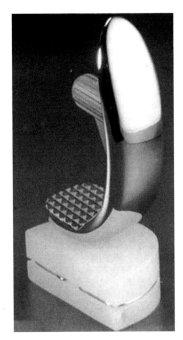

FIGURE 40-1 All-polyethylene implant.

Chondrocalcinosis

Chondrocalcinosis and radiographic signs of calcium within the cartilage or meniscus are not contraindications to UKA. However, clinical inflammatory disease with popliteal cyst and/or synovitis effusion demonstrating of an active pathology is a contraindication.[10]

Lateral Posttraumatic Arthritis

Posttraumatic arthritis secondary to lateral tibial plateau fracture malunion causes pain and limited function for patients who are often relatively younger than the degenerative population, and UKA potentially allows correction of the intra-articular deformation due to the tibia's fracture. Lustig et al[11] reported, in lateral UKA, improvement of knee pain, function, and an excellent survivorship at 5 to 10 years, with 80% good results at 15 years. Despite the limited number of indications and the technical challenge, lateral UKA could be an efficient option to treat lateral arthritis secondary to fractures with malunion, relieve knee pain, and restore knee function. Furthermore, implant survival rates seem to be comparable or close to those obtained for lateral UKA implanted for primary osteoarthritis.

patella or in cases of lateral patellar subluxation, implanting medial UKA is contraindicated. Other conditions of the patellofemoral joint such as spurring and intraoperative degenerative aspect of the medial facet or trochlea, anterior knee pain on physical examination are not considered as contraindications in the knee with AMOA.[7,8] Konan et al[9] found that UKA improved pain and function in all patients, with medial patellofemoral disease not affecting outcomes, contrary to central or lateral grade III patellofemoral disease having lower scores.

Absolute Contraindication

Joint infection and inflammatory disease should be considered as contraindication to UKA.

In case of previous high tibial osteotomy (HTO) leading to an extra-articular deformity, the risk of overcorrection exists when the intra-articular varus deformity is corrected with UKA and may generate early failure of the lateral compartment.[12]

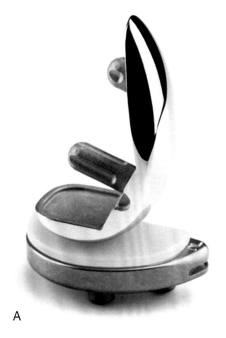

A

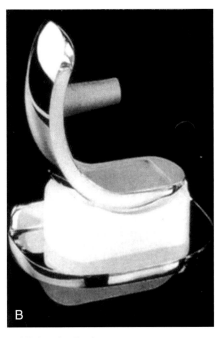

B

FIGURE 40-2 **A:** Fixed- and **B:** mobile-bearing implants.

Thickness of cartilage <25% in lateral and patellofemoral compartments may demonstrate global osteoarthritis in the knee with an increased risk of early failure due to progression of the disease.

ACL deficiency is not an absolute contraindication. Some authors reported good results and mid-term survivorship for medial UKA performed in ACL-deficient knee or with a concomitant ACL reconstruction.[13,14] The laxity is evaluated clinically as well as on lateral X-rays with anterior stress. An anterior translation, on stress views, greater than 10 mm or a posterior saucer-shaped indentation, reflecting ACL deficiency, can be an indication to perform an ACL reconstruction at the time of the UKA in young patients. In those special cases of knees associated to anterior laxity, UKA may still be considered if the osteoarthritis disease is localized to the medial compartment without a posterior wear pattern and the frontal deformity is fully reducible. The surgical technique in those cases could be modified with reduction of the tibial posterior slope during the tibial cut to reduce the anterior tibial laxity.

Extra-articular Deformity

Osteoarthritis secondary to lower limb malalignment due to an extra-articular deformity is a contraindication to UKA. The extra-articular deformity can be secondary to a metaphyseal or diaphyseal fracture or due to a congenital deformity of the distal femur (essentially for valgus with hypoplasia of the lateral condyle) or the proximal tibia.

In cases where there are no or minimal intra-articular deformity, UKA might overcorrect the bone wear leading to early failure on the opposite compartment and on the implant due to excessive force. In the case of monocompartmental osteoarthritis associated to an extra-epiphyseal deformity, HTO is recommended to correct the lower limb malalignment.

The Ideal Patient

To resume indications of UKA, the "ideal" patient should have osteoarthritis or avascular necrosis localized to a single compartment, with a reducible intra-articular deformity (<10° in varus, <15° in valgus, and no flexion contracture > 15°). Age and weight have no impact in cases of modern metal-backed implant. In cases of AMOA, if preoperative investigations find spurring and arthritis of the medial facet and/or trochlea, UKA can be implanted. For the special case of ACL deficiency in patients describing no A/P instability, UKA is still a good option if the osteoarthritis is localized to the medial compartment without any posterior wear pattern. UKA is reserved for patients with an advanced osteoarthritis (grade III or IV). Studies have demonstrated poorer outcomes and survival when medial UKA is used in patients with milder stages of osteoarthritis with partial-thickness cartilage loss.[15]

IMPLANT DESIGNS

Mobile- Versus Fixed-Bearing UKA

Theoretical advantages of mobile-bearing UKA, which is free to slide only in the anteroposterior axis, are based on an increased area of femorotibial contact during flexion producing a lower load stress transmission to the polyethylene, and then a more durable implant fixation over time. However, some disadvantages such as technical difficulty with regard to ligament balance and alignment, an increased risk of dislocation, and impingement have been described.

In the literature, several meta-analyses, systematic reviews, or randomized studies have compared the clinical outcomes of fixed- versus mobile-bearing UKA. They found no significant differences in clinical and functional outcomes between the two implants. They did not identify any significant difference in the relative risks for aseptic loosening, painful progression of osteoarthritis, periprosthetic fractures, and revision rates.[16-18]

The main reasons for revision in fixed-bearing UKA are progression of OA and wear, while mobile-bearing UKAs are often revised because of aseptic loosening, progression of OA, and dislocation.[19] Time to failure could be shorter for mobile-bearing UKA perhaps due to a greater susceptibility of mobile-bearing outcomes to technical errors.[20]

Concerning polyethylene backside wear due to the mobility of the bearing surfaces, Burton et al,[21] using a displacement-controlled simulator, found a significantly greater volumetric wear rate for medial and lateral mobile-bearing UKA as compared to the fixed-bearing design.

In conclusion, fixed-bearing UKA has similar excellent outcomes and at least equivalent survivorship to the mobile-bearing implants without the risk of dislocation, allowing the surgeon to focus on gap-balancing while ensuring slight undercorrection.

With fixed-bearing UKA, a greater degree of undercorrection is tolerated giving the surgeon a wider margin of error. Even if mobile-bearing UKA may better replicate a native knee kinematics, both implant designs have similar functional outcomes.

Cemented Versus Cementless

Cemented implants are still the gold standard in UKA, but the proportion of cementless prosthesis is growing. The advantages of cementless implant include reduced surgical time, reduced incidence of tibial radiolucencies, avoiding cementation errors leading to impingement, or wear from third-body cement particles. Cementless coatings could be composed of hydroxyapatite alone (Unix UKA, Stryker, Mahwah, NJ, USA), porous titanium with hydroxyapatite (Oxford UKA), or tritanium (Tritanium UKA, Stryker Orthopaedics, Mahwah, NJ, USA).

Few studies in the literature have compared cementless versus cemented implants from the same manufacturers. Schlueter-Brust et al[22] compared 152 cemented medial Uniglide UKAs versus 78 uncemented and 10 hybrid UKAs. The cementless group had a 97.4% 10-year survival rate versus 95.4% (and no significant difference) for the cemented group. Inversely, Panzram et al[23] found a similar 5-year implant survival of 94.1% for cemented group compared to 89.7% for uncemented (no statistical difference) in the incidence of radiolucent lines at 5 years. The New Zealand Joint Registry (Eighteen Year report January 1999 to December 2016. Wellington, New Zealand; 2017) reported a low revision rate of 0.8/100 component years for the uncemented Oxford UKA, but the lowest revision rate was for the cemented ZUK Zimmer UKA at 0.54/100 component years. Randomized control trials reported lower incidence of radiolucent lines[24,25] and better Knee Society Functional Scores for cementless UKA group versus cemented UKA.[24]

A biomechanical study showed that cementless UKA bears a higher risk of periprosthetic tibial plateau fractures as compared to cemented implant UKA (in cases of extended vertical saw cuts and reduced bone mineral density), but no difference was observed in clinical settings.[26]

All-Polyethylene Versus Metal-Backed

The theoretical advantages of all-polyethylene implants are greater bone preservation for insert thickness <9 to 10 mm (which is approximately total thickness of the thinnest metal-backed fixed-bearing UKA), and reduced backside wear and implant cost.[27] Disadvantages are a worse stresses and strains transmission to the underlying bone with 1.8 to 6 times greater microdamage compared to the metal-backed designs[28] which could lead to increased risk of aseptic loosening and pain. The clinical outcomes of all-polyethylene UKA are mixed, with several studies showing excellent mid- to long-term survivorship, while other studies found inferior outcomes compared to metal-backed designs.[29,30]

KINEMATICS OF THE NATIVE KNEE AND UKA

The biomechanics and kinematics differ between the lateral and the medial knee compartments. It is essential to understand these variations explaining the differences between indications and surgical techniques, which are the keys to perform a successful UKA.

The knee joint kinematics consists of a progressive femoral external rotation relative to the tibia with knee flexion and posterior displacement of the lateral femoral condyle (up to 10 mm) with respect to the medial condyle (slight posterior translation of 2 mm). The femur starts its motion from a neutral rotation, reaching about an average 7° of external rotation in mid-flexion.

Compared to the healthy knee, the femur in medial unicompartmental osteoarthritis has less external rotation during the whole range of motion. The femoral condyle translation on the medial tibial plateau seems to be strictly dependent on ACL integrity.[31] Cartilage erosion on arthritic knees with intact cruciate ligaments occurred in the central to medial region of the medial plateau, while osteoarthritic knees develop larger posterior wear in case of ACL rupture. Inversely, the relative motion of the lateral condyle on the tibial plateau seems to be independent of osteoarthritic degeneration and ACL integrity.

At the end of knee extension, between full extension and 20° of knee flexion, external rotation of the tibia occurs and results in tightening of both cruciate ligaments, which locks the knee. The tibia is then in the position of maximal stability with respect to the femur. This phenomenon, called the "screw-home" mechanism, is believed to be a key element for knee stability in upright standing. Surgeons must keep in mind that a good femoral implant position in flexion of the lateral compartment may lead to an excessive internal rotation in extension and impingement on the tibial spine eminence. Therefore, the positioning in flexion should exaggerate the lateral rotation and the lateral positioning (almost on the lateral osteophytes to obtain a satisfactory position in extension).

A CT scan study[32] evaluating femorotibial rotation reported that the femur tended to be in a relatively internally rotated position in knee with severe osteoarthritis. This functional limitation is probably attributable to cartilage degeneration, osteophytes, and menisci disease related to arthritic changes.

Casino et al[33] carried out kinematic tests with 3D navigation system performed before and after surgery and included varus/valgus stress at 0° and 30° and passive range of motion. They found that varus/valgus laxity in extension was significantly reduced from 7.7° to 4.0° after UKA. The axial rotation during the passive range of motion was similar in osteoarthritic knees (17.9°) and knees after UKA (15.8°). During flexion, the medial compartment displaced posteriorly 9 mm while the lateral compartment showed a mean posterior translation of 18.3 mm, confirming the medial pivot concept in which the medial compartment bears knee stability when the lateral compartment bears knee mobility as demonstrated during *in vivo* kinematic study.[34]

PREOPERATIVE PREPARATION

Physical Examination Criteria

Preserved range of motion, meaning minimum 100° of flexion, and no lack of extension are required to perform UKA. The coronal and sagittal laxities have to be evaluated, especially in the posttraumatic valgus knee. During

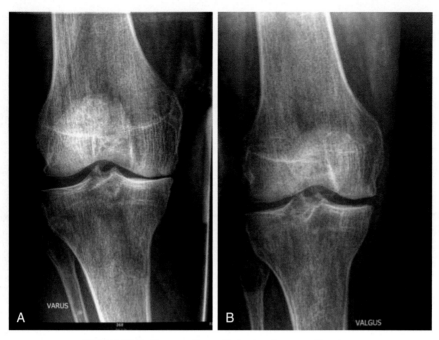

FIGURE 40-3   Preoperative radiographs: **A:** varus, **B:** valgus.

the varus/valgus stress test, the coronal deformation should be fully correctible. Assessment of the ACL should be interpreted with caution, as the pivot shift test may be limited due to pain and swelling in an arthritic knee (**Fig. 40-3**).

Varus >10° and valgus >15° are usually considered as contraindications for UKA. In cases where the deformity is not fully correctable, soft-tissue releases are required and thus a TKA should be performed. UKA implants are only dedicated to fill the gap left by the worn cartilage and restore natural tension of the collateral ligament.

Knee pain should be localized in one compartment and potentially being showed precisely by the patient ("finger sign").

Imaging

The radiological analysis systematically includes anteroposterior (AP) and lateral views of the knee, full-length radiographs in bipodal and single-leg stance, varus and valgus stress radiographs, and a skyline view at 45° of knee flexion. Radiographs assess full-thickness cartilage loss in the involved compartment and intact cartilage thickness in the unaffected compartment, and confirm that the deformity is fully reducible. The lateral view of the joint confirms the absence of anterior tibial translation greater than 10 mm (referencing the posterior edge of the tibial plateau) and also shows that tibial erosion is limited to the anterior and mid-portions of the tibial plateau, confirming that the ACL is competent. A skyline view of patellofemoral joint should also be completed to ensure that there is

no lateral joint space narrowing at 45° of flexion. The presence of periarticular osteophytes is not an absolute contraindication for a UKA.

Patient Expectations

It is important to understand why patients are undergoing UKA. If the main motivation is to return to high-level sporting activities, then a UKA is not the appropriate solution.[35] Resistant pain and limitations in the daily activities are the only reasons to justify surgery, particularly for young and active patients. Patients must be prepared for surgery, including both physical and psychological preparation. The physical preparation includes maintaining range of motion to limit the risk of a postoperative knee contracture and to prepare the patient for the postoperative rehabilitation program. In addition, it is essential to optimize the quadriceps' and hamstrings' strength at the time of surgery. Each step of the postoperative days and goals of the rehabilitation have to be presented to the patients preoperatively in an effort to manage their expectations and include them in a fast-track recovery program reducing the length of stay.

SURGICAL POSITIONING

The procedure can be performed under epidural or general anesthesia. The operative limb will be positioned according to the preference of the operator. The limb could be supported by a padded posterior thigh allowing the leg to hang freely at 110° during the procedure or supported with lateral leg-holder of the thigh and placed at 90° flexion. Tourniquet is not obligatory according to the surgeon preference.

THE SURGICAL STEPS FOR MEDIAL UNICOMPARTMENTAL KNEE ARTHROPLASTY

Main Principles in Medial UKA

* Undercorrection of lower limb alignment

Performing a successful UKA requires a slight undercorrection of the limb alignment and to provide optimal soft-tissue balancing restoration (2 mm of medial laxity) in flexion and extension. The mechanical axis should pass between the middle of the resurfaced compartment and the tibial spines.

* Correct congruency between components

Restoring an anatomical alignment is the key to prevent implant loosening and polyethylene wear. The objective is to ensure congruency between the femoral component and the surface of the polyethylene in both flexion and extension without overhang that can lead to edge loading, especially between 20° and 60° of flexion when maximum forces occur during weight bearing.

* Restoring tension of the soft tissues

This allows the knee to remain stable and improve the implant's survival.

* Tibial slope

Excessive slope increases tension on the ACL and the risk of tibial loosening. Insufficient slope leads to limitation of flexion. The objective is to match the patient's native natural slope, and the final target is a slope of 5° to 7°.

* Component sizing

On the tibia, the largest size that can be accommodated without overhang is desired to place the component on the cortical rim.

Operative Technique

This technique is adaptable to a mobile-bearing or a fixed-bearing medial UKA.

* Approach

The skin incision starts medially to the superior pole of the patella and ends medial to the tibial tubercle, with two-thirds above the joint line and one-third below (**Fig. 40-4**). A medial arthrotomy is performed through a para-patellar approach.

Anterior horn of the medial meniscus and a portion of the fat pad are removed to facilitate intra-articular visualization. Caution has to be paid during deep medial dissection to not damage the deep fibers of the MCL. Inspection of the lateral compartment and patellofemoral joint and testing of the ACL can be performed (**Fig. 40-5**). Osteophytes of the medial femur and of the intercondylar notch are removed.

* Tibial preparation

Objectives of the tibial component position are orthogonal to the tibial mechanical axis and 5° of tibial slope. The rotation position is aligned to the flexion axis of the native knee kinematics.

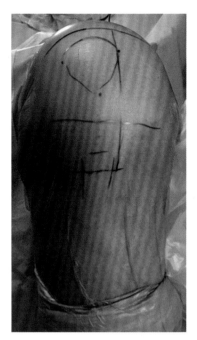

FIGURE 40-4 Skin incision on a right knee.

The horizontal bone cut is performed with an extramedullary guide and has to be the minimal amount needed to fit the tibial tray. The extramedullary guide is aligned to the anterior tibial crest with a neutral varus-valgus alignment (**Fig. 40-6**).

A thin curved retractor is helpful to protect the MCL from the saw blade during the tibial cut.

A risk during the tibial cut is to place too much tibial slope, especially for obese patients with thickness of soft tissues.

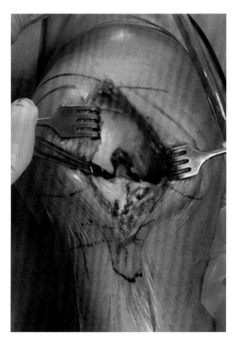

FIGURE 40-5 Inspection of the lateral compartment and patellofemoral joint and testing of the ACL.

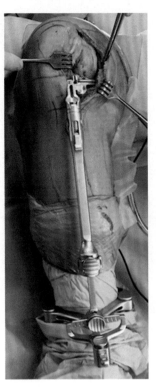

FIGURE 40-6 The extramedullary guide is aligned to the anterior tibial crest with a neutral varus–valgus alignment.

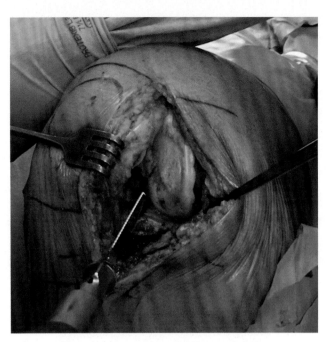

FIGURE 40-7 The sagittal bone cut is made medially to the apex of the medial spine, in the same plane as the flexion axis of the knee from 40° to 100° of flexion.

The sagittal bone cut is made medially to the apex of the medial spine, in the same plane as the flexion axis of the knee from 40° to 100° of flexion (**Fig. 40-7**).

The spacer block, set to the appropriate thickness, is easily inserted in flexion to confirm adequate tibial bone resection depth (**Fig. 40-8**). If it is tight, posterior medial osteophytes should be removed and a small amount of posterior femoral cartilage has to be removed, before concluding that bone resection is not enough.

• Femoral preparation

The femoral implant size can be preoperatively determined by x-ray planning, but most of the time during surgery with progressive size increments.

The distal femoral cut could be performed using two different techniques first, with the help of an intramedullary guide (independent cut). The entrance hole of the intramedullary guide is medially above the roof of the intercondylar notch. A second technique is with a cutting guide that relies on the tibial cut (dependent cut) with correction of the deformity (**Fig. 40-9**).

The distal femoral cut should be minimal to allow a resurfacing cut, and adapted to the thickness of the femoral component. The extension space is then checked using a dedicated spacer block.

Next, the posterior femoral cut and chamfers are completed with the appropriately sized cutting block when the rotation is set (**Fig. 40-10**).

• Extension and flexion gap balancing

The remaining medial meniscus is removed and the ligament's tension with the trial components is tested.

The range of motion is analyzed. A flexion at 120° has to be obtained as well as full extension. The knee has to be "locked" in extension and conserve a slight medial laxity of 1 or 2 mm during the flexion. This "security" laxity confirms there is no overcorrection and only the intra-articular deformity was treated.

Any impingement in maximal flexion and full extension between implants and bone has to be detected at this step to prevent polyethylene wear, especially for mobile-bearing implants.

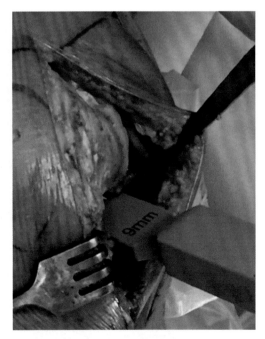

FIGURE 40-8 The spacer block is confirming adequate tibial bone resection depth.

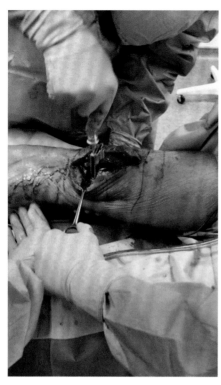

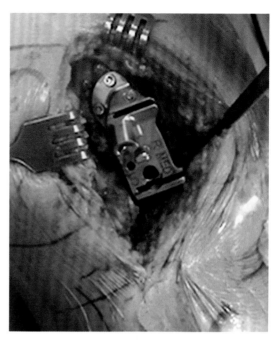

FIGURE 40-10 The posterior femoral cut and chamfers performed with appropriately sized cutting block.

FIGURE 40-9 The extramedullary distal femoral cutting guide is inserted to correct the deformity.

After removal of the trial components, all the bony foreign bodies and osteophytes, particularly behind the posterior femoral condyle, are resected.

• Tibial preparation

Ideally, the component should be fully supported by the cortex without any overhang more than 1 mm (**Fig. 40-11**). Occasionally, the vertical tibial cut should

be redone 1 or 2 mm more laterally to avoid undersizing the tibial implant. The posterior border of the tibial trial should be aligned with the posterior cortex. It is pinned in place and the keel slot is fashioned.

• Cementation of implants

In case of sclerotic surfaces, perforation with a drill can facilitate the cementation. Tibia is cemented first and excess cement is removed, especially posteriorly. The femoral implant is then cemented, excess cement removed, and both components are compressed together at 45° of

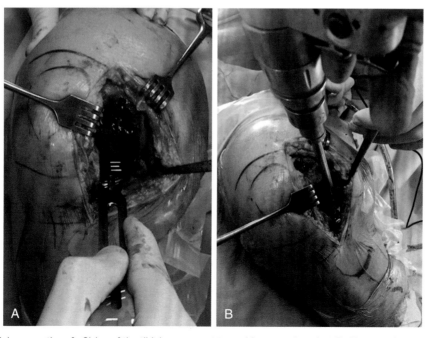

FIGURE 40-11 Tibial preparation. **A:** Sizing of the tibial component to avoid any overhanging. **B:** Fixation of the trial tibial component.

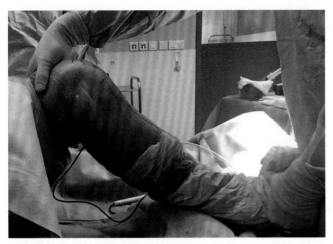

FIGURE 40-12 Component's compression at 45° of flexion until cement is hard.

flexion until cement is hard (**Fig. 40-12**). The polyethylene bearing is inserted in flexion around 100°.

- Cementless fixation

Indications are the same between cemented and cementless fixations except for very few patients who would need an extra-small tibial component. For those, it is better to use cemented fixation.[36] The surgical techniques for cemented and cementless are nearly similar. In cementless technique, care has to be taken with the holes permitting good primary fixation and secondly osteointegration. The cementless tibial component is partially inserted with the introducer, and soft tissue between the component and the implant is removed before the component is fully impacted with a light hammer. The femoral component is impacted in press-fit too with the hammer.

THE SURGICAL STEPS FOR LATERAL UNICOMPARTMENTAL KNEE ARTHROPLASTY

Lateral UKA represents the minority of UKA and amounts for less than 10% of UKA performed for osteoarthritis.[37]

Due to this rarity, the specific indications, the anatomic characteristics of the lateral compartment, and the kinematics, lateral UKA remains a technically demanding surgery.

The literature results of UKA for isolated lateral osteoarthritis are not always as good as for isolated medial OA. The most significant factor leading to reoperation is progression of medial disease. Lateral arthritis is typically well-tolerated for a longer period of time than medial arthritis.

Anatomy

The tibial plateau on the lateral side is convex. A congenital hypoplastic lateral femoral condyle is often associated.

The congruency between the femoral condyle and the tibial plateau heavily depends on the presence of the meniscus and on its form. If this is removed, stability is lost and degenerate changes can occur rapidly explaining the significant numbers of fairly young patients who develop lateral arthritis after lateral meniscectomy.

Whereas on the medial side the pathological changes initially occur anteriorly, on the lateral side the changes start posteriorly. This particularity is important to orientate the imaging diagnostic. On the lateral side since the cartilage wear is posterior, it is only by taking a Rosenberg view that the true severity of the condition can be appreciated.

Indications

The indications are based on clinical and radiological criteria. The main indication is lateral osteoarthritis due to pathological loading with valgus knee deformity (under 15°) and/or a hypoplastic lateral femoral condyle. Other indications are AVN of the femoral condyle, and posttraumatic or postlateral meniscectomy.

Age is no longer a contraindication for UKA, especially in case of posttraumatic OA in young patients. A lateral UKA can be proposed to patients who are younger than 60 years.[11,38] For young and active patients, with a low-grade unicompartmental osteoarthritis, alternatives to treat lateral osteoarthritis due to valgus axial malalignment are the distal femoral and/or high tibial varus-producing osteotomy. However, outcomes and survival of a varus-producing osteotomy are generally less predictable and the surgical techniques are more challenging compared with a high tibial valgus osteotomy; the recovery time after osteotomy is longer when compared to UKA.

Biomechanically, a dynamic varus moment in full weight bearing exists in many valgus knees. If the alignment is less than 15° of valgus, the load applied on the knee in stance phase passes through the medial compartment, so that the postoperative forces on the lateral compartment and on the prosthesis are low.

Clinical and radiological signs of osteoarthritis in the medial or patellofemoral compartments are contraindications for lateral UKA. Occasional exceptions can be made for asymptomatic patellofemoral osteoarthritis in selected patients (over 70 years old, significant comorbidities, low activity levels). A lateral facetectomy can be performed with UKA and provide relief for isolated lateral patellar osteoarthritis.

Specificity of Preoperative Planning for Lateral UKA

The preoperative investigations determine the origin of the valgus knee and differentiate situations:

- Lateral condylar dysplasia
- A posttraumatic valgus knee related to a fracture of the tibial plateau or of the lateral condyle

- A postlateral meniscectomy valgus knee
- A valgus knee secondary to an underlying coxofemoral pathology, with or without a prosthesis
- An axial deviation by congenital valgus tibial curvature

The lateral femoral hypoplasia is the most common indication. Position of the femoral component must be adapted to the dysplasia's severity. When condylar dysplasia is severe, the femoral component has to be positioned more distal and more posterior. This technique corrects the dysplasia at its original site both in the sagittal and the coronal planes and restores an anatomical joint space.

In the posttraumatic or postmeniscectomy valgus knee, there is no compensation for femoral dysplasia. The poor subchondral bone quality and a comminution and depression of the lateral tibial plateau have to be anticipated and may require the possibility of bone graft or reinforcing screws in the transverse plane. Preoperative planning with CT scans might be useful in these cases. The last two situations are less frequent and likely best treated with TKA or osteotomies.

Approach

A lateral parapatellar approach is preferred for this procedure but some authors have used a medial parapatellar approach.[39]

The upper limit of the incision is at the superior pole of the patella, and the distal limit is 2 cm below the joint line toward the lateral side of the tibial tuberosity. A lateral arthrotomy is performed to open the joint. To improve the exposure, the patella will be retracted medially and an additional resection of the lateral facet treating a localized patellar spurring can be associated. Thereafter, the lateral portion of the fat pad is excised to visualize the condyle, ACL, and corresponding lateral tibial plateau.

It is important to note that the principles of ligament balancing cannot be applied to a lateral UKA and the collateral ligaments should not be balanced or released. The iliotibial band is not released from its tibial insertion.

The patellofemoral compartment, the medial femorotibial compartment, and the ACL are checked to confirm the isolated lateral compartment osteoarthritis and the absence of anterior laxity. The osteophytes in the intercondylar notch should be removed to avoid late impingement with the ACL.

The osteophytes on the lateral femoral condyle should be preserved to help for the positioning of the femoral compartment.[40] The femoral component should be as lateral as possible when the knee is in flexion, sometimes bordering on the lateral osteophytes. The anterior contact point between the anterior part of the femoral condyle and the anterior part of the tibial plateau represents the anterior limit of the femoral component. It is important to identify and mark this point before the bone cuts.

Release of the lateral tibial margin should be minimal to respect the peripheral ligamentous structures. This is an essential aspect during UKA and a security of a final undercorrection during the ligamentous tension testing.[41]

First Step: Tibial Cut

The tibial cut should be performed using an extramedullary guide to obtain an orthogonal (90°) cut to the tibial mechanical axis. The bone resection should be minimal (2-4 mm maximum), because the disease more often affects the femoral side.[41] It is important to keep the depth of the tibial cut as conservative as possible to take advantage of the strength of the tibial cortex with a large contact area proximally. If the surgeon would like to keep some degree of valgus, it should not be done with the tibial cut but rather with the femoral cut.

The natural slope on the lateral compartment, which is around 0°, should be reproduced to avoid being tight in flexion (anterior slope) and to protect the ACL (high posterior slope).

To finish, the sagittal cut should be performed respecting the tibial spine eminence, being near to but not involving them. The cut has to follow the line joining the most medial point of the mid-portion of lateral plateau (posterior to the ACL insertion) seen in flexion and the most medial border of the lateral plateau of the anterior part of the lateral plateau (anterior to the ACL insertion) seen in extension. Due to the natural orientation of lateral tibial plateau in external rotation ("screw-home mechanism"), this line crosses the patellar tendon which is then in the way of the saw blade. Thus the sagittal tibial cut should be internally rotated.[41] A careful retraction of the tendon helps make this sagittal cut freehand possible.

Second Step: Femoral Cuts

Each prosthesis has its specific technique, but the principles and major steps are similar between the different implants. The distal femoral cut could be performed using two different techniques.

First, with the help of an intramedullary guide (independent cut). The entrance hole of the intramedullary guide is centered above the roof of the intercondylar notch. The distal femoral cut can be made based upon the angle between the anatomic and mechanical axis (usually 4°-6°). Second, the technique with a cutting guide that relies on the tibial cut (dependent cut), as for medial UKA. The distal femoral cut should be minimal to allow for a distalized femoral implant to compensate the femoral wear. The extension space is then checked using a dedicated spacer block.

Next, the posterior femoral cut and chamfers are completed with the appropriately sized cutting block when the rotation is set.

The posterior cut should be minimal to compensate for the posterior offset and to obtain a similar gap in flexion and extension. Through this technique, femoral resurfacing implant does not reproduce the anatomy but is used to augment and compensate in case of lateral condylar hypoplasia.

Rotation of the cutting blocks is essential. The lateral aspect of the femoral cutting block should follow the lateral aspect of the condyle to avoid any excessive internal rotation in extension due to the screw-home mechanism related to the natural divergence of the lateral femoral condyle (compared to the medial condyle). The size of the cutting block is determined by searching for the best compromise between an anatomically centered position on the femoral condyle and a long axis perpendicular to the resected tibial plateau. Particular care should be given to avoid oversizing of the femoral component. The anterior edge of the femoral component should be located at the mark of the anterior contact point identified at the beginning of the surgery. This landmark is localized 1 to 2 mm below the cartilage–bone interface that was created by making the distal cut avoiding a potential notch between the femoral implant and the patella.

Once the posterior cut and chamfers have been made and the cutting guide is removed, removal of any posterior osteophytes, or any bony or soft-tissue remnant, is crucial to obtain good range of flexion to avoid any posterior impingement with the polyethylene in high flexion.

Third Step: Positioning of the Implant

The size of the tibia is chosen after all cuts are made and result in the best compromise between maximal tibial coverage, but without any overhang in the sagittal and coronal planes.

The tibial implant should be as close as possible to the tibial eminences and should have 10° to 15° of internal rotation. The femoral implant positioning in flexion should exaggerate the external rotation and be positioned as laterally as possible, almost on the lateral osteophytes to obtain an ideal contact with the tibia without impingement on the tibial eminences.

The knee is then brought into maximal flexion and internally rotated to facilitate the final preparation of the tibia with the appropriate guide with the underlying keel impacted into the subchondral bone. The knee should be tested in flexion–extension with the trial components in place and inserting a trial polyethylene liner. At that step, it is important to search for any impingement of the femur against the tibial spine eminences in extension due to a lack of external rotation in flexion. In flexion and in extension, the medial part of the femoral component should be in line with the middle of the tibial component. The testing of the flexion–extension gaps allows the surgeon to choose the appropriate height of polyethylene liner. The polyethylene insert

is often thicker here than for the medial side due to femoral dysplasia.

However, it is essential to undercorrect the deformity in lateral UKAs to avoid any overstuffing of the unresurfaced medial compartment, which is essential for successful long-term results.[38] The philosophy of lateral UKA is that it is a resurfacing procedure correcting only the intraarticular wear and respecting any extra-articular deformity. This is not a deformity-correcting procedure. At the end, the surgeon should confirm the presence of residual laxity on the lateral side through a varus stress test at 15° flexion (unlocked knee).

The final cemented tibial component is inserted first with the knee in full flexion and internally rotated to improve the exposure of the lateral compartment. Once the femoral implant has been inserted, bringing the knee close to extension helps to remove any posterior cement. Finally, the polyethylene can be inserted in flexion after the cleaning and the drying of the metal-backed tibial implant.

Common Surgical Errors Leading to Failure in Lateral UKA

Overcorrection of a valgus deformity to varus will cause overload of the medial compartment and development of medial osteoarthritis.

The anatomical divergence of the lateral femoral condyle in flexion should be taken in consideration to avoid impingement of the tibial spine in extension.

Caution should be taken during the tibial cut to prevent an excessive tibial slope and affecting the ligament balancing.

The tibial component should be internally rotated 15° to 20° on the sagittal plane and aligned to the natural tibial slope.

Conclusion

With careful patient selection and appropriate surgical technique (correct implant position and size selection), avoiding overcorrection of the preoperative valgus deformity, lateral UKA can provide a durable construct with long-term success and reliable pain relief (**Fig. 40-13**).

According to the anatomical differences and the biomechanical characteristics of the medial and lateral compartments, some surgical considerations must be underlined for lateral compartment UKA.

Considering lateral UKA as a resurfacing procedure and not as a deformity-correcting procedure reduces the complication of medial compartment osteoarthritis progression.

Due to the increased mobility of the lateral compartment, a fixed-bearing prosthesis should be implanted.

Lateral UKA demonstrates equivocal implant survival and outcomes in properly selected patients when compared with medial UKA.

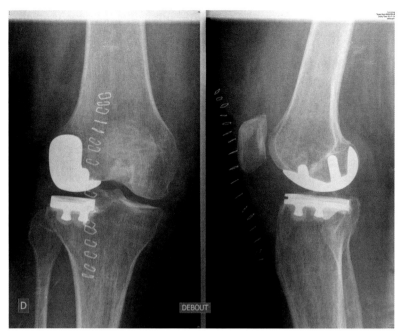

FIGURE 40-13 Lateral unicompartmental knee arthroplasty.

RESULTS AND SURVIVAL OF UKA

Recent studies demonstrate very good survival for modern UKA with 10-year survivorship at 90% or greater,[42,43] and it would be relatively easier to revise in case of failure.[44] Revision of a failed UKA had better results with more satisfied patients than revision TKA.

Results of Medial UKA for Osteoarthritis

Long-term studies found 15-year survival rate of 92% for UKA performed for medial osteoarthritis even if radiolucent lines around tibia component are often observed during the follow-up,[45] considered with mobile-bearing UKA of a specific design (Oxford; Biomet; Warsaw, IN) as reactive lines.

For fixed-bearing metal-backed tibia UKA, the two most common causes of failures were progression of arthritis in the uninvolved compartments (65%) and polyethylene wear (25%).[46,47] The average time for conversion to TKA or addition of a patellofemoral implant was 13 years (range, 3 months to 21 years). According to Kaplan-Meier analysis, the 20-year survival free of revision for any reason was 74% ± 7%.

Niinimäki et al[48] compared UKA versus TKA results performed for primary osteoarthritis. They reported on 27-year data from the Finnish joint registry, and provided comparative outcomes between those two strategies. Kaplan-Meier survivorship of UKAs was 89% at 5 years, 81% at 10 years, and 70% at 15 years. The corresponding rates for TKAs were 96%, 93%, and 88%, respectively.

UKAs had inferior long-term survivorship compared with cemented TKAs, even after adjusting for the age and sex of the patients (hazard ratio [HR] = 2.2; P < .001), but populations were not comparable in terms of indications, implant designs, and patient demographics. Despite these limitations, their conclusions outlined that UKA offers tempting advantages compared with a TKA, especially regarding functional outcomes. However, long-term revision risks are higher with a UKA,[48] but it is also well known that UKAs are also more often revised due to ease of revision compared to TKA.

Results of Medial UKA in Young Patients

In a study evaluating the results of UKA in patients younger than 50 years, our results suggested that, first, UKA for unicompartmental arthritis improved function in them and allowed a return to previous level of activities.[7] Second, satisfying radiological results can be achieved in terms of implant fixation and alignment, and third, survivorship was acceptable but lower than the survivorship for older patients. In fact, revisions for polyethylene wear or progression of arthritis in the patellofemoral joint remain important concerns in altering the survivorship of the implant in this group of patients in which conventional polyethylene was used. Our experience showed that knee function can be restored after UKA in patients younger than 50 years and UKA may be a reliable option for middle-aged patients; however, wear after 10 years remains a problem in this category of patients.[7] More recently, Walker et al[49] observed that UKA allowed patients younger than 60 years to return to regular physical activities with almost two-thirds of the patients reaching a high activity level (UCLA ≥ 7).

Results of Medial UKA in Old Patients (Older Than 75 years)

Due to the lower morbidity and mortality, UKA represents an interesting solution for older patients with unicompartmental arthritis as an alternative to TKA providing higher function and better forgotten joint scores with similar survivorship. Fabre-Aubrespy et al[50] compared, in a retrospective matched-pair study, 101 patients who underwent UKA versus patients who underwent TKA for primary osteoarthritis or osteonecrosis of the knee. Patients were matched one-to-one with a TKA group based on age, gender, BMI, and preoperative Knee Society Score (KSS).

At the last follow-up, compared with those in the TKA group, patients from UKA group had better KSS, higher Knee Injury Osteoarthritis Outcome Scores, and a better rate of forgotten knees. The 16-year survivorships free from revision for any reason were similar in the two groups.

Results of Lateral UKA

Lateral UKA can provide satisfying long-term clinical and radiological results, and the survivorship at 10, 16, and 22 years is comparable to the survivorship obtained for medial UKA.[40] Recent studies reported a very low failure rate when the results of older series were more controversial. A significant improvement of the results over time is observed and this is probably linked also to an improvement of the patient's selection.

The results of our series concerning the group of patients operated after 1989 were comparable with those reported recently and compare favorably with the results of medial UKA.[40]

Results of UKA for Avascular Osteonecrosis of the Knee

In a retrospective study,[2] we analyzed the results of UKA for osteonecrosis using a modern implant and strict inclusion criteria (limitation of the osteonecrosis to one compartment of the knee, status of the uninvolved compartment, of the patellofemoral articulation, and of the ACL, fully correctable deformity on stress radiographs). The data suggested that the UKA is an efficient procedure in osteonecrosis to improve pain and function, restoring proper lower-limb mechanical axis, and achieve a durable survivorship at 12 years.[3] Inversely, in a review of the literature, Myers et al[51] showed better outcomes after TKA for spontaneous osteonecrosis of the knee than outcomes with UKA. However, they noted an improvement

in outcome scores for the most recent series of UKA for osteonecrosis of the knee with strict selection criteria. The outcomes of UKA reported in our study[2] for osteonecrosis are comparable with the average results of TKA for osteonecrosis with a revision rate of 3%, a mean global knee score of 85 points, and 96.7% survival at 12 years.

These data suggested that UKA is reliable in osteonecrosis for relieving pain and improving function, restoring the lower-limb mechanical axis, and achieving durable survivorship.

FAILURES AND REVISION OF UKA

Introduction

The main causes of revision UKA are progression of osteoarthritis in the other compartments, aseptic loosening of the components and polyethylene (PE) wear, impingement, bearing dislocation in mobile-bearing implants, periprosthetic fracture, infection, stiffness, and unexplained pain.[52,53] The etiology of failure had to be precisely identified before the revision surgery. Early failure in UKA is mostly due to surgical mistake.[54] Postoperative hip–knee–ankle angle (HKA) is a determinant factor. A malalignment of the component with HKA greater than 3° in varus or greater than 7° of valgus has been found to lead to early failure.[55]

Progression of Osteoarthritis in the Other Compartments

Overcorrection alignment of the limb with UKA will cause overloading on the nonprosthetic compartment and generate degenerative changes.

Concerning the patellofemoral compartment, osteoarthritis changes could be linked to an oversized and/or malrotated femoral component with impingement with the femoropatellar joint. It can also be related to progression of osteoarthritis in the patellofemoral joint, especially laterally.

Treatment options are an isolated replacement of the newly involved compartment or conversion to TKA.

Aseptic Loosening

Risk factors of aseptic loosening are younger age, obesity, residual varus deformity, excessive posterior slope, ACL instability, and tibial PE wear.[52] PE wear is more frequent with fixed-bearing and is associated with component malposition, undercorrection of the preoperative deformity, quality and processing of the PE, and thickness of the PE < 6 mm. Treatment relies on the conversion to TKA. In rare cases of PE wear with well-fixed components and correct alignment of the limb, and no osteolysis or metallosis, a new modular tibial insert can be proposed with encouraging continued follow-up.[56]

Bearing Dislocation in Mobile-Bearing Implants

Bearing dislocation is a complication of mobile-bearing UKA and could be secondary to unbalanced flexion and extension gaps, impingements of the mobile insert, component malposition, or instability due to knee laxity.[57]

Bearing dislocation in lateral UKA is due to laxity of the lateral collateral ligament in flexion. Bearing dislocation in medial UKA is due to laxity of the medial collateral ligament.

It can be treated with bearing exchange to a thicker bearing or revision to TKA in case of significant laxity.

Periprosthetic Fracture

Periprosthetic fracture is an uncommon complication with incidence of less than 1%[58] and occurs more frequently on the tibial plateau below the tibial component. It can be related to a mechanical mistake with a deeper tibial cut or excessive pinning of the guide, or secondary to osteolysis and bone resorption due to PE wear or a direct knee trauma.

If the components are well fixed and in appropriate alignment, osteosynthesis could be appropriate. If the fracture is associated with component loosening, malalignment, or bone loss, a revision to TKA is recommended.

Infection

Incidence of infection following UKA is lower than after TKA. In case of acute infection of cemented UKA, irrigation and débridement associated with intravenous antibiotic therapy is recommended.[59] For the cementless prosthesis, implant removal is easier and a one-stage revision to a cemented implant associated to irrigation, débridement, and antibiotics therapy could be considered.

For chronic cases with failure of irrigation treatment or chronic infection, two-stage revision to TKA is recommended.

Stiffness

Stiffness due to arthrofibrosis is lower for UKA. It has been associated with oversizing of the femoral and tibial component or patellofemoral impingement.

If the components are appropriately sized and positioned, a manipulation under anesthesia can be performed within the first 6 weeks. Past this period, an arthroscopic arthrolysis is required. When the components are malpositioned or oversized or in case of patellofemoral impingement, revision to TKA is necessary.

Unexplained Pain

Proportion of postoperative unexplained pain is reported to be more frequent after UKA than after TKA.[60] Without a precise etiology for the failure, a revision UKA has a very high risk for persisting pain with the following TKA.[61] In these cases of unexplained pain, magnetic resonance imaging can serve to evaluate osteoarthritis progression, and arthroscopic exploration with biopsies can complete the work-up.

Preoperative Evaluation

An exhaustive evaluation should be made before revision surgery including physical examination, radiographs and CT scans, serologies, and articular aspiration to track infection. Bone scintigraphy is not a reliable test to determinate infection or loosening in the first 2 years after UKA.[61]

As in any revision surgery, a precise preoperative evaluation is required to determine the exposure and the implant of choice depending on bone loss and ligament integrity. Primary components could be utilized in some cases with minimal bone loss. Revision components with metal augments and stem extensions should be available for cases with important bone loss and have to be planned.

Revision Strategies

Due to bone defects and potential ligamentous insufficiencies, revision of UKA can be technically challenging and all the difficulties have to be anticipated. Mostly, UKA can be revised to a primary TKA. In 8%, UKAs were revised to a hinged system due to deep tibial resection damaging the MCL.[62]

In rare cases, revision UKA to a UKA can be performed. The only etiology permitting that strategy is an isolated loosened femoral or tibial component without any bone loss and ligamentous insufficiency. Several studies have shown that this procedure is associated with a three- to fourfold increased re-revision rate.[63,64]

The first step of revision strategy is to eliminate an infection in order to set a one- versus two-stage procedure. In case of failed medial UKA, the existing approach can be used and a medial capsulotomy performed. For failed lateral UKA, the more lateral skin incision has to be used. Then, according to the preference of the operator, a medial or a lateral capsulotomy can be made. The tibial plateau can be placed in external rotation and partially anteriorly dislocated to improve exposure. During implant removal, care should be taken to preserve the bone stock. All cement, necrotic, and granulomatous tissue have to be removed. The bone defect, tibial and femoral, should be compensated for restoring the initial joint line. The change of the joint line should not exceed 4 mm.[65] For minor epiphyseal defects less than 5 mm, cement or autologous bone can be used. For all defect reconstruction procedures, a stem extension is recommended. Bone defects between 5 and 8 mm can be reconstructed with autologous bone from the nonprosthetic tibial plateau and be protected with a short tibial stem extension (length

30 mm). Bone defects greater than 8 mm have to be reconstructed with metal augments or wedges. The recent use of metaphyseal trabecular metal cones has reduced the need for additional long tibial stems.

After having prepared the tibial component, the flexion gap should be prepared first. The first step is to restore the correct rotation of the femoral component, avoiding internal rotation. After having set the rotation, the size of the flexion gap has to be controlled. In case of a large flexion gap, the largest femoral component and/or posterior condyle metal augments are used. The next step is the extension gap. The distal femoral cut has to reproduce the space of the gap flexion.

Finally, testing with the trial components in place allows one to check coronal stability over the full range of motion and patellofemoral tracking.

In case of a deficiency of the ipsilateral collateral ligament, instability, or inability to balance the flexion-extension gaps, a constrained implant should be implanted.

Results of Revision UKA

- Re-revision rate

Compared to primary TKA, revised TKA after UKA had a re-revision rate 4 times higher, and revised UKA with a UKA had a re-revision rate 13 times higher.[63] This is confirmed with the data from the Australian Registry which found a higher re-revision rate for revision UKA to UKA compared to revision UKA to TKA, excluding septic complications. The cumulative percent revision rates for UKA at 5, 10, and 15 years were 8.1%, 14.6%, and 22.1%, respectively, against 3.6%, 5.3%, and 7.4%, respectively, for TKA.[66].

- Clinical outcomes

Contrary to primary UKA having better functional results than primary TKA, UKA revised to TKA had a significantly worse outcome.[63] The mean Oxford knee score after revision UKA resembles that after revised TKA. The reason for revision is an important factor for satisfaction in revision of surgery for UKA,[61] especially for unexplained pain.

- Bone loss

Revision UKA is accompanied with less bony defects than revision of TKA. In only 50% of revision UKAs, a primary TKA could be implanted without any stems or bone grafts or augments. The height of polyethylene inlay tends to be thicker than in primary TKA.[67]

Conclusion

Revision UKA to TKA is not comparable to primary TKA with worse clinical outcomes. Revision UKA to TKA is technically easier than revision TKA. A failed UKA should not be revised to another UKA. The reason for failure has to be clearly identified before revision, influencing the outcomes and technical aspects.

PROCESS OPTIMIZATION IN PERIOPERATIVE MANAGEMENT

Perioperative Management

By applying local infiltration anesthesia, an efficient optimization of pain therapy is possible,[68] as well as involving the patient in a multimodal process of pain control. The standardized use of tranexamic acid is a proven coagulation therapy resulting in reduction of swelling and hematoma formation.[69] This postoperative pain reduction will reduce the length of stay, improve rehabilitation, and allow quick recovery. The use of a tourniquet can be limited to the time of the cementing in order to reduce muscle damage.[70]

Rehabilitation and Postoperative Care

Chemical thromboembolic prophylaxis is important for minimizing the incidence of deep venous thrombosis. Liddle et al[71] reported a lower rate of thromboembolic complications following UKA compared to TKA. Patients are allowed to bear full weight as tolerated and are instructed to ambulate beginning the day of surgery. An assistive device, typically a cane or walker, is used for 1 to 2 weeks. Outpatient physical therapy sessions and home exercise programs focus on quadriceps strengthening and range of motion exercises.

A recent study[72] had suggested that self-directed exercises may be appropriate for most patients following UKA. Formal outpatient physical therapy could be still indicated for selected patients.

Conclusion

UKA is a highly effective treatment option for unicompartmental advanced degenerative disease, particularly for young and active patients, offering several advantages over TKA. The 10-year survival has been reported to be similar to TKA with proper patient selection and surgical principles.

The advantages of UKA include preservation of bone stock, better functional results, a faster recovery time, greater range of motion, preservation of normal knee's kinematics, lower postoperative infection rate, and shorter hospital stay. For young and active patients, a modern UKA represents a valid alternative to bridge the gap between HTO and TKA.

Component loosening, progression of arthritis in the remaining compartments, and polyethylene wear remain a problem, particularly in young, active, and heavy patients. Correct implant orientation and alignment are essential to reduce edge loading, contact stresses, and wear. In a similar manner, overstuffing the unresurfaced compartment leads to rapid progression of arthritis in the other compartments.

Recent evolutions in terms of surgical technique and implant designs have made UKA the gold standard for patients with severe monocompartmental intra-articular deformities secondary to osteoarthritis.

REFERENCES

1. Marmor L. Unicompartmental arthroplasty for osteonecrosis of the knee joint. *Clin Orthop Relat Res.* 1993;294:247-253.

2. Parratte S, Argenson J-NA, Dumas J, Aubaniac J-M. Unicompartmental knee arthroplasty for avascular osteonecrosis. *Clin Orthop Relat Res.* 2007;464:37-42. doi:10.1097/BLO.0b013e31812f7821.

3. Ollivier M, Jacquet C, Lucet A, Parratte S, Argenson J-N. Long-term results of medial unicompartmental knee arthroplasty for knee avascular necrosis. *J Arthroplasty.* 2018;34(3):465-468. doi:10.1016/j.arth.2018.11.010.

4. Lum ZC, Crawford DA, Lombardi AV, et al. Early comparative outcomes of unicompartmental and total knee arthroplasty in severely obese patients. *Knee.* 2018;25(1):161-166. doi:10.1016/j.knee.2017.10.006.

5. Berend KR, Berend ME, Dalury DF, Argenson J-N, Dodd CA, Scott RD. Consensus statement on indications and contraindications for medial unicompartmental knee arthroplasty. *J Surg Orthop Adv.* 2015;24(4):252-256.

6. Price AJ, Dodd Ca. F, Svard UGC, Murray DW. Oxford medial unicompartmental knee arthroplasty in patients younger and older than 60 years of age. *J Bone Joint Surg Br.* 2005;87(11):1488-1492. doi:10.1302/0301-620X.87B11.16324.

7. Parratte S, Argenson J-NA, Pearce O, Pauly V, Auquier P, Aubaniac J-M. Medial unicompartmental knee replacement in the under-50s. *J Bone Joint Surg Br.* 2009;91(3):351-356. doi:10.1302/0301-620X.91B3.21588.

8. Berend KR, Lombardi AV, Morris MJ, Hurst JM, Kavolus JJ. Does preoperative patellofemoral joint state affect medial unicompartmental arthroplasty survival? *Orthopedics.* 2011;34(9):e494-e496. doi:10.3928/01477447-20110714-39.

9. Konan S, Haddad FS. Does location of patellofemoral chondral lesion influence outcome after Oxford medial compartmental knee arthroplasty? *Bone Joint J.* 2016;98-B(10 suppl B):11-15. doi:10.1302/0301-620X.98B10.BJJ-2016-0403.R1.

10. Hernigou P, Pascale W, Pascale V, Homma Y, Poignard A. Does primary or secondary chondrocalcinosis influence long-term survivorship of unicompartmental arthroplasty? *Clin Orthop Relat Res.* 2012;470(7):1973-1979. doi:10.1007/s11999-011-2211-5.

11. Lustig S, Parratte S, Magnussen RA, Argenson J-N, Neyret P. Lateral unicompartmental knee arthroplasty relieves pain and improves function in posttraumatic osteoarthritis. *Clin Orthop Relat Res.* 2012;470(1):69-76. doi:10.1007/s11999-011-1963-2.

12. Valenzuela GA, Jacobson NA, Buzas D, et al. Unicompartmental knee replacement after high tibial osteotomy: invalidating a contraindication. *Bone Joint J.* 2013;95-B(10):1348-1353. doi:10.1302/0301-620X.95B10.30541.

13. Boissonneault A, Pandit H, Pegg E, et al. No difference in survivorship after unicompartmental knee arthroplasty with or without an intact anterior cruciate ligament. *Knee Surg Sports Traumatol Arthrosc.* 2013;21(11):2480-2486. doi:10.1007/s00167-012-2101-8.

14. Weston-Simons JS, Pandit H, Jenkins C, et al. Outcome of combined unicompartmental knee replacement and combined or sequential anterior cruciate ligament reconstruction: a study of 52 cases with mean follow-up of five years. *J Bone Joint Surg Br.* 2012;94(9):1216-1220. doi:10.1302/0301-620X.94B9.28881.

15. Hamilton TW, Pandit HG, Inabathula A, et al. Unsatisfactory outcomes following unicompartmental knee arthroplasty in patients with partial thickness cartilage loss: a medium-term follow-up. *Bone Joint J.* 2017;99-B(4):475-482. doi:10.1302/0301-620X.99B4.BJJ-2016-1061.R1.

16. Smith TO, Hing CB, Davies L, Donell ST. Fixed versus mobile bearing unicompartmental knee replacement: a meta-analysis. *Orthop Traumatol Surg Res.* 2009;95(8):599-605. doi:10.1016/j.otsr.2009.10.006.

17. Li MG, Yao F, Joss B, Ioppolo J, Nivbrant B, Wood D. Mobile vs. fixed bearing unicondylar knee arthroplasty: a randomized study on short term clinical outcomes and knee kinematics. *Knee.* 2006;13(5):365-370. doi:10.1016/j.knee.2006.05.003.

18. Emerson RH, Hansborough T, Reitman RD, Rosenfeldt W, Higgins LL. Comparison of a mobile with a fixed-bearing unicompartmental knee implant. *Clin Orthop Relat Res.* 2002;404:62-70.

19. Parratte S, Pauly V, Aubaniac J-M, Argenson J-NA. No long-term difference between fixed and mobile medial unicompartmental arthroplasty. *Clin Orthop Relat Res.* 2012;470(1):61-68. doi:10.1007/s11999-011-1961-4.

20. Peersman G, Stuyts B, Vandenlangenbergh T, Cartier P, Fennema P. Fixed- versus mobile-bearing UKA: a systematic review and meta-analysis. *Knee Surg Sports Traumatol Arthrosc.* 2015;23(11):3296-3305. doi:10.1007/s00167-014-3131-1.

21. Burton A, Williams S, Brockett CL, Fisher J. In vitro comparison of fixed- and mobile meniscal-bearing unicondylar knee arthroplasties: effect of design, kinematics, and condylar lift-off. *J Arthroplasty.* 2012;27(8):1452-1459. doi:10.1016/j.arth.2012.02.011.

22. Schlueter-Brust K, Kugland K, Stein G, et al. Ten year survivorship after cemented and uncemented medial Uniglide® unicompartmental knee arthroplasties. *Knee.* 2014;21(5):964-970. doi:10.1016/j.knee.2014.03.009.

23. Panzram B, Bertlich I, Reiner T, Walker T, Hagmann S, Gotterbarm T. Cementless Oxford medial unicompartimental knee replacement: an independent series with a 5-year-follow-up. *Arch Orthop Trauma Surg.* 2017;137(7):1011-1017. doi:10.1007/s00402-017-2696-9.

24. Pandit H, Liddle AD, Kendrick BJL, et al. Improved fixation in cementless unicompartmental knee replacement: five-year results of a randomized controlled trial. *J Bone Joint Surg Am.* 2013;95(15):1365-1372. doi:10.2106/JBJS.L.01005.

25. Kendrick BJL, Kaptein BL, Valstar ER, et al. Cemented versus cementless Oxford unicompartmental knee arthroplasty using radiostereometric analysis: a randomised controlled trial. *Bone Joint J.* 2015;97-B(2):185-191. doi:10.1302/0301-620X.97B2.34331.

26. Seeger JB, Haas D, Jäger S, Röhner E, Tohtz S, Clarius M. Extended sagittal saw cut significantly reduces fracture load in cementless unicompartmental knee arthroplasty compared to cemented tibia plateaus: an experimental cadaver study. *Knee Surg Sports Traumatol Arthrosc.* 2012;20(6):1087-1091. doi:10.1007/s00167-011-1698-3.

27. Saenz CL, McGrath MS, Marker DR, Seyler TM, Mont MA, Bonutti PM. Early failure of a unicompartmental knee arthroplasty design with an all-polyethylene tibial component. *Knee.* 2010;17(1):53-56. doi:10.1016/j.knee.2009.05.007.

28. Scott CEH, Eaton MJ, Nutton RW, Wade FA, Evans SL, Pankaj P. Metal-backed versus all-polyethylene unicompartmental knee arthroplasty: proximal tibial strain in an experimentally validated finite element model. *Bone Joint Res.* 2017;6(1):22-30. doi:10.1302/2046-3758.61.BJR-2016-0142.R1.

29. Lustig S, Paillot J-L, Servien E, Henry J, Ait Si Selmi T, Neyret P. Cemented all polyethylene tibial insert unicompartmental knee arthroplasty: a long term follow-up study. *Orthop Traumatol Surg Res.* 2009;95(1):12-21. doi:10.1016/j.otsr.2008.04.001.

30. Hutt JRB, Farhadnia P, Massé V, LaVigne M, Vendittoli P-A. A randomised trial of all-polyethylene and metal-backed tibial components in unicompartmental arthroplasty of the knee. *Bone Joint J.* 2015;97-B(6):786-792. doi:10.1302/0301-620X.97B6.35433.

31. Du PZ, Markolf KL, Boguszewski DV, McAllister DR. Femoral contact forces in the anterior cruciate ligament deficient knee: a robotic study. *Arthroscopy.* 2018;34(12):3226-3233. doi:10.1016/j.arthro.2018.06.051.

32. Matsui Y, Kadoya Y, Uehara K, Kobayashi A, Takaoka K. Rotational deformity in varus osteoarthritis of the knee: analysis with computed tomography. *Clin Orthop Relat Res.* 2005;433:147-151.

33. Casino D, Martelli S, Zaffagnini S, et al. Knee stability before and after total and unicondylar knee replacement: in vivo kinematic evaluation utilizing navigation. *J Orthop Res.* 2009;27(2):202-207. doi:10.1002/jor.20746.

34. Argenson J-NA, Komistek RD, Aubaniac J-M, et al. In vivo determination of knee kinematics for subjects implanted with a unicompartmental arthroplasty. *J Arthroplasty.* 2002;17(8):1049-1054. doi:10.1054/arth.2002.34527.

35. Lo Presti M, Costa GG, Cialdella S, et al. Return to sports after unicompartmental knee arthroplasty: reality or utopia? A 48-month follow-up prospective study. *J Knee Surg.* 2018;32(2):186-191. doi:10.1055/s-0038-1635111.

36. Pandit H, Jenkins C, Beard DJ, et al. Cementless Oxford unicompartmental knee replacement shows reduced radiolucency at one year. *J Bone Joint Surg Br.* 2009;91(2):185-189. doi:10.1302/0301-620X.91B2.21413.

37. Parratte S, Ollivier M, Lunebourg A, Abdel MP, Argenson J-N. Long-term results of compartmental arthroplasties of the knee: long term results of partial knee arthroplasty. *Bone Joint J.* 2015;97-B(10 suppl A):9-15. doi:10.1302/0301-620X.97B10.36426.

38. Lustig S, Lording T, Frank F, Debette C, Servien E, Neyret P. Progression of medial osteoarthritis and long term results of lateral unicompartmental arthroplasty: 10 to 18 year follow-up of 54 consecutive implants. *Knee.* 2014;21(suppl 1):S26-S32. doi:10.1016/S0968-0160(14)50006-3.

39. Sah AP, Scott RD. Lateral unicompartmental knee arthroplasty through a medial approach. Surgical technique. *J Bone Joint Surg Am.* 2008;90 suppl 2(Pt 2):195-205. doi:10.2106/JBJS.H.00257.

40. Argenson J-NA, Parratte S, Bertani A, Flecher X, Aubaniac J-M. Long-term results with a lateral unicondylar replacement. *Clin Orthop Relat Res.* 2008;466(11):2686-2693. doi:10.1007/s11999-008-0351-z.

41. Ollivier M, Abdel MP, Parratte S, Argenson J-N. Lateral unicondylar knee arthroplasty (UKA): contemporary indications, surgical technique, and results. *Int Orthop.* 2014;38(2):449-455. doi:10.1007/s00264-013-2222-9.

42. Vasso M, Del Regno C, Perisano C, D'Amelio A, Corona K, Schiavone Panni A. Unicompartmental knee arthroplasty is effective: ten year results. *Int Orthop.* 2015;39(12):2341-2346. doi:10.1007/s00264-015-2809-4.

43. Pandit H, Jenkins C, Gill HS, Barker K, Dodd CAF, Murray DW. Minimally invasive Oxford phase 3 unicompartmental knee replacement: results of 1000 cases. *J Bone Joint Surg Br.* 2011;93(2):198-204. doi:10.1302/0301-620X.93B2.25767.

44. Lunebourg A, Parratte S, Ollivier M, Abdel MP, Argenson J-NA. Are revisions of unicompartmental knee arthroplasties more like a primary or revision TKA? *J Arthroplasty.* 2015;30(11):1985-1989. doi:10.1016/j.arth.2015.05.042.

45. Price AJ, Waite JC, Svard U. Long-term clinical results of the medial Oxford unicompartmental knee arthroplasty. *Clin Orthop Relat Res.* 2005;435:171-180.

46. Argenson J-NA, Parratte S, Flecher X, Aubaniac J-M. Unicompartmental knee arthroplasty: technique through a mini-incision. *Clin Orthop Relat Res.* 2007;464:32-36. doi:10.1097/BLO.0b013e3180986da7.

47. Argenson J-NA, Blanc G, Aubaniac J-M, Parratte S. Modern unicompartmental knee arthroplasty with cement: a concise follow-up, at a mean of twenty years, of a previous report. *J Bone Joint Surg Am.* 2013;95(10):905-909. doi:10.2106/JBJS.L.00963.

48. Niinimäki T, Eskelinen A, Mäkelä K, Ohtonen P, Puhto A-P, Remes V. Unicompartmental knee arthroplasty survivorship is lower than TKA survivorship: a 27-year Finnish registry study. *Clin Orthop Relat Res.* 2014;472(5):1496-1501. doi:10.1007/s11999-013-3347-2.

49. Walker T, Streit J, Gotterbarm T, Bruckner T, Merle C, Streit MR. Sports, physical activity and patient-reported outcomes after medial unicompartmental knee arthroplasty in young patients. *J Arthroplasty.* 2015;30(11):1911-1916. doi:10.1016/j.arth.2015.05.031.

50. Fabre-Aubrespy M, Ollivier M, Pesenti S, Parratte S, Argenson J-N. Unicompartmental knee arthroplasty in patients older than 75 results in better clinical outcomes and similar survivorship compared to total knee arthroplasty. A matched controlled study. *J Arthroplasty.* 2016;31(12):2668-2671. doi:10.1016/j.arth.2016.06.034.

51. Myers TG, Cui Q, Kuskowski M, Mihalko WM, Saleh KJ. Outcomes of total and unicompartmental knee arthroplasty for secondary and spontaneous osteonecrosis of the knee. *J Bone Joint Surg Am.* 2006;88 suppl 3:76-82. doi:10.2106/JBJS.F.00568.

52. Kim KT, Lee S, Lee JI, Kim JW. Analysis and treatment of complications after unicompartmental knee arthroplasty. *Knee Surg Relat Res.* 2016;28(1):46-54. doi:10.5792/ksrr.2016.28.1.46.

53. Kim S-J, Postigo R, Koo S, Kim JH. Causes of revision following Oxford phase 3 unicompartmental knee arthroplasty. *Knee Surg Sports Traumatol Arthrosc.* 2014;22(8):1895-1901. doi:10.1007/s00167-013-2644-3.

54. Fehring TK, Odum SM, Masonis JL, Springer BD. Early failures in unicondylar arthroplasty. *Orthopedics.* 2010;33(1):11. doi:10.3928/01477447-20091124-10.

55. Perkins TR, Gunckle W. Unicompartmental knee arthroplasty: 3- to 10-year results in a community hospital setting. *J Arthroplasty.* 2002;17(3):293-297.

56. Lunebourg A, Parratte S, Galland A, Lecuire F, Ollivier M, Argenson J-N. Is isolated insert exchange a valuable choice for polyethylene wear in metal-backed unicompartmental knee arthroplasty? *Knee Surg Sports Traumatol Arthrosc.* 2016;24(10):3280-3286. doi:10.1007/s00167-014-3392-8.

57. Pandit H, Hamilton TW, Jenkins C, Mellon SJ, Dodd CAF, Murray DW. The clinical outcome of minimally invasive Phase 3 Oxford unicompartmental knee arthroplasty: a 15-year follow-up of 1000 UKAs. *Bone Joint J.* 2015;97-B(11):1493-1500. doi:10.1302/0301-620X.97B11.35634.

58. Brown NM, Engh G, Fricka K. Periprosthetic fracture following partial knee arthroplasty. *J Knee Surg.* 2018;32(10):947-952. doi:10.1055/s-0038-1672204.

59. Labruyère C, Zeller V, Lhotellier L, et al. Chronic infection of unicompartmental knee arthroplasty: one-stage conversion to total knee arthroplasty. *Orthop Traumatol Surg Res.* 2015;101(5):553-557. doi:10.1016/j.otsr.2015.04.006.

60. Baker PN, Petheram T, Avery PJ, Gregg PJ, Deehan DJ. Revision for unexplained pain following unicompartmental and total knee replacement. *J Bone Joint Surg Am.* 2012;94(17):e126. doi:10.2106/JBJS.K.00791.

61. Kerens B, Boonen B, Schotanus M, Lacroix H, Emans PJ, Kort N. Revision from unicompartmental to total knee replacement: the clinical outcome depends on reason for revision. *Bone Joint J.* 2013;95-B:1204-1208. doi:10.1302/0301-620X.95B9.31085.

62. Khan Z, Nawaz SZ, Kahane S, Esler C, Chatterji U. Conversion of unicompartmental knee arthroplasty to total knee arthroplasty: the challenges and need for augments. *Acta Orthop Belg.* 2013;79(6):699-705.

63. Pearse AJ, Hooper GJ, Rothwell A, Frampton C. Survival and functional outcome after revision of a unicompartmental to a total knee replacement: the New Zealand National Joint Registry. *J Bone Joint Surg Br.* 2010;92(4):508-512. doi:10.1302/0301-620X.92B4.22659.

64. Hang JR, Stanford TE, Graves SE, Davidson DC, de Steiger RN, Miller LN. Outcome of revision of unicompartmental knee replacement. *Acta Orthop.* 2010;81(1):95-98. doi:10.3109/17453671003628731.

65. Kowalczewski JB, Labey L, Chevalier Y, Okon T, Innocenti B, Bellemans J. Does joint line elevation after revision knee arthroplasty affect tibio-femoral kinematics, contact pressure or collateral ligament lengths? An in vitro analysis. *Arch Med Sci.* 2015;11(2):311-318. doi:10.5114/aoms.2014.46078.

66. Davidson MD, De Steiger PR, Lewis MP, et al. Australian Orthopaedic Association National Joint Replacement Registry. Annual Report 2016. Hip, Knee & Shoulder Arthroplasty.

67. Dudley TE, Gioe TJ, Sinner P, Mehle S. Registry outcomes of unicompartmental knee arthroplasty revisions. *Clin Orthop Relat Res.* 2008;466(7):1666-1670. doi:10.1007/s11999-008-0279-3.

68. Hu B, Lin T, Yan S-G, et al. Local infiltration analgesia versus regional blockade for postoperative analgesia in total knee arthroplasty: a meta-analysis of randomized controlled trials. *Pain Physician.* 2016;19(4):205-214.

69. Samujh C, Falls TD, Wessel R, Smith L, Malkani AL. Decreased blood transfusion following revision total knee arthroplasty using tranexamic acid. *J Arthroplasty.* 2014;29(9 suppl):182-185. doi:10.1016/j.arth.2014.03.047.

70. Pfitzner T, von Roth P, Voerkelius N, Mayr H, Perka C, Hube R. Influence of the tourniquet on tibial cement mantle thickness in primary total knee arthroplasty. *Knee Surg Sports Traumatol Arthrosc.* 2016;24(1):96-101. doi:10.1007/s00167-014-3341-6.

71. Liddle AD, Judge A, Pandit H, Murray DW. Adverse outcomes after total and unicompartmental knee replacement in 101,330 matched patients: a study of data from the National Joint Registry for England and Wales. *Lancet.* 2014;384(9952):1437-1445. doi:10.1016/S0140-6736(14)60419-0.

72. Fillingham YA, Darrith B, Lonner JH, Culvern C, Crizer M, Della Valle CJ. Formal physical therapy may not be necessary after unicompartmental knee arthroplasty: a randomized clinical trial. *J Arthroplasty.* 2018;33(7S):S93-S99.e3. doi:10.1016/j.arth.2018.02.049.

chapter 41

Robotic Application of Unicompartmental Knee Arthroplasty

Joost A. Burger, MD | Andrew D. Pearle, MD

INTRODUCTION

Unicompartmental knee arthroplasty (UKA) has become a reliable treatment for isolated unicompartmental knee osteoarthritis (OA) that has a quicker recovery, improved function, less morbidity, lower risk of infection, and less blood loss compared to total knee arthroplasty.[1,2] However, longevity of the UKA remains a concern, which contributes in preventing widespread acceptance. While high-volume UKA surgeons have reported comparable long-term survivorship to TKA, less specialized surgeons have shown inferior survival rates.[3] Current registry-based studies have shown that surgeons, as well as hospital volume, influence survivorship for UKA.[4,5]

With the increased utilization of UKA, the understanding of the surgical factors influencing UKA outcomes has advanced. Lower limb alignment, implant positioning, implant size, and knee stability have all been shown to influence function and survivorship after UKA.[6] When using a conventional technique, consistency of these surgical variables remains difficult in UKA, even when it is done by highly experienced surgeons.[7] In addition, current surgeons often perform UKA with a minimally invasive technique to reduce soft-tissue and bone trauma, making the procedure even more demanding.[8]

Over almost 3 decades, technological advances have developed to control essential surgical variables to optimize UKA outcomes. In 1992, the first robotic system was used for joint arthroplasty. It was an autonomous system, meaning that the robot performed a predefined operative plan independent of any surgeon. Device-specific complications and the autonomous nature of the system led to concerns about the safety, resulting in initial rejection.[9] Another technology used in the orthopedic operating room is computer-assisted navigation. This is classified as a passive device since it assists the surgeon in creating an operative plan and provides visual guidance while using surgical tools. Although this is a powerful visual aid, the outcome of the procedure still relies on conventional tools, which can limit the accuracy of the bone cuts. For this reason, semi-autonomous robotic systems were developed. In contrast to computer-assisted surgery, which provides passive guidance and feedback, these systems provide restraints for surgical bone resection within a predefined operative plan by feedback and safety controls. This prevents inadvertent bone removal and has been shown to be more accurate regarding implant placement than conventional techniques.[10] In 2001, the first semi-autonomous robotic system was used in TKA, expanding later to UKA.[11] Cobb et al studied the results of this system in UKA and showed that tibiofemoral alignment in the coronal plane was within 2° of the surgical plan in 100% of UKA patients using the semi-autonomous robotic system compared to 40% using a conventional technique.[12] This led to growing interest and increase development of so-called robotic-assisted systems.

Currently, two robotic-assisted systems are commercially available for UKA. The Mako system (Stryker, Mahwah, NJ, USA) initially obtained FDA clearance in November 2008 and was first CE marked in January 2008. The Navio system (Smith & Nephew, Memphis, TN, USA) initially received FDA and CE Mark approval in February and December 2012, respectively. This chapter gives an overview of these systems and their performances in the setting of UKA, with the pearls and pitfalls of these systems being discussed.

MAKO SYSTEM

Registration and Planning Procedure

The Mako robot is an image-based system; therefore, a preoperative CT scan is acquired to generate a patient-specific 3D model of the knee. The system allows the surgeon to template the femoral and tibial component on the generated model, preoperatively, based on alignment parameters (**Fig. 41-1**). Before the patient arrives in the operation room, the Mako system is positioned. When the patient is positioned and sterilely draped, small incisions are used to place optical tracker pins into the tibia and femur, which helps the robotic system determine where the leg is in space. Next, an incision for the UKA procedure is made and anatomical landmarks are registered. The hip rotation center is located by rotating the femur in a clockwise fashion and an optically tracked pointer is used to capture ankle and knee landmarks (**Fig. 41-2**). The surgeon then registers several mapping points on the tibial and femoral bone surface, allowing the robotic system to merge the preoperative 3D model with the actual anatomy of the knee (**Fig. 41-3**). A virtual plan

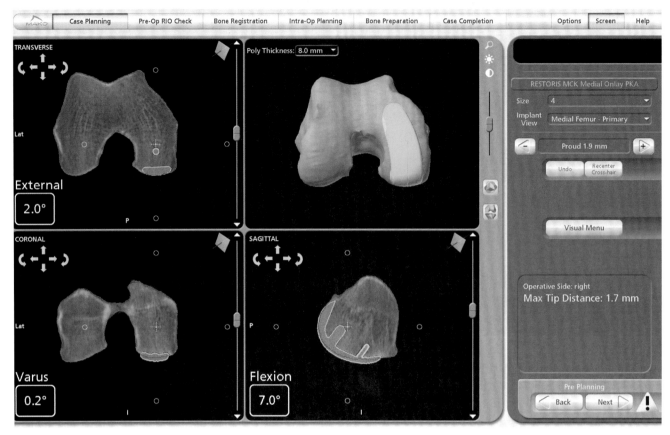

FIGURE 41-1   Mako example: preoperative planning of the femoral component on top of the CT-based patient-specific 3D model of the knee.

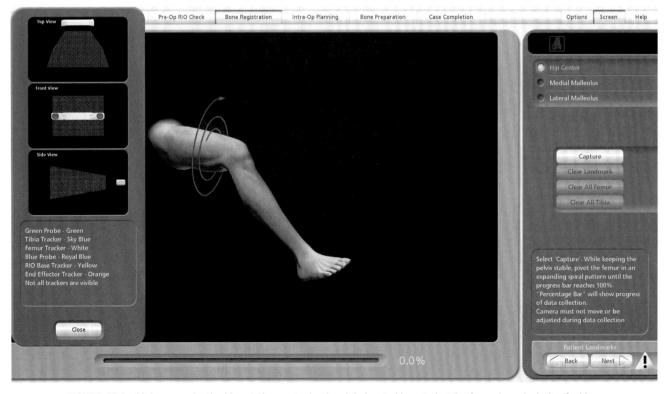

FIGURE 41-2   Mako example: the hip rotation center landmark is located by rotating the femur in a clockwise fashion.

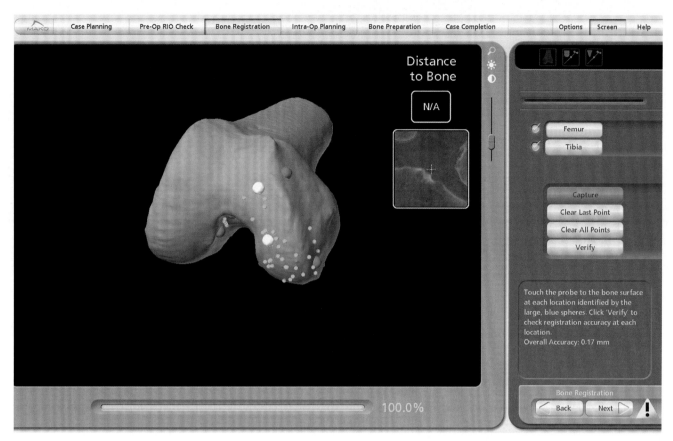

FIGURE 41-3   Mako example: the surgeon uses an optically tracked pointer to register several mapping points (green dots) to merge the CT-based 3D bone model with the actual anatomy of knee, which is then checked for accuracy (white and blue dots).

is generated after the knee is put through a full range of flexion while valgus (medial UKA) or varus (lateral UKA) load is applied to restore collateral ligament tension. At this point the system provides the surgeon with implant tracking and gap-distance information throughout the entire range of flexion (**Fig. 41-4**). With these data, the surgeon will optimize the preoperative plan by adjusting component positioning and size, so that proper patient-specific kinematics can be restored and the Mako system can determine the final required bone resection areas.

Plan Execution

To begin bone preparation in accordance with the surgeon's plan, the high-speed saline-cooled burr employed by the robotic arm is placed in the surgical field. The robotic arm and burr are under direct control of the surgeon. During execution of the predefined plan, movement and bone resection with the burr is virtually visible on the monitor (**Fig. 41-5**). When the surgeon reaches the virtual resection boundaries, the system provides auditory and tactile feedback, restricting bone cuts outside predefined resection areas. In addition, the burr automatically stops if the surgeon goes outside the area or when rapid movement of the patient's anatomy occurs. After the bone is properly prepared, trial implants are placed to test kinematics of the knee. Finally, the cemented UKA

components are implanted and the appropriate polyethylene insert is chosen (**Fig. 41-6**). The Mako system has a closed-implant platform, allowing only one UKA implant design to be used during the procedure.

Accuracy and Reproducibility

The majority of the literature regarding accuracy and reproducibility of the Mako robot has shown promising results for UKA. A randomized controlled trial by Bell et al compared the accuracy of component positioning in the axial, coronal, and sagittal plane between 62 Mako and 58 conventional UKAs using postoperative CT scans. Root mean squared (RMS) errors were lower using robotic UKA in all component parameters ($P < .01$). The number of patients with implant positioning within 2° of the target position was significantly higher for all tibial and femoral planes using the Mako system.[7] Lonner and colleagues retrospectively reviewed 27 conventional and 31 Mako UKAs. They found that RMS error of the tibial slope was 3.1° in the conventional group and 1.9° in the robotic-assisted group, with 2.6 times greater variability for the conventional group ($P = .02$). In the coronal plan, RMS error was 3.4° with the conventional technique and 1.8° with the Mako system ($P < .0001$).[13] Earlier findings by Coon et al found similar results, comparing 44 conventional and 33 robotic UKAs.[14] Citak et al

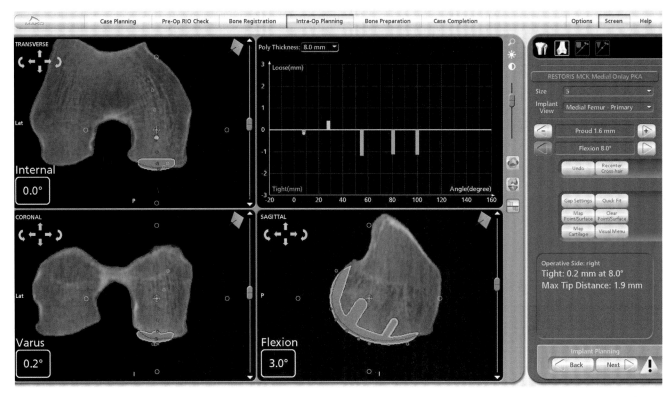

FIGURE 41-4 Mako example: Adjusting implant positioning and size in transverse, coronal, and sagittal plane based on alignment values, implant tracking (red and orange dots) and gap distance information (graph in the upper right quandrant).

used cadavers to compare implant positioning between Mako (6 knees) and conventional UKAs (12 knees). The authors found that translation and angular RMS errors for implant orientation were better using Mako than the conventional UKA. RMS error differences between the two techniques were 3.5 mm and 6.5° for femoral component placement; and 4.3 mm and 14.2° for tibial component placement.[15]

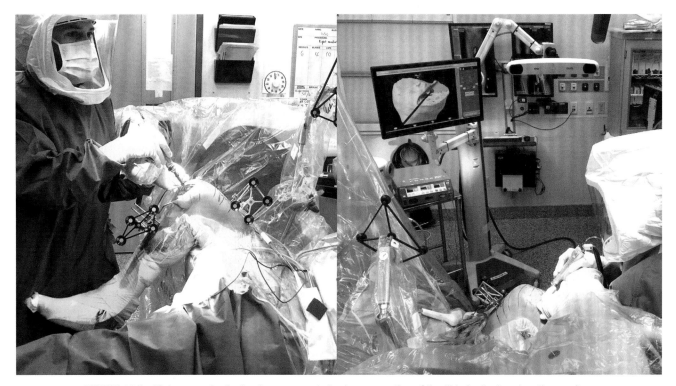

FIGURE 41-5 Mako example: the burring process during bone resection of the tibia is displayed on the monitor.

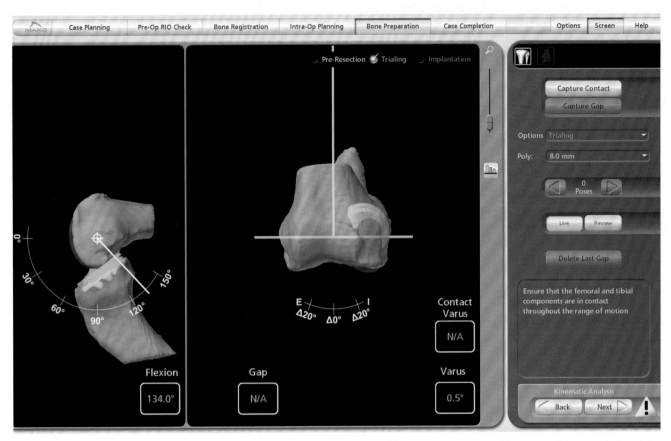

FIGURE 41-6   Mako example: an appropiate polyethylene thickness is chosen to restore proper patient specific kinematics of the knee during trialing. (Image reprinted with permission from Stryker Corporation. Copyright © 2019 Stryker Corporation. All rights reserved.)

A noncomparative study by Dunbar et al reported accuracy of implant placement in 50 Mako UKA patients. The authors showed that translation and angular RMS error was within 1.6 mm and 3.0°, respectively, for both the femoral component and tibial component in all planes.[16] Khamaisy et al showed improved congruence and restored joint space width of the lateral compartment after robotic medial UKA.[17] Comparable findings were noted for robotic lateral UKAs.[18] A study by Plate et al examined soft-tissue balancing in 52 UKA patients through a full range of flexion angles (0°, 30°, 60°, 90°, 110°). They observed soft-tissue balancing was accurate up to 0.53 mm compared to the preoperative plan, with 83% of the patients within 1 mm.[19]

Despite the aforementioned results favoring the Mako system, one retrospective study reported little to no radiographic differences between the Mako and conventional UKA.[20] In addition, a prospective study by MacCallum et al compared tibial positioning of 87 Mako with 177 conventional UKAs using postoperative radiographs. Tibial baseplate positioning in the coronal plane was significantly more accurate with the Mako system than with the conventional technique; however, the conventional UKA was more accurate in the sagittal plane.[21]

Clinical Outcomes

Due to the relative recency of the Mako development, mid- to long-term data are not widely available yet. As this system is utilized more for UKA procedures, the available data pool will become larger and more mature. At this moment, Pearle et al have examined survivorship in a multicenter cohort of 1080 robotic UKAs with a minimum follow-up of 2 years (mean 2.5 years).[22] A survival rate of 98.8% and a satisfaction rate of 92% were reported. Kleeblad et al studied survivorship and patient satisfaction as well, including 432 robotic UKAs with a minimum follow-up of 5 years (mean 5.7 years). They found a survival rate of 97.5% and reported that 91% patients were satisfied with their overall knee function.[23] These findings seem to be higher than other large cohorts, including conventional UKAs.[22,24]

With regard to functional outcomes, a retrospective study by Hansen et al found greater range of movement at 2 weeks follow-up in the conventional than the Mako group. However, the authors reported that Mako UKA patients had a shorter length of stay in the hospital and earlier clearance of physical therapy.[20] An RCT by Blyth et al showed faster decrease of postoperative pain scores in the Mako than the conventional group. In addition, the authors found significantly higher AKKS scores at 3 months follow-up for the robotic UKA patients, although this significant difference was no longer observed at 1 year.[25] Interestingly, comparative studies analyzing gait demonstrated that the Mako UKA resulted in a more normal gait pattern than conventional UKA at short- and mid-term follow-up.[26,27] Although the literature is highly supportive of the Mako system's accuracy when compared to conventional UKA, more evidence is needed in order to confidently evaluate the clinical benefits of each method.

NAVIO SYSTEM

Registration and Planning Procedure

The registration and planning process of the Navio system is fairly similar to the Mako system for UKA. However, instead of using a CT scan to generate a 3D model of the patient's knee, a mapping procedure with an optically tracked pointer is used. Therefore, the Navio system is classified as an imageless system. Similar to the Mako system, optical tracker pins are fixed to the femur and tibia for spatial orientation, landmarks (rotation of the hip center, knee, and ankle) are registered, and the incision for the approach to the knee is made. The surgeon will then move the pointer over the bony surface of the hemitibial plateau and the femoral hemi-condyle (**Fig. 41-7**). This "painting" procedure allows the system to create a 3D model of the medial (medial UKA) or lateral knee (lateral UKA). A gap-balancing process comparable to the Mako system is then initiated to provide the surgeon with tracking and gap-distance information throughout the entire range of flexion (**Fig. 41-8**). Based on these data and lower limb alignment, implant size and position are

determined by the system. Final adjustment can be made by the surgeon prior to bone resection for proper patient-specific kinematics (**Fig. 41-9**).

Plan Execution

To burr the predefined resection area, a lightweight hand-held tool, rather than a robotic arm, is controlled by the surgeon (**Fig. 41-10**). Furthermore, unlike the Mako system that provides haptic constraints through the robotic arm, the hand-held burr prevents inadvertent bone resection by speed and exposure control safeguards. Each safeguard functions based on the tool's position in relation to the predefined resection area. When the surgeon moves the tool closer to the boundaries of the resection area, the exposure mode will automatically begin to retract the burr back within the tool's guard while the speed mode begins to decrease burr speed. Each mode operates in a gradual manner and places greater restriction on the tool as it is moved closer to the boundaries of the preplanned area. After bone preparation, implant installation and verification can be established. In design, the Navio system was to be an open-implant platform. However, when acquired by Smith and Nephew in 2014, the Navio system was converted to a semiclosed-implant platform allowing multiple different Smith and Nephew implant designs to be used.

Accuracy and Reproducibility

Studies reporting accuracy of implant positioning after Navio UKA are increasing. A study by Khare et al compared implant orientation of the Navio and conventional UKA using pre- and postoperative CT scans of 12 cadaver

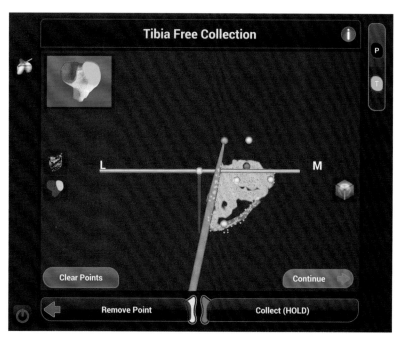

FIGURE 41-7   Navio example: "painting process" of the tibia with the optically tracked pointer to generated a 3D model of the patient-specific knee.

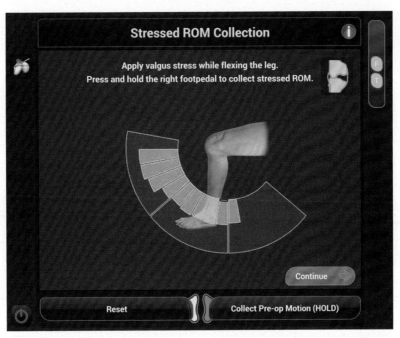

FIGURE 41-8 Navio example: the surgeon puts the patient's knee through a full range of flexion while valgus (medial UKA) load is applied to restore collateral ligament tension. The system tracks the movement of the limb to generate implant tracking and gap distance information.

specimens. The maximum RMS femoral implant orientation was for the robotic approach 2.81° and for the conventional approach 7.52°. The maximum RMS tibial implant orientation was 2.96° and 4.05°, respectively.[28] Lonner et al found similar angular results using the Navio UKA in 25 cadavers. Femoral implant angular RMS within 2.28° and translation RMS errors within 1.62 mm for all planes was reported. Tibial implant angular and translation RMS errors were within 2.43° and 1.60 mm, respectively.[29]

Gregori et al examined the mechanical axis alignment on radiographs of 92 patients who underwent Navio UKA. The authors found that the planned and the postoperative coronal alignment was within 3° in 89% of the patients, with an RMS error of 1.98°. The RMS error between the implant plan and the postoperative coronal position of the femoral and tibial component, and tibial slope was within 2.9°.[30] Herry et al showed that planning of the implant positioning and the accuracy resulted in improved joint-line restitution, comparing 40 Navio UKA patients with 40 conventional UKA patients. Mean joint line height difference was 1.5 mm after Navio UKA and 4.6 mm after the conventional technique, meaning that the joint line was distalized more in the conventional group (P < .05).[31] Batailler et al performed a case-control trial to compare the limb alignment, tibial implant position, and revision rate between 80 Navio UKAs (57 medial and 23 lateral) and 80 matched conventional UKAs. Significantly less outliers were reported for limb alignment, as well as for coronal and sagittal tibial position in the robotic lateral and medial UKA (P < .05). Furthermore, component malposition or limb malalignment were the main reasons for revision in the conventional group (86%), compared to none in the robotic group.[32]

Overall, precision of implant positioning with the Navio system appears to be similar to the Mako system; however, the Navio technology still needs more clinical assessment to confirm these results.

Clinical Outcomes

The Navio system was commercially available 4 years after the Mako system, and therefore time is needed to develop a larger base of supporting literature. A study by Parra et al reported a single-center case series of 47 patients using the Navio. They reported significantly improvement of quality of life and function during sport and recreational activities, as well as reduced pain after robotic UKA.[33] Gonzales showed that 18 patients reported preoperative OKS scores of 22, which improved to 37 at 6 weeks after surgery.[34] Another study by Canetti reported reduce time to return to sport after Navio UKA (11 knees) compared to conventional UKA (17 knees) (P < .01).[35] Furthermore, a study by Battenberg et al reported early survivorship of 99.2% at 2 years follow-up, including 128 Navio UKA patients. Further mid- and long-term studies are necessary to show whether patients experience continued benefit from procedures using the Navio.[34]

PEARLS AND PITFALLS

Bone Preservation

Literature has shown that the extent of tibial bone resection is less with robotic than conventional UKA. Ponzio and Lonner found that tibial inserts ≥10 mm were used in 6.4% of robotic UKAs and 15.5% in conventional

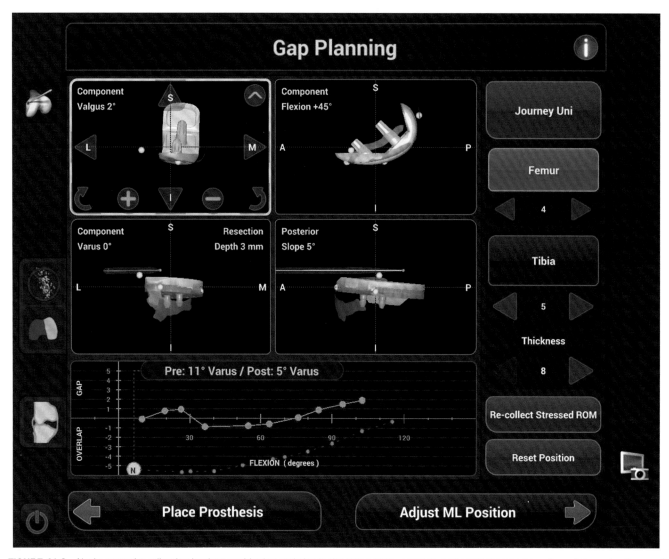

FIGURE 41-9 Navio example: adjusting implant positioning and size in the transverse, coronal, and sagittal plane based on alignment values and gap distance information (the graph in the bottom quandrant). Implant tracking information is shown during the next step ("Adjust ML position").

UKAs. No significant difference in tibial polyethylene thickness was seen between the Mako and Navio robot.[36] Minimizing bone resection is important as it is associated with less postoperative pain, faster recovery, and less bone edema.[36,37] In addition, aggressive resections can avoid challenging revision procedures with augments and/or stems.[38] Finally, more aggressive resections reduce the surface of the tibial plateau. This can lead to usage of smaller tibial components, causing increased strain.[39] Several authors have suggested that higher stress on a smaller surface may lead to earlier aseptic loosening.[40] Therefore, minimizing bone resection may have a biomechanical advantageous as well.

Complications

Complications associated specifically with robotic UKA are related to optically tracker pin placement. Tracking pins required for robotic UKA have shown minimal added complication risk. Although these complications are rare, superficial infection around the pin, osteomyelitis (probably due to thermal necrosis after pin placement), neurovascular injury, and stress fractures need to be kept in mind.[41–43] When focusing on preventing stress fractures, some have advocated for unicortical and metaphyseal placement of pins.[44] For reducing the risk for infection, it has been suggested to avoid transcortical placement.[43] However, the choice of pin placement remains controversial.[41–43] Other concerns when using robotic systems in UKA are prolonged operation time and case conversion as a result of software or hardware problems.

With regard to soft-tissue injuries, studies have reported complications with autonomous robotic technologies, although this is not described with semi-autonomous robotics in UKA.[9] In addition, a study by Sultan et al reported that robotic assistance in TKA using controlled oscillating saws reduces the risk of soft-tissue complications compared to conventional techniques.[45]

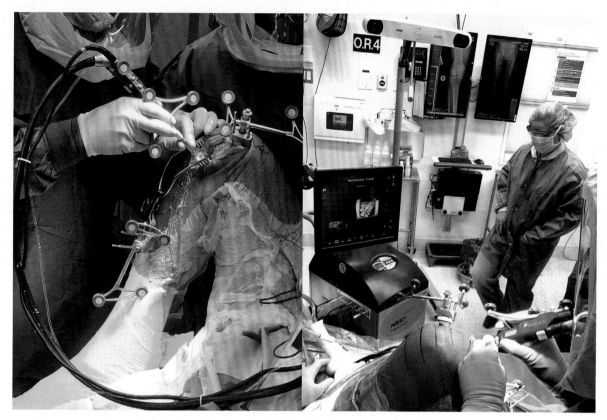

FIGURE 41-10   Navio example: the burring process during bone resection of the femur is displayed on the monitor. (Courtesy of Smith & Nephew, Inc.)

When extrapolating these results, a manually controlled oscillating saw in conventional UKAs may have higher risk of soft-tissue complications compared to the controlled burr used in robotic UKA.

Despite the concerns, robotic UKA has the potential to decrease the risk of component loosening, polyethylene wear, progressive osteoarthritis of the contralateral compartment of the knee, and instability compared to conventional UKA, as a result of the more accurate and reproducible implant placement.[6] Therefore, robotic systems may provide significant value to decrease the complication risk of UKA.

Image-Based and Imageless

Robotic UKA can be either imaged-based or imageless. The former allows the surgeon to preplan implant size and positioning based on alignment parameters before stepping into the operation room. Moreover, the surgeon can assess ACL tunnels, subchondral bone bed, osteophytes, cystic formations and regions of avascular necrosis. However, disadvantages of imaged-based robotic UKA are the additional cost of the CT scan, patient inconvenience, extra time needed for preoperative planning, and the higher radiation exposure.[46] With regard to radiation doses, future technology may change the radiation exposure of CT scans, as imaging industries are constantly developing new methods. Furthermore, current scanning protocols can deliver high-quality scans with low radiation doses.[47]

While image-based systems merge a detailed preoperative CT scan of the patient's knee with the intraoperative registered mapping points of the surgeon, imageless systems depend entirely on the accuracy of the intraoperative "painting" procedure. It must be noted that incorrect "painting" can lead to an incorrect predefined plan. Although the imageless Navio seems to show similar results as the image-based Mako regarding accuracy and reproducibility, comparative studies are necessary to evaluate whether accuracy and safety are compromised by imageless robotic UKA.

Learning Curve and Operation Time

Integrating new technology in the operating room is associated with prolonged operation times and increased learning curves to achieve favorable outcomes. Early results of Coon showed that short learning curves could be expected with the Mako in UKA. After an initial 10 cases, the tourniquet time remained under 60 minutes.[48] Jinnah et al showed similar results with the Mako robot. They examined UKA cases performed by 11 surgeons and found a steady state surgical time after 13 surgeries with no increased risk for the patient during the learning phase.[49]

The surgical time of the Navio robot was studied by Wallace et al. Five surgeons performed the procedure, two of which had prior experience with another robotic-assisted device. The authors reported that eight surgeries were required to have two consecutive surgeries completed within the 95% confidence interval of the steady state surgical time (tracker placement to implant trial acceptance). The average of the steady state surgical time was 50 minutes (range 37-55 minutes).[50]

Another study by Kayani et al studied the number of Mako UKAs needed for achieving operating times and surgical-team confidence levels equivalent to those of conventional UKAs. The transition from the conventional technique to robotic UKA was associated with a learning curve of six cases with an average operation time of 87.3 minutes (initial surgical incision to final wound closure). The average operation time after the six cases was 61.7 minutes, which was similar to the conventional UKA. Additionally, the authors reported improved accuracy of the implant positioning, however, without a learning curve. Furthermore, no added complications using the Mako robot were described.[51]

Although similar operation times in robotic and conventional UKA are reported, MacCallum et al and Hansen et al noted that robotic assistance added extra time to the surgical procedure, as a result of the registration process.[20,21] In addition, setup time of the robot is often not reported in studies and needs to be considered.[52] Overall, this new technology can be integrated safely without lengthy learning curves and additional risks for UKA patients, even when used by inexperienced surgeons.[53,54]

Cost-Effectiveness

One of the main obstacles is the high initial cost of robotic UKA. Most of these relatively new devices require extensive marketing, research, and development. Therefore, high prices are needed to be commercially viable for companies. To date, the Mako robot costs approximately one million dollars and the Navio system costs around half that price. Besides the initial investment, robotic systems come with maintenance costs and image-based systems require preoperative preparation with added cost to the patient, which are sometimes non-reimbursable.[55,56] However, increasing implementation and competition can result in reduced overall cost. In addition, some hospitals have chosen to share the Navio system for UKA to mitigate overall costs. Furthermore, as the Navio and Mako system can also be used for total knee arthroplasty, and additionally Mako for total hip arthroplasty, there is a greater potential opportunity to be cost-effective.

When reviewing the literature, cost-effectiveness studies are currently lacking. A study by Swank et al applied cost estimates of robotic technology for UKA. They reported that robotic investments of $800,000 for high-volume hospitals can easily see a return in a period of 2 years.[56] Another study by Moschetti et al compared cost-effectiveness of robotic UKA with conventional UKA using a Markov decision analysis. The authors based their robotic data on the Mako system, including initial and service costs, as well as cost for preoperative CT scans. Two-year revision rates for robotic UKA were set at 1.2% and 3.1% for conventional UKA. Taken together, they found that robotic UKA compared to the conventional procedure can be cost-effective at high-volume hospitals with more than 94 cases per year. The authors reported that robotic systems need to cost <$100.000 to be cost-effective at medium-volume centers (3-12 procedures per year).[55]

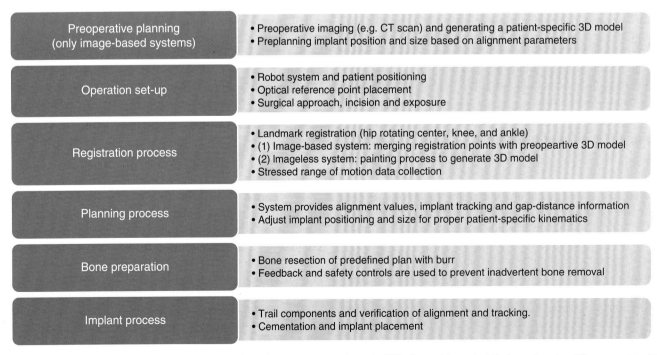

FIGURE 41-11 The general order of the process of semi-autonomous systems in UKA. It must be noted that small order differences may be present from surgeon to surgeon.

Cool et al evaluated short-term revision and the associated costs of matched robotic (246 knees) and conventional UKA patients (492 knees). They found lower revision rates and shorter length of stays during the revision procedure with lower associated costs for robotic UKA. For the index procedure, shorter length of stay and lower associated cost were also reported for robotic UKA. The mean cost of index plus revision procedures was 7.06% less for robotic compared to conventional UKA.[57] These findings are in line with Kayani et al, who showed that robotic UKA was associated with decreased postoperative pain, shorter length of stay, decreased opiate requirements, and improved early functional rehabilitation compared to conventional UKA.[37] Although no cost calculations were done by the authors, it can be expected that these findings reduce the cost of a robotic UKA procedure.

Generally, concerns regarding price remain as the benefit from improved accuracy and reproducibility of implantation have yet to show widespread clinical efficacy. If widespread clinical efficacy is shown, any additional costs will be justifiable as improved patient outcomes may lead to less healthcare expenditure in the long term.

CONCLUSION

Technological advancements of robotic-assisted surgery within the orthopedic field have given surgeons a high level of control and precision during surgery (**Fig. 41-11**). Current semi-autonomous systems for UKA enhance control for implant positioning, soft-tissue balance, and limb alignment, leading to more predictable and consistent results compared to using conventional techniques. Furthermore, the ability to quantify surgical variables and accurately control those variables has the potential to improve UKA outcomes for less experienced surgeons. While emerging mid- to long-term results and cost-effectiveness analysis are necessary to evaluate the real benefit of robotic-assisted systems, current findings are promising. If these results are continued, and more convincing clinical outcomes are shown, robotic-assisted UKA may lead to increased acceptance of UKA surgery.

REFERENCES

1. Liddle AD, Judge A, Pandit H, Murray DW. Adverse outcomes after total and unicompartmental knee replacement in 101330 matched patients: a study of data from the National Joint Registry for England and Wales. *Lancet.* 2014;384(9952):1437-1445.
2. Liddle AD, Pandit H, Judge A, Murray DW. Patient-reported outcomes after total and unicompartmental knee arthroplasty: a study of 14 076 matched patients from the National Joint Registry for England and Wales. *Bone Joint J.* 2015;97-B(6):793-801.
3. Newman J, Pydisetty RV, Ackroyd C. Unicompartmental or total knee replacement: the 15-year results of a prospective randomised controlled trial. *J Bone Joint Surg Br.* 2009;91(1):52-57.
4. Baker P, Jameson S, Critchley R, Reed M, Gregg P, Deehan D. Center and surgeon volume influence the revision rate following unicondylar knee replacement. *J Bone Joint Surg Am.* 2013;95(8):702-709.
5. Badawy M, Espehaug B, Indrekvam K, Havelin LI, Furnes O. Higher revision risk for unicompartmental knee arthroplasty in low-volume hospitals. *Acta Orthop.* 2014;85(4):342-347.
6. Christ AB, Pearle AD, Mayman DJ, Haas SB. Robotic-assisted unicompartmental knee arthroplasty: state-of-the art and review of the literature. *J Arthroplasty.* 2018;33(7):1994-2001.
7. Bell SW, Anthony I, Jones B, MacLean A, Rowe P, Blyth M. Improved accuracy of component positioning with robotic-assisted unicompartmental knee arthroplasty. *J Bone Joint Surg.* 2016;98(8):627-635.
8. Fisher DA, Watts M, Davis KE. Implant position in knee surgery: a comparison of minimally invasive, open unicompartmental, and total knee arthroplasty. *J Arthroplasty.* 2003;18(7 suppl 1):2-8.
9. Honl M, Dierk O, Gauck C, et al. Comparison of robotic-assisted and manual implantation of a primary total hip replacement: a prospective study. *J Bone Joint Surg Am.* 2003;85(8):1470-1478.
10. Jacofsky DJ, Allen M. Robotics in arthroplasty: a comprehensive review. *J Arthroplasty.* 2016;31(10):2353-2363.
11. Jakopec M, Harris SJ, Rodriguez y Baena F, Gomes P, Cobb J, Davies BL. The first clinical application of a "hands-on" robotic knee surgery system. *Comput Aided Surg.* 2001;6(6):329-339.
12. Cobb J, Henckel J, Gomes P, et al. Hands-on robotic unicompartmental knee replacement. *J Bone Joint Surg Br.* 2006;88-B(2):188-197.
13. Lonner JH, John TK, Conditt MA. Robotic arm-assisted UKA improves tibial component alignment: a pilot study. *Clin Orthop Relat Res.* 2010;468(1):141-146.
14. Coon TM, Driscoll MD, Conditt MA. Robotically assisted UKA is more accurate than manually instrumented UKA. *Orthop Proc.* 2018;92-B(suppl_I):157.
15. Citak M, Suero EM, Citak M, et al. Unicompartmental knee arthroplasty: is robotic technology more accurate than conventional technique? *Knee.* 2013;20(4):268-271.
16. Dunbar NJ, Roche MW, Park BH, Branch SH, Conditt MA, Banks SA. Accuracy of dynamic tactile-guided unicompartmental knee arthroplasty. *J Arthroplasty.* 2012;27(5):803-808.e1.
17. Khamaisy S, Zuiderbaan HA, van der List JP, Nam D, Pearle AD. Medial unicompartmental knee arthroplasty improves congruence and restores joint space width of the lateral compartment. *Knee.* 2016;23(3):501-505.
18. Zuiderbaan HA, Khamaisy S, Thein R, Nawabi DH, Pearle AD. Congruence and joint space width alterations of the medial compartment following lateral unicompartmental knee arthroplasty. *Bone Joint J.* 2015;97-B(1):50-55.
19. Plate JF, Mofidi A, Mannava S, et al. Achieving accurate ligament balancing using robotic-assisted unicompartmental knee arthroplasty. *Adv Orthop.* 2013;2013:1-6.
20. Hansen DC, Kusuma SK, Palmer RM, Harris KB. Robotic guidance does not improve component position or short-term outcome in medial unicompartmental knee arthroplasty. *J Arthroplasty.* 2014;29(9):1784-1789.
21. MacCallum KP, Danoff JR, Geller JA. Tibial baseplate positioning in robotic-assisted and conventional unicompartmental knee arthroplasty. *Eur J Orthop Surg Traumatol.* 2016;26(1):93-98.
22. Pearle AD, van der List JP, Lee L, Coon TM, Borus TA, Roche MW. Survivorship and patient satisfaction of robotic-assisted medial unicompartmental knee arthroplasty at a minimum two-year follow-up. *Knee.* 2017;24(2):419-428.
23. Kleeblad LJ, Borus TA, Coon TM, Dounchis J, Nguyen JT, Pearle AD. Midterm survivorship and patient satisfaction of robotic-arm-assisted medial unicompartmental knee arthroplasty: a multicenter study. *J Arthroplasty.* 2018;33(6):1719-1726.
24. Kleeblad LJ, van der List JP, Zuiderbaan HA, Pearle AD. Larger range of motion and increased return to activity, but higher revision rates following unicompartmental versus total knee arthroplasty in patients under 65: a systematic review. *Knee Surg Sports Traumatol Arthrosc.* 2018;26(6):1811-1822.

25. Blyth MJG, Anthony I, Rowe P, Banger MS, MacLean A, Jones B. Robotic arm-assisted versus conventional unicompartmental knee arthroplasty: exploratory secondary analysis of a randomised controlled trial. *Bone Joint Res*. 2017;6(11):631-639.

26. Motesharei A, Rowe P, Blyth M, Jones B, Maclean A. A comparison of gait one year post operation in an RCT of robotic UKA versus traditional Oxford UKA. *Gait Posture*. 2018;62:41-45.

27. Millar LJ, Banger M, Rowe PJ, Blyth M, Jones B, Maclean A. O 017 – a five-year follow up of gait in robotic assisted vs conventional unicompartmental knee arthroplasty. *Gait Posture*. 2018;65(6):31-32.

28. Khare R, Jaramaz B, Hamlin B, Urish KL. Implant orientation accuracy of a hand-held robotic partial knee replacement system over conventional technique in a cadaveric test. *Comput Assist Surg*. 2018;23(1):8-13.

29. Lonner JH, Smith JR, Picard F, Hamlin B, Rowe PJ, Riches PE. High degree of accuracy of a novel image-free handheld robot for unicondylar knee arthroplasty in a cadaveric study. *Clin Orthop Relat Res*. 2015;473(1):206-212.

30. Gregori A, Picard F, Lonner J, Smith J, Jaramaz B. Accuracy of imageless robotically assisted unicondylar knee arthroplasty. Paper presented at: 15th Annual Meeting of CAOS; 2015.

31. Herry Y, Batailler C, Lording T, Servien E, Neyret P, Lustig S. Improved joint-line restitution in unicompartmental knee arthroplasty using a robotic-assisted surgical technique. *Int Orthop*. 2017;41(11):2265-2271.

32. Batailler C, White N, Ranaldi FM, Neyret P, Servien E, Lustig S. Improved implant position and lower revision rate with robotic-assisted unicompartmental knee arthroplasty. *Knee Surg Sports Traumatol Arthrosc*. 2018;27(4):1232-1240.

33. Vega Parra P, Palacios Barajas J, Márquez Ambrosi R, Duarte J. Reemplazo parcial de rodilla mediante el sistema robótico NAVIO: resultados clínicos postquirúrgicos evaluados mediante Knee injury Osteoarthritis Outcome Score. *Rev Chil Ortop Traumatol*. 2017;58(01):007-012.

34. Evidence Communications, Clinical Scientific & Medical Affairs, Smith & Nephew. Evidence in focus: compendium of evidence. 2018. Available at http://www.smith-nephew.com/documents/education%20and%20evidence/literature/2018/15298-us-en%20v1%20navio%20compendium%20of%20evidence%200918.pdf Accessed June 9, 2019.

35. Canetti R, Batailler C, Bankhead C, Neyret P, Servien E, Lustig S. Faster return to sport after robotic-assisted lateral unicompartmental knee arthroplasty: a comparative study. *Arch Orthop Trauma Surg*. 2018;138(12):1765-1771.

36. Ponzio DY, Lonner JH. Robotic technology produces more conservative tibial resection than conventional techniques in UKA. *Am J Orthop*. 2016;45(7):E465-E468.

37. Kayani B, Konan S, Tahmassebi J, Rowan FE, Haddad FS. An assessment of early functional rehabilitation and hospital discharge in conventional versus robotic-arm assisted unicompartmental knee arthroplasty. *Bone Joint J*. 2019;101-B(1):24-33.

38. Schwarzkopf R, Mikhael B, Li L, Josephs L, Scott RD. Effect of initial tibial resection thickness on outcomes of revision UKA. *Orthopedics*. 2013;36(4):e409-e414.

39. Small SR, Berend ME, Rogge RD, Archer DB, Kingman AL, Ritter MA. Tibial loading after UKA: evaluation of tibial slope, resection depth, medial shift and component rotation. *J Arthroplasty*. 2019;28(9):179-183.

40. Woods CJ, Heller MO, Browne M. Assessing the effect of unicondylar knee arthroplasty on proximal tibia bone strains using digital image correlation. *Int J Biomed Eng Sci*. 2017;4(3):1-6.

41. Beldame J, Boisrenoult P, Beaufils P. Pin track induced fractures around computer-assisted TKA. *Orthop Traumatol Surg Res*. 2010;96(3):249-255.

42. Berning ET, Fowler RM. Thermal damage and tracker-pin track infection in computer-navigated total knee arthroplasty. *J Arthroplasty*. 2011;26(6):977.e21-977.e24.

43. Kamara E, Berliner ZP, Hepinstall MS, Cooper HJ. Pin site complications associated with computer-assisted navigation in hip and knee arthroplasty. *J Arthroplasty*. 2017;32(9):2842-2846.

44. Thomas A, Pemmaraju G, Nagra G, Bassett J, Deshpande S. Complications resulting from tracker pin-sites in computer navigated knee replacement surgery. *Acta Orthop Belg*. 2015;81(4):708-712.

45. Sultan AA, Piuzzi N, Khlopas A, Chughtai M, Sodhi N, Mont MA. Utilization of robotic-arm assisted total knee arthroplasty for soft tissue protection. *Expert Rev Med Devices*. 2017;14(12):925-927.

46. Ponzio DY, Lonner JH. Preoperative mapping in unicompartmental knee arthroplasty using computed tomography scans is associated with radiation exposure and carries high cost. *J Arthroplasty*. 2015;30(6):964-967.

47. Henckel J, Richards R, Lozhkin K, et al. Very low-dose computed tomography for planning and outcome measurement in knee replacement: the imperial knee protocol. *J Bone Joint Surg Br*. 2006;88-B(11):1513-1518.

48. Coon TM. Integrating robotic technology into the operating room. *Am J Orthop*. 2009;38(2):7-9.

49. Jinnah R, Lippincott CJ, Horowitz S, Conditt MA. The learning curve of robotically-assisted UKA. Paper presented at: 56th Annual Meeting of the Orthopaedic Research Society. Paper no. 407.

50. Wallace D, Gregori A, Picard F, et al. The learning curve of a novel handheld robotic system for unicondylar knee arthroplasty. *Orthop Proc*. 2014;96-B(suppl 16):13.

51. Kayani B, Konan S, Pietrzak JRT, Huq SS, Tahmassebi J, Haddad FS. The learning curve associated with robotic-arm assisted unicompartmental knee arthroplasty. *Bone Joint J*. 2018;100B(8):1033-1042.

52. Pearle AD, O'Loughlin PF, Kendoff DO. Robot-assisted unicompartmental knee arthroplasty. *J Arthroplasty*. 2010;25(2):230-237.

53. Simons M, Riches P. The learning curve of robotically-assisted unicondylar knee arthroplasty. *Orthop Proc*. 2014;96-B(suppl 11):152.

54. Karia M, Masjedi M, Andrews B, Jaffry Z, Cobb J. Robotic assistance enables inexperienced surgeons to perform unicompartmental knee arthroplasties on dry bone models with accuracy superior to conventional methods. *Adv Orthop*. 2013;2013:1-7.

55. Moschetti WE, Konopka JF, Rubash HE, Genuario JW. Can robot-assisted unicompartmental knee arthroplasty be cost-effective? A Markov decision analysis. *J Arthroplasty*. 2016;31(4):759-765.

56. Swank ML, Alkire M, Conditt M, Lonner JH. Technology and cost-effectiveness in knee arthroplasty: computer navigation and robotics. *Am J Orthop*. 2009;38(2 suppl):32-36.

57. Cool CL, Needham KA, Coppolecchia A, Khlopas A, Mont MA. Revision analysis of robotic-arm assisted and manual unicompartmental knee arthroplasty. *J Arthroplasty*. 2019;34(5):926-931.

chapter 42

Osseous Deficiencies in Total Knee Replacement

Robert A. Sershon, MD | Kevin B. Fricka, MD | Nancy L. Parks, MS | C. Anderson Engh Jr, MD

BACKGROUND

Osseous deficiencies in complex primary and revision total knee arthroplasty (TKA) settings can pose significant surgical challenges. Causes of bone loss are broad and often multifactorial, including periprosthetic osteolysis, subsidence of loose implants, fracture, stress shielding, osteonecrosis, or infection.

Bone loss can involve the femur and/or the tibia. The extent of bone loss ranges from minimal to the loss of the entire metaphysis. Reconstruction is dictated primarily by the amount of bone loss and secondarily by ligamentous integrity. Tools available to reconstruct bone loss include particulate or bulk allograft, solid metal augments, porous metal augments, and segmental solid implants. For increasing defect size, intramedullary stems become necessary to offload the metaphyseal construct. Interface management is critical to successful bone reconstruction.

When a bone defect is repaired, the once "single" host–implant interface turns into a "double" interface: host-augment-implant. The interface between the host bone and the graft or porous augment must be supportive and healthy enough for graft healing or ingrowth fixation to a porous surface. The counter-face must allow cement fixation to the implant. The final goal is to achieve a well-functioning final construct that possesses structural stability, appropriate balancing, and proper alignment.

When bone loss is anticipated or encountered intraoperatively, a classification system allows for a methodological approach to managing the deficiency. A classification system should allow preoperative prediction and preparation for surgical reconstruction, realizing that radiographs likely underestimate the amount of bone loss. The classification also guides intraoperative decision-making. It is imperative to prepare for severe deficiencies in order to have the necessary equipment and components available for any scenario.

In this chapter, we present a systematic approach for management of osseous deficiencies in TKA, encompassing preoperative assessment, implant removal, description of existing classification systems, and reconstruction options based upon the Anderson Orthopaedic Research Institute (AORI) classification for bone loss in the setting of revision knee arthroplasty.

PREOPERATIVE ASSESSMENT

Preoperatively, the surgeon should attempt to establish the mechanism of implant failure, gauge ligamentous stability, estimate bone loss, and plan for the upcoming reconstruction. The most common causes of failure for modern TKA implants include aseptic loosening, infection, instability, fracture, and stiffness. The frequency of wear, osteolysis, and patellofemoral complications has decreased substantially since the 1990s and early 2000s due to changes in surgical technique, polyethylene processing, sterilization techniques, and implant design.[1,2] Irrespective of failure mode, revision arthroplasty must correct the factors that led to failure of the primary arthroplasty.

Essential elements of the physical exam include gait assessment, skin integrity and evidence of prior incisions, range of motion with the presence or absence of contracture, extensor mechanism competency, ligament competency, neurovascular exam, and spine and hip examination.[3] Laboratory tests include a screening erythrocyte sedimentation rate and C-reactive protein level, with possible fluid aspiration including cell count, culture, D-dimer, and alpha-defensin assay to differentiate septic from aseptic loosening.[4]

In most instances, radiographs are the major source of preoperative information regarding the mechanism of failure and degree of bone loss. Comparisons should be made with prior imaging studies when available. Recommended views include standing anteroposterior, lateral, Merchant, and standing full-length views of the bilateral lower extremities. These views allow for evaluation of femoral and tibial implant position and size, assessment of current bone stock, interface fixation, critique of patellar height and coronal position, and coronal alignment. Rarely, fluoroscopically guided spot views can also be obtained to better evaluate the status of the bone–cement or bone–implant interface for tibial and femoral components.[5] Routine use of MRI or CT is not recommended due to increased cost and failure to significantly alter management.[6] X-rays of the contralateral knee can identify the joint line relationship to bony landmarks, such as the femoral epicondyles for the femur and the fibular head for the tibia.

Bone loss encountered at the time of revision surgery generally exceeds the preoperative radiographic estimation.[7] This is especially true in the case of osteolysis, in which the remaining bone is often of such poor quality as to be structurally incompetent; when it is adequately debrided, a much larger defect than predicted must be reconstructed.

When evaluating the femur radiographically, careful scrutiny of the distal femoral interface and the posterior condylar interface, which are the most common sites for interface loosening and bone loss, is warranted. Bone deficits involving the medial or lateral femoral metaphysis may indicate ligamentous deficiency. Femoral bone defects tend to be larger in posterior cruciate-substituting designs, hinged implants, and stemmed implants. When evaluating the tibia, a careful assessment of the integrity of the tibial tuberosity, the remaining bone stock with reference to the fibular head, quality of the metaphyseal bone, and the tibial slope is required (**Fig. 42-1A** to C). Tibiofemoral, distal femoral, and proximal tibial anatomic angles should be measured and compared to prior radiographs if available.

IMPLANT REMOVAL

It is important to identify the manufacturer and design of the prosthesis preoperatively in the event that design-specific disassembly or removal tools are required. Following adequate exposure, the foremost goal of implant removal is to retain bone stock. The sequence of component removal depends on exposure, implant stability, and surgeon preference. The polyethylene insert is removed first to decrease tension and enhance exposure. The tibial tray is often easier to remove next because the tibial interface consists of a two-dimensional interface, compared to the multiple interface planes of the femur.

Circumferential exposure of the tibia prior to attempted component extraction prevents excessive bone loss, fracture, ligamentous, or neurovascular injury. Extraction of the tibial component should begin at the medial implant - cement interface, with the use of microsaws, hi-speed pencil-tipped burrs, and osteotomes. The central metaphyseal cancellous bone often cannot be accessed and will be sacrificed. Peripheral bone support is typically maintained, resulting in a contained central defect that is easier to reconstruct compared to an uncontained or segmental defect. Rarely, a long, well-fixed stemmed tibial component is present that requires a tibial tubercle osteotomy for removal. Following extraction of the tibial implant and stem, any remaining cement is removed using reverse curette and cement-splitting osteotomes. The trial tibial component aligned by the intramedullary canal is inserted to protect the remaining bone stock and becomes the initial reference for flexion and extension gaps.

Removing the femoral component also requires adequate exposure and disruption of the implant–bone (cementless fixation) or implant–cement (cemented fixation) interface. The anterior, medial, lateral, and posterior implant interfaces are freed with osteotomes, microsaws, or a pencil-tip burr. In some cementless femurs, a Gigli saw is used. The femoral notch interfaces are then released with curved and straight osteotomes. The femoral implant is extracted with a universal extraction device, using force judiciously to avoid damaging the remaining bone stock.

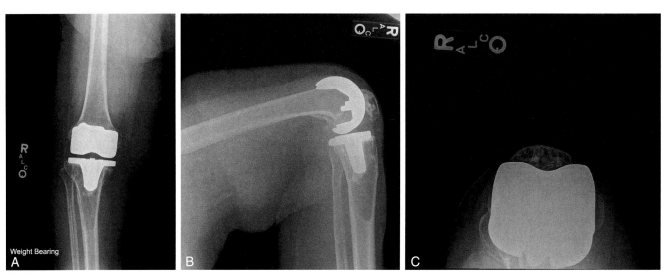

FIGURE 42-1 Standard radiographs (AP **(A)**, lateral **(B)**, and sunrise **(C)**) identify a cruciate retaining cementless femur with cemented tibia. The patella is stable with probable osteolysis. The tibia has varus alignment suggestive of loosening with extensive metaphyseal osteolysis and cement-implant radiolucencies.

BONE DEFECT CLASSIFICATION

Several bone defect classifications have been described. The most helpful classifications are easy to use, reproducible, and guide reconstruction.[8]

Massachusetts General Hospital Classification

The Massachusetts General Hospital femoral-only defect classification system separates osseous defects into major and minor categories and then further into contained or uncontained defects.[9] It classifies femoral defects into major and minor types according to the epicondylar level (above versus below), volume (>1 or ≤1 cm³), and containment (contained vs uncontained). Contained defects have cancellous bone loss only, with no significant cortical loss. Uncontained defects have cortical bone loss that results in lack of support for a portion of the implant. Condylar dissociations are categorized as uncontained.

University of Pennsylvania Classification

The University of Pennsylvania (UPENN) classification quantifies bone loss on a continuous numerical scale from 1 to 100 points.[10] The system is set up as a finite element grid based on standard preoperative (AP) and lateral knee radiographs. The classification is intended to anticipate and accurately quantify bone loss preoperatively and has been found to be valid and reliable.[7] While the UPENN system is precise, quantitative, and readily allows for comparisons of bone loss severity, it lacks the therapeutic recommendations present in other classification systems.

Huff and Sculco Classification

The Huff and Sculco classification is based on the Anderson Orthopedic Research Institute (AORI) bone defect classification.[11] The basic patterns of bone loss are cystic, epiphyseal, cavitary, and segmental. Cystic defects are small defects in the trabecular bone that do not affect implant stability. Epiphyseal defects involve cortical bone loss in the epiphyseal/metaphyseal regions, often compromising implant stability and requiring augmentation with stems. Cavitary defects consist of massive, intracortical, metaphyseal defects that require bulk allograft reconstruction or metaphyseal filling cones or sleeves with stems. Segmental defects are a combination of epiphyseal and cavitary defects, with a large extent of bone loss that may involve collateral ligament attachments. Reconstruction options again include bulk allograft or prosthetic reconstruction with stems and often require hinge-type revision prostheses.

Anderson Orthopaedic Research Institute Classification

We prefer the AORI classification system, which is the reconstructive template for this chapter. Bone deficiency is assessed intraoperatively after the prosthesis is removed (**Fig. 42-2**). Three aspects define the classification:
1. femoral ("F") or tibial ("T") location
2. severity of bone loss—minimal, moderate, severe, defined as type 1, 2, or 3, respectively
3. single or both condyle/plateaus, defined as A or B, respectively.[12]

SURGICAL RECONSTRUCTION

Reconstruction options for bony defects can be guided according to the AORI classification system. In order to achieve a stable knee that possesses structural stability, appropriate balancing, and proper alignment, the axial and rotational alignment as well as the joint line must be restored. Cement augmentation, modular metal augmentation, and bone grafting replace lost metaphyseal bone. Intramedullary stems determine axial alignment and offload the metaphyseal reconstruction. After removal of components, the tibial reconstruction is addressed first. The joint line is recreated with trial components. Component rotation, flexion–extension gaps, and the need for constraint are then assessed. As an overview, type 1 defects possess intact metaphyseal bone with a relatively normal joint line. These can typically be treated with a primary implant, with or without modular augmentation. Type 1 defects may require a longer stem. Type 2 defects demonstrate damaged metaphyseal cancellous bone that requires revision components with augmentation (bone graft, modular augments, metaphyseal sleeves, or trabecular metal cones) and stem fixation to offload stress and support the metaphyseal reconstruction. Type 3 defects universally require structural allografts or large porous metal augments, often necessitating segmental replacements secondary to the ligamentous insufficiency. Type 3 defects by definition often have ligament deficiency and require higher levels of constraint or hinged implants (**Table 42-1**).

AORI Type 1 Defect ("Intact" Metaphysis)

A type 1 defect indicates that there is adequate metaphyseal cancellous bone to support the implant and the joint line has not been substantially altered.[12] Revision style components are not typically needed, and stems are optional. These defects may only require a particulate allograft, cement with screws, or small solid augments attached to the component.

Although bony defects may be minimal, close attention must be paid to restoring the joint line and correcting

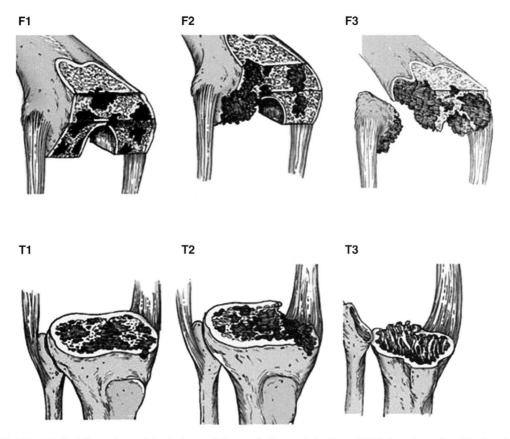

FIGURE 42-2 Medical illustrations of the Anderson Orthopaedic Research Institute (AORI) Bone Loss Classification System.

any previous malrotation of components. Joint line aberrations following knee arthroplasty are associated with worse clinical outcomes, mid-flexion instability, and altered patellofemoral mechanics.[13,14] The native joint line is located 10 to 15 mm proximal to the fibular head and 25 to 30 mm distal to the medial epicondyle.[15,16] These landmarks can be used as rough predictors of joint line restoration in all revisions.

Cement and Screws

Small defects involving one condyle or plateau can be managed with bone cement in isolation or with axially aligned screws for additional support and cement.[6,17-19]

Bone cement with screws is easy to employ, cost-effective, and appropriate in patients with small osseous defects. Supportive screws should be introduced perpendicular to the implant, serving as support pillars. The surgeon must ensure that the screw heads are not sitting proud to the intact cut surface in order to avoid unintentional implant misalignment (**Fig. 42-3**).

Particulate Graft

A particulate autograft or allograft is most often utilized for contained AORI type 1 or 2 defects, where the bone graft can be captured.[19] When impacted, particulate graft, peripheral host bone support, and a stem create a

TABLE 42-1   Overview of the Anderson Orthopaedic Research Institute (AORI) Bone Defect Classification System

Bone	Tibia	Femur	Joint Line	Reconstruction	Stemmed Component	Ligaments	Constraint
Intact	T1	F1	Normal	Cement	Optional	Intact	Unconstrained
Damaged	T2	F2	Uneven	Bone graft, solid augments, occasional porous augments	Yes	Variable damage	Variable constraint
Deficient	T3	F3	Altered	Allograft, segmental replacement, sleeve/cone	Yes	Often compromised	Required, often hinged

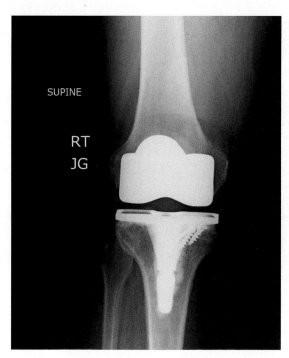

FIGURE 42-3 Postoperative AP radiograph showing a cruciate retaining (CR) total knee replacement with use of cement and screws to fill a bony defect.

stable reconstruction. Although cost-effective when compared to metal augments, widespread use of particulate bone grafting for defects larger than type 1 bone loss has diminished in North America.[20-23] Our current indication for the use of the particulate allograft is in small to moderate sized, contained defects in younger patients who may require future revisions.

AORI Type 2 Defect ("Damaged" Metaphysis)

Type 2 defects affect one condyle/plateau (type 2A) or both condyles/plateaus (type 2B) and are characterized by moderate areas of bone loss. Type 2 bone loss includes femoral metaphyseal loss distal to the femoral epicondyles and tibial loss proximal to the tibial tubercle. The metaphyseal bone stock is "damaged" but not completely deficient. Unlike type 1 defects, type 2 bone defects provide inadequate support for an implant without the use of stems. The tibia is prepared first, since its position will establish the flexion–extension gaps and assist in setting the rotation of the femoral component. For type T2A defects that have a minimally damaged contralateral plateau, the tibial cut is made perpendicular to the tibial axis at the level of the intact plateau (**Fig. 42-4**). For tibial defects in the range of 10 mm in depth, the gap can be filled with a solid augment on the undersurface of the implant. Porous cones and sleeves can be used for smaller defects but are more commonly employed in the setting of tibial plateau defects greater than 10 mm.[6,18,24,25] Porous augments are not cemented

to the host bone, allowing for eventual osseointegration. The tibial component is cemented to the porous augment.

Type T2B defects lack a bony reference for the joint line. Defects less than 10 mm in thickness can be restored with a thicker tibial tray or medial/lateral augments as previously described. Larger type 2B tibial defects will require porous cones or sleeves (**Fig. 42-5**). Both cones and sleeves provide a large surface area for biologic fixation and are accompanied by a tibial stem. Cones are not integral to the stem and thus allow greater freedom in placing cones in position for maximal host–cone contact. Further, the final orientation of the tibial stem is not dictated by the placement of the cone. However, smaller cones may limit the diameter of the stem and often require fully cemented stem reconstruction. In contrast, sleeves are directly attached and sized to the tibial stem, allowing metaphyseal cementless sleeve and press-fit diaphyseal stem fixation. The downside of sleeves is that the proximal position of the tibial tray is dictated by the tibial intramedullary canal. When the position of the tibial tray dictated by the canal is found to be suboptimal, smaller diameter, shorter stems can be cemented through the metaphyseal augment or offset stems can be utilized.[6]

Once the tibial joint line is reconstructed, femoral bone defects are addressed. Intramedullary femoral guides typically determine the distal femoral resection. Type F2A defects rely on the reconstructed tibia and contralateral intact femoral condyle to determine the level of distal resection and assist with femoral component rotation. When using a gap-balancing technique, if ligament damage prevents determination of femoral rotation, the epicondylar axis can be used as the main reference for rotation. The deficient femoral condyle is augmented with solid metal augments. Larger type F2A defects with scant metaphyseal bone can be treated with porous metal augments. Alternatively, deficient single femoral condyles can be reconstructed with the use of intramedullary aligned femoral sleeves combined with solid metal augments. The choice of porous augments or sleeves is based on surgeon preference. Porous augments and sleeves attached to stems have essentially replaced bulk allograft in all but the youngest patients with type 2 defects.

Type F2B femoral defects, by definition, require posterior and distal augmentation (**Fig. 42-6**). The effects of augments on flexion and extension spaces are similar to those encountered in primary arthroplasty.[26] Spacer blocks referencing the tibial reconstruction can identify differences in the flexion–extension gaps and relative defect sizes. Typically, the extension space is tighter than the flexion space. Increasing femoral component size can address the flexion space until the femoral component becomes excessively wide in the medial–lateral dimension. In this scenario, a small amount of flexion laxity can be addressed with increased constraint or slight elevation of the joint line. Type F2 defects do not typically necessitate

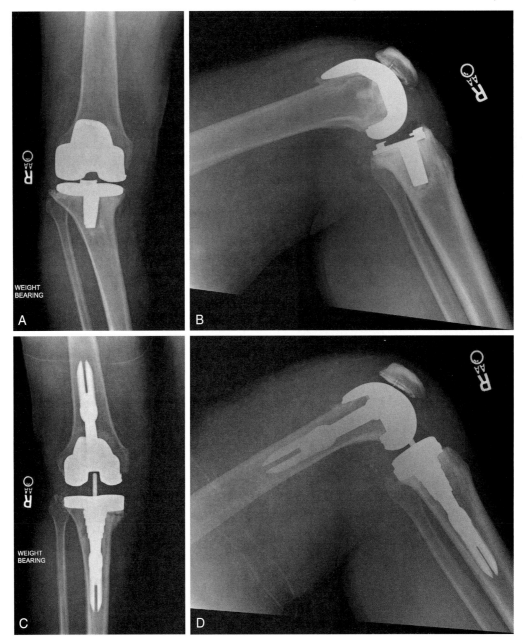

FIGURE 42-4 Preoperative AP **(A)** and lateral **(B)** radiographs of type T2A/F2A defects. Post-revision AP **(C)** and lateral **(D)** radiographs. The surgeon chose a solid metal augment, off-loaded by a cementless sleeve and diaphyseal-engaging stem for the tibia. The femur depicts a standard revision implant design with distal and posterior augments and a press-fit stem.

a hinge reconstruction. Small defects 1 cm³ or less are easily filled with solid metal augments. Larger defects require porous cones fitted to the defect or metaphyseal sleeves attached to an intramedullary stem.

Traditionally, larger type 2B and type 3 defects were treated with bulk allografts.[12,20,22] The availability of porous metal augments and sleeves in multiple shapes and sizes from several manufacturers has greatly decreased the need for bulk allografts in all but the youngest patients.[27-30] Whether allograft, porous augments, or sleeves are chosen, the important principle is that the bone with which they come into contact is healthy, strong, and conforming to the reconstruction choice. This allows a durable junction to the host bone either by bony ingrowth or fibrous fixation. The counter-face of the allograft or porous metal is cemented to the femoral implant and stem. When sleeves are chosen, the sleeve has a direct mechanical coupling to the stem and implant. As with tibial constructs, the position of the stem within the canal dictates the medial or lateral position of the femoral component when utilizing press-fit diaphyseal fixation with sleeves. With porous cones, larger diameter press-fit femoral stems may not pass through the cone and may require full cement fixation of a smaller diameter and shorter stem.

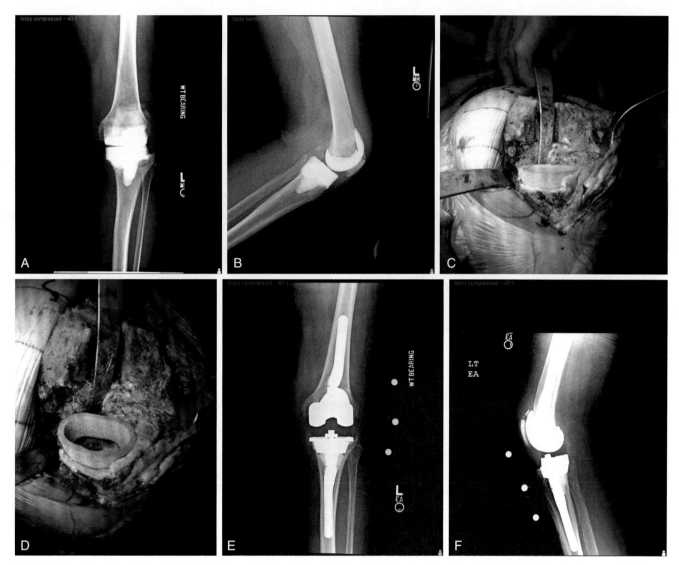

FIGURE 42-5 Example of a type T2B defect. Preoperative radiographs (**A** and **B**). Intraoperative photos show tibial metaphysis severely damaged requiring a metaphyseal cone and stem for support (**C** and **D**). Postoperative radiographs showing hybrid fixation of the tibial component with an offset, press-fit stem. The femur depicts a standard revision implant design with distal and posterior augments and an offset press-fit stem (**E** and **F**).

AORI Type 3 Defect ("Deficient" Metaphysis)

Type 3 AORI osseous defects occur when bone loss compromises a major portion of the condyles or the plateau, rendering the metaphysis "deficient."[12] Such defects are commonly the result of a failed revision TKA, periprosthetic fracture, or massive osteolysis. Type 3 defects require diaphyseal stems to off-load and align large metaphyseal porous metal augments, structural allografts or allograft-prosthetic composite, and occasionally distal femoral replacements (**Fig. 42-7**). On the femoral side, type F3 defects are often associated with collateral ligament insufficiency. On the tibia, although rare, a type T3 defect can compromise the tibial tubercle with the resultant need for extensor mechanism reconstruction. Consequently, type 3 bone deficiencies require stability beyond what a standard varus–valgus constrained

implant is capable of providing, resulting in the use of hinged implants, megaprostheses, or allograft-prosthetic composite reconstruction.

Constrained Condylar and Hinged Devices

Varying degrees of prosthesis constraint are available to address instability in the setting of severe bone loss, often seen with AORI type 3 defects. Higher degrees of constraint, such as unlinked constrained prosthesis, are reserved for patients with mild to moderate varus–valgus laxity. Hinged implants should be available for all cases with anticipated flexion instability, excessive hyperextension, or global instability (**Fig. 42-8**). While an unlinked varus–valgus constrained knee may appear stable intraoperatively, in a very short period of time flexion, instability or hyperextension can develop leading to instability requiring conversion to a hinged component. Multiple

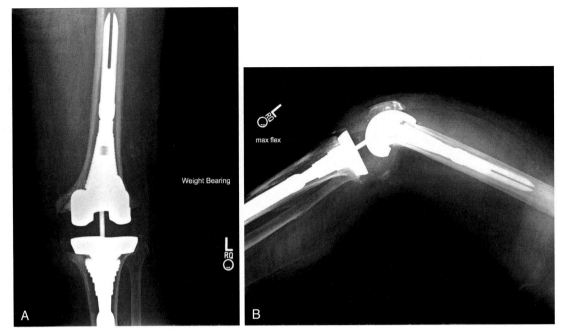

FIGURE 42-6 **A** and **B:** Example of types T2B and F2B defect reconstruction in the setting of a previously infected TKA. A thick tibial tray and distal femoral augments were used to restore the joint line. Posterior femoral augments were used to restore the flexion gap. Metaphyseal sleeves restored metaphyseal bone loss on both the tibia and femur. Press-fit stems were used on both the femoral and tibial sides to enhance construct stability.

authors have shown successful outcomes with the use of both unlinked constraint and hinged implants with metal or bony allograft augmentation in the setting of AORI types 2 to 3 bone loss.[27-38]

Endoprostheses and Allograft-Prosthesis Composites

In the setting of massive bone loss resulting from multiple prior revisions, periprosthetic fracture, or tumors rendering joint reconstruction impractical with hinged devices, endoprostheses are used to replace the entire distal femur or proximal tibia (**Fig. 42-9**). Although implantation of these devices makes up a small portion of knee arthroplasty procedures, reports have shown patients gain significant improvement in functional outcomes and Knee Society scores at medium to long-term follow-up.[39,40] Perhaps the best indication for an endoprosthesis is the very distal periprosthetic femoral fracture in an elderly patient. The ability to weight-bear as tolerated with a stable implant and comparatively rapid recovery is a substantial advantage in an elderly patient compared to open reduction and internal fixation methods.

Allograft prosthesis composites (APCs) have been used for over 30 years and are an alternative to endoprosthesis that have demonstrated reasonable results.[23,41,42] Use of modern implant reconstruction implant designs can eliminate the risks associated with APCs, including disease transmission, nonunion, and instability. Furthermore, this construct is rarely necessary in all but the very young patient.

Extensor Mechanism Deficiency

Rarely, type 3 tibial defects present with or develop intraoperative disruption of the distal patellar insertion. Reattachment of the patellar tendon has been described in the tumor and arthroplasty literature, consisting of augmentation with synthetic mesh material, allograft tendon, or autograft reconstruction with gastrocnemius augmentation.[43-45]

RESULTS

Bulk Allograft

Structural bone grafting in the setting of knee revision has good results at short- to medium-term follow-up, with 75% to 90% survival at 10 years.[12,20,22,46] This construct allows for axial loading at the graft–host junction, which possibly enhances graft–host union[20,22](**Fig. 42-10**). A systematic review comparing the use of structural allograft vs porous metal cones in patients with AORI type 2 or 3 defects demonstrated yearly revisions rates of 1.2% for cones and 2.6% for allografts.[47] Although the overall revision rates were not statistically significant, there was a trend toward favoring cones. The use of structural allograft has diminished since the arrival of modular porous metal augmentation for moderately large defects, which avoids the disadvantages of longer surgical time, nonunion, graft resorption, and collapse.[6,18,25] Because shaping and implantation of a structural allograft is a technically demanding and time-consuming technique, we reserve its use for younger patients in an effort to restore bone stock when future reconstructions are imminent.[20]

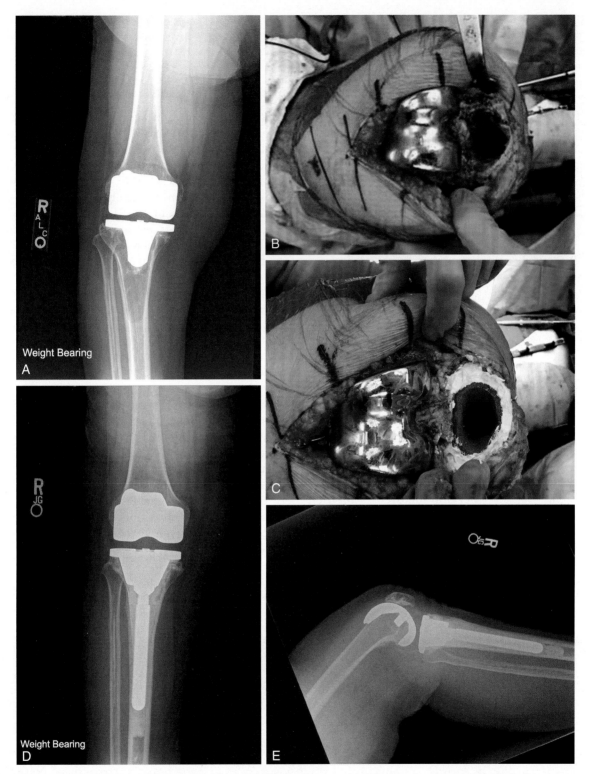

FIGURE 42-7 Preoperative radiograph of a type T3 tibial defect **(A)**. The femur and patella were found to have stable fixation. Intraoperative T3 defect following implant removal and débridement **(B)**. Placement of a porous tibial cone to fill the deficient metaphyseal bone **(C)**. Postoperative radiographs demonstrating a tibial cone with offset press-fit tibial stem **(D** and **E)**.

Metal Augments

Unilateral or bilateral tibial augments can consistently restore the anatomic joint line in AORI type 1 or 2 defects. Prosthetic augments can be porous or solid, rectangular or wedge-shaped, and can be affixed to the femoral or tibial implant with the use of cement or screws to allow up to 20 mm of segmental bone loss to be restored.[6,18,48]

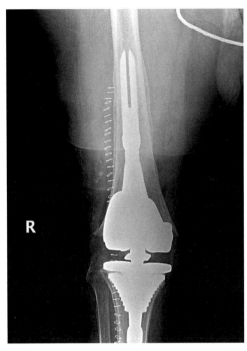

FIGURE 42-8 Postoperative X-ray of a hinged revision implant used to provide stability in a type 3 reconstruction.

Multiple investigations have demonstrated excellent success with the use of modular metal block or wedge augmentation to bony defects on both the tibial and femoral sides, when combined with cemented or press fit stems.[6,18,25,48,49] Patel et al followed 79 revision total knee patients with AORI type 2 defects treated with metal augments, reporting a survival rate of 92% at 11 years.[25] In this cohort, only 4% required subsequent revision for aseptic loosening, with 15% of cases demonstrating stable radiolucent lines. In less severe type 1 defects, which are often encountered in

the setting of revision UKA, modular metal augments and stems have been shown to successfully reconstruct the joint line.[50,51]

Porous Metaphyseal Sleeves and Cones

Metaphyseal cones and sleeves have become increasingly popular due to their ease of use, modularity, structural stability, and potential for ingrowth. Porous metaphyseal cones are optimally used in the setting of large AORI type 2 metaphyseal defects.[6,18,48,52] Recent reports have also proven their value in the setting of a completely deficient metaphysis, as seen in AORI type 3 defects[28,29,32,33,35,37] (**Fig. 42-11**). Watters et al reported the outcomes of AORI type 2 and 3 bone defects treated with porous-coated sleeves in 108 patients with a mean follow-up of 5.3 years (range 2 to 9 years).[30] The authors reported a 16% reoperation rate, most commonly for recurrent infection, with two patients (1.5%) requiring sleeve removal. Only one sleeve demonstrated radiographic evidence of failed osseointegration. Klim et al reported on the use of metaphyseal sleeves in 56 patients undergoing a two-stage revision TKA with a minimum 2-year follow-up (mean 5.3 years).[53] Nine patients (16%) were re-revised for reinfection, with no patients requiring revision for aseptic loosening.

With the use of tibial cones, Kamath et al reported on 66 patients treated for AORI type 2 or 3 tibial defects with a mean follow-up of 5.8 years.[28] The authors reported greater than 95% survivorship at final follow-up, with three patients undergoing revisions (infection, aseptic loosening, and fracture) and two patients having radiolucencies. Potter et al followed 159 patients with femoral cones used for severe femoral bone loss and demonstrated a 5-year survivorship over 95% when the end point was revision of the cone for aseptic loosening.[29] However, the survivorship decreased to 84% when revision of the cone

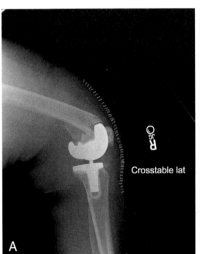
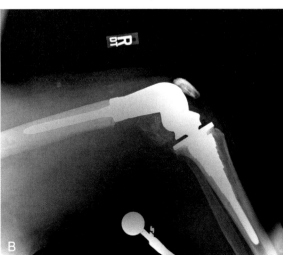
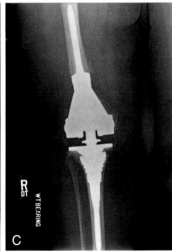

FIGURE 42-9 Lateral X-ray showing distal femur fracture in the presence of a total knee arthroplasty **(A)**. Postoperative lateral X-ray showing a distal femoral endoprosthesis **(B)**. Postoperative anteroposterior X-ray showing a distal femoral endoprosthesis **(C)**.

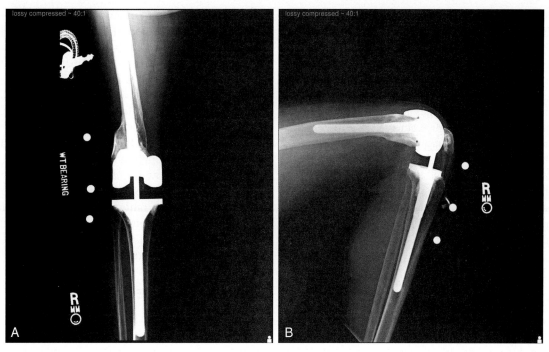

FIGURE 42-10   Anteroposterior **(A)** and lateral **(B)** X-rays of F3 reconstruction using an entire distal femoral allograft with a long stem. 5 years postoperatively, the graft–host union is healed.

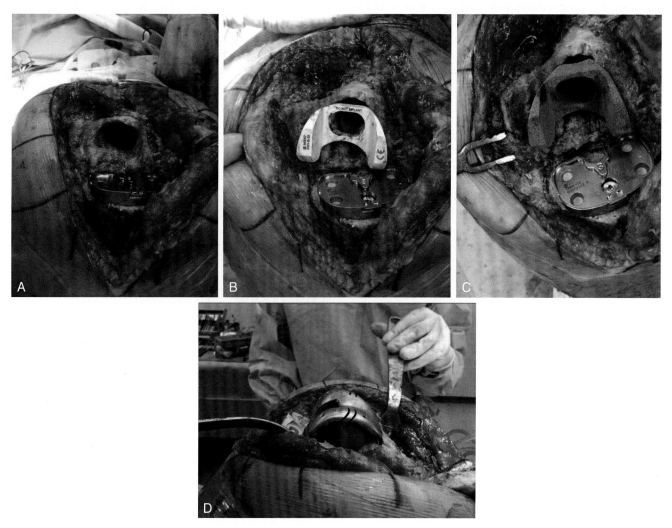

FIGURE 42-11   Intraoperative view of a type F3 bone defect. Deficient distal femur **(A)**; trial augment in place **(B)**; porous metaphyseal augment in place **(C)**; and femoral component in place on augment **(D)**.

occurred for any reason. All six revisions for aseptic loosening of the cone occurred in patients with hinged TKAs and AORI type 3 defects, leading the authors to suggest development of implants with different shapes, sizes, and methods of preparation be considered for type 3 femoral defects.

Metaphyseal sleeves and cones result in clinically relevant Knee Society score improvements at 3 to 5 years postoperatively, with radiographic stability consistently above 90%, and 5 to 10 year survivorship ranging from 84% to 99%.[27-30,32,33,35,37] For these reasons, we have adopted the use of porous cones and sleeves over bulk allograft in the setting of AORI type 2 to 3 defects, with the most recent use of a bulk allograft occurring at our institution in 2012.

Stems

The use of stems at revision surgery restores coronal alignment and confers stability to the reconstruction through stable fixation with load transfer from the components to host bone. Historically, there has been a debate over cemented stem fixation compared to press fit diaphyseal fixation. Cemented stems have demonstrated survivorship near 95% for aseptic loosening at 8 to 9 year follow-up.[54,55] Diaphyseal-engaging press-fit stems have also shown low revision rates (3%-6%) for aseptic loosening at 8 to 12 years follow-up.[56-58]

The advent of porous augments and sleeves has somewhat changed the debate about cemented or cementless stems. The type of metaphyseal reconstruction chosen can dictate the choice between cemented or press-fit stems. When porous cones are chosen, the position of the cone can conflict with a diaphyseal-engaging stem. This is especially true in the setting of larger diameter stems that do not readily pass through cones. In this scenario, smaller diameter stems can be passed through the cone, fixed with cement, and confer immediate implant stability. Current studies using porous cones with predominantly cemented stems have demonstrated revision rates for aseptic loosening to be lower than 5% at 5 to 10 years follow-up.[28,29,59] When sleeves are chosen for metaphyseal reconstruction, diaphyseal-engaging press-fit stems determine the final position of the revision construct. This technique is relatively straightforward to perform and requires minimal customization during bone preparation. Results using sleeves in the setting of press-fit stems have demonstrated revision rates for aseptic loosening to be lower than 5% at 5 to 12 years follow-up.[56-58]

Constraint

Increasing constraint requirements should follow an algorithmic approach, which consists of three generalizable options: (1) condylar implants with a posterior-stabilized or constrained condylar inserts in cases of isolated posterior cruciate ligament insufficiency, (2) unlinked constrained condylar implants for mild instability, and (3) linked hinged implants or endoprosthesis in cases of severe ligamentous instability or massive bone loss resulting in collateral ligament compromise.[31,36]

Investigators have shown greater than 90% survivorship at 5 to 12 years following revision TKA with the use of varus–valgus constrained implants.[27-33,35,56,58,60] The use of sleeves and cones in the setting of hinged devices has shown acceptable outcomes, with survival rates as high as 90% at mean follow-up of 5 to 7.5 years; however, two investigators have reported inferior results with the use of hinged devices with tantalum femoral cones for revision for aseptic loosening in type 3 defects, suggesting preferential use of unlinked implants when feasible or sleeved devices if hinged constraint is required.[29,30,38]

AORI EXPERIENCE

We have used the AORI defect classification system in revising and reconstructing over 2000 total knee replacements. It has proven easy to implement, effectively describes the degree of bone loss and guides management of the defects. Tibial and femoral defects are independent of one another. For example, of the revisions with an F1 defect, no tibial defect was found in 14%, T1 defect in 54%, T2 defect in 30%, and T3 defect in 2%. The most commonly encountered defects are T1 and F1, with nearly 40% of revisions falling into those categories. For 99% of cases with these smaller defects, it was a first-time revision.

About 25% of all revisions fell into the T2A or F2A category, requiring a solid metal augment or autograft to fill the defect. T2B defects were present in 18% of revised tibial components and F2B defects in 20% of revised femoral components. T3 and F3 defects are the least commonly encountered, with fewer than 15% of revision cases reaching that level of severity. These occurred most often in cases of osteolysis, infection, and loose components. These extensive reconstructions had the highest failure rate (14%).

CONCLUSION

When performing revision total knee arthroplasty, surgeons must be able to deal with bone defects on the tibia and the femur. Preoperative exam and radiographic review will allow the surgeon to identify the reasons for implant failure, determine ligamentous stability, estimate bone loss, and plan for the upcoming reconstruction. Reconstructive options for significant bone loss have evolved since the last version of this chapter. Allograft (particulate and bulk) reconstruction was common in the past. Now, metaphyseal defects are usually reconstructed with porous metal cones or sleeves that have potential for osseointegration and long-term fixation. This requires viable and supportive bone to provide a durable junction for long-term fixation. Both of these methods use a stemmed implant, which offloads metaphyseal stress and transfers load to the diaphysis.

A classification system for knee bone loss can guide preparation for surgery and the intraoperative reconstruction. Currently available systems can address a range of bone defects. When there is minimal metaphyseal bone loss, the reconstruction does not require porous metaphyseal fixation. With increasing metaphyseal bone loss, the same systems offer metaphyseal porous augments and cones or porous sleeves. These cases always require either cemented or press-fit stems. More severe defects and some periprosthetic fractures can be managed with an endoprosthesis. Hinged implants must be available and are reserved for cases with residual instability.

REFERENCES

1. Sharkey PF, Lichstein PM, Shen C, Tokarski AT, Parvizi J. Why are total knee arthroplasties failing today—has anything changed after 10 years? *J Arthroplasty*. 2014;29(9):1774-1778.
2. Delanois RE, Mistry JB, Gwam CU, Mohamed NS, Choksi US, Mont MA. Current epidemiology of revision total knee arthroplasty in the United States. *J Arthroplasty*. 2017;32(9):2663-2668.
3. McDowell M, Park A, Gerlinger TL. The painful total knee arthroplasty. *Orthop Clin North Am*. 2016;47(2):317-326.
4. Parvizi J, Tan TL, Goswami K, et al. The 2018 definition of periprosthetic hip and knee infection: an evidence-based and validated criteria. *J Arthroplasty*. 2018;33(5):1309-1314.e2.
5. Chalmers BP, Sculco PK, Fehring KA, Taunton MJ, Trousdale RT. Fluoroscopically assisted radiographs improve sensitivity of detecting loose tibial implants in revision total knee arthroplasty. *J Arthroplasty*. 2017;32(2):570-574.
6. Sheth NP, Bonadio MB, Demange MK. Bone loss in revision total knee arthroplasty: evaluation and management. *J Am Acad Orthop Surg*. 2017;25(5):348-357.
7. Mulhall KJ, Ghomrawi HM, Engh GA, Clark CR, Lotke P, Saleh KJ. Radiographic prediction of intraoperative bone loss in knee arthroplasty revision. *Clin Orthop Relat Res*. 2006;446:51-58.
8. Qiu YY, Yan CH, Chiu KY, Ng FY. Bone defect classifications in revision total knee arthroplasty. *J Orthop Surg*. 2011;19(2):238-243.
9. Hoeffel DP, Rubash HE. Revision total knee arthroplasty: current rationale and techniques for femoral component revision. *Clin Orthop Relat Res*. 2000;380:116-132.
10. Nelson CL, Lonner JH, Rand JA, Lotke PA. Strategies of stem fixation and the role of supplemental bone graft in revision total knee arthroplasty. *J Bone Joint Surg Am*. 2003;85-A(suppl 1):S52-S57.
11. Huff TW, Sculco TP. Management of bone loss in revision total knee arthroplasty. *J Arthroplasty*. 2007;22(7 suppl 3):32-36.
12. Engh GA. Bone defect classification. In: Engh GA, Roraback CH, eds. *Revision Total Knee Arthroplasty*. 1st ed. Baltimore, MD: Williams and Wilkins;1997:63-120, chap 5.
13. Hofmann AA, Kurtin SM, Lyons S, Tanner AM, Bolognesi MP. Clinical and radiographic analysis of accurate restoration of the joint line in revision total knee arthroplasty. *J Arthroplasty*. 2006;21(8):1154-1162.
14. Porteous AJ, Hassaballa MA, Newman JH. Does the joint line matter in revision total knee replacement? *J Bone Joint Surg Br*. 2008;90(7):879-884.
15. Pereira GC, von Kaeppler E, Alaia MJ, et al. Calculating the position of the joint line of the knee using anatomical landmarks. *Orthopedics*. 2016;39(6):381-386.
16. Laskin RS. Joint line position restoration during revision total knee replacement. *Clin Orthop Relat Res*. 2002;404:169-171.
17. Ritter MA, Harty LD. Medial screws and cement: a possible mechanical augmentation in total knee arthroplasty. *J Arthroplasty*. 2004;19(5):587-589.
18. Daines BK, Dennis DA. Management of bone defects in revision total knee arthroplasty. *J Bone Joint Surg Am*. 2012;94(12):1131-1139.
19. Lotke PA, Carolan GF, Puri N. Impaction grafting for bone defects in revision total knee arthroplasty. *Clin Orthop Relat Res*. 2006;446:99-103.
20. Engh GA, Ammeen DJ. Use of structural allograft in revision total knee arthroplasty in knees with severe tibial bone loss. *J Bone Joint Surg Am*. 2007;89(12):2640-2647.
21. Parks NL, Engh GA. The Ranawat Award. Histology of nine structural bone grafts used in total knee arthroplasty. *Clin Orthop Relat Res*. 1997;345:17-23.
22. Engh GA, Herzwurm PJ, Parks NL. Treatment of major defects of bone with bulk allografts and stemmed components during total knee arthroplasty. *J Bone Joint Surg Am*. 1997;79(7):1030-1039.
23. Stockley I, McAuley JP, Gross AE. Allograft reconstruction in total knee arthroplasty. *J Bone Joint Surg Br*. 1992;74(3):393-397.
24. Fehring TK, Peindl RD, Humble RS, Harrow ME, Frick SL. Modular tibial augmentations in total knee arthroplasty. *Clin Orthop Relat Res*. 1996;327:207-217.
25. Patel JV, Masonis JL, Guerin J, Bourne RB, Rorabeck CH. The fate of augments to treat type-2 bone defects in revision knee arthroplasty. *J Bone Joint Surg Br*. 2004;86(2):195-199.
26. Rand JA. Bone deficiency in total knee arthroplasty. Use of metal wedge augmentation. *Clin Orthop Relat Res*. 1991;271:63-71.
27. Chalmers BP, Desy NM, Pagnano MW, Trousdale RT, Taunton MJ. Survivorship of metaphyseal sleeves in revision total knee arthroplasty. *J Arthroplasty*. 2017;32(5):1565-1570.
28. Kamath AF, Lewallen DG, Hanssen AD. Porous tantalum metaphyseal cones for severe tibial bone loss in revision knee arthroplasty: a five to nine-year follow-up. *J Bone Joint Surg Am*. 2015;97(3):216-223.
29. Potter GD III, Abdel MP, Lewallen DG, Hanssen AD. Midterm results of porous tantalum femoral cones in revision total knee arthroplasty. *J Bone Joint Surg Am*. 2016;98(15):1286-1291.
30. Watters TS, Martin JR, Levy DL, Yang CC, Kim RH, Dennis DA. Porous-coated metaphyseal sleeves for severe femoral and tibial bone loss in revision TKA. *J Arthroplasty*. 2017;32(11):3468-3473.
31. Azzam K, Parvizi J, Kaufman D, Purtill JJ, Sharkey PF, Austin MS. Revision of the unstable total knee arthroplasty: outcome predictors. *J Arthroplasty*. 2011;26(8):1139-1144.
32. Derome P, Sternheim A, Backstein D, Malo M. Treatment of large bone defects with trabecular metal cones in revision total knee arthroplasty: short term clinical and radiographic outcomes. *J Arthroplasty*. 2014;29(1):122-126.
33. Graichen H, Scior W, Strauch M. Direct, cementless, metaphyseal fixation in knee revision arthroplasty with sleeves-short-term results. *J Arthroplasty*. 2015;30(12):2256-2259.
34. Jones RE, Skedros JG, Chan AJ, Beauchamp DH, Harkins PC. Total knee arthroplasty using the S-ROM mobile-bearing hinge prosthesis. *J Arthroplasty*. 2001;16(3):279-287.
35. Lachiewicz PF, Watters TS. Porous metal metaphyseal cones for severe bone loss: when only metal will do. *Bone Joint J*. 2014;96-B(11 suppl A):118-121.
36. Luttjeboer JS, Benard MR, Defoort KC, van Hellemondt GG, Wymenga AB. Revision total knee arthroplasty for instability-outcome for different types of instability and implants. *J Arthroplasty*. 2016;31(12):2672-2676.
37. Rao BM, Kamal TT, Vafaye J, Moss M. Tantalum cones for major osteolysis in revision knee replacement. *Bone Joint J*. 2013;95-B(8):1069-1074.
38. Shen C, Lichstein PM, Austin MS, Sharkey PF, Parvizi J. Revision knee arthroplasty for bone loss: choosing the right degree of constraint. *J Arthroplasty*. 2014;29(1):127-131.
39. Harrison RJ Jr, Thacker MM, Pitcher JD, Temple HT, Scully SP. Distal femur replacement is useful in complex total knee arthroplasty revisions. *Clin Orthop Relat Res*. 2006;446:113-120.

40. Springer BD, Sim FH, Hanssen AD, Lewallen DG. The modular segmental kinematic rotating hinge for nonneoplastic limb salvage. *Clin Orthop Relat Res.* 2004;421:181-187.

41. Dennis DA, Little LR. The structural allograft composite in revision total knee arthroplasty. *Orthopedics.* 2005;28(9):1005-1007.

42. Harris AI, Poddar S, Gitelis S, Sheinkop MB, Rosenberg AG. Arthroplasty with a composite of an allograft and a prosthesis for knees with severe deficiency of bone. *J Bone Joint Surg Am.* 1995;77(3):373-386.

43. Browne JA, Hanssen AD. Reconstruction of patellar tendon disruption after total knee arthroplasty: results of a new technique utilizing synthetic mesh. *J Bone Joint Surg Am.* 2011;93(12):1137-1143.

44. Calori GM, Mazza EL, Vaienti L, et al. Reconstruction of patellar tendon following implantation of proximal tibia megaprosthesis for the treatment of post-traumatic septic bone defects. *Injury.* 2016;47(suppl 6):S77-S82.

45. Springer BD, Della Valle CJ. Extensor mechanism allograft reconstruction after total knee arthroplasty. *J Arthroplasty.* 2008;23(7 suppl):35-38.

46. Bauman RD, Lewallen DG, Hanssen AD. Limitations of structural allograft in revision total knee arthroplasty. *Clin Orthop Relat Res.* 2009;467(3):818-824.

47. Beckmann NA, Mueller S, Gondan M, Jaeger S, Reiner T, Bitsch RG. Treatment of severe bone defects during revision total knee arthroplasty with structural allografts and porous metal cones—a systematic review. *J Arthroplasty.* 2015;30(2):249-253.

48. Radnay CS, Scuderi GR. Management of bone loss: augments, cones, offset stems. *Clin Orthop Relat Res.* 2006;446:83-92.

49. Sah AP, Scott RD, Springer BD, Bono JV, Deshmukh RV, Thornhill TS. Custom-made angled inserts for tibial coronal malalignment in total knee arthroplasty. *J Arthroplasty.* 2009;24(2):288-296.

50. Lewis PL, Davidson DC, Graves SE, de Steiger RN, Dònnelly W, Cuthbert A. Unicompartmental knee arthroplasty revision to TKA: are tibial stems and augments associated with improved survivorship? *Clin Orthop Relat Res.* 2018;476(4):854-862.

51. Chou DT, Swamy GN, Lewis JR, Badhe NP. Revision of failed unicompartmental knee replacement to total knee replacement. *Knee.* 2012;19(4):356-359.

52. Barnett SL, Mayer RR, Gondusky JS, Choi L, Patel JJ, Gorab RS. Use of stepped porous titanium metaphyseal sleeves for tibial defects in revision total knee arthroplasty: short term results. *J Arthroplasty.* 2014;29(6):1219-1224.

53. Klim SM, Amerstorfer F, Bernhardt GA, et al. Septic revision total knee arthroplasty: treatment of metaphyseal bone defects using metaphyseal sleeves. *J Arthroplasty.* 2018;33(12):3734-3738.

54. Gililland JM, Gaffney CJ, Odum SM, Fehring TK, Peters CL, Beaver WB. Clinical & radiographic outcomes of cemented vs. diaphyseal engaging cementless stems in aseptic revision TKA. *J Arthroplasty.* 2014;29(9 suppl):224-228.

55. Wang C, Pfitzner T, von Roth P, Mayr HO, Sostheim M, Hube R. Fixation of stem in revision of total knee arthroplasty: cemented versus cementless—a meta-analysis. *Knee Surg Sports Traumatol Arthrosc.* 2016;24(10):3200-3211.

56. Greene JW, Reynolds SM, Stimac JD, Malkani AL, Massini MA. Midterm results of hybrid cement technique in revision total knee arthroplasty. *J Arthroplasty.* 2013;28(4):570-574.

57. Gross TP, Liu F. Total knee arthroplasty with fully porous-coated stems for the treatment of large bone defects. *J Arthroplasty.* 2013;28(4):598-603.

58. Wood GC, Naudie DD, MacDonald SJ, McCalden RW, Bourne RB. Results of press-fit stems in revision knee arthroplasties. *Clin Orthop Relat Res.* 2009;467(3):810-817.

59. Fleischman AN, Azboy I, Fuery M, Restrepo C, Shao H, Parvizi J. Effect of stem size and fixation method on mechanical failure after revision total knee arthroplasty. *J Arthroplasty.* 2017;32(9 suppl):S202-S208.e1.

60. Heesterbeek PJ, Wymenga AB, van Hellemondt GG. No difference in implant micromotion between hybrid fixation and fully cemented revision total knee arthroplasty: a randomized controlled trial with radiostereometric analysis of patients with mild-to-moderate bone loss. *J Bone Joint Surg Am.* 2016;98(16):1359-1369.

chapter 43

The Varus Knee: Considerations for Alignment and Balance

David W. Anderson, MD, MS | Kelly J. Hendricks, MD | Cameron K. Ledford, MD

Primary osteoarthritis develops in a slow, progressive fashion and can affect one or all three of the major joint compartments of the knee. Varus deformity is the most common anatomic deformity encountered by surgeons performing knee replacements for patients with advanced arthritis of the knee. Severe varus deformity may lead to premature failure of total knee arthroplasties because of the technical difficulties associated with satisfactory alignment and ligament balance. All varus knees, however, should not necessarily be treated the same with regard to a standard formal release. Clinical outcomes and complication rates of total knee arthroplasty can be optimized with appropriate surgical planning and understanding of the balancing techniques associated with and required for surgical treatment of the arthritic varus knee.

Soft-tissue balance and implant alignment are essential components when understanding the complexities of primary total joint surgery. This includes an understanding of restoration of neutral mechanical alignment and the concept of anatomic restoration with respect to natural patient anatomy, which has gained interest among knee surgeons. Recent studies have also shown that the historical problem of polyethylene wear has been overtaken by other failure mechanisms such as aseptic loosening, instability, malalignment, and periprosthetic infection as more common reasons for revision.[1] Even with continuing technologic advancement, including computer-based technology and robotics, and improved appreciation for biomechanics, revision rates have not significantly decreased.

The purpose of either partial or total knee arthroplasty is to replace the damaged cartilage and bone with an artificial implant that compensates for this pathologic process. Restoration of a neutral mechanical alignment is typically the goal of this procedure. Historically, most surgeons use a measurement based on intramedullary access to the canals of the femur and tibia. Extramedullary techniques have also been available. Computer-based navigation and robotics offer alternatives to standard intramedullary techniques as well. A leg is neutrally aligned (or has a neutral mechanical axis) in the coronal plane when a line drawn from the center of the femoral head to the center of the ankle mortise passes through the center of the knee joint. Localization of the femoral head is often difficult and inaccurate during surgery, which makes intraoperative measurement of the mechanical axis difficult. When

an anatomic axis measurement system is used, the range of 4° to 9° of valgus is considered neutral alignment. Any coronal alignment of less than 4° of valgus is considered varus.

TYPES OF VARUS DEFORMITY

Greater than half of the patients older than 65 years have radiographic changes in the knee consistent with osteoarthritis.[2] Knee deformities in the arthritic patient can be classified into intra-articular and extra-articular deformity and further divided into three types. *Flexible* deformities are those that can be passively corrected into a neutral leg alignment. *Fixed* deformities are those that cannot be passively corrected. *Mixed* deformities may be partially correctable but are still partially fixed. Extra-articular deformity can be metaphyseal or diaphyseal. The ability to correct extra-articular deformity will depend on the magnitude of the deformity and the distance from the joint. Full-leg standing radiographs with the use of various mechanical and anatomic angles can be measured to assist in planning for these extra-articular deformities.

Pain may preclude the examiner for making a proper evaluation during the physical examination as to the nature of the patient's deformity. Final determination as to whether the deformity is fixed or flexible should be made with the patient under anesthesia. When a large series of patients undergoing knee replacement were evaluated, less than one-third of the varus deformities that appeared fixed preoperatively were indeed fixed when the patient was anesthetized. It was only the fixed deformities that required soft-tissue releases. If a surgeon were to erroneously perform a soft-tissue release for a varus deformity that was not truly fixed, the outcome could lead to knee instability postoperatively.

Many patients with fixed varus deformities have a concomitant inability to fully extend the knee passively. Laskin noted that over 75% of patients who underwent total knee arthroplasty with a fixed varus deformity also had a fixed flexion contracture in a 10-year period of patients studied.[3] Su estimated that up to 60% of the total patients undergoing total knee arthroplasty had some degree of knee flexion contracture.[4] There is no appreciated correlation between the exact magnitude of the varus deformity and the magnitude of the flexion deformity.

CAUSES OF VARUS DEFORMITY

Some patients have a varus deformity of the leg secondary to angulation of the femoral or tibial shaft at some distance from the knee. This is considered to be an extra-articular malalignment. Causes of this may include a malunited fracture, Paget disease, or a congenital deformity such as Blount disease or fibrous dysplasia. Other more rare underlying metabolic processes may also contribute to these deformities. Although such deformities must be taken into account when assessing overall leg alignment and surgical planning, the majority of knee deformity exists because of a pathologic process that is intra-articular or immediately adjacent to the knee joint.

The basic intra-articular cause a varus deformity is an asymmetric loss of articular cartilage or bone that is greater from the medial side than from the lateral side of the knee. Loss of cartilage often occurs from medial mechanical overload and/or a knee with abnormal kinematics. The two most common conditions are insufficient anterior cruciate ligament or prior medial meniscus surgery, such as a partial or total meniscectomy. Meniscal tears are the most common knee injury, with approximately 700,000 partial meniscectomies performed in the United States yearly.[5-7] Degenerative meniscal tears are more common in patients aged 42 to 65 years and can occur from gradual loss of inherent meniscal stability, chronic wear, athletic activities, activities of daily living, and traumatic twisting injuries.[8] The injured meniscus has an impaired ability to distribute load and resisted tibial translation. Partial or complete loss of the meniscus and meniscus stability promotes early development of chondromalacia and osteoarthritis.[9] Medial overload may also occur in the leg with a varus hip alignment, bowing of the femoral shaft, or varus collapse after a high tibial osteotomy.

Regardless of the mechanism, the physiological process of cartilage loss medially results in increased stress to the underlying bone of the tibial plateau resulting in subchondral sclerosis. The stiffness of the subchondral bone can result in elevated stresses in the articular cartilage, naturally evolving into wear/chondromalacia and further joint line collapse. With fraying and wear of the cartilage, the synovial fluid can be pressurized into the bone surface potentially causing cystic changes to occur. Periarticular osteophytes can form as the joint degenerates, increasing the surface area through which the joint distributes force. Unlike a valgus knee, which can be associated with hypoplasia or dysgenesis of the posterior lateral and distal aspects of the lateral femoral condyle, there does not appear to be a significant difference in the shape or extent of the posterior portion of the medial femoral condyle when varus knees are compared with knees in a neutral or valgus alignment.

In addition to bony changes, the medial soft tissue around the knee also endures changes. Initially, the medial soft tissues in a patient with a varus deformity will remain relatively normal. Thus the deformity remains flexible. Through the natural progression of the varus deformity, the soft tissues medially can become contracted or pseudo-contracted, which makes the joint no longer correctable and a fixed deformity. The contracture can be accentuated by peripheral osteophyte formation both medially and posteriorly. Fixed deformity requires surgical correction techniques for adequate soft tissue balance.

PREOPERATIVE EVALUATION AND RELEVANT ANATOMY

Careful preoperative evaluation and planning can lead to successful management of a degenerative varus knee. Surgeons should obtain a detailed history and perform a physical exam that includes evaluation of the hip, knee, ankle, and overall limb alignment. This should also include an assessment of the quality of the soft tissue envelope surrounding the knee including the presence and location of previous incisions, stability to varus and valgus stress throughout the range of motion, the presence of flexion contracture, and the ability to correct the coronal deformity at 30° of flexion. A complete set of knee radiographs including a weight-bearing anteroposterior view, a lateral view, and a sunrise/merchant view should also be evaluated. Particular attention should be given for the presence of subchondral sclerosis, cystic changes, and osteophytes. Medial and posterior osteophytes may give indication that there is impinging soft tissue that can confound a physical examination. Consideration should be given in the preoperative planning and intraoperative surgical technique to address these medial and posterior osteophytes. Additional discussion with the patient and planning should be undertaken with options to address previous retained hardware as well as options to treat defects found from previous ligament reconstruction, for example, bone tunnels from previous ACL reconstructions.

While full-length weight-bearing films are not necessary in preoperative planning, these can assist in determining the distal valgus resection angle and the level of bony resection at both the distal femur and proximal tibia. The authors find full-length films particularly useful in patients with previous posttraumatic deformity and in short- or tall-statured individuals. Special attention should be paid to lateral radiographs with regard to the patella and tibial tuberosity. With patella baja, patellar abnormality, or prominent tibial tuberosity, surgical exposure of the knee could be more challenging due to difficulty with the version or subluxation of the patella. Consideration should be given in preoperative planning and choice of surgical instrumentation with these types of patients. It is the recommendation of these authors that surgeons use an appropriate physical examination

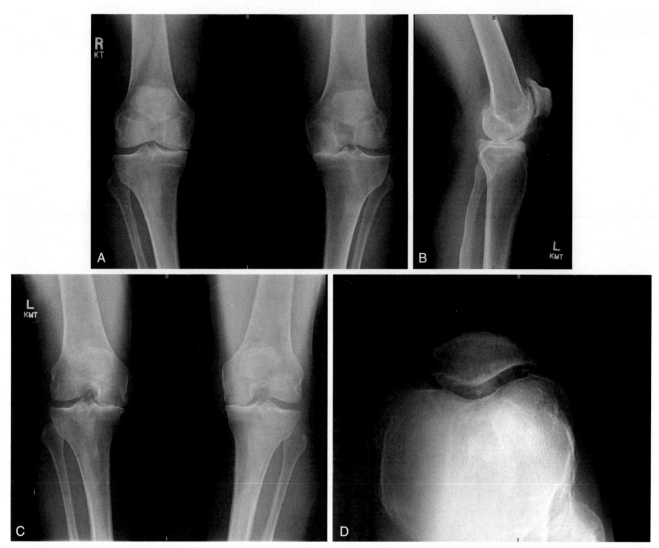

FIGURE 43-1   Standard radiographic evaluation of the adult knee. **A:** Weight-bearing AP view for evaluation of the tibiofemoral joint space including formation of osteophytes on the joint margin or on the tibial spines, narrowing of the joint cartilage with sclerosis of subchondral bone, presence or absence of small cystic or pseudocystic areas with sclerotic walls in the subchondral bone, and/or altered shape of the distal femur or proximal tibia. **B:** Lateral view taken in slight flexion (around 30°) allows for radiographic assessment of the patellofemoral joint, patellar position (alta or baja), and tibial slope. **C:** Weight-bearing 45° PA (Rosenberg) flexion view to evaluate for early tibiofemoral arthritis and posterior wear not always evident on standard AP view. **D:** Merchant or sunrise view to evaluate patellofemoral space, tilt, and alignment.

and radiographic evaluation (**Figs. 43-1 and 43-2**) when determining implant type for the planned total knee arthroplasty and always have options available for a more constrained device if needed due to significant bony deformity, ligamentous laxity, or soft-tissue imbalance.

When performing a total knee arthroplasty on a varus knee, the medial soft tissues are typically tight. Balancing therefore relies on appropriate understanding and potential release of the medial soft-tissue structures. Static stabilizers include the superficial fibers of the medial collateral ligament, posterior oblique ligament, posterior cruciate ligament, and posterior capsule. Dynamic stabilizers include the pes anserine tendons and the semimembranosus tendon. Release of anterior structures primarily affects the flexion gap, while release of posterior structures affects the extension gap.

TREATMENT OF INTRA-ARTICULAR VARUS DEFORMITY

Insall and Ranawat described the traditional method for correction of a combined varus and flexion deformity of the knee in the 1970s.[10,11] The correction of a varus deformity during total knee arthroplasty should be gradual and progressive, as aggressive and immediate releases can lead to an imbalance of both the extension and flexion spaces. Soft-tissue releases do not always affect flexion and extension equally and symmetrically.[12,13] Careless releases of the medial or lateral structures can lead to early, mid-, and late-term knee instability. The authors encourage appropriate templating prior to total knee arthroplasty, even for the most routine of cases. This typically involves utilizing an anteroposterior view radiograph with a

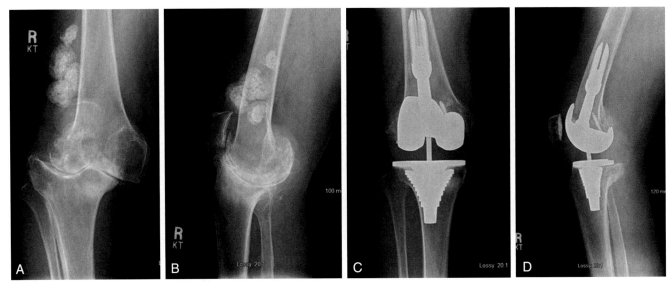

FIGURE 43-2 **A** and **B:** AP and lateral view of a 73-year-old man with severe degenerative changes including severe erosion of the tibia, lateral and axial migration of his tibia in relation to his femur, varus deformity, severe dishing and erosion of his tibia with pronounced posterior slope, and multiple loose bodies in the patellofemoral pouch. **C** and **D:** 1 year postoperative AP and lateral radiographs after semi-constrained total knee arthroplasty, which was preferred by the authors due to ligament imbalance found at the time of surgery for this complex deformity.

vertical line drawn down the center of the femoral and tibial shafts. On the tibial shaft, a perpendicular line is drawn to the first line at the level of the tibial plateau with consideration of the relative amount of the bony resection, which can be determined based on the deformity and the ratio of the lateral to medial resection. In general, approximately 2 mm is estimated to be removed from the most involved side on the tibial plateau. On the femoral side, a horizontal line is drawn that is approximately 5° of valgus from the vertical line that was drawn previously. The valgus angle is taken into consideration with the stature of the patient and overall length of the femur. This more horizontal line passes through the most proximal point of the intracondylar notch to give an idea of the bony resection needed from the medial and lateral femoral condyles. The lateral view should be inspected for any posterior osteophytes. Osteophytes are taken in consideration for removal during the exposure, particularly paying attention to how these might affect the extension stability as well as achieving full extension considering capsular tightness from the posterior capsule. The lateral view may also be used for sizing the femoral component as part of the templating process.

Prior to making an incision, the surgeon should evaluate the coronal ligamentous stability of the knee in order to determine if the deformity is flexible or fixed. If, under anesthesia, the limb can be corrected to a neutral alignment, the surgeon should consider performing minimal soft-tissue releases during the surgical approach.

The standard surgical approach includes a longitudinal anterior incision with full thickness flaps followed by a standard medial parapatellar arthrotomy. This is followed by elevation of the soft tissues from the anteromedial tibial plateau. This elevation begins at the medial

border of the patellar tendon insertion and progresses around the medial tibia to a degree such that the joint can be easily accessed with the appropriate retraction to remove the bony resections and place the instrumentation. Technically, this exposure is most easily performed with the knee in slight flexion and with gradual external rotation of the lower leg using cautery to release the tissue in a subperiosteal fashion taking care not to aggressively cauterize the tissue (**Fig. 43-3**). With the knee held in slight external rotation, a Cobb elevator or curved periosteal elevator is passed posteriorly at the joint line just beyond the mid-coronal line (**Fig. 43-4**). During this portion of the procedure, the anteromedial osteophytes are removed, either with a rongeur or with an osteotome (**Fig. 43-5**). To properly visualize the tibial plateau surface, the tibia must be subluxed anterior to the femur. The surgeon needs a soft-tissue "window" that is of appropriate size through which to deliver the resected bone and to place the instruments to perform the procedure, in addition to consideration for appropriate placement of the final components later in the procedure, regardless of whether they are cemented, cementless, or hybrid components. Forcible attempts to perform this procedure through a soft-tissue window that is not of the appropriate size can lead to inadvertent tearing of the medial capsular structures, inappropriate bony resections, unintended retention of soft tissue/bone/cement debris, or malposition of final components.

After full exposure of the knee, basic bone cuts of the distal femur and tibia are performed to establish the extension space. The timing of remaining cuts of the femur (anterior/posterior femur and chamfer cuts) may be performed based upon surgeon-preferred technique (measured resection vs gap balance) and will largely affect the

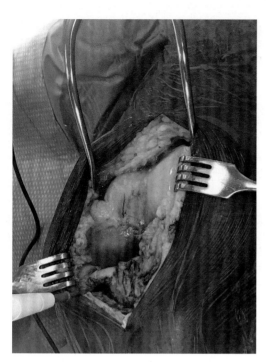

FIGURE 43-3 Elevation of the anteromedial capsule with cautery.

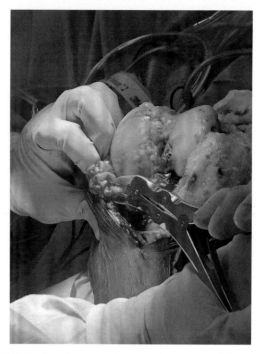

FIGURE 43-5 Use of a rongeur to remove the anteromedial osteophytes.

flexion space. The surgeon is also to remove any excessive osteophytes from the tibia and femoral condyles. At this point, it is possible to begin assessing ligamentous balance in extension, if there are no impinging posterior structures such as large osteophytes. (It is typically not possible to easily remove large posterior osteophytes from the posterior tibia and posterior femur prior to final bone cuts; thus consideration should be given on the

impact of such osteophytes on the extension space.) Once cuts are completed, an appropriate assessment should be made regarding the knee balance of both the extension and flexion gap and if soft-tissue releases will be required.

A variety of methods are available to determine ligament balancing and the presence of residual medial contracture. The simplest method involves using lamina spreaders with large flat paddles (**Fig. 43-6**). With the knee fully extended, the spreaders are placed between the cut surfaces of the distal femur and proximal tibia. These are gently extended until a firm endpoint is obtained on both the medial and lateral surfaces of the joint. The distance between the cut surfaces is then measured. In equally balanced medial and lateral compartments, the distances should be equal if tension was applied appropriately. The knee may also be brought into 90° of flexion

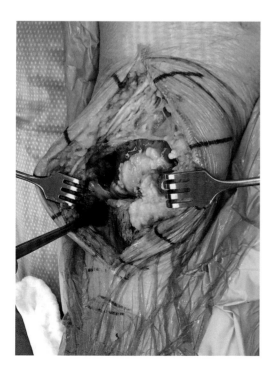

FIGURE 43-4 Use of a Cobb elevator to elevate the medial structures.

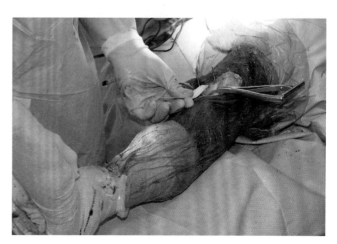

FIGURE 43-6 Measurement of the extensor space with lamina spreaders and a ruler.

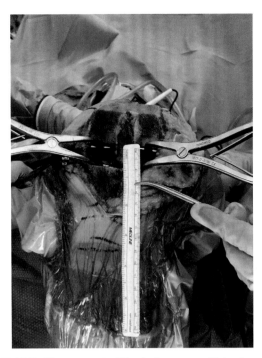

FIGURE 43-7 Measurement of the flexion space with lamina spreaders and a ruler.

and a similar technique applied with the spreaders placed on the medial and lateral posterior condyles. These can then be gradually and gently extended until a firm endpoint is obtained. The joint space may then be measured with a ruler and this measurement compared to the extension measurement for an assessment of the overall joint balance (**Fig. 43-7**).

Another simple method uses spacer blocks (**Fig. 43-8**). These blocks are available in most implant sets in a variety of thicknesses. They may be progressively placed into the extension space until the space is filled. The knee can then be stressed into varus and valgus. There should be less than 2 mm of gapping, but more importantly any

such gapping should be equal medially and laterally. Spacer blocks may also be used with the knee at 90° of flexion and similarly the knee may be stressed to evaluate for gapping. The flexion and extension spaces as determined by the spacer blocks are used to evaluate appropriate ligamentous balancing in full extension and flexion.

A third method of determining balance is through the use of a graduated tension device (**Fig. 43-9**), also known as a gap-balancing technique. Modern design changes have made these graduated tension devices more amenable to use in less invasive surgery, as previous versions could be considered somewhat bulky or cumbersome. One of the authors (K.H.) prefers to utilize the trial implants and then applying a varus and valgus force in both flexion and extension as part of the algorithm for determining appropriate soft-tissue releases.

There are a variety of computerized navigation methods and robotic techniques available to surgeons which may improve precision of resections and overall joint balance. Additionally, such methods avoid femoral canal cannulation, thus avoiding the potential associated risks of fat emboli. Perhaps of most interest with computerized technology is the availability of live feedback for implant position and joint stability. This information may potentially improve the decision-making process for potential necessary releases or corrections that can be made intraoperatively removing reliance on this portion of procedure from "surgeon feel." The effect of intraoperative releases can be immediately visualized with some of these technologies by applying a varus or valgus stress in the respective flexion range. This feedback can also be coupled with the utilization of previously discussed lamina

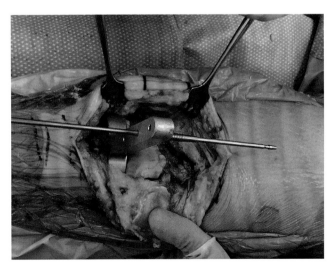

FIGURE 43-8 Measurement of the extensor space with a spacer block and alignment rod.

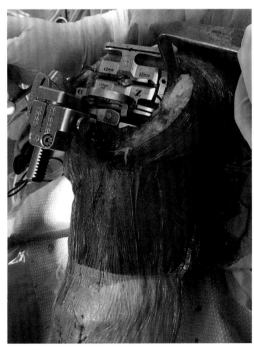

FIGURE 43-9 Measurement of the extensor space with a tension device.

spreaders, spacer blocks, or trial components. The long-term results of these technologies compared to standard instrumentation have yet to be fully determined, however should certainly be taken into consideration with current technique and future surgeon training.

SOFT-TISSUE RELEASES IN THE VARUS KNEE

There are two different preferred techniques regarding total knee arthroplasty balancing: measured resection and gap balancing. In general, measured resection requires balancing the soft tissues after the bony resections have been completed. Gap balancing, on the other hand, uses the tension of native soft tissues and ligaments to determine the appropriate level of the bony resection. It is the experience and opinion of the authors that most surgeons use a combination of both techniques to achieve balance in a total knee arthroplasty.

Following accurate femoral and tibial bony resections and addressing easily accessible anteromedial osteophytes, the surgeon should consider soft-tissue balance with the goal of creating symmetric rectangular flexion and extension gaps. As discussed previously, there are multiple techniques and devices available for this balancing. For the majority of varus knee deformity in a knee with moderate to severe arthritis, a thorough removal of medial osteophytes in conjunction with minimal soft tissue medial sleeve release will result in a well-balanced knee. However, there are times when the medial structures are tight enough, or the lateral structures lax enough, to lead to unequal flexion and/or extension gaps.

Caution should be used and it is not advisable to resect additional bone from the distal femur or proximal tibia as a means to achieve soft-tissue balance. These additional bone resections can alter the mechanical alignment of the total knee arthroplasty and lead to early failure. Increased distal femoral resection will raise the joint line and can lead to mid flexion instability due to the laxity of the collateral ligaments throughout the range of motion. If a surgeon finds themselves increasing the thickness of the polyethylene from the initial planned resection on a consistent basis, they should reevaluate their surgical technique to ensure there is not distortion of the joint line causing instability.

If the surgeon finds that the knee does not have the appropriate balance to proceed, the surgeon must first ensure that the bony resections made were accurate and have appropriate alignment. After ensuring appropriate bone resections, the surgeon may consider proceeding with additional medial soft-tissue releases. The authors recommend addressing extension stability first. Removal of any anteromedial osteophytes will functionally lengthen the medial collateral ligament due to potential tethering of the medial soft tissues. This can improve the medial coronal balance in full extension. If additional

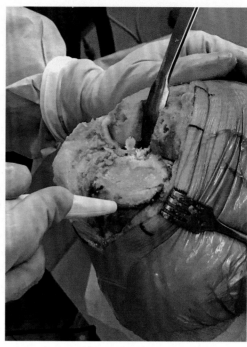

FIGURE 43-10 Release of the posterior structures with use of a Cobb elevator. The knee can be externally rotated through the tibia to access the insertion of the semimembranosus tendon on the posteromedial tibia if needed as part of the sequential release.

soft-tissue releases are required, the next step is to continue around the posterior medial corner to include the deep MCL, the posterior oblique ligament, the posterior medial capsule, and the fibers of the semimembranosus insertion (**Fig. 43-10**). This step is particularly useful with fixed varus deformity including the presence of a flexion contracture. The knee should be externally rotated and the insertion of the semimembranosus tendon on the posteromedial tibia identified. The insertion is then gently released in a subperiosteal fashion utilizing electrocautery or a subperiosteal/Cobb elevator. The joint should then be reassessed for balance in extension to determine if further soft-tissue releases required.

If residual varus deformity/contracture is still present, consideration should be given to addressing the posterior cruciate ligament, whether through recession with a cruciate-retaining component or with removal and utilization of a posterior-stabilized component. There is continuing debate among orthopedic surgeons as to the retention of the PCL during total knee arthroplasty surgery. It can be considered that in severe varus deformity, particularly with flexion contracture, that the PCL is part of the deformity, potentially requiring complete release. The availability of conforming bearing surfaces and medial congruent cruciate-retaining bearing surfaces has made this debate more interesting as mid-term and long-term results slowly become available. Regardless of the surgeon's particular preference for how to treat the PCL, these authors feel that posterior-stabilized and semi-constrained implants should be available during the surgeries in the event it is found that they are needed to optimize the stability joint and also patient outcomes. The PCL may be released from either the femoral or tibial insertion, or sectioned in its mid-substance. Release from the proximal tibia in a subperiosteal fashion will allow the ligament to retract proximally, thereby retaining the bulk of the ligament posteriorly and avoiding excess bleeding from a branch of the middle geniculate artery. This can be seen when the ligament is excised completely. If release of the semimembranosus and PCL is still not sufficient to correct the fixed varus deformity, the next step is subperiosteal elevation (or recession) of the insertion of the pes anserinus tendons and the superficial medial collateral ligament. This release is not equivalent to a transection of the capsule at the joint line, as the capsule is still tethered posteriorly. Subperiosteal elevation in this manner can progress distally as far as necessary to affect a complete release medially and allow sliding of the medial structures more proximally. Thoughtful and gradual releases in this manner and order should be able to correct any varus knee deformity as long as the appropriate bony resections have been made. Any further ligament imbalance found after these releases may need to be addressed with further constraint in the implant, particularly in the coronal plane.

Once coronal plane balancing has been achieved in extension, the next step would be to confirm equal balance in flexion. Multiple etiologies and corrections can be helpful if flexion space is assessed as not equal to the extension space. First, inaccurate posterior femoral condylar cuts should be considered as a potential cause for imbalance at 90° of flexion. An internally rotated cut/component will result in medial flexion tightness. If cuts are assessed to be accurate, alternative balancing techniques include pie crusting of the medial collateral ligament. This involves either making a small horizontal incision in the ligament or making multiple puncture holes using a large diameter hypodermic needle. Another technique is to downsize the tibial component by resecting a portion of the medial tibial plateau for further MCL functional lengthening. Prior to proceeding with this technique, the presence of any remaining osteophytes should be considered. In addition, there may be limitations with implant sizing of any particular system, and correlation of tibial to femoral component sizing must be confirmed prior to employing such technique.

POSTOPERATIVE PROTOCOL

Preoperative physical therapy can be thought of as the beginning of the postoperative protocol, as many studies support improved outcomes with a good preoperative therapy program. Nonetheless, with a well-balanced and stable knee, there is no contraindication to allowing patients to become full weight bearing and perform range of motion as tolerated immediately following surgery. In the setting of an iatrogenic medial collateral ligament rupture, or in instances where the superficial medial collateral ligament has been pie-crusted, the operative extremity can be braced in a hinged knee brace with unrestricted range of motion. Active and active-assist range of motion should be considered for the first 2 weeks while the wound is healing, with emphasis placed on obtaining full extension. Aggressive passive range of motion should be avoided during the wound-healing phase. Additionally, patients should be counseled on the use of assistive device and risk of falling during their early recovery. Routine postoperative antibiotics and anticoagulation based on current evidence-based medicine protocols should also be utilized.

RESULTS OF SOFT-TISSUE RELEASES IN THE VARUS KNEE

A prospective study by Peters et al[14] recorded soft-tissue releases required to produce balanced flexion and extension gaps during primary total knee arthroplasty over an 8-year period. 855 out of 1216 patients had a varus deformity in this study. Among the varus knees, 37% required zero releases, 55% required one or two releases, and 7.5% required three or more releases. Patients with greater preoperative deformity required a greater number releases to achieve a balanced knee at the time of primary total knee arthroplasty. For varus knees, the selective release most commonly included the posterior oblique or the anterior portion of the MCL. Clinical outcomes as measured were improved independent of the degree of deformity.

Early techniques promoted a more global release of soft-tissue structures prior to bone resections.[10] Whiteside et al have described the concept of selective soft-tissue release and a cadaveric model with subsequent clinical study. This study demonstrated that a high percentage of varus knees required release of the posterior oblique and anterior portions of the MCL due to tightness of the extension and flexion space, respectively.[15]

When the medial capsule is recessed, there is an increase in the size of the extension and flexion spaces. If the PCL requires release or removal as well, the flexion space will increase even further. An alternative to medial release for a varus contracture is advancement and tightening of the lateral soft tissues as described by Mihalko and Krackow[16] and Pritsch et al.[17] This technique is likely more of historical significance, with the potential disadvantage of these procedures being limitation of postoperative range of motion while the ligament advancement heels, and the potential for restriction of flexion.

The "inside-out" technique for correction of varus deformities has been described by Meftah et al.[18] This technique includes also performing a posterior medial capsulotomy at the level of the tibial cut and incising the superficial medial collateral ligament in a piecrust manner in extension, followed by serial manipulation with a valgus stress. The authors concluded this technique was a safe, reproducible, and effective manner to treat combined varus and flexion deformity of the knee during total knee arthroplasty without the risk of overrelease of the medial collateral ligament or need for constrained implants. This technique has been validated in a biomechanical cadaver study comparing "pie-crusting" to traditional released to determine the effects on flexion and extension gaps.[19] Valgus laxity was increased in traditional release specimens at 90° of flexion compared to "pie-crusting" alone. "Pie-crusting" of the anterior or posterior aspect of the medial soft-tissue sleeve can affect changes more in flexion than extension. Complete traditional release produces more effect in flexion than in stay extension compared to "pie-crusting." Similarly, Mehdikhani et al[20] reported that an algorithmic "pie-crusting" release technique results in significant reduction in the use of constrained inserts with no detrimental effects and clinical results, joint function, and stability in total knee arthroplasties performed with a posterior-stabilized cemented implant for patients with a preoperative varus deformity.

Recent popularity of kinematic alignment and constitutional varus can cause a surgeon to leave the overall alignment in varus after total knee arthroplasty. A retrospective review of 361 consecutive primary total knee arthroplasties was performed with a minimum of 1 year follow-up to review outcomes of leaving residual varus alignment after total knee arthroplasty.[21] This study found at 25% of limbs were left in residual varus. Outcome scores showed no difference between groups left in neutral, varus, or valgus alignment. The findings failed to support the notion that leaving varus knees in residual varus will improve outcomes or pain. However, residual varus alignment does not appear to increase varus laxity at a minimum of 5 years follow-up after total knee arthroplasty with a cruciate-retaining total knee arthroplasty.[22]

CONCLUSION

Varus knee deformity remains the most common deformity encountered prior to total knee arthroplasty. Selective soft-tissue release in the primary total knee arthroplasty through a variety of techniques can lead to excellent clinical and radiographic results regardless of preoperative alignment. Consistent soft-tissue balance and coronal plane alignment can be achieved with the use of standard measured bone resection, gap-balancing techniques, or combining these two techniques. Results may be improved with regard to surgical technique, implant positioning, limb alignment, joint function, and patient outcomes with the utilization of computer-based options in the future as surgeons become more familiar with these advancing technologies. Current literature supports techniques which will hopefully avoid subsequent flexion instability and decrease the need for revision due to early and mid-term instability.

REFERENCES

1. Thiele K, Perka C, Matziolis G, Mayr HO, Sostheim M, Hube R. Current failure mechanisms after knee arthroplasty have changed: polyethylene wear is less common in revision surgery. *J Bone Joint Surg Am.* 2015;97(9):715-720.
2. Deshpande BR, Katz JN, Solomon DH, et al. Number of persons with symptomatic knee osteoarthritis in the US: impact of race and ethnicity, age, sex, and obesity. *Arthritis Care Res.* 2016;68:1743-1750.
3. Laskin RS. The Genesis total knee prosthesis: a 10-year followup study. *Clin Orthop Relat Res.* 2001;388:95-102.
4. Su EP. Fixed flexion deformity and total knee arthroplasty. *J Bone Joint Surg Br.* 2012;94-B(11 suppl A):112-115.
5. McDermott ID, Amis AA. The consequences of meniscectomy. *J Bone Joint Surg Br.* 2006;88:1549-1556.
6. Brophy RH, Matava MJ. Surgical options for meniscal replacement. *J Am Acad Orthop Surg.* 2012;20:265-272.
7. Sihvonen R, Paavola M, Malmivaara A, et al. Arthroscopic partial meniscectomy versus sham surgery for a degenerative meniscal tear. *N Engl J Med.* 2013;369:2515-2524.
8. Greis PE, Bardana DD, Holmstrom MC, Burks RT. Meniscal injury: I. Basic science and evaluation. *J Am Acad Orthop Surg.* 2002;10:168-176.
9. Rao AJ, Erickson BJ, Cvetanovich GL, Yanke AB, Bach BR, Cole BJ. The meniscus-deficient knee: biomechanics, evaluation, and treatment options. *Orthop J Sports Med.* 2015;3(10):1-14. doi:10.1177/2325967115611386.
10. Insall J, Ranawat CS, Scott WN, Walker P. Total condylar knee replacement: preliminary report. *Clin Orthop Relat Res.* 1976;120:149-154.
11. Insall J, Scott WN, Ranawat CS. The total condylar knee prosthesis. A report of two hundred and twenty cases. *J Bone Joint Surg Am.*1979;61(2):173-180.
12. Krackow KA, Mihalko WM. Flexion-extension joint gap changes after lateral structure release for valgus deformity correction in total knee arthroplasty: a cadaveric study. *J Arthroplasty.* 1999;14:994-1004.
13. Krackow KA, Mihalko WM. The effect of medial release on flexion and extension gaps in cadaveric knees: implications for soft-tissue balancing in total knee arthroplasty. *Am J Knee Surg.* 1999;12:222-228.
14. Peters CL, Jimenez C, Erickson J, Anderson MB, Pelt CE. Lessons learned from selective soft-tissue release for gap balancing in primary total knee arthroplasty: an analysis of 1216 consecutive total knee arthroplasties: AAOS exhibit selection. *J Bone Joint Surg Am.* 2013;95(20):e152.
15. Whiteside LA, Saeki K, Mihalko WM. Functional medical ligament balancing in total knee arthroplasty. *Clin Orthop Relat Res.* 2000;380:45-57.
16. Mihalko WM, Krackow KA. Posterior cruciate ligament effects on the flexion space and total knee arthroplasty. *Clin Orthop Relat Res.* 1999;360:243-250.
17. Pritsch M, Fitzgerald RH, Bryan RS. Surgical treatment of ligamentous instability after total knee arthroplasty. *Arch Orthop Trauma Surg.* 1984;102:154-160.
18. Meftah M, Blum YC, Raja D, Ranawat AS, Ranawat CS. Correcting fixed varus deformity with flexion contracture during total knee arthroplasty: the "inside-out" technique. AAOS exhibit selection. *J Bone Joint Surg Am.* 2012;94(10):e66.
19. Mihalko WM, Woodard EL, Hebert CT, Crockarell JR, Williams JL. Biomechanical validation of medial pie-crusting for soft-tissue balancing in knee arthroplasty. *J Arthroplasty.* 2015;30(2):296-299.

20. Mehdikhani KG, Moreno BM, Reid JJ, de Paz Nieves A, Lee YY, Della Valle AG. An algorithmic, pie-crusting medial soft tissue release reduces the need for constrained inserts patients with severe varus deformity undergoing total knee arthroplasty. *J Arthroplasty.* 2016;31(7):1465-1469.

21. Meneghini RM, Grant TW, Ishmael MK, Ziemba-Davis M. Leaving residual varus alignment after total knee arthroplasty does not improve patient outcomes. *J Arthroplasty.* 2017;32(9):S171-S176.

22. Hatayama K, Terauchi M, Saito K, Higuchi H. Does residual varus alignment cause increasing varus laxity at a minimum of five years after total knee arthroplasty? *J Arthroplasty.* 2017;32(6):1808-1813.

chapter 44

The Valgus Knee: Considerations for Alignment and Balance

Matthew J. Dietz, MD | Arbi Nazarian, MD

The goal of total joint replacement is the improvement of pain and function through the restoration of joint surfaces and improvements in angular deformity. Addressing these issues in a reproducible fashion can be more challenging in the valgus knee. It is encountered less frequently than varus knees which account for approximately 90% of total knees in the United States. The 10% of knees presenting with a valgus deformity require special considerations in preoperative planning and intraoperative surgical steps, but when performed well can provide a successful outcome with excellent longevity.

In addition to the limited experience some surgeons have with valgus knee deformities, the inherent challenges are the resultant bone loss, involving primarily the lateral femoral condyle (**Fig. 44-1**A to E) and lateral tibial plateau, the contracted lateral soft tissues and resulting laxity of medial soft tissues, and overall angular deformities that are often underappreciated.[1-3]

Once conservative nonoperative measures have been exhausted, consideration is given to correction of the valgus malalignment and resurfacing of the arthritic surfaces with total knee arthroplasty. In this chapter, we will outline the steps taken to safely restore the mechanical axis and achieve ligamentous balance when approaching a valgus knee during total knee arthroplasty.

PREOPERATIVE EVALUATION

History and Physical Examination

A careful patient history is always important but may be even more so in the case of treating a patient with valgus knee arthritis. Patients may report slow, steady symptom progression occurring over years, whereas a more rapid progression raises concerns for gross incompetence of structures on the medial side of the knee. A history can also provide an etiology of the valgus angulation be it from prior trauma or lateral meniscectomy. In both instances, previous incisions should be accounted for in the preoperative plan.

While physical examination is important in diagnosing osteoarthritis, it is critical to understanding and planning for surgery. The following steps are part of our critical examination of patients being evaluated for end-stage arthritis. The patient's gait should be routinely assessed. The range of motion is measured, and the presence or absence of any flexion contracture should be noted as patients with a preoperative flexion contracture in addition to valgus angulation are at much higher risk for postoperative peroneal nerve palsy.[4] Patellofemoral articulation is evaluated along with the status of the extensor mechanism; assessment of the collaterals in full extension, mid-flexion, and 90° of flexion will provide a more complete assessment of the ligaments, eliminating the tight posterior capsule which may provide a false sense of stability. The ability to correct the valgus deformity is also noted. This information is important as it provides the surgeon an indication as to whether the angulation will be easily correctable (full correction obtained on examination), require releases (partially correctable), or may require a more extensive release and possibly the use of a constrained prosthesis in the setting of fixed valgus angulation. The assessment is concluded with a thorough neurovascular examination. When treating valgus knee arthritis with primary knee arthroplasty, the risk of peroneal nerve palsy exists; sensory and motor function of the superficial and deep peroneal nerves should be assessed and documented. Additionally, as in all patients, assessment of the back, hips, and feet should be performed. Patients with valgus angulation will often have a pes planovalgus deformity of the foot.[5,24] There is no consensus on whether the foot and ankle deformities should be addressed prior to knee arthroplasty. Most would agree that the surgeon and patient should consider which joint is more symptomatic and if the hindfoot angulation is flexible or fixed. Several studies have documented conflicting reports of alterations in the mechanical axis after correction of knee varus or valgus angulation after a total knee arthroplasty. In some instances where a flexible foot deformity exists there may be sufficient correction through the knee to affect ankle or foot alignment, and may be performed first.[6,7]

However, contrary to this, Meding et al highlighted a series of total knee arthroplasty failures related to uncorrected pes planus deformities.[8] The degree of expected correction, risk for wound complications, expected compliance with foot and ankle orthosis, and

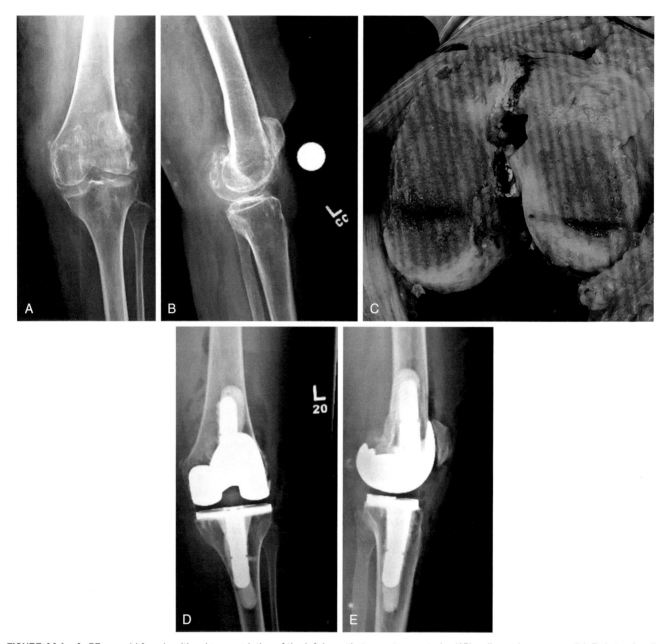

FIGURE 44-1   A: 57-year-old female with valgus angulation of the left knee that on anteroposterior (AP) radiograph appears mild. **B:** Lateral radiograph provides an indication of the relative lateral femoral condyle hypoplasia. This severe condylar hypoplasia was confirmed intraoperatively **(C)** and accounted for when making femoral rotational alignments and femoral cutting block sizing. **D** and **E:** AP and lateral radiographs postoperatively demonstrated a constrained condylar component with short, fully cemented stems.

concern for longevity of the implant should all be factors considered when planning total knee arthroplasty in this situation.

Radiographic Examination

Standard weight-bearing and flexion anteroposterior, lateral, Merchant, and alignment radiographs are obtained. Fluoroscopic examination or stress radiographs may provide more information as to the degree of correction obtainable but are not routinely done at our institution. The anteroposterior (AP) radiographs are critically evaluated for deformity, joint space narrowing, osteophytes, cysts, and subchondral sclerosis (**Fig. 44-2**A to D). In certain instances, the AP view may underrepresent the degree of wear present which may only be seen on the lateral view. On the lateral view, the lateral femoral condyle is evaluated, which may demonstrate possible hypoplasia (**Fig. 44-1**C) or a large posterolateral defect in the tibia may be evident.

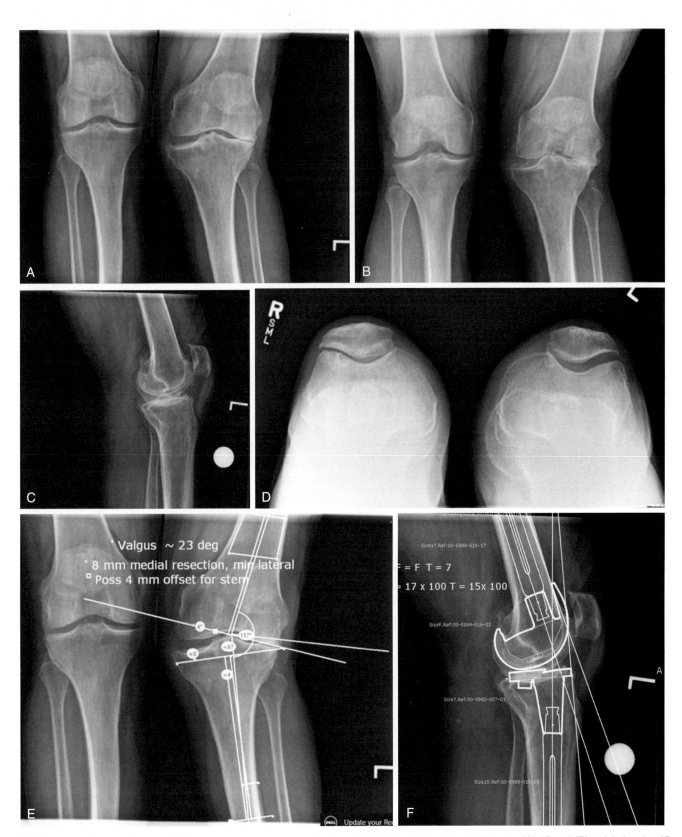

FIGURE 44-2 63-year-old male with 20 + year history of pain related to sports injury. Preoperative radiographs **(A)** AP and **(B)** weight-bearing AP demonstrate a severe valgus angulation of the left knee. **C:** lateral radiograph provides indication of the severe wear of the lateral tibial plateau. **D:** Merchant view. **E:** AP templating radiograph provides indication of level of resection of distal femur and proximal tibia. **F:** lateral radiograph indicates sizing of components and planned stem insertion. Final constrained condylar implants **(G)** AP and **(H)** lateral with follow-up at 5 y.

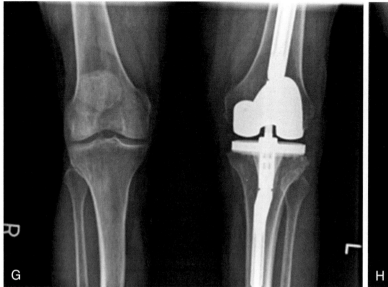
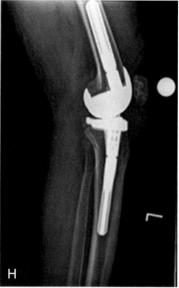

FIGURE 44-2 *Continued*

Templating

Templating, often used for sizing of components, can be extremely useful in planning bony resections (**Fig. 44-2E**) and can provide additional information regarding restoration of mechanical alignment. A line is drawn down the femoral and tibial shafts. A perpendicular line to the tibial shaft line is drawn at the level of the more involved tibial plateau (typically the lateral tibial plateau). This line represents the anatomic and mechanical tibial axis as both coincide which gives the surgeon an estimation as to the amount of tibial resection on the lateral and medial aspects of the tibial plateau. On the femoral side, another horizontal line is drawn with 3° to 5° of valgus alignment from the anatomic axis vertical femoral line. This measurement allows for correction of the mechanical axis. Typically, this line passes just medial to the center of the knee which is a starting point for an intramedullary guide in varus knees. However, particular attention should be paid to the femoral starting site which may need to be moved more lateral to avoid unintentional entry into the medial cortex of the femoral shaft when using an intramedullary guide.

The lateral view is commonly used for sizing purposes. Keeping posterior osteophytes in mind, the posterior aspect of the femoral condyles is outlined and used for sizing. The lateral views are especially important if the surgeon is considering the use of stems in the surgical construct (**Fig. 44-2F**).

Implant Considerations

In preparation for a successfully executed total knee arthroplasty of the valgus knee, it is important to give some consideration to implant selection. Excellent results can be achieved utilizing a cruciate retaining implant when operating on a valgus knee. Cruciate retaining implants are bone conserving and have an excellent track record. Choosing an unconstrained implant may limit the perioperative risks for the patient due to smaller bone resection; it may also reduce blood loss and surgery time.[9] However, the posterior stabilized implant (cruciate sacrificing) offers many advantages as the resection of the posterior cruciate ligament (PCL) allows the surgeon to bypass a major deforming force of the valgus knee and can make balancing the knee considerably easier. If balance is unable to be achieved, a constrained implant should always be available. It should be noted that most posterior stabilized implants do not offer varus and valgus constraint. The use of constrained implants in the setting of severe valgus knee deformity (often defined as > 15°) has been well studied in the literature and found to be successful.[10] However, constrained and stemmed implants increase intramedullary material; the preparation for these implants can, in turn, increase the risk of periprosthetic fractures. Another consideration is the financial savings offered by using primary implants. Anderson et al described using constrained condylar implants without stems to decrease cost with no adverse effects in the short- and mid-term results.[11] However, long-term follow-up is necessary to evaluate for potential aseptic loosening. Nonetheless, when increased constraint is necessary, one option is to use stemmed, constrained condylar knees, which have shown excellent long-term outcomes. In general, a condylar constrained prosthesis is chosen if medial or lateral laxity greater than 3 to 5 mm is detected after concerted effort to obtain balance (**Fig. 44-3A to F**).[12] Constrained condylar designs are useful for instability where a collateral ligament is still present

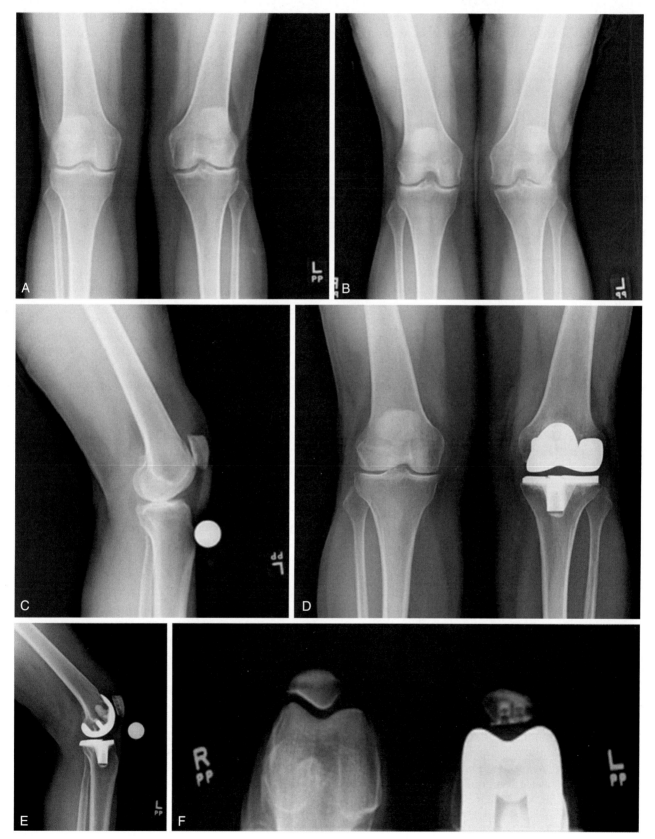

FIGURE 44-3   67-year-old female with lateral and anterior knee pain with correctable valgus angulation and severe wear seen on **(A)** AP, **(B)** AP weight-bearing, and **(C)** lateral radiographs. Excellent balance, stability, and patella tracking were achieved with a cruciate retaining total knee arthroplasty **(D-F)**.

although lax; they typically provide stability allowing for only 1° to 2° of accepted laxity. However, in cases where the collateral ligaments are absent or damaged and there is significant bone loss (i.e., rheumatoid arthritis, Charcot arthropathy), a rotating hinge device may provide additional and necessary stability (**Fig. 44-4**A to D). Although loads to the bone/implant interface will be greater in these designs, overall results have been encouraging.[13] While all implant constraints have been shown to be usable in the valgus knee, surgeons should understand the need for added constraint to achieve balance within the knee and have implants available to make necessary adjustments intraoperatively.

Patient Positioning

The patient is brought into the operating room and transferred onto a regular operating table. We prefer spinal anesthesia, typically 0.5% bupivacaine, at our institution unless contraindicated. If utilizing femoral and sciatic nerve blocks, one may consider delaying dosing of the sciatic catheter until after completion of the surgery and postoperative assessment of peroneal nerve function. Once spinal anesthesia is administered, the patient is positioned supine on the operating table. A thigh tourniquet is placed and the operative site is shaved. Multiple knee positioning devices exist depending on surgeon preference. The senior author prefers keeping the leg/foot free and uses the lateral thigh post at the level of the tourniquet to prevent excessive external rotation during the course of surgery. A flat foot positioner is also used at the distal end of the table at a level that coincides with 90° flexion of the knee. The foot rests on top of this post during steps that require flexion of the knee.

Surgical Technique

Once the patient is positioned on the operating table, the operative leg is prepped and draped in the usual sterile manner. Prophylactic intravenous (IV) antibiotics and IV tranexamic acid are administered prior to incision. If there is a contraindication to IV tranexamic acid, a topical form is injected into the wound at the end of the procedure after capsular closure and prior to skin closure. An esmark is used to exsanguinate the limb and the tourniquet is inflated to 250 mmHg. The authors prefer a medial parapatellar approach, although a lateral parapatellar approach has been described with success. There are certain unique challenges associated with the valgus knee which have been extensively cited in the literature, such as surgeon unfamiliarity, obtaining proper rotational alignment, soft-tissue balancing, and patellar tracking. The incision, which extends from

4 to 5 cm above the superior pole of the patella to 2 to 3 cm distal and just medial to the tibial tubercle, is marked. The size of the incision varies depending on the patient's body habitus; knees with a bigger soft-tissue envelope require longer incisions for safe and effective exposures.

After the skin incision, curved mayo scissors are used to dissect deeper tissue down to the fascial layer overlying the quadriceps tendon, vastus medialis oblique, patella, and patellar tendon. Some dissection of the medial skin flap aids in exposure. Attempts should be made to limit undermining the lateral skin; however, lateral skin flap undermining may be necessary to aid in exposure in obese knees. The arthrotomy is performed by incising the quadriceps tendon proximally, keeping a 1 to 2 mm tendinous sleeve on the medial aspect attached to the vastus medialis oblique (VMO), which becomes important during arthrotomy closure and aids in patellar tracking. The incision is carried along the medial aspect of the patella, again leaving a 1 to 2 mm soft-tissue attachment on the patella and further down along the medial aspect of the patellar tendon and ending subperiosteally 2 to 3 cm distal to the tibial tubercle.

The medial soft tissue along the tibia is released using a knife or electrocautery. This soft-tissue sleeve is not as extensive as in a varus knee exposure. However, a medial peel is still required to provide safe exposure. Therefore, a medial peel to the midsagittal plane exposing 1 to 1.5 cm distal to the joint line should provide adequate exposure without insulting the superficial medial collateral ligament (MCL) which typically inserts 5 cm distal to the joint line. The medial peel should not be extensive due to the valgus nature of the knee, which creates medial soft-tissue–ligamentous complex attenuation and compromises the surgeon's ability to easily balance the knee.[14] Retractors are placed to expose the knee further. The author removes a portion of the infrapatellar fat pad and synovium from the anterior aspect of the femur to improve exposure. The knee is then flexed, and the lateral meniscus is incised allowing placement of a lateral retractor that provides exposure and holds the patella in a subluxed position. Surgeon preference dictates the order of the next steps and whether the surgeon prefers a gap-balancing or measured resection technique. While the senior author prefers the measured resection technique, the importance of obtaining a well-balanced knee cannot be overstated.

Depending on the condition of the PCL and the implant decision, the anterior cruciate and possibly the PCL or their remnants are excised. Peripheral osteophytes are removed to aid in exposure unless utilizing a patient-specific guide.

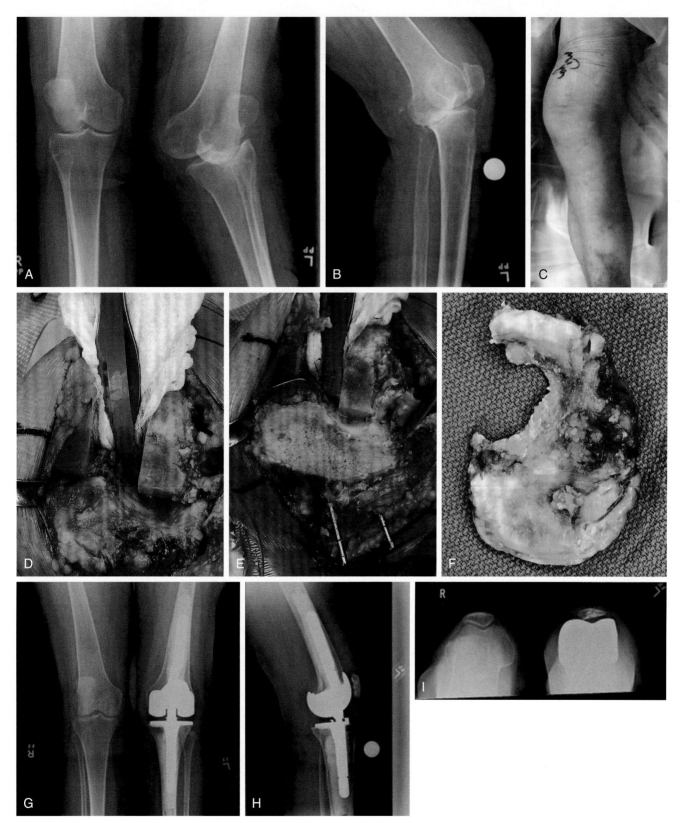

FIGURE 44-4 66-year-old active female with debilitating knee pain and instability. **A:** AP and **(B)** lateral radiographs demonstrate a nearly dislocated knee with incompetence of the medial collateral ligament and severe wear of the lateral tibial plateau. Intraoperative findings (video) confirm radiographic findings with no competent MCL in place. **C:** Intraoperative images demonstrate severe wear of the lateral tibial plateau with resection to the base of the defect **(D)** and image of the resected tibial bone **(E)**. Given the significant findings and chronic attenuation **(G-I)**, the patient was treated with a fully cemented rotating hinge-type knee and has now returned to work **(F-H)**.

SPECIAL CONSIDERATIONS IN THE VALGUS KNEE

Distal Femoral Resection

When an intramedullary guide is used to plan the distal femoral resection, care should be taken when using the opening reamer to gain access to the femoral canal. The entry point is 1 cm anterior and slightly medial to the PCL. Care should be taken not to deviate from the entry point as excessive medial/lateral starting points can lead to excessive varus/valgus resections, respectively. In addition, a posterior starting point will lead to a distal femoral resection that is in flexion; an intramedullary guide that is inserted too deep and contacts the proximal femoral cortex risks resection with extension deformity and possible notching. An entry reamer with a correct starting point should preferably not contact the femoral cortices. Changes to the distal femur may lead to valgus angulation which can lead to the intramedullary guide impinging the medial femoral cortex. Careful attention to the preoperative template can aid in avoiding this issue.

Depending on the extent of the valgus deformity, the valgus angle on the cutting guide is set between 3° and 5° of valgus. Leaving patients in 5° of valgus will often leave concern that they are "undercorrected," and some authors propose a distal cut at 3° to counteract any tendency for valgus recurrence.[15] If a flexion contracture was noted preoperatively, an additional 2 mm are taken off the distal femur for approximately every 9° of flexion contracture.[16]

Femoral Sizing

A traditional femoral sizer can be used to both obtain the size of and determine rotation of the femoral component. The presence of a hypoplastic lateral condyle does not preclude the use of anterior or posterior referencing femoral cutting guides but, if not appreciated, can lead to underestimation of planned external rotation and resultant internal rotation of the femoral component. A small osteotome can act as shim to account for this relative hypoplasia. Some systems allow for rotation to be dialed into the femoral guide. Most importantly, we routinely use the transepicondylar axis and a secondary check using the anteroposterior axis (Whiteside's line) which has equally been shown to be accurate in determining rotational alignment in a valgus knee (**Fig. 44-1C**).[17] A guide to perform the anterior, posterior, and chamfer resections is used. This guide can also provide an estimate to the degree of soft-tissue imbalance in the flexed position.

Tibia Resection

If a cruciate retaining arthroplasty is being performed, care should be taken to place a blunt retractor along the medial aspect of the PCL to further expose the tibial plateau and avoid the neurovascular bundle. The menisci are excised to improve exposure. The knee is then flexed and maximally externally rotated to fully expose the tibial surface. We routinely use an extramedullary tibial guide as valgus knees tend to have a tibia valga deformity.[18] The clamp is positioned just proximal to the malleoli and slightly on the medial aspect of the ankle in line with the second ray of the foot on AP view and along the tibial crest. Care should be taken not to excessively externally or internally rotate the foot which can lead to varus and valgus tibial resections, respectively.

The tibial cutting guide is raised to the level of the plateaus and aligned with the medial third of the tibial tubercle. The exact level of resection is based on preoperative templating, ligamentous laxity, and surgeon preference in using either the lateral or medial plateau. However, an appropriate level of resection can make obtaining a balanced knee much simpler. The cutting guide is firmly placed against the tibia. An alignment rod is used to check slope and alignment again.

As a general rule in varus knees, a 10 mm resection is made based on the higher and less involved side, the lateral plateau. In valgus knees, a smaller 2 to 4 mm resection is made based on the lower and involved side, the lateral plateau. In a severely worn knee, a resection of 1 to 2 mm will provide a thin tibial cut that is just below the sclerotic bone. A cut that is too large will require more extensive lateral releases and a larger polyethylene component to balance the laxity on the medial side. A smaller or larger resection is made based on preoperative flexion contracture or coronal ligamentous laxity. An alignment rod is used to check alignment once again prior to making any bony resections. Of note, tibial guides have varying degrees of tibial slope built into the device, and one should exercise caution when checking alignment on the lateral view. The extension gap is evaluated using a 10 mm spacer block. At this point, adequate resection may be present medially but still tight laterally indicating sufficient bony resection but the need for additional soft-tissue release later in the procedure.

The tibia is then exposed and the tibia tray is sized and positioned based on the rotation of the tibial tubercle. It is important to obtain proper tibial rotation especially with the use of a constrained condylar device as improper rotation will transmit significant stresses across the polyethylene and implant interfaces. A trial femoral component is then inserted with lateral placement that still allows for sufficient support by both condyles but will provide improved patella tracking.

Once the trial femoral component and tibial components are in place, a trial polyethylene can be inserted and the flexion and extension gaps assessed.

Evaluation of the Flexion and Extension Gaps

The goal of total knee arthroplasty is to obtain equal and symmetric gaps in both extension and flexion. If a trapezoidal gap is encountered in extension, appropriate soft-tissue releases are made to obtain a rectangular gap. Bony resections beyond what is required to obtain a balanced knee should be avoided as the joint line could be impacted and the components could be placed in soft metaphyseal bone. During the process of achieving ligamentous balance, a series of steps are employed depending on the severity of angulation and degree of correction required.

Lateral Ligament Release for Fixed Valgus Deformity

1. Remove remaining peripheral osteophytes
2. Release posterior lateral capsule from the posterior femur
3. Release posterolateral capsule transversely, generally using electrocautery from the posterior margin of the iliotibial (IT) band to just lateral to the PCL
4. Pie-crust the IT band with an 18 gauge needle or a 15 blade for tight extension gaps; if the deformity is severe, the IT band can be fully released. The authors prefer the use of an 18 gauge needle on a small hemostat to provide adequate/controlled release. The multiple stab holes are made in a staggered fashion to avoid inadvertent creation of multiple holes in line that may propagate and lead to complete tears. The depth of any release should be made with care not to exceed 5 mm to protect the peroneal nerve
5. Release the popliteus tendon if there is a tight flexion gap
6. Release the lateral collateral ligament (LCL) lastly (depending on surgeon preference, this structure can be resected first; it should be noted that if both the popliteus tendon and the LCL are released, the knee may be rendered unstable; a constrained component may be considered)

At this point, the patella is subluxed and prepared. All trial components are inserted, and the knee is critically evaluated by checking alignment and taking it through range of motion. Varus and valgus stresses are applied and both bony and soft-tissue tensions are tested. Once satisfied with component position, alignment, and range of motion, the tourniquet is deflated and patella tracking is evaluated. Valgus knees are known to have the problem of patella maltracking.[19] Therefore, care at all steps ensuring proper rotation and placement of components to improve tracking should be made. Occasionally, a small lateral retinacular release can be performed if the patella tracking is deemed to be unsatisfactory and tibial and femoral components are appropriately positioned. A cruciform release can be done for more extensive lateral release.[20] Historically, the lateral release rates have been as high as 41%, but perhaps with our continued understanding of component orientation as well as improvements in implant design, current release rates may be lower.[21,22] Whenever a release is performed, it is important to pay attention to preserving the superior lateral geniculate artery.

The knee is thoroughly irrigated and the tibial, femoral, and patella components are cemented into place. A trial polyethylene component is inserted, and the knee is placed in extension until the cement is hardened. Once the cement is cured, the knee is ranged and stability is checked again. Slight laxity on the medial side of up to 1 to 2 mm can be acceptable with excellent clinical and long-term results.[23] Prior to the insertion of the final polyethylene liner, we inject the capsule and surrounding soft-tissue structures with a multimodal cocktail consisting of ropivacaine, ketorolac, epinephrine, and clonidine. A total volume of 100 mL is injected. Special care is taken not to inject in the posterolateral capsule to avoid a transient common peroneal nerve palsy.

The knee is again irrigated and the wound is closed in layers. We do not routinely use drains; however, if an extensive release was performed, the surgeon may wish to deflate the tourniquet prior to closure and achieve hemostasis to prevent a large hematoma. A sterile dressing is placed and the patient is awakened and taken to recovery.

Postoperative Course

Immediately postoperatively, the pulses are checked to ensure adequate perfusion is present. If palpation is difficult, a Doppler is employed. Patients in our institution routinely undergo spinal anesthesia, but peroneal nerve function is closely monitored and tested as soon as the effects of the spinal have diminished.

Physical therapy is initiated the same day with full weight-bearing, quadriceps, and range-of-motion exercises. Patients use assistive devices such as a front wheel walker or cane for the first 1 to 2 weeks and are transitioned to ambulation without assistance. We do not recommend continuous passive motion machines as literature has shown no difference in long-term range of motion; use of these machines may have unintentional consequences such as peroneal nerve palsy from compression of the nerve within the machine due to excessive external rotation of the leg.[4]

Patients typically stay in the hospital overnight for observation after elective total knee arthroplasty.

Patients are encouraged to get up for meals, go to the bathroom, and get out of bed—all with assistance. They continue to have therapy, and activity levels are continuously assessed and increased. Intravenous fluids are discontinued once the patient tolerates oral intake. Discharge planning is initiated when patients are consented for surgery. Discharge planners work with patients to arrange for home health needs, physical therapy, in home safety tips, and any specific needs individualized for each patient to make their transition back home more convenient.

Complications

Total knee arthroplasty is a highly effective procedure that immeasurably improves patients' quality of life. Complications and adverse events, however rare, are associated with medical and surgical treatments. Complications specific to total knee arthroplasty include bleeding, infection, thromboembolic events, neural deficits, periprosthetic fracture, need for reoperation or revision, readmission, wound complications, instability, and stiffness.

Specific to the valgus knee, two complications are well described and documented in the orthopedic literature and relate to peroneal nerve palsy and patella maltracking.[4,15,22] A most devastating complication is injury to the common peroneal nerve, which has been reported to be 0.5% to 1% and as high as 3% in knees with preoperative valgus alignment and flexion contracture.[24-26] Sensory or motor deficits are usually evident once the spinal has worn off within the first 24 hours. The first step in a patient with peroneal nerve compromise is to loosen the dressings and flex the extremity to relieve pressure and take traction off the nerve. However, if deficits persist, an ankle–foot orthosis is recommended to prevent equines deformity of the foot due to Achilles tendon contracture. About 50% or more improve in time without additional treatment. If nerve function has not recovered by 3 months postoperatively, most surgeons recommend electrodiagnostic testing, and, if results are abnormal, the surgeon may consider surgical nerve release or other surgical intervention such as a tendon transfer.[27,28]

As previously discussed, patella tracking is a known complication in total knee arthroplasty, especially in valgus knees; it can be avoided by appropriate implant positioning and soft-tissue manipulation. By appropriately externally rotating the femoral and tibial components, lateralizing the femoral component, and positioning the patella button, the need for a lateral retinacular release may be avoided.

Intraoperative (recognized/unrecognized) or postoperative medial femoral condyle fracture is a rare but concerning complication seen in chronic valgus knee where relative osteopenia in the medial femoral condyle occurs (**Fig. 44-5**). The fracture can occur within the metaphyseal bone and lead to subsidence of the femoral component as seen in **Fig. 44-5C and E**. This nontraumatic fracture pattern has been described by Vestermark et al; this group suggests consideration for a prophylactic stemmed femoral component in female patients with poor bone quality. Any need for revision of the femoral component should be delayed until fracture healing allows for implant removal with less significant bone loss.[29]

Discussion

The valgus knee consists of both bony and soft-tissue deformities that should be addressed. There are many techniques described in the literature in the approach to the valgus knee.[14,30,31] Equivalent results can be obtained by using a medial or lateral parapatellar approach, but the lateral approach is often cited as being more difficult.[1,32] If general principles are adhered to and the mechanical axis of the knee is restored, results are, by and large, good and patients benefit from excellent long-term function.[33]

Great caution should be exercised in each step of the procedure, especially considering more extensive posterolateral releases due to the proximity of the peroneal nerve to the posterolateral corner (12 mm).[34] Soft-tissue releases should be performed in a carefully titrated fashion to obtain a stable knee without sacrificing integrity of the remaining soft-tissue restraint. In fixed valgus deformities, a lateral epicondylar osteotomy can be an alternative to extensive soft-tissue release.[33,35] Alternatively, some authors advocate reconstruction of the MCL.[20]

In general, mild, moderate, and severe deformities can be adequately addressed by cruciate retaining implants and soft-tissue releases, but as deformity becomes severe, a posterior stabilized, condylar constrained, or hinged implant and more extensive soft-tissue releases may be necessary.[36] The literature has shown good to excellent outcomes for all of the aforementioned implants when chosen appropriately for a given deformity. The unique challenges presented by the valgus knee can be managed and overcome by proper planning, adherence to well-established principles, and surgical mastery of described techniques.

ACKNOWLEDGMENTS

The authors would like to thank Adam E. Klein, MD, and Benjamin M. Frye, MD, for contributing patient radiographs and images for this chapter.

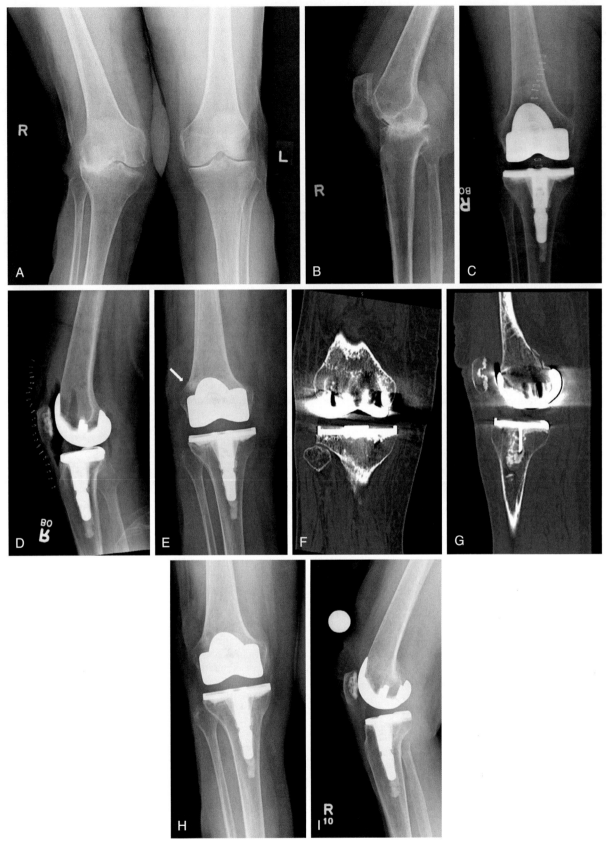

FIGURE 44-5 82-year-old female with severe valgus knee osteoarthritis with angulation of approximately 29°. **A:** AP and **(B)** lateral radiographs demonstrate severe posterolateral wear. Immediate postoperative images **(C)** and **(D)** demonstrate well-sized components with a short-stemmed tibial component, cruciate retaining femoral component, and medial congruent polyethylene bearing. Six weeks postoperatively, the patient began experiencing increased pain and was found to have a nondisplaced transverse periprosthetic femur fracture **(E)** and while the fracture line was most evident laterally (white arrow), there was subsidence of her femoral component into varus angulation (comparing **C** and **E**). This fracture was confirmed on CT scan **(F)** and **(G)**. The patient was treated with a hinged knee brace and made non–weight-bearing. At 6 mo postoperatively, the patient's fractures have healed and she is asymptomatic without further subsidence of her implants **(H)** and **(I)**.

REFERENCES

1. Kahlenberg CA, Trivellas M, Lee YY, Padgett DE. Preoperative valgus alignment does not predict inferior outcome of total knee arthroplasty. *HSS J.* 2018;14(1):50.
2. Satish BR, Ganesan JC, Chandran P, Basanagoudar PL, Balachandar D. Efficacy and mid term results of lateral parapatellar approach without tibial tubercle osteotomy for primary total knee arthroplasty in fixed valgus knees. *J Arthroplasty.* 2013;28(10):1751.
3. Xie K, Lyons ST. Soft tissue releases in total knee arthroplasty for valgus deformities. *J Arthroplasty.* 2017;32(6):1814.
4. Idusuyi OB, Morrey BF. Peroneal nerve palsy after total knee arthroplasty. Assessment of predisposing and prognostic factors. *J Bone Joint Surg Am.* 1996;78(2):177.
5. Gross KD, Felson DT, Niu J, et al. Association of flat feet with knee pain and cartilage damage in older adults. *Arthritis Care Res.* 2011;63(7):937.
6. Jeong BO, Kim TY, Baek JH, Jung H, Song SH. Following the correction of varus deformity of the knee through total knee arthroplasty, significant compensatory changes occur not only at the ankle and subtalar joint, but also at the foot. *Knee Surg Sports Traumatol Arthrosc.* 2018;26(11):3230.
7. Mullaji A, Shetty GM. Persistent hindfoot valgus causes lateral deviation of weightbearing axis after total knee arthroplasty. *Clin Orthop Relat Res.* 2011;469(4):1154.
8. Meding JB, Keating EM, Ritter MA, Faris PM, Berend ME, Malinzak RA. The planovalgus foot: a harbinger of failure of posterior cruciate-retaining total knee replacement. *J Bone Joint Surg Am.* 2005;87(suppl 2):59.
9. Berman AT, Geissele AE, Bosacco SJ. Blood loss with total knee arthroplasty. *Clin Orthop Relat Res.* 1988;234:137.
10. Easley ME, Insall JN, Scuderi GR, Bullek DD. Primary constrained condylar knee arthroplasty for the arthritic valgus knee. *Clin Orthop Relat Res.* 2000;380:58.
11. Anderson JA, Baldini A, MacDonald JH, Tomek I, Pellicci PM, Sculco TP. Constrained condylar knee without stem extensions for difficult primary total knee arthroplasty. *J Knee Surg.* 2007;20(3):195.
12. Maynard LM, Sauber TJ, Kostopoulos VK, Lavigne GS, Sewecke JJ, Sotereanos NG. Survival of primary condylar-constrained total knee arthroplasty at a minimum of 7 years. *J Arthroplasty.* 2014;29(6):1197.
13. Barrack RL. Evolution of the rotating hinge for complex total knee arthroplasty. *Clin Orthop Relat Res.* 2001;392:292.
14. Lombardi AV Jr, Dodds KL, Berend KR, Mallory TH, Adams JB. An algorithmic approach to total knee arthroplasty in the valgus knee. *J Bone Joint Surg Am.* 2004;86-A(suppl 2):62.
15. Keblish PA. The lateral approach to the valgus knee. Surgical technique and analysis of 53 cases with over two-year follow-up evaluation. *Clin Orthop Relat Res.* 1991;271:52.
16. Bengs BC, Scott RD. The effect of distal femoral resection on passive knee extension in posterior cruciate ligament-retaining total knee arthroplasty. *J Arthroplasty.* 2006;21(2):161.
17. Arima J, Whiteside LA, McCarthy DS, White SE. Femoral rotational alignment, based on the anteroposterior axis, in total knee arthroplasty in a valgus knee. A technical note. *J Bone Joint Surg Am.* 1995;77(9):1331.
18. Alghamdi A, Rahme M, Lavigne M, Masse V, Vendittoli PA. Tibia valga morphology in osteoarthritic knees: importance of preoperative full limb radiographs in total knee arthroplasty. *J Arthroplasty.* 2014;29(8):1671.

19. Lee SS, Lee H, Lee DH, Moon YW. Slight under-correction following total knee arthroplasty for a valgus knee results in similar clinical outcomes. *Arch Orthop Trauma Surg.* 2018;138(7):1011-1019.
20. Politi J, Scott R. Balancing severe valgus deformity in total knee arthroplasty using a lateral cruciform retinacular release. *J Arthroplasty.* 2004;19(5):553.
21. Clarke HD, Fuchs R, Scuderi GR, Scott WN, Insall JN. Clinical results in valgus total knee arthroplasty with the "pie crust" technique of lateral soft tissue releases. *J Arthroplasty.* 2005;20(8):1010.
22. Laskin RS. Lateral release rates after total knee arthroplasty. *Clin Orthop Relat Res.* 2001;392:88.
23. Matsuda S, Ito H. Ligament balancing in total knee arthroplasty-Medial stabilizing technique. *Asia Pac J Sports Med Arthrosc Rehabil Technol.* 2015;2(4):108.
24. Clarke HD, Schwartz JB, Math KR, Scuderi GR. Anatomic risk of peroneal nerve injury with the "pie crust" technique for valgus release in total knee arthroplasty. *J Arthroplasty.* 2004;19(1):40.
25. Park JH, Restrepo C, Norton R, Mandel S, Sharkey PF, Parvizi J. Common peroneal nerve palsy following total knee arthroplasty: prognostic factors and course of recovery. *J Arthroplasty.* 2013;28(9):1538.
26. Bruzzone M, Ranawat A, Castoldi F, Dettoni F, Rossi P, Rossi R. The risk of direct peroneal nerve injury using the Ranawat "inside-out" lateral release technique in valgus total knee arthroplasty. *J Arthroplasty.* 2010;25(1):161.
27. Schinsky MF, Macaulay W, Parks ML, Kiernan H, Nercessian OA. Nerve injury after primary total knee arthroplasty. *J Arthroplasty.* 2001;16(8):1048.
28. Zywiel MG, Mont MA, McGrath MS, Ulrich SD, Bonutti PM, Bhave A. Peroneal nerve dysfunction after total knee arthroplasty: characterization and treatment. *J Arthroplasty.* 2011;26(3):379.
29. Vestermark GL, Odum SM, Springer BD. Early femoral condyle insufficiency fractures after total knee arthroplasty: treatment with delayed surgery and femoral component revision. *Arthroplast Today.* 2018;4(2):249.
30. Krackow KA, Jones MM, Teeny SM, Hungerford DS. Primary total knee arthroplasty in patients with fixed valgus deformity. *Clin Orthop Relat Res.* 1991;273:9.
31. Elkus M, Ranawat CS, Rasquinha VJ, Babhulkar S, Rossi R, Ranawat AS. Total knee arthroplasty for severe valgus deformity. Five to fourteen-year follow-up. *J Bone Joint Surg Am.* 2004;86-A(12):2671.
32. Gunst S, Villa V, Magnussen R, Servien E, Lustig S, Neyret P. Equivalent results of medial and lateral parapatellar approach for total knee arthroplasty in mild valgus deformities. *Int Orthop.* 2016;40(5):945.
33. Mullaji AB, Shetty GM. Lateral epicondylar osteotomy using computer navigation in total knee arthroplasty for rigid valgus deformities. *J Arthroplasty.* 2010;25(1):166.
34. Jenkins MJ, Farhat M, Hwang P, Kanawati AJ, Graham E. The distance of the common peroneal nerve to the posterolateral structures of the knee. *J Arthroplasty.* 2016;31(12):2907.
35. Conjeski JM, Scuderi GR. Lateral femoral epicondylar osteotomy for correction of fixed valgus deformity in total knee arthroplasty: a technical note. *J Arthroplasty.* 2018;33(2):386.
36. Ritter MA, Faris GW, Faris PM, Davis KE. Total knee arthroplasty in patients with angular varus or valgus deformities of > or = 20 degrees. *J Arthroplasty.* 2004;19(7):862.

chapter 45

Managing Fixed Flexion Before and After Total Knee Arthroplasty: Maximizing Range of Motion

Vinay K. Aggarwal, MD | James I. Huddleston III, MD

INTRODUCTION

Total knee arthroplasty (TKA) is an incredibly successful procedure at alleviating pain in patients with advanced arthritis of the knee. The goal of the procedure is to relieve pain and improve function by restoring motion to a diseased joint. A variety of patient conditions, both systemic and local, can lead to bony destruction, soft-tissue contraction, and ultimately a fixed flexion deformity (FFD). To begin this chapter, we will highlight the key anatomic features of the normal knee joint that become compromised in patients with FFD and outline some of the causes that lead to decreased movement in the knee.

Once pain is severe enough and lack of motion begins to affect a patient's quality of life, TKA is ultimately one of the only viable options remaining. In patients with significant FFD, special considerations must be given to the intraoperative and postoperative courses, which we discuss in detail in this chapter. Great care must be taken in the surgical technique, the prosthesis choice and positioning, and rehabilitation protocol chosen for the patient following TKA. While the results of TKA are extremely encouraging, these patients still pose a particular challenge for arthroplasty surgeons. Much has been studied in terms of predicting patients' postoperative range of motion (ROM) after TKA, and these predictors will be discussed further in patients with and without preoperative FFD.

Even in spite of the best preoperative and intraoperative planning, some patients are unable to achieve a functional ROM. These patients must be counseled closely as to their expected outcomes and followed frequently to monitor for gains in postoperative ROM. There are several strategies that can be employed to help patients with FFD after index TKA in order to gain or restore their motion and achieve the level of functionality and satisfaction they were hoping for at the outset. These management options will be reviewed toward the end of the chapter with a particular focus on revision TKA for patients with unrelenting stiffness.

NATIVE KNEE JOINT MOTION AND KINEMATICS

The normal knee joint involves a complex interplay between bony geometry and ligamentous stabilization, both of which contribute greatly to the kinematic behavior of the knee. In addition to contributions from the surrounding musculature, the structure of the bones and ligaments allows for harmonious three-dimensional motion. This motion translates into seamless function for activities of daily living and recreational or athletic endeavors. While TKA consistently provides high levels of pain relief, the procedure continues to evolve even now with regard to the quest to emulate this normal knee motion.

Anatomic Features of the Native Knee

The bony geometry of the knee joint plays a large role in normal joint ROM and function. The distal femoral anatomy is such that the medial and lateral condyles are asymmetric with respect to their radii of curvature and overall diameters.[1] The nondiseased proximal tibia has approximately 5° to 10° of posterior slope.[2] Finally, the posterior condylar offset of the femur cannot be understated in its importance in allowing for adequate flexion. Without the posterior condyles being offset from the posterior femoral cortex, the posterior tibia would impinge on the posterior cortex of the femur in flexion, thereby preventing deep flexion.[1] In design of TKA implants and reconstruction of the knee, the offset from the posterior condyles must be recreated and not reduced significantly in size. In addition to bony clearance in deep flexion, this posterior condylar offset allows for soft tissues to clear up to approximately 150°, although this is increasingly seen as a significant source of motion restriction in the growing population of obese individuals. These patients who are experiencing thigh-calf impingement can pose specific challenges for surgeons performing TKA, as stiffness is a significant postoperative concern.

The ligaments and soft tissues of the knee are too many to review in detail here but suffice it to say they all play significant roles in the kinematics of the joint. Normal joint motion is afforded by the dynamic interplay between compliant capsular tissue, cruciate and collateral ligaments, and mobile musculature that can lengthen and contract to their full extent.

When the anterior cruciate ligament (ACL) and posterior cruciate ligament (PCL) function normally, they allow for the geometry of the distal femur and proximal tibia to interact in flexion–extension as well as rotation during the course of the gait cycle. With pathologic processes leading to either ACL or PCL deficiency, development of arthritis and subsequent contractures about the knee occur.[3,4] For example, with PCL deficiency, there is decreased femoral rollback on the plateaus leading to earlier impingement from the tibia and therefore limited knee flexion.[5]

Perhaps more important than the cruciate ligaments are the collateral ligaments when it comes to knee joint contracture and stiffness. Coronal plane soft-tissue balancing may involve selective releases of the medial and/or lateral collateral ligaments (MCLs, LCLs). One study by Mihalko et al evaluated the soft-tissue release or bone resection maneuvers performed during TKA to achieve balance and full motion in patients with flexion contracture.[6] They report that only MCL- or LCL-balancing procedures were necessary to correct FFD in 35.9% of patients—thereby implicating the collaterals as the most likely primary structure contributing to the original contracture. Nonetheless, the etiology of stiffness in knees is multifactorial, and despite properly functioning ACL, PCL, MCL, and LCL, tightness in the posterior capsule, extensor mechanism, and bony deformity can lead to coronal and sagittal plane deformities in the long run.[7]

Knee Joint Range of Motion and Classification

Despite attempts at defining a normal knee joint arc of motion (AOM), it is important to point out that individual factors will all dictate a person's everyday knee range in a nonarthritic state. These factors include genetic predisposition and patient factors such as age as well as external influences such as cultural environment, body habitus, and engagement in activities or exercise.[8-10] Studies evaluating normal joint motion have shown that with age, flexion certainly decreases but should stay above 130°, while extension may slightly increase and remain between 1° and 2° by age 69 years.[11]

As far as required ROM for normal activities of daily life, studies have reported that at least 90° of knee flexion and even up to 135° may be needed for comfortable execution of many activities including stair climbing, sitting on chairs, toileting, and getting into a bathtub safely.[12,13] Particularly in non-Western cultures, individuals may need up to 165° of knee flexion in their everyday lives such as during squatting, kneeling, or sitting cross-legged during prayer or other activities.[12]

These deep flexion activities further exaggerate the posterior femoral rollback that was discussed earlier. Past 135° of knee flexion, several studies have shown that the lateral femur rolls posteriorly up to 31 mm from the center of the knee and even translates completely off of the lateral tibial plateau.[5,14,15] Stability of the knee joint is maintained at these extreme angles by the lateral meniscus, which as mentioned earlier is mobile and translates with the femur as it rolls back, as well as by the musculature including the contraction of the quadriceps muscle.[5] Without normal knee kinematics and resultant flexion contractures greater than 15°, the energy expended by the musculature during walking has been measured to be significantly increased in both healthy patients and those who underwent TKA.[16]

The amount of motion in a knee is significant as far as function is concerned; however, it is equally important when trying to discuss patient motion in the clinical and research settings. Classification of knee ROM has been performed in a myriad of ways in the literature with not much universal agreement.[17] Sculco defined limitations of motion as mild, moderate, or severe based on the total ROM arc.[18] His classification quantified severe ROM as an arc of less than 30° to 45°, moderate with an arc of 45° to 70°, and mild with a motion arc of 70° to 90°. This classification allowed for an assessment of contracture severity prior to undergoing TKA and even helped dictate the type and amount of soft-tissue releases needed to be performed at the time of operation.[18]

Scoring systems used in evaluating patients with both acute and chronic injuries of the knee are several and vary based on the goals of assessment.[17,19] One of the main objective criteria in several of these scoring systems is the degree of flexion contracture and the arc of normal knee ROM. In the Knee Society Score (KSS), 25 points out of a possible 100 are achieved through amount of knee flexion (one for every 5° motion) and presence of flexion contracture.[20] The amount of knee motion has been further shown by Ritter to affect other aspects of KSS assessment including the walking ability score and stair climbing score.[21] The Hospital for Special Surgery (HSS) Knee Score meanwhile delegates 18 points out of 100 for ROM component (one for every 8°).

The importance of developing a good classification system for knee joint motion is common to all good classification systems in orthopedics: that is, the system allows for a common language in the clinical and research settings and also provides either diagnostic or prognostic information, thereby ultimately guiding clinical treatment. Jain et al classified preoperative FFD into two groups and reported on the surgical considerations intraoperatively as well as the postoperative outcomes in ROM improvement after TKA for each group.[22] This allows for a discussion with the patient as to what ROM category they are in preoperatively and what to expect after a surgical intervention. Similarly, ROM classification after TKA has been shown by Quah et al to predict expected improvement in flexion contracture following surgery over the course of 2 years.[23] In their study, both groupings (FFD 5°-15° vs. >15°) improved significantly over 2 years; however, the first group had complete resolution of FFD, whereas the second group had residual mean contracture of 3° postoperatively.

Recreation of the normal knee joint motion is the goal of any knee surgery including TKA for arthritis. Restoration of biomechanical principals to normal knee kinematics has evolved over several decades, yet it still remains a challenge for arthroplasty surgeons. Much debate regarding the optimal method to restore joint anatomy and motion continues; however, there is no question that joint motion plays a large role in patient satisfaction and reported outcomes after treatment. Therefore, classification and scoring systems utilizing motion as a predictor for success and guide for treatment are useful and necessary tools.

FIXED FLEXION BEFORE TOTAL KNEE ARTHROPLASTY

A large percentage of patients undergoing TKA will have altered biomechanics and ROM as a result of their underlying disease process leading to a painful knee joint. There are a number of conditions that contribute to contractures and FFDs about the knee. These conditions can affect the bony geometry, the soft-tissue structure and compliance, or both. Here we review some of the causes of fixed flexion about the knee and the options to manage the stiffness before a potential TKA.

Etiology of Preoperative Fixed Flexion Deformities

The most common joint disorder of the knee in the United States is osteoarthritis.[24] Symptomatic knee osteoarthritis is said to affect 10% of men and 13% of women age 60 years or older, and the vast majority of TKA patients are diagnosed as having osteoarthritis.[25] Risk factors for the development of osteoarthritis of the knee include systemic and local factors such as genetic predisposition, obesity, age, female gender, and muscle weakness as well as sports participation, prior knee injury, and occupational exposures.[24,25]

Due to its overwhelming prevalence, osteoarthritis is then logically one of the most common reasons for flexion contracture in patients indicated for TKA.[7] The preoperative FFD is due to a multitude of factors but usually includes a combination of stiff collateral and cruciate ligaments, tightened posterior capsule, and posterior osteophyte formation. A study by Fishkin et al evaluated

the changes in the medial and lateral collateral ligaments with osteoarthritis by evaluating and comparing the stiffness in a group of osteoarthritic patients undergoing TKA with a group of osteoarthritic cadavers and a group of normal control nonarthritic cadavers. As expected, when strain was applied and assessed, the osteoarthritic groups (patients and cadavers) had statistically significantly increased stiffness measurements than the normal controlled group of cadaver knees (60.7 vs. 21.4 N/mm in medial compartment, 29.2 vs. 19.5 N/mm in the lateral compartment, $P < .05$).[26] The recommendation therefore in patients undergoing TKA with FFD due to osteoarthritis is to take special care to release and balance the collateral ligaments carefully in addition to performing adequate capsular release, posterior osteophyte excision, and bony resection.[7]

Rheumatoid arthritis (RA) is a classically described cause of severe preoperative FFD with additional deformities of valgus and external rotation of the knee joint.[27] With the advent of disease-modifying antirheumatic drugs (DMARDs), TKA performed for RA was thought to diminish significantly. However, epidemiological data from the Nationwide Inpatient Sample prove the rate of TKA being performed for RA to remain stable from 2002 to 2013.[28] The incidence in 2002 was 3.3% versus that in 2013 was actually 3.5%, suggesting a slight increase, likely due to the aging United States population as well as the overall increase in utility of the operation for all patients across the board.

Several studies have evaluated the degree of flexion contracture in patients with RA undergoing TKA and have documented the amount of correction attainable at final follow-up.[29-32] Wang et al describe a series of 38 patients undergoing bilateral TKA for moderate to severe FFD with mean contracture of 38° and mean ROM of 49°. They were able to completely correct the contracture in 33 patients, with only 5 patients having residual contracture of 5° to 10° after TKA.[29] They and other authors advocate the use of careful soft-tissue release rather than bony overresection to avoid complication and need for significant constraint during primary TKA.[29,32]

Severe contracture occurs due to frank ankylosis of the knee joint, which can be caused by bony disease or significant fibrous tissue between the distal femur and proximal tibia. These patients are often resting in significant flexion or extension with minimal arcs of motion and have been reported on in the United States and in Asia as well.[33-35] Interestingly, because the patients have often lived with their severe contracture for so long, pain is often a secondary issue relative to functional deficits in these patients. The preoperative ROM is usually between 0° and 10° with severe flexion contractures of up to a mean of 105° in one study.[35] Kim and colleagues were able to achieve a correction to mean FFD of 6° after TKA with motion of 97° in their series of 27 patients.[35] The most important consideration in treating patients with bony ankylosis with TKA is recognizing and avoiding potential complications. Reported complications include patellar tendon avulsion, patellar fracture, peroneal nerve palsy, hematoma, and deep joint infection.[33,34] Infection must be ruled out in these patients as undiagnosed chronic septic arthritis of the native knee joint leading to severe contracture can be catastrophic if TKA is undertaken.

Hemophilia is a more rarely encountered reason for undergoing primary TKA; however, it is one of the most commonly reported reasons for flexion contracture in the arthroplasty literature.[36-44] Hemophiliacs experience fixed flexion as a result of extrinsic tightness from quadriceps contractures and surrounding fibrous ankylosis over the course of years.[39,41] Patients with hemophilia undergoing TKA have inferior outcomes compared to those with primary osteoarthritis.[37,42] Traditionally this was due to a significantly higher complication rate including hemarthrosis, deep joint infection, MCL injury, and periprosthetic fracture.[42,43]

Careful surgical technique and management of preoperative expectations regarding ultimate ROM have led to encouraging results with TKA in hemophilia patients with FFD.[44]

Kubes et al report on 72 TKAs done in patients with hemophilia types A and B and showed an improvement in mean flexion contracture from 17° preoperatively to 7° postoperatively.[42] They report that TKA in hemophiliacs increases extension more so than flexion and that patients should be operated on prior to surpassing a flexion contracture of greater than 22° to obtain satisfactory improvement in extension. Similarly Atilla et al state based on a receiver operator curve analysis that a preoperative flexion contracture of 27.5° is an important threshold in predicting whether hemophilia patients will significantly improve their amount of extension.[36]

Although the list of potential diagnoses (including several other inflammatory arthropathies that we would not detail in this chapter) leading to flexion contracture prior to TKA is lengthy, several miscellaneous causes of stiffness that are less reported in the literature should be mentioned. An obvious etiology is prior surgical intervention on the knee joint leading to scar formation and ultimately stiffness either in flexion, extension, or both. While arthroscopic procedures such as ACL reconstruction can result in significant swelling of the joint and eventual stiffness, open procedures are more likely to result in the scarring, leading to an eventual flexion contracture. Specifically, procedures on the extensor mechanism such as quadriceps or patellar tendon rupture repair and patellar fracture fixation can lead to shortened extensors, adhesions in the musculature or retinaculum, and ultimately a lack of full knee joint extension.[7]

Trauma to the knee joint resulting in either a fracture or soft-tissue injury will often result in deformity and contracture as well. This can be due to fracture malunion, scar tissue formation, or actual development of arthritis.

Often referred to as posttraumatic arthritis, Blagojevic showed in a meta-analysis that previous knee trauma resulted in 3.86 odds ratio of developing osteoarthritis of the knee.[45] Finally, the presence of pain in the knee itself is often enough to cause joint stiffness, and if left long enough without motion, eventual flexion contracture of the knee. Much is written about pain as a consequence of osteoarthritis and the inflammatory cascade that occurs within the knee joint.[46] However, pain as a cause of stiffness is more difficult to prove yet intuitively makes clinical sense. Often seen with patients in the clinical setting both before and after surgery, pain in the knee leads to a refusal to move the joint and, as such, an eventual stiffness and contracture of the surrounding ligaments and muscles about the knee.

Dealing With Stiffness Before TKA: What are the Options?

Due to the success in correcting flexion contracture deformity during the actual TKA procedure itself, treating stiffness before TKA is not often pursued. Unlike sports medicine procedures such as ACL reconstruction in which optimal postoperative outcomes are usually the result of close to normal preoperative knee joint ROM, patients undergoing TKA rarely are able to achieve normal knee kinematics before their TKA.

Nonetheless, there has been significant evaluation of physical therapy (PT) prior to TKA in efforts to improve postoperative outcomes. Termed "prehabilitation," several studies have evaluated the efficacy of preoperative education and exercise treatment or evaluation on functional recovery and disability after TKA.[47-50] One study by Mizner et al finds preoperative quadriceps strength to be a good predictor of postoperative functional ability up to 1 year after TKA.[47] Meanwhile a cohort study evaluated three groups for effects of preoperative exercise (Group 1 control, Group 2 strengthening and ROM group, Group 3 cardiovascular exercise group) on knee function scores after TKA found no difference between the three with regard to all measurement scales utilized.[49]

Debate exists regarding the efficacy of prehabilitation on TKA outcomes as is seen from the results of a Cochrane review and systematic review in the literature.[51,52] In one of the only randomized studies, Swank et al found patients with severe osteoarthritis undergoing usual care and exercise prior to TKA had better strength and function after surgery compared to those patients only undergoing usual care protocols.[53] However, even based on the multitude of studies, it is still difficult to draw any definitive conclusions or make recommendations for or against the use of preoperative PT and education due to the large variety of protocols, small numbers of patients, and lack of randomization in most of them.

Surgical options for degenerative arthritis leading to stiffness prior to TKA are truly limited to arthroscopic interventions such as meniscal débridement and synovectomy. Two landmark papers including randomization to arthroscopic intervention or placebo-type surgery both showed no advantage to either arthroscopic lavage or débridement in patients with degenerative joint disease.[54,55] This has led to significant change with regard to the indications for knee arthroscopy in alleviating joint pain and stiffness in patients with existing arthritic changes. Interestingly, however, one paper from Japan reports on the unique use of an arthroscopic posteromedial release in patients with medial osteoarthritis and flexion contracture.[56] They report in 58 knees with Kellgren and Lawrence grades of 3 or 4 that the mean improvement in functional and pain scores was significantly increased after intervention, suggesting a possible role for less invasive surgery in temporizing patients with FFD prior to TKA. Even so, it is difficult to endorse this intervention in this uncontrolled study, and so much of the management of FFD can and should be done with the use of TKA as will be discussed below.

INTRAOPERATIVE MANAGEMENT OF FIXED FLEXION DURING TKA

The optimal time to manage FFD of the knee joint is during the index TKA itself. Studies have shown residual flexion contracture after TKA to be associated with poorer functional outcomes and scores, with a resulting risk of leaving these contractures to become permanent.[7] As discussed earlier, the goal during TKA is to alleviate pain and restore function. Traditionally, this starts with the surgical approach, continues with soft-tissue balancing and bony cuts to achieve symmetric flexion and extension gaps, and concludes with optimal component positioning to restore posterior condylar offset and mechanical alignment of the limb.[7,57,58]

Surgical Technique

The surgical technique in patients with severe deformity always begins with special attention to the approach starting with placement of the incision. Old surgical scars must be mapped out to determine if utilizable, and the location of the incision should be extensile in the event as additional exposure is required. In general, the most lateral skin incision should be used. The skin may be thick and adherent to the underlying extensor mechanism from resting in a flexed position for prolonged periods of time. The specific comparisons of a median parapatellar approach versus a midvastus or subvastus approach will not be discussed here, but even in the noncontracted patient, several randomized studies have failed to show a definitive difference in postoperative motion, knee scores, or final quad strength.[59-61]

Once an arthrotomy is undertaken, exposure of the tibiofemoral joints may require removal of patellar osteophytes, or if significantly contracted and adherent to the underlying femur, osteotomy of the patellar undersurface and a lateral release for aid with mobilization. When FFD is so severe that patellar mobilization is not possible in spite of these efforts, significant proximal and distal extension of the incision may be required for potential use of a quadriceps snip, V-Y turndown, or tibial tubercle osteotomy (TTO).[18] The TTO can be used with soft-tissue attachment laterally and secured at the end of the TKA with wire fixation with good postoperative outcomes and high rates of bony union.[62] We have no experience with a V-Y turndown. The need for a TTO is rare, as most knees can be safely exposed with a quadriceps snip and an extensive medial peel on the tibia, aided by tibial external rotation and an anterior drawer maneuver.

A discussion on posterior cruciate retaining versus substituting implant design will not be provided in this chapter. However, it should be noted that there remains debate as to the effects of the PCL on restoring normal knee joint kinematics after TKA.[63,64] Nonetheless, in general, the retention or substitution of the PCL has not shown to significantly affect postoperative ROM, functional outcomes, proprioception, or strength in most studies to date.[65-67] In patients with severe FFD and contracture, we feel as though the PCL will likely be pathologic in function regardless and can be safely excised during the initial approach to further allow for improved exposure and subluxation of the tibia from the femur.

Regarding the distal femoral cut, there are varying philosophies as to initial intraoperative management in a patient with FFD. Initial additional distal femoral resection can lead to joint line elevation, patella baja, and midflexion instability—all of which can lead to problems of their own after complex TKA.[2] It has been shown that an additional 3.5 mm of distal femoral resection is needed to completely correct 10° of FFD.[68] On the contrary, not resecting enough distal femur initially will inevitably lead to flexion contracture after TKA in patients already presenting with severe preoperative FFD. Tanzer et al report a series in which they evaluate the natural history of flexion contracture after TKA where they avoided excessive bony resection of the distal femur. Patients had a mean preoperative FFD of 12.9° and immediate postoperative FFD of 14.8°, yet they found at final follow-up of just over 1 year, patients had FFD of 2.9° suggesting that flexion contracture can significantly improve after TKA and does not require excessive distal femoral resection.

Similarly, the tibial cut can greatly affect the knee range in both flexion and extension. Avoiding significant bony cuts will make a potential revision surgery easier and can avoid excessive use of constrained implants when possible. Recreation of tibial slope is one of the more important technical features and may be influenced by the surgeon's choice of posterior cruciate substituting or retaining implant design.[2] In a three-dimensional model by Walker et al, tibial slope was found to be the most important surgical variable in optimizing knee flexion with posterior tilt of 10° accounting for an improved flexion of 30°.[69]

Additionally, to avoid excessive bony resection to correct flexion contracture, it is imperative to address the contracted posterior capsule as well as osteophytes that tent the capsule preventing full extension.[70] Careful release of the capsule from the distal femoral condyles and proximal tibial surface using a combination of periosteal elevators, osteotomes, and electrocautery has been described to be both safe and efficacious.[18,71] In addition to posterior capsular release, excision of posterior osteophytes tenting the capsule is important in achieving maximal extension. In a study of over 800 cases with flexion contracture between 5° and 30°, Bellemans et al describe a stepwise algorithmic approach to achieving full extension that involved (1) mediolateral ligament balancing with resection of all osteophytes and overresection of the distal femur by 2 mm, (2) progressive posterior capsular release and osteophyte removal, (3) additional resection of the distal femur up to a maximum of 4 mm, and (4) hamstring tenotomy. They report 98.6% of cases achieved correction of the contracture with only steps 1 and 2 of their approach.[72] Fig. 45-1 demonstrates a severe varus knee with large posterior osteophytes and preoperative FFD of 25° corrected after resection of osteophytes and coronal plane balancing with a constrained TKA (**Fig. 45-1**).

In order to achieve symmetric flexion and extension gaps, a gap-balancing or measured resection technique can be employed, and the limb can be aligned in either mechanical (MA) or kinematic alignment (KA). Regardless of the technique used, the gaps must be balanced to avoid persisting contracture or laxity and instability of the joint through the arc of knee motion. In an interesting analysis of two comparable groups of TKA performed using either MA versus KA philosophy, the authors found the KA group to achieve the same sagittal deformity correction with less total bony resection and less ligament release required, allowing for bone stock preservation and minimizing soft-tissue trauma.[73] Howell et al have also studied KA in TKA extensively and have found similar advantages in the flexion–extension plane with regard to bony resection translating in acceptable mid-term follow-up results.[74,75]

One final potential contribution of surgical technique on FFD during TKA to consider and prevent residual contracture is the closure of the arthrotomy and wound. In theory, closing the knee in flexion should allow for additional flexion motion. It is unclear, however, how this clinically affects extension movement as there is a natural trade-off. There are equivocal studies by Emerson and Masri showing conflicting results with regard to benefits of capsular and wound closure in flexion; however, it is clear that with adequate rehabilitation, the long-term results and ultimate residual deformity after TKA are not affected by closure technique.[76,77]

Implant Factors

Since the first implanted TKA in 1968, there have been significant evolutionary changes to the prosthesis design which has led to an overall improvement in pain relief and long-term survivorship. Nonetheless, the fact that there continues to be constant change to implant geometry and that there are hundreds of knee designs on the market reveals the concept that surgeons and engineers have been unable to perfectly replicate the normal knee kinematics and motion that lead to seamless function and ultimately patient satisfaction.

The geometry of the TKA components plays a large role in recreating knee ROM and preventing a stiff knee, particularly in flexion. Particularly the shape of the femoral components medial and lateral condyles has been linked to motion in the sagittal plane. Some designs employ a symmetric medial and lateral condyle, whereas others utilize asymmetric profiles in efforts to mimic axial knee rotation with flexion and extension.[2] Furthermore, the radius of curvature between the distal femoral condyles and posterior condyles has been adjusted with some implant models to allow for reproduction of native knee femoral rollback and flexion.[78] The smaller radius of curvature of the posterior condyle and change in center of curvature allowed for 10° of increased flexion in one study.[79] The posterior femoral offset must be recreated to achieve full flexion; however, it is important to note that excessive posterior offset can actually paradoxically limit knee extension by tenting the posterior capsule and shortening the posterior soft tissues.[80] Regarding achievement of full extension, prosthetic design changes have been fewer; however, the tibial component slope, the shape of the anterior polyethylene liner, and the cam-post mechanism in cruciate substituting femoral components all play a role in preventing residual FFD after TKA.[81]

Prosthesis positioning certainly affects TKA ROM as well. Several studies including biomechanical analysis by Walker et al showed how both tibial and femoral position can limit flexion.[69] Tibial rotation must be appropriate for patellofemoral tracking and to avoid overhang and pain from impingement. However, Walker showed displacement of the baseplate from anterior to posterior by 5 mm improved knee flexion by 10°.[69] Likewise, femoral displacement posteriorly by 2.5 mm decreased knee flexion by 10° due to reduction in PCL tension in cruciate retaining models. Berger et al showed femoral component internal rotation affected knee flexion by tightening the medial flexion space and limited room for ultimate flexion.[82]

The question of femoral sizing in the anterior–posterior dimension is a critical technical factor as well. Clearly the femur size affects the flexion space, and it is critical that the appropriately sized implant for patient anatomy be chosen to obtain maximum flexion.[2] In cases where the femur is undersized, there will be reduced posterior condylar offset, bony impingement in flexion, mid-flexion

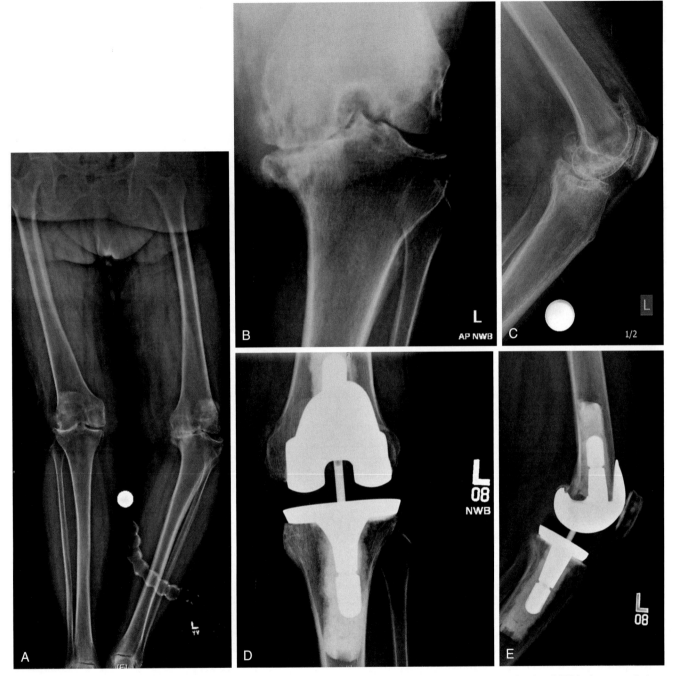

FIGURE 45-1   A: Standing limb alignment AP radiograph demonstrating a patient with severe varus left knee deformity of 30° in the coronal plane. **B:** AP view of the knee without weight-bearing, showing how the varus deformity can be underestimated without long leg films. **C:** Lateral view showing large posterior osteophytes leading to a preoperative fixed flexion deformity (FFD) of 25°. **D** and **E:** Patient's coronal plane and sagittal plane deformities were corrected after resection of osteophytes and varus–valgus balancing with a constrained TKA designed implant.

instability, and decreased femoral rollback—all of which lead to less flexion and poorly functioning TKA. In cases where the femur is oversized, there will be overstuffing of both the flexion space and the patellofemoral joint leading to decreased flexion as well. Increasing the thickness of the metal in the posterior condyles was thought to add flexion with some designs to help with posterior clearance and offset; however, clinical studies have not borne out with definitive results.[2,83] Regarding the best choice when

between femoral sizes, there are conflicting preferred techniques in the literature. Some advocate choosing the smaller femoral size, recutting the distal femur, and using a thicker polyethylene liner to balance the gaps.[2] Whereas Whiteside et al report especially in cases of flexion contracture, choosing the larger femoral size to overstuff the flexion space, recutting the tibia to balance the gaps, and performing additional soft-tissue releases as needed with good results.[84] One of the only studies comparing outcomes between knees left a little too tight versus too loose (fixed flexion versus genu recurvatum) concluded that surgeons should err on the side of FFD if neutral alignment cannot be achieved because TKAs in this group did better with regard to outcome scores and ultimate ROM at 2 years postoperatively.[85]

POSTOPERATIVE CONSIDERATIONS FOR STIFFNESS AFTER TKA

Despite efforts to correct FFD during index TKA, some patients are left with a residual deformity after surgery. In patients with prior flexion contracture, this result may be expected; however, in patients who have no preoperative flexion contracture, the consequence can be devastating. Regardless of preoperative ROM, there is no question that postoperative motion is a prime determinant of patient functional outcome and satisfaction after TKA. Here we discuss how to manage preoperative expectations for patients undergoing TKA based on some literature data regarding stiffness.

Prevalence and Causes of Postoperative Stiffness

The literature reports on stiffness after TKA must be interpreted with careful attention to the authors' definition of stiffness as well as the preoperative function of the patients. There are varying definitions for stiffness in each article with no consensus in the clinical or research setting: Nelson et al report limited motion following TKA as flexion contracture >15° or maximum flexion of <75°; Yercan et al describe stiffness as postoperative ROM of less than 10° to 90°; and Gandhi et al define arthrofibrosis as flexion of less than 90° at 1 year post TKA.[86-88] In these series, the authors have reported on consecutive patients with reported prevalence of stiffness as follows: Nelson et al 1.3% at 32 months post-op (total of 1000 patients studied); Yercan et al 5.3% at 31 months post-op (total of 1188 patients studied); and Gandhi et al 3.7% at 12 months post-op (1216 patients studied).[86-88]

A separate group of studies examines the incidence of flexion contracture after TKA in patients who were presenting with preoperative FFD.[23,89,90] In Lam's cohort of 284 TKAs with FFD, they report an incidence of 6.3% (18 knees) that resulted in unsatisfactory motion at 12 months—seven patients had FFD>10°, six patients had flexion<90°, and five patients had both.[89] In general, these studies all report significant improvement in knee functional scores and ROM after TKA and a residual improvement in knee flexion contracture up to 5 years postoperatively.

Several studies have evaluated revision TKA to determine the different failure modes of TKA and reasons for revision surgery. Interestingly, in a 2014 article by Sharkey et al, the most common reasons for revision TKA in 781

revisions performed were loosening (39.9%) and infection (27.4%) by a significant majority.[91] Arthrofibrosis only made up 4.5% of the revisions done in the study cohort, and this number had decreased from their prior study performed 10 years earlier. Meanwhile, Le et al reviewed their group of 253 first-time revision TKAs and found stiffness to be the reason for revision in 14% to 18% of cases, the third most commonly encountered etiology for revision TKA after infection and instability.[92]

In the largest database study on revision TKA in the United States, Delanois et al report on 337,597 procedures and again reported infection and loosening to be the most common etiologies for revision TKA at 20.4% and 20.3%, respectively.[93] In their study of the Nationwide Inpatient Sample database, however, there is no ICD-9 (International Classification of Diseases-9) code for arthrofibrosis included, and so many of the revisions for stiffness may be inaccurately categorized under an umbrella diagnosis of "other mechanical complication of prosthetic implant" or "other complication due to internal joint prosthesis." Therefore, database studies are often inaccurate with regard to capturing the true incidence of revision TKA performed due to postoperative FFD.

Much has been written about the causes of stiffness after primary TKA; however, the most important factor which has been shown to predict postoperative ROM time and again in the literature is preoperative ROM.[86,89,94-96] Lam et al showed in a multivariate analysis the only preoperative variable predictive of poor outcome after TKA was high FFD ($P < .001$), and that the overall flexion achieved at 12 months was directly related to the preoperative flexion.[89] In another logistic regression model, Aderinto et al found preoperative FFD was predictive of postoperative FFD > 10° at 1 week ($P = .006$) and 6 months following TKA ($P = .003$).[94] Yet, they along with Quah et al found that a gradual correction in FFD can be expected up to 2 to 3 years after TKA. Regardless of the severity of preoperative FFD, most patients were found to have absent or very mild contracture at midterm follow-up, and this did cause functional deficit.[23,94] Furthermore, severity of the flexion deficit preoperatively was shown to actually lead to better outcomes in Lam's cohort, as those knees with <90° of preoperative flexion gained a mean of 29.3°, whereas those knees with greater than 130° of flexion lost 15.2°.[89]

Aside from preoperative ROM, other factors may be involved in causing stiffness after TKA. Gender has been implicated, with men being significantly more likely than women to have fixed flexion contracture both in the short term and at up to 2 years postoperatively.[94,96] Older age may also be associated with postoperative FFD; however, interestingly in this same series, obesity was not a risk factor for flexion contracture after TKA.[96] While there is no CPT code for conversion TKA, prior knee surgery is certainly another risk factor for postoperative stiffness due to scar formation and adhesions under the extensor mechanism often leading to a shortened quadriceps and FFD.

Just as in the case of causes of preoperative FFD, post-operative contracture can often be caused by a painful joint and refusal to move or engage in PT exercises. A common cause of pain after TKA is postoperative hemarthrosis and swelling. Therefore, special attention must be given to achieving adequate hemostasis intraoperatively and postoperative anticoagulation regimens. Patients with hemophilia as discussed previously have a significant risk for both preoperative and postoperative FFD, and so focused PT regimens for these patients have even been described.[41] In a group of 874 primary TKAs performed in Australia, a comparison of arthrofibrosis rates and need for manipulation under anesthesia (MUA) was performed in patients receiving postoperative warfarin versus low-molecular-weight heparin. The authors found statistically significantly higher rates of arthrofibrosis requiring MUA in the warfarin group (26% vs. 8%, $P < .0001$).[97]

Finally, it should be briefly mentioned that in addition to patient factors, implant factors certainly play a role in causing postoperative stiffness after TKA. As was discussed in the section regarding intraoperative management of TKA to avoid postoperative stiffness, the femoral, tibial, and patellofemoral preparation can all affect the flexion, extension ROM, as well as general stability of the joint. The anteroposterior dimensions of the femoral component mainly affect flexion ROM. The tibial cut will affect both flexion and extension, and so the thickness of the polyethylene liner will greatly influence the ultimate flexion contracture after TKA. While there continues to be much debate regarding how much laxity is optimal in achieving maximal postoperative ROM, one author recommends leaving the extension space with a minimum of 1 mm laxity to avoid postoperative flexion contracture.[98]

Outcomes and Predictors for Postoperative Range of Motion

Expected ROM after contemporary TKA has been well-studied and has plateaued somewhere around an average of 120° AOM even with modern designs.[99] Here we will discuss the expected outcomes for patients with FFD undergoing TKA and conclude with a summary of predictors for postoperative ROM.

A study from France detailed the expected ROM improvement in their series of 107 patients undergoing TKA with flexion contracture of at least 20°. Forty-six of these patients had concomitant flexion of less than 90°. They found that total ROM improved by a mean of 39° overall, extension improved by 21°, and mean residual flexion contracture was 7°.[100] On the opposite end of the spectrum, a study from India analyzed ROM improvements in two groups of patients with nearly ankylosed joints with stiffness in either extension (SE) or in flexion (SF). They reported on 115 TKAs and found the AOM to improve similarly and dramatically in both groups: SE group mean preoperative AOM 10.9 to postoperative AOM 86.5°; SF group mean AOM 8.7 to postoperative AOM 92.2°. The KSSs in both groups of patients improved dramatically; however, it is important to note that complications from TKA including infection, extensor mechanism disruption, and residual stiffness were higher in this severely contracted group of patients at 20.9% incidence.[101]

The functional outcomes of severely ankylosed patients are affected by a clearly higher rate of complications and overall lower outcome scores than patients without this type of ankylosis undergoing TKA. However, when a lower threshold of severity of contracted patients (FFD>10°) was compared to a matched group of control patients undergoing TKA without FFD, Cheng et al showed that both groups had equivalent outcomes with regard to residual extension, total ROM, and KSSs.[102] This is one of the only long-term studies evaluating ROM in this group of contracted patients, with a follow-up of 10 years after index TKA. Nevertheless, several authors agree that the initial correction in FFD achieved at time of TKA is the most important time to prevent residual contracture and ensure optimal outcome.[100,101,103] In fact Mitsuyasu, performed an analysis and found that when extension at 3 months was correlated with long-term results, if there was contracture of greater than 15° at this time point then it was unlikely to improve in the mid-term follow-up period.[103]

A final important point when discussing outcomes after TKA in patients with FFD is that regardless of their ultimate ROM and functional scores, achieving postoperative stability is of paramount importance to ensuring a good long-term result. Therefore, the type of implant utilized to achieve stability is an equally important consideration as Berend et al point out. In their review of 52 TKAs with flexion contracture greater than 20°, they obtained 94% success with residual contracture of less than 10°.[104] In their series, they utilized a cruciate retaining device in 31 knees, a posterior stabilized design in 14 knees, a condylar constrained design in 5 knees, and a rotating hinge in 2 knees.

Assessment of ROM can be done via active patient ROM, passive ROM, or measurement of flexion against gravity. In the authors' experience, we recommend along with others to utilize flexion against gravity as the optimal method for predicting postoperative ROM and as a guide for patient expectation setting in the office setting. This value should be recorded at time of surgery and used as a goal for the PT program that the patient will be on in the postoperative period.[105]

We have already reviewed many of the causes and factors that affect postoperative ROM after TKA including preoperative ROM, underlying diagnosis, age, gender, weight, and intraoperative factors such as flexion–extension gap balancing, prosthetic design and sizing, and wound closure. Of these, preoperative ROM has been shown over the course of several decades to be the best predictor of postoperative ROM.[96,106,107] Interestingly, patients with the least preoperative ROM can expect to gain the most motion, whereas those with significant preoperative ROM may be at risk to lose motion after TKA. The last section will discuss postoperative management of TKA and its influence on stiffness.

MANAGEMENT OF FIXED FLEXION AFTER TKA

The management of an FFD after TKA includes nonoperative and operative treatment modalities. The most conservative of these strategies has been discussed previously and includes observation for the flexion contracture to gradually improve with time. However, active nonoperative treatment approaches include medication management and rehabilitation methods such as the use of continuous passive motion (CPM) and MUA. Operative interventions include use of arthroscopy and ultimately revision TKA to address persisting stiffness after index surgery.

Medication Effects on Stiffness After TKA

Medications can have a significant effect on development of arthrofibrosis after TKA. The most commonly studied of these includes anticoagulation use and its effect on ROM after TKA. In a very large study of 32,320 patients, Kahlenberg et al evaluated the type of anticoagulant used in a nationwide database of unilateral primary TKA and the subsequent rates of MUA.[108] They found significant higher rates of MUA in patients receiving oral warfarin, direct factor Xa inhibitors (e.g., rivaroxaban), and fondaparinux in comparison to patients receiving aspirin or low-molecular-weight heparin for venous thromboembolism (VTE) prophylaxis.

Rehabilitation and Manipulation

The efficacy of using CPM machines after TKA has been debated for several decades with evidence supporting both the use and disuse of these machines. The machines were developed to improve ROM in the early postoperative period and also potentially aid with achieving discharge goals earlier in the hospital stay. Over the years, the practice of CPM has seemingly fallen out of favor and rapid rehabilitation PT protocols have replaced the machines to aid in early recovery, ROM obtainment, and even same-day surgery TKA discharge.

In the early 1990s, a randomized trial by Johnson et al reported CPM led to earlier discharge from hospital and significantly improved early and late knee flexion by 10° at 12 months without increasing complications.[109] A meta-analysis of 14 studies by Brosseau et al found that active knee flexion and analgesia use at 2 weeks were lower in the groups of patients who received physiotherapy and CPM versus those who received physiotherapy alone. They also noted a decrease in hospital length of stay as well as need for MUA after TKA in the studies that were analyzed. Yet the authors concluded further research would need to evaluate these benefits against inconvenience and expense of CPM.

Regarding cost of CPM usage, the estimated added cost per patient has been reported to be from approximately $235 to $286.[110,111] Worland et al actually performed a randomized trial comparing using CPM alone including at home against using professional physical therapists and found no difference in knee scores or ROM at 6 months but an increase in cost of nearly $300 per patient with the professional PT group.[110] Meanwhile, a newer prospective randomized control trial from Hospital for Special Surgery reported on CPM plus PT versus just PT alone and found no benefit from the CPM machine in achieving excellent knee ROM (120° at 3 months) with an added cost of the machine at $235 per patient.[111]

There have been several other prospective clinical trials that have failed to show an advantage of CPM over PT alone in optimizing ROM and avoiding FFD after TKA.[112,113] Aside from providing no benefit and increasing costs per patient, there is concern that CPM use may have actual harmful effects on outcome after TKA. Pope et al found no ROM benefits at 1 year in their CPM groups yet had added postoperative complications of increased bloody wound drainage as well as analgesia requirements in patients receiving CPM from 0° to 70°.[114] In addition to increased wound drainage, Maloney et al even found higher rates of superficial and deep joint infection when they used CPM and, as a result, altered their CPM protocol to start later in the postoperative course to allow the wound to first properly heal.[115]

As mentioned previously, the push for early discharge from the hospital has led to sweeping implementation of "rapid rehabilitation" protocols designed to promote early recovery after TKA beginning in the postanesthesia care unit itself. While twice-a-day PT has long become the norm at most institutions, the combination of preoperative patient education and multimodal pain control pathways has transformed patient outcomes after TKA from a functional (including ROM goals) and satisfaction perspective. Femoral nerve blocks have been abandoned in favor of local intra-articular infiltrations and adductor canal blocks to allow for unimpeded ambulation early on and ultimately obtainment of maximal motion and avoidance of stiffness in the long run.[116] Nonetheless, even more novel methods of postoperative recovery involve the use of patient education materials and home instructional video applications without formal outpatient PT, and these programs have proven to be equally effective in appropriately selected patients.[117]

If prevention of stiffness is not possible after TKA with early postoperative interventions, there have been rare instances where knee immobilization has been used to hole the limb in an extended position to treat FFD. These are typically patients with severe preoperative flexion contracture that was unable to be fully corrected at time of surgery. A hinged cast brace, knee immobilizer, dynamic splinting, or serial casting have all been described to treat these FFD after TKA with varying levels of success.[7,118-120]

Other nonoperative interventions termed local modalities are performed by physical therapists or rehabilitation physicians to improve motion and other deficits after TKA in patients with problems such as flexion contracture, muscle weakness, and nerve entrapment. These modalities can include braces, shoe lifts, and orthoses as well as electrical stimulation, peroneal nerve release, and intramuscular botulinum toxin injections.[121,122] To evaluate the efficacy of botulinum toxin type A on flexion contracture following TKA, Smith et al performed a prospective double-blinded randomized controlled trial between Botox and placebo saline injections into the contracted hamstring tendons at 6 weeks postoperatively.[123] The Botox group started with mean flexion contracture of 19°, whereas the placebo group started with a mean of 13°. Both groups improved by 1 year postoperatively to a contracture of 1° suggesting that Botox may add no additional value to existing physiotherapy regimens. Finally, myofascial release and Astym therapy are two newer practices by rehabilitation specialists in treating flexion contracture after TKA. Initial series have reported positive results; however, no controlled studies exist to verify an added benefit of these therapies over home exercises and time.[124,125]

A final method to alleviate FFD and stiffness after TKA prior to surgical reintervention is use of MUA. Much has been written regarding the optimal timing of MUA with studies essentially all in agreement that the greatest efficacy results if the procedure is undertaken within the first 12 weeks after index arthroplasty.[126-129] Pagoti et al studied 62 MUAs out of a total of 7423 TKAs performed at their institution (a rate of 0.84%) and found when divided into groups by timing, patients undergoing MUA within 90 days of TKA gained significantly more flexion at both 6 weeks and 1 year than those undergoing MUA after 180 days from TKA.[127]

Likewise, Issa et al analyzed 144 MUAs out of 2128 TKAs and categorized early and late manipulations as those performed within 12 weeks of TKA and those after 12 weeks from index TKA.[126] Compared to patients undergoing late MUA, those in the early group had significantly higher mean gain in flexion (36.5° vs. 17°), high final ROM (110° vs. 95°), and higher Knee Society function scores (88 vs. 83 points). In a multivariate analysis, they confirmed that early manipulation correlated significantly with higher outcome scores.

Unfortunately for patients presenting with postoperative FFD, MUA has had less reported success for gains in extension than for gains in flexion. The majority of studies in the literature demonstrate obvious improvement of flexion ROM; however, we were unable to find any studies focusing on gains in extension with MUA performed after index TKA. Only one study evaluated the use of manipulation for flexion contracture, and this was an intraoperative manipulation performed while measuring the force of manipulation and the amount of gap formed in extension. Authors concluded that manipulation for flexion contracture is ineffective in opening the extension joint space and therefore FFD should be treated either with surgical soft-tissue release, additional bone cuts, or component exchange/tibial insert downsizing.[130] **Fig. 45-2** demonstrates the significant improvement in flexion after MUA compared to extension.

Proper technique for MUA is extremely important especially in cases with severe contracture and stiffness to avoid one of several complications that have been reported. Position of the manipulators hands should be as close to the joint as possible and over the tibial tubercle to decrease the lever arm and therefore the amount of torque applied to the femur and tibia, as this may result in periprosthetic fracture, loosening of components, or extensor mechanism rupture.[131] While some patients undergoing early MUA within 6 weeks have had outcomes reported similar to those of a primary TKA, patients suffering complications after MUA will never regain such function and satisfaction.[129] In general, avoidance of complications after MUA can be achieved by careful attention to appropriate indications and timing as well as technique for closed manipulation.[131]

Surgical Interventions

When nonoperative management of fixed flexion after TKA fails and the patient continues to suffer from poor functional outcome and persisting pain, surgical options must be explored. The least invasive of these is through the use of arthroscopy. Although technically more challenging than arthroscopy of the native knee due to poor visualization and metal reflection, arthroscopic lysis of adhesions (LOA) can lead to significant improvements in both flexion and extension ROM. In order to obtain additional extension, adhesions can be lysed from the patella and quadriceps, whereas to obtain additional flexion, the retinaculum can be divided and the PCL, if still present, can be released. Three separate series reviewing LOA after stiff TKA report their mean degrees of motion improved in both extension and flexion: Djian et al performed LOA at an average of 24 months after index TKA and went from 9° to 2.5° extension deficit and from 70° to 100° of flexion by 3 months; Bodendorfer et al performed LOA at an average of 4 months after index TKA and similarly improved extension by 6° and flexion by

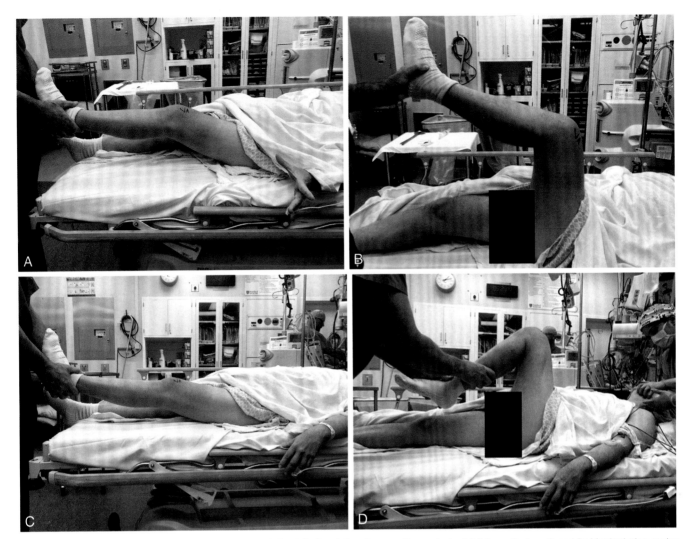

FIGURE 45-2 **A** and **B:** Patient who underwent TKA with fixed flexion deformity as well as a lack of full knee flexion. **C** and **D:** Manipulation under anesthesia (MUA) demonstrates the significant improvement in flexion as compared to the mild gain extension.

29°, and finally Tjoumakaris et al performed LOA and reduced extension deficit from 16° to 4° and flexion deficit from 79° to 103°.[132-134]

When FFD cannot be managed with nonoperative modalities alone, arthroscopic LOA provides a good alternative to improving ROM deficits and can even precede an MUA to prevent the complications with this procedure mentioned previously.[132] A last resort prior to undertaking revision TKA with actual femoral or tibial component exchange is the use of an open approach knee arthrotomy, débridement, and LOA.[135] Importantly, aggressive rehabilitation protocols must be employed immediately following such a surgical procedure to maintain the joint motion obtained at time of débridement. Keeney et al report on a limited approach protocol to treat contracted TKA patients using soft-tissue releases, component retention, and tibial insert downsizing. They compared this cohort of patients to those receiving true revision TKA with exchange of both components and found patients in the limited approach protocol to have significantly better improvements in mean knee ROM, mean clinical score, and mean functional scores.[136] Although the authors recognize this in their discussion, a main critique of this paper was the significant selection bias involved as patients with increased severity of contracture were less likely to be in the limited approach group, therefore significantly skewing the results in favor of this subset of patients.

The final topic we cover in this chapter is the use of revision TKA in addressing residual flexion contracture after index arthroplasty for patients who have persisting pain and dissatisfaction with their functional result. The incidence of revision TKA for stiffness was mentioned in the previous section but in general is cited to account for 4.5% to 18% of revisions performed in the United States.[91,92] The results and technical factors of these revisions surgeries are discussed here.

Overall, the outcomes of revision TKA for stiffness are quite satisfactory in improving ROM as well as patient function. Christensen et al reviewed their series of 11 revision TKAs performed in patients with painful and stiff knees with ROM<70°. They found a significant improvement in ROM from 39.7° to 83.2° and a decrease in flexion contracture from 13.2° to 0.9° at mean follow-up of 37.6 months (minimum 2 years).[137] Furthermore, all 11 of their patients had pain scores improved significantly and were all left with high satisfaction after revision TKA. Authors from The Rothman Institute reviewed their 39 cases of revision TKA for stiffness and had similar improvement in motion: overall ROM went from 68° to 90° and flexion contracture diminished from 14° to 5° at mid-term follow-up (74.4 months).[138] However, they were faced with a rerevision rate of 25.6% (10 patients required a second revision) and were unable to find any predictors of failure for these cases. Like the Rothman group, Nicholls et al also expressed revision TKA to have good results with respect to pain relief and were less than optimistic in achieving high functional outcome ratings. They noted predictors for poor outcome to be revision in patients with patella baja and inflammatory arthropathies and good outcomes of revision to be in patients with osteoarthritis and malposition of components.[139]

Regarding the surgical factors themselves, revision TKA with component exchange can be necessary due to poor flexion–extension gap balancing, underresection of bone, or malposition of components. In addition to a thorough open débridement of scar tissue and performing soft-tissue releases as necessary, component exchange can often lead to good outcomes in the appropriately indicated patients. In their study of 14 patients undergoing revision TKA for painful flexion contracture of at least 15°, Fehring et al found a significant improvement in postrevision ROM and pain scores but not function scores.[140] They reported eight of their patients were found to have what they termed a Type 1 error (flexion/extension mismatch); five of their patients had a Type 2 error (inadequate tibial bone resection); and nearly all of their patients required removal of the femoral component.

In one of the largest series of revision TKA performed for stiffness, Hug et al discuss a protocol-driven approach to revision with either component retention and insert exchange, single component revision, or complete component revision.[141] They studied 69 revision TKAs and found that in patients with both components revised, the mean AOM increase was greatest at 45°, in patients with just tibial insert exchange, motion increase was 32°, and in patients with either femoral or tibial component exchange, and average motion increase was 29°. It is difficult to know the reason for this difference in motion achieved with each group other than the fact that the most severely stiff patients were in the complete component revision group. At the least, this would suggest that poorly placed components can certainly lead to the most significant deficits when it comes to knee motion.

Lastly, an important consideration in revision TKA for stiffness is the type of implant utilized after soft-tissue releases, additional bone cuts, and ligament rebalancing has occurred. The use of constrained implants with mid-level and higher levels of constraint is becoming increasingly popular.[142] This is particularly the case when the tibial polyethylene insert is downsized significantly to achieve increased sagittal plane laxity with flexion and extension.[143]

Furthermore, Bingham et al have recently written about the use of rotating-hinge–type implants, conferring the highest levels of constraint, in treatment of severe arthrofibrosis after TKA.[144] These implants were used in the revision setting and allowed for the highest level of soft-tissue release to maximize flexion–extension arcs of motion. The authors matched 34 patients undergoing revision TKA with rotating hinge to 68 patients without hinged revision TKA. They found a larger increase in ROM in the hinge group (20° vs. 12°, $P = .048$) and a lower rate of MUA in the hinge group as well.

No matter how well indicated the patient or technically proficient the surgeon is in performing the revision TKA, however, there is no question that even with the biggest improvements in functional scores and ROM, outcomes do not approach those of a well-done primary TKA.

CONCLUSION

TKA is an exceptionally successful procedure providing dramatic improvements in pain and function for patients with advanced arthritis. The procedure has evolved over the course of several decades in efforts to mimic the natural kinematics of the native knee joint and maximize ROM. Patients with preoperative FFD pose challenges for surgeons undertaking TKA; however, these patients generally do quite well with significant improvements in their motion and function. Those patients who are left with postoperative stiffness are among the most difficult to treat by arthroplasty surgeons. The armamentarium of treatment options should include an initial foray into nonoperative modalities including additional rehabilitation, PT modalities, nonsteroidal anti-inflammatory medications, and in early instances MUA. If these are unsuccessful, surgical intervention must be attempted with varying degrees of success in the literature. Revision TKA in combination with newer early rehabilitation programs and pain control protocols has had encouraging success in treating these patients moving forward.

REFERENCES

1. Iwaki H, Pinskerova V, Freeman MA. Tibiofemoral movement 1: the shapes and relative movements of the femur and tibia in the unloaded cadaver knee. *J Bone Joint Surg Br.* 2000;82(8):1189-1195.
2. Guoan L, Schule S, Maloney W, Rubash H. *Improving flexion in total knee arthroplasty.* In: *The Adult Knee.* Vol 1. 1st ed. Philadelphia: Lippincott Williams & Wilkins; 2003:1234-1242.
3. Van de Velde SK, Bingham JT, Hosseini A, et al. Increased tibiofemoral cartilage contact deformation in patients with anterior cruciate ligament deficiency. *Arthritis Rheum.* 2009;60(12):3693-3702. doi:10.1002/art.24965.
4. Sanders TL, Pareek A, Barrett IJ, et al. Incidence and long-term follow-up of isolated posterior cruciate ligament tears. *Knee Surg Sports Traumatol Arthrosc.* 2017;25(10):3017-3023. doi:10.1007/s00167-016-4052-y.

5. Li G, Zayontz S, DeFrate LE, Most E, Suggs JF, Rubash HE. Kinematics of the knee at high flexion angles: an in vitro investigation. *J Orthop Res.* 2004;22(1):90-95. doi:10.1016/S0736-0266(03)00118-9.

6. Mihalko WM, Whiteside LA. Bone resection and ligament treatment for flexion contracture in knee arthroplasty. *Clin Orthop Relat Res.* 2003;406:141-147. doi:10.1097/01.blo.0000030512.43495.74.

7. Su EP. Fixed flexion deformity and total knee arthroplasty. *J Bone Joint Surg Br.* 2012;94(11 suppl A):112-115. doi:10.1302/0301-620X.94B11.30512.

8. Hallaçeli H, Uruç V, Uysal HH, et al. Normal hip, knee and ankle range of motion in the Turkish population. *Acta Orthop Traumatol Turc.* 2014;48(1):37-42. doi:10.3944/AOTT.2014.3113.

9. Roaas A, Andersson GB. Normal range of motion of the hip, knee and ankle joints in male subjects, 30-40 years of age. *Acta Orthop Scand.* 1982;53(2):205-208.

10. Roach KE, Miles TP. Normal hip and knee active range of motion: the relationship to age. *Phys Ther.* 1991;71(9):656-665.

11. Soucie JM, Wang C, Forsyth A, et al. Range of motion measurements: reference values and a database for comparison studies. *Haemophilia.* 2011;17(3):500-507. doi:10.1111/j.1365-2516.2010.02399.x.

12. Mulholland SJ, Wyss UP. Activities of daily living in non-Western cultures: range of motion requirements for hip and knee joint implants. *Int J Rehabil Res.* 2001;24(3):191-198.

13. Rowe PJ, Myles CM, Walker C, Nutton R. Knee joint kinematics in gait and other functional activities measured using flexible electrogoniometry: how much knee motion is sufficient for normal daily life? *Gait Posture.* 2000;12(2):143-155.

14. Hefzy MS, Kelly BP, Cooke TD, al-Baddah AM, Harrison L. Knee kinematics in-vivo of kneeling in deep flexion examined by biplanar radiographs. *Biomed Sci Instrum.* 1997;33:453-458.

15. Nakagawa S, Kadoya Y, Todo S, et al. Tibiofemoral movement 3: full flexion in the living knee studied by MRI. *J Bone Joint Surg Br.* 2000;82(8):1199-1200.

16. Murphy MT, Skinner TL, Cresswell AG, Crawford RW, Journeaux SF, Russell TG. The effect of knee flexion contracture following total knee arthroplasty on the energy cost of walking. *J Arthroplasty.* 2014;29(1):85-89. doi:10.1016/j.arth.2013.04.039.

17. Mont MA, Banerjee S, Jauregui JJ, Cherian JJ, Kapadia BH. What outcome metrics do the various knee rating systems for assessment of outcomes following total knee arthroplasty measure? A systematic review of literature. *Surg Technol Int.* 2015;26:269-274.

18. Sculco T. *Management of the stiff knee.* In: *The Adult Knee.* 1st ed. Philadelphia: Lippincott Williams & Wilkins; 2003:1333-1338.

19. Bach CM, Nogler M, Steingruber IE, et al. Scoring systems in total knee arthroplasty. *Clin Orthop Relat Res.* 2002;399:184-196.

20. Insall JN, Dorr LD, Scott RD, Scott WN. Rationale of the Knee Society clinical rating system. *Clin Orthop Relat Res.* 1989;248:13-14.

21. Ritter MA, Campbell ED. Effect of range of motion on the success of a total knee arthroplasty. *J Arthroplasty.* 1987;2(2):95-97.

22. Jain JK, Sharma RK, Agarwal S. Total knee arthroplasty in patients with fixed flexion deformity: treatment protocol and outcome. *Curr Orthop Pract.* 2013;24(6):659. doi:10.1097/BCO.0000000000000031.

23. Quah C, Swamy G, Lewis J, Kendrew J, Badhe N. Fixed flexion deformity following total knee arthroplasty. A prospective study of the natural history. *Knee.* 2012;19(5):519-521. doi:10.1016/j.knee.2011.09.003.

24. Zhang Y, Jordan JM. Epidemiology of osteoarthritis. *Clin Geriatr Med.* 2010;26(3):355-369. doi:10.1016/j.cger.2010.03.001.

25. Heidari B. Knee osteoarthritis prevalence, risk factors, pathogenesis and features: Part I. *Casp J Intern Med.* 2011;2(2):205-212.

26. Fishkin Z, Miller D, Ritter C, Ziv I. Changes in human knee ligament stiffness secondary to osteoarthritis. *J Orthop Res.* 2002;20(2):204-207. doi:10.1016/S0736-0266(01)00087-0.

27. Hwang YS, Moon KP, Kim KT, Kim JW, Park WS. Total knee arthroplasty for severe flexion contracture in rheumatoid arthritis knees. *Knee Surg Relat Res.* 2016;28(4):325-329. doi:10.5792/ksrr.16.020.

28. Harb MA, Solow M, Newman JM, et al. Have the annual trends of total knee arthroplasty in rheumatoid arthritis patients changed? *J Knee Surg.* 2018;31(9):841-845. doi:10.1055/s-0037-1615822.

29. Wang W, Niu D. Balancing of soft tissues in total knee arthroplasty for patients with rheumatoid arthritis with knee flexion contracture. *Zhongguo Xiu Fu Chong Jian Wai Ke Za Zhi.* 2008;22(10):1173-1176.

30. Lu H, Mow CS, Lin J. Total knee arthroplasty in the presence of severe flexion contracture: a report of 37 cases. *J Arthroplasty.* 1999;14(7):775-780.

31. Abe S, Kohyama K, Yokoyama H, et al. Total knee arthroplasty for rheumatoid knee with bilateral, severe flexion contracture: report of three cases. *Mod Rheumatol.* 2008;18(5):499-506. doi:10.1007/s10165-008-0079-3.

32. Yan D, Yang J, Pei F. Total knee arthroplasty treatment of rheumatoid arthritis with severe versus moderate flexion contracture. *J Orthop Surg.* 2013;8:41. doi:10.1186/1749-799X-8-41.

33. Lü H, Li H, Guan Z, Sun T, Yuan Y. Total knee arthroplasty for extension ankylosing deformity. *Zhonghua Wai Ke Za Zhi.* 2007;45(6):405-408.

34. Montgomery WH, Insall JN, Haas SB, Becker MS, Windsor RE. Primary total knee arthroplasty in stiff and ankylosed knees. *Am J Knee Surg.* 1998;11(1):20-23.

35. Kim YH, Cho SH, Kim JS. Total knee arthroplasty in bony ankylosis in gross flexion. *J Bone Joint Surg Br.* 1999;81(2):296-300.

36. Atilla B, Caglar O, Pekmezci M, Buyukasik Y, Tokgozoglu AM, Alpaslan M. Pre-operative flexion contracture determines the functional outcome of haemophilic arthropathy treated with total knee arthroplasty. *Haemophilia.* 2012;18(3):358-363. doi:10.1111/j.1365-2516.2011.02695.x.

37. Strauss AC, Schmolders J, Friedrich MJ, et al. Outcome after total knee arthroplasty in haemophilic patients with stiff knees. *Haemophilia.* 2015;21(4):e300-e305. doi:10.1111/hae.12698.

38. Strauss AC, Goldmann G, Schmolders J, et al. Impact of preoperative knee stiffness on the postoperative outcome after total knee arthroplasty in patients with haemophilia. *Z Orthop Unfall.* 2015;153(5):526-532. doi:10.1055/s-0035-1557768.

39. Rodriguez-Merchan EC. Correction of fixed contractures during total knee arthroplasty in haemophiliacs. *Haemophilia.* 1999;5(suppl 1):33-38.

40. Chiang CC, Chen PQ, Shen MC, Tsai W. Total knee arthroplasty for severe haemophilic arthropathy: long-term experience in Taiwan. *Haemophilia.* 2008;14(4):828-834. doi:10.1111/j.1365-2516.2008.01693.x.

41. Kamath AF, Horneff JG, Forsyth A, Nikci V, Nelson CL. Total knee arthroplasty in hemophiliacs: gains in range of motion realized beyond twelve months postoperatively. *Clin Orthop Surg.* 2012;4(2):121-128. doi:10.4055/cios.2012.4.2.121.

42. Kubeš R, Salaj P, Hromádka R, et al. Range of motion after total knee arthroplasty in hemophilic arthropathy. *BMC Musculoskelet Disord.* 2018;19(1):162. doi:10.1186/s12891-018-2080-0.

43. Song SJ, Bae JK, Park CH, Yoo MC, Bae DK, Kim KI. Mid-term outcomes and complications of total knee arthroplasty in haemophilic arthropathy: a review of consecutive 131 knees between 2006 and 2015 in a single institute. *Haemophilia.* 2018;24(2):299-306. doi:10.1111/hae.13383.

44. Moore MF, Tobase P, Allen DD. Meta-analysis: outcomes of total knee arthroplasty in the haemophilia population. *Haemophilia.* 2016;22(4):e275-e285. doi:10.1111/hae.12885.

45. Blagojevic M, Jinks C, Jeffery A, Jordan KP. Risk factors for onset of osteoarthritis of the knee in older adults: a systematic review and meta-analysis. *Osteoarthr Cartil.* 2010;18(1):24-33. doi:10.1016/j.joca.2009.08.010.

46. Trouvin A-P, Perrot S. Pain in osteoarthritis. Implications for optimal management. *Joint Bone Spine*. 2018;85(4):429-434. doi:10.1016/j.jbspin.2017.08.002.

47. Mizner RL, Petterson SC, Stevens JE, Axe MJ, Snyder-Mackler L. Preoperative quadriceps strength predicts functional ability one year after total knee arthroplasty. *J Rheumatol*. 2005;32(8):1533-1539.

48. Beaupre LA, Lier D, Davies DM, Johnston DBC. The effect of a preoperative exercise and education program on functional recovery, health related quality of life, and health service utilization following primary total knee arthroplasty. *J Rheumatol*. 2004;31(6):1166-1173.

49. D'Lima DD, Colwell CW, Morris BA, Hardwick ME, Kozin F. The effect of preoperative exercise on total knee replacement outcomes. *Clin Orthop Relat Res*. 1996;326:174-182.

50. Crowe J, Henderson J. Pre-arthroplasty rehabilitation is effective in reducing hospital stay. *Can J Occup Ther*. 2003;70(2):88-96. doi:10.1177/000841740307000204.

51. McDonald S, Hetrick S, Green S. Pre-operative education for hip or knee replacement. *Cochrane Database Syst Rev*. 2004;(1):CD003526. doi:10.1002/14651858.CD003526.pub2.

52. Ackerman IN, Bennell KL. Does pre-operative physiotherapy improve outcomes from lower limb joint replacement surgery? A systematic review. *Aust J Physiother*. 2004;50(1):25-30.

53. Swank AM, Kachelman JB, Bibeau W, et al. Prehabilitation before total knee arthroplasty increases strength and function in older adults with severe osteoarthritis. *J Strength Cond Res*. 2011;25(2):318-325. doi:10.1519/JSC.0b013e318202e431.

54. Moseley JB, O'Malley K, Petersen NJ, et al. A controlled trial of arthroscopic surgery for osteoarthritis of the knee. *N Engl J Med*. 2002;347(2):81-88. doi:10.1056/NEJMoa013259.

55. Sihvonen R, Paavola M, Malmivaara A, et al. Arthroscopic partial meniscectomy versus sham surgery for a degenerative meniscal tear. *N Engl J Med*. 2013;369(26):2515-2524. doi:10.1056/NEJMoa1305189.

56. Moriya H, Sasho T, Sano S, Wada Y. Arthroscopic posteromedial release for osteoarthritic knees with flexion contracture. *Arthroscopy*. 2004;20(10):1030-1039. doi:10.1016/j.arthro.2004.08.018.

57. Andriacchi TP, Galante JO. Retention of the posterior cruciate in total knee arthroplasty. *J Arthroplasty*. 1988;3 suppl:S13-S19.

58. An VVG, Scholes CJ, Fritsch BA. Factors affecting the incidence and management of fixed flexion deformity in total knee arthroplasty: a systematic review. *Knee*. 2018;25(3):352-359. doi:10.1016/j.knee.2018.03.008.

59. Keating EM, Faris PM, Meding JB, Ritter MA. Comparison of the midvastus muscle-splitting approach with the median parapatellar approach in total knee arthroplasty. *J Arthroplasty*. 1999;14(1):29-32.

60. Matsueda M, Gustilo RB. Subvastus and medial parapatellar approaches in total knee arthroplasty. *Clin Orthop Relat Res*. 2000;371:161-168.

61. Parentis MA, Rumi MN, Deol GS, Kothari M, Parrish WM, Pellegrini VD. A comparison of the vastus splitting and median parapatellar approaches in total knee arthroplasty. *Clin Orthop Relat Res*. 1999;367:107-116.

62. Bruce WJ, Rooney J, Hutabarat SR, Atkinson MC, Goldberg JA, Walsh WR. Exposure in difficult total knee arthroplasty using coronal tibial tubercle osteotomy. *J Orthop Surg*. 2000;8(1):61-65. doi:10.1177/230949900000800111.

63. Banks SA, Markovich GD, Hodge WA. In vivo kinematics of cruciate-retaining and -substituting knee arthroplasties. *J Arthroplasty*. 1997;12(3):297-304.

64. Li G, Zayontz S, Most E, Otterberg E, Sabbag K, Rubash HE. Cruciate-retaining and cruciate-substituting total knee arthroplasty: an in vitro comparison of the kinematics under muscle loads. *J Arthroplasty*. 2001;16(8 suppl 1):150-156.

65. Han CW, Yang IH, Lee WS, Park KK, Han CD. Evaluation of postoperative range of motion and functional outcomes after cruciate-retaining and posterior-stabilized high-flexion total knee arthroplasty. *Yonsei Med J*. 2012;53(4):794-800. doi:10.3349/ymj.2012.53.4.794.

66. Shoji H, Wolf A, Packard S, Yoshino S. Cruciate retained and excised total knee arthroplasty. A comparative study in patients with bilateral total knee arthroplasty. *Clin Orthop Relat Res*. 1994;305:218-222.

67. Becker MW, Insall JN, Faris PM. Bilateral total knee arthroplasty. One cruciate retaining and one cruciate substituting. *Clin Orthop Relat Res*. 1991;271:122-124.

68. Liu DW, Reidy JF, Beller EM. The effect of distal femoral resection on fixed flexion deformity in total knee arthroplasty. *J Arthroplasty*. 2016;31(1):98-102. doi:10.1016/j.arth.2015.07.033.

69. Walker PS, Garg A. Range of motion in total knee arthroplasty. A computer analysis. *Clin Orthop Relat Res*. 1991;262:227-235.

70. Zhen P, Li S-S, Li X-S, Ren M, Shao H-B. Posterior capsule releasing in total knee arthroplasty for patients with rheumatoid arthritis with stiff knees in flexion. *Zhongguo Gu Shang*. 2015;28(3):272-275.

71. Pinter Z, Staggers R, Lee S, Bergstresser S, Shah A, Naranje S. Open posterior capsular release with an osteotome in total knee arthroplasty does not place important neurovascular structures at risk. *Knee Surg Sports Traumatol Arthrosc*. 2019;27(7):2120-2123. doi:10.1007/s00167-019-05399-1.

72. Bellemans J, Vandenneucker H, Victor J, Vanlauwe J. Flexion contracture in total knee arthroplasty. *Clin Orthop Relat Res*. 2006;452:78-82. doi:10.1097/01.blo.0000238791.36725.c5.

73. An VVG, Twiggs J, Leie M, Fritsch BA. Kinematic alignment is bone and soft tissue preserving compared to mechanical alignment in total knee arthroplasty. *Knee*. 2019;26(2):466-476. doi:10.1016/j.knee.2019.01.002.

74. Paschos NK, Howell SM, Johnson JM, Mahfouz MR. Can kinematic tibial templates assist the surgeon locating the flexion and extension plane of the knee? *Knee*. 2017;24(5):1006-1015. doi:10.1016/j.knee.2017.07.008.

75. Howell SM, Shelton TJ, Hull ML. Implant survival and function ten years after kinematically aligned total knee arthroplasty. *J Arthroplasty*. 2018;33(12):3678-3684. doi:10.1016/j.arth.2018.07.020.

76. Masri BA, Laskin RS, Windsor RE, Haas SB. Knee closure in total knee replacement: a randomized prospective trial. *Clin Orthop Relat Res*. 1996;331:81-86.

77. Emerson RH, Ayers C, Higgins LL. Surgical closing in total knee arthroplasty. A series followup. *Clin Orthop Relat Res*. 1999;368:176-181.

78. Maloney WJ, Schurman DJ. The effects of implant design on range of motion after total knee arthroplasty. Total condylar versus posterior stabilized total condylar designs. *Clin Orthop Relat Res*. 1992;278:147-152.

79. Walker PS, Sathasivam S. Design forms of total knee replacement. *Proc Inst Mech Eng H*. 2000;214(1):101-119. doi:10.1243/0954411001535282.

80. Onodera T, Majima T, Nishiike O, Kasahara Y, Takahashi D. Posterior femoral condylar offset after total knee replacement in the risk of knee flexion contracture. *J Arthroplasty*. 2013;28(7):1112-1116. doi:10.1016/j.arth.2012.07.029.

81. Meng F, Jaeger S, Sonntag R, Schroeder S, Smith-Romanski S, Kretzer JP. How prosthetic design influences knee kinematics: a narrative review of tibiofemoral kinematics of healthy and joint-replaced knees. *Expert Rev Med Devices*. 2019;16(2):119-133. doi:10.1080/17434440.2019.1564037.

82. Berger RA, Crossett LS, Jacobs JJ, Rubash HE. Malrotation causing patellofemoral complications after total knee arthroplasty. *Clin Orthop Relat Res*. 1998;356:144-153.

83. Most E, Li G, Schule S, et al. The kinematics of fixed- and mobile-bearing total knee arthroplasty. *Clin Orthop Relat Res*. 2003;416:197-207. doi:10.1097/01.blo.0000092999.90435.d1.

84. Whiteside LA, Mihalko WM. Surgical procedure for flexion contracture and recurvatum in total knee arthroplasty. *Clin Orthop Relat Res.* 2002;404:189-195.

85. Koo K, Silva A, Chong HC, et al. Genu recurvatum versus fixed flexion after total knee arthroplasty. *Clin Orthop Surg.* 2016;8(3):249-253. doi:10.4055/cios.2016.8.3.249.

86. Nelson CL, Kim J, Lotke PA. Stiffness after total knee arthroplasty. *J Bone Joint Surg Am.* 2005;87 suppl 1(pt 2):264-270. doi:10.2106/JBJS.E-00345.

87. Yercan HS, Sugun TS, Bussiere C, Ait Si Selmi T, Davies A, Neyret P. Stiffness after total knee arthroplasty: prevalence, management and outcomes. *Knee.* 2006;13(2):111-117. doi:10.1016/j.knee.2005.10.001.

88. Gandhi R, de Beer J, Leone J, Petruccelli D, Winemaker M, Adili A. Predictive risk factors for stiff knees in total knee arthroplasty. *J Arthroplasty.* 2006;21(1):46-52. doi:10.1016/j.arth.2005.06.004.

89. Lam LO, Swift S, Shakespeare D. Fixed flexion deformity and flexion after knee arthroplasty. What happens in the first 12 months after surgery and can a poor outcome be predicted? *Knee.* 2003;10(2):181-185.

90. Cheng K, Dashti H, McLeod G. Does flexion contracture continue to improve up to five years after total knee arthroplasty? *J Orthop Surg.* 2007;15(3):303-305. doi:10.1177/230949900701500312.

91. Sharkey PF, Lichstein PM, Shen C, Tokarski AT, Parvizi J. Why are total knee arthroplasties failing today – has anything changed after 10 years? *J Arthroplasty.* 2014;29(9):1774-1778. doi:10.1016/j.arth.2013.07.024.

92. Le DH, Goodman SB, Maloney WJ, Huddleston JI. Current modes of failure in TKA: infection, instability, and stiffness predominate. *Clin Orthop Relat Res.* 2014;472(7):2197-2200. doi:10.1007/s11999-014-3540-y.

93. Delanois RE, Mistry JB, Gwam CU, Mohamed NS, Choksi US, Mont MA. Current epidemiology of revision total knee arthroplasty in the United States. *J Arthroplasty.* 2017;32(9):2663-2668. doi:10.1016/j.arth.2017.03.066.

94. Aderinto J, Brenkel IJ, Chan P. Natural history of fixed flexion deformity following total knee replacement: a prospective five-year study. *J Bone Joint Surg Br.* 2005;87(7):934-936. doi:10.1302/0301-620X.87B7.15586.

95. McAuley JP, Harrer MF, Ammeen D, Engh GA. Outcome of knee arthroplasty in patients with poor preoperative range of motion. *Clin Orthop Relat Res.* 2002;404:203-207.

96. Goudie ST, Deakin AH, Ahmad A, Maheshwari R, Picard F. Flexion contracture following primary total knee arthroplasty: risk factors and outcomes. *Orthopedics.* 2011;34(12):e855-e859. doi:10.3928/01477447-20111021-18.

97. Walton NP, Jahromi I, Dobson PJ, Angel KR, Lewis PL, Campbell DG. Arthrofibrosis following total knee replacement; does therapeutic warfarin make a difference? *Knee.* 2005;12(2):103-106. doi:10.1016/j.knee.2004.06.004.

98. Okamoto S, Okazaki K, Mitsuyasu H, et al. Extension gap needs more than 1-mm laxity after implantation to avoid post-operative flexion contracture in total knee arthroplasty. *Knee Surg Sports Traumatol Arthrosc.* 2014;22(12):3174-3180. doi:10.1007/s00167-014-2858-z.

99. Seo JG, Moon Y-W, Chang MJ, et al. Design modifications of high-flexion TKA do not improve short term clinical and radiographic outcomes. *BMC Musculoskelet Disord.* 2014;15:433. doi:10.1186/1471-2474-15-433.

100. Massin P, Petit A, Odri G, et al. Total knee arthroplasty in patients with greater than 20 degrees flexion contracture. *Orthop Traumatol Surg Res.* 2009;95(4 suppl 1):S7-S12. doi:10.1016/j.otsr.2009.04.001.

101. Rajgopal A, Panda I, Dahiya V. A comparative study on the long-term outcome of total knee arthroplasty performed for knees stiff in extension and those stiff in flexion. *J Arthroplasty.* 2017;32(11):3396-3403. doi:10.1016/j.arth.2017.06.027.

102. Cheng K, Ridley D, Bird J, McLeod G. Patients with fixed flexion deformity after total knee arthroplasty do just as well as those without: ten-year prospective data. *Int Orthop.* 2010;34(5):663-667. doi:10.1007/s00264-009-0801-6.

103. Mitsuyasu H, Matsuda S, Miura H, Okazaki K, Fukagawa S, Iwamoto Y. Flexion contracture persists if the contracture is more than 15° at 3 months after total knee arthroplasty. *J Arthroplasty.* 2011;26(4):639-643. doi:10.1016/j.arth.2010.04.023.

104. Berend KR, Lombardi AV, Adams JB. Total knee arthroplasty in patients with greater than 20 degrees flexion contracture. *Clin Orthop Relat Res.* 2006;452:83-87. doi:10.1097/01.blo.0000238801.90090.59.

105. Lee DC, Kim DH, Scott RD, Suthers K. Intraoperative flexion against gravity as an indication of ultimate range of motion in individual cases after total knee arthroplasty. *J Arthroplasty.* 1998;13(5):500-503.

106. Lizaur A, Marco L, Cebrian R. Preoperative factors influencing the range of movement after total knee arthroplasty for severe osteoarthritis. *J Bone Joint Surg Br.* 1997;79(4):626-629.

107. Harvey IA, Barry K, Kirby SP, Johnson R, Elloy MA. Factors affecting the range of movement of total knee arthroplasty. *J Bone Joint Surg Br.* 1993;75(6):950-955.

108. Kahlenberg CA, Richardson SS, Schairer WW, Sculco PK. Type of anticoagulant used after total knee arthroplasty affects the rate of knee manipulation for postoperative stiffness. *J Bone Joint Surg Am.* 2018;100(16):1366-1372. doi:10.2106/JBJS.17.01110.

109. Johnson DP, Eastwood DM. Beneficial effects of continuous passive motion after total condylar knee arthroplasty. *Ann R Coll Surg Engl.* 1992;74(6):412-416.

110. Worland RL, Arredondo J, Angles F, Lopez-Jimenez F, Jessup DE. Home continuous passive motion machine versus professional physical therapy following total knee replacement. *J Arthroplasty.* 1998;13(7):784-787.

111. Joshi RN, White PB, Murray-Weir M, Alexiades MM, Sculco TP, Ranawat AS. Prospective randomized trial of the efficacy of continuous passive motion post total knee arthroplasty: experience of the hospital for special surgery. *J Arthroplasty.* 2015;30(12):2364-2369. doi:10.1016/j.arth.2015.06.006.

112. Chen B, Zimmerman JR, Soulen L, DeLisa JA. Continuous passive motion after total knee arthroplasty: a prospective study. *Am J Phys Med Rehabil.* 2000;79(5):421-426.

113. MacDonald SJ, Bourne RB, Rorabeck CH, McCalden RW, Kramer J, Vaz M. Prospective randomized clinical trial of continuous passive motion after total knee arthroplasty. *Clin Orthop Relat Res.* 2000;380:30-35.

114. Pope RO, Corcoran S, McCaul K, Howie DW. Continuous passive motion after primary total knee arthroplasty. Does it offer any benefits? *J Bone Joint Surg Br.* 1997;79(6):914-917.

115. Maloney WJ, Schurman DJ, Hangen D, Goodman SB, Edworthy S, Bloch DA. The influence of continuous passive motion on outcome in total knee arthroplasty. *Clin Orthop Relat Res.* 1990;256:162-168.

116. Nakagawa S, Arai Y, Inoue H, et al. Comparative effects of peri-articular multimodal drug injection and single-shot femoral nerve block on pain following total knee arthroplasty and factors influencing their effectiveness. *Knee Surg Relat Res.* 2016;28(3):233-238. doi:10.5792/ksrr.2016.28.3.233.

117. Rajan RA, Pack Y, Jackson H, Gillies C, Asirvatham R. No need for outpatient physiotherapy following total knee arthroplasty: a randomized trial of 120 patients. *Acta Orthop Scand.* 2004;75(1):71-73. doi:10.1080/00016470410001708140.

118. Finger E, Willis FB. Dynamic splinting for knee flexion contracture following total knee arthroplasty: a case report. *Cases J.* 2008;1(1):421. doi:10.1186/1757-1626-1-421.

119. Karam MD, Pugely A, Callaghan JJ, Shurr D. Hinged cast brace for persistent flexion contracture following total knee replacement. *Iowa Orthop J.* 2011;31:69-72.

120. He Q, Xiao L, Ma J, Zhao G. A case report of successful treatment of 90° knee flexion contracture in a patient with adult-onset Still's disease. *BMC Surg.* 2016;16:7. doi:10.1186/s12893-016-0122-9.

121. Ulrich SD, Bhave A, Marker DR, Seyler TM, Mont MA. Focused rehabilitation treatment of poorly functioning total knee arthroplasties. *Clin Orthop Relat Res.* 2007;464:138-145.

122. Seyler TM, Jinnah RH, Koman LA, et al. Botulinum toxin type A injections for the management of flexion contractures following total knee arthroplasty. *J Surg Orthop Adv.* 2008;17(4):231-238.

123. Smith EB, Shafi KA, Greis AC, Maltenfort MG, Chen AF. Decreased flexion contracture after total knee arthroplasty using Botulinum toxin A: a randomized controlled trial. *Knee Surg Sports Traumatol Arthrosc.* 2016;24(10):3229-3234. doi:10.1007/s00167-016-4277-9.

124. Silva DCCMe, de Andrade Alexandre DJ, Silva JG. Immediate effect of myofascial release on range of motion, pain and biceps and rectus femoris muscle activity after total knee replacement. *J Bodyw Mov Ther.* 2018;22(4):930-936. doi:10.1016/j.jbmt.2017.12.003.

125. Chughtai M, Mont MA, Cherian C, et al. A novel, nonoperative treatment demonstrates success for stiff total knee arthroplasty after failure of conventional therapy. *J Knee Surg.* 2016;29(3):188-193. doi:10.1055/s-0035-1569482.

126. Issa K, Banerjee S, Kester MA, Khanuja HS, Delanois RE, Mont MA. The effect of timing of manipulation under anesthesia to improve range of motion and functional outcomes following total knee arthroplasty. *J Bone Joint Surg Am.* 2014;96(16):1349-1357. doi:10.2106/JBJS.M.00899.

127. Pagoti R, O'Brien S, Blaney J, Doran E, Beverland D. Knee manipulation for reduced flexion after total knee arthroplasty. Is timing critical? *J Clin Orthop Trauma.* 2018;9(4):295-299. doi:10.1016/j.jcot.2017.11.017.

128. Gu A, Michalak AJ, Cohen JS, Almeida ND, McLawhorn AS, Sculco PK. Efficacy of manipulation under anesthesia for stiffness following total knee arthroplasty: a systematic review. *J Arthroplasty.* 2018;33(5):1598-1605. doi:10.1016/j.arth.2017.11.054.

129. Newman ET, Herschmiller TA, Attarian DE, Vail TP, Bolognesi MP, Wellman SS. Risk factors, outcomes, and timing of manipulation under anesthesia after total knee arthroplasty. *J Arthroplasty.* 2018;33(1):245-249. doi:10.1016/j.arth.2017.08.002.

130. Matsui Y, Minoda Y, Fumiaki I, Nakagawa S, Okajima Y, Kobayashi A. Intraoperative manipulation for flexion contracture during total knee arthroplasty. *Orthopedics.* 2016;39(6):e1070-e1074. doi:10.3928/01477447-20160421-04.

131. Smith EL, Banerjee SB, Bono JV. Supracondylar femur fracture after knee manipulation: a report of 3 cases. *Orthopedics.* 2009;32(1):18.

132. Djian P, Christel P, Witvoet J. Arthroscopic release for knee joint stiffness after total knee arthroplasty. *Rev Chir Orthop Reparatrice Appar Mot.* 2002;88(2):163-167.

133. Bodendorfer BM, Kotler JA, Zelenty WD, Termanini K, Sanchez R, Argintar EH. Outcomes and predictors of success for arthroscopic lysis of adhesions for the stiff total knee arthroplasty. *Orthopedics.* 2017;40(6):e1062–e1068. doi:10.3928/01477447-20171012-06.

134. Tjoumakaris FP, Tucker BC, Post Z, Pepe MD, Orozco F, Ong AC. Arthroscopic lysis of adhesions for the stiff total knee: results after failed manipulation. *Orthopedics.* 2014;37(5):e482-e487. doi:10.3928/01477447-20140430-60.

135. Scuderi GR, Kochhar T. Management of flexion contracture in total knee arthroplasty. *J Arthroplasty.* 2007;22(4 suppl 1):20-24. doi:10.1016/j.arth.2006.12.110.

136. Keeney JA, Clohisy JC, Curry M, Maloney WJ. Revision total knee arthroplasty for restricted motion. *Clin Orthop Relat Res.* 2005;440:135-140.

137. Christensen CP, Crawford JJ, Olin MD, Vail TP. Revision of the stiff total knee arthroplasty. *J Arthroplasty.* 2002;17(4):409-415.

138. Kim GK, Mortazavi SMJ, Parvizi J, Purtill JJ. Revision for stiffness following TKA: a predictable procedure? *Knee.* 2012;19(4):332-334. doi:10.1016/j.knee.2011.06.016.

139. Nicholls DW, Dorr LD. Revision surgery for stiff total knee arthroplasty. *J Arthroplasty.* 1990;5 suppl:S73-S77.

140. Fehring TK, Odum SM, Griffin WL, McCoy TH, Masonis JL. Surgical treatment of flexion contractures after total knee arthroplasty. *J Arthroplasty.* 2007;22(6 suppl 2):62-66. doi:10.1016/j.arth.2007.03.037.

141. Hug KT, Amanatullah DF, Huddleston JI III, Maloney WJ, Goodman SB. Protocol-driven revision for stiffness after total knee arthroplasty improves motion and clinical outcomes. *J Arthroplasty.* 2018;33(9):2952-2955. doi:10.1016/j.arth.2018.05.013.

142. Farid YR, Thakral R, Finn HA. Low-dose irradiation and constrained revision for severe, idiopathic, arthrofibrosis following total knee arthroplasty. *J Arthroplasty.* 2013;28(8):1314-1320. doi:10.1016/j.arth.2012.11.009.

143. Donaldson JR, Tudor F, Gollish J. Revision surgery for the stiff total knee arthroplasty. *Bone Joint J.* 2016;98-B(5):622-627. doi:10.1302/0301-620X.98B5.35969.

144. Bingham JS, Bukowski BR, Wyles CC, Pareek A, Berry DJ, Abdel MP. Rotating-hinge revision total knee arthroplasty for treatment of severe arthrofibrosis. *J Arthroplasty.* 2019;34(7S):S271-S276. doi:10.1016/j.arth.2019.01.072.

chapter 46

Managing Osteotomies and Extra-articular Deformity and Retained Hardware in Total Knee Arthroplasty

Kevin Hug, MD | Nicholas J. Giori, MD, PhD

INTRODUCTION

Total knee arthroplasty (TKA) is a successful and reproducible surgery that improves pain, function, and limb alignment in knees that have developed arthritis and deformity. Most limb deformity in osteoarthritic knees arises intra-articularly, from asymmetric wear of the joint surfaces over time. Malalignment and associated ligament imbalance are most commonly corrected in TKA with appropriate bone resection and soft-tissue balancing. However, some patients with knee arthritis have an accompanying extra-articular deformity (EAD) of the femur and/or tibia. These deformities can be due to congenital conditions, trauma, metabolic disorders, or from previous surgery.

EAD poses technical challenges to TKA that must often be addressed with supplemental corrections of limb alignment, rotation, and soft-tissue balance at the time of knee replacement. These corrections can be made at the time of TKA or can be done as a separate procedure prior to TKA. Correction of EAD can be done either with modification of intra-articular bone cuts at the time of TKA or with extra-articular osteotomies, commonly at the site of deformity. Numerous techniques have been described for addressing EAD, and the recent popularization of surgical navigation has further expanded the toolkit available to surgeons. However, each EAD is fundamentally unique and often requires custom solutions tailored to the specific deformity. This chapter aims to characterize techniques for overcoming EAD in TKA by emphasizing principles that can be tailored by the surgeon to each patient's specific deformity.

FEMORAL DEFORMITY

Developmental femoral shaft bowing in the coronal plane is the most common EAD encountered in candidates for TKA, especially in Asian and Indian populations.[1,2] Posttraumatic femoral deformities often arise after femoral shaft fractures that heal in a malunited position. Many femoral fractures, especially those that do not undergo open reduction and internal fixation, heal with varying degrees of shortening, translation, rotation, and malalignment any point along the length of the femur, with deformities of the distal femur close to the site of the TKA being particularly difficult to manage. Previous corrective osteotomies can change the bony anatomy of the femur. Like fractures, these prior osteotomies are commonly close to the knee joint and involve hardware, making them more complex to manage. Standing 36-inch radiographs of the entire limb aid in evaluating translation and angulation but provide little information on rotational deformities. CT scans and intraoperative visualization remain the best tools for assessing malrotation.

TIBIAL DEFORMITY

Tibial deformities affecting TKA can also be present at any point along the length of the leg but are most commonly found at the tibial metaphysis. These are often a result of previous tibial plateau fractures or high-tibial osteotomies (HTOs). When assessing previous HTO, it is vital to recall and understand that proximal tibial slope and translation are frequently changed as a result of the osteotomy. For this reason, intraoperative visual referencing using the tibial plateau may be inaccurate and lead to incorrect final alignment or issues with the tibial stem component contacting the metaphyseal endosteal cortex. Offset tibial stems or well-designed implants with multiple smaller pegs may be useful in this situation.

As in the femur, hardware is often present in the proximal tibia and must be addressed in sequential or simultaneous fashion. The tibial tubercle and extensor mechanism are of vital importance to the success of a TKA, and their competency must be preserved. Previous injury, surgery, or fixation may have changed the orientation or integrity of these structures. Any evidence of extensor lag on examination or patella baja/alta on preoperative imaging should be identified and incorporated into the surgical plan. Additionally, hardware removal around the tibial tubercle at the time of surgery may create bone voids that act as stress risers, increasing the fracture risk of this structure.

RETAINED HARDWARE

Retained hardware is often a complicating factor in patients with EAD. Plates, screws, staples, and nails can be present both in the periparticular region or along the femoral or tibial shafts. There is no single correct way to deal with retained hardware, as each case poses unique issues and challenges. In general, if the hardware does not impede intraoperative instrumentation or implant insertion, it can be left in place and ignored (as long as it does not compromise potential future surgical options). If hardware interferes with TKA implantation, it must be removed.[3] Acceptable options include removing hardware selectively or entirely. As a last resort, difficult-to-remove hardware can be burred or cut with appropriate metal-cutting tools.[4] The surgeon can choose to perform hardware removal in staged fashion prior to TKA or simultaneously at the time of TKA. If there is a large burden of hardware that will leave significant stress risers or if there is concern for previous infection, staged removal and culture as needed is preferred. Otherwise, single-stage TKA is performed, and hardware obstructing insertion of the prosthesis is removed as it is encountered. In single-stage TKA, bone voids from removed hardware must be anticipated and addressed with bone graft and/or supplemental fixation such as stems, augments, and cones/sleeves.[5,6]

It is important to remember that even hardware distant from the joint can interfere with TKA if it impedes access to the intramedullary canal. Full-length femoral nails and distal interlocking screws can interfere with stemmed revision femoral components and can occasionally even interfere with primary implants. Femoral arthroplasty components from different manufactures each possess their own specific geometry. In general, cruciate-retaining and sacrificing, but not substituting, femoral components do not have a femoral box and rarely interfere with previous femoral nails. Conversely, cruciate-substituting and varus–valgus–constrained implants can have larger box geometries and may interfere with a previous femoral nail, even without placing a stem. Numerous references exist to help determine the exact geometry and dimensions of most implants on the market.[7] Additionally, even short femoral nails or long-stemmed hip replacement components can affect intramedullary referencing even though their location can be quite proximal to the knee joint. If an intramedullary component at the hip is present at or distal to the femoral isthmus, using an intramedullary alignment jig may be inaccurate or impossible. In these cases, we do not recommend short intramedullary alignment rods as they do not provide accurate alignment. Extramedullary alignment jigs with intraoperative radiographic assistance, custom cutting jigs designed from preoperative three-dimensional imaging, or surgical navigation should be employed.

Lastly, an evaluation of retained hardware prior to TKA should always include attention to previous incisions and any soft-tissue defects. Previous incisions should be used when possible. Incisions can be lengthened or connected at nonacute angles as long as the flaps are sufficiently large. In general, choosing the most lateral of the previous incisions is least likely to compromise skin viability and healing. If soft-tissue redundancy allows, scars can be excised to promote more cosmetic rehealing, but tension-free approximation should not be compromised to accomplish this. Previous gastrocnemius rotational flaps or other soft-tissue abnormalities/defects should be identified, especially at the proximal-medial tibia where coverage is often the most tenuous. Plastic surgery consultation preoperatively may be helpful in determining the best plan for the surgical approach and exposure.

PREOPERATIVE PLANNING

Preoperative planning begins with a thorough history and physical examination. The surgeon should understand the cause of the EAD from the history, particularly if prior trauma was involved. The physical examination should focus on clinical alignment, skin quality, prior incisions, muscle strength, and ligamentous assessment. A long-lasting deformity can result in excessive ligament stress and stretching that may not be evident on imaging. Deformity can also result in secondary patellar maltracking.

Preoperative imaging is critical in cases of deformity. A full-length hip-to-ankle standing radiograph is of vital importance in planning for a case with EAD (**Fig. 46-1**). The radiograph should be evaluated both for EAD, as well as intra-articular deformities such as asymmetric bone loss at the joint line, commonly seen in advanced osteoarthritis. Both types of deformities must be accounted for in planning for correction of alignment. Lateral X-rays should be viewed for deformities in the sagittal plane, and patellar integrity should be evaluated with a Merchant view of the knee. Supplemental advanced imaging such as a CT scan can be helpful for evaluating bone loss in three dimensions and is also sometimes required for various types of surgical navigation or patient-specific instrumentation.[8]

With previous surgeries and retained hardware, an index of suspicion for infection is warranted, and screening laboratory tests with possible aspiration prior to definitive surgery should be considered.

The spectrum of EAD and retained hardware often requires careful planning for specific instruments required during that case. When considering retained hardware, consider having broken hardware-removal trays, implant-specific (or universal) extraction devises, metal cutting burrs, and intraoperative fluoroscopy available. When considering EAD, consider having revision-constrained instrumentation with augments/cones/stems, extra-articular navigation, computer navigation, patient-specific instrumentation, saws, angle-measuring guides, plates, screws, nails, and custom implants available.[9-11]

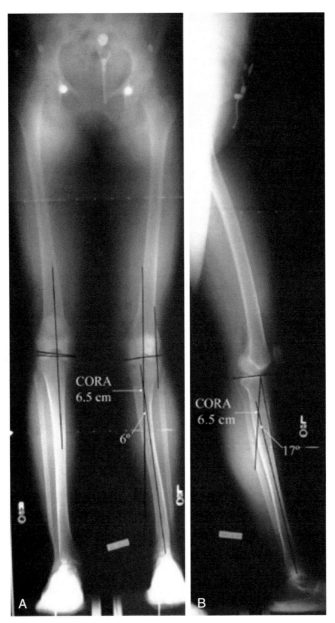

FIGURE 46-1 A 28-year-old woman presented with complaints of her leg "going out" and her knee hyperextending. **A:** A 51-inch AP alignment radiograph reveals a 6-degree apex medial deformity with the CORA 6.5 cm distal to the proximal tibial joint orientation line and **B:** the lateral alignment radiograph shows a 17-degree apex posterior angulation with a CORA 6.5 cm distal to the proximal tibial joint orientation line. This patient has an oblique plane angular deformity without translation. (From Tornetta P. *Rockwood and Greens Fractures in Adults.* Philadelphia: Wolters Kluwer; 2020.)

SURGICAL TECHNIQUE, INTRA-ARTICULAR CORRECTION

Preoperatively, a hip-to-ankle radiograph is evaluated to plan deformity correction. A line is drawn along the mechanical axis of the femur, from the center of the femoral head to the center of the knee. Another line is drawn perpendicular to this mechanical axis line at the distal femur, demonstrating the proposed distal femoral resection in the coronal plane. If this resection line violates the origin of either the medial collateral ligament or lateral collateral ligament, a corrective extra-articular osteotomy is recommended. In general, femoral deformities <20° in the coronal plane can be corrected intra-articularly without the need for a supplemental osteotomy.[12,13]

Similarly, tibial deformity is also assessed with a hip-to-ankle radiograph. A line is drawn along the shaft of the tibia, starting from the center of the ankle and moving proximally. If the line exits the tibia below the articular surface, a supplemental extra-articular osteotomy is recommended. Another line is drawn perpendicular to this mechanical axis line at the proximal

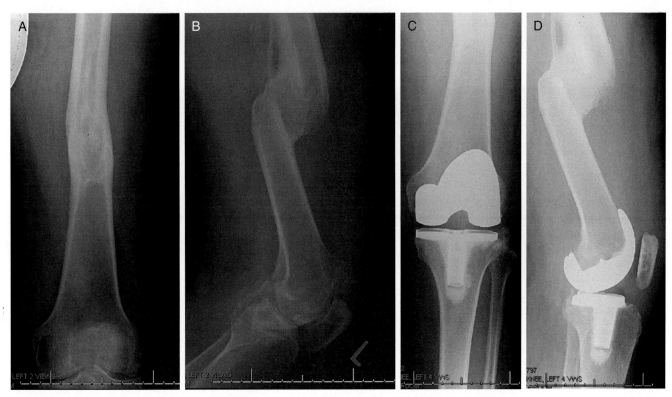

FIGURE 46-2   A and **B:** show the leg of a 57-year-old man who sustained a femur fracture 40 years prior, treated with bed rest in traction, now with end-stage knee arthritis. Despite his significant deformity at the femoral mid-shaft, he met criteria for TKA with intra-articular correction. As a femoral intramedullary alignment guide would be unreliable, this case was performed with surgical navigation (**C** and **D**).

tibia, demonstrating the bone resection in the coronal plane. In general, tibial deformities <30° in the coronal plane can be corrected with an intra-articular osteotomy alone.[12,14]

If the femoral deformity or previous implanted hardware is distal to the isthmus of the femoral shaft, a shorter guide rod can be used if intramedullary alignment is attempted, but one must be aware that short guide rods are not accurate and intraoperative X-ray is recommended for confirmation. Alternately extramedullary alignment, surgical navigation, or patient-specific instrumentation can be used (**Fig. 46-2**). Significant soft-tissue deformities often accompany long-standing EAD and must be addressed during TKA. Conservative bone cuts and standard stepwise soft-tissue releases are employed with evaluation of the flexion and extension gaps, including medial tibial reduction osteotomies or femoral condylar sliding osteotomies in rare cases.[15] If soft tissues are insufficient, additional prosthetic constraint can be used to obtain sufficient stability of the knee (**Fig. 46-3**). With greater constraint, stems are required to augment prosthetic fixation to the associated bone. In some cases, offset couplers between the stems and articular hardware for either the femoral or tibial components can help to centralize the prosthesis at the joint line in complex deformity cases.

SURGICAL TECHNIQUE, EXTRA-ARTICULAR CORRECTION

When a limb deformity does not meet criteria for intra-articular correction, additional osteotomies away from the knee joint must be performed in addition to TKA.[16,17]

The correction osteotomy can either be performed in simultaneous or staged fashion with the TKA, depending on the specifics of the osteotomy and fixation strategies employed. Osteotomies that utilize fixation requiring limited weight-bearing postoperatively or those that require separate surgical approaches from a TKA are more likely to benefit from a staged correction (**Fig. 46-4**). Conversely, osteotomies that can withstand immediate full weight-bearing and those that can be performed through the same incision as TKA are more appealing candidates for single-stage correction.[18,19]

Numerous strategies and technique guides exist for performing lower extremity osteotomies. Each case is unique, requiring somewhat customized fixation constructs depending on the specific goals of surgery. The ideal location for deformity correction is directly at the site of the deformity itself, known as the CORA (center of rotation and angulation). However, various anatomic and post-surgical factors can sometimes make this impossible. The surgeon should understand that deformity correction distant from the CORA introduces secondary deformities that

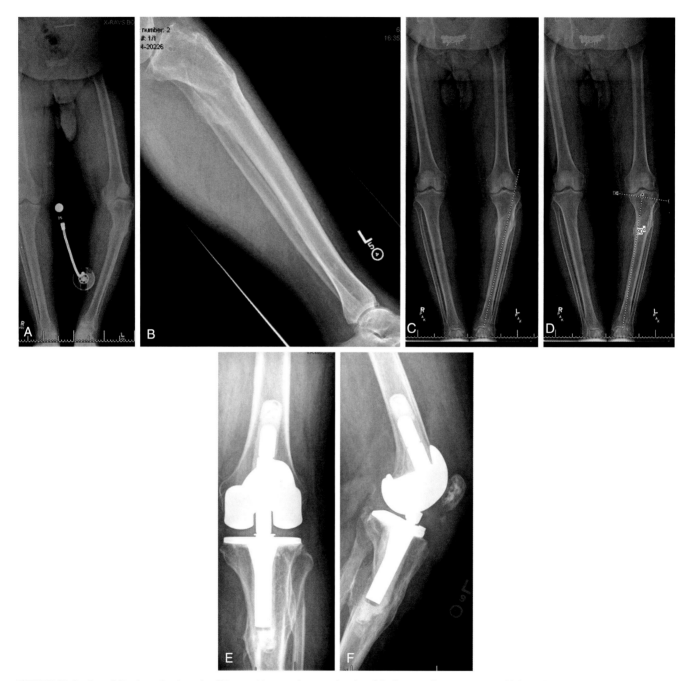

FIGURE 46-3   A and **B:** show the leg of a 65-year-old man who sustained a tibia fracture from a motor vehicle collision decades prior. He was treated nonoperatively, and the fracture healed in varus and flexion. He went on to develop end-stage knee arthritis. **C:** shows a line drawn from the center of the ankle mortise up the shaft of the distal part of the tibia below the deformity. One can see that the extension of this line passes within the breadth of the tibial plateau. He thus met criteria for an intra-articular correction. **D:** shows the planned resection, which is perpendicular to the mechanical axis of the tibia. The patient required a complete release of medial structures including the medial collateral ligament (MCL), medial gastrocnemius, medial posterior capsule, medial hamstrings, and pes anserinus in order to have enough medial gap to place a prosthesis. Due to the extensive release required, a rotating hinge knee prosthesis was implanted with successful result **(E** and **F).**

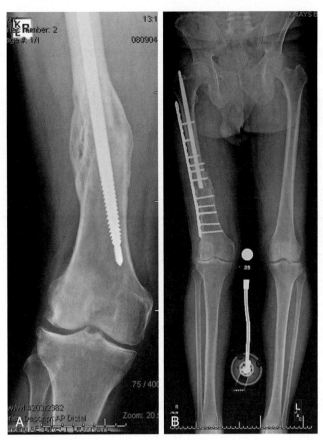

FIGURE 46-4   A: shows a 60-year-old male who sustained a femoral shaft fracture 30 years prior, treated with an early version of a femoral intramed-ullary nail that is extremely difficult to remove. He healed with a significant valgus deformity in the coronal plane through his fracture. The CORA was exposed, and an osteotomy perpendicular to the proximal shaft was performed. This exposed the nail, allowing for it to be transected with a metal cut-ting burr. The distal segment of the nail was removed with trephines, as it could interfere with subsequent TKA. The proximal portion of the nail was left in place to avoid the trauma associated with nail removal. The distal osteotomy was performed in identical fashion, and a lateral plate was implanted. After successful healing of this staged procedure, he is now able to undergo a TKA with an intra-articular correction, utilizing standard implants **(B)**.

must be accounted for.[20] Deformities can also be uniplanar or multiplanar, and correction strategies must address the deformity in all planes.[21] Techniques including opening- and closing-wedge osteotomies, dome osteotomies, and Ilizarov/thin wire spatial frames have all been described for complex deformity correction in the lower extremity.[22-24]

The goal of every extra-articular osteotomy is to restore the mechanical axis of the limb to as close to normal as possible, thus allowing for any supplemental intra-articular correction to take place at the time of TKA, as detailed above. In metaphyseal regions, opening and clos-ing techniques with plate fixation are usually preferred. These often require careful angular measurements and cor-rection. In diaphyseal areas, intramedullary nails can be very useful for recreating normal anatomy and osteotomies can be made at the CORA. Any surgical osteotomy plan prior to TKA must include provisions for how the inserted osteotomy hardware will affect TKA component insertion, and individualized solutions are often required. **Fig. 46-5** demonstrates a clinical example of this technique.

CONCLUSION

EAD and retained hardware present unique challenges to performing a successful TKA. Many deformities can be corrected with intra-articular techniques utilizing bone cuts and soft-tissue releases at the time of TKA, while other deformities require supplemental osteotomies in simultaneous or staged fashion. Similarly, retained hardware can either be partially removed during TKA as it is encountered or more formally removed in a staged procedure prior to TKA. The surgeon must also consider alternative referencing techniques including extramedullary referencing, computer navigation, or patient-specific instrumentation, as well as alternative TKA implants including offset couplers, stemless com-ponents, or increased constraint on a case-by-case basis. As long as the mechanical axis of the limb is recreated, patients with even the most complex deformities can achieve long-term satisfactory results after TKA and alignment correction.

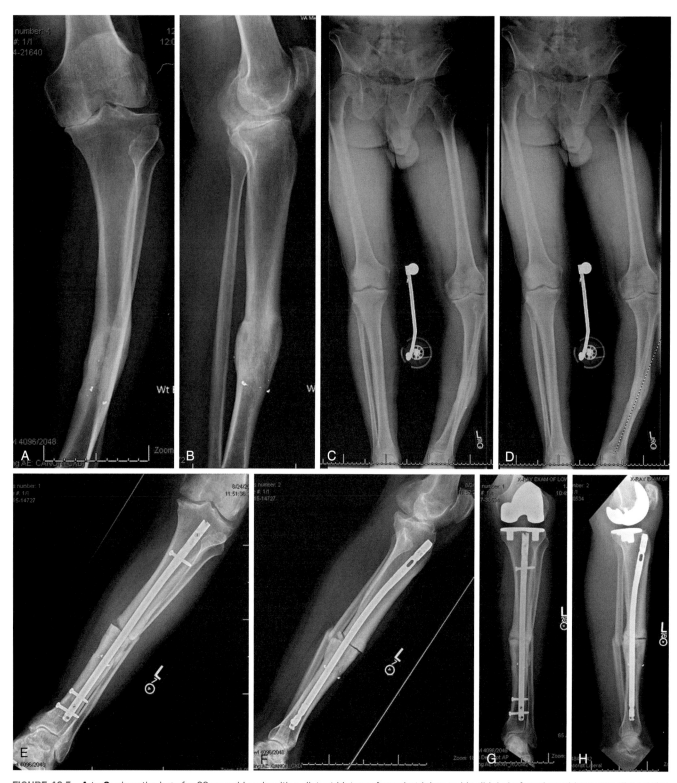

FIGURE 46-5 **A** to **C:** show the leg of a 69-year-old male with a distant history of gunshot injury to his tibial shaft and resulting varus tibial deformity, now with end-stage knee arthritis. **D:** shows that a line drawn through the long axis of his tibial shaft does not exit through his articular margin, so a staged, extra-articular osteotomy was planned. The CORA was exposed, and osteotomy cuts were made perpendicular to the long axis of each shaft segment. The fibula was also osteotomized. A standard tibial nail was inserted (**E** and **F**). In staged fashion, he then underwent a TKA utilizing a press-fit stemless tibial baseplate to accommodate the tibial nail (**G** and **H**).

REFERENCES

1. Mullaji AB, Marawar SV, Mittal V. A comparison of coronal plane axial femoral relationships in Asian patients with varus osteoarthritic knees and healthy knees. *J Arthroplasty.* 2009;24(6):861-867.
2. Lasam MP, Lee KJ, Chang CB, Kang YG, Kim TK. Femoral lateral bowing and varus condylar orientation are prevalent and affect axial alignment of TKA in Koreans. *Clin Orthop Relat Res.* 2013;471(5):1472-1483.
3. Morsi E, Habib ME, Hadhoud M. Comparison between results of high tibial osteotomy above and below tibial tubercle in relation to future total knee arthroplasty. *J Arthroplasty.* 2014;29:2087-2090.
4. Georgiadis GM, Skakun WC. Total knee arthroplasty with retained tibial implants: the role of minimally invasive hardware removal. *Am J Orthop.* 2016;45(7):E481-E486.
5. Yoshino N, Takai S, Watanabe Y, Nakamura S, Kubo T. Total knee arthroplasty with long stem for treatment of nonunion after high tibial osteotomy. *J Arthroplasty.* 2004;19(4):528-531.
6. Niinimaki T, Eskelinen A, Ohtonen P, Puhto AP, Mann BS, Leppilahti J. Total knee arthroplasty after high tibial osteotomy: a registry-based case-control study of 1,036 knees. *Arch Orthop Trauma Surg.* 2014;134:73-77.
7. Thompson SM, Lindisfarne EA, Bradley N, Solan M. Periprosthetic supracondylar femoral fractures above a total knee replacement: compatibility guide for fixation with a retrograde intramedullary nail. *J Arthroplasty.* 2014;29(8):1639-1641.
8. Paley D, Tetsworth K. Mechanical axis deviation of the lower limbs. *Clin Orthop Relat Res.* 1992;280:48-64.
9. Bottros J, Klika AK, Lee HH, Polousky J, Barsoum WK. The use of navigation in total knee arthroplasty for patients with extra-articular deformity. *J Arthroplasty.* 2008;23(1):74-78.
10. Hazratwala K, Matthews B, Wilkinson M, Barroso-Rosa S. Total knee arthroplasty in patients with extra-articular deformity. *Arthroplasty Today.* 2016;2(1):26-36.
11. Mullaji A, Shetty GM. Computer-assisted total knee arthroplasty for arthritis with extra-articular deformity. *J Arthroplasty.* 2009;24(8):1164-1169.
12. Wang JW, Wang CJ. Total knee arthroplasty for arthritis of the knee with extra-articular deformity. *J Arthoplasty.* 2002;84(10):1769-1774.
13. Wang JW, Chen WS, Lin PC, Hsu CS, Wang CJ. Total knee replacement with intra-articular resection of bone after malunion of a femoral fracture: can sagittal angulation be corrected? *J Bone Joint Surg Br.* 2010;92-B:1392-1396.
14. Xiao-Gang Z, Shahzad K, Li C. One-stage total knee arthroplasty for patients with osteoarthritis of the knee and extra-articular deformity. *Int Orthop.* 2012;36:2457-2463.
15. Paredes-Carnero X, Escobar J, Galdo JM, Babé JG. Total knee arthroplasty for treatment of osteoarthritis associated with extra-articular deformity. *J Clin Orthop Trauma.* 2018;9(2):125-132.
16. Wolff AM, Hungerford DS, Pepe CL. The effect of extraarticular varus and valgus deformity on total knee arthroplasty. *Clin Orthop Relat Res.* 1991;271:135-151.
17. Hungerford DS. Extra-articular deformity is always correctable intra-articularly: to the contrary. *Orthopedics.* 2009;32:677.
18. Lonner JH, Siliski JM, Lotke PA. Simultaneous femoral osteotomy and total knee arthroplasty for treatment of osteoarthritis associated with severe extra-articular deformity. *J Bone Joint Surg Am.* 2000;82:342-348.
19. Radke S, Radke J. Total knee arthroplasty in combination with a one-stage tibial osteotomy: a technique for correction of a gonarthrosis with a severe (>15 degrees) tibial extra-articular deformity. *J Arthroplasty.* 2002;17(5):533-537.
20. Paley D. *Principles of Deformity Correction.* New York: Springer; 2002.
21. Wagner R, Luedke C. Total knee arthroplasty with concurrent femoral and tibial osteotomies in osteogenesis imperfecta. *Am J Orthop.* 2014;43(1):37-42.
22. Dabis J, Templeton-Ward O, Lacey AE, Narayan B, Trompeter A. The history, evolution, and basic science of osteotomy techniques. *Strategies Trauma Limb Reconstr.* 2017;12(3):169-180.
23. Fletcher MD. Single stage tibial osteotomy and long stem total knee arthroplasty to correct adverse consequences of unequal tibial lengthening with an Ilizarov circular fixator. *J Orthop Case Rep.* 2015;5(3):9-11.
24. Meehan JP, Khadder MA, Jamali AA, Trauner KB. Closing wedge retrotubercular tibial osteotomy and TKA for posttraumatic osteoarthritis with angular deformity. *Orthopedics.* 2009;32(5):360.

chapter 47

Total Knee Replacement in Special Situations

Tyler J. Vovos, MD | Paul F. Lachiewicz, MD

INTRODUCTION

The vast majority of total knee arthroplasties (TKA) are performed for primary osteoarthritis, but there are numerous rheumatologic, hematologic, metabolic, and neurologic disorders that may contribute to knee dysfunction. In these "special situations," the surgeon and supportive consultants should be cognizant of unique features that may influence clinical decision making and treatment. Preoperative optimization, postoperative care, technical aspects of the procedure, and component design should be considered. This chapter reviews several of the less common conditions with which the arthroplasty surgeon should be familiar.

PAGET DISEASE OF BONE

Paget disease of bone is a chronic disorder of unknown etiology characterized by increased bone resorption, bone formation, and remodeling.[1] In the United States, the prevalence ranges from 1.5% to 3% in people older than 60 years and it is more common in men.[1,2] Osteoclasts mediate the early stage of the disease, which is characterized by excessive bone resorption and marked elevation of serum alkaline phosphatase.[3] This is followed by a mixed phase of both osteoclastic and osteoblastic activity, during which there is increased deposition of abnormal bone. Finally, a chronic sclerotic phase occurs, during which bone formation predominates, leading to osseous enlargement, trabecular thickening, sclerosis, and replacement of bone marrow with vascular and fibrous tissue.

The diagnosis of Paget disease of bone, which may be associated with localized bone pain or may be incidental, is confirmed by radiographs or laboratory studies.[1] Monoostotic and polyostotic variants exist, and the pelvis, lumbosacral spine, proximal or distal femur, and tibial plateau or diaphysis are most commonly affected.[1] When symptomatic, constant poorly localized bone pain at rest is typical.[1] Patients may also present with deformity, pathologic stress fractures, secondary arthropathy in adjacent joints, skin temperature changes, or compressive neurologic complications in the spine or skull.[1] Involvement of the hip is more common than the knee, but 10% to 12% of patients with Paget disease of bone in the knee area develop symptomatic arthritis.[4] Radiographs parallel histologic changes and may show diffuse osteopenia, or more frequently a mixed or sclerotic picture (**Fig. 47-1**).[1] A bone scan, if obtained, shows increased isotope uptake in involved bone and may be used as a screening tool during evaluation of patients. However, a bone scan may be "cold" during early osteolytic stages of the disease.[1,5] Medical treatment of bone pain may include bisphosphonates or calcitonin to relieve symptoms and prevent potential complications and may be helpful in differentiating arthritic joint pain from pain due to the underlying disorder.[1,6]

Total knee arthroplasty may be indicated and helpful for patients with Paget disease of bone and debilitating gonarthrosis.[4,7,8] Most patients are in the sclerotic or relatively inactive phase of disease when presenting for arthroplasty.[1] An evaluation to exclude high-output cardiac failure should be considered, especially in patients with polyostotic disease. Two studies have reported no difference in perioperative blood loss between those patients who received preoperative bisphosphonate therapy and those who did not.[4,8] Varus and anterior bowing of an enlarged distal femur are common radiographic findings (**Fig. 47-2**), and full-length hip–knee–ankle radiographs in both planes may assist in preoperative planning.[1,4] An intramedullary femoral instrument may result in a flexed or varus alignment of the distal femur resection and should be used in conjunction with preoperative planning and/or extramedullary cutting guides.[4,8] When anterior tibial bowing is present, the proximal tibial resection performed with the standard extramedullary tibial guide may result in excessive anterior bone resection or compromise of the extensor mechanism.[1] When there is a severe extra-articular deformity, the choices include correcting the deformity inside the knee joint by asymmetric bone resections (often requiring a varus–valgus constrained component) or an extra-articular osteotomy prior to or in conjunction with total knee arthroplasty. Metaphyseal or diaphyseal osteotomies have been performed and usually are fixed with intramedullary rod or plate fixation.[9,10] Medial bone loss and cysts in the proximal tibia can result in a fixed varus deformity. Arthroplasty of the knee with Paget disease of bone is usually performed with posterior-stabilized or constrained condylar components, depending on bone quality and depth of bone resection, and the ligament releases required (**Fig. 47-3**).[1,4,11] Pathologic

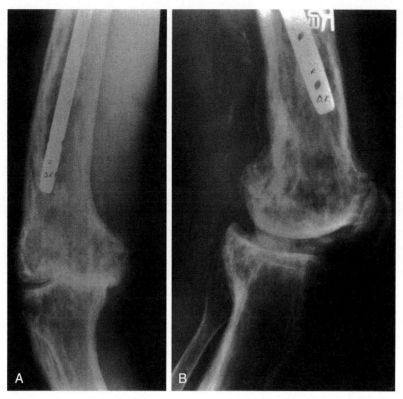

FIGURE 47-1 **A** and **B:** Preoperative radiographs of a patient with Paget disease about the knee.

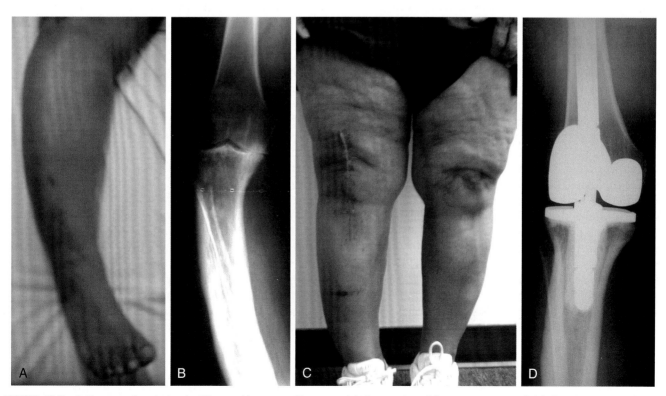

FIGURE 47-2 **A:** Preop supine photo of a 58-year-old woman with severe right knee pain and limp, severe varus of right leg, due to anterolateral bowing of tibia; **B:** preoperative standing AP radiograph shows loss of medial joint space and Paget disease of the tibia only; **C:** 2-year postoperative standing photo; **D:** 2-year postoperative standing AP radiograph, showing CCK prosthesis used, as well as deformity of limb corrected through knee joint.

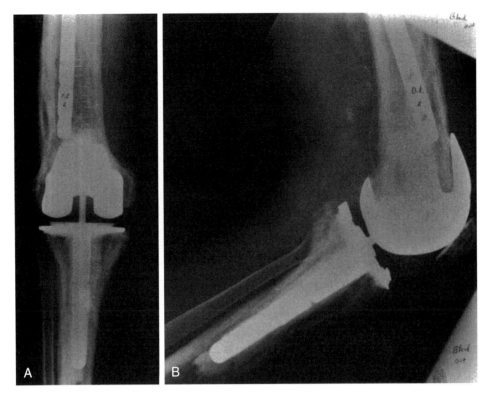

FIGURE 47-3 **A** and **B:** Postoperative radiographs after total knee arthroplasty in a patient with Paget disease.

fractures through pagetic bone are not uncommon, and the senior author recommends cement fixation of all components and use of variable length stem extensions.[4]

Lee et al.[8] reported the results of 20 consecutive primary knees in patients with Paget disease of the bone. The mean Knee Society scores for pain improved from 41 to 97 points, and function score from 36 to 67 points postoperatively. A mismatch between the size of the femoral and tibial components was noted in 15 of 21 knees (71%), with the bone affected by Paget disease requiring the larger size component. Difficulty with exposure of the knee was common and partial detachment of the patellar tendon was required in three of four knees in which the patella could not be everted. Ligament balancing was difficult in three knees, with one requiring proximal release and reattachment of the medial collateral ligament, one had complete distal release of the medial collateral ligament, and one had a lateral ligament "reefing" to achieve balance. For these difficult arthritic knees with Paget disease of bone, the senior author prefers an elongated quadriceps tendon incision (or "quad snip" procedure) for exposure, and the use of constrained condylar components rather than collateral ligament release and reattachment or reefing.

POLIOMYELITIS

Although the prevalence of poliomyelitis has decreased due to vaccination programs, there may occasionally be patients with the neuromuscular sequelae and severe symptomatic knee arthritis and instability. Total knee arthroplasty in these patients is technically difficult due to the combination of deformity, lower extremity weakness, and frequent multiaxial ligament instability. A recurvatum deformity may be present, as well as external rotation deformity of the tibia, excessive valgus deformity, and hindfoot abnormalities.[12] As a result of profound quadriceps weakness, patients may develop a dependence on locking the knee in hyperextension for stability.[12] This propensity to "back-knee" in the stance phase of gait alters joint mechanics, likely increasing osteoarthritic changes and progressive recurvatum.[12] Although the use of a full extremity drop-lock, hinged knee–ankle–foot brace may provide symptomatic relief, this orthosis is usually not well tolerated for prolonged use and ambulation.

If total knee arthroplasty is performed, recurvatum may be corrected by underresection of the distal femur or distal augmentation of the femoral component.[12,13] This technique reduces the knee extension gap to take advantage of the cam effect of the collateral ligaments and the geometry of the femoral component. As this procedure may generate 5 to 10 degrees of flexion contracture, "buckling" or instability of the knee may occur, as patients lose the ability to stabilize their knee through hyperextension. Patients considering total knee arthroplasty should be counseled that a brace may still be required postoperatively to permit ambulation. Another option would be to perform the arthroplasty leaving the knee with 5 to 10 degrees of recurvatum, but this may increase the risk of component loosening and instability.[14]

Cemented posterior-stabilized or constrained condylar components with stem extensions can provide stability, can decrease the risk of early component loosening, and are recommended.[12,15-17] Rarely, an extra-articular deformity may be so severe that intra-articular bone resection and soft-tissue releases may result in excessive bone loss and ligament instability. Extra-articular osteotomies have been reported for these situations[18]; however, it may be preferable to implant a rotating-hinge prosthesis with custom recurvatum cutting guides.[16,19]

Several studies report, that with careful preoperative planning and component selection, good outcomes of total knee arthroplasty in patients with poliomyelitis. Gan et al.[15] reported 16 arthroplasties performed in patients with polio-affected knees with a minimum 18 months follow-up. There were eight posterior-stabilized, six cruciate-retaining, and two constrained condylar components. Modest improvements in Knee Society scores, Oxford Knee scores, and SF-36 scores were reported, with a low rate of complications. Only one patient with aseptic loosening and acquired hyperextension deformity required revision. Tigani et al.[16] reported the results of 10 patients using one posterior-stabilized, two constrained condylar, and seven rotating-hinge components. Knee Society scores improved in all patients. One patient had revision for infection, and one patient, with a constrained condylar component, had a recurrent recurvatum deformity. A rotating-hinge prosthesis was recommended for these patients to permit hyperextension and compensate for loss of quadriceps strength. Jordan et al.[17] reported the results of 17 primary knees in poliomyelitis patients between 1991 and 2001. The components implanted were eight posterior-stabilized, eight constrained condylar, and one rotating-hinge component. The Knee Society scores improved from 45 to 87 points, and stability was satisfactory in all patients, including four with severe quadriceps weakness. The postoperative complications included one patient with deep vein thrombosis and two knees had a manipulation for stiffness.

PARKINSON DISEASE

Parkinson disease affects approximately 4 million people worldwide and is the second most common neurodegenerative disorder following Alzheimer disease.[20] In this disorder, the basal ganglia (substantia nigra) undergo progressive degeneration. Patients lose motor coordination, have muscle tremors, and may have varying degrees of mental impairment. Medical treatment includes dopamine and dopaminergic agonists.

Patients with Parkinson disease who are considered for total knee arthroplasty should have some capacity for ambulation preoperatively and mental capacity to follow postoperative instructions. Relative contraindications include preoperative delirium, inability to undergo regional anesthesia, absence of a multidisciplinary team

(neurologist, pain specialist, and physiatrist), a Hoehn and Yahr rating $\geq$ 3, a knee flexion contracture > 25 degrees, and lack of response to preoperative bupivacaine injection.[21] Preoperative optimization and physical therapy for these patients is problematic due to the musculoskeletal rigidity, tremor, contracture, and gait instability.[21] A multidisciplinary approach, with perioperative neurologic consultation, is helpful to decrease length of hospital stay, improve Unified Parkinson's Disease Rating Scale scores, and improve Knee Society Pain and Function scores.[22] These patients are particularly susceptible to postoperative knee flexion contractures, which may be treated with injections of botulinum toxin type A into the hamstring and gastrocnemius muscles, with static progressive extension bracing and rigorous physical therapy.[23] Intraoperatively, these patients may often require the use of constrained condylar or rotating-hinge prostheses for stability, and a postoperative femoral nerve block should be avoided as this may contribute to a flexion contracture.[21]

Several studies have reported that patients with Parkinson disease have improvements in short-term function and pain after total knee arthroplasty comparable to that in the general population.[24-26] Wong et al.[24] compared outcomes of 43 knees in patients with Parkinson disease to age- and gender-matched controls and reported no difference in range of motion (change from baseline), Oxford Knee Scores, or complications at 1 year follow-up. Tinning et al.[25] compared outcomes of 32 knees in patients with Parkinson disease to age-matched controls and reported no difference in 1 year Knee Society scores, pain, or range of motion between the groups. However, there was a significant decrease in Knee Society Function scores at 5 years in the affected patients. Rondon et al.[26] reported a higher rate of revision of knees in patients with Parkinson disease, compared to control patients, in 52 total hip arthroplasties and 71 total knee arthroplasties, with 23.6% requiring revision at average follow-up of 5.3 years. There was an increased rate of infection in patients with Parkinson disease. There is progressive decline in ambulation and overall function in patients with Parkinson disease, and patients and families should be counseled preoperatively. Ashraf et al.[27] reported that patients with Parkinson disease have similar knee function up to 3 years postoperatively, but functional outcomes deteriorate with longer follow-up times.

NEUROPATHIC ARTHRITIS

Neuropathic arthritis, or Charcot arthropathy of the knee, is characterized by joint degeneration associated with a loss of sensation or impaired proprioception in the affected limb. The modern associated disorders are severe diabetes mellitus and congenital indifference to pain, with tertiary syphilis and chronic cervical disk herniation now less common.[28-30] The Eichenholz classification describes the clinical and radiographic progression of the Charcot joint from the acute phase (dissolution), through the healing phase (coalescence), to the resolution phase.[30] Clinically, the knee joint has effusion and instability with relatively little pain considering the degree of destruction. However, approximately half of patients with neuropathic joints have moderate to severe pain with weight-bearing. The differential diagnosis includes low-grade septic arthritis, chronic crystalline arthritis, or pauci-articular rheumatoid arthritis. Radiographic joint destruction may be excessive, and progressive angular deformity is common (**Fig. 47-4**).[28] Nonoperative treatment with a long-leg brace and bisphosphonate therapy has been attempted.[30]

Historically, neuropathic arthritis of the knee was considered an absolute contraindication for any knee arthroplasty. Knee arthrodesis, once recommended, has generally been abandoned due to poor clinical results.[31] Over the last decade, total knee arthroplasty has been reconsidered for the neuropathic knee in the coalescence or resolution phases. Preoperatively, a complete medical and neurologic evaluation is recommended, to determine a possible treatable cause of the neuropathic knee, including testing for syphilis, diabetes mellitus, and anemias associated with vitamin B12 or thiamine deficiency. Despite extensive testing, the etiology of many cases remains unknown. There are numerous difficulties in performing total knee arthroplasty in this disorder, including fixed deformity, bone loss, poor bone quality, and collateral ligament insufficiency. Bone loss in the proximal tibia may be severe and require a metal augment, long stems, bone grafting, or highly porous cone for reconstruction (**Fig. 47-5**).[32-34] A posterior-stabilized component may be attempted, but a constrained condylar or rotating-hinge prosthesis is usually necessary for stability.[32-35] A higher risk of periprosthetic fracture has also been reported.[34]

A relatively high rate of complications has been reported after total knee arthroplasty in patients with neuropathic arthropathy. Parvizi et al.[32] reported the techniques and outcomes of 40 knees at a mean of 7.9 years clinical follow-up and 6.4 years radiographic follow-up. Thirty-eight of 40 knees had bone deficiency treated by an augment in 10, autograft in 17, and allograft in 2 knees. A long stem was used in 27 knees and a rotating hinge in 5 knees. There were six reoperations for periprosthetic fracture, aseptic loosening, instability, and deep infection. Bae et al.[35] reported the results of 11 rotating-hinge knees at a mean of 12 years follow-up. The mean knee score increased from 45 to 95 points and mean function score increased from 45 to 94 points, and there were three major complications (two dislocations and one infection).[35] Tibbo et al.[34] reported the outcomes of 37 knees, predominantly with constrained condylar or rotating-hinge components, and 7 with a metaphyseal cone for bone loss. At 10 years, 88% of patients were free of aseptic revision and 70% were free of any revision.

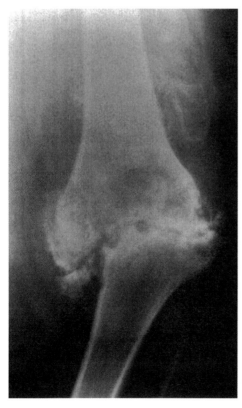

FIGURE 47-4   Preoperative bone deficiency in a patient with Charcot arthropathy.

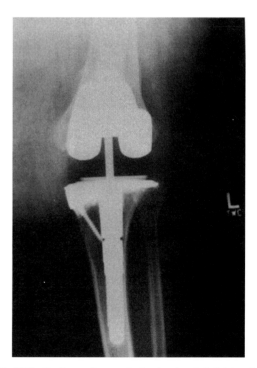

FIGURE 47-5   Postoperative radiograph showing joint alignment restoration with wedges and bone cement in a patient with Charcot arthropathy.

Six (16%) revisions were performed: four for infection, one for tibial component loosening, and one for global instability. Three patients had an intraoperative fracture.

HEMOPHILIA

Hemophilia is a disorder of blood coagulation caused by inherited x-linked recessive clotting factor deficiencies.[36] The most common forms of hemophilia are classic hemophilia or hemophilia A, with factor VIII deficiency, and Christmas disease or hemophilia B, with factor IX deficiency.[36] Recurrent hemarthrosis most commonly affects the knee and there is an immune-mediated arthritis due to chronic exposure of the synovium and articular cartilage to metabolites of blood.[36] Chronic synovitis leads to further intra-articular bleeding and high-grade chondral loss, subchondral bone destruction, and joint contractures (**Fig. 47-6**).[36] Radiographs typically show squaring of the patella (Jordan sign), widening of the intercondylar notch, and enlarged femoral condyles, which result in femoral–tibial mismatch.[36] Initial management of hemarthrosis includes intravenous clotting factor replacement therapy, and occasionally aspiration and splinting.[36,37] Synovectomy, either open, arthroscopic or with radioactive isotopes, may slow the progression of synovitis to joint destruction.[37,38]

For symptomatic end-stage arthritis, total knee arthroplasty can provide relief of pain and improvement in function. The preoperative assessment should be multidisciplinary and include measurement of Factor VIII and inhibitor levels. Preoperative transfusion should result in factor levels of 100% of normal. Each unit of factor infused per kilogram of body weight should result in a 2% increase in factor levels.[39] Patients with inhibitors are resistant to conventional therapy, and special techniques that overwhelm the inhibitor with high doses of factor may allow surgery to be performed safely. Historically, the prevalence of human immunodeficiency virus 1 (HIV-1) infection has ranged from 33% to 92% in patients with hemophilia A, and from 14% to 52% in patients with hemophilia B.[40] However, these rates have decreased with modern HIV awareness and treatment.[40] Screening for HIV is recommended in these patients, and antiretroviral therapy may mitigate the previously high risk of prosthetic joint infection.[41,42] Perioperatively, surgical drains are not recommended as these result in greater blood loss and do not alter the rate of wound complications, length of stay, or functional outcomes.[43] A multimodal blood loss prevention protocol including use of tranexamic acid can decrease perioperative blood loss, need for transfusions, and costs of factor VIII administration.[44]

Total knee arthroplasty in this disorder is very difficult, due to joint soft-tissue fibrosis, severe deformity, poor bone quality, and altered bony anatomy (**Fig. 47-7**). Exposure may require an extended quadriceps tendon incision or quadriceps snip procedure.[45,46] The senior author has never had to perform a quadriceps tendon turndown or tibial tubercle osteotomy. A flexion contracture associated with valgus and external rotation deformities are most commonly seen. Posterior-stabilized components, with additional stems or metal augments, are frequently used.[47] Computer navigation was reported in one study to help restore the mechanical axis with improved accuracy of component orientation in patients with hemophilic arthropathy.[48] Robotic-assisted total knee arthroplasty has also been reported in this disorder.[49] Cement fixation of all components is generally performed (**Fig. 47-8**).[50,51]

There are numerous reports of good functional outcomes of total knee arthroplasty in patients with hemophilic arthropathy.[45] Goddard et al.[52] reviewed 60 knees at 9.2 years mean follow-up, and 57 (95%) had a good or excellent result. With infection and aseptic loosening as endpoints, the survival at 20 years was reported as 94%.

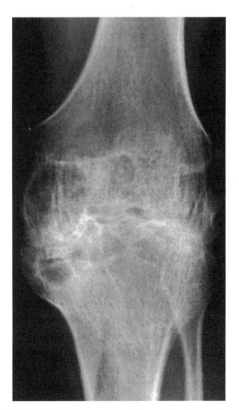

FIGURE 47-7 Hemophilic arthropathy. Note cysts.

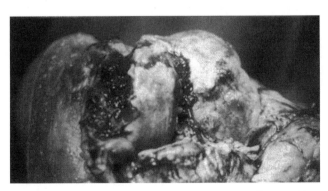

FIGURE 47-6 Distal femur in a patient with hemophilic synovitis.

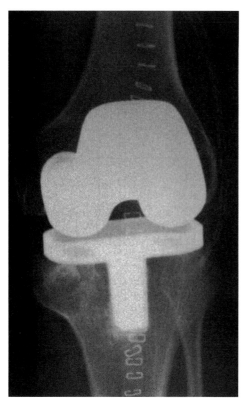

FIGURE 47-8 Postoperative radiograph showing bone graft in cysts in a patient with hemophilic arthropathy.

Although patients with severe preoperative knee flexion contractures may have improvement in motion and function after knee arthroplasty,[46] the amount of preoperative flexion contracture may predict postoperative residual flexion contracture.[53] One study[53] reported that a preoperative flexion contracture threshold of 27.5 degrees predicted a flexion contracture of more than 15 degrees at final follow-up. Some studies have reported a high rate of postoperative complications in hemophilic patients having knee arthroplasty. In a meta-analysis study of 336 knees, Moore et al.[54] reported a complication rate of 31.5%, most commonly bleeding (9%) and infection (7%). The rate of revision was 6.3%. Recurrent hemarthrosis is an infrequent late complication of knee arthroplasty, occurring in approximately 1.6% of patients. This has been previously treated by open or arthroscopic synovectomy, but embolization has been reported to be safe and effective in these patients.[55]

DIABETES MELLITUS

Diabetes mellitus is a systemic disorder affecting 2% to 4% of the population in the United States.[56] The rate of total knee arthroplasty is reported to be over twice as high in diabetic patients as in the general population.[57] Although diabetes may affect almost any organ system, the effect on the vascular system, especially small vessels, is of greatest concern with regard to wound healing, the risk of infection, and the patient's ability to tolerate the

stress of surgery. The extent of impairment correlates with both the duration of disease and adequacy of control of blood glucose level. The preoperative evaluation of cardiac and renal function is important, as cardiac ischemia and impaired renal function may be present without symptoms.

Patients with diabetes mellitus have been reported to have worse functional outcome and less improvement in range of motion than patients without diabetes.[58,59] High rates of postoperative complications are reported in diabetic patients after knee arthroplasty, and even greater with poorly controlled diabetes.[60,61] These complications include pneumonia, stroke, urinary tract infection, ileus, postoperative hemorrhage, transfusion, surgical site infection, and death.[59-64] Patients with uncontrolled diabetes have also been reported to have longer lengths of hospital stay, fewer routine discharges, and increased rates of 30-day readmission following TKA.[60,61,65]

Most importantly, patients with diabetes have an increased risk of both deep and superficial infections after total knee arthroplasty, possibly due to impaired phagocytosis.[66-72] There are conflicting reports of a higher association of elevated preoperative hemoglobin A1c with prosthetic joint infection.[68-71,73] Two studies have recommended that total knee arthroplasty should be delayed until the Hb A1c is less than 7 to 8.[70,71]

Bone strength and fracture healing are adversely affected by hyperglycemia, and one study reported an association of diabetes mellitus with an increased risk of periprosthetic fracture and aseptic loosening.[59] Maradit-Kremers et al.[74] reported that higher preoperative glucose values on the day of surgery were significantly associated with both the overall risk of revisions and revisions for aseptic loosening. Some surgeons have noted reduced complications with the use of sliding scale insulin in the perioperative period. Patients with insulin dependence should be counseled preoperatively that there is an increased risk for reoperation and decreased 10-year implant survivorship compared to nondiabetic patients.[75]

INFLAMMATORY ARTHROPATHIES

Inflammatory arthropathies, including rheumatoid arthritis, juvenile rheumatoid arthritis, and spondyloarthropathy, now account for only 2.7% of lower extremity arthroplasties performed in the United States.[76] Total knee arthroplasty has been reported to decrease health care costs and improve health status in patients with these disorders.[77] Over the last several decades, the rates of total knee arthroplasty have decreased, and the average age at time of surgery has increased among these patients.[76] This is likely due to an improvement in biologic treatments.[78,79]

When total knee arthroplasty is indicated in these patients, a multidisciplinary approach is warranted, as cardiac and pulmonary involvement are frequent.[80] In patients with polyarticular disease, the preoperative evaluation should include assessment of multiple joints, including the cervical spine. The impact of immune modulating medications on outcomes after total knee arthroplasty is very controversial. The effects of biologics on wound healing and infection appear to be less notable than high-dose systemic glucocorticoids.[81,82] In one study,[81] the use of infliximab within 4 weeks of elective knee or hip arthroplasty was not associated with a higher risk of short- or long-term infection compared to withholding infliximab for longer time periods. However glucocorticoid use, especially greater than 10 mg/day, was associated with an increased risk of infection. Another study[82] reported that a diagnosis of rheumatoid arthritis and prescriptions for prednisone, colchicine, or allopurinol were predictive of postoperative infection following lower extremity arthroplasty, but not among patients prescribed specific disease-modifying antirheumatic drugs and TNF-α inhibitors. The American College of Rheumatology and the American Association of Hip and Knee Surgeons have developed evidence-based guidelines for the perioperative management of antirheumatic drug therapy in adult patients with inflammatory arthropathies having elective total hip and total knee arthroplasty with the timing of withholding and restarting medications in the perioperative period based upon the dosing frequency of the drug.[83]

Several analyses of databases reported that these patients are at increased risk for complications after total knee arthroplasty, including pneumonia, bleeding, requirement for blood transfusion, longer length of hospital stay, readmission, and revision.[65,84,85] Two studies reported no difference in major noninfectious perioperative complications or mortality after total knee arthroplasty between patients with rheumatoid arthritis and osteoarthritis.[86,87] There seems to be consensus that there is an increased risk of periprosthetic joint infection in patients with inflammatory arthritis.[87-90] Those patients who develop prosthetic joint infection are also more likely to have antibiotic-resistant organisms.[91] The reason for increased rate of postoperative infection is not fully understood but is likely multifactorial.

Total knee arthroplasty can be technically challenging in these patients due to poor bone quality, valgus deformity, flexion contracture, and collateral ligament laxity. The senior author recommends routine fixation of posterior-stabilized components with antibiotic loaded cement. However, several recent studies reported good results with cementless and hybrid components.[92-94] In one study of 47 patients who had knee arthroplasty with sintered metal bead surfaces,[92] 98.4% survival at 10 years was reported. There is controversy over the routine need for posterior-stabilized components in patients with rheumatoid arthritis. In a study of 119 cruciate-retaining knees in 75 patients with rheumatoid arthritis with minimum follow-up of 15 years, Lee et al.[95] reported overall survival rates of 98.7% at 10 years with no revisions for posterior instability or patellofemoral problems.

Patients with juvenile inflammatory arthritis may be challenging due to the small size of the knee, contractures, and psychosocial problems. Parvizi et al.[96] reported the results of 25 knees in patients with juvenile arthritis younger than 20 years with a mean 10.7 years clinical follow-up. There was good relief of pain, with increase in mean Knee Society scores (27.6 to 88.3 points), but modest improvements in mean Knee Society function scores (14.8 to 39.2 points) and range of motion. Symptomatic loosening was seen in two knees (8%), and one was revised. Palmer et al. reported the results of 15 knees in patients with juvenile arthritis at a minimum of 12 years postoperatively, and noted good relief of pain and restoration of function. Three knees (20%) had revision for loosening.[97]

POSTTRAUMATIC ARTHRITIS

There are numerous factors to consider in patients with posttraumatic arthritis considering total knee arthroplasty, including nonunion, malunion, bone deficiency, malalignment, latent infection, retained hardware, arthrofibrosis, and a compromised soft-tissue envelope.[98] These patients tend to be male, younger, more active, and, if employed, have more physically demanding jobs. Thus, patient expectations and the demands placed on the knee arthroplasty are usually greater than in patients with primary osteoarthritis. The patients should be counseled preoperatively that the procedure will be more complicated and has a higher risk of prosthetic joint infection. The preoperative examination should include evaluation for low-grade infection, deformity, ligament competence, range of motion, peripheral pulses, and previous incisions in the knee.[98] Long-standing weight-bearing radiographs are recommended and computed tomography scan may be helpful to assess bone quality and defects.[98] The evaluation for infection should include at least an ESR and CRP, and if the clinical suspicion is high, a preoperative knee joint aspiration for cell count and culture is recommended.[98] In patients with one or more periarticular plate and screws, it may be reasonable to first, as a separate procedure, remove the hardware and obtain multiple cultures of the plate and surrounding tissues.

Poor range of motion of the knee is common in these patients, and the surgical approach may be challenging.[98] Previous skin incisions, scars, and burn injuries should be considered in planning the skin incision. Incisions should be as far apart as possible and if they must intersect, a right angle is preferable to an acute angle. If the skin bridge between two incisions is longer than the length of the incision, circulation should be sufficient for healing.[99] All flaps should include the full subcutaneous layer, as the plexus feeding the skin and adipose tissue lies above this.[100] Most of the deep perforators arise medially, and the most lateral incision that can be made without compromising exposure should be considered.[99] If there have been multiple

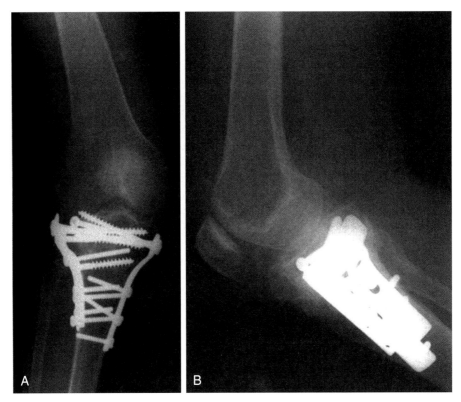

FIGURE 47-9 **A** and **B:** Posttraumatic arthritis with valgus deformity and retained hardware.

incisions, a preoperative consultation with a plastic surgeon may be considered for tissue expanders, flap coverage, or a sham incision. In rare situations, a planned gastrocnemius flap, or even a distally based vastus lateralis flap, may be considered.[101,102] A medial parapatellar or Insall approach is usually performed, but occasionally a quadriceps snip may be necessary for exposure.[103]

These knees may have intra- or extra-articular deformities, and preoperative planning may be helpful to determine whether the deformities can be corrected through the intra-articular bone resections or if an extra-articular osteotomy is required.[98] Revision knee instruments and components, computer navigation, or patient specific instruments may rarely be considered in cases with severe deformities.[104,105] These procedures may include the use of augments, stems, or intramedullary rods of various lengths to bypass cortical defects from previous screw holes (**Fig. 47-9**).[98,106] The senior author usually uses a posterior-stabilized component. If ligament incompetence is present or the knee is unable to be balanced, a varus–valgus constrained component can provide satisfactory clinical and functional outcomes (**Fig. 47-10**).[107] Although rare, when complete ligament incompetence or extensive bone loss is present, a rotating-hinge or tumor prosthesis should be considered.[108] Finally, our preference is to generally remove retained plates, screws, and nails as a separate initial procedure, and obtain cultures of the retained hardware and surrounding tissue.

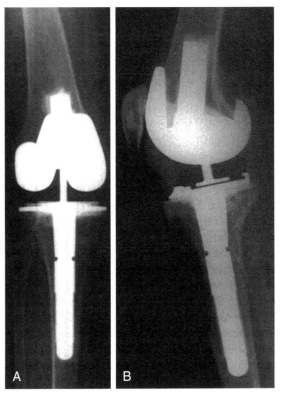

FIGURE 47-10 **A** and **B:** Postoperative radiographs showing long-stemmed constrained implant in patient with posttraumatic arthritis.

There are higher rates of complications, including infection, and generally worse outcomes of total knee arthroplasty in patients with posttraumatic arthritis.[90,109-117] Scott et al.[109] compared 31 patients with posttraumatic arthritis to age- and gender-matched primary osteoarthritis patients and reported a higher rate of complications in patients with posttraumatic arthritis, but no difference in patient-reported outcomes or satisfaction between groups. The most common complications were wound problems (13%) and stiffness (10%). Saleh et al.[115] reviewed 16 studies of total knee arthroplasty for posttraumatic arthritis, and noted a 20.9% rate of superficial infection (62/296 total patients) and 16.5% rate of deep infection (67/405 total patients). In a study of the Medicare database from 2005 to 2012, Bala et al.[110] identified 3509 patients with posttraumatic arthritis and 257,611 with primary osteoarthritis, and reported a higher rate of deep infection, cellulitis or seroma, wound complications, and revision in patients with posttraumatic arthritis. Another database study by Jamsen et al.[90] noted higher rate of infection in patients with posttraumatic arthritis. Ge et al.[112] reported that, compared to patients with soft-tissue knee trauma, a history of fracture has a higher association with surgical site complications and 90-day readmissions after total knee arthroplasty. Suzuki et al.[111] reported risk factors for infection in this patient population include a history of fracture fixation and presence of retained fixation hardware.

Functional outcomes have been noted to be worse in posttraumatic arthritis. Lunebourg et al.[117] compared functional outcomes of 33 patients with a history of periarticular fracture with 407 primary arthritis controls. At mean 11 years follow-up, there were worse improvements in range of motion and knee osteoarthritis outcome scores (KOOS) in posttraumatic arthritis patients. Implant survival in patients with this diagnosis may be lower than in those with primary osteoarthritis. El-Galaly et al.[116] in a study of the Danish Knee Arthroplasty Registry reported a higher rate of revisions in patients with posttraumatic arthritis within the first 5 years after surgery (hazard ratio 1.5 to 2.4 between age categories), but no difference in risk of revision after 5 years. Abdel et al.[113] reported 96% 15-year survival free from revision for aseptic loosening in 62 patients with total knee arthroplasty after a prior tibial plateau fracture. Of the 21 complications, most occurred less than 2 years after surgery. Putman et al.[114] reported 89% 10-year survival in 263 patients with total knee arthroplasty after knee trauma or prior surgery.

ARTHROPLASTY AFTER HIGH TIBIAL OSTEOTOMY

High tibial osteotomy was formerly a common surgical option for the treatment of medial osteoarthritis with varus deformity in young and active patients. These may be either closing or opening wedge, usually with plate fixation. With lateral compartment arthritis and valgus deformity, distal femoral osteotomy with plate fixation is used. The clinical results of knee osteotomies deteriorate over time, with 5-year survival rates ranging from 71% to 95% and 10-year survival rates ranging from 51% to 98%.[118-120] Factors associated with survival include age, gender, BMI, range of motion, severity of preoperative arthritis, postoperative correction angle, and choice of opening or closing wedge osteotomy.[118-120]

These osteotomies have been performed using both longitudinal or transverse incisions.[121,122] Closing wedge tibial osteotomy may result in a change of position of the patella (patella baja) and joint line. This is generally not seen after distal femoral osteotomies.[123] Although the medial opening wedge osteotomy has become more frequently used, Han et al.,[124] in a review of published studies, reported no difference in clinical or radiographic outcomes, or rates of revision between closing and opening wedge osteotomies. However, a quadriceps snip, tibial tubercle osteotomy, and lateral soft-tissue release were more frequently used in total knee arthroplasty after closing wedge osteotomy. In addition, impingement of a tibial component stem may occur after closing wedge osteotomy. The authors use a posterior-stabilized component in all knees with prior osteotomy, as ligament balancing is difficult or impossible.

Several technical challenges may be seen in the conversion of previous proximal tibial osteotomy to a total knee arthroplasty.[118] There may be difficulty in exposure of the knee due to patella baja and a quadriceps snip may be needed.[125] Retained hardware may be removed to permit component placement (**Fig. 47-11**), but this may not always be necessary.[122,126] Sclerotic bone at the osteotomy may impinge on a central stem. Small tibial defects can be treated with cement or metal augment, but a larger defect may require an autograft or, rarely, an allograft femoral head.[118] The tibial component and stem should be placed as medially as possible to avoid lateral overhang and stem cortical impingement or perforation. Rarely, a custom offset tibial stem may be needed in knees with severe tibial deformity.[127] The location of the tibial tubercle may not be a reliable guide for tibial component rotation in these knees.[128]

Conversion of a high tibial osteotomy to total knee arthroplasty has been reported to have worse or similar clinical and radiographic results, and rates of revision and complications compared to primary total knee arthroplasty (**Fig. 47-12**). This may be related to several factors, including anatomic deformity, ligament stability, components required, surgical techniques, and duration of follow-up.[118] In a systematic review, van Raaij et al.[129] reported that previous high tibial osteotomy does not compromise the results of total knee arthroplasty, but the quality of evidence was low. There are two retrospective studies reporting a higher risk of both complications and revisions secondary to patellar instability, infection,

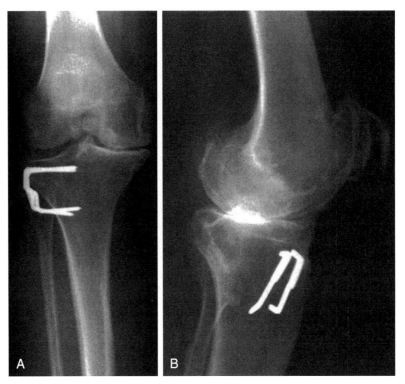

FIGURE 47-11 **A** and **B:** Knee after proximal tibial osteotomy.

stiffness, and aseptic loosening.[130,131] In a matched control study, Kazakos et al.[132] reported clinical results comparable to osteoarthritic primary knees at 4.5 years follow-up in a series of 38 knees, despite a higher rate of a variety of complications. Bae et al.[125] compared the outcomes of 32 conversion knees to matched controls and reported no differences in Knee Society scores, WOMAC scores, range of motion, or radiographic alignment between cohorts.

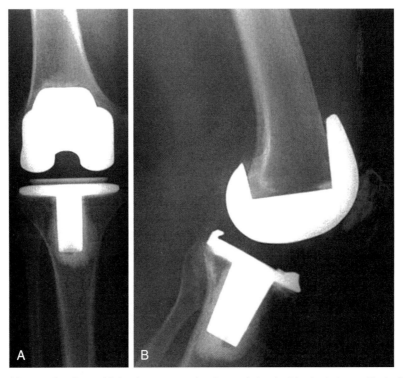

FIGURE 47-12 **A** and **B:** Total knee arthroplasty with hardware removal and use of standard implants in a patient with previous tibial osteotomy.

ARTHROPLASTY AFTER PRIOR ARTHRODESIS OR ANKYLOSIS

Patients may uncommonly have spontaneous ankylosis or arthrodesis due to posttraumatic conditions, inflammatory arthropathy, or infection.[133,134] This has usually been considered an absolute contraindication for knee arthroplasty. However, due to the social and functional limitations of a knee arthrodesis, conversion to arthroplasty has been recently considered.[135] The great technical difficulties of this procedure include difficulty with exposure, bone loss, insufficient skin and subcutaneous tissue, ligament incompetence, and atrophy or absence of the extensor mechanism.[135] When conversion to total knee arthroplasty is considered, the surgeon should have reasonable assurance that the quadriceps mechanism is intact (the ability to perform a straight leg raise is necessary, but not sufficient). Lack of extensor function requires locking in hyperextension during the stance phase of gait, which leads to increased stress on the prosthesis and failure due to loosening and wear.[136]

Conversion of an arthrodesis or ankylosed knee to a knee arthroplasty places a notable stretch and compromise on the soft tissues and skin around the knee. Consultation with a plastic surgeon and the use of skin grafting, vascularized gastrocnemius flaps, or tissues expanders may be considered.[137] Exposure of the joint will be difficult, and the patella may be ankylosed to the femur requiring a tibial tubercle osteotomy[135,137] or other extensile approaches, such as quadriceps snip or turndown to prevent patellar tendon avulsion.[135] The femoral component is placed as posteriorly as possible to decrease anterior joint overstuffing.[135] As the collateral ligaments may be absent or incompetent, constrained condylar or rotating-hinge prostheses are usually necessary.[133,135,137]

There are relatively few studies of the results of conversion of knee arthrodesis to total knee arthroplasty. Patients should be counseled preoperatively about the high risk of complications. In a study of eight patients, Clemens et al.[133] reported that five patients had reoperation, including two with recurrent infection resulting in amputation and one with a chronic draining sinus. In five knees available for evaluation of knee function, flexion ranged from 90 to 120 degrees with an extension lag of 10 to 40 degrees. Kovalak et al.[134] reported six patients who had total knee arthroplasty after spontaneous ankylosis, and, at 86 months follow-up, mean knee flexion was 85 degrees, HSS knee scores improved 38 points, and WOMAC score improved 22.7 points. There were two infections, one treated by débridement and one by arthrodesis. In a review of the literature, Kernkamp et al.[135] reported outcomes in six studies with 123 knee arthrodeses converted to arthroplasty. In five studies with 105 knees, there was a mean gain in flexion of 80 degrees.[133,138-141] Two studies reported a mean improvement in HSS score of 20 points in a total of 43 knees.[140,141] In three studies including 76 patients, 18% had moderate to severe pain postoperatively.[139-141] In three studies all 61 patients were satisfied with the procedure.[133,138,141] In another study, five of seven patients were satisfied.[140] Finally, in a study of 37 knees, satisfaction was achieved in only 10 patients (29%), but this was defined as no pain and able to ambulate unlimited distance.[139] Complications were frequent, occurring in 65% (80 of 123) knee arthrodesis converted to arthroplasty. The most frequent complications reported were skin necrosis (25%), arthrofibrosis (13%), infection (11%), and revision (11%). The major complications of revision arthrodesis, amputation, and death occurred in less than 5% of knees.

GENU RECURVATUM

Severe recurvatum of the knee has traditionally been considered a contraindication to total knee arthroplasty, as it has been associated with serious neurological disorders. In considering knee arthroplasty in such a patient, an attempt to determine the cause of the deformity should be considered.[142] These include fixed ankle equinus, severe quadriceps weakness, and malunion of fracture of the proximal tibia.[143] If the cause is determined and correctable, this should be considered preoperatively.[142] Genu recurvatum related to polio has already been described.[12,144] Krackow and Weiss reported transposing the collateral ligaments posteriorly on the femur for genu recurvatum.[13] If the recurvatum is due to anterior tibial bowing, an increase in the angle of the tibial cut (up to 15 degrees) could be considered.[142] In patients with a neuromuscular disorder the use of a rotating-hinge component is recommended.[142]

There are few studies of the results of knee arthroplasty in severe genu recurvatum. Wang et al.[145] reported the outcomes of 12 patients with a mean recurvatum of 11 degrees (range 6 to 15 degrees) due to femoral fracture malunion treated by intra-articular resection and soft-tissue balancing. At mean 93 months follow-up, the mean recurvatum was 3 degrees (range 0 to 6 degrees), and there were notable increases in Knee Society knee and function scores. Meding et al.[146] reported the results of 57 posterior-stabilized components performed in knees with a mean preoperative recurvatum deformity of 11 degrees (range 5 to 20 degrees). At 4.5 years follow-up, Knee Society knee, function, and pain scores improved by 40, 37, and 30 points, respectively. The mean postoperative extension was 0 degree, and only two patients both with preoperative recurvatum of 10 degrees, had hyperextension deformity. Computer navigation has also been reported to be helpful for knees with recurvatum deformity.[147,148]

CUSTOM COMPONENTS

Historically, custom implants have been used for unusual cases, in which standard size components would not be appropriate due to extremes of anatomic size or morphology, such as in patient with juvenile rheumatoid arthritis.[149] Custom components have also been used in revisions, and in cases with severe bone loss.[149] The current impetus for the fabrication of custom components in primary total knee arthroplasty for patients without anatomic abnormalities is related to the high rate of persistent pain and patient dissatisfaction with standard knee components.[149] It has been suggested that a mismatch between the patient's anatomy and the size of noncustom components may contribute to pain and dissatisfaction. Mahoney et al.[150] reported that femoral component overhang over 3 mm increased the risk for persistent pain at 2 years postoperatively. Another goal of modern custom knee components is to restore the alignment of the arthritic knee to the predisease state, corrected for any loss of bone and cartilage.[149]

The majority of "custom" knee replacements now available involve fabrication of customized cutting jigs for the specific patient, using standard off-the-shelf knee components. A CT or MRI scan, required preoperatively, permits the implant manufacturer's engineer to design specific instruments for preplanned axial and coronal alignment.[149] Nobel et al.[151] reported that custom instrumentation may reduce operative time, decrease incision length, decrease number of instruments used, and increase hospital efficiency. Other studies have reported that custom instrumentation results in similar or better component alignment and accurately templates component size.[152] A least one manufacturer, ConforMIS Inc. (Burlington, MA), has taken the concept further by providing both patient matched instruments and implant components. With this system, the patient's knee is imaged preoperatively by a CT scan, and individual 3D models of the distal femur and proximal tibia are fabricated and used for fitting of virtual total knee components.[153] Included in the preoperative imaging and planning are the centers of the femoral head and talus, which allow for placement of components perpendicular to the mechanical axis and for the correction of coronal deformities.[153] The actual components are then fabricated with traditional materials. Following the principle of component alignment along the mechanical axis,[153] the patient's distal femoral condylar angle is reproduced and transferred to the tibial polyethylene, which inserts into a tibial component placed perpendicular to the mechanical axis.[153] Theoretically, this system allows for an endless number of sizes and shapes to match a specific patient's bony geometry, while reducing the total number of instruments and trays needed in stock.[153]

There are few published studies of custom components in primary TKA. The cost of these components is obviously greater than standard components, but it is possible that this may be mitigated by a decrease in costs of inventory and instrument sterilization, and improved outcomes.[154,155] In a matched controlled study of 100 custom TKAs, Ivie et al.[156] reported that custom TKAs were 1.8 times more likely to be within the desired ±3 degrees from

the neutral mechanical axis than standard components. Zeller et al., using mobile fluoroscopy to assess kinematics in custom and noncustom cruciate-retaining knees, reported that patients with custom knee components had kinematics more similar to a normal knee.[157] Other studies have noted less favorable results of custom components. White et al. reported that custom components had decreased range of motion, higher rates of manipulation, and worse satisfaction and KSS pain scores than "off the shelf" components.[158] In a study of custom unicompartmental knees, Talmo et al. reported a relatively high rate of short- to intermediate-term failure with early aseptic loosening, especially of the femoral component.[159] Larger cohort studies with longer follow-up are required before widespread use of these custom fabricated components and instruments can be routinely recommended.

DWARFISM

There are numerous metabolic and genetic etiologies for short stature, including growth hormone deficiency, congenital hypothyroidism, idiopathic short stature, achondroplasia, Morquio disease, and spondylo-epiphyseal dysplasia.[160] Although underlying genotypes vary, phenotypes are similar and pose specific challenges for knee arthroplasty.[160] When arrested epiphyseal development results in delayed endochondral ossification, the unsupported cartilage surface leads to degeneration of the loaded joint, with progressive varus or valgus deformities.[160,161] In young patients, osteotomies may be a temporizing solution, but progressive joint destruction may require knee arthroplasty.[160]

Total knee arthroplasty in these patients is challenging due to severe deformity, hypotonia, ligamentous laxity, and limited motion with flexion contracture.[160,162-167] With severe deformities, femoral osteotomy before or at the time of arthroplasty has been reported.[164,165,168] Computer navigation has been reported when intramedullary instrumentation is prohibited by large deformities or femoral bowing.[163] The deformity and severe soft-tissue contractures may require a quadriceps snip for exposure.[163,166] Soft-tissue releases are often required for ligament balancing and patellar tracking.[162,163,165,166] Standard size knee components and instruments may not be appropriate in patients with dwarfism, and custom fabricated components and instruments have been reported.[163,166] With severe deformity, ligament deficiency, or hypotonia, custom constrained or hinged components can provide good results. Sewell et al.,[162] in a series of 11 custom rotating-hinge knees in patients with severe deformities and ligamentous laxity due to dwarfism, reported good outcomes at mean follow-up of 7 years with 44 and 30 point improvements in Knee Society clinical and function scores, respectively. There were four complications: one patella fracture, one periprosthetic tibia fracture, one revision for aseptic loosening of the femoral component, and one patient with persistent anterior knee pain.

Patients with achondroplasia typically have wide, flared metaphyses and metaphyseal angulation, lateral collateral ligament laxity, and limited motion with flexion contractures.[163] There are few case reports of knee arthroplasty in patients with achondroplasia.[160,163,164] Kim et al.[163] reported five knees in patients with achondroplasia and preoperative varus deformity ranging from 5 to 30 degrees, and all had improvements in deformity, motion, Knee Society scores (35.9 to 82.9), and average function scores (47.9 to 96.7).[162,163,165,166,169] Ling et al.[166] reported two knees with Grade III Kashin–Beck disease with skeletal dysplasia, complex knee deformity, and functional limitation treated by staged arthroplasty. Detailed preoperative planning of bone resection and soft-tissue balancing resulted in correct alignment, and improved pain and function. De Waal et al.[165] reported two knee arthroplasties in patients with Morquio disease and one with hereditary spondylo-epiphyseal dysplasia. Guenther et al.[160] reported that 138 total knee arthroplasties in patients with dwarfism (height ≤ 150 cm) of various etiologies had notable improvements in HSS score and function score at 1- and 5-year follow-up. Revision was performed in one knee at 1-year follow-up, and three knees at 5-year follow-up.

OSTEOGENESIS IMPERFECTA

This is an inheritable group of collagen-related disorders affecting up to 50,000 people in the United States.[170] There is an abnormality in type 1 collagen secondary to mutations in the COL1A1 and COL1A2 genes, with both abnormal collagen cross-linking and decreased production of collagen molecules.[163] In adults, orthopedic manifestations include kyphoscoliosis, spondylolisthesis, and posttraumatic and accelerated degenerative joint disease.[170] Patients are susceptible to long bone fractures usually treated nonoperatively, and high rates of nonunion, malunion, and deformity are seen in cases of both closed and open treatment.[170]

Total knee arthroplasty in patients with osteogenesis imperfecta and painful knee arthritis is challenging due to bone fragility, prior fractures, and deformity.[163,170] The use of conventional intramedullary instruments may not be possible, and the use of computer navigation has been reported.[171] The Ilizarov method has been reported to correct severe deformity preoperatively,[172] but concurrent femoral and/or tibial osteotomies with knee arthroplasty has also been reported. Wagner et al.[173] reported three knee arthroplasties with concurrent femoral and/or tibial osteotomies in two patients followed for a mean of 6 years. One patient had nonunion of the tibial osteotomy treated with fixation and iliac crest bone graft. The second patient, with staged bilateral procedures, had two-level tibial osteotomy with right knee arthroplasty which healed uneventfully and resulted in pain-free, unassisted ambulation. However, the left knee arthroplasty with two-level tibial osteotomy had several complications, including nonunion of the proximal site and valgus malunion of the distal site, and required reoperation.

There are few case reports of the outcome of total knee arthroplasty in these patients.[163,174] Papagelopoulos noted good results in three knees.[174] Kim et al.[163] reported two knees in two patients with this disorder. One patient, with a 25 degrees varus deformity and motion from 5 to 45 degrees, had a soft-tissue expander preoperatively, and then a posterior-stabilized knee with medial ligament release. The second patient, with a 17 degrees valgus deformity, had a semi-constrained prosthesis with lateral retinacular release. There were no complications and both patients were pain free with improved function.

CONCLUSION

Although total knee arthroplasty is usually challenging in patients with these "special" medical conditions, careful preoperative, often multispecialty, evaluation and optimization of the patient is important for a successful outcome. Careful preoperative planning for exposure, bone preparation, ligament balancing, and specific knee components for those patients with anatomic abnormalities or prior surgical procedures is equally important for success of total knee arthroplasty.

REFERENCES

1. Klein GR, Parvizi J. Surgical manifestations of Paget's disease. *J Am Acad Orthop Surg.* 2006;14(11):577-586.
2. Lyles KW, Siris ES, Singer FR, Meunier PJ. A clinical approach to diagnosis and management of Paget's disease of bone. *J Bone Miner Res.* 2001;16(8):1379-1387. doi:10.1359/jbmr.2001.16.8.1379.
3. Demulder A, Takahashi S, Singer FR, Hosking DJ, Roodman GD. Abnormalities in osteoclast precursors and marrow accessory cells in Paget's disease. *Endocrinology.* 1993;133(5):1978-1982. doi:10.1210/endo.133.5.7691583.
4. Gabel GT, Rand JA, Sim FH. Total knee arthroplasty for osteoarthrosis in patients who have Paget disease of bone at the knee. *J Bone Joint Surg Am Vol.* 1991;73a(5):739-744. doi:10.2106/00004623-199173050-00013.
5. Whitehouse RW. Paget's disease of bone. *Semin Musculoskelet Radiol.* 2002;6(4):313-322. doi:10.1055/s-2002-36730.
6. Lozano-Calderon SA, Colman MW, Raskin KA, Hornicek FJ, Gebhardt M. Use of bisphosphonates in orthopedic surgery: pearls and pitfalls. *Orthop Clin North Am.* 2014;45(3):403-416. doi:10.1016/j.ocl.2014.03.006.
7. Broberg MA, Cass JR. Total knee arthroplasty in Paget's disease of the knee. *J Arthroplasty.* 1986;1(2):139-142.
8. Lee GC, Sanchez-Sotelo J, Berry DJ. Total knee arthroplasty in patients with Paget's disease of bone at the knee. *J Arthroplasty.* 2005;20(6):689-693. doi:10.1016/j.arth.2004.11.007.
9. Tsaridis E, Sarikloglou S, Papasoulis E, Lykoudis S, Koutroumpas I, Avtzakis V. Correction of tibial deformity in Paget's disease using the Taylor spatial frame. *J Bone Joint Surg Br.* 2008;90(2):243-244. doi:10.1302/0301-620X.90B2.19412.
10. Parvizi J, Frankle MA, Tiegs RD, Sim FH. Corrective osteotomy for deformity in Paget disease. *J Bone Joint Surg Am Vol.* 2003;85-A(4):697-702.
11. Schai PA, Scott RD, Younger AS. Total knee arthroplasty in Paget's disease: technical problems and results. *Orthopedics.* 1999;22(1):21-25.

12. Patterson BM, Insall JN. Surgical management of gonarthrosis in patients with poliomyelitis. *J Arthroplasty*. 1992;7 suppl: 419-426.

13. Krackow KA, Weiss AP. Recurvatum deformity complicating performance of total knee arthroplasty. A brief note. *J Bone Joint Surg Am Vol*. 1990;72(2):268-271.

14. Moran MC. Functional loss after total knee arthroplasty for poliomyelitis. *Clin Orthop Relat Res*. 1996;323:243-246.

15. Gan Z-WJ, Pang HN. Outcomes of total knee arthroplasty in patients with poliomyelitis. *J Arthroplast*. 2016;31(11):2508-2513. doi:10.1016/j.arth.2016.04.019.

16. Tigani D, Fosco M, Amendola L, Boriani L. Total knee arthroplasty in patients with poliomyelitis. *Knee*. 2009;16(6):501-506. doi:10.1016/j.knee.2009.04.004.

17. Jordan L, Kligman M, Sculco TP. Total knee arthroplasty in patients with poliomyelitis. *J Arthroplast*. 2007;22(4):543-548.

18. Moyad TF, Estok D. Simultaneous femoral and tibial osteotomies during total knee arthroplasty for severe extra-articular deformity. *J Knee Surg*. 2009;22(1):21-26.

19. Rahman J, Hanna SA, Kayani B, et al. Custom rotating hinge total knee arthroplasty in patients with poliomyelitis affected limbs. *Int Orthop*. 2015;39(5):833-838. doi:10.1007/s00264-014-2572-y.

20. Huse DM, Schulman K, Orsini L, Castelli-Haley J, Kennedy S, Lenhart G. Burden of illness in Parkinson's disease. *Mov Disord*. 2005;20(11):1449-1454. doi:10.1002/mds.20609.

21. Macaulay W, Geller JA, Brown AR, Cote LJ, Kiernan HA. Total knee arthroplasty and Parkinson disease: enhancing outcomes and avoiding complications. *J Am Acad Orthop Surg*. 2010;18(11):687-694.

22. Mehta S, Vankleunen JP, Booth RE, Lotke PA, Lonner JH. Total knee arthroplasty in patients with Parkinson's disease: impact of early postoperative neurologic intervention. *Am J Orthop (Belle Mead NJ)*. 2008;37(10):513-516.

23. Shah SN, Hornyak J, Urquhart AG. Flexion contracture after total knee arthroplasty in a patient with Parkinson's disease: successful treatment with botulinum toxin type A. *J Arthroplast*. 2005;20(8):1078-1080.

24. Wong EH, Oh LJ, Parker DA. Outcomes of primary total knee arthroplasty in patients with Parkinson's disease. *J Arthroplasty*. 2018;14(18):30159-30161. doi:10.1016/j.arth.2018.02.028.

25. Tinning CG, Cochrane LA, Singer BR. Primary total knee arthroplasty in patients with Parkinson's disease: analysis of outcomes. *Acta Orthopaedica Belgica*. 2013;79(3):301-306.

26. Rondon AJ, Tan TL, Schlitt PK, Greenky MR, Phillips JL, Purtill JJ. Total joint arthroplasty in patients with Parkinson's disease: survivorship, outcomes, and reasons for failure. *J Arthroplasty*. 2018;33(4):1028-1032. doi:10.1016/j.arth.2017.11.017.

27. Ashraf M, Priyavadhana S, Sambandam SN, Mounasamy V, Sharma OP. Total knee arthroplasty in patients with Parkinson's disease- a critical analysis of available evidence. *Open Orthop J*. 2017;11:1087-1093. doi:10.2174/1874325001711011087.

28. Gupta R. A short history of neuropathic arthropathy. *Clin Orthop*. 1993;296(296):43-49.

29. Nakajima H, Uchida K, Oki H, et al. Rapidly progressive neuropathic arthropathy of the knee in possible association with a huge extruded cervical intervertebral disc herniation. *Rheumatol Int*. 2010;30(6):811-815. doi:10.1007/s00296-009-0999-z.

30. Kucera T, Urban K, Sponer P. Charcot arthropathy of the knee. A case-based review. *Clin Rheumatol*. 2011;30(3):425-428. doi:10.1007/s10067-010-1617-x.

31. Drennan DB, Fahey JJ, Maylahn DJ. Important factors in achieving arthrodesis of the Charcot knee. *J Bone Joint Surg Am Vol*. 1971;53(6):1180-1193.

32. Parvizi J, Marrs J, Morrey BF. Total knee arthroplasty for neuropathic (Charcot) joints. *Clin Orthop Relat Res*. 2003;(416):145-150. doi:10.1097/01.blo.0000081937.75404.ed.

33. Kim YH, Kim JS, Oh SW. Total knee arthroplasty in neuropathic arthropathy. *J Bone Joint Surg Br*. 2002;84(2):216-219.

34. Tibbo ME, Chalmers BP, Berry DJ, Pagnano MW, Lewallen DG, Abdel MP. Primary total knee arthroplasty in patients with neuropathic (Charcot) arthropathy: contemporary results. *J Arthroplasty*. 2018;9(18):30351-30356. doi:10.1016/j.arth.2018.04.003.

35. Bae DK, Song SJ, Yoon KH, Noh JH. Long-term outcome of total knee arthroplasty in Charcot joint: a 10- to 22-year follow-up. *J Arthroplasty*. 2009;24(8):1152-1156. doi:10.1016/j.arth.2009.05.003.

36. Carvajal Alba JA, Jose J, Clifford PD. Hemophilic arthropathy. *Am J Orthop (Belle Mead NJ)*. 2010;39(11):548-550.

37. Rodriguez-Merchan EC. The knee in severe haemophilia with special emphasis on surgical/invasive procedures. *Thromb Res*. 2014;134(3):545-551. doi:10.1016/j.thromres.2014.05.033.

38. Rodriguez-Merchan EC, Gomez-Cardero P. Arthroscopic knee debridement can delay total knee replacement in painful moderate haemophilic arthropathy of the knee in adult patients. *Blood Coagul Fibrinolysis*. 2016;27(6):645-647. doi:10.1097/MBC.0000000000000443.

39. Greene WB, DeGnore LT, White GC. Orthopaedic procedures and prognosis in hemophilic patients who are seropositive for human immunodeficiency virus. *J Bone Joint Surg Am Vol*. 1997;(72):2-11.

40. Stehr-Green JK, Jason JM, Evatt BL. Geographic variability of hemophilia-associated AIDS in the United States: effect of population characteristics. Hemophilia-Associated AIDS Study Group. *Am J Hematol*. 1989;32(3):178-183.

41. Chalmers BP, Abdel MP, Taunton MJ, Trousdale RT, Pagnano MW. Mid-term results of total hip and total knee arthroplasty in patients with human immunodeficiency virus. *Orthopedics*. 2017;40(4):e699-e702. doi:10.3928/01477447-20170522-03.

42. Enayatollahi MA, Murphy D, Maltenfort MG, Parvizi J. Human immunodeficiency virus and total joint arthroplasty: the risk for infection is reduced. *J Arthroplast*. 2016;31(10):2146-2151. doi:10.1016/j.arth.2016.02.058.

43. Mortazavi SMJ, Firoozabadi MA, Najafi A, Mansouri P. Evaluation of outcomes of suction drainage in patients with haemophilic arthropathy undergoing total knee arthroplasty. *Haemophilia*. 2017;23(4):e310-e315. doi:10.1111/hae.13224.

44. Rodriguez-Merchan EC, Romero-Garrido JA, Gomez-Cardero P. Multimodal blood loss prevention approach including intra-articular tranexamic acid in primary total knee arthroplasty for patients with severe haemophilia A. *Haemophilia*. 2016;22(4):e318-e320. doi:10.1111/hae.12942.

45. Mortazavi SMJ, Haghpanah B, Ebrahiminasab MM, Baghdadi T, Toogeh G. Functional outcome of total knee arthroplasty in patients with haemophilia. *Haemophilia*. 2016;22(6):919-924. doi:10.1111/hae.12999.

46. Strauss AC, Schmolders J, Friedrich MJ, et al. Outcome after total knee arthroplasty in haemophilic patients with stiff knees. *Haemophilia*. 2015;21(4):e300-e305. doi:10.1111/hae.12698.

47. Innocenti M, Civinini R, Carulli C, Villano M, Linari S, Morfini M. A modular total knee arthroplasty in haemophilic arthropathy. *Knee*. 2007;14(4):264-268.

48. Cho KY, Kim KI, Khurana S, Cho SW, Kang DG. Computer-navigated total knee arthroplasty in haemophilic arthropathy. *Haemophilia*. 2013;19(2):259-266. doi:10.1111/hae.12063.

49. Kim KI, Kim DK, Juh HS, Khurana S, Rhyu KH. Robot-assisted total knee arthroplasty in haemophilic arthropathy. *Haemophilia*. 2016;22(3):446-452. doi:10.1111/hae.12875.

50. Lachiewicz PF. Total joint replacement in special medical conditions. In: Callaghan JJ, Dennis DA, Paprosky WG, eds. *Orthopaedic Knowledge Update-Hip and Knee Reconstruction*. Chicago: American Academy of Orthopaedic Surgeons; 1995:79-86.

51. Kjaersgaard-Andersen P, Christiansen SE, Ingerslev J, Sneppen O. Total knee arthroplasty in classic hemophilia. *Clin Orthop Relat Res*. 1990;(256):137-146.

47 / TOTAL KNEE REPLACEMENT IN SPECIAL SITUATIONS   **707**

SECTION 6 / PRIMARY TOTAL KNEE ARTHROPLASTY

52. Goddard NJ, Mann HA, Lee CA. Total knee replacement in patients with end-stage haemophilic arthropathy: 25-year results. *J Bone Joint Surg Br.* 2010;92(8):1085-1089. doi:10.1302/0301-620X.92B8.23922.

53. Atilla B, Caglar O, Pekmezci M, Buyukasik Y, Tokgozoglu AM, Alpaslan M. Pre-operative flexion contracture determines the functional outcome of haemophilic arthropathy treated with total knee arthroplasty. *Haemophilia.* 2012;18(3):358-363. doi:10.1111/j.1365-2516.2011.02695.x.

54. Moore MF, Tobase P, Allen DD. Meta-analysis: outcomes of total knee arthroplasty in the haemophilia population. *Haemophilia.* 2016;22(4):e275-e285. doi:10.1111/hae.12885.

55. Kolber MK, Shukla PA, Kumar A, Zybulewski A, Markowitz T, Silberzweig JE. Endovascular management of recurrent spontaneous hemarthrosis after arthroplasty. *Cardiovasc Intervent Radiol.* 2017;40(2):216-222. doi:10.1007/s00270-016-1511-2.

56. Cahill GF. Disorders of carbohydrate metabolism. In: Wyngaarden JB, Smith LH, eds. *Cecil Textbook of Medicine.* Philadelphia: WB Saunders; 1982:1053-1071.

57. King KB, Findley TW, Williams AE, Bucknell AL. Veterans with diabetes receive arthroplasty more frequently and at a younger age. *Clin Orthop.* 2013;471(9):3049-3054. doi:10.1007/s11999-013-3026-3.

58. Wada O, Nagai K, Hiyama Y, Nitta S, Maruno H, Mizuno K. Diabetes is a risk factor for restricted range of motion and poor clinical outcome after total knee arthroplasty. *J Arthroplast.* 2016;31(9):1933-1937. doi:10.1016/j.arth.2016.02.039.

59. Yang Z, Liu H, Xie X, Tan Z, Qin T, Kang P. The influence of diabetes mellitus on the post-operative outcome of elective primary total knee replacement: a systematic review and meta-analysis. *Bone Joint J.* 2014;96-B(12):1637-1643. doi:10.1302/0301-620X.96B12.34378.

60. Marchant MH Jr, Viens NA, Cook C, Vail TP, Bolognesi MP. The impact of glycemic control and diabetes mellitus on perioperative outcomes after total joint arthroplasty. *J Bone Joint Surg Am Vol.* 2009;91(7):1621-1629. doi:10.2106/JBJS.H.00116.

61. Bolognesi MP, Marchant MH Jr, Viens NA, Cook C, Pietrobon R, Vail TP. The impact of diabetes on perioperative patient outcomes after total hip and total knee arthroplasty in the United States. *J Arthroplast.* 2008;23(6 suppl 1):92-98. doi:10.1016/j.arth.2008.05.012.

62. Bohl DD, Saltzman BM, Sershon RA, Darrith B, Okroj KT, Della Valle CJ. Incidence, risk factors, and clinical implications of pneumonia following total hip and knee arthroplasty. *J Arthroplast.* 2017;32(6):1991-1995.e1. doi:10.1016/j.arth.2017.01.004.

63. Belmont PJ Jr, Goodman GP, Waterman BR, Bader JO, Schoenfeld AJ. Thirty-day postoperative complications and mortality following total knee arthroplasty: incidence and risk factors among a national sample of 15,321 patients. *J Bone Joint Surg Am Vol.* 2014;96(1):20-26. doi:10.2106/JBJS.M.00018.

64. Wang S, Zhao Y. Diabetes mellitus and the incidence of deep vein thrombosis after total knee arthroplasty: a retrospective study. *J Arthroplast.* 2013;28(4):595-597. doi:10.1016/j.arth.2012.07.023.

65. Siracuse BL, Ippolito JA, Gibson PD, Ohman-Strickland PA, Beebe KS. A preoperative scale for determining surgical readmission risk after total knee arthroplasty. *J Bone Joint Surg Am Vol.* 2017;99(21):e112. doi:10.2106/JBJS.16.01043.

66. Menon TJ, Thjellesen D, Wroblewski BM. Charnley low-friction arthroplasty in diabetic patients. *J Bone Joint Surg Br.* 1983;65(5):580-581.

67. Wong RY, Lotke PAS, Ecker ML. Factors influencing wound healing after total knee arthroplasty. *Orthop Trans.* 1986;10:497.

68. Iorio R, Williams KM, Marcantonio AJ, Specht LM, Tilzey JF, Healy WL. Diabetes mellitus, hemoglobin A1C, and the incidence of total joint arthroplasty infection. *J Arthroplast.* 2012;27(5):726-729.e1. doi:10.1016/j.arth.2011.09.013.

69. Maradit Kremers H, Lewallen LW, Mabry TM, Berry DJ, Berbari EF, Osmon DR. Diabetes mellitus, hyperglycemia, hemoglobin A1C and the risk of prosthetic joint infections in total hip and knee arthroplasty. *J Arthroplast.* 2015;30(3):439-443. doi:10.1016/j.arth.2014.10.009.

70. Cancienne JM, Werner BC, Browne JA. Is there an association between hemoglobin A1C and deep postoperative infection after TKA? *Clin Orthop.* 2017;475(6):1642-1649. doi:10.1007/s11999-017-5246-4.

71. Tarabichi M, Shohat N, Kheir MM, et al. Determining the threshold for HbA1c as a predictor for adverse outcomes after total joint arthroplasty: a multicenter, retrospective study. *J Arthroplast.* 2017;32(9S):S263-S267.e1. doi:10.1016/j.arth.2017.04.065.

72. Namba RS, Inacio MCS, Paxton EW. Risk factors associated with deep surgical site infections after primary total knee arthroplasty: an analysis of 56,216 knees. *J Bone Joint Surg Am Vol.* 2013;95(9):775-782. doi:10.2106/JBJS.L.00211.

73. Harris AHS, Bowe TR, Gupta S, Ellerbe LS, Giori NJ. Hemoglobin A1C as a marker for surgical risk in diabetic patients undergoing total joint arthroplasty. *J Arthroplast.* 2013;28(8 suppl):25-29. doi:10.1016/j.arth.2013.03.033.

74. Maradit Kremers H, Schleck CD, Lewallen EA, Larson DR, Van Wijnen AJ, Lewallen DG. Diabetes mellitus and hyperglycemia and the risk of aseptic loosening in total joint arthroplasty. *J Arthroplast.* 2017;32(9S):S251-S253. doi:10.1016/j.arth.2017.02.056.

75. Watts CD, Houdek MT, Wagner ER, Abdel MP, Taunton MJ. Insulin dependence increases the risk of failure after total knee arthroplasty in morbidly obese patients. *J Arthroplast.* 2016;31(1):256-259. doi:10.1016/j.arth.2015.08.026.

76. Mertelsmann-Voss C, Lyman S, Pan TJ, Goodman SM, Figgie MP, Mandl LA. US trends in rates of arthroplasty for inflammatory arthritis including rheumatoid arthritis, juvenile idiopathic arthritis, and spondyloarthritis. *Arthritis Rheumatol.* 2014;66(6):1432-1439. doi:10.1002/art.38384.

77. March LM, Barcenilla AL, Cross MJ, Lapsley HM, Parker D, Brooks PM. Costs and outcomes of total hip and knee joint replacement for rheumatoid arthritis. *Clin Rheumatol.* 2008;27(10):1235-1242. doi:10.1007/s10067-008-0891-3.

78. Harty L, O'Toole G, FitzGerald O. Profound reduction in hospital admissions and musculoskeletal surgical procedures for rheumatoid arthritis with concurrent changes in clinical practice (1995-2010). *Rheumatology.* 2015;54(4):666-671. doi:10.1093/rheumatology/keu340.

79. Asai S, Takahashi N, Funahashi K, et al. Concomitant methotrexate protects against total knee arthroplasty in patients with rheumatoid arthritis treated with tumor necrosis factor inhibitors. *J Rheumatol.* 2015;42(12):2255-2260. doi:10.3899/jrheum.150410.

80. Goodman SM, Figgie M. Lower extremity arthroplasty in patients with inflammatory arthritis: preoperative and perioperative management. *J Am Acad Orthop Surg.* 2013;21(6):355-363. doi:10.5435/JAAOS-21-06-355.

81. George MD, Baker JF, Hsu JY, et al. Perioperative timing of infliximab and the risk of serious infection after elective hip and knee arthroplasty. *Arthritis Care Res.* 2017;69(12):1845-1854. doi:10.1002/acr.23209.

82. Salt E, Wiggins AT, Rayens MK, et al. Moderating effects of immunosuppressive medications and risk factors for post-operative joint infection following total joint arthroplasty in patients with rheumatoid arthritis or osteoarthritis. *Semin Arthritis Rheum.* 2017;46(4):423-429. doi:10.1016/j.semarthrit.2016.08.011.

83. Goodman SM, Springer B, Guyatt G, et al. 2017 American College of Rheumatology/American Association of Hip and Knee Surgeons guideline for the perioperative management of antirheumatic medication in patients with rheumatic diseases undergoing elective total hip or total knee arthroplasty. *J Arthroplast.* 2017;32(9):2628-2638. doi:10.1016/j.arth.2017.05.001.

84. Jauregui JJ, Kapadia BH, Dixit A, et al. Thirty-day complications in rheumatoid patients following total knee arthroplasty. *Clin Rheumatol.* 2016;35(3):595-600. doi:10.1007/s10067-015-3037-4.

85. Cancienne JM, Werner BC, Browne JA. Complications of primary total knee arthroplasty among patients with rheumatoid arthritis, psoriatic arthritis, ankylosing spondylitis, and osteoarthritis. *J Am Acad Orthop Surg.* 2016;24(8):567-574. doi:10.5435/JAAOS-D-15-00501.

86. Izumi M, Migita K, Nakamura M, et al. Risk of venous thromboembolism after total knee arthroplasty in patients with rheumatoid arthritis. *J Rheumatol.* 2015;42(6):928-934. doi:10.3899/jrheum.140768. [Erratum appears in *J Rheumatol.* 2016 Mar;43(3):681; PMID: 26932996].

87. Stundner O, Danninger T, Chiu Y-L, et al. Rheumatoid arthritis vs osteoarthritis in patients receiving total knee arthroplasty: perioperative outcomes. *J Arthroplast.* 2014;29(2):308-313. doi:10.1016/j.arth.2013.05.008.

88. Kong L, Cao J, Zhang Y, Ding W, Shen Y. Risk factors for periprosthetic joint infection following primary total hip or knee arthroplasty: a meta-analysis. *Int Wound J.* 2017;14(3):529-536. doi:10.1111/iwj.12640.

89. Carroll K, Dowsey M, Choong P, Peel T. Risk factors for superficial wound complications in hip and knee arthroplasty. *Clin Microbiol Infect.* 2014;20(2):130-135. doi:10.1111/1469-0691.12209.

90. Jamsen E, Huhtala H, Puolakka T, Moilanen T. Risk factors for infection after knee arthroplasty. A register-based analysis of 43,149 cases. *J Bone Joint Surg Am Vol.* 2009;91(1):38-47. doi:10.2106/JBJS.G.01686.

91. Tan TL, Gomez MM, Kheir MM, Maltenfort MG, Chen AF. Should preoperative antibiotics Be tailored according to patient's comorbidities and susceptibility to organisms? *J Arthroplast.* 2017;32(4):1089-1094.e3. doi:10.1016/j.arth.2016.11.021.

92. Vigano R, Whiteside LA, Roy M. Clinical results of bone ingrowth TKA in patients with rheumatoid arthritis. *Clin Orthop.* 2008;466(12):3071-3077. doi:10.1007/s11999-008-0394-1.

93. Hotfiel T, Carl H-D, Eibenberger T, et al. Cementless femoral components in bicondylar hybrid knee arthroplasty in patients with rheumatoid arthritis: a 10-year survivorship analysis. *J Orthop Surg (Hong Kong).* 2017;25(2):2309499017716252. doi:10.1177/2309499017716252.

94. Sharma S, Nicol F, Hullin MG, McCreath SW. Long-term results of the uncemented low contact stress total knee replacement in patients with rheumatoid arthritis. *J Bone Joint Surg Br.* 2005;87(8):1077-1080.

95. Lee JK, Kee YM, Chung HK, Choi CH. Long-term results of cruciate-retaining total knee replacement in patients with rheumatoid arthritis: a minimum 15-year review. *Can J Surg.* 2015;58(3):193-197.

96. Parvizi J, Lajam CM, Trousdale RT, Shaughnessy WJ, Cabanela ME. Total knee arthroplasty in young patients with juvenile rheumatoid arthritis. *J Bone Joint Surg Am Vol.* 2003;85-A(6):1090-1094.

97. Palmer DH, Mulhall KJ, Thompson CA, Severson EP, Santos ERG, Saleh KJ. Total knee arthroplasty in juvenile rheumatoid arthritis. *J Bone Joint Surg Am Vol.* 2005;87(7):1510-1514.

98. Benazzo F, Rossi SM, Ghiara M, Zanardi A, Perticarini L, Combi A. Total knee replacement in acute and chronic traumatic events. *Injury.* 2014;45 suppl 6:S98-S104. doi:10.1016/j.injury.2014.10.031.

99. Younger AS, Duncan CP, Masri BA. Surgical exposures in revision total knee arthroplasty. *J Am Acad Orthop Surg.* 1998;6(1):55-64.

100. Haertsch PA. The blood supply to the skin of the leg: a post-mortem investigation. *Br J Plast Surg.* 1981;34(4):470-477.

101. Patnaik S, Nayak B, Mishra L, Sahoo AK. Complex primary total knee replacement (TKR) using prophylactic gastrocnemius flap and rotating-hinge knee in post-traumatic, infective arthritis of the knee – a case report. *J Orthop Case Rep.* 2015;5(4):40-43. doi:10.13107/jocr.2250-0685.342.

102. Auregan JC, Begue T, Tomeno B, Masquelet AC. Distally-based vastus lateralis muscle flap: a salvage alternative to address complex soft tissue defects around the knee. *Orthop Traumatol Surg Res.* 2010;96(2):180-184. doi:10.1016/j.rcot.2010.02.013.

103. Massin P, Bonnin M, Paratte S, et al. Total knee replacement in post-traumatic arthritic knees with limitation of flexion. *Orthop Traumatol Surg Res.* 2011;97(1):28-33. doi:10.1016/j.otsr.2010.06.016.

104. Begue T, Mebtouche N, Levante S. One-stage procedure for total knee arthroplasty in post-traumatic osteoarthritis of the knee with wound defect. Usefulness of navigation and flap surgery. *Knee.* 2012;19(6):948-950. doi:10.1016/j.knee.2012.03.012.

105. Schotanus MG, van Haaren EH, Hendrickx RP, Jansen EJ, Kort NP. Accuracy of CT-based patient-specific guides for total knee arthroplasty in patients with post-traumatic osteoarthritis. *Eur J Orthop Surg Traumatol.* 2015;25(8):1313-1320. doi:10.1007/s00590-015-1677-3.

106. Reis MD. Prophylactic intramedullary femoral rod during total knee arthroplasty with simultaneous femoral plate removal. *J Arthroplasty.* 1998;13(6):718-721.

107. Rai S, Liu XZ, Feng XB, et al. Primary total knee arthroplasty using constrained condylar knee design for severe deformity and stiffness of knee secondary to post-traumatic arthritis. *J Orthop Surg Res.* 2018;13(1):67. doi:10.1186/s13018-018-0761-x.

108. Baker P, Critchley R, Gray A, et al. Mid-term survival following primary hinged total knee replacement is good irrespective of the indication for surgery. *Knee Surg Sport Traumatol Arthrosc.* 2014;22(3):599-608. doi:10.1007/s00167-012-2305-y.

109. Scott CE, Davidson E, MacDonald DJ, White TO, Keating JF. Total knee arthroplasty following tibial plateau fracture: a matched cohort study. *Bone Joint J.* 2015;97-B(4):532-538. doi:10.1302/0301-620X.97B4.34789.

110. Bala A, Penrose CT, Seyler TM, Mather RC III, Wellman SS, Bolognesi MP. Outcomes after total knee arthroplasty for post-traumatic arthritis. *Knee.* 2015;22(6):630-639. doi:10.1016/j.knee.2015.10.004.

111. Suzuki G, Saito S, Ishii T, Motojima S, Tokuhashi Y, Ryu J. Previous fracture surgery is a major risk factor of infection after total knee arthroplasty. *Knee Surg Sport Traumatol Arthrosc.* 2011;19(12):2040-2044. doi:10.1007/s00167-011-1525-x.

112. Ge DH, Anoushiravani AA, Kester BS, Vigdorchik JM, Schwarzkopf R. Preoperative diagnosis can predict conversion total knee arthroplasty outcomes. *J Arthroplast.* 2018;33(1):124-129. doi:10.1016/j.arth.2017.08.019.

113. Abdel MP, von Roth P, Cross WW, Berry DJ, Trousdale RT, Lewallen DG. Total knee arthroplasty in patients with a prior tibial plateau fracture: a long-term report at 15 years. *J Arthroplasty.* 2015;30(12):2170-2172. doi:10.1016/j.arth.2015.06.032.

114. Putman S, Argenson JN, Bonnevialle P, et al; Societe francaise de chirurgie orthopedique et traumatologie. Ten-year survival and complications of total knee arthroplasty for osteoarthritis secondary to trauma or surgery: a French multicentre study of 263 patients. *Orthop Traumatol Surg Res.* 2018;104(2):161-164. doi:10.1016/j.otsr.2017.11.019.

115. Saleh H, Yu S, Vigdorchik J, Schwarzkopf R. Total knee arthroplasty for treatment of post-traumatic arthritis: systematic review. *World J Orthop.* 2016;7(9):584-591. doi:10.5312/wjo.v7.i9.584.

116. El-Galaly A, Haldrup S, Pedersen AB, Kappel A, Jensen MU, Nielsen PT. Increased risk of early and medium-term revision after post-fracture total knee arthroplasty. *Acta Orthopaedica.* 2017;88(3):263-268. doi:10.1080/17453674.2017.1290479.

117. Lunebourg A, Parratte S, Gay A, Ollivier M, Garcia-Parra K, Argenson JN. Lower function, quality of life, and survival rate after total knee arthroplasty for posttraumatic arthritis than for primary arthritis. *Acta Orthopaedica.* 2015;86(2):189-194. doi:10.3109/17453674.2014.979723.

118. Song SJ, Bae DK, Kim KI, Lee CH. Conversion total knee arthroplasty after failed high tibial osteotomy. *Knee Surg Relat Res.* 2016;28(2):89-98. doi:10.5792/ksrr.2016.28.2.89.

119. Kim JH, Kim HJ, Lee DH. Survival of opening versus closing wedge high tibial osteotomy: a meta-analysis. *Sci Rep.* 2017;7(1):7296. doi:10.1038/s41598-017-07856-8.

120. Khoshbin A, Sheth U, Ogilvie-Harris D, et al. The effect of patient, provider and surgical factors on survivorship of high tibial osteotomy to total knee arthroplasty: a population-based study. *Knee Surg Sports Traumatol Arthrosc.* 2017;25(3):887-894. doi:10.1007/s00167-015-3849-4.

121. Kelley MA. *Nonprosthetic Management of the Arthritic Knee. Orthopaedic Knowledge Update-Hip and Knee Reconstruction.* Chicago: American Academy of Orthopaedic Surgeons; 1995:245-249.

122. Johnson BP, Dorr LD. Total knee arthroplasty after high tibial osteotomies. In: Lotke PA, ed. *Master Techniques in Orthopaedic Surgery, Knee Arthroplasty.* New York: Raven Press; 1995:177-192.

123. Coventry MB, Ilstrup DM, Wallrichs SL. Proximal tibial osteotomy. A critical long-term study of eighty-seven cases. *J Bone Joint Surg Am Vol.* 1993;75(2):196-201.

124. Han JH, Yang JH, Bhandare NN, et al. Total knee arthroplasty after failed high tibial osteotomy: a systematic review of open versus closed wedge osteotomy. *Knee Surg Sports Traumatol Arthrosc.* 2016;24(8):2567-2577. doi:10.1007/s00167-015-3807-1.

125. Bae DK, Song SJ, Park CH, Liang H, Bae JK. Comparison of midterm results between conversion total knee arthroplasties following closed wedge high tibial osteotomy and primary total knee arthroplasties: a matched pair study including patellar symptom and position. *J Orthop Sci.* 2017;22(3):495-500. doi:10.1016/j.jos.2016.12.019.

126. Windsor RE, Insall JN, Vince KG. Technical considerations of total knee arthroplasty after proximal tibial osteotomy. *J Bone Joint Surg Am Vol.* 1988;70(4):547-555.

127. Nagamine R, Inoue S, Miura H, Matsuda S, Iwamoto Y. Femoral shaft bowing influences the correction angle for high tibial osteotomy. *J Orthop Sci.* 2007;12(3):214-218. doi:10.1007/s00776-007-1112-7.

128. Meding JB, Keating EM, Ritter MA, Faris PM. Total knee arthroplasty after high tibial osteotomy. A comparison study in patients who had bilateral total knee replacement. *J Bone Joint Surg Am Vol.* 2000;82(9):1252-1259.

129. van Raaij TM, Bakker W, Reijman M, Verhaar JA. The effect of high tibial osteotomy on the results of total knee arthroplasty: a matched case control study. *BMC Musculoskelet Disord.* 2007;8:74. doi:10.1186/1471-2474-8-74.

130. Parvizi J, Hanssen AD, Spangehl MJ. Total knee arthroplasty following proximal tibial osteotomy: risk factors for failure. *J Bone Joint Surg Am Vol.* 2004;86-A(3):474-479.

131. Farfalli LA, Farfalli GL, Aponte-Tinao LA. Complications in total knee arthroplasty after high tibial osteotomy. *Orthopedics.* 2012;35(4):e464-e468. doi:10.3928/01477447-20120327-21.

132. Kazakos KJ, Chatzipapas C, Verettas D, Galanis V, Xarchas KC, Psillakis I. Mid-term results of total knee arthroplasty after high tibial osteotomy. *Arch Orthop Trauma Surg.* 2008;128(2):167-173. doi:10.1007/s00402-007-0488-3.

133. Clemens D, Lereim P, Holm I, Reikeras O. Conversion of knee fusion to total arthroplasty: complications in 8 patients. *Acta Orthopaedica.* 2005;76(3):370-374.

134. Kovalak E, Can A, Stegemann N, Erdogan AO, Erdogan F. Total knee arthroplasty after osseous ankylosis of the knee joint. *Acta Orthop Traumatol Turc.* 2015;49(5):503-507. doi:10.3944/AOTT.2015.14.0304.

135. Kernkamp WA, Verra WC, Pijls BG, Schoones JW, van der Linden HM, Nelissen RG. Conversion from knee arthrodesis to arthroplasty: systematic review. *Int Orthop.* 2016;40(10):2069-2074. doi:10.1007/s00264-016-3150-2.

136. van Krieken FM, den Heeten GJ, Pedersen DR, Brand RA, Crowninshield RD. Prediction of muscle and joint loads after segmental femur replacement for osteosarcoma. *Clin Orthop Relat Res.* 1985;198(198):273-283.

137. Cho SH, Jeong ST, Park HB, Hwang SC, Kim DH. Two-stage conversion of fused knee to total knee arthroplasty. *J Arthroplasty.* 2008;23(3):476-479. doi:10.1016/j.arth.2007.06.013.

138. Cameron HU, Hu C. Results of total knee arthroplasty following takedown of formal knee fusion. *J Arthroplasty.* 1996;11(6):732-737.

139. Naranja RJ, Lotke PA, Pagnano MW. Total knee arthroplasty in a previously ankylosed or arthrodesed knee. *Clin Orthop.* 1996;(331):234-237.

140. Henkel TR, Boldt JG, Drobny TK, Munzinger UK. Total knee arthroplasty after formal knee fusion using unconstrained and semiconstrained components: a report of 7 cases. *J Arthroplasty.* 2001;16(6):768-776. doi:10.1054/arth.2001.24375.

141. Kim YH, Oh SH, Kim JS. Conversion of a fused knee with use of a posterior stabilized total knee prosthesis. *J Bone Joint Surg Am Vol.* 2003;85-A(6):1047-1050.

142. Baldini A, Castellani L, Traverso F, Balatri A, Balato G, Franceschini V. The difficult primary total knee arthroplasty: a review. *The bone & joint journal.* 2015;97-B(10 suppl A):30-39. doi:10.1302/0301-620X.97B10.36920.

143. Meding JB, Keating EM, Ritter MA, Faris PM, Berend ME. Genu recurvatum in total knee replacement. *Clin Orthop Relat Res.* 2003;(416):64-67. doi:10.1097/01.blo.0000092988.12414.18.

144. Whiteside LA, Mihalko WM. Surgical procedure for flexion contracture and recurvatum in total knee arthroplasty. *Clin Orthop Relat Res.* 2002;(404):189-195.

145. Wang JW, Chen WS, Lin PC, Hsu CS, Wang CJ. Total knee replacement with intra-articular resection of bone after malunion of a femoral fracture: can sagittal angulation be corrected? *J Bone Joint Surg Br.* 2010;92(10):1392-1396. doi:10.02/0301-620X.92B10.24551.

146. Meding JB, Keating EM, Ritter MA, Faris PM, Berend ME. Total knee replacement in patients with genu recurvatum. *Clin Orthop Relat Res.* 2001;(393):244-249.

147. Mullaji A, Lingaraju AP, Shetty GM. Computer-assisted total knee replacement in patients with arthritis and a recurvatum deformity. *J Bone Joint Surg Br.* 2012;94(5):642-647. doi:10.1302/0301-620X.94B5.27211.

148. Seo SS, Kim CW, Lee CR, Seo JH, Kim DH, Kim OG. Outcomes of total knee arthroplasty in degenerative osteoarthritic knee with genu recurvatum. *Knee.* 2018;25(1):167-176. doi:10.1016/j.knee.2017.10.008.

149. Slamin J, Parsley B. Evolution of customization design for total knee arthroplasty. *Curr Rev Musculoskelet Med.* 2012;5(4):290-295. doi:10.1007/s12178-012-9141-z.

150. Mahoney OM, Kinsey T. Overhang of the femoral component in total knee arthroplasty: risk factors and clinical consequences. *J Bone Joint Surg Am Vol.* 2010;92(5):1115-1121. doi:10.2106/JBJS.H.00434.

151. Noble JW Jr, Moore CA, Liu N. The value of patient-matched instrumentation in total knee arthroplasty. *J Arthroplasty.* 2012;27(1):153-155. doi:10.1016/j.arth.2011.07.006.

152. Ng VY, Arnott L, Li J, et al. Comparison of custom to standard TKA instrumentation with computed tomography. *Knee Surg Sport Traumatol Arthrosc.* 2014;22(8):1833-1842. doi:10.1007/s00167-013-2632-7.

153. Fitz W, Buttacavoli FA. Custom-made knee replacements. In: Scott WN, Diduch DR, Long WJ, eds. *Insall & Scott Surgery of the Knee.* 6th ed. Philadelphia, PA: Elsevier; 2018:1519-1525.

154. Culler SD, Jevsevar DS, Shea KG, Wright KK, Simon AW. The incremental hospital cost and length-of-stay associated with treating adverse events among Medicare beneficiaries undergoing TKA. *J Arthroplasty.* 2015;30(1):19-25. doi:10.1016/j.arth.2014.08.023.

155. Culler SD, Martin GM, Swearingen A. Comparison of adverse events rates and hospital cost between customized individually made implants and standard off-the-shelf implants for total knee arthroplasty. *Arthroplasty today.* 2017;3(4):257-263. doi:10.1016/j.artd.2017.05.001.

156. Ivie CB, Probst PJ, Bal AK, Stannard JT, Crist BD, Sonny Bal B. Improved radiographic outcomes with patient-specific total knee arthroplasty. *J Arthroplasty.* 2014;29(11):2100-2103. doi:10.1016/j.arth.2014.06.024.

157. Zeller IM, Sharma A, Kurtz WB, Anderle MR, Komistek RD. Customized versus patient-sized cruciate-retaining total knee arthroplasty: an in vivo kinematics study using mobile fluoroscopy. *J Arthroplasty.* 2017;32(4):1344-1350. doi:10.1016/j.arth.2016.09.034.

158. White PB, Ranawat AS. Patient-specific total knees demonstrate a higher manipulation rate compared to "off-the-shelf implants". *J Arthroplasty.* 2016;31(1):107-111. doi:10.1016/j.arth.2015.07.041.

159. Talmo CT, Anderson MC, Jia ES, Robbins CE, Rand JD, McKeon BP. High rate of early revision after custom-made unicondylar knee arthroplasty. *J Arthroplasty.* 2018;33(7S):S100–S104. doi:10.1016/j.arth.2018.03.010.

160. Guenther D, Kendoff D, Omar M, et al. Total knee arthroplasty in patients with skeletal dysplasia. *Arch Orthop Trauma Surg.* 2015;135(8):1163-1167. doi:10.1007/s00402-015-2234-6.

161. Stanescu R, Stanescu V, Muriel MP, Maroteaux P. Multiple epiphyseal dysplasia, Fairbank type: morphologic and biochemical study of cartilage. *Am J Med Genet.* 1993;45(4):501-507. doi:10.1002/ajmg.1320450420.

162. Sewell MD, Hanna SA, Al-Khateeb H, et al. Custom rotating-hinge primary total knee arthroplasty in patients with skeletal dysplasia. *J Bone Joint Surg Br.* 2012;94(3):339-343. doi:10.1302/0301-620X.94B3.27892.

163. Kim RH, Scuderi GR, Dennis DA, Nakano SW. Technical challenges of total knee arthroplasty in skeletal dysplasia. *Clin Orthop.* 2011;469(1):69-75. doi:10.1007/s11999-010-1516-0.

164. Walter SG, Schwering T, Preiss S. Two-staged bilateral, femoral alignment osteotomy with concomitant total knee arthroplasty in an achondroplasia patient – a case report. *J Orthop Case Rep.* 2017;7(2):33-36. doi:10.13107/jocr.2250-0685.738.

165. de Waal Malefijt MC, van Kampen A, van Gemund JJ. Total knee arthroplasty in patients with inherited dwarfism–a report of five knee replacements in two patients with Morquio's disease type A and one with spondylo-epiphyseal dysplasia. *Arch Orthop Trauma Surg.* 2000;120(3-4):179-182.

166. Ling M, Wu X, Chang Y, et al. Staged total knee arthroplasty for bilateral complex knee deformities from Kashin-Beck disease and skeletal dysplasia. *Knee.* 2017;24(3):692-698. doi:10.1016/j.knee.2016.11.011.

167. Oh K-J, Yoon J-R, Yang J-H. Total knee arthroplasty in a pseudoachondroplastic dwarfism patient with bilateral patellar dislocation. *The Knee.* 2013;20(1):45-48. doi:10.1016/j.knee.2012.10.012.

168. Shirley ED, Ain MC. Achondroplasia: manifestations and treatment. *J Am Acad Orthop Surg.* 2009;17(4):231-241.

169. Jamil W, Allami MK, Mbakada N, Kluge W. Total knee arthroplasty in a patient with Hardcastle syndrome. *Orthopedics.* 2009;32(12):916. doi:10.3928/01477447-20091020-20.

170. Roberts TT, Cepela DJ, Uhl RL, Lozman J. Orthopaedic considerations for the adult with osteogenesis imperfecta. *J Am Acad Orthop Surg.* 2016;24(5):298-308. doi:10.5435/JAAOS-D-15-00275.

171. Nishimura A, Hasegawa M, Kato K, Fukuda A, Sudo A, Uchida A. Total knee arthroplasty in osteogenesis imperfecta: case report. *Knee.* 2008;15(6):494-496. doi:10.1016/j.knee.2008.07.005.

172. Ring D, Jupiter JB, Labropoulos PK, Guggenheim JJ, Stanitsky DF, Spencer DM. Treatment of deformity of the lower limb in adults who have osteogenesis imperfecta. *J Bone Joint Surg Am Vol.* 1996;78a(2):220-225. doi:10.2106/00004623-199602000-00008.

173. Wagner R, Luedke C. Total knee arthroplasty with concurrent femoral and tibial osteotomies in osteogenesis imperfecta. *Am J Orthop (Belle Mead NJ).* 2014;43(1):37-42.

174. Papagelopoulos PJ, Morrey BF. Hip and knee replacement in osteogenesis imperfecta. *J Bone Joint Surg Am Vol.* 1993;75(4):572-580.

Perioperative Management in Total Knee Replacement

JAMES I. HUDDLESTON III

chapter 48

Preoperative and Perioperative Medical Management

Vignesh K. Alamanda, MD | Bryan D. Springer, MD

This chapter acquaints the reader with an approach to the patient undergoing knee replacement and describes strategies for modifying both preoperative and perioperative risk factors that can help minimize the risk of periprosthetic joint infection.

SCOPE OF PROBLEM

Periprosthetic joint infection (PJI) remains a significant, expensive and morbid complication of total knee arthroplasty (TKA). It has a measurable impact on all parties involved including the patient, surgeon, as well as the healthcare system.[1] PJI is projected to have an economic burden in excess of 1.62 billion dollars by the year 2020.[2] This is especially important to address since estimates currently project large increases in demand for total knee arthroplasties. By the year 2030, the demand for total knee arthroplasties is projected to grow by 673%.[3] The demand for revisions will also follow a similar trend.[3]

The incidence of deep periprosthetic infection after primary total hip and knee replacements has been reported in the literature to range anywhere from 0.5% to 2%.[1,4] In examining total knee revision procedures, Bozic et al showed that infection was the leading cause of revisions comprising 25% of all failures in TKA.[5] Other studies have also reported infection to be an important reason for patients undergoing revision in the total knee population with rates ranging from 33% to 38%.[6,7] Kurtz et al have also shown that infection is on the rise as a reason for revisions and will continue to be the dominant reason for revisions.[8,9] The Centers for Disease Control and Prevention (CDC) provided new guidelines that had important updates and additional recommendations for the prevention of surgical site infections. However, as noted by Parvizi et al, the lack of evidence in many of the areas prevents it from being a comprehensive guide.[10]

Thus, it is important that we attempt to further understand and minimize the risk factors in both the preoperative and perioperative settings which can play a role in the development of PJI. In particular, modifiable risk factors from the patient perspective can help with decreasing the overall risk of developing a PJI.

PATIENT MODIFIABLE RISK FACTORS

Diabetes Mellitus

Diabetes has been associated with increased risk of surgical site infection in a variety of surgical procedures.[11,12] Additionally, the incidence of diabetes is continuing to rise in the United States.[13] Diabetes has been shown to be a positive predictor of PJI in multiple studies. Analysis of these studies has shown diabetes to increase the odds ratio by 2.28 times in one of the largest series (Table 48-1).

Hemoglobin A1c (Hgb A1c) is frequently used as a marker of long-term glycemic control and may take 3 months to change. Patients with optimal glycemic control should have Hgb A1C levels less than 7.0. Hgb A1c has frequently been used a routine screening test as it is a simple test which allows the provider to gain insight of the patient's glycemic control over the past 3 months.[21,22] However, it appears that perioperative glucose levels have an increased ability to predict PJI as opposed to Hgb A1c alone.[23,24]

Surgical stress increases the production of hormones that antagonize insulin and predisposes patients to hyperglycemia. In particular, perioperative glycemic control needs to be strictly enforced as surgical stress–related postoperative hyperglycemia, even in patients without a diagnosis of diabetes, has been found to be an independent risk factor for the development of surgical site

TABLE 48-1 Diabetes and Periprosthetic Joint Infection

Authors	Sample Size	OR (Confidence Interval)
Jamsen et al[14]	7181	2.3 (1.1-4.7)
Wu et al[15]	297	5.47 (1.77-16.97)
Lee et al[16]	1133	6.07 (1.43-25.75)
Bozic et al[17]	8301	1.19 (1.06-1.34)
Yang et al[18]	110, 923	1.61 (1.38-1.88)
Kunutsor et al[19]	512,508	1.74 (1.45-2.09)
Marchant et al[20]	751, 340	2.28 (1.36-3.81)
Stryker et al[21]	1702	3.75 (1.25-11.22)

infection in a dose-related relationship.[25-27] Thus, it is recommended that blood glucose levels be maintained between 110 and 180 mg/dL in the perioperative period to help minimize the risks associated with hyperglycemia. This can be achieved with frequent blood sugar checks and initiation of diabetic management protocols in the postoperative period. Alternatively, other markers such as serum fructosamine have also been proposed to serve as an adjunct to measuring glycemic control.[28]

Obesity

Similar to diabetes, the prevalence of obesity has also significantly increased. Obesity has been shown to significantly contribute to a higher rate of osteoarthritis and eventual increased use of arthroplasty.[29] While studies have shown that patient satisfaction and functional improvement in the obese patient population are similar to the nonobese group, obese patients are, nonetheless, at higher risk of postoperative complications, specifically PJI.[30] Multiple studies have correlated increased body mass index (BMI) with increased rates of wound infection[31-33] (Table 48-2).

Obesity predisposes patients to higher surgical times with increased surgical dissections needed to gain exposure. Additionally, the poor vascularization of adipose tissue further compounds this problem. A workgroup of the American Association of Hip and Knee Surgeons (AAHKS) evidence-based committee came up with a consensus opinion that consideration should be given to delaying total joint arthroplasty in a patient with a BMI > 40, especially when associated with other comorbid conditions, such as poorly controlled diabetes or malnutrition.[29]

Additionally, surgeons should also have an index of suspicion for metabolic syndrome in those with obesity. Metabolic syndrome is composed of a cluster of conditions arising from insulin resistance that impairs normal leukocyte function. It is defined as having a BMI >30 kg/m^2 with central obesity, as well as two of the following: hyperlipidemia, hyperglyceridemia, hypertension, or diabetes.[38] Zmistowski et al have shown increased risk of PJI (14.3% vs. 0.8%) in those with uncontrolled metabolic syndrome compared to those with controlled disease/healthy cohort.[39] Thus, patients with obesity should also be screened to ensure that they do not have other features that define metabolic syndrome. Patients with obesity or metabolic syndrome should have their elective TKA delayed till their BMI <40 and should be directed appropriately such as being referred to a dietician in order to accomplish that goal.

Malnutrition

An often underappreciated facet of obesity involves malnutrition or so-called paradoxical malnutrition in obese patients that have high-caloric but nutritionally poor diets. A prospective study evaluating the role of malnutrition in total joint arthroplasty found that malnutrition was present in 42.9% of obese patients.[40] Additionally, the geriatric population, patients with gastrointestinal problems, patients with a history of alcohol abuse, and those with cancer are also at increased risk of malnutrition. Multiple studies have implicated malnutrition as a contributing factor in increasing the risk of a PJI.[41,42] Specifically, patients with malnutrition were found to have five to seven times greater risk of developing a major wound complication.[43] Malnutrition has also been associated with increased risks of infection after undergoing revision total joint arthroplasty.[44] Similarly, Bohl et al have also reported increased odds of PJI for patients with malnutrition.[45]

Simple and immediately available laboratory tests can help to identify patients at risk for malnutrition. These include a total lymphocyte count of less than 1500 cells/mm^3, a serum albumin of less than 3.5 g/dL, or a transferrin level of less than 200 mg/dL.[41] Patients with preoperative malnutrition should be encouraged to work with a dietician to improve their nutritional intake and help prepare them for the catabolic demands required in the postsurgical period.

Smoking

Smoking, and its primary offending component, nicotine, has been associated with microvascular constriction and decreased oxygen delivery to tissues.[46,47] In particular when analyzing the effects of smoking on total joint arthroplasty, Duchman et al reported increased risk of wound complication with both current as well as former smokers in a large national database study with current smokers having higher rate of wound complications than former smokers.[48,49] Additional studies have also corroborated the deleterious effects of smoking as it pertains to PJI[50] (Table 48-3).

It has been shown that a smoking cessation program can help decrease complications associated with the use of nicotine even if it is introduced as late as 4 weeks before

TABLE 48-2	Obesity and Periprosthetic Joint Infection	
Authors	**Sample Size**	**OR (Confidence Interval)**
Kunutsor et al[19]	512,508	3.68 (2.25-6.01)
Jamsen et al[14]	7181	6.4 (1.7-24.6)
Everhart et al[34]	1, 875	5.28 (1.38-17.1)
Maoz et al[35]	4078	4.13 (1.3-12.88)
Jung et al[36]	9, 481	1.94 (0.63-5.70)
George et al[37]	150,934	2.14 (1.48-3.1)

TABLE 48-3 Smoking and Periprosthetic Joint Infection		
Authors	Sample Size	OR (Confidence Interval)
Singh et al[51]	33, 336	1.41(1.16-1.72)
Singh[52]	1185	3.42 (0.69-16.85)
Duchman et al[48]	78,191	1.47 (1.21-1.78)
Teng et al[50]	8,181	3.71 (1.86-7.41)

TABLE 48-4 *Staphylococcus aureus* Screening and Reduction in Periprosthetic Joint Infection		
Authors	Sample Size	RR (Confidence Interval)
Baratz et al[62]	3434	0.74 (0.44-1.21)
Gottschalk et al[63]	178	0.14(0.03-0.65)
Hacek et al[64]	1495	0.45(0.17-1.17)
Hadley et al[65]	2058	0.88(0.36-2.17)
Lamplot et al[66]	1224	0.22(0.08-0.63)
McDonald et al[67]	305	0.36(0.08-1.59)
Rao et al[61]	2071	0.52 (0.24-1.14)
Rao et al[68]	3346	1.59 (0.83-3.05)
Sankar et al[69]	395	0.24(0.01-5.79)
Schweizer et al[70]	43, 087	0.48 (0.28-0.82)

surgery.[53] Thus, it is our recommendation that patient undergoing total joint arthroplasty has a minimum period of 4 weeks of smoking cessation prior to their surgery. Smoking cessation can be confirmed via easily available laboratory test, the serum cotinine assay (normal value of ≤10 ng/d).[54]

Vitamin D

Vitamin D, as measured by serum 25-hydroxyvitamin D, has long been known to play a crucial role in bone hemostasis.[55] Vitamin D deficiency, defined by a serum 25-hydroxyvitamin D concentration ≤20 ng/mL), is unfortunately quite common in the US population with an overall prevalence reported at 41.6%.[56] Studies have shown vitamin D levels to be severely low in patients with PJI.[57,58] Animal models have also shown that while deficiency of vitamin D results in increased risk of PJI, this can be reversed with preoperative repletion.[58]

Studies have shown vitamin D levels to be severely low in patients with PJI.[57,58] New mice data seem to suggest that restoring vitamin D levels can improve periprosthetic infection rates in a mice model study.[58] Thus, it is our recommendation that vitamin D levels be obtained preoperatively and if deficient, <20 ng/mL, supplementation be instituted.

Staphylococcus Aureus Screening

The prevalence of *Staphylococcus aureus* and methicillin-resistant *Staphylococcus aureus* (MRSA) colonization in patients admitted to hospitals is increasing.[59] Nasal swab rapid polymerase chain reaction has allowed physicians to identify patients who are colonized. This allows for the elimination of the bacteria from the patient's nasal flora prior to surgery. Kim et al have found that implementing an institution-wide prescreening program allows for the identification of carrier status of *Staphylococcus aureus* among patients and leads to significant reduction in postoperative rates of surgical site infections.[60] Similarly, Rao et al noted that implementation of an institutional decolonization protocol helped to decrease overall infection rate and resulted in significant economic gains for the hospital[61] (**Table 48-4**).

It is our recommendation that patients undergoing elective total joint arthroplasty undergo screening for *S. aureus* through nasal swabs. If they are positive, we recommend that they undergo application of mupirocin nasal ointment twice daily to both nares and bathe with chlorhexidine daily for 5 days immediately prior to the scheduled surgery. In addition, patients who screen positive for MRSA should also receive a single dose of vancomycin along with standard perioperative antibiotics. Patients can also be treated prophylactically with routine nasal decolonization protocol as an alternative to routine screening. Several options exist including application of mupirocin as noted above, as well as the use of povidone-iodine and chlorohexidine and alcohol-based solution.[71,72] The use of alcohol-based and povidone-iodine agents also has the added advantage of preventing antibiotic resistance and shorter duration of administration.[10]

Inflammatory Arthropathies

Patients with inflammatory arthropathies such as rheumatoid arthritis or systemic lupus erythematosus are often at increased risk of postoperative infection.[73,74] Multiple systematic reviews have been performed by other authors which appear to confirm the correlation between inflammatory arthropathies such as rheumatoid arthritis and periprosthetic infection. Setor et al pooled 13 studies involving 177, 618 patients and showed that rheumatoid arthritis increases the relative risk of PJI by 1.70 (95% confidence interval 1.37, 2.11).[19] Similarly, Kong et al also pooled 12 studies to show that rheumatoid arthritis increases the odds of PJI by 1.57.[75] Many of these patients are on complex drug regimen that includes a variety of immunomodulators. These medications often have deleterious effects on wound healing and infections. For example, tumor necrosis factor (TNF) alpha inhibitors are tremendously helpful adjuncts in the management of these diseases. However, they place patients at significant risk for developing opportunistic infections. Momohara et al reported patients on TNF alpha inhibitors to be at higher risk for surgical site infections.[76]

A recent guideline published jointly by the American College of Rheumatology and American Association of Hip and Knee Surgeons used available evidence to make recommendation on which medications should be stopped in elective total joint arthroplasty and if withheld, when they should be restarted.[77] In general, traditional disease-modifying antirheumatic medications (DMARDs) such as methotrexate, do not need to be withheld prior to surgery. Biologicals, however, place patients at increased risk for development of PJI and should be withheld one dosing cycle prior to surgery. The medication can be restarted following surgery once surgical wounds have healed and in the absence of signs of infection.

Urinary Tract Infection

A common nosocombial infection, urinary tract infections (UTIs), creates a reservoir of pathogens and potentially increases patient morbidity during surgical intervention. The role of UTI in the development of PJI, however, remains controversial. Some authors have noted the development of PJI in patients with UTI,[78] while others have shown no association between UTI and PJI.[79]

It is our recommendation that if the patient has symptoms of UTI such as dysuria, urgency, frequency, etc and has more than 1×10^5 colony forming units (CFUs)/mL of urine, surgery should be postponed. However, if the patient is asymptomatic but has 1×10^5 or more CFU/mL of urine, we recommend not withholding surgery and treating their UTI with a routine course of postoperative oral antibiotic.

Poor Oral Health

Total joint replacement patients tend to have good dental hygiene in general.[80] However, there is not a lot of literature on the role of preoperative screening as well as the association between poor dental hygiene and PJI. Recent studies have questioned the need to obtain routine preoperative dental screening for hip and knee arthroplasty patients.[81] In general, we recommend a common-sense approach—patients should have a dental exam and clearance if they have evidence of decayed teeth, abscess, gingivitis, or periodontitis and should have routine cleanings done prior to surgical intervention.

PERIOPERATIVE MODIFIABLE RISK FACTORS

Surgical Site Preparation and Irrigant Options

Current evidence recommends the use of chlorhexidine gluconate–based solutions for surgical site preparations, and it has been found to be superior to the use

of iodophor-based solutions as well as other ion-based solution at reducing the burden of microbes at the surgical site. Chlorhexidine gluconate acts by disrupting the cellular membranes of bacteria and is longer acting than iodophors. While chlorhexidine gluconate and povidone-iodine both reduce bacterial counts on contact, the effect is much longer with chlorhexidine.[82,83] Additionally, iodophors can be inactivated by serum proteins and should be allowed to dry in order to maximize their antimicrobial action.[82] Alcohol is also a potent antimicrobial. However, it lacks residual activity after application. Chlorohexidine has also been used in the preoperative setting to help further decrease rates of PJI. In a randomized clinical trial performed by Kapadia et al, the use of chlorohexidine-impregnated cloth the night before and morning of surgery was found to decrease rate of PJI as compared to the control cohort of soap and water.[84,85] Similar results were also reported by Zywiel et al.[86]

The use of various irrigants has also been explored to help with reduction in PJI. Brown et al have reported significant improvements in rates of infection after incorporating dilute betadine lavage before closure.[87] Dilute betadine is now being used in multiple protocols to help in the reduction of PJI.[88] Frisch et al compared the use of intraoperative dilute chlorhexidine with the use of dilute betadine and found similar results in helping minimize PJI.[89] Chlorhexidine irrigation with concentrations as low as 2% has also been found to be effective at treating MRSA biofilm.[90]

Our recommendation is the use of a combination agent that involves both chlorhexidine gluconate as well as isopropyl alcohol. Hair removal is another facet of surgical site preparation that can potentially play a role in increasing surgical site infections. We recommend that hair removal be minimized and if necessary that electric clippers be used rather than shavers in accordance with the CDC guidelines.[91]

Based on the current literature available, we recommend the use of either dilute betadine lavage or chlorhexidine lavage at the conclusion of the procedure. If using betadine, we recommend diluting approximately 17.5 mL of 10% sterile povidone-iodine with 500 cc of normal saline to generate a 3.5% solution and to irrigate the wound with this solution for 3 minutes. The wound is to be then thoroughly irrigated with normal saline prior to wound closure. Interestingly, recent retrospective reports have shown no significant advantage in reducing PJI with the use of betadine lavage in primary or revision arthroplasty.[92,93] However, these preliminary results will have to be confirmed through large-scale, prospective, randomized studies.

Antibiotic Prophylaxis

Preoperative antibiotic prophylaxis is effective in reducing rates of surgical site infections and has been incorporated in many surgical checklists.[47] Routine prophylactic antibiotics should be dosed in accordance with the patient's weight and should include a first-generation cephalosporin such as cefazolin. Patients allergic to beta-lactam antibiotic should receive vancomycin or clindamycin in a timely fashion. Prophylactic antibiotics should be administered ideally as close to the time of the incision as possible. First-generation cephalosporin and clindamycin should be administered within 1 hour and vancomycin should be administered within 2 hours of incision. We recommend that a single dose of vancomycin be considered in addition to standard preoperative antibiotics for those who have been shown to be colonized with MRSA or those who had a prior infection with MRSA.

Administration of preoperative antibiotic prophylaxis is effective in reducing rates of surgical site infections.[94] Routine prophylactic antibiotics, dosed in accordance with the patient's weight, should include a first-generation cephalosporin such as cefazolin. Patients who are allergic to beta-lactam antibiotic should receive clindamycin or vancomycin. However, timing is also equally important as the choice of antibiotic. Prophylactic antibiotics should be administered ideally as near to the time of the incision as possible, but within 60 minutes prior to the incision for a first-generation cephalosporin or clindamycin and within 2 hours of incision for vancomycin. We recommend that vancomycin be considered for those who have been shown to be colonized with MRSA or those who had a prior infection with MRSA. Additionally, we recommend that antibiotics be discontinued within 24 hours after the surgical procedure.

Operating Room Environment

Several operating room variables have been studied to see if rates of infection could be decreased in total joint replacement patients. These include the use of ultraviolet light, laminar flow, body exhaust suits, etc. However, maintaining a disciplined operating room by limiting operating room traffic has been shown to decrease the rate of surgical site infections.[95,96] Thus, it is crucial that traffic into and out of the operating room through both the sterile core as well as the common corridor be limited during arthroplasty procedures to decrease the risk of surgical site infections.

It is imperative that traffic into and out of the operating be limited during arthroplasty procedures to decrease the risk of surgical site infections. Multiple studies have strongly correlated the operating room microbial load with movement and number of personnel in the operating room.[97-99]

Avoidance of Aggressive Anticoagulation

Aggressive anticoagulation in the postoperative period can lead to bleeding and hematoma formation in the postoperative period at the surgical site. Hemarthrosis in the immediate postsurgical period provides an excellent culture media for potential growth of bacteria.[100] De Jong et al have shown that hematoma formation following hemiarthroplasty for

femoral neck fracture leads to increased odds of developing a PJI.[101] Huang et al, likewise, have shown up to a 13.7 times increase in the odds of developing PJI with administration of warfarin as compared to the administration of aspirin for venous thromboembolism (VTE) prophylaxis.[102] Systematic reviews have evaluated the role of aspirin as a suitable agent for VTE prophylaxis due to its low cost and suitable risk profile.[103] Parvizi et al have also shown noninferiority of low-dose aspirin for VTE prophylaxis as compared to high-dose aspirin.[104]

Aggressive anticoagulation can lead to postoperative hemarthrosis that can increase the risk of developing PJI as well as wound complications. Multiple studies have shown aspirin to be a safe and effective agent for VTE prophylaxis with a favorable risk profile.[105] It is our recommendation that aggressive anticoagulation be avoided expect in at-risk patients and that low-dose aspirin be instituted for patients undergoing routine arthroplasty.

CONCLUSION

While PJI may not be completely eliminated in the coming years, surgeons should make use of available evidence-based guidelines, such as the ones proposed above, to help improve patient and perioperative modifiable risk factors to minimize risk of PJI. This can ensure that patients are in optimal medical condition prior to undergoing their proposed surgery.

REFERENCES

1. Bozic KJ, Ries MD. The impact of infection after total hip arthroplasty on hospital and surgeon resource utilization. *J Bone Joint Surg Am.* 2005;87(8):1746-1751.
2. Kurtz SM, Lau E, Watson H, Schmier JK, Parvizi J. Economic burden of periprosthetic joint infection in the United States. *J Arthroplasty.* 2012;27(8 suppl):61-65.e1.
3. Kurtz S, Ong K, Lau E, Mowat F, Halpern M. Projections of primary and revision hip and knee arthroplasty in the United States from 2005 to 2030. *J Bone Joint Surg Am.* 2007;89(4):780-785.
4. Sculco TP. The economic impact of infected total joint arthroplasty. *Instr Course Lect.* 1993;42:349-351.
5. Bozic KJ, Kurtz SM, Lau E, et al. The epidemiology of revision total knee arthroplasty in the United States. *Clin Orthop Relat Res.* 2010;468(1):45-51.
6. Fehring TK, Odum S, Griffin WL, Mason JB, Nadaud M. Early failures in total knee arthroplasty. *Clin Orthop Relat Res.* 2001;392:315-318.
7. Vessely MB, Whaley AL, Harmsen WS, Schleck CD, Berry DJ. The Chitranjan Ranawat Award: long-term survivorship and failure modes of 1000 cemented condylar total knee arthroplasties. *Clin Orthop Relat Res.* 2006;452:28-34.
8. Kurtz SM, Lau E, Schmier J, Ong KL, Zhao K, Parvizi J. Infection burden for hip and knee arthroplasty in the United States. *J Arthroplasty.* 2008;23(7):984-991.
9. Kurtz SM, Ong KL, Lau E, Bozic KJ, Berry D, Parvizi J. Prosthetic joint infection risk after TKA in the Medicare population. *Clin Orthop Relat Res.* 2010;468(1):52-56.
10. Parvizi J, Shohat N, Gehrke T. Prevention of periprosthetic joint infection: new guidelines. *Bone Joint J.* 2017;99-B(4 suppl B):3-10.
11. Golden SH, Peart-Vigilance C, Kao WH, Brancati FL. Perioperative glycemic control and the risk of infectious complications in a cohort of adults with diabetes. *Diabetes Care.* 1999;22(9):1408-1414.

12. Dryden M, Baguneid M, Eckmann C, et al. Pathophysiology and burden of infection in patients with diabetes mellitus and peripheral vascular disease: focus on skin and soft-tissue infections. *Clin Microbiol Infect.* 2015;21(suppl 2):S27-S32.

13. Klonoff DC. The increasing incidence of diabetes in the 21st century. *J Diabetes Sci Technol.* 2009;3(1):1-2.

14. Jamsen E, Nevalainen P, Eskelinen A, Huotari K, Kalliovalkama J, Moilanen T. Obesity, diabetes, and preoperative hyperglycemia as predictors of periprosthetic joint infection: a single-center analysis of 7181 primary hip and knee replacements for osteoarthritis. *J Bone Joint Surg Am.* 2012;94(14):e101.

15. Wu C, Qu X, Liu F, Li H, Mao Y, Zhu Z. Risk factors for periprosthetic joint infection after total hip arthroplasty and total knee arthroplasty in Chinese patients. *PLoS One.* 2014;9(4):e95300.

16. Lee QJ, Mak WP, Wong YC. Risk factors for periprosthetic joint infection in total knee arthroplasty. *J Orthop Surg.* 2015;23(3):282-286.

17. Bozic KJ, Lau E, Kurtz S, Ong K, Berry DJ. Patient-related risk factors for postoperative mortality and periprosthetic joint infection in medicare patients undergoing TKA. *Clin Orthop Relat Res.* 2012;470(1):130-137.

18. Yang Z, Liu H, Xie X, Tan Z, Qin T, Kang P. The influence of diabetes mellitus on the post-operative outcome of elective primary total knee replacement: a systematic review and meta-analysis. *Bone Joint J.* 2014;96-B(12):1637-1643.

19. Kunutsor SK, Whitehouse MR, Blom AW, Beswick AD, Team I. Patient-related risk factors for periprosthetic joint infection after total joint arthroplasty: a systematic review and meta-analysis. *PLoS One.* 2016;11(3):e0150866.

20. Marchant MH Jr, Viens NA, Cook C, Vail TP, Bolognesi MP. The impact of glycemic control and diabetes mellitus on perioperative outcomes after total joint arthroplasty. *J Bone Joint Surg Am.* 2009;91(7):1621-1629.

21. Stryker LS, Abdel MP, Morrey ME, Morrow MM, Kor DJ, Morrey BF. Elevated postoperative blood glucose and preoperative hemoglobin A1C are associated with increased wound complications following total joint arthroplasty. *J Bone Joint Surg Am.* 2013;95(9):808-814,S1-2.

22. Dronge AS, Perkal MF, Kancir S, Concato J, Aslan M, Rosenthal RA. Long-term glycemic control and postoperative infectious complications. *Arch Surg.* 2006;141(4):375-380; discussion 80.

23. Iorio R, Williams KM, Marcantonio AJ, Specht LM, Tilzey JF, Healy WL. Diabetes mellitus, hemoglobin A1C, and the incidence of total joint arthroplasty infection. *J Arthroplasty.* 2012;27(5):726-729.e1.

24. Chrastil J, Anderson MB, Stevens V, Anand R, Peters CL, Pelt CE. Is hemoglobin A1c or perioperative hyperglycemia predictive of periprosthetic joint infection or death following primary total joint arthroplasty? *J Arthroplasty.* 2015;30(7):1197-1202.

25. Latham R, Lancaster AD, Covington JF, Pirolo JS, Thomas CS Jr. The association of diabetes and glucose control with surgical-site infections among cardiothoracic surgery patients. *Infect Control Hosp Epidemiol.* 2001;22(10):607-612.

26. Richards JE, Kauffmann RM, Obremskey WT, May AK. Stress-induced hyperglycemia as a risk factor for surgical-site infection in nondiabetic orthopedic trauma patients admitted to the intensive care unit. *J Orthop Trauma.* 2013;27(1):16-21.

27. Ata A, Lee J, Bestle SL, Desemone J, Stain SC. Postoperative hyperglycemia and surgical site infection in general surgery patients. *Arch Surg.* 2010;145(9):858-864.

28. Shohat N, Tarabichi M, Tischler EH, Jabbour S, Parvizi J. Serum fructosamine: a simple and inexpensive test for assessing preoperative glycemic control. *J Bone Joint Surg Am.* 2017;99(22):1900-1907.

29. Workgroup of the American Association of Hip and Knee Surgeons Evidence Based Committee. Obesity and total joint arthroplasty: a literature based review. *J Arthroplasty.* 2013;28(5):714-721.

30. Mason JB, Callaghan JJ, Hozack WJ, Krebs V, Mont MA, Parvizi J. Obesity in total joint arthroplasty: an issue with gravity. *J Arthroplasty.* 2014;29(10):1879.

31. Malinzak RA, Ritter MA, Berend ME, Meding JB, Olberding EM, Davis KE. Morbidly obese, diabetic, younger, and unilateral joint arthroplasty patients have elevated total joint arthroplasty infection rates. *J Arthroplasty.* 2009;24(6 suppl):84-88.

32. Winiarsky R, Barth P, Lotke P. Total knee arthroplasty in morbidly obese patients. *J Bone Joint Surg Am.* 1998;80(12):1770-1774.

33. Olsen LL, Moller AM, Brorson S, Hasselager RB, Sort R. The impact of lifestyle risk factors on the rate of infection after surgery for a fracture of the ankle. *Bone Joint J.* 2017;99-B(2):225-230.

34. Everhart JS, Altneu E, Calhoun JH. Medical comorbidities are independent preoperative risk factors for surgical infection after total joint arthroplasty. *Clin Orthop Relat Res.* 2013;471(10):3112-3119.

35. Maoz G, Phillips M, Bosco J, et al. The Otto Aufranc Award: modifiable versus nonmodifiable risk factors for infection after hip arthroplasty. *Clin Orthop Relat Res.* 2015;473(2):453-459.

36. Jung P, Morris AJ, Zhu M, Roberts SA, Frampton C, Young SW. BMI is a key risk factor for early periprosthetic joint infection following total hip and knee arthroplasty. *N Z Med J.* 2017;130(1461):24-34.

37. George J, Piuzzi NS, Ng M, Sodhi N, Khlopas AA, Mont MA. Association between body mass index and thirty-day complications after total knee arthroplasty. *J Arthroplasty.* 2018;33(3):865-871.

38. Gage MJ, Schwarzkopf R, Abrouk M, Slover JD. Impact of metabolic syndrome on perioperative complication rates after total joint arthroplasty surgery. *J Arthroplasty.* 2014;29(9):1842-1845.

39. Zmistowski B, Dizdarevic I, Jacovides CL, Radcliff KE, Mraovic B, Parvizi J. Patients with uncontrolled components of metabolic syndrome have increased risk of complications following total joint arthroplasty. *J Arthroplasty.* 2013;28(6):904-907.

40. Huang R, Greenky M, Kerr GJ, Austin MS, Parvizi J. The effect of malnutrition on patients undergoing elective joint arthroplasty. *J Arthroplasty.* 2013;28(8 suppl):21-24.

41. Ellsworth B, Kamath AF. Malnutrition and total joint arthroplasty. *J Nat Sci.* 2016;2(3):e179.

42. Courtney PM, Rozell JC, Melnic CM, Sheth NP, Nelson CL. Effect of malnutrition and morbid obesity on complication rates following primary total joint arthroplasty. *J Surg Orthop Adv.* 2016;25(2):99-104.

43. Greene KA, Wilde AH, Stulberg BN. Preoperative nutritional status of total joint patients. Relationship to postoperative wound complications. *J Arthroplasty.* 1991;6(4):321-325.

44. Yi PH, Frank RM, Vann E, Sonn KA, Moric M, Della Valle CJ. Is potential malnutrition associated with septic failure and acute infection after revision total joint arthroplasty? *Clin Orthop Relat Res.* 2015;473(1):175-182.

45. Bohl DD, Shen MR, Kayupov E, Cvetanovich GL, Della Valle CJ. Is hypoalbuminemia associated with septic failure and acute infection after revision total joint arthroplasty? A study of 4517 patients from the National Surgical Quality Improvement Program. *J Arthroplasty.* 2016;31(5):963-967.

46. Moller AM, Pedersen T, Villebro N, Munksgaard A. Effect of smoking on early complications after elective orthopaedic surgery. *J Bone Joint Surg Br.* 2003;85(2):178-181.

47. Sorensen LT, Jorgensen S, Petersen LJ, et al. Acute effects of nicotine and smoking on blood flow, tissue oxygen, and aerobe metabolism of the skin and subcutis. *J Surg Res.* 2009;152(2):224-230.

48. Duchman KR, Gao Y, Pugely AJ, Martin CT, Noiseux NO, Callaghan JJ. The effect of smoking on short-term complications following total hip and knee arthroplasty. *J Bone Joint Surg Am.* 2015;97(13):1049-1058.

49. Cherian JJ, Mont MA. Where There Is Smoke, There Is Fire! Commentary on an article by Kyle R. Duchman, MD, et al.: "The effect of smoking on short-term complications following total hip and knee arthroplasty". *J Bone Joint Surg Am.* 2015;97(13):e53.

50. Teng S, Yi C, Krettek C, Jagodzinski M. Smoking and risk of prosthesis-related complications after total hip arthroplasty: a meta-analysis of cohort studies. *PLoS One.* 2015;10(4):e0125294.

51. Singh JA, Houston TK, Ponce BA, et al. Smoking as a risk factor for short-term outcomes following primary total hip and total knee replacement in veterans. *Arthritis Care Res.* 2011;63(10):1365-1374.

52. Singh JA. Smoking and outcomes after knee and hip arthroplasty: a systematic review. *J Rheumatol.* 2011;38(9):1824-1834.

53. Lindstrom D, Sadr Azodi O, Wladis A, et al. Effects of a perioperative smoking cessation intervention on postoperative complications: a randomized trial. *Ann Surg.* 2008;248(5):739-745.

54. Pirkle JL, Flegal KM, Bernert JT, Brody DJ, Etzel RA, Maurer KR. Exposure of the US population to environmental tobacco smoke: the Third national health and nutrition Examination survey, 1988 to 1991. *J Am Med Assoc.* 1996;275(16):1233-1240.

55. St-Arnaud R. The direct role of vitamin D on bone homeostasis. *Arch Biochem Biophys.* 2008;473(2):225-230.

56. Forrest KY, Stuhldreher WL. Prevalence and correlates of vitamin D deficiency in US adults. *Nutr Res.* 2011;31(1):48-54.

57. Maier GS, Horas K, Seeger JB, Roth KE, Kurth AA, Maus U. Is there an association between periprosthetic joint infection and low vitamin D levels? *Int Orthop.* 2014;38(7):1499-1504.

58. Hegde V, Dworsky EM, Stavrakis AI, et al. Single-dose, preoperative vitamin-D supplementation decreases infection in a mouse model of periprosthetic joint infection. *J Bone Joint Surg Am.* 2017;99(20):1737-1744.

59. Goyal N, Aggarwal V, Parvizi J. Methicillin-resistant Staphylococcus aureus screening in total joint arthroplasty: a worthwhile endeavor. *J Knee Surg.* 2012;25(1):37-43.

60. Kim DH, Spencer M, Davidson SM, et al. Institutional prescreening for detection and eradication of methicillin-resistant *Staphylococcus aureus* in patients undergoing elective orthopaedic surgery. *J Bone Joint Surg Am.* 2010;92(9):1820-1826.

61. Rao N, Cannella B, Crossett LS, Yates AJ Jr, McGough R III. A preoperative decolonization protocol for staphylococcus aureus prevents orthopaedic infections. *Clin Orthop Relat Res.* 2008;466(6):1343-1348.

62. Baratz MD, Hallmark R, Odum SM, Springer BD. Twenty percent of patients may remain colonized with methicillin-resistant *Staphylococcus aureus* despite a decolonization protocol in patients undergoing elective total joint arthroplasty. *Clin Orthop Relat Res.* 2015;473(7):2283-2290.

63. Gottschalk MB, Johnson JP, Sadlack CK, Mitchell PM. Decreased infection rates following total joint arthroplasty in a large county run teaching hospital: a single surgeon's experience and possible solution. *J Arthroplasty.* 2014;29(8):1610-1616.

64. Hacek DM, Robb WJ, Paule SM, Kudrna JC, Stamos VP, Peterson LR. *Staphylococcus aureus* nasal decolonization in joint replacement surgery reduces infection. *Clin Orthop Relat Res.* 2008;466(6):1349-1355.

65. Hadley S, Immerman I, Hutzler L, Slover J, Bosco J. *Staphylococcus aureus* decolonization protocol decreases surgical site infections for total joint replacement. *Arthritis.* 2010;2010:924518.

66. Lamplot JD, Luther G, Mawdsley EL, Luu HH, Manning D. Modified protocol decreases surgical site infections after total knee arthroplasty. *J Knee Surg.* 2015;28(5):395-403.

67. McDonald LT, Clark AM, Landauer AK, Kuxhaus L. Winning the war on surgical site infection: evidence-based preoperative interventions for total joint arthroplasty. *AORN J.* 2015;102(2):182.e1-182.e11.

68. Rao N, Cannella BA, Crossett LS, Yates AJ Jr, McGough RL III, Hamilton CW. Preoperative screening/decolonization for Staphylococcus aureus to prevent orthopedic surgical site infection: prospective cohort study with 2-year follow-up. *J Arthroplasty.* 2011;26(8):1501-1507.

69. Sankar B, Hopgood P, Bell KM. The role of MRSA screening in joint-replacement surgery. *Int Orthop.* 2005;29(3):160-163.

70. Schweizer ML, Chiang HY, Septimus E, et al. Association of a bundled intervention with surgical site infections among patients undergoing cardiac, hip, or knee surgery. *J Am Med Assoc.* 2015;313(21):2162-2171.

71. Steed LL, Costello J, Lohia S, Jones T, Spannhake EW, Nguyen S. Reduction of nasal *Staphylococcus aureus* carriage in health care professionals by treatment with a nonantibiotic, alcohol-based nasal antiseptic. *Am J Infect Control.* 2014;42(8):841-846.

72. Anderson MJ, David ML, Scholz M, et al. Efficacy of skin and nasal povidone-iodine preparation against mupirocin-resistant methicillin-resistant *Staphylococcus aureus* and *S. aureus* within the anterior nares. *Antimicrob Agents Chemother.* 2015;59(5):2765-2773.

73. Ravi B, Croxford R, Hollands S, et al. Increased risk of complications following total joint arthroplasty in patients with rheumatoid arthritis. *Arthritis Rheumatol.* 2014;66(2):254-263.

74. Ravi B, Escott B, Shah PS, et al. A systematic review and meta-analysis comparing complications following total joint arthroplasty for rheumatoid arthritis versus for osteoarthritis. *Arthritis Rheum.* 2012;64(12):3839-3849.

75. Kong L, Cao J, Zhang Y, Ding W, Shen Y. Risk factors for periprosthetic joint infection following primary total hip or knee arthroplasty: a meta-analysis. *Int Wound J.* 2017;14(3):529-536.

76. Momohara S, Kawakami K, Iwamoto T, et al. Prosthetic joint infection after total hip or knee arthroplasty in rheumatoid arthritis patients treated with nonbiologic and biologic disease-modifying antirheumatic drugs. *Mod Rheumatol.* 2011;21(5):469-475.

77. Goodman SM, Springer B, Guyatt G, et al. 2017 American College of Rheumatology/American Association of Hip and Knee Surgeons guideline for the perioperative management of antirheumatic medication in patients with rheumatic diseases undergoing elective total hip or total knee arthroplasty. *J Arthroplasty.* 2017;32(9):2628-2638.

78. David TS, Vrahas MS. Perioperative lower urinary tract infections and deep sepsis in patients undergoing total joint arthroplasty. *J Am Acad Orthop Surg.* 2000;8(1):66-74.

79. Koulouvaris P, Sculco P, Finerty E, Sculco T, Sharrock NE. Relationship between perioperative urinary tract infection and deep infection after joint arthroplasty. *Clin Orthop Relat Res.* 2009;467(7):1859-1867.

80. Wood TJ, Petruccelli D, Piccirillo L, Staibano P, Winemaker M, de Beer J. Dental hygiene in maintaining a healthy joint replacement: a survey of Canadian total joint replacement patients. *Curr Orthop Pract.* 2016;27(5):515-519.

81. Lampley A, Huang RC, Arnold WV, Parvizi J. Total joint arthroplasty: should patients have preoperative dental clearance? *J Arthroplasty.* 2014;29(6):1087-1090.

82. Fletcher N, Sofianos D, Berkes MB, Obremskey WT. Prevention of perioperative infection. *J Bone Joint Surg Am.* 2007;89(7):1605-1618.

83. Bosco JA III, Slover JD, Haas JP. Perioperative strategies for decreasing infection: a comprehensive evidence-based approach. *J Bone Joint Surg Am.* 2010;92(1):232-239.

84. Kapadia BH, Elmallah RK, Mont MA. A randomized, clinical trial of preadmission chlorhexidine skin preparation for lower extremity total joint arthroplasty. *J Arthroplasty.* 2016;31(12):2856-2861.

85. Kapadia BH, Jauregui JJ, Murray DP, Mont MA. Does preadmission cutaneous chlorhexidine preparation reduce surgical site infections after total hip arthroplasty? *Clin Orthop Relat Res.* 2016;474(7):1583-1588.

86. Zywiel MG, Daley JA, Delanois RE, Naziri Q, Johnson AJ, Mont MA. Advance pre-operative chlorhexidine reduces the incidence of surgical site infections in knee arthroplasty. *Int Orthop.* 2011;35(7):1001-1006.

87. Brown NM, Cipriano CA, Moric M, Sporer SM, Della Valle CJ. Dilute betadine lavage before closure for the prevention of acute postoperative deep periprosthetic joint infection. *J Arthroplasty.* 2012;27(1):27-30.

88. Heller S, Rezapoor M, Parvizi J. Minimising the risk of infection: a peri-operative checklist. *Bone Joint J.* 2016;98-B(1 suppl A):18-22.

89. Frisch NB, Kadri OM, Tenbrunsel T, Abdul-Hak A, Qatu M, Davis JJ. Intraoperative chlorhexidine irrigation to prevent infection in total hip and knee arthroplasty. *Arthroplast Today.* 2017;3(4):294-297.

90. Smith DC, Maiman R, Schwechter EM, Kim SJ, Hirsh DM. Optimal irrigation and debridement of infected total joint implants with chlorhexidine gluconate. *J Arthroplasty.* 2015;30(10):1820-1822.

91. Bratzler DW, Hunt DR. The surgical infection prevention and surgical care improvement projects: national initiatives to improve outcomes for patients having surgery. *Clin Infect Dis.* 2006;43(3):322-330.

92. Hernandez NM, Hart A, Taunton MJ, et al. Use of povidone-iodine irrigation prior to wound closure in primary total hip and knee arthroplasty: an analysis of 11,738 cases. *J Bone Joint Surg Am.* 2019;101(13):1144-1150.

93. Hart A, Hernandez NM, Abdel MP, Mabry TM, Hanssen AD, Perry KI. Povidone-iodine wound lavage to prevent infection after revision total hip and knee arthroplasty: an analysis of 2,884 cases. *J Bone Joint Surg Am.* 2019;101(13):1151-1159.

94. Fernandez AH, Monge V, Garcinuno MA. Surgical antibiotic prophylaxis: effect in postoperative infections. *Eur J Epidemiol.* 2001;17(4):369-374.

95. Allo MD, Tedesco M. Operating room management: operative suite considerations, infection control. *Surg Clin North Am.* 2005;85(6):1291-1297,xii.

96. Babkin Y, Raveh D, Lifschitz M, et al. Incidence and risk factors for surgical infection after total knee replacement. *Scand J Infect Dis.* 2007;39(10):890-895.

97. Taaffe K, Lee B, Ferrand Y, et al. The influence of traffic, area location, and other factors on operating room microbial load. *Infect Control Hosp Epidemiol.* 2018;39(4):1-7.

98. Weiser MC, Shemesh S, Chen DD, Bronson MJ, Moucha CS. The effect of door opening on positive pressure and airflow in operating rooms. *J Am Acad Orthop Surg.* 2018;26(5):e105-e113.

99. Stauning MT, Bediako-Bowan A, Andersen LP, et al. Traffic flow and microbial air contamination in operating rooms at a major teaching hospital in Ghana. *J Hosp Infect.* 2017;99(3):263-270.

100. Kapadia BH, Berg RA, Daley JA, Fritz J, Bhave A, Mont MA. Periprosthetic joint infection. *Lancet.* 2016;387(10016):386-394.

101. de Jong L, Klem T, Kuijper TM, Roukema GR. Factors affecting the rate of surgical site infection in patients after hemiarthroplasty of the hip following a fracture of the neck of the femur. *Bone Joint J.* 2017;99-B(8):1088-1094.

102. Huang RC, Parvizi J, Hozack WJ, Chen AF, Austin MS. Aspirin is as effective as and safer than warfarin for patients at higher risk of venous thromboembolism undergoing total joint arthroplasty. *J Arthroplasty.* 2016;31(9 suppl):83-86.

103. An VV, Phan K, Levy YD, Bruce WJ. Aspirin as thromboprophylaxis in hip and knee arthroplasty: a systematic review and meta-analysis. *J Arthroplasty.* 2016;31(11):2608-2616.

104. Parvizi J, Huang R, Restrepo C, et al. Low-dose aspirin is effective chemoprophylaxis against clinically important venous thromboembolism following total joint arthroplasty: a preliminary analysis. *J Bone Joint Surg Am.* 2017;99(2):91-98.

105. Wilson DG, Poole WE, Chauhan SK, Rogers BA. Systematic review of aspirin for thromboprophylaxis in modern elective total hip and knee arthroplasty. *Bone Joint J.* 2016;98-B(8):1056-1061.

chapter 49

Pathways for the Episode of Care

Jorge A. Padilla, MD | Hayeem Rudy, BA | James Slover, MD, MS

INTRODUCTION

Given the rising costs of healthcare in recent decades, increasing emphasis is being placed on transitioning to a system of value-based care, where patient-centered outcomes are maximized and expenditures are minimized. To this end, healthcare organizations have sought to design innovative methods for delivery of care. Standardization is one strategy for increasing efficiency. Clinical pathways for the delivery of care to patients with a given diagnosis have been used to improve resource utilization, workflow efficiency, and quality of care through an increase in standardization.

A clinical pathway is a standardized system designed for patients with a specific clinical diagnosis, which establishes a pragmatic plan for the sequence, timing, and delivery of care throughout the entire episode.[1-3] Clinical pathways are a multidisciplinary approach, designed to optimize patient-centered care, with emphasis on evidence-based medicine.[2,3] They may take the form of protocols, algorithms, care continuums, practice parameters, integrated care pathways, care maps, and guidelines. In recent years, improvement in standardized clinical pathways has been one of the principle driving forces for cost containment and quality enhancement initiatives as they organize the procedures and optimize the use of resources that would otherwise be uncoordinated and wasteful.[4] Standardized pathways provide the patient and the care team with direction and predictability that will ultimately assist patients navigate in the direction of the planned health outcome. This chapter discusses standardized clinical pathways for the episode of care (EOC) in total knee arthroplasty (TKA), a surgical procedure with significant opportunity for standardization and evidence-based practice.

VALUE AND CLINICAL PATHWAYS

TKA is widely recognized as an efficacious treatment method for patients with degenerative disease of the knee, uncontrollable pain, and unacceptable physical function. In 2014, TKA was among the procedures with the most substantial inpatient expenditures, contributing largely to the economic unsustainability of the current US healthcare system.[5,6] Despite its success, a substantial number of TKA patients have suboptimal outcomes or complications, and inefficiencies in care delivery are prevalent. As the framework for healthcare shifts from a volume-based model to a value-based one, physicians and healthcare institutions must align their efforts to integrate evidence-based medicine into clinical practice for the purpose of creating added value. Standardization of care in the form of clinical pathways has been demonstrated as a robust approach for achieving these goals in orthopedic surgery.

Standardized pathways can be designed to reliably incorporate important quality metric measures and patient-reported outcomes, which have been emphasized by the Centers for Medicare and Medicaid Services (CMS).[7-9] Adherence to standardized clinical care pathways provides uniformity among cases in a fashion designed to improve communication, decrease error, improve patient outcomes, and reduce outcome variation. The benefits of creating a standardized clinical care pathway for the EOC relating to TKA are myriad.[4,10] Standardization creates a streamlined workflow for physicians and care providers to follow throughout the continuum of care and allows for effective planning. Well-designed standardized care pathways promote interdisciplinary collaborative practice, which has been demonstrated to effectively reduce waste by obviating circuitous and oftentimes unnecessary variations in the delivery of care that inefficiently consume healthcare resources.[2,8,9,11] The predictability of standardized care pathways also allows for more precise cost tracking for healthcare organizations, improving decision-making regarding the distribution of resources.[2,11,12] Clinical pathways have been found to be most advantageous for high-volume procedures that lack substantial unexpected events, such as TKA.[2,13]

DEVELOPING PATHWAYS

The process of developing a standardized clinical care pathway begins with the assembly of a multidisciplinary panel comprised of stakeholders and caregivers who will participate in reviewing and refining of evidenced-based practices for incorporation or exclusion in the pathway.[14,15] The members of the panel may include orthopedic surgeons, anesthesiologists, internists, hospital administrators, nurses, social workers, patients, and safety and quality leaders. The panel must set a goal for the pathway and identify current practices and the potential areas for improvement of the current care delivery model. For each individual component (e.g., procedure or test), the panel reviews and discusses evidence-based practices and implementation strategies. The panel then develops a track with detailed steps that will guide clinicians and caregivers across the care continuum. Routine tests or procedures deemed unnecessary by the panel are discarded from the standardized pathway. After finalizing the pathway, an implementation plan should be developed to test the feasibility and impact on overall hospital costs and patient outcomes.

The multidisciplinary effort allows for incorporation of diverse input and may provide mechanisms for dissemination of the pathway to caregivers as well. It is important to recognize that the pathway is continuously evolving, and as medical technology and evidence advances, the pathway will change. Therefore, it remains important to periodically and critically reevaluate the pathway to update it to reflect new evidence and clinical practices. We offer a summarized iteration of our 2-day TKA clinical care pathway as an example and discuss certain important elements of its current iteration in this chapter (**Table 49-1**).

THE EPISODE OF CARE

The EOC can be broadly defined as the collection of services provided to a patient to completely treat a discrete clinical condition. Time components of the EOC may include the preoperative, acute care, and the post–acute care period (**Fig. 49-1**).[2] For example, the Comprehensive Care for Joint Replacement (CJR), an alternative payment model (APM) for the EOC associated with total joint arthroplasty (TJA), developed by the CMS, defines the EOC as all services provided beginning upon admission for a Medicare Severity Diagnosis Related Group (MS-DRG) 469 or 470 and ending 90 days post discharge.[16]

Care coordinators are an early innovation that may play an important role in future care pathways for total knee replacement in the acute care period and beyond, as they help manage the patient's entire EOC and are responsible for achieving a smooth transition through the preoperative, acute care, and postoperative care periods.[15] The presence of care coordinators facilitates interdisciplinary communication between providers and patients throughout the continuum of care, which has been shown to contain the overall expenditures of TKA by preventing unnecessary use of resources in the hospital and after discharge.[15,17] Care coordinators achieve this by addressing the patients' needs and expectations during the preoperative period and ensuring the delivery of essential services throughout the entire EOC.[15,18] However, they are associated with additional cost, and coordination through leverage in technology and other innovative mechanisms are likely to proliferate in the future as a means to reduce these costs while simultaneously increasing care coordination. Perhaps the most valuable contribution from care coordinators is the facilitation of post hospital care, a common barrier to even the most well-intentioned discharge plans.

Preoperative Period

The preoperative period is a significant time for patients who may feel overwhelmed at the prospect of undergoing surgical intervention. To manage this, it has been demonstrated that standardizing preoperative patient education programs improve patient understanding and satisfaction, as well as specific factors such as discharge disposition, the rate of postoperative complications, and inpatient hospital length of stay (LOS).[19-25] An increased rate of discharge to home instead of discharge to an inpatient facility with a preoperative education program has also been reported.[19] Other studies substantiate these findings and further demonstrated a reduced rate of short-term postoperative falls following the implementation of a standardized patient education protocol.[25] In addition to effectively addressing the information needs of a patient, a properly designed preoperative patient education program can help manage and organize the postoperative care and discharge planning.[19,21-26] Patients who are properly educated about the intervention and their role in the recovery process have also been demonstrated to take a more proactive role in their rehabilitation.[20] All of these factors enhance patient experience, streamline costs, and improve outcomes. Other studies evaluating the effects of preoperative education as part of standardized care pathways in TKA have had similar positive results, which makes the importance of beginning to address recovery during the preoperative period absolutely clear.[21-24]

The preoperative period also serves as a time when the health of patients with multiple medical comorbidities and psychosocial difficulties can be adequately optimized for surgical intervention and improved recovery. Previous studies have reported worse outcomes following TKA in patients who failed to receive proper medical treatment for their comorbidities prior to surgery.[27] A multidisciplinary preoperative assessment and meticulous health optimization program has been shown to reduce morbidity and mortality following TKA.[28] Bernstein et al demonstrated significantly higher quality of care and lower resource utilization in patients who underwent a preoperative optimization protocol as part of a standardized pathway in hip and knee arthroplasty.[29] However, overuse of routine preadmission testing may lead to unnecessary expenditures, and therefore, preoperative evaluations and testing must be carefully scrutinized. For example, one analysis investigated the effects of obviating routine preoperative studies including urinalyses, prothrombin time, partial thromboplastin time, and international normalized ration measurements and demonstrated increased cost savings with no impact on clinical and patient-reported outcomes following TKA.[15] Incorporating preoperative assessment and medical optimization into a standardized clinical pathway in TKA, careful evidence-based evaluation of the value of preoperative test with elimination of those that do not provide value can improve resource utilization, interdisciplinary collaboration, and workflow efficiency.[30-33]

TABLE 49-1 Two-Day Total Knee Arthroplasty Clinical Care Pathway

	Preoperative Period	POD 0	POD 1	POD 2
MD/NP	• Medical clearance • Anesthesia clearance • Discharge planning	• Monitor HGB/HCT • Monitor O₂ Sat, and vitals • Pain management • Dressing/drainage	• Assess physiological stability of patient • Fluid balance and electrolytes • Monitor HGB/HCT and determine the need for blood transfusion • Prescription for anticoagulation treatment • Adequate pain meds and reassessment • Assess wound • Initiate bowel regimen • Inform patient of D/C between 10 and 11 • Finalize anticoagulation plan	• Check HGB/HCT • Medicine reconciliation • Scripts • Discharge orders • Check for equipment • Instructions for follow-up of surgical and primary MD for anticoagulation and medication management
Nursing	• Preadmission testing admit assessment • Class or DVD	• Routine vitals monitoring as per standard • Pain management assessment as per standard • Continuous passive motion • Cryotherapy • OOB 30 min	• Obtain anticoagulation prescription • Routine vitals monitoring as per standard • Pain management assessment as per standard • Continuous passive motion • Cryotherapy • Instructions of new medications and side effects • 24-h notice given • Encourage incentive spirometer • Encourage oral fluids/advance diet as tolerated • OOB all meals for 1 h • Mobilize per PT	• Pain management assessment as per standard • Continuous passive motion • Cryotherapy • Complete anticoagulant teaching • Inform patient they may receive survey • Complete instructions on new medications and side effects • Routine postop monitoring • Bathing independent in bathroom with assistive devices • LE dressings with aids as needed • Instructions on signs and symptoms of infection • Activity at home • OOB all meals • Bowel regimen ongoing for home • Follow-up visits • Inform patient may receive discharge call
CM	• Guided patient services preadmission completed 1-2 wk before surgery • Preoperative counseling regarding discharge needs and expectations		• Complete psychosocial assessment with discharge planning and insurance review • Confers with PT for activity level and progress • Reviews and confirms discharge plan and transport needs with patient and/or caregiver • Refers to home care/subacute/acute rehab • Finalizes transport mode with patient or caregiver • Performs admission UR • Confirm selected anticoagulant • Receives script for anticoagulant and begins process if an injectable • Follow-up of anticoagulant for availability, accessibility, and affordability	• Performs discharge UR • Reviews and finalizes discharge plans and transport with patient and/or caregivers • Reviews and finalizes services, equipment, and transportation with patient and/or caregivers
PT	Bed mobility	Moderate assist	Minimal assist/independent	Independent
	Supine ↔ sit	Dependent/maximum assist	Minimal assist/independent	Independent
	Sit ↔ stand	2 person/maximum assist	Minimal assist/independent	Independent

(Continued)

TABLE 49-1	**Two-Day Total Knee Arthroplasty Clinical Care Pathway—Continued**			
	Preoperative Period	**POD 0**	**POD 1**	**POD 2**
	Ambulation	0-5 ft maximum/moderate assist with AD	40-100 ft up/down supervised	40-100 ft up/down supervised
	Stairs		4 steps up/down minimal assist in afternoon	4 Steps up/down independent
	CPM	As per MD protocol	As per MD protocol	As per MD protocol
	Active and/or passive ROM	As tolerated by patient	0°-75°	0°-90°
OT	Toilet transfer		Moderate assist in AM. Minimal assist in PM.	Minimal assist/independent in AM. Independent in PM.
	Toileting		Minimal assist in AM. Supervision in the PM.	Supervision/independent in AM. Independent in PM.
	Dressing		Maximum/moderate assist with equipment in AM. Minimal assist with no equipment in PM.	Minimal assist with no equipment in AM. Supervision/independent with no equipment in PM.

CM, care manager; HCT, hematocrit; HGB, hemoglobin; O$_2$ Sat, oxygen saturation; OOB, out of bed; OT, occupational therapy; POD, postoperative day; PT, physical therapy.

Acute Care Period

The acute care period includes all services provided from the surgical procedure to the time of discharge. This is a critical time within the EOC as it has been demonstrated that 80% of the total hospital expenditures for TKA are generated during the first 48 hours of admission in the acute care period.[34] Therefore, interventions by healthcare institutions to increase the value of care provided in this period has been shown to substantially reduce resource wasting, unnecessary hospital services, and LOS.[2,15,18,34]

Components of a standardized clinical care pathway in the postoperative period may address several facets of care including prophylactic antibiotic cessation, pain management strategies, wound care, medical comorbidity management, and physical therapy. A review of outcomes in patients who did and did not undergo a postoperative care pathway that included these elements found significantly improved quality metrics including reduced overall cost and lower 90-day complication rates in patients who were part of a standardized pathway.[35] In order for clinical pathways to create value through an evidence-based approach, the routine use of hospital resources must be vigorously scrutinized, and physicians should make efforts to reduce unnecessary practices. During the acute care period, discontinuing the use of routine practices such as urinary catheterization, intraoperative pathology specimen evaluation, postoperative radiographic imaging, and surveillance venous duplex in TKA patients treated prophylactically have all been proven to improve value by reducing the overall cost while simultaneously maintaining patient outcomes.[15,36-38]

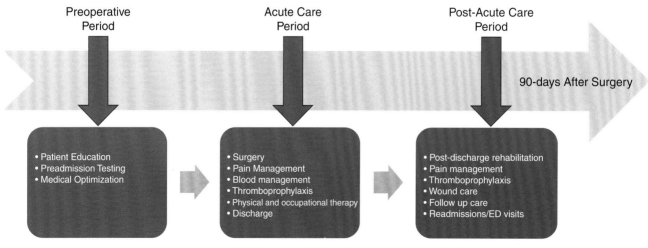

FIGURE 49-1 90-d episode of care for total knee arthroplasty.

LOS is a key cost driver in the acute care period that has received much attention in the effort to improve the value of care. In early discussions concerning shortening LOS, there was hesitation that a reduction in inpatient hospital time would compromise patient outcomes.[13] Numerous studies have since demonstrated that this is not the case and that a reduction in LOS may in fact have a positive impact on patient-reported outcomes and patient satisfaction.[2,7,15,17,18,34,39,40] However, discharge to home, rather than an inpatient rehabilitation facility, is more important for savings than LOS, and increasing LOS by a small number of days to accomplish this is cost-effective.[15,18]

Optimal pain management is critical throughout the EOC for several reasons. Suboptimal pain control can delay postoperative mobility and discharge and worsen patient satisfaction.[41,42] Moreover, given the current state of crisis relating to the opioid epidemic in the United States, there is a pressing need to curb overuse of these types of pain medications.[43] The inclusion of standardized multimodal pain protocols in clinical pathways has proven beneficial for the TKA candidate allowing shorter LOS, more rapid mobilization, and decreased opioid use.[15,42] Studies have demonstrated that programs that incorporate early postoperative rehabilitation into clinical pathways results in shorter hospital LOS and more rapid attainment of short-term functional outcomes when compared to a more delayed rehabilitation program.[44,45] Furthermore, ambulation as early as 2 to 4 hours following surgery reduces the risk of thromboembolic events and the need for pharmacological prophylactic treatment post discharge.[11]

Blood management is a vital component during the perioperative period as blood loss and allogenic blood transfusions can result in a substantial increase in LOS, complications, and total hospital cost.[46] Due to the potential risk of complications associated with blood loss and transfusions, it is imperative to integrate blood management strategies into clinical care pathways. The use of tranexamic acid (TXA) in TJA patients is a safe and effective intervention for reducing intraoperative blood loss and postoperative transfusion rates by enhancing coagulation without increasing the rate of thromboembolic events.[46-48] Studies have shown that incorporation of TXA into clinical care pathways effectively reduces discharge to inpatient facilities and total hospital cost per episode as well.[15,18,47,48] Standardization of anticoagulation regimens has also been found to lead to significant reduction in the rates of pulmonary embolism. The study reported a statistically significant reduction in total cost per patient by 2% each year that the protocol was in place as well. The use of a tourniquet intraoperatively allows for a bloodless surgical field, which some have suggested may reduce surgical time and improve cementation.[49] However, recent studies have reported that the use of a tourniquet resulted in no additional benefits regarding blood management

and in fact may delay recovery time, decrease short-term range of motion, and increase pain and the rate of thromboembolic events. Therefore, discontinuation of tourniquets may allow for a more rapid discharge and decrease opioid use, and further study of this is needed.[46,50] It is important to point out that any conclusions drawn from these studies are often limited given the difficulty of quantifying total blood loss as well as nonuniform indications for blood transfusion.

Post–Acute Care Period

One of the fastest growing expense categories for Medicare has been the cost associated with the post–acute care period, which includes readmissions, routine follow-up appointments, rehabilitation, and discharge to inpatient facilities.[51] Discharging a patient to an inpatient post–acute care facility is one of the largest components of the financial burden of the postoperative period, which can reach greater than 40% the total cost for the entire TKA episode.[52,53] Therefore, avoidance of use of these facilities whenever safe and feasible is paramount. Standardized clinical care pathways that routinely emphasize discharge to home versus inpatient rehabilitation facilities, unless specifically indicated, have been shown to significantly reduce the cost of the EOC surrounding TKA.[54,55] Despite concerns of increasing readmission in patients who are discharged earlier and directly home as part of a standardized clinical pathway, the literature suggests that readmission rates have remained the same and, in fact, improved in several studies when patients are discharged directly home.[13,56,57]

OUTCOMES

Clinical pathways have successfully decreased the LOS and readmission rates and improved discharge disposition, with increased discharge to home versus inpatient rehabilitation facility.[15,18] They included increased utilization of multimodal analgesia protocols focused on pain control for early ambulation postoperatively and discontinued the use of non-value-adding practices such as autologous blood donation, radiofrequency bipolar sealer, and routine urinary catheterization to increase cost-effectiveness while maintaining or improving patient outcomes. At our institution, multiple clinical care coordinators were hired to maintain communication with patients and caregivers in order to maximize communication and coordination and minimize readmissions and unnecessary emergency department or office visits. Following implementation of the clinical pathway with these elements, the LOS was reduced from 4.27 to 2.96 days, discharge to inpatient rehabilitation facilities from 71% to 28%, and 90-day readmission from 13% to 8%. A total savings of 30% compared to expenditures before implementation of the pathway was accrued.[15,18]

Other pathways have demonstrated similar success.[2] In one study, 56 primary TKA patients whose EOC was not part of a standardized pathway program were compared with 103 primary TKA patients who received their operation after the implementation of a clinical pathway.[2] Patients were similar in terms of age, pain score on visual analog scale, clinical knee scores, surgical approach, and operating room time. As part of this program, a knee-implant standardization program was implemented to reduce variation in knee-implant selection and reduce costs in this area. Compared to patients who received care as part of a nonstandardized program, patients who were part of the standardized clinical pathway had shorter LOS (4.16 days vs. 6.79 days, $P < .0001$), mean actual hospital cost ($8747.18 vs. $10,043.11, $P < .0001$), and lower mean inflation-adjusted hospital cost ($8747.18 vs. $10,804.98, $P < .0001$).[2] At 8 years follow-up, there were no significant differences with respect to the need for manipulation, revision surgery for any reason, and hospital readmission rates.[2] The results of this study demonstrated that combined with an effort to reduce variability within the cost of knee implants, standardized clinical pathways can significantly improve healthcare quality measures, including LOS and cost, compared to a system without a standardized clinical pathway, with decreased cost and no long-term decrease in outcomes.

The importance of data analysis in these efforts has also been demonstrated. Data from an institutional total joint registry have been shown to improve decision-making.[2,58] One study allowed for each surgeon to be a given copy of the utilization data for TJA for each member of the department.[58] In addition, data on patient complications for each member of the department were collected and distributed to surgeons. The dissemination of these data was used to improve the pathway and compliance and was reviewed monthly to discuss clinical complications and cost utilization. This was done for 3 years, at which point the data were reviewed. Upon analysis, mean LOS following knee and hip arthroplasty was significantly reduced compared to LOS prior to the program. In addition, variability in total hospital LOS was reduced from ±6 days to ±3 days in the study period. The study also found a reduction in mortality, but no differences in infection and readmission rates.[58] This demonstrates that robust and accurate data collection continues to be critical for the assessment of compliance, outcomes, and continuous improvement initiatives and provides an objective way to demonstrate to providers the impact of change in behavior, practice, and care strategies.

TECHNOLOGY

The incorporation of technologies into clinical pathways has contributed to their effectiveness in several ways. The electronic medical record (EMR) is a ubiquitous technological advancement that has enhanced communication between care providers and they have been incorporated into clinical pathways to facilitate care processes.[59] One study demonstrated that the use of an EMR as integrated into a clinical pathway for TKA significantly improved the time from initiation of surgical analgesia to arrival in the postanesthesia care unit, Visual Analogue Scale pain scores, and the volume of patient-controlled epidural analgesia required to control pain.[60] In addition to EMR platforms, newer experimental technologies may find themselves incorporated in clinical care pathways to facilitate care coordination and other aspects of preparation and recovery. Novel electronic-based rehabilitation platforms have also been developed, which provide patients with improved access to postoperative recovery protocols.[61,62] Mobile web-based applications provide patients with audiovisual information to enhance care coordination regarding the perioperative course, wound care, and self-rehabilitation protocols.[61] Additionally, patient-reported outcome measurements and communications between providers and patients are available through the application.[63] Previous studies have demonstrated non-inferiority in functional and patient-reported outcomes upon implementation of electronic-based rehabilitation instruments.[61-64] Furthermore, the financial burden of such tools is substantially reduced in comparison to home health services.[61] Virtual reality is another emerging technology that has demonstrated some promise as an alternative, immersive rehabilitation program following TJA.[65] As newer technologies gain acceptance within the orthopedic community, further comparisons with conventional methods are warranted prior to their incorporation into standardized clinical pathways, but they will likely play an important role as efforts to increase value by improving outcomes and decreasing costs continue.

LIMITATIONS

Care pathways do have limitations and potential negative consequences. Physicians may experience decreases in their autonomy if excessively stringent pathways are enforced, which may limit morale and productivity. For this reason and others, physicians should have a stake in the development and continuous improvement of standardized clinical pathways. More importantly, unwavering standardization may stifle innovation and the ability to personalize the care plan to the patient with specific needs. While the guidelines put in place by standardized care pathways may be evidence-based and thus suited to best address the typical TJA patient, patients with unique characteristics who fall outside of the "range" of those best-served by standardized pathways may require alternative treatment strategies.

Another challenge for the implementation of evidence-based standardized clinical pathways is the large upfront capital required.[66] Small community-based hospitals may experience difficulties gathering the funds required to properly develop and apply a value-based protocols across an entire institution. However, in the long run, these efforts will be cost saving. In 2015, a group of 19 orthopedic surgeons developed and applied a standardized clinical pathway which had an upfront cost of $220,000 which included administrative expenses, employment of new personnel, and increased personnel work hours.[53] Despite the initial difficulties encountered, their practice saved greater than $1.9 million during the first year, therefore recovering and generating value through the pathway over time, demonstrating the value that can be generated by employing standard clinical pathways.

CONCLUSION

Standardized clinical pathways for TKA offer a pragmatic, reliable approach to improve value for the TKA EOC by improving outcomes and decreasing the overall cost per episode. Cost containment is achieved through optimization of the patient and efficiency of resources used throughout the episode, while maintaining or improving patient outcomes. Patient outcomes are improved with the use of proper education, evidence-based interventions, increased care coordination, and reduction in complications, readmissions, and optimized discharge disposition. Furthermore, standardized clinical pathways improve multidisciplinary collaboration by offering a structured plan of care for decreasing resource waste, improving care coordination, and patient-provider communication, and they provide the framework for data collection and analysis that can be used for monitoring care variation and the impact of future improvement efforts.

REFERENCES

1. Kim TK, Chang MJ, Kim SJ, Song YD, Kim SK. Continuous improvements of a clinical pathway increased its feasibility and improved care providers' perception in TKA. *Knee Surg Relat Res.* 2014;26(4):199-206. doi:10.5792/ksrr.2014.26.4.199.

2. Healy W, Iorio R, Ko J, Appleby D, David L. Impact of cost reduction programs on short-term patient outcome and hospital cost of total knee arthroplasty. *J Bone Joint Surg Am.* 2002;84(3):348-353.

3. Hertog A, Gliesche K, Timm J, Mühlbauer B, Zebrowski S. Pathway-controlled fast-track rehabilitation after total knee arthroplasty: a randomized prospective clinical study evaluating the recovery pattern, drug consumption, and length of stay. *Arch Orthop Trauma Surg.* 2012;132(8):1153-1163. doi:10.1007/s00402-012-1528-1.

4. Bozic KJ, Maselli J, Pekow PS, Lindenauer PK, Vail TP, Auerbach AD. The influence of procedure volumes and standardization of care on quality and efficiency in total joint replacement surgery. *J Bone Joint Surg Am.* 2010;92(16):2643-2652. doi:10.2106/JBJS.I.01477.

5. Stranges E, Russo A, Friedman B. Procedures with the most rapidly increasing hospital costs, 2004-2007. *Value Heal.* 2010;13(3):A89. doi:10.1016/S1098-3015(10)72424-4.

6. HCUP National Inpatient Sample (NIS). Rockville, MD; 2014. Available at http://hcupnet.ahrq.gov/. Accessed 7, 2019.

7. Pilot P, Bogie R, Draijer WF, Verburg AD, van Os JJ, Kuipers H. Experience in the first four years of rapid recovery; is it safe? *Injury.* 2006;37:S37-S40. doi:10.1016/S0020-1383(07)70010-4.

8. Pinzur MS, Gurza E, Kristopaitis T, et al. Hospitalist–orthopedic co-management of high-risk patients undergoing lower extremity reconstruction surgery. *Orthopedics.* 2009;32(7):495-501. doi:10.3928/01477447-20090527-14.

9. Larsen K, Hvass KE, Hansen TB, Thomsen PB, Søballe K. Effectiveness of accelerated perioperative care and rehabilitation intervention compared to current intervention after hip and knee arthroplasty. A before-after trial of 247 patients with a 3-month follow-up. *BMC Musculoskelet Disord.* 2008;9(1):59. doi:10.1186/1471-2474-9-59.

10. Scranton PE. The cost effectiveness of streamlined care pathways and product standardization in total knee arthroplasty. *J Arthroplasty.* 1999;14(2):182-186. doi:10.1016/S0883-5403(99)90123-7.

11. Husted H, Holm G. Fast track in total hip and knee arthroplasty - experiences from Hvidovre University Hospital, Denmark. *Injury.* 2006;37:S31-S35. doi:10.1016/S0020-1383(07)70009-8.

12. Walter FL, Bass N, Bock G, Markel DC. Success of clinical pathways for total joint arthroplasty in a community hospital. *Clin Orthop Relat Res.* 2006;457:133-137. doi:10.1097/01.blo.0000246567.88585.0a.

13. Duggal S, Flics S, Cornell CN. *Introduction of clinical pathways in orthopedic surgical care: the experience of the hospital for special surgery.* In: *Perioperative Care of the Orthopedic Patient.* New York, NY: Springer; 2014:365-371. doi:10.1007/978-1-4614-0100-1_31.

14. Van Citters AD, Fahlman C, Goldmann DA, et al. Developing a pathway for high-value, patient-centered total joint arthroplasty. *Clin Orthop Relat Res.* 2014;472(5):1619-1635. doi:10.1007/s11999-013-3398-4.

15. Iorio R, Clair AJ, Inneh IA, Slover JD, Bosco JA, Zuckerman JD. Early results of medicare's bundled payment initiative for a 90-day total joint arthroplasty episode of care. *J Arthroplasty.* 2016;31(2):343-350. doi:10.1016/j.arth.2015.09.004.

16. U.S. Centers for Medicare & Medicaid Services. Bundled Payments for Care Improvement (BPCI) initiative: general information. 2019. https://innovation.cms.gov/initiatives/bundled-payments/. Accessed July 27, 2019.

17. Preston JS, Caccavale D, Smith A, Stull LE, Harwood DA, Kayiaros S. Bundled payments for care improvement in the private sector: a win for everyone. *J Arthroplasty.* 2018;33(8):1-6. doi:10.1016/j.arth.2018.03.007.

18. Dundon JM, Bosco J, Slover J, Yu S, Sayeed Y, Iorio R. Improvement in total joint replacement quality metrics. *J Bone Joint Surg.* 2016;98(23):1949-1953. doi:10.2106/JBJS.16.00523.

19. Yoon RS, Nellans KW, Geller JA, Kim AD, Jacobs MR, Macaulay W. Patient education before hip or knee arthroplasty lowers length of stay. *J Arthroplasty.* 2010;25(4):547-551. doi:10.1016/J.ARTH.2009.03.012.

20. Mertes SC, Raut S, Khanduja V. Integrated care pathways in lower-limb arthroplasty: are they effective in reducing length of hospital stay? *Int Orthop.* 2013;37(6):1157-1163. doi:10.1007/s00264-013-1829-1.

21. Moulton LS, Evans PA, Starks I, Smith T. Pre-operative education prior to elective hip arthroplasty surgery improves postoperative outcome. *Int Orthop.* 2015;39(8):1483-1486. doi:10.1007/s00264-015-2754-2.

22. Crowe J, Henderson J. Pre-arthroplasty rehabilitation is effective in reducing hospital stay. *Can J Occup Ther.* 2003;70(2):88-96. doi:10.1177/000841740307000204.

23. Huang S-W, Chen P-H, Chou Y-H. Effects of a preoperative simplified home rehabilitation education program on length of stay of total knee arthroplasty patients. *Orthop Traumatol Surg Res.* 2012;98(3):259-264. doi:10.1016/J.OTSR.2011.12.004.

24. Tait MA, Dredge C, Barnes CL. Preoperative patient education for hip and knee arthroplasty: financial benefit? *J Surg Orthop Adv.* 2015;24(4):246-251. doi:10.3113/JSOA.2015.0246.

25. Clarke HD, Timm VL, Goldberg BR, Hattrup SJ. Preoperative patient education reduces in-hospital falls after total knee arthroplasty. *Clin Orthop Relat Res.* 2012;470(1):244-249. doi:10.1007/s11999-011-1951-6.

26. Padilla JA, Feng JE, Anoushiravani AA, Hozack WJ, Schwarzkopf R, Macaulay W. Modifying patient expectations can enhance total hip arthroplasty postoperative satisfaction. *J Arthroplasty.* 2019;34(7 suppl):S209-S214. doi:10.1016/j.arth.2018.12.038.

27. Bass AR, Rodriguez T, Hyun G, et al. Myocardial ischaemia after hip and knee arthroplasty: incidence and risk factors. *Int Orthop.* 2015;39(10):2011-2016. doi:10.1007/s00264-015-2853-0.

28. Kamal T, Conway RM, Littlejohn I, Ricketts D. The role of a multidisciplinary pre-assessment clinic in reducing mortality after complex orthopaedic surgery. *Ann R Coll Surg Engl.* 2011;93(2):149-151. doi:10.1308/003588411X561026.

29. Bernstein DN, Liu TC, Winegar AL, et al. Evaluation of a preoperative optimization protocol for primary hip and knee arthroplasty patients. *J Arthroplasty.* 2018;33(12):3642-3648. doi:10.1016/j.arth.2018.08.018.

30. Sayeed Z, El-Othmani MM, Anoushiravani AA, Chambers MC, Saleh KJ. Planning, building, and maintaining a successful musculoskeletal service line. *Orthop Clin North Am.* 2016;47(4):681-688. doi:10.1016/j.ocl.2016.05.010.

31. Barbieri A, Vanhaecht K, Van Herck P, et al. Effects of clinical pathways in the joint replacement: a meta-analysis. *BMC Med.* 2009;7:32. doi:10.1186/1741-7015-7-32.

32. Kee JR, Edwards PK, Barnes CL. Effect of risk acceptance for bundled care payments on clinical outcomes in a high-volume total joint arthroplasty practice after implementation of a standardized clinical pathway. *J Arthroplasty.* 2017;32(8):2332-2338. doi:10.1016/J.ARTH.2017.03.007.

33. Gooch K, Marshall DA, Faris PD, et al. Comparative effectiveness of alternative clinical pathways for primary hip and knee joint replacement patients: a pragmatic randomized, controlled trial. *Osteoarthr Cartil.* 2012;20(10):1086-1094. doi:10.1016/J.JOCA.2012.06.017.

34. Healy WL, Iorio R, Richards JA, Lucchesi C. Opportunities for control of hospital costs for total joint arthroplasty after initial cost containment. *J Arthroplasty.* 1998;13(5):504-507. doi:10.1016/S0883-5403(98)90048-1.

35. Featherall J, Brigati DP, Faour M, Messner W, Higuera CA. Implementation of a total hip arthroplasty care pathway at a high-volume health system: effect on length of stay, discharge disposition, and 90-day complications. *J Arthroplasty.* 2018;33(6):1675-1680. doi:10.1016/J.ARTH.2018.01.038.

36. Glaser D, Lotke P. Cost-effectiveness of immediate postoperative radiographs after uncomplicated total knee arthroplasty. *J Arthroplasty.* 2000;15(4):475-478. doi:10.1054/arth.2000.4338.

37. Kocher MS, Erens G, Thornhill TS, Ready JE. Cost and effectiveness of routine pathological examination of operative specimens obtained during primary total hip and knee replacement in patients with osteoarthritis. *J Bone Joint Surg Am.* 2000;82(11):1531-1535.

38. Quick RC, Kwolek CJ, Minion DJ. Surveillance venous duplex is not clinically useful after total joint arthroplasty when effective deep venous thrombosis prophylaxis is used. *Ann Vasc Surg.* 2004;18(2):193-198.

39. Schwarzkopf R, Zamansani T, Houng M, Bridgeman T. The effect of a clinical pathway strategy for managing care in total joint replacement: the impact on perioperative outcomes. *J Clin Exp Orthop.* 2016;2(1):11. doi:10.4172/2471-8416.100011.

40. Specht K, Kjaersgaard-Andersen P, Kehlet H, Wedderkopp N, Pedersen BD. High patient satisfaction in 445 patients who underwent fast-track hip or knee replacement. *Acta Orthop.* 2015;86(6):702-707. doi:10.3109/17453674.2015.1063910.

41. Horlocker T, Kopp S, Pagnano M, Hebl J. Analgesia for total hip and knee arthroplasty: a multimodal pathway featuring peripheral nerve block. *J Am Acad Orthop Surg.* 2006;14(3):126-135.

42. Duellman TJ, Gaffigan C, Milbrandt JC, Allan DG. Multi-modal, pre-emptive analgesia decreases the length of hospital stay following total joint arthroplasty. *Orthopedics.* 2009;32(3):167.

43. Smith SR, Bido J, Collins JE, Yang H, Katz JN, Losina E. Impact of preoperative opioid use on total knee arthroplasty outcomes. *J Bone Joint Surg.* 2017;99(10):803-808. doi:10.2106/JBJS.16.01200.

44. Munin MC, Rudy TE, Glynn NW, Crossett LS, Rubash HE. Early inpatient rehabilitation after elective hip and knee arthroplasty. *JAMA.* 1998;279(11):847-852. doi:10.1001/jama.279.11.847.

45. Pour AE, Parvizi J, Sharkey PF, Hozack WJ, Rothman RH. Minimally invasive hip arthroplasty: what role does patient preconditioning play? *J Bone Joint Surg Am.* 2007;89(9):1920-1927. doi:10.2106/JBJS.F.01153.

46. Lu Q, Peng H, Zhou G, Yin D. Perioperative blood management strategies for total knee arthroplasty. *Orthop Surg.* 2018;10(1):8-16. doi:10.1111/os.12361.

47. Evangelista PJ, Aversano MW, Koli E, et al. Effect of tranexamic acid on transfusion rates following total joint arthroplasty: a cost and comparative effectiveness analysis. *Orthop Clin North Am.* 2017;48(2):109-115. doi:10.1016/j.ocl.2016.12.001.

48. Whiting DR, Duncan CM, Sierra RJ, Smith HM. Tranexamic acid benefits total joint arthroplasty patients regardless of preoperative hemoglobin value. *J Arthroplasty.* 2015;30(12):2098-2101. doi:10.1016/J.ARTH.2015.05.050.

49. Levine B, Haughom B, Strong B, Hellman M, Frank R. Blood management strategies for total knee arthroplasty. *J Am Acad Orthop Surg.* 2014;22(6):361-371.

50. Yin D, Delisle J, Banica A, et al. Tourniquet and closed-suction drains in total knee arthroplasty. No beneficial effects on bleeding management and knee function at a higher cost. *Orthop Traumatol Surg Res.* 2017;103(4):583-589. doi:10.1016/J.OTSR.2017.03.002.

51. Chandra A, Dalton MA, Holmes J, et al. Large increases in spending on postacute care in Medicare point to the potential for cost savings in these settings. *Health Aff.* 2013;151(6):414-420. doi:10.1097/CCM.0b013e31823e986a.A.

52. Braithwaite RS, Col NF, Wong JB. Estimating hip fracture morbidity, mortality and costs. *J Am Geriatr Soc.* 2003;51(3):364-370. doi:10.1046/j.1532-5415.2003.51110.x.

53. Althausen PL, Mead L. Bundled payments for care improvement. *J Orthop Trauma.* 2016;30(12):S50-S53. doi:10.1097/BOT.0000000000000715.

54. Weiser MC, Kim KY, Anoushiravani AA, Iorio R, Davidovitch RI. Outpatient total hip arthroplasty has minimal short-term complications with the use of institutional protocols. *J Arthroplasty.* 2018;33(11):3502-3507. doi:10.1016/j.arth.2018.07.015.

55. Froemke CC, Wang L, DeHart ML, Williamson RK, Ko LM, Duwelius PJ. Standardizing care and improving quality under a bundled payment initiative for total joint arthroplasty. *J Arthroplasty.* 2015;30(10):1676-1682. doi:10.1016/j.arth.2015.04.028.

56. Pitter FT, Jørgensen CC, Lindberg-Larsen M, Kehlet H, Lundbeck Foundation Center for Fast-track Hip and Knee Replacement Collaborative Group. Postoperative morbidity and discharge destinations after fast-track hip and knee arthroplasty in patients older than 85 years. *Anesth Analg.* 2016;122(6):1807-1815. doi:10.1213/ANE.0000000000001190.

57. Yanik JM, Bedard NA, Hanley JM, Otero JE, Callaghan JJ, Marsh JL. Rapid recovery total joint arthroplasty is safe, efficient, and cost-effective in the veterans administration setting. *J Arthroplasty.* 2018;33(10):3138-3142. doi:10.1016/j.arth.2018.07.004.

58. Amadio PC, Naessens JM, Rice RL, Ilstrup DM, Evans RW, Morrey BF. Effect of feedback on resource use and morbidity in hip and knee arthroplasty in an integrated group practice setting. *Mayo Clin Proc.* 1996;71(2):127-133. doi:10.1016/S0025-6196(11)64504-7.

59. Singer A, Duarte Fernandez R. The effect of electronic medical record system use on communication between pharmacists and prescribers. *BMC Fam Pract.* 2015;16(1):155. doi:10.1186/s12875-015-0378-7.

60. Urban MK, Chiu T, Wolfe S, Magid S. Electronic ordering system improves postoperative pain management after total knee or hip arthroplasty. *Appl Clin Inform.* 2015;6(3):591-599. doi:10.4338/ACI-2014-12-RA-0114.

61. Davidovitch RI, Anoushiravani AA, Feng JE, et al. Home health services are not required for select total hip arthroplasty candidates: assessment and supplementation with an electronic recovery application. *J Arthroplasty.* 2018;33(7S):S49-S55. doi:10.1016/j.arth.2018.02.048.

62. Fleischman AN, Crizer MP, Tarabichi M, et al. 2018 John N. Insall Award. Recovery of knee flexion with unsupervised home exercise is not inferior to outpatient physical therapy after TKA: a randomized trial. *Clin Orthop Relat Res.* 2019;477(1):60-69. doi:10.1097/CORR.0000000000000561.

63. Padilla JA, Rudy HL, Gabor JA, et al. Relationship between the patient-reported outcome measurement information system and traditional patient-reported outcomes for osteoarthritis. *J Arthroplasty.* 2019;34(2):265-272. doi:10.1016/J.ARTH.2018.10.012.

64. Fillingham YA, Darrith B, Lonner JH, Culvern C, Crizer M, Della Valle CJ. Formal physical therapy may not be necessary after unicompartmental knee arthroplasty: a randomized clinical trial. *J Arthroplasty.* 2018;33(7):S93-S99.e3. doi:10.1016/J.ARTH.2018.02.049.

65. Lee M, Suh D, Son J, Kim J, Eun S-D, Yoon B. Patient perspectives on virtual reality-based rehabilitation after knee surgery: importance of level of difficulty. *J Rehabil Res Dev.* 2016;53(2):239-252. doi:10.1682/JRRD.2014.07.0164.

66. Pelt CE, Anderson MB, Erickson JA, Gililland JM, Peters CL. Adding value to total joint arthroplasty care in an academic environment: the Utah experience. *J Arthroplasty.* 2018;33(6):1636-1640. doi:10.1016/j.arth.2018.01.028.

chapter 50

Preventing Thromboembolism in Total Knee Arthroplasty

Venus Vakhshori, MD | Mary Kate Erdman, MD | Jay R. Lieberman, MD

Total knee arthroplasty (TKA) is effective in relieving pain, increasing mobility, and improving quality of life for patients. Despite the overall success of this procedure, patients undergoing TKA are at risk for developing symptomatic venous thromboembolic disease. Since total joint arthroplasty is usually an elective procedure performed in relatively healthy individuals, pulmonary embolism (PE) may be a devastating complication. In some cases, the first manifestation of venous thromboembolic disease may be a symptomatic or fatal PE. Therefore, selection of an effective method of prophylaxis is an essential part of the care of patients undergoing arthroplasty.[1] Despite the completion of a number of well-designed clinical trials that have assessed the efficacy and safety of a variety of modalities for prophylaxis, the ideal method of prophylaxis is still to be determined. The selection of a prophylactic regimen is influenced not only by its ability to prevent symptomatic venous thromboembolism (VTE) without causing bleeding complications, but also by decreased duration of hospital stay.[1]

TKA differs from total hip arthroplasty (THA) with regard to VTE in a number of critical elements. First, the overall deep vein thrombosis (DVT) rate is higher in patients undergoing TKA than in those undergoing THA without prophylaxis.[1-3] This may be secondary to the routine use of a tourniquet and intraoperative flexion of the knee.[4] Second, it is more difficult to suppress venous thrombus formation in patients undergoing TKA than in those undergoing THA despite the use of the same prophylactic regimens.[5-7] Finally, a postoperative hematoma is more likely to require reoperation in a TKA patient than in a THA patient, making this bleeding complication more costly in the setting of TKA.[1,8,9] In this chapter, we review the available data on VTE prophylaxis after TKA.

PATHOGENESIS

The triad of venous stasis, hypercoagulability, and endothelial injury is associated with thrombus formation and is present in the perioperative period in patients undergoing TKA.[10,11] Histologically, thrombi originate near a region of reduced venous flow. They are composed of alternating "red" layers, composed of fibrin and red blood cells, which have been implicated in thrombus origination, and "white" layers, composed of platelets and neutrophils,

which play a major role in thrombus propagation.[11-13] Venous stasis often occurs in these patients as a result of the use of a tourniquet on the thigh, persistent knee flexion, and reduced postoperative mobility.[1,8,9,14] After tourniquet deflation, there are increased levels of thrombosis markers, including prothrombin fragment 1.2, plasmin/alpha2-antiplasmin complex, D-dimer, fibrinopeptide A, and thrombin–antithrombin complexes.[15-17] The trauma of the procedure itself can result in a sustained activation of tissue factor and other clotting factors, which then localizes at the sites of vascular injury and areas of venous stasis.[11,18,19] These changes are evident as early as 4 hours after surgery, suggesting that venous thrombosis occurs intraoperatively or in the immediate postoperative period, and may benefit from early prophylaxis.[15-17] In addition, postoperative reduction in antithrombin III levels and inhibition of the endogenous fibrinolytic system may allow for continued thrombus growth (**Fig. 50-1**).[1,11,14,20,21]

EPIDEMIOLOGY

The literature demonstrates that without prophylaxis, the prevalence of asymptomatic, venographically verified postoperative DVT is 40% to 80% and 0.3% to 3.0% for PE following TKA.[1,8,9,22] Factors associated with the development of VTE include prior VTE, prolonged immobilization, varicose veins, obesity, advanced age, and cardiac dysfunction (**Table 50-1**).[11,23,24] Even in the absence of these risk factors, however, all patients undergoing a TKA are at increased risk for development of DVT or PE.[9,14,25] A majority of venographically documented DVT occurs within 24 hours after surgery.[26] Proximal venous thrombi, even those that are nonocclusive and asymptomatic, show an association with proximal DVT extension and symptomatic or fatal PE.[14,27,28] In contrast, most distal thrombi, found in veins located below the knee, are small, clinically insignificant, and usually do not require treatment with therapeutic anticoagulation.[29-31] Thrombosis of the veins in the calf is generally an asymptomatic, self-limiting process that spontaneously resolves, but in some cases there will be proximal clot propagation. There is low risk of development of chronic venous insufficiency.[29,30] However, complications of a distal thrombus may occur more frequently in patients who have had a total joint arthroplasty.[14,28,32] Using duplex ultrasonography to

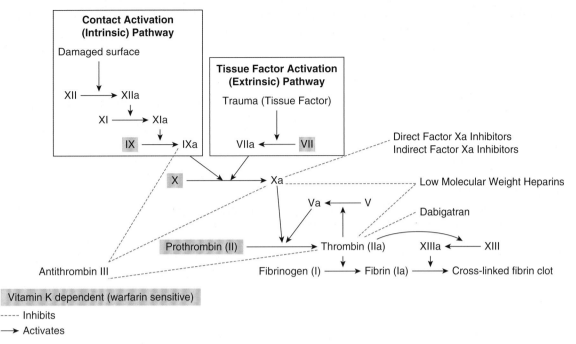

FIGURE 50-1 Coagulation pathways. Both the contact activation (intrinsic) and tissue factor activation (extrinsic) pathways converge, which leads to activation of factor X and the subsequent formation of thrombin. The prothrombin time (PT) measures the function of the extrinsic and common pathways. The partial thromboplastin time (PTT) measures the function of the intrinsic and common pathways.

TABLE 50-1	Risk Factors for Venous Thromboembolic Disease
Clinical risk factors	Prior venous thromboembolic disease
	Paralysis or prolonged immobility
	Obesity
	Advanced age
	Fractures of the pelvis, hip, femur, or tibia
	Varicose veins
	Surgery involving the abdomen, pelvis, lower extremities
	Congestive heart failure
	Myocardial infarction
	Diabetes mellitus
	Stroke
	Smoking
Hemostatic abnormalities	Antithrombin III deficiency
	Protein C deficiency
	Protein S deficiency
	Dysfibrinogenemia
	Presence of lupus anticoagulant and antiphospholipid antibodies
	Myeloproliferative disorders
	Heparin-induced thrombocytopenia
	Disorders of plasminogen and plasminogen activation

screen patients who had arthroplasty, Oishi et al found that within 2 weeks after surgery, 17% of patients with a distal DVT had proximal propagation of their thrombus.[28] Due to the high risk of DVT and the risk of fatality in the case of pulmonary embolism, postoperative VTE prophylaxis is essential in limiting thrombus formation and preventing propagation and embolism.

RISK STRATIFICATION

Providing effective VTE prophylaxis while reducing the risk of bleeding events in elective total joint arthroplasty patients has triggered significant interest in risk stratification paradigms. Despite potent anticoagulants, early-mobilization protocols, and advancements in regional anesthesia, the rate of symptomatic PE following TKA has held constant over time.[33] Cote et al performed a systematic review including 18 multicenter prospective randomized controlled trials assessing the efficacy of VTE prophylaxis regimens after elective TKA. In an analysis of pooled data comparing rates of symptomatic PE in studies published before 2006 versus studies published in 2006 or later, the estimated rate of symptomatic PE increased by 0.0006% ($P > .999$) despite all the advances associated with TKA during that time period.[33] These results suggest that a cohort of patients possess nonmodifiable risk factors, and PE after TKA is not a "never event" even with the most potent prophylaxis regimen. Accurate assessment of a TKA patient's risk profile and tailoring of their postoperative VTE prophylaxis regimen accordingly defines the principle of risk stratification, a critical concept in the future of arthroplasty.

There have been multiple attempts to identify TJA patients with higher risk profiles for VTE events; however, no validated risk assessment tool currently exists.[34-37] Bohl et al utilized the American College of Surgeons National Surgical Quality Improvement Program (NSQIP) database to identify independent risk factors in elective TJA patients for the development of symptomatic PE; these risk factors were subsequently assigned a point value which helped define thresholds between low-, medium-, and high-risk patients.[37] This was validated against a single-center registry of TJA patients. The patients thought to be at increased risk for VTE were older than 70 years, female, obese, and undergoing a TKA. There are notable limitations to this instrument: the NSQIP database does not contain data on personal history of symptomatic VTE and there are no specific recommendations for prophylaxis for low-, medium-, and high-risk patients. Despite these limits, it does equip the provider with a means by which to stratify a patient's risk for developing symptomatic PE in the postoperative setting. In the absence of robust, validated risk stratification instruments that

provide recommendations for specific VTE prophylaxis regimens, a safe and effective plan must be made through shared decision making between the patient and physician.

VTE PROPHYLAXIS AFTER TKA

A variety of pharmacologic and mechanical approaches have been used to decrease the risk of VTE after TKA. Pharmacologic options include aspirin, vitamin K antagonists, unfractionated heparin, low-molecular-weight heparin (LMWH), fondaparinux, direct factor Xa inhibitors, and dabigatran. Mechanical approaches have included early mobilization, use of graded compression stockings, and use of sequential intermittent pneumatic compression boots. The most recent American Academy of Orthopaedic Surgeons (AAOS) clinical practice guidelines for VTE prevention were released in 2011.[38-40] This update to the 2007 guidelines included a more comprehensive statistical analysis and increased granularity in the grading schema (**Table 50-2**). Ultimately, however, no specific prophylactic regimen was

TABLE 50-2 Summary of AAOS Guidelines Regarding Venous Thromboembolism (VTE) Prevention[38-40]

American Academy of Orthopaedic Surgeons (AAOS) 2011 Guidelines for Preventing Venous Thromboembolism Before Elective Hip or Knee Arthroplasty[38,39]

Recommendation	Grade
1. Recommend against the use of routine postoperative duplex ultrasonography screening of patients who undergo elective hip or knee arthroplasty	Strong
2. Recommend assessment of the risk of VTE by determining whether these patients had a previous VTE	Weak
3. Cannot recommend for or against routinely assessing patients for risk factors other than a history of previous thromboembolism	Inconclusive
4. Recommend assessment for known bleeding disorders like hemophilia and the presence of active liver disease which increase risk for bleeding and bleeding-associated complications	Consensus
5. Cannot recommend for or against routinely assessing patients for risk factors for bleeding and bleeding-associated complications other than a known bleeding disorder or active liver disease	Inconclusive
6. Recommend discontinuation antiplatelet agents (e.g., aspirin, clopidogrel) before undergoing elective hip or knee arthroplasty	Moderate
7. Recommend the use of pharmacologic agents and/or mechanical compressive devices for the prevention of VTE in patients undergoing elective hip or knee arthroplasty, and who are not at elevated risk beyond that of the surgery itself for VTE or bleeding	Moderate
8. Cannot recommend for or against specific prophylactic options	Inconclusive
9. Recommend patients and physicians discuss the duration of prophylaxis	Consensus
10. Recommend pharmacologic prophylaxis and mechanical compressive devices in patients undergoing elective hip or knee arthroplasty and who have also had a previous VTE	Consensus
11. Recommend mechanical compressive devices in patients undergoing elective hip or knee arthroplasty and who also have a known bleeding disorder and/or active liver disease	Consensus
12. Recommend early mobilization for patients following elective hip and knee arthroplasty	Consensus
13. Recommend neuraxial anesthesia for patients undergoing hip and knee arthroplasty to help limit blood loss	Moderate
14. Cannot recommend for or against use of inferior vena cava filters to prevent PE in patients undergoing elective hip and knee arthroplasty who also have a contraindication to chemoprophylaxis and/or known residual venous thromboembolic disease	Inconclusive

Readers are strongly encouraged to consult the full guidelines and evidence report for this information and create individualized treatment decisions for each patient.

TABLE 50-3 **Summary of ACCP Guidelines Regarding Venous Thromboembolism Prevention[41]**

American College of Chest Physicians (ACCP) 2012 Guidelines for Prevention of Venous Thromboembolism in Orthopaedic Surgery Patients[41]

Recommendation	Grade
In patients undergoing THA or TKA, one of the following agents should be used for a minimum of 10-14 days, rather than providing no antithrombotic prophylaxis.	
• Low-molecular-weight heparin (LMWH)	1B
• Fondaparinux	1B
• Apixaban	1B
• Dabigatran	1B
• Rivaroxaban	1B
• Low-dose unfractionated heparin	1B
• Adjusted-dose vitamin K antagonist	1B
• Aspirin	1B
• Intermittent pneumatic compression device (IPCD)	1C
In patients undergoing THA or TKA, regardless of IPCD use or the length of treatment, LMWH should be used in preference to other alternative agents	2B
In patients undergoing major orthopedic surgery, thromboprophylaxis should be extended in the outpatient period for up to 35 d from the day of surgery rather than for only 10-14 d.	2B

THA, total hip arthroplasty; TKA, total knee arthroplasty.
Readers are strongly encouraged to consult the full guidelines and evidence report for this information and create individualized treatment decisions for each patient. (1B = strong recommendation, moderate-quality evidence. 1C = strong recommendation, low-quality evidence. 2B = weak recommendation, moderate-quality evidence.)

able to be recommended at that time given the available evidence. Partly in response to criticism from the orthopedic community, the American College of Chest Physicians (ACCP) published guidelines in 2012 focused on the reduction of *symptomatic* VTE events.[41] Although the ACCP guidelines favored LMWH for its safety and efficacy profile, a wide variety of pharmacologic agents and home compression devices were considered reasonable alternatives in TJA patients compared to no prophylaxis at all (**Table 50-3**).

Aspirin

The use of aspirin for thromboprophylaxis after TKA has been increasing.[42] Aspirin irreversibly inactivates cyclooxygenase (COX)-1, inhibits prostaglandin H_2 formation, inhibits platelets, and acetylates coagulation proteins including fibrinogen, promoting fibrinolysis.[43] Platelet inactivation by aspirin subsequently inhibits the release of multiple factors involved in venous thrombosis, including fibrinogen, thrombospondin, and von Willebrand factor, and prevents thrombin formation catalyzed by the calcium ion–dependent complex of tissue factor and activated factor VII.[43]

The Pulmonary Embolism Prevention (PEP) trial assessed 4088 patients undergoing hip and knee arthroplasty (including 1440 TKA patients) and 13,356 patients undergoing hip fracture surgery, randomized to either 160 mg of aspirin daily or placebo. In hip fracture patients, symptomatic VTE events were reduced by 36%. However, no statistically significant differences were seen in the arthroplasty group.[44] The rate of symptomatic DVT in the arthroplasty group given aspirin was 0.73%, compared to 0.93% in the placebo group. The rate of PE was 0.43% in patients receiving aspirin, and 0.49% in those receiving placebo.[44] There was no difference in bleeding rates as defined by evacuation of a hematoma (0.4% with aspirin vs. 0.4% with placebo).[44] There were statistical limitations to this study including that 24% of patients randomized to the aspirin group received aspirin or another nonsteroidal anti-inflammatory drug (NSAID) within the 48 hours prior to randomization.

In a large registry study evaluating 41,537 patients undergoing TKA receiving no chemo-thromboprophylaxis, aspirin only, anticoagulant only (LMWH, warfarin, or factor Xa inhibitors), or both aspirin and anticoagulant, aspirin was found to be noninferior to other anticoagulants in terms of VTE (no chemo-thromboprophylaxis = 4.79%, aspirin only = 1.16%, anticoagulant only = 1.42%, aspirin and anticoagulant = 1.31%) and bleeding events (no chemo-thromboprophylaxis = 1.50%, aspirin only = 0.90%, anticoagulant only = 1.14%, aspirin and anticoagulant = 1.35%).[45] In a prospective, cross-over study, 4651 TJA patients received either 325 mg or 81 mg of aspirin twice daily with a subsequent switch to the alternative dosing regimen during their therapy course. Preliminary analysis showed no statistical difference in VTE rates between lower- and higher-dose groups (0.1% vs. 0.3%, respectively). There was a slightly lower, but not statistically significant, difference, in rates of gastrointestinal bleeding or ulceration between lower- and higher-dose groups (0.3% vs. 0.4%, respectively).[46] This study provides support for the use of lower-dose aspirin in patients without significant risk factors for the development of postoperative VTE.

A recent multicenter, double-blind, randomized, controlled trial was conducted with TKA and THA patients to determine if extended prophylaxis with aspirin was safe and effective. All patients received 5 days of once-daily 10 mg of rivaroxaban. The patients were then randomized to either an additional 9 days (for TKA patients) of once-daily 10 mg of rivaroxaban or a control group that received once-daily 81 mg of aspirin. In the TKA patients, there was no difference in the rate of VTE (0.86% with rivaroxaban vs. 0.87% with aspirin; $P = 1.00$). There was also no difference in major bleeding in the TKA patients (0.25% with rivaroxaban vs. 0.62% with aspirin; $P = .29$).[2] Other trials have shown similarly low rates of VTE and bleeding with aspirin, especially when used in conjunction with early ambulation and pneumatic compression boots.[47-54]

Aspirin has multiple advantages, including its oral administration, no requirement for monitoring, low cost, lower bleeding risk, and high patient compliance.[47-55] Long-term high-dose aspirin use may lead to epigastric pain, heartburn, nausea, or gastrointestinal bleeding.[56] The major limitation with determining the true efficacy of aspirin is the need for data from multicenter, randomized trials comparing the efficacy and safety of aspirin versus the new, more potent anticoagulant agents (e.g., rivaroxaban, dabigatran, or apixaban).

Vitamin K Antagonists

Warfarin, a potent anticoagulant, has a long track record in preventing VTE after TKA. It functions by blocking the transformation of vitamin K in the liver, and thereby inhibiting production of vitamin K–dependent clotting factors II, VII, IX, and X (**Fig. 50-1**).[57] The rate of symptomatic PE with the use of warfarin prophylaxis is between 0.31% and 0.9%.[58] Multiple randomized trials comparing warfarin to LMWH have shown that while LMWH was more effective in limiting asymptomatic thrombi and overall DVT formation, there was no difference in rates of post discharge symptomatic events, including PE. Higher rates of bleeding were seen with the use of LMWH.[5,59-65]

The major advantages of warfarin prophylaxis include a proven track record, oral administration, low cost, and adjustable dosing. The magnitude of anticoagulation can be titrated for each patient based on the international normalized ratio (INR). A target INR of 2.0 (range 1.8-2.5) provides effective prophylaxis and limits bleeding complications. Disadvantages of warfarin use include frequent laboratory monitoring of the INR, interaction with many other medications and foods complicating the ability to maintain a therapeutic level, and the delayed onset of its anticoagulant effect which may leave a patient vulnerable to VTE.[1,8,57,66] Despite close monitoring, patients receiving

warfarin for chemical thromboprophylaxis are within their targeted INR range for approximately half the duration of their treatment course.[67] Additionally, there is a 0.4% to 5% incidence of major bleeding.[1,5,8,59,60,63-65,68] If the INR needs to be returned to normal, such as in the case of life-threatening bleeding, prothrombin complex concentrates, fresh frozen plasma, or intravenous or oral vitamin K may be required.[69] Warfarin reversal via transfusion can quickly reverse the anticoagulation properties of warfarin, but it is also associated with immunologic reactions, infection, and transfusion related injuries.[70]

Heparin and Low-Molecular-Weight Heparins

Standard unfractionated heparin is a heterogeneous mixture of glycosaminoglycans. The pentasaccharide sequence of heparin binds antithrombin III, forming a ternary complex, leading to inhibition of thrombin, factor IX, and factor Xa.[71] Heparin can be fractionated to separate LMWH which contains fewer than 18-saccharide units. Due to this structure, LMWH is unable to induce thrombin inhibition as it cannot bind to both thrombin and antithrombin simultaneously (**Fig. 50-2**).[14,72] Therefore, LMWH primarily functions by indirectly inhibiting factor Xa.[73] Additionally, LMWH induces less bleeding than standard heparin because of reduced inhibition of platelet function and decreased microvascular permeability. LMWH has a bioavailability of at least 90%, with a substantially reduced ability to bind to plasma proteins, vascular endothelium, or other circulating cells.[74] Due to these differences, LMWH is used more frequently than unfractionated heparin in total joint arthroplasty.

LMWH provides highly effective prevention of DVT and PE. The risk reduction in total DVT is up to 71% with enoxaparin compared to placebo.[75] A large meta-analysis

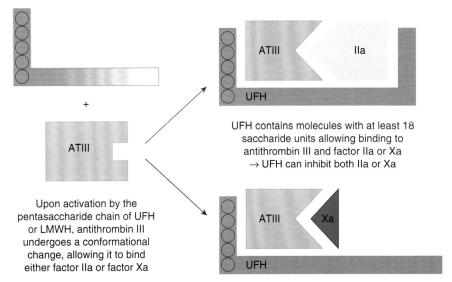
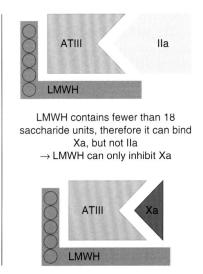

FIGURE 50-2 Heparins must bind antithrombin III (ATIII) via the high-affinity pentasaccharide (denoted by five circles), which induces a conformational change in ATIII. Both unfractionated heparin (UFH) and low-molecular-weight heparin (LMWH) bind ATIII and factor Xa, leading to the inactivation of factor Xa. However, to inactivate thrombin (factor IIa), an additional 13-saccharide unit is required to form a ternary complex. LMWH molecules that do not contain 18-saccharide units bind to ATIII but not to thrombin. Therefore, UFN leads to thrombin inactivation, but LMWH does not.[72]

comparing LMWH with warfarin revealed lower rates of proximal DVT (5.9% with LMWH vs. 10.2% with warfarin) and symptomatic PE (0.2% with LMWH vs. 0.4% with warfarin).[76] However, LMWH leads to higher rates of major bleeding events (2.4% with LMWH vs. 1.3% with warfarin).[76] In a trial comparing 778 patients who received an initial 10 days of LWMH that were randomized to receive either LMWH or aspirin for the following 28 days, 1.3% of patients receiving LMWH and 0.3% of patients receiving aspirin had a VTE event. Clinically significant bleeding occurred in 1.3% of those receiving LMWH and 0.5% of patients receiving aspirin, demonstrating that aspirin was noninferior to LMWH.[77]

The use of LMWH has several advantages. The prolonged half-life of LMWH allows for once- to twice-daily dosing and no laboratory monitoring is required.[14,67,73] However, subcutaneous injections are necessary, which may limit patient compliance.[73] The bleeding risk with LMWH is higher than warfarin and aspirin.[78] LMWH may be partially reversed in an emergency situation with the use of protamine.[79] LMWH is metabolized in the kidney, and modifications in dosing are necessary in patients with renal insufficiency. Both unfractionated heparin and LMWH can lead to heparin-induced thrombocytopenia (HIT). The risk is much lower with LMWH (0.2%) compared to unfractionated heparin (2.6%), but this risk should be considered prior to use.[80]

Fondaparinux

Fondaparinux sodium is a synthetic pentasaccharide that is structurally related to the antithrombin binding site of heparin. The pentasaccharide selectively binds to antithrombin III, causing a rapid indirect inhibition of factor Xa, a key enzyme in the coagulation pathway.[81] In several large randomized controlled trials, the rate of symptomatic VTE when using fondaparinux was found to be 3.2% to 8.5%, with a bleeding rate of 1.8% to 4.1%.[82-86] The rate of symptomatic VTE was 47% lower with the use of fondaparinux compared to LMWH. However, fondaparinux was associated with a 64% higher rate of major bleeding than LMWH.[83] Although fondaparinux is FDA approved for use in hip fracture patients, because of the concerns regarding bleeding, it has been used on a limited basis for TKA patients in the United States.

There are several advantages to fondaparinux. It has a highly predictable response and is 100% bioavailable, with a rapid onset of action and only once-daily dosing which does not require laboratory testing.[81] Fondaparinux does not cross-react with heparin antibodies and is safe for use in patients with HIT.[81] However, it requires subcutaneous injection, which may limit patient compliance. In addition, although effects may be reversed with prothrombin complex concentrates, this may be associated with allergic reactions, HIT, stroke, myocardial infarction, and disseminated intravascular coagulation.[86]

Factor Xa Inhibitors

Direct factor Xa inhibitors ("xabans") are another class of oral anticoagulants, the most popular of which are rivaroxaban, apixaban, and edoxaban.[81] These medications are highly selective competitive inhibitors of factor Xa and inhibit both free and clot-bound factor Xa to prolong clotting times.[87-89] Multiple randomized controlled trials have demonstrated that factor Xa inhibitors are effective and safe in preventing VTE after arthroplasty (**Table 50-4**).[90-93] In the RECORD3 trial, 2531 patients undergoing TKA were randomized to 10 mg rivaroxaban or 40 mg enoxaparin, and total VTE or death in 9.6% of those receiving rivaroxaban and 18.9% of those receiving enoxaparin ($P < .001$) were shown. There was also a lower rate of symptomatic VTE in the rivaroxaban group (0.7% with rivaroxaban vs. 2.0% with enoxaparin, $P = .005$). There were equivalent rates of major bleeding in both groups (0.6% with rivaroxaban vs. 0.5% with enoxaparin; $P = .77$).[90] The RECORD4 trial randomized 3148 patients receiving TKA to either 10 mg rivaroxaban once daily or 30 mg enoxaparin twice daily, and demonstrated a 6.7% rate of total VTE or mortality in the rivaroxaban group compared to 9.3% in the enoxaparin group ($P = .0118$), and a symptomatic VTE rate of 0.7% in the rivaroxaban group compared to 1.2% in the enoxaparin group ($P = .1868$). There were equivalent major bleeding rates in both groups (0.7% with rivaroxaban vs. 1.2% with enoxaparin; $P = .11$).[91]

Several randomized trials have compared apixaban to enoxaparin, demonstrating the safety and efficacy of apixaban after THA or TKA (**Table 50-4**).[94-96] The ADVANCE-1 trial randomized 3195 patients undergoing TKA to 2.5 mg apixaban twice daily or 30 mg enoxaparin twice daily, and showed an equivalent total VTE and mortality rate (9.0% with apixaban vs. 8.8% with enoxaparin). When comparing the incidence of symptomatic VTE (defined as the aggregation of symptomatic DVT and nonfatal and fatal PE), apixaban did not satisfy criteria to be deemed noninferior to enoxaparin (1.2% with apixaban vs. 0.8% with enoxaparin). However, there was statistically significantly less major bleeding with apixaban (0.7% with apixaban vs. 1.4% with enoxaparin, $P = .05$).[94] The ADVANCE-2 trial randomized 3057 patients undergoing elective TKA to 2.5 mg apixaban twice daily or 40 mg enoxaparin once daily, showing superior efficacy with total VTE and mortality rate of 15% in apixaban group versus 24% in enoxaparin group ($P < .001$). There was a symptomatic VTE rate of 0.46% in the apixaban group versus 0.46% in the enoxaparin group ($P = 1.00$). There were similar rates of major bleeding in both groups (0.6% with apixaban vs. 0.9% with enoxaparin; $P = .3014$).[95]

In the evaluation of edoxaban in the setting of TKA, one randomized trial showed its safety and efficacy. The STARS E-3 trial randomized 716 patients undergoing TKA to 30 mg edoxaban once daily or 20 mg enoxaparin

TABLE 50-4	Summary of Randomized Trials Evaluating Factor Xa Inhibitors					
Trial	**Intervention**	**VTE Events**	**P-value**	**Major Bleeding Events**	**P-value**
RECORD1[92] (THA)	Rivaroxaban 10 mg daily Enoxaparin 40 mg daily	18/1595 (1.1%) 58/1558 (3.7%)	<.001	6/2209 (0.3%) 2/2224 (0.1%)	.18
RECORD2[93] (THA)	Rivaroxaban 10 mg daily Enoxaparin 40 mg daily	17/864 (2.0%) 81/869 (9.3%)	<.001	1/1228 (<0.1%) 1/1229 (<0.1%)	Not listed
RECORD3[90] (TKA)	Rivaroxaban 10 mg daily Enoxaparin 40 mg daily	79/824 (9.6%) 166/878 (18.9%)	<.001	7/1220 (0.6%) 6/1239 (0.5%)	.77
RECORD4[91] (TKA)	Rivaroxaban 10 mg daily Enoxaparin 30 mg BID	58/864 (6.7%) 82/878 (9.3%)	.0362	10/1526 (0.7%) 4/1508 (0.3%)	.1096
ADVANCE-1[94] (TKA)	Apixaban 2.5 mg BID Enoxaparin 30 mg BID	104/1157 (9.0%) 100/1130 (8.8%)	.06	11/1596 (0.7%) 22/1588 (1.4%)	.05
ADVANCE-2[95] (TKA)	Apixaban 2.5 mg BID Enoxaparin 40 mg daily	147/976 (15.1%) 243/997 (24.4%)	<.001	9/1501 (0.6%) 14/1508 (0.9%)	.3014
ADVANCE-3[96] (THA)	Apixaban 2.5 mg BID Enoxaparin 40 mg daily	27/1949 (1.4%) 74/1917 (3.9%)	<.001	22/2673 (0.8%) 18/2659 (0.7%)	.54
STARS E-3[97] (TKA)	Edoxaban 30 mg daily Enoxaparin 20 mg BID	22/299 (7.4%) 41/295 (13.9%)	.010	4/354 (1.1%) 1/349 (0.3%)	.373

THA, total hip arthroplasty; TKA, total knee arthroplasty; VTE, venous thromboembolism.

twice daily and compared rates of symptomatic PE and asymptomatic or symptomatic DVT. Edoxaban was shown to be superior to enoxaparin in efficacy (7.4% incidence of primary efficacy outcome in the edoxaban group compared to 13.9% in the enoxaparin group, $P = .010$ for superiority). There was a similar incidence of major bleeding events in both groups (1.1% with edoxaban vs. 0.3% with enoxaparin; $P = .373$).[97]

There are several benefits to the use of oral direct factor Xa inhibitors, which provide potent anticoagulation via oral administration with once- or twice-daily dosing, and no requirement for lab monitoring.[81] Additionally, the FDA has recently approved andexanet alfa for urgent reversal of rivaroxaban and apixaban in the event of life-threatening bleeding.[98] As with any chemical anticoagulant, there is a risk of bleeding events, but factor Xa

inhibitors have not shown a significant increase in the rates of bleeding compared to other commonly used anticoagulants.[81] However, most surgeons administer these agents 18 to 24 hours after the surgical procedure to limit bleeding.

Dabigatran

Dabigatran is a competitive direct inhibitor of thrombin.[99] It is a synthetic, reversible, orally available thrombin inhibitor, which inhibits both free thrombin, fibrin-bound forms of thrombin, and thrombin-induced platelet aggregation.[99] Several randomized clinical trials support the use of dabigatran for VTE prophylaxis after arthroplasty (Table 50-5).[100-103] In the pooled analysis of three randomized controlled trials comparing dabigatran

TABLE 50-5	Summary of Randomized Trials Comparing Dabigatran to Enoxaparin[101-103]					
Trial	**Intervention**	**VTE Events**	**P-value**	**Major Bleeding Events**	**P-value**
RE-NOVATE[100] (THA)	Dabigatran 220 mg daily Dabigatran 150 mg daily Enoxaparin 40 mg daily	53/880 (6.0%) 75/874 (8.6%) 60/897 (6.7%)	<.0001 <.0001	23/1146 (2.0%) 15/1163 (1.3%) 18/1154 (1.6%)	.44 .60
RE-NOVATE II[101] (THA)	Dabigatran 220 mg daily Enoxaparin 40 mg daily	61/792 (7.7%) 69/785 (8.8%)	<.0001	14/1010 (1.4%) 9/1003 (0.9%)	.40
RE-MOBILIZE[103] (TKA)	Dabigatran 220 mg daily Dabigatran 150 mg daily Enoxaparin 30 mg BID	188/604 (31.1%) 219/649 (33.7%) 163/643 (25.3%)	.0243 .0009	5/857 (0.6% 5/871 (0.6%) 12/868 (1.4%)	not listed
RE-MODEL[102] (TKA)	Dabigatran 220 mg daily Dabigatran 150 mg daily Enoxaparin 40 mg daily	183/503 (36.4%) 213/526 (40.5%) 193/512 (37.7%)	.38 .82	10/679 (1.5%) 9/703 (1.3%) 9/694 (1.3%)	.82 1.00

THA, total hip arthroplasty; TKA, total knee arthroplasty; VTE, venous thromboembolism.

and enoxaparin in patients undergoing TKA or THA, patients were randomized to either dabigatran 220 mg daily (2033 patients), dabigatran 150 mg daily (2071 patients), or enoxaparin (40 mg once daily or 30 mg twice daily) (2096 patients).[104] The rate of VTE-related death, PE, and proximal DVT was 3.0% in the dabigatran 220 mg group, 3.8% in the dabigatran 150 mg group, and 3.3% in the enoxaparin group ($P = .20$ and $P = .91$, compared to enoxaparin). The major bleeding rate was 1.4% for those receiving dabigatran 220 mg, 1.1% in those receiving dabigatran 150 mg, and 1.4% in those receiving enoxaparin ($P = .61$ and $P = .16$, compared to enoxaparin).[104] The current dosing recommendation for VTE prophylaxis is 220 mg daily.[105,106]

The major advantages of dabigatran include once-daily oral dosing which does not require laboratory testing. Currently, no interactions with other medications have been identified.[99] In the event of life-threatening bleeding, idarucizumab may be used for rapid and safe dabigatran reversal.[107] However, gastrointestinal side effects, including nausea, vomiting, and constipation, have been described. Additionally, dabigatran is 10 to 30 times more expensive than warfarin.[99]

Mechanical Methods

Intermittent pneumatic compression devices (IPCDs) are a mechanical method that has been shown to be efficacious in limiting clot formation after TKA. They can be applied to either the calf or the foot. IPCDs function to prevent DVT formation by increasing the velocity of venous blood flow in the extremities, decreasing venous stasis, and enhancing endogenous fibrinolytic activity.[108,109] The appeal of these types of devices is that they do not require any laboratory monitoring, there is no potential for bleeding, and they are generally well tolerated by patients. These mechanical methods of prophylaxis seem to be particularly well-suited for patients undergoing TKA in view of concerns about the effects of bleeding and the influence of hematoma formation on postoperative range of motion.[14,110] The results of several randomized trials performed more than two decades ago demonstrated that intermittent pneumatic compression provides effective prophylaxis in patients undergoing TKA.[111-114] Combined with aspirin, the incidence of symptomatic DVT and PE can be as low as 1.5% and 0.5% respectively.[115] Calf compression in conjunction with low-molecular-weight heparin (LMWH) leads to a lower incidence of DVT than with LMWH alone, suggesting that mechanical compression may augment the efficacy of chemoprophylaxis.[116,117] Intermittent plantar compression of the foot simulates the hemodynamic effects that occur during normal walking, increasing venous return, and has been shown to decrease the incidence of DVT.[112,118-122]

The problem with IPCD is that with shorter hospital length of stays or even same day discharge, they can only be used for a short period of time. Recently, portable mechanical compression devices have been assessed, and show decreased rates of major bleeding events with equivalent DVT rates compared to chemoprophylactic agents.[113,123] To our knowledge, there are no large, multicenter, randomized trials assessing the efficacy of home mechanical compression devices compared to chemoprophylaxis in TKA patients. Colwell et al randomized 410 patients undergoing THA to receive prophylaxis with a mobile compression device or LMWH for 10 days, with a total VTE rate of 5% in the compression group and 5% in the LMWH group ($P = .935$), and 0% major bleeding in the mobile compression group compared to 6% in the LMWH group ($P = .0004$).[123] In a subsequent study, Colwell et al reviewed a large registry assessing the use of mobile compression devices in 3060 patients undergoing THA or TKA, showing similar efficacy compared to previously published VTE rates for other prophylactic options.[113] In both of these studies, approximately 60% of the patients combined aspirin with home mechanical compression. The potential efficacy of these devices is limited by patient compliance; there is a lack of therapeutic benefit when the device is not being used. In addition, there are concerns about the cost of these devices.[124]

In the past it has been hypothesized that compression stockings or use of continuous passive motion machines can reduce symptomatic clots, but this has not been demonstrated in the literature.[125-141]

IVC Filters

In patients who are at high risk for VTE due to hypercoagulable state or prior VTE, preoperatively placed inferior vena cava (IVC) filters may offer an additional method of preventing PE by mechanically capturing DVT prior to embolization to the lungs, without systemic risk of bleeding complications. The placement and potential removal of IVC filters may result in procedural complications.[142] Therefore, there is limited justification for the use of IVC filters in elective TKA patients, even those with a history of PE or DVT. The recent ACCP guidelines specifically recommended against their use for these patients.[41] IVC filters may reduce the risk of subsequent PE, but do not reduce the risk of DVT.[143-145] Few studies have shown IVC filters are safe and beneficial in preventing PE in patients undergoing total joint arthroplasty, and further research is needed.[146,147]

DURATION OF PROPHYLAXIS

Postoperative prophylaxis to prevent DVT formation is the standard of care after TKA; however, the optimal duration of thromboprophylaxis remains unclear. Previous studies have demonstrated that routine duplex ultrasonographic screening for asymptomatic DVT before hospital discharge is not effective.[148,149] The ACCP guidelines suggest a minimum of 10 to 14 days, and up to 35 days, of postoperative thromboprophylaxis after major orthopedic surgery, including TKA.[41] The average length of stay after a TKA has decreased significantly, limiting the availability of inpatient lab monitoring and ease of wound assessment. These factors may affect a surgeon's choice of anticoagulation.[150] The AAOS does not recommend a specific duration of VTE prophylaxis.[39] A 2016 Cochrane review showed inconclusive

evidence supporting extended-duration anticoagulation to prevent VTE after TKA.[151] While extended-duration thromboprophylaxis may decrease the incidence of VTE, there is an associated increased risk of bleeding events.[152] Hematoma, wound drainage, and INR greater than 1.5 are significant risk factors for periprosthetic infection.[153] A recent study showed that patients receiving warfarin, direct factor Xa inhibitors, and fondaparinux were more likely to require manipulation under anesthesia after

TABLE 50-6   Summary of Mechanism of Action, Advantages, and Disadvantages of Common Prophylaxis Regimens

Method	Mechanism	Advantages	Disadvantages
Aspirin	Platelet inhibition Inhibits prostaglandin and thromboxane production	Oral Inexpensive No lab monitoring High patient compliance Beneficial effects in preventing cardiovascular disease, stroke, certain cancers	Gastrointestinal bleeding and discomfort Less potent anticoagulant
Vitamin K antagonists	Blocks the synthesis of vitamin K–dependent clotting factors	Oral Inexpensive	Lab monitoring Delayed onset and reversal Reversal with FFP is rapid but requires allogenic transfusion; reversal with vitamin K is slow Multiple drug interactions
Unfractionated heparin	Enhances antithrombin III ability to inhibit factors IIa (thrombin) and Xa	Reversal with protamine Rapid onset and clearance	Heparin-induced thrombocytopenia Subcutaneous injection multiple times per day May require lab monitoring Bleeding
Low-molecular-weight heparin	Enhances antithrombin III ability to inhibit factor Xa	Fixed dosing No lab monitoring Partial reversal with protamine Rapid onset and clearance	Renal dosing is required Heparin-induced thrombocytopenia Subcutaneous injection Bleeding
Fondaparinux	Enhances antithrombin III ability to inhibit factor Xa	No lab monitoring Rapid onset and clearance	Subcutaneous injection Reversal requires prothrombin complex concentrates Bleeding
Dabigatran	Direct thrombin inhibition	Oral Relatively inexpensive No lab monitoring Reversal with idarucizumab	Gastrointestinal side effects Bleeding
Factor Xa inhibitors (rivaroxaban, apixaban, edoxaban)	Direct factor Xa inhibition	Oral Relatively inexpensive No lab monitoring Reversal with andexanet alfa	Bleeding
Mechanical (e.g., pneumatic compression boots, foot pumps)	Mechanical, prevent venous stasis	No bleeding risk	Requires patient compliance Patient discomfort Stockings may create reverse gradients
IVC filters	Prevents thrombus embolization to lungs	Can be used in patients who are unable to use chemical prophylaxis	Requires procedural placement (and possible removal) Does not prevent DVT

DVT, deep vein thrombosis; FFP, fresh frozen plasma; IVC, inferior vena cava.

total knee replacement than patients receiving aspirin or LMWH.[154] Surgeons must carefully weigh the risks and benefits of anticoagulation. In addition, surgeons must address the patient's ability to mobilize when determining the duration of prophylaxis. It is possible that early mobilization and rapid discharge from the hospital will limit VTE rates in the future, but this needs to be determined by studying a large population of patients.

RECOMMENDATIONS

Patients undergoing TKA are at high risk of developing DVT and PE. Primary prophylaxis with an effective regimen is mandatory in these patients. The selection of a prophylaxis regimen is a balance between efficacy and safety. Although none of the modalities for prophylaxis available today is without limitations and risks, there are a variety of agents that provide effective and safe prophylaxis (**Table 50-6**). Risk stratification may assist surgeons in providing the most appropriate anticoagulation options. For patients undergoing TKA, aspirin, dabigatran, factor Xa inhibitors, fondaparinux, LMWH, or warfarin, and home mechanical compression are effective in reducing the prevalence of PE and proximal clot formation. Although home compression devices have been shown to be effective, there are concerns about cost and compliance. In patients with higher risk for VTE, such as those with history of VTE, active malignancy, hypercoagulable states, morbid obesity, multiple medical comorbidities, family history of DVT or PE, and limited mobility, surgeons may consider more aggressive thromboprophylaxis regimens.[37] The optimal duration of prophylaxis for patients undergoing TKA has not yet been determined, but the ACCP guidelines recommend a minimum of 10 days and up to 35 days of postoperative thromboprophylaxis. The various prophylaxis regimens have differing efficacy and safety profiles and should be tailored to each individual patient.

REFERENCES

1. Lieberman JR, Geerts WH. Prevention of venous thromboembolism after total hip and knee arthroplasty. *J Bone Joint Surg Am.* 1994;76(8):1239-1250.
2. Anderson DR, Dunbar M, Murnaghan J, et al. Aspirin or rivaroxaban for VTE prophylaxis after hip or knee arthroplasty. *N Engl J Med.* 2018;378(8):699-707. doi:10.1056/NEJMoa1712746.
3. Stringer MD, Steadman CA, Hedges AR, Thomas EM, Morley TR, Kakkar VV. Deep vein thrombosis after elective knee surgery. An incidence study in 312 patients. *J Bone Joint Surg Br.* 1989;71(3):492-497.
4. Mori N, Kimura S, Onodera T, Iwasaki N, Nakagawa I, Masuda T. Use of a pneumatic tourniquet in total knee arthroplasty increases the risk of distal deep vein thrombosis: a prospective, randomized study. *Knee.* 2016;23(5):887-889. doi:10.1016/j.knee.2016.02.007.
5. Hull R, Raskob G, Pineo G, et al. A comparison of subcutaneous low-molecular-weight heparin with warfarin sodium for prophylaxis against deep-vein thrombosis after hip or knee implantation. *N Engl J Med.* 1993;329(19):1370-1376. doi:10.1056/NEJM199311043291902.
6. Dua A, Desai SS, Lee CJ, Heller JA. National trends in deep vein thrombosis following total knee and total hip replacement in the United States. *Ann Vasc Surg.* 2017;38:310-314. doi:10.1016/j.avsg.2016.05.110.
7. O'Reilly RF, Burgess IA, Zicat B. The prevalence of venous thromboembolism after hip and knee replacement surgery. *Med J Aust.* 2005;182(4):154-159.
8. Lieberman JR. Warfarin prophylaxis after total knee arthroplasty. *Am J Knee Surg.* 1999;12(1):49-53.
9. Geerts WH, Bergqvist D, Pineo GF, et al. Prevention of venous thromboembolism: American College of Chest Physicians Evidence-Based Clinical Practice Guidelines (8th Edition). *Chest.* 2008;133(6 suppl):381S-453S. doi:10.1378/chest.08-0656.
10. Cushman M. Epidemiology and risk factors for venous thrombosis. *Semin Hematol.* 2007;44(2):62-69. doi:10.1053/j.seminhematol.2007.02.004.
11. Gordon RJ, Lombard FW. Perioperative venous thromboembolism: a review. *Anesth Analg.* 2017;125(2):403-412. doi:10.1213/ANE.0000000000002183.
12. Bovill EG, van der Vliet A. Venous valvular stasis-associated hypoxia and thrombosis: what is the link? *Annu Rev Physiol.* 2011;73:527-545. doi:10.1146/annurev-physiol-012110-142305.
13. Sevitt S. The structure and growth of valve-pocket thrombi in femoral veins. *J Clin Pathol.* 1974;27(7):517-528.
14. Lieberman JR. Prevention of deep venous thromboembolism following primary and revision hip and knee arthroplasty. In: Bono J, McCarthy J, Thornhill TS, eds. *Revision Total Hip Arthroplasty.* New York: Springer-Verlag; 1999:401-417.
15. Sharrock NE, Go G, Sculco TP, Ranawat CS, Maynard MJ, Harpel PC. Changes in circulatory indices of thrombosis and fibrinolysis during total knee arthroplasty performed under tourniquet. *J Arthroplasty.* 1995;10(4):523-528.
16. Reikeras O, Clementsen T. Thrombosis markers in hip versus knee arthroplasty: a pilot study. *J Orthop Surg.* 2009;17(3):291-295. doi:10.1177/230949900901700309.
17. Reikerås O, Clementsen T. Time course of thrombosis and fibrinolysis in total knee arthroplasty with tourniquet application. Local versus systemic activations. *J Thromb Thrombolysis.* 2009;28(4):425-428. doi:10.1007/s11239-008-0299-6.
18. Mackman N. New insights into the mechanisms of venous thrombosis. *J Clin Invest.* 2012;122(7):2331-2336. doi:10.1172/JCI60229.
19. Mackman N. Role of tissue factor in hemostasis, thrombosis, and vascular development. *Arterioscler Thromb Vasc Biol.* 2004;24(6):1015-1022. doi:10.1161/01.ATV.0000130465.23430.74.
20. Francis CW, Ricotta JJ, Evarts CM, Marder VJ. Long-term clinical observations and venous functional abnormalities after asymptomatic venous thrombosis following total hip or knee arthroplasty. *Clin Orthop Relat Res.* 1988;232:271-278.
21. Stulberg BN, Francis CW, Pellegrini VD, et al. Antithrombin III/low-dose heparin in the prevention of deep-vein thrombosis after total knee arthroplasty. A preliminary report. *Clin Orthop Relat Res.* 1989;248:152-157.
22. Kim Y-H, Kim JS. Incidence and natural history of deep-vein thrombosis after total knee arthroplasty. A prospective, randomised study. *J Bone Joint Surg Br.* 2002;84(4):566-570.
23. Zhang J, Chen Z, Zheng J, Breusch SJ, Tian J. Risk factors for venous thromboembolism after total hip and total knee arthroplasty: a meta-analysis. *Arch Orthop Trauma Surg.* 2015;135(6):759-772. doi:10.1007/s00402-015-2208-8.
24. White RH, Henderson MC. Risk factors for venous thromboembolism after total hip and knee replacement surgery. *Curr Opin Pulm Med.* 2002;8(5):365-371.
25. Fisher WD. Impact of venous thromboembolism on clinical management and therapy after hip and knee arthroplasty. *Can J Surg.* 2011;54(5):344-351. doi:10.1503/cjs.007310.
26. Maynard MJ, Sculco TP, Ghelman B. Progression and regression of deep vein thrombosis after total knee arthroplasty. *Clin Orthop Relat Res.* 1991;273:125-130.

27. Lee JS, Moon T, Kim TH, et al. Deep vein thrombosis in patients with pulmonary embolism: prevalance, clinical significance and outcome. *Vasc Specialist Int.* 2016;32(4):166-174. doi:10.5758/vsi.2016.32.4.166.

28. Oishi CS, Grady-Benson JC, Otis SM, Colwell CW, Walker RH. The clinical course of distal deep venous thrombosis after total hip and total knee arthroplasty, as determined with duplex ultrasonography. *J Bone Joint Surg Am.* 1994;76(11):1658-1663.

29. Righini M. Is it worth diagnosing and treating distal deep vein thrombosis? No. *J Thromb Haemost.* 2007;5(suppl 1):55-59. doi:10.1111/j.1538-7836.2007.02468.x.

30. Righini M, Paris S, Le Gal G, Laroche J-P, Perrier A, Bounameaux H. Clinical relevance of distal deep vein thrombosis. Review of literature data. *Thromb Haemost.* 2006;95(1):56-64.

31. Yun W-S, Lee KK, Cho J, Kim H-K, Kyung H-S, Huh S. Early treatment outcome of isolated calf vein thrombosis after total knee arthroplasty. *J Korean Surg Soc.* 2012;82(6):374-379. doi:10.4174/jkss.2012.82.6.374.

32. Bosque J, Coleman SI, Di Cesare P. Relationship between deep vein thrombosis and pulmonary embolism following THA and TKA. *Orthopedics.* 2012;35(3):228-233; quiz 234-235. doi:10.3928/01477447-20120222-12.

33. Cote MP, Chen A, Jiang Y, Cheng V, Lieberman JR. Persistent pulmonary embolism rates following total knee arthroplasty even with prophylactic anticoagulants. *J Arthroplasty.* 2017;32(12):3833-3839. doi:10.1016/j.arth.2017.06.041.

34. Parvizi J, Huang R, Raphael IJ, Arnold WV, Rothman RH. Symptomatic pulmonary embolus after joint arthroplasty: stratification of risk factors. *Clin Orthop Relat Res.* 2014;472(3):903-912. doi:10.1007/s11999-013-3358-z.

35. González Della Valle A, Serota A, Go G, et al. Venous thromboembolism is rare with a multimodal prophylaxis protocol after total hip arthroplasty. *Clin Orthop Relat Res.* 2006;444:146-153. doi:10.1097/01.blo.0000201157.29325.f0.

36. Vulcano E, Gesell M, Esposito A, Ma Y, Memtsoudis SG, Gonzalez Della Valle A. Aspirin for elective hip and knee arthroplasty: a multimodal thromboprophylaxis protocol. *Int Orthop.* 2012;36(10):1995-2002. doi:10.1007/s00264-012-1588-4.

37. Bohl DD, Maltenfort MG, Huang R, Parvizi J, Lieberman JR, Della Valle CJ. Development and validation of a risk stratification system for pulmonary embolism after elective primary total joint arthroplasty. *J Arthroplasty.* 2016;31(9 suppl):187-191. doi:10.1016/j.arth.2016.02.080.

38. Mont MA, Jacobs JJ, Boggio LN, et al. Preventing venous thromboembolic disease in patients undergoing elective hip and knee arthroplasty. *J Am Acad Orthop Surg.* 2011;19(12):768-776. doi:10.5435/00124635-201112000-00007.

39. Lieberman JR. The new AAOS clinical practice guidelines on venous thromboembolic prophylaxis: how to adapt them to your practice. *J Am Acad Orthop Surg.* 2011;19(12):717-721.

40. Lieberman JR, Heckmann N. Venous thromboembolism prophylaxis in total hip arthroplasty and total knee arthroplasty patients: from guidelines to practice. *J Am Acad Orthop Surg.* 2017;25(12):789-798. doi:10.5435/JAAOS-D-15-00760.

41. Falck-Ytter Y, Francis CW, Johanson NA, et al. Prevention of VTE in orthopedic surgery patients: antithrombotic therapy and prevention of thrombosis, 9th ed: American College of Chest Physicians Evidence-Based Clinical Practice Guidelines. *Chest.* 2012;141(2 suppl):e278S-e325S. doi:10.1378/chest.11-2404.

42. Parvizi J, Ceylan HH, Kucukdurmaz F, Merli G, Tuncay I, Beverland D. Venous thromboembolism following hip and knee arthroplasty: the role of aspirin. *J Bone Joint Surg Am.* 2017;99(11):961-972. doi:10.2106/JBJS.16.01253.

43. Mekaj YH, Daci FT, Mekaj AY. New insights into the mechanisms of action of aspirin and its use in the prevention and treatment of arterial and venous thromboembolism. *Ther Clin Risk Manag.* 2015;11:1449-1456. doi:10.2147/TCRM.S92222.

44. Prevention of pulmonary embolism and deep vein thrombosis with low dose aspirin: Pulmonary Embolism Prevention (PEP) trial. *Lancet.* 2000;355(9212):1295-1302.

45. Hood BR, Cowen ME, Zheng HT, Hughes RE, Singal B, Hallstrom BR. Association of aspirin with prevention of venous thromboembolism in patients after total knee arthroplasty compared with other anticoagulants: a noninferiority analysis. *JAMA Surg.* 2018;154(1):65-72. doi:10.1001/jamasurg.2018.3858.

46. Parvizi J, Huang R, Restrepo C, et al. Low-dose aspirin is effective chemoprophylaxis against clinically important venous thromboembolism following total joint arthroplasty: a preliminary analysis. *J Bone Joint Surg Am.* 2017;99(2):91-98. doi:10.2106/JBJS.16.00147.

47. Cusick LA, Beverland DE. The incidence of fatal pulmonary embolism after primary hip and knee replacement in a consecutive series of 4253 patients. *J Bone Joint Surg Br.* 2009;91(5):645-648. doi:10.1302/0301-620X.91B5.21939.

48. Kim YH, Choi IY, Park MR, Park TS, Cho JL. Prophylaxis for deep vein thrombosis with aspirin or low molecular weight dextran in Korean patients undergoing total hip replacement. A randomized controlled trial. *Int Orthop.* 1998;22(1):6-10.

49. Reitman RD, Emerson RH, Higgins LL, Tarbox TR. A multimodality regimen for deep venous thrombosis prophylaxis in total knee arthroplasty. *J Arthroplasty.* 2003;18(2):161-168. doi:10.1054/arth.2003.50026.

50. Dorr LD, Gendelman V, Maheshwari AV, Boutary M, Wan Z, Long WT. Multimodal thromboprophylaxis for total hip and knee arthroplasty based on risk assessment. *J Bone Joint Surg Am.* 2007;89(12):2648-2657. doi:10.2106/JBJS.F.00235.

51. Bozic KJ, Vail TP, Pekow PS, Maselli JH, Lindenauer PK, Auerbach AD. Does aspirin have a role in venous thromboembolism prophylaxis in total knee arthroplasty patients? *J Arthroplasty.* 2010;25(7):1053-1060. doi:10.1016/j.arth.2009.06.021.

52. Lotke PA, Palevsky H, Keenan AM, et al. Aspirin and warfarin for thromboembolic disease after total joint arthroplasty. *Clin Orthop Relat Res.* 1996;324:251-258.

53. Lotke PA, Lonner JH. The benefit of aspirin chemoprophylaxis for thromboembolism after total knee arthroplasty. *Clin Orthop Relat Res.* 2006;452:175-180. doi:10.1097/01.blo.0000238822.78895.95.

54. Azboy I, Barrack R, Thomas AM, Haddad FS, Parvizi J. Aspirin and the prevention of venous thromboembolism following total joint arthroplasty. *Bone Joint J.* 2017;99-B(11):1420-1430. doi:10.1302/0301-620X.99B11.BJJ-2017-0337.R2.

55. McKenna R, Galante J, Bachmann F, Wallace DL, Kaushal PS, Meredith P. Prevention of venous thromboembolism after total knee replacement by high-dose aspirin or intermittent calf and thigh compression. *Br Med J.* 1980;280(6213):514-517.

56. Sutcliffe P, Connock M, Gurung T, et al. Aspirin for prophylactic use in the primary prevention of cardiovascular disease and cancer: a systematic review and overview of reviews. *Health Technol Assess.* 2013;17(43):1-253. doi:10.3310/hta17430.

57. Fiore L, Deykin D. Anticoagulant therapy. In: Beutler E, ed. *Williams Hematology.* New York: McGraw-Hill; 1995:1562-1583.

58. Dager WE. Warfarin for venous thromboembolism prophylaxis after elective hip or knee arthroplasty: exploring the evidence, guidelines, and challenges remaining. *Ann Pharmacother.* 2012;46(1):79-88. doi:10.1345/aph.1P626.

59. RD heparin compared with warfarin for prevention of venous thromboembolic disease following total hip or knee arthroplasty. RD Heparin Arthroplasty Group. *J Bone Joint Surg Am.* 1994;76(8):1174-1185.

60. Hamulyák K, Lensing AW, van der Meer J, Smid WM, van Ooy A, Hoek JA. Subcutaneous low-molecular weight heparin or oral anticoagulants for the prevention of deep-vein thrombosis in elective hip and knee replacement? Fraxiparine Oral Anticoagulant Study Group. *Thromb Haemost.* 1995;74(6):1428-1431.

61. Colwell CW, Collis DK, Paulson R, et al. Comparison of enoxaparin and warfarin for the prevention of venous thromboembolic disease after total hip arthroplasty. Evaluation during hospitalization and three months after discharge. *J Bone Joint Surg Am.* 1999;81(7):932-940.

62. Francis CW, Pellegrini VD, Totterman S, et al. Prevention of deep-vein thrombosis after total hip arthroplasty. Comparison of warfarin and dalteparin. *J Bone Joint Surg Am.* 1997;79(9):1365-1372.

63. Leclerc JR, Geerts WH, Desjardins L, et al. Prevention of venous thromboembolism after knee arthroplasty. A randomized, double-blind trial comparing enoxaparin with warfarin. *Ann Intern Med.* 1996;124(7):619-626.

64. Heit JA, Berkowitz SD, Bona R, et al. Efficacy and safety of low molecular weight heparin (ardeparin sodium) compared to warfarin for the prevention of venous thromboembolism after total knee replacement surgery: a double-blind, dose-ranging study. Ardeparin Arthroplasty Study Group. *Thromb Haemost.* 1997;77(1):32-38.

65. Fitzgerald RH, Spiro TE, Trowbridge AA, et al. Prevention of venous thromboembolic disease following primary total knee arthroplasty. A randomized, multicenter, open-label, parallel-group comparison of enoxaparin and warfarin. *J Bone Joint Surg Am.* 2001;83-A(6):900-906.

66. Shorr RI, Ray WA, Daugherty JR, Griffin MR. Concurrent use of nonsteroidal anti-inflammatory drugs and oral anticoagulants places elderly persons at high risk for hemorrhagic peptic ulcer disease. *Arch Intern Med.* 1993;153(14):1665-1670.

67. Nam D, Sadhu A, Hirsh J, Keeney JA, Nunley RM, Barrack RL. The use of warfarin for DVT prophylaxis following hip and knee arthroplasty: how often are patients within their target INR range? *J Arthroplasty.* 2015;30(2):315-319. doi:10.1016/j.arth.2014.08.032.

68. Lieberman JR, Sung R, Dorey F, Thomas BJ, Kilgus DJ, Finerman GA. Low-dose warfarin prophylaxis to prevent symptomatic pulmonary embolism after total knee arthroplasty. *J Arthroplasty.* 1997;12(2):180-184.

69. Hanley JP. Warfarin reversal. *J Clin Pathol.* 2004;57(11):1132-1139. doi:10.1136/jcp.2003.008904.

70. Jackson CM. Mechanism of heparin action. *Baillieres Clin Haematol.* 1990;3(3):483-504.

71. Hirsh J, Warkentin TE, Shaughnessy SG, et al. Heparin and low-molecular-weight heparin: mechanisms of action, pharmacokinetics, dosing, monitoring, efficacy, and safety. *Chest.* 2001;119(1 suppl):64S-94S.

72. Hirsh J, Levine MN. Low molecular weight heparin. *Blood.* 1992;79(1):1-17.

73. Young E, Venner T, Ribau J, Shaughnessy S, Hirsh J, Podor TJ. The binding of unfractionated heparin and low molecular weight heparin to thrombin-activated human endothelial cells. *Thromb Res.* 1999;96(5):373-381.

74. Leclerc JR, Geerts WH, Desjardins L, et al. Prevention of deep vein thrombosis after major knee surgery – a randomized, double-blind trial comparing a low molecular weight heparin fragment (enoxaparin) to placebo. *Thromb Haemost.* 1992;67(4):417-423.

75. Westrich GH, Haas SB, Mosca P, Peterson M. Meta-analysis of thromboembolic prophylaxis after total knee arthroplasty. *J Bone Joint Surg Br.* 2000;82(6):795-800.

76. van Veen JJ, Maclean RM, Hampton KK, et al. Protamine reversal of low molecular weight heparin: clinically effective? *Blood Coagul Fibrinolysis.* 2011;22(7):565-570. doi:10.1097/MBC.0b013e3283494b3c.

77. Anderson DR, Dunbar MJ, Bohm ER, et al. Aspirin versus low-molecular-weight heparin for extended venous thromboembolism prophylaxis after total hip arthroplasty: a randomized trial. *Ann Intern Med.* 2013;158(11):800-806. doi:10.7326/0003-4819-158-11-201306040-00004.

78. Suen K, Westh RN, Churilov L, Hardidge AJ. Low-molecular-weight heparin and the relative risk of surgical site bleeding complications: results of a systematic review and meta-analysis of randomized controlled trials of venous thromboprophylaxis in patients after total joint arthroplasty. *J Arthroplasty.* 2017;32(9):2911-2919.e6. doi:10.1016/j.arth.2017.04.010.

79. Martel N, Lee J, Wells PS. Risk for heparin-induced thrombocytopenia with unfractionated and low-molecular-weight heparin thromboprophylaxis: a meta-analysis. *Blood.* 2005;106(8):2710-2715. doi:10.1182/blood-2005-04-1546.

80. Bauer KA. Fondaparinux sodium: a selective inhibitor of factor Xa. *Am J Health Syst Pharm.* 2001;58(suppl 2):S14-S17.

81. Venker BT, Ganti BR, Lin H, Lee ED, Nunley RM, Gage BF. Safety and efficacy of new anticoagulants for the prevention of venous thromboembolism after hip and knee arthroplasty: a meta-analysis. *J Arthroplasty.* 2017;32(2):645-652. doi:10.1016/j.arth.2016.09.033.

82. Bauer KA, Eriksson BI, Lassen MR, Turpie AG, Steering Committee of the Pentasaccharide in Major Knee Surgery Study. Fondaparinux compared with enoxaparin for the prevention of venous thromboembolism after elective major knee surgery. *N Engl J Med.* 2001;345(18):1305-1310. doi:10.1056/NEJMoa011099.

83. Eriksson BI, Bauer KA, Lassen MR, Turpie AG, Steering Committee of the Pentasaccharide in Hip-Fracture Surgery Study. Fondaparinux compared with enoxaparin for the prevention of venous thromboembolism after hip-fracture surgery. *N Engl J Med.* 2001;345(18):1298-1304. doi:10.1056/NEJMoa011100.

84. Turpie AGG, Bauer KA, Eriksson BI, Lassen MR, PENTATHALON 2000 Study Steering Committee. Postoperative fondaparinux versus postoperative enoxaparin for prevention of venous thromboembolism after elective hip-replacement surgery: a randomised double-blind trial. *Lancet.* 2002;359(9319):1721-1726. doi:10.1016/S0140-6736(02)08648-8.

85. Lassen MR, Bauer KA, Eriksson BI, Turpie AGG, European Pentasaccharide Elective Surgery Study (EPHESUS) Steering Committee. Postoperative fondaparinux versus preoperative enoxaparin for prevention of venous thromboembolism in elective hip-replacement surgery: a randomised double-blind comparison. *Lancet.* 2002;359(9319):1715-1720. doi:10.1016/S0140-6736(02)08652-X.

86. Franchini M, Lippi G. Prothrombin complex concentrates: an update. *Blood Transfus.* 2010;8(3):149-154. doi:10.2450/2010.0149-09.

87. Samama MM. The mechanism of action of rivaroxaban–an oral, direct Factor Xa inhibitor–compared with other anticoagulants. *Thromb Res.* 2011;127(6):497-504. doi:10.1016/j.thromres.2010.09.008.

88. Agrawal A, Manna B. *Apixaban.* In: *StatPearls.* Treasure Island, FL: StatPearls Publishing; 2018. Available at http://www.ncbi.nlm.nih.gov/books/NBK507910/. Accessed October 23, 2018.

89. Stacy ZA, Call WB, Hartmann AP, Peters GL, Richter SK. Edoxaban: a comprehensive review of the pharmacology and clinical data for the management of atrial fibrillation and venous thromboembolism. *Cardiol Ther.* 2016;5(1):1-18. doi:10.1007/s40119-016-0058-2.

90. Lassen MR, Ageno W, Borris LC, et al. Rivaroxaban versus enoxaparin for thromboprophylaxis after total knee arthroplasty. *N Engl J Med.* 2008;358(26):2776-2786. doi:10.1056/NEJMoa076016.

91. Turpie AGG, Lassen MR, Davidson BL, et al. Rivaroxaban versus enoxaparin for thromboprophylaxis after total knee arthroplasty (RECORD4): a randomised trial. *Lancet.* 2009;373(9676):1673-1680. doi:10.1016/S0140-6736(09)60734-0.

92. Eriksson BI, Borris LC, Friedman RJ, et al. Rivaroxaban versus enoxaparin for thromboprophylaxis after hip arthroplasty. *N Engl J Med.* 2008;358(26):2765-2775. doi:10.1056/NEJMoa0800374.

93. Kakkar AK, Brenner B, Dahl OE, et al. Extended duration rivaroxaban versus short-term enoxaparin for the prevention of venous thromboembolism after total hip arthroplasty: a double-blind, randomised controlled trial. *Lancet*. 2008;372(9632):31-39. doi:10.1016/S0140-6736(08)60880-6.

94. Lassen MR, Raskob GE, Gallus A, Pineo G, Chen D, Portman RJ. Apixaban or enoxaparin for thromboprophylaxis after knee replacement. *N Engl J Med*. 2009;361(6):594-604. doi:10.1056/NEJMoa0810773.

95. Lassen MR, Raskob GE, Gallus A, et al. Apixaban versus enoxaparin for thromboprophylaxis after knee replacement (ADVANCE-2): a randomised double-blind trial. *Lancet*. 2010;375(9717):807-815. doi:10.1016/S0140-6736(09)62125-5.

96. Lassen MR, Gallus A, Raskob GE, et al. Apixaban versus enoxaparin for thromboprophylaxis after hip replacement. *N Engl J Med*. 2010;363(26):2487-2498. doi:10.1056/NEJMoa1006885.

97. Fuji T, Wang C-J, Fujita S, et al. Safety and efficacy of edoxaban, an oral factor Xa inhibitor, versus enoxaparin for thromboprophylaxis after total knee arthroplasty: the STARS E-3 trial. *Thromb Res* 2014;134(6):1198-1204. doi:10.1016/j.thromres.2014.09.011.

98. Andexxa—an antidote for apixaban and rivaroxaban. *J Am Med Assoc*. 2018;320(4):399-400. doi:10.1001/jama.2018.9257.

99. Dubois EA, Cohen AF. Dabigatran etexilate. *Br J Clin Pharmacol*. 2010;70(1):14-15. doi:10.1111/j.1365-2125.2010.03644.x.

100. Eriksson BI, Dahl OE, Rosencher N, et al. Dabigatran etexilate versus enoxaparin for prevention of venous thromboembolism after total hip replacement: a randomised, double-blind, non-inferiority trial. *Lancet*. 2007;370(9591):949-956. doi:10.1016/S0140-6736(07)61445-7.

101. Eriksson BI, Dahl OE, Huo MH, et al. Oral dabigatran versus enoxaparin for thromboprophylaxis after primary total hip arthroplasty (RE-NOVATE II*). A randomised, double-blind, non-inferiority trial. *Thromb Haemost*. 2011;105(4):721-729. doi:10.1160/TH10-10-0679.

102. Eriksson BI, Dahl OE, Rosencher N, et al. Oral dabigatran etexilate vs. subcutaneous enoxaparin for the prevention of venous thromboembolism after total knee replacement: the RE-MODEL randomized trial. *J Thromb Haemost*. 2007;5(11):2178-2185. doi:10.1111/j.1538-7836.2007.02748.x.

103. RE-MOBILIZE Writing Committee, Ginsberg JS, Davidson BL, Comp PC, et al. Oral thrombin inhibitor dabigatran etexilate vs North American enoxaparin regimen for prevention of venous thromboembolism after knee arthroplasty surgery. *J Arthroplasty*. 2009;24(1):1-9. doi:10.1016/j.arth.2008.01.132.

104. Friedman RJ, Dahl OE, Rosencher N, et al. Dabigatran versus enoxaparin for prevention of venous thromboembolism after hip or knee arthroplasty: a pooled analysis of three trials. *Thromb Res*. 2010;126(3):175-182. doi:10.1016/j.thromres.2010.03.021.

105. Leung LL. Direct oral anticoagulants and parenteral direct thrombin inhibitors: dosing and adverse effects. In: Mannucci PM, ed. *UpToDate*. Waltham, MA; 2018. Available at https://www.uptodate.com/contents/direct-oral-anticoagulants-and-parenteral-direct-thrombin-inhibitors-dosing-and-adverse-effects. Accessed January 7, 2019.

106. van Ryn J, Stangier J, Haertter S, et al. Dabigatran etexilate—a novel, reversible, oral direct thrombin inhibitor: interpretation of coagulation assays and reversal of anticoagulant activity. *Thromb Haemost*. 2010;103(6):1116-1127. doi:10.1160/TH09-11-0758.

107. Pollack CV, Reilly PA, van Ryn J, et al. Idarucizumab for dabigatran reversal–full cohort analysis. *N Engl J Med*. 2017;377(5):431-441. doi:10.1056/NEJMoa1707278.

108. Allenby F, Boardman L, Pflug JJ, Calnan JS. Effects of external pneumatic intermittent compression on fibrinolysis in man. *Lancet*. 1973;2(7843):1412-1414.

109. Weitz J, Michelsen J, Gold K, Owen J, Carpenter D. Effects of intermittent pneumatic calf compression on postoperative thrombin and plasmin activity. *Thromb Haemost*. 1986;56(2):198-201.

110. Pierce TP, Cherian JJ, Jauregui JJ, Elmallah RK, Lieberman JR, Mont MA. A current review of mechanical compression and its role in venous thromboembolic prophylaxis in total knee and total hip arthroplasty. *J Arthroplasty*. 2015;30(12):2279-2284. doi:10.1016/j.arth.2015.05.045.

111. Hull R, Delmore TJ, Hirsh J, et al. Effectiveness of intermittent pulsatile elastic stockings for the prevention of calf and thigh vein thrombosis in patients undergoing elective knee surgery. *Thromb Res*. 1979;16(1-2):37-45.

112. Haas SB, Insall JN, Scuderi GR, Windsor RE, Ghelman B. Pneumatic sequential-compression boots compared with aspirin prophylaxis of deep-vein thrombosis after total knee arthroplasty. *J Bone Joint Surg Am*. 1990;72(1):27-31.

113. Colwell CW, Froimson MI, Anseth SD, et al. A mobile compression device for thrombosis prevention in hip and knee arthroplasty. *J Bone Joint Surg Am*. 2014;96(3):177-183. doi:10.2106/JBJS.L.01031.

114. Hardwick ME, Pulido PA, Colwell CW. A mobile compression device compared with low-molecular-weight heparin for prevention of venous thromboembolism in total hip arthroplasty. *Orthop Nurs*. 2011;30(5):312-316. doi:10.1097/NOR.0b013e31822c5c28.

115. Lachiewicz PF, Soileau ES. Mechanical calf compression and aspirin prophylaxis for total knee arthroplasty. *Clin Orthop Relat Res*. 2007;464:61-64. doi:10.1097/BLO.0b013e3181468951.

116. Eisele R, Kinzl L, Koelsch T. Rapid-inflation intermittent pneumatic compression for prevention of deep venous thrombosis. *J Bone Joint Surg Am*. 2007;89(5):1050-1056. doi:10.2106/JBJS.E.00434.

117. Pavon JM, Williams JW, Adam SS, et al. *Effectiveness of Intermittent Pneumatic Compression Devices for Venous Thromboembolism Prophylaxis in High-Risk Surgical and Medical Patients*. Washington, DC: Department of Veterans Affairs (US); 2015. Available at http://www.ncbi.nlm.nih.gov/books/NBK333230/. Accessed October 12, 2018.

118. Westrich GH, Sculco TP. Prophylaxis against deep venous thrombosis after total knee arthroplasty. Pneumatic plantar compression and aspirin compared with aspirin alone. *J Bone Joint Surg Am*. 1996;78(6):826-834.

119. Gardner AM, Fox RH. The venous footpump: influence on tissue perfusion and prevention of venous thrombosis. *Ann Rheum Dis*. 1992;51(10):1173-1178.

120. Stannard JP, Harris RM, Bucknell AL, Cossi A, Ward J, Arrington ED. Prophylaxis of deep venous thrombosis after total hip arthroplasty by using intermittent compression of the plantar venous plexus. *Am J Orthop*. 1996;25(2):127-134.

121. Fordyce MJ, Ling RS. A venous foot pump reduces thrombosis after total hip replacement. *J Bone Joint Surg Br*. 1992;74(1):45-49.

122. Warwick D, Harrison J, Glew D, Mitchelmore A, Peters TJ, Donovan J. Comparison of the use of a foot pump with the use of low-molecular-weight heparin for the prevention of deep-vein thrombosis after total hip replacement. A prospective, randomized trial. *J Bone Joint Surg Am*. 1998;80(8):1158-1166.

123. Colwell CW, Froimson MI, Mont MA, et al. Thrombosis prevention after total hip arthroplasty: a prospective, randomized trial comparing a mobile compression device with low-molecular-weight heparin. *J Bone Joint Surg Am*. 2010;92(3):527-535. doi:10.2106/JBJS.I.00047.

124. Nicolaides A, Goldhaber SZ, Maxwell GL, et al. Cost benefit of intermittent pneumatic compression for venous thromboembolism prophylaxis in general surgery. *Int Angiol*. 2008;27(6):500-506.

125. Hui AC, Heras-Palou C, Dunn I, et al. Graded compression stockings for prevention of deep-vein thrombosis after hip and knee replacement. *J Bone Joint Surg Br*. 1996;78(4):550-554.

126. Cohen AT, Skinner JA, Warwick D, Brenkel I. The use of graduated compression stockings in association with fondaparinux in surgery of the hip. A multicentre, multinational, randomised, open-label, parallel-group comparative study. *J Bone Joint Surg Br*. 2007;89(7):887-892. doi:10.1302/0301-620X.89B7.18556.

SECTION 7 / PERIOPERATIVE MANAGEMENT IN TKR

127. Sarmiento A, Goswami AD. Thromboembolic prophylaxis with use of aspirin, exercise, and graded elastic stockings or intermittent compression devices in patients managed with total hip arthroplasty. *J Bone Joint Surg Am*. 1999;81(3):339-346.

128. Silbersack Y, Taute BM, Hein W, Podhaisky H. Prevention of deep-vein thrombosis after total hip and knee replacement. Low-molecular-weight heparin in combination with intermittent pneumatic compression. *J Bone Joint Surg Br*. 2004;86(6):809-812.

129. Best AJ, Williams S, Crozier A, Bhatt R, Gregg PJ, Hui AC. Graded compression stockings in elective orthopaedic surgery. An assessment of the in vivo performance of commercially available stockings in patients having hip and knee arthroplasty. *J Bone Joint Surg Br*. 2000;82(1):116-118.

130. Sigel B, Edelstein AL, Savitch L, Hasty JH, Felix WR. Type of compression for reducing venous stasis. A study of lower extremities during inactive recumbency. *Arch Surg*. 1975;110(2):171-175.

131. Lynch AF, Bourne RB, Rorabeck CH, Rankin RN, Donald A. Deep-vein thrombosis and continuous passive motion after total knee arthroplasty. *J Bone Joint Surg Am*. 1988;70(1):11-14.

132. He ML, Xiao ZM, Lei M, Li TS, Wu H, Liao J. Continuous passive motion for preventing venous thromboembolism after total knee arthroplasty. *Cochrane Database Syst Rev*. 2014;(7):CD008207. doi:10.1002/14651858.CD008207.pub3.

133. Alkire MR, Swank ML. Use of inpatient continuous passive motion versus no CPM in computer-assisted total knee arthroplasty. *Orthop Nurs*. 2010;29(1):36-40. doi:10.1097/NOR.0b013e3181c8ce23.

134. Bruun-Olsen V, Heiberg KE, Mengshoel AM. Continuous passive motion as an adjunct to active exercises in early rehabilitation following total knee arthroplasty – a randomized controlled trial. *Disabil Rehabil*. 2009;31(4):277-283. doi:10.1080/09638280801931204.

135. Chen B, Zimmerman JR, Soulen L, DeLisa JA. Continuous passive motion after total knee arthroplasty: a prospective study. *Am J Phys Med Rehabil*. 2000;79(5):421-426.

136. Denis M, Moffet H, Caron F, Ouellet D, Paquet J, Nolet L. Effectiveness of continuous passive motion and conventional physical therapy after total knee arthroplasty: a randomized clinical trial. *Phys Ther*. 2006;86(2):174-185.

137. Harms M, Engstrom B. Continuous passive motion as an adjunct to treatment in the physiotherapy management of the total knee arthroplasty patient. *Physiotherapy*. 1991;77(4):301-307. doi:10.1016/S0031-9406(10)61768-3.

138. Johnson DP, Eastwood DM. Beneficial effects of continuous passive motion after total condylar knee arthroplasty. *Ann R Coll Surg Engl*. 1992;74(6):412-416.

139. Lenssen TAF, van Steyn MJA, Crijns YHF, et al. Effectiveness of prolonged use of continuous passive motion (CPM), as an adjunct to physiotherapy, after total knee arthroplasty. *BMC Musculoskelet Disord*. 2008;9:60. doi:10.1186/1471-2474-9-60.

140. McInnes J, Larson MG, Daltroy LH, et al. A controlled evaluation of continuous passive motion in patients undergoing total knee arthroplasty. *J Am Med Assoc*. 1992;268(11):1423-1428.

141. Montgomery F, Eliasson M. Continuous passive motion compared to active physical therapy after knee arthroplasty: similar hospitalization times in a randomized study of 68 patients. *Acta Orthop Scand*. 1996;67(1):7-9.

142. Bass AR, Mattern CJ, Voos JE, Peterson MGE, Trost DW. Inferior vena cava filter placement in orthopedic surgery. *Am J Orthop*. 2010;39(9):435-439.

143. Bikdeli B, Chatterjee S, Desai NR, et al. Inferior vena cava filters to prevent pulmonary embolism: systematic review and meta-analysis. *J Am Coll Cardiol*. 2017;70(13):1587-1597. doi:10.1016/j.jacc.2017.07.775.

144. Khansarinia S, Dennis JW, Veldenz HC, Butcher JL, Hartland L. Prophylactic Greenfield filter placement in selected high-risk trauma patients. *J Vasc Surg*. 1995;22(3):231-235; discussion 235-236.

145. Obeid FN, Bowling WM, Fike JS, Durant JA. Efficacy of prophylactic inferior vena cava filter placement in bariatric surgery. *Surg Obes Relat Dis*. 2007;3(6):606-608; discussion 609-610. doi:10.1016/j.soard.2007.08.005.

146. Agarwal S, Rana A, Gupta G, Raghav D, Sharma RK. Total knee arthroplasty in a diagnosed case of deep vein thrombosis – our experience and review of literature. *J Orthop Case Rep*. 2017;7(1):16-19. doi:10.13107/jocr.2250-0685.668.

147. Dhand S, Stulberg SD, Puri L, Karp J, Ryu RK, Lewandowski RJ. The role of potentially retrievable inferior vena cava filters in high-risk patients undergoing joint arthroplasty. *J Clin Diagn Res*. 2015;9(12):TC01-TC03. doi:10.7860/JCDR/2015/11397.6890.

148. Robinson KS, Anderson DR, Gross M, et al. Ultrasonographic screening before hospital discharge for deep venous thrombosis after arthroplasty: the post-arthroplasty screening study. A randomized, controlled trial. *Ann Intern Med*. 1997;127(6):439-445.

149. Ciccone WJ, Fox PS, Neumyer M, Rubens D, Parrish WM, Pellegrini VD. Ultrasound surveillance for asymptomatic deep venous thrombosis after total joint replacement. *J Bone Joint Surg Am*. 1998;80(8):1167-1174.

150. Molloy IB, Martin BI, Moschetti WE, Jevsevar DS. Effects of the length of stay on the cost of total knee and total hip arthroplasty from 2002 to 2013. *J Bone Joint Surg Am*. 2017;99(5):402-407. doi:10.2106/JBJS.16.00019.

151. Forster R, Stewart M. Anticoagulants (extended duration) for prevention of venous thromboembolism following total hip or knee replacement or hip fracture repair. *Cochrane Database Syst Rev*. 2016;(3):CD004179. doi:10.1002/14651858.CD004179.pub2.

152. Barrellier M-T, Lebel B, Parienti J-J, et al. Short versus extended thromboprophylaxis after total knee arthroplasty: a randomized comparison. *Thromb Res*. 2010;126(4):e298-304. doi:10.1016/j.thromres.2010.07.018.

153. Parvizi J, Ghanem E, Joshi A, Sharkey PF, Hozack WJ, Rothman RH. Does "excessive" anticoagulation predispose to periprosthetic infection? *J Arthroplasty*. 2007;22(6 suppl 2):24-28. doi:10.1016/j.arth.2007.03.007.

154. Kahlenberg CA, Richardson SS, Schairer WW, Sculco PK. Type of anticoagulant used after total knee arthroplasty affects the rate of knee manipulation for postoperative stiffness. *J Bone Joint Surg Am*. 2018;100(16):1366-1372. doi:10.2106/JBJS.17.01110.

chapter 51

Blood Management

Ugonna N. Ihekweazu, MD | Geoffrey Westrich, MD

INTRODUCTION

Total knee arthroplasty (TKA) is one of the most commonly performed orthopedic procedures worldwide. Historically, TKA has been associated with a substantial amount of blood loss, with an average of up to 1.5 L of total blood loss and up to 38% of TKA patients requiring allogenic blood transfusion (ABT).[1-3] Significant blood loss and ABT can result in a number of complications including infection, transfusion reactions, delayed physical recovery, prolonged hospital stays, and increased mortality.[3,4] In addition to the risks associated with significant blood loss and ABT, the costs associated with these complications can be substantial. Therefore, proactive blood management strategies are essential in TKA patients to mitigate the amount of blood loss and limit the need for ABT.

The goal of blood management is to maintain the patient's hemoglobin at the highest possible level, while simultaneously diminishing the risk for ABT. Blood loss is a multifactorial issue, as described below. Therefore, a management strategy must include a multidisciplinary approach. Efforts to appropriately manage blood loss should start preoperatively. Patients at high risk for bleeding, or those in whom postoperative anemia would be poorly tolerated, should be identified, worked up, and treated when appropriate. Intraoperatively, a variety of surgical, pharmacologic, and anesthetic factors influence blood loss and should be addressed. Finally, during the postoperative period, there remain several opportunities for effective management of blood loss and prevention of ABT. The purpose of this chapter is to review the latest blood management strategies reported in the literature. These strategies will be presented in order, from the initial preoperative assessment and intervention to intraoperative techniques and finally postoperative care.

PREOPERATIVE

Effective perioperative blood management begins during the initial preoperative visit. Assessment should occur at least 3 weeks prior to surgery, to allow time for further workup and intervention when necessary.[5] A thorough examination should include assessment of the patient's overall physiologic status, including nutritional state, body habitus, and past medical history, with a particular focus on history of cardiovascular disease.[5] Preoperative screening should also include the patient's personal and family history of bleeding and an accounting of all medications taken at home. Preoperative laboratory investigations may include a complete blood count with differential, serum ferritin, transferrin saturation index, vitamin B_{12}, folic acid, serum creatinine, and c-reactive protein as a marker of inflammation.[6,7]

Male sex, body mass index <27 kg/m^2, and preoperative hemoglobin <11 g/dL are known risk factors for perioperative ABT.[8] Anemia, defined by the World Health Organization as a hemoglobin concentration of <13.0 g/dL for men and <12.0 g/dL for women,[9] is prevalent among patients undergoing TKA, as 24% to 44% of patients undergoing the procedure are reported to be anemic preoperatively.[4] There are many causes for anemia, and when identified additional workup should be completed, including consultation with a hematologist or other specialist when appropriate. Optimization of preoperative hemoglobin to a level above 12 g/dL is ideal as levels below this have been associated with a higher risk of perioperative ABT.[8] Ultimately, the goal is to identify anemia, nutritional, or metabolic deficiencies and appropriately treat such modifiable risk factors when present, prior to surgical intervention.

Vitamin Deficiency

Iron, vitamin B_{12}, and folate are integral to the development of red blood cells (RBCs), and deficiencies in these compounds have been associated with anemia.[7] In particular, iron deficiency anemia has been reported to account for up to 50% of patients with hemoglobin levels below 12 g/dL.[10] Patients with anemia due to nutritional causes, including iron deficiency anemia, can be treated with a healthy diet and nutritional supplementation with vitamin B_{12}, folate, and oral or intravenous (IV) iron, depending on the cause of anemia. A variety of treatment plans and algorithms are found in the literature. Cuenca et al demonstrated that preoperative supplementation with iron (256 mg/d), vitamin C (1000 mg/d), and folate (5 mg/d) 30 to 45 days prior to surgery significantly decreased the need for ABT when compared with patients who did not receive preoperative supplementation (5.8% and 32%, respectively).[11] This study demonstrates the importance of nutritional health prior to surgery and the impact of correction of nutritional deficiencies on perioperative outcomes.

With respect to iron deficiency anemia, both IV and oral administration can be beneficial in the appropriate setting.[11-13] However, IV administration appears to be superior to oral in terms of efficacy.[14] In a prospective study, Theusinger et al demonstrated that administration of IV iron over a 3-week period prior to surgical intervention resulted in maximum increase in preoperative hemoglobin levels without adverse events related to oral iron treatments.[15] Iron administration should be performed judiciously, as supplementation in the absence of iron deficiency has been associated with constipation, heartburn, and abdominal pain.[16]

Erythropoietin

Erythropoietin (EPO) is a naturally occurring glycoprotein produced from renal pericapillary cells in response to hypoxic conditions resulting from physiologic states such as anemia or chronic obstructive pulmonary disease.[17] When produced, EPO acts on the bone marrow to increase RBC differentiation, maturation, and ultimately total RBC mass. The role of EPO in blood management is frequently discussed in arthroplasty literature, as its use leads to significant reductions in ABTs in patients receiving surgery.[18,19] EPO in its recombinant form, epoetin-α, causes the same physiologic results and has been routinely used in chronic anemia patients with renal disease and those undergoing chemotherapy.[7] Perioperative administration for arthroplasty procedures has been performed alone, in conjunction with preoperative autologous donation (PAD), and postoperatively.[20]

A variety of dosing regimens have been described;[21] however, three or four weekly preoperative subcutaneous injections (600 IU/kg) are most frequently used and may deliver the best results.[20,22,23] EPO supplementation leads to a mean rise in preoperative hemoglobin of 1.9 g/dL,[24] and multiple studies have demonstrated a significant benefit of preoperative EPO supplementation when compared to placebo, PAD, and reinfusion systems.[20,24,25]

A major limitation to routine EPO use is cost, as the average price per patient is equivalent to two to three units of PAD or three to four units of allogenic blood.[26] Given this fact, it is not surprising that routine use of EPO as a blood management strategy was found to lack cost effectiveness.[26] Selective use of preoperative EPO is considered most appropriate in scenarios where significant amounts of blood loss are anticipated, such as complex primary TKA, simultaneous bilateral TKA, and revision TKA.[27] EPO supplementation should also be considered in patients diagnosed with preoperative anemia, those with low body weight (<50 kg), and in scenarios where ABT is especially undesirable such as in Jehovah's Witnesses population.

Management of Outpatient Medications

The treatment team must appreciate the impact that outpatient medications have on blood management throughout a TKA episode of care. Cardiovascular disease is common among patients undergoing TKA, and antiplatelet therapies are routinely used to manage these conditions. Furthermore, a subset of patients with cardiovascular disease has previously undergone percutaneous coronary interventions (PCI) with stent placements. Dual antiplatelet therapies are common in this patient population and typically consist of aspirin and a $P2Y_{12}$ inhibitor (e.g., clopidogrel). Current guidelines for dual antiplatelet therapy in patients with coronary artery disease (CAD) vary and depend upon on a number of factors including the length of time since the PCI and the type of stent that was implanted.[28] From a surgical perspective, blood loss can be substantial when surgery is performed in a patient taking antiplatelet medications.[29] These patients can also be more challenging to the anesthesiologist, as excessive bleeding can occur when neuraxial anesthesia is attempted.[30]

Increased perioperative bleeding may also result from nonsteroidal antiinflammatory drug (NSAID) use. NSAIDs are widely used as an analgesic in the management of degenerative joint disease. NSAIDs reduce inflammation by impeding prostaglandin production via inhibition of cyclooxygenase enzymes. Nonselective NSAIDs (COX-1 and COX-2 inhibitors) are known to impair platelet aggregation and prolong bleeding time due to their blockade of the COX-1 enzyme. Alternatively, COX-2 selective medications such as celecoxib can relieve pain and reduce inflammation without impacting bleeding time or platelet aggregation and therefore can be safely used perioperatively.

Other common agents that may increase perioperative risk in patients planning elective TKA include warfarin, factor Xa inhibitors, and herbal supplements such as gingko biloba. As previously mentioned, a thorough accounting of all perioperative medications should be performed prior to elective TKA, including nonprescription medications and supplements. The benefit of stopping any medication should be weighed against its risks and should be done in collaboration with the prescribing physician. Ultimately, an individualized approach should be taken during the perioperative period with multidisciplinary input to maximize patient safety and surgical outcome.

Preoperative Autologous Donation

Preoperative autologous blood donation (PAD) programs were developed in the late 1980s to combat the newly recognized risk of viral transmission of diseases such as HIV associated with ABT.[31] The goal of PAD programs was to provide patients with a safe source of blood prior to major procedures such as TKA. PAD is performed 3 weeks prior to a planned surgery where major blood loss was expected. The ideal candidate is a patient who weighs more than 110 lbs and has hemoglobin greater than 11 g/dL.[32] The technique involves procurement of one to two units of the patients own blood prior to surgery. The procured blood is then processed, stored, and ultimately transfused back to the patient either intraoperatively or postoperatively. In 1992, PAD accounted for nearly 8.5% of all blood collected in the United States.[33] While the literature has demonstrated significant reductions in ABT when PAD programs were utilized,[7] a consensus has yet to be reached with regard to its efficacy.

The logistics of PAD programs can be challenging and may present opportunities for complications to occur. Storage of donated blood requires advanced planning, storage, and preparation and as a result introduces the risk for clerical error, bacterial contamination, and infection.[5,32] Additionally, mismanagement of donated blood may result in underutilization of product, with reports suggesting a >50% incidence of unused blood.[5,32] PAD has also been associated with fluid overload.[5,32] To be considered for PAD, patients must have a baseline hemoglobin level >11 g/dL; therefore, many of the patients most at risk for ABT (those with preoperative anemia) are excluded from consideration. Finally, cost is an additional factor which limits the use of PAD. For all of these reasons, routine use of PAD has fallen out of favor for primary TKA, especially with the routine use of tranexamic acid (TXA).

Acute Normovolemic Hemodilution

Acute normovolemic hemodilution (ANH) involves the removal of whole blood from a patient, while circulating blood volume is maintained with crystalloid fluid.[34,35] Typically, two to three units of blood is collected from the patient 1 hour prior to the operation and total blood volume is maintained with IV fluids. Postoperatively, the stored blood units are reinfused to the patient. While some studies have shown that this technique can be efficacious in reducing the need for ABT,[34] other studies have demonstrated otherwise.[36,37] Similar to PAD, logistical problems concerning the timing, storage, and usage of donated units of blood exist with this technique. However, ANH may be useful in the Jehovah's Witnesses population when substantial blood loss is anticipated, but ABT is undesirable.

INTRAOPERATIVE

A variety of techniques are available for limiting intraoperative blood loss. Options include the use of a tourniquet, hypotensive epidural anesthesia (HEA), ANH, antifibrinolytic use, topical fibrin sealants, cell salvage, and reinfusion and periarticular injections, to name a few. The challenge that the surgical team must weigh is whether the risk and costs associated with each of the available treatment modalities is appropriate when considering the benefit that the patient may receive. Nevertheless, general principles of meticulous surgical technique should be upheld, including exposure through avascular tissue planes, limitation of surgical exposure to what is required

for safe execution of the procedure, and maintenance of careful hemostasis throughout the operation.

Tourniquet

Tourniquets are commonly used in TKA as they allow for a technically easier surgery, with enhanced visualization through a bloodless field, improved cement interdigitation, and decrease in surgical time.[38] When utilized, tourniquets are typically inflated to a level 100 to 150 mm Hg greater than the patient's systolic blood pressure. While the majority of surgeons commonly use tourniquets during TKA, their routine use is somewhat controversial. Within minutes of the applied pressure, local ischemia ensues, resulting in reactive hyperemia and the potential for local muscle damage, neurapraxia, thigh pain, delayed wound healing, thrombosis, increased joint swelling, and stiffness.[39]

Thorey et al randomized knees in 20 patients undergoing simultaneous bilateral TKA to either have the tourniquet released prior to wound closure or after wound closure.[40] A significant reduction in surgical time was reported with delayed tourniquet release compared to release prior to wound closure (51 and 58 minutes, respectively). No differences were noted in perioperative blood loss or complications at 6 months follow-up. In a nonrandomized prospective cohort study of 90 patients undergoing TKA, Huang et al divided patients into three groups: tourniquet used the whole surgery until after wound closure, tourniquet deflated prior to wound closure, and tourniquet used only during cementation.[41] They found that use of a tourniquet only during cementation resulted in lower levels of serum markers of inflammation and muscle damage. However, there were no observed differences between the groups with regard to Hospital for Special Surgery knee score, range of motion (ROM), estimated blood loss, swelling ratio, visual analog scale pain score, and hospital stay.

In 2011, Tai et al performed a meta-analysis of 8 randomized controlled trials (RCTs) and 3 high-quality prospective studies involving 634 knees, where clinical outcomes of TKA with and without tourniquet use were compared.[39] They found that TKA without tourniquet use had better clinical outcomes, fewer complications, and better ROM in the early postoperative period. Additionally, their results demonstrated that the true blood loss in TKA was not reduced with tourniquet use, as reactive hyperemia due to ischemic conditions may result in greater hidden blood loss during the postoperative period. It is important to point out that challenges associated with quantifying total blood loss and nonuniform indications for blood transfusion may limit the conclusions that can be drawn from these data.

At this time, the literature does not provide definitive guidance regarding the time and use of tourniquet use during TKA. Nevertheless, the treatment team should weigh the benefits of its use against the perceived disadvantages. Additionally, patients with risk factors for arterial complications such as a history of vascular claudication, radiographic evidence of calcification, absent pedal pulses, or a history of vascular procedures should be screened and consultation with a vascular surgeon should be performed prior to consideration of tourniquet use. In most of the above scenarios, tourniquet use is typically avoided to prevent embolization of arterial plaque distally and potential vascular occlusion.

Hypotensive Epidural Anesthesia

HEA is a technique introduced by Nigel Sharrock, whereby blood loss is reduced by maintaining a low mean arterial blood pressure (typically 50 to 55 mm Hg) throughout the surgical procedure.[42] An epidural dermatome block at the T2 level results in a decrease in the conduction of the cardioacceleratory fibers of the sympathetic chain, ultimately leading to a reduction in arterial pressure. While HEA has been shown to limit intraoperative blood loss in the TKA,[43,44] most of the literature has focused on its total hip arthroplasty applications. Additionally, concerns about tissue hypoperfusion, bradycardia, and other serious cardiopulmonary sequelae have been documented in the literature.[44,45] However, studies suggest that HEA is safe even in high-risk patient populations, including patients with poor cardiac or renal function.[46] Ultimately, an interdisciplinary approach should be taken when deciding to use this approach.

Periarticular Injections

Replacement of traditional methods of postoperative pain control with multimodal approaches, which include periarticular injections, has led to improvements in many quality measures, Hospital Consumer Assessment of Healthcare Providers and Systems (HCAHPS) pain scores, and cost-effectiveness.[47] Epinephrine, a known agent of hemostasis due to its effects as a vasoconstrictor, has been added to certain periarticular pain cocktails as an adjunct to decrease blood loss. Anderson et al injected bupivacaine and epinephrine into a series of patients undergoing TKA just prior to wound closure. When compared to a control, the periarticular injection group had 32% less drain output; however, no statistical differences were noted in ABT between the two groups.[48] While potentially promising, more high-quality studies are needed to further assess its efficacy in reducing ABT prior to recommending its routine use in TKA.

Antifibrinolytic Agents

Perhaps the most significant advancement in the management of blood loss in orthopedics over the past decade has been the introduction of antifibrinolytic agents to everyday practice. These medications function as clot stabilizers by decreasing the rate of fibrinolysis, ultimately resulting in a more stable hemostasis. TXA, ε-aminocaproic acid (EACA), and aprotinin are the most commonly recognized agents in this class of medications. Aprotinin, a nonlysine antifibrinolytic agent, while exceedingly efficient at decreasing blood loss, had a significant cardiovascular risk profile and has been removed from the market.[49] While EACA and TXA have similar efficacy in the reduction of perioperative bleeding and ABT, EACA is significantly more expensive.[50]

Of the two available antifibrinolytics on the market, TXA is the most widely used and studied agent in the orthopedic literature. TXA functions as a clot stabilizer as it competitively binds to the lysine-binding site on plasminogen, preventing fibrin from binding to the plasminogen–plasmin tissue activator complex, thereby inhibiting fibrin clot degradation and bleeding.[51] TXA is known to rapidly penetrate into the synovial fluid and membranes, reaching the same concentration as in plasma within 15 minutes and peak concentration within 1 hour after IV administration.[51] TXA is primarily renally excreted; therefore, the IV dose should be reduced in patients with renal impairment. The dose should be decreased by 50% for a glomerular filtration rate (GFR) of 0.5 mL/min, 25% for a GFR of 10 to 50 mL/min, and 10% for a GFR of 10 mL/min.[51] Absolute contraindications to TXA use include known allergies to the medication, ongoing acute arterial or venous thrombosis, subarachnoid hemorrhage, and an intrinsic risk or history of thrombosis or thromboembolism.[8] Relative contraindications include cardiac or peripheral vascular disease, seizures, and acute renal failure. Conversely, the literature has demonstrated that TXA can safely be administered with all deep venous thrombosis (DVT) prophylaxis regimens, does not increase perioperative complications, does not alter prothrombin time or activate partial thromboplastin time, and is not associated with increased rates of DVT or pulmonary embolism.[52,53] However, additional research is required to more definitively outline its risk profile, as TXA may particularly beneficial in certain "high-risk" populations where the benefits of improved blood management may outweigh the perceived risks of thrombosis.

TXA is very effective at limiting blood loss in TKA. In 2003, Good et al randomized patients undergoing TKA to receive TXA or a placebo and found that TXA decreased total blood loss by 30%, reduced the drainage volume by nearly 50%, and decreased the transfusion requirement by 47%.[54] Over the past decade, the literature has become replete with well-conducted studies that overwhelmingly endorse the routine use of TXA for blood management in TKA.[55-58] The benefits realized from improved blood management also translate to enhanced functional outcomes. During the immediate postoperative period, TXA has been shown to improve arc of motion and enhance patient participation in inpatient physical therapy following TKA.[59,60] Serrano et al demonstrated that the benefits of topical TXA use extended beyond the hospitalization period, with significant improvements in knee function demonstrated during the first 6 postoperative weeks.[61]

A variety of TXA dosing regimens and routes exist, and at this time no consensus has been reached on the optimal protocol. TXA can be administered via IV, topically, or orally, with time to peak plasma concentration differing by route (5 to 15 minutes, 30 minutes, and 2 hours, respectively).[62] Despite these differences, benefits for each route of administration have been reported in the literature.[63-65] While some have touted the cost savings associated with oral dosing,[65] the logistics involved with administering an oral dose 2 hours prior to incision has made it difficult for some centers to adopt this protocol. For the patient in whom IV or oral TXA use would be undesirable, a 2 to 4 g topical dose of TXA can safely be used and has been found to have clinical outcomes comparable to IV administration.[64] However, the IV form of administration is most common. A typical dosing regimen recommends either 10 to 20 mg/kg or simply 1 g administered IV prior to incision with an optional additional dose given roughly 3 hours after the initial dose. Still, alternative dosing protocols exist. Some authors have found that the combination of IV and topical TXA is more effective than either regimen used independently,[66,67] leading to higher postoperative hemoglobin levels without influencing drug safety in TKA patients.

TXA can also be administered with an additive such as epinephrine. Recently, Zeng et al performed a placebo-controlled trial in which 179 patients undergoing primary TKA were randomized to receive IV low-dose epinephrine plus TXA, topical epinephrine plus TXA, or TXA alone. They found that combined administration of low-dose epinephrine and TXA demonstrated a reduction in perioperative blood loss and the inflammatory response compared with TXA alone.[68]

TXA has been shown to be cost-effective when compared to other agents,[69] preoperative 3-week iron supplementation, a 1-week EPO regimen,[70] reinfusion drains,[71] and autologous blood donation.[72] At this time, a specific evidence-based recommendation cannot be given due to the lack of consensus in the literature. At our institution, if able to be tolerated, either 1 g or 10 mg/kg of TXA is given prior to elevation of the tourniquet and an additional dose is given 3 hours after the initial dose. When unable to be given IV, a single topical dose of 1 g (which may be diluted in 30 mL of normal saline) is given after cementation and prior to wound closure.

Cell Salvage

Intraoperative cell salvage involves recovering blood lost during surgery, filtering and washing the recovered blood, and subsequently reinfusing the blood to the patient shortly thereafter. Many devices and techniques have been developed after it was originally popularized for use in major thoracic and abdominal procedures.[73] While some reports have demonstrated reductions in ABT,[74] the literature regarding its orthopedic applications, in particular its use in TKA, is extremely limited. One issue is that a significant amount of blood needs to be collected in order to perform the filtering and washing procedure, and the smaller blood loss associated with a routine TKA today, especially when TXA is utilized, makes it hard to justify its use. Future research will need to further define the safety, efficacy, and cost-effectiveness of this technique in the modern era. At this time, intraoperative cell salvage is not routinely used in our institution.

Surgical Accessories

In addition to the aforementioned techniques for management of intraoperative blood loss, a number of adjuncts may be of use to the surgeon, including topical hemostatic agents, electrocautery, argon beam coagulation (ABC), and bone wax. As with most devices, the relative cost associated with use of these adjuncts must be weighed against the potential benefits.

Several topical hemostatic agents have been shown to reduce blood loss in TKA, including fibrin sealants, plant-derived cellulose, platelet-rich plasma (PRP), collagen agents, and thrombin. Currently, the literature describing application of these agents in TKA is sparse, with the fibrin sealants being the most studied. Topical fibrin sealants (such as glues and tissue adhesives) are typically composed of fibrinogen, factor XIII, thrombin, and antifibrinolytic agents such as aprotinin or TXA. Local hemostasis is achieved by mimicking the final step of the coagulation pathway, thereby forming a stable fibrin seal. In a meta-analysis of 8 RCTs, involving 641 patients, Wang et al found that while use of fibrin sealants significantly reduced postoperative drainage, ROM, and blood transfusion rates, no substantial differences were found in total blood loss.[75] Additionally, there were no significant differences in any adverse events, fever, infection, or hematoma. Fibrin sealants may cost upward of $450 per case[17]; therefore, additional studies should explore its cost-effectiveness when applied to TKA. Floseal (Baxter International) is a thrombin-based sealant that is applied in spray form. In a study from our institution, Kim et al randomized 196 patients undergoing TKA to receive the topical spray intraoperatively compared to a control group treated without topical hemostatic agents.[76] There were no significant differences in postoperative drain outputs, change in hemoglobin, transfusion rates, or postoperative complications between the groups. The role of PRP as a promising orthopedic tool continues to be explored; however, the literature regarding its efficacy in TKA blood management is limited and of poor quality. At this time, topical hemostatic agents are not routinely used in our institution.[77]

Monopolar electrocautery is a pen-like device that delivers electric current to the patient's tissues to aid in hemostasis. On the other hand, bipolar sealers deliver radiofrequency energy combined with continuous flow saline in order to maintain cool temperatures, causing less damage to the surrounding tissues. While some studies have demonstrated benefits of bipolar sealants as compared to monopolar electrocautery in terms of reduced blood loss, change in hemoglobin, and ABT,[78] others have found no significant differences between the two devices.[79] With regard to bipolar sealants, cost should be a consideration as they can add an additional $400 per case.[17] Alternatively, if the surgeon desires a cheaper supplementary form of cautery, an ABC device may be considered. With ABC use, radiofrequency cautery is delivered to tissues via ionized argon gas. The argon gas displaces blood from the surgical field to improve visibility, while simultaneously reducing the amount of eschar formation and tissue damage. ABC devices are inexpensive, roughly $4 per disposable pencil; however, there is no literature regarding its use in arthroplasty. Therefore, recommendations cannot be made until further research is performed.

Finally, two relatively simple tools that may aid in the reduction of blood loss during TKA are the use of a femoral bone plug and application of bone wax. In conventional TKA, when navigation or robotics is not utilized, femoral alignment is typically obtained with the use of an intramedullary (IM) alignment rod. The IM rod violates the medullary canal, damaging cancellous bone and the endosteal circulation, resulting in blood loss. Autologous bone graft obtained from bone cuts performed later in the procedure can be fashioned into plugs that can seal the canal. Most of the available literature shows potentially less blood loss, but no difference in transfusion rates with or without plugging the canal with bone and/or cement.[80-85] As the placement of an autologous bone plug into the femoral canal is simple, safe, not time-consuming, and free, we do recommend this technique as routine practice.

Alternatively, bone wax, which is a mixture of beeswax, paraffin, and isopropyl palmitate, is an inexpensive substance that is used to mechanically control bleeding from bone surfaces. In a prospective RCT that included 100 patients undergoing primary unilateral TKA, Moo et al found that the application of bone wax to uncovered bleeding bone surfaces significantly reduced total blood loss and maintained higher postoperative hemoglobin compared to a control group not treated with bone wax. However, allergic reactions, inflammation, and foreign body reactions have been reported with bone wax use; therefore, the surgeon should apply this judiciously.[86]

POSTOPERATIVE

Following wound closure, bleeding into the knee joint continues to occur. A variety of tools and techniques are available to the surgeon and the treatment team to mitigate this form of blood loss. Postoperative strategies to reduce the burden of ABT include cryotherapy, limb position, and reinfusion systems. Cryotherapy involves the application of cold, which may be achieved using bags of ice or cooled water or any manufactured cooling therapy device. The cold temperature penetrates the local soft tissues and when applied over a joint reduces intra-articular temperatures with the ability to reduce local blood flow in addition to other benefits.[87] While cryotherapy may provide theoretical benefits, Adie et al found no discernible benefits with cryotherapy after conducting a systematic review and meta-analysis.[87]

A potentially inexpensive option for minimizing blood loss following TKA is maintaining the knee in a flexed position, during the immediate postoperative period. While knee flexion in the immediate postoperative period may seem counterintuitive due to concerns for development of postoperative flexion contracture, wound healing, and venous thromboembolism (VTE), some studies have demonstrated tangible benefits to blood management. In a recent meta-analysis of RCTs, Wu et al found that maintenance of the knee in a high flexion significantly reduced transfusion requirements and improved ROM following TKA, while also avoiding complications related to wound healing and VTE.[88] While these findings are promising, the severity of the potential complications that may occur due to maintaining the postoperative knee in a flexed position is substantial; therefore, additional research into this technique is needed before definitive recommendations can be made.

Autologous Reinfusion Drains

The postoperative reinfusion technique is similar to intraoperative cell salvage, including the collection of shed blood from the knee joint and the subsequent filtering, washing, and reinfusion of the blood into the patient 6 to 8 hours later. Although reinfusion systems have been shown to be a safe and efficacious method of transfusion, while also reducing the burden of ABT, the literature remains conflicted. Moonen et al randomly assigned 160 patients undergoing total hip arthroplasty (THA) and TKA to receive either a reinfusion system or regular drain and found a statistically significant reduction in ABT when the reinfusion system was used (6%) compared with the regular drain group (19%, $P = .015$).[89] In a recent meta-analysis of prospective RCTs on the use of reinfusion systems, the authors found a significant reduction in the need for ABT when the results were pooled.[90] Although a potentially attractive option, the perceived benefits of this technique must be weighed against concerns regarding its efficacy, risk of coagulopathy, contamination, and expense. In a prospective RCT, Al-Zahid et al found that when comparing reinfusion drains to closed suction drains and no drains, no differences were found in postoperative hemoglobin level, ABT rates, or American Knee Society Score.[91] Coagulopathy secondary to reinfusion is thought to occur as a result of the altered composition of the rein-fused blood, with demonstrated elevations in fibrin split products and inflammatory cytokines.[92] Cost is an additional factor, as the unit cost of a reinfusion system has been reported as $581, which is substantially greater than alternative means of blood management such as TXA.[71] Due to the conflicting results in the literature and the relative high cost associated with reinfusion systems compared to alternative practices, we do not recommend routine use of this technique following primary TKA.

Allogeneic Blood Transfusion

The majority of the chapter has been devoted to reducing the incidence of ABT following TKA. However, in spite of our greatest efforts, blood loss following TKA is inevitable and in the susceptible patient, ABT may be necessary. The risks involved with transfusion are substantial and have been well-described.[5,7,8,17,32] Briefly, the potential complications may be infectious with disease transmission, cardiopulmonary with fluid overload or acute lung injury, and/or systemic with transfusion reaction or anaphylaxis.[17] The relative cost of ABT should also be considered, as expenses associated with the logistics of executing the transfusion of one unit of allogeneic blood have been estimated to be approximately $787.[72] Nichols et al performed a retrospective chart review of patients undergoing unilateral and bilateral primary TKA as well as those undergoing revision TKA. In their comparative risk evaluation, they found that patients who required ABT had increased incremental total hospitalization costs at $2,477 (12%), $4,235 (15%), and $8,594 (35%) higher for primary TKA, bilateral TKA, and revision TKA, respectively.

With these concerns in mind, the treatment team should have an appreciation for the appropriate scenarios for when an ABT is indicated. The "transfusion trigger" concept has been popular for decades and historically called for transfusion of allogeneic blood according to the so-called "10/30" rule: give a transfusion when the patient's hemoglobin or hematocrit fell below 10 g/dL or 30%, respectively. As our understanding of the deleterious effects of ABT has matured, recommendations for more restrictive transfusion triggers have followed. Guidelines for more restrictive transfusion triggers have been developed by both the American Association of Blood Banks (AABB)[93] and the American Society of Anesthesiologists Task Force on Perioperative Blood Transfusion and Adjuvant Therapies.[94] The relative safety of more restrictive transfusion strategies has been demonstrated.[95,96] After instituting a restrictive protocol limiting consideration of ABT to values less than 8 g/dL, Carson et al retrospectively reviewed transfusion patterns in 8787 patients who were surgically treated for hip fracture. They found transfusion to have no effect on mortality in patients with hemoglobin levels as low as 8 g/dL.[95] In a small study of healthy patients, Weiskopf

et al demonstrated that hemoglobin levels as low as 5 g/dL could be tolerated as long as circulating volume was appropriately maintained with replacement fluids.[96]

Current guidelines suggest that thresholds for transfusion should not only consider absolute hemoglobin level but also clinical symptoms of anemia as well as the volume status of the patient. The treatment team should evaluate the patient for signs such as tachycardia, malaise, and dizziness. In addition, the team must take into account the patient's comorbidities, such as CAD, severity of illness, and amount of surgical blood loss. At this time, evidence-based guidelines recommend transfusing postsurgical patients who demonstrate clinical symptoms of anemia when hemoglobin levels are lower than 7 to 8 g/dL.[93,94] Many hospital systems have enacted institutional policies and have demonstrated success with these protocols. After implementation of an individualized patient blood management protocol, Loftus et al reported a 44% decrease in transfusion rate and a significant reduction in complications, readmissions, and length of hospital stay.[97] Based on the available evidence in the literature, institutions should enact a restrictive transfusion trigger protocol, whereby clinical symptoms are considered in conjunction with absolute hemoglobin and hematocrit values. When practical evidence-based guidelines are implemented, it is possible to reduce transfusion-associated complications and significantly improve ABT rates following TKA while also improving outcomes and costs associated with the procedure.

Conclusions

Blood management is essential in knee surgery, especially when considering the large blood loss and the risks involved with ABT. Blood loss following TKA is inevitable; therefore, consideration of the blood management tools available is integral to the treatment plan of a TKA patient.

In addition to avoidance of ABT, a sound blood management protocol must also place an emphasis on maintenance of ample blood volume. Consequently, this chapter has evaluated the various preoperative, intraoperative, and postoperative measures that the surgeon and the treatment team can take to meet these goals. The most significant advancement in blood management over the last decade has been the implementation of routine TXA use. When incorporated into the perioperative blood management protocol, this medication has not only been proven to reduce blood loss and decrease the need for ABT but has also been shown to be relatively cheap and cost-effective as a blood management agent. Future studies will need to further define which populations of patients can tolerate TXA, as despite its safe clinical record, there is a reluctance to use this medication in patients with certain medical comorbidities. Furthermore, the ideal dose and methods of administration of TXA need further clarification. Despite several lingering questions, the routine use of TXA as well as the implementation of restrictive transfusion triggers has reduced the transfusion rate after primary TKA to nearly zero.

As a result of the success of TXA, routine use of other costlier and/or logistically challenging methods, such as EPO, PAD, topical hemostatic agents, and intraoperative cell salvage, has fallen out of favor. Nevertheless, there may be unique scenarios where the patient would benefit from one of these other techniques. Therefore, the treatment team should maintain an appreciation of these methods as options when necessary. As discussed, blood management techniques are multifaceted, and with many treatment options available, a multidisciplinary approach which includes the surgeon, anesthesiologist, internist, and hematologist should be utilized. With a team-based approach, the relative advantages and disadvantages of all treatment options can be weighed, yielding a sound treatment plan for bleeding management before, during, and after the patient's TKA.

REFERENCES

1. Sehat KR, Evans RL, Newman JH. Hidden blood loss following hip and knee arthroplasty. Correct management of blood loss should take hidden loss into account. *J Bone Joint Surg Br*. 2004;86:561-565. doi:10.1302/0301-620X.86B4.14508.
2. Kalairajah Y, Simpson D, Cossey AJ, Verrall GM, Spriggins AJ. Blood loss after total knee replacement. *J Bone Joint Surg Br*. 2005;87-B:1480-1482. doi:10.1302/0301-620X.87B11.16474.
3. Bong MR, Patel V, Chang E, Issack PS, Hebert R, Di Cesare PE. Risks associated with blood transfusion after total knee arthroplasty. *J Arthroplasty*. 2004;19:281-287. doi:10.1016/j.arth.2003.10.013.
4. Spahn DR. Anemia and patient blood management in hip and knee surgery. *Anesthesiology*. 2010;113:482-495. doi:10.1097/ALN.0b013e3181e08e97.
5. Stulberg BN, Zadzilka JD. Blood management issues. Using blood management strategies. *J Arthroplasty*. 2007;22:95-98. doi:10.1016/j.arth.2007.03.002.
6. Shander A, Knight K, Thurer R, Adamson J, Spence R. Prevalence and outcomes of anemia in surgery: a systematic review of the literature. *Am J Med*. 2004;116:58-69. doi:10.1016/j.amjmed.2003.12.013.
7. Themistoklis T, Theodosia V, Konstantinos K, Georgios D. Perioperative blood management strategies for patients undergoing total knee replacement: where do we stand now? *World J Orthop*. 2017;8:441-454.
8. Kirane Y, Cushner F. Blood management. Orthopedic Knowledge Update. *Hip Knee Reconstr*. 2017;5:27-43.
9. Domenica Cappellini M, Motta I. Anemia in clinical practice-definition and classification: does hemoglobin change with aging? *Semin Hematol*. 2015;52:261-269. doi:10.1053/j.seminhematol.2015.07.006.
10. Guralnik JM, Eisenstaedt RS, Ferrucci L, Klein HG, Woodman RC. Prevalence of anemia in persons 65 years and older in the United States : evidence for a high rate of unexplained anemia. *Blood*. 2004;104:2263-2268. doi:10.1182/blood-2004-05-1812.Three.
11. Cuenca J, García-Erce JA, Martínez F, Cardona R, Pérez-Serrano L, Muñoz M. Preoperative haematinics and transfusion protocol reduce the need for transfusion after total knee replacement. *Int J Surg*. 2007;5:89-94. doi:10.1016/j.ijsu.2006.02.003.
12. Andrews CM, Lane DW, Bradley JG. Iron pre-load for major joint replacement. *Transfus Med*. 1997;7:281-286.
13. Petis SM, Lanting BA, Vasarhelyi EM, Naudie DDR, Ralley FE, Howard JL. Is there a role for preoperative iron supplementation in patients preparing for a total hip or total knee arthroplasty? *J Arthroplasty*. 2017;32:2688-2693. doi:10.1016/j.arth.2017.04.029.
14. Onken JE, Bregman DB, Harrington RA, et al. A multicenter, randomized, active-controlled study to investigate the efficacy and safety of intravenous ferric carboxymaltose in patients with iron deficiency anemia. *Transfusion*. 2014;54:306-315. doi:10.1111/trf.12289.
15. Theusinger OM, Leyvraz P-F, Schanz U, Seifert B, Spahn DR. Treatment of iron deficiency anemia in orthopedic surgery with intravenous iron: efficacy and limits. *Anesthesiology*. 2007;107:923-927. doi:10.1097/01.anes.0000291441.10704.82.
16. Lachance K, Savoie M, Bernard M, et al. Oral ferrous sulfate does not increase preoperative hemoglobin in patients scheduled for hip or knee arthroplasty. *Ann Pharmacother*. 2011;45:764-770. doi:10.1345/aph.1P757.
17. Levine BR, Haughom B, Strong B, Hellman M, Frank RM. Blood management strategies for total knee arthroplasty abstract. *J Am Acad Orthop Surg*. 2014;22:361-371. doi:10.5435/JAAOS-22-06-361.
18. Kopolovic I, Ostro J, Tsubota H, et al. CME article a systematic review of transfusion-associated graft-versus-host disease. *Blood*. 2015;126:406-415. doi:10.1182/blood-2015-01-620872.I.K.
19. Bierbaum BE, Callaghan JJ, Galante JO, Rubash HE, Tooms RE, Welch RB. An analysis of blood management in patients having a total hip or knee arthroplasty. *J Bone Joint Surg Am*. 1999;81:2-10.
20. Bezwada HP, Nazarian DG, Henry DH, Booth RE Jr. Preoperative use of recombinant human erythropoietin before total joint arthroplasty. *J Bone Joint Surg Am*. 2003;85-A:1795-1800.
21. Kourtzis N, Pafilas D, Kasimatis G. Blood saving protocol in elective total knee arthroplasty. *Am J Surg*. 2004;187:261-267. doi:10.1016/j.amjsurg.2003.11.022.
22. So-Osman C, Nelissen RG, Koopman-van Gemert AW, et al. Patient blood management in elective total hip- and knee-replacement surgery (Part 2). *Anesthesiology*. 2014;120:852-860. doi:10.1097/ALN.0000000000000135.
23. Moonen AFCM, Thomassen BJW, Knoors NT, van Os JJ, Verburg AD, Pilot P. Pre-operative injections of epoetin-alpha versus post-operative retransfusion of autologous shed blood in total hip and knee replacement: a prospective randomised clinical trial. *J Bone Joint Surg Br Vol*. 2008;90-B:1079-1083. doi:10.1302/0301-620X.90B8.20595.
24. Weber EWG, Slappendel R, Hémon Y, et al. Effects of epoetin alfa on blood transfusions and postoperative recovery in orthopaedic surgery: the European Epoetin Alfa Surgery Trial (EEST). *Eur J Anaesthesiol*. 2005;22:249-257. doi:10.1017/S0265021505000426.
25. Stowell C, Chandler H, Jove M, Guilfoyle M, Wacholtz M. An open-label, randomized study to compare the safety and efficacy of perioperative epoetin alfa with preoperative autologous blood donation in total joint arthroplasty. *Orthopedics*. 1999;22:s105-s112.
26. Bedair H, Yang J, Dwyer MK, McCarthy JC. Preoperative erythropoietin alpha reduces postoperative transfusions in THA and TKA but may not be cost-effective. *Clin Orthop Relat Res*. 2014;473:590-596. doi:10.1007/s11999-014-3819-z.
27. Pierson J, Hannon T, Earles D. A blood-conservation algorithm to reduce blood transfusions after total hip and knee arthroplasty. *J Bone Joint Surg*. 2004;86:1512-1518.
28. Levine GN, Bates ER, Bittl JA, et al. 2016 ACC/AHA guideline focused update on duration of dual antiplatelet therapy in patients with coronary artery disease: a report of the American College of Cardiology/American Heart Association task force on clinical practice guidelines. *J Am Coll Cardiol*. 2016;68:1082-1115. doi:10.1016/j.jacc.2016.03.513.
29. Chassot PG, Delabays A, Spahn DR. Perioperative use of antiplatelet drugs. *Best Pract Res Clin Anaesthesiol*. 2007;21:241-256. doi:10.1016/j.bpa.2007.02.002.

30. Vandermeulen EP, Van Aken H, Vermylen J. Anticoagulants and spinal-epidural anesthesia. *Anesth Analg.* 1994;79:1165-1177. doi:10.1213/00000539-199412000-00024.

31. Giordano G, Dockery J, Wallace B, et al. An autologous blood program coordinated by a regional blood center: a 5-year experience. *Transfusion.* 1991;31:509-512. doi:10.1046/j.1537-2995. 1991.31691306247.x.

32. Bezwada HR, Nazarian DG, Henry DH, Booth RE Jr, Mont MA. Blood management in total joint arthroplasty. *Am J Orthop (Belle Mead NJ).* 2006;35(10):458-464.

33. Goodnough LT, Brecher M, Kanter M, AuBuchon J. Transfusion medicine. First of two parts–blood transfusion. *N Engl J Med.* 1999;340:438-447.

34. Olsfanger D, Fredman B, Goldstein B, Shapiro A, Jedeikin R. Acute normovolaemic haemodilution decreases postoperative allogeneic blood transfusion after total knee replacement. *Br J Anaesth.* 1997;79:317-321. doi:10.1093/bja/79.3.317.

35. Gillon J, Thomas MJ, Desmond MJ. Consensus conference on autologous transfusion. Acute normovolaemic haemodilution. *Transfusion.* 1996;36:640-643.

36. Goodnough LT, Despotis GJ, Merkel K, Monk TG. A randomized trial comparing acute normovolemic hemodilution and preoperative autologous blood donation in total hip arthroplasty. *Transfusion.* 2000;40:1054-1057.

37. Mielke LL, Entholzner EK, Kling M, et al. Preoperative acute hypervolemic hemodilution with hydroxyethylstarch: an alternative to acute normovolemic hemodilution? *Anesth Analg.* 1997;84:26-30. doi:10.1097/00000539-199701000-00005.

38. Whitehead DJ, MacDonald SJ. TKA sans tourniquet: let it bleed: opposes. *Orthopedics.* 2011;34:497-500. doi:10.3928/01477447-20110714-44.

39. Tai T-W, Lin C-J, Jou I-M, Chang C-W, Lai K-A, Yang C-Y. Tourniquet use in total knee arthroplasty: a meta-analysis. *Knee Surg Sports Traumatol Arthrosc.* 2011;19:1121-1130. doi:10.1007/s00167-010-1342-7.

40. Thorey F, Stukenborg-Colsman C, Windhagen H, Wirth CJ. The effect of tourniquet release timing on perioperative blood loss in simultaneous bilateral cemented total knee arthroplasty: a prospective randomized study. *Technol Health Care.* 2008;16:85-92.

41. Huang ZY, Pei FX, Ma J, et al. Comparison of three different tourniquet application strategies for minimally invasive total knee arthroplasty: a prospective non-randomized clinical trial. *Arch Orthop Trauma Surg.* 2014;134:561-570. doi:10.1007/s00402-014-1948-1.

42. Sharrock N, Mineo C, Robert M, Urquhart C, Barbara R. Hemodynamic effects of low dose epinephrine and sodium nitroprusside during epidural hypotensive anesthesia. *Reg Anesth.* 1989;14.

43. Kiss H, Raffl M, Neumann D, Hutter J, Dorn U. Epinephrine-augmented hypotensive epidural anesthesia replaces tourniquet use in total knee replacement. *Clin Orthop Relat Res.* 2005(436):184-189. doi:10.1097/01.blo.0000161825.90633.12.

44. Juelsgaard P, Larsen UT, Sorensen JV, Madsen F, Soballe K. Hypotensive epidural anesthesia in total knee replacement without tourniquet: reduced blood loss and transfusion. *Reg Anesth Pain Med.* 2001;26(2):105-110. doi:10.1053/rapm.2001.21094.

45. Danninger T, Stundner O, Ma Y, Bae JJ, Memtsoudis SG. The impact of hypotensive epidural anesthesia on distal and proximal tissue perfusion in patients undergoing total hip arthroplasty. *J Anesth Clin Res.* 2013;4:366. doi:10.4172/2155-6148.1000366.

46. Sharrock NE, Beksac B, Flynn E, Go G, Della Valle AG. Hypotensive epidural anaesthesia in patients with preoperative renal dysfunction undergoing total hip replacement. *Br J Anaesth.* 2006;96:207-212. doi:10.1093/bja/aei308.

47. Kim K, Elbuluk A, Yu S, Iorio R. Cost-effective peri-operative pain management: assuring a happy patient after total knee arthroplasty. *Bone Joint J.* 2018;100B:55-61. doi:10.1302/0301-620X.100B1. BJJ-2017-0549.R1.

48. Anderson LA, Engel GM, Bruckner JD, Stoddard GJ, Peters CL. Reduced blood loss after total knee arthroplasty with local injection of bupivacaine and epinephrine. *J Knee Surg.* 2009;22:130-136. doi:10.1055/s-0030-1247737.

49. Mangano DT, Tudor IC, Dietzel C. The risk associated with aprotinin in cardiac surgery. *N Engl J Med.* 2006;354:353-365. doi:10.1056/NEJMoa051379.

50. Sepah YJ, Umer M, Ahmad T, Nasim F, Chaudhry MU, Umar M. Use of tranexamic acid is a cost effective method in preventing blood loss during and after total knee replacement. *J Orthop Surg Res.* 2011;6:22. doi:10.1186/1749-799X-6-22.

51. Kim C, Park SS-H, Davey JR. Tranexamic acid for the prevention and management of orthopedic surgical hemorrhage: current evidence. *J Blood Med.* 2015;6:239-244. doi:10.2147/JBM.S61915.

52. Lee SH, Cho K-Y, Khurana S, Kim K-I. Less blood loss under concomitant administration of tranexamic acid and indirect factor Xa inhibitor following total knee arthroplasty: a prospective randomized controlled trial. *Knee Surg Sports Traumatol Arthrosc.* 2013;21:2611-2617. doi:10.1007/s00167-012-2213-1.

53. Yang Z-G, Chen W-P, Wu L-D. Effectiveness and safety of tranexamic acid in reducing blood loss in total knee arthroplasty: a meta-analysis. *J Bone Joint Surg Am.* 2012;94:1-7. doi:10.1016/S0021-9355(12)70269-2.

54. Good L, Peterson E, Lisander B. Tranexamic acid decreases external blood loss but not hidden blood loss in total knee replacement. *Br J Anaesth.* 2003;90:596-599. doi:10.1093/bja/aeg.

55. Seo JG, Moon YW, Park SH, Kim SM, Ko KR. The comparative efficacies of intra-articular and IV tranexamic acid for reducing blood loss during total knee arthroplasty. *Knee Surg Sports Traumatol Arthrosc.* 2013;21:1869-1874. doi:10.1007/s00167-012-2079-2.

56. Hsu C-H, Lin P-C, Kuo F-C, Wang J-W. A regime of two intravenous injections of tranexamic acid reduces blood loss in minimally invasive total hip arthroplasty: a prospective randomised double-blind study. *Bone Joint Lett J.* 2015;97-B:905-910. doi:10.1302/0301-620X.97B7.35029.

57. Drosos GI, Ververidis A, Valkanis C, et al. A randomized comparative study of topical versus intravenous tranexamic acid administration in enhanced recovery after surgery (ERAS) total knee replacement. *J Orthop.* 2016;13:127-131. doi:10.1016/j.jor.2016.03.007.

58. Tzatzairis TK, Drosos GI, Kotsios SE, Ververidis AN, Vogiatzaki TD, Kazakos KI. Intravenous vs topical tranexamic acid in total knee arthroplasty without tourniquet application: a randomized controlled study. *J Arthroplasty.* 2016;31:2465-2470. doi:10.1016/j.arth.2016.04.036.

59. Grosso MJ, Trofa DP, Danoff JR, et al. Tranexamic acid increases early perioperative functional outcomes after total knee arthroplasty. *Arthroplast Today.* 2018;4:74-77. doi:10.1016/j.artd.2017.05.009.

60. Dorweiler M, Boin M, Froehle A, Lawless M, May J. Improved early postoperative range of motion in total knee arthroplasty using tranexamic acid: a retrospective analysis. *J Knee Surg.* 2019;32(2):160-164.

61. Serrano Mateo L, Goudarz Mehdikhani K, Cáceres L, Lee Y yu, Gonzalez Della Valle A. Topical tranexamic acid may improve early functional outcomes of primary total knee arthroplasty. *J Arthroplasty.* 2016;31:1449-1452. doi:10.1016/j.arth.2016.01.009.

62. Benoni G, Bjorkman S, Fredin H. Application of pharmacokinetic data from healthy volunteers for the prediction of plasma concentrations of tranexamic acid in surgical patients. *Clin Drug Investig.* 1995;10:280-287.

63. Sun X, Dong Q, Zhang Y-G. Intravenous versus topical tranexamic acid in primary total hip replacement: a systemic review and meta-analysis. *Int J Surg.* 2016;32:10-18. doi:10.1016/j.ijsu.2016.05.064.

64. Meena S, Benazzo F, Dwivedi S, Ghiara M. Topical versus intravenous tranexamic acid in total knee arthroplasty. *J Orthop Surg.* 2017;25:2309499901668430. doi:10.1177/2309499016684300.

65. Fillingham YA, Kayupov E, Plummer DR, Moric M, Gerlinger TL, Della Valle CJ. The James A. Rand Young Investigator's Award: a randomized controlled trial of oral and intravenous tranexamic acid in total knee arthroplasty: the same efficacy at lower cost? *J Arthroplasty.* 2016;31:26-30. doi:10.1016/j.arth.2016.02.081.

66. Lin SY, Chen CH, Fu YC, Huang PJ, Chang JK, Huang HT. The efficacy of combined use of intraarticular and intravenous tranexamic acid on reducing blood loss and transfusion rate in total knee arthroplasty. *J Arthroplasty.* 2015;30:776-780. doi:10.1016/j.arth.2014.12.001.

67. Adravanti P, Di Salvo E, Calafiore G, Vasta S, Ampollini A, Rosa MA. A prospective, randomized, comparative study of intravenous alone and combined intravenous and intraarticular administration of tranexamic acid in primary total knee replacement. *Arthroplast Today.* 2018;4:85-88. doi:10.1016/j.artd.2017.08.004.

68. Zeng W, Liu J, Wang F, Chen C, Zhou Q, Yang L. Low-dose epinephrine plus tranexamic acid reduces early postoperative blood loss and inflammatory response: a randomized controlled trial. *J Bone Joint Surg.* 2018;100:295-304.

69. Ramkumar DB, Ramkumar N, Tapp SJ, Moschetti WE. Pharmacologic hemostatic agents in total joint arthroplasty—a cost-effectiveness analysis. *J Arthroplasty.* 2018;33(7):2092-2099.e9. doi:10.1016/j.arth.2018.02.068.

70. Phan DL, Ani F, Schwarzkopf R. Cost analysis of tranexamic acid in anemic total joint arthroplasty patients. *J Arthroplasty.* 2016;31(3):579-582. doi:10.1016/j.arth.2015.10.001.

71. Springer BD, Odum SM, Fehring TK. What is the benefit of tranexamic acid vs reinfusion drains in total joint arthroplasty? *J Arthroplasty.* 2016;31:76-80. doi:10.1016/j.arth.2015.08.006.

72. Tuttle JR, Ritterman SA, Cassidy DB, Anazonwu WA, Froehlich JA, Rubin LE. Cost benefit analysis of topical tranexamic acid in primary total hip and knee arthroplasty. *J Arthroplasty.* 2014;29:1512-1515. doi:10.1016/j.arth.2014.01.031.

73. Bridgens JP, Evans CR, Dobson PMS, Hamer AJ. Intraoperative red blood-cell salvage in revision hip surgery: a case-matched study. *J Bone Joint Surg Am.* 2007;89:270-275. doi:10.2106/JBJS.F.00492.

74. Blatsoukas KS, Drosos GI, Kazakos K, et al. Prospective comparative study of two different autotransfusion methods versus control group in total knee replacement. *Arch Orthop Trauma Surg.* 2010;130:733-737. doi:10.1007/s00402-010-1062-y.

75. Wang H, Shan L, Zeng H, Sun M, Hua Y, Cai Z. Is fibrin sealant effective and safe in total knee arthroplasty? A meta-analysis of randomized trials. *J Orthop Surg.* 2014;9:36.

76. Kim HJ, Fraser MR, Kahn B, Lyman S, Figgie MP. The efficacy of a thrombin-based hemostatic agent in unilateral total knee arthroplasty: a randomized controlled trial. *J Bone Joint Surg Am.* 2012;94:1160-1165. doi:10.2106/JBJS.K.00531.

77. Gardner MJ, Demetrakopoulos D, Klepchick PR, Mooar PA. The efficacy of autologous platelet gel in pain control and blood loss in total knee arthroplasty: an analysis of the haemoglobin, narcotic requirement and range of motion. *Int Orthop.* 2007;31:309-313. doi:10.1007/s00264-006-0174-z.

78. Suarez JC, Slotkin EM, Szubski CR, Barsoum WK, Patel PD. Prospective, randomized trial to evaluate efficacy of a bipolar sealer in direct anterior approach total hip arthroplasty. *J Arthroplasty.* 2015;30:1953-1958. doi:10.1016/j.arth.2015.05.023.

79. Nielsen CS, Gromov K, Jans Ø, Troelsen A, Husted H. No effect of a bipolar sealer on total blood loss or blood transfusion in nonseptic revision knee arthroplasty—a prospective study with matched retrospective controls. *J Arthroplasty.* 2017;32:177-182. doi:10.1016/j.arth.2016.06.037.

80. Ko PS, Tio MK, Tang YK, Tsang WL, Lam JJ. Sealing the intramedullary femoral canal with autologous bone plug in total knee arthroplasty. *J Arthroplasty.* 2003;18:6-9. doi:10.1054/arth.2003.50001.

81. Li X, Qi XB, Han X, et al. Effects of sealing the intramedullary femoral canal in total knee arthroplasty. *Medicine (Baltimore).* 2017;96:e7388. doi:10.1097/MD.0000000000007388.

82. Batmaz AG, Kayaalp ME, Oto O, Bulbul AM. Sealing of femoral tunnel with autologous bone graft decreases blood loss. *Acta Chir Orthop Traumatol Cech.* 2016;83:348-350.

83. Vulcano E, Regazzola GMV, Murena L, Ronga M, Cherubino P, Surace MF. Femoral bone plug in total knee replacement. *Orthopedics.* 2015;38:617-618. doi:10.3928/01477447-20151002-03.

84. Torres-Claramunt R, Hinarejos P, Pérez-Prieto D, et al. Sealing of the intramedullar femoral canal in a TKA does not reduce postoperative blood loss: a randomized prospective study. *Knee.* 2014;21:853-857. doi:10.1016/j.knee.2014.03.010.

85. Protzman NM, Buck NJ, Weiss CB. Autologous bone plugs in unilateral total knee arthroplasty. *Indian J Orthop.* 2013;47:182-187. doi:10.4103/0019-5413.108914.

86. Solomon LB, Guevara C, Büchler L, Howie DW, Byard RW, Beck M. Does bone wax induce a chronic inflammatory articular reaction? *Clin Orthop Relat Res.* 2012;470:3207-3212. doi:10.1007/s11999-012-2457-6.

87. Adie S, Naylor JM, Harris IA. Cryotherapy after total knee arthroplasty. A systematic review and meta-analysis of randomized controlled trials. *J Arthroplasty.* 2010;25:709-715. doi:10.1016/j.arth.2009.07.010.

88. Wu Y, Yang T, Zeng Y, Si H, Li C, Shen B. Effect of different postoperative limb positions on blood loss and range of motion in total knee arthroplasty: an updated meta-analysis of randomized controlled trials. *Int J Surg.* 2017;37:15-23. doi:10.1016/j.ijsu.2016.11.135.

89. Moonen AFCM, Knoors NT, Van Os JJ, Verburg AD, Pilot P. Retransfusion of filtered shed blood in primary total hip and knee arthroplasty: a prospective randomized clinical trial. *Transfusion.* 2007;47:379-384. doi:10.1111/j.1537-2995.2007.01127.x.

90. Zhao H, Jiang Y, Ma B, Guo M, Fan Q. Post-operative autotransfusion in total hip or knee arthroplasty: a meta-analysis of randomized controlled trials. *PLoS One.* 2013;8:e55073. doi:10.1371/journal.pone.0055073.

91. Al-Zahid S, Davies AP. Closed suction drains, reinfusion drains or no drains in primary total knee replacement? *Ann R Coll Surg Engl.* 2012;94:347-350. doi:10.1308/003588412X13171221590098.

92. Matsuda K, Nozawa M, Katsube S, Maezawa K, Kurosawa H. Activation of fibrinolysis by reinfusion of unwashed salvaged blood after total knee arthroplasty. *Transfus Apher Sci.* 2010;42:33-37. doi:10.1016/j.transci.2009.10.005.

93. Carson JL, Grossman BJ, Kleinman S, et al. Red blood cell transfusion: a clinical practice guideline from the AABB. *Ann Intern Med.* 2012;157:49-58. doi:10.7326/0003-4819-157-1-201206190-00429.

94. American Society of Anesthesiologists Task Force on Perioperative Blood Transfusion and Adjuvant Therapies. Practice guidelines for perioperative blood transfusion and adjuvant therapies: an updated report by the American Society of Anesthesiologists task force on perioperative blood transfusion and adjuvant therapies. *Anesthesiology.* 2006;105:198-208. doi:10.1097/00000542-200607000-00030.

95. Carson JL, Duff A, Berlin JA, et al. Perioperative blood transfusion and postoperative mortality. *J Am Med Assoc.* 1998;279:199-205. doi:10.1001/jama.279.3.199.

96. Weiskopf RB, Viele MK, Feiner J, et al. Human cardiovascular and metabolic response to acute, severe isovolemic anemia. *J Am Med Assoc.* 1998;279:217-221. doi:10.1001/jama.279.3.217.

97. Loftus TJ, Spratling L, Stone BA, Xiao L, Jacofsky DJ. A patient blood management program in prosthetic joint arthroplasty decreases blood use and improves outcomes. *J Arthroplasty.* 2016;31:11-14. doi:10.1016/j.arth.2015.07.040.

chapter 52

Outpatient Total Knee Arthroplasty

Carl B. Wallis, MD | David A. Crawford, MD | Keith R. Berend, MD |
Adolph V. Lombardi Jr, MD, FACS

INTRODUCTION

As techniques and design of total knee arthroplasty (TKA) have been refined over the years, postoperative patient care practices too have evolved dramatically. Historically, patients were admitted for 7 to 10 days after TKA.[1] The first night was spent in a mini-intensive care unit and strict bed rest was observed. Knees were immobilized and wrapped in bulky Jones dressings, and patients would finally be allowed to stand on postoperative day 2 or 3. With the advent of in-hospital skilled nursing facilities (SNFs), patients soon would spend the latter 5 to 7 days of their stay in these units. Then, as less-invasive surgical techniques began to emerge, the status quo of patient recovery began to be challenged. Rapid recovery protocols quickly took hold, and the average length of stay (LOS) has since been declining. Now, it is common for patients to stay 1 or 2 nights after a TKA procedure with full weight-bearing the day of surgery and discharge to home. The next frontier that has increasingly been adopted is outpatient TKA.

While the move to outpatient TKA is in keeping with the ultimate goal for elective surgery to provide patients with consistently excellent results and the best possible experience, it is also motivated by pressure for cost reduction, particularly in light of escalating demand for the procedure.[2] This drive to reduce costs by eliminating inpatient admissions has to be balanced by the potential increase in postoperative complications and readmissions. Traditionally, patients have required inpatient admission due to concerns for postoperative pain and decreased mobility. However, with improved postoperative protocols, these challenges can and have been addressed. This chapter discusses these specific challenges and the pathways that have been developed to make outpatient TKA a reality.

SURGICAL FACILITY

Outpatient TKA truly can be performed in any setting, from a large tertiary referral hospital to a stand-alone ambulatory surgery center (ASC). There are advantages and disadvantages to either setting. In the hospital setting, there is a safety net of medical consultants and intensive care unit (ICU) resources should a complication arise. Additionally, larger hospitals may have greater access to

a broad inventory of implants and instrumentation that a smaller facility may not readily carry. Perhaps one of the biggest disadvantages to a larger facility is the surgeon's lack of direct management of perioperative staff. The surgeon often must work with hospital administration to enact changes, which may prove challenging and obstructive. In an ASC or even in some specialty-specific hospitals, the surgeon is likely to have more input in making changes necessary to improve efficiency and enact outpatient protocols.

What is more important than the actual facility is the culture of the staff. To perform outpatient TKA safely requires more than the surgeon simply deciding to discharge his or her patients on same day as surgery. It requires an entire team to be on the same page and to have the vision of rapid recovery and safe, early discharge to home. The surgeon needs buy-in from nursing, anesthesiology, physical therapy, and administration in order to accomplish the goal of same-day discharge. This is not a transition done overnight. It often requires a gradual reduction of length of stay until the average stay is one overnight. Then certain patients may be selected for same-day discharge. This practice allows a gradual assimilation of perioperative staff to the culture of outpatient TKA and permits the surgeon and others to safely identify and address challenges along the way without significant disruption to the overall mission.

Our experience has mirrored the above pathway of gradual transition. The authors of this chapter developed a musculoskeletal specialty hospital where a rapid recovery pathway was implemented. With direct oversight of staff and the execution of this protocol, length of stay was gradually reduced to an average of 1.5 days. The transition was then made to same-day discharge, which influenced the development of a separate ASC following the same rapid recovery clinical pathway.

PATIENT SELECTION

All patients presenting for TKA may be considered as candidates for outpatient surgery. As rapid recovery protocols and medical optimization improve, what was once an option only for healthy, highly motivated patients is now being offered to mainstream patients. Still, care must be exercised to ensure that patients are medically optimized and that key comorbidities are identified. This begins with the patient's initial visit to the surgeon's clinic. A brief survey of the patient's medical history may be all that is necessary to preclude a patient from outpatient surgery. The outpatient TKA candidate must have appropriate medical insurance. While age is not an independent contraindication for outpatient TKA, most patients aged 65 years and older have their insurance through Medicare, which did not support outpatient TKA in the ASC prior to January 1, 2020.

The preoperative medical evaluation is another important step in this process. This involves a comprehensive history and physical, appropriate laboratory and/or other testing, and referral to a medical specialist if needed. Meding et al observed that preoperative medical evaluations for elective total joint arthroplasty (TJA) procedures identified a substantial number of new diagnoses, and that 2.5% of patients were considered unacceptable surgical candidates as a result of these visits.[3] In addition, general medical specialists can provide medication reconciliation along with instructions on which medications to discontinue prior to surgery as well as the proper dosing of other medications on the day of surgery.

There is a difference in opinion as to what if any firm selection and exclusion criteria should be established for outpatient TKA, such as restrictions on BMI, age, comorbidities, etc. Pollock et al conducted a review of the literature regarding outpatient arthroplasty and found that the mean age for those undergoing outpatient total and unicompartmental knee arthroplasty was 55 to 68 years, whereas the overall age of knee arthroplasty patients nationally averaged 66.1 years. Mean BMI also varied from 27.5 to 30.8 kg/m^2 with many authors not reporting their values.[4] Interestingly, the majority of studies in this review showed a predominance of males in the outpatient cohort in spite of an annual higher proportion nationwide of females receiving TKA (61.6% in 2014). Some centers have worked in collaboration with internal medicine teams to establish outpatient selection protocols or scoring systems. Meneghini et al developed the Outpatient Arthroplasty Risk Assessment (OARA) score, which records a patient's specific comorbidities and predicts the likelihood of that patient being safe for same-day discharge after a joint arthroplasty procedure.[5] This would allow the internist, during the patient's preoperative medical examination, to filter the patient into either an outpatient or inpatient pathway depending on their calculated score. Courtney et al retrospectively reviewed 1012 patients who underwent hip and knee arthroplasty to evaluate which risk factors were associated with postoperative complications.[6] They observed that 6.9% of patients developed a complication requiring physician intervention, and of those 84% occurred more than 24 hours after surgery. They concluded that chronic obstructive pulmonary disease (COPD), congestive heart failure (CHF), coronary artery disease (CAD), and liver cirrhosis were independent risk factors for developing late (>24 hours) complications.

In a separate study, Courtney et al queried the American College of Surgeons, National Surgical Quality Improvement Program (ACS-NSQIP) database, to compare complications between outpatient and inpatient TJA and identify risk factors associated with these events.[7] Out of 169,406 patients, 1220 were identified as outpatient (0.7%). The study found that the outpatient and inpatient groups had overall complication rates of 8% and 16%, respectively. Risk factors for readmission and complications were age older than 70 years, malnutrition, cardiac history, smoking history, or diabetes mellitus. Of note, outpatient surgery alone did not account for an increased risk of readmission or reoperation.

Whatever criteria are used to select patients, utilizing a consistent group of physicians to perform medical evaluations is essential to enhance the process and ensure that the surgeon's and internist's goals are aligned. Frequent feedback and collaboration between the surgeon and the medical team will fine-tune the process and maximize efficiency in patient care.

PREOPERATIVE EDUCATION

As important as it is to exclude those patients who are not safe for outpatient TKA, it is also important to identify and include those patients who are otherwise good candidates but may be anxious about a same-day discharge. This requires careful patient education from the initial clinical visit. Because TKA is a highly utilized procedure, patients come to their surgeon with certain expectations, built up from the collective experiences of their peers. The surgeon must carefully and compassionately cut through these expectations and forge his or her own prescribed experience for the patient. Keys to this pathway are ensuring adequate social support, thoroughly answering all questions regarding the procedure, and providing substantial written and/or audiovisual resources for the patient. When these expectations are firmly rooted early, the patient is more likely to have a positive experience throughout their personal TKA journey.

Even more importantly, all team members throughout the clinical pathway must be united in their communications, messaging, goals, and expectations for same-day discharge. If the surgeon sets the expectation, then each team member must be trusted to maintain that expectation throughout the patient's journey. This includes clinical receptionists, nurses, schedulers, preoperative medical consultants, perioperative nurses, anesthesiology providers, and physical therapists. This multidisciplinary approach not only ensures a consistent expectation but also empowers other staff members to participate in the patient's instruction and thus eases the burden on the surgeon for thoroughly educating the patient. Dowsey et al prospectively randomized 163 patients into either a clinical pathway or control group prior to TJA.[8] They reported that the clinical pathway group had a significant reduction in hospital LOS, earlier ambulatory ability, decreased readmission rate, and more accurate matching of the patient's discharge destination (i.e., home versus SNF). These results support that clinical pathways are not only important in preparing a patient for same-day discharge, but they can also contribute to reducing complications and improving overall outcomes.

Even if the entire team shares the same vision for outpatient TKA, patients will still have questions and anxieties leading up to surgery. Comprehensive educational resources such as pamphlets, brochures, and DVDs can be a valuable tool in reinforcing and maintaining the patient's expectations and answering important questions. Many centers also employ "joint camps" or multidisciplinary meetings to allow patients to get acquainted with the setting and personnel they will encounter on the day of surgery. This preoperative encounter also allows physical therapists to address medical equipment needs, teach the patient how to adapt to activities of daily living, and instruct caregivers on how they can best help the patient in the immediate postoperative period. Nurses can use this platform to educate patients and caregivers on wound management and common complications. Ideally, these instructional sessions may be arranged in conjunction with the patient's preoperative medical assessment to reduce the patient's travel burdens. Familiarity with these concepts will help alleviate the fears and anxieties of the patient and contribute to a smooth and efficient recovery process.[9-11]

PERIOPERATIVE PAIN MANAGEMENT

One of the biggest roadblocks to outpatient TKA is postoperative pain. However, heavy narcotics and deep general anesthetics can leave the patient oversedated and with disruptive side effects such as nausea and vomiting, prolonging the acute recovery period and postponing the patient's participation in physical therapy. Rapid recovery pathways overcome this challenge in three specific ways: perioperative multimodal pain management, regional analgesia, and periarticular injections. Preoperative education yet again can be a useful tool in managing a patient's expectations prior to surgery, this time in regard to perioperative pain, and before any pharmacologic agent is administered. Working in connection with the anesthesiology team, the surgeon, and anesthetist can play a vital role in preparing the patient for the reality of postoperative pain and reassuring him or her that pain after surgery is normal, even after adequate administration of pain medications. If the patient is adequately prepared for this reality, then it will help mitigate the anxiety and fear that may arise upon awakening in the recovery room.[12]

Multimodal Pain Management

Multimodal pain management involves using several different pain medications throughout the perioperative period to control pain through different biochemical pathways. Paramount to this is the concept of preemptive analgesia. Multimodal pain management works based on the distinction between peripheral neurogenic pain and its resultant stimulation of the inflammatory cascade. Surgical trauma stimulates peripheral nociceptors, which in turn release cytokines, prostaglandins, and other chemical mediators that induce an inflammatory reaction. This inflammatory reaction compounds the patient's perception of pain. Additionally, the surgical trauma will cause central sensitization or increased excitability of spinal neurons, thus reducing the patient's pain tolerance.[13] Historically, a patient's pain was treated upon demand, after all these processes had been initiated, thus requiring high doses of narcotics to quell the pain response. This strategy leaves the patient constantly playing "catch-up" and precludes safe discharge home on the day of surgery. Effective multimodal pain management and preemptive analgesia involve minimizing the peripheral sensitization of nociceptors by treating the patient pre- and intraoperatively, heading off the resultant stimulation of the inflammatory cascade and ultimately limiting central sensitization.[13] A variety of medications have proven successful in this process.

Nonsteroidal anti-inflammatory drugs (NSAIDs) are frequently employed in multimodal pain regimens to limit the patient's inflammatory response. Cyclooxygenase-2 (COX-2)-inhibiting nonsteroidal medications are increasingly used due to their reportedly decreased frequency of gastrointestinal side effects. Mallory et al performed a study evaluating the effect of adding a COX-2 inhibitor to the pain regimen of patients undergoing TJA with spinal or epidural anesthesia and reported a significant reduction in postoperative pain as well as less postoperative confusion and nausea.[14]

Gabapentin and pregabalin, which are anticonvulsant drugs used to treat neuropathic pain, are another important type of medication used to minimize need for narcotics. These medications not only work to minimize postoperative pain on the day of surgery but also have been shown to reduce later onset of neuropathic pain. Buvanendran et al performed a randomized double-blinded study of 240 patients undergoing TKA.[15] One group was given 300 mg of pregabalin for 14 days postoperatively, and the other was given a placebo. The authors found that the incidence of neuropathic pain was none at both 3 and 6 months in the pregabalin group, while in the placebo group, it was 8.7% and 5.2%, respectively. They also found that patients treated with pregabalin used fewer epidural opioids, required less oral opioid pain medications during their hospitalization, and had greater active knee flexion over the first 30 days postoperatively.

Acetaminophen is another pain medication added to multimodal pain regimens both pre- and postoperatively and can be administered orally or intravenously (IV). A recent randomized controlled trial showed no difference in postoperative opioid consumption or mean pain scores at 24 hours postoperative between those receiving acetaminophen orally versus IV.[16]

In addition to pain medications, other medications are frequently administered to preemptively mitigate potential side effects, mainly nausea, pruritis, and sedation. These include dexamethasone, metoclopramide, ondansetron, and scopolamine patches. Furthermore, side effects can be reduced simply by adequate hydration. Patients often receive 1000 mL of crystalloid prior to surgery and additional fluids as deemed appropriate intraoperatively.

The exact multimodal pain regimen varies between different centers, but the concept remains the same. Pain and potential side effects are treated preemptively and through various pharmacological remedies to limit narcotic consumption and allow patients to mobilize quickly.

Epidural and Regional Anesthesia

The goal of epidural and regional anesthesia is twofold: first, it allows for reduced administration of powerful sedatives required for a general anesthetic, thereby reducing postoperative sedation and promoting earlier mobilization; second, it functions to limit afferent nerve transmission to central receptors, limiting the effects of central sensitization discussed earlier. Epidural anesthesia has been shown to be effective in decreasing postoperative narcotic use.[17] In addition, Williams-Russo et al showed that epidural anesthesia allowed more rapid achievement of in-hospital postoperative rehabilitation goals compared to general anesthesia.[18] Side effects of epidural anesthesia include hypotension and urinary retention, which can prolong postoperative rehabilitation efforts.

Regional anesthetics offer advantages similar to epidurals but in a more focused area and with diminished risk of hypotension or urinary retention. Compared to traditional pain regimens, regional analgesia has been shown to reduce the side effects of parenteral narcotics, improve pain control, allow earlier functional recovery, and reduce LOS. One study showed that femoral nerve blocks in patients undergoing TKA lowered risk of readmission.[19] However, femoral nerve blocks are notorious for inducing quadriceps weakness, significantly increasing fall risk, and challenging early discharge pathways. Adductor canal blocks are more attractive in that they offer the same sensory blockade as a femoral nerve block with much less risk of motor weakness. Jaeger et al performed a double-blind randomized study proving that quadriceps strength as a percentage of baseline was significantly higher in the adductor canal block group compared to the femoral nerve block group.[20] Typically, the adductor canal block is performed under ultrasound guidance with 12 to 15 mL of 0.5% ropivacaine.

A newer regional anesthetic technique that has been adopted is blockade in the interspace of the popliteal artery and posterior capsule of the knee (IPACK) block.

Like other regional analgesia techniques, IPACK blocks are done under ultrasound guidance and have been shown to provide substantial sensory blockade to the posterior knee without affecting the common peroneal nerve. Sankineani et al performed a prospective study comparing 120 patients undergoing TKA who either received both adductor canal and IPACK blocks or an adductor canal block alone.[21] Their results showed that patients who received both the adductor canal and IPACK blocks had significantly better visual analog scale (VAS) pain scores at 8 hours postoperatively and on postoperative days 1 and 2. Additionally, these patients had better knee ROM and were able to ambulate farther.

Periarticular Injections

The last approach to perioperative pain control involves direct injection of local anesthetics into the periarticular soft tissues during surgery. This practice helps block immediate transmission of pain signals and, depending on what agent is used, can provide prolonged pain control. There are a variety of combinations of local anesthetics agents such as bupivacaine or ropivacaine utilized with other agents such as opioid narcotics, epinephrine, and ketorolac. One study at the current authors' center showed that a combination of 0.25% bupivacaine, epinephrine, and a long-acting narcotic injected during TKA significantly reduced the need for breakthrough narcotics on the day of surgery.[22] The study also showed that patients receiving this treatment had reduced blood loss, reduced postoperative confusion, and greater knee ROM. The injection cocktail was later modified to eliminate the opioid narcotic.

Pain management represents one of the biggest hurdles to successful outpatient TKA. Multimodal preemptive regimens, regional analgesia, and periarticular injections all work in concert to minimize postoperative pain and side effects that preclude early mobilization and discharge. In establishing new protocols, it is essential that the surgeon develop strong working relationships with anesthesia and nursing in order to better understand current practices and offer suggestions and changes that will catalyze rapid recovery.

SURGICAL APPROACH

The idea of outpatient TKA was only entertained after the development of less-invasive surgical approaches to the knee. Patients recovered much more quickly due to the diminished soft-tissue trauma afforded by these new approaches. TKA traditionally has been performed utilizing a medial parapatellar approach to the knee. In this approach, the quadriceps tendon is incised just lateral to the vastus medialis. The arthrotomy continues distally, curving around the patella and ending just medial to the tibial tubercle. The limited medial parapatellar arthrotomy simply reduces the length of the standard medial parapatellar approach and eliminates eversion of the patella. Alternative approaches have been developed in an attempt to spare the quadriceps tendon, reduce postoperative pain, and promote a quicker recovery. These techniques include the subvastus, midvastus, and quadriceps sparing techniques described by Berger et al.[23]

Berger was one of the first to describe outpatient TKA and only after he had developed his quadriceps sparing approach. In this technique the arthrotomy starts at the superior pole of the patella and follows the medial border of the patella distally to the joint line. The patella is not dislocated, and all bone cuts are performed *in situ*.[23] The subvastus approach follows the same orientation as the medial parapatellar approach distally, but instead of cutting into the quadriceps tendon, it instead curves medially along the medial border of the entire vastus medialis. The vastus medialis is then peeled off the medial intermuscular septum. The midvastus approach is similar, though the superior portion dissects through the intermuscular fibers of the vastus medialis. Again, the distal exposure is identical to the medial parapatellar approach. There is conflict among experts on the utility of these less-invasive approaches with some studies showing decreased postoperative pain and improved function and others showing no difference in outcomes.[24]

Perhaps more important than the type of arthrotomy that is used is the care taken to minimize soft-tissue trauma while simultaneously carefully protecting important structures. This is the only part of the outpatient pathway for which the surgeon is solely responsible, so care must be taken to ensure that the surgeon delivers his or her best product, yet moves through the case in an efficient and streamlined manner.

BLOOD MANAGEMENT

Controlling blood loss is another key challenge to outpatient TKA. Postoperative anemia will not only limit a patient's ability to mobilize and safely return home, but it can also be a frequent cause of emergency department visits or readmissions. A study by Lovecchio et al showed that of 492 outpatient TJA patients queried from the ACS-NSQIP database, 6.3% had postdischarge complications.[25] This was compared to 1476 fast-track (<2 day LOS) patients who had a 1.1% postdischarge complication rate. The study found that most of the postdischarge complications in the outpatient group were due to bleeding requiring transfusion, but this occurred at similar rates overall in the two groups.[25] These findings suggest the increased importance of careful blood management in outpatient TKA.

The first step in blood management is identifying patients who are at risk for postoperative anemia. The patient's preoperative hemoglobin level is one of the best predictors of postoperative hemoglobin level. If the preoperative hemoglobin level is less than 13 g/dL, the patient's risk of blood transfusion is four times higher.[26] Once identified preoperatively, a patient at risk for postoperative blood transfusion may either be diverted to an inpatient-based pathway or treated with iron and erythropoietin in an attempt to address their anemia.[27]

Hypotensive anesthesia techniques have been present for many years to minimize intraoperative blood loss and subsequent need for blood transfusions. These techniques attempt to keep the mean arterial pressure at or below 60 mmHg.[28] Again, this requires collaboration with anesthesiology providers to clearly define goals and expectations if such techniques are not already in use.

More recently, tranexamic acid (TXA) has been incorporated into clinical pathways to reduce the need for postoperative transfusions. TXA is a synthetic lysine antifibrinolytic that functions to reduce clot breakdown by limiting fibrin degradation.[29] TXA has been shown in numerous studies to reduce the need for blood transfusions without increasing the risk of venous thromboembolism.[29-31] It is available in IV, topical, and oral routes, all of which have been shown to significantly reduce postoperative anemia.[30,31] IV administration of TXA is typically dosed with 1 g prior to incision and a second 1 g dose given at closure or in the recovery room. For topical application, 2 to 3 g of TXA is mixed with 50 to 100 mL of saline and applied during wound closure. The advent of TXA, along with other blood management strategies, has certainly helped to make outpatient TKA a safe and successful reality.

POSTOPERATIVE CARE

Once the patient arrives in the postanesthesia recovery unit, the recovery room nursing staff and physical therapists become the next critical component for successful outpatient TKA. At this point, the preemptive multimodal pain protocol employed throughout the perioperative period should have minimized the need for postoperative narcotics and curtailed the side effects of sedation and nausea. The goal now is for the patient to awaken promptly from anesthesia and be ready to participate in physical therapy.

Epidural catheters, if used, are pulled 1 to 4 hours postop, and Foley catheters, if needed, are removed at 2 hours. Oral and IV multimodal pain medications are administered according to the prescribed regimen. Physical therapy is initiated once the patient is alert and oriented, usually within a few hours after surgery. To discharge home, just as in inpatient stays, therapists ensure that patients meet certain criteria. These usually include demonstrating the ability to independently move from a supine to standing position and likewise return from a standing to a supine position, and being able to independently transfer to and from a chair and to a standing position. After these initial criteria are met, patients may be expected to ambulate approximately 100 feet as well as ascend and descend a limited set of stairs. Other standard discharge criteria are frequently used, including stable vital signs and ability to tolerate a regular diet. Prior to discharge, the staff again ensures that the patient has adequate pain control on oral medications to minimize readmission for pain control issues.

It is imperative that arrangements be made prior to surgery to ensure the patient has support at home along with a plan for postoperative therapy and monitoring of any early complications. Discharge instructions are clearly discussed between the nurse, therapist, patient, and caregiver prior to discharge and all questions are thoroughly answered. The patient and caregiver should also be sent home with plenty of written instructions to make the transition home as seamless as possible. Therapy regimens vary with some patients receiving in-home therapy sessions for the first week to reduce travel and others immediately starting outpatient therapy. In a study by Warren et al, outpatient therapy protocols alone were compared with home health protocols followed by outpatient therapy in a group of patients who underwent TKA.[32] They found that there was no difference in Knee Osteoarthritis and Outcome Score (KOOS), 6-minute walk test, or knee ROM between the two groups at 2 months. They did find, however, that those who received outpatient therapy alone completed therapy on average 20 days sooner, and that they underwent just as many therapy sessions as the group who had home health first.[32] These findings would suggest that home health initially does not provide any added benefit versus simply starting outpatient therapy upon discharge. This is certainly an important finding, given the added cost of a home health regimen.

It is important that the patient and any caregiver be given explicit instructions on monitoring for signs of surgical site infection, deep vein thrombosis, and other common early complications. It is the authors' preference to close TKA incisions with a running subcuticular stitch and occlusive skin glue to minimize wound drainage. Dressings are left in place for 2 days and then the incision can be open to air. If persistent wound drainage occurs, then patients need to return promptly to the office for evaluation. Patients should also be instructed on the tenets of proper pain control, with an eye toward minimizing narcotic consumption. Other methods for early surveillance are to have a clinic nurse, mid-level provider, or the surgeon himself call the patient on postoperative day 1 or every few days to follow the patient's progress. If there are any concerns or problems, these should be addressed in detail either over the phone or in the office as appropriate.

OUTCOMES

Studies looking at the success of outpatient TKA are numerous. Berger first described his outcomes of outpatient TKA in a group of 50 selected patients.[23] Strict exclusion criteria were followed including history within 1 year of myocardial infarction, pulmonary embolism, or any anticoagulation therapy. Additionally, patients with a BMI >40 kg/m^2 or more than three medical comorbidities were excluded from the outpatient pathway. All included patients had their surgery done as the first TKA of the day. Of the 50 patients, 96% were able to discharge home the same day. There were three readmissions. One patient was readmitted 8 days after surgery for gastric bleeding, one at 21 days for subcutaneous infection, and one at 9 weeks for a manipulation under anesthesia.[23]

Berger had a follow-up study in 2006 with the addition of 50 more patients with the same selection criteria. None of these patients required overnight stay, bringing the success of same-day discharge of these selected 100 patients to 98%.[33]

Given the success of selected patients, Berger examined the feasibility of outpatient arthroplasty in an unselected group of patients.[34] This study included both total and unicondylar knee arthroplasties with the only exclusion criteria being surgery after 12:00 pm. In this study, 104 of 111 patients (94%) were discharged home on the day of surgery. In the first 3 months after surgery, there were a total of eight patients (7.2%) readmitted, all of whom had had a TKA. Of importance for selection criteria, they found no differences in patients who required an overnight stay and those treated as an outpatient with regard to average age, body weight, BMI, or medical comorbidities.

In a more recent study by Springer et al, patients who underwent outpatient TJA were retrospectively compared with those who underwent inpatient TJA with regard to 30-day complications, including all unplanned care episodes (readmissions, ED/urgent care visits, etc.).[35] A total of 137 patients who underwent outpatient TJA were reviewed and compared with 148 patients who underwent inpatient TJA. It was found that the outpatient group had an 11.7% rate of unplanned care episodes within 30 days compared with 6.6% in the inpatient group. Of note, these rates did not reach statistical significance ($p = .18$).[35]

In a systematic review of the literature, Pollock et al found 17 articles that compared readmission and complication rates among outpatient TKA patients.[4] They found that there was no difference in readmission and complication rates among outpatient and inpatient groups in each of these studies. Additionally, they found that studies assessing satisfaction reported a high level of satisfaction for the majority of patients. It would appear from these studies that outpatient TKA can be performed safely and effectively given the appropriate clinical pathways.[4]

Multiple studies have also reported on the financial advantages of outpatient arthroplasty.[36-39] One study conducted a detailed cost analysis between inpatient and outpatient TKAs and found that outpatient TKAs yielded a median cost savings of approximately 30%.[38] They reported no return to hospital or readmission encounters in this small group. By avoiding costly inpatient facility fees, a high volume procedure such as TKA has the potential to save the healthcare industry a significant amount when extrapolated on a larger scale.

The authors of this chapter have extensive experience in outpatient TKA. Between June 2013 and December 2017, 4744 patients underwent 6000 hip and knee arthroplasty procedures performed by authors at an ambulatory surgery center, including 2237 primary total knee arthroplasties in 1754 patients. Forty-two percent of patients were males (741) and 58% were females (1013). Mean age was 59.0 years (SD 6.1, range 25-87) and mean BMI was 35.0 kg/m² (SD 7.6, range 17-66). Of the 2237 primary TKA procedures, patients in 2054 (92%) went home the same day while 9 (0.4%) were transferred to an acute facility, and 174 (7.8%) required an overnight stay, with 47 of those staying for convenience related to travel distance or later operative time. Of the 118 patients who stayed overnight for a medical reason or 9 patients transferred, the most common reasons were respiratory issues, nausea/vomiting, undiagnosed obstructive sleep apnea, or inability to void.

Twenty-six (1.2%) patients, including the 9 patients transferred, suffered a major complication within 48 hours; 31 (1.4%) patients had an unplanned care episode between 48 hours and 90 days postoperatively; 21 (0.9%) patients suffered a surgical complication requiring operative intervention within 90 days; and 226 (10.1%) patients required a manipulation within 90 days postoperatively. These results prove that outpatient TKA can be performed safely and efficiently with at least 92% of patients successfully discharging on the day of surgery.

CONCLUSION

Outpatient TKA has been successfully implemented and is growing rapidly among many centers around the world. The transition to an outpatient arthroplasty center requires a change in the culture and vision of the perioperative staff. Any facility can foster this change. Patient expectations are established early, and the patient is given consistent education throughout the perioperative journey. The surgeon must exercise mindful patient selection in close collaboration with the consulting medical assessment and anesthesiology teams. Multimodal pain management regimens have revolutionized rapid recovery in TKA and truly made outpatient surgery a reality. As clinical pathway techniques continue to improve and evolve, the outreach of outpatient TKA will grow and expand across centers throughout the world.

REFERENCES

1. Lombardi AV Jr, Barrington JW, Berend KR, et al. Outpatient arthroplasty is here now. *Instr Course Lect.* 2016;65:531-546.
2. Crawford DA, Berend KR, Lombardi AV Jr. Techniques and eligibility for same day/next day discharge of TKA. In: Scott WN, ed. *Insall and Scott Surgery of the Knee.* 6th ed. Philadelphia: Elsevier; 2018:2001-2006, chap 184.
3. Meding JB, Klay M, Healy A, Ritter MA, Keating EM, Berend ME. The prescreening history and physical in elective total joint arthroplasty. *J Arthroplasty.* 2007;22(6 suppl 2):21-23.
4. Pollock M, Somerville L, Firth A, Lanting B. Outpatient total hip arthroplasty, total knee arthroplasty, and unicompartmental knee arthroplasty: a systematic review of the literature. *JBJS Rev.* 2016;4(12). pii:01874474-201612000-00004.
5. Meneghini RM, Ziemba-Davis M, Ishmael MK, Kuzma AL, Caccavallo P. Safe selection of outpatient joint arthroplasty patients with medical risk stratification: the "Outpatient Arthroplasty Risk Assessment Score". *J Arthroplasty.* 2017;32(8):2325-2331.
6. Courtney PM, Rozell JC, Melnic CM, Lee GC. Who should not undergo short stay hip and knee arthroplasty? Risk factors associated with major medical complications following primary total joint arthroplasty. *J Arthroplasty.* 2015;30(9 suppl):1-4.
7. Courtney PM, Boniello AJ, Berger RA. Complications following outpatient total joint arthroplasty: an analysis of a national database. *J Arthroplasty.* 2017;32(5):1426-1430.
8. Dowsey M, Kilgour ML, Santamaria NM, Choong PFM. Clinical pathways in hip and knee arthroplasty: a prospective randomised controlled study. *Med J Aust.* 1999;170(2):59-62.
9. Berend K, Lombardi AV Jr, Mallory TH. Rapid recovery protocol for peri-operative care of total hip and total knee arthroplasty patients. *Surg Technol Int.* 2004;13:239-247.
10. Lombardi AV Jr, Berend KR, Adams JB. A rapid recovery program: early home and pain free. *Orthopedics.* 2010;33(9):656.
11. Lombardi AV Jr, Viacava AJ, Berend KR. Rapid recovery protocols and minimally invasive surgery help achieve high knee flexion. *Clin Orthop Relat Res.* 2006;452:117-122.
12. Lee A, Gin T. Educating patients about anaesthesia: effects of various modes on patient's knowledge, anxiety and satisfaction. *Curr Opin Anaesthesiol.* 2005;18(2):205-208.
13. Woolf CJ, Chong MS. Preemptive analgesia – treating postoperative pain by preventing the establishment of central sensitization. *Anesth Analg.* 1993;77:362-379.
14. Mallory TH, Lombardi AV Jr, Fada RA, Dodds KL, Adams JB. Pain management for joint arthroplasty: preemptive analgesia. *J Arthroplasty.* 2002;17(4 suppl 1):129-133.
15. Buvanendran A, Kroin JS, Della Valle CJ, Kari M, Moric M, Tuman KJ. Perioperative oral pregabalin reduces chronic pain after total knee arthroplasty: a prospective, randomized, controlled trial. *Anesth Analg.* 2010;110(1):199-207.
16. Hickman SR, Mathieson KM, Bradford LM, Garman CD, Gregg RW, Lukens DW. Randomized trial of oral versus intravenous acetaminophen for postoperative pain control. *Am J Health Syst Pharm.* 2018;75(6):367-375.
17. Mallory TH, Lombardi AV Jr, Fada RA, Dodds KL. Anesthesia options: choices and caveats. *Orthopedics.* 2000;23(9):919-920.
18. Williams-Russo P, Sharrock NE, Haas SB, et al. Randomized trial of epidural versus general anesthesia; outcome after primary total knee replacement. *Clin Orthop Relat Res.* 1996;331:199-208.
19. Fowler SJ, Symons J, Sabato S, Myles PS. Epidural analgesia compared with peripheral nerve blockade after major knee surgery: a systematic review and meta-analysis of randomized trials. *Br J Anaesth.* 2008;100(2):154-164.
20. Jaeger P, Nielsen ZJ, Henningsen MH, Hilsted KL, Mathiesen O, Dahl JB. Adductor canal block versus femoral nerve block and quadriceps strength: a randomized, double-blind, placebo-controlled, crossover study in healthy volunteers. *Anesthesiology.* 2013;118(2):409-415.
21. Sankineani SR, Reddy ARC, Eachempati KK, Jangale A, Gurava Reddy AV. Comparison of adductor canal block and IPACK block (interspace between the popliteal artery and the capsule of the posterior knee) with adductor canal block alone after total knee arthroplasty: a prospective control trial on pain and knee function in immediate postoperative period. *Eur J Orthop Surg Traumatol.* 2018;28(7):1391-1395.

22. Lombardi AV Jr, Berend KR, Mallory TH, Dodds KL, Adams JB. Soft tissue and intra-articular injection of bupivacaine, epinephrine, and morphine has a beneficial effect after total knee arthroplasty. *Clin Orthop Relat Res.* 2004;428:125-130.

23. Berger RA, Sanders S, Gerlinger T, Della Valle C, Jacobs JJ, Rosenberg AG. Outpatient total knee arthroplasty with a minimally invasive technique. *J Arthroplasty.* 2005;20(7 suppl 3):33-38.

24. Liu HW, Gu WD, Xu NW, Sun JY. Surgical approaches in total knee arthroplasty: a meta-analysis comparing the midvastus and subvastus to the medial peripatellar approach. *J Arthroplasty.* 2014;29(12):2298-2304.

25. Lovecchio F, Alvi H, Sahota S, Beal M, Manning D. Is outpatient arthroplasty as safe as fast-track inpatient arthroplasty? A propensity score matched analysis. *J Arthroplasty.* 2016;31(9 suppl):197-201.

26. Salido J, Marín LA, Gómez LA, Zorrilla P, Martínez C. Preoperative hemoglobin levels and the need for transfusion after prosthetic hip and knee surgery: analysis of predictive factors. *J Bone Joint Surg Am.* 2002;84-A(2):216-220.

27. Spahn DR. Anemia and patient blood management in hip and knee surgery: a systematic review of the literature. *Anesthesiology.* 2010;113(2):482-495.

28. Eroglu A, Uzunlar H, Erciyes N. Comparison of hypotensive epidural anesthesia and hypotensive total intravenous anesthesia on intraoperative blood loss during total hip replacement. *J Clin Anesth.* 2005;17(6):420-425.

29. Duncan CM, Gillette BP, Jacob AK, Sierra RJ, Sanchez-Sotelo J, Smith HM. Venous thromboembolism and mortality associated with tranexamic acid use during total hip and knee arthroplasty. *J Arthroplasty.* 2015;30(2):272-276.

30. Gilbody J, Dhotar HS, Perruccio AV, Davey JR. Topical tranexamic acid reduces transfusion rates in total hip and knee arthroplasty. *J Arthroplasty.* 2014;29(4):681-684.

31. Han X, Gong G, Han N, Liu M. Efficacy and safety of oral compared with intravenous tranexamic acid in reducing blood loss after primary total knee and hip arthroplasty: a meta-analysis. *BMC Musculoskelet Disord.* 2018;19(1):430.

32. Warren M, Kozik J, Cook J, Prefontaine P, Ganley K. A Comparative study to determine functional and clinical outcome differences between patients receiving outpatient direct physical therapy versus home physical therapy followed by outpatient physical therapy after total knee arthroplasty. *Orthop Nurs.* 2016;35(6):382-390.

33. Berger RA, Sanders S, D'Ambrogio E, et al. Minimally invasive quadriceps-sparing TKA: results of a comprehensive pathway for outpatient TKA. *J Knee Surg.* 2006;19(2):145-148.

34. Berger RA, Kusuma SK, Sanders SA, Thill ES, Sporer SM. The feasibility and perioperative complications of outpatient knee arthroplasty. *Clin Orthop Relat Res.* 2009;467(6):1443-1449.

35. Springer BD, Odum SM, Vegari DN, Mokris JG, Beaver WB Jr. Impact of inpatient versus outpatient total joint arthroplasty on 30-day hospital readmission rates and unplanned episodes of care. *Orthop Clin North Am.* 2017;48(1):15-23.

36. Aynardi M, Post Z, Ong A, Orozco F, Sukin DC. Outpatient surgery as a means of cost reduction in total hip arthroplasty: a case-control study. *HSS J.* 2014;10(3):252-255.

37. Bertin KC. Minimally invasive outpatient total hip arthroplasty. *Clin Orthop Relat Res.* 2005;435:154-163.

38. Huang A, Ryu JJ, Dervin G. Cost savings of outpatient versus standard inpatient total knee arthroplasty. *Can J Surg.* 2017;60(1):57-62.

39. Richter DL, Diduch DR. Cost comparison of outpatient versus inpatient unicompartmental knee arthroplasty. *Orthop J Sports Med.* 2017;5(3):2325967117694352.

Complications of Total Knee Replacement

BRETT R. LEVINE

HANY S. BEDAIR

chapter 53

Intraoperative Complications During Total Knee Arthroplasty

David W. Fitz, MD | Brett Mulawka, MD | Christopher M. Melnic, MD

INTRODUCTION

Total knee arthroplasty (TKA) is a highly successful and cost-effective operation.[1,2] Registry data consistently report excellent 10-year survival rates, with 96% in the Swedish Arthroplasty Registry and 94% in the Australian registrar.[3] Patient satisfaction is also high, typically reported as >80% having good or excellent outcomes.[4-6] Such success, in part, has driven the annual incidence of TKA to increase in developed countries.[7] In the United States, the demand for TKA is projected to rise by 673% to 3.48 million by 2030 and in revision TKA by 601%.[8] Additionally, this increase in demand is expected to be driven by patients aged <65 years.[8] Coupled with an aging population, increasing obesity, and the importance of maintaining an active lifestyle, the rise in failed TKAs is inevitable and the burden of revision TKAs will increase.

Compared with primary TKA, revision procedures are more technically demanding and have a higher risk of complications. Extensive scarring can complicate exposure and extensile approaches may be indicated. Local anatomy may be altered and delineation of important structures can be difficult. Component removal, if indicated, must be done with care as to minimize bone loss and fracture. The removal of cement should be done meticulously, as well, to avoid maligning the new implants, creating bone defects and preventing fractures (both on cement removal and implant insertion). Osteolysis and stress shielding can be encountered in the revision setting which can exacerbate the risk of fracture or avulsion of important structures. Stemmed components may be indicated and can lead to iatrogenic fracture.

To minimize complications, a thorough knowledge of anatomy and appropriate surgical technique is essential. Not only does it allow for effective surgical planning, but enables the surgeon to be proactive and anticipate potential complications before they occur. In this chapter, potential intraoperative complications will be described as well as the management and methods to avoid encountering them in the first place.

INTRAOPERATIVE FRACTURE

While intraoperative fractures during primary TKA are well reported in the literature, thankfully they are rare, with an incidence of less than 1%.[9-12] During revision surgery, like all other complications, the risk increases, with a reported incidence of 3%.[13-15] Knee periprosthetic fractures, postoperative and intraoperative, are associated with high morbidity and mortality, with mortality rates as high as 17% at 6 months and 30% at 1 year.[16,17] Although rare compared to other complications, they are a challenging problem and can lead to significant morbidity and expense. Periprosthetic fractures and infections are associated with the greatest length of stay and cost for revision TKA.[18]

Various classification systems have been devised to describe and guide treatment of periprosthetic TKA fractures. In general, these systems focus on a specific anatomic region: distal femur, proximal tibia, and patella. Depending on the system, further details are included such as fracture pattern, chronology, bone quality, treatment recommendations, and outcomes. Currently, the most widely used and cited systems are those described by Lewis and Rorabeck for distal femur fractures, by Felix for tibial fractures, and by Ortiguera and Berry for patella fractures.[19-24] These will be described in detail in the upcoming sections.

In an attempt to standardize and modernize periprosthetic fracture management, the Arbeitsgemeinschaft für Osteosynthesefragen, AO, Foundation developed a comprehensive classification system for all periprosthetic fractures, the United Classification System (UCS).[25] The UCS is based on the established Vancouver classification of proximal femur periprosthetic fractures and utilizes the core principles of fracture location, component fixation, and bone stock.[26] The UCS has been validated and has substantial inter- and intraobserver reliability for periprosthetic fractures associated with TKA.[27,28] **Table 53-1** summarizes this approach.

With either primary or revision TKA, fractures can occur at any point during the procedure, from initial exposure to final implantation, and in either the femur, tibia, patella, or combination of all three. Risk factors for periprosthetic fractures include those both patient- and procedure- related. Patient-related risk factors involve conditions that result in osteopenia, including rheumatoid arthritis, advanced age, female gender, malnutrition, osteoporosis, neuromuscular disorders, dementia, and chronic corticosteroid use.[29-33] Procedure-related risk factors include component removal, intramedullary

TABLE 53-1   Unified Classification System for Periprosthetic Fractures: Knee

		V Knee		
		V.3 **Distal Femur**	**V.4** **Proximal Tibia**	**V.34** **Patella**
A *Apophyseal* or extra-articular/ periarticular	A1	Lateral epicondyle	Medial or lateral plateau, nondisplaced	Disrupted extensor mechanism, proximal pole
	A2	Medial epicondyle	Tibial tubercle	Disrupted extensor mechanism, distal pole
B *Bed* of the implant or around the implant	B1	Proximal to stable component, good bone	Stem and component stable, good bone	Intact extensor mechanism, implant stable, good bone
	B2	Proximal to loose component, good bone	Loose stem/component, good bone	Loose implant, good bone
	B3	Proximal to loose component, poor bone/defect	Loose stem/component, poor bone/defect	Loose implant, poor bone
C *Clear* or distal to the implant	–	Proximal to the implant and cement mantle	Distal to the implant and cement mantle	–
D *Dividing* the bone between two implants or interprosthetic or intercalary	–	Between hip and knee arthroplasties, close to knee	Between ankle and knee arthroplasties, close to knee	–
E *Each* of two bones supporting one arthroplasty or polyperiprosthetic	–	Femur and tibia/patella		
F *Facing* and articulating with a hemiarthroplasty	–	Fracture of the femoral condyle articulating with tibial hemiarthroplasty	–	Fracture of the patella that has no surface replacement and articulates with the femoral component of the total knee arthroplasty (TKA)

instrumentation, central box preparation, and trialing of components.[9,13-15] Understanding and anticipating these risk factors is critical to success and avoiding intraoperative complications.

INTRAOPERATIVE FRACTURE: FEMUR

In both the primary and revision setting, fractures of the femur are the most common, with the medial femoral condyle being the most common femoral location.[9,13] Fractures, however, have been reported in the cortices of the diaphysis, lateral condyle, medial and lateral epicondyle, as well as the supracondylar area. Like all periprosthetic fractures, osteopenic bone, whether from a systemic condition, medication, osteolysis, or iatrogenic weakening, will increase the risk of an intraoperative fracture.

CLASSIFICATION

Lewis and Rorabeck developed the first widely used classification scheme, accounting for both the integrity of the prosthesis and the location of the fracture.[20] Type I fractures are nondisplaced with a stable prosthesis. Type II fractures have a displaced fracture but a stable prosthesis. Type III

fractures are those with a radiographically or clinically loose prosthesis regardless of the fracture displacement.

Anatomy

A thorough understanding of the femoral anatomy is essential for a successful revision TKA. Native anatomic differences in the diaphysis and metaphysis must be assessed as well as alterations to these areas from the prior surgeries. Extra-articular deformity from prior fractures may alter the geometry of the femoral canal. Cortical thickness can be attenuated in osteopenic bone, and surgeons should take extra care when instrumenting the canal. Hardware and/or cement from previous surgeries should be noted preoperatively and planned for accordingly. If removal is necessitated, the surgeon should address potential stress risers from explanted hardware.

The femoral diaphysis has an anterior bow, and femoral morphology can vary greatly between different races and genders, with increased bowing seen in Asians and females.[34,35] There is a risk for fracture or cortical perforation with canal preparation or insertion of diaphyseal-engaging stems. Iatrogenic changes to the femoral diaphysis can also increase the risk of fracture, in particular femoral notching. In both biomechanical and clinical studies, anterior notching has been documented to compromise the strength for the distal femur and contribute to periprosthetic fractures.[29,36-39] Anterior notching of as little as 3 mm can decrease the mean torsional strength of the distal femur by 29% to 39% and bending strength decreased 18% with full-thickness notching.[37,38] Notching, however, may not always predispose to fracture. Ritter et al reviewed 670 primary TKAs and observed notching ≥3 mm in 138 (20.5%) of cases, but only 2 (0.3%) developed a supracondylar femur fracture.[36] Osseous remodeling over time may protect against fracture with the risk following notching to be minimized by 6 months postoperatively.[36] Nevertheless, the surgeon should avoid notching, especially the anterior-medial cortex, to prevent excessive stress in the distal femur.[40] The surgeon should be aware of preoperative notching or intraoperative notching and bypass accordingly with stems if encountered.

Metaphyseal anatomy must also be considered in revision TKA. Individuals of small stature and females can have a narrow distal femur. Revision femoral components often have a wider and deeper box cut than primary posterior-stabilized components. With a smaller medial–lateral dimension of the distal femur, the cut is proportionally larger and deeper. The bridge of bone between the proximal corner of the box and the metaphyseal flare can significantly narrow, especially medially. Additionally, positioning the cutting guide too far medial or lateral can further exacerbate this problem. Even with precise surgical technique, box preparation can potentially result in a femoral condyle fracture.

Prevention

Risk of intraoperative fracture can be minimized through proper preoperative planning and evaluation. Prior incisions should be documented and the soft-tissue envelope assessed. As the blood supply to the skin on the anterior knee is predominantly from medial vessels, the most lateral incision should be chosen. Radiographs should include weight-bearing AP, lateral, and merchant views. The anterior bow of the femur is best visualized on the lateral view and should be utilized for stemmed components. Whole-femur views from the hip to knee should be available as well to assess cortical thickness, extra-articular deformity, and previous hardware. Bone loss and osteolysis can be visualized on radiographs, yet are typically underestimated and underappreciated. The surgeon should have a low threshold to obtain a computed tomography (CT) scan to further delineate the extent and severity of bone loss.

Various steps carry an increased risk for intraoperative fracture during a TKA, and the surgeon should be vigilant at these times to prevent this complication. Fractures have been reported to occur during exposure, component removal, instrumentation, and trialing.[13,14] Extensile exposures, which are described in detail in a separate chapter, may be needed to safely expose the knee. During removal of implants, a small oscillating saw or flexible osteotome should be used to carefully disengage the component from the native bone with a goal of minimizing bone loss. If cement remains, this too should be carefully removed, respecting the remaining bone. Residual cement in the femoral canal can deviate intramedullary instrumentation, such as drill bits or reamers, and lead to canal perforation. Preexisting deformity, reactive bone formation, or prior hardware can have a similar effect. Trialing of components should be done carefully in the revision setting, especially if significant bone loss is encountered. A flexion–extension gap mismatch can potentiate an epicondylar avulsion fracture if the knee is brought into extension with a tight extension gap or vice versa. Impaction of trial or final components can cause a fracture as impaction force is critical. If difficulty is encountered during insertion, impaction force should not be increased. Rather, the surgeon should reassess and ensure the distal femur can accommodate the component. There should be a low threshold for obtaining an intraoperative radiograph to assess fit and position, especially if diaphyseal-engaging stems are used.

Stemmed implants have become a mainstay in revision TKA to augment prosthetic stability if metaphyseal bone is compromised. Biomechanical studies have shown that stems increase the mechanical stability by transferring load over a larger area, reducing strain at the bone–component interface.[41-43] Both cemented and cementless stem options are available. Cementless, or press-fit, stems must be compatible with the dimensions of the patient's diaphysis as mismatch can lead to a fracture. Diaphyseal-engaging stems tend to be longer, generally ≥75 mm in length. Slotted, or "clothes-pin," stems decrease stress at the end of the stem tip.[44,45] Slotted stems also are more forgiving in a highly bowed femur. The stem should be inserted so that the axis of the slot parallels the bow of the femur. Longer stems (≥150 mm) are available with bows to match the natural bow of the femur.

Management

The goals of managing an intraoperative fracture are similar to those of managing any fracture: achieve anatomic reduction with rigid internal fixation that affords early range of motion activities. Intraoperative fractures should be addressed upon identification and if in question radiographs should be obtained during the procedure to identify the fracture. Exposure often needs to be extended to adequately visualize the fracture and for fixation. Excessive soft-tissue stripping, however, should be avoided to not devascularize the fracture fragments and optimize the possibility of union.

Various fixation strategies exist for managing periprosthetic femur fractures that can be employed for intraoperative fractures. These include condylar blade plates, locking and nonlocking plates, interfragmentary lag screws, or intramedullary fixation. Retrograde intramedullary nails are a viable solution for periprosthetic diaphyseal femur fractures, but do require an open box design. In a revision TKA, this is rarely an option given the use of stemmed components and closed box.

Condylar blade plates historically were the mainstay treatment for periprosthetic femur fractures,[31,46,47] but their use has diminished with the advent of modern plating systems (locked and nonlocked). Rigid distal fixation was unpredictable with blades, especially in osteoporotic bone and distal fracture patterns. Significant failure rates, upwards of 80%, were reported in osteoporotic bone and comminuted fractures.[48] Attempts to enhance fixation were attempted and included various allograft solutions and polymethylmethacrylate.[46,47,49] Currently, its use should be reserved for minimally comminuted, displaced fractures in patients with good bone stock.[30]

Modern plating systems employ locking screw technology to create rigid fixed-angle constructs and have become the mainstay of treatment for periprosthetic femur fractures (**Fig. 53-1**). In most plating systems, strategically placed screws have the option to be rigidly secured to the plate at a fixed angle, similar to the condylar blade. The use of multiple fixed-angle screws in the distal segment increases fixation and stability.[50] Toggle of the screw at its interface with the plate is prevented, providing a rigid internal scaffold for the fragments. Locking plates also afford the benefit of including unicortical locking screws. A large intercondylar box or femoral diaphyseal stem can preclude the ability to use bicortical fixation, but a unicortical locking screw can still provide support. Some plating systems have also incorporated polyaxial screw options, incorporating screw angulation

with locking technology. Screws can be inserted in a 15-degree cone around a central axis and still lock into the plate, allowing the surgeon more options to gain fixation into optimal bone and around the prosthesis.[51] Other plate designs accommodate cables, which can be useful in the diaphyseal segment if stemmed components are in place or an ipsilateral total hip arthroplasty is present. Favorable results have been reported with locking plates with a recent systematic review reporting 87% union rates.[52] There are potential disadvantages to locking plates including nonunion/malunion, hardware failure, and infection, but the reported complication rate is lower than other fixation methods.[52]

Bypassing a distal femur fracture with a longer diaphyseal-engaging stem, is a possible treatment option and is supported in the literature.[19,32,53,54] The stem should bypass the fracture by at least two cortical diameters. Cables can be used for additional fixation if significant deformity is present.

Condyle fractures are the most common intraoperative femur fracture encountered during revision surgery.[13,14] For these as well as epicondylar fractures, interfragmentary lag screw fixation may be acceptable in non- and minimally displaced fractures.[54] A diaphyseal-engaging stem is indicated in comminuted and displaced fractures to off-load forces at the fracture.[54] Washers can be used in cases of poor bone quality. In condylar fractures, a buttress plate can be added to resist shear forces.

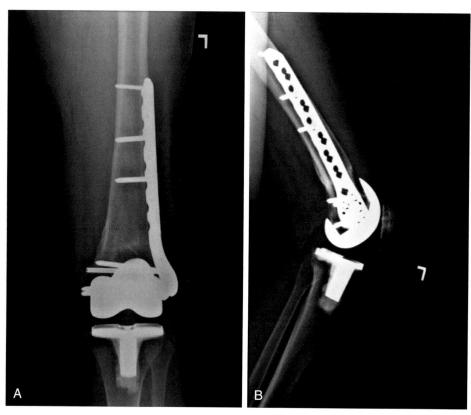

FIGURE 53-1 AP (**A**) and lateral (**B**) radiographs 1 year following a revision arthroplasty. A lateral locking plate was employed for fracture fixation.

Bone grafting may be considered to augment healing. Healy et al reported improved union rates with addition of bone graft (autogenous iliac crest or femoral head allograft).[46] Cement should be used judiciously around the fracture, limited to being placed at or proximal to the fracture line, so as to avoid interference with bone healing.

Postoperatively, weight-bearing and range of motion should be dictated by fixation. If rigid fixation is achieved, range of motion should be started immediately to prevent stiffness. Protected weight-bearing should be considered for 4 to 6 weeks when an intraoperative distal femur fracture is encountered. In a review of intraoperative fractures during aseptic revision TKA, Sassoon et al reported weight-bearing limitations in 22% of patients.[13]

INTRAOPERATIVE FRACTURE: TIBIA

Compared to periprosthetic femur fractures, periprosthetic tibia fractures are rare in both the primary and revision setting.[9,13,14] With diaphyseal-engaging press-fit stems, however, tibial fractures are more common than femur fractures.[15] Like femoral fractures, the risk is increased in the revision setting. Felix et al reported over a five times greater risk during revision surgery.[21] Intraoperative tibia fractures can occur throughout the bone with fractures reported in the medial and lateral tibial plateaus as well as the anterior, posterior, medial, and lateral cortices of the diaphysis.[9,13-15] Patient-related risk factors for tibia fractures are similar to those of femoral fractures and include anything that weakens the bone. In the revision setting, this includes osteolysis and stress shielding.

Classification

Felix, Stuart, and Hanssen's Mayo classification for periprosthetic tibial fractures is the most commonly used system.[21] It characterizes fractures based upon three characteristics: anatomic location, implant stability, and timing. Type I fractures are at the level of the tibial plateau and involve the implant baseplate–bone interface. Type II fractures are more distal at the diaphyseal–metaphyseal junction and involve the implant stem–bone interface. Type III fractures occur distal to the tibial stem or keel. Type IV fractures involve the tibial tubercle. These fractures are further subclassified whether the implant is radiographically stable (subclass A) or loose (subclass B) and whether the fracture occurred intraoperatively (subclass C).

Anatomy

Like the femur, understanding the anatomy of the tibia is essential for successful revision surgery. Whether from prior surgery, trauma, or anatomic variance, metaphyseal–diaphyseal distortion is of particular importance,

especially if intramedullary instrumentation and stem components are to be used. Offset trays or stems may be indicated if there is significant distortion. Attention should also be paid to cortical thickness as this can be attenuated in osteopenic bone and press-fit stems can cause iatrogenic type IIC fractures.[15] Prior hardware can create stress risers, and the surgeon should be prepared to address such challenges.

Prevention

Careful preoperative planning and surgical technique can minimize intraoperative complications. Extensile exposures, including a tibial tubercle osteotomy, may be needed. Preoperative weight-bearing radiographs should be obtained and the entire tibia should be visualized.

Like femoral fractures, tibial fractures can occur at any step throughout the procedure from exposure to component impaction, but typically occur with retractor placement, medullary preparation, stem and component insertion, or from torsional stress placed on the leg.[9,15,22] Retractors should be placed by the surgeon with care and ideally under direct visualization. Blind or careless retractor placement can create a divot in the tibial metaphysis, especially in osteopenic bone. To improve visualization of the tibia, the deep medial collateral ligament (MCL), semimembranosus, and posterior capsule can be sequentially released subperiosteally to the posteromedial tibia. This will allow the tibia to hyperflex and externally rotate and provide complete access to the medial aspect of the tibia.

The tibial component must be removed judiciously and completely. A combination of oscillating or reciprocating saws and flexible osteotomes can be used. Premature attempts at removal of the tibial component can create unnecessary bone loss or create iatrogenic fractures of the tibia and femur. Adequate clearance of the distal femur must be ensured before the tibial component is removed. Removal of the distal femoral component prior to the tibia can also aid in visualization and increase working room.

Cement removal can also lead to fractures, usually type IC or IIC.[21] Cement should be removed in a piecemeal fashion instead of en-block. Proximal cement can be mosaicized with an osteotome or high-speed burr for careful removal. After fracture with an osteotome, the cement fragments should be levered toward the canal to avoid perforation. Care should be taken while removing cement from the canal to avoid cortical perforation as well. A distal cement plug may be encountered and can be addressed by drilling through the plug. The plug can then be removed with a threaded T-handle or fractured with dedicated cement removal tools and removed piece-meal.

Like the femur, implant selection must be chosen with the patient's anatomy in mind. Long-stemmed components can create type IIC fractures during reaming and impaction.[15] Use of offset couplers can aid in addressing metaphyseal–diaphyseal distortion. The stem should fill the canal; however, as stem fill has been shown to be the strongest predictor of failure.[55] If either patient anatomy or bone stock precludes the use of an appropriate press-fit stem, a shorter, fully cemented stem can be considered. Excellent midterm results have been shown for both cementless and cemented stem revision TKA constructs.[56-61]

Management

Treatment of intraoperative tibial fractures is based on pattern and location with the Mayo classification guiding treatment. Type IC fractures are typically minimally displaced split or depression fractures of the tibial plateau. Often, these fractures can be stabilized with cancellous or cortical bone screws prior to final implant impaction or with longer stem to bypass the fracture.[21] Small contained defects, <5 mm, can be addressed with a cement or bone graft.[62] Modular augments, screw and cement fixation, or structural allograft can be used for larger defects.[63-68]

Type IIC fractures typically occur in conjunction with stems, either removal or insertion, and canal preparation.[15,22] Treatment can include a longer stem to bypass the fracture. If nondisplaced, they can be treated with protected weight-bearing and early motion.[15]

Type IIIC fractures occur distal to the stem, and treatment depends on displacement. If displaced, they require open reduction and internal fixation.[54] Locking plates with either unicortical or polyaxial locking screws may be beneficial in these settings, providing options for fixation around the tibial prosthesis proximally.[50] Nondisplaced fractures can be treated conservatively, with either non–weight-bearing or protected weight-bearing.[15,54]

Type IVC, which involve the tibial tubercle, are devastating complications and usually related to difficult exposure and osteoporotic bone. Techniques to minimize tension on the tubercle will be discussed in the next section. Repair with screw fixation can be attempted through the fragment, but residual displacement is common.[69]

INTRAOPERATIVE FRACTURE: PATELLA

Patellar fractures are the second most common periprosthetic fracture around the knee, with a reported incidence of 0.12% to 3.9%.[16] Intraoperatively, patella fractures are uncommon in either the primary or revision setting, although the risk is increased in revision TKA. Alden et al reported no intraoperative patella fractures in his review of 17,389 primary TKAs,[9] while Sassoon et al reported three patella fractures during 894 septic revisions and 5 during aseptic revisions.[13,14]

Classification

The most commonly cited classification system was described by Ortiguera and Berry.[24] Type I fractures have stable implants and an intact extensor mechanism. Type

II fractures cause a disruption of the extensor mechanism with or without a stable implant. Type III fractures have an intact extensor mechanism, but an unstable implant. Type III fractures are further subdivided based on bone stock. Type IIIa have reasonable bone stock. Type IIIb have poor bone stock defined by less than 10 mm thickness or severe comminution.

Anatomy

The patella is the largest sesamoid bone in the body and is embedded in the tendon of quadriceps femoris, lying anterior to the distal femur (femoral condyles). It is flat, distally tapered and proximally curved, and has anterior and articular surfaces, three borders and an apex, which is the distal end of the bone.[70]

The arterial supply of the patella is derived from the genicular anastomosis, particularly from the genicular branches of the popliteal artery and from the anterior tibial recurrent artery.[70] The patella has both an extraosseous and intraosseous blood supply. Following a typical medial parapatellar approach and total meniscectomy routinely performed in TKA, the superior genicular artery is the only remaining major vessel providing a significant blood supply to the patella.[71] Lateral retinacular release used to improve tracking may further compromise the blood supply and has been associated with increased risk of patellar fracture.[72,73]

Prevention

Patient and surgical factors can contribute to the intraoperative risk of patella fractures. Osteopenic bone, for any reason, can predispose to patella fracture. Iatrogenic fractures may start with the use or towel clips when holding the patella during bony preparation or resection. It is imperative when using this technique to not grab the proximal or distal poles with the towel clips and initiate a potential fracture. Fracture risk, however, is most associated with the mechanical strength of the patella. Patellar thickness <25 mm and postresection thickness <15 mm significantly increase the strain and fracture risk.[74] In primary setting, calipers should be used to measure the patella before preparation. During revision, component removal can create a significant reduction in thickness of the patella, leaving only a cortical shell. Additionally, the residual vascular supply may be damaged, contributing to further weakening.

Initial exposure should be adequate to reduce the strain on the extensor mechanism. With poor exposure, excessive force may be needed to evert or sublux the patella laterally. In an osteoporotic or osteolytic patella, retractor leverage may create a fracture. In the revision setting, the surgeon should decide whether revising the patella is necessary and whether revision can be done safely. If the patellar button is to be removed, the surgeon should employ similar care and technique as with the femur and tibia. Once resected, a trial component or protector can be used to disperse the force over a larger surface area.

Management

Intraoperative fractures are usually identified prior to final fixation. Once identified, adequate exposure should be ensured to both visualize and address the fracture. A quadriceps snip may be necessary to reduce stress on the extensor mechanism and prevent further injury. In management of an intraoperative fracture, continuity of the extensor mechanism takes priority over resurfacing. A vertical fracture is typically stable, providing the extensor mechanism is intact, and can be managed with observation. The transverse fracture, however, is problematic and needs to be addressed to restore extensor mechanism function. A tension-band construct is reliable method of fixation if possible.[71] If the fragments cannot be adequately reduced or the patella is severely comminuted, partial patellectomy with tendon advancement or total patellectomy may be necessary.[71,75] Following internal fixation, the ability of the patella to be resurfaced should be assessed. If adequate bone stock remains (>13 mm), the patella may be resurfaced at this time.[75,76] With compromised bone stock, resurfacing should not be undertaken. If the patient heals the fracture and becomes symptomatic, resurfacing at a later date can be considered with a biconvex patella component, patellar bone grafting, or porous metal implant.[77,78]

EXTENSOR MECHANISM INJURY

The true incidence of patellar tendon disruption has been reported between 0.1% and 3%[69,79,80] although it remains difficult to determine the true incidence of intraoperative patellar tendon injury. Sources of disruption can be associated with exposure, anatomic constraints, iatrogenic injury from saw blades, or during implantation or explantation of components. Risk factors, such as previous surgeries, preoperative contractures, and obesity should be considered. Patellar tendon injuries can occur as an avulsion from the tibial tubercle or distal pole of the patella. Midsubstance injuries to the patellar tendon may be caused by errant saw blade technique.

Quadriceps tendon rupture after TKA is noted to have a prevalence of 0.1%.[81] The incidence of rupture intraoperatively is unknown. Risk factors for intraoperative rupture include systemic disorders, excessive patella resection, and prior quadriceps snip or V-Y turndown.[80]

Anatomy

Extensor mechanism components consist of the quadriceps muscles, quadriceps tendon, patella, patellar tendon, retinaculum, and tibial tubercle. The blood supply, although originally circumferential from genicular arteries, is often disrupted from surgical approaches. The commonly used medial parapatellar arthrotomy disrupts the descending genicular, superior and inferior genicular arteries. Excision of the infrapatellar fat pad, meniscus, and lateral release can damage lateral genicular blood supply. The disrupted vascularity limits potential healing after injury.[82]

Prevention

Poor results with extensor mechanism injury (EMI) emphasize the importance in preventing these devastating injuries. Previous surgeries, such as previous arthroplasty, tibial tubercle osteotomy, or high tibial osteotomies, increase the complexity of the exposure and risk intraoperative damage to the extensor mechanism. Adhesions and scar tissue can make revision knee surgery challenging and increase risk to the extensor mechanism during exposure and implantation of components. Host factors, such as comorbidities, obesity, previous trauma, and preoperative contractures, must be taken into consideration to prevent damaging the extensor mechanism. Adequate releases and excision of previous scar tissue may help aid in exposure in the complicated TKA and revision knee arthroplasty.

Prophylactic fixation of the patellar tendon may prevent intraoperative disruption. Placement of a smooth 1/8 inch pin into the tibia tubercle may decrease chances of patellar tendon propagation and avulsion from the tubercle.[83] When the proximal extensor mechanism is withholding exposure, quadriceps snip may be performed with limited postoperative consequences.[84,85] This technique involves carrying the typical medial parapatellar arthrotomy across the quadriceps tendon proximally to increase exposure of the knee. Typically, repair is performed in the usual fashion and postoperative rehabilitation remains unchanged.[84]

Management

Treatment of intraoperative patellar tendon disruption can be categorized into repair, repair with augmentation, and reconstruction. Observation and acute fusion, though relevant in chronic extensor mechanism injuries, has no role in the acute complete disruption. Mechanism of injury, host factors, and available constructs must all be taken into consideration when deciding which method to pursue after intraoperative injury.

Direct primary repair may be performed with sutures, staples, or wires when adequate tissue is available. Being mindful during exposure to keep a healthy medial cuff of tissue during medial release may allow repairing the patellar tendon directly to the medial sleeve of tissue and augmenting with sutures anchors or staples. Though direct primary repair has shown successful results in native knees, literature regarding direct primary repair in the setting of TKA has not proven as effective.[69,86,87]

Courtney et al studied direct repair in 58 patients with patella tendon ruptures, 45% which were within 2 weeks of the index procedure. They noted a 26% reoperation rate and 33% with poor outcomes.[88]

When direct primary repair does not produce adequate fixation or strength, intraoperative augmentation of the repair should be considered. Augmentation with autograft, allograft, or synthetic grafts may be considered. Autograft hamstring tendon augmentation has been shown to produce a stronger repair than fascia or free grafts.[79,89,90] Leaving the semitendinosus attached to the proximal tibia, the proximal tendon is harvested. This can then be run up the medial side of the patellar tendon remnant and sutured side to side. The tendon can then be brought down the lateral aspect of the patellar tendon after anchoring to the inferior pole of the patella. One should be mindful to not overtighten the reconstruction and risk patella baja. Checking safe intraoperative range of motion can help with postoperative restrictions.[83]

Courtney et al report on their experience of direct patella tendon repairs versus augmentation of EMI. Complications rates were reported upwards of 63% and continued extensor lags of 30° were often present.[88] The distinction of outcomes between acute and chronic injuries was not delineated.

Complete ruptures of the quadriceps necessitate repair with or without augmentation. Surgical primary repair of the quadriceps tendon has had poor results, with 33% to 36% rerupture rates.[80,81,91] Augmentation with autografts, synthetic grafts, or allografts should be considered.[81]

COLLATERAL LIGAMENT INJURY

TKA coronal balance and stability relies on MCL integrity. Revision for instability is often due to poor function of this important structure. Intraoperative injury to the MCL is reported in the literature between 0.5% and 8%.[92-94] This is generally noted to be an iatrogenic intraoperative complication.

Anatomy

The MCL is composed of the deep and superficial layers. It is the largest structure on the medial side of the knee.[95] The superficial MCL has one femoral and two tibial attachments. The femoral insertion is located approximately 3.2 mm proximal and 4.8 mm posterior to the medial epicondyle.[95] Distally, the superficial MCL attaches at two points. The proximal site is not a direct attachment to bone, but instead to soft tissue. The distal attachment site is broad and located just anterior to the posteromedial tibial crest. The deep MCL is a thickening of the joint capsule and runs mostly parallel to the superficial MCL. It is composed of the meniscofemoral and meniscotibial ligaments.[95]

Prevention

The MCL is vulnerable during medial capsule release, resection of the medial meniscus, distal and posterior femoral cuts, and the medial tibia cut.[83] Careful protection of the MCL during these surgical steps is of utmost importance to prevent iatrogenic injury. Subluxation of the tibia during exposure can also cause avulsion-type injuries to the MCL. Challenging anatomical variances and obesity may increase the risk.

Management

Currently, no consensus on how to manage intraoperative MCL injuries has been reached. Primary repair with or without postoperative bracing, repair with augmentation, and increasing component constraint are reported in the literature.

Numerous authors have described primary repair with postoperative bracing and had successful results up to 4 years out from surgery.[92,93] Postoperative stiffness was a common complication of this technique. Primary repair may be done with sutures, anchors, or transosseous tunnels. The decision is dependent upon the quality of tissue and location of the injury. Primary end-to-end repair for midsubstance injury can be performed while utilizing a trial spacer that is smaller than the final polyethylene by approximately 2 mm. This will allow for tensioning of the MCL repair after insertion of the final polyethylene.[83] A running, locking, nonabsorbable, and braided suture is recommended.[96] For avulsion of the MCL, two running and locking sutures are utilized from the damaged end of the tendon and back to create four free ends. The free ends are then anchored to bone utilizing suture anchors, bone tunnels, or screw with washers. Tensioning in midflexion is recommended.[96] When quality primary repair is not achievable, augmentation should be considered. Two common techniques reported are hamstring and partial quadriceps autograft.[97]

Bohl et al report their outcomes with 48 total knees with intraoperative MCL injury treated with primary repair and bracing. Patients were treated in an unlocked hinged brace for 6 weeks postoperatively. Five required further surgery for stiffness (4 MUA), two for aseptic loosening, and the authors conclude MCL repair and bracing to be an acceptable option.[96] Jung et al reported on utilizing quadriceps tendon autograft in five cases where the MCL tissue was not amenable to primary repair and demonstrated no complications with the extensor mechanism and no residual coronal instability at 16 months postoperatively.[97]

Increased constraint may be considered when MCL injury is experienced in TKA. Some have advocated the "internal brace" that a varus/valgus constraining TKA can provide.[94] With this technique, the MCL is repaired in the usual fashion, and the increased varus/valgus constraint is utilized to protect the repair during healing. The benefit to this technique is that the protection of the MCL repair is indefinite. This technique does increase the cost and complexity of the surgery and is thought to increase the polyethylene wear and stresses at the implant interfaces.[98] The additional morbidity of the surgery from increased bone cuts and stems should be considered before pursuing this option.

VASCULAR INJURY

Major vascular injury is a rare but potentially devastating complication of TKA. For this section, major vascular injury will refer to the popliteal system. Geniculate injuries and damage to the small periarticular vessels are relatively common during TKA, reported to occur in 38% of all primary TKAs, and do not have such drastic consequences.[99] Major arterial complications can lead to wound healing problems, infection, and amputation. The incidence of major vascular injury is 0.017% to 0.05% depending on series,[100-103] and revision surgery is a known risk factor.[104] Mechanisms of injury include tourniquet-related occlusion or thrombosis, direct injury, or traction injury.[105]

Anatomy

The popliteal artery descends obliquely as a continuation of the superficial femoral artery from the adductor hiatus medially to the crural intraosseous space laterally where it divides into the anterior and posterior tibial arteries.[106] As the artery courses distally from the medial border of the femur to the laterally placed interosseous space, it crosses the knee joint line, closely opposed to the posterior capsule of the knee placing it at risk of injury during TKA. The popliteal artery is slightly lateral to the midsagittal plane of the tibia at the level of the joint.[107] When the knee is flexed, the popliteal artery falls posteriorly, allowing some measure of protection from direct injury.[108,109] In the revision setting, however, the protective effect of flexion is lost as there is no significant difference in the position of the artery in either flexion or extension.[110]

Prevention

Assessing a patient's risk for vascular complication is critical portion of the preoperative evaluation. A careful history must be taken to determine if there is a history of prior vascular surgery, arterial insufficiency, or peripheral vascular disease. On physical examination, asymmetric or absent pedal pulses should be documented and the popliteal fossa should be palpated as an aneurysm may present as pulsatile mass. Radiographs should be scrutinized for calcified vessels. If there is any concern for vascular compromise, a preoperative vascular consultation should be obtained.

For patients with vascular risk factors, the surgeon should consider abandoning the tourniquet. Assistants should be instructed to avoid compressing the popliteal fossa as this may displace the neurovascular structures anteriorly. Retractors should be placed medial to the posterior cruciate ligament (PCL). Care must be taken while working in the back of the knee, especially during meniscal excision, removal of osteophytes, débridement, and posterior capsular release. Adequate visualization, including appropriate exposure and lighting, is essential. If a tourniquet is employed, it should be deflated prior to polyethylene insertion, so hemostasis in the posterior compartment can be obtained.

Management

Any concern for an intraoperative vascular injury warrants an immediate vascular surgery consultation for potential intervention.

Nerve Injury

Neurologic injuries following TKA can include brachial plexus neuropathy, sacral plexus neuropathy, sciatic neuropathy, and infrapatellar branch of the saphenous nerve (ISN) injuries,[111-115] but the focus of this section will be peroneal nerve injuries. The incidence of peroneal nerve injury ranges from 0.3% to 1.3% depending on the study.[116-119] Risk factors include preoperative flexion contractures, valgus deformities, prolonged tourniquet use, and preexisting neuropathic conditions.[120] Revision surgery as well increases the risk for peroneal nerve palsy. In a Mayo Clinic study, 0.6% of revision TKA sustained a nerve injury compared to only 0.2% of primary TKA.[117]

Anatomy

The common peroneal nerve (CPN) enters the popliteal fossa on the lateral side of the tibial nerve and runs distally along the medial side of the biceps tendon. It passes between the biceps femoris tendon and the lateral head of the gastrocnemius and runs distally posterior to the fibular head. It next winds superficially across the lateral aspect of the neck of the fibula before piercing the peroneus longus through a fibrous tunnel and dividing into the superficial peroneal and deep peroneal nerves.[121] Anatomic and magnetic resonance studies place the CPN on average 13.5 to 14.9 mm from the posterolateral corner of the tibial plateau and 35.8 mm from the posterior border of the iliotibial band.[121,122]

Prevention

Given the association of nerve injuries with preexisting neuropathic conditions and preoperative deformities, the preoperative history and physical are critical. A careful history of neuropathic or radicular symptoms should be assessed. On examination, asymmetric or diminished sensation in the sural, saphenous, deep peroneal, superficial peroneal, and tibial distributions should be assessed and documented. Sagittal and coronal deformities should be noted as well.

Intraoperative concerns focus primarily on prevention. Longer tourniquet times have been associated with an increased incidence of neurologic complications.[123] The tourniquet should not be inflated for more than 120 minutes. If additional tourniquet is required, a reperfusion of 20 minutes is recommended. A longer deflation time prior to reinflation was also found to reduce neurologic injury.[123]

Although identification of an intraoperative peroneal nerve injury would be atypical, there are portions of the TKA in which the risk is increased. During balancing of the valgus knee, the lateral structures may need to be released. Ranawat et al has described a "pie-crusting" technique when the extension gap remains unbalanced after intra-articular release: the iliotibial band is lengthened in a controlled manner as necessary from inside with use of multiple oblique stab incisions 1 cm above the joint line.[124] The surgeon should perform such a maneuver with caution, given the proximity of the CPN to the posterolateral corner.

Management

Identification of a laceration or direct injury to the peroneal nerve would warrant immediate neurosurgical or microvascular consultation for repair. More commonly, attention should be paid to the patient postoperatively, especially in high-risk patients. Immediate treatment for a peroneal palsy should consist of removal of constricting dressings and positioning of the knee in 20° to 30° of flexion with the hip extended.[116,117] Patients with partial palsies have a good prognosis with multiple studies showing greater than 50% progressing to complete recovery.[117-119,125] An ankle–foot orthosis should be considered for those patients lack dorsiflexion to prevent an equinus contracture of the ankle. For patients failing to recover, exploration and decompression of peroneal is recommended for any patient whose palsy, especially if severe, does not improve after 3 months as evidenced by clinical assessment or electromyography (EMG).[126,127]

CONCLUSION

Complications are unavoidable in surgery, and this is especially true in revision TKA. Minimizing these risks, however, is paramount. Careful preoperative planning is critical to success and allows the surgeon to anticipate challenges in the operating room. Anatomy is the basis of our profession and is essential to safely embark on revision surgery. Not only should the surgeon know the normal anatomy, but, they must understand the individual

patient's variants as well as the distortions created from prior surgery. Teamwork and communication are fundamental as well when planning and executing these cases. All efforts should be made prior to surgery to minimize the risks for the benefit of the patient, and if a complication does arise, the preparation and anticipation can aid in a successful outcome.

REFERENCES

1. Ethgen O, Bruyere O, Richy F, Dardennes C, Reginster JY. Health-related quality of life in total hip and total knee arthroplasty. A qualitative and systematic review of the literature. *J Bone Joint Surg Am.* 2004;86-A:963-974.
2. Jenkins PJ, Clement ND, Hamilton DF, Gaston P, Patton JT, Howie CR. Predicting the cost-effectiveness of total hip and knee replacement: a health economic analysis. *Bone Joint J.* 2013;95-B:115-121.
3. Hamilton DF, Howie CR, Burnett R, Simpson AH, Patton JT. Dealing with the predicted increase in demand for revision total knee arthroplasty: challenges, risks and opportunities. *Bone Joint J.* 2015;97-B:723-728.
4. Hamilton D, Henderson GR, Gaston P, MacDonald D, Howie C, Simpson AH. Comparative outcomes of total hip and knee arthroplasty: a prospective cohort study. *Postgrad Med J.* 2012;88:627-631.
5. Dennis DA, Clayton ML, O'Donnell S, Mack RP, Stringer EA. Posterior cruciate condylar total knee arthroplasty. Average 11-year follow-up evaluation. *Clin Orthop Relat Res.* 1992(281):168-176.
6. Ranawat CS, Luessenhop CP, Rodriguez JA. The press-fit condylar modular total knee system. Four-to-six-year results with a posterior-cruciate-substituting design. *J Bone Joint Surg Am.* 1997;79:342-348.
7. Kurtz SM, Ong KL, Lau E, et al. International survey of primary and revision total knee replacement. *Int Orthop.* 2011;35:1783-1789.
8. Kurtz S, Ong K, Lau E, Mowat F, Halpern M. Projections of primary and revision hip and knee arthroplasty in the United States from 2005 to 2030. *J Bone Joint Surg Am.* 2007;89:780-785.
9. Alden KJ, Duncan WH, Trousdale RT, Pagnano MW, Haidukewych GJ. Intraoperative fracture during primary total knee arthroplasty. *Clin Orthop Relat Res.* 2010;468:90-95.
10. Pinaroli A, Piedade SR, Servien E, Neyret P. Intraoperative fractures and ligament tears during total knee arthroplasty. A 1795 posterostabilized TKA continuous series. *Orthop Traumatol Surg Res.* 2009;95:183-189.
11. Mardian S, Wichlas F, Schaser KD, et al. Periprosthetic fractures around the knee: update on therapeutic algorithms for internal fixation and revision arthroplasty. *Acta Chir Orthop Traumatol Cech.* 2012;79:297-306.
12. Lombardi AV Jr, Mallory TH, Waterman RA, Eberle RW. Intercondylar distal femoral fracture. An unreported complication of posterior-stabilized total knee arthroplasty. *J Arthroplasty.* 1995;10:643-650.
13. Sassoon AA, Wyles CC, Norambuena Morales GA, Houdek MT, Trousdale RT. Intraoperative fracture during aseptic revision total knee arthroplasty. *J Arthroplasty.* 2014;29:2187-2191.
14. Sassoon AA, Nelms NJ, Trousdale RT. Intraoperative fracture during staged total knee reimplantation in the treatment of periprosthetic infection. *J Arthroplasty.* 2014;29:1435-1438.
15. Cipriano CA, Brown NM, Della Valle CJ, Moric M, Sporer SM. Intra-operative periprosthetic fractures associated with press fit stems in revision total knee arthroplasty: incidence, management, and outcomes. *J Arthroplasty.* 2013;28:1310-1313.
16. Toogood PA, Vail TP. Periprosthetic fractures: a common problem with a disproportionately high impact on healthcare resources. *J Arthroplasty.* 2015;30:1688-1691.

17. Whitehouse MR, Mehendale S. Periprosthetic fractures around the knee: current concepts and advances in management. *Curr Rev Musculoskelet Med*. 2014;7:136-144.

18. Bozic KJ, Kamath AF, Ong K, et al. Comparative epidemiology of revision arthroplasty: failed THA poses greater clinical and economic burdens than failed TKA. *Clin Orthop Relat Res*. 2015;473:2131-2138.

19. Rorabeck CH, Taylor JW. Periprosthetic fractures of the femur complicating total knee arthroplasty. *Orthop Clin North Am*. 1999;30:265-277.

20. Rorabeck CH, Taylor JW. Classification of periprosthetic fractures complicating total knee arthroplasty. *Orthop Clin North Am*. 1999;30:209-214.

21. Felix NA, Stuart MJ, Hanssen AD. Periprosthetic fractures of the tibia associated with total knee arthroplasty. *Clin Orthop Relat Res*. 1997;(345):113-124.

22. Stuart MJ, Hanssen AD. Total knee arthroplasty: periprosthetic tibial fractures. *Orthop Clin North Am*. 1999;30:279-286.

23. Hanssen AD, Stuart MJ. Treatment of periprosthetic tibial fractures. *Clin Orthop Relat Res*. 2000;(380):91-98.

24. Ortiguera CJ, Berry DJ. Patellar fracture after total knee arthroplasty. *J Bone Joint Surg Am*. 2002;84-A:532-540.

25. Duncan CP, Haddad FS. The Unified Classification System (UCS): improving our understanding of periprosthetic fractures. *Bone Joint J*. 2014;96-B:713-716.

26. Duncan CP, Masri BA. Fractures of the femur after hip replacement. *Instr Course Lect*. 1995;44:293-304.

27. Van der Merwe JM, Haddad FS, Duncan CP. Field testing the Unified Classification System for periprosthetic fractures of the femur, tibia and patella in association with knee replacement: an international collaboration. *Bone Joint J*. 2014;96-B:1669-1673.

28. Vioreanu MH, Parry MC, Haddad FS, Duncan CP. Field testing the Unified Classification System for peri-prosthetic fractures of the pelvis and femur around a total hip replacement: an international collaboration. *Bone Joint J*. 2014;96-B:1472-1477.

29. Rorabeck CH, Angliss RD, Lewis PL. Fractures of the femur, tibia, and patella after total knee arthroplasty: decision making and principles of management. *Instr Course Lect*. 1998;47:449-458.

30. Althausen PL, Lee MA, Finkemeier CG, Meehan JP, Rodrigo JJ. Operative stabilization of supracondylar femur fractures above total knee arthroplasty: a comparison of four treatment methods. *J Arthroplasty*. 2003;18:834-839.

31. Bezwada HP, Neubauer P, Baker J, Israelite CL, Johanson NA. Periprosthetic supracondylar femur fractures following total knee arthroplasty. *J Arthroplasty*. 2004;19:453-458.

32. Dennis DA. Periprosthetic fractures following total knee arthroplasty. *Instr Course Lect*. 2001;50:379-389.

33. Gross AE. Periprosthetic fractures of the knee: puzzle pieces. *J Arthroplasty*. 2004;19:47-50.

34. Noble PC, Alexander JW, Lindahl LJ, Yew DT, Granberry WM, Tullos HS. The anatomic basis of femoral component design. *Clin Orthop Relat Res*. 1988;(235):148-165.

35. Hoaglund FT, Low WD. Anatomy of the femoral neck and head, with comparative data from Caucasians and Hong Kong Chinese. *Clin Orthop Relat Res*. 1980;(152):10-16.

36. Ritter MA, Faris PM, Keating EM. Anterior femoral notching and ipsilateral supracondylar femur fracture in total knee arthroplasty. *J Arthroplasty*. 1988;3:185-187.

37. Lesh ML, Schneider DJ, Deol G, Davis B, Jacobs CR, Pellegrini VD Jr. The consequences of anterior femoral notching in total knee arthroplasty. A biomechanical study. *J Bone Joint Surg Am*. 2000;82-A:1096-1101.

38. Culp RW, Schmidt RG, Hanks G, Mak A, Esterhai JL Jr, Heppenstall RB. Supracondylar fracture of the femur following prosthetic knee arthroplasty. *Clin Orthop Relat Res*. 1987;(222):212-222.

39. Shawen SB, Belmont PJ Jr, Klemme WR, Topoleski LD, Xenos JS, Orchowski JR. Osteoporosis and anterior femoral notching in periprosthetic supracondylar femoral fractures: a biomechanical analysis. *J Bone Joint Surg Am*. 2003;85-A:115-121.

40. Haddad FS, Masri BA, Garbuz DS, Duncan CP. The prevention of periprosthetic fractures in total hip and knee arthroplasty. *Orthop Clin North Am*. 1999;30:191-207.

41. Bertin KC. Tibial component fixation in total knee arthroplasty: a comparison of pegged and stemmed designs. *J Arthroplasty*. 2007;22:670-678.

42. Rawlinson JJ, Peters LE, Campbell DA, Windsor R, Wright TM, Bartel DL. Cancellous bone strains indicate efficacy of stem augmentation in constrained condylar knees. *Clin Orthop Relat Res*. 2005;440:107-116.

43. Conlisk N, Gray H, Pankaj P, Howie CR. The influence of stem length and fixation on initial femoral component stability in revision total knee replacement. *Bone Joint Res*. 2012;1:281-288.

44. Barrack RL, Stanley T, Burt M, Hopkins S. The effect of stem design on end-of-stem pain in revision total knee arthroplasty. *J Arthroplasty*. 2004;19:119-124.

45. Barrack RL, Rorabeck C, Burt M, Sawhney J. Pain at the end of the stem after revision total knee arthroplasty. *Clin Orthop Relat Res*. 1999;(367):216-225.

46. Healy WL, Siliski JM, Incavo SJ. Operative treatment of distal femoral fractures proximal to total knee replacements. *J Bone Joint Surg Am*. 1993;75:27-34.

47. Zehntner MK, Ganz R. Internal fixation of supracondylar fractures after condylar total knee arthroplasty. *Clin Orthop Relat Res*. 1993;(293):219-224.

48. Figgie MP, Goldberg VM, Figgie HE III, Sobel M. The results of treatment of supracondylar fracture above total knee arthroplasty. *J Arthroplasty*. 1990;5:267-276.

49. Tani Y, Inoue K, Kaneko H, Nishioka J, Hukuda S. Intramedullary fibular graft for supracondylar fracture of the femur following total knee arthroplasty. *Arch Orthop Trauma Surg*. 1998;117:103-104.

50. Haidukewych GJ, Jacofsky DJ, Hanssen AD. Treatment of periprosthetic fractures around a total knee arthroplasty. *J Knee Surg*. 2003;16:111-117.

51. Hanschen M, Aschenbrenner IM, Fehske K, et al. Mono- versus polyaxial locking plates in distal femur fractures: a prospective randomized multicentre clinical trial. *Int Orthop* 2014;38:857-863.

52. Ebraheim NA, Kelley LH, Liu X, Thomas IS, Steiner RB, Liu J. Periprosthetic distal femur fracture after total knee arthroplasty: a systematic review. *Orthop Surg*. 2015;7:297-305.

53. Cain PR, Rubash HE, Wissinger HA, McClain EJ. Periprosthetic femoral fractures following total knee arthroplasty. *Clin Orthop Relat Res*. 1986;(208):205-214.

54. Engh GA, Ammeen DJ. Periprosthetic fractures adjacent to total knee implants: treatment and clinical results. *Instr Course Lect*. 1998;47:437-448.

55. Huang Y, Zhou Y, Shao H, Gu J, Tang H, Tang Q. What is the difference between modular and nonmodular tapered fluted titanium stems in revision total hip arthroplasty. *J Arthroplasty*. 2017;32:3108-3113.

56. Mabry TM, Vessely MB, Schleck CD, Harmsen WS, Berry DJ. Revision total knee arthroplasty with modular cemented stems: long-term follow-up. *J Arthroplasty*. 2007;22:100-105.

57. Murray PB, Rand JA, Hanssen AD. Cemented long-stem revision total knee arthroplasty. *Clin Orthop Relat Res*. 1994;(309):116-123.

58. Peters CL, Erickson J, Kloepper RG, Mohr RA. Revision total knee arthroplasty with modular components inserted with metaphyseal cement and stems without cement. *J Arthroplasty*. 2005;20:302-308.

59. Peters CL, Erickson JA, Gililland JM. Clinical and radiographic results of 184 consecutive revision total knee arthroplasties placed with modular cementless stems. *J Arthroplasty*. 2009;24:48-53.

60. Shannon BD, Klassen JF, Rand JA, Berry DJ, Trousdale RT. Revision total knee arthroplasty with cemented components and uncemented intramedullary stems. *J Arthroplasty*. 2003;18:27-32.

61. Wood GC, Naudie DD, MacDonald SJ, McCalden RW, Bourne RB. Results of press-fit stems in revision knee arthroplasties. *Clin Orthop Relat Res*. 2009;467:810-817.

62. Gross AE. Revision total knee arthroplasty of bone grafts versus implant supplementation. *Orthopedics*. 1997;20:843-844.

63. Hockman DE, Ammeen D, Engh GA. Augments and allografts in revision total knee arthroplasty: usage and outcome using one modular revision prosthesis. *J Arthroplasty*. 2005;20:35-41.

64. Reichel H, Hube R, Birke A, Hein W. Bone defects in revision total knee arthroplasty: classification and management. *Zentralbl Chir*. 2002;127:880-885.

65. Ritter MA. Screw and cement fixation of large defects in total knee arthroplasty. *J Arthroplasty*. 1986;1:125-129.

66. Ritter MA, Keating EM, Faris PM. Screw and cement fixation of large defects in total knee arthroplasty. A sequel. *J Arthroplasty*. 1993;8:63-65.

67. Bush JL, Wilson JB, Vail TP. Management of bone loss in revision total knee arthroplasty. *Clin Orthop Relat Res*. 2006;452:186-192.

68. Engh GA, Herzwurm PJ, Parks NL. Treatment of major defects of bone with bulk allografts and stemmed components during total knee arthroplasty. *J Bone Joint Surg Am*. 1997;79:1030-1039.

69. Rand JA, Morrey BF, Bryan RS. Patellar tendon rupture after total knee arthroplasty. *Clin Orthop Relat Res*. 1989;(244):233-238.

70. Standring S. Knee. In: Standring S, ed. *Gray's Anatomy: The Anatomical Basis of Clinical Practice*. 41st ed. New York: Elsevier Limited; 2016:xviii, 1562.

71. Adigweme OO, Sassoon AA, Langford J, Haidukewych GJ. Periprosthetic patellar fractures. *J Knee Surg*. 2013;26:313-317.

72. Goldberg VM, Figgie HE III, Inglis AE, et al. Patellar fracture type and prognosis in condylar total knee arthroplasty. *Clin Orthop Relat Res* 1988(236):115-122.

73. Healy WL, Wasilewski SA, Takei R, Oberlander M. Patellofemoral complications following total knee arthroplasty. Correlation with implant design and patient risk factors. *J Arthroplasty*. 1995;10:197-201.

74. Reuben JD, McDonald CL, Woodard PL, Hennington LJ. Effect of patella thickness on patella strain following total knee arthroplasty. *J Arthroplasty*. 1991;6:251-258.

75. Parvizi J, Kim KI, Oliashirazi A, Ong A, Sharkey PF. Periprosthetic patellar fractures. *Clin Orthop Relat Res*. 2006;446:161-166.

76. Pagnano MW, Scuderi GR, Insall JN. Patellar component resection in revision and reimplantation total knee arthroplasty. *Clin Orthop Relat Res*. 1998(356):134-138.

77. Hanssen AD. Bone-grafting for severe patellar bone loss during revision knee arthroplasty. *J Bone Joint Surg Am*. 2001;83-A:171-176.

78. Hanssen AD, Pagnano MW. Revision of failed patellar components. *Instr Course Lect*. 2004;53:201-206.

79. Cadambi A, Engh GA. Use of a semitendinosus tendon autogenous graft for rupture of the patellar ligament after total knee arthroplasty. A report of seven cases. *J Bone Joint Surg Am*. 1992;74:974-979.

80. Lynch AF, Rorabeck CH, Bourne RB. Extensor mechanism complications following total knee arthroplasty. *J Arthroplasty*. 1987;2:135-140.

81. Dobbs RE, Hanssen AD, Lewallen DG, Pagnano MW. Quadriceps tendon rupture after total knee arthroplasty. Prevalence, complications, and outcomes. *J Bone Joint Surg Am*. 2005;87:37-45.

82. Nam D, Abdel MP, Cross MB, et al. The management of extensor mechanism complications in total knee arthroplasty. AAOS exhibit selection. *J Bone Joint Surg Am* 2014;96:e47.

83. Scott RD. *Total Knee Arthroplasty*. 1st ed. Philadelphia, PA: Saunders Elsevier; 2005:148.

84. Garvin KL, Scuderi G, Insall JN. Evolution of the quadriceps snip. *Clin Orthop Relat Res*. 1995(321):131-137.

85. Rand JA, Ries MD, Landis GH, Rosenberg AG, Haas S. Intraoperative assessment in revision total knee arthroplasty. *J Bone Joint Surg Am*. 2003;85-A(suppl 1):S26-S37.

86. Kim TW, Kamath AF, Israelite CL. Suture anchor repair of quadriceps tendon rupture after total knee arthroplasty. *J Arthroplasty*. 2011;26:817-820.

87. Schoderbek RJ Jr, Brown TE, Mulhall KJ, et al. Extensor mechanism disruption after total knee arthroplasty. *Clin Orthop Relat Res*. 2006;446:176-185.

88. Courtney PM, Edmiston TA, Pflederer CT, Levine BR, Gerlinger TL. Is there any role for direct repair of extensor mechanism disruption following total knee arthroplasty? *J Arthroplasty*. 2018;33:S244-S248.

89. Ecker ML, Lotke PA, Glazer RM. Late reconstruction of the patellar tendon. *J Bone Joint Surg Am*. 1979;61:884-886.

90. Gustilo R, Thompson R: Quadriceps and patellar tendon ruptures following total knee arthroplasty. In: Rand JA, Dorr LD, Knee Society (U.S.), eds. *Total Arthroplasty of the Knee: Proceedings of the Knee Society, 1985-1986*. Rockville, MD: Aspen Publishers; 1986:xviii, 325.

91. Yun AG, Rubash HE, Scott RD, Laskin RS. Quadriceps rupture associated with a proximal quadriceps release in total knee arthroplasty. A report of three cases. *J Bone Joint Surg Am*. 2003;85-A:1809-1811.

92. Leopold SS, McStay C, Klafeta K, Jacobs JJ, Berger RA, Rosenberg AG. Primary repair of intraoperative disruption of the medial collateral ligament during total knee arthroplasty. *J Bone Joint Surg Am*. 2001;83-A:86-91.

93. Siqueira MB, Haller K, Mulder A, Goldblum AS, Klika AK, Barsoum WK. Outcomes of medial collateral ligament injuries during total knee arthroplasty. *J Knee Surg*. 2016;29:68-73.

94. Lee GC, Lotke PA. Management of intraoperative medial collateral ligament injury during TKA. *Clin Orthop Relat Res*. 2011;469:64-68.

95. LaPrade RF, Engebretsen AH, Ly TV, Johansen S, Wentorf FA, Engebretsen L. The anatomy of the medial part of the knee. *J Bone Joint Surg Am*. 2007;89:2000-2010.

96. Bohl DD, Wetters NG, Del Gaizo DJ, Jacobs JJ, Rosenberg AG, Della Valle CJ. Repair of intraoperative injury to the medial collateral ligament during primary total knee arthroplasty. *J Bone Joint Surg Am*. 2016;98:35-39.

97. Jung KA, Lee SC, Hwang SH, Jung SH. Quadriceps tendon free graft augmentation for a midsubstance tear of the medial collateral ligament during total knee arthroplasty. *Knee*. 2009;16:479-483.

98. Callaghan JJ, O'Rourke MR, Liu SS. The role of implant constraint in revision total knee arthroplasty: not too little, not too much. *J Arthroplasty*. 2005;20:41-43.

99. Statz JM, Ledford CK, Chalmers BP, Taunton MJ, Mabry TM, Trousdale RT. Geniculate artery injury during primary total knee arthroplasty. *Am J Orthop (Belle Mead NJ)*. 2018;47(10). doi:10.12788/ajo.2018.0097.

100. Rand JA. Vascular complications of total knee arthroplasty. Report of three cases. *J Arthroplasty*. 1987;2:89-93.

101. Parvizi J, Pulido L, Slenker N, Macgibeny M, Purtill JJ, Rothman RH. Vascular injuries after total joint arthroplasty. *J Arthroplasty*. 2008;23:1115-1121.

102. Bernhoff K, Rudstrom H, Gedeborg R, Bjorck M. Popliteal artery injury during knee replacement: a population-based nationwide study. *Bone Joint J*. 2013;95-B:1645-1649.

103. Ko LJ, DeHart ML, Yoo JU, Huff TW. Popliteal artery injury associated with total knee arthroplasty: trends, costs and risk factors. *J Arthroplasty*. 2014;29:1181-1184.

104. Saleh KJ, Hoeffel DP, Kassim RA, Burstein G. Complications after revision total knee arthroplasty. *J Bone Joint Surg Am*. 2003;85-A(suppl 1):S71-S74.

105. Kumar SN, Chapman JA, Rawlins I. Vascular injuries in total knee arthroplasty. A review of the problem with special reference to the possible effects of the tourniquet. *J Arthroplasty*. 1998;13:211-216.

106. Williams PL, Warwick R, Dyson M, Bannister L. Angiology. In: Williams PL, ed. *Gray's Anatomy.* 37th ed. Edinburgh, New York: C. Livingstone; 1989:785.

107. Ninomiya JT, Dean JC, Goldberg VM. Injury to the popliteal artery and its anatomic location in total knee arthroplasty. *J Arthroplasty.* 1999;14:803-809.

108. Yoo JH, Chang CB. The location of the popliteal artery in extension and 90 degree knee flexion measured on MRI. *Knee.* 2009;16:143-148.

109. Farrington WJ, Charnley GJ: The effect of knee flexion on the popliteal artery and its surgical significance. *J Bone Joint Surg Br.* 2003;85:1208; author reply 1208.

110. Abdel Karim MM, Anbar A, Keenan J. Position of the popliteal artery in revision total knee arthroplasty. *Arch Orthop Trauma Surg.* 2012;132:861-865.

111. Gunston FH, MacKenzie RI. Complications of polycentric knee arthroplasty. *Clin Orthop Relat Res.* 1976(120):11-17.

112. Eggers KA, Asai T. Postoperative brachial plexus neuropathy after total knee replacement under spinal anaesthesia. *Br J Anaesth.* 1995;75:642-644.

113. Myers MA, Harmon RL. Sacral plexopathy and sciatic neuropathy after total knee arthroplasty. *Electromyogr Clin Neurophysiol.* 1998;38:423-426.

114. Tennent TD, Birch NC, Holmes MJ, Birch R, Goddard NJ. Knee pain and the infrapatellar branch of the saphenous nerve. *J R Soc Med.* 1998;91:573-575.

115. Kachar SM, Williams KM, Finn HA. Neuroma of the infrapatellar branch of the saphenous nerve a cause of reversible knee stiffness after total knee arthroplasty. *J Arthroplasty.* 2008;23:927-930.

116. Rose HA, Hood RW, Otis JC, Ranawat CS, Insall JN. Peroneal-nerve palsy following total knee arthroplasty. A review of The Hospital for Special Surgery experience. *J Bone Joint Surg Am.* 1982;64:347-351.

117. Asp JP, Rand JA. Peroneal nerve palsy after total knee arthroplasty. *Clin Orthop Relat Res.* 1990(261):233-237.

118. Idusuyi OB, Morrey BF. Peroneal nerve palsy after total knee arthroplasty. Assessment of predisposing and prognostic factors. *J Bone Joint Surg Am.* 1996;78:177-184.

119. Schinsky MF, Macaulay W, Parks ML, Kiernan H, Nercessian OA. Nerve injury after primary total knee arthroplasty. *J Arthroplasty.* 2001;16:1048-1054.

120. Nercessian OA, Ugwonali OF, Park S. Peroneal nerve palsy after total knee arthroplasty. *J Arthroplasty.* 2005;20:1068-1073.

121. Bruzzone M, Ranawat A, Castoldi F, Dettoni F, Rossi P, Rossi R. The risk of direct peroneal nerve injury using the Ranawat "inside-out" lateral release technique in valgus total knee arthroplasty. *J Arthroplasty.* 2010;25:161-165.

122. Clarke HD, Schwartz JB, Math KR, Scuderi GR. Anatomic risk of peroneal nerve injury with the "pie crust" technique for valgus release in total knee arthroplasty. *J Arthroplasty.* 2004;19: 40-44.

123. Horlocker TT, Hebl JR, Gali B, et al. Anesthetic, patient, and surgical risk factors for neurologic complications after prolonged total tourniquet time during total knee arthroplasty. *Anesth Analg.* 2006;102:950-955.

124. Ranawat AS, Ranawat CS, Elkus M, Rasquinha VJ, Rossi R, Babhulkar S. Total knee arthroplasty for severe valgus deformity. *J Bone Joint Surg Am.* 2005;87(suppl 1):271-284.

125. Webster DA, Murray DG. Complications of variable axis total knee arthroplasty. *Clin Orthop Relat Res.* 1985(193):160-167.

126. Krackow KA, Maar DC, Mont MA, Carroll C IV. Surgical decompression for peroneal nerve palsy after total knee arthroplasty. *Clin Orthop Relat Res.* 1993(292):223-228.

127. Mont MA, Dellon AL, Chen F, Hungerford MW, Krackow KA, Hungerford DS. The operative treatment of peroneal nerve palsy. *J Bone Joint Surg Am.* 1996;78:863-869.

chapter 54

The Stiff Total Knee

Ivan De Martino, MD I Vanni Strigelli, MD I Peter K. Sculco, MD I Thomas P. Sculco, MD

INTRODUCTION

Total knee arthroplasty (TKA) has been demonstrated to be an efficacious and cost-effective solution for end-stage osteoarthritis (OA) of the knee. One of the most common complications within the early postoperative period is reduced knee range of motion (ROM). Stiffness following TKA is a challenge for patients and surgeons alike and occurs in approximately 5% of patients post surgery.[1,2] The definition of what constitutes a stiff knee and the overall severity varies across studies.[2-9] A recent classification system provided by the International consensus of the definition and classification of fibrosis categorizes knee stiffness according to loss of movement based on the deviation from full flexion or extension as mild, moderate, and severe extension restriction (5° to 10°, 11° to 20°, >20°) or flexion range (90° to 100°, 70° to 89°, <70°).[10] However, what is considered as total stiffness is probably best related to the preoperative knee ROM. Flexion of 90° is considered unsatisfactory when presented with an initial preoperative flexion of 120°. Yet, in a patient presenting with a preoperative flexion of 60°, reaching 90° can be considered a promising outcome. The evaluation of the stiff knee after TKA must be approached in a systematic fashion as the underlying etiology may be biologic, psychosocial, or mechanical, and the treatment plan must be modified based on these data. Further, several potential reasons for knee stiffness include primary arthrofibrosis, component malrotation, component overstuffing, instability, coronal malalignment, pain catastrophizing, and kinesophobia.[10] In addition, severe preoperative knee stiffness and prior open surgical procedures increase the risk of reduced ROM post TKA.

Developing stiffness can be frustrating for the patient: walking requires 65° of flexion, rising from a chair requires 70°, and descending stairs around 100° depending on the stair height. When a patient has severe stiffness, almost every activity of daily living is negatively impacted, with the most basic tasks requiring a minimum of 60° of flexion.[8,11] For this reason, stiffness after TKA leads to inferior patient-reported outcomes scores and inferior general health scores. Proper patient education and evaluation are integral in optimizing patient satisfaction following TKA.[12] To date, the best predictors of ROM post TKA are preoperative motion and the passive motion achieved at time of surgery.[2,9] The aim of this chapter is to outline the specific causes of stiffness in the setting of TKA and provide surgical management tailored to the underlying etiology.

EPIDEMIOLOGY

The prevalence of stiffness post TKA ranges from 1.3% to 14%.[6,7,9,13] However, the definition of stiffness is variable among these studies. Gandhi et al reported an incidence of 3.7%, using a definition of stiffness as flexion less than 90°,[6] while Yercan reported an incidence of 5.3% with a definition of 10° or more of extension and/or less than 95° of flexion.[7] Le et al showed stiffness as the third most common reason for TKA failure, behind infection and instability.[13] Zmistowski et al further demonstrated that postoperative stiffness following TKA is one of the most common causes of readmission within the first 90 days after surgery and for revision TKA.[14] Regardless of the selected study, stiffness post TKA is one of the more commonly encountered early complications requiring conservative and possibly operative management.

ETIOLOGIES

Knee stiffness can be categorized as intrinsic (anatomically localized in the knee) or extrinsic (outside of the knee joint). Intrinsic etiologies include severe reduction in preoperative ROM, low-grade infection, aseptic loosening, or poor surgical technique.[9] Extrinsic etiologies include hip or spine disease, neurologic injury, abnormal inflammatory response, complex regional pain syndrome (CPRS), patient motivation, and improper indication for the TKA.[9] Among these, perhaps the most significant risk factor is a preoperative reduction in ROM, as a stiff knee is more likely to yield postoperative stiffness after a knee replacement. Vince further categorized etiologies of stiffness into five groups: pathology, patient, rehab, surgical technique, and implant design.[17] Among those five, some etiologies are more commonly associated with early stiffness after TKA, while others have a strong affinity with late-onset stiffness. Etiologies more commonly associated with early stiffness after TKA include component malposition, arthrofibrosis, and CPRS. Etiologies seen in late stiffness include synovitis, tendinitis, aseptic loosening, or prosthetic breakage. Periprosthetic joint infections (PJIs) have been known to cause both early and late reductions in ROM.

Intrinsic Causes

Poor surgical technique is one of the leading causes of stiffness in the postoperative period. Femoral or tibial malalignment or malrotation can lead to pain and stiffness post TKA. Malalignment results in asymmetry of the extension gap, while malrotation can result in asymmetry of the flexion gap and additional patellar tracking issues. Tibial malrotation can also cause increased medial collateral ligament (MCL) ligament tension during flexion which could also impede early motion. Other intrinsic causes of stiffness post TKA include overstuffing of the patellofemoral joint, mismatch of the flexion and extension gaps, inaccurate ligament balancing, oversized components, joint line elevation, and excessive tightening of the extensor mechanism. In these circumstances, the most appropriate course of treatment is a revision surgery. While not generally attributable to poor surgical technique, aseptic loosening (can yield recurrent effusions and pain) is a prominent cause of stiffness following TKA.[18,19]

A postoperative hemarthrosis or large effusion can decrease early ROM. Increased intra-articular tension secondary to hemarthrosis causes a mechanical restriction of flexion, in addition to pain. If motion remains limited for 4 to 6 weeks, fibrosis may develop, resulting in permanent ROM reduction and a stiff knee. In a similar fashion, recurrent hemarthrosis secondary to hypervascular and hypertrophied synovium, impingement of the hypertrophied synovium, repetitive trauma, pigmented villonodular synovitis, anticoagulation, vascular disorders, and hemophilia can all cause delayed postoperative stiffness.[20] However, the incidence remains low, with a previously reported rate of 0.3% to 0.7%.[20]

Uncontrolled pain in the postoperative period can negatively impact early ROM. The inability to perform basic range-of-motion exercises can limit the patient from achieving full extension and an optimal level of flexion. Other intrinsic causes of increased knee pain in the postoperative period include synovitis, popliteal tendon impingement, and femoropatellar maltracking with irritation of the lateral facet of the patella.[19,21]

Infection

Periprosthetic joint infection (PJI) following TKA is one of the most devastating complications seen, often resulting in revision surgery. PJI can manifest as a painful or stiff knee, as the inflammatory reaction to the infecting agent can lead to development of intra-articular fibrosis. Due to its devastating nature, a surgeon should always exclude PJI as a potential diagnosis in a patient presenting with a stiff knee, particularly in a TKA that has delayed loss of motion in the setting of increasing pain.

Overstuffing

Overstuffing of a joint can result from insufficient bone resection or oversized implants and can involve the patellafemoral or tibiafemoral joint. Overstuffing the patellafemoral joint can commonly be seen in two conditions: an anteriorly displaced femoral component or an underresected patellar (combination of patella bone and button is greater than the original thickness).[9,15,22]

The anterior displacement of the femur can be a consequence of insufficient anterior femoral bone resection or from oversizing of the femoral component. The first scenario results in an anterior translation of a femoral component of appropriate size. In the second condition, a larger than required femoral component size is chosen, and the anterior flange is anterior to the anterior cut surface of the femur.[15] Anterior displacement of the femur is most often a potential problem regarding posterior referencing instruments and must always be considered during the anterior resection.[22] The junction of the anterior cut and anterior cortex should lay on the same coronal plane and be inspected and palpated. The thickness of the anterior femur bone resection should not be less than the thickness of the anterior flange of the femoral implant, when possible. The risk of overstuffing anteriorly has decreased as anterior–posterior size differential has decreased from 4 mm to around 2 mm for most contemporary knee systems concomitant with an increase in the number of femoral sizes available.

Similarly, the cumulative patella bone–patella button thickness can be excessively thick if the patella resection is insufficient. The thickness of the patellar resection should be at least equal to the thickness of the patellar component. Failure to do so would inadvertently increase the total thickness of the patella following implant insertion. Prior to resection, the patella can be measured in order to ensure the appropriate bone and cartilage removal. If patella overstuffing occurs, knee flexion can be limited due to a tight patellafemoral joint.[22]

Lastly, Vince found internal rotation of the tibial component to be one of the most common causes of stiff TKA revisions.[17] An internal rotation of the tibia may cause maltracking and lateralization of the patella, with a risk of dislocation moving from an extended position to a flexed position. This subsequently may result in a painful stiff TKA. In addition, internal rotation of the tibial component increases MCL tension which will also negatively influence knee motion. On the femoral side, an excess of internal rotation of the femur can also be a cause of patella maltracking, pain, and reduced knee ROM.

Overstuffing the tibiafemoral joint is most commonly seen when insufficient bone is removed from the tibia or distal femur, when the femoral component is larger than the femoral anteroposterior dimension and it is translated posteriorly or in the presence of an upslope in tibial resection.

Failure to recreate native tibial slope in a cruciate retaining (CR) knee can lead to an overly tight posterior cruciate ligament (PCL) and reduced ROM. For cruciate-sacrificing, posterior-substituting (PS) implant designs, decreasing the posterior slope of the tibia during preparation of the proximal tibia may also lead to an overly tight flexion gap and reduced knee flexion. Some surgeons prefer to set the posterior slope of the tibial cut at 0° or 3°, which is a relatively low angle compared with the natural posterior slope of the tibia. Some PS-TKA manufacturers also recommend this in their surgical procedure manuals. However, the extent to which the decreased posterior slope affects the flexion gap with PS-TKA remains unclear.[24] In case of reverse tibial slope, an overly tight flexion gap can be created in PS-TKA.

Posterior osteophytes, both on the tibia or femur, can also result in reduced knee extension and flexion if not adequately addressed at time of TKA. Large posterior femoral osteophytes can increase tension on the posterior capsule, and this can prevent full extension. Retained osteophytes behind the femoral component can also impinge against the posterior tibia or tibial component during flexion, preventing full flexion. Osteophytes on the tibia are usually removed with tibial resection, while posterior femoral osteophytes must be extracted. In order to do so, the knee is positioned in 90° of flexion with a laminar spreader and then removed with a curved osteotome and/or curette. In patients with a preoperative flexion contracture, additional stripping/release of the posterior capsule may be necessary.

Additional sources of impingement include native bone overhang from either behind the posterior condyles of the femoral component or posterior portion of the proximal tibia. The residual bone in these areas may cause impingement and limit flexion.[22] Utilization of a small tibial component or poor positioning in the anterior aspect can afford a similar effect, resulting in uncovered bone in the posterior knee. The uncovered posterior cortex of the tibia can lead to a contact between the posterior femur and tibia as the knee is flexed, potentially increasing the risk of impingement and stiffness.

Implant Design

When a posterior cruciate ligament–preserving knee (CR) implant is used, careful evaluation of the balance must be done in order to avoid limited flexion. Tightness of the PCL may lead to limited knee flexion, while overrelease of the PCL may limit flexion due to paradoxical anterior translation prior to rollback.[12,15]

When trial components have been inserted and passive knee flexion performed, if the polyethylene liner trial lifts off anteriorly with deeper flexion, then a tight PCL should be suspected.[25] The PCL may also be pathologic and may contribute to the overall mechanical deformity. For example, Laskin et al showed that in patients with a preoperative varus contracture of at least 15°, the PCL is most likely involved.[23] In these patients, a PCL release is often necessary to achieve adequate balance. It is important to distinguish between a tight flexion gap and excessive roll back due to an overly tensioned PCL.[23]

EXTRINSIC CAUSES

Knee stiffness can arise due to extrinsic causes outside of the knee joint as well. Patient factors (including preoperative ROM), body habitus, and patient personality have

all previously been implicated with stiffness.[15] Patients that are obese may have limited ROM secondary to posterior soft-tissue impingement as the knee flexes,[15] and some studies have shown a direct relationship between BMI and reduced ROM.[26] Interestingly, patients with low BMI may be at increased risk for reduced ROM as well.[17]

Demographic risk factors that have been reported in the literature include age and ethnicity. Younger age at time of TKA has been associated with increased risk of stiffness post TKA.[17] Springer et al reported that patients younger than 45 years and of African-American ethnicity were twice as likely to undergo a manipulation under anesthesia (MUA).[27] Patient comorbidities may also contribute to the risk of developing stiffness. For example, the diagnosis of diabetes mellitus has been associated with reduced ROM and risk for arthrofibrosis. Other patient factors that may limit ROM include poor patient motivation which may compromise postoperative rehabilitation protocols and overall compliance with postoperative exercises.[6] In addition, previous open surgical procedures on the affected knee have been suggested as a risk factor for arthrofibrosis after TKA.[5,28]

Other extrinsic causes that can lead to knee stiffness include any muscular or nervous system disorder that prevents normal knee motion. Central or peripheral nervous system disorders that may lead to spasticity might negatively influence final ROM. Parkinson disease, not well pharmacologically controlled, results in increased spasticity, cogwheel rigidity, and knee stiffness. Additionally, tight quadriceps or hamstring muscles secondary to muscle injury, heterotopic ossification (HO), or long-standing juvenile inflammatory conditions limiting knee ROM prior to the completion of skeletal growth may be an extrinsic source of knee stiffness.[9] Problems affecting other joints can influence TKA outcome. Pain originated at the hip radiating to the knee should be evaluated such as radiculopathy. Moreover, flexion deformity of the ipsilateral hip can develop into a compensatory flexion deformity of the knee. A patient with severe valgus or varus OA of both knees who undergo a TKA in one of the affected joints, after the surgery, would have a leg length discrepancy resulting in longer operated limb versus the nonoperated one. The patient may balance the leg length discrepancy by bending the operated knee resulting in a potential flexion contracture. The two possible solutions are the use of a shoe lift on the nonoperated limb or to perform a simultaneous bilateral TKA. In addition, spine deformity, such as dorsal or lumbar kyphosis, can lead to knee flexion.[12] Finally, improper surgical indications for TKA might lead to a painful and/or stiff TKA. Evaluation of preoperative radiographs may confirm this suspicion, and caution must be taken when considering surgery for patients with severe pain but minimal preoperative radiographic degenerative changes.[29]

Arthrofibrosis

Arthrofibrosis is an abnormal inflammatory response. In the literature, fibrosis after TKA ranges from 1% to 15%.[10] However, this high variability can be contributed in part by the lack of a preexisting precise definition.[10] Arthrofibrosis is characterized by excessive intra-articular deposit of thick fibrous tissue, made of extracellular matrix components, between the extensor mechanism and anterior femoral cortex, involving medial and lateral gutters and posterior capsule. Recent efforts have been made to achieve a clear definition: postsurgical fibrosis of the knee was defined as limited ROM of the knee, in flexion and/or extension, that is not attributable to a bony or prosthetic block to movement from malaligned or mispositioned components, hardware, ligament reconstruction, infection (septic arthritis), pain, complex regional pain, or other specific causes, and is due to fibrosis of the soft tissues which was not present preoperatively. Pain is a possible cause of stiffness; this can be demonstrated by examination under anesthesia.[10] Therefore, when fibrosis occurs in association with another pathology causing stiffness, this was not considered true postsurgical fibrosis. Knee arthrofibrosis is diagnosed primarily on clinical assessment after exclusion of all the other causes of stiffness and ultimately confirmed with histopathologic analysis.

Arthrofibrosis is usually accompanied by a combined loss of extension and flexion and associated pain. Isolated loss of extension is relatively rare and is typically found in patients with a significant preoperative flexion contracture. Isolated loss of flexion occurs more frequently due to suprapatellar pouch pathology.[30] Patellar clunk syndrome has been defined as parapatellar fibrous nodules on the undersurface of the quadriceps; patient's experience a painful clunk when extending the knee from a flexed position but is usually not a cause of reduced ROM. Patellofemoral synovial hyperplasia is characterized by a more diffuse proliferation of tissue proximal to the patella. It includes pain and crepitus, not clunk, and occurs usually during active knee extension from a flexed position; again ROM is often not affected.[31]

Focal fibroses of the fat pad can be commonly encountered during surgery, yet it does not typically cause severe ROM limitations. Sometimes it can be related to the infrapatellar contracture syndrome (IPCS) with related limited ROM and patellar entrapment.[32] During the surgical procedure, direct visualization of fibrosis can support the clinical diagnosis. Biopsy is not required to make a diagnosis; furthermore, fibrotic tissue in arthrofibrosis may not be discernible from scar tissue. Tissue taken at the time of surgery may be analyzed to have histopathological evidence of fibrosis, but today the ultimate diagnosis remains clinical.[10]

The pathological mechanism of fibrosis is unknown but seems to be an abnormal inflammatory response mediated by myofibroblast cells and transforming growth factor (TGF) 1-β. TGF-β plays a key role in the pathogenesis of arthrofibrosis due to an increased inflammatory reaction with infiltration of inflammatory cells.[33,35] Pftzner et al showed that another protein called bone morphogenetic protein 2 (BMP-2) could have a role in arthrofibrosis and inflammatory reaction, demonstrating an overexpression of BMP-2 in the synovial fluid in arthrofibrotic TKAs.[35] Pftzner et al have been able to show that there is a connection between BMP-2 concentration in the synovial fluid and soft-tissue density of the anterior joint capsule.[36] Freeman et al have showed that arthrofibrotic tissue is composed of a dense fibroblastic region.[34] They suggest that increased inflammatory-associated oxidative stress affords an accumulation of mast cells secreting FGF (fibroblast growth factor), driving fibroblast proliferation and creating avascular regions of hypoxia.

Fibroblasts react to the hypoxic environment and undergo metaplastic transformation to fibrocartilage, followed by HO. Hypoxia and oxidative stress are being considered as potential therapeutic targets for fibrosis. Unterhauser et al described the fibrotic tissue as composed of solid extracellular matrix of collagen fiber network with α-smooth muscle actin (ASMA)-containing fibroblasts. In arthrofibrosis, tissue fibroblast contraction may be involved in tissue fibrosis and contraction with consecutive loss of motion; myofibroblasts could be a future therapeutic target of antifibrosis agents.[37] Brown et al demonstrated that intra-articular injection of Anakinra, an interleukin-1 receptor (IL-1R) antagonist, into patients who developed arthrofibrosis following TKA developed an improvement in ROM and pain with 75% of patients able to return to prior activity levels.[38] The hypothesis mechanism is that IL-1α/β will drive an inflammatory phenotype in fibroblasts isolated from the knee. Dixon et al showed that stimulation with IL-1α/β induced a proinflammatory phenotype in fibroblasts that might have a role in arthrofibrosis.[39]

Complex Regional Pain Syndrome

CRPS is a regional posttraumatic disorder that results in knee pain and stiffness. It is also known as reflex sympathetic dystrophy (RSD). There are two types of CRPS: (type I) without a primary nerve lesion and (type II) resulting of a nerve lesion and characterized by pain in combination with sensory, autonomic, trophic, and motor abnormalities.[40-42] Schutzer and Gossling have defined RSD as an exaggerated response of an extremity to an injury.[43] This response is manifested by four characteristics: (1) intense or unduly prolonged pain, (2) vasomotor disturbances, (3) delayed functional recovery, and (4) trophic changes in the soft tissues. Clinical symptoms of CRPS type I are increased skin temperature, edema, skin color changes, continuous pain, pseudomotor, and motor trophic disturbances.[44,45] It is more common in the upper extremities and, thus, may be underreported in lower extremity cases. Furthermore, any additional surgery performed in this situation, usually, aggravates symptoms. The diagnosis must be confirmed as soon as possible in order to avoid surgical intervention. The molecular mechanism is unclear; prostaglandins and cytokines as well as nervous system play important roles. Prostaglandins are involved in vasoactive processes, pain, and inflammation.[42] Cytokines activate osteoblasts and osteoclasts, which explains the osteoporosis, and drive to sensitization of peripheral nociceptors facilitating the release of neuropeptides from nociceptors.[46] Various criteria sets have been used over time in diagnosing CRPS; currently, the use of the Budapest criteria set is recommended and laboratory tests and radiology are mainly used to exclude another diagnosis.[42,43] A lot of different treatments are mentioned in the literature. Most authors agree that glucocorticoids, NSAIDs, biphosphonates, and dimethylsulfoxide cream can help.[46-48] Metamizole, indomethacin, and diclofenac seem to be more effective than other NSAIDs; paracetamol is not suggested.[42] Antineuropathic pain drugs can be recommended empirically based on the assumption that the pain may be neuropathic. Intravenous long-term ketamine administration has shown efficacy and offers temporary relief from severe pain.[46] The lumbar sympathetic ganglia block has been used to treat chronic pain in CRPS. In a series of 662 primary TKAs, RSD was diagnosed in five patients (0.8%), four of whom demonstrated marked limitation of flexion requiring manipulation during the early postoperative period. Limitation of flexion, along with excessive pain and cutaneous hypersensitivity, should alert the surgeon to the possibility of RSD.[49] Burns et al showed excellent results in patients with CRPS developed after a TKA.[50] All patients received NSAIDs and physiotherapy and, if needed, MUA. Goals of physiotherapy are restoration of ranges of motion, improving strength, and improving function of the affected limb. The patient should be encouraged to bear weight and use the affected limb. Adequate analgesia is mandatory to allow patients to participate in physical therapy, and, if necessary, an opioid should be added. Physiotherapy should start with gentle massage and desensitization treatment. Exercises of isometric strengthening and flexibility should be done to achieve, later, more aggressive range-of-motion exercises and isotonic strengthening.[51] Early diagnosis and treatment of CRPS increase the successful outcome. Patients with clinical signs and symptoms of CRPS should be referred as soon as possible to a physician with expertise in evaluating and treating this condition; multidisciplinary teams (rheumatologists, physical, and occupational therapists) should be involved with these patients.

Heterotopic Ossification

Severe heterotopic ossification (HO) following TKA is rare. Minor HO without clinical symptoms is probably more common but typically does not result in a stiff knee. Toyoda showed that 25 of 63 primary knee replacements

(39%) had postoperative HO, mainly in the region anterior to the distal femur,[52] maybe, due to damage to the cortex or periosteum occurring during the anterior femoral osteotomy. In a second paper, 500 patients undergoing total knee replacement, the incidence of HO was 15%. Only in a small group of patients (1%) with HO was there a significant clinical impact.[53] Furia and Pellegrini reviewed 98 TKAs and found an incidence of minor HO in 26% of cases.[54] For all patients with HO, mean lumbar spine bone mineral density was significantly elevated compared with a matched control group. HO following primary TKA correlates with a limitation of postoperative knee flexion.[54] Daluga noted HO in 17 of the 60 patients (28.3%) whose knees were manipulated and in 1 of the 28 patients in the control group (3.7%). Thirteen of the 17 patients with HO had bilateral procedures performed, but only three had HO in both knees. When compared the bilateral knee scores of the 10 patients with HO, the knee with heterotopic bone did as well or better as the knee without heterotopic bone in 7 of the 10 bilateral cases.[28] Hasegawa et al found HO around the distal femur in 10 (5%) of 221 knees after primary cementless TKA.[55] Lovelock et al found HO in 10% of their 224 knees. However, HO did not cause pain or limitation of motion. Only two patients experienced pain due to its presence in the extensor mechanism (quadriceps).[56] Harwin et al reviewed 158 primary TKAs and found six cases (3.8%) of HO. They recognized two main risk factors: hypertrophic OA and previous HO and suggested prophylactic irradiation or indomethacin treatment in these cases.[57] Rader et al showed HOs in 54 (9%) of 615 cases after TKA.[58] The largest ossifications were located in the anterior distal femur. In 12 cases, smaller ossifications were found in other knee regions. The development of HO showed a positive correlation with hypertrophic arthrosis and a negative correlation with rheumatoid arthritis. Only four patients (four knees) had clinical symptoms; two were successfully operated with removal of the ossification.[58] The cellular mechanism remains still unknown despite the multiple proposed hypotheses.[59,60] The diagnosis is easily made after the radiographic appearance of ossification and usually it does not appear before 6 weeks. The treatment is conservative, mostly physiotherapy aimed to recover ROM. Only in severe cases, with large bony fragments, is surgical removal necessary.

SURGICAL MANAGEMENT

History and physical examination are important to understand the causes of stiffness and to plan the surgery. ROM should be documented in order to characterize the knee joint stiffness in extension or in flexion. Posterior impingement, anterior adhesions, patella baja, or retraction of soft tissue such as joint capsule, quadriceps, and patellar retinaculum can be responsible for limited flexion. Anterior impingement, contracture of anterior and posterior cruciate ligament, or contracture of the posterior capsule may be responsible for limited knee extension.[61] Radiographic preoperative images must include anteroposterior, lateral, and patellar views. Long-axis AP images can be used to measure the mechanical axis of the extremity. Clinical and radiographic data are mandatory in order to achieve a thoughtful surgical plan, to determine the bone stock, the surgical exposure, the quality of soft tissue, and to choose the right implant. In knees affected by flexion contracture, a standard AP radiograph will alter the apparent remaining joint space because the X-ray beams would not be parallel to the joint line. The tibial plateau should be parallel to the X-rays in order to have a true AP position.[62]

SURGICAL EXPOSURE

Exposure begins with the skin incision. An anterior midline skin incision is the best approach, and it should be done with the knee in flexion. If there has been prior surgery, prior scars must be taken into consideration. The bloody supply from the femoral artery passes from medial to lateral across the knee, and in case of multiple prior incisions, the most lateral one would be the safer to use.[63] In case of prior incisions, it is important to not create a short skin bridge between them. A skin bridge between two parallel incisions should be at least 5 to 6 cm.[64] Old transverse incisions can be safety transected at 90°.[65,66] Creating an acute-angle skin flap between to the two incisions, less than 60°, increases the risk of skin necrosis and, when it is possible, should be avoided.[67] Care must be taken not to devascularize the skin edges by excessive retraction and undermining of the skin.

The most common approach to the knee is the medial parapatellar capsule's incision because it can easily be converted in a quadriceps snip or in a V-Y quadriceps-splasty. If the patella is adherent to the distal femur, it can be osteotomized and separated. If necessary, lateral facetectomy can help, in addition to a lateral release. The patella may be everted or merely subluxated laterally without eversion, achieving a good view of the knee in flexion. Everting the patella during the flexion may increase the risk of injury to the patellar tendon, and it is usually not necessary.[16] A headed pin on the patellar tendon insertion can help to avoid the tendon avulsion.[25] Once the capsule has been entered, the medial and lateral gutters must be free from the scar tissue and from the thickened synovial tissue. Wide resection of any fibrous adhesions in the medial and lateral gutter such as in the suprapatellar pouch must be done to achieve a good exposure of the joint. Soft tissue from the posterior aspect of the patellar tendon is removed, and then ligaments and capsular release can be performed in a sequential fashion starting with a subperiosteal release of the MCL. Cruciate ligaments are removed if present because they are often shortened, and posterior-stabilized implants are preferred.[68] The goal is to obtain a knee flexion of 90°

in order to perform appropriate bone cuts on the tibia, femur, and patella to allow insertion of trial components.[25] The general rules for balanced and symmetrical flexion and extension gaps are applied. The aim of the surgery is to create a stable knee with a good ROM.

Patients with flexion contractures will have a normal flexion gap but a narrow gap in extension. This can be corrected by releasing the soft tissue, resecting more distal femur or a combination of bone resecting and tissue release. In contracted knees, a posterior release of the capsule from the posterior tibia and femur can be done. With the knee in flexion, the tibia can be subluxated anteriorly and the capsule is released from the posterior tibial surface using electrocautery for a distance of approximately 1 cm. In the same way, the gastrocnemius and the medial and lateral hamstring can be released. The soft tissues can be released from the posterior aspect of the distal femur using a periosteal elevator. The posterior capsule can be elevated in a proximal direction from the posterior femur, starting from the intercondylar area, and posterior osteophytes behind the posterior condyles are removed with a curve osteotome.

In severely contracted knees, mobilization of the adherent soft tissues must be radical before flexion of the knee, in order to avoid fractures and patellar tendon avulsion. In case of flexion contracture knees, additional bone may be resected from the distal femur to increase the extension gap without a commitment increase in the flexion gap, but it would elevate the joint line and the patella is moved distally.[16,69,70] In general, for each 10° of flexion contracture, an additional 2 mm resection can be taken,[68] and with a posterior-stabilized implant, the joint line can be elevated up to 6 to 10 mm without hindering performance.[16,68] Furthermore, a decrease in the posterior slope of the tibial cut will help in the correction, since every degree of posterior slope equals a degree of residual flexion contracture.[68] Soft-tissue release from the posterior aspect of the knee and a modest proximal migration of the joint line would correct most of flexion contracture deformities.[71,72]

In knees that are stiff in extension, the extensor mechanism is usually contracted and a quadriceps snip or a Coones-Adams inverted V-Y quadricepsplasty may be required in order to obtain a good exposure.[69] Quadriceps snip provides a good exposure, with minimal risk of iatrogenic damage to the extensor mechanism, and it helps to flex the knee during surgery, without alteration in postoperative ROM or weight-bearing. Furthermore, it can be easily extended into a quadriceps V-Y turndown. Coones-Adams inverted V-Y quadricepsplasty is primarily used to lengthen the quadriceps tendon; however, the knee must be immobilized postoperatively, with restricted flexion for 6 weeks, and it is associated with a higher degree of extensor lag.[73] An anterior tibial tuberosity osteotomy (TTO) does not deal with extensor pathology; it can be useful in case of patella baja to raise the patella resulting in a greater flexion.[3,73] TTO does not require restricted flexion if the fixation is stable, but it requires weight-bearing protection with crutches, and it is not recommended for ankylosed knee in which physical therapy or manipulation could lead to complications such as nonunion, fragmentation, would problem over the fixation devices.

Sometimes, in case of excessive release, coronal or flexion instability can be observed due to a greater space in flexion than in extension. Balance in coronal instability should be achieved by additional release on the tighter side of the joint, but, if asymmetrical laxity persists, a constrained implant can be considered. In the stiff knee, extensive posterior soft-tissue release may lead to a flexion instability, which can be addressed by different methods: using a constrained condylar implant, increasing the femoral component size, translating the femoral component posteriorly, or using posterior condylar augments. Simply increasing the thickness of the tibial component makes the knee tight in extension, resulting in a flexion contracture. In the most extreme circumstance, such as in case of preoperative flexion contracture of >30°, in which there is complete instability due to ligaments insufficiency, a rotating hinge prosthesis may be necessary.[68]

Assessing Flexion and Extension at Surgery

Decreased flexion may be associated with a tight flexion gap. Decreased extension may result from a tight extension gap. In a situation in which posterior condyles are underresected or the distal femoral condyles are overresected, the gap will be larger in extension that in flexion. In this scenario, stabilizing the knee in extension with an appropriate thick tibial component will led to a tight knee in flexion. The correct approach should be downsizing the femoral component to open the flexion space and use a thicker tibial insert or use a thinner tibial insert in conjunction with distal femoral augments. The opposite situation would be consequent to a distal femur underresection or a posterior condyle overresection, creating a gap in flexion larger than the gap in extension. In this scenario, stabilizing the knee in flexion will determine a tight knee in extension, and a flexion contracture will be present after the surgery. The correct approach should be performing an additional bone resection of the distal femur. A posterior capsular release could be performed as well in case of preoperative flexion contracture.[12,22]

Restoring posterior tibial slope is necessary to recover the normal anatomy and failure to do so may predispose to tightness in flexion. An oversized femoral component can result in flexion tightness, but the result could also occur with a correct femoral size if it is implanted posteriorly and excessively tightens the flexion gap.[17] In addition, an oversized and posteriorized femoral component can also tension the posterior capsule which can

limit terminal extension. The external rotation of the femoral component may affect flexion gap. Positioning the femoral component along the epicondylar axis creates a rectangular space in flexion. If external rotation is not enough, it can result in a smaller space, during flexion, in the medial compartment, although an excess of external rotation can lead to medial instability in flexion. Achieving a good mechanical axis of the knee is important too. A residual varus or valgus deformity can be consequent of inadequate release of capsular and ligaments structures but also can be consequent of improper bone cuts. This residual deformity may affect the ROM.

Elevation of the joint line can occur with overresection of distal femur and underresection of the tibia. When excessive, it may result to pseudopatella baja that is associated with loss of flexion and patellar pain.[74]

POSTOPERATIVE TKA STIFFNESS TREATMENT

The treatment for stiffness following TKA is guided by its etiology and chronicity. Current methods to improve ROM after TKA include intensive physiotherapy, MUA, arthroscopic or open lysis of adhesions (LOA), and revision TKA. In general, treatment of stiffness in the early postoperative period (6 weeks) favors noninvasive options, such as physical therapy with or without continuous passive motion devices. Failure of these modalities results in utilization of MUA. For patients that suffer with persistent stiffness (>6 months), arthroscopic or open LOA in conjunction with repeat MUA is often considered. Lastly, revision surgery remains the final line of treatment, for patients that have failed all previous other modalities or have component malposition or overstuffing as the determined etiology.

Physical Therapy

Physical therapy rehabilitation remains an integral component of the postoperative care after TKA. The arthrofibrotic knee represents a difficult challenge for the therapist, requiring careful attention and skill to improve functional outcomes. With stiff patients, ROM is the typical limiting factor. As such, the interventions need to prioritize range-of-motion deficits early in order to diminish the chance that fibrotic tissue matures and becomes resistant. An aggressive physical therapy regimen is favorable, as current literature has found aggressive physical therapy is the most influential factor for postoperative flexion.[75,76] A variety of specific physical therapy regimens and adjunctive treatments have been previously described, including usage of NSAIDs, the rest-ice-compression-elevation (RICE) method, continuous passive motion devices, bracing, neuromuscular electrical stimulation, and soft-tissue mobilization.[77]

Manipulation Under Anesthesia

Manipulation under anesthesia (MUA) remains a commonly performed procedure for early-onset postoperative stiffness. Often, MUA is performed multiple times before moving on to another treatment modality. MUA often increases ROM greatly, with a recent systematic review showing an average gain in flexion of 32° and overall gain of 36° ROM before and after MUA.[78] This is in conjunction with a less than 1% complication rate, pooling over 900 patients.[78] In that same review, Gu et al determined the optimal time of MUA performance should be between 4 and 12 weeks following TKA.[78]

MUA should be performed under regional anesthesia, only exerting mild to moderate flexion force. During the manipulation, it is important that the cephalad force exertion occurs under the thigh in order to allow the tibial component to roll beneath the femoral component during knee flexion. This repetitive and progressive flexion should be performed until adhesions are disrupted, with a knee flexion of 120° obtained. While 120° of knee flexion may not be possible based upon the existing preoperative knee flexion, maximal effort should be made to optimize motion during the procedure.[25]

Revision Surgery

In patients that fail previous interventions like an MUA and do not have a mechanical cause of stiffness, LOA is typically the next considered treatment modality. The reported incidence of LOA is 0.8%.[79] The purpose of the procedure is to release adhesions within the suprapatellar pouch, lateral and medial gutters, and the intercondylar notch.[80] However, performance of LOA for an indication of stiffness is not particularly common. In a survey of 82 surgeons, 55% mentioned that they do not perform open or arthroscopic LOA, with only 4% responding that they routinely performed LOA for stiffness.[81] While the rationale for limited performance is most likely multifactorial, one common aspect is the similar gain in ROM seen in patients that receive LOA versus MUA. Prior studies have shown a flexion ROM improvement of 24° to 34°,[5,79,82,83] similar to that gained in MUA. LOA, while widely considered a safe treatment modality, still has risks associated with the procedure.[84]

Lastly, revision TKA is the final treatment option for improving knee functionality in patients with stiffness after primary TKA. A revision TKA is when one or both components are replaced. The previous incidence of revision for arthrofibrosis has been documented as high as 10%.[85] A recent systematic review found that revision surgery results in significant improvement in ROM, functional scores, and pain, but that overall complications rates are high and patients should be advised appropriately.[86]

CONCLUSION

The underlying causes of a stiff knee both before and after TKA are often multifactorial. A combination of patient demographic factors, knee-specific factors, and surgical factors can all contribute to reduced ROM after TKA. A careful patient history and physical, meticulous surgical technique regarding implant sizing and rotation, and ligament balancing are essential to optimizing clinical outcomes. For those patients who develop postsurgical fibrosis, early intervention within 3 months with an MUA appears to be successful in the majority (85%) of patients. For those who do not improve, arthroscopic versus open procedures can be considered, and, for those recalcitrant cases or when malrotation has been identified, revision surgery can be considered. Further research is needed regarding the molecular pathways involved in abnormal scarring and fibrosis so patients can ideally be identified prior to surgery in order to prevent stiffness. These patients may be best managed with pharmacologic adjuncts when additional interventions are needed post TKA.

REFERENCES

1. Abdel MP, Ledford CK, Kobic A, Taunton MJ, Hanssen AD. Contemporary failure aetiologies of the primary, posterior-stabilised total knee arthroplasty. *Bone Joint J.* 2017;99-B(5):647-652. doi:10.1302/0301-620X.99B5.BJJ-2016-0617.R3.
2. Kim JM, Moon MS. Squatting following total knee arthroplasty. *Clin Orthop Relat Res.* 1995;313:177-186.
3. Krackow KA. *Flexion contracture.* In: *The Techniques of Total Knee Arthroplasty.* St. Louis: Mosby; 1990:282-294.
4. Krackow KA. Postoperative period. In: Krackow KA, ed. *The Technique of Total Knee Arthroplasty.* St. Louis: C.V. Mosby; 1990:385-424.
5. Scranton PE Jr. Management of knee pain and stiffness after total knee arthroplasty. *J Arthroplasty.* 2001;16:428-435.
6. Gandhi R, de Beer J, Leone J, Petruccelli D, Winemaker M, Adili A. Predictive risk factors for stiff knees in total knee arthroplasty. *J Arthroplasty.* 2006;21(1):46-52.
7. Yercan HS, Sugun TS, Bussiere C, Ait Si Selmi T, Neyret P. Stiffness after total knee arthroplasty. *J Lyon Chir Genou.* 2004;11:327-336.
8. Christensen CP, Crawford JJ, Olin MD, Vail TP. Revision of the stiff total knee arthroplasty. *J Arthroplasty.* 2002;17(4):409-415.
9. Nelson CL, Kim J, Lotke PA. Stiffness after total knee arthroplasty. *J Bone Joint Surg Am.* 2005;87 suppl 1(pt 2):264-270.
10. Kalson NS, Borthwick LA, Mann DA, et al. International consensus on the definition and classification of the fibrosis of the definition and classification of fibrosis of the knee joint. *Bone Joint J.* 2016;98-B(11):1479-1488.
11. Kurosaka M, Yoshiya S, Mizuno K, et al. Maximizing knee flexion after total knee arthroplasty: the need and the pitfalls. *J Arthroplasty.* 2002;17:59.
12. Manrique J, Gomez MM, Parvizi J. Stiffness after total knee arthroplasty. *J Knee Surg.* 2015;28(2):119-126. doi:10.1055/s-0034-1396079.
13. Le DH, Goodman SB, Maloney WJ, Huddleston JJ. Current modes of failure in TKA: infection, instability, and stiffness predominate. *Clin Orthop Relat Res.* 2014;472(7):2197-2200.
14. Zmistowski B, Restrepo C, Hess J, Adibi D, Cangoz S, Parvizi J. Unplanned readmission after total joint arthroplasty: rates, reasons, and risk factors. *J Bone Joint Surg Am.* 2013;95(20):1869-1876.
15. Scuderi GR. The stiff total knee arthroplasty: causality and solution. *J Arthroplasty.* 2005;20(4 suppl 2):23-26.

16. Scuderi GR, Kochhar T. Management of flexion contracture in total knee arthroplasty. *J Arthroplasty.* 2007;22(4 suppl 1):20-24.

17. Vince KG. The stiff total knee arthroplasty: causes and cures. *J Bone Joint Surg Br.* 2012;94(11 suppl A):103-111. doi:10.1302/0301-620X.94B11.30793.

18. Sharkey PF, Lichstein PM, Shen C, Tokarski AT, Parvizi J. Why are total knee arthroplasty failing today – has anything changed after 10 years? *J Arthroplasty.* 2014;29(9):1774-1778. doi:10.1016/j.arth.2013.07.024.

19. Alves WM Jr, Migon EZ, Zabeu JL. Pain following total knee arthroplasty – a systematic approach. *Rev Bras Ortop.* 2015;45(5):384-391. doi:10.1016/S2255-4971(15)30424-9.

20. Yoo JH, Oh HC, Park SH, Lee S, Lee Y, Kim SH. Treatment of recurrent hemarthrosis after total knee arthroplasty. *Knee Surg Relat Res.* 2018;30(2):147-152. doi:10.5792/ksrr.17.059.

21. Bonnin MP, de Kok A, Verstraete M, et al. Popliteus impingement after TKA may occur with well-sized prostheses. *Knee Surg Sports Traumatol Arthrosc.* 2017;25(6):1720-1730. doi:10.1007/s00167-016-4330-8.

22. Laskin RS, Beksac B. Stiffness after total knee arthroplasty. *J Arthroplasty.* 2004;19(4 suppl 1):41-46.

23. Laskin RS. The Insall Award. Total knee replacement with posterior cruciate ligament retention in patients with a fixed varus deformity. *Clin Orthop Relat Res.* 1996;331:29-34.

24. Okazaki K, Tashiro Y, Mizu-uchi H, Hamai S, Doi T, Iwamoto Y. Influence of the posterior tibial slope on the flexion gap in total knee arthroplasty. *Knee.* 2014;21(4):806-809. doi:10.1016/j.knee.2014.02.019.

25. Sculco TP. *Management of the stiff knee.* In: *The Adult Knee First Edition.* Philadelphia: Lippincott Williams & Wilkins; 2003: 1333-1340.

26. Bonnefoy-Mazure A, Martz P, Armand S, et al. Influence of body mass index on sagittal knee range of motion and gait speed recovery 1-year after total knee arthroplasty. *J Arthroplasty.* 2017;32(8):2404-2410. doi:10.1016/j.arth.2017.03.008.

27. Springer BD, Odum SM, Nagpal VS, et al. Is socioeconomic status a risk factor for stiffness after total knee arthroplasty? A multicenter case-control study. *Orthop Clin North Am.* 2012;43(5):e1-e7.

28. Daluga D, Lombardi AV Jr, Mallory TH, Vaughn BK. Knee manipulation following total knee arthroplasty. Analysis of prognostic variables. *J Arthroplasty.* 1991;6(2):119-128.

29. Dowsey MM, Nikpour M, Dieppe P, Choong PFM. Associations between pre- operative radiographic changes and outcomes after total knee joint replacement for osteoarthritis. *Osteoarthr Cartil.* 2012;20:1095-1102.

30. Klein W, Shan N, Gassen A. Arthroscopic management of postoperative arthrofibrosis of the knee joint: indication, technique, and results. *Arthroscopy.* 1994;10(6):591-597.

31. Dajani KA, Stuart MJ, Dahm DL, Levy AL. Arthroscopic treatment of patellar clunk and synovial hyperplasia after total knee arthroplasty. *J Arthroplasty.* 2010;25(1):97-103.

32. Paulos LE, Rosenberg TD, Drawbert J, Manning J, Abbott P. Infrapatellar contracture syndrome. An unrecognized cause of knee stiffness with patella entrapment and patella infera. *Am J Sports Med.* 1987;15:331-341.

33. Freeman TA, Parvizi J, Della Valle CJ, Steinbeck MJ. Reactive oxygen and nitrogen species induce protein and DNA modifications driving arthrofibrosis following total knee arthroplasty. *Fibrogenesis Tissue Repair.* 2009;2(1):5.

34. Freeman TA, Parvizi J, Dela Valle CJ, Steinbeck MJ. Mast cells and hypoxia drive tissue metaplasia and heterotopic ossification in idiopathic arthrofibrosis after total knee arthroplasty. *Fibrogenesis Tissue Repair.* 2010;3:17.

35. Pfitzner T, Geissler S, Duda G, Perka C, Matziolis G. Increased BMP expression in arthrofibrosis after TKA. *Knee Surg Sports Traumatol Arthrosc.* 2012;20(9):1803-1808.

36. Pfitzner T, Röhner E, Krenn V, Perka C, Matziolis G. BMP-2 dependent increase of soft tissue density in arthrofibrotic TKA. *Open Orthop J.* 2012;6:199-203.

37. Unterhauser FN, Bosch U, Zeichen J, Weiler A. Alpha-smooth muscle actin containing contractile fibroblastic cells in human knee arthrofibrosis tissue. Winner of the AGA-DonJoy Award 2003. *Arch Orthop Trauma Surg.* 2004;124:585-591.

38. Brown CA, Toth AP, Magnussen B. Clinical benefits of intra-articular anakinra for arthrofibrosis. *Orthopedics.* 2010;33:877.

39. Dixon D, Coates J, del Carpio Pons A, et al. A potential mode of action for Anakinra in patients with arthrofibrosis following total knee arthroplasty. *Sci Rep.* 2015;5:16466. doi:10.1038/srep16466.

40. Harden RN, Bruehl S, Stanton-Hicks M, Wilson PR. Proposed new diagnostic criteria for complex regional pain syndrome. *Pain Med.* 2007;8:326-331.

41. Marinus J, Moseley GL, Birklein F, et al. Clinical features and pathophysiology of complex regional pain syndrome. *Lancet Neurol.* 2011;10:637-648.

42. Van der Veen P. CRPS: a contingent hypothesis with prostaglandins as crucial conversion factor. *Med Hypotheses.* 2015;85(5):568-575.

43. Schutzer SF, Gossling HR. The treatment of reflex sympathetic dystrophy syndrome. *J Bone Joint Surg Am.* 1984;66(4):625-629.

44. Van Bussel CM, Stronks DL, Huygen FJ. Complex regional pain syndrome type I of the knee: a systematic literature review. *Eur J Pain.* 2014;18(6):766-773.

45. Schlereth T, Drummond PD, Birklein F. Inflammation in CRPS: role of the sympathetic supply. *Auton Neurosci.* 2014;182:102-107.

46. Żyluk A, Puchalski P. Effectiveness of complex regional pain syndrome treatment: a systematic review. *Neurol Neurochir Pol.* 2018;52(3):326-333. pii:S0028-3843(18) 30017-3.

47. Birklein F, Dimova V. Complex regional pain syndrome-up-to-date. *Pain Rep.* 2017;2(6):e624.

48. Robinson JN, Sandom J, Chapman PT. Efficacy of pamidronate in complex regional pain syndrome type I. *Pain Med.* 2004;5(3):276-280.

49. Katz MM, Hungerford DS, Krackow KA, Lennox DW. Reflex sympathetic dystrophy as a cause of poor results after total knee arthroplasty. *J Arthroplasty.* 1986;1(2):117-124.

50. Burns AW, Parker DA, Coolican MR, Rajaratnam K. Complex regional pain syndrome complicating total knee arthroplasty. *J Orthop Surg.* 2006;14(3):280-283.

51. Rho RH, Brewer RP, Lamer TJ, Wilson PR. Complex regional pain syndrome. *Mayo Clin Proc.* 2002;77(2):174-180.

52. Toyoda T, Matsumoto H, Tsuji T, Kinouchi J, Fujikawa K. Heterotopic ossification after total knee arthroplasty. *J Arthroplasty.* 2003;18(6):760-764.

53. Dalury DF, Jiranek WA. The incidence of heterotopic ossification after total knee arthroplasty. *J Arthroplasty,* 2004;19(4):447-452.

54. Furia JP, Pellegrini VD. Heterotopic ossification following primary total knee arthroplasty. *J Arthroplasty.* 1995;10(4):413-419, .

55. Hasegawa M, Ohashi T, Uchida A. Heterotopic ossification around distal femur after total knee arthroplasty. *Arch Orthop Trauma Surg.* 2002;122(5):274-278. doi:10.1007/s00402-001-0377-0.

56. Lovelock JE, Griffiths HJ, Silverstein AM, Anson PS. Complications of total knee replacement. *AJR Am J Roentgenol.* 1984;142:985-992.

57. Harwin SF, Stein AJ, Stern RE, Kulick RG. Heterotopic ossification following primary total knee arthroplasty. *J Arthroplasty.* 1993;8(2):113-116.

58. Rader CP, Berthel T, Haase M, Scheidler M, Eulert J. Heterotopic ossification after total knee arthroplasty. 54/615 cases after 1-6 years' follow-up. *Acta Orthop Scand.* 1997;68(1):46-50.

59. Jowsey J, Coventry MB, Robins PR. Heterotopic ossification: theoretical considerations, possible etiologic factors, and a clinical review of total hip arthroplasty patients exhibiting this phenomenon. In: Murray WR, ed. *The Hip: Proceedings of the Fifth Open Scientific Meeting of the Hip Society.* St. Louis: CV Mosby; 1977:210-221.

60. Tornkvist H, Nilsson OS, Bauer FC, Lindholm TS. Experimentally induced heterotopic ossification in rats influenced by anti-inflammatory drugs. *Scand J Rheumatol.* 1983;12:177-180.

61. Pujol N, Bisrenoult P, Beaufils P. Post-traumatic stiffness: surgical techniques. *Orthop Traumatol Surg Res.* 2015;101(1 suppl):S179-S186. doi:10.1016/j.otsr.2014.06.026.

62. Lotke PA, Simon RG. *Flexion contracture in total Knee arthroplasty.* In: *Knee Arthroplasty Handbook.* USA: Springer Verlag; 2006:57-69.

63. Colombel M, Mariz Y, Dahhan P, Kénési C. Arterial and lymphatic supply of the knee integuments. *Surg Radiol Anat.* 1998;20(1):35-40.

64. Stern SH, Moeckel BH, Insall JN. Total knee arthroplasty in valgus knee. *Clin Orthop Relat Res.* 1991;273:5-8.

65. Windsor RE, Insall JN, Vince KG. Technical considerations of total knee arthroplasty after proximal tibial osteotomy. *J Bone Joint Surg Am.* 1988;70(4):547-555.

66. Vaishya R, Vijay V, Demesugh DM, Agarwal AK. Surgical approaches for total knee arthoroplasty. *J Clin Orthop Trauma.* 2016;7(2):71-79. doi:10.1016/j.jcot.2015.11.003.

67. Della Valle CJ, Berger RA, Rosenberg AG. Surgical exposures in revision total knee arthroplasty. *Clin Orthop Relat Res.* 2006;446:59-68.

68. Su EP. Fixed flexion deformity and total knee arthroplasty. *J Bone Joint Surg Br.* 2012;94(11 suppl A):112-115. doi:10.1302/0301-620X.94B11.30512.

69. Mihalko WM, Whiteside LA. Bone resection and ligament treatment for flexion contracture in knee arthroplasty. *Clin Orthop Relat Res.* 2003;406:141-147.

70. Debette C, Lusting S, Servien E, et al. Total knee arthroplasty of the stiff knee: three hundred and four cases. *Int Orthop.* 2014;38(2):285-289. doi:10.1007/s00264-013-2252-3.

71. Whiteside LA, Mihalko WM. Surgical procedure for flexion contracture and recurvatum in total knee arthroplasty. *Clin Orthop Relat Res.* 2002;404:189-195.

72. Bellemans J, Vendenneucker H, Victor J, Vanlauwe J. Flexion contracture in total knee arthroplasty. *Clin Orthop Relat Res.* 2006;452:78-82.

73. Thienpont E. Revision knee surgery technique. *Effort Open Rev.* 2016;1(5):233-238. doi:10.1302/2058-5241.1.000024.

74. Chonko DJ, Lombardi AV Jr, Berend KR. Patella baja and total knee arthroplasty (TKA): etiology, diagnosis, and management. *Surg Technol Int.* 2004;12:231-238.

75. Shoji H, Solomonow M, Yoshino S, D'Ambrosia R, Dabezies E. Factors affecting postoperative flexion in total knee arthroplasty. *Orthopedics.* 1990;13:643-649.

76. Mauerhan DR, Mokris JG, Ly A, Kiebzak GM. Relationship between length of stay and manipulation rate after total knee arthroplasty. *J Arthroplasty.* 1998;13:896-900.

77. Cheuy VA, Foran JRH, Paxton RJ, Bade MJ, Zeni JA, Stevens-Lapsley JE. Arthrofibrosis associated with total knee arthroplasty. *J Arthroplasty.* 2017;32(8):2604-2611. doi:10.1016/j.arth.2017.02.005.

78. Gu A, Michalak AJ, Cohen JS, Almeida ND, McLawhorn AS, Sculco PK. Efficacy of manipulation under anesthesia for stiffness following total knee arthroplasty: a systematic review. *J Arthroplasty.* 2018;33(5):1598-1605. doi:10.1016/j.arth.2017.11.054.

79. Tjoumakaris FP, Tucker BS, Post Z, Pepe MD, Orozco F, Ong AC. Arthroscopic lysis of adhesions for the stiff total knee: results after failed manipulation. *Orthopedics.* 2014;37:e482-e487.

80. Hegazy AM, Elsoufy MA. Arthroscopic arthrolysis for arthrofibrosis of the knee after total knee replacement. *HSS J* 2011;7:130-133.

81. Vun SH, Shields DW, Sen A, Shareef S, Sinha S, Campbell AC. A national questionnaire survey on knee manipulation following total knee arthroplasty. *J Orthop.* 2015;12:193-196.

82. Jerosch J, Aldawoudy AM. Arthroscopic treatment of patients with moderate arthrofibrosis after total knee replacement. *Knee Surg Sports Traumatol Arthrosc.* 2007;15:71-77.

83. Schwarzkopf R, William A, Deering RM, Fitz W. Arthroscopic lysis of adhesions for stiff total knee arthroplasty. *Orthopedics.* 2013;36:e1544-e1548.

84. Enad JG. Arthroscopic lysis of adhesions for the stiff total knee arthroplasty. *Arthrosc Tech.* 2014;3:e611-e614.

85. Schroer WC, Berend KR, Lombardi AV, et al. Why are total knees failing today? Etiology of total knee revision in 2010 and 2011. *J Arthroplasty.* 2013;28:116-119.

86. Cohen JC, Gu A, Lopez NS, Park MS, Fehring KA, Sculco PK. Efficacy of revision surgery for the treatment of stiffness after total knee arthroplasty: a systematic review. *J Arthroplasty.* 2018;33:3049-3055.

chapter 55

Preventing Wound Complications After Total Knee Arthroplasty

Fred D. Cushner, MD I Shazaan F. Hushmendy, MD

Proper wound healing is essential for a successful total knee arthroplasty (TKA). Should wound failure occur, complications such as prosthetic infection or wound defects requiring a complex plastic surgery reconstruction may occur. This often results in lengthy hospital stays, decreased function, and failed expectations of both the patient and physician. This chapter focuses on the prevention of wound failure, detection, and treatment options.

VASCULAR SUPPLY TO THE KNEE

Under normal circumstances, the blood supply to the anterior aspect of the knee consists of a random plexus of perforating blood vessels. These vessels, the extraosseous parapatellar anastomotic ring,[1-5] are formed by six main perforating arteries originating from the popliteal artery (**Fig. 55-1**). In addition, three extrinsic vessels contribute to the blood supply of the knee. (1) The first extrinsic vessel consists of branches of the profunda femoris and the vessel supplying the rectus femoris, vastus intermedius, and vastus lateralis that via a dermal plexus supplies the inferior aspect of the knee. (2) Supreme genicular vessels originate from the superficial femoral artery and develop into the musculoarticular branch and the saphenous artery. The musculoarticular branch supplies the medial aspect of the joint as well as the medial superior skin and the saphenous artery terminates to supply the area of skin just below the medial plateau. (3) The third extrinsic vessel is a recurrent branch of the anterior tibial artery that supplies the skin lateral to the patellar tendon.

PREVENTION OF WOUND COMPLICATIONS

Based on the anatomy described above, the skin surrounding the knee has both a medial and lateral vascular distribution. The musculoarticular branches supply the medial skin, whereas the anterior tibial artery has a lateral distribution. A random, plentiful blood supply exists, and under most circumstances, the skin around the knee can tolerate a single midline incision such as that required for TKA. However, many factors exist that can compromise proper wound healing. These factors can be divided into patient systemic factors, local factors, surgical technique factors, and postoperative factors.

Systemic Factors

A thorough history and physical examination are required before performing the indicated TKA. Although emphasis is often placed upon the patient's cardiac or pulmonary status, equally important is the wound healing potential of the individual patient. Of utmost importance is the vascular status of the involved limb. Because of the ambulatory limitations of an arthritic knee, claudication symptoms may not be present despite significantly impaired blood flow. Therefore, physical examination should include evaluation of the skin around the knee and a thorough vascular examination of the limb should be performed. Atrophic changes, decreased hair growth, inadequate pulses, and presence of skin discoloration should be noted. The preoperative X-rays may also provide a clue of vascular compromise through the identification of calcified blood vessels and evidence of arterial sclerosis. A vascular surgery consult may be necessary to evaluate for the potential of vascular reconstruction. Changes in normal TKA protocols may also be required, for example, the use of an arterial tourniquet may be contraindicated or preoperative intravenous heparin may be required to aid in maintaining the patency of previously reconstructed vessels. In other instances, preoperative arteriograms may be required to document adequate blood flow or normal anatomy as is the case in congenital absence of the patella.

Large vessel arterial calcifications identified on preoperative radiographs are of important significance for ischemic complications in patients undergoing a TKA such as an increased risk for protracted wound healing and arterial thrombosis. If identified, it is important to consider performing a TKA without the use of a tourniquet. There is contentious debate in literature as to whether the use of a tourniquet will adversely affect the patient's TKA. Rupture of preexisting plaques, potential occlusion of peripheral arteries and possible intimal tear of large vessels is a concern; however, many studies have shown no deterioration in ankle-brachial indices (ABIs) of patient with peripheral vascular disease with the use of a tourniquet.[6]

Another factor to consider before surgery is anemia. Although debatable, anemia has been thought to play a role in wound healing,[7,8] with wounds in patients

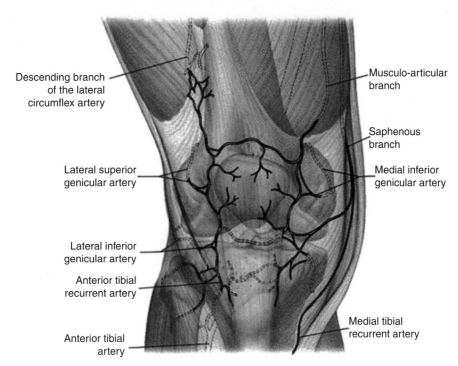

Descending branch
of the lateral
circumflex artery

Musculo-articular
branch

Saphenous
branch

Lateral superior
genicular artery

Medial inferior
genicular artery

Lateral inferior
genicular artery

Anterior tibial
recurrent artery

Medial tibial
recurrent artery

Anterior tibial
artery

FIGURE 55-1   Blood supply of the knee demonstrating the extraosseous parapatellar anastomotic ring.

with a hematocrit less than 35% thought to be in jeopardy[9] because of a decrease in oxygen tension at the skin edges of the surgical wound.[9,10] Heughan et al concluded that anemia is well tolerated and that mild to moderate anemia does not adversely impair oxygen delivery in wound healing[11]; however, this does not mean that preoperative anemia should be ignored. In fact, it is now protocol in our institution to evaluate a patient's hemoglobin level before performing the indicated TKA and those with preoperative anemia receiving erythropoietin supplementation before surgery. Patients with hemoglobin levels of more than 10 and less than 13 receive 40,000 units of erythropoietin for 1 to 3 weeks before surgery in conjunction with iron supplementation (**Fig. 55-2**). This approach is an attempt to maximize preoperative blood levels, thus limiting exposure to allogeneic transfusions. Furthermore, by limiting transfusion requirements, there may also play a role in avoiding wound complications and surgical site infections.[12]

Preexisting medical conditions should also be of concern to the treating physician. Not only should conditions such as chronic venostasis be noted on physical examination, but also a history of venous ulceration. Diagnosis of human immunodeficiency virus infection should also be recorded.[13] Lehman et al noted increased infection in human immunodeficiency virus patients undergoing total joint arthroplasty.[14] Although human immunodeficiency virus should not prevent TKA, discussion should take place before TKA regarding increased evidence of wound failure potential.

A patient's nutritional status may play a role in wound healing potential. Albumin levels (less than 3.5 g per dL) as well as total lymphocyte count (less than 1500) may make a patient more prone to wound failure.[15,16] Once a decreased nutritional status is documented, these deficiencies should be corrected before surgery. Furthermore, it is important to realize that obese patients can demonstrate laboratory criteria of malnutrition and potential wound complications,[17-20] due to excess caloric intake of nutrient-poor foods. Moreover, surgical exposure in a morbidly obese patient is technically more difficult because of the abundant adipose tissue as well as physical limitations on knee flexion and joint exposure. Because

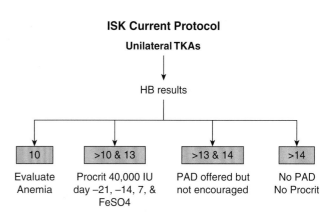

ISK Current Protocol

Unilateral TKAs

HB results

10	>10 & 13	>13 & 14	>14
Evaluate Anemia	Procrit 40,000 IU day −21, −14, 7, & FeSO4	PAD offered but not encouraged	No PAD No Procrit

FIGURE 55-2   Preoperative protocol currently recommended at the author's institution. An emphasis is made on maximizing the patient's blood levels before surgery. FeSO$_4$, ferrous sulfate; HB, hemoglobin; ISK, Insall-Scott-Kelly; PAD, preoperative autologous donations; TKA, total knee arthroplasty. (Procrit: Janssen Pharmaceuticals, Titusville, NJ.)

of these limitations, more vigorous skin retraction may be required. The relationship between body mass index (BMI) and prosthetic joint injection from wound issues has been well studied in the literature.[18,21] Obese patients have demonstrated increased wound drainage postoperatively.[22,23] In 2014, a prospective study by Dowsey and Choong demonstrated that patients with a BMI >40 kg/m^2 has a nine-time greater risk of periprosthetic joint infection (PJI).[24] Despite these findings, obesity is not a contraindication for TKA. Stern and Insall[25] showed no difference in wound complications with TKA and obese patients. This same cohort of patients was examined at a 10-year follow-up, and once again, no increase in wound difficulties was noted.[26] It should be mentioned that even though anthropometric measurements have been established for malnutrition, their use is still limited with no standardized parameters. An emphasis should be on proper tissue handling in the obese patient during surgery. Heavy-tooth forceps and crushing clamps should be avoided, as should excessive skin retraction. Retraction should be intermittent, when applied, to avoid local edema, which may complicate blood flow to the wound edges.

One modifiable risk factor that can be controlled is cigarette smoking. By inhibiting skin microcirculation, cigarette smoking can compromise skin circulation.[27-29] Furthermore, multiple studies describe the detrimental effects of smoking with its increase in reoperation rates, implant loosening, deep infections, and mortality.[30] Because of the lengthy vasoconstrictor effects, cessation of smoking must occur more than 4 weeks before surgery for some benefit to occur.[27-29] After cessation for 4 weeks, the patient's metabolic and immune functions start to normalize, which helps decrease the morbidity and mortality compared to a patient that continues to smoke.[31-33] Postoperatively, the patient should continue to be a nonsmoker by attending smoking cessations programs or counseling sessions. These programs have shown to reduce the rate of smoking before and up to 6 months after surgery which can help reduce the incidence of postoperative complications.[34-36]

Certain medical comorbidities may interfere with wound healing. Wong et al demonstrated delay in wound healing in the diabetic patient, with increased wound separation, erythema, and swelling noted.[37] These healing delays may be secondary to delayed collagen synthesis that results in delayed wound tensile strength. Peripheral vasoconstriction in both large and small vessels may also contribute. Wilson et al found no increased risk for infection after TKA in diabetic patients.[22] Controversy also exists with regard to wound healing and rheumatoid arthritis patients. Although Wong and associates[37] found a 30% complication rate in rheumatoid arthritis compared with osteoarthritic patients, this conflicts with the data of Garner and associates,[38] in which no delay in wound healing was noted. It is unclear whether corticosteroids

used to treat rheumatoid arthritis interfered with wound healing rather than the disease itself. Wilson et al demonstrated wound healing difficulty in rheumatoid arthritis patients but only in those treated with corticosteroids.[22] No difference in wound healing was reported when corticosteroids were not used. It has been our experience that rheumatoid arthritis skin is fragile, and caution should be exercised in tissue handling as well as with the placement and removal of adherent drapes.

Recognition of systemic factors before surgery can aid in their correction, thus improving wound healing potential.

Local Factors

Wound healing potential includes not only the location of previously placed skin incisions but other factors such as the degree of deformity, rotational element of deformity, skin adherence, or history of previous trauma such as burns. Multiple studies have shown increased wound healing problems in knees with numerous incisions.[39,40] Problems arise when an avascular bridge exists between the new and previous incision. Not all complications occur in knees with multiple incisions. Any knee with decreased subcutaneous tissue, in particular the hypodermis layer which contains loose connective tissue and fat lobules, has decreased skin elasticity, which may put a wound at risk. This includes patients with significant long bone trauma or a history of burns. Large rotary deformities may also place a patient at risk for wound failure, with inadequate skin available for closure after the rotary and varus–valgus deformities are corrected.

Surgical Technique Factors

Although local factors can be identified but not always modified, surgical technique factors can be modified to enhance wound healing potential. To begin, an adequate skin exposure should be chosen. Even though the patient and physician want to avoid long incisions, the incision should be extensive enough to avoid excessive skin retraction. In addition, the skin should be handled gently to preserve the subcutaneous fascial layer. Large flaps should be avoided, and no lateral flaps should be required though occasionally adhesions may be present in the subcutaneous layer of valgus deformities that require release. This should be done only on an as-needed basis. If a flap becomes necessary, it should be minimal and as deep as possible to help preserve the blood flow to this dermal plexus.

A lateral release during a TKA is not a benign procedure. Many studies have shown that patients having a lateral release have a decrease in the skin oxygen at the wound healing edges resulting in wound healing complications.[10] With the use of proper component position, appropriate patella thickness, and correct component rotation, the lateral release rate can be decreased. Despite this, a lateral release may be required that can result in the disruption of the superior genicular vessels. Johnson and Eastwood[10] noted a decrease in skin oxygen tension when the lateral release was performed. As a result of this lateral release, the rate of superficial drainage and infection rates were also increased in those patients. At the author's institution, if a lateral release is required, a lateral flap is avoided. We prefer an all-inside approach from the middle flap to help seal the postoperative hematoma inside the joint. If a large flap is performed in conjunction with a lateral release, the postoperative hematoma is allowed egress through the lateral release site underneath the subcutaneous level. This may present increased pressure on the skin and may lead to prolonged postoperative drainage, and in these cases, a subcutaneous drain should be considered.

With no previous incision, the midline approach is preferred. Johnson[41] and Dennis[42] evaluated skin oxygen tension for a variety of incisions (midline, medial parapatellar, medial curved) and concluded that a medial-side circulation predominance existed in the cutaneous circulation. The lateral aspect of the skin incision demonstrated lower skin oxygen tension throughout the postoperative period. By postoperative day 8, preoperative skin oxygen levels returned to normal, which is another factor why a lateral incision should be avoided. Previously placed skin incisions make initial incisions more difficult. If avoidance is not possible, we attempt to incorporate the new incision within the old. If parallel incisions exist, choose the most lateral one. Transverse incisions can be crossed, in most instances at 90° angles with really no threat to the local skin blood supply.[2,42,43] If a wide scar with minimal subcutaneous tissue is present, the knee may be at risk because it disrupts the underling dermal plexus.[42] If this occurs, treatment should include soft tissue expanders. Of importance during surgical technique is the distance between previous incisions. If the skin bridge is less than 2.5 cm, tissue expanders should be considered. Skin bridges of less than 2 cm may result in tissue necrosis between the previous incisions and the new incision (**Fig. 55-3**). Other technical factors include repair of the medial retinaculum. It is commonplace in our institution to perform flexion of the knee after closing the retinaculum to evaluate the suture integrity. If the sutures break under direct visualization, these can be replaced before closure of the more superficial layers. If this is difficult at the time of surgery, new skin closure systems are available that may be helpful (**Fig. 55-4**). Currently, a variety of skin closure methods are being used. Surgeons can choose between skin staples, monocryl, and monoderm (quill suture device). Utilization of skin glue after a monoderm skin closure is routine practice in our institution.

Postoperative Factors

As with surgical factors, postoperative factors can be manipulated to aid in wound healing potential. Avoiding hemarthrosis is of utmost concern, as a large hematoma

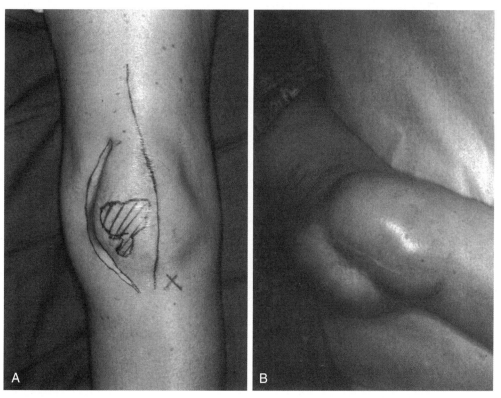

FIGURE 55-3 Fifty-year-old woman with numerous previous incisions as well as a potential avascular skin bridge. **A:** Patient before tissue expander. **B:** Tissue expander in place.

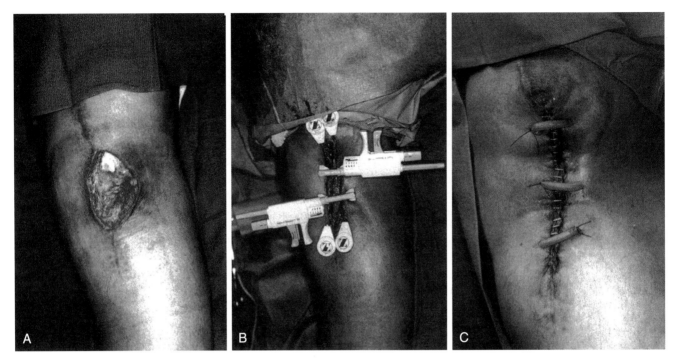

FIGURE 55-4   Use of wound stretching device to aid in closure. **A:** Skin defect with exposed extensor tendons. **B:** Stretching device applying traction to the skin edges. **C:** Closure obtained without excessive tension.

can serve as a culture medium for infection and may also lead to local skin compromise because of the tension placed on the subcutaneous tissue. In an attempt to avoid hemarthrosis, some authors deflate the tourniquet before the closure while other authors have concluded that intraoperative tourniquet deflation actually leads to increased blood loss compared with a tourniquet deflated at the close of the case.[42]

Postoperative drains may also play a role in preventing postoperative drainage. Holt and coworkers examined blood loss and wound problems in both drained and undrained TKAs.[4] In this study, 40% of the undrained knees and 0% of the drained knees required dressing reinforcement. The undrained knees also had a higher incidence of ecchymosis, and these authors concluded that drains are effective in preventing the accumulation of blood in the surrounding soft tissues. Crevoisier and colleagues[44] concluded that after they examined 32 patients, there was no advantage of closed-suction drainage, though this was a small study of only 32 patients and probably of insufficient size to derive a conclusion on the risk of wound infections. Ovadia and associates evaluated 58 patients after TKA placed into drained and undrained groups.[45] Although there was little difference in the rate of infection, there was more serous discharge in the undrained group. At our institution, we use postoperative drainage, which we believe not only avoids hemarthrosis but also provides reinfusion benefits. With the use of reinfusion drains, the allogeneic transfusion rate has been reduced to approximately 2% to 3% for the unicompartmental knee.[46] The drain is removed on postoperative day 1, and postoperative antibiotics are

used for the first 24 hours while the drain is in place. This is important as Drinkwater and Neil have shown an increase in bacterial colonization with drains left in for longer than 24 hours.[47]

Concerns have been raised over bleeding complications with postoperative deep venous thrombosis prophylaxis. It should be noted that bleeding complications occurred even before low-molecular-weight heparins were used for deep venous thrombosis prophylaxis. For example, Stulberg and associates,[48] looking at 638 TKAs, saw a wound complication rate of 18.1% and a drainage rate of 10.6%. Studies using low-molecular-weight heparin note bleeding complication rates of 2% to 5% in the literature.[49-51] It should be noted that bleeding problems are multifactorial. Some wound complications can be avoided with careful hemostasis, proper dosing of anticoagulation agents, and meticulous closure. Review of these papers shows that the bleeding complications are poorly defined and are often not stratified with regard to presence or absence of lateral release, presence or absence of varus release, timing of medications, and the dose. In our experience with a watertight closure in the subcutaneous layer in conjunction with aggressive stapling of the skin edges, postoperative hematoma and wound complications have not been a problem even with the use of low-molecular-weight heparin (enoxaparin) when this was our choice for deep vein thrombosis (DVT) prophylaxis.

Another postoperative modality that has raised concern for wound healing potential is the continuous passive motion (CPM) machine. Benowitz and Jacob[27] showed a decrease in oxygen tension when the CPM machine was past 40° during the first 3 days.[52] Although skin oxygen tension was noted to be decreased, our experience with an aggressive CPM protocol showed no increase in wound complications. Yashar[53] also found no increase in problems with an accelerated flexion program. In this case, 70° to 100° was used immediately in the recovery room with no increase in wound complications noted. Although the average patient can probably tolerate a CPM machine on a high-flexion program, in a patient with a history of potential wound complications, perhaps CPM machine use should be modified. Currently, the use of a CPM machine for routine TKA's has been largely abandoned, and this is mentioned for historic review.

Finally, a major contribution to the field of joint arthroplasty has been the use of tranexamic acid (TXA), an antifibrinolytic agent. There is no shortage of studies describing its effectiveness with reduction of blood loss, hemoglobin level and blood transfusion requirements.[54-56] Multiple randomized control trials have demonstrated the use of perioperative intravenous TXA comparable to topical and more recently oral form of the drug.[55,57] Currently, the orthopedic community has published a set of guidelines to try and standardize the use of TXA in arthroplasty procedures. Fillingham et al published eight recommendations (**Table 55-1**) to demonstrate how TXA has become the "standard of care" in arthroplasty surgery.[58]

With the use of TXA reducing blood loss, it will be important to see its effect on postoperative hematoma and wound complications. A study by Kim et al describes the combinative use of TXA with rivaroxaban showing a decrease in wound complications when compared to rivaroxaban without TXA use.[59]

Wound complications can be prevented or decreased by understanding the local vascular anatomy and by manipulating systemic, local, surgical, and postoperative factors. Maximizing each of these factors will lead to prevention of wound healing problems.

TREATMENT

Treatment of wound healing failures depends on the etiology and conditions noted. Despite optimizing all systemic and local factors and initiating postoperative protocols to enhance wound healing, a small number of patients still demonstrate wound healing failure. When this occurs, the surgeon is left with treating the wound complication and maintaining a functional prosthesis. Wound complications are divided into serous drainage, tense hematoma, superficial tissue necrosis, and full-thickness necrosis. These conditions can occur with or without the presence of infection or with or without prosthesis exposure. When dealing with any wound compromise, infection must be ruled out or treated before picking coverage options.

Because not all factors can be corrected before surgery, even the best of surgeons cannot erase the effects of previously placed incisions or local changes from previous trauma. Therefore, prevention at our institution often involves the use of a soft tissue expander, and we reported our initial results.[60] The skin was gradually expanded for an average of 64.5 days before the indicated TKA. All wounds healed without incident. A long-term follow-up of the use of soft tissue expanders around the knee was recently reported by Manifold et al.[61] In this study, soft tissue expanders were used on 29 knees in 27 patients before TKA and followed up at 34 and 44 months. The average Knee Society score for these patients was 83.7. Although one major wound complication occurred during tissue expansion, necessitating abandonment of the planned arthroplasty, no major wound complications occurred in those patients who underwent knee arthroplasty. Based on this study, we continue to use soft tissue expanders when the potential for wound healing failure exists, such as knees with numerous previous incisions, significant varus rotational angulations, posttraumatic

TABLE 55-1	**Summary of TXA Guidelines**[58]	
Number	**Questions**	**Strength of Recommendation**
1	Systemic, local, and oral tranexamic acid (TXA) administration is effective in reducing blood loss and transfusion requirement	Strong
2	Systemic, local, and oral delivery of TXA are equivalent in efficacy	Strong
3	Efficacy proven for various doses and topical application	Strong
4	No benefit of multiple or additional doses	Strong
5	TXA is more efficacious when given prior to skin incision	Moderate
6	No increased deep vein thrombosis (DVT) rate in patients without a known history of venous thromboembolism (VTE) for all forms of dosing	Strong
7	Patients with higher comorbidity burden do not have increased risk of developing adverse events with DVT dosing	Moderate
8	All forms of dosing do not increase the risk of developing an arterial thromboembolic event (ATE)	Moderate

injury, decreased skin elasticity, or decreased subcutaneous tissue. In short, we use this technique in any knee we think has a potential to fail. During this long-term study, we began using subcutaneous drains at the time of TKA because two knees were taken back for hematoma. The drain evacuation was left in place until the drainage significantly decreased. Since adding this to our protocol, no further evacuation of postoperative hematoma has been needed. The criteria of soft tissue expanders may be subjective, but any patient with adherent immobile skin or anyone with a previous skin incision is considered a candidate for this procedure. Only mild complications have been noted using this technique, and it continues to be our mainstay for those knees with high wound failure potential.

Before development of this technique, a sham incision was used. This was reported in the past for those patients thought to have high wound necrosis potential. This incision consists of a midline incision to the depth of the subcutaneous tissue. Skin flaps were elevated, and the wound closed in a standard fashion. The wound was then observed to see if skin healed without incident. It was thought that if the wound could heal without incident, a TKA could be performed safely. Obviously, if the wound failed, local measures could be used to obtain healing without the increased pressure of an exposed prosthesis. The sham incision is mentioned for historical reasons and is no longer used at our institution.

TECHNIQUE OF TISSUE EXPANSION

For those patients who would benefit from soft tissue expansion, this procedure is performed before performing the TKA in the operating room (**Fig. 55-5**). The first step is to inject the subcutaneous space with fluid. This hydrodissection separates the subcutaneous planes from the skin above. We currently use a mixture of lidocaine (Xylocaine) (0.05%) and 1/1,000,000 epinephrine. Usually, 300 mL is injected into the subcutaneous space. Injection is continued until the subcutaneous tissue is noted to blanch. A small incision is then made in line with the planned TKA. Based on the location of the adherent skin or previous incisions, two tissue expanders are used. If two expanders are used, they can be placed at 90° angles to each other, and each expander typically has a 200-mm capacity. The placement of the tissue expanders can be adjusted according to the patient's specific needs. Using blunt dissection, a subcutaneous pocket is created, and the expander balloon is inserted. Currently, we admit the patient for 24 hours and place the patient in a knee

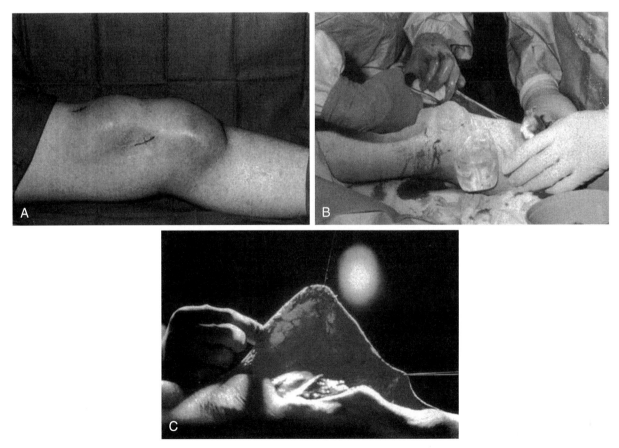

FIGURE 55-5   Sixty-seven-year-old woman after completing the tissue expansion process. **A:** Expander in place. **B:** Expander easily removed at the time of total knee arthroplasty. **C:** Abundant skin with enhanced vasculature noted.

immobilizer for 1 week. When this week is completed, gradual expansion is started, and on an average, 10% of the expanded volume is injected weekly. Injection speed is based on the patient's comfort as well as the presence of capillary refill of 5 seconds or less over the expander surface. As long as the patient tolerates the expansion, expander volume can be increased. Surgery is performed 2 weeks after the last expansion injection. These expanders do not present a problem when removed at the time of surgery (**Fig. 55-6**). Based on previous experience, our current recommendations are the placement of drains in the deep, as well as subcutaneous pouches left by the tissue expander. With regard to skin incision and expansion,

the choice exists of using the old incision or creating a new one. When possible, the incision deemed more adequate is used. We have found that tissue expanders enhance a vascularity of the flap in the old incision; if the prior incision is not adequate, a new longitudinal incision is chosen. If excessive skin is present after tissue expansion, the remaining edges are reapproximated. We have often found this is necessary. Certainly, the elastic skin contracts with time and in most cases no skin débridements are required.

This technique has been reported by other authors, mostly in case reports with revision TKA.[3,62] While allowing primary closure without tension, standard TKA

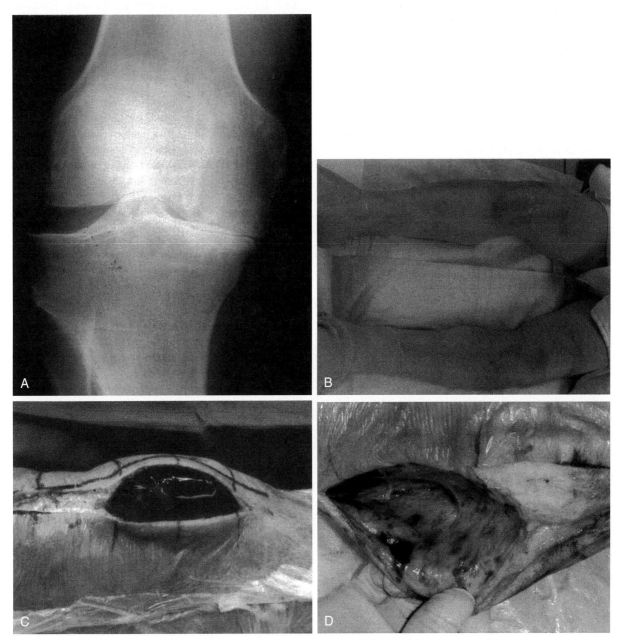

FIGURE 55-6   A: Preoperative X-rays demonstrating rotational varus deformity. **B:** Clinical appearance of limb demonstrating a rotary deformity as well as varus alignment. **C:** Preoperative photo after tissue expander placement. **D:** Pseudomembrane that forms secondary to tissue expander use.

protocols can be followed with the emphasis on postoperative range of motion and function. More importantly, invasive procedures such as free flaps can be avoided. Although potential complications such as hematoma and infection of prosthesis, as well as prosthesis failure exist with this technique, they can be limited. Benefits of tissue expansion include primary closure without tension, immediate range of motion, ability to use CPM, and the avoidance of disfiguring and reconstructive procedures such as flap coverage.

TREATMENT OF A POSTOPERATIVE DRAINING WOUND

One type of wound failure noted after TKA is prolonged serous drainage. The question that remains for all surgeons is when to explore a chronically draining wound. If excessive erythema or purulence is not present, the wounds can initially be observed. The etiology of this prolonged drainage may be secondary to a large hematoma, but if drainage is not resolved in 5 to 7 days, evacuation may become necessary. It is thought that hematoma can adversely affect the wound, placing increased tension on the skin edges. Possible breakdown of the hematoma may also play a role in wound healing. When prolonged drainage occurs, physical therapy and CPM may be limited or halted. Suspicion always exists for infection because 17% to 50% of chronically draining wounds show later evidence of infection.[63-65] It is for this reason that not all authors agree with the observation of prolonged draining of wounds. Weiss and Krackow[64] reported on early intervention with eight draining TKAs. These authors concluded that with early intervention, infection could perhaps be avoided.[66] Multiple papers have demonstrated an increase in PJI with a persistent draining wound.[23,67] There continues to be a lack of consensus over the treatment of persistent wound drainage after total joint arthroplasty surgery.

With a lack of strict algorithm, clinical acumen plays a critical role. Currently, the International Consensus Meeting on Periprosthetic Joint Infection has a strong recommended that a draining wound 5 to 7 days postoperatively should be treated surgically with an irrigation and débridement with modular component exchange. Patel et al showed that each additional day of wound drainage increased the risk of infection in total hip arthroplasty (THA) and TKA (42% and 29%, respectively).[68] In parallel, other studies similarly conclude that wound drainage >5 days shows an increase in the development of deep infection.[69,70] But even with this recommendation, there is ample variability in practices when it comes to using conservative modalities vs when to perform a surgical débridement. Parvizi et al found that the procrastination of surgical débridement (POD 22 vs POD 14) lead to an increased likelihood of explanation and antibiotic suppression.[23] Another study by Reich and Ezzet suggest that the use of aspiration with sealing of the draining wound

site can be used to prevent unnecessary reoperations.[67] With all these different recommendations, the operative surgeon should be proactive and aggressive in treating a draining arthroplasty.

Recently, there have been questions on the use of negative pressure wound therapy (NPWT) on primary arthroplasty incisions to prevent postoperative wound drainage and further deep infections. The use of NPWT was originally seen in reconstructive plastic surgery because of its direct mechanism of modulating inflammation, angiogenesis, and granulation tissue.[71] These benefits have shown to be beneficial in the reconstruction field by preventing seromas and even possibly resolving postoperative wound drainage.[72,73] Cooper and Bas preformed a retrospective study on comparing antimicrobial dressings (108 patients) to incisional NPWT (30 patients) in revision arthroplasty patients. Even with a bias of applying NPWT in higher risk patients, there was an overall less wound complication (6.9% vs 26.9%, $P = .024$) and surgical site infections (3.3% vs 18.5% $P = .045$) in the NPWT cohort.[74] Furthermore, he performed a similar retrospective study in periprosthetic fractures in THA and TKA patients. Again, the NPWT cohort showed fewer wound complications (4% vs 35%, $P = .002$), fewer deep infections (0% vs 25%, $P = .004$) and fewer reoperations (4% vs 25%, $P = .021$) compared to the antimicrobial hydrofiber dressing cohort.[75] Despite the lack of large prospective standardized studies to validate the use of NPWT, there is increased acceptance for its use in revision surgeries and PJIs.

DEEP TISSUE HEMATOMA

When a deep hematoma that is not draining occurs, the patient can be observed. With any signs of local skin compromise, increased pain, or limited range of motion, surgical exploration may become necessary. In our experience, early intervention for painful, limiting hematomas often allows a patient an early return to normal TKA protocols.

SUPERFICIAL SOFT TISSUE NECROSIS

Superficial necrosis is a vague term encompassing numerous conditions. It can describe a benign stitch abscess that improves with suture débridement and dressing changes and may even be used to describe the superficial soft tissue infection secondary to cellulitis. The term *superficial* is essentially used to describe complications that do not extend to the level of the prosthesis and bone. These superficial infections should be treated aggressively, and cultures should be obtained before initiating any antibiotic treatment. Should a superficial infection or soft tissue necrosis occur, CPM as well as physical therapy should be discontinued until wound appearance improves. It is difficult to differentiate from a deep necrosis and superficial necrosis, so surgical exploration may be needed to appropriately treat the lesion.

With aggressive treatment of superficial infections, skin necrosis can still occur. It is thought that skin necrosis smaller than 3 cm in size can be treated with local débridements and limb immobilization.[76] Paramount to successful treatment of these infections is adequate débridement. Necrotic and nonviable tissue must be removed at the time of surgical exploration and débridement. If at the time of surgical exploration, the infection is noted to be superficial, local wound débridements may be effective, and prosthesis salvage remains possible. If the prosthesis becomes exposed during the débridement, necrosis is no longer just superficial, and treatment for a major skin necrosis should be initiated.

Treatment of a superficial necrosis begins with local wound care. Local wound care techniques range from wet-to-dry saline dressing changes, hydrogels, hydrocolloids, iodine to protease-modulating agents. Depending on the severity of the necrosis, a surgeon can utilize any of these methods with consultation of a wound care clinic or plastic surgeon. Sometimes the degree of skin necrosis requires local débridement as well as appropriate antibiotic coverage.[39] Often, eschars are noted to develop on the anterior aspect of the leg, with no evidence of infection. This eschar can be observed until it is separated from the surrounding skin edges. Contracture occurs during this time, and eventual coverage may be less of a burden due to the constricting nature of the wound. Although small wounds may be allowed to heal by secondary intention, this allows the benefit of not undergoing another surgical procedure and continued range of motion once the wound appearance is stabilized. Skin grafting is indicated when the time for the untreated healing is longer than the healing of a routine skin grafting in the postoperative 5 to 7 days that accompany it. Once the skin graft is placed, the knee immobilizer is required to allow penetration of the vascular buds and the underlying wound. Obviously, infection should be controlled for a skin graft to be effective. Skin grafts are effective for treating soft tissue defects. For coverage of prosthesis, tendon, or bone, this is not successful.

A third option in treatment for superficial necrosis is local fasciocutaneous flap. Hallock[76] reported on six patients in whom coverage was successfully performed using this fasciocutaneous technique. Once again, the diagnosis of infection must be ruled out for this technique to be effective.

FULL-THICKNESS SOFT TISSUE NECROSIS

Full-thickness soft tissue necrosis is the most serious of wound complications. This involves deep penetration of the soft tissue and includes exposure of not only the bone and joint below, but also of the prosthesis that was placed, requiring coverage options and major surgical reconstructions. Although these major reconstructions are successful in maintaining the limb in an established prosthesis, there is a toll with regard to function. Adam et al[77] reported long-term functional results of an exposed TKA treated by flap coverage. Although the wound was essentially covered, in 76% of the cases, functional score was not as good as those with primary wound healing. Other options include advancement of local tissue or the transfer of distant tissue in the form of free flap.[63,64] However, because of the complex nature of this problem, the prosthesis is often removed to treat the soft tissue difficulties, and early intervention from plastic surgery consultation cannot be overemphasized.[78] The use of the gastrocnemius flap is well described in the orthopedic and plastic surgery literature.[79-82] Using this technique, the medial head of the gastrocnemius muscle is used because of its wide arc of motion. It is detached from its insertion on the Achilles and then rotated proximally. The lateral gastrocnemius can also be used for lateral wound difficulties, but it is the medial gastrocnemius that is used for defects around the patella and tibial tubercle. These flaps are effective for covering the two-thirds of the tibia, whereas distal coverage requires free flap, free muscle transfer.

In cases in which gastrocnemius flaps are inadequate, a free muscle transfer, such as one using the latissimus dorsi muscle, the rectus abdominis muscle, or a scapular free flap, may be used. All these methods are well described and are reliable in obtaining coverage.[39] Gerwin and coworkers[83] describe 12 patients who had an exposed prosthesis with a medial gastrocnemius flap, and 90% healing was achieved. Markovich et al noted similar experience with muscle flap coverage.[84] These authors described the results of five latissimus dorsi free flaps, six medial gastrocnemius rotational flaps, and two rectus abdominis free flaps, with 100% wound vascularization noted. In this series, prosthesis retention was achieved in 83% of the cases. In evaluating the results, decreased knee function was noted when an infection along with necrosis occurred. Recently, Nahabedian and associates described their 10-year results with 35 complex TKA wounds.[85] These patients were treated with aggressive wound management, and a 97% limb salvage rate was achieved. These authors emphasize the success of an aggressive approach to wound failures; secondary plastic procedures were required in 23% of patients, and secondary orthopedic procedures were required in 15% of the patients.

CONCLUSION

Wound problems are not always avoided with TKA procedures. Despite meticulous surgical technique and appropriate closure, wound failure can occur. The key to prevention of these lesions is twofold. By identifying those patients at risk, many wound failures can be avoided. When wound failure does occur, aggressive treatment is needed. With this approach, the prosthesis can be retained, and an acceptable long-term function can be achieved.

REFERENCES

1. Cruse PJ, Foord R. A five-year prospective study of 23,649 surgical wounds. *Arch Surg.* 1973;107(2):206-210.

2. Windsor RE, Insall JN, Vince KG. Technical considerations of total knee arthroplasty after proximal tibial osteotomy. *J Bone Joint Surg Am.* 1988;70(4):547-555. Available at http://www.embase.com/search/results?subaction=viewrecord&from=export&id=L18126413%0A; http://rd8hp6du2b.search.serialssolutions.com?sid=EMBASE&issn=00219355&id=doi:&atitle=Technical+considerations+of+total+knee+arthroplasty+after+proximal+tibial+osteotomy&. Accessed 5 November, 2018.

3. Namba RS, Diao E. Tissue expansion for staged reimplantation of infected total knee arthroplasty. *J Arthroplasty.* 1997;12(4):471-474. doi:10.1016/S0883-5403(97)90208-4.

4. Holt BT, Parks NL, Engh GA, Lawrance JM. Comparison of closed-suction drainage and no drainage after primary total knee arthroplasty. *Orthopedics.* 1997;20(12):1121-1125. Available at http://ovidsp.ovid.com/ovidweb.cgi?T=JS&PAGE=reference&D=med4&NEWS=N&AN=9415907%0A; http://onlinelibrary.wiley.com/o/cochrane/clcentral/articles/398/CN-00146398/frame.html%0A; http://ovidsp.ovid.com/ovidweb.cgi?T=JS&PAGE=reference&D=emed7&NEWS=N&AN=27521665. Accessed 5 November, 2018

5. Waisbrod H, Treiman N. Intra-osseous venography in patellofemoral disorders. A preliminary report. *J Bone Joint Surg Br.* 1980;62-B(4):454-456. Available at http://www.ncbi.nlm.nih.gov/entrez/query.fcgi?cmd=Retrieve&db=PubMed&dopt=Citation&list_uids=7430223. Accessed 5 November, 2018.

6. Woelfle-Roos JV, Dautel L, Wernerus D, Woelfle KD, Reichel H. Vascular calcifications on the preoperative radiograph: predictor of ischemic complications in total knee arthroplasty? *J Arthroplasty.* 2016;31(5):1078-1082. doi:10.1016/j.arth.2015.11.033.

7. Arey L. Wound healing. *Physiol Rev.* 1966;16:327.

8. Glenn F, Moore SW. The disruption of abdominal wounds. *Surg Gynecol Obs.* 1941;72:1041-1046.

9. Achauer BM, Black KS, Litke DK. Transcutaneous PO2 in flaps: a new method of surgical prediction. *Plast Reconstr Surg.* 1980;65:738-745.

10. Johnson DP, Eastwood DM. Lateral patellar release in knee arthroplasty: effect on wound healing. *J Arthroplasty.* 1992;7(407):427-431. doi:10.1016/S0883-5403(07)80035-0.

11. Heughan C, Grisilis G, Hunt T. The effect of anemia on wound healing. *Ann Surg.* 1974;179(2):163-167. doi:10.1097/00000658-197402000-00009.

12. Frisch NB, Wessell NM, Charters MA, Yu S, Jeffries JJ, Silverton CD. Predictors and complications of blood transfusion in total hip and knee arthroplasty. *J Arthroplasty.* 2014;29(9 suppl):189-192. doi:10.1016/j.arth.2014.03.048.

13. Boylan MR, Basu N, Naziri Q, Issa K, Maheshwari AV, Mont MA. Does HIV infection increase the risk of short-term adverse outcomes following total knee arthroplasty? *J Arthroplasty.* 2015;30(9):1629-1632. doi:10.1016/j.arth.2015.03.018.

14. Lehman CR, Ries MD, Paiement GD, Davidson AB. Infection after total joint arthroplasty in patients with human immunodeficiency virus or intravenous drug use. *J Arthroplasty.* 2001;16(3):330-335. doi:10.1054/arth.2001.21454.

15. Ecker ML, Lotke PA. Postoperative care of the total knee patient. *Orthop Clin North Am.* 1989;20(1):55-62. Available at http://www.ncbi.nlm.nih.gov/entrez/query.fcgi?cmd=Retrieve&db=PubMed&dopt=Citation&list_uids=2919079. Accessed 9 November, 2018.

16. Dickhaut SC, DeLee JC, Page CP. Nutritional statistics. Importance in predicting wound healing after amputation. *J Bone Joint Surg Am.* 1984;66(1):71-75.

17. Via M. The malnutrition of obesity: micronutrient deficiencies that promote diabetes. *ISRN Endocrinol.* 2012;2012:103472. doi:10.5402/2012/103472.

18. Yi PH, Frank RM, Vann E, Sonn KA, Moric M, Della Valle CJ. Is potential malnutrition associated with septic failure and acute infection after revision total joint arthroplasty? *Clin Orthop Relat Res.* 2015;473(1):175-182. doi:10.1007/s11999-014-3685-8.

19. Kaidar-Person O, Person B, Szomstein S, Rosenthal RJ. Nutritional deficiencies in morbidly obese patients: a new form of malnutrition? Part A: Vitamins. *Obes Surg.* 2008;18(7):870-876.

20. Kaidar-Person O, Person B, Szomstein S, Rosenthal RJ. Nutritional deficiencies in morbidly obese patients: a new form of malnutrition? Part B: Minerals. *Obes Surg.* 2008;18(8):1028-1034. doi:10.1007/s11695-007-9350-5.

21. George DA, Drago L, Scarponi S, Gallazzi E, Haddad FS, Romano CL. Predicting lower limb periprosthetic joint infections: a review of risk factors and their classification. *World J Orthop.* 2017;8(5):400-411. doi:10.5312/wjo.v8.i5.400.

22. Wilson MG, Kelley K, Thornhill TS. Infection as a complication of total knee-replacement arthoplasty. *J Bone Joint Surg Am.* 1990;72-A(6):878-883. Available at http://citeseerx.ist.psu.edu/viewdoc/download?doi=10.1.1.894.1251&rep=rep1&type=pdf. Accessed 11 November, 2018.

23. Jaberi FM, Parvizi J, Haytmanek CT, Joshi A, Purtill J. Procrastination of wound drainage and malnutrition affect the outcome of joint arthroplasty. *Clin Orthop Relat Res.* 2008;466(6):1368-1371. doi:10.1007/s11999-008-0214-7.

24. Dowsey MM, Choong PFM. Obese diabetic patients are at substantial risk for deep infection after primary TKA. *Clin Orthop Relat Res.* 2009;467(6):1577-1581. doi:10.1007/s11999-008-0551-6.

25. Stern S, Insall J. Total knee arthroplasty in obese patients. *J Bone Joint Surg Am.* 1990;72(9):1400-1404.

26. Griffin FM, Scuderi GR, Insall JN, Colizza W. Total knee arthroplasty in patients who were obese with 10 years followup. *Clin Orthop Relat Res.* 1998;356:28-23. doi:10.1097/00003086-199811000-00006.

27. Benowitz NL, Jacob P III. Daily intake of nicotine during cigarette smoking. *Clin Pharmacol Ther.* 1984;35(4):499-504. doi:10.1038/clpt.1984.67.

28. Benowitz NL, Kuyt F, Jacob P. Influence of nicotine on cardiovascular and hormonal effects of cigarette smoking. *Clin Pharmacol Ther.* 1984;36(1):74-81. doi:10.1038/clpt.1984.142.

29. Benowitz NL, Kuyt F, Jacob P, Jones RT, Osman AL. Cotinine disposition and effects. *Clin Pharmacol Ther.* 1983;34(5):604-611. doi:10.1038/clpt.1983.222.

30. Singh JA. Smoking and outcomes after knee and hip arthroplasty: a systematic review. *J Rheumatol.* 2011;38(9):1824-1834. doi:10.3899/jrheum.101221.

31. Springer BD. Modifying risk factors for total joint arthroplasty: strategies that work nicotine. *J Arthroplasty.* 2016;31(8):1628-1630. doi:10.1016/j.arth.2016.01.071.

32. Villebro NM, Pedersen T, Møller AM, Tønnesen H. Long-term effects of a preoperative smoking cessation programme. *Clin Respir J.* 2008;2(3):175-182. doi:10.1111/j.1752-699X.2008.00058.x.

33. Lindström D, Azodi OS, Wladis A, et al. Effects of a perioperative smoking cessation intervention on postoperative complications: a randomized trial. *Ann Surg.* 2008;248(5):739-745. doi:10.1097/SLA.0b013e3181889d0d.

34. Cropley M, Theadom A, Pravettoni G, Webb G. The effectiveness of smoking cessation interventions prior to surgery: a systematic review. *Nicotine Tob Res.* 2008;10(3):407-412. doi:10.1080/14622200801888996.

35. Zaki A, Abrishami A. Interventions in the preoperative clinic for long term smoking cessation: a quantitative systematic review. *Can J Anaesth.* 2008;55(1):11-21.

36. Thomsen T, Villebro N, Møller AM. Interventions for preoperative smoking cessation. *Cochrane Database Syst Rev.* 2014;(3). doi:10.1002/14651858.CD002294.pub4.

37. Wong R, Lotke P, Ecker M. Factors influencing wound healing after total knee arthroplasty. *Orthop Trans.* 1986;10:497.

38. Garner R, Mowot A, Hazleman B. Factors influencing wound healing after total knee arthroplasty. *J Bone Joint Surg.* 1973;55:134-144.

39. Craig SM. Soft tissue considerations in the failed total knee arthroplasty. In: Scott WN, ed. *The Knee*. Vol. 2. St. Louis, MO: Mosby-Yearbook; 1994:1279-1295.

40. Gorgan TJ, Dorey F, Rollins J, Amstutz HC. Deep sepsis following total knee arthroplasty. *J Bone Joint Surg Am*. 1986;68(2):226-234.

41. Johnson DP. Midline or parapatellar incision for knee arthroplasty. A comparative study of wound viability. *J Bone Joint Surg Br*. 1988;70(4):656-658. Available at http://www.ncbi.nlm.nih.gov/entrez/query.fcgi?cmd=Retrieve&db=PubMed&dopt=Citation&list_uids=3403619. Accessed 18 November, 2018.

42. Dennis D. Wound complications in total knee arthroplasty. *Knee Arthroplast*. 1997;46(165):163-169. doi:10.1016/S0010-0277(97)00004-8.

43. Ecker ML, Lotke PA. Wound healing complications. In: Rand JA, ed. *Total Knee Arthroplasty*. New York, NY: Raven Press; 1993:403-407.

44. Crevoisier XM, Reber P, Noesberger B. Is suction drainage necessary after total joint arthroplasty? *Arch Orthop Trauma Surg*. 1998;117(3):121-124. doi:10.1007/s004020050210.

45. Ovadia D, Luger E, Bickels J, Menachem A, Dekel S. Efficacy of closed wound drainage after total joint arthroplasty: a prospective randomized study. *J Arthroplasty*. 1997;12(3):317-321. Available at http://ovidsp.ovid.com/ovidweb.cgi?T=JS&PAGE=reference&D=emed4&NEWS=N&AN=1999016397. Accessed 18 November, 2018.

46. Cushner FD, Scott WN. Evolution of blood transfusion management for a busy knee practice. *Orthopedics*. 1999;22:s145. doi:10.1016/j.hrtlng.2017.08.008.

47. Drinkwater CJ, Neil MJ. Optimal timing of wound drain removal following total joint arthroplasty. *J Arthroplasty*. 1995;10(2):185-189. doi:10.1016/S0883-5403(05)80125-1.

48. 48 Stulberg B, Insall J, Williams G, Ghelman B. Deep-vein thrombosis following total knee replacement. An analysis of six hundred and thirty-eight arthroplasties. *J Bone Joint Surg Am*. 1984;66-A(2):194-201. Available at http://jbjs.org/content/jbjsam/66/2/194.full.pdf. Accessed 9 November, 2018.

49. Levine MN, Gent M, Hirsh J, et al. Ardeparin (low-molecular-weight heparin) vs graduated compression stockings for the prevention of venous thromboembolism: a randomized trial in patients undergoing knee surgery. *Arch Intern Med*. 1996;156(8):851-856. doi:10.1001/archinte.156.8.851.

50. Leclerc JR, Geerts WH, Desjardins L, et al. Prevention of venous thromboembolism (VTE) after knee arthroplasty - a randomized, double-blind trial, comparing enoxaparin to warfarin sodium. *Haemostasis*. 1994;24(suppl 1):231. Available at https://www.cochranelibrary.com/central/doi/10.1002/central/CN-00236089/full. Accessed 13 November, 2018.

51. Spiro TE, Fitzgerald RH, Trowbridge A. Enoxaparin (a low molecular weight heparin) and warfarin for the prevention of venous thromboembolic disease after elective knee replacement surgery [Abstract no: 970]. *Blood*. 1994;84:246a. Available at https://www.cochranelibrary.com/central/doi/10.1002/central/CN-00236051/full. Accessed 21 October, 2018.

52. Lotke PA, Faralli VJ, Orenstein EM, Ecker ML. Blood loss after total knee replacement. Effects of tourniquet release and continuous passive motion. *J Bone Joint Surg Am*. 1991;73(7):1037-1040.

53. Yashar AA, Venn-Watson E, Welsh T, Colwell CW Jr, Lotke P. Continuous passive motion with accelerated flexion after total knee arthroplasty. *Clin Orthop Relat Res*. 1997;345:38-43. Available at http://www.ncbi.nlm.nih.gov/entrez/query.fcgi?cmd=Retrieve&db=PubMed&dopt=Citation&list_uids=9418619. Accessed 19 November, 2018.

54. Yi Z, Bin S, Jing Y, Zongke Z, Pengde K, Fuxing P. Tranexamic acid administration in primary total hip arthroplasty: a randomized controlled trial of intravenous combined with topical versus single-dose intravenous administration. *J Bone Joint Surg Am*. 2016;98(12):983-991. doi:10.2106/JBJS.15.00638.

55. Luo ZY, Wang HY, Wang D, Zhou K, Pei FX, Zhou ZK. Oral vs intravenous vs topical tranexamic acid in primary hip arthroplasty: a prospective, randomized, double-blind, controlled study. *J Arthroplasty*. 2018;33(3):786-793. doi:10.1016/j.arth.2017.09.062.

56. Ponnusamy KE, Kim TJ, Khanuja HS. Perioperative blood transfusions in orthopaedic surgery. *J Bone Joint Surg Am*. 2014;96(21):1836-1844. doi:10.2106/JBJS.N.00128.

57. Aggarwal AK, Singh N, Sudesh P. Topical vs intravenous tranexamic acid in reducing blood loss after bilateral total knee arthroplasty: a prospective study. *J Arthroplasty*. 2016;31(7):1442-1448. doi:10.1016/j.arth.2015.12.033.

58. Fillingham YA, Ramkumar DB, Jevsevar DS, et al. Tranexamic acid use in total joint arthroplasty: the clinical practice guidelines endorsed by the American Association of Hip and Knee Surgeons, American Society of Regional Anesthesia and Pain Medicine, American Academy of Orthopaedic Surgeons, Hip Society, and Knee Society. *J Arthroplasty*. 2018;33(10):3065-3069. doi:10.1016/j.arth.2018.08.002.

59. Kim SM, Moon YW, Lim SJ, Kim DW, Park YS. Effect of oral factor Xa inhibitor and low-molecular-weight heparin on surgical complications following total hip arthroplasty. *Thromb Haemost*. 2016;115(3):600-607. doi:10.1160/TH15-07-0527.

60. Gold DA, Craig Scott S, Scott WN. Soft tissue expansion prior to arthroplasty in the multiply-operated knee. *J Arthroplasty*. 1996;11(5):512-521. doi:10.1016/S0883-5403(96)80102-1.

61. Manifold SG, Cushner FD, Craig-Scott S, Scott WN. Long-term results of total knee arthroplasty after the use of soft tissue expanders. *Clin Orthop Relat Res*. 2000;380:133-139. doi:10.1097/00003086-200011000-00017.

62. Santore RF, Kaufman D, Robbins AJ, Dabezies EJJr. Tissue expansion prior to revision total knee arthroplasty. *J Arthroplasty*. 1997;12(4):475-478. doi:10.1016/S0883-5403(97)90209-6.

63. Bergstorm S, Kruston K, Lidgren I. Treatment of infected knee arthroplasty. *Clin Orthop Relat Res*. 1989;245:173.

64. Weiss AP, Krackow KA. Persistent wound drainage after primary total knee arthroplasty. *J Arthroplasty*. 1993;8(3):285-289. Available at http://ovidsp.ovid.com/ovidweb.cgi?T=JS&PAGE=reference&D=emed6&NEWS=N&AN=23173321. Accessed 23 October, 2018.

65. Insall J, Aglietti P. A five to seven-year of unicondylar arthroplasty. *J Bone Joint Surg Am*. 1980;62:1329-1337. doi:10.1051/acarologia/20142134.

66. Sculco T. Local wound complications after total knee arthroplasty. In: Ranawat C, ed. *Total Condylar Knee Arthroplasty*. New York, NY: Springer;1985.

67. Reich MS, Ezzet KA. A nonsurgical protocol for management of postarthroplasty wound drainage. *Arthroplast Today*. 2018;4(1):71-73. doi:10.1016/j.artd.2017.03.009.

68. Patel VP, Walsh M, Sehgal B, Preston C, DeWal H, Di Cesare PE. Factors associated with prolonged wound drainage after primary total hip and knee arthroplasty. *J Bone Joint Surg Am*. 2007;89(1):33-38. doi:10.2106/JBJS.F.00163.

69. Lonner JH, Lotke PA. Aseptic complications after total knee arthroplasty. *J Am Acad Orthop Surg*. 1999;7(5):311-324. doi:10.5435/00124635-199909000-00004.

70. Saleh K, Olson M, Resig S, et al. Predictors of wound infection in hip and knee joint replacement: results from a 20 year surveillance program. *J Orthop Res*. 2002;20(3):506-515. doi:10.1016/S0736-0266(01)00153-X.

71. Siqueira MB. Role of negative pressure wound therapy in total hip and knee arthroplasty. *World J Orthop*. 2016;7(1):30-37. doi:10.5312/wjo.v7.i1.30.

72. Pachowsky M, Gusinde J, Klein A, et al. Negative pressure wound therapy to prevent seromas and treat surgical incisions after total hip arthroplasty. *Int Orthop*. 2012;36(4):719-722. doi:10.1007/s00264-011-1321-8.

73. Hansen E, Durinka JB, Costanzo JA, Austin MS, Deirmengian GK. Negative pressure wound therapy is associated with resolution of incisional drainage in most wounds after hip arthroplasty. *Clin Orthop Relat Res*. 2013;471(10):3230-3236. doi:10.1007/s11999-013-2937-3.

74. Cooper HJ, Bas MA. Closed-incision negative-pressure therapy versus antimicrobial dressings after revision hip and knee surgery: a comparative study. *J Arthroplasty*. 2016;31(5):1047-1052. doi:10.1016/j.arth.2015.11.010.

75. Cooper HJ, Roc GC, Bas MA, et al. Closed incision negative pressure therapy decreases complications after periprosthetic fracture surgery around the hip and knee. *Injury.* 2018;49(2):386-391. doi:10.1016/j.injury.2017.11.010.

76. Hallock GG. Salvage of total knee arthroplasty with local fasciocutaneous flaps. *J Bone Joint Surg Am.* 1990;72(8):1236-1239. doi:10.2106/00004623-199072080-00017.

77. Adam RF, Watson SB, Jarratt JW, Noble J, Watson JS. Outcome after flap cover for exposed total knee arthroplasties - a report of 25 cases. *J Bone Joint Surg Br.* 1994;76B(5):750-753.

78. Bengtson S, Carlsson Å, Relander M, Knutson K, Lidgren L. Treatment of the exposed knee prosthesis. *Acta Orthop.* 1987;58(6): 662-665. doi:10.3109/17453678709146510.

79. Hemphill ES, Ebert FR, Muench AG. The medial gastrocnemius muscle flap in the treatment of wound complications following total knee arthroplasty. *Orthopedics.* 1992;15(4):477-480. Available at http://ovidsp.ovid.com/ovidweb.cgi?T=JS&PAGE=reference&D=med3&NEWS=N&AN=1565583%0A; http://ovidsp.ovid.com/ovidweb.cgi?T=JS&PAGE=reference&D=emed5&NEWS=N&AN=22160103. Accessed 23 October, 2018.

80. Eckhardt J, Lesavoy M, Dubrow T. Exposed endo-prosthesis. *Clin Orthop Relat Res.* 1990;251:220.

81. Peled IJ, Frankl U, Wexler MR. Salvage of exposed knee prosthesis by gastrocnemius myocutaneous flap coverage. *Orthopedics.* 1983;6(10):1320-1322. doi:10.3928/0147-7447-19831001-11.

82. Salibian A, Sanford H. Salvage of an infected total knee prosthesis with medial and lateral gastrocnemius muscle flaps. *J Bone Joint Surg Am.* 1983;65(5):681-684.

83. Gerwin M, Rothaus KO, Windsor RE, Brause BD, Insall JN. Gastrocnemius muscle flap coverage of exposed or infected knee prostheses. *Clin Orthop Relat Res.* 1993;286:64-70. Available at http://ovidsp.ovid.com/ovidweb.cgi?T=JS&PAGE=reference&D=emed6&NEWS=N&AN=23059469. Accessed 25 November, 2018.

84. Markovich G, Dorr L, Klein N, McPherson E, Vince K. Muscle flaps in total knee arthroplasty. *Clin Orthop Relat Res.* 1995;321:122-130.

85. Nahabedian MY, Orlando JC, Delanois RE, Mont MA, Hungerford DS. Salvage procedures for complex soft tissue defects of the knee. *Clin Orthop Relat Res.* 1998;356:119-124. doi:10.1097/00003086-199811000-00017.

chapter 56

Extensor Mechanism Complications After Total Knee Arthroplasty

Douglas A. Dennis, MD I Lindsay T. Kleeman-Forsthuber, MD

Total knee arthroplasty (TKA) is an effective surgical treatment for patients with symptomatic end-stage knee arthritis. A well-functioning knee replacement relies on an intact, functional extensor mechanism. The extensor mechanism consists of the quadriceps muscles, quadriceps tendon, patella, patellar tendon with its associated tibial tubercle insertion site, and the medial and lateral retinacular soft tissues that help facilitate central patellar tracking. There are several unique complications related to the extensor mechanism following TKA that cumulatively accounts for up to 50% of all TKA complications.[1] These complications include mechanical abnormalities such as patellofemoral instability, patellar crepitus and clunk, patellar component loosening, and component failure or more devastating injuries such as extensor mechanism disruption. There is continued debate on whether to leave the patella nonresurfaced considering all the potential complications associated with resurfacing. However, leaving the patella nonresurfaced has shown to have relatively high rates of anterior knee pain and need for revision.[2-7] Here we review the various complications related to the extensor mechanism following TKA along with treatment options and preventative strategies.

PATELLOFEMORAL INSTABILITY

Proper central tracking of the patella within the trochlear groove requires a complicated balance of forces and is influenced by soft-tissue integrity, patellar resection, component positioning, and implant design. Revision rate for TKA related to patellofemoral complications is around 8%[2,8]; however, recent studies indicate that patellofemoral complications may be decreasing with modern implants and improved surgical technique.[9,10] Patient factors that can predispose to patellofemoral instability include medial retinacular laxity, traumatic disruption of the medial patellofemoral ligament, lateral retinacular contracture, weakness of the vastus medialis oblique muscle, and trochlear hypoplasia.[11] The medial soft tissue structures are needed to counterbalance the more lateral vector pull of the quadriceps and decrease the functional Q-angle. Patients with a valgus knee deformity or lateralized tibial tubercle are predisposed to patellar instability due to an increased functional Q-angle.[12] If any of these

factors are identified, they must be addressed at the time of surgery to ensure proper patella tracking.

Proper surgical technique is paramount to achieving patellofemoral stability. The patellar osteotomy should be a symmetric resection such that the remaining medial and lateral patella facet thicknesses are the same. A proper resection will remove more of the medial facet since the native medial facet is typically thicker than the lateral facet.[13] The resection should remove enough bone to accommodate the thickness of the patellar button without overstuffing. Patellar tracking is optimized when the patellar component is medialized as far as possible and the femoral and tibial components are rotated appropriately. If the femoral component is internally rotated relative to the transepicondylar line or if the tibial component is internally rotated relative to the tibial tubercle, the patella will track laterally and be at higher risk for dislocation (**Fig. 56-1**). One should avoid medial translation of both the femoral and tibial components as these errors result in lateralization of the tibial tubercle and a lateral force vector force on the patella.

Advancements in implant designs have greatly improved patellofemoral stability. Previous prostheses with high patellofemoral complication rates typically had a shallow trochlear groove, short and narrow anterior flange, and a small radius of curvature.[14] Newer implant features that have improved patellar tracking include a more laterally oriented trochlear groove, heightened lateral flange, and deepened intercondylar notch. Use of rotating tibial platform (or mobile bearing) implant has shown to improve patellar tracking with less lateral patellar tilt, lower patellofemoral contact stresses, and decreased need for a lateral retinacular release when compared to fixed tibial bearings.[15,16] Several different types of patellar component designs exist, including a dome-shaped button and conforming biconcave patellar component (also known as an anatomic patella). Cadaveric studies have shown increased inferosuperior shear forces with the domed patella component compared to biconcave components[17]; however, this has not shown to affect clinical outcomes thus far.[18,19] Anatomic patellar designs have sagittal plane kinematics that more closely resemble a nonresurfaced patella when surveilled under fluoroscopy during a deep knee bend.[20] However, because of the bicondylar ridge, the patellar component must be

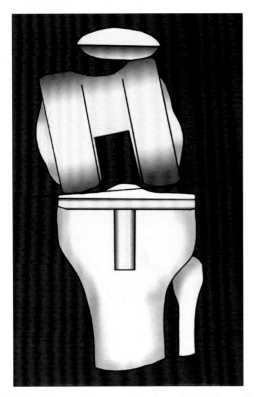

FIGURE 56-1 Diagram demonstrating the effect of femoral component malrotation on patellofemoral tracking. The femoral component is excessively internally rotated relative to the posterior femoral condylar axis. This excessive rotation prevents the patellar component from tracking centrally in the trochlear groove and predisposes to patellar subluxation or dislocation.

precisely rotated for appropriate tracking in the trochlear groove, whereas the dome component with its symmetric 360° conformity is more forgiving to malrotation.

Instability of the patellofemoral joint should be identified and addressed at the time of surgery. The knee is tested through full range of motion during implant trialing and then again before capsular closure to ensure the patella tracks centrally without lateral tilt or subluxation. The tourniquet should be released at this stage to eliminate the binding effect of the extensor mechanism which can alter patellar tracking.[21,22] One can use the "no thumb" technique to assess tracking, in which the medial border of the patella should make contact with the medial femoral condyle through knee range of motion without the surgeon having to manually reduce it. This technique has shown to overestimate the number of cases needing lateral release,[23,24] with some preferring the towel clip technique in which a clip is used to hold the quadriceps to the superior patella pole to mimic arthrotomy closure. The senior author prefers the "no thumb" technique to avoid overtightening the extensor mechanism during arthrotomy closure, which can have adverse effects on postoperative knee flexion and patella contact pressures. If patellar tilt or instability is noted, the etiology should be identified and addressed. The most likely causes for instability include imbalance of extensor mechanism soft

tissues, component malposition, or anatomic abnormalities. For extensor mechanism imbalance, a lateral retinacular release can be performed to improve tracking.[25] The lateral release should be performed at least 1 cm lateral to patellar periphery to protect the superolateral geniculate artery that perfuses the patella.[26] Advancement of the vastus medialis muscle or medial retinacular tissues during capsular closure via imbrication can also be performed.[27] For patients with severe valgus deformities or a lateralized tibial tubercle, a medial tibial tubercle transfer can be performed. If proper tracking cannot be achieved with any of these realignment procedures, sometimes revision and repositioning of the components may be necessary to improve rotation and tracking.

PATELLAR COMPONENT LOOSENING

Loosening of the patellar component accounts for a low percentage of TKA failures, which is reported between 3% and 4.8%.[9,28,29] Early patellar component designs were associated with higher patellar loosening rates, particularly cementless metal-backed patellar components, with revision rates as high as 13.5%.[29] Other factors associated with increased risk for patellar loosening include body mass index over 30 kg/m^2, preoperative valgus knee alignment of 10° or more, preoperative knee flexion of 100° or more, osteopenia and tibial component thickness 12 mm or greater.[28] Certain surgical techniques that have been associated with loosening include component malposition, joint line elevation, performing a lateral retinacular release, uneven patellar resection, limited patellar bone stock, patellar subluxation, loosening of other components, and patellar avascular necrosis.[29,30]

Diagnosing patellar component loosening can be challenging, as patients can present with subtle symptoms.[30] Initial evaluation of symptomatic patellofemoral pain should always include radiographic imaging and infectious work-up. Most standard knee radiograph series used to evaluate the patellofemoral joint include a flexed lateral and Merchant view in which the knee is flexed and the patella component is compressed against the trochlea (**Fig. 56-2**). If loosening has occurred at the cement–implant interface, this position of compression can reduce a loose patellar component and potentially mask loosening[31] (**Fig. 56-3**). If patellar component loosening is suspected but not able to be diagnosed radiographically, a bone scan or arthroscopic evaluation may be required to confirm the diagnosis.

Patients with patellar loosening do not always require treatment, as shown by Berend et al who reviewed 180 loose all-polyethylene patellar implants and found that only 0.3% required revision.[30] For those needing operative treatment, options include component revision (assuming there is enough bone stock to support another implant), bone graft augmentation, patellar resection arthroplasty (patelloplasty), gull-wing osteotomy (**Fig. 56-4**), use of a

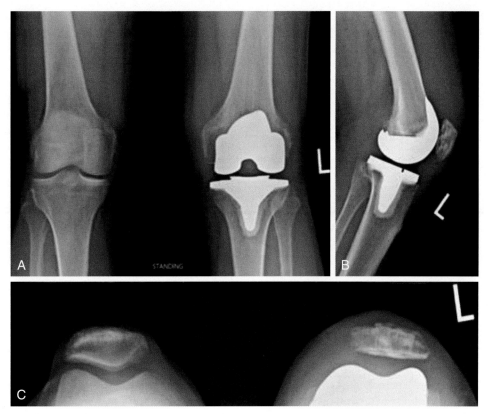

FIGURE 56-2 Standard radiographic series to evaluate painful patellofemoral joint following total knee arthroplasty. Images include **(A)** standing anterior–posterior view, **(B)** standing lateral view at 30° of flexion, and **(C)** Merchant view of the patellofemoral joint.

porous tantalum metal component, or complete patellectomy.[32] Revision with an all-polyethylene cemented patellar component can be considered if the remaining patellar thickness is a minimum of 10 to 12 mm, no fracture is present, and patellar vascularity is preserved.[33] Designs with three peripheral lugs are often useful when revising central lug designs, in which bone loss is typically central. A circular, three-lug design is also often selected when

revising a failed three-lug device. In this situation, rotation of the component from its original position often provides adequate bone for fixation of the new patellar component. Outcomes following isolated patellar component revision have shown poor outcomes overall, with high complication rates (up to 45%) and need for reoperation.[34,35] Complications reported from isolated revision include patellar fracture, patellofemoral instability, infection, extensor lag, and polyethylene wear.[35,36] Considering this, all other etiologies for failure of the patellofemoral component need to be assessed and addressed, including lateral retinacular contracture and femoral/tibial component malposition. Component malposition is best assessed with a computed tomography scan so that rotation of the components relative to anatomic landmarks can be determined. In summary, isolated patellofemoral

FIGURE 56-3 Radiographic example of a loose patellar component. White arrow indicates the patellar component which has visible lucency at the bone–cement interface and dissociation from the patella. The patellar component remains within the trochlear groove on this image while the patella is subluxated laterally.

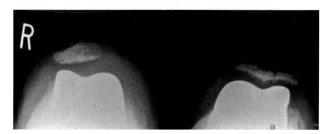

FIGURE 56-4 Radiographic example of a gull-wing osteotomy on the left performed for a failed patellar component without enough bone stock to support another patellar component at the time of revision.

component revision should be done with caution and high index of suspicion for other contributing factors. If the patellar component is well-fixed, has no evidence of damage or wear, and tracks appropriately, the patellar component can be safely retained even if revision of other components is being performed.[37]

PATELLAR COMPONENT WEAR

Patellar component failure due to polyethylene wear is a complication most commonly reported with metal-backed patellar components, with a reported incidence of 4.7%.[29] Metal-backed patellar components can also have polyethylene dissociation, seen as early as 14 months after TKA.[38] By nature of their design, metal-backed patellar components have an overall thinner polyethylene-bearing surface than the all-polyethylene implants which predispose to increased wear. The polyethylene is thinnest along the peripheral edge with the metal backing not entirely extending to the periphery of the polyethylene. This creates a sharp cutting edge and bending moment that can result in polyethylene dissociation or excessive wear (**Fig. 56-5**). Patients at highest risk for these complications include active males with increased body weight and knee flexion greater than 115°.[38,39] Patellar tilting, subluxation, increased composite patellofemoral thickness, or a flexed femoral component can further predispose to patellar component failure. If the polyethylene wear is excessive enough, metal-on-metal wear between the patellar component metal plate and femoral component can occur resulting in significant damage.[39] One should be prepared to revise all components any time revision of a metal-backed patellar component is needed if there is evidence of destructive wear.

Osteolysis secondary to polyethylene wear should also be assessed. In the absence of other findings, isolated revision of a metal-backed patellar component to a cemented all-polyethylene component has been associated with good clinical outcomes and low complication rates.[40,41] Wear of an all-polyethylene patellar components is usually well-tolerated. This is often associated with some polyethylene deformation which can improve contact mechanics.

PATELLOFEMORAL CREPITUS/CLUNK

Patellofemoral crepitus and patellar clunk syndrome are frustrating complications following TKA that can result in significant patient dissatisfaction. The reported incidence varies widely from 0% to 18% and is primarily seen with posterior-stabilized (PS) femoral implants that have a large intercondylar box.[42,43] Both conditions result from proliferation of peripatellar fibrosynovial tissue at the superior pole of the patella (**Fig. 56-6**). Patellar clunk occurs when a discrete fibrosynovial nodule develops and gets entrapped within the intercondylar box of the femoral component during knee flexion producing a painful, audible "clunk" as the knee is extended (**Fig. 56-7**). Patellofemoral crepitus can have subtle clinical exam findings with either asymptomatic or symptomatic crepitation during knee motion. Dennis et al performed a retrospective multicenter case-controlled study of 60 patients requiring surgery for symptomatic patellar crepitus and identified several risk factors including previous knee surgery, use of smaller patellar components, decreased composite patellar thickness, shortened patellar tendon length, smaller femoral components, increased posterior

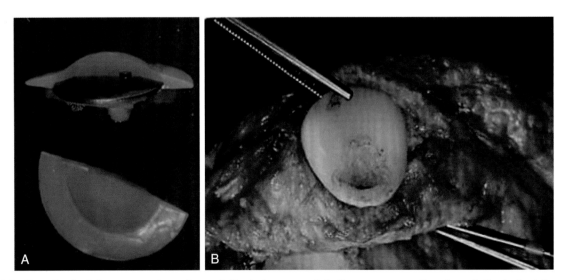

FIGURE 56-5 Example of patellar component wear in a metal-backed component. **A:** Shows a cross section of a metal-backed patellar component. The polyethylene is thinnest around the periphery with the metal backing not extending to edge of the component. This results in a sharp cutting edge and bending moment that can result in either polyethylene dissociation or excess wear **(B)**. Here the polyethylene remains associated with the metal backing, but it has worn through the polyethylene at the periphery resulting in exposed metal backing that can articulate against the femoral component.

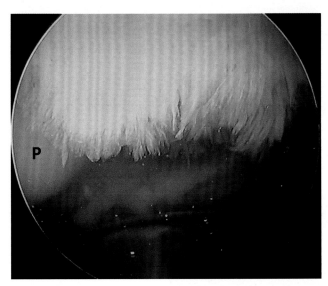

FIGURE 56-6 Knee arthroscopy image of a patient following total knee arthroplasty demonstrating proliferation of fibrosynovial tissue on the undersurface of the quadriceps tendon at the superior patellar pole responsible for causing patellar clunk syndrome and crepitus. The resurfaced patella is labeled "P" and the metal femoral component is labeled "F." This nodule of tissue can be successfully removed arthroscopically to alleviate the conditions.

femoral condylar offset, flexed positioning of the femoral component, and thicker polyethylene inserts. The condition typically develops within 1 year of surgery with range of 3 to 21 months.[44-46]

Nonoperative treatment with avoidance of high patellofemoral loading activities (such as walking stairs or squatting) and use of antiinflammatory medications will suffice in most cases. Many patients with patellar crepitus require no treatment and are often unaware that they have developed this condition.[47] Some patients with symptomatic patellar crepitus will have resolution of their symptoms within 1 year of symptom onset without surgical intervention.[45] For patients requiring surgical treatment, either arthroscopic or open synovial débridement can be performed with satisfactory outcomes reported.[44] Arthroscopic débridement has shown to successfully treat both patellar clunk and crepitus with several studies showing improved pain and functional scores and low recurrence rates.[43,48,49]

While patients do well with both conservative and surgical treatments of patellofemoral crepitus, prevention should be a primary focus. Smaller femoral components should be avoided whenever possible and care should be taken to avoid flexing the femoral component during implantation.[46] Native patella baja can be identified preoperatively, but it can also occur iatrogenically by elevating the joint line with an excessive distal femoral resection. Patients with native patella baja should be counseled on an increased risk for patellofemoral crepitus and care should be taken to avoid elevating the joint line with a minimized distal femoral resection. Patellar resection should be enough to accommodate the thickness of the patellar component without overstuffing and the component should be positioned as superior as possible. Contact between the trochlea and patella shifts superior on the patella as the knee goes into deeper flexion, so superior placement of the patellar component will avoid any contact between the trochlea and nonresurfaced bone.[42] Removing any exposed bone along the periphery of the patellar component (particularly the lateral facet) has also shown to lower incidence of crepitus.[50] Any excessive synovial tissue on the posterior aspect of the quadriceps tendon should also be excised as this is the tissue that proliferates to cause these conditions (**Fig. 56-8**).[42]

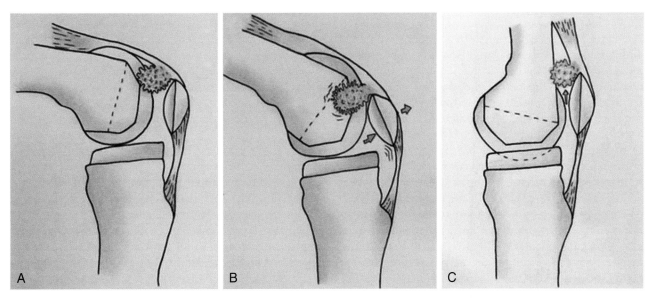

FIGURE 56-7 Diagram demonstrating the pathogenesis of patellar clunk syndrome. Synovial tissue on the undersurface of the distal quadriceps tendon can proliferate and form a well-defined nodule of tissue (**A**). When a posterior-stabilized femoral component with a box is used, this nodule of fibrosynovial tissue can become entrapped within the intercondylar box of the femoral component as the knee goes from full flexion (**A**) into mid-flexion (**B**). This causes a painful audible and palpable "clunk" as the knee goes into terminal extension (**C**).

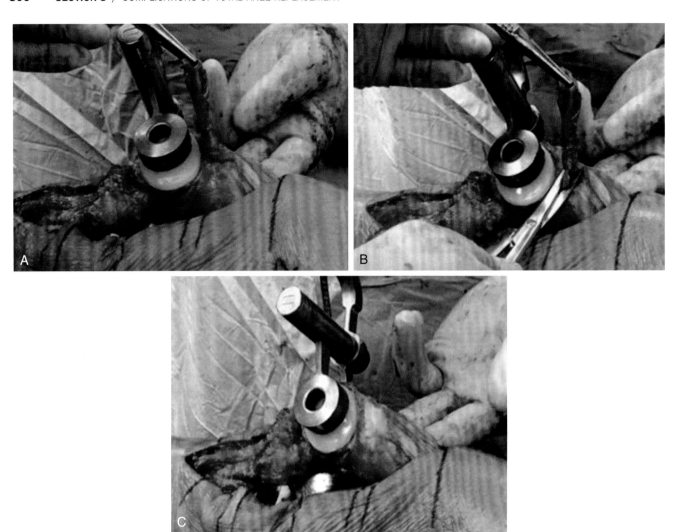

FIGURE 56-8 Images demonstrating excision of excess soft tissue on undersurface of quadriceps tendon during primary total knee arthroplasty to prevent patellar crepitus and patellar clunk syndrome. Excessive fibrosynovial tissue on the undersurface of the quadriceps tendon is identified at the junction of the distal quadriceps and proximal pole of the patella prior to arthrotomy closure **(A)**. This excess tissue is sharply excised with care to protect the underlying quadriceps fibers **(B)**. The cleaned undersurface of the quadriceps is visualized with all the tendon fibers preserved **(C)**.

Implant design features can affect the incidence of patellar crepitus. Fukunaga et al[51] described the intercondylar box ratio, defined as the ratio of the intercondylar box height to the anterior–posterior height of the femoral component (**Fig. 56-9**). Many second- and third-generation PS femoral components have been designed with a decreased intercondylar box ratio resulting in a decreased incidence of patellar clunk and crepitus.[51-56] Notably, those prostheses with an intercondylar box ratio less than 0.7 were found to have no patellar clunk.[51] Femoral components with a high intercondylar box ratio allow contact of the distal quadriceps tendon earlier in flexion than components with a lower ratio. The authors concluded that this design feature may be responsible for the high incidence of patellofemoral crepitus and clunk with certain prostheses. Martin et al demonstrated a lower incidence of patellofemoral crepitus with use of a modern PS implant that had a thinner and narrower anterior flange as well as a smaller femoral intercondylar

box ratio.[47] With further improvements in implant design and surgical technique, incidence of symptomatic clunk or crepitus will hopefully continue to decrease.

EXTENSOR MECHANISM DISRUPTION

Injury to the extensor mechanism is a rare but devastating complication following TKA with historically poor outcomes and high complication rates.[57,58] It can occur at any point along the extensor mechanism including the quadriceps tendon, patella, patellar tendon, or tibial tubercle. There are unique risk factors associated with injuries at the various locations and a variety of surgical techniques described for treatment.

Quadriceps Rupture

Quadriceps rupture following TKA is a rare phenomenon, with a reported incidence ranging from 0.1% to 1.1%.[59-61]

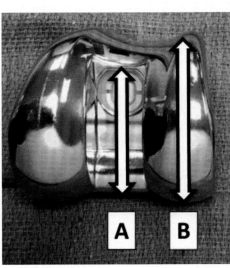
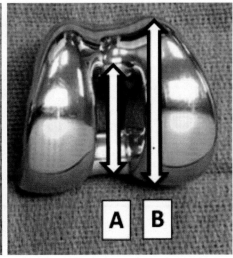

FIGURE 56-9 Diagram comparing the intercondylar box ratio between two different types of posterior-stabilized femoral components. The component on the left has a large intercondylar box distance (A) making its intercondylar box ratio (A/B) higher than the intercondylar box ratio for the component on the right, which has a smaller A distance. Femoral components with an intercondylar box ratio higher than 0.7 (like the one on the left) have been associated with higher rates of crepitus and patellar clunk syndrome.[18] Modern implants (like the component on the right) have smaller intercondylar boxes and have demonstrated lower rates of patellar clunk.[19]

There is a higher incidence of quadriceps injury reported in patients with rheumatoid arthritis[59] and patients undergoing knee manipulation for arthrofibrosis. Iatrogenic injury to the quadriceps tendon has also been implicated, particularly in stiff knees with difficult exposure that requires a rectus snip or V-Y turndown.[61,62] Quadriceps disruption can also occur postoperatively due to trauma or prior vascular insult. Specifically, injury to the superior lateral genicular artery during a lateral retinacular release has been proposed as a possible risk factor.[61]

Treatment of quadriceps tendon ruptures depends on whether the tear is complete or partial. Incomplete or partial tendon tears can be managed nonoperatively with overall good results.[59] Patients are usually placed into a knee brace locked in extension or long leg cast to help facilitate healing with graduated increase in range of motion. Bracing is also a suitable option for patients with complete ruptures who are not good surgical candidates, such as elderly or low-demand patients with severe medical comorbidities. While several surgical treatment options have been described for quadriceps tendon ruptures, outcomes overall are usually marginal and associated with high complication rates. Primary repair of a complete quadriceps tendon tear has shown to have quite poor outcomes[63] with a 40% re-rupture rate reported.[59] Some studies have shown better results with primary repair if the quadriceps injury occurs in the acute postoperative period (within 90 days) and is treated early.[60] Others have described use of a semitendinosus or gracilis tendon autograft or allograft incorporated into a primary repair to help reenforce the construct when poor vascular supply is present or for chronic ruptures[64] (**Fig. 56-10**). For quadriceps ruptures with severe tendon retraction or tissue loss, options include using a medial gastrocnemius

flap,[65] Achilles tendon allograft, or reconstruction with a complete extensor mechanism allograft (EMA) (**Fig. 56-11**).[66] These same techniques are commonly used for patellar tendon disruptions with many studies reporting collective outcomes for both injuries. Results with allografts for both quadriceps and patellar tendon injuries have relatively poor clinical outcomes.[63,66-68] Lim et al showed improved pain and functional scores following allograft reconstruction but with an average extensor lag of 14° at 2-year follow-up with one-third of patients having an extensor lag over 30°.[67] Brown et al demonstrated similarly poor results in their series of 57 patients treated with EMA with 38% of their entire series failing due to infection, poor Knee Society scores (KSS), or extensor lag greater than 30° at mean follow-up duration of 57.6 months.[66] Another study by Ricciardi et al showed EMA survivorship of 69% at mean of 68 months; however, the reoperation rate was 58% with these patients having worse outcomes.[68] One explanation for the lower success rates with EMA could be surgical technique. Burnett et al demonstrated significantly better outcomes and lower postoperative extensor lag when the graft was fully tensioned in extension as opposed to minimally tensioned (mean extensor lag of 4.3° vs. 59°).[69] There was no difference in knee flexion observed between groups, indicating full tensioning is not detrimental to knee flexion.

More recently, use of a synthetic Marlex mesh has been described for complex extensor mechanism disruptions. The mesh consists of a nonabsorbable polypropylene sheet which is tubularized, sandwiched between two layers of soft tissue, and secured with nonabsorbable sutures (**Fig. 56-12**). Postoperatively, the author's preference is for leg immobilization in full extension for 3 months (first 6 weeks in a cast) with slow progressive increase in

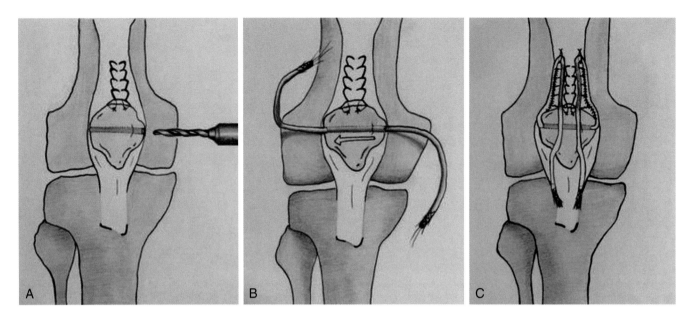

FIGURE 56-10 Diagram demonstrating use of a semitendinosus and gracilis autograft for augmentation of a quadriceps tendon rupture repair. After débridement of the quadriceps ruptured tendon edges, a primary repair of the tendon is performed with a Krackow stitch using heavy non-absorbable sutures. The semitendinosus and gracilis tendons are harvested from the patient, stripped of muscle and the tendon edges are then approximated and secured using a Krackow whipstitch technique to add length to the graft. A transverse tunnel is drilled through the patella to accommodate the thickness of the graft **(A)**. The graft is then passed through a predrilled transverse tunnel in the patella **(B)** and incorporated proximally to the quadriceps tendon on each side of the patella using a running Krackow stitch with heavy nonabsorbable suture. The free tendon ends are then secured distally into the patellar tendon in similar fashion **(C)**.

motion of 15° to 20° every 2 weeks for an additional 4 to 6 weeks. Patient compliance is critical to achieve optimal outcomes with this procedure. Results in the literature for the synthetic polypropylene mesh technique are variable with many showing improvement in pain and functional scores, but persistent extensor lag between 5° and 40°.[70] Abdel et al reviewed results of 27 quadriceps ruptures treated with Marlex synthetic mesh as part of a series of other extensor mechanism injuries and found overall 89% survivorship at 2-year follow-up with a mean extensor lag of 9° at final follow-up.[71] The most common complications included infection, arthrofibrosis, and wound healing issues that were treated conservatively. A recent meta-analysis comparing synthetic mesh to EMA for extensor mechanism disruption found similar success rates between groups with about 25% failure in both groups.[72] The benefits of synthetic mesh over EMA included lower cost, no risk for disease transmission, easier availability, and potentially lower risk for graft stretch out over time.[72] Synthetic mesh offers promising outcomes for this patient population with more long-term studies needed to better understand patient outcomes.

Patella Fracture

Fracture of the patella is an uncommon complication following TKA with a reported incidence between 0.3% and 5.4%.[61,73] One of the largest series from the Mayo Clinic showed an incidence of 0.68% with the majority of fractures occurring within 2 years of the initial surgery.[74] Several risk factors have been identified (**Table 56-1**) including patient-specific factors, perioperative

technique, and postoperative events. Errors in patellar resection (both over- and underresection) during resurfacing can predispose to patellar fracture. Overresection of the patella with residual bone thickness less than 15 mm results in increased anterior patellar strain and increased risk for fracture.[75] Conversely, underresection of the patellar component and overstuffing will increase the joint reactive force on the patella and increases risk for fracture. Restoring the composite patellar height to its native thickness is critical to avoid these complications. Several studies have identified single central peg components as having a higher risk of fracture as it is more disruptive to the central patellar blood supply.[76,77] Whenever possible, the authors favor use of a three-peg component. Disruption of the blood supply to the patella can cause avascular necrosis and increased risk for fracture (**Fig. 56-13**). Vascular supply to the patella comes from four main extraosseous vessels as well as a network of intraosseous vessels.[78] A standard medial parapatellar approach will disrupt the extraosseous superior and inferior medial geniculate arteries, while a lateral meniscectomy may disrupt the lateral inferior genicular artery.[78,79] The superior lateral genicular artery is typically the only remaining extraosseous vessel following standard medial parapatellar approach for TKA but it becomes at risk during lateral retinacular release.[26] Performing a lateral release has been identified in several studies as a significant risk factor for patellar fracture.[80,81] The intraosseous blood supply comes from both the quadriceps tendon and the retropatellar fat pad, so excessive fat pad resection can compromise this blood supply.[26] Only enough fat pad to allow for exposure should be removed to preserve this blood supply.

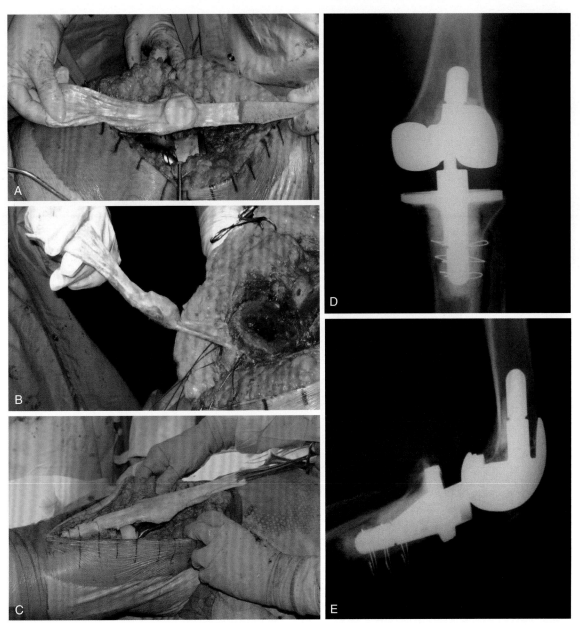

FIGURE 56-11 Example of extensor mechanism allograft (EMA) reconstruction technique for extensor mechanism disruption after total knee arthroplasty. The allograft consists of a large tibial tubercle bone block (approximately 2 cm in depth x 6-8 cm in width x 6-8 cm in height) with the patellar tendon, patella, and quadriceps tendon all attached as shown in **(A)**. Special care should be taken to choose a graft with abundant quadriceps tendon length. Prior to insertion, the proximal aspect of the allograft bone block is beveled into a dovetail configuration as shown in **(A)** so that it can engage the bone at the tibial recipient site. The patient's native tibial tubercle is removed with osteotomes to create a bed for the allograft bone block with a reverse dovetail configuration to engage the dovetail shape of the allograft when it is pulled superiorly. This technique provides inherent bone stability to avoid graft migration and allows a snug press-fit between tibia and allograft. The bone block can be secured into the tibia using thin wires drilled through the tibia as shown in **(B)** or with lag screws, however wires tend to have lower rates of iatrogenic fracture in the frozen cadaveric bone. The EMA is then tensioned with the knee in full extension as shown in **(C)** and secured proximally to the native quadriceps tendon using strong nonabsorbable sutures. Special care is taken to appropriately restore the joint line. **D and E:** Demonstrate AP and lateral postoperative radiographs showing the EMA in place following complete healing. (Images are courtesy of Robert E. Booth, Jr., MD.)

Patellar fractures can be classified using several different classification systems. The classification described by Ortiguera and Berry is based on the integrity of the extensor mechanism and implant stability.[74] Type I fractures have a stable implant and intact extensor mechanism. Type II fractures have an associated disruption of the extensor mechanism, either with or without a loose component. Type III fractures involve a loose patellar component but with intact extensor mechanism and are

subcategorized based on quality of the remaining bone. Type IIIA fractures have good bone stock, while type IIIB fractures have poor bone stock defined by less than 10 mm of remaining bone thickness or comminution.

Treatment for patellar fractures depends on the integrity of the extensor mechanism and patellar component stability. For patients with a nondisplaced fracture, stable patellar component, and no extensor lag, treatment can consist of immobilization in a cast or brace in full extension until the

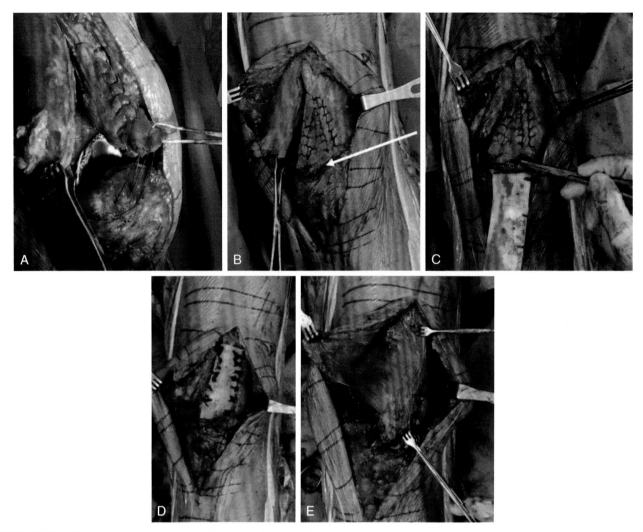

FIGURE 56-12   Clinical intraoperative images of the author's preferred technique for a synthetic Marlex mesh reconstruction of a traumatic quadriceps rupture following total knee arthroplasty. A running Krackow stitch with nonabsorbable suture is performed and passed through the quadriceps tendon **(A)**. The sutures are passed through the patella via longitudinal drill holes and tensioned tightly in full extension to reapproximate the torn edge of the tendon to the superior pole of the patella **(B)**. The synthetic mesh is then positioned to bridge the zone of the repair **(C)**. The mesh is secured proximally to the quadriceps tendon and distally to peripatellar tissues using nonabsorbable sutures in full extension **(D)**. The vastus medialis oblique (VMO) muscle is then mobilized to provide superficial coverage of the mesh **(E)**. The VMO is further secured with nonadditional sutures. At completion, there is no exposed mesh superficially and the skin can be safely closed in standard fashion. The entire leg is immobilized in a long leg cast for up to 12 weeks with graduated progressive knee range of motion initiated at 12 weeks.

fracture has healed. If patients have a grossly intact extensor mechanism with mild extensor lag, nonoperative treatment can also be considered with good results reported.[74,82] When the extensor mechanism is disrupted, surgical repair or reconstruction should be considered. Fractures with adequate bone stock should be treated with open reduction and internal fixation, whereas those with insufficient bone stock may require a partial or total patellectomy with possible soft tissue augmentation. Fragment excision can be considered for displaced pole fractures without extensor

TABLE 56-1 **Risk Factors for Patellar Fracture**		
Patient Factors	**Surgical Factors**	**Postoperative Factors**
Male[1-3]	Patella resurfacing[5,9]	Avascular necrosis[17]
Obesity[1]	Improper patella resection[5,10]	Trauma[5]
High activity[1]	Component malpositioning[10]	Excessive early flexion[1]
Osteoporosis[4]	Lateral retinacular release[10-14]	Arthrofibrosis requiring manipulation
Revision total knee arthroplasty (TKA)[5]	Patellar maltracking[5,10]	
Rheumatoid arthritis[6]	Press-fit patella component	
Initial thickness ≤18 mm[7]	Hinged TKA[15]	
Preoperative varus >15°[8]	Central peg component[10,16]	

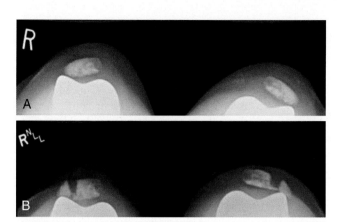

FIGURE 56-13 Merchant radiographic views of patient at 5 **(A)** and 9 **(B)** months postoperatively with bilateral patellar avascular necrosis resulting in bilateral patella fractures in the absence of any trauma. Patient clinically had full active knee motion with no extensor lag bilaterally. The right knee was symptomatic with patellofemoral pain and was treated surgically with patellar component removal and partial patellectomy. The left side was asymptomatic and has been treated conservatively with a satisfactory outcome.

mechanism disruption.[82] If the patellar component is loose, component revision should be performed whenever possible. Total patellectomy is typically reserved for severely comminuted fractures or failed prior interventions.[82]

Unfortunately, outcomes following operative treatment of patellar fractures are poor with high complication rates and need for reoperation.[74] Ortiguera and Berry[75] reported on one of the largest series of patella fractures following TKA. Eleven patients underwent surgical intervention for a type II patellar fracture with six patients having complications and five patients needing reoperation. Twenty patients underwent surgery for a type III fracture (with a loose patellar component) with nine patients having significant complications and four patients needing revision.[76] Other series have shown that patients with displaced patella fractures treated with open reduction and internal fixation have high rates of nonunion, with rates ranging as high as 90% to 100%.[1,74,76,81,82] Infection rates following operative treatment are similarly high ranging from 6% to 31%.[62,73,74,83] Patients treated with patellectomy for comminuted patella fractures can achieve good pain control and function. Chang et al showed improved pain in nine patients treated with patellectomy for comminuted patellar fractures, all with an extensor lag of less than 10°. However, functional results were inferior to those following initial arthroplasty.[84] Patients undergoing surgical treatment for patellar fractures should be extensively counseled on risks and outcomes following treatment.

Patellar Tendon Rupture

Patellar tendon rupture is another devastating injury yet with a low incidence between 0.17% and 0.56%.[29,57,85] Due to the low incidence, it has been difficult to identify risk factors for its occurrence. Some have identified certain medical conditions which predispose patients to patellar tendon injuries, including rheumatoid arthritis,

diabetes mellitus, or collagen vascular disease.[86] Others have demonstrated that patients with chronic steroid use are at increased risk. Some studies have shown a higher incidence with use of hinged prostheses, presumably due to the higher constraint of these implants.[87] Other factors contributing to this injury include a previous patellofemoral realignment procedure,[88] revision surgery,[57] multiple prior surgeries,[61,89] infection, trauma, and chronic patellar tendonitis.[89]

Several treatment options exist for patellar tendon injuries. In cases where the patellar tendon peels off the tibial tubercle during surgery, the tendon can be reattached using drill holes or a suture anchor as long as the periosteal sleeve remains intact. Primary repair of chronic ruptures or avulsions often have unfavorable results. Rand et al reported poor outcomes with both suture anchor and staple repair for his series of 18 patellar tendon ruptures, with 4 patients developing a deep infection.[57] Gilmore et al similarly found poor outcomes with primary repair of post-TKA patellar tendon ruptures with best results achieved when using autogenous augmentation of the repair with structures such as the medial gastrocnemius[90] or semitendinosus tendon autograft.[86,89] Use of allogenic grafts had the highest rates of re-rupture.[89] Crossett et al used an Achilles tendon allograft in nine patients and had two patients with early graft failures requiring revision.[91] Emerson et al described a technique using an EMA containing a cemented patellar component in 10 patients. Two patients experienced a graft rupture, one patient with patellar loosening and one patient with a patellar fracture.[92,93] Successful outcomes have been shown with use of a medial gastrocnemius flap, particularly when used as a salvage procedure for failed prior repairs;[65,90] however, these series are small with limited follow-up duration. The use of synthetic polypropylene meshes is gaining interest for use of patellar tendon ruptures, with promising early results as described previously.[61,72] More quality long-term studies are needed to better understand outcomes with this technique for this challenging complication.

RESURFACED VERSUS NONRESURFACED PATELLA

Whether or not to resurface the patella at the time of TKA remains a controversial topic with an impressive amount of literature supporting both sides of the debate. Leaving the patella nonresurfaced has become a popular trend in the United States over the past few decades, based on European literature showing minimal impact on outcomes or revision rates with nonresurfacing.[94] Patellar resurfacing has been associated with higher risks for certain complications including patella fracture, devascularization, component loosening or failure, patellofemoral instability, injury to the extensor mechanism, and patellar clunk syndrome.[30,42,95] The major issue with leaving the patella nonresurfaced is persistent anterior knee pain that may require a secondary resurfacing procedure. Some studies from the United States have demonstrated that the TKA revision rates to resurface a nonresurfaced patellar have increased over the past decade,[2] accounting for around 4% of all TKA failures.[9] Quality studies have shown conflicting results on the topic. Burnett et al performed a randomized controlled trial (RCT) of 90 patients with a minimum 10-year follow-up duration and found no significant difference in revision rates or clinical outcomes between patients with resurfaced and nonresurfaced patellae.[96] They found no correlation between patellar cartilage integrity at the time of initial surgery and the need for revision. Other studies have found higher rates of reoperation in the nonresurfaced group, but no difference in pain or functional outcomes.[3,4] Several meta-analyses have demonstrated inferior outcomes with nonresurfacing of the patella.[3-7,97] Parvizi et al performed a meta-analysis of RCTs, which revealed a higher instance of anterior knee pain and need for revision in nonresurfaced patellae, with the revision rate being 8.7%.[6] Another meta-analysis and systematic review revealed better pain and function scores in the resurfaced group with a lower incidence of revision (1% reoperation vs. 6.9% in the nonresurfaced group).[7] Pilling et al in another meta-analysis of RCTs showed significantly higher reoperation rates in the nonresurfaced group and higher rates of anterior knee pain in the nonresurfaced group (24% vs. 13%), but this did not reach statistical significance. Patellofemoral-related complications were also higher in the nonresurfaced group.[5] Further evaluation has shown patella resurfacing to be economically favorable, assuming that revision rates for secondary resurfacing remain above 0.77%.[98] Cumulatively, the literature seems to support resurfacing the patella; however, there is a recognized bias toward higher reoperation in the nonresurfaced group as secondary resurfacing is a surgical option to treat persistent anterior knee pain that could falsely increase revision rates. Additionally, many comparative studies are historical and evaluated designs with a trochlear groove which poorly accommodated native patellar anatomy. Whiteside and Nakamura described improved results with nonresurfacing using a femoral component with a modern, "patella-friendly" trochlear design.[99]

When leaving the patella nonresurfaced, there are several surgical techniques described, including leaving the patella alone entirely, performing osteophyte excision, peripheral electrocautery denervation, and soft tissue débridement. Some advocate for drilling or microfracture of the patella when eburnated bone is present.[100-104] A meta-analysis of prospective RCTs by Findlay et al reviewed the various different nonresurfacing techniques and found no difference in pain scores between the various nonresurfacing techniques and no difference compared to patellar resurfacing.[100] While some studies have shown early benefit with electrocautery denervation of a nonresurfaced patella,[101] other studies have failed to find any significant impact on outcomes at 2 to –5 years follow-up duration.[101-104]

If revision for secondary patellar resurfacing is required, appropriate patient education is needed as studies have shown inferior outcomes following secondary resurfacing compared to subjects in which the patella was resurfaced primarily.[105-109] Parvizi et al studied outcomes in 39 patients who underwent secondary resurfacing at average of 29 months following the initial TKA. All patients had improved pain and functional scores; however, eight patients were dissatisfied with their outcomes.[105] Another study showed that out of 232 patients undergoing secondary resurfacing, only 64% had satisfactory outcomes and there was no significant improvement in pain scores following revision.[107] The most common complications included infection, wound healing issues, patellofemoral instability, and patella fracture.[107] Similarly, Toro-Ibarguen et al showed only 59% of patients had improvement in their pain following secondary resurfacing and 65% of patients remained unsatisfied.[106] Using the Trent and Wales Arthroplasty Registrar, Thomas et al found only 44% had resolution of their knee pain following secondary resurfacing with only 40% of patients having satisfactory outcomes.[110]

There may be a cohort of patients that do well with a nonresurfaced patella. Shih et al evaluated nonresurfaced patellae at average of 8.5 years following TKA and found normal patellofemoral tracking and articular surface in about 60% of patients. In the remaining patients, the most common issues encountered were radiographic patellar degenerative changes and maltracking. They found that patients with patellar maltracking prior to TKA were at higher risk for these abnormalities, and thus patients with preoperative maltracking may benefit from resurfacing at the time of the initial TKA.[111] This has been supported by other studies showing that patients with patella tilt or patellar dysplasia are at increased risk for secondary resurfacing.[112,113] Another variable associated with poor outcomes following nonresurfacing was shorter patellar height. In their series of 119 knees in patients with rheumatoid arthritis, Fern et al found that patients with patellar height 15 mm or higher above the joint line had significantly lower rates of anterior knee pain following TKA with a nonresurfaced patella. They suggested that patellar height less than 15 mm may be a useful variable to decide who should undergo resurfacing to reduce the risk of anterior knee pain. Further evidence is needed to help guide surgeons in developing a selective resurfacing protocol.

PREVENTATIVE TECHNIQUE

Avoiding the various complications related to the extensor mechanism following TKA can be achieved with good surgical technique and patient education. Proper handling of the patella is critical. Cumulatively, the literature demonstrates lower rates of anterior knee pain and lower revision rates with patellar resurfacing. The patellar resection should be enough to accommodate the thickness of the patellar component with care to avoid over- or under-resection. The cut should be flush to create uniform facet thickness which typically involves more resection of the thicker medial facet. The patellar component should be placed superiorly to lower rates of crepitus and medially to improve patellar tracking. Lateral releases can be performed to improve soft tissue balance for tracking but with care to protect the patellar vascular supply. Patellar vascularity can be preserved with a minimal fat pad excision and lateral release at least 1 cm from the patellar periphery. Any excess soft tissue along the undersurface of the quadriceps should be sharply excised to lower the incidence of patellar crepitus and clunk. Proper rotational positioning of the femoral and tibial components, particularly avoided internal rotation or medial shifting, is crucial for proper patellar tracking. Flexed posturing of the femoral component should be avoided to lower the incidence of extensor mechanism irritation or disruption. When using a PS femoral component, implants with narrow flange and a smaller intercondylar box ratio are preferred to lower the incidence of crepitus. Postoperatively, patients should work on graduated knee motion avoiding excessive flexion in the early postoperative period to avoid arthrotomy repair disruption, but progressive enough motion to avoid arthrofibrosis. With appropriate preoperative planning, good surgical technique, use of modern implants, and patient compliance, the risk for potentially devastating complications of the extensor mechanism will hopefully continue to decrease.

CONCLUSION

Complications related to the extensor mechanism following TKA remain some of the most challenging issues for arthroplasty surgeons to manage. There are various treatment options available for extensor complications, however prevention is paramount. Most of these complications can be minimized by recognizing and addressing contributing factors along with good surgical technique. Improvements in implant design have helped to decrease the incidence of some complications, yet careful surgical execution is still critical. There is continued debate on whether the patella should be resurfaced in all cases with further literature needed on selective resurfacing. Surgeons should be mindful of the various complications that can arise related to the extensor mechanism and make every effort to avoid them when possible.

REFERENCES

1. Brick GW, Scott RD. The patellofemoral component of total knee arthroplasty. *Clin Orthop Relat Res.* 1988;(231):163-178.
2. Sharkey PF, Hozack WJ, Rothman RH, Shastri S, Jacoby SM. Insall Award paper. Why are total knee arthroplasties failing today? *Clin Orthop Relat Res.* 2002;(404):7-13.
3. Pavlou G, Meyer C, Leonidou A, As-Sultany M, West R, Tsiridis E. Patellar resurfacing in total knee arthroplasty: does design matter? *J Bone Joint Surg Am.* 2011;93:1301-1309.
4. He J-Y, Jiang L-S, Dai L-Y. Is patellar resurfacing superior than nonresurfacing in total knee arthroplasty? A meta-analysis of randomized trials. *Knee.* 2011;18:137-144.
5. Pilling RD, Moulder E, Allgar V, Messner J, Sun Z, Mohsen A. Patellar resurfacing in primary total knee replacement. *J Bone Joint Surg Am.* 2012;94:2270-2278.
6. Parvizi J, Rapuri VR, Saleh KJ, Kuskowski MA, Sharkey PF, Mont MA. Failure to resurface the patella during total knee arthroplasty may result in more knee pain and secondary surgery. *Clin Orthop Relat Res.* 2005;438:191-196.
7. Longo UG, Ciuffreda M, Mannering N, D'Andrea V, Cimmino M, Denaro V. Patellar resurfacing in total knee arthroplasty: systematic review and meta-analysis. *J Arthroplast.* 2018;33:620-632.
8. Kwon Y, Lombardi AV, Jacobs JJ, Fehring TK, Lewis CG, Cabanela ME. Risk stratification algorithm for management of patients with metal-on-metal hip arthroplasty. *J Bone Joint Surg.* 2014;4:1-6.
9. Sharkey PF, Lichstein PM, Shen C, Tokarski AT, Parvizi J. Why are total knee arthroplasties failing today—has anything changed after 10 years? *J Arthroplasty.* 2014;29:1774-1778.
10. Dalury DF, Pomeroy DL, Gorab RS, Adams MJ. Why are total knee arthroplasties being revised? *J Arthroplast.* 2013;28:120-121.
11. Sakai N, Luo ZP, Rand JA, An KN. The influence of weakness in the vastus medialis oblique muscle on the patellofemoral joint: an in vitro biomechanical study. *Clin Biomech.* 2000;15:335-339.
12. Merkow RL, Soudry M, Insall JN. Patellar dislocation following total knee replacement. *J Bone Joint Surg Am.* 1985;67:1321-1327.
13. Baldwin JL, House CK. Anatomic dimensions of the patella measured during total knee arthroplasty. *J Arthroplast.* 2005;20:250-257.
14. Theiss SM, Kitziger KJ, Lotke PS, Lotke PA. Component design affecting patellofemoral complications after total knee arthroplasty. *Clin Orthop Relat Res.* 1996;(326):183-187.
15. Sawaguchi N, Majima T, Ishigaki T, Mori N, Terashima T, Minami A. Mobile-bearing total knee arthroplasty improves patellar tracking and patellofemoral contact stress: in vivo measurements in the same patients. *J Arthroplast.* 2010;25:920-925.
16. Yang CC, McFadden LA, Dennis DA, Kim RH, Sharma A. Lateral retinacular release rates in mobile- versus fixed-bearing TKA. *Clin Orthop Relat Res.* 2008;466:2656-2661.
17. Singerman R, Gabriel SM, Maheshwer CB, Kennedy JW. Patellar contact forces with and without patellar resurfacing in total knee arthroplast. *J Arthroplast.* 1999;14(5):603-609.
18. Smith AJ, Wood DJ, Li M-G. Total knee replacement with and without patellar resurfacing. *Bone Joint J.* 2008;90-B:43-49.
19. Holt GE, Dennis DA. The role of patellar resurfacing in total knee arthroplasty. *Clin Orthop Relat Res.* 2003;(203):76-83. doi:10.1097/01.blo.0000092991.90435.fb.
20. Stiehl JB, Komistek RD, Dennis DA, Keblish PA. Kinematics of the patellofemoral joint in total knee arthroplasty. *J Arthroplast.* 2001;16:706-714.
21. Husted H, Jensen TT. Influence of the pneumatic tourniquet on patella tracking in total knee arthroplasty. *J Arthroplasty.* 2005;20:694-697.
22. Marson BM, Tokish JT. The effect of a tourniquet on intraoperative patellofemoral tracking during total knee arthroplasty. *J Arthroplasty.* 1999;14:197-199.
23. Cho W-S, Woo J-H, Park H-Y, Youm Y-S, Kim B-K. Should the 'no thumb technique' be the golden standard for evaluating patellar tracking in total knee arthroplasty? *Knee.* 2011;18:177-179.
24. Bindelglass DF, Vince KG. Patellar tilt and subluxation following subvastus and parapatellar approach in total knee arthroplasty. Implication for surgical technique. *J Arthroplasty.* 1996;11:507-511.
25. Hsu HC, Luo ZP, Rand JA, An KN. Influence of lateral release on patellar tracking and patellofemoral contact characteristics after total knee arthroplasty. *J Arthroplasty.* 1997;12:74-83.

26. Kayler DE, Lyttle D. Surgical interruption of patellar blood supply by total knee arthroplasty. *Clin Orthop Relat Res.* 1988;(229):221-227.

27. Shelbourne K, Urch S, Gray T. Results of medial retinacular imbrication in patients with unilateral patellar dislocation. *J Knee Surg.* 2012;25:391-396.

28. Meding JB, Fish MD, Berend ME, Ritter MA, Keating EM. Predicting patellar failure after total knee arthroplasty. *Clin Orthop Relat Res.* 2008;466:2769-2774.

29. Healy WL, Wasilewski SA, Takei R, Oberlander M. Patellofemoral complications following total knee arthroplasty. Correlation with implant design and patient risk factors. *J Arthroplast.* 1995;10:197-201.

30. Berend ME, Ritter MA, Keating EM, Faris PM, Crites BM. The failure of all-polyethylene patellar components in total knee replacement. *Clin Orthop Relat Res.* 2001;(388):105-111.

31. Rath NK, Dudhniwala AG, White SP, Forster MC. Aseptic loosening of the patellar component at the cement–implant interface. *Knee.* 2012;19:823-826.

32. Garcia RM, Kraay MJ, Conroy-Smith PA, Goldberg VM. Management of the deficient patella in revision total knee arthroplasty. *Clin Orthop Relat Res.* 2008;466:2790-2797.

33. Rand JA. Treatment of the patella at reimplantation for septic total knee arthroplasty. *Clin Orthop Relat Res.* 2003;416:105-109.

34. Leopold SS, Silverton CD, Barden RM, Rosenberg AG. Isolated revision of the patellar component in total knee arthroplasty. *J Bone Joint Surg Am.* 2003;85-A:41-47.

35. Berry DJ, Rand JA. Isolated patellar component revision of total knee arthroplasty. *Clin Orthop Relat Res.* 1993;(286):110-115.

36. Berend ME, Harty LD, Ritter MA, Stonehouse DM. Excisional arthroplasty for patellar loosening in total knee arthroplasty. *J Arthroplast.* 2003;18:668-671.

37. Lonner JH, Mont MA, Sharkey PF, Siliski JM, Rajadhyaksha AD, Lotke PA. Fate of the unrevised all-polyethylene patellar component in revision total knee arthroplasty. *J Bone Joint Surg Am.* 2003;85-A:56-59.

38. Stulberg SD, Stulberg BN, Hamati Y, Tsao A. Failure mechanisms of metal-backed patellar components. *Clin Orthop Relat Res.* 1988;(236):88-105.

39. Bayley JC, Scott RD, Ewald FC, Holmes GB. Failure of the metal-backed patellar component after total knee replacement. *J Bone Joint Surg Am.* 1988;70:668-674.

40. Garcia RM, Kraay MJ, Goldberg VM. Isolated all-polyethylene patellar revisions for metal-backed patellar failure. *Clin Orthop Relat Res.* 2008;466:2784-2789.

41. Burke WV, Ammeen DJ, Engh GA. Isolated revision of failed metal-backed patellar components. *J Arthroplast.* 2005;20:998-1001.

42. Conrad DN, Dennis DA. Patellofemoral crepitus after total knee arthroplasty: etiology and preventive measures. *Clin Orthop Surg.* 2014;6:9.

43. Choi WC, Ryu K-J, Lee S, Seong SC, Lee MC. Painful patellar clunk or crepitation of contemporary knee prostheses. *Clin Orthop Relat Res.* 2013;471:1512-1522.

44. Koh Y-G, Kim S-J, Chun Y-M, Kim Y-C, Park Y-S. Arthroscopic treatment of patellofemoral soft tissue impingement after posterior stabilized total knee arthroplasty. *Knee.* 2008;15:36-39.

45. Hwang B-H, Nam C-H, Jung K-A, Ong A, Lee S-C. Is further treatment necessary for patellar crepitus after total knee arthroplasty? *Clin Orthop Relat Res.* 2013;471:606-612.

46. Dennis DA, Kim RH, Johnson DR, Springer BD, Fehring TK, Sharma A. The John Insall award: control-matched evaluation of painful patellar crepitus after total knee arthroplasty. *Clin Orthop Relat Res.* 2011;469:10-17.

47. Martin JR, Jennings JM, Watters TS, Levy DL, McNabb DC, Dennis DA. Femoral implant design modification decreases the incidence of patellar crepitus in total knee arthroplasty. *J Arthroplast.* 2017;32:1310-1313.

48. Lucas TS, DeLuca PF, Nazarian DG, Bartolozzi AR, Booth RE. Arthroscopic treatment of patellar clunk. *Clin Orthop Relat Res.* 1999;(367):226-229.

49. Dajani KA, Stuart MJ, Dahm DL, Levy BA. Arthroscopic treatment of patellar clunk and synovial hyperplasia after total knee arthroplasty. *J Arthroplast.* 2010;25:97-103.

50. Meftah M, Jhurani A, Bhat JA, Ranawat AS, Ranawat CS. The effect of patellar replacement technique on patellofemoral complications and anterior knee pain. *J Arthroplasty.* 2012;27:1075-1080.e1.

51. Fukunaga K, Kobayashi A, Minoda Y, Iwaki H, Hashimoto Y, Takaoka K. The incidence of the patellar clunk syndrome in a recently designed mobile-bearing posteriorly stabilised total knee replacement. *J Bone Joint Surg Br.* 2009;91-B:463-468.

52. Clarke HD, Fuchs R, Scuderi GR, Mills EL, Scott WN, Insall JN. The influence of femoral component design in the elimination of patellar clunk in posterior-stabilized total knee arthroplasty. *J Arthroplasty.* 2006;21:167-171.

53. Ip D, Wu WC, Tsang WL. Comparison of two total knee prostheses on the incidence of patella clunk syndrome. *Int Orthop.* 2002;26:48-51.

54. Yau W-P, Wong JWK, Chiu K-Y, Ng T-P, Tang W-M. Patellar clunk syndrome after posterior stabilized total knee arthroplasty. *J Arthroplasty.* 2003;18:1023-1028.

55. Maloney WJ, Schmidt R, Sculco TP. Femoral component design and patellar clunk syndrome. *Clin Orthop Relat Res.* 2003;410:199-202.

56. Ranawat AS, Ranawat CS, Slamin JE, Dennis DA. Patellar crepitation in the P.F.C. sigma total knee system. *Orthopedics.* 2006;29:S68-S70.

57. Rand JA, Morrey BF, Bryan RS. Patellar tendon rupture after total knee arthroplasty. *Clin Orthop Relat Res.* 1989;(244):233-238.

58. Leopold SS, Greidanus N, Paprosky WG, Berger RA, Rosenberg AG. High rate of failure of allograft reconstruction of the extensor mechanism after total knee arthroplasty. *J Bone Joint Surg Am.* 1999;81:1574-1579.

59. Dobbs RE, Hanssen AD, Lewallen DG, Pagnano MW. Quadriceps tendon rupture after total knee arthroplasty. *J Bone Joint Surg.* 2005;87:37-45.

60. Chhapan J, Sankineani SR, Chiranjeevi T, Reddy MV, Reddy D, Gurava Reddy AV. Early quadriceps tendon rupture after primary total knee arthroplasty. *Knee.* 2018;25:192-194.

61. Lynch AF, Rorabeck CH, Bourne RB. Extensor mechanism complications following total knee arthroplasty. *J Arthroplasty.* 1987;2:135-140.

62. Grace JN, Sim FH. Fracture of the patella after total knee arthroplasty. *Clin Orthop Relat Res.* 1988;(230):168-175.

63. Courtney PM, Edmiston TA, Pflederer CT, Levine BR, Gerlinger TL. Is there any role for direct repair of extensor mechanism disruption following total knee arthroplasty? *J Arthroplasty.* 2018;33:S244-S248.

64. Rosenberg AG. Management of extensor mechanism rupture after TKA. *J Bone Joint Surg Br.* 2012;94-B:116-119.

65. Whiteside LA. Surgical technique: muscle transfer restores extensor function after failed patella-patellar tendon allograft. *Clin Orthop Relat Res.* 2014;472:218-226.

66. Brown NM, Murray T, Sporer SM, Wetters N, Berger RA, Della Valle CJ. Extensor mechanism allograft reconstruction for extensor mechanism failure following total knee arthroplasty. *J Bone Joint Surg Am.* 2015;97:279-283.

67. Lim CT, Amanatullah DF, Huddleston JI, et al. Reconstruction of disrupted extensor mechanism after total knee arthroplasty. *J Arthroplast.* 2017;32:3134-3140.

68. Ricciardi BF, Oi K, Trivellas M, Lee Y, Della Valle AG, Westrich GH. Survivorship of extensor mechanism allograft reconstruction after total knee arthroplasty. *J Arthroplasty.* 2017;32:183-188.

69. Burnett RSJ, Berger RA, Paprosky WG, Della Valle CJ, Jacobs JJ, Rosenberg AG. Extensor mechanism allograft reconstruction after total knee arthroplasty. A comparison of two techniques. *J Bone Joint Surg Am.* 2004;86-A:2694-2699.

70. Nodzo SR, Rachala SR. Polypropylene mesh augmentation for complete quadriceps rupture after total knee arthroplasty. *Knee.* 2016;23:177-180.

71. Abdel MP, Salib CG, Mara KC, Pagnano MW, Perry KI, Hanssen AD. Extensor mechanism reconstruction with use of Marlex mesh. *J Bone Joint Surg.* 2018;100:1309-1318.

72. Shau D, Patton R, Patel S, Ward L, Guild G. Synthetic mesh vs. allograft extensor mechanism reconstruction in total knee arthroplasty—a systematic review of the literature and meta-analysis. *Knee*. 2018;25:2-7.

73. Keating EM, Haas G, Meding JB. Patella fracture after post total knee replacements. *Clin Orthop Relat Res*. 2003;416:93-97.

74. Ortiguera CJ, Berry DJ. Patellar fracture after total knee arthroplasty. *J Bone Joint Surg Am*. 2002;84-A:532-540.

75. Reuben JD, McDonald CL, Woodard PL, Hennington LJ. Effect of patella thickness on patella strain following total knee arthroplasty. *J Arthroplast*. 1991;6:251-258.

76. Chalidis BE, Tsiridis E, Tragas AA, Stavrou Z, Giannoudis PV. Management of periprosthetic patellar fractures. *Injury*. 2007;38:714-724.

77. Goldberg VM, Figgie HE, Inglis AE, et al. Patellar fracture type and prognosis in condylar total knee arthroplasty. *Clin Orthop Relat Res*. 1988;(236):115-122.

78. Brick GW, Scott RD. Blood supply to the patella. Significance in total knee arthroplasty. *J Arthroplast*. 1989;4 suppl:S75-S79.

79. Bonutti PM, Miller BG, Cremens MJ. Intraosseous patellar blood supply after medial parapatellar arthrotomy. *Clin Orthop Relat Res*. 1998;(352):202-214.

80. Tria AJ, Harwood DA, Alicea JA, Cody RP. Patellar fractures in posterior stabilized knee arthroplasties. *Clin Orthop Relat Res*. 1994;(299):131-138.

81. Scott RD, Turoff N, Ewald FC. Stress fracture of the patella following duopatellar total knee arthroplasty with patellar resurfacing. *Clin Orthop Relat Res*. 1982;(170):147-151.

82. Hozack WJ, Goll SR, Lotke PA, Rothman RH, Booth RE. The treatment of patellar fractures after total knee arthroplasty. *Clin Orthop Relat Res*. 1988;(236):123-127.

83. Parvizi J, Kim K-I, Oliashirazi A, Ong A, Sharkey PF. Periprosthetic patellar fractures. *Clin Orthop Relat Res*. 2006;446:161-166.

84. Chang MA, Rand JA, Trousdale RT. Patellectomy after total knee arthroplasty. *Clin Orthop Relat Res*. 2005;440:175-177.

85. Boyd AD, Ewald FC, Thomas WH, Poss R, Sledge CB. Long-term complications after total knee arthroplasty with or without resurfacing of the patella. *J Bone Joint Surg Am*. 1993;75:674-681.

86. Cadambi A, Engh GA. Use of a semitendinosus tendon autogenous graft for rupture of the patellar ligament after total knee arthroplasty. A report of seven cases. *J Bone Joint Surg Am*. 1992;74:974-979.

87. Hui FC, Fitzgerald RH. Hinged total knee arthroplasty. *J Bone Joint Surg Am*. 1980;62:513-519.

88. Grace JN, Rand JA. Patellar instability after total knee arthroplasty. *Clin Orthop Relat Res*. 1988;(237):184-189.

89. Gilmore JH, Clayton-Smith ZJ, Aguilar M, Pneumaticos SG, Giannoudis PV. Reconstruction techniques and clinical results of patellar tendon ruptures: evidence today. *Knee*. 2015;22:148-155.

90. Jaureguito JW, Dubois CM, Smith SR, Gottlieb LJ, Finn HA. Medial gastrocnemius transposition flap for the treatment of disruption of the extensor mechanism after total knee arthroplasty. *J Bone Joint Surg*. 1997;79:866-873.

91. Crossett LS, Sinha RK, Sechriest VF, Rubash HE. Reconstruction of a ruptured patellar tendon with achilles tendon allograft following total knee arthroplasty. *J Bone Joint Surg Am*. 2002;84-A:1354-1361.

92. Emerson RH, Head WC, Malinin TI. Reconstruction of patellar tendon rupture after total knee arthroplasty with an extensor mechanism allograft. *Clin Orthop Relat Res*. 1990;(260):154-161.

93. Emerson RH, Head WC, Malinin TI. Extensor mechanism reconstruction with an allograft after total knee arthroplasty. *Clin Orthop Relat Res*. 1994;(303):79-85.

94. Ali A, Lindstrand A, Nilsdotter A, Sundberg M. Similar patient-reported outcomes and performance after total knee arthroplasty with or without patellar resurfacing. *Acta Orthop*. 2016;87:274-279.

95. Barrack RL, Bertot AJ, Wolfe MW, Waldman DA, Milicic M, Myers L. Patellar resurfacing in total knee arthroplasty. A prospective, randomized, double-blind study with five to seven years of follow-up. *J Bone Joint Surg Am*. 2001;83-A:1376-1381.

96. Burnett RS, Haydon CM, Rorabeck CH, Bourne RB. Patella resurfacing versus nonresurfacing in total knee arthroplasty: results of a randomized controlled clinical trial at a minimum of 10 years' followup. *Clin Orthop Relat Res*. 2004;(428):12-25.

97. Tang X-B, Wang J, Dong P-L, Zhou R. A meta-analysis of patellar replacement in total knee arthroplasty for patients with knee osteoarthritis. *J Arthroplast*. 2018;33:960-967.

98. Meijer KA, Dasa V. Is resurfacing the patella cheaper? An economic analysis of evidence based medicine on patellar resurfacing. *Knee*. 2015;22:136-141.

99. Whiteside LA, Nakamura T. Effect of femoral component design on unresurfaced patellas in knee arthroplasty. *Clin Orthop Relat Res*. 2003;410:189-198.

100. Findlay I, Wong F, Smith C, Back D, Davies A, Ajuied A. Non-resurfacing techniques in the management of the patella at total knee arthroplasty: a systematic review and meta-analysis. *Knee*. 2016;23:191-197.

101. van Jonbergen HPW, Scholtes VAB, Poolman RW. A randomised, controlled trial of circumpatellar electrocautery in total knee replacement without patellar resurfacing. *Bone Joint J*. 2014;96-B:473-478.

102. Baliga S, McNair CJ, Barnett KJ, MacLeod J, Humphry RW, Finlayson D. Does circumpatellar electrocautery improve the outcome after total knee replacement? *J Bone Joint Surg Br*. 2012;94-B:1228-1233.

103. Gupta S, Augustine A, Horey L, Meek RMD, Hullin MG, Mohammed A. Electrocautery of the patellar rim in primary total knee replacement: beneficial or unnecessary? *J Bone Joint Surg Br*. 2010;92-B:1259-1261.

104. Kwon SK, Nguku L, Han CD, Koh Y-G, Kim D-W, Park KK. Is electrocautery of patella useful in patella non-resurfacing total knee arthroplasty?: a prospective randomized controlled study. *J Arthroplast*. 2015;30:2125-2127.

105. Parvizi J, Mortazavi SMJ, Devulapalli C, Hozack WJ, Sharkey PF, Rothman RH. Secondary resurfacing of the patella after primary total knee arthroplasty. *J Arthroplast*. 2012;27:21-26.

106. Toro-Ibarguen AN, Navarro-Arribas R, Pretell-Mazzini J, Prada-Cañizares AC, Jara-Sánchez F. Secondary patellar resurfacing as a rescue procedure for persistent anterior knee pain after primary total knee arthroplasty: do our patients really improve? *J Arthroplast*. 2016;31:1539-1543.

107. van Jonbergen H-PW, Boeddha AV, M van Raaij JJA. Patient satisfaction and functional outcomes following secondary patellar resurfacing. *Orthopedics*. 2016;39:e850-e856.

108. Bhattee G, Moonot P, Govindaswamy R, Pope A, Fiddian N, Harvey A. Does malrotation of components correlate with patient dissatisfaction following secondary patellar resurfacing? *Knee*. 2014;21:247-251.

109. Muoneke HE, Khan AM, Giannikas KA, Hägglund E, Dunningham TH. Secondary resurfacing of the patella for persistent anterior knee pain after primary knee arthroplasty. *J Bone Joint Surg Br*. 2003;85:675-678.

110. Thomas C, Patel V, Mallick E, Esler C, Ashford RU. The outcome of secondary resurfacing of the patella following total knee arthroplasty: results from the Trent and Wales Arthroplasty Register. *Knee*. 2018;25:146-152.

111. Shih H-N, Shih L-Y, Wong Y-C, Hsu RW-W. Long-term changes of the nonresurfaced patella after total knee arthroplasty. *J Bone Joint Surg*. 2004;86-A:935-939.

112. Roessler PP, Moussa R, Jacobs C, et al. Predictors for secondary patellar resurfacing after primary total knee arthroplasty using a "patella-friendly" total knee arthroplasty system. *Int Orthop*. 2019;43(3):611-617. doi:10.1007/s00264-018-4075-8.

113. Franck F, Ouanezar H, Jacquel A, Pibarot V, Wegrzyn J. The predictive factors of secondary patellar resurfacing in computer-assisted total knee arthroplasty. A prospective cohort study. *Int Orthop*. 2018;42:1051-1060.

chapter 57

Periprosthetic Fractures

James R. Berstock, MBChB, MRCS, FRCS (T&O), MD, PGCert Med Ed |
Donald S. Garbuz, MD, MHSc, FRCS | Bassam A. Masri, MD, FRCS

INTRODUCTION

The incidence of periprosthetic fractures (PPFs) around a total knee arthroplasty (TKA) is rising and is believed to have quadrupled between 2000 and 2008 in the United States.[1] This is likely due to increasing numbers of TKAs within an aging, more osteoporotic population.[2] Approximately 1 in 40 patients who undergo primary TKA will sustain a PPF.[3] It has been estimated that intraoperative PPFs occur during approximately 4% of TKAs, often involving the medial femoral condyle.[4] A study of the Scottish National Database revealed a postoperative 5-year incidence of 0.6% after primary TKA and 1.7% after revision TKA.[5] PPFs around a TKA may occur in the femur, tibia, or patella and have been defined as occurring within 15 cm of the joint surface or within 5 cm of an intramedullary stem.[6-8] Distal femoral fractures are the most common PPF occurring in 0.3% to 2.5% of TKAs.[9-13] Patellar fractures occurred in 0.68% in a series from the Mayo clinic,[14] and others report fractures in 0.15% to 21% of resurfaced patellae and 0.05% of nonresurfaced patellae after a TKA.[14-19] The least commonly observed are tibial PPFs, reported in 0.4% to 1.7% of TKAs.[20]

Most fractures result from a low-velocity injury.[21] Risk factors include inflammatory arthropathy, steroid use, age > 70 years, poor bone stock, neurological disorders, and revision arthroplasty.[5,22] Prosthesis-related factors include loosening and osteolysis secondary to polythene wear.[21] Notching during the surgical preparation of the femoral component no longer appears to be a significant risk factor for PPF.[23]

Patients presenting with knee PPFs are more likely to be medically comorbid, female, and older when compared with patients undergoing revision TKA for other reasons.[24] Consequently, the 1-year mortality following a distal femoral PPF has been reported at 20.6%.[25] Complications following the treatment of this complex problem are also common. In a recent review of 58 distal femoral PPFs, readmission within 90 days of treatment occurred in over 20% of patients.[24] In a prospective study of 37 PPFs around a TKA, only 68% reached their prefracture mobility by 1 year and 22% had undergone surgical revision for various reasons. Additionally, nonoperative complications occurred in 16%.[26]

The financial implications of PPFs around TKAs have also been studied. The costs of treatment with revision arthroplasty were on average $37,680, with readmissions each costing $16,806 in 2013. Fracture fixation costs $25,539, with readmissions costing an average of $15,269.[24]

The goal of treatment is to expeditiously restore function while avoiding complications. This involves restoration of limb alignment, length, and rotation while enabling early mobilization. The treatment of knee PPFs may be challenging because of poor bone quality and the presence of components (proximally and distally), which may or may not be loose. Operative management has demonstrated benefits over nonoperative management of distal femoral fractures without a prosthesis,[27] and for the same reasons it forms the mainstay of treatment in PPFs after TKA.

DISTAL FEMORAL PERIPROSTHETIC FRACTURES

Classification

Historic classifications of distal femoral PPFs such as those from Neer et al in 1967,[28] DiGioia et al in 1991,[29] and Chen et al in 1994[30] concern themselves with fracture displacement and provide guidance as to the suitability of nonoperative management or surgical fixation. With the evolution of fixation and revision arthroplasty techniques, a modern group of classifications attempts to direct specific surgical treatment for each fracture type.

Rorabeck and Taylor acknowledged the important role of revision arthroplasty and described three types of fracture in 1997 (**Table 57-1**).[31,32] Type 1 represents a nondisplaced fracture with a well-fixed femoral component, type 2 describes a displaced fracture with a well-fixed femoral component, and type 3 is reserved for a loose or failed component. This classification promotes the use of revision arthroplasty for the treatment for type 3 fractures and remains highly influential today.

Su et al classified distal femoral fractures according to location, with a view to guiding the use of retrograde or antegrade nail fixation.[33] Kim et al considered bone stock, component fixation, and fracture reducibility in developing their classification system.[34] Further, Backstein et al sought to determine the feasibility of retrograde nailing.[35] Frenzel et al include consideration of the timing of treatment after injury.[36] Fakler and colleagues integrate femoral component design into their 2017 classification to create 16 fracture types.[37]

TABLE 57-1 Rorabeck Classification

Type	Description	Treatment
Type 1	Nondisplaced; component intact	Fixation or nonoperative
Type 2	Displaced; component intact	Fixation (nail or plate)
Type 3	Displaced; component loose or failing	Revision arthroplasty

The Unified Classification System (UCS), based on the Vancouver classification of PPFs of the proximal femur, provides a pragmatic guide to treatment while considering fracture location, implant loosening, bone stock, and other implants (**Table 57-2**).[38] Within the UCS, the most important categories with reference to the presence of a knee replacement are types B1, B2, and B3. The type D fracture (interprosthetic) requires special consideration because of the presence of a hip stem/implant within the proximal femur. Type E fractures can be managed as individual fractures of each bone, which should be classified individually.

Nonoperative Management

Deforming forces from the gastrocnemius which cause posterior angulation and rotation of the distal femur are compounded by the shortening forces from the quadriceps and are challenging to control with casting and bracing techniques alone. Malunion occurred in all displaced fractures treated nonoperatively in a series by Moran et al.[39] Nonoperative management is therefore reserved for completely nondisplaced fractures with inherent fracture stability and for the frailest of patients who are unlikely to survive surgery. Where appropriate, we recommend 12 weeks of hinged knee bracing with non–weight-bearing for a minimum of 6 weeks and regular radiographic assessment.

Fixation (Retrograde Nailing or Plating)

Distal femoral fractures with a well-fixed femoral component (B1 fractures, e.g., **Figs. 57-1** and **57-2**) may be treated satisfactorily with internal fixation (**Fig. 57-3**). The 2008 systematic review of 415 distal femoral PPFs by Herrera et al included data from 29 case series of patients treated with either retrograde intramedullary nailing (RIMN) or plate fixation. They identified an overall non-union rate of 9%, fixation failure of 4%, infection in 3%, and revision surgery in 13%. This review reports an 87% relative risk reduction of nonunion and a 70% relative risk reduction of revision surgery when RIMN is used when compared with traditional nonlocking plating.[40]

However, there was a nonsignificant trend toward benefit from emerging modern locking compression plate (LCP) technology.[40]

A systematic review of the modern era of treatment by Ebraheim et al in 2015 analyzed all treatments for distal femoral PPFs, with displaced B1 fractures being the most common pattern identified.[41] Ebraheim et al concluded that the most successful treatments were LCP (union rate 87%, complication rate 35%) and intramedullary nail (union rate 84%, complication rate 53%).[41] The most common complications in both groups were nonunion, malunion, delayed union, and the need for revision surgery.

The meta-analysis by Shin et al in 2017 included eight randomized controlled trials comparing RIMN with LCP for distal femoral PPFs. Postoperative Knee Society Scores, time to union, nonunion rates, and revision surgery requirements were not significantly different between LCP and RIMN treatment groups.[42]

RIMN may have theoretical biomechanical advantages over LCP due to it being coaxial with the anatomical axis of the femur and therefore providing greater stiffness under axial loading than a unilateral locking plate. This may be particularly beneficial when there is medial comminution. However, RIMN can only be used in open-box knee designs where the notch limits the nail diameter

TABLE 57-2 Unified Classification System

Type		Example	Treatment
A (apophyseal)		Tibial tuberosity Inferior pole fracture of the patella Epicondylar avulsion fracture	Operative or nonoperative depending on displacement
B (bed of implant)	B1: Well fixed	Distal femur fracture	Fixation (nail or plate)
	B2: Implant loose	Distal femur fracture	Revision
	B3: Implant loose and poor bone stock	Distal femur fracture	Complex revision
C (clear of implant bed)		Femoral diaphysis fracture	Fixation (nail or plate)
D (dividing)		Fracture diving the supporting bone between a THA and TKA.	Plating
E (each of two bones supporting an arthroplasty)		Femur and tibial fracture	Manage each on its merit
F (facing an implant)		Fracture of an unresurfaced patella	Manage individual fracture

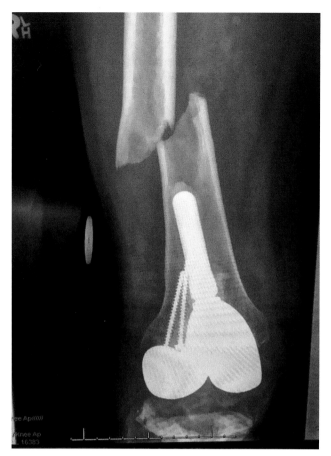

FIGURE 57-1 AP radiograph of B1 distal femoral periprosthetic fracture with well-fixed femoral component.

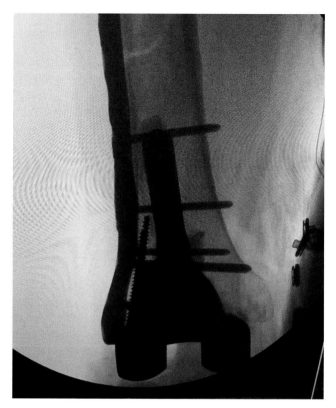

FIGURE 57-3 Locking plate fixation for B1 distal femoral periprosthetic fracture.

and influences the nail entry point which may be more posterior than required, leading to fracture hyperextension.[43] Compatibility studies of common TKA and RIMN designs are reported in the literature.[44,45] The presence of

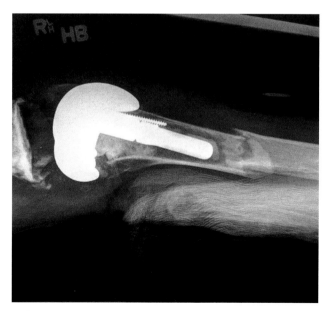

FIGURE 57-2 Lateral of B1 distal femoral periprosthetic fracture with well-fixed femoral component.

a proximal implant may induce a stress riser at the junction between implants. There also needs to be sufficient bone distally for solid fixation with the distal locking screws. As a result of these limitations and depending on the particular case, LCP might be preferable to RIMN. Also, lateral translation of the femoral component may force an incorrect intraarticulations entry point for nail, forcing the fracture to drift into malalignment, usually in too much valgus.

We recommend a direct lateral approach to the distal femur for plating with the patient supine and the knee flexed to 30° on a bolster. The locking plate can be passed submuscularly under the vastus lateralis until the distal contours match those of the distal femur. A wire, parallel to the knee joint, is used to provisionally hold the plate to the distal fragment. With the fracture reduced, the proximal femur and plate should be controlled temporarily with either a wire, bone clamp, or screw. Distal locking screws should then be inserted to gain good purchase of the distal fragment. Stab incisions are used to insert proximal screws percutaneously. Screws are not placed into areas of comminution to reduce construct stiffness and therefore promote union. Five proximal screws (~10 cortices) should be adequate. In general, a long plate should be used with screws placed away from the fracture site. Bicortical fixation is preferred to unicortical fixation, unless it is impossible to use bicortical fixation due to the presence of bulky stems.

Polyaxial Versus Monoaxial Locking Plates

Polyaxial plates allow screws to be directed into the best bone before locking into the plate and can also help by avoiding the femoral component. A pilot randomized controlled trial of polyaxial versus monoaxial locking plate fixation in 40 patients with supracondylar distal femoral fractures with stable femoral components did not demonstrate any advantage to either technique in 2018.[46]

In a recent series of polyaxial plate fixation for distal femoral PPFs, union was achieved in 35 of 45 fractures (78%) 6 months after the index procedure.[47] The time to union reported in the literature has generally led to a cautious approach regarding weight-bearing status after plate fixation. However, allowing immediate full weight-bearing using modern lateral locking distal femoral plates was not associated with a higher rate of failure of fixation in a series of 127 nonperiprosthetic distal femur fractures from the United Kingdom in 2017.[48] From a technical point of view, polyaxial plate fixation may be easier than monoaxial locking fixation.

Nail Plate Combinations

The combination of using a nail with a plate to fix osteoporotic distal femoral fractures is gaining interest. This may afford patients earlier weight-bearing and improved ambulation.[49] NPCs have been used with good results in the setting of distal femoral nonunions.[50] In a series of nine patients with PPFs treated with a retrograde nail and locking plate combination, patients were all permitted to bear weight as tolerated immediately after surgery. The mean union time in this series was 20 weeks.[51]

Other Fixation Methods

The use of a supplementary medial plate and far cortical locking plates is a promising development in the field of fixation of distal femoral PPFs but with little supporting evidence currently.[52] However, there are certain fracture patterns that benefit from a supplemental medial plate. An oblique fracture pattern from proximomedial to distolateral may predispose the distal fragment to displace medially. The addition of a short medial plate through a limited subvastus approach can prevent this problem. **Fig. 57-4** shows a nonunion secondary to a failed open reduction and internal fixation (ORIF) of a B1 distal femoral PPF with medial displacement of the distal femur. The plate was revised, and a supplemental medial plate was applied with resultant radiographic union (**Figs. 57-5** and **57-6**). Polymethylmethacrylate augmentation and cortical allograft struts have also been used as adjuvants to fixation with varying levels of success.

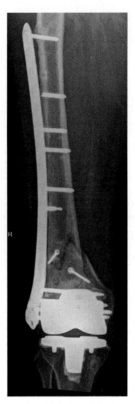

FIGURE 57-4 Nonunion secondary to a failed open reduction and internal fixation (ORIF) of a B1 distal femoral periprosthetic fracture with medial displacement of the distal femur. (Image courtesy of Prof. Karl Stoffel, Kantonsspital Baselland, University of Basel, Switzerland.)

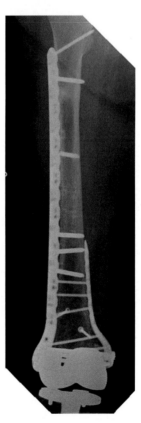

FIGURE 57-5 AP radiograph 12 wk following revision open reduction and internal fixation (ORIF) with supplemental medial plating. (Image courtesy of Prof. Karl Stoffel, Kantonsspital Baselland, University of Basel, Switzerland.)

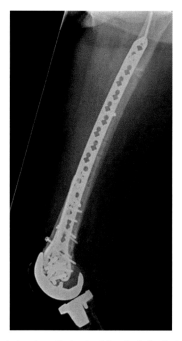

FIGURE 57-6 Lateral radiograph 12 wk following revision open reduction and internal fixation (ORIF) with supplemental medial plating. (Image courtesy of Prof. Karl Stoffel, Kantonsspital Baselland, University of Basel, Switzerland.)

Revision Arthroplasty

If fixation is likely to fail, revision arthroplasty should be considered. Indications include a loose component, inadequate distal bone for fixation, and failed fixation despite multiple attempts to gain union.[53] These will require revision arthroplasty implants or distal femoral replacement (DFR) with a tumor prosthesis.[54] The decision largely depends on the extent of the fracture, quality of bone stock, and involvement of the epicondyles or collateral ligaments. We recommend positioning and draping to enable an extensile surgical approach if required, with according consideration of a sterile tourniquet. Where multiple scars exist, use of the most lateral usually promotes better wound healing. A tibial tubercle osteotomy may enhance exposure of the proximal tibia.[53]

Distal Femoral Replacement

The reduction in mortality observed with early mobilization of hip fracture patients has led some to advocate DFR instead of operative fixation as a treatment for PPFs around a TKA in the elderly. **Fig. 57-7** shows a highly comminuted distal femoral PPF in osteoporotic bone treated with DFR. Good results have been achieved using DFR

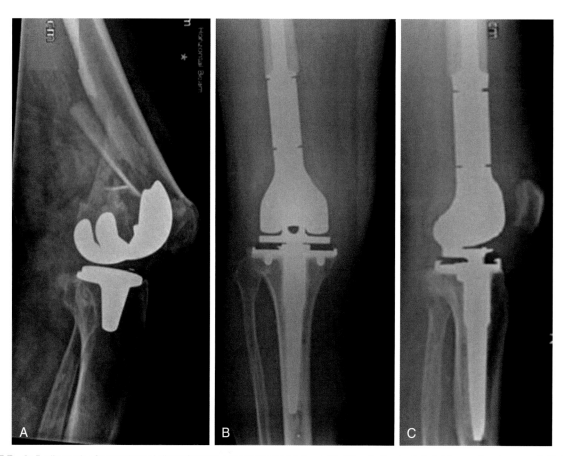

FIGURE 57-7 **A:** Radiograph of comminuted distal femoral periprosthetic fracture. **B:** AP radiograph of distal femoral replacement. **C:** Lateral radiograph of distal femoral replacement.

for PPFs in recent series.[55,56] In a series of 17 distal femur replacements for fracture, acceptable functional outcomes were achieved, although 2 out of 17 required further revision surgery.[57] In the retrospective study of distal femoral PPFs by Gan et al, a series of patients were treated with either tumor prosthesis or locking plate. While complication rates and clinical outcomes were similar between the groups, the mean time to return to weight-bearing in the tumor prosthesis group was 2.9 days compared to 18.9 weeks in the locking plate group.[58]

In another series, LCP and DFR had similar mortality at 90 days (9% vs. 4%) and 365 days (22% vs. 10%), need for additional surgery (9% vs. 3%), and survivors maintaining ambulation (77% vs. 81%).[59] Retrospective comparison of patients treated with either fixation or DFR revealed less reliance on aids following DFR in one series,[60] but no difference in another.[25] Results are currently awaited from the UK-based KFORT feasibility trial of fixation or replacement for nonperiprosthetic distal femoral fractures in the elderly and may be extrapolated to displaced B1 fractures in the elderly in lieu of other evidence.

Interprosthetic—UCS Type D Fractures

Polyaxial locking plate fixation is usually adequate when both components are well fixed. When one component is loose, revision arthroplasty is necessary. In this scenario, custom-made implants such as femoral sleeves or couplers can be designed to link the well-fixed component to the revision component.[53] If both components are loose, total femoral replacement is required. Viable femoral bone can be scaffolded around the prosthesis to reconstitute some bone stock around the implant.

Timing of Surgery

No difference in mortality was found in a series of 69 patients with periprosthetic knee fractures operated either within or after 48 hours of admission with a PPF. In this series, the overall 1 year mortality was 4.3%.[61] In a series of patients treated with LCP or DFR, waiting 3 or more days after presentation had similar mortality risk to those whose surgery was completed within 3 days of the injury.[59] However, in a larger series of 283 elderly patients with nonperiprosthetic distal femur patients, delays to surgical treatment of more than 2 days after injury was associated with increased patient mortality.[62] Clearly planning the appropriate treatment of these complex injuries is important and must be weighed against surgical delay, while keeping in mind that many of these patients may need to be transferred to a tertiary care center for a more specialized level of care.

TIBIAL PERIPROSTHETIC FRACTURES

Classification

The most commonly used classification of tibial PPFs is that of Felix et al from 1997 and is based on four distinct

TABLE 57-3 Felix et al Classification of Tibial Periprosthetic Fractures

Type	Description
Type I	Fracture of tibial plateau
Type II	Fracture adjacent to tibial stem
Type III	Fracture of the tibial shaft, distal to component
Type IV	Fracture of tibial tubercle

categories (**Table 57-3**).[20] These may be further subdivided into three types: subtype A represents a well-fixed prosthesis, subtype B represents component loosening, and subtype C refers to intraoperative fractures. Similar to femoral PPFs, the UCS classification is also helpful for considering the fate of the component.

Treatment

Treatment is largely dictated by the stability of the tibial component. Nondisplaced or minimally displaced fractures with a well-fixed tibial component may be treated nonoperatively. **Figs. 57-8** and **57-9** demonstrate an undisplaced tibial B1 fracture which was treated nonoperatively. Plate fixation is used for plateau and shaft fractures, and screws for tibial tubercle fractures. Stemmed revision arthroplasty is reserved for loose or failed implants. The use of metal augments, sleeves, or cones depends on the adequacy of remaining bone.

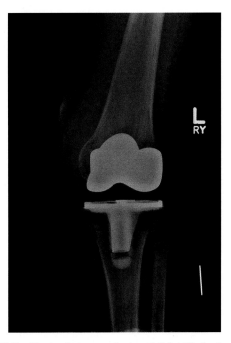

FIGURE 57-8 AP showing an undisplaced tibial B1 fracture treated nonoperatively.

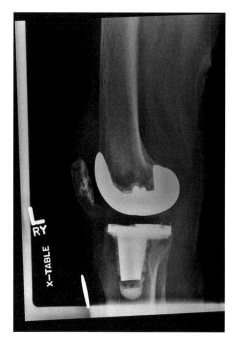

FIGURE 57-9   Lateral showing an undisplaced tibial B1 fracture treated nonoperatively.

Although there is limited prognostic data, complications are also common after tibial PPF management. In a series of nine patients with tibial PPFs treated with ORIF (*n* = 6), revision arthroplasty (*n* = 1), arthrodesis (*n* = 1), and amputation (*n* = 1), the rate of adverse events and revision was 55.6%. This included impaired wound healing, infection, and failure of fixation. Additional surgical procedures for failure included soft-tissue management, arthrodesis, amputation, and repeat osteosynthesis.[63]

PATELLAR PERIPROSTHETIC FRACTURES

Patellar fractures may be due to direct trauma, intraoperative injury to the proximal or distal pole, or fatigue.[19,64] Unlike femoral and tibial PPFs, patellar PPFs are more frequent in males.[65] This may be due to activities generating greater knee extension forces in heavier males.[14] Risk factors include revision surgery, malalignment, patellar maltracking and patellar osteonecrosis, asymmetric resection, overresection, and underresection increasing the patellofemoral joint reaction force.[14,19,64,66] Design, placement, and size of patellar component pegs (e.g., a large central peg) may also weaken the underlying bone.[67]

Classification

Goldberg et al[64] describe four types according to the fracture configuration, stability of the patellar component, and integrity of the extensor mechanism (**Table 57-4**).

Treatment

Nonoperative treatment is acceptable for fractures where the extensor mechanism is intact, and the patellar

TABLE 57-4   Goldberg Classification of Patellar Periprosthetic Fractures

Type	Description
Type I	Fracture not involving implant/cement interface or quadriceps mechanism
Type II	Fracture involving implant/cement interface and/or quadriceps mechanism
Type III A	Inferior pole fracture with patellar ligament rupture
Type III B	Inferior pole fracture without patellar ligament rupture
Type IV	All types with fracture dislocations

component remains well-fixed.[14,53,64] We recommend knee bracing fixed in extension for the first 2 weeks followed by a gradual increase in knee range of motion protected within a brace for 6 weeks. In the series by Ortiguera and Berry, 97% of Goldberg I fractures were successfully treated with nonoperative methods.[14] Surgical management of other Goldberg types (extensor mechanism repair, open reduction and internal fixation of the patella with or without removal or revision of the patellar component, and partial patellectomy) resulted in a 41% complication rate, most commonly including revision surgery.[14] This remains a challenging group to treat. Accordingly, for comminuted fractures, nonsurgical treatment or partial patellectomy and patellar tendon or quadriceps tendon reattachment may be advisable.[7,14] If the implant is loose and bone stock permits, the patellar component may be revised. When bone stock is inadequate, partial or complete patellectomy is recommended over revision TKA. **Figs. 57-10 to 57-13**

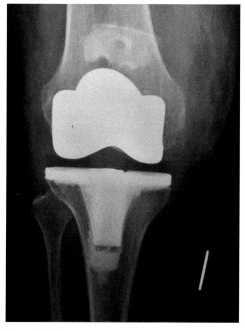

FIGURE 57-10   AP showing a displaced patella periprosthetic fracture.

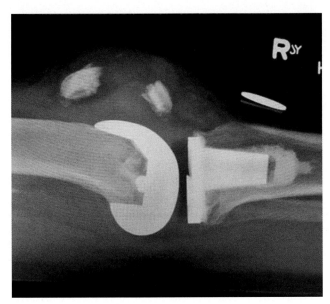

FIGURE 57-11 Lateral showing displaced patella periprosthetic fracture.

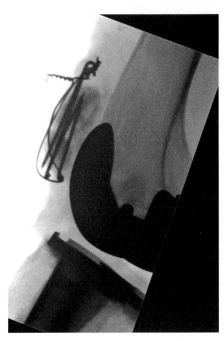

FIGURE 57-13 Fluoroscopy image showing removal of the patellar component and open reduction and internal fixation (ORIF) with tension band wiring.

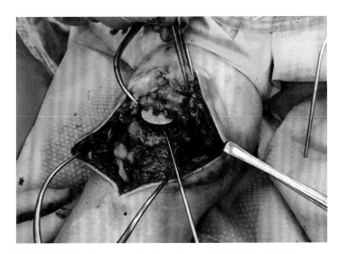

FIGURE 57-12 Intraoperative image showing a loose patella button.

CONCLUSION

The successful management of the majority of periprosthetic fractures around the knee can be achieved after consideration of implant stability and fracture characteristics.

show a patella fracture with a loose button treated with removal of the implant and ORIF with a tension band wire technique.

In view of the complications associated with surgical management, nonoperative treatment can be considered in all patients with mild symptoms and good knee function.[65] Many patients with patellar fracture in the series from the Mayo clinic were identified on routine follow-up and presented with no or mild pain. In these instances, 4 to 6 weeks of joint immobilization may lead to acceptable results.[7,14,64]

REFERENCES

1. Barnes CL, Vail TP, Takemoto SK. Where do knee revisions for infection, fracture, and other revisions get treated? *J Arthroplasty.* 2013;28(3):423-428.
2. Kurtz S, Ong K, Lau E, Mowat F, Halpern M. Projections of primary and revision hip and knee arthroplasty in the United States from 2005 to 2030. *J Bone Joint Surg Am.* 2007;89(4): 780-785.
3. Della Rocca GJ, Leung KS, Pape HC. Periprosthetic fractures: epidemiology and future projections. *J Orthop Trauma.* 2011;2(25 suppl):S66-S70.
4. Alden KJ, Duncan WH, Trousdale RT, Pagnano MW, Haidukewych GJ. Intraoperative fracture during primary total knee arthroplasty. *Clin Orthop Relat Res.* 2010;468(1):90-95.
5. Meek RM, Norwood T, Smith R, Brenkel IJ, Howie CR. The risk of peri-prosthetic fracture after primary and revision total hip and knee replacement. *J Bone Joint Surg Br.* 2011;93(1):96-101.
6. Cordeiro EN, Costa RC, Carazzato JG, Silva Jdos S. Periprosthetic fractures in patients with total knee arthroplasties. *Clin Orthop Relat Res.* 1990;252:182-189.
7. Dennis DA. Periprosthetic fractures following total knee arthroplasty. *Instr Course Lect.* 2001;50:379-389.
8. Culp RW, Schmidt RG, Hanks G, Mak A, Esterhai JL Jr, Heppenstall RB. Supracondylar fracture of the femur following prosthetic knee arthroplasty. *Clin Orthop Relat Res.* 1987;222:212-222.
9. Healy WL, Siliski JM, Incavo SJ. Operative treatment of distal femoral fractures proximal to total knee replacements. *J Bone Joint Surg Am.* 1993;75(1):27-34.

10. Inglis AE, Walker PS. Revision of failed knee replacements using fixed-axis hinges. *J Bone Joint Surg Br.* 1991;73(5):757-761.
11. Merkel KD, Johnson EW Jr. Supracondylar fracture of the femur after total knee arthroplasty. *J Bone Joint Surg Am.* 1986;68(1):29-43.
12. Ritter MA, Faris PM, Keating EM. Anterior femoral notching and ipsilateral supracondylar femur fracture in total knee arthroplasty. *J Arthroplasty.* 1988;3(2):185-187.
13. Schroder HM, Berthelsen A, Hassani G, Hansen EB, Solgaard S. Cementless porous-coated total knee arthroplasty: 10-year results in a consecutive series. *J Arthroplasty.* 2001;16(5):559-567.
14. Ortiguera CJ, Berry DJ. Patellar fracture after total knee arthroplasty. *J Bone Joint Surg Am.* 2002;84-A(4):532-540.
15. Keating EM, Haas G, Meding JB. Patella fracture after post total knee replacements. *Clin Orthop Relat Res.* 2003;416:93-97.
16. Parvizi J, Kim KI, Oliashirazi A, Ong A, Sharkey PF. Periprosthetic patellar fractures. *Clin Orthop Relat Res.* 2006;446:161-166.
17. Chang MA, Rand JA, Trousdale RT. Patellectomy after total knee arthroplasty. *Clin Orthop Relat Res.* 2005;440:175-177.
18. Grace JN, Sim FH. Fracture of the patella after total knee arthroplasty. *Clin Orthop Relat Res.* 1988;230:168-175.
19. Windsor RE, Scuderi GR, Insall JN. Patellar fractures in total knee arthroplasty. *J Arthroplasty.* 1989;(4 suppl):S63-S67.
20. Felix NA, Stuart MJ, Hanssen AD. Periprosthetic fractures of the tibia associated with total knee arthroplasty. *Clin Orthop Relat Res.* 1997;345:113-124.
21. Nagwadia H, Joshi P. Outcome of osteosynthesis for periprosthetic fractures after total knee arthroplasty: a retrospective study. *Eur J Orthop Surg Traumatol.* 2018;28(4):683-690.
22. Cain PR, Rubash HE, Wissinger HA, McClain EJ. Periprosthetic femoral fractures following total knee arthroplasty. *Clin Orthop Relat Res.* 1986;208:205-214.
23. Ritter MA, Thong AE, Keating EM, et al. The effect of femoral notching during total knee arthroplasty on the prevalence of postoperative femoral fractures and on clinical outcome. *J Bone Joint Surg Am.* 2005;87(11):2411-2414.
24. Reeves RA, Schairer WW, Jevsevar DS. Costs and risk factors for hospital readmission after periprosthetic knee fractures in the United States. *J Arthroplasty.* 2018;33(2):324-330.e1.
25. Ruder JA, Hart GP, Kneisl JS, Springer BD, Karunakar MA. Predictors of functional recovery following periprosthetic distal femur fractures. *J Arthroplasty.* 2017;32(5):1571-1575.
26. Eschbach D, Buecking B, Kivioja H, et al. One year after proximal or distal periprosthetic fracture of the femur -two conditions with divergent outcomes? *Injury.* 2018;49(6):1176-1182.
27. Butt MS, Krikler SJ, Ali MS. Displaced fractures of the distal femur in elderly patients. Operative versus non-operative treatment. *J Bone Joint Surg Br.* 1996;78(1):110-114.
28. Neer CS II, Grantham SA, Shelton ML. Supracondylar fracture of the adult femur. A study of one hundred and ten cases. *J Bone Joint Surg Am.* 1967;49(4):591-613.
29. DiGioia AM III, Rubash HE. Periprosthetic fractures of the femur after total knee arthroplasty. A literature review and treatment algorithm. *Clin Orthop Relat Res.* 1991;271:135-142.
30. Chen F, Mont MA, Bachner RS. Management of ipsilateral supracondylar femur fractures following total knee arthroplasty. *J Arthroplasty.* 1994;9(5):521-526.
31. Rorabeck CH, Taylor JW. Classification of periprosthetic fractures complicating total knee arthroplasty. *Orthop Clin North Am.* 1999;30(2):209-214.
32. Rorabeck CH, Angliss RD, Lewis PL. Fractures of the femur, tibia, and patella after total knee arthroplasty: decision making and principles of management. *Instr Course Lect.* 1998;47:449-458.
33. Su ET, DeWal H, Di Cesare PE. Periprosthetic femoral fractures above total knee replacements. *J Am Acad Orthop Surg.* 2004;12(1):12-20.
34. Kim KI, Egol KA, Hozack WJ, Parvizi J. Periprosthetic fractures after total knee arthroplasties. *Clin Orthop Relat Res.* 2006;446:167-175.
35. Backstein D, Safir O, Gross A. Periprosthetic fractures of the knee. *J Arthroplasty.* 2007;22(4 suppl 1):45-49.
36. Frenzel S, Vecsei V, Negrin L. Periprosthetic femoral fractures–incidence, classification problems and the proposal of a modified classification scheme. *Int Orthop.* 2015;39(10):1909-1920.
37. Fakler JKM, Ponick C, Edel M, et al. A new classification of TKA periprosthetic femur fractures considering the implant type. *BMC Musculoskelet Disord.* 2017;18(1):490.
38. Duncan CP, Haddad FS. The Unified Classification System (UCS): improving our understanding of periprosthetic fractures. *Bone Joint J.* 2014;96-B(6):713-716.
39. Moran MC, Brick GW, Sledge CB, Dysart SH, Chien EP. Supracondylar femoral fracture following total knee arthroplasty. *Clin Orthop Relat Res.* 1996;324:196-209.
40. Herrera DA, Kregor PJ, Cole PA, Levy BA, Jonsson A, Zlowodzki M. Treatment of acute distal femur fractures above a total knee arthroplasty: systematic review of 415 cases (1981-2006). *Acta Orthop.* 2008;79(1):22-27.
41. Ebraheim NA, Kelley LH, Liu X, Thomas IS, Steiner RB, Liu J. Periprosthetic distal femur fracture after total knee arthroplasty: a systematic review. *Orthop Surg.* 2015;7(4):297-305.
42. Shin YS, Kim HJ, Lee DH. Similar outcomes of locking compression plating and retrograde intramedullary nailing for periprosthetic supracondylar femoral fractures following total knee arthroplasty: a meta-analysis. *Knee Surg Sports Traumatol Arthrosc.* 2017;25(9):2921-2928.
43. Service BC, Kang W, Turnbull N, Langford J, Haidukewych G, Koval KJ. Influence of femoral component design on retrograde femoral nail starting point. *J Orthop Trauma.* 2015;29(10):e380-e384.
44. Thompson SM, Lindisfarne EA, Bradley N, Solan M. Periprosthetic supracondylar femoral fractures above a total knee replacement: compatibility guide for fixation with a retrograde intramedullary nail. *J Arthroplasty.* 2014;29(8):1639-1641.
45. Jones MD, Carpenter C, Mitchell SR, Whitehouse M, Mehendale S. Retrograde femoral nailing of periprosthetic fractures around total knee replacements. *Injury.* 2016;47(2):460-464.
46. Kanakaris NK, Obakponovwe O, Krkovic M, et al. Fixation of periprosthetic or osteoporotic distal femoral fractures with locking plates: a pilot randomised controlled trial. *Int Orthop.* 2018;43(5):1193-1204.
47. Lotzien S, Hoberg C, Hoffmann MF, Schildhauer TA. Clinical outcome and quality of life of patients with periprosthetic distal femur fractures and retained total knee arthroplasty treated with polyaxial locking plates: a single-center experience. *Eur J Orthop Surg Traumatol.* 2019;29(1):189-196.
48. Poole WEC, Wilson DGG, Guthrie HC, et al. 'Modern' distal femoral locking plates allow safe, early weight-bearing with a high rate of union and low rate of failure: five-year experience from a United Kingdom major trauma centre. *Bone Joint J.* 2017;99-B(7):951-957.
49. Bascı O, Karakasli A, Kumtepe E, Guran O, Havitcioglu H. Combination of anatomical locking plate and retrograde intramedullary nail in distal femoral fractures: comparison of mechanical stability. *Eklem Hastalik Cerrahisi.* 2015;26(1):21-26.
50. Attum B, Douleh D, Whiting PS, et al. Outcomes of distal femur nonunions treated with a combined nail/plate construct and autogenous bone grafting. *J Orthop Trauma.* 2017;31(9):e301-e304.
51. Hussain MS, Dailey SK, Avilucea FR. Stable fixation and immediate weight-bearing after combined retrograde intramedullary nailing and open reduction internal fixation of noncomminuted distal interprosthetic femur fractures. *J Orthop Trauma.* 2018;32(6):e237-e240.
52. Tosounidis TH, Giannoudis PV. What is new in distal femur periprosthetic fracture fixation? *Injury.* 2015;46(12):2293-2296.

53. Konan S, Sandiford N, Unno F, Masri BS, Garbuz DS, Duncan CP. Periprosthetic fractures associated with total knee arthroplasty: an update. *Bone Joint J.* 2016;98-B(11):1489-1496.

54. Jassim SS, McNamara I, Hopgood P. Distal femoral replacement in periprosthetic fracture around total knee arthroplasty. *Injury.* 2014;45(3):550-553.

55. Girgis E, McAllen C, Keenan J. Revision knee arthroplasty using a distal femoral replacement prosthesis for periprosthetic fractures in elderly patients. *Eur J Orthop Surg Traumatol.* 2018;28(1):95-102.

56. Marczak D, Kowalczewski J, Czubak J, Okon T, Synder M, Sibinski M. Short and mid term results of revision total knee arthroplasty with Global Modular Replacement System. *Indian J Orthop.* 2017;51(3):324-329.

57. Rahman WA, Vial TA, Backstein DJ. Distal femoral arthroplasty for management of periprosthetic supracondylar fractures of the femur. *J Arthroplasty.* 2016;31(3):676-679.

58. Gan G, Teo YH, Kwek EBK. Comparing outcomes of tumor prosthesis revision and locking plate fixation in supracondylar femoral periprosthetic fractures. *Clin Orthop Surg.* 2018;10(2):174-180.

59. Hoellwarth JS, Fourman MS, Crossett L, et al. Equivalent mortality and complication rates following periprosthetic distal femur fractures managed with either lateral locked plating or a distal femoral replacement. *Injury.* 2018;49(2):392-397.

60. Hart GP, Kneisl JS, Springer BD, Patt JC, Karunakar MA. Open reduction vs distal femoral replacement arthroplasty for comminuted distal femur fractures in the patients 70 years and older. *J Arthroplasty.* 2017;32(1):202-206.

61. Sellan ME, Lanting BA, Schemitsch EH, MacDonald SJ, Vasarhelyi EM, Howard JL. Does time to surgery affect outcomes for periprosthetic femur fractures? *J Arthroplasty.* 2018;33(3):878-881.

62. Myers P, Laboe P, Johnson KJ, et al. Patient mortality in geriatric distal femur fractures. *J Orthop Trauma.* 2018;32(3):111-115.

63. Schreiner AJ, Schmidutz F, Ateschrang A, et al. Periprosthetic tibial fractures in total knee arthroplasty - an outcome analysis of a challenging and underreported surgical issue. *BMC Musculoskelet Disord.* 2018;19(1):323.

64. Goldberg VM, Figgie HE III, Inglis AE, et al. Patellar fracture type and prognosis in condylar total knee arthroplasty. *Clin Orthop Relat Res.* 1988;236:115-122.

65. Yoo JD, Kim NK. Periprosthetic fractures following total knee arthroplasty. *Knee Surg Relat Res.* 2015;27(1):1-9.

66. Wetzner SM, Bezreh JS, Scott RD, Bierbaum BE, Newberg AH. Bone scanning in the assessment of patellar viability following knee replacement. *Clin Orthop Relat Res.* 1985;199:215-219.

67. Goldstein SA, Coale E, Weiss AP, Grossnickle M, Meller B, Matthews LS. Patellar surface strain. *J Orthop Res.* 1986;4(3):372-377.

chapter 58

Instability After Total Knee Arthroplasty

Jason H. Oh, MD | Giles R. Scuderi, MD, FACS

INTRODUCTION

Instability has been found to be the cause of 10% to 24% of total knee arthroplasty (TKA) revisions[1-4] and is the second most common cause of both early and late revisions, trailing behind infection in the early subgroup and aseptic loosening in the later subgroup.[5,6] With the expansion of the aging population and increasing access to orthopedic care, the demand for TKA and subsequent revision arthroplasty has been increasing at an historic rate. With projections for primary TKA as high as 1.26 million to 1.68 million per year in the United States alone by 2030[7] and annual increases in the numbers of revision TKA on the order of 13.5% annually,[8] it is imperative for the surgeon to be able to effectively diagnose instability as the cause of TKA failure and then to make appropriate management decisions.

Upon initial patient evaluation, the clinician must bear in mind that the patient's subjective complaint of "instability" may be completely unrelated to true mechanical instability. For example, buckling-type symptoms can commonly be attributed to pain or quadriceps weakness. Frank dislocation is rare, comprising only 0.5% to 3.3% of all revision TKA cases.[9-11] Patients with true instability are more likely to complain of anterior knee pain, multifocal areas of soft tissue tenderness, recurrent effusions, and difficulty walking or climbing steps.

Obtaining a comprehensive history is paramount to success in accurate diagnosis and management of the problem. Elements of the history that should be reviewed include the initial diagnosis that necessitated the primary arthroplasty procedure, prior knee injuries and surgeries, the presence of preoperative deformity and/or contractures, the date of the primary procedure, and the type of implants used. Ideally, the operative report should be obtained and carefully reviewed. Any history of connective tissue disorder or other risk factors for generalized ligamentous laxity should be elucidated. It is important to establish whether the arthroplasty was initially satisfactory and then went on to develop instability symptoms or whether the knee was persistently problematic from the initial procedure. The patient should be asked about any significant fluctuations in weight since the procedure, especially if there was a dramatic weight loss following bariatric surgery.

Upon physical examination, the patient's gait should be carefully observed with attention to gait on both level ground, as well as while ascending and descending steps. Reliance on ambulatory aids should be noted. Muscular weakness should be graded, especially if associated with observable muscular atrophy. The integrity of the extensor mechanism should be confirmed. Stability testing for varus/valgus and anterior/posterior (AP) laxity should be performed at full extension, 30°, and 90°. The total range of motion should be recorded, with special attention to hyperextension or above-average hyperflexion. If an effusion is present, consider aspiration since a sterile hemarthrosis is a common finding associated with instability, with an average synovial red blood cell count of 65,000 per cubic millimeter found in one study.[12]

Full-length AP weight-bearing radiographs including the hip, knee, and ankle are helpful to establish the mechanical alignment of the limb. High-quality lateral views are important to accurately assess the tibial slope and femoral posterior condylar offset. Axial patellofemoral views (e.g., sunrise or Merchant views) should be obtained to assess patellofemoral alignment. The sizing and positioning of the components should be scrutinized, as should any evidence of component wear or breakage. Manual stress radiographs may be considered to gain additional information. Three-dimensional computed tomography imaging can be considered for cases of suspected subtle component malrotation or in preparation for revision surgery with significant bone loss. In all cases, infection must be ruled out prior to undertaking operative intervention.

Surgical treatment is warranted for most cases of symptomatic instability. The specific intervention should be tailored to the mechanism of failure, with the goal of achieving a stable knee with the level of constraint dependent upon the integrity of the collateral ligaments. Constrained implants (Fig. 58-1) have intrinsic stability because the enhanced tibial post provides varus–valgus stability. For cases with severe incompetence of the medial and lateral collateral ligaments, a rotating hinge knee prosthesis may be indicated (Fig. 58-2). While various methods of ligament repair and reconstruction have been described for ligament instability, we have found that good outcomes can be predictably attained with the use of constrained implants that substitute for the loss of ligament integrity (Table 58-1). Implantation of a constrained

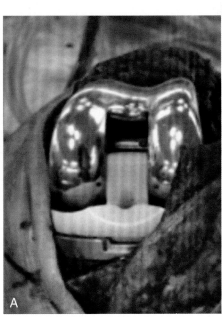

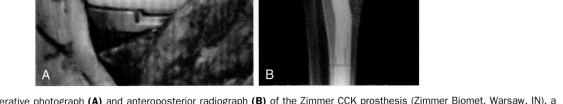

FIGURE 58-1 Intraoperative photograph **(A)** and anteroposterior radiograph **(B)** of the Zimmer CCK prosthesis (Zimmer Biomet, Warsaw, IN), a type of constrained prosthesis.

prosthesis or rotating hinge should follow the principles of revision TKA, including the use of modular augmentation to address bone defects and stem fixation to transfer loads away from the prosthesis–bone interface to the diaphysis.

TIBIOFEMORAL INSTABILITY

Flexion Instability

Flexion instability is characterized by an inappropriately large flexion space that leads to painful episodes of tibiofemoral subluxation or frank dislocation (**Fig. 58-3**) while in flexion. Flexion instability is a risk factor for accelerated wear of the polyethylene insert and recurrent effusions. Symmetric flexion instability is associated with a rectangular flexion gap while asymmetric flexion instability is associated with a trapezoidal flexion gap. The diagnosis of flexion instability may be challenging because the main symptom is pain and radiographs are likely to demonstrate well-fixed, reasonably positioned components on weight-bearing views. However, careful attention while taking the history and physical examination can help elucidate the diagnosis of flexion instability, as well as the subtype and underlying etiology. Symmetric flexion instability is more common than asymmetric flexion instability. In general, symmetrical flexion instability is due to choosing a tibial articular surface that fills the extension gap, but it is too thin to fill the flexion gap. This is usually due to overresection of the posterior condyles with failure to restore the posterior condylar offset or underresection of the distal femur.

Asymmetrical flexion instability is characterized by a trapezoidal flexion gap. This condition may arise from inappropriate femoral component rotation (i.e., deviation from anatomic landmarks such as the epicondylar axis or femoral AP axis), isolated collateral ligament attenuation, or iatrogenic collateral ligament injury. The clinical ramifications of asymmetric flexion instability have been less well-studied than those of symmetric flexion instability; however, reports

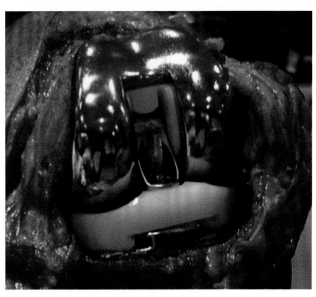

FIGURE 58-2 Intraoperative photograph of a rotating hinge prosthesis.

TABLE 58-1	Constraint—When Is It Needed?					
	3 Ligament Knee	2 Ligament Knee		1 Ligament Knee		0 Ligament Knee
	CR	UC	PS	VVC	VVC	Hinged
Posterior cruciate ligament	X	–	–	–	–	–
Lateral collateral ligament	X	X	X	X	–	–
Medial collateral ligament	X	X	X	–	X	–

CR, posterior cruciate ligament–retaining; PS, posterior cruciate ligament–substituting; UC, ultracongruent; VVC, varus–valgus constrained.

have demonstrated improved range of motion and less pain with a rectangular flexion gap as opposed to a trapezoidal flexion gap.[13]

Etiology

As mentioned above, symmetric flexion instability can arise either from surgical errors or from postoperative complications. Surgical errors in femoral preparation can be subdivided into failure to restore the femoral posterior condylar offset, overstuffing of the distal condylar offset, or a combination of the two. Similarly, symmetric flexion instability may be created on the tibial side by resecting the tibia with excessive posterior slope (**Fig. 58-4**). In addition, when cruciate-retaining implants are implanted, flexion instability may occur if the posterior cruciate ligament (PCL) is inadvertently damaged intraoperatively. A cruciate-retaining TKA that is well-balanced intraoperatively can still develop flexion instability postoperatively from PCL attenuation or rupture, which may be due to a trauma

(e.g., a fall directly onto the flexed knee) or chronic attritional injury. Undiagnosed or subclinical rheumatic disease may play a role in chronic attritional pathology. PCL-substituting (PS) implant designs are protected against posterior tibial subluxation by the cam-post mechanism; however, even PS implants may be prone to painful and debilitating anterior subluxation in flexion, as well as accelerated wear of the polyethylene post, if left inappropriately balanced.

Late instability may be the result of gradual posterior, usually posteromedial, polyethylene wear. Radiographic review may reveal thinning of the tibial polyethylene insert, approaching proximity of the femoral and tibial components or subtle osteolysis.

Evaluation

In the initial evaluation of an unsatisfied patient with a TKA, it is important to maintain a high index of suspicion for flexion instability because the symptoms may be vague and subtle. The chief complaint is usually anterior

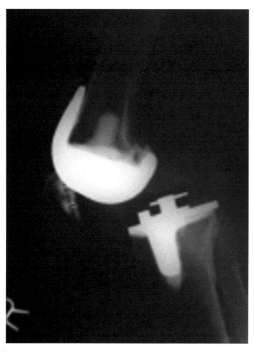

FIGURE 58-3 Lateral radiograph demonstrating posterior tibiofemoral dislocation in a total knee arthroplasty with flexion instability.

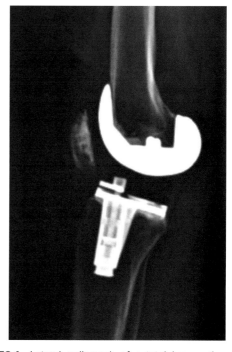

FIGURE 58-4 Lateral radiograph of a total knee arthroplasty with excessive tibial slope.

knee pain, including retinacular pain and/or pain at the tibial insertion of the pes anserinus tendons.[14] Other common complaints include buckling, recurrent knee effusions, difficulty rising from a seated position, and difficulty managing stairs, especially on stair descent. Patients may also report that they feel dependent upon ambulation aids because of a sensation that they cannot trust the knee from "slipping out" underneath them.

On the physical examination, the patient's gait must be observed both on a level surface and contrasted against the gait ascending and descending steps. Excessive caution when rising from a seated position should be noted. An effusion may be present; if so, aspiration and synovial fluid analysis can be considered to assess for the presence of hemarthrosis, as well as to rule out infection. Patients with isolated flexion instability will usually be stable to manual varus and valgus stress applied in full extension and 30° of flexion. AP drawer testing performed at 90° of flexion, with the leg in a dependent position hanging unsupported off the examination table, may demonstrate excessive translation. The absolute threshold of anteroposterior translation that may signify pathologic laxity will vary somewhat between different patients and different implant designs, though greater than 5 mm of translation has been identified as abnormal in some studies. The posterior sag sign noted at 90° is indicative of flexion instability in cruciate-retaining knees. In such cases, the quadriceps active test should be performed as an adjunct. Dial testing for posterolateral rotatory instability should be performed to assess the competency of the posterolateral corner structures. Lateral radiographs should be carefully assessed for posterior tibial subluxation. Posterior condylar offsets may also be measured and compared to the contralateral side.

Treatment and Outcomes

Conservative treatment for symptomatic flexion instability has limited indications. For the first instance of acute postoperative dislocation of a PS implant, closed reduction and bracing with adjunctive quadriceps strengthening has been described with maintenance of reduction in approximately 60% to 75% of cases.[10,15-17] In cases of chronic instability without dislocation, a trial of quadriceps strengthening with or without bracing, with the use of symptomatic treatment for focal pain and swelling, may be used.

However, the mainstay of treatment for most cases of recurrent and symptomatic flexion instability should be surgical. While it may be appealing to revise the tibial polyethylene to a thicker size in order to stabilize the flexion space, if the femoral component is already appropriately sized, then the extension gap will become too tight and a flexion contracture may ensue. Careful intraoperative assessment must be performed to ensure flexion/extension space balancing and symmetry in order

to prevent the recurrence of the same issue. If the cause of instability is determined to be an undersized femoral component, then the femur should be revised to an appropriately larger implant with the use of posterior condylar augments to restore the posterior condylar offset (**Figs. 58-5** and **58-6**). Alternatively, if an appropriately sized femoral component was placed upon an inadequate distal resection, the femur should be revised with proximal migration of the same sized component, thereby increasing the extension gap to match the flexion gap. A thicker tibial polyethylene insert should then be inserted. In both cases, the joint line should be restored to its anatomic location following the revision procedure.

If PCL rupture or attenuation is diagnosed as the root cause of flexion instability with a cruciate retaining implant, the knee should be revised to an ultracongruent or PS design. In cases of excessive tibial posterior slope, the tibia should recut with an appropriate degree of slope. The PCL insertion may be compromised in these cases and the use of a PS implant should be strongly considered.

Multiple small single-center studies have reported 90% satisfaction rates following revision surgeries for isolated flexion instability when equal and symmetric flexion and extension gaps were achieved.[4,18] **Table 58-2** details our management paradigms for flexion instability.

MEDIAL-LATERAL INSTABILITY

Etiology

Medial-lateral instability is characterized by excessive varus or valgus gapping and can occur in both extension and flexion. Medial-lateral pseudo-instability may be due to component loosening and/or osteolysis, and treatment algorithms detailing the management of bone loss and revision principles are discussed in other chapters. In contrast, true medial-lateral instability arises from collateral ligament injury or imbalance. Medial-lateral

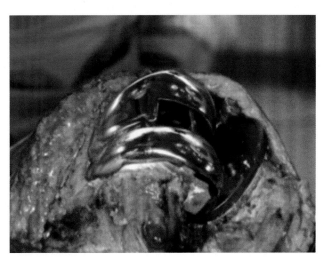

FIGURE 58-5 Intraoperative photograph of posterior condylar augmentation.

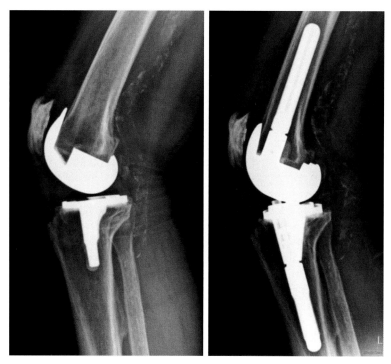

FIGURE 58-6 Preoperative and postoperative radiographs demonstrating the restoration of appropriate posterior condylar offset with augments.

instability patterns are related to preoperative coronal plane malalignment and subsequent overcorrection or, more commonly, undercorrection of coronal deformity at the time of the index arthroplasty.

The most typical scenario leading to varus instability occurs with the preoperative varus knee. Underrelease of the medial collateral ligament with a fixed varus deformity leaves the medial side tighter than the lateral side. This results in residual varus malalignment and causes progressive stretching and attenuation of the lateral supporting soft-tissue structures. Frank varus deformity may gradually recur over time, and medial tibial polyethylene wear and/or catastrophic fracture can be seen late.

Conversely, postoperative valgus instability is most commonly associated with preoperative valgus knees. Trepidation over injury to the common peroneal nerve, or postoperative traction palsy, leads to an inadequate lateral soft tissue release and the knee is ultimately left imbalanced. With continuous loading over time, the medial collateral ligament (MCL) continues to stretch,

leading to recurrence of valgus deformity. Valgus tibiofemoral instability may also contribute to concurrent lateral patellofemoral instability as the medial patellofemoral ligament and retinaculum also undergo progressive stretching and attenuation.

Iatrogenic injury to the collateral ligaments must also be considered when evaluating the coronally unstable knee. Symptomatic instability is more likely with medial rather than lateral collateral ligament injury since there are no stabilizing forces other than the MCL on the medial side, whereas the iliotibial band and posterolateral corner structures provide lateral stability of the knee. MCL injury may be due to direct laceration (usually with an oscillating saw while performing the proximal tibial cut) or excessive loading of the MCL when evaluating final stability. Traumatic injury to the MCL may also occur following a fall with a valgus stress resulting in symptomatic instability (**Fig. 58-7**). With a lack of MCL integrity, revision with a constrained prosthesis may be necessary (**Fig. 58-8**).

TABLE 58-2	Management Paradigms for Tibiofemoral Flexion Instability
Root Cause	**Treatment**
Undersized femoral component	Revision to larger femoral component with use of posterior condylar augments
Excessively distalized femoral component	Revision of femoral component with additional bone resection from distal femur; thicker tibial polyethylene insert
Excessive posterior tibial slope	Revision of tibial component with less slope. Consider conversion to posterior stabilized system if any posterior cruciate ligament (PCL) incompetence
PCL attenuation or rupture	Revise to PCL-substituting implant with cam-post mechanism

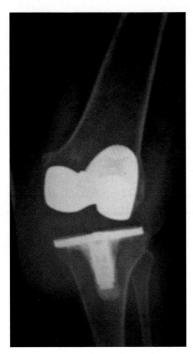

FIGURE 58-7 Anteroposterior radiograph of a total knee arthroplasty with traumatic rupture of the medial collateral ligament.

Evaluation

The diagnosis of medial-lateral instability can usually be established on physical examination with direct manual stress. If the knee is examined in full extension, the tension of the posterior capsule may mask collateral ligament incompetence. Therefore, it is usually preferable to

examine the knee in approximately 15° to 30° of flexion to isolate the collateral ligaments. During gait analysis, the patient may also display a varus or valgus thrust. Supine AP radiographs may or may not demonstrate asymmetric opening and therefore weight-bearing or stress radiographs should be performed.

Treatment and Outcomes

If a medial collateral ligament laceration is detected during the implantation of a cruciate retaining TKA with a competent PCL, good outcomes have been achieved with direct suture repair of the ligament with or without hamstring tendon augmentation.[19] In the case of MCL avulsion from bone, suture anchor reattachment can be performed. Constrained implants are not required if secure MCL repair has been attained. A hinged knee brace providing coronal plane stability is recommended for up to 6 weeks postoperatively, with no limitations upon range of motion.

If, however, acute MCL injury is recognized during a PS TKA procedure, then additional constraint is warranted. Lee and Lotke[20] reported on a series of 37 cases of intraoperative MCL injury, in which 30 patients were managed with constrained designs, while the remaining 7 patients received standard PS implants. The patients in the constrained group had higher Knee Society scores than those in the nonconstrained group. Furthermore, none of the constrained patients required reoperation for instability through early to mid-term follow-up, whereas four out of seven nonconstrained patients required revision for instability.

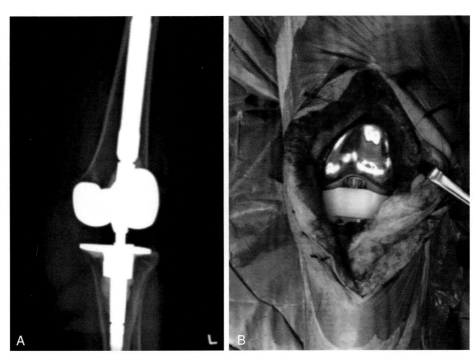

FIGURE 58-8 Anteroposterior radiograph **(A)** and intraoperative photograph **(B)** of the same patient from **Fig. 58-7**, following revision to a rotating hinge design.

In cases of chronic or progressive coronal plane instability, surgical correction is required. Following extensile exposure, the tibial polyethylene insert should be carefully examined for wear or breakage. For the persistent fixed varus knee, a subperiosteal medial release should be performed as described by Insall,[21] continuing until medial and lateral balance are achieved. Once this step has been accomplished, the flexion and extension gaps should be assessed; if equal, then the procedure can be completed with the insertion of an appropriately sized—most likely thicker—tibial polyethylene insert. Otherwise, femoral component revision may need to be undertaken to produce balanced gaps. If medial-lateral balance cannot be achieved even after a complete subperiosteal medial release, some have recommended lateral collateral ligament advancement via osteotomy and proximal advancement of the lateral epicondyle.[22] However, we have not addressed residual instability in this manner and usually resort to a more constrained implant. In low-demand, elderly patients, some degree of medial-lateral imbalance can be accepted with the conversion to constrained components, relying on the implant constraint to provide stability. Constraint may also be necessary in cases of severe lateral soft tissue attenuation in which adequate soft tissue tensioning and stability cannot be obtained.

For the fixed valgus deformity, several approaches have been developed over the past several decades for the optimal release of the lateral soft tissues. The progressive "inside-out" lateral soft tissue releases initially described by Insall[20] and subsequent adaptations of algorithmic lateral soft tissue releases have gradually fallen out of favor due to risk of overcorrection.[23-26] Our preferred technique is the updated Insall "lateral pie crust" technique, in which the extension gap is tensioned with a laminar spreader and a #15 scalpel is used to selectively release only those lateral soft tissues that are tightest upon direct palpation following careful release of the posterolateral capsule.[27] Care should be taken during the release not to overcorrect the deformity. Further lateral collateral ligament release via lateral epicondylar osteotomy may be necessary when dealing with high degrees of fixed valgus deformity or a valgus deformity associated with a flexion contracture.[28] Although anatomic studies have demonstrated the safety of this algorithm with respect to direct peroneal nerve injury,[29] the fact remains that sudden large corrections of valgus malalignment, especially with associated flexion contracture, can lead to postoperative peroneal nerve palsy. If this is a major concern, the surgeon can consider leaving the lateral tissues slightly underreleased and implant a constrained prosthesis. As mentioned above, this approach should be reserved for elderly, low-demand patients. Medial collateral ligament laxity may be addressed with proximal MCL advancement techniques, but we prefer implantation of a more constrained implant.[24] **Table 58-3** below details our management paradigms for medial-lateral instability.

GLOBAL INSTABILITY

Etiology

Global instability is characterized by combined AP and varus–valgus laxity that occurs both in flexion and extension. Causes for global instability can be subdivided into three major categories. The first category is due to extensor mechanism disruption, including traumatic injuries, postpatellectomy status, and intrinsic or acquired deficits of the femoral nerve and quadriceps musculature. Neuromuscular disorders leading to quadriceps dysfunction, although increasingly rare after the eradication of polio, have historically been recognized as the cause of an important subtype of global instability marked by recurvatum deformity of the knee. This deformity is likely to recur following TKA due to progressive forceful stretching of the posterior capsule and collateral ligaments.[30,31] Progressive hyperextension has also been noted in patients with connective tissue disorders and hyperelasticity such as Ehlers-Danlos Syndrome.[32,33] Second, global instability may also arise from apparent collateral ligament lengthening, as in cases with severe polyethylene wear or component subsidence. In these cases, the collateral ligaments are actually intact but

TABLE 58-3	Management Paradigms for Tibiofemoral Medial-Lateral Instability	
Etiology	**Management**
Intraoperative medial collateral ligament (MCL) injury	Acute suture repair +/− hamstring tendon augmentation; supplement with knee brace for a posterior cruciate ligament (PCL)–retaining prosthesis or revision to CCK Revision to CCK prosthesis for a PCL-substituting prosthesis
Underreleased MCL	Subperiosteal medial release, polyethylene exchange +/− femoral component revision
Underreleased lateral tissues	Lateral soft tissue pie-crusting +/− lateral epicondylar osteotomy, polyethylene exchange +/− femoral component revision
Attenuated lateral tissues	Lateral epicondyle advancement or constrained implants
Attenuated MCL	Medial epicondyle advancement or constrained implants

due to bone loss and component subsidence, there is a pseudolaxity of the collateral ligaments. Finally, global instability may develop in cases of true collateral ligament lengthening, as in certain traumatic injuries, as well as metabolic conditions such as severe obesity, diabetes mellitus, and progressive rheumatologic or connective tissue disorders.[9,34]

Evaluation

The clinical picture of a globally unstable patient will include elements of both anteroposterior and varus–valgus instability. Pain and recurrent effusions are common findings, as well as complaints of buckling and difficulty changing positions (e.g., from seated to standing). On physical examination, the knee may be in recurvatum with hyperextension and may be able to attain unusually high degrees of terminal flexion. Subluxation or frank dislocation may be present (**Fig. 58-9**), especially if there is severe polyethylene wear, component subsidence, and loss of the inherent stability of the implant design. If neuromuscular dysfunction leading to quadriceps weakness is a factor, the patient may exhibit a classic "quadriceps gait," in which the upper body pitches forward with each step of the affected leg in order to offset the quadriceps' inability to provide eccentric contraction. Extensor lag will oftentimes be present, with complete inability to overcome gravity if the extensor mechanism has been disrupted. Imaging and synovial fluid studies are likely to demonstrate a combination of the abnormalities of other manifestations of tibiofemoral instability.

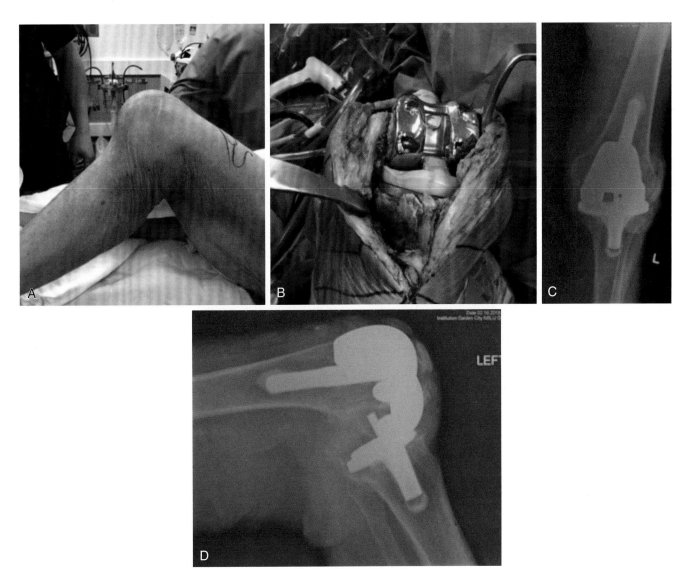

FIGURE 58-9 Preoperative **(A)** and intraoperative **(B)** photographs as well as anteroposterior **(C)** and lateral **(D)** radiographs of a total knee arthroplasty with global instability.

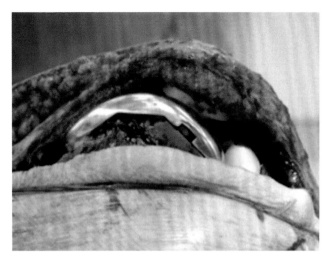

FIGURE 58-10 Intraoperative photograph demonstrating the use of a distal femoral augment.

Treatment and Outcomes

Surgical treatment is the mainstay of management for the globally unstable TKA. Conservative treatment with a hinged knee brace and the use of ambulatory assistive devices should be reserved only for patients who are not able to undergo surgery.

If recurvatum or hyperextension deformity is identified as the primary problem, the surgeon must first distinguish whether neuromuscular dysfunction is the root cause. If so, the problem should be assumed to be progressive and more aggressive corrective measures will need to be taken. Affected patients should be counseled accordingly. The corrective plan should include femoral revision with distal augmentation (**Fig. 58-10**) to lower the joint line and increase tension upon the posterior capsule and collateral ligaments, with the acceptance of some degree of flexion contracture at the end of the procedure, especially in cases with known connective tissue disorders.[31,35] When hyperextension is associated with global instability, revision to a thicker tibial articular component may be adequate to correct the instability. In patients with connective tissue disorders or neuromuscular disease, it is our recommendation to accept a mild flexion contracture since the posterior capsule and collateral ligaments will stretch over time and gradually bring the knee to full extension. In severe cases of global instability, it may be necessary to convert to a hinged prosthesis with an intrinsic extension bumper to ensure that recurvatum will not recur (**Fig. 58-11**). Such cases should be kept under careful surveillance with attention toward possible early component loosening or internal disassociation.[36,37] Continued hyperextension during gait can also lead to tibial polyethylene wear with failure of the hyperextension bumper, requiring revision of the tibial insert. Patients who experience these complications may require knee arthrodesis.

In cases due to traumatic extensor mechanism disruption, historically poor outcomes have been noted

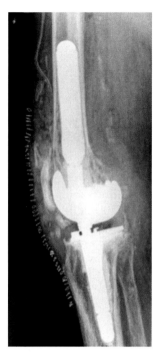

FIGURE 58-11 Lateral radiograph of the same patient from **Fig. 58-9** following revision to a hinged prosthesis.

after direct repair, with failure rates as high as 63% at medium-term follow-up.[38,39] Extensor mechanism reconstruction with allograft or synthetic mesh is preferred, though success rates with modern techniques are still no higher than 65% to 75%.[40-43] Some degree of extensor lag should be expected even in the best case scenario, and patients should be extensively counseled regarding the high likelihood of failure secondary to deep infection or excessive extensor lag. Refractory cases may need to be salvaged with resection arthroplasty or knee arthrodesis, particularly when persistent infection is present. Knee arthrodesis should also be considered in the case of severe neuromuscular dysfunction.

Cases of isolated polyethylene wear with well-balanced flexion and extension gaps may be managed with tibial polyethylene exchange when there is not evidence of component loosening, subsidence, or osteolysis. Component subsidence or loosening should be managed with complete revision. Degeneration of the collateral ligaments secondary to obesity or certain metabolic conditions may be successfully managed with revision to constrained components, though severe cases may require conversion to hinged components. In all revision situations, basic principles should still be followed with the reestablishment of the anatomic joint line and creation of equal and symmetric flexion and extension gaps. By following these principles, the surgeon can reduce the need for additional unnecessary constraint. **Table 58-4** below details our management paradigms for global instability.

For information on patellofemoral instability, please see Chapter 30.

TABLE 58-4   Management Paradigms for Tibiofemoral Global Instability

Root Cause	Treatment
Extensor mechanism disruption	Extensor mechanism reconstruction with allograft or mesh
Neuromuscular dysfunction of quadriceps	Femoral revision with distal augmentation; if recalcitrant, then convert to hinged components or knee arthrodesis
Tibial polyethylene wear	Tibial polyethylene exchange
Component subsidence	Component revision
Diffuse collateral ligament attenuation	Conversion to constrained or hinged design

CONCLUSION

Instability is an often under-recognized and under-diagnosed source of pain and disability following total knee arthroplasty, and represents a significant portion of the revision burden in the United States. The various forms of instability detailed in this chapter must be systematically ruled out in the evaluation of patients complaining of persistent pain or swelling following knee arthroplasty. Prosthetic knee instability can be prevented through meticulous primary surgical planning and execution with regards to accurate bony resections and careful soft tissue management. In the revision setting, any compromise of the posterior cruciate and/or collateral ligaments must be appropriately addressed with the judicious use of constraint. In every case, fundamental anatomic and biomechanical principles must be followed in order to obtain a stable, well-balanced knee.

REFERENCES

1. Cottino U, Sculco PK, Sierra RJ, Abdel MP. Instability after total knee arthroplasty. *Orthop Clin N Am.* 2016;47(2):311-316. doi:10.1016/j.ocl.2015.09.007.
2. Jun Song S, Detch RC, Maloney WJ, Goodman SB, Huddleston JI III. Causes of instability after total knee arthroplasty. *J Arthroplast.* 2014;29(2):360-364. doi:10.1016/j.arth.2013.06.023.
3. Le DH, Goodman SB, Maloney WJ, et al. Current modes of failure in TKA: infection, instability, and stiffness predominate Clinical Orthopaedics and Related Research ® A Publication of the Association of Bone and Joint Surgeons®. *Clin Orthop Relat Res.* 2014;472:2197-2200. doi:10.1007/s11999-014-3540-y.
4. Parratte S, Pagnano MW. Instability after total knee arthroplasty. *J Bone Joint Surg Am.* 2008;90(1):184-194.
5. Hossain F, Patel S, Haddad FS. Midterm assessment of causes and results of revision total knee arthroplasty. *Clin Orthop Relat Res.* 2010;468:1221-1228. doi:10.1007/s11999-009-1204-0.
6. Lombardi AV, Berend KR, Adams JB. Why knee replacements fail in 2013: patient, surgeon, or implant?. *Bone Joint J.* 2014;96-B(11 suppl A):101-104. doi:10.1302/0301-620X.96B11.34350.
7. Sloan M, Premkumar A, Sheth NP. Projected volume of primary total joint arthroplasty in the U.S., 2014 to 2030. *J Bone Joint Surg Am.* 2018;100(17):1455-1460. doi:10.2106/JBJS.17.01617.
8. Kurtz S, Ong K, Lau E, Mowat F, Halpern M. Projections of primary and revision hip and knee arthroplasty in the United States from 2005 to 2030. *J Bone Joint Surg.* 2007;89(4):780. doi:10.2106/JBJS.F.00222.
9. Jethanandani RG, Maloney WJ, Huddleston JI, Goodman SB, Amanatullah DF. Tibiofemoral dislocation after total knee arthroplasty. *J Arthroplast.* 2016;31(10):2282-2285. doi:10.1016/j.arth.2016.03.010.
10. Lombardi AV, Mallory TH, Vaughn BK, et al. Dislocation following primary posterior-stabilized total knee arthroplasty. *J Arthroplast.* 1993;8(6):633-639. doi:10.1016/0883-5403(93)90012-S.
11. Saleh KJ, Dykes DC, Tweedie RL, et al. Functional outcome after total knee arthroplasty revision. *J Arthroplast.* 2002;17(8):967-977. doi:10.1054/arth.2002.35823.
12. Fehring TK, Valadie AL. Knee instability after total knee arthroplasty. *Clin Orthop Relat Res.* 1994;(299):157-162. Available at http://www.ncbi.nlm.nih.gov/pubmed/8119011.
13. Laskin RS. Flexion space configuration in total knee arthroplasty. *J Arthroplast.* 1995;10(5):657-660. doi:10.1039/C39900001100.
14. Pagnano MW, Hanssen AD, Lewallen DG, Stuart MJ. Flexion instability after primary posterior cruciate retaining total knee arthroplasty. *Clin Orthop Relat Res.* 1998;(356):39-46. Available at http://www.ncbi.nlm.nih.gov/pubmed/9917666.
15. Conti A, Camarda L, Mannino S, Milici L, D'Arienzo M. Anterior dislocation in a total knee arthroplasty: a case report and literature review. *J Orthop.* 2015;12:S130-S132. doi:10.1016/j.jor.2014.06.014.
16. Gebhard JS, Kilgus DJ. Dislocation of a posterior stabilized total knee prosthesis. A report of two cases. *Clin Orthop Relat Res.* 1990;(254):225-229. Available at http://www.ncbi.nlm.nih.gov/pubmed/2323136.
17. Sharkey PF, Hozack WJ, Booth RE, Balderston RA, Rothman RH. Posterior dislocation of total knee arthroplasty. *Clin Orthop Relat Res.* 1992;(278):128-133. Available at http://www.ncbi.nlm.nih.gov/pubmed/1563142.
18. Schwab JH, Haidukewych GJ, Hanssen AD, Jacofsky DJ, Pagnano MW. Flexion instability without dislocation after posterior stabilized total knees. *Clin Orthop Relat Res.* 2005;440:96-100. Available at http://www.ncbi.nlm.nih.gov/pubmed/16239790.
19. Leopold SS, McStay C, Klafeta K, Jacobs JJ, Berger RA, Rosenberg AG. Primary repair of intraoperative disruption of the medial collateral ligament during total knee arthroplasty. *J Bone Joint Surg Am.* 2001;83-A(1):86-91. Available at http://www.ncbi.nlm.nih.gov/pubmed/11205863.
20. Lee G-C, Lotke PA. Management of intraoperative medial collateral ligament injury during TKA. *Clin Orthop Relat Res.* 2011;469:64-68. doi:10.1007/s11999-010-1502-6.
21. Insall JN, Binazzi R, Soudry M, Mestriner LA. Total knee arthroplasty. *Clin Orthop Relat Res.* 1985;(192):13-22. Available at http://www.ncbi.nlm.nih.gov/pubmed/3967412.
22. Jain JK, Agarwal S, Sharma RK. Ligament reconstruction/advancement for management of instability due to ligament insufficiency during total knee arthroplasty: a viable alternative to constrained implant. *J Orthop Sci.* 2014;19(4):564-570. doi:10.1007/s00776-014-0564-9.

23. Buechel FF. A sequential three-step lateral release for correcting fixed valgus knee deformities during total knee arthroplasty. *Clin Orthop Relat Res*. 1990;(260):170-175. Available at http://www.ncbi.nlm.nih.gov/pubmed/2225620.

24. Healy WL, Iorio R, Lemos DW. Medial reconstruction during total knee arthroplasty for severe valgus deformity. *Clin Orthop Relat Res*. 1998;(356):161-169. Available at http://www.ncbi.nlm.nih.gov/pubmed/9917681.

25. Kanamiya T, Whiteside LA, Nakamura T, Mihalko WM, Steiger J, Naito M. Ranawat Award paper. Effect of selective lateral ligament release on stability in knee arthroplasty. *Clin Orthop Relat Res*. 2002;(404):24-31. Available at http://www.ncbi.nlm.nih.gov/pubmed/12439233.

26. Krackow KA, Mihalko WM. Flexion-extension joint gap changes after lateral structure release for valgus deformity correction in total knee arthroplasty: a cadaveric study. *J Arthroplast*. 1999;14(8):994-1004. doi:10.1016/S0883-5403(99)90016-5.

27. Clarke HD, Fuchs R, Scuderi GR, Scott WN, Insall JN. Clinical results in valgus total knee arthroplasty with the "pie crust" technique of lateral soft tissue releases. *J Arthroplast*. 2005;20(8):1010-1014. doi:10.1016/j.arth.2005.03.036.

28. Conjeski JM, Scuderi GR. Lateral femoral epicondylar osteotomy for correction of fixed valgus deformity in total knee arthroplasty: a technical note. *J Arthroplast*. 2018;33(2):386-390. doi:10.1016/j.arth.2017.09.018.

29. Clarke HD, Schwartz JB, Math KR, Scuderi GR. Anatomic risk of peroneal nerve injury with the "pie crust" technique for valgus release in total knee arthroplasty. *J Arthroplast*. 2004;19(1):40-44. Available at http://www.ncbi.nlm.nih.gov/pubmed/14716649.

30. Krackow KA, Weiss AP. Recurvatum deformity complicating performance of total knee arthroplasty. A brief note. *J Bone Joint Surg Am Vol*. 1990;72(2):268-271. Available at http://www.ncbi.nlm.nih.gov/pubmed/2303513.

31. Meding JB, Keating EM, Ritter MA, Faris PM, Berend ME. Genu recurvatum in total knee replacement. *Clin Orthop Relat Res*. 2003;416(416):64-67. doi:10.1097/01.blo.0000092988.12414.18.

32. Farid A, Beekhuizen S, van der Lugt J, Rutgers M. Knee joint instability after total knee replacement in a patient with Ehlers-Danlos syndrome: the role of insert changes as practical solution. *BMJ Case Rep*, 2018;2018, bcr-2017-223395. doi:10.1136/bcr-2017-223395.

33. Rose PS, Johnson CA, Hungerford DS, Mcfarland EG. Total knee arthroplasty in ehlers-danlos syndrome. *J Arthroplasty*. 2004;19(2):190-196. doi:10.1016/j.arth.2003.03.001.

34. Can A, Erdogan F, Erdogan AO. Tibiofemoral instability after primary total knee arthroplasty: posterior-stabilized implants for obese patients. *Orthopedics*. 2017;40(5):e812-e819. doi:10.3928/01477447-20170608-02.

35. Jordan L, Kligman M, Sculco TP. Total knee arthroplasty in patients with poliomyelitis. *J Arthroplast*. 2007;22(4):543-548. doi:10.1016/j.arth.2006.03.013.

36. Giori NJ, Lewallen DG. Total knee arthroplasty in limbs affected by poliomyelitis. The Journal of Bone and Joint Surgery. *J Bone Joint Surg Am*. 2002;84–A(7):1157-1161. Available at http://www.ncbi.nlm.nih.gov/pubmed/12107315.

37. Tigani D, Fosco M, Amendola L, Boriani L. Total knee arthroplasty in patients with poliomyelitis. *Knee*. 2009;16(6):501-506. doi:10.1016/j.knee.2009.04.004.

38. Courtney PM, Edmiston TA, Pflederer CT, Levine BR, Gerlinger TL. Is there any role for direct repair of extensor mechanism disruption following total knee arthroplasty? *J Arthroplast*. 2018;33(7):S244-S248. doi:10.1016/j.arth.2017.11.045.

39. Maffulli N, Spiezia F, La Verde L, Rosa MA, Franceschi F. The management of extensor mechanism disruption after total knee arthroplasty. *Sport Med Arthrosc Rev*. 2017;25(1):41-50. doi:10.1097/JSA.0000000000000139.

40. Brown NM, Murray T, Sporer SM, Wetters N, Berger RA, Della Valle CJ. Extensor mechanism allograft reconstruction for extensor mechanism failure following total knee arthroplasty. *J Bone Joint Surg*. 2015;97(4):279-283. doi:10.2106/JBJS.N.00759.

41. Lim CT, Amanatullah DF, Huddleston JI, et al. Reconstruction of disrupted extensor mechanism after total knee arthroplasty. *J Arthroplast*. 2017;32(10):3134-3140. doi:10.1016/j.arth.2017.05.005.

42. Ricciardi BF, Oi K, Trivellas M, Lee Y, Della Valle AG, Westrich GH. Survivorship of extensor mechanism allograft reconstruction after total knee arthroplasty. *J Arthroplast*. 2017;32(1):183-188. doi:10.1016/j.arth.2016.06.031.

43. Shau D, Patton R, Patel S, Ward L, Guild G. Synthetic mesh vs. allograft extensor mechanism reconstruction in total knee arthroplasty – a systematic review of the literature and meta-analysis. *Knee*. 2018;25(1):2-7. doi:10.1016/j.knee.2017.12.004.

chapter 59

Patellofemoral Problems in Total Knee Arthroplasty

Nicholas B. Frisch, MD, MBA | Richard A. Berger, MD

Patellofemoral complications are among the most common postoperative problem associated with the current design of total knee prostheses and are a major cause of revision surgery.[1-9] Patellofemoral complications affect up to 12% of all total knee replacements done in the United States. Although there is evidence that patellofemoral complications have diminished somewhat over the past decade,[10] they are still a common reason for pain and dysfunction after total knee arthroplasty.[11,12] In some series, up to 50% of the revisions performed were for a problem related to the patellofemoral articulation,[6] and those that were revised for patellofemoral complications have a high risk of reoperation.[13]

This chapter addresses patellofemoral complications from two perspectives. First, they are considered as they relate to primary total knee arthroplasty, to enable the surgeon to optimize patellofemoral tracking and minimize complications. The various aspects of primary total knee arthroplasty that affect the patellofemoral joint are covered so that these common complications may be avoided. In the second half of this chapter, the diagnosis and management of patellofemoral complications after total knee arthroplasties are addressed.

PATELLOFEMORAL JOINT IN PRIMARY TOTAL KNEE ARTHROPLASTY

Patellofemoral complications are the most common complications in total knee arthroplasty that can be avoided. Patellar tilt is a common radiographic finding and can range from minimal to dramatic. When patellar tilt is associated with a metal-backed patellar component, this can lead to eccentric wear and delamination with the possibility of eventual scoring of the femoral component, which necessitates complete revision surgery (**Fig. 59-1**). As the problems of the patellofemoral joint progress, subluxation and frank dislocation can occur. Patellar maltracking leads to shear forces over time that can result in either debonding of the patellar prosthesis from the native patella or shearing off of the prosthesis from the fixation lugs (**Fig. 59-2**). These shear forces on the patella over time can also lead to patella fragmentation or fracture.

The Tight Lateral Retinaculum

It has been the conventional wisdom that patellofemoral maltracking is secondary to a tight lateral retinaculum and, therefore, that the solution to this problem is a lateral retinacular release. Once a lateral retinacular release is performed, however, patellar tracking usually does not improve substantially. A few well-placed towel clips, however, can lead to the false conclusion that the patella is tracking appropriately. In these cases, it is often found postoperatively that the patella is not tracking well, and with time, patellofemoral maltracking and failure occur.

In most total knee arthroplasties with patellofemoral maltracking, a tight lateral retinaculum is not the sole problem; it is really only a symptom indicating that, in some way, the patellofemoral articulation has been altered. Occasionally, such as in a knee with a valgus deformity, real lateral retinacular tightness is identified either preoperatively (**Fig. 59-3**) or intraoperatively after the arthrotomy has been performed. In these cases, the solution is a lateral retinacular release, which allows the patella to track in a more anatomic position in the trochlear groove. The majority of knees that require total knee arthroplasty are associated with a varus deformity, however, and in the majority of these cases, the patella tracks quite well before arthroplasty. Furthermore, implant designs have evolved to create a more anatomic patellofemoral relationship to improve tracking and minimize patellofemoral complications.[14,15] Thus, if the patellar trochlear relationship is recreated, appropriate patellar tracking will result. If that relationship is altered, however poor tracking ensues and manifests as lateral patellar tracking, subluxation, or frank dislocation. Thus, a tight lateral retinaculum is rarely the problem; it is only a symptom that intraoperatively the patellar trochlear relationship has been altered.

Resection of the Patellofemoral Joint

As with the tibiofemoral articulation, the surgeon should take care in resecting the patellofemoral joint. In general, the resected patella should be restored millimeter for millimeter with polyethylene.[16-18] Thus, the amount of bone resected should precisely equal the thickness of the patellar component to be implanted so that the final thickness

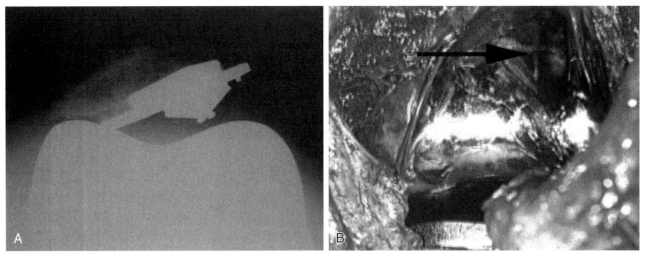

FIGURE 59-1 Patellar tilt associated with a metal-backed patella. **A:** Radiograph. **B:** Intraoperative view of the femoral component that has been scored by the metal-backed patella (*arrow*) and requires revision.

of the patella–prosthesis composite is equivalent to the thickness of the native patella (**Fig. 59-4**). This is accomplished by first measuring the thickness of the native patella and then cutting it in the coronal plane, removing an amount of patellar bone that is equivalent to the thickness of the component to be inserted. The amount of bone resected is typically between 8 and 10 mm, which should correspond to the thickness of the patella component used. In general, at least 12 mm of patella should be left after resection.

It is important to resect the patella parallel to the coronal plane so that the patellar prosthesis is not tilted on the native patella. This can be accomplished by resecting some of the synovium around the patella so that the patellar tendon is exposed and the cut parallel to it. Booth et al[19] have described the patellar nose as also a useful landmark for resecting the patella. A useful rule of thumb is that the thickness of the final patella–prosthesis composite should be on the order of 21 to 23 mm for smaller patients and 24 to 26 mm for larger patients. Thought

and care should be taken when the combined thickness of the native patella and the patellar prosthesis is outside this range. There are several different techniques for patellar resurfacing,[20] but whether a patellar clamp, a patellar reamer, or a plain saw is used, it is important to adhere to these principles. Achieving a composite thickness that closely approximates the native thickness is associated with greater improvement in quality of life, physical measures, and Western Ontario and McMaster Universities Arthritis Index stiffness scores.[21]

The consequences of not properly restoring the patellofemoral joint are significant.[22-25] If patellar resection is excessive, so that the final construct of prosthesis plus native patella is significantly less than the native thickness, the quadriceps musculature is put at a substantial mechanical disadvantage, as the patella contributes approximately 30% to the extensor mechanism's moment arm.[26,27] In addition, it is important to note that small differences in the final height of the patella are quite important. For example, if the patella before arthroplasty

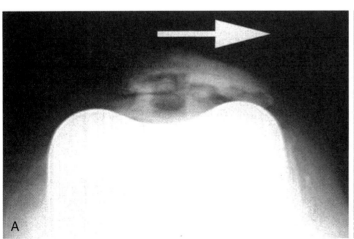
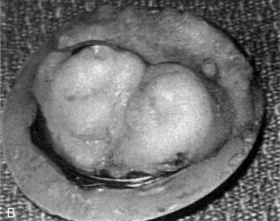

FIGURE 59-2 **A:** Patellar maltracking has led to failure of the cemented patellar component secondary to shear forces (*arrow*). **B:** Failed metal-backed patellar component that has debonded from the surrounding cement mantle.

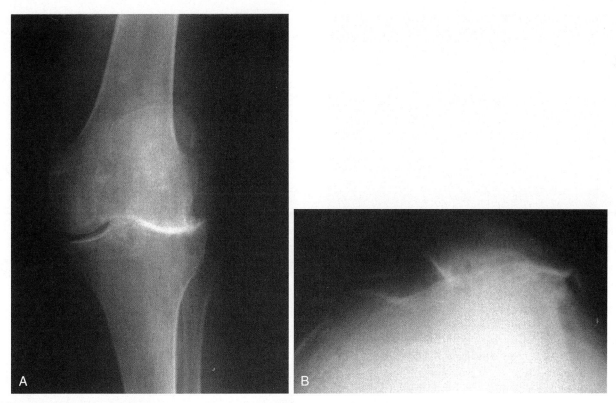

FIGURE 59-3 Preoperative anteroposterior **(A)** and patellar view **(B)** of a knee with a valgus deformity with lateral patellar tracking noted preoperatively.

measures 25 mm and the final thickness of the resected patella plus the patellar implant is only 20 mm, the overall reduction in patellar thickness is 20%. Therefore, in this particular situation, 5 mm corresponds to a 20% reduction in patellar thickness, which will substantially affect quadriceps function.[26]

Overstuffing the patellofemoral joint, although it improves quadriceps function, increases the resultant patellofemoral force and lateralizes the Q-angle force; this results in a tightened lateral retinaculum and lateral maltracking.[28] As the patellofemoral joint is overstuffed with either too thick a patella or an oversized femoral component, the lateral retinaculum is stretched.[29] The result is lateral patellar tracking, subluxation, and potentially dislocation.[23] In addition to a tight lateral retinaculum secondary to overstuffing of the patellofemoral joint, other patellofemoral problems occur, many of which are associated with an increased Q angle, which further raises the resultant force that tends to pull the patella laterally.[24,28,30]

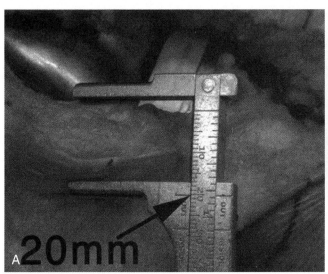
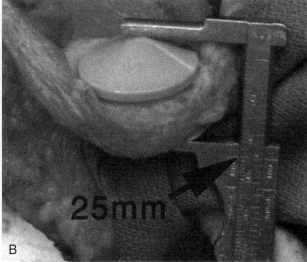

FIGURE 59-4 **A:** Measurement of patellar thickness before resurfacing; the thickness is 20 mm. **B:** After resurfacing, with the trial component in place, the thickness is 25 mm. If additional bone is not resected, overstuffing of the patellofemoral joint will occur.

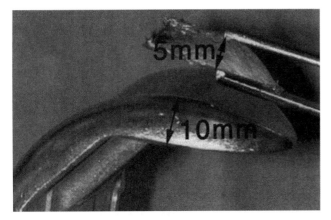

FIGURE 59-5 The thickness of the anterior flange of the femoral component is 10 mm, whereas the bone resected from the anterior femur is only 5 mm in thickness. This can lead to overstuffing of the patellofemoral joint.

The patellofemoral joint can also be overstuffed by failure to resect enough anterior femur.[24] Most femoral components are 10 mm thick anteriorly, and in some patients, particularly women, the anterior trochlea that has been resected is not as thick as the component that replaces it (**Fig. 59-5**). In addition, the fear of notching the anterior femur has led many surgeons not to resect as much trochlea anteriorly as is being replaced by the component. This further leads to overstuffing of the patellofemoral joint. These problems can be avoided by carefully measuring the amount of bone resected from the trochlear groove and by ensuring that cutting guides are positioned appropriately.

Oversizing of the femoral component can also cause overstuffing of the patellofemoral joint.[10,24] This is because, in flexion, the anteroposterior dimension of the femur contributes to the patellofemoral joint (**Fig. 59-6**). This problem is more commonly seen with posterior-stabilized

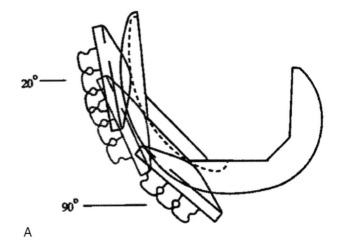

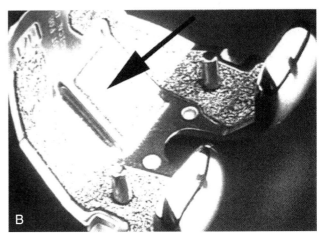

FIGURE 59-7 **A** and **B:** Femoral component with a deepened trochlear groove (*arrow*).

than with cruciate-retaining total knee arthroplasties, secondary to the tendency to upsize the femoral component, which makes it larger than the native anteroposterior diameter of the femur. This also tightens the retinaculum and makes it more likely that patellofemoral tracking problems will occur. Additionally increasing the position of the femoral component anteriorly can result in an increased extensor mechanism arc and therefore result in decreased flexion.[31]

Many modern femoral components now have a deepened trochlear groove anteriorly, which prevents overstuffing of the joint (**Fig. 59-7**).[15,32,33] It is important to remember, however, that this should be thought of as adjunctive treatment for the patellofemoral joint, and care still must be taken to not overstuff it.

Femoral Component

Femoral component design, size, rotation, and placement all play an important role in patellofemoral tracking.[30,32,34,35] The trochlear groove, being part of the femoral component, is related to placement and rotation of the femoral component itself. With the advent of the measured resection technique[36] in total knee arthroplasty,

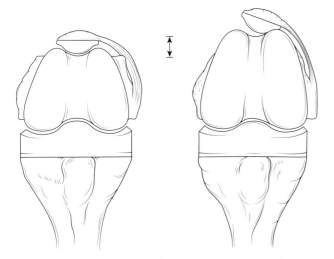

FIGURE 59-6 The correct femoral component size (left) will allow appropriate patellar tracking. Use of a larger femoral component (right) leads to overstuffing of the patellofemoral joint and creates the potential for patellar maltracking. (From Krackow KA. *The Technique of Total Knee Arthroplasty*. St. Louis, MO: Mosby; 1990:215, Fig. 6-25, with permission.)

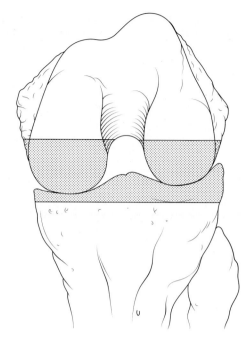

FIGURE 59-8 Resection of equal amounts of bone from the posterior femoral condyles leads to internal rotation of the femoral component and poor patellar tracking. (From Krackow KA. *The Technique of Total Knee Arthroplasty*. St. Louis, MO: Mosby; 1990:131, with permission.)

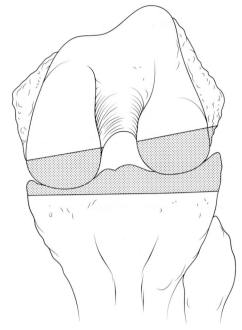

FIGURE 59-9 Appropriate resection of bone from the posterior femoral condyles to avoid internal rotation of the femoral component. The cut is parallel to the epicondylar axis, with more bone being removed form the posteromedial than from the posterolateral condyle. (From Krackow KA. *The Technique of Total Knee Arthroplasty*. St. Louis, MO: Mosby; 1990:131, with permission.)

the initial thought was to remove equal amounts of bone from the medial and lateral posterior condyles (**Fig. 59-8**). However, when equal amounts of posterior condyle are resected in combination with a nonanatomic tibial cut (removing more lateral tibial bone than medial tibial bone), the femoral component is internally rotated on the tibia, which increases the Q angle of the knee and leads to patellar maltracking.[32,34,37] To avoid this problem, in the majority of knees, more bone needs to be resected from the posterior medial femoral condyle than from the posterolateral femoral condyle (**Fig. 59-9**). In many modern total knee systems, the surgical protocols recommend cutting the femoral component with some external rotation relative to the posterior condyles to optimize patellar tracking. Although external femoral rotation relative to the posterior condyles is helpful, a more accurate method of rotating the femoral component is to align the component parallel to the surgical epicondylar axis (**Fig. 59-10**).

The epicondylar axis can be found by identifying the lateral prominence of the lateral epicondyle and the medial sulcus of the medial epicondyle (**Fig. 59-10**).[38,39] If the medial sulcus is difficult to identify, the entire medial condyle is easy to palpate and is in essence a large prominence. If the center of that large prominence is then identified, that also corresponds to the sulcus of the medial epicondyle.[22] The medial sulcus is the insertion point of the deep medial collateral ligament, and overlying this is the fan-like insertion of the superficial medial collateral ligament. These landmarks can be seen and felt intraoperatively in the majority of cases and routinely used to confirm appropriate femoral bone resection and component rotation.

Most surgeons and most instrumentation systems, however, still use the posterior femoral condyles as a reference point for femoral component alignment. Therefore, it is important to know the relationship between the posterior femoral condyles and the epicondylar axis. This has been shown to be approximately 3° of external rotation, and thus many instrumentation systems rotate the femoral cutting block in 3° of external rotation relative to the posterior femoral condyles (**Fig. 59-11**).

In most varus knees, using either the posterior condyles as a reference point for femoral component rotation

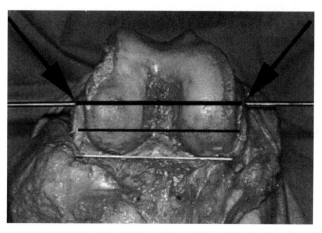

FIGURE 59-10 The epicondylar axis has been marked by pins placed in the center of the medial and lateral epicondyles (*arrows*). The femoral cut is then made parallel to this line (*lower line*). Note that more bone will be resected from the medial than from the lateral condyle.

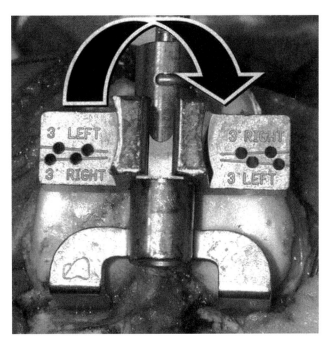

FIGURE 59-11 Initial femoral guide for the NexGen total knee system as seen on a left knee. The guide orients the cutting block for the femoral component in 3° of external rotation relative to the posterior condyles (*arrow*). Although this guide is accurate in the majority of knees, appropriate external rotation should always be confirmed using either the epicondylar axis or the Whiteside line.

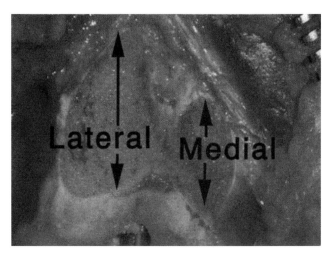

FIGURE 59-12 View of the cut anterior surface of the distal femur (right knee). The exposed bone is substantially longer on the lateral side than on the medial side, which indicates appropriate external rotation of the femoral cuts.

works reasonably well. This is not true in valgus knees, however. Most valgus knees have hypoplasia of the lateral condyle that is present distally as well as posteriorly. Therefore, in the valgus knee, referencing the posterior condyles results in substantial internal rotation of the femoral component leading to extremely poor patellofemoral tracking. In the valgus knee, even though the lateral retinaculum is sometimes tight, correcting the axial deformity and properly aligning the components decreases the Q angle and improves patellar tracking. If this is done properly, a lateral release is rarely required.

A useful intraoperative sign to ensure that appropriate femoral cuts have been made is the anterior trochlear groove. In the normal femur, the lateral side of the trochlear groove is more prominent than the medial side. Therefore, when the anterior surface of the trochlear groove is cut, more bone should be removed from the lateral than from the medial side of the trochlear groove. When viewed from above, the exposed bone on the medial side should be much shorter in length than the exposed bone on the lateral side (**Fig. 59-12**). This is often referred to as the "piano sign" or the "boot sign" with the toe on the medial side and the heel and shank on the lateral side. If the exposed bone on the medial side is equal or longer in length than on the lateral side, then the femoral component is internally rotated and the epicondylar axis should be identified and rotation reassessed and corrected.

In addition to the epicondylar axis and the posterior femoral condyles, a third landmark, which was described by Whiteside and Arima,[40] is also useful. The Whiteside

line, which is the deepest part of the trochlear recess, should be perpendicular to the epicondylar axis and is a useful final check to ensure that the femoral cutting block is oriented appropriately (**Fig. 59-13**).

In addition to rotation of the femoral component, mediolateral placement of the femoral component can also affect patellofemoral tracking.[32] A component that is placed too far medially moves the entire trochlear groove medially, which results in relative lateral tracking of the patella (**Fig. 59-14**). Although, on most femora, the mediolateral dimension of the component comes close to covering the exposed femur, oftentimes there are a few millimeters of uncovered femur. The femur should be placed as close to the lateral edge of the exposed bone as possible. This helps in patellofemoral tracking by lateralizing the trochlear groove. It is important, however, not to excessively lateralize the femoral component. If the

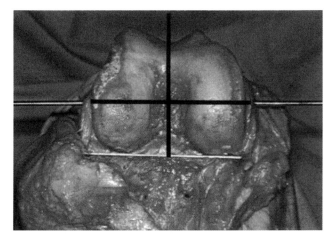

FIGURE 59-13 Whiteside line is drawn in the deepest part of the trochlear recess and is perpendicular to the epicondylar axis, which has been marked with pins in the center of the medial and lateral epicondyles.

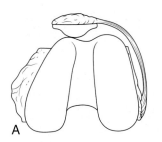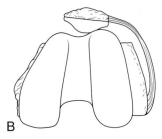

FIGURE 59-14 Lateral placement of the femoral component **(A)** optimizes patellar tracking compared with medial placement **(B)**. (From Krackow KA. *The Technique of Total Knee Arthroplasty.* St. Louis, MO: Mosby; 1990:139, Fig. 5-12, with permission.)

component overhangs the femoral condyle laterally this tends to tent the retinaculum and results in a tightening of the lateral retinaculum with associated pain and poor patellar tracking.

Tibial Component in Primary Total Knee Arthroplasty

Just as femoral component rotation is extremely important in patellofemoral tracking, so is tibial component rotation. Internally rotating the tibial component increases the Q angle and therefore increases the resultant force, which tends to dislocate the patella laterally. Externally rotating the tibial component decreases the Q angle, which reduces the resultant force that tends to dislocate the component laterally and results in improved patellar tracking.[23] It must be stated, however, that excessive external rotation of the tibial component can lead to intoeing, with subsequent problems such as tripping and cosmetic deformity.

It has been suggested that the proper rotational orientation of the tibial component is alignment with the center of the medial one-third of the tibial tubercle. However, this is a difficult landmark to assess. A better landmark is to use the tip of the tibial tubercle. Berger et al[37] have described a technique to align the rotation of the tibial component. A pin is placed in the tibial tubercle at the tip and aimed toward the posterior cruciate ligament. This determines the orientation of the tibia. Then, the component is placed 18° internal to the tip of the tibial tubercle (this is 3 minutes on a clock face). This point then corresponds roughly with the center of the medial one-third; however, it is a much more reproducible mark (**Fig. 59-15**). An alternative method to check proper rotation of the tibial component is to align the anterior edge of the component with the anterior edge of the native tibia.[22]

Appropriate rotation of the tibial component is complicated by the asymmetric nature of the proximal tibia. With most symmetric tibial components, when they are placed on the tibia such that posterolaterally the tibial component is flush with the bone, some posteromedial bone will remain uncovered. This represents the proper tibial component rotation (**Fig. 59-16**). If, however, the component is too large and the surgeon tries to obtain

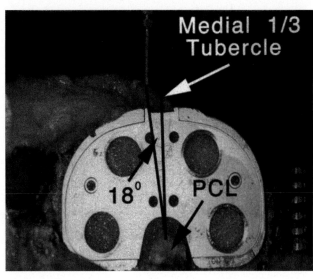

FIGURE 59-15 Guidelines for obtaining appropriate external rotation of the tibial component. A pin is placed in the tibial tubercle at the tip and aimed toward the posterior cruciate ligament (PCL). This determines the orientation of the tibia. The component is then placed 18° internal to the tip of the tibial tubercle (3 min on a clock face). This point corresponds roughly with the center of the medial one-third of the tibial tubercle.

perfect tibial coverage, internal rotation of the tibial component occurs due to the attempt to cover the exposed posteromedial bone. It should be noted that this is also true with asymmetric tibial components, as they too may not fully cover the tibia if placed in an appropriate amount of external rotation. Therefore, the rotation of the tibial component should be determined independent of tibial coverage.

In addition, mediolateral tibial component placement can also affect the patellofemoral articulation and patellofemoral tracking. Lateral placement of the tibial tray decreases the Q angle and improves patellofemoral tracking. Therefore, it is recommended that the tibial tray

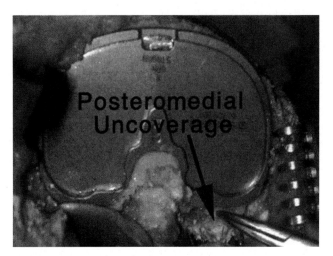

FIGURE 59-16 When the tibial component has been externally rotated appropriately, the posteromedial portion of the proximal tibia is uncovered.

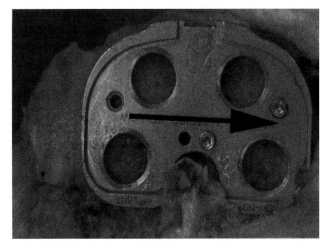

FIGURE 59-17 View of the tibial trial appropriately positioned on a right knee. The component is placed as far lateral as is possible (*arrow*) to optimize patellar tracking, leaving medial bone uncovered. It is important to clear away adequate soft tissue to visualize the lateral border of the tibia and to place a retractor in this space to keep the patella retracted laterally.

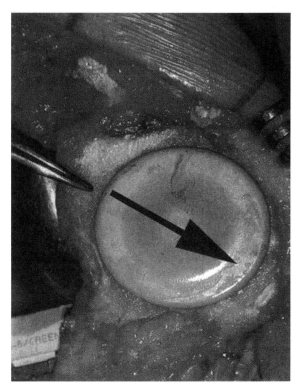

FIGURE 59-18 The patellar button is placed medially on the native patella to optimize patellar tracking (*arrow*).

be placed as far lateral as possible; it is thus important to clear enough soft tissue around the lateral edge of the tibia for it to be appropriately visualized (**Fig. 59-17**). As the majority of arthritic knees have a varus deformity, the small amount of proximal tibia that is uncovered on the medial side of the knee can then be removed, which aids in obtaining appropriate ligamentous balance by effectively lengthening the medial collateral ligament.

Patellar Component

In addition to recreating appropriate patellar thickness, mediolateral patellar component placement also plays a role in patellofemoral tracking. Most patellae are oblong with a larger medial-to-lateral distance than superior–inferior distance. The patellar button can be placed either medially or laterally on the patella. Placing the patellar button medially on the native patella results in a decreased Q angle, whereas placing it laterally results in an increased Q angle (**Fig. 59-18**). Therefore, medial positioning helps patellofemoral tracking.[33,41,42] In addition, it has been shown by Hofmann[41] that the normal center of the patella lies approximately 3 mm medial to the center of the underlying bone, and thus the center of the patellar button should be placed at least 3 mm medial to the center of the remaining bone. Further work by Miller et al[30] found that patellar kinematics were improved with placement of the patellar component 3.75 mm medial to the geometric center of the patella. Any remaining bone on the lateral side of the native patella should be removed as this bone can overgrow, causing patellofemoral impingement and pain. In addition, this small amount of bone tends to tent the retinaculum on the lateral side, tightening it with resultant poor patellofemoral tracking.

Conclusion

Multiple factors affect the patellofemoral joint in primary total knee arthroplasty. Avoidance of overstuffing the patellofemoral joint and properly sizing the femoral component are critical. Overstuffing the joint with the normal Q angle of the knee results in tightening of the lateral retinaculum and the resultant force tends to dislocate the patella laterally.

Lateral placement of the femoral component on the femur and lateral placement of the tibial component on the tibia also decrease the Q angle, as does medialization of the patellar component on the native patella. Appropriate patellofemoral tracking is based upon proper femoral and tibial component rotation. Internal rotation of the femoral or tibial component results in poor patellofemoral tracking, whereas appropriate external rotation of the femoral and tibial components optimizes patellofemoral tracking.[43] The femoral component should be rotated parallel to the epicondylar axis and the tibial component should be rotated 18° internally from the tip of the tibial tubercle.

After all of the components are in place, a trial reduction should be performed to assess patellofemoral tracking. This assessment should be done without towel clips in the retinaculum using the "no thumb" technique. If there is any concern about patellofemoral tracking, the tourniquet can be released, as this can affect patellofemoral tracking by binding of the

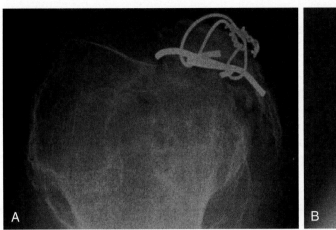
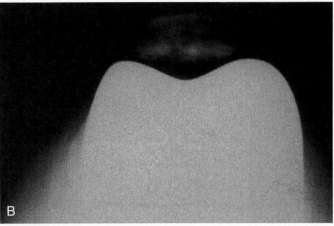

FIGURE 59-19 **A:** Preoperative patellar view of a knee with severe lateral maltracking. The procedure was performed without a retinacular release but with special attention to appropriate component position. **B:** Postoperative patellar view.

quadriceps musculature. If the patella is still not tracking properly, attention should be directed to the components to determine if their rotation and position are optimal. A lateral retinacular release should be performed only if the lateral retinaculum was tight preoperatively. If the lateral retinaculum was not tight preoperatively, then the trochlear patellar relationship has been disrupted and therefore must be corrected. With today's modern total knee systems, the most common problem is internal rotation of the femoral or tibial components. In conclusion, with attention to detail, alignment, rotation, and position, even the most complex patellofemoral joint can be handled and can track well postoperatively (**Fig. 59-19**).

REVISION TOTAL KNEE ARTHROPLASTY FOR PATELLAR MALTRACKING

As has been discussed earlier, it is important to strive to avoid patellofemoral complications by proper component rotation and alignment with attention to soft-tissue balance. Patellofemoral complications do occur after total knee arthroplasty and the following section addresses the diagnosis and treatment of these problems.

Once patellofemoral problems occur, it is important to identify and address the underlying cause. Although it is appealing to believe that a simple lateral release will correct a subluxing or dislocating patella, if the underlying cause of the subluxation or dislocation is not identified, a lateral release merely provides a transient solution. Lateral releases with or without medial reefing should be considered only when the lateral retinaculum was tight preoperatively and was not released. The most commonly identified cause of patellar maltracking is internal rotation of the femoral or tibial component or both.

Assessment of Patellofemoral Maltracking

When patellofemoral problems are assessed, it is important to obtain a complete set of radiographs that include a Merchant or skyline view. A long mechanical axis view should also be obtained to assess axial alignment. Although patellofemoral problems can result from axial malalignment, the problem is often improper rotation of the tibial or femoral component or both.

Berger et al[37] have described a technique to allow for assessing component rotation preoperatively using noninvasive computed tomographic (CT) scanning methods. With this technique, the femoral component can be evaluated using a single cut through the epicondylar axis. The epicondylar axis is drawn from the lateral prominence to the medial sulcus and a second line is drawn in reference to the posterior condyles. The difference between these two angles is the femoral component rotation (**Fig. 59-20**). The femoral component should be parallel to the epicondylar axis, and any internal rotation may result in patellofemoral problems.

Tibial component rotation can also be assessed using this method. Three cuts through the tibia are obtained: one through the tibial tubercle, one through the proximal tibial plateau, and one through the tibial component. These three cuts are then superimposed. The geometric center of the tibial plateau is found, and this point is connected to the tip of the tibial tubercle. This defines the orientation of the tibial tubercle. A second line is made in the anteroposterior axis of the tibial component. The difference between these two lines defines tibial component rotation (**Fig. 59-21**). Through previous studies, we have determined that appropriate component rotation using this method should be 18°.[37] If the tibial component rotation is more than 18°, the tibial component is too internally rotated and patellofemoral problems are likely.

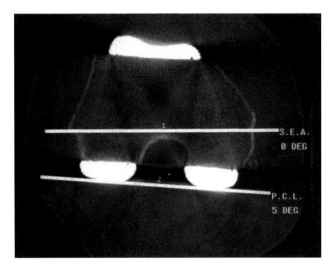

FIGURE 59-20 Computed tomographic scan through the epicondylar axis of a right knee. The epicondylar axis (*upper line*) is compared with the position of the posterior condyles of the femoral component (*lower line*) to determine femoral component rotation. The component pictured is internally rotated 5°. P.C.L., posterior condylar line; S.E.A., surgical epicondylar axis.

We have shown in a study of 20 well-functioning total knee arthroplasties and 30 total knee arthroplasties with patellofemoral maltracking that the severity of patellofemoral problems in an otherwise well-aligned, well-balanced knee is related to the amount of overall internal rotation of the femoral component plus the tibial component (**Fig. 59-22**).[37] More severe complications were associated with greater amounts of combined internal rotation of the femoral or the tibial component or both. Subsequent authors have confirmed the accuracy of traditional CT scanning for identifying femoral and tibial component rotation.[44] More recently there have been investigations of tibial component rotation using

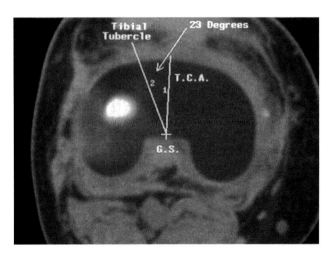

FIGURE 59-21 Computed tomographic scan to determine tibial component rotation. A line is drawn from the tip of the tibial tubercle to the geometric center of the tibia and is compared to a line marking the anteroposterior axis of the tibial component. Appropriate rotation is 18°. The component shown is internally rotated 5°. G.S., geometric center; T.C.A., tibial component axis.

three-dimensional reconstructions to address potential challenges associated with the use of two-dimensional CT scans.[45-48] Roper et al describe a specific protocol for assessing tibial component rotation using an stepwise protocol with 3D reconstructions.[49] They suggest that using a standardized protocol with 3D reconstructions provides excellent intra- and interobserver reliability. With minor patellofemoral problems, only a mild amount of malrotation is likely to be present. With more serious patellofemoral problems, however, significant malrotation of both components is suspected.

Using CT, the amount and location of component malrotation can be easily assessed. If the problem lies with only one component, then an isolated component revision can be contemplated. If the problem is isolated tibial component internal rotation, an alternative to revising the tibial component is to have a custom externally rotated polyethylene liner made. This can be specially ordered from the manufacturer and has been successfully used in our experience to correct patellofemoral maltracking in the face of isolated internal rotation of the tibial component.

In addition to preoperative CT scans, an intraoperative assessment of component rotation can be made. When femoral component rotation is assessed, the epicondylar axis can be easily identified using the lateral prominence and the medial sulcus. Tibial component rotation can be assessed intraoperatively by noting where the center of the tibial component is located relative to the tip of the tubercle (**Fig. 59-23**). Although intraoperative assessment is important, it is strongly recommended that CT scans be used, as often anatomic variations, which initially lead to abnormal rotation of the components, will still be present and can fool the revision surgeon, particularly if exposure is difficult.

Extensor Mechanism Disruption

Other extensor mechanism problems exist that may or may not be related to tibiofemoral component rotation. One of the more devastating complications after total knee arthroplasty is extensor mechanism disruption, which has been reported to occur in as many as 2.5% of cases.[50] Although normally an acute quadriceps rupture can be easily repaired primarily,[8] a much more difficult situation develops with chronic quadriceps or patellar tendon ruptures.[51]

Extensor mechanism disruptions manifest clinically as loss of active extension. When the quadriceps tendon is disrupted, a defect is often palpable proximal to the patella (**Fig. 59-24**). Radiographs often confirm the diagnosis of an extensor mechanism disruption, with the patella seen in a far more proximal or distal position than normal (**Fig. 59-25**), and a skyline or Merchant view shows that the patella is not present in the trochlear groove (**Fig. 59-26**). The "rising moon" sign, in which the patella is seen riding above the level of the top of the femoral component on the

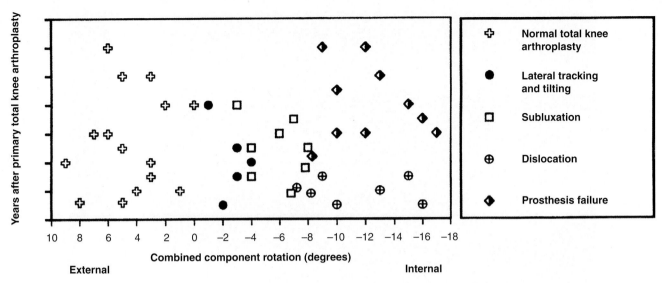

FIGURE 59-22 Graphic representation of the results of combined femoral and tibial rotation on patellar tracking after total knee arthroplasty. With greater amounts of combined internal rotation, patellar maltracking and the risk of ultimate patellar failure increase with time. (From Berger RA, Crossett LS, Jacobs JJ, et al. Malrotation causing patellofemoral complications after total knee arthroplasty. *Clin Orthop Relat Res*. 1998;356:144-153, Fig. 7, with permission.)

anteroposterior projection (**Fig. 59-27**), has been described for patellar tendon ruptures. On the lateral radiograph, the Insall-Salvati ratio can be used to assess the integrity of the patellar tendon (**Fig. 59-28**).[52] This is the ratio between the length of the patellar tendon (as measured from the insertion on the tibial tubercle to the insertion on the base of the patella) divided by the length of the patella. The normal ratio is approximately 1.2; values above this indicate patellar tendon disruption.

Patellar tendon ruptures can be divided into two broad categories: acute and chronic. Although the acute patellar tendon rupture can be addressed by primary repair with or without augmentation from a semitendinosus graft, chronic ruptures are more difficult to treat. When

considering isolated extensor mechanism reconstruction it critical to assess component orientation. Underlying component malposition or malrotation will predispose isolated reconstruction to failure and must be addressed concurrently. Treatment of this catastrophic complication using primary direct repair or xenograft was associated with failure in 11 of 17 cases in one series.[51] Alternative

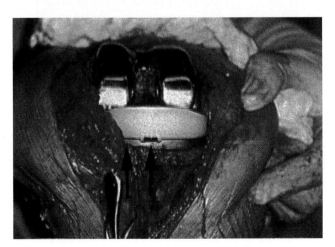

FIGURE 59-23 Intraoperative assessment of tibial component rotation in a right knee. The center of the tibial component (*right arrow*) lies medial to the medial third of the tibial tubercle (*left arrow*) and, thus, is internally rotated. The tibial tubercle has a towel clamp placed around it, and the center of the tubercle is marked with an elevator.

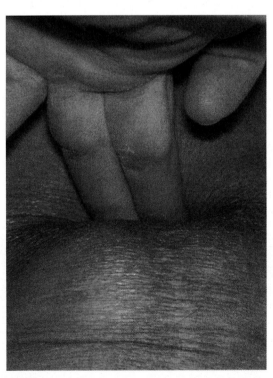

FIGURE 59-24 Clinical photograph of the knee of a patient with a quadriceps tendon rupture after a total knee arthroplasty. There is a palpable defect proximal to the patella.

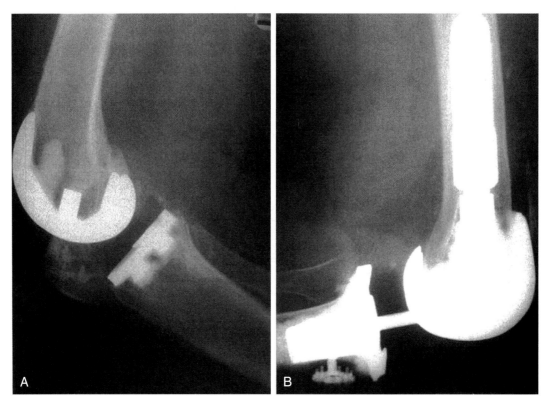

FIGURE 59-25 **A:** Lateral radiograph of a quadriceps tendon rupture. The patella is seen to lie distal to its normal position. **B:** Lateral radiograph of a patellar tendon rupture showing the patella far proximal to its normal position. Note the hardware in the region of the tibial tubercle, which indicates that a portion of or the entire patellar tendon was damaged at the time of the revision surgery, and an attempt was made to repair the tendon using a soft-tissue washer.

surgical techniques for management include reconstruction with autogenous semitendinosus tendon,[50] medial gastrocnemius muscle transposition flap,[53] achilles tendon allograft,[54] synthetic mesh,[55] or extensor mechanism allograft.[56-59]

Emerson et al reported initial optimistic results in a group of 13 knees treated with a complete allograft extensor mechanism reconstruction, including the tibial tubercle, patellar tendon, patella, and quadriceps tendon for patellar tendon ruptures that occurred during or after total knee arthroplasty.[56] They found reliable osseous union at the junction of the distal allograft bone plug (at the inferior portion of the allograft patellar tendon) and

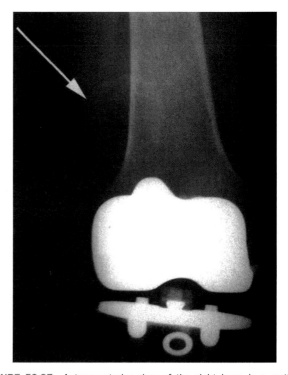

FIGURE 59-27 Anteroposterior view of the right knee in a patient with a patellar tendon rupture. The "rising moon" sign is seen with the patella far proximal to its normal position, as depicted here by the white arrow demonstrating the patella position. Note the metallic hardware present in the region of the tibial tubercle, indicative of an attempt to repair a partially or entirely detached patellar tendon at the time of the primary knee arthroplasty with a soft-tissue washer.

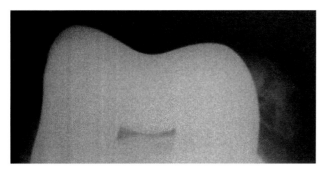

FIGURE 59-26 Skyline or Merchant view of the right knee showing dislocation of the patella from the trochlea in a patient with a quadriceps tendon rupture.

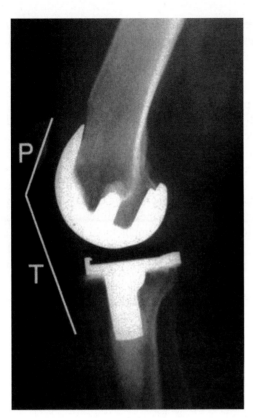

FIGURE 59-28 Lateral radiograph of the knee of a patient with a patellar tendon disruption. The Insall ratio is determined by dividing the length of the patellar tendon (T) by the length of the patella (P). The normal value is 1, with values greater than 1.2 indicative of a patellar tendon disruption.

the host tibial tubercle, and no patient had an extensor lag of more than 20°. A subsequent follow-up of the same group, however, found that three of the nine remaining patients had unacceptable extensor lags of 20° to 40°.[57] Using the original technique as described by Emerson, in which the graft was tensioned to allow for 60° of flexion "without excessive tightness," our group previously reported poor results, with seven out of seven reconstructions having failed clinically at a mean of 39 months.[58]

Better results were reported by Nazarian and Booth[59] in a series of 40 patients when the surgical technique was modified to include suturing the quadriceps anastomoses in full extension under maximal tension. Using this technique, we have found that the rate of recurrent extensor lag is greatly decreased, and we currently use an extensor mechanism allograft for patients with chronic extensor mechanism disruptions, severe patella baja, and patellar fragmentation, and for patients who have previously had a patellectomy with poor extensor mechanism function.

Our present surgical technique includes the use of fresh frozen allografts and tensioning of the graft in full extension. The patellar tendon insertion and tibial bone block are placed into a tight-fitting trough in the native tibia with fixation using multiple wires around the allograft; a bicortical screw is used if additional fixation is needed (**Fig. 59-29**). The native extensor tissue is oversewn with the allograft using heavy nonabsorbable suture, and the patella is not resurfaced (**Fig. 59-30**). An alternative

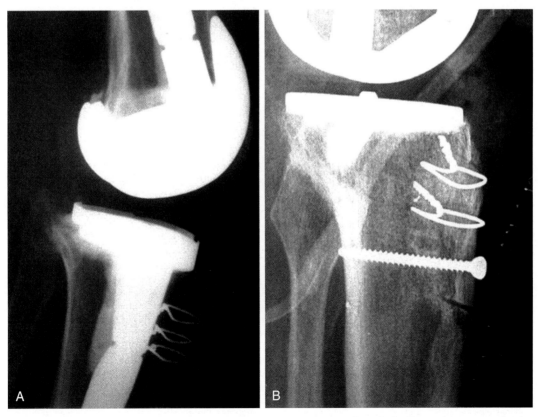

FIGURE 59-29 Fixation methods for the tibial bone block of an extensor mechanism allograft. **A:** Six-month postoperative lateral radiograph showing a healed junction between the tibial bone block and the native tibia. The bone block was held in place using three wires. **B:** Immediately postoperative lateral radiograph after an extensor mechanism allograft in which adjunctive fixation was achieved using a bicortical screw.

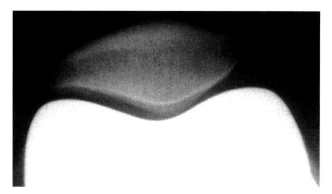

FIGURE 59-30   Merchant view after an extensor mechanism allograft. The patella is not resurfaced and is seen tracking centrally.

is reconstruction with a fresh frozen Achilles tendon allograft with an os calcis bone block using similar surgical technique and principles.[54,60] Crossett et al showed

reliable reconstruction of patellar tendon rupture with Achilles tendon allograft. In the nine patients studied, the average extensor lag decreased from 44° preoperatively to 3° postoperatively.[54]

Another technique that has gained popularity for managing patellar tendon disruption is the use of synthetic mesh to aid in the reconstruction. Browne et al describe this technique by inserting a mesh graft into a tibial trough and securing with polymethylmethacrylate and a transfixion screw.[55] The mesh is then incorporated into the repair in a pants-over-vest fashion (**Fig. 59-31**). They demonstrated a postoperative extensor lag less than 10° in 9 of 13 patients at a mean follow-up of 42 months.

Postoperative management includes the use of a brace locked in extension for 6 to 8 weeks followed by gentle active flexion exercises. Active extension is allowed at approximately 10 weeks postoperatively, and in our experience, flexion slowly improves over the subsequent

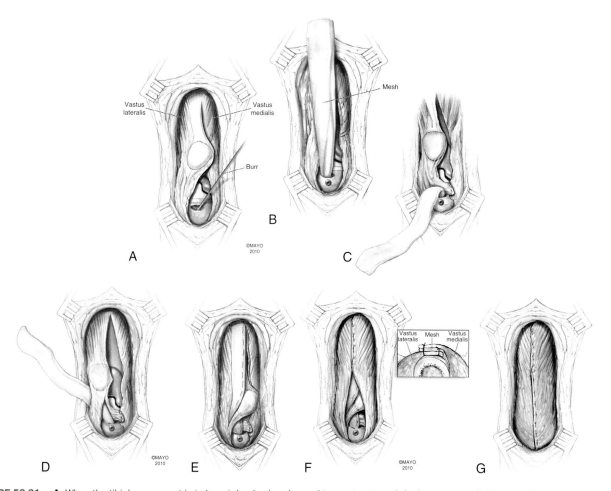

FIGURE 59-31   **A:** When the tibial component is to be retained, a burr is used to create a trough in the anteromedial aspect of the tibia to accept the mesh graft. **B:** The mesh graft is inserted into the tibial trough and secured with polymethylmethacrylate and a transfixion screw and washer. **C:** A laterally based flap of host tissue is elevated and interposed between the mesh graft and the polyethylene. This soft tissue is secured to the medial soft tissue in addition to the undersurface of the mesh. **D:** A portal is created in the lateral soft tissues to allow delivery of the graft from deep to superficial in relation to the extensor retinaculum and patella. **E:** The patella and the quadriceps tendon are mobilized and advanced to restore the appropriate patellar height. The graft is then secured with suture to the lateral retinaculum, vastus lateralis, and quadriceps tendon. Redundant mesh may be removed proximally. **F:** The vastus medialis muscle and medial retinaculum are mobilized to allow these medial soft tissues to advance in a so-called pants-over-vest manner over the mesh graft. The cross-sectional image demonstrates the envelopment of the mesh graft with the vastus lateralis (deep) and the vastus medialis (superficial) at the level of the distal part of the femur. This construct is then secured with a suture. **G:** The distal arthrotomy is closed tightly to completely cover the mesh graft with host soft tissue. (Reproduced from Browne JA, Hanssen AD. Reconstruction of patellar tendon disruption after total knee arthroplasty: results of a new technique utilizing synthetic mesh. *J Bone Joint Surg Am.* 2011;93(12):1137-1143.)

3 to 6 months. It is imperative that appropriate tibiofemoral component alignment and rotation be assessed both preoperatively and intraoperatively to prevent recurrence of extensor mechanism dysfunction, and in our experience, component revision is often necessary.

CONCLUSION

Once patellofemoral problems occur and become clinically significant, it is important to identify and address the underlying cause of the malfunctioning patella; a simple lateral release alone merely results in a transient solution. Multiple factors may contribute to patellofemoral problems in the failed total knee arthroplasty. The most common cause of patellar maltracking, however, is internal rotation of the femoral or tibial component or both. Preoperatively, CT scans can assess and quantify this malrotation. Intraoperatively, the rotation of the femoral component can be assessed using the epicondylar axis and the tibial component's rotation can be assessed using the tibial tubercle. The offending component or components must be revised.

After all of the revision components are in place, a trial reduction should be performed to assess patellofemoral tracking. This assessment should be done without towel clips in the retinaculum using the "no thumb" technique. Subsequent alterations in the components can be performed until the patella tracks properly. When these techniques are used and attention is given to detail, alignment, rotation, and position, even the most complex patellofemoral joint problem can be handled, and the patella can track well postoperatively.

REFERENCES

1. Aglietti P, Buzzi R, Bassi PB. Arthroscopic partial meniscectomy in the anterior cruciate deficient knee. *Am J Sports Med.* 1988;16(6):597-602.
2. Aglietti P, Buzzi R, Gaudenzi A. Patellofemoral functional results and complications with the posterior stabilized total condylar knee prosthesis. *J Arthroplasty.* 1988;3(1):17-25.
3. Brick GW, Scott RD. The patellofemoral component of total knee arthroplasty. *Clin Orthop Relat Res.* 1988;231:163-178.
4. Bryan RS, Rand JA. Revision total knee arthroplasty. *Clin Orthop Relat Res.* 1982;170:116-122.
5. Clayton ML, Thirupathi R. Patellar complications after total condylar arthroplasty. *Clin Orthop Relat Res.* 1982;170:152-155.
6. Doolittle KH II, Turner RH. Patellofemoral problems following total knee arthroplasty. *Orthop Rev.* 1988;17(7):696-702.
7. Insall JN, Binazzi R, Soudry M, Mestriner LA. Total knee arthroplasty. *Clin Orthop Relat Res.* 1985;192:13-22.
8. Lynch AF, Rorabeck CH, Bourne RB. Extensor mechanism complications following total knee arthroplasty. *J Arthroplasty.* 1987;2(2):135-140.
9. Webster DA, Murray DG. Complications of variable axis total knee arthroplasty. *Clin Orthop Relat Res.* 1985;193:160-167.
10. Kelly MA. Patellofemoral complications following total knee arthroplasty. *Instr Course Lect.* 2001;50:403-407.
11. Sierra RJ, Cooney WP, Pagnano MW, Trousdale RT, Rand JA. Reoperations after 3200 revision TKAs: rates, etiology, and lessons learned. *Clin Orthop Relat Res.* 2004;425:200-206.
12. Eisenhuth SA, Saleh KJ, Cui Q, Clark CR, Brown TE. Patellofemoral instability after total knee arthroplasty. *Clin Orthop Relat Res.* 2006;446:149-160.
13. WPt C, Sierra RJ, Trousdale RT, Pagnano MW. Revision total knees done for extensor problems frequently require reoperation. *Clin Orthop Relat Res.* 2005;440:117-121.
14. Martin JR, Jennings JM, Watters TS, Levy DL, McNabb DC, Dennis DA. Femoral implant design modification decreases the incidence of patellar crepitus in total knee arthroplasty. *J Arthroplasty.* 2017;32(4):1310-1313.
15. Webb JE, Yang HY, Collins JE, Losina E, Thornhill TS, Katz JN. The evolution of implant design decreases the incidence of lateral release in primary total knee arthroplasty. *J Arthroplasty.* 2017;32(5):1505-1509.
16. Hsu HC, Luo ZP, Rand JA, An KN. Influence of patellar thickness on patellar tracking and patellofemoral contact characteristics after total knee arthroplasty. *J Arthroplasty.* 1996;11(1):69-80.
17. Marmor L. Technique for patellar resurfacing in total knee arthroplasty. *Clin Orthop Relat Res.* 1988;230:166-167.
18. Oishi CS, Kaufman KR, Irby SE, Colwell CW Jr. Effects of patellar thickness on compression and shear forces in total knee arthroplasty. *Clin Orthop Relat Res.* 1996;331:283-290.
19. Booth RE Jr. *The patellar nose: an anatomic guide for patellar resurfacing.* In: *Knee Society Combined Specialty Day Meetings.* Orlando, FL: American Academy of Orthopaedic Surgeons; 2000.
20. Camp CL, Martin JR, Krych AJ, Taunton MJ, Spencer-Gardner L, Trousdale RT. Resection technique does affect resection symmetry and thickness of the patella during total knee arthroplasty: a prospective randomized trial. *J Arthroplasty.* 2015;30(12):2110-2115.
21. Alcerro JC, Rossi MD, Lavernia CJ. Primary total knee arthroplasty: how does residual patellar thickness affect patient-oriented outcomes? *J Arthroplasty.* 2017;32(12):3621-3625.
22. Insall JEM. Surgical technique and instrumentation in total knee arthroplasty. In: Insall JSW, ed. *Surgery of the Knee.* New York: Churchill Livingston; 2001:1553.
23. Merkow RL, Soudry M, Insall JN. Patellar dislocation following total knee replacement. *J Bone Joint Surg Am.* 1985;67(9):1321-1327.
24. Rand JA. The patellofemoral joint in total knee arthroplasty. *J Bone Joint Surg Am.* 1994;76(4):612-620.
25. Reuben JD, McDonald CL, Woodard PL, Hennington LJ. Effect of patella thickness on patella strain following total knee arthroplasty. *J Arthroplasty.* 1991;6(3):251-258.
26. Kaufer H. Patellar biomechanics. *Clin Orthop Relat Res.* 1979;144:51-54.
27. Wendt PP, Johnson RP. A study of quadriceps excursion, torque, and the effect of patellectomy on cadaver knees. *J Bone Joint Surg Am.* 1985;67(5):726-732.
28. Huberti HH, Hayes WC. Patellofemoral contact pressures. The influence of q-angle and tendofemoral contact. *J Bone Joint Surg Am.* 1984;66(5):715-724.
29. Briard JL, Hungerford DS. Patellofemoral instability in total knee arthroplasty. *J Arthroplasty.* 1989;(4 suppl):S87-S97.
30. Miller MC, Zhang AX, Petrella AJ, Berger RA, Rubash HE. The effect of component placement on knee kinetics after arthroplasty with an unconstrained prosthesis. *J Orthop Res.* 2001;19(4):614-620.
31. Mihalko W, Fishkin Z, Krackow K. Patellofemoral overstuff and its relationship to flexion after total knee arthroplasty. *Clin Orthop Relat Res.* 2006;449:283-287.
32. Rhoads DD, Noble PC, Reuben JD, Tullos HS. The effect of femoral component position on the kinematics of total knee arthroplasty. *Clin Orthop Relat Res.* 1993;286:122-129.
33. Yoshii I, Whiteside LA, Anouchi YS. The effect of patellar button placement and femoral component design on patellar tracking in total knee arthroplasty. *Clin Orthop Relat Res.* 1992;275:211-219.
34. Anouchi YS, Whiteside LA, Kaiser AD, Milliano MT. The effects of axial rotational alignment of the femoral component on knee stability and patellar tracking in total knee arthroplasty demonstrated on autopsy specimens. *Clin Orthop Relat Res.* 1993;287:170-177.

35. Miller MC, Berger RA, Petrella AJ, Karmas A, Rubash HE. Optimizing femoral component rotation in total knee arthroplasty. *Clin Orthop Relat Res.* 2001;392:38-45.

36. Hungerford DS, Krackow KA. Total joint arthroplasty of the knee. *Clin Orthop Relat Res.* 1985;192:23-33.

37. Berger RA, Crossett LS, Jacobs JJ, Rubash HE. Malrotation causing patellofemoral complications after total knee arthroplasty. *Clin Orthop Relat Res.* 1998;356:144-153.

38. Berger RA, Rubash HE, Seel MJ, Thompson WH, Crossett LS. Determining the rotational alignment of the femoral component in total knee arthroplasty using the epicondylar axis. *Clin Orthop Relat Res.* 1993;286:40-47.

39. Poilvache PL, Insall JN, Scuderi GR, Font-Rodriguez DE. Rotational landmarks and sizing of the distal femur in total knee arthroplasty. *Clin Orthop Relat Res.* 1996;331:35-46.

40. Whiteside LA, Arima J. The anteroposterior axis for femoral rotational alignment in valgus total knee arthroplasty. *Clin Orthop Relat Res.* 1995;321:168-172.

41. Hofmann AA, Tkach TK, Evanich CJ, Camargo MP, Zhang Y. Patellar component medialization in total knee arthroplasty. *J Arthroplasty.* 1997;12(2):155-160.

42. Anglin C, Brimacombe JM, Wilson DR, et al. Biomechanical consequences of patellar component medialization in total knee arthroplasty. *J Arthroplasty.* 2010;25(5):793-802.

43. Berger RA, Rubash HE. Rotational instability and malrotation after total knee arthroplasty. *Orthop Clin North Am.* 2001;32(4):639-647, ix.

44. Jazrawi LM, Birdzell L, Kummer FJ, Di Cesare PE. The accuracy of computed tomography for determining femoral and tibial total knee arthroplasty component rotation. *J Arthroplasty.* 2000;15(6):761-766.

45. Konigsberg B, Hess R, Hartman C, Smith L, Garvin KL. Inter- and intraobserver reliability of two-dimensional CT scan for total knee arthroplasty component malrotation. *Clin Orthop Relat Res.* 2014;472(1):212-217.

46. Amanatullah DF, Ollivier MP, Pallante GD, et al. Reproducibility and precision of CT scans to evaluate tibial component rotation. *J Arthroplasty.* 2017;32(8):2552-2555.

47. Hirschmann MT, Konala P, Amsler F, Iranpour F, Friederich NF, Cobb JP. The position and orientation of total knee replacement components: a comparison of conventional radiographs, transverse 2D-CT slices and 3D-CT reconstruction. *J Bone Joint Surg Br.* 2011;93(5):629-633.

48. De Valk EJ, Noorduyn JC, Mutsaerts EL. How to assess femoral and tibial component rotation after total knee arthroplasty with computed tomography: a systematic review. *Knee Surg Sports Traumatol Arthrosc.* 2016;24(11):3517-3528.

49. Roper GE, Bloemke AD, Roberts CC, Spangehl MJ, Clarke HD. Analysis of tibial component rotation following total knee arthroplasty using 3D high definition computed tomography. *J Arthroplasty.* 2013;28(8 suppl):106-111.

50. Cadambi A, Engh GA. Use of a semitendinosus tendon autogenous graft for rupture of the patellar ligament after total knee arthroplasty. A report of seven cases. *J Bone Joint Surg Am.* 1992;74(7):974-979.

51. Rand JA, Morrey BF, Bryan RS. Patellar tendon rupture after total knee arthroplasty. *Clin Orthop Relat Res.* 1989;244:233-238.

52. Insall J, Salvati E. Patella position in the normal knee joint. *Radiology.* 1971;101(1):101-104.

53. Jaureguito JW, Dubois CM, Smith SR, Gottlieb LJ, Finn HA. Medial gastrocnemius transposition flap for the treatment of disruption of the extensor mechanism after total knee arthroplasty. *J Bone Joint Surg Am.* 1997;79(6):866-873.

54. Crossett LS, Sinha RK, Sechriest VF, Rubash HE. Reconstruction of a ruptured patellar tendon with achilles tendon allograft following total knee arthroplasty. *J Bone Joint Surg Am.* 2002;84-a(8):1354-1361.

55. Browne JA, Hanssen AD. Reconstruction of patellar tendon disruption after total knee arthroplasty: results of a new technique utilizing synthetic mesh. *J Bone Joint Surg Am.* 2011;93(12):1137-1143.

56. Emerson RH Jr, Head WC, Malinin TI. Reconstruction of patellar tendon rupture after total knee arthroplasty with an extensor mechanism allograft. *Clin Orthop Relat Res.* 1990;260:154-161.

57. Emerson RH Jr, Head WC, Malinin TI. Extensor mechanism reconstruction with an allograft after total knee arthroplasty. *Clin Orthop Relat Res.* 1994;303:79-85.

58. Leopold SS, Greidanus N, Paprosky WG, Berger RA, Rosenberg AG. High rate of failure of allograft reconstruction of the extensor mechanism after total knee arthroplasty. *J Bone Joint Surg Am.* 1999;81(11):1574-1579.

59. Nazarian DG, Booth RE Jr. Extensor mechanism allografts in total knee arthroplasty. *Clin Orthop Relat Res.* 1999;367:123-129.

60. Sinha RK, Crossett LS, Rubash HE. Extensor mechanism disruption after total knee arthroplasty. In: Insall JN, Scott WN, eds. *Surgery of the Knee.* New York: Churchill Livingstone; 2001.

chapter 60

Persistent Effusions and Recurrent Hemarthrosis After Total Knee Arthroplasty

Stuart B. Goodman, MD, PhD, FRCSC, FACS, FBSE, FICORS | Jiri Gallo, MD, PhD

PART 1. PERSISTENT EFFUSIONS AFTER TOTAL KNEE ARTHROPLASTY

Introduction

A patient's expectation after total knee arthroplasty (TKA) is a knee that is painless and functional in terms of movement, strength, and endurance without signs of inflammation. This section will focus predominantly on patients with an early chronic effusion of unknown etiology after TKA.

Definition

A chronic effusion is defined as occurrence of a *significant amount of joint fluid in the TKA after the first 3 months postoperatively*. Conversely, a small amount of joint fluid is a normal finding after TKA. Although no data are available, we propose *that repeated aspirations for swelling of the TKA indicate that the TKA is not functioning normally and should be further investigated*. For the diagnosis of simple recurrent effusion, the aspirated joint fluid *should not be bloody (indicative of hemarthrosis)*. If the data including the appearance/content of joint fluid support the diagnosis of prosthetic-joint infection (PJI), the case is reclassified from chronic effusion to PJI. Similarly, bloody fluid requires a different diagnostic and therapeutic approach (see below).

Epidemiology

There are two peaks in the incidence of chronic effusion post TKA; the first is *early postoperatively* (usually up to 2 years). The second peak, more common occurrence, is *late* and begins between the 10th and 20th year postoperatively at which time aseptic loosening or polyethylene wear becomes a concern.

True data for "chronic effusion of unknown etiology," including the cases with effusion associated with hypersensitivity, are not known, but these are generally rare. The cumulative percent revision of primary TKA at 3 years is between 0.9% and 3.0% depending on age and gender according to the 2018 Annual Report of the Australian Orthopaedic Association National Joint Replacement Registry.[1] The incidence of early chronic effusion as a reason of revision is included in this interval. Less than 5% of all the reasons for reoperation of TKA performed between 2006 and 2015 were so-called "other reasons" (meaning other than infection, loosening, wear, fracture, femoropatellar problems, and instability), according to the Swedish Knee Arthroplasty Register Annual Report for 2017.[2] According to data from the Czech national registry of TKA, 0.85% of TKAs (period 2015-2018) were reoperated due to chronic effusion of unknown etiology as of October 18, 2018.[3]

Etiology of Persistent Effusion

An effective and individualized strategy for treatment is based on the correct diagnosis for the chronic effusion. There are multiple etiologies that can lead to a chronic effusion after TKA (**Table 60-1**). Generally, an increased amount of joint fluid in the TKA is associated with *mechanical and/or biological stimuli*. Compared to the mechanical causes, the biological etiologies have clear pathogenic mechanisms leading to overproduction of joint fluid.

Biological Reasons

First, *PJI* must be excluded as the cause of failure. With infection, the pseudosynovial cells are stimulated as part of the host complex response to microbial invasion. A significant amount of fluid can be transported into the joint cavity via alteration of the vessel network in the synovial subintima as part of septic inflammation by the mechanism of "plasma-leakage."[4] Unfortunately, even if the joint fluid is clear and standard diagnostic tests are negative, microorganisms might still be the cause of a chronic joint effusion after TKA.

The process of *aseptic loosening* can be also accompanied by persistent effusion of the TKA (see Chapter 62). Briefly, prosthetic by-products from implant surfaces due to wear or corrosion interact with cells in the pseudosynovium, triggering an inflammatory response that leads to hyperproduction of joint fluid.[5] A chronic effusion

TABLE 60-1	Classification of Chronic Effusions After TKA According to Etiology (Modified by Niki et al[23])
Type of Effusion	**Description**
Infected	The patient's knee joint fulfills the MSIS criteria for PJI based on the results of clinical, serological, joint fluid, tissue, and implant examinations.
Wear-induced	PJI has been excluded; prosthetic by-products of wear can be isolated in the joint fluid or periprosthetic tissues; the cellular/biochemical/immunological characteristics of joint fluid are consistent with particle-induced synovitis.
Associated with instability	Exclusion of the abovementioned conditions; effusion without inflammation in combination with clinical instability; aspirate is usually clear, yellow (straw yellow).
Associated with metal sensitivity	Still controversial; skin/tissue signs of late hypersensitivity are unreliable; lymphocytes predominate in the cellular profile; unpredictable behavior of stimulation tests (e.g., lymphocyte transformation test).
Rheumatic	Criteria for a particular rheumatic disease confirmed by a rheumatologist; the appearance of the joint fluid may be cloudy and depends on the activity of the disease.
Miscellaneous	There still are cases that have an effusion of unknown cause after repeated aspiration and clinical/laboratory examinations.

MSIS, Musculoskeletal Infection Society; PJI, prosthetic-joint infection; TKA, total knee arthroplasty.

after TKA may predate the clinically evident pathology by months and years, however is very rare early after surgery.

Hypersensitivity to implant metals and products of corrosion[6] is linked to the type IV (delayed) type of immune response mediated by lymphocytes. This could induce chronic inflammation associated with chronic effusion. Surprisingly, there still are relatively few conclusions available for clinical practice despite extensive research.[7]

In addition, persistent effusion after TKA can be associated with the primary disease that led to TKA surgery, such as an *increase in the activity of rheumatoid arthritis.* The pathogenic mechanism leading to effusion and joint destruction in rheumatoid arthritis is inflammation due to autoimmune synovitis.[8-10] Similarly, urate crystals or calcium pyrophosphate dihydrate crystal deposition disease can lead to increased joint fluid after TKA.[11] The aspirate is typically cloudy and opaque, and may be colored raising the possibility of PJI.[12]

Pigmented villonodular synovitis (PVNS) can occur also after primary TKA in either a localized or diffuse form. The true incidence of this association is not known as only case reports have been documented in the literature.[13] A proliferative disease of the pseudosynovium could be associated with the inflammatory host response to prosthetic by-products. However, there is a question of the border between "normal" and abnormal proliferation of the pseudosynovium, as all patients who undergo exposure to prosthesis by-products (the difference is only in the amount) exhibit morphological transformation of the pseudosynovium.

Finally, *repetitive blood leakage into TKA* can induce synovitis and chronic effusion (recurrent hemarthrosis) as is seen in hemophilic diseases.[14]

Mechanical Reasons

There is a wide range of knee instability that could be associated with pain and persistent effusion after TKA.[15]

The mechanism by which joint fluid is produced in unstable knees has not been fully elucidated at this time. It is thought to be associated with traumatization of the synovium when it is repetitively stretched during usage of an unstable TKA which may cause repetitive subclinical bleeding into the joint cavity. Also, an excessive and asymmetric wear of polyethylene associated with instability might contribute to overproduction of joint fluid.

The Tissues That Produce the Synovial Fluid After TKA

Histological studies of tissues retrieved from TKA cases describe *synovium-like tissue* (also called *pseudosynovium*) covering the inner part of the TKA capsule.[16] In a stable, functional, and nonirritated TKA, the pseudosynovial tissue is thin and discrete (**Fig. 60-1**). On the other hand, pseudosynovium can vary widely in morphology, structure, and size with instability or aseptic loosening (**Fig. 60-2**).

Surprisingly, this tissue has not been extensively analyzed, compared to what has been accomplished with total hip arthroplasty.[5,17,18] This is peculiar as the amount of joint fluid is much higher in TKA than in THA, and the tissue is easily available at the time of surgery. Thus, one must deduce the morphological and functional characteristics of the synovium after TKA from the studies of native knees. Despite that, the biological signals directing the development/homeostasis of the pseudosynovium are different compared to the native or osteoarthritic joint.

A surface layer consisting of pseudosynovial macrophage-like cells (analogous to Type A cells) and fibroblast-like cells (analogous to Type B cells) is on the inner surface of the pseudosynovium (**Fig. 60-3**). A fibrous tissue layer, whose size and structure depends on the age of the TKA, is located immediately beneath the surface layer and is analogous to the supporting sublining layer in native joint synovium. When a TKA is healthy

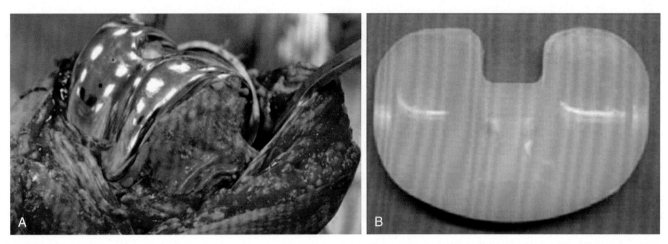

FIGURE 60-1 **A:** This shows a pseudosynovial membrane covering the distal femur around a right stable TKA 23 years after the index surgery. **B:** The polyethylene liner retrieved during the same surgery shows minor wear combined with oxidative degradation of the polyethylene surface. TKA, total knee arthroplasty.

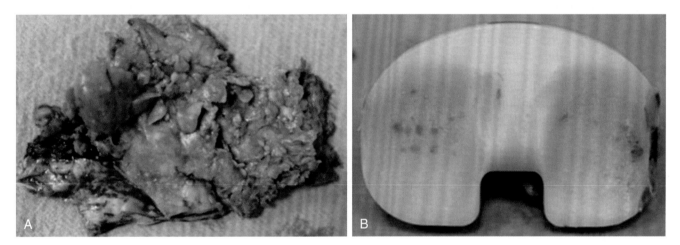

FIGURE 60-2 **A:** This shows hypertrophic changes in the pseudosynovial tissue retrieved from a left TKA with aseptic loosening 18 years after the index surgery. **B:** The polyethylene liner retrieved during the same surgery shows gross polyethylene damage combining pitting, burnishing, and delamination. TKA, total knee arthroplasty.

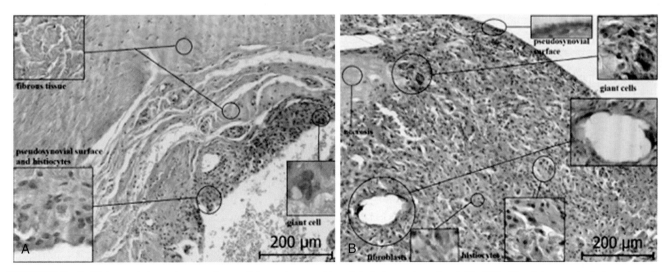

FIGURE 60-3 **A:** Histomorphology of a pseudosynovial membrane retrieved during a surgery of a stable TKA without gross polyethylene damage. **B:** Histomorphology of a pseudosynovial membrane retrieved during a surgery for aseptically loosened TKA. H & E. Scale bar: 200 μm. TKA, total knee arthroplasty.

and stable, this sublining tissue consists of a thin but relatively well-organized fibrous tissue containing fibroblasts, capillaries, and small arterioles/venules, as well as sympathetic and sensory nerves similar to the native joint. Alternatively, a hypertrophic and proliferative fibrous tissue layer with signs of degradation, including zones of necrosis, is typical for the aseptic loosening (**Fig. 60-3**).

In response to inflammatory or mechanical signals, an inflammatory macrophage population differentiates from monocytes. These are attracted to the joint by specific chemokines from the pseudosynovial circulatory network. In the case of late effusions, specific pro-inflammatory chemokines are expressed as a part of host response to prosthetic by-products (mainly wear particles).[19] Contrary, an early chronic effusion after TKA is poorly understood.

Inflammatory macrophages and other immune cells produce a broad range of pro-inflammatory substances including those stimulating surface pseudosynovial cells to excessive production of joint fluid and/or opening an influx of plasma ultrafiltrate into the joint cavity. Their local counterpart are *resident-tissue macrophages* that are able to resolve inflammation, restore tissue organization, and maintain the "healthy" native joint.[20] However, this regulatory action is insufficient and not fully understood in the case of chronic effusion after TKA.

Clinical Picture

There is no clinical picture specific for "chronic effusion" after TKA. Generally, the knee can be asymptomatic in the early stages. With an increasing amount of fluid, there are subjective symptoms like pain, pressure in the joint, and a feeling of joint fullness during function.

Diagnostic Workup

A systematic approach to diagnosis of an effusion after TKA is important. Evaluation consists of a thorough history and physical examination, laboratory tests (examination of blood, joint fluid, and pseudosynovium), and imaging. Effusions occurring very early suggest infection or instability. Late effusions are often associated with mechanical loosening, residual/late instability, or wear.

Aspiration of Joint Fluid

Aspiration is the key step for diagnosis. It should be done under strictly aseptic conditions. Generally, joint fluid aspirated from a stable and healthy TKA is not significantly different from that obtained from a native knee joint.[21] However, there can be a wide difference among the patients with TKA in terms of cellular and biochemical content.[22]

JOINT FLUID EXAMINATION

Regardless of the time after the surgery, the critical task of diagnostic workup is to *exclude infection/aseptic loosening/instability* as a cause of persistent effusion.

If infection is excluded, the following methods could contribute to the etiology of persistent effusion (**Table 60-2**). Analysis of joint fluid can distinguish between noninfective inflammatory and noninflammatory causes. One study presents a role for a *fluorescence-activated cell sorter* for phenotypic characteristics of joint fluid cells.[23] The authors were able to distinguish between aseptic/septic signals as well as to identify cases of hypersensitivity and effusions associated with an increased activity of rheumatoid arthritis.

New more precise techniques are available for detailed analysis. Flow cytometry allows simultaneous quantification of many surface proteins using fluorescently labeled antibodies. In addition, sophisticated computational techniques are needed to analyze, visualize, integrate, and interpret these datasets.[24,25] Single-cell flow and mass cytometry analysis has been developed, allowing examination of tiny amounts of joint fluid.[26] In addition, synovial fluid metabolites might help differentiate between low-grade and high-grade inflammatory joint pathologies.[27]

TABLE 60-2   List of Methods Contributing to Identification of Persistent Effusion After TKA; Methods Intended for Infection are Excluded

Method	Findings
SF cell count	Low/high cell count fluid, predominance of neutrophils/lymphocytes, account for monocytes/eosinophils/basophils
SF microscopy	Ranging from prosthetic by-products through finding of phagocytes, urate/pyrophosphate crystals to very rare findings like LE cells
Biochemical analysis	Set of biomarkers including particular metabolites could help discriminate a particular noninfectious pattern of persistent effusion (difficult interpretation to date)
Flow/mass cytometry	Very exact description of cell subtypes including their activation status (difficult interpretation to date)
Microarray	Reports transcription levels of thousands of genes in parallel (difficult interpretation to date)
Biopsy	Synovitis score, foreign body reaction, hypersensitivity, other granulomatous inflammation, pigmented villonodular synovitis
Immunological tests	Can play a role in identification of rheumatic diseases, reactive arthritis as well as hypersensitivity

LE, lupus erythematosus; SF, synovial fluid; TKA, total knee arthroplasty.

BIOPSY

Pseudosynovium can be easily and safely obtained by means of the arthroscopic techniques (there are no data supporting fine-needle biopsy in this case). Small parts of tissue are taken with the grasping forceps under direct visual control. Generally accepted rules for tissue sampling in terms of number or place are lacking. Usually, places with hypertrophic pseudosynovium are sampled. After removal, small tissue samples are put in transport containers filled with a fixation solution, usually formalin (10% mixture of water and formaldehyde). Special solutions (e.g., for RNA analysis etc.) are required for immunogenetic examination.

A number of studies evaluated the contribution of histopathological examination in distinguishing between septic and nonseptic causes of TKA failure. In addition, there are protocols proposed for the classification of synovitis[28,29] characterizing tissue samples as low- or high-grade synovitis. However, there is no study specific for interpreting biopsies from patients suffering from chronic noninfective effusion after TKA.

IMMUNOLOGICAL TESTS

A plethora of immunological tests analyzing serum/joint fluid/tissue samples have been described.[30] These may help identify differences between noninfectious causes of persistent effusion after TKA as the pathophysiology of joint effusion and its chronicity is tightly associated either with immune reaction on the stimuli from prosthetic by-products or the inability to control the immune response to prosthetic by-products. In general, the inflammatory response is coordinated by hundreds of genes, a large number of cells, cytokines and other substances. Currently there is not a single test available that could characterize a particular immune response *in toto*. Only small parts of the immune response can be detected by a particular test, and we begin to understand what benefits the results of diagnostic immunology might provide using bioinformatics. Levels of inflammatory mediators (cytokines, enzymes, eicosanoids) can be determined in blood synovial fluid samples. Particular functions of neutrophils, lymphocytes can be assessed separately as well as the type of immune response (Th1, Th2, Th17 etc.). There is also diagnostic potential in detection of basophils, eosinophils, macrophages, and other immune cells. Quantification of a particular immune population can be readily accomplished by flow cytometry that has become a standard test in the sorting of leukocyte populations/subpopulations (including their state of differentiation, activation, clonality etc.). Clinical immunophenotyping could open a new avenue for better understanding of the previously homogenous set of non-infected and/or non-rheumatologic joint fluids including those associated with an implant pathology. Importantly, diagnostic rheumatology and immunology can also help differentiate other infection-related diseases like mycobacterial arthritis, Lyme borreliosis or other reactive arthritis. A gene expression signature that occurs as a result of an altered or unaltered immunopathology including persistent production of synovial joint fluid can be determined in the future. Together, these tests should stay in hands of clinical immunologists and rheumatologists.

IMAGING STUDIES

Radiography is important in the diagnostic workup for a TKA complication. Imaging can detect loosening of the implant, gross instability, periprosthetic osteolysis as well as other implant-related pathology.

Detailed evaluation of the bone–implant interface can be assessed on *computed tomography* using metal reduction reconstruction algorithms, and dual-energy data acquisition combined with postprocessing techniques in order to reduce metal artifacts.[31] *Magnetic resonance* can identify both the periprosthetic bone defects[32] and pathology of periprosthetic soft tissues.[33] Thickening of pseudosynovium and low-to-intermediate signal intensity similar to skeletal muscle is typical of polyethylene wear–induced synovitis.[34] One large retrospective study reported that magnetic resonance imaging can distinguish between pseudosynovium induced by infection, prosthetic by-products, and other stimuli.[35] It can also be clinically useful in patients with recurrent hemarthrosis and vascular complications.

Bone scintigraphy including *FDG-PET* (fluoro-D-glucose positron emission tomography) can help identify the cause of symptomatic knee often when other methods have failed.[36,37]

Treatment

An algorithmic approach is presented (**Fig. 60-4**). If there is a suspicion that an infection could be the cause of persistent effusion, one should follow the recent guidelines for the PJI therapy. Generally, modifiable causes should be targeted via reoperation (**Table 60-3**).

Persistent Effusion of Unknown/Unmodifiable Etiology

There is lack of evidence on the approach to persistent effusion after TKA of unknown etiology. This occurs when the knee (TKA) feels stable, the bone bed is intact, function is acceptable, but the effusion reoccurs.

Considering the pathogenic mechanisms underlying chronic inflammation in periprosthetic pseudosynovium, *anti-inflammatory strategies* might be used to resolve persistent effusion after TKA. These strategies could direct the functional state of pseudosynovium macrophages and fibroblasts into M2 anti-inflammatory phenotype as well as reduce the number or activity of neutrophils.[38] In this way, anti-inflammatory, homeostatic macrophages/fibroblasts as well as resident-tissue cells could resolve the sterile inflammation without surgery. Unfortunately, the majority of these approaches have not been studied in patients after TKA (**Table 60-4**).

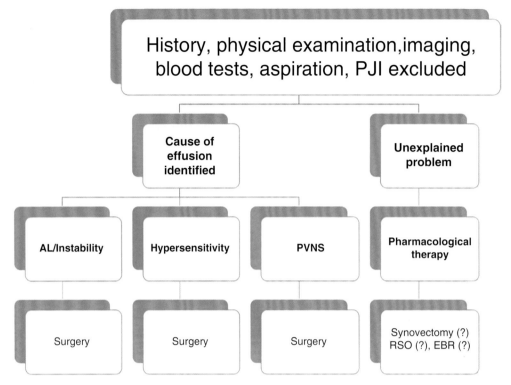

FIGURE 60-4   Algorithm for approaching persistent noninfective effusion after TKA. AL, aseptic loosening; EBR, external beam radiotherapy; PVNS, pigmented villonodular synovitis; RSO, radiosynoviorthesis; TKA, total knee arthroplasty.

PHARMACOLOGICAL INTERVENTIONS

Intra-articular injection of corticosteroids seems to be the most direct way to resolution of sterile inflammatory synovitis.[39] However, there is a concern for the efficacy as well as potential harms with this intervention. Several studies question the long-term efficacy of corticosteroid injection even in osteoarthritic synovitis.[40,41] A recent study examining the effect of corticosteroid injection into TKA[42] reported a 0.16% risk of acute infection within 3 months, or 1 infection per 625 injections. The senior author of this study limits indications for intra-articular injection of corticosteroids in patients after TKA to those undergoing manipulation under anesthesia and those with chronic serous or bloody effusions with a negative infection workup.

NSAIDs (nonsteroidal anti-inflammatory drugs) might be effective for treatment of persistent effusion after TKA. In the case of osteoarthritis, diclofenac 150 mg/day has good documentation for the relief of pain, and reduction of stiffness and disability.[43] However, one concern for long-term administration is the risk of gastrointestinal bleeding.[44] COX-2 selective NSAIDs can be offered to patients with an increased risk of gastrointestinal events or NSAIDs can be combined with gastrointestinal protective drugs. To date there is no such study available after TKA.

Recently, biological therapy has become the gold standard in many systemic autoimmune inflammatory diseases.[45] There are few studies examining the effect of

TABLE 60-3	**Approaches to Known Etiology of Persistent Effusion**
Cause	**Strategy**
Infection	One-, two-stage reimplantation[a] depending on the stage of PJI as well as pathogen and host parameters
Instability	Revision surgery correcting the instability is required
Aseptic loosening	Débridement, reimplantation of new implants
Hypersensitivity	More controversial, revision surgery consisting of débridement, partial/total synovectomy, and reimplantation of a hypoallergic implant might prove useful
Flare of rheumatic disease	Treatment of the underlying disease
PVNS	Synovectomy
Unknown etiology	Pharmacological resolution, synovectomy

[a]Chronicity of infection in this case excludes dair (débridement, antibiotics and implant retention) from the choice.
PVNS, pigmented villonodular synovitis.

TABLE 60-4   List of Methods Potentially Suitable for Resolution of Persistent Synovitis and Their Efficacy to Persistent Effusion After TKA

Method	Evidence for TKA Persistent Effusion
Injection of corticosteroids	Very low
NSAIDs	No
Methotrexate	No
Biological therapy	No
Lipid mediators	No
Radiosynovectomy	No
Low-dose external beam radiotherapy	No
Surgical synovectomy	Low

This table shows the directions for further research.
NSAIDs, nonsteroidal anti-inflammatory drugs; TKA, total knee arthroplasty.

TNF-alpha antagonists particularly on chronic synovitis in these diseases.[46] The effect of Anakinra (a recombinant human interleukin-1 receptor antagonist; IL-1Ra) on chronic knee synovitis has been reported also.[47] To date there is no such study available for knees after TKA.

Lipid mediators are a promising group of substances that direct the resolution process in the tissues/organs.[48-50] To date it is not known which of the pro-resolving molecules (lipoxins, resolvins, protectins, maresins) might be effective in the reduction of inflammatory/dysregulated pseudosynovium in a preexisting TKA. Which cells orchestrate the resolution of inflammation, and the specific molecular pathways (IL-4, 9, 10, 22, TGF-beta) and metabolic conditions are also unknown. In addition, the appropriate vehicle for an intra-articular delivery of the "resolution molecules" has yet to be developed and clinically tested in adequate trials.[51] To date there is no study available for the treatment of persistent effusion after TKA.

RADIOSYNOVECTOMY

The surface layer of pseudosynovium up to 1.0 to 1.2 mm in depth can be eradicated with beta-irradiation.[52] This treatment produces necrotizing proliferative hypertrophy of the pseudosynovium in TKA. Therefore, a persistent synovitis can be targeted by radioactive Yttrium (^{90}Y). This might be combined with surgical synovectomy in order to prevent recurrence of the disease.[53,54] One study reported promising results of lutetium-177 tin colloid in patients with knee inflammatory synovitis refractory to the conventional treatment.[55] Rhenium-188 tin colloid radiosynovectomy was also proposed for the same indication.[56] However, the overall evidence for these treatments is still insufficient and in relation to the knee with a preexisting TKA currently none exists. Contraindications to this procedure including pregnancy, breast feeding, and age under 20 years are very rare among the patients undergoing TKA.

EXTERNAL BEAM RADIOTHERAPY

Recently, a review was published summarizing the orthopedic indications for external beam radiotherapy,[57] including tumor/other proliferative processes. Several studies report the outcomes of external beam radiotherapy in patients with PVNS applied either separately or after surgery.[53,58-60] However, there are no reports of this treatment for persistent effusion after TKA. In non-TKA indications, this approach is applied on the whole circumference of the affected knee with 3000 to 4000 rad.[58] Contraindications to this therapy include absence of a definitive diagnosis, open epiphyses, infection or malignant tumor.[57,61] A risk of secondary cancer development must be communicated to the patient.[62]

SURGICAL SYNOVECTOMY

Partial synovectomy is a routine part of TKA surgeries despite the fact that no meta-analysis has demonstrated the effect of this procedure on the final clinical outcome.[63] Nevertheless, removal of the pseudosynovium during revision TKA is a useful step contributing to the overall success of the procedure.[64] Therefore, a stable TKA in patients with a negative diagnostic workup and only persistent effusion could benefit from partial synovectomy. However, there are little data on the efficacy of this procedure in this particular situation. Several studies report long-term evidence for either surgical synovectomy with or without radiosynoviorthesis in non-TKA patients.[65,66] With regard to technique, there is a concern that arthroscopic synovectomy may not ensure complete removal of hypertrophic synovium even in the hands of an experienced surgeon.[67] There may be injury to the prosthesis also. Furthermore, the surgeon cannot address instability and perform a polyethylene exchange during an arthroscopic procedure.

PVNS is particularly challenging, as it tends to recur even when the surgery is performed.[13,68] In the diffuse-type of PVNS, total synovectomy combined with restoration of TKA stability may be a successful strategy.[13] In some patients, total synovectomy may be difficult to achieve even after TKA. In these cases, a combination of synovectomy with external beam radiation might be an alternative to surgery alone. If there is a recurrence of PVNS after a surgery, external beam radiation may be an option to stop the local recurrence of PVNS.[53]

PART 2. RECURRENT HEMARTHROSIS AFTER TOTAL KNEE ARTHROPLASTY

Incidence and Causation

Minor and limited bleeding within the joint after TKA is expected. However, when a larger hemarthrosis causes excessive pain and swelling that interfere with rehabilitation, then the hemarthrosis is of greater significance and requires appropriate diagnosis and treatment. If the hemarthrosis is acute, i.e., occurs within a few hours after surgery, then direct injury to a major vessel should be considered, and immediate steps taken to reexamine the patient and obtain vascular surgery consultation as necessary (see Chapter 62). Recurrent hemarthrosis appearing weeks, months, or even years after TKA is more common than acute vascular injury; however, chronic hemarthrosis is still infrequent, with an incidence between 0.17% and 1.6% of TKA cases.[69,70] The interval between TKA and bleeding is an average of 32.2 months (range of 1 month to 10 years).[70]

These delayed bleeding events may be due to repetitive trauma to the hypertrophied synovium; residual synovial inflammation or entrapment; local proliferative diseases such as PVNS; mechanical factors including knee instability, prosthetic loosening, or impingement of the soft tissues by the prosthesis or cement; blood dyscrasias such as hemophilia, other factor deficiencies, or platelet

disorders; medications including anticoagulants and antiplatelet drugs; or systemic disease that is associated with excessive fragility of vessels, e.g., diabetes, hypertension, or atherosclerosis[69,71,72] (**Fig. 60-5**). Rarely, recurrent hemarthrosis is due to pseudoaneurysm, arteriovenous fistula, or other vascular abnormality.[69,71,73]

Clinical Diagnosis

The history and physical examination are important to the diagnosis and treatment of hemarthrosis after TKA. The history should include the timing of prior knee surgery (or surgeries), the number and frequency of hemarthroses and how they were addressed, and whether there are any predisposing local or general medical conditions. A history of

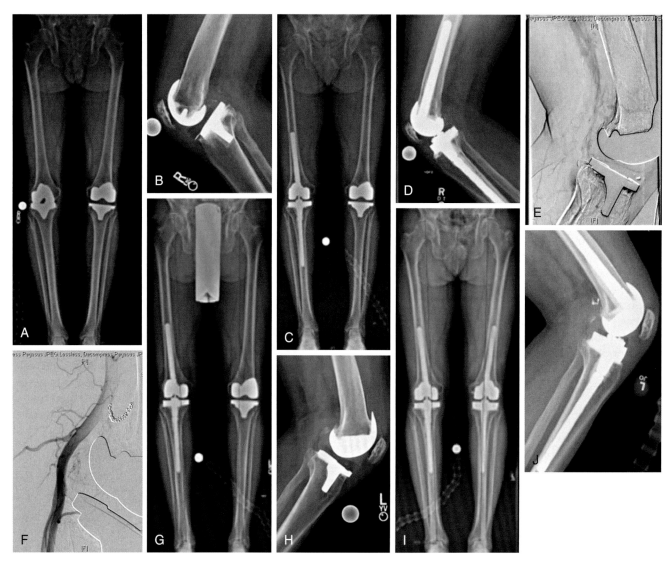

FIGURE 60-5 Bilateral TKAs with recurrent hemarthrosis. Preoperative three-foot standing (**A**) and right lateral (**B**) radiographic views show right posterior tibial subluxation, a loose migrated tibial component, and a disengaged polyethylene liner. The right knee was revised to a more constrained TKA (**C** and **D**). Several years later, the contralateral left knee began having recurrent hemarthrosis with mild flexion instability. Vascular surgery consultation with subsequent selective angiogram of the knee showed a large posterior feeding artery associated with a vascular blush (**E**), which underwent occlusion with a coil (**F**). Unfortunately, the instability progressed with continued recurrent hemarthroses (**G** and **H** taken just before the coiling procedure). The left knee was revised to a more constrained prosthesis and extensive synovectomy was performed (**I** and **J**); TKA, total knee arthroplasty.

trauma or use of anticoagulants and other medications is also relevant. The patient should be asked how the knee was functioning prior to the occurrence of the bleeding episodes, including any pain, catching, or giving way, and whether the knee felt stable or loose subjectively. Low-grade fever, redness, warmth, and swelling may occur with large hemarthroses; however, the diagnosis of acute or chronic infection should also be kept in mind. Thus, the use of antibiotics for a prolonged period postoperatively or wound healing problems after primary TKA should be inquired, as this practice could mask an ongoing, partially suppressed infection.

The physical examination should include a general assessment of the patient and entire limb including documentation of any signs of infection and inflammation. The wound should be inspected, and the extent of healing, redness, swelling, warmth, tenderness, and active movement of the knee determined. Vascular assessment of the limb should ideally include evaluation of warmth and capillary filling of the foot, palpation of foot and popliteal pulses, and if suspected, the presence of bruits around the knee, especially in the popliteal fossa. A brief neurological examination of the limb is also important.

Radiographs and Laboratory Investigations

Radiographs of the knee will help assessing whether implant loosening, malposition, or periprosthetic fracture is present, as well as the existence of any protruding or loose pieces of cement, prosthesis, or bone. Pseudoaneurysm after TKA can be identified with either ultrasound or magnetic resonance angiography.[74] A diffuse periarticular blush with tortuous or hypertrophied feeding vessels can be seen angiographically in cases with pseudosynovial hypervascularity.[70]

Bloodwork should include a complete blood count, indices of possible blood dyscrasia including prothrombin time (PT), partial thromboplastin time (PTT), and international normalized ratio (INR); erythrocyte sedimentation rate (ESR) and C reactive protein (CRP) to rule out infection; and any other test appropriate for treatment of systemic disease.

Diagnostic Joint Aspiration

Joint aspiration should be performed with strict sterile technique. The character of the aspirate should be bloody and the amount should be documented. If the aspirate is frank blood, then performing a cell count may not be as useful; in these cases, the aspirate should be sent for aerobic and anaerobic culture, especially if infection is suspected.

The Next Steps: Conservative Management Versus Advanced Imaging

When a significant hemarthrosis first occurs after the perioperative period post TKA, the knee is usually aspirated for diagnostic purposes and pain relief, and a conservative course is then undertaken.[69,75] Anticoagulants are stopped (if nonessential) for a period of time, and the limb elevated and rested. Local application of ice and a compression dressing may prove useful. Prolonged immobilization is contraindicated, as this leads to stiffness, muscle atrophy, and functional loss. After the period of conservative treatment (usually lasting several days), the knee is gently remobilized with physical therapy. This approach was effective in more than 82% (14/17) of patients with hemarthrosis after TKA in one study.[72]

If the hemarthrosis is recurrent, advanced imaging is the next step. There are two generally preferred options for this investigation: angiography of the vasculature around the knee[69-71,73,76-81] and magnetic resonance angiography (MRA).[82] Selective trans-arterial angiography is the more commonly used method (**Fig. 60-5**). This technique can be used in the acute or chronic situation and identifies aneurysms, pseudoaneurysms, arteriovenous fistulas, or more commonly, a localized synovial vascular "blush" emanating from one of the geniculate arteries. The most common discrete source of bleeding identified by angiography is from the superior lateral geniculate artery.[72,75,83] However, the most frequent angiographic abnormality observed is hypervascular synovium.[70]

The standard angiographic technique is both diagnostic and therapeutic: the localized hypervascular synovial area can be identified, and then embolized using polyvinyl alcohol or other particles, microspheres, and/or coils.[71,73,75-77,79] The particles and microspheres are usually 200 to 700 µm in diameter, large enough to interrupt the blood flow of the branches of the responsible geniculate artery.[69,73] Smaller particles/spheres can occlude the end arterioles servicing the skin, which may lead to skin necrosis.[73,77] If larger, more proximal vessels need to be occluded, coils measuring 2 to 3 mm are used. Most series reporting the results of selective transarterial angiography and embolization are small, with less than 10 patients.[69] An American series of 13 patients who received a unicompartmental or total primary or revision knee arthroplasty reported clinical success in 12 of 13 patients (92.3%) undergoing embolization.[75] Two of the 13 patients had transient cutaneous ischemia. A series from the Netherlands reported 24 embolization procedures in 14 patients, in which the first attempt was deemed technically successful in all cases.[77] However, the clinical success rate was only 50% after one procedure; four and three patients underwent second and third embolization procedures, respectively, due to recurrent hemarthrosis. The final success rate (absence of further bleeding after an average of about 2 years) was 86% (12 of 14 patients). Another American series described the outcome of 10 patients who had knee procedures (9 arthroplasty related) and subsequent hemarthrosis requiring embolization.[71] Fourteen procedures were performed; four patients required a second procedure of which only two were successful in controlling the recurrent bleeding. Two patients had minor localized skin ischemia. A larger series has recently been reported, but this series also included native knees. This Austrian series of 35 knees (18 of which were arthroplasty cases) reported a 100% success rate in identification and embolization of vascular structures, but only a 93.4% clinical success rate (two patients had recurrent episodes of bleeding).[76] Although the above studies are limited, they suggest that an initial attempt at embolization is warranted if conservative management of recurrent hemarthrosis fails. A recent systematic review reports on 91 patients with recurrent spontaneous hemarthrosis who underwent 99 embolization procedures (particulate embolics, coils, or gelfoam).[70] The angiography interventions were associated with two major and six minor complications. Recurrent hemarthrosis after the embolization procedure was observed in 11% (10/91 patients).

MRA is a less invasive diagnostic technique compared to selective transarterial angiography. MRA is first used to anatomically localize the hyperemic synovium and feeding vessel(s), which can then be selectively embolized, without performing a more extensive and invasive angiographic procedure.[82] MRA is accomplished by obtaining rapid sequential T1-weighted three-dimensional gradient-echo MRI (magnetic resonance imaging) images of the knee after an intravenous bolus of 0.2 mmol/kg gadodiamide. Using a subtraction technique in which mask images are first obtained without contrast, a three-dimensional model of the vasculature is obtained from the popliteal artery to the trifurcation below the knee. In a series of 13 cases with failed conservative (11) or surgical (synovectomy) management, 12 cases had an identifiable feeding artery to the hypervascular synovium using MRA. Seven of nine patients who underwent subsequent angiographic embolization had no recurrent bleeding. Two patients who failed embolization were treated conservatively thereafter. Four other patients who underwent MRA subsequently had synovectomy instead of embolization, with successful results. Two patients who had MRA, then synovectomy that failed to control the recurrent bleeding, had successful embolization. Thus, MRA is a minimally invasive diagnostic procedure that can serve as a guide for a less extensive angiographic procedure. Both selective transarterial angiography and MRA use contrast agents, and caution must be taken in patients who have specific allergies to these agents or have renal or liver disease. The safety profile for the above imaging techniques seems to favor MRA. Furthermore, MRA facilitates an assessment of the prosthesis interface and areas of osteolysis.[33]

Surgical and Radiographic Synovectomy

Once the diagnosis of delayed hemarthrosis after TKA has been made clinically, conservative management is first instituted, if there are no obvious indications for surgical management (e.g., instability, loosening, or malposition of the knee components). If the conservative approach is unsuccessful due to continued bleeding (**Fig. 60-6**),

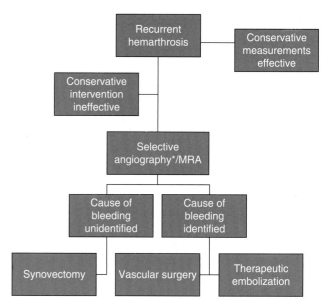

FIGURE 60-6 Algorithm for approaching recurrent hemarthrosis after TKA. Note that diagnostic angiography could be followed immediately by therapeutic embolization at some institutions. In the case of recurrent hemarthrosis, therapeutic embolization can be repeated or open surgical procedures performed. MRA, magnetic resonance angiography.

or if the hemarthrosis is recurrent, then investigation with advanced imaging, namely selective transarterial angiography or magnetic resonance angiography, is performed next. The success rate of the angiographic techniques is quite acceptable, as outlined above. In some cases, however, angiography is either unsuccessful (even when repeated), or the patient or surgeon prefer a surgical option. The latter decision may be selected, for example, when there is chronic synovial thickening and bogginess, or when the diagnosis of residual mechanical impingement is made.[84]

Although surgical synovectomy can be performed arthroscopically or in open fashion, an open approach is preferable due to a higher success rate of over 90%.[85,86] The open surgical technique facilitates a full assessment of the knee components with respect to alignment and stability; aids in the exposure of the knee to examine for loose or foreign bodies, meniscal remnants, and areas of direct soft tissue impingement; and avoids scuffing of the components by arthroscopic instruments. When an open synovectomy is performed currently, it is guided by the results of the prior angiographic study, as a definite source of hemarthrosis has not been identified during open synovectomy.[85] Electrocautery is used to perform the synovectomy, and to thermally obliterate remaining vessels within the inflamed synovium. The tourniquet should be released prior to closure of the capsule to ensure no active bleeding vessels remain. A drain should be placed in the knee joint prior to closure, and the knee mobilized so as not to avoid postoperative stiffness.

Rarely, in recalcitrant cases in which the knee does not respond to angiographic embolization or surgical synovectomy, radioactive synovectomy could lead to resolution of the recurrent hemarthrosis.[87,88] A radioisotope of yttrium has been used to ablate the inflamed synovium. Yttrium-90 penetrates up to 11 mm, with a mean penetration of 3.6 mm.[87] Contraindications to this procedure include pregnancy, breast feeding, age less than 20, and ongoing local infection. Osteonecrosis and malignancy are potential risks of this treatment but have not been reported in the scenario of TKA.

CONCLUSION

Chronic effusion is an unacceptable and frustrating complication of TKA. The diagnostic workup must exclude PJI as a cause of persistent effusion. An algorithmic approach is presented. If PJI is excluded, then surgical removal of the pseudosynovium is the first surgical treatment option. Refractory cases can be treated in combination with radiosynovectomy.

Late or recurrent hemarthrosis after TKA is a rare phenomenon. The majority of cases are due to impingement of hypertrophic and hypervascular synovium. When the diagnosis is first made, reversible and potentially modifiable risk factors (such as anticoagulation) should be acted upon. A conservative plan is instituted, and if unsuccessful, advanced imaging is undertaken, with the plan for embolization of the feeding vessels from the responsible geniculate artery. Open surgical synovectomy is performed if there is clinical failure after one or more attempts at embolization. The clinical outcomes are excellent in general, even if more advanced techniques and treatments are necessary.

REFERENCES

1. Australian Orthopaedic Association National Joint Replacement Registry. *Hip, Knee & Shoulder Arthroplasty: Annual Report 2018.*Adelaide, SA; 2018:250.
2. *S.K.A. Register, Annual Report 2017.* Sweden: Lund University; 2017:41-49.
3. CSOT. *National Joint Replacement Registry: Knee Arthroplasty.* Prague: Registers of Ministry of Health Czech Republic; 2018.
4. Finsterbusch M, Voisin MB, Beyrau M, Williams TJ, Nourshargh S. Neutrophils recruited by chemoattractants in vivo induce microvascular plasma protein leakage through secretion of TNF. *J Exp Med.* 2014;211(7):1307-1314.
5. Gallo J, Goodman SB, Konttinen YT, Wimmer MA, Holinka M. Osteolysis around total knee arthroplasty: a review of pathogenetic mechanisms. *Acta Biomater.* 2013;9(9):8046-8058.
6. Akil S, Newman JM, Shah NV, Ahmed N, Deshmukh AJ, Maheshwari AV. Metal hypersensitivity in total hip and knee arthroplasty: current concepts. *J Clin Orthop Trauma.* 2018;9(1):3-6.
7. Teo WZW, Schalock PC. Metal hypersensitivity reactions to orthopedic implants. *Dermatol Ther.* 2017;7(1):53-64.
8. Buckley CD, McGettrick HM. Leukocyte trafficking between stromal compartments: lessons from rheumatoid arthritis. *Nat Rev Rheumatol.* 2018;14(8):476-487.
9. Sohrabian A, Mathsson-Alm L, Hansson M, et al. Number of individual ACPA reactivities in synovial fluid immune complexes, but not serum anti-CCP2 levels, associate with inflammation and joint destruction in rheumatoid arthritis. *Ann Rheum Dis.* 2018;77(9):1345-1353.
10. Orr C, Vieira-Sousa E, Boyle DL, et al. Synovial tissue research: a state-of-the-art review. *Nat Rev Rheumatol.* 2017;13(8):463-475.
11. Yahia SA, Zeller V, Desplaces N, et al. Crystal-induced arthritis after arthroplasty: 7 cases. *Joint Bone Spine.* 2016;83(5):559-562.
12. Oliviero F, Scanu A, Galozzi P, et al. Prevalence of calcium pyrophosphate and monosodium urate crystals in synovial fluid of patients with previously diagnosed joint diseases. *Joint Bone Spine.* 2013;80(3):287-290.
13. Camp CL, Yuan BJ, Wood AJ, Lewallen DG. Pigmented villonodular synovitis diagnosed during revision total knee arthroplasty for flexion instability and patellar fracture. *Knee.* 2016;23(2):338-341.
14. Cooke EJ, Zhou JY, Wyseure T, et al. Vascular permeability and remodelling coincide with inflammatory and reparative processes after joint bleeding in factor VIII-deficient mice. *Thromb Haemost.* 2018;118(6):1036-1047.
15. Wilson CJ, Theodoulou A, Damarell RA, Krishnan J. Knee instability as the primary cause of failure following total knee arthroplasty (TKA): a systematic review on the patient, surgical and implant characteristics of revised TKA patients. *Knee.* 2017;24(6):1271-1281.
16. Tomankova T, Kriegova E, Fillerova R, Luzna P, Ehrmann J, Gallo J. Comparison of periprosthetic tissues in knee and hip joints: differential expression of CCL3 and DC-STAMP in total knee and hip arthroplasty and similar cytokine profiles in primary knee and hip osteoarthritis. *Osteoarthr Cartil.* 2014;22(11):1851-1860.
17. Goldring SR, Jasty M, Roelke MS, Rourke CM, Bringhurst FR, Harris WH. Formation of a synovial-like membrane at the bone-cement interface. Its role in bone resorption and implant loosening after total hip replacement. *Arthritis Rheum.* 1986;29(7):836-842.
18. Gallo J, Vaculova J, Goodman SB, Konttinen YT, Thyssen JP. Contributions of human tissue analysis to understanding the mechanisms of loosening and osteolysis in total hip replacement. *Acta Biomater.* 2014;10(6):2354-2366.
19. Dyskova T, Gallo J, Kriegova E. The role of the chemokine system in tissue response to prosthetic by-products leading to periprosthetic osteolysis and aseptic loosening. *Front Immunol.* 2017;8:1026.
20. Kurowska-Stolarska M, Alivernini S. Synovial tissue macrophages: friend or foe? *RMD Open.* 2017;3(2):e000527.
21. Chalmers PN, Walton D, Sporer SM, Levine BR. Evaluation of the role for synovial aspiration in the diagnosis of aseptic loosening after total knee arthroplasty. *J Bone Joint Surg Am.* 2015;97(19):1597-1603.
22. Galandakova A, Ulrichova J, Langova K, et al. Characteristics of synovial fluid required for optimization of lubrication fluid for biotribological experiments. *J Biomed Mater Res B Appl Biomater.* 2017;105(6):1422-1431.
23. Niki Y, Matsumoto H, Otani T, et al. Phenotypic characteristics of joint fluid cells from patients with continuous joint effusion after total knee arthroplasty. *Biomaterials.* 2006;27(8):1558-1565.
24. Hu Z, Glicksberg BS, Butte AJ. Robust prediction of clinical outcomes using cytometry data. *Bioinformatics.* 2018;35(7):1197-1203.
25. Saeys Y, Van Gassen S, Lambrecht BN. Computational flow cytometry: helping to make sense of high-dimensional immunology data. *Nat Rev Immunol.* 2016;16(7):449-462.
26. Stavrakis S, Holzner G, Choo J, deMello A. High-throughput microfluidic imaging flow cytometry. *Curr Opin Biotechnol.* 2018;55:36-43.
27. Anderson JR, Chokesuwattanaskul S, Phelan MM, et al. ^{1}H NMR metabolomics identifies underlying inflammatory pathology in osteoarthritis and rheumatoid arthritis synovial joints. *J Proteome Res.* 2018;17(11):3780-3790.
28. Krenn V, Perino G, Ruther W, et al. 15 years of the histopathological synovitis score, further development and review: a diagnostic score for rheumatology and orthopaedics. *Pathol Res Pract.* 2017;213(8):874-881.
29. Najm A, le Goff B, Venet G, et al. IMSYC immunologic synovitis score: a new score for synovial membrane characterization in inflammatory and non-inflammatory arthritis. *Joint Bone Spine.* 2018;86(1):77-81.

30. Miller LE. Autoimmunity. In: Stevens CD, Miller LE, eds. *Clinical Immunology and Serology. A Laboratory Perspective*. Philadelphia: F.A.Davis Company; 2017:233-262.
31. Khodarahmi I, Fishman EK, Fritz J. Dedicated CT and MRI techniques for the evaluation of the postoperative knee. *Semin Musculoskelet Radiol*. 2018;22(4):444-456.
32. Minoda Y, Yamamura K, Sugimoto K, Mizokawa S, Baba S, Nakamura H. Detection of bone defects around zirconium component after total knee arthroplasty. *Knee*. 2017;24(4):844-850.
33. Sneag DB, Bogner EA, Potter HG. Magnetic resonance imaging evaluation of the painful total knee arthroplasty. *Semin Musculoskelet Radiol*. 2015;19(1):40-48.
34. Fritz J, Lurie B, Potter HG. MR imaging of knee arthroplasty implants. *RadioGraphics*. 2015;35(5):1483-1501.
35. Li AE, Sneag DB, Greditzer HG IV, Johnson CC, Miller TT, Potter HG. Total knee arthroplasty: diagnostic accuracy of patterns of synovitis at MR imaging. *Radiology*. 2016;281(2):499-506.
36. Niccoli G, Mercurio D, Cortese F. Bone scan in painful knee arthroplasty: obsolete or actual examination? *Acta Biomed*. 2017;88(2-S):68-77.
37. Verberne SJ, Sonnega RJ, Temmerman OP, Raijmakers PG. What is the accuracy of nuclear imaging in the assessment of periprosthetic knee infection? *Clin Orthop Relat Res*. 2017;475(5):1395-1410.
38. Kampylafka E, d'Oliveira I, Linz C, et al, Resolution of synovitis and arrest of catabolic and anabolic bone changes in patients with psoriatic arthritis by IL-17A blockade with secukinumab: results from the prospective PSARTROS study. *Arthritis Res Ther*. 2018;20(1):153.
39. Rice DA, McNair PJ, Lewis GN, Dalbeth N. The effects of joint aspiration and intra-articular corticosteroid injection on flexion reflex excitability, quadriceps strength and pain in individuals with knee synovitis: a prospective observational study. *Arthritis Res Ther*. 2015;17:191.
40. McAlindon TE, LaValley MP, Harvey WF, et al. Effect of intra-articular triamcinolone vs saline on knee cartilage volume and pain in patients with knee osteoarthritis: a randomized clinical trial. *J Am Med Assoc*. 2017;317(19):1967-1975.
41. Juni P, Hari R, Rutjes AW, et al. Intra-articular corticosteroid for knee osteoarthritis. *Cochrane Database Syst Rev*. 2015;(10):CD005328.
42. Mills ES, Elman MB, Foran JRH. The risk of acute infection following intra-articular corticosteroid injection into a pre-existing total knee arthroplasty. *J Arthroplasty*. 2018;33(1):216-219.
43. da Costa BR, Reichenbach S, Keller N, et al. Effectiveness of non-steroidal anti-inflammatory drugs for the treatment of pain in knee and hip osteoarthritis: a network meta-analysis. *Lancet*. 2017;390(10090):e21-e33.
44. Garcia-Rayado G, Navarro M, Lanas A. NSAID induced gastrointestinal damage and designing GI-sparing NSAIDs. *Expert Rev Clin Pharmacol*. 2018;11(10):1031-1043.
45. Emery P, Pope JE, Kruger K, et al. Efficacy of monotherapy with biologics and JAK inhibitors for the treatment of rheumatoid arthritis: a systematic review. *Adv Ther*. 2018;35(10):1535-1563.
46. Mathiessen A, Conaghan PG. Synovitis in osteoarthritis: current understanding with therapeutic implications. *Arthritis Res Ther*. 2017;19(1):18.
47. Brown C, Toth A, Magnussen R. Clinical benefits of intra-articular anakinra for persistent knee effusion. *J Knee Surg*. 2011;24(1):61-65.
48. Schett G, Neurath MF. Resolution of chronic inflammatory disease: universal and tissue-specific concepts. *Nat Commun*. 2018;9(1):3261.
49. Dalli J, Serhan CN. Identification and structure elucidation of the pro-resolving mediators provides novel leads for resolution pharmacology. *Br J Pharmacol*. 2018;176(8):1024-1037.
50. Serhan CN, Levy BD. Resolvins in inflammation: emergence of the pro-resolving superfamily of mediators. *J Clin Invest*. 2018;128(7):2657-2669.
51. Barden AE, Moghaddami M, Mas E, Phillips M, Cleland LG, Mori TA. Specialised pro-resolving mediators of inflammation in inflammatory arthritis. *Prostaglandins Leukot Essent Fatty Acids*. 2016;107:24-29.
52. Kampen WU, Brenner W, Kroeger S, Sawula JA, Bohuslavizki KH, Henze E. Long-term results of radiation synovectomy: a clinical follow-up study. *Nucl Med Commun*. 2001;22(2):239-246.
53. Capellen CF, Tiling R, Klein A, et al. Lowering the recurrence rate in pigmented villonodular synovitis: a series of 120 resections. *Rheumatology*. 2018;57(8):1448-1452.
54. Shabat S, Kollender Y, Merimsky O, et al. The use of surgery and yttrium 90 in the management of extensive and diffuse pigmented villonodular synovitis of large joints. *Rheumatology*. 2002;41(10):1113-1118.
55. Jha P, Arora G, Shamim SA, et al. Lutetium-177 tin colloid radiosynovectomy in patients with inflammatory knee joint conditions intractable to prevailing therapy. *Nucl Med Commun*. 2018;39(9):803-808.
56. Shamim SA, Kumar R, Halanaik D, et al. Role of rhenium-188 tin colloid radiosynovectomy in patients with inflammatory knee joint conditions refractory to conventional therapy. *Nucl Med Commun*. 2010;31(9):814-820.
57. Gross CE, Frank RM, Hsu AR, Diaz A, Gitelis S. External beam radiation therapy for orthopaedic pathology. *J Am Acad Orthop Surg*. 2015;23(4):243-252.
58. Nassar WA, Bassiony AA, Elghazaly HA. Treatment of diffuse pigmented villonodular synovitis of the knee with combined surgical and radiosynovectomy. *HSS J*. 2009;5(1):19-23.
59. Horoschak M, Tran PT, Bachireddy P, et al. External beam radiation therapy enhances local control in pigmented villonodular synovitis. *Int J Radiat Oncol Biol Phys*. 2009;75(1):183-187.
60. Park G, Kim YS, Kim JH, et al. Low-dose external beam radiotherapy as a postoperative treatment for patients with diffuse pigmented villonodular synovitis of the knee: 4 recurrences in 23 patients followed for mean 9 years. *Acta Orthop*. 2012;83(3):256-260.
61. Ganesh V, Chan S, Raman S, et al. A review of patterns of practice and clinical guidelines in the palliative radiation treatment of uncomplicated bone metastases. *Radiother Oncol*. 2017;124(1):38-44.
62. Mazonakis M, Tzedakis A, Lyraraki E, Damilakis J. Organ-specific radiation-induced cancer risk estimates due to radiotherapy for benign pigmented villonodular synovitis. *Phys Med Biol*. 2016;61(17):6400-6412.
63. Zhao ZQ, Xu J, Wang RL, Xu LN. The efficacy of synovectomy for total knee arthroplasty: a meta-analysis. *J Orthop Surg Res*. 2018;13(1):51.
64. Abdel MP, Della Valle CJ. The surgical approach for revision total knee arthroplasty. *Bone Joint J*. 2016;98-B(1 suppl A):113-115.
65. Auregan JC, Klouche S, Bohu Y, Lefevre N, Herman S, Hardy P. Treatment of pigmented villonodular synovitis of the knee. *Arthroscopy*. 2014;30(10):1327-1341.
66. Oztemur Z, Bulut O, Korkmaz M, et al. Surgical synovectomy combined with yttrium 90 in patients with recurrent joint synovitis. *Rheumatol Int*. 2013;33(5):1321-1326.
67. Chalmers PN, Sherman SL, Raphael BS, Su EP. Rheumatoid synovectomy: does the surgical approach matter? *Clin Orthop Relat Res*. 2011;469(7):2062-2071.
68. Patel KH, Gikas PD, Pollock RC, et al. Pigmented villonodular synovitis of the knee: a retrospective analysis of 214 cases at a UK tertiary referral centre. *Knee*. 2017;24(4):808-815.
69. Saksena J, Platts AD, Dowd GS. Recurrent haemarthrosis following total knee replacement. *Knee*. 2010;17(1):7-14.
70. Kolber MK, Shukla PA, Kumar A, Zybulewski A, Markowitz T, Silberzweig JE. Endovascular management of recurrent spontaneous hemarthrosis after arthroplasty. *Cardiovasc Intervent Radiol*. 2017;40(2):216-222.
71. Guevara CJ, Lee KA, Barrack R, Darcy MD. Technically successful geniculate artery embolization does not equate clinical success for treatment of recurrent knee hemarthrosis after knee surgery. *J Vasc Interv Radiol*. 2016;27(3):383-387.

72. Yoo JH, Oh HC, Park SH, Lee S, Lee Y, Kim SH. Treatment of recurrent hemarthrosis after total knee arthroplasty. *Knee Surg Relat Res.* 2018;30(2):147-152.

73. Kalmar PI, Leithner A, Ehall R, Portugaller RH. Is embolization an effective treatment for recurrent hemorrhage after hip or knee arthroplasty? *Clin Orthop Relat Res.* 2016;474(1):267-271.

74. Daniels SP, Sneag DB, Berkowitz JL, Trost D, Endo Y. Pseudoaneurysm after total knee arthroplasty: imaging findings in 7 patients. *Skelet Radiol.* 2018;48(5):699-706.

75. Weidner ZD, Hamilton WG, Smirniotopoulos J, Bagla S. Recurrent hemarthrosis following knee arthroplasty treated with arterial embolization. *J Arthroplasty.* 2015;30(11):2004-2007.

76. Waldenberger P, Chemelli A, Hennerbichler A, et al. Transarterial embolization for the management of hemarthrosis of the knee. *Eur J Radiol.* 2012;81(10):2737-2740.

77. van Baardewijk LJ, Hoogeveen YL, van der Geest ICM, Schultze Kool LJ. Embolization of the geniculate arteries is an effective treatment of recurrent hemarthrosis following total knee arthroplasty that can be safely repeated. *J Arthroplasty.* 2018;33(4):1177-1180.e1.

78. Pham TT, Bouloudian S, Moreau PE, et al. Recurrent hemarthrosis following total knee arthroplasty. Report of a case treated with arterial embolization. *Joint Bone Spine.* 2003;70(1):58-60.

79. Ogilvie ME, Tutton SM, Neilson JC, Rilling WS, Hohenwalter EJ. Geniculate artery embolization for management of recurrent hemarthrosis: a single-center experience. *J Vasc Interv Radiol.* 2016;27(7):1097-1099.

80. Karataglis D, Marlow D, Learmonth DJ. Atraumatic haemarthrosis following total knee replacement treated with selective embolisation. *Acta Orthop Belg.* 2006;72(3):375-377.

81. Bagla S, Rholl KS, van Breda A, Sterling KM, van Breda A. Geniculate artery embolization in the management of spontaneous recurrent hemarthrosis of the knee: case series. *J Vasc Interv Radiol.* 2013;24(3):439-442.

82. Hash TW II, Maderazo AB, Haas SB, Saboeiro GR, Trost DW, Potter HG. Magnetic resonance angiography in the management of recurrent hemarthrosis after total knee arthroplasty. *J Arthroplasty.* 2011;26(8):1357-1361.e1.

83. Katsimihas M, Robinson D, Thornton M, Langkamer VG. Therapeutic embolization of the genicular arteries for recurrent hemarthrosis after total knee arthroplasty. *J Arthroplasty.* 2001;16(7):935-937.

84. Kawata M, Inui H, Taketomi S, Nakamura K, Nakagawa T, Tanaka S. Recurrent hemarthrosis after total knee arthroplasty caused by the impingement of a remnant lateral meniscus: a case report. *Knee.* 2014;21(2):617-619.

85. Kindsfater K, Scott R. Recurrent hemarthrosis after total knee arthroplasty. *J Arthroplasty.* 1995;10 suppl:S52-S55.

86. Ohdera T, Tokunaga M, Hiroshima S, Yoshimoto E, Matsuda S. Recurrent hemarthrosis after knee joint arthroplasty: etiology and treatment. *J Arthroplasty.* 2004;19(2):157-161.

87. Fine S, Klestov A. Recurrent hemarthroses after TKA treated with an intraarticular injection of yttrium-90. *Clin Orthop Relat Res.* 2016;474(3):850-853.

88. Kapetanos GA, Papavasiliou KA, Makris V, Nikolaides AP, Kirkos JM, Symeonides PP. Recurrent spontaneous hemarthrosis after total knee arthroplasty successfully treated with synoviorthesis. *J Arthroplasty.* 2008;23(6):931-933.

chapter 61

Metal Allergy and Management

Nicholas B. Frisch, MD, MBA | Joshua J. Jacobs, MD

Metal allergy is a highly controversial topic as it pertains to knee arthroplasty. There are some who even question its existence. Those that do acknowledge the existence of metal allergy as a real clinical entity also acknowledge the diagnostic challenges and lack of evidence on optimal management. Should screening for metal allergy be routine? If a patient reports a metal allergy, what is the appropriate workup? Should "hypoallergenic" implants be used in patients with suspected metal allergy? These are some of the many questions facing adult reconstructive orthopedic surgeons that will be addressed in this chapter.

INTRODUCTION

The prevalence of metal allergy in the general population has been estimated to range between 10% and 15%.[1] About 14% of the population are actually sensitive to nickel if you use patch testing as the diagnostic tool. As it pertains to total knee arthroplasty (TKA) there is controversy over whether or not clinically significant metal allergy truly exists. The literature supports the presence of allergic reactions to other commonly used medical devices. These include those used in cardiovascular surgery,[2-4] neurology,[5] plastic surgery,[6,7] and dentistry.[8-10] Implantation of other orthopedic devices have similarly demonstrated immune reactions.[11-18] Case reports exist within the arthroplasty literature to support the presence of allergic reactions as well.[19-26] With a growing body of literature around this topic, it is impossible to ignore. At a minimum, it is important to create an algorithm for addressing metal allergy in the clinical setting when the issue does arise.

ALLERGIC REACTIONS TO METAL IMPLANTS

Allergic responses to metal implants are generally thought to be type IV hypersensitivity reactions.[13,17,27-31] These are cell-mediated, delayed-type hypersensitivity reactions that occur when sensitized T lymphocytes recognize an antigen and initiate a cascade that ultimately results in the release of cytokines that perpetuate an inflammatory response. Metal debris, both particulate and ionic, are generated from metal components, typically from a combination of wear and corrosion. It is known that all metals, when placed in contact with biologic systems, will experience some degree of corrosion.[27] Released metal ions can complex with local serum proteins to activate the immune response. In addition to these type IV hypersensitivity reactions, there is also a concomitant innate immune response to implant-derived wear and corrosion debris. This involves a nonspecific reaction, which is immediate and largely macrophage driven.[31]

CLINICAL PRESENTATION

When a patient presents as a candidate for arthroplasty, it is informative to determine if the patient has a previous history of a presumed metal allergy. Most surgeons routinely ask patients if they have allergies to medications or other environmental factors, but may not specifically inquire about a history of metal allergy. Nam et al reported on 1495 patients undergoing total hip and total knee arthroplasty (THA and TKA, respectively), of whom 1.7% self-reported a history of metal allergy. When specifically asked about a history of metal allergy, this number increased to 4%. Those with a reported metal allergy were associated with decreased functional outcomes after TKA and decreased mental health scores after THA when compared with patients not reporting a metal allergy.[32] An additional, albeit potentially controversial, topic to consider is the psychological factors that may adversely impact clinical outcomes after TKA. Otero et al performed a prospective study on 446 patients undergoing THA and TKA and demonstrated that patients who report allergies have lower postoperative outcome scores.[33] Although this study did not specifically address the issue of metal allergies, this suggests that patients who report multiple allergies may be predisposed to have higher dissatisfaction after joint replacement. However, it was noted that there was a similar increase in Physical Component Summary (PCS) and Mental Component Summary (MCS), which also shows that even if they have a lower satisfaction rate, they still experience comparable improvement to patients who did not report any allergies.

Diagnosing a patient with metal allergy can be challenging and the symptoms may be vague. Typically, there will be a dermatitis (cutaneous reaction), urticaria, or vasculitis.[24,34-36] In the immediate postoperative period it should be noted that patients may develop a reaction involving the skin adjacent to the surgical incision (**Fig. 61-1**). Often these reactions represent a superficial contact dermatitis in response to the dressing adhesive or the 2-octyl cyanoacrylate adhesive.[37-39] In these cases,

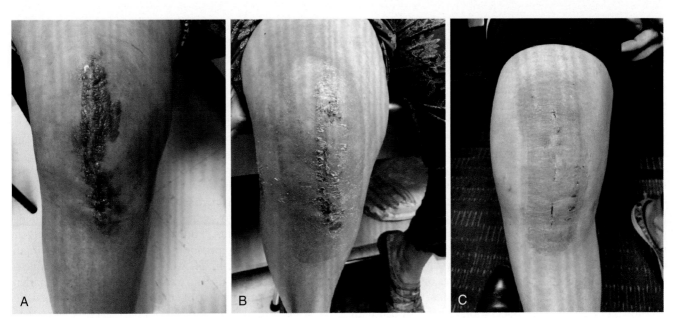

FIGURE 61-1 Cutaneous reactions to surgical dressings including: **(A)** Dermabond applied over the surgical incision at the time of closure, **(B)** hydrocolloid dressing, and **(C)** surgical mesh dressing.

removal of the offending dressing or adhesive is required as well as routine surveillance. An oral antihistamine may also be helpful. In more severe cases, referral to a dermatologist is recommended; in general, however, these will resolve over time. In some instances the use of a topical or oral corticosteroid has been advised to facilitate resolution of the skin reaction.[39]

The diagnosis of metal allergy is particularly challenging in patients with nonspecific symptoms such as pain, chronic effusion, stiffness, or loss of function. These patients require a comprehensive workup since there is a broad differential diagnosis that includes periprosthetic joint infection, aseptic component loosening, mid-flexion instability, component malalignment with patellar maltracking, complex regional pain syndrome, crystalline arthropathy, or potentially a psychological disorder.[40,41] It is essential to obtain with a detailed history and physical examination. Appropriate laboratory tests to rule out infection should be obtained including an erythrocyte sedimentation rate (ESR) and a C-reactive protein (CRP); if these tests are abnormal, an arthrocentesis should be performed for a synovial white blood cell count and differential, crystal analysis to rule out crystalline arthropathy, and culture. Cultures can be held for longer time (greater than 2 weeks) to rule out infections with fastidious organisms. Imaging studies should include with routine plain radiographs. If there is concern for component malalignment, consider advanced imaging with CT scan to properly measure component rotation. A technetium bone scan can be used to better assess potential aseptic component loosening, provided that the patient is a minimum of 1 year postoperative.

After excluding other causes of chronic pain, a specific workup for metal allergy can be considered; however, the diagnostic and predictive value of currently available testing modalities has not been established in patients with symptomatic total knee replacements. The two most commonly used tests include cutaneous patch testing and *in vitro* lymphocyte transformation testing.

PATCH TESTING

Patch testing has historically been the test of choice for diagnosing metal allergies. A common panel typically contains nickel sulfate and cobalt dichloride. Other metals can be added to these panels including molybdenum, vanadium, and palladium. The advantages of patch testing are that it can be routinely performed by dermatologists without a special facility and that it is suitable for large-scale screening allowing simultaneous evaluation of many different potential antigens substances.[34,42] The disadvantages of patch testing are multiple:

1. The interpretation of the skin reactions is subjective and qualitative.
2. The testing evaluates reactions of the skin which has specialized antigen presenting cells (Langerhans cells) which are not present in the deep tissues.[34,40] Thus, it is unclear whether skin testing reflects the propensity for a deep tissue reaction.
3. There is a subset of patients who are anergic and will not respond to anything.
4. There is a question regarding how well the challenging agent (typically a metal salt) represents the actual metal/protein antigens *in situ*.
5. There is the theoretical possibility that patch testing, particularly if repeated, may induce metal allergy.

Granchi et al performed patch testing on 20 candidates for TKA, 27 patients with well-functioning TKA, and 47 patients with loosening of TKA components to evaluate the frequency of metal allergy in patients after TKA.[43] The frequency of a positive skin reaction to metals increased significantly after TKA, regardless of implant stability. Additionally, they found a fourfold increase in TKA failure in patients who had a history of metal allergy before implantation. Bravo et al retrospectively compared 161 TKA after skin patch testing for history of metal allergy to 161 TKA patients without any prior history of metal allergy and no patch testing to determine the relationship between positive patch testing results and complications, clinical outcomes, and clinical survivorship.[44] They found no difference in complication rates between patients with positive or negative patch testing. They found no difference in postoperative Knee Society Scores or survivorship free of reoperation and revision at mean 5.3 year follow-up. They did find an association between those with a reported history of metal allergy and a negative patch test with arthrofibrosis. However, none of these patients required revision.

LYMPHOCYTE TRANSFORMATION TEST

The lymphocyte transformation test (LTT) is an alternative to skin patch testing. *In vitro* testing takes advantage of the fact lymphocytes will proliferate when exposed to an antigen that they are sensitized to. The advantage of LTT testing is that circulating lymphocytes and monocytes are assayed, thereby bypassing the skin and avoiding the confounding responses of epidermal Langerhans cells as well as obviating the potential for sensitization with serial tests. Furthermore, these results are quantitative, which can be helpful in analysis. Compared to skin testing, LTT may have higher sensitivity.[16] However, LTT testing has many of the same cons as patch testing, including the uncertainty of the applicability of challenge agents, the lack of robust clinical validation.[1,16,34,40] In addition, LTT testing may not be readily available in some clinical settings.

CLINICAL MANAGEMENT

Awareness of the potential for metal allergy has increased in the population and among surgeons. Several review articles have been published in recent years to highlight this growing concern for potential metal allergy.[1,27,45-47] Despite this increased awareness, there appears to be a limited implementation of the two available diagnostic tests. Hallock et al performed a survey of orthopedic surgeons regarding the question of metal allergy to orthopedic implants. Only 6.8% of respondents reported they always screen for metal allergy and only 4.5% often screen, compared to 50% who rarely do.[48] Similarly, Razak et al performed a survey regarding metal allergy

screening prior to joint arthroplasty and reported that 69% of respondents do not perform routine screening. Even if the patch test came back positive, 44% of surgeons would continue with standard implants.[49] While both of these surveys suffer from poor surgeon response, they demonstrate that there is no real consensus regarding the clinical significance of metal allergy and therefore there is a low propensity to perform either patch testing or the LTT.

Given the current state of the art, metal allergy is a diagnosis of exclusion. There is no agreed upon clinically validated protocol for metal allergy testing. Some have attempted to create diagnostic criteria for allergy to metallic implants,[50] but little consensus exists and the lack of large-scale prospective studies leaves many unanswered questions. In TKA candidates, it is reasonable to consider preoperative metal allergy testing if the patient has a significant history of cutaneous sensitivity to jewelry or a purported history of an allergic reaction to a previous metal implant. Such testing may guide implant selection. In postoperative patients with nonspecific symptoms such as persistent pain, swelling, dissatisfaction, or loss of function, remember to first perform a thorough diagnostic workup to rule out the most common etiologies. If there is still concern for metal allergy, particularly if there are cutaneous manifestations, metal hypersensitivity testing can be employed, but these tests are difficult to interpret and should not be used as a sole indication for revision surgery. Given the aforementioned pros and cons of patch testing and LTT, some authors advocate combining tests to improve diagnostic accuracy.[15,18] Thomas et al advocate for a combined assessment including patch testing, LTT, and periprosthetic histologic and cytokine assessment.[12] Regardless, robust clinical validation of these approaches is lacking and the patient needs to be informed of the uncertainty of the diagnosis.

If preoperative testing is positive for cobalt and/or chromium sensitivity, there are a number of materials to choose from which either do not contain these elements or minimize the release of these elements. These include titanium alloy, zirconium–niobium alloy, or other ceramicized surface components (**Fig. 61-2**). A cobalt- and chromium-free femoral component can also be used in conjunction with an all-polyethylene tibial component. This approach eliminates or minimizes exposure to metals to which the patient has demonstrated sensitivity via patch testing and/or *in vitro* testing and result in exposure to less reactive metals. If preoperative testing is positive for nickel sensitivity (found in approximately 15% of the general population), the issue is less clear. Standard cobalt-alloy implants contain <1% nickel, which is present in the bulk alloy and is not present in a bioavailable state. While one can avoid even this small amount of nickel by using titanium alloy or zirconium–niobium alloy components, some believe that standard cobalt chromium and stainless steel implants are appropriate regardless of positive metal

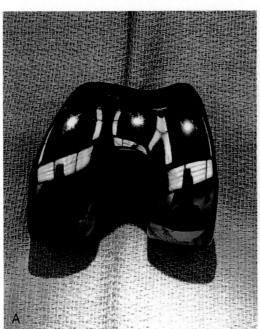 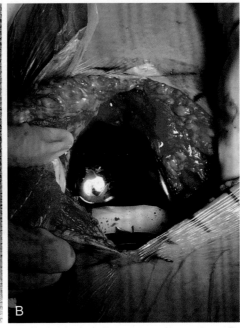

FIGURE 61-2   Alternative bearing surfaces. **A:** Oxinium femoral component. **B:** All titanium total knee implant.

allergy testing.[47,49] The assertion is that standard components use will result in more predictable results and that these implants have proven longevity in clinical practice. In addition, the use of an implant system in which the surgeon is unaccustomed could have a deleterious effect on outcomes. Furthermore, cost profiles may vary with such implants being more expensive, which remains a relevant concern for the sustainability of our healthcare system.

Munch et al reviewed the Danish Knee Arthroplasty Registry cross-referenced with a contact allergy patch test database to evaluate the association between metal allergy and revision surgery.[51] 327 patients were identified who had both primary TKA and metal allergy patch testing. They did not find an association between metal allergy and revision surgery. Interestingly they noted that those patients who underwent two or more revisions had a higher prevalence of metal allergy, which they attributed to increased release of metal from wear and corrosion. There is no large study available to demonstrate that using "hypoallergenic implants" improves long-term outcomes. Ultimately it is at the discretion of the surgeon and the patients as they engage in a shared decision-making process.

In our practice, standard cobalt-alloy bearings are avoided when possible in patients with suspected sensitivity to Co, Cr, and/or Ni. Although no large study demonstrates superiority of "hypoallergenic implants" in comparison to cobalt-alloy femoral components, there are several smaller studies that suggest good results.[23,52] Innocenti et al reported on 24 patients with suspected metal allergy treated with Oxinium (oxygen diffusion-hardened zirconium–niobium alloy) femoral components and all-poly tibial components.[52] They performed detailed medical histories, patch testing, and lab assays,

ultimately showing 20.8% of patients were considered to have metal allergy. At mean follow-up of 79.2 months, no patients reported any allergic reactions and there were no reported implant failures or patient-reported anterior knee pain. Furthermore, experience with revision surgery in both THA and TKA for presumed or documented metal allergy with noncobalt alloy bearings has resulted in improved outcomes.[21,22,53]

Since there are only anecdotal case reports or small case series supporting revision surgery for metal allergy, revision surgery should only be considered a last resort for the persistently symptomatic patient with no evidence of loosening, infection, malrotation, instability, or chronic regional pain syndrome who has failed other nonoperative interventions. The informed consent process needs to convey that the outcome of such revisions is unpredictable. Trials of antihistamines and corticosteroids for skin reactions should be considered first. Revision surgery can be very challenging especially with well-fixed components; bone loss carries with it additional postoperative risks. Furthermore, the use of noncobalt alloy components does not address the issue of the debris shed from the stainless steel surgical tools which contain approximately 10% to 14% nickel. Currently, non–stainless steel surgical tools are not readily available and the use of stainless steel instrumentation certainly exposes tissue to metal debris generated during bone preparation and implantation (**Fig. 61-3**).

In summary, metal hypersensitivity to orthopedic implants remains a challenging and poorly understood clinical entity. The true prevalence is unknown, but clinically significant symptomatology is very rare in total knee replacements. Clinical presentation typically involves a cutaneous reaction; the presence of nonspecific

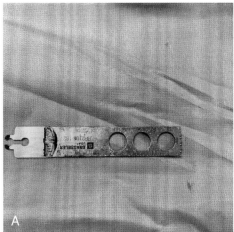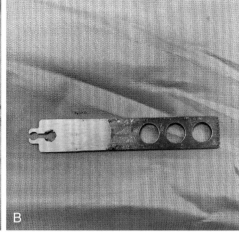

FIGURE 61-3 Stainless steel saw blade demonstrating routine wear after total knee arthroplasty on the **(A)** front and **(B)** back of the blade.

symptoms such as pain and swelling is not helpful in the differential diagnosis. Current diagnostic methods have not been clinically validated, so in isolation they should be used with caution. Initially, conservative management is indicated. In rare cases implant removal and replacement with a hypoallergenic implant may be undertaken, but should be considered a last resort with unpredictable outcomes. Finally, preoperative testing prior to a primary knee arthroplasty may be indicated when there is a patient-reported history of intolerance to jewelry or of a previous reaction to a metal implant to help guide implant selection. However, routine lab screening is not currently supported by the literature and is not recommended.

REFERENCES

1. Lachiewicz PF, Watters TS, Jacobs JJ. Metal hypersensitivity and total knee arthroplasty. *J Am Acad Orthop Surg.* 2016;24(2):106-112.
2. Kataoka Y, Kapadia SR, Puri R, et al. Suspected hypersensitivity reaction following drug-eluting stent implantation. Novel insights with optical coherence tomography. *JACC: Cardiovasc Interv.* 2012;5(7):e21-e23.
3. Nakajima Y, Itoh T, Morino Y. Metal allergy to everolimus-eluting cobalt chromium stents confirmed by positive skin testing as a cause of recurrent multivessel in-stent restenosis. *Catheter Cardiovasc Interv.* 2016;87(4):E137-E142.
4. D'Arrigo G, Giaquinta A, Virgilio C, Davi A, Pierfrancesco V, Veroux M. Nickel allergy in a patient with a nitinol stent in the superficial femoral artery. *J Vasc Interv Radiol.* 2014;25(8):1304-1306.
5. Lobotesis K, Mahady K, Ganesalingam J, et al. Coiling-associated delayed cerebral hypersensitivity: is nickel the link? *Neurology.* 2015;84(1):97-99.
6. Alijotas-Reig J, Garcia-Gimenez V. Delayed immune-mediated adverse effects related to hyaluronic acid and acrylic hydrogel dermal fillers: clinical findings, long-term follow-up and review of the literature. *J Eur Acad Dermatol Venereol.* 2008;22(2):150-161.
7. Cantisani C, Cigna E, Grieco T, et al. Allergic contact dermatitis to synthetic rubber following breast augmentation. *Eur Ann Allergy Clin Immunol.* 2007;39(6):185-188.
8. Hosoki M, Nishigawa K, Miyamoto Y, Ohe G, Matsuka Y. Allergic contact dermatitis caused by titanium screws and dental implants. *J Prosthodont Res.* 2016;60(3):213-219.

9. Pigatto PD, Brambilla L, Ferrucci S, Zerboni R, Somalvico F, Guzzi G. Systemic allergic contact dermatitis associated with allergy to intraoral metals. *Dermatol Online J.* 2014;20(10).
10. Chow M, Botto N, Maibach H. Allergic contact dermatitis caused by palladium-containing dental implants. *Dermatitis.* 2014;25(5): 273-274.
11. Merritt K, Rodrigo JJ. Immune response to synthetic materials. Sensitization of patients receiving orthopaedic implants. *Clin Orthop Relat Res.* 1996;326:71-79.
12. Thomas P, von der Helm C, Schopf C, et al. Patients with intolerance reactions to total knee replacement: combined assessment of allergy diagnostics, periprosthetic histology, and peri-implant cytokine expression pattern. *BioMed Res Int.* 2015; 2015:910156.
13. Hallab NJ, Caicedo M, Finnegan A, Jacobs JJ. Th1 type lymphocyte reactivity to metals in patients with total hip arthroplasty. *J Orthop Surg Res.* 2008;3:6.
14. Lalor PA, Revell PA, Gray AB, Wright S, Railton GT, Freeman MA. Sensitivity to titanium. A cause of implant failure? *J Bone Joint Surg Br.* 1991;73(1):25-28.
15. Vermes C, Kuzsner J, Bardos T, Than P. Prospective analysis of human leukocyte functional tests reveals metal sensitivity in patients with hip implant. *J Orthop Surg Res.* 2013;8:12.
16. Hallab NJ, Anderson S, Stafford T, Glant T, Jacobs JJ. Lymphocyte responses in patients with total hip arthroplasty. *J Orthop Res.* 2005;23(2):384-391.
17. Hallab NJ, Caicedo M, Epstein R, McAllister K, Jacobs JJ. In vitro reactivity to implant metals demonstrates a person-dependent association with both T-cell and B-cell activation. *J Biomed Mater Res A.* 2010;92(2):667-682.
18. Frigerio E, Pigatto PD, Guzzi G, Altomare G. Metal sensitivity in patients with orthopaedic implants: a prospective study. *Contact Dermatitis.* 2011;64(5):273-279.
19. Earll MD, Earll PG, Rougeux RS. Wound drainage after metal-on-metal hip arthroplasty secondary to presumed delayed hypersensitivity reaction. *J Arthroplasty.* 2011;26(2):338.e5-338.e7.
20. Biant LC, Bruce WJ, van der Wall H, Walsh WR. Infection or allergy in the painful metal-on-metal total hip arthroplasty? *J Arthroplasty.* 2010;25(2):334.e11-334.e16.
21. Kosukegawa I, Nagoya S, Kaya M, Sasaki K, Sasaki M, Yamashita T. Revision total hip arthroplasty due to pain from hypersensitivity to cobalt-chromium in total hip arthroplasty. *J Arthroplasty.* 2011;26(6):978.e1-3.
22. Perumal V, Alkire M, Swank ML. Unusual presentation of cobalt hypersensitivity in a patient with a metal-on-metal bearing in total hip arthroplasty. *Am J Orthop.* 2010;39(5):E39-E41.

23. Bergschmidt P, Bader R, Mittelmeier W. Metal hypersensitivity in total knee arthroplasty: revision surgery using a ceramic femoral component. A case report. *Knee*. 2012;19(2):144-147.

24. Verma SB, Mody B, Gawkrodger DJ. Dermatitis on the knee following knee replacement: a minority of cases show contact allergy to chromate, cobalt or nickel but a causal association is unproven. *Contact Dermatitis*. 2006;54(4):228-229.

25. Handa S, Dogra S, Prasad R. Metal sensitivity in a patient with a total knee replacement. *Contact Dermatitis*. 2003;49(5):259-260.

26. Peat F, Coomber R, Rana A, Vince A. Vanadium allergy following total knee arthroplasty. *BMJ Case Rep*. 2018;2018:1-4.

27. Hallab N, Merritt K, Jacobs JJ. Metal sensitivity in patients with orthopaedic implants. *J Bone Joint Surg Am*. 2001;83(3):428-436.

28. Hallab N, Jacobs JJ, Black J. Hypersensitivity to metallic biomaterials: a review of leukocyte migration inhibition assays. *Biomaterials*. 2000;21(13):1301-1314.

29. Hallab NJ, Jacobs JJ. Biologic effects of implant debris. *Bull NYU Hosp Jt Dis*. 2009;67(2):182-188.

30. Willert HG, Buchhorn GH, Fayyazi A, et al. Metal-on-metal bearings and hypersensitivity in patients with artificial hip joints. A clinical and histomorphological study. *J Bone Joint Surg Am*. 2005;87(1):28-36.

31. Athanasou NA. The pathobiology and pathology of aseptic implant failure. *Bone Joint Res*. 2016;5(5):162-168.

32. Nam D, Li K, Riegler V, Barrack RL. Patient-reported metal allergy: a risk factor for poor outcomes after total joint arthroplasty? *J Arthroplasty*. 2016;31(9):1910-1915.

33. Otero JE, Graves CM, Gao Y, et al. Patient-reported allergies predict worse outcomes after hip and knee arthroplasty: results from a prospective cohort study. *J Arthroplasty*. 2016;31(12):2746-2749.

34. Mitchelson AJ, Wilson CJ, Mihalko WM, et al. Biomaterial hypersensitivity: is it real? Supportive evidence and approach considerations for metal allergic patients following total knee arthroplasty. *BioMed Res Int*. 2015;2015:137287.

35. Rostoker G, Robin J, Binet O, et al. Dermatitis due to orthopaedic implants. A review of the literature and report of three cases. *J Bone Joint Surg Am*. 1987;69(9):1408-1412.

36. Teo WZ, Schalock PC. Metal hypersensitivity reactions to orthopedic implants. *Dermatol Ther*. 2016;7(1):53-64.

37. Knackstedt RW, Dixon JA, O'Neill PJ, Herrera FA. Rash with DERMABOND PRINEO Skin Closure System use in bilateral reduction mammoplasty: a case series. *Case Rep Med*. 2015;2015:642595.

38. Chalmers BP, Melugin HP, Sculco PK, et al. Characterizing the diagnosis and treatment of allergic contact dermatitis to 2-octyl cyanoacrylate used for skin closure in elective orthopedic surgery. *J Arthroplasty*. 2017;32(12):3742-3747.

39. Chan FJ, Richardson K, Kim SJ. Allergic dermatitis after total knee arthroplasty using the Prineo wound-closure device: a report of three cases. *JBJS Case Connect*. 2017;7(2):e39.

40. WMMihalko, SBGoodman, MAmini, NHallab. Metal Sensitivity Testing and Associated Total Joint Outcomes. Paper presented at: American Academy of Orthopaedic Surgeons Annual Meeting; 2013; Chicago, IL.

41. Park CN, White PB, Meftah M, Ranawat AS, Ranawat CS. Diagnostic algorithm for residual pain after total knee arthroplasty. *Orthopedics*. 2016;39(2):e246-e252.

42. Granchi D, Cenni E, Trisolino G, Giunti A, Baldini N. Sensitivity to implant materials in patients undergoing total hip replacement. *J Biomed Mater Res B*. 2006;77(2):257-264.

43. Granchi D, Cenni E, Tigani D, Trisolino G, Baldini N, Giunti A. Sensitivity to implant materials in patients with total knee arthroplasties. *Biomaterials*. 2008;29(10):1494-1500.

44. Bravo D, Wagner ER, Larson DR, Davis MP, Pagnano MW, Sierra RJ. No increased risk of knee arthroplasty failure in patients with positive skin patch testing for metal hypersensitivity: a matched cohort study. *J Arthroplasty*. 2016;31(8):1717-1721.

45. Akil S, Newman JM, Shah NV, Ahmed N, Deshmukh AJ, Maheshwari AV. Metal hypersensitivity in total hip and knee arthroplasty: current concepts. *J Clin Orthop Trauma*. 2018;9(1):3-6.

46. Faschingbauer M, Renner L, Boettner F. Allergy in total knee replacement. Does it exist? *HSS J*. 2017;13(1):12-19.

47. Middleton S, Toms A. Allergy in total knee arthroplasty: a review of the facts. *Bone Joint J*. 2016;98-B(4):437-441.

48. Hallock K, Vaughn NH, Juliano P, Marks JG Jr. Metal hypersensitivity and orthopedic implants: survey of orthopedic surgeons. *Dermatitis*. 2017;28(1):76-80.

49. Razak A, Ebinesan AD, Charalambous CP. Metal allergy screening prior to joint arthroplasty and its influence on implant choice: a Delphi consensus study amongst orthopaedic arthroplasty surgeons. *Knee Surg Relat Res*. 2013;25(4):186-193.

50. Schalock PC, Thyssen JP. Patch testers' opinions regarding diagnostic criteria for metal hypersensitivity reactions to metallic implants. *Dermatitis*. 2013;24(4):183-185.

51. Munch HJ, Jacobsen SS, Olesen JT, et al. The association between metal allergy, total knee arthroplasty, and revision: study based on the Danish Knee Arthroplasty Register. *Acta Orthop*. 2015;86(3):378-383.

52. Innocenti M, Carulli C, Matassi F, Carossino AM, Brandi ML, Civinini R. Total knee arthroplasty in patients with hypersensitivity to metals. *Int Orthop*. 2014;38(2):329-333.

53. Gupta R, Phan D, Schwarzkopf R. Total knee arthroplasty failure induced by metal hypersensitivity. *Am J Case Rep*. 2015;16:542-547.

Revision Total Knee Arthroplasty

ROBERT L. BARRACK

SECTION **9**

chapter 62

Evaluation of the Symptomatic Total Knee Replacement

David C. Ayers, MD | Matthew E. Deren, MD

Total knee replacement (TKR) is a reliable surgical procedure that provides predictable pain relief and restoration of knee function for the vast majority of patients. A minority of patients have persistent symptoms after surgery or develop new postoperative symptoms. A comprehensive history and thorough physical examination are crucial to accurately diagnose the cause of a patient's symptoms.[1] Often, it is helpful to examine the patient on more than one occasion to ensure consistency in the history and physical findings. Some patients have symptoms severe enough to define the knee replacement as a failure. Radiographs are a routine part of the evaluation of a failed TKR.[2] Selective use of diagnostic tests supplements the information gathered from the history, physical examination, and routine radiographs and typically allows for an accurate diagnosis in patients with a symptomatic TKR.[1] A specific diagnosis and treatment plan are mandatory before undertaking any additional surgical procedure.[1,3]

HISTORY

A comprehensive history is crucial when evaluating patients with complaints after TKR. All problems that preceded the knee replacement should be documented, including antecedent operations, date of the index TKR, and any perioperative problems or delays in recovery or rehabilitation. Persistent swelling or drainage after the knee replacement raises the index of suspicion for infection.[4] It is important to determine whether primary wound healing occurred and whether the patient had an initial period of pain relief after the TKR surgery. It is helpful to determine whether the patient's presenting symptoms are the same as the symptoms before the TKR. If the patient's current symptoms are identical to the preoperative symptoms, the original diagnosis of the knee being the cause of the patient's pain must be carefully reevaluated. Medical comorbidities should be determined, including the presence of diabetes mellitus, a neurologic or vascular disease, a septic focus, and an immunocompromised state.

One must initially establish the exact nature of the patient's complaint. Although pain is typically given as the chief complaint, specific questioning may reveal that the problem is actually weakness, giving way, or swelling. Giving way may be a sign of ligamentous instability, patellofemoral instability, component malalignment, or muscle weakness or inhibition. Weakness may be a result of spinal stenosis or muscle atrophy. After pain has been established as the principal problem, the exact location of the pain should be sought and localized as precisely as possible. Radicular pain may arise from lumbar spine disease. Medial knee pain may result from hip disease. Pain in the thigh or calf can be of vascular or neurologic origin. Pain that is well localized to the anterior portion of the knee is often of patellofemoral origin. Posterior knee pain may be related to a popliteal cyst, deep venous thrombosis, or pseudoaneurysm. Pain that is consistently localized to a small area may result from a neuroma[5] or chronic bursitis. Typically the pain is described as related to the knee joint in the region of the medial and lateral joint lines.

Factors that aggravate or alleviate the pain should be sought. Pain associated with weight-bearing activities may indicate mechanical loosening. Pain that is constant, that is unrelated to activity, and that occurs at night may be related to infection. Start-up pain that worsens with the first few steps is typical of loosening and may represent inadequate ingrowth of a cementless prosthesis or early loosening of a cemented prosthesis. Pain associated with inadequate ingrowth of a cementless prosthesis is often present within the first year, whereas pain associated with loosening of a well-aligned noninfected cemented prosthesis occurs much later.[6]

The patient should be questioned regarding functional activities. The distance or time a patient reports being able to walk should be recorded, along with the use of ambulatory devices. It is helpful to ask about the patient's ability to ascend and descend stairs and to know which leg is used to go up or down first. The ability of the patient to arise from a chair and symptoms typical of instability during walking are important to question the patient about.

The patient should be queried regarding his or her expectations after knee replacement. The patient's problems preoperatively should be compared with his or her anticipated results and current symptoms and function. The patient's employment history should be recorded and taken into consideration. Patients receiving workers' compensation benefits have been reported to have less predictable results after TKR. Any ongoing or pending legal action regarding the patient's knee condition should be questioned and recorded. Underlying depression or psychiatric disease should be evaluated. Current or previous treatment with antidepressants or other neuropsychiatric medications should be recorded. Patients with a preoperative mental composite score of less than 50 on the Short Form-36 Questionnaire are at increased risk for less improvement in their physical function score after TKR.

PHYSICAL EXAMINATION

A thorough physical examination of the patient with pain after TKR should not be limited to the knee, as knee pain can be associated with lumbar spine, hip, or retroperitoneal pathology. Therefore, examination of the spine, hip, and abdomen is necessary in addition to the knee. It is useful to begin with the examination of the extrinsic causes of knee pain. Careful examination of the lumbar spine is particularly important if there is any radicular component to the patient's pain. Examination of the hip is mandatory and should include range of motion and whether motion of the hip reproduces pain in the knee. Gait abnormalities, limb length inequality, hip girdle weakness, or fixed deformity of the hip should be sought. If range of motion of the hip is limited or other aspects of the hip examination are abnormal, radiographic examination of the hip is required. In some instances, injection of local anesthetic into the hip and determining whether this alleviates the patient's knee pain can be helpful. Examination of the patient's feet should include evaluation for evidence of peripheral neuropathy. Hypersensitivity of the limb associated with cool, shiny skin may indicate reflex sympathetic dystrophy. Absence of ankle deep tendon reflexes may indicate lumbar spine disease. Absent pulses may indicate peripheral vascular disease and often warrant noninvasive arterial duplex scanning. Finally, be sure to examine the foot and ankle alignment, as hindfoot or forefoot deformities can place increased stresses on the knee.

Examination of the knee joint often begins while observing the patient's walk with and without supportive aids. Varus or valgus alignment of the knee may indicate ligamentous instability, component loosening or subsidence, or component malpositioning. Patients with hyperextension when weight-bearing may have posterior cruciate insufficiency or excessive wear of the posterior aspect of the polyethylene insert. The knee should be evaluated for erythema, edema, or an intra-articular effusion. Point tenderness to palpation at the joint line may be indicative of impingement of an underlying prominence such as an unresected osteophyte, a cementophyte, or an overhanging implant. Point tenderness and inflammation about the medial aspect of the tibia are often indicative of pes anserine bursitis. Point tenderness away from the joint line, with a positive Tinel sign and elimination of the point tenderness by a local injection indicates a neuroma.[5]

Active and passive range of motion of the knee replacement should be recorded. The maximum flexion and extension should be compared with preoperative values measured before the index knee replacement. The presence of crepitus with motion should be noted. The knee should be examined for a fixed flexion contracture or an extensor lag. An audible pop that occurs as the knee moves from flexion into extension is termed *patellar clunk syndrome* and results from a soft-tissue nodule at the superior pole of the patella.[7] The audible pop results from the soft-tissue nodule popping into the trochlear groove.[7]

Knee stability is determined by static ligament testing. A TKR typically approximates the stability of a normal knee with mild anterior cruciate instability.[8] Ligament competence in full extension and at 30° and 90° of flexion should be evaluated. Laxity to stress testing is typically recorded as 1+, 2+, and 3+, with notation of whether there is a firm end point. Sagittal plane laxity (anterior and posterior translation of the tibia on the femur to stress) should also be evaluated. Pseudolaxity is created by component collapse and should not be confused with ligament insufficiency.

In patients with symptoms after TKR, a detailed examination of the patellofemoral joint is important because patellofemoral pathology is the most common cause of additional surgery after TKR.[9] Determine the competence of the extensor mechanism by evaluating the strength of knee extension and the presence of an extensor lag. Patellar tracking should be observed during passive motion and active motion. The presence of patellar tilting, crepitus, or clunking should be sought. Patellar mobility should be assessed in full extension and slight flexion. A positive apprehension sign is indicative of patellar instability, whereas decreased patellar mobility may be associated with patella baja or fibrosis and scar formation. The medial and lateral aspects of the patella should be palpated for patellar tenderness. Rotational abnormal alignment of the femoral or tibial components may be difficult to observe during examination of the knee.[10] If present, malrotation of the components may be manifested by patellofemoral instability.

RADIOGRAPHIC EXAMINATION

A complete radiographic evaluation is necessary to assess a painful TKR. The patient's preoperative radiographs may be helpful as TKR for early-stage osteoarthritis is a known risk factor for continued pain and lower satisfaction following arthroplasty.[11] Initial postoperative radiographs should be reviewed for radiolucent lines at the bone–cement interface or the implant–bone interface. A careful review of sequential radiographs is an important part of evaluating a symptomatic TKR. Radiolucent lines are a common finding after cemented TKR.[12] Radiolucent lines that are noncircumferential and observed over only

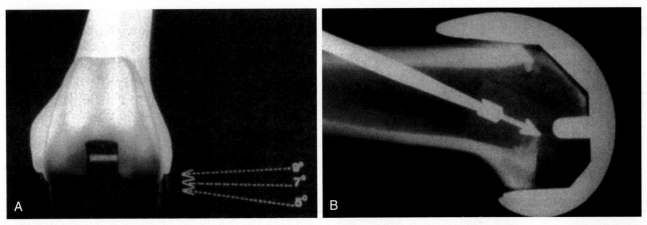

FIGURE 62-1   A: Distal fluoroscopic examination must consider the angle of the distal femoral cut. The X-ray beam must be angled accordingly to evaluate the distal femoral interface. **B:** A lateral fluoroscopic view of the distal femoral interface. The arrow indicates the radiolucency between the distal femur and the implant. (From Fehring TK, McAvoy GM. Fluoroscopic evaluation of the painful total knee arthroplasty. *Clin Orthop Relat Res.* 1996;331:226-233, with permission.)

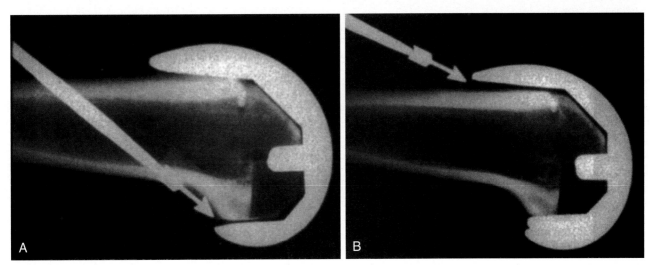

FIGURE 62-2   A: Lateral fluoroscopic view of the posterior condylar interface. The arrow indicates the radiolucency between the posterior runner and the posterior condyle. **B:** A lateral fluoroscopic view of the anterior femoral interface. The arrow indicates the radiolucency between the implant and the anterior femur. (From Fehring TK, McAvoy GM. Fluoroscopic evaluation of the painful total knee arthroplasty. *Clin Orthop Relat Res.* 1996;331:226-233, with permission.)

a minority of the interface are not diagnostic of loosening.[12] Radiographic evidence of loosening is defined as a radiolucency that is progressive in serial X-rays or circumferential and larger than 2 mm at either the cement–prosthesis or bone–cement interface. Component subsidence or change in position is diagnostic of implant loosening. A radiolucent line that is present at only a portion of the interface (especially in zones I and IV of the tibial component), is less than 1 mm in width, and is not progressive on serial radiographs does not indicate loosening of the prosthesis and is most likely not the etiology of the patient's pain. A radiolucency that has developed and progressed over a short period has an entirely different meaning than one that was present on the immediate postoperative X-ray and has not progressed.

Routine radiographic examination should include a minimum of three views: a coronal anteroposterior (AP) view obtained with the patient bearing weight on the limb, a lateral view taken with the knee flexed approximately 30°, and a patellar axial view with the knee flexed between 30° and 45°. The femoral interface is examined best in the lateral view, whereas both the AP and lateral views can be helpful when examining the tibial interface. Many believe that the bone–implant interface is more difficult to assess in cementless TKRs. Fluoroscopic examinations can be quite helpful to ensure optimal visualization of the interface by placing the X-ray beam tangential to the interface being examined (**Fig. 62-1**).[13] The location of the X-ray beam differs in the lateral plane when examining the femoral interface and the tibial interface.[14] Some authors have advocated using fluoroscopy to realign the X-ray beam when examining the interface at the anterior femoral flange and the posterior condyles interface (**Fig. 62-2**).[13] Fluoroscopic

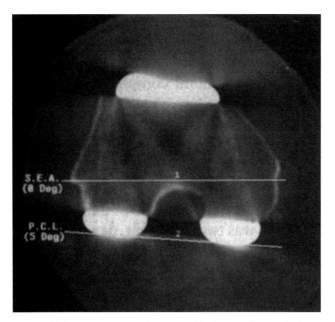

FIGURE 62-3 Axial computed tomographic image of the right femur through the epicondylar axis. The surgical epicondylar axis (SEA) connects the lateral epicondylar prominence and the medial sulcus of the medial epicondyle. The posterior condylar line (PCL) connects the medial and lateral prosthetic posterior condylar surfaces. Deg, degrees. (From Berger RA, Crossett LS, Jacobs JJ, et al. Malrotation causing patellofemoral complications after total knee arthroplasty. *Clin Orthop Relat Res*. 1998;356:144-153, with permission.)

examination is also helpful to examine the tibial bone interface in the AP plane.

Alignment of the limb and each individual component should be radiographically determined and may be best evaluated on long-leg, standing hip-knee-ankle radiographs. These may be particularly helpful if malalignment of the components is suspected in the coronal plane. The femoral component should ideally be aligned 90° to the mechanical axis of the limb. The tibial component should be oriented at 90° to the anatomic axis of the tibia. The anterior flange of the femoral component on the lateral radiograph should be parallel to the anterior cortex of the femur. The orientation of the tibial component on the lateral view differs based on the type of component used. In a posterior cruciate–retaining component, the tibial component typically has approximately 7° of posterior slope. In a cruciate-substituting component, the tibial component is implanted between 0° and 3° of posterior slope. The rotational alignment of the prosthetic components is difficult to determine with plain radiographic examinations. If malrotation of the femoral or tibial component is suspected, obtaining a computed tomographic scan of the knee can be quite helpful.[10] The rotational alignment of the femoral component in relation to the transepicondylar axis (**Fig. 62-3**) and the tibial component in relation to the tibial tubercle can be determined.[10] This technique provides a noninvasive method for quantitatively determining the rotational alignment of the tibial and femoral components on a standard computed tomographic

scanner and can be useful for patients with patellofemoral instability.[10]

The lateral radiograph yields much information pertinent to the evaluation of a painful TKR. The size (AP diameter) of the femoral component can be measured and compared with the AP diameter of the contralateral femur. An increase in the AP diameter of the femur may be associated with poor range of motion and stiffness. A decrease in the AP diameter of the femur may be associated with flexion instability. Elevation of the joint line resulting in an acquired patella baja can be detected on the lateral view. An acquired patella baja may result in restriction of flexion of the TKR. The point of contact between the femur and tibial insert is visualized on the lateral radiograph. Excessive rollback of the femoral component may be related to tightness of the posterior cruciate ligament and resultant pain and poor flexion of the TKR. The thickness of the patellar remnant can be assessed on the lateral radiograph. A thick patellar remnant that results in an increased lateral diameter of the patellar can result in decreased knee flexion.

The patellar axial view is particularly useful for evaluating tracking of the patellofemoral joint.[9] Patellar tilt or instability is visualized in this view (**Fig. 62-4**). Occasionally, radiographs in varying degrees of flexion are useful. In addition, problems related to the polyethylene of the patellar component can often be visualized such as wear-through of metal-backed components or polyethylene dissociation.[9] Stress fractures of the patella can also be seen in the skyline view.

The AP radiograph with the patient bearing weight gives information regarding the polyethylene thickness of the tibial insert and ligament balance. Varus and valgus stress views are useful if the patient is unable to bear weight on the limb and for documenting ligamentous instability.[8]

NUCLEAR MEDICINE EXAMINATION

After a thorough history, physical examination, and study of serial X-rays, occasionally there still may be uncertainty regarding the fixation of the prosthetic components in a patient with a painful TKR. Radionucleotide studies may be used to aid in the diagnosis of loosening and infection.[15-17] One must bear in mind that in asymptomatic knees, increased activity on diphosphonate scanning can be expected for at least 1 year after surgery. Increased activity of the diphosphonate scan after 1 year is present in 89% of tibial and 63% of femoral components in asymptomatic knee replacements.[2,16,18] Bone scans must therefore be carefully interpreted as an additional data point in conjunction with the data obtained from the history, the physical examination, and the radiographs (**Fig. 62-5**).[19] A negative bone scan is in many respects more helpful than a positive scan. If a diphosphonate scan has normal uptake in a patient with a painful TKR, the pain is unlikely

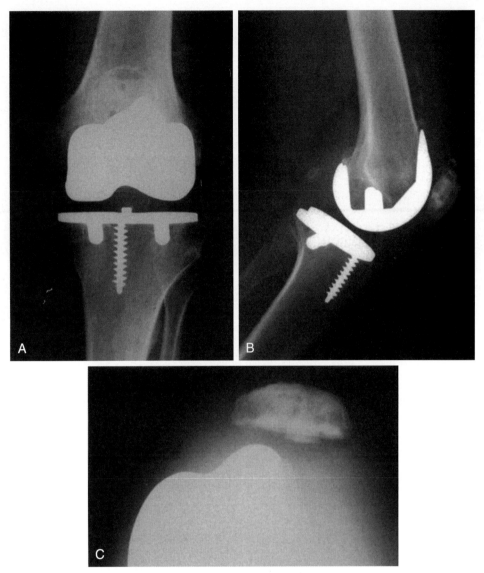

FIGURE 62-4 Anteroposterior **(A)** and lateral **(B)** radiographs of a 76-year-old man, 8 y after cementless total knee replacement returned for knee instability after exchange of tibial insert and revision of patellar component. The patellar component was lateralized, resulting in patellar instability seen on the patellar axial view **(C)**.

to originate from loosening or infection. Conversely, if there is increased uptake about the TKR, the patient does not necessarily have infection or loosening. Other causes of accelerated bone turnover in addition to infection and loosening include trauma and tumor. Technetium diphosphonate scan has a sensitivity of 95% in detecting infection; its specificity is only 20%.[15,20]

Gallium citrate is a radioisotope that accumulates in areas of inflammation. On intravenous injection, gallium binds to serum transferrin and is carried to the extracellular space, including sites of infection. Gallium scan sensitivity is high, and a negative scan can reliably rule out infection. However, because gallium may show increased uptake at uninfected sites of bone remodeling, the positive predictive value is 70% to 75%.[21-23]

Scans using indium (indium-111) may improve the diagnostic accuracy of radionucleotide scans for infection.[18]

A sample of the patient's blood is drawn, and the white cells in it are labeled with indium-111. These labeled cells are reinfused. Local areas of increased white cell accumulation in bone as seen on a subsequent scan are suggestive of infection. Using indium-111 to diagnose infection has a reported accuracy of 84%, sensitivity of 83%, and specificity of 85% (**Fig. 62-6**).[24] False-positives have been seen in patients with rheumatoid arthritis or osteolysis. An accuracy of 95% has been reported for diagnosing infection in TKR when using indium-111 in combination with technetium diphosphonate scans.[22] If both of these nuclear studies are normal, further diagnostic studies, continued observation, and referral for a second opinion are all appropriate treatment options.[20,23] In the author's practice, nuclear medicine studies are used to confirm when subtle loosening of a component is suspected based on

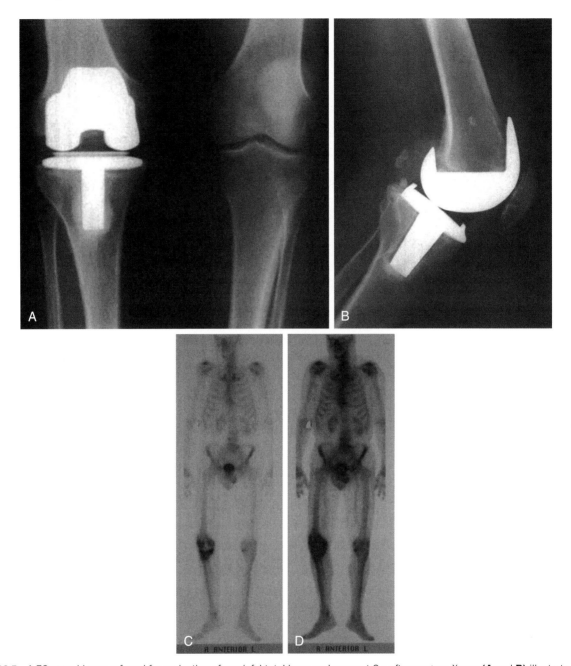

FIGURE 62-5 A 73-year-old man referred for evaluation of a painful total knee replacement 2 y after surgery. X-rays (**A** and **B**) illustrate loosening of the femoral and tibial components. Bone scans (**C** and **D**) illustrate increased uptake at both the distal femur and proximal tibia. Aspiration was negative for infection. Cultures obtained at revision surgery were positive for coagulase-negative *Staphylococcus aureus*.

radiographs. For radiographs that demonstrate clear loosening of the components, bone scan is often not needed for the diagnosis.

COMPUTED TOMOGRAPHY

Computed tomography (CT) can be a useful adjunct, particularly when evaluating the rotation of the femoral and tibial components. CT can be used in cases with patellar instability to evaluate the rotation of the tibial component compared to the tibial tubercle and posterior condyles of the tibial plateau. The femoral component rotation can be compared to the epicondylar axis. A CT

of both knees may be helpful in cases with a contralateral knee with minimal arthritis or a well-functioning total knee arthroplasty (TKA). Considerable variation in the component rotation, size, and alignment from the contralateral knee may indicate a problem with component position contributing to the painful TKR.

MAGNETIC RESONANCE IMAGING

Some centers have developed specific protocols to limit metal artifact while performing magnetic resonance imaging (MRI) of a total knee arthroplasty.[25] The appearance of the synovium and surrounding soft tissues has been

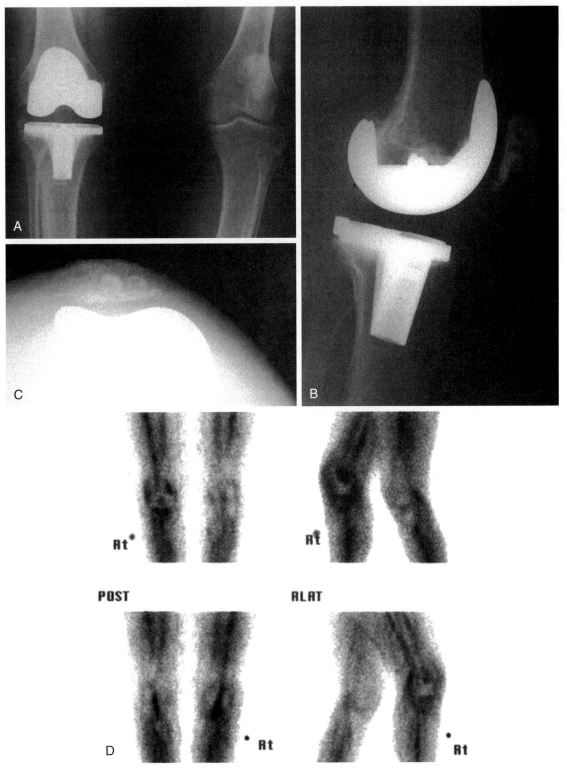

FIGURE 62-6   A 78-year-old woman referred for evaluation of painful total knee replacement 16 mo after surgery. X-rays **(A to C)** show no evidence of implant loosening. Indium-111 scan is positive **(D)**, with increased uptake at distal femur and proximal tibia. Cultures obtained during revision total knee replacement grew *streptococcus*.

assessed through MRI, with three major categories established: frondlike and hypertrophic synovium; lamellated and hyperintense; and homogeneous effusion.[26] Frondlike appearance of the synovium has been correlated with the degree of polyethylene surface damage in a study of

61 patients with total knee arthroplasty who had MRI performed prior to revision surgery.[27] In one study of 28 infected TKA compared to noninfected TKA, lamellated hyperintense synovitis on MRI had a sensitivity of 0.85 to 0.92 and a specificity of 0.85 to 0.87 in detecting

infected TKA.[28] The ability to reproduce these results outside of specialized centers has yet to be established. In the author's practice, MRI is rarely performed but may be useful in cases in which an injury is suspected to the posterior cruciate ligament, the collateral ligaments, or the extensor mechanism. In cases of recurrent hemarthrosis following TKR without evidence of instability, MRI can be useful to diagnosis synovitis which may contribute.

LABORATORY EVALUATION

Blood studies commonly used to evaluate patients with a painful TKR include a blood cell count and differential, erythrocyte sedimentation rate (ESR), and C-reactive protein. These studies are intended to serve as screening tests for infection.[19,29] The white blood cell count is the least useful and is elevated in a minority of patients with an infected TKR.[19,29] The sedimentation rate has a sensitivity of 60% to 80% when 30 mm per hour is used as the cutoff level for diagnosing infection.[19,29,30] An elevated sedimentation rate is an extremely nonspecific finding, and the ESR may remain elevated for several months after surgery in asymptomatic, noninfected TKRs. The C-reactive protein returns to a normal level sooner than the ESR and is therefore more helpful in evaluating a patient with a painful TKR within 3 months of the index surgical procedure.[19,30]

Analysis of fluid aspirated from the painful TKR is the standard of care to determine if a prosthetic infection is present. A synovial fluid white blood cell count of greater than 25,000 per μL or a differential with more than 75% polymorphonuclear leukocytes is highly suggestive of infection.[20,31-33] Laboratory culture of the joint aspirate can also identify the bacterial species causing the infection and its antibiotic sensitivities.[34] A finding of elevated protein and low glucose levels in the aspirated fluid is consistent with deep prosthetic infection.[19,34,35] It is important to determine whether the patient had been on antibiotics at the time of the aspirate or in the immediate past, as antibiotic use is a major factor in obtaining false-negative cultures from fluid aspirated from infected TKRs. In patients who have not been on antibiotics, aspiration has been found to be 75% sensitive in detecting infection.[31] If a high index of suspicion for infection exists, a second knee aspirate can increase the sensitivity to 85%.[31] False-negative aspirates are not uncommon and a single negative aspiration does not rule out infection. Aspiration of a TKR must be performed under sterile conditions and without the use of local anesthetics. The preservative added to lidocaine is bactericidal to many bacteria and may lead to false-negative cultures of the aspirated fluid.

Synovial biomarkers have gained interest as a method of diagnosing prosthetic joint infection in painful TKR. Alpha-defensin is released by neutrophils and serves a broad-spectrum antimicrobial action against pathogens within the joint.[35] It has been studied as a biomarker for prosthetic joint infection in fluid aspirated from the

joint.[36] In one study of 39 aspirations of TKR and total hip replacement with an equivocal diagnosis of prosthetic joint infection, synovial fluid alpha-defensin had a sensitivity of 82%, specificity of 82%, negative predictive value of 92%, and positive predictive value of 64%.[37] Alpha-defensin has a role as an additional data point to help determine the likelihood of a prosthetic joint infection in a painful TKR.[38]

Molecular biologic techniques may aid greatly in our ability to diagnose infection in TKRs. Polymerase chain reaction (PCR) testing of fluid aspirated from a painful TKR is the most sensitive test to detect bacteria in the specimen.[39] This test is based on the fact that nearly all bacteria that cause infections after TKR have a gene that encodes the 16S RNA of a small ribosomal subunit of the bacteria. A set of primers is used to target this gene and amplify the production of DNA from these bacteria. The type of bacterial DNA can then be identified. This study is extremely sensitive and may have a high false-positive rate in laboratories not expert in this technique.[39] In one multicentered study using PCR to detect prosthetic joint infection in revision cases, PCR was compared to the consensus definition considered to be the gold standard.[40] PCR to detect infection had a sensitivity of 97.4%, specificity of 100%, positive predictive value of 100%, and negative predictive value of 98.7%. This laboratory investigation is not currently in routine clinical use and is not quantitative but qualitative. Nonetheless this test may be an invaluable aid in diagnosing periprosthetic infections in the future, and it has the added benefit that it is not affected by the presence of antibiotics in the synovial fluid.

In the author's practice, all patients undergoing a revision TKR are aspirated in the clinic prior to surgery. This fluid is sent routinely for alpha-defensin to provide more data points to help in the diagnosis of an occult periprosthetic joint infection. The authors do not routinely send for PCR but consider the test in cases with negative culture but elevated synovial markers concerning for infection as another data point to help with the diagnosis. If no fluid is obtained, then synovial fluid is aspirated intraoperatively and sent for immediate cell count.

TOTAL KNEE REPLACEMENT FAILURES

TKR provides the arthritic patient with predictable pain relief and restoration of function of the arthritic joint. There are patients who do not obtain this predictable result, and this group can be divided into two categories. The first group contains failures that occur early in the postoperative period, within the first 5 years. The second group, or late failures, includes patients in whom failure occurs after 10 years.

Early failures after TKR are of great concern, as both patients and surgeons have come to expect results far superior to this, with 10 to 15 years of prosthetic function before revision is necessary. A group of 440 patients in whom the index replacement failed and revision was necessary were studied.[6] Of the 440 patients evaluated, 279 (63%) had revision surgery within 5 years of their index replacement. In this cohort, 105 of the 279 patients (38%) had revision surgery because of infection; 74 (27%) had revision surgery because of instability; 37 (13%) had revision surgery because of patellofemoral problems; and 21 (7%) had revision surgery because of wear or osteolysis.[6] In only 8 (3%) patients, there was an early revision due to aseptic loosening of the prosthesis. Two major causes of early failure of TKR ultimately requiring revision surgery seen in this series were the failure of cementless fixation and prosthetic instability.[6] If all the knee replacements had been cemented routinely and the ligaments balanced carefully, the number of early revisions would have decreased by approximately 40%, and the overall failures would have been reduced by 25%.[6] Special care must be given to the soft-tissue aspects of the knee replacement procedure to avoid early revision for instability by ensuring careful equalization of the flexion and extension gaps.

No patient with a painful TKR should be offered revision surgery without a diagnosis as to the cause of the patient's pain.[1] There is little place for surgical exploration of the painful total knee, either arthroscopically or through an open incision.[3] One can determine the etiology of the pain in the vast majority of patients with pain after TKR by carrying out a complete history and a thorough physical examination, reviewing serial and current radiographs, ordering appropriate laboratory examinations, and obtaining occasional radionucleotide scans when appropriate.[1,3]

REFERENCES

1. Ayers DC, Dennis DA, Johanson NA, et al. Common complications of total knee arthroplasty. *J Bone Joint Surg Am.* 1997;79:278-311.
2. Schneider R, Soudry M. Radiographic and scintigraphic evaluation of total knee arthroplasty. *Clin Orthop Relat Res.* 1986;205:108-112.
3. Mont MA, Serna FK, Krackow KA. Exploration of radiographically normal total knee replacements for unexplained pain. *Clin Orthop Relat Res.* 1996;331:216-219.
4. Rand JA. Sepsis following total knee arthroplasty. In: Rand JA, ed. *Total Knee Arthroplasty.* New York: Raven Press; 1993:349-375.
5. Dellon AL, Mont MA, Krackow KA, et al. Partial denervation for persistent neuroma pain after total knee arthroplasty. *Clin Orthop Relat Res.* 1995;316:145-150.
6. Fehring TK, Odum S, Griffin WL. Early failures in total knee arthroplasty. *Clin Orthop Relat Res.* 2001;392:315-318.
7. Beight JL, Yao B, Hozack WJ, et al. The patellar "clunk" syndrome after posterior stabilized total knee arthroplasty. *Clin Orthop Relat Res.* 1994;299:139-142.
8. Fehring TK, Valadie AL. Knee instability after total knee arthroplasty. *Clin Orthop Relat Res.* 1994;299:157-162.
9. Rand JA. The patellofemoral joint in total knee arthroplasty. *J Bone Joint Surg Am.* 1994;76:612-620.
10. Berger RA, Crossett LS, Jacobs JJ, et al. Malrotation causing patellofemoral complications after total knee arthroplasty. *Clin Orthop Relat Res.* 1998;356:144-153.
11. Drosos GI, Triantafilidou T, Ververidis A, et al. Persistent postsurgical pain and neuropathic pain after total knee replacement. *World J Orthop.* 2015;6(7):528-536.
12. Hunter JC, Jattner RS, Murray WR. Loosening of the total knee replacement: correlation with pain and radiolucent lines. A prospective study. *Invest Radiol.* 1987;22:891-894.
13. Fehring TK, McAvoy G. Fluoroscopic evaluation of the painful total knee arthroplasty. *Clin Orthop Relat Res.* 1996;331:226-233.
14. Mintz AD, Pilkington DA, Howie DW. A comparison of plain and fluoroscopically guided radiographs in the assessment of arthroplasty of the knee. *J Bone Joint Surg Am.* 1989;71:1343-1347.
15. Davis LP. Nuclear imaging in the diagnosis of the infected total joint arthroplasty. *Semin Arthroplasty.* 1994;5:147-152.
16. Kantor SG, Schneider R, Insall JN. Radionuclide imaging of asymptomatic versus symptomatic total knee arthroplasties. *Clin Orthop Relat Res.* 1990;260:118-123.
17. Morrey BF, Westholm F, Schoifet S. Long-term results of various treatment options for infected total knee arthroplasty. *Clin Orthop Relat Res.* 1989;248:120-128.
18. Rosenthall L, Lepanto L, Raymone F. Radiophosphate uptake on asymptomatic knee arthroplasty. *J Nucl Med.* 1987;28:1546-1549.
19. Levitsky KA, Hozack WJ, Balderston RA. Evaluation of the painful prosthetic joint: relative value of bone scan, sedimentation rate and joint aspiration. *J Arthroplasty.* 1991;6:237-244.
20. Hansen AD, Rand JA. Evaluation and treatment of infection at the site of a total hip or knee arthroplasty. *J Bone Joint Surg Am.* 1998;80:910-922.
21. Magnuson JE, Brown ML, Hausen JF. In-111 labeled leukocyte scintigraphy in suspected orthopedic prosthesis infection: comparison with other imaging modalities. *Radiology.* 1988;168:235-239.
22. Merkel KD, Brown ML, Dewangee MK. Comparison of indium-labeled-leukocyte imaging with sequential technetium-gallium scanning in the diagnosis of low-grade musculoskeletal sepsis: a prospective study. *J Bone Joint Surg Am.* 1985;67:465-476.
23. Windsor RE, Insall JN. Management of the infected total knee arthroplasty. In: Insall JN, ed. *Surgery of the Knee.* Vol. 2. New York: Churchill Livingstone; 1993:47-71.
24. Rand JA, Brown ML. The value of indium 111 leukocyte scanning in the evaluation of painful or infected total knee arthroplasties. *Clin Orthop Relat Res.* 1990;259:179-182.
25. Li AE, Sneag DB, Greditzer HG, et al. Total knee arthroplasty: diagnostic accuracy of patterns of synovitis at MR imaging. *Radiology.* 2016;281(2):499-506.
26. Li AE, Johnson CC, Sneag DB, et al. Frondlike synovitis on MRI and correlation with polyethylene surface damage of total knee arthroplasty. *AJR Am J Roentgenol.* 2017;209(4):W231-W237.
27. Plodkowski AJ, Hayter CL, Miller TT, et al. Lamellated hyperintense synovitis: potential MR imaging sign of an infected knee arthroplasty. *Radiology.* 2013;266(1):256-260.
28. Aslto K, Osterman K, Peltola H. Changes in erythrocyte sedimentation rate and C-reactive protein after total hip arthroplasty. *Clin Orthop Relat Res.* 1984;184:118-120.
29. Carlsson AS. Erythrocyte sedimentation rate in infected and non-infected total hip arthroplasties. *Acta Orthop Scand.* 1978;49:287-291.
30. Barrack RL, Jennings RW, Wolfe MW, et al. The value of preoperative aspiration before total knee revision. *Clin Orthop Relat Res.* 1997;345:8-16.
31. Duff GP, Lachiewicz PL, Kelly SS. Aspiration of the knee joint before revision arthroplasty. *Clin Orthop Relat Res.* 1996;331:132-139.
32. O'Neill DA, Harris WH. Failed total hip replacement: assessment by plain radiographs, arthrograms, and aspiration of the hip joint. *J Bone Joint Surg Am.* 1984;66:540-546.
33. Chimento GF, Finger S, Barrack RL. Gram stain detection of infection during revision arthroplasty. *J Bone Joint Surg Br.* 1996;78:828-839.
34. Windsor RE, Insall JN, Urs WK. Two-stage reimplantation for the salvage of total knee arthroplasty complicated by infection: further follow-up and refinement of indications. *J Bone Joint Surg Am.* 1990;72:272-278.

35. Ganz T, Selsted ME, Szklarek D, et al. Defensins. Natural peptide antibiotics of human neutrophils. *J Clin Invest.* 1985;76(4):1427-1435.

36. Deirmengian C, Kardos K, Kilmartin P, et al. Diagnosing periprosthetic joint infection: has the era of the biomarker arrived? *Clin Orthop Relat Res.* 2014;472(11):3254-3262.

37. Kelly MP, Darrith B, Hannon CP, et al. Synovial fluid alpha-defensin is an adjunctive tool in the equivocal diagnosis of periprosthetic joint infection. *J Arthroplasty.* 2018;33(11):3537-3540.

38. Parvizi J, Tan TL, Goswami K, et al. The 2018 definition of periprosthetic hip and knee infection: an evidence-based and validated criteria. *J Arthroplasty.* 2018;33(5):1309-1314.

39. Marian BD, Martin DS, Levine MJ. Polymerase chain reaction detection of bacterial infection in total knee arthroplasty. *Clin Orthop Relat Res.* 1996;331:11-22.

40. Moshirabadi A, Razi M, Arasteh P, et al. Polymerase chain reaction assay using the restriction fragment length polymorphism technique in the detection of prosthetic joint infections: a multi-centered study. *J Arthroplasty.* 2019;34(2):359-364.

chapter 63

Preoperative Planning for Revision Total Knee Arthroplasty

Daniel J. Berry, MD

Careful preoperative planning for a complex operation like revision knee replacement provides tremendous benefits to the patient and surgeon by improving the quality and efficiency of the surgery and by reducing the potential for operative complications. At its best, preoperative planning involves more than just advance consideration of the tools required to remove failed implants and consideration of the design and size of implants that will be implanted: Preoperative planning involves consideration of all the resources that will be needed during surgery and in the postoperative period; preoperative planning involves a mental rehearsal of the planned operation from start to finish, which allows the surgeon to consider the order of steps in which the operation will be performed and the techniques that he or she must be familiar with to complete each step; and preoperative planning involves considering contingencies for problems that might arise during surgery. Thorough and thoughtful preoperative planning helps the surgeon to have on hand all of the materials necessary for an optimal reconstruction and allows the surgeon to become familiar with and have access to techniques, implants, and tools that could be needed to overcome potential problems. The chance of needing to compromise because a specific implant or tool was not available or because the surgeon was not familiar with a specific useful technique is reduced. Finally, detailed preoperative planning helps the surgeon predict problems that are important to discuss with the patient in advance. The patient, then, is better informed about the risks of surgery and potential problems that may compromise the surgical outcome; such an understanding leads to more realistic patient expectations and ultimately to greater patient satisfaction with the entire process of surgery, regardless of the outcome.

PREOPERATIVE EVALUATION

Patient History and Physical Examination

Identify problems by history and physical examination that will influence what procedure is done and how it is done. Determine if the patient has a history or physical findings of hip problems such as pain or stiffness, known arthritis, or previous fracture or osteotomy of the hip or femur. Determine if the patient has an ipsilateral tibial

deformity or ankle or foot problems. These pieces of information are important to optimize the mechanical axis of the limb at operation. Learn as much as possible about the patient's failed knee replacement. Identify the implant manufacturer, implant design, and implant sizes. Accurate and specific implant identification can be made by reviewing stickers from the actual implants that are placed in the patient's medical record. If part of the knee implant will be retained intact at operation, all this information is essential to ensure that matching parts are available. Learn whether special design-specific instruments are available for implant extraction or disassembly. Review whether there is anything in the history or examination to suggest infection of the failed total knee arthroplasty (TKA). If so, consider preoperative evaluation with measurement of C-reactive protein level, erythrocyte sedimentation rate, knee aspiration,[1,2] and radionuclide scans.

Evaluate the skin and previous skin incisions and find out if the patient has ever had problems with wound healing. Measure the knee range of motion and consider whether stiffness may make an extensile exposure necessary. Determine if there is evidence of ligamentous deficiency or knee instability. Test extensor mechanism power. Evaluate the patient's vascular status. If significant peripheral vascular disease is a concern by history or examination, consider a preoperative vascular medicine or vascular surgery consult, or preoperative noninvasive arterial studies, or both. Ask if the patient has a history of venous thromboembolic problems; if so, plan accordingly for venous thromboembolism prophylaxis and consider whether preoperative evaluation by an internist, vascular medicine specialist, or thrombosis expert would be helpful. Consider the patient's overall medical situation. Make arrangements for an appropriate preoperative medical evaluation and for postoperative support by specialists in internal medicine, cardiology, pulmonology, nephrology, or other medical disciplines if needed. If a large procedure is planned, and if the patient has numerous medical problems, make preoperative arrangements for a postoperative intensive care unit bed. Determine if the patient has experienced unusual bleeding or blood loss problems that may require preoperative hematologic evaluation and special arrangements with the blood bank. By having the patient evaluated in advance by specialists in other disciplines, such as plastic surgery, vascular surgery, or internal medicine, some problems may be avoided. Equally important, if problems do occur intra- or postoperatively, the consultants can deal with them more effectively because they already know the patient. Likewise, the patient is more likely to take the problem in stride because the potential for such problems was anticipated.

Radiographs

Knee radiographs should include anteroposterior standing films, lateral films, and patellar skyline views, and a long-standing radiograph from hips to ankles (**Fig. 63-1**).[3,4] Stress films occasionally may be helpful to determine the degree of ligament competence. Fluoroscopically positioned radiographs provide views that are perfectly tangential to the implant interface and provide the most detailed information of implant fixation status (**Fig. 63-2**). Combine the radiographic information with the rest of the preoperative evaluation to determine the mechanism of previous implant failure. Understanding the failure mechanism helps determine what needs to be done to correct the problem. Determine if the previous implants appear to be well-fixed or loose. Determine if the implants are well-positioned or malpositioned on an anteroposterior radiograph. Use the radiographs to determine the proper angle of femoral and tibial resection needed to restore the mechanical axis of the limb (**Fig. 63-3**). Use templates to estimate the bone resections needed to place the tibial and femoral components in optimal orientation (**Fig. 63-4**). Acetate overlay templates have mostly now been replaced by digital templates which have been shown to be effective and provide additional tools to measure angles, lengths, and alignment.[5,6] Use templates over the anteroposterior and lateral radiographs to determine the approximate tibial or femoral implant sizes that will be needed. Evaluate the location and severity of tibial and femoral bone loss. Use templates to determine whether metal prosthetic augmentation or bone grafts will be needed (**Fig. 63-5**). Examine the distal femur carefully for subtle signs of osteolysis of the condyles, especially posteriorly (**Fig. 63-6**). Consider the severity of femoral and tibial bone loss and how long-term fixation will be obtained and maintained. Metaphyseal fixation with porous coated sleeves or highly porous metal cones can help achieve these goals by providing biologic fixation and a stronger implant foundation in deficient bone.[7-14] If metaphyseal fixation will be used, template the size and configuration of possible sleeves or cones (**Fig. 63-7**). Use templates to determine the length and diameter of planned tibial and femoral implant stems (**Fig. 63-8**). Determine whether offset stems are likely to be needed to compensate for unusual bone shape or bone deformity (**Fig. 63-9**).

Evaluate the patella. Is the implant metal backed or all polyethylene? Is it loose or well-fixed? If the patella needs to be removed, consider whether adequate bone stock

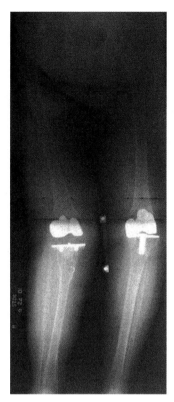

FIGURE 63-1 Long-standing hip-to-ankle radiograph of both lower extremities.

remains to allow another implant to be placed. Consider whether there is evidence of tibial or femoral implant malrotation or of patellar maltracking. If the major problem is patellofemoral maltracking, consider evaluating rotation of the implants with a computed tomographic scan.[15]

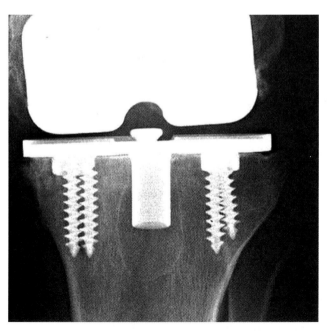

FIGURE 63-2 Fluoroscopically positioned radiograph of an uncemented tibial component demonstrates a complete radiolucent line at the implant–bone interface and osteolysis around the stem of the implant. The implant was not bone ingrown at revision.

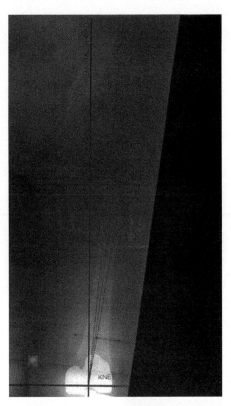

FIGURE 63-3 Template over a long hip-to-ankle radiograph demonstrates that a 7° valgus cut on the femur (in combination with a 0° cut on the tibia) will restore the mechanical axis of the limb to neutral.

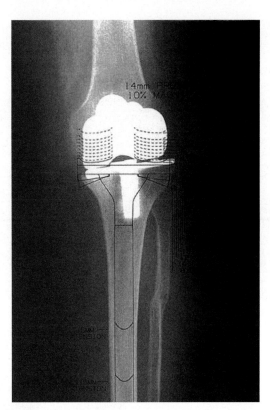

FIGURE 63-5 Template over anteroposterior radiograph of the tibia. The template demonstrates that a medial tibial metal augmentation wedge will be needed to compensate for medial tibial bone defect.

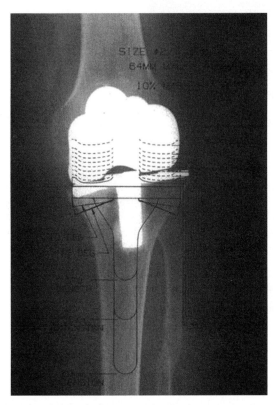

FIGURE 63-4 Template over anteroposterior radiograph of the tibia demonstrating the axis of a 0° tibial cut needed to restore the mechanical axis of the limb to neutral. Note that the real tibial resection line would be more superior and would remove less bone (see **Fig. 63-6**).

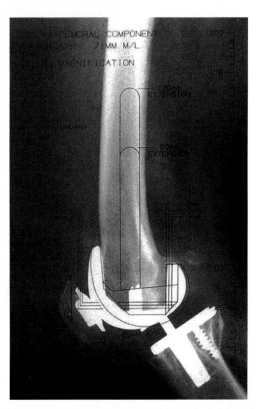

FIGURE 63-6 Osteolysis of the posterior femoral condyles. The femoral template also demonstrates that an offset femoral stem will be needed to avoid impingement of the stem against the posterior femoral cortex.

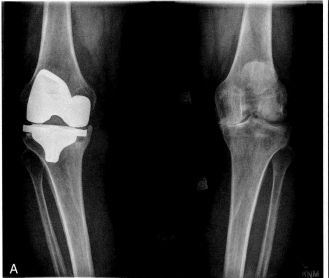
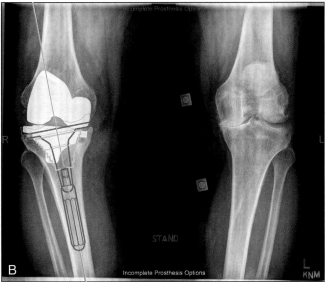
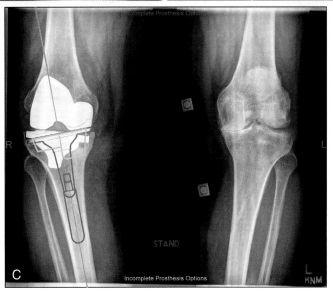

FIGURE 63-7   **A:** Radiograph of patient with notable proximal tibial bone loss. **B:** Template showing possible reconstruction with metaphyseal fixation employing a metaphyseal sleeve and uncemented stem. **C:** Template showing possible reconstruction with metaphyseal fixation employing a metaphyseal cone and cemented stem.

After obtaining a careful history and physical examination and good radiographs, it is helpful to consider each issue that will affect the operation in a methodical and organized manner. Systematic review of each subject is useful for three reasons: First, it forces the surgeon to consider every aspect of the planned operation—this makes it less likely that a tool or implant will be needed that was not anticipated and therefore is not available. Second, it forces the surgeon to review the planned steps of the operation—in doing so, the surgeon can move through the actual procedure more efficiently. Having conceived the plan in advance, the surgeon will have less need to pause to think about options during surgery. A careful plan forces the surgeon to think through how a decision at one point in the operation will affect the requirements for the rest of the procedure. Finally, by considering each

step of the procedure, the surgeon should have in mind a plan A, a plan B, and a plan C for each contingency: Anticipating challenges and problems blunts their negative impact should they occur at operation.

STEP-BY-STEP PREOPERATIVE CONSIDERATIONS

Skin

Consider the scars already present. If a single midline vertical incision is present, plan to use it. If there are multiple scars, plan which will be best to use. Because much of the cutaneous blood supply comes from medially, in general, the most lateral usable previous incision is best. If the risk of skin slough seems high even if precautions are taken,

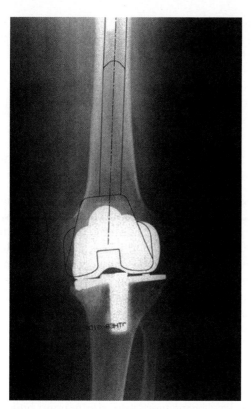

FIGURE 63-8   Template over anteroposterior radiograph of the femur to estimate planned diameter of a press-fit femoral stem.

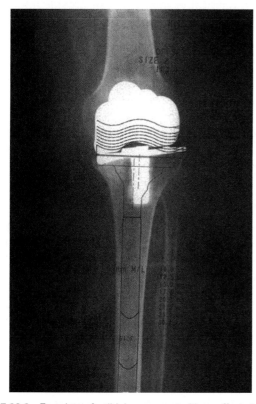

FIGURE 63-9   Template of a tibial component with an offset stem over anteroposterior radiograph of the tibia. Use of an offset stem eliminates the medial overhang of the tibial component seen in **Fig. 63-5** (the same case without an offset stem).

consider having the patient evaluated by a plastic surgeon preoperatively. The plastic surgeon may have useful ideas about how to prevent problems and, if a problem does occur, the patient will have been seen and evaluated in advance. If muscle flaps from previous surgery will be elevated, get information about the location of the vascular pedicle to the flap and consider plastic surgery consultation.

Peripheral Vascular Supply

If the patient has evidence by history or physical examination of significant peripheral vascular disease, consider consultation with a vascular surgeon or vascular medicine expert. Consider noninvasive vascular studies and transcutaneous oximetry to determine if wound healing at the knee level is likely to be a problem. If the patient has marked peripheral vascular disease or previous vascular reconstruction, consider doing most of the procedure, with the exception of exposure and implant cementation, without a tourniquet inflated.[16] When the knee is flexed, bleeding often is minimal.

Neurologic Status

Make sure the preoperative neurologic status is evaluated and carefully documented. For patients at high risk for nerve palsy after surgery, set in place a preoperative plan to reduce that risk. Patients with large flexion contractures, valgus knee deformities, and particularly a combination of the two are at risk when the deformity is corrected and the peroneal nerve is placed under tension.[17] Avoid the use of long-lasting regional anesthesia or nerve blocks that will make postoperative evaluation of nerve function difficult. A preoperative plan to keep the knee flexed postoperatively until neurologic status is verified is reasonable, and a plan can be set in place to gradually extend the knee while the clinical status of the nerve is evaluated postoperatively.

Exposure

Even though the need for an extensile knee exposure can never be determined with certainty until the operation itself is under way, frequently it can be predicted in advance. The most common situation that requires an extensile exposure is the very stiff knee. The main extensile exposures to the knee are proximal quadriceps snip, V-Y quadricepsplasty, and tibial tubercle osteotomy.[18] Extensile knee exposures are discussed in detail in Chapter 64.

Implant Removal

One of the most important issues to address by preoperative planning is removal of previous implants. Identify the manufacturer, implant design, and size of the failed knee implants. Keep in mind that some implant designs have several design iterations, some of which look remarkably similar radiographically.

It is important to know the type of implant for several reasons. First, if some of the previous components will be retained, compatible components (tibia, femur, patella, tibial insert, tibial insert locking pins, etc.) need to be available. Second, knowing the type of implants in place allows the surgeon to have implant-specific extractors available. Finally, the surgeon can learn in advance about implant-specific methods of disassembly or reassembly.

Consider what tools may be needed to remove the implants from the bone. For cemented implants, have osteotomes, saws, or ultrasonic instruments[19-21] available to cut the prosthesis–cement interface. Have extractors available to remove implants. If the implants have stems, have special instruments available to remove the stem from the canal. Be aware that for stemmed implants, the condylar portion of the implant may detach from the stem during removal, and having stem-specific extractors can speed and simplify stem extraction. If there are large cement columns in the femur or tibia, have special instruments available to remove cement. The instruments designed for cement removal in revision hip arthroplasty are particularly useful. These include hand instruments, cannulated cement removal systems, and ultrasonic cement removal systems.

If the implants are uncemented, have oscillating and/or reciprocating saws available to cut the bone–implant interfaces. Metal-cutting instruments may be needed when there are well-fixed implant stems or pegs that need to be cut free of the implant before extraction.[22]

Bone Defects and Templating

Consider the location, severity, and geometry of bone loss. Use templates to determine the planned implant position and implant size. Templating may help predict the optimal entry point to the medullary canal for a specific implant system. Also use templates to plan for bone defect management. Have metal augmentation for femoral and tibial components available. Have appropriate bone grafts available if they may be needed. Have metaphyseal fixation devices, either sleeves or cones, available for most cases with notable distal femoral or proximal tibial bone loss (**Fig. 63-7**). For extremely large defects of the femur or tibia, structural distal femoral grafts or proximal tibial grafts may be needed. Have available internal fixation materials to fix grafts in place.

Consider the implant stems needed to provide added fixation, to off-load stress, and to bypass bone defects. In general, larger defects require longer stems to off-load stress. Cemented and uncemented stems both have advantages and disadvantages, and there is a role for both in contemporary revision knee arthroplasty.[23-26] When

possible, bone defects that could lead to fracture, including old screw holes, should be bypassed.

Finally, with templates, determine if any bone deformities will make difficult or compromise ideal implant placement. Determine if offset implant stems or special custom stems may be needed to optimize positioning and sizing of the implants and stems.

Flexion–Extension Gap Balancing and Joint Line Restoration

Consider what will be necessary to balance flexion and extension gaps. When possible, the simultaneous goals of the operation are to balance the flexion and extension gaps and to restore the joint line to a normal level. There is growing understanding, however, that in practice sometimes these two goals are mutually exclusive. Not rarely in revision TKA, the flexion gap is considerably larger than the extension gap, and some elevation of the joint line is necessary to balance the knee in flexion and extension.

Study the preoperative radiographs to determine the relative amounts of posterior femoral bone loss and distal femoral bone loss that are present. More posterior femoral bone loss means more posterior femoral buildup will be needed to fill the flexion gap. If there is a great deal of distal femoral bone loss, as measured from the epicondyles, more distal femoral augmentation probably will be required. Physical examination can provide information on the likely relative sizes of the flexion and extension gaps. If the knee is loose in flexion but tight in extension (as evidenced by a flexion contracture), the flexion gap probably will be larger than the extension gap. Likewise, if the knee hyperextends, is lax in extension, or has an extension contracture, then the extension gap may be larger than the flexion gap. Understanding the probable relative sizes of flexion and extension gaps in advance allows the surgeon to consider the measures that will be required to equalize the gaps.

Stability and Ligament Defects

Information obtained by history and the physical examination is important to solve ligament problems. Successful management of ligament problems falls into several categories.

1. Optimization of the limb and implant alignment: This requires viewing long-standing hip-to-ankle films to determine the optimal tibial femoral angle (and thus the angle of the distal femur cut). If the knee has medial ligament insufficiency, make sure not to leave the mechanical axis of the knee lateral to the center of the knee; if the knee has lateral ligament insufficiency, make sure not to leave the mechanical axis medial to the center of the knee.

2. Implant constraint level: For revision TKA, different levels of constraint are needed for different problems. The general tenet is to use the least constraint necessary to solve the problem effectively. Although excessively constrained implants are not desirable, providing a marginally adequate level of constraint often is not in the patient's best interest, particularly if the patient is elderly and cannot tolerate repetitive procedures. Most situations of moderate ligament laxity can be treated with release of tight ligaments coupled with tensioning of loose ligaments. When these measures are not sufficient, use of constrained condylar implants generally can solve the problem. Infrequently, profound ligament deficiency or failure of previous procedures to stabilize an unstable knee requires the use of rotating hinge implants.

Extensor Mechanism

Good function of the extensor mechanism is important for the overall function of the knee.

Determine from physical examination if the extensor mechanism is intact. If it is grossly deficient, consider whether revision TKA is appropriate. Alternatives include external bracing with a drop lock brace or knee arthrodesis. If revision TKA is deemed appropriate, extensor mechanism reconstruction will be necessary, typically with polymer mesh augmentation or an allograft (either an Achilles tendon allograft with a bone block or a bone–patellar tendon–patella quadriceps tendon allograft) or rarely in acute cases with repair and autogenous tissue augmentation (such as semitendinosus and/or gracilis tendon).[27] Due to their specialized nature, such allograft materials usually need to be ordered in advance, even in hospitals with a standard bone bank.

Consider how the patella will be managed. Well-functioning patellar implants usually should be preserved. Most dome-shaped patellar components do not need to be removed—even if the new tibial and femoral implants being placed are from a different manufacturer—because the small incongruences that arise from intermanufacturer implant geometry differences usually do not justify the risks of patellar revision. If the patellar implant is loose, determine if sufficient bone remains for patellar reimplantation. When the bone appears too deficient to consider reimplantation, consider other options for patellar management: resection arthroplasty with patelloplasty or impaction grafting of the patella.

Review the patellar skyline radiographs and consider whether efforts to improve patellar or extensor mechanism tracking will be needed.

Closure

Anticipate whether closure is likely to be problematic. Most commonly, wound closure is problematic when patients have extremely woody tissue, a foreshortened limb that will be lengthened (such as one with a long-standing resection arthroplasty), or a limb with a great deal of deformity. Preoperative evaluation by a plastic surgeon can be helpful in these circumstances.

POSTOPERATIVE ISSUES

Venous Thromboembolic Disease

Preoperatively, consider whether the patient is at high risk for postoperative venous thromboembolism. For patients at especially high risk, consider a preoperative vascular medicine consultation. Determine in advance the plan for postoperative venous thromboembolism prophylaxis.

Medical Issues

Determine whether special medical problems require special medical management after surgery. Patients with major medical problems and patients anticipated to have extremely large operations may require a postoperative intensive care unit bed, which may be arranged in advance. Make preoperative arrangements to have specific postoperative consultations and support from cardiology, pulmonary, or other groups if the patient has major medical problems in these areas.

Pain Management

Consider whether special pain management measures will be needed postoperatively. Discussion with the anesthesia team before the operation can be helpful, and sometimes regional nerve blocks may be used.

Dismissal Plan

Before surgery, discuss the plan for care after the hospitalization with the patient and patient's family. Determine the level of support available in the patient's own home. If the patient will require help beyond that available at home, arrange for a bed in a rehabilitation facility. Securing a bed in advance can optimize the postoperative recovery environment.

REFERENCES

1. Duff G, Lachiewicz P, Kelley S. Aspiration of the knee joint before revision arthroplasty. *Clin Orthop Relat Res*. 1996;331:132.
2. Windsor R, Bono J. Infected total knee replacements. *J Am Acad Orthop Surg*. 1994;2:44.
3. Patel DV, Ferrus BD, Aichroth PM. Radiological study of alignment after total knee replacement: short radiographs or long radiographs? *Int Orthop*. 1991;15:209.
4. Petersen TL, Engh GA. Radiographic assessment of knee alignment after total knee arthroplasty. *J Arthroplasty*. 1988;3:67-72.
5. Jamali AA. Digital templating and preoperative deformity analysis with standard imaging software. *Clin Orthop Relat Res*. 2009;467:2695-2704.

6. Savov P, Windhagen H, Haasper C, Ettinger M. Digital templating of rotating hinge revision and primary total knee arthroplasty. *Orthop Rev.* 2018;10:7811.

7. Barnett SL, Mayer RR, Gondusky JS, Choi L, Patel JJ, Gorab RS. Use of stepped porous titanium metaphyseal sleeves for tibial defects in revision total knee arthroplasty: short term results. *J Arthroplasty.* 2014;29:1219-1224.

8. Bohl DD, Brown NM, McDowell MA, et al. Do porous tantalum metaphyseal cones improve outcomes in revision total knee arthroplasty? *J Arthroplasty.* 2018;33:171-177.

9. Chalmers BP, Desy NM, Pagnano MW, Trousdale RT, Taunton MJ. Survivorship of metaphyseal sleeves in revision total knee arthroplasty. *J Arthroplasty.* 2017;32:1565-1570.

10. Denehy KM, Abhari S, Krebs VE, et al. Excellent metaphyseal fixation using highly porous cones in revision total knee arthroplasty. *J Arthroplasty.* 2019;34(10):2439-2443. doi: 10.1016/j.arth.2019.03.045.

11. Haidukewych GJ, Hanssen A, Jones RD. Metaphyseal fixation in revision total knee arthroplasty: indications and techniques. *J Am Acad Orthop Surg.* 2011;19:311-318.

12. Potter GD III, Abdel MP, Lewallen DG, Hanssen AD. Midterm results of porous tantalum femoral cones in revision total knee arthroplasty. *J Bone Joint Surg.* 2016;98:1286-1291.

13. Sculco PK, Abdel MP, Hanssen AD, Lewallen DG. The management of bone loss in revision total knee arthroplasty: rebuild, reinforce, and augment. *Bone Joint J.* 2016;98B(1 suppl A):120-124.

14. Watters TS, Martin JR, Levy DL, Yang CC, Kim RH, Dennis DA. Porous-coated metaphyseal sleeves for severe femoral and tibial bone loss in revision TKA. *J Arthroplasty.* 2017;32:3468-3473.

15. Berger RA, Crossett LS, Jacobs JJ, et al. Malrotation causing patellofemoral complications after total knee arthroplasty. *Clin Orthop Relat Res.* 1998;356:144-153.

16. Rush JH, Vidovich JD, Johnson MA. Arterial complications of total knee replacement: the Australian experience. *J Bone Joint Surg Br.* 1987;69:400.

17. Asp JPL, Rand JA. Peroneal nerve palsy after total knee arthroplasty. *Clin Orthop Relat Res.* 1990;261:233.

18. Roehrig G, Kang M, Scuderi G. Surgical exposure for the complex revision total knee arthroplasty. *Tech Knee Surg.* 2009;8:154-160. doi:10.1097/BTK.0b013e3181b57fd6.

19. Caillouette JT, Gorab RS, Klapper RC, et al. Revision arthroplasty facilitated by ultrasonic tool cement removal. *Orthop Rev.* 1991;20:353-440.

20. Klapper RC, Caillouette JT. The use of ultrasonic tools in revision arthroplasty procedures. *Contemp Orthop.* 1990;20:273-279.

21. Klapper RC, Caillouette JT, Callaghan JJ, et al. Ultrasonic technology in revision joint arthroplasty. *Clin Orthop Relat Res.* 1992;285:147-154.

22. Berry DJ. Component removal during revision total knee arthroplasty. In: Lotke PA, Garino JP, eds. *Revision Total Knee Arthroplasty.* Philadelphia: Lippincott–Raven Publishers; 1998.

23. Fleischman AN, Azboy I, Fuery M, Restrepo C, Shao H, Parvizi J. Effect of stem size and fixation method on mechanical failure after revision total knee arthroplasty. *J Arthroplasty.* 2017;32:S202-S208.

24. Heesterbeek PJ, Wymenga AB, van Hellemondt GG. No difference in implant micromotion between hybrid fixation and fully cemented revision total knee arthroplasty: a randomized controlled trial with radiostereometric analysis of patients with mild-to-moderate bone loss. *J Bone Joint Surg.* 2016;98:1359-1369.

25. Kosse NM, van Hellemondt GG, Wymenga AB, Heesterbeek PJ. Comparable stability of cemented vs press-fit placed stems in revision total knee arthroplasty with mild to moderate bone loss: 6.5 results from a randomized controlled trial with radiostereometric analysis. *J Arthroplasty.* 2017;32:197-201.

26. Dennis DA, Berry DJ, Engh G, et al. Revision total knee arthroplasty. *J Am Acad Orthop Surg.* 2008;16:442-454.

27. Emerson RH Jr, Head WC, Malinin TI. Reconstruction patellar tendon rupture after total knee arthroplasty with an extensor mechanism allograft. *Clin Orthop Relat Res.* 1990;260:154.

chapter 64

Surgical Approaches in Revision

Blake J. Schultz, MD | Nicholas J. Giori, MD, PhD | James I. Huddleston III, MD

INTRODUCTION

Revision total knee arthroplasty (TKA) can be technically challenging with potential complications including compromised wound healing, extensor mechanism disruption, intraoperative fracture, bone loss, arthrofibrosis, instability, and increased risk of infection.[1-4] Adequate exposure and proper soft tissue management can help reduce complications, though this can be challenging in revision surgery. While the standard medial parapatellar approach may be adequate, there are several specific surgical techniques that aid the wide exposure necessary for a successful operation. With all techniques, an algorithmic approach will facilitate optimal results.

SKIN INCISIONS

Selection of the proper skin incision is crucial to optimize healing. In most cases, the previous skin incision can be utilized. In cases where multiple incisions are present, skin necrosis is a possible devastating complication. Skin bridges should be maximized when possible. The blood supply to the skin of the anterior knee arises medially from branches of the saphenous artery (**Fig. 64-1**). As a general rule, the most lateral incision should be utilized.[5] This is an "intervascular plane" and thus more likely to heal.[6] (**Fig. 64-2**). Extension of the incision proximally and distally into normal tissue is often necessary. The subcutaneous tissue and skin flaps should be kept as thick as possible to decrease the risk of wound healing problems.[2]

In complex cases, the "sham incision" approach can be used. This method calls for making a skin incision, elevating subcutaneous flaps, and then closing. It is thought that the healing of the skin incision creates a "delay phenomenon," whereby subsequent tissue survival is increased through the recruitment of new vessels.[7] Tissue expansion is an additional option in cases of compromised skin.[8] In general, the surgeon should have a low threshold to consult a plastic surgeon preoperatively.

MEDIAL PARAPATELLAR APPROACH

The medial parapatellar approach provides adequate exposure in most revision TKA cases. A methodical, stepwise approach is necessary to minimize damage to the extensor mechanism. After the arthrotomy has been made, the scar tissue should be excised from the suprapatellar pouch as well as from the medial and lateral gutters. The scar tissue should then be debrided from the peripatellar and infrapatellar regions, completing a tenolysis of the extensor mechanism.[9] Surgeons should have a low threshold to avoid patellar eversion in an effort to minimize potential catastrophic damage to the extensor mechanism.[10] Alternatively, a smooth pin can be placed in the center of the patellar ligament into the tibial tubercle, acting as a stress reliever to help prevent complete avulsion of the patellar tendon.[11] If additional exposure is needed, various techniques can be utilized.

MEDIAL PEEL

A medial tibial peel can be performed for added exposure by releasing the deep medial collateral ligament and semimembranosus tendon. This should allow for the tibia to be delivered anteriorly with increasing external rotation. As the tibial tubercle continues to rotate laterally, the entire extensor mechanism moves laterally, facilitating access to the lateral tibial plateau (▶ Video 64-1).

An additional arthrotomy can be made laterally to allow exposure to the anterior aspect of the lateral tibial plateau. Care should be taken to limit the proximal extent of the lateral arthrotomy to the level of the inferior portion of the patella, as this will avoid disruption of the superior lateral genicular artery, the only remaining blood supply to the patella in most cases.

QUADRICEPS SNIP

The quadriceps snip evolved from the quadriceps turndown approach, which Insall modified by using a less acute angle with the goal of preserving the superior lateral genicular artery[5] (**Fig. 64-3**). The quadriceps tendon is incised at a 45° angle at its most proximal aspect, transecting the rectus femoris tendon near its musculotendinous junction. Combining the medial tibial peel and the quadriceps snip allows lateral mobilization of the extensor mechanism both proximally and distally. This combination is very powerful and can be used to gain adequate exposure in the vast majority of TKA revisions. Even with the combined techniques, no modification of postoperative rehab is needed. If patella eversion remains difficult, you can add a lateral retinacular release or convert the quadriceps incision to a turndown, though this is rarely needed. The quadriceps snip provides excellent exposure

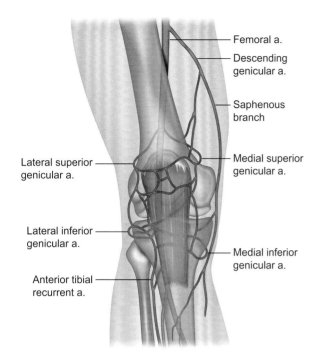

FIGURE 64-1   Blood supply to the patella. Note the contribution of the saphenous branch to the blood supply of the anterior knee.

without having to modify postoperative rehabilitation protocols. We perform a quadriceps snip in nearly all revision cases.

V-Y QUADRICEPS TURNDOWN

The V-Y quadriceps turndown was initially described by Coonse and Adams in 1943 with a distally based inverted V with the apex centered at the proximal limit of the quadriceps tendon[12] (**Fig. 64-4**). One benefit of the V-Y quadriceps turndown is that it allows for lengthening of the quadriceps tendon, reducing tension on the extensor mechanism and increasing postoperative flexion. This is particularly important for stiff or ankylosed knees. The additional flexion may come at a high cost though, as clinical experience has shown subsequent increases in muscle weakness and extensor lag with this technique.[1,13-18] Additionally, the vascular supply to the patella is severely compromised, increasing the risk of avascular necrosis. Scott and Siliki describe taking the lateral limb of the inverted V distally and laterally, creating exposure through the lateral parapatellar scar and taking care to preserve the lateral superior genicular artery.[13] The tendon can be repaired with heavy, nonabsorbable sutures, with attention to recreating the appropriate amount of tension. A good guide is an anatomic approximation that allows

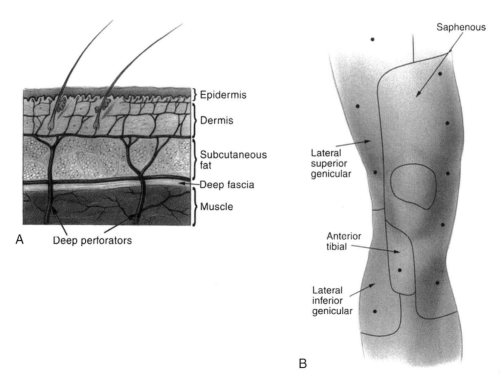

FIGURE 64-2   **A:** Microvascular anatomy of the skin of the thigh. The vessels just superficial to the deep fascia form an anastomosis. The skin blood supply arises from this anastomosis, with little communication in the subcutaneous tissues. The deep perforators supply the anastomosis about the deep fascia. **B:** Areas supplied by the deep vessels (solid circles indicate approximate position of deep perforators). Most of the blood supply comes from the medial side, so when multiple incisions are present the most lateral incision should be utilized. This is more likely to be an "intervascular plane" and thus more likely to heal.

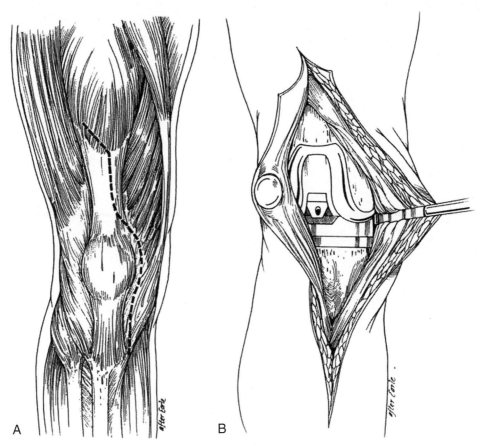

FIGURE 64-3 Quadriceps snip. A medial parapatellar incision is used **(A)**, with further exposure of the knee being obtained by snipping the quadriceps muscle proximally, with extension of the incision laterally **(B)**. A greater degree of exposure will be obtained with a more distal and transverse cut.

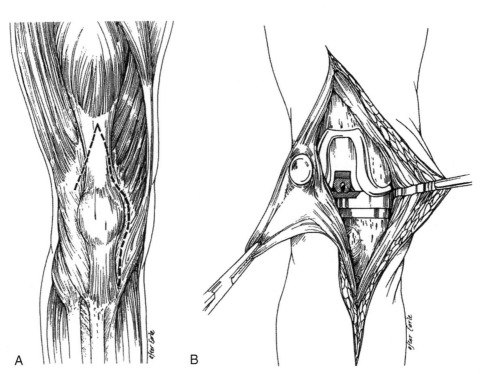

FIGURE 64-4 V-Y turndown. The incision **(A)** and exposure obtained **(B)** with the patella turndown. The quadriceps tendon should be repaired with the use of a nonabsorbable suture and should be protected postoperatively.

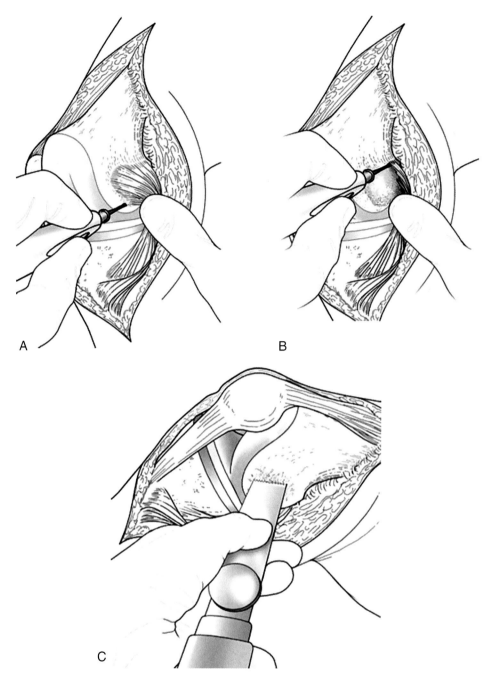

FIGURE 64-5 Femoral peel. Beginning **(A)** and completion **(B)** of release of the medial collateral ligament with cautery. **C:** Using a saw to "freshen up" the bony origins of the MCL insertion site. (Reproduced with permissions from Lavernia C, Contreras JS, Alcerro JC. The peel in total knee revision: exposure in the difficult knee. *Clin Orthop Relat Res*. 2011;469:146-153.)

flexion to 90°. It is imperative to avoid overlengthening of the tendon, as this can lead to extensor lag. Because of these potential complications, especially the extensor lag, the V-Y turndown is mostly historic and is rarely utilized by the current generation of arthroplasty surgeons. Initial rehabilitation protocols called for 2 weeks of postoperative immobilization. Modern practice is for 0° to 30° with active flexion but only passive extension and toe-touch weight-bearing in a knee immobilizer for the first week. After that, patients are encouraged to advance flexion by 10° daily until the maximum passive flexion achieved

intraoperatively is reached. Active extension is commenced at 6 to 8 weeks postoperatively.[19] In our experience, this technique is rarely, if ever, utilized.

EXTENSIVE FEMORAL PEEL

The extensive femoral peel was first described by Windsor and Insall in 1988 and involves complete subperiosteal peel of the femur, including origins of medial and lateral collateral ligaments, representing a "skeletonization" of the distal femur.[20,21] The concern with this extensive release is severe knee instability that may require hinge-type implants.[22,23] Lavernia and Alcerro studied a modified extensive femoral peel using dissection with electrocautery[24] (**Fig. 64-5**). After reconstruction, they use an oscillating saw in a "brushlike fashion" to remove the surface layer of fibrous tissue and cortical bone on the origin and insertion of the ligaments. In 116 revisions with a minimum of 2-year follow-up, they showed improved Knee Society Scores, Hospital for Special Surgery Knee Scores, quality of well-being, and Western Ontario and McMaster Universities Osteoarthritis Index scores. They were able to use a constrained condylar device in most reconstructions. The peel allowed them to avoid major tendon or muscle disruption and the potential complications associated with tibial tubercle osteotomy (TTO). The postoperative protocol involves a knee immobilizer until the patient can perform a straight leg raise without assistance. Physical therapy was started postoperative day 1 with assisted continuous passive range of motion from 0° to 30°. Flexion was gradually increased to 90°, usually by day 3, and maintained here for 8 weeks.

MEDIAL EPICONDYLAR OSTEOTOMY

The medial epicondylar osteotomy can be used to correct soft tissue contractures associated with varus and flexion deformities. Engh popularized this technique, citing the increased exposure of the posterior capsule without extensive ligament stripping.[25] The capsule is incised through a medial arthrotomy and reflected from the medial tibial metaphysis to the mid-coronal plane. The medial epicondyle is osteotomized with the knee flexed to 90°, preserving the adductor magnus tendon and medial collateral ligament insertion sites (**Fig. 64-6**). A cortical bridge is maintained between the osteotomized medial femoral condyle and the anterior femoral bone resection. Posterior displacement of the osteotomy provides access to the posterior compartment, allowing for further releases, including the posteromedial capsule, if necessary. The osteotomy can be repaired with heavy, nonabsorbable sutures, reliably restoring knee stability in the author's experience. As long as this fixation is stable, postoperative rehab does not need to be restricted. Potential downsides of this approach are heterotrophic bone and fibrous union around the osteotomy site and potential fragmentation of the osteotomized segment if it is made too thin.

THE "BANANA PEEL" EXPOSURE

The "banana peel" exposure involves peeling the patellar tendon off the tibial tubercle, leaving lateral and distal tendon and soft tissue hinges to keep the extensor mechanism intact. This prophylactically relieves tension on the extensor mechanism to avoid iatrogenic avulsion and is always combined with a proximal quadriceps snip[4] (**Fig. 64-7**). A standard midline incision is used and extended distally to expose the distal extent of the peel. A medial parapatellar arthrotomy and a quadriceps snip are performed, followed by a careful peel on the patella tendon in a continuous sleeve, which exposes the anterior tibia

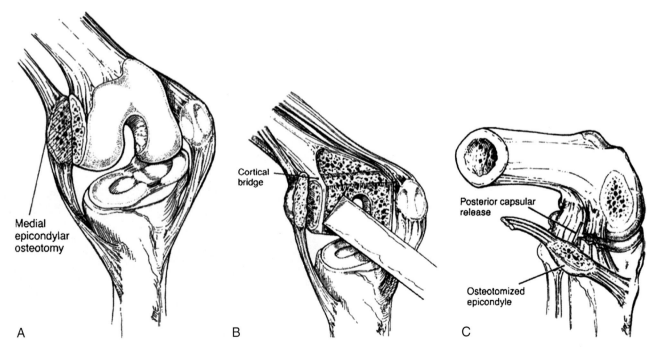

A
B
C

FIGURE 64-6 Medial epicondylar osteotomy. **A:** The osteotomized epicondyle with intact adductor magnus tendon and collateral ligaments is displaced posterior to the medial femoral condyle. Exposure is enhanced by the external rotation and varus angulation of the knee in a flexed position. **B:** A cortical bridge is established between the anterior femoral bone resection and the osteotomized medial femoral epicondyle. Sutures are passed beneath this bridge of cortical bone to anchor the repair of the epicondyle. **C:** The posteromedial capsule, including fibers of the posterior oblique ligament, is released with cautery to fully correct varus deformity and flexion contracture of the knee.

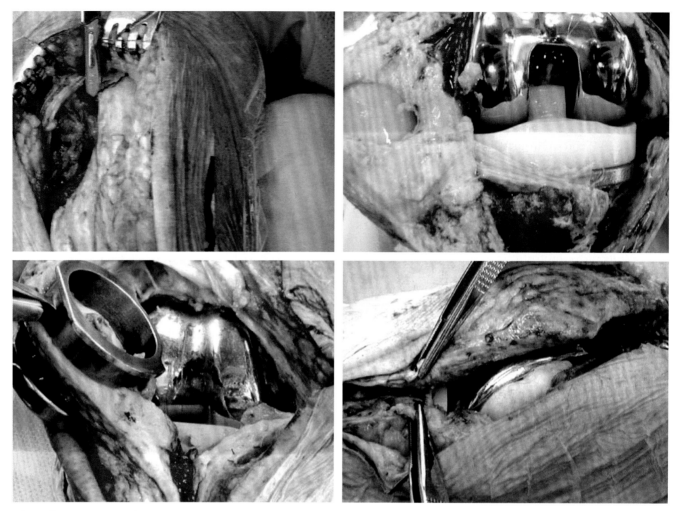

FIGURE 64-7 Banana peel exposure showing the standard quadriceps snip, with exposure of the anterior tibia as the patella is manually everted. Elevation in a single sleeve facilitates closure. (Reproduced with permission from Lahav A, Hofmann AA. The "banana peel" exposure method in revision total knee arthroplasty. *Am J Orthop.* 2007;36:526-529; discussion 529.)

as the patella is manually everted. Eversion of a single sleeve, while maintaining the distal and lateral patella tendon and soft tissue attachments, is vital. Posteromedially, a subperiosteal sleeve is elevated for full exposure of the joint. The advantage of this approach is that it does not involve bony work. Disadvantages include disruption of the extensor mechanism. Lahav and Hofmann retrospectively reviewed 97 patients with a minimum of 2-year follow up, showing no extensor lag and mean ROM of 106°. They reported no patients with pain over the tibial tubercle. This success has not been reproduced in the literature, and in our experience, this technique has never been utilized.

TIBIAL TUBERCLE OSTEOTOMY

TTO is indicated when adequate exposure has not been achieved after a quadriceps snip and extensive medial peel on the tibia. It was originally described by Whiteside in 1990.[26,27] In addition to extensile exposure, TTO allows for access to the intramedullary canal and in some cases

proximal translation of the patellar insertion to mitigate patella baja. Massive tibial osteolysis that may jeopardize fixation is an absolute contraindication to TTO. An 8 to 10 cm bony fragment with minimum thickness of 1 cm proximally is desired. A bony bridge is left proximally to prevent proximal migration of the osteotomized

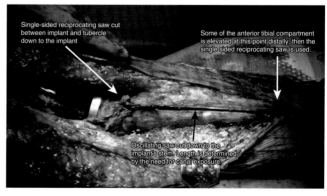

FIGURE 64-8 Description of the different saw cuts used for a tibia tubercle osteotomy.

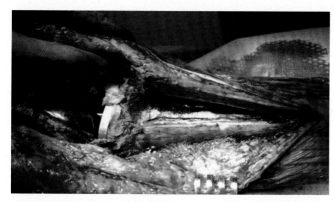

FIGURE 64-9 Broad osteotomes are used to crack the lateral cortex. The blood supply to the tubercle fragment is maintained from the lateral musculature.

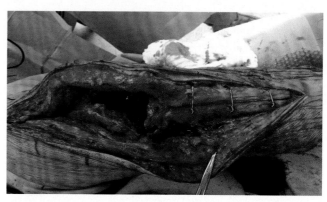

FIGURE 64-11 Closure of the osteotomy is achieved with wires and/or screws.

bone. It is desirable to leave periosteum and soft tissue attachments intact laterally to facilitate osseous healing. (**Figs. 64-8 to 64-11**) This can be achieved by using osteotomes to crack the lateral cortex. At the conclusion of the operation, the osteotomy is fixed with multiple wires and/or screws (▶ Video 64-2). There are data that support not modifying postoperative rehabilitation protocols after TTO.[26,28,29] Some surgeons advocate this approach when there is not any obvious motion at the osteotomy site through a range of motion after fixation. However, given what is at stake if the extensor mechanism is compromised, our opinion is that surgeons should have a low threshold to protect weight-bearing and to limit flexion to 90° if there are any concerns about fixation or anticipated osseous healing. In these cases, we will remove all

restrictions at 6 weeks postoperatively, assuming radiographs show signs of union. Further study is warranted to determine which specific postoperative limitations, if any, are needed after TTO.

SUMMARY

There are many different techniques available for revision TKA. It is important for the surgeon to be aware of the pros and cons of each and to match these with their patient's specific needs. For any exposure, a stepwise approach is essential. Always select the most lateral skin incision if possible and start with the standard medial parapatellar approach. While obtaining wide exposure, it is imperative to beware of patellar tendon avulsion, as disruption of the extensor mechanism is a devastating complication. Débridement of the fibrous tissue in the medial and lateral gutters and suprapatellar pouch allows for improvement visualization, as does an extensive medial peel and externally rotating the tibia. A quadriceps snip combined with extensive medial peel provides adequate exposure in most cases, but a TTO is also a proven option when needed.

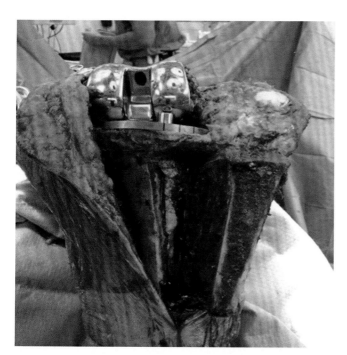

FIGURE 64-10 This osteotomy provides fantastic exposure of the knee joint and exposure of the entire cement mantle in the tibia.

REFERENCES

1. Aglietti P, Windsor RE, Buzzi R, Insall JN. Arthroplasty for the stiff or ankylosed knee. *J Arthroplasty.* 1989;4:1-5.
2. Garbedian S, Sternheim A, Backstein D. Wound healing problems in total knee arthroplasty. *Orthopedics.* 2011;34:e516-e518.
3. Ritter MA, Carr K, Keating EM, Faris PM, Meding JB. Tibial shaft fracture following tibial tubercle osteotomy. *J Arthroplasty.* 1996;11:117-119.
4. Lahav A, Hofmann AA. The "banana peel" exposure method in revision total knee arthroplasty. *Am J Orthop.* 2007;36:526-529; discussion 529.
5. Insall J. *Surgical approaches to the knee.* In: *Insall & Scott Surgery of the Knee.* Philadelphia, PA: Elsevier/Churchill Livingstone; 1984:41-54.
6. Younger AS, Duncan CP, Masri BA. Surgical exposures in revision total knee arthroplasty. *J Am Acad Orthop Surg.* 1998;6:55-64.
7. Callegari PR, Taylor GI, Caddy CM, Minabe T. An anatomic review of the delay phenomenon: I. Experimental studies. *Plast Reconstr Surg.* 1992;89:397-407; discussion 417-418.

8. Long WJ, Wilson CH, Scott SMC, Cushner FD, Scott WN. 15-year experience with soft tissue expansion in total knee arthroplasty. *J Arthroplasty.* 2012;27:362-367.

9. Sharkey PF, Homesley HD, Shastri S, Jacoby SM, Hozack WJ, Rothman RH. Results of revision total knee arthroplasty after exposure of the knee with extensor mechanism tenolysis. *J Arthroplasty.* 2004;19:751-756.

10. Fehring TK, Odum S, Griffin WL, Mason JB. Patella inversion method for exposure in revision total knee arthroplasty. *J Arthroplasty.* 2002;17:101-104.

11. Laskin RS, Riegèr MA. The surgical technique for performing a total knee replacement arthroplasty. *Orthop Clin North Am.* 1989;20:31-48.

12. Coonse K, Adams J. A new operative approach to the knee joint. *Surg Gynecol Obstet.* 1943;77(4):344-347.

13. Scott RD, Siliski JM. The use of a modified V-Y quadricepsplasty during total knee replacement to gain exposure and improve flexion in the ankylosed knee. *Orthopedics.* 1985;8:45-48.

14. Trousdale RT, Hanssen AD, Rand JA, Cahalan TD. V-Y quadricepsplasty in total knee arthroplasty. *Clin Orthop Relat Res.* 1993;286:48-55.

15. Rajgopal A, Ahuja N, Dolai B. Total knee arthroplasty in stiff and ankylosed knees. *J Arthroplasty.* 2005;20:585-590.

16. Tsukamoto N, Miura H, Matsuda S, Mawatari T, Kato H, Iwamoto Y. Functional evaluation of four patients treated with V-Y quadricepsplasty in total knee arthroplasty. *J Orthop Sci.* 2006;11:394-400.

17. Smith PN, Parker DA, Gelinas J, Rorabeck CH, Bourne RB. Radiographic changes in the patella following quadriceps turndown for revision total knee arthroplasty. *J Arthroplasty.* 2004;19:714-719.

18. Barrack RL, Smith P, Munn B, Engh G, Rorabeck C. The Ranawat Award. Comparison of surgical approaches in total knee arthroplasty. *Clin Orthop Relat Res.* 1998;356:16-21.

19. Yuenyongviwat V, Windsor R. *V-Y quadriceps turndown.* In: *Techniques in Revision Hip and Knee Arthroplasty.* Philadelphia, PA: Elsevier Saunders; 2015:45-48.

20. Thomas H, Russell W. Difficult exposure in total knee arthroplasty: the femoral peel. *Curr Orthop Pract.* 2008;19:272-275.

21. Windsor R, Insall J. Exposure in revision total knee arthroplasty: the femoral peel. *Tech Orthop.* 1988;3(2):2-4.

22. Barrack RL. Evolution of the rotating hinge for complex total knee arthroplasty. *Clin Orthop Relat Res.* 2001;392:292-299.

23. Whiteside LA. Ligament balancing in revision total knee arthroplasty. *Clin Orthop Relat Res.* 2004;423:178-185.

24. Lavernia C, Contreras JS, Alcerro JC. The peel in total knee revision: exposure in the difficult knee. *Clin Orthop Relat Res.* 2011;469:146-153.

25. Engh G, McCauley J. *Joint line restoration and flexion-extension balance with revision total knee arthroplasty.* In: *Revision Total Knee Arthroplasty.* Philadelphia, PA: Lippincott Williams & Wilkins;1997:235-251.

26. Whiteside LA. Exposure in difficult total knee arthroplasty using tibial tubercle osteotomy. *Clin Orthop Relat Res.* 1995;321:32-35.

27. Whiteside LA, Ohl MD. Tibial tubercle osteotomy for exposure of the difficult total knee arthroplasty. *Clin Orthop Relat Res.* 1990;260:6-9.

28. Ries MD, Richman JA. Extended tibial tubercle osteotomy in total knee arthroplasty. *J Arthroplasty.* 1996;11:964-967.

29. Chalidis BE, Ries MD. Does repeat tibial tubercle osteotomy or intramedullary extension affect the union rate in revision total knee arthroplasty? A retrospective study of 74 patients. *Acta Orthop.* 2009;80:426-431.

chapter 65

Implant Removal in Revision Total Knee Arthroplasty

Brent A. Lanting, MD, FRCSC, MSc | Steven J. MacDonald, MD, FRCSC

Revision of a total knee replacement is a challenging procedure that is comprised of a number of steps. Achieving a good exposure and removing the components with minimal destruction is a critical aspect of the revision. To achieve a reconstruction that is stable and durable, reconstruction can be best performed if the surgeon understands the objectives of each step and the variety of techniques necessary to achieve good exposure and remove the implants and cement efficiently and safely.

The goal of this chapter is to provide the revision knee surgeon with an organized approach to remove the prior implants and retained cement with minimal trauma to the patient. The chapter will begin by exploring how to expose the joint to gain access to the knee. We will then discuss the range of specific tools and techniques for removal of the femoral, tibial, and patellar components for both cemented and cementless components.

EXPOSURE

To be able to remove the components in an efficient and safe way, a good exposure is critical. The medial parapatellar approach is certainly the workhorse for revision scenarios and can be maximized by performing a complete extensor mechanism tenolysis. To make this approach more extensile, a quadriceps snip or tibial tubercle osteotomy (TTO) can be performed. The turn down, while previously described, is no longer indicated as the quadriceps snip and TTO provide excellent exposure when needed. The decision of exposure techniques such as the TTO or snip should be considered in light of the clinical need. For example, in cases of inadequate exposure with a long cemented tibial component, a TTO may be helpful to address both challenges.

An important concept is developing planes both above and below the quadriceps. After performing the medial parapatellar arthrotomy, a synovectomy should be performed. In particular, aggressive resection of all scar tissues in the lateral gutter as well as the undersurface of the patellar and quadriceps tendons should be performed. The often thickened and fibrosed patellar tendon should be dissected free and mobilized to clearly identify the attachment to the tibia. To maximize the extensor mechanism mobility as well as the exposure of the tibial component, this débridement at the level of the proximal tibia should continue laterally beyond the patellar tendon insertion. After addressing the extensor mechanism, the fibrotic tissue and proliferative synovium can be removed from the lateral gutter by dissecting it from the extensor mechanism using cautery. Resection should proceed until the normal lateral gutter volume has been restored. It is also important to dissect and define the lateral border of the patella to improve patellar mobilization. It may be helpful to remove excess bone lateral to the patellar button to assist with the mobilization of the patella. When there is an extensor scarring, adhesions between the quadriceps and the anterior femur should be broken down, even proximal to the capsule. In rare circumstances, a cobb may be needed to breakdown adhesions of the quadriceps to the anterior femur.

After this aggressive dissection, the patella can be mobilized effectively. If required and possible, the patella is usually readily everted, which allows direct access to the component–bone interfaces of the femur, particularly on the harder to reach lateral side. When eversion is not possible, lateral subluxation is usually sufficient if adequate flexion can be achieved.[1] Although use of a pin in the patellar tendon close to the tibial tubercle to prevent avulsion has been described, it does not remove the possibility of avulsion.

TOOLS

To be able to perform a successful removal of implants and retained cement, the surgeon needs to understand the full range of tools and instruments required as well as which ones are required for the particular revision about to be performed. This includes tools required for cemented or cementless components as well as the cement itself. It is important to understand the surgical team's unique skill set and preferences, as several different instruments and techniques can be applied equally well for the same purpose. The surgeon should have a clear consideration of the steps of the procedure as well as the equipment needed for the primary plan as well as potentially needed adjunct plans. Generic and industry partner revision systems should be considered to achieve successful extraction.

Component-Specific Tools

The majority of revision total knee arthroplasties can be performed successfully with the use of universal extraction devices, which are designed to be applied to a variety of different components. Manufacturer-specific extraction devices may be available and can greatly reduce operative time and effort. Obtaining the operative note for the index procedure can be helpful in determining the implant manufacturer and design as well as in understanding unique challenges of the implant to be removed. At times it may be helpful to discuss with a colleague or industry representative to understand implant features that may not be familiar to the revision surgeon.

Hand and Power Tools

The instruments described in the following subsections should be available during all revision total knee arthroplasties. Their specific use is mentioned briefly in this section and is elaborated on in the sections dealing with femoral, tibial, and patellar component removal.

Osteotomes

Osteotomes are one of the most effective and widely used instruments for component removal. Gently curved osteotomes, straight osteotomes, and flexible and angled osteotomes are available in a variety of widths. These are used at the cement–metal interface to remove the implant and subsequently to remove the cement. Care must be exercised to combat the tendency to damage the softer cancellous bone or pathologic bone either by misdirecting the osteotome or by prying on this soft bone.[2] Ensuring the osteotomes are in good condition as well as ensuring the geometry of the curved osteotome is consistent is helpful.

Power Saw

Power saws can be used in a fashion similar to osteotomes to disrupt the component interface. Used in a similar environment as osteotomes, a range of widths should be available. Thin saw blades are recommended to minimize bone loss, but care should be taken to ensure there is minimal deflection during use. The blade should abut the component surface to minimize bone loss, and irrigation should be considered to avoid thermal damage to the bone. In addition, power saws can be used to readily remove an all-polyethylene component, exposing the underlying cement. For cementless implants, saw blade widths should be appropriate to the unique metal geometries of these constructs, particularly for tibial components where the keel has gaps to allow the saw blades to pass beyond the keel to access the posterior aspect of the tibial plateau. The saw can also be important in cutting through porous metal (such as pegs). It is recommended to be familiar with a range of saw blades for both oscillating and reciprocating applications. Multiple saw blades may be needed and should be available.

Power Burr

A power burr is another critical tool for all revisions. Both metal-cutting and fine pencil tips should be available. These burrs can be used to define the prosthesis–bone or prosthesis–cement interface. Burrs are also useful for removal of residual cement, polyethylene, or sclerotic bone once the implant has been removed. In rare circumstances, a metal-cutting burr may be needed to remove components by sectioning them or cutting off porous aspects of the implant when required. This may include cutting off the stem of the implant in certain circumstances, but this may be conducted more easily with high-speed instruments.

Gigli Saw

Although not commonly used, a Gigli saw can be used to expediently remove well-fixed cemented and cementless femoral components.[1] The Gigli saw is placed at the most proximal edge of the trochlear flange and directed distally and anteriorly. As with other instruments, the saw is kept against the component to minimize bone loss. If the maneuver is performed properly, the saw is in constant contact with the metal prosthesis, resulting in the need for several wires to be available. The distal and posterior femoral component interfaces are more difficult to access using a Gigli saw due to their geometries. For the posterior condyles, a Gigli saw can be used and potentiated by drilling a hole adjacent to the component and directed toward the notch[1] and then passing the wire through this hole. As the Gigli saws break readily, a number of these devices should be available.

High-Speed Instruments

Although metal-cutting burrs can be used, alternative methods for cutting the prosthesis include high-speed cutting tools. The ability to cut the prosthesis is important during revision scenarios such as the need to cut the prosthesis to gain access to well-fixed distal stems or for implants with ingrowth potential. Very rarely, sectioning the implant may be needed. Diamond-tipped wheels can be very helpful in these scenarios and are uniquely helpful when removing well-fixed metal-backed patellar components. Several manufacturers make high-speed tools with metal-cutting tips. These tools should be used with care as they can be destructive of the bone or soft tissues due to their aggressive construct and high-speed nature. Irrigation should also be considered to prevent thermal necrosis of the bone as required. To contain the spread of metal debris, a wet surgical sponge should be placed on the surrounding tissue.

Ultrasonic Tools

The ultrasonic device converts electrical energy to mechanical energy, which can be applied to a specially designed tip.[2] Methylmethacrylate selectively absorbs this energy, which causes the cement to soften and facilitates its removal. The ultrasonic tip provides both tactile and auditory feedback when cortical bone is contacted instead of cement and resists progress of the tip. These features enable ultrasonic tools to be used to safely and selectively remove cement with minimal damage to surrounding bone.[3] While important for revision hip replacements, they are less important during knee arthroplasty revisions, as the surgeon often has direct access to the cement.

REMOVAL OF COMPONENTS

The order in which components should be removed depends, in part, on the amount of exposure that one is able to obtain. In general, it is advised to remove the polyethylene component first. This relaxes the soft tissues and allows for greater exposure of the femoral and tibial components. Prior to the case, it is important to review the device "stickers" rather than operative notes as the operative notes may not have the degree of accuracy needed for surgical plans. Reviewing the implants to understand the characteristics of the polyethylene and if specialized instruments are needed is helpful, especially in scenarios of more constrained constructs. As part of the implant review, understanding when specialized equipment is available and helpful is important. Some systems have extraction tools that thread into the implants, greatly facilitating the surgeon's ability to control and extract the implants. Also, some implants can be dissociated with unique tools that need to be available prior to initiating the surgery. Following polyethylene removal, the femoral component is removed next. Removing the femoral component first allows access to the underlying tibial component and significantly facilitates removal of the tibial component. Care should always be taken not to damage the softer bone exposed by removal of the total knee components by aggressive retraction.

Femoral Component

For both cemented and cementless femoral components, the objectives and principles of removal are the same. Time must be spent to carefully disrupt the entire component interface (prosthesis–bone or prosthesis–cement) while causing minimal bone damage. Failure to completely dissociate the femoral component from the underlying bone before implant extraction can result in significant bone loss or in fracture, making the reconstruction of the knee very challenging.[4]

To remove the femoral component, the anterior, medial, and lateral margins of the component should be débrided of all soft tissues. Once the interfaces are adequately visualized, a straight or curved narrow osteotome can be used to debond the implant from the underlying bone or cement (**Fig. 65-1**). It is important to protect the softer cancellous bone under the implant by carefully angling the osteotome toward the metal prosthesis at all

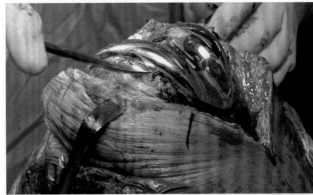
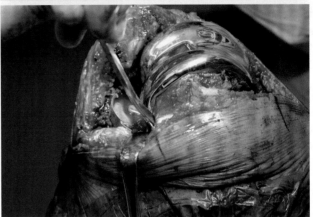

FIGURE 65-1 Intraoperative photographs showing femoral component removal with an osteotome.

times. This can be achieved by using a curved osteotome angled toward the implant or the bevel directed toward the bone. A curved osteotome is typically the best instrument to disrupt the fixation of the posterior condyle either through the notch if open or from the lateral or medial aspect of the knee as appropriate.

A power saw equipped with a thin blade may be used in place of osteotomes and in many cases will actually be more protective of the underlying host bone than can be achieved with osteotomes. As with the osteotome, the saw blade must be kept adjacent to the prosthesis at all times, and the operator must carefully resist the tendency for the saw blade to deflect into the soft bone (**Fig. 65-2**). Thin saw blades remove less bone but are more prone to deflection. The use of osteotomes may still be necessary as saw blades do not work well adjacent to changes in implant geometry such as pegs or abrupt angular changes and in particular at the location of the posterior condyles.

Another technique for femoral component removal has been described using a Gigli saw, as described previously. Angling the saw anteriorly ensures contact with the prosthesis at all times, which minimizes the amount of bone resected. The posterior condylar interfaces are disrupted with a combination of the Gigli saw and osteotomes.

When all of the interfaces have been adequately disrupted, the femoral component can be removed by impact loading through a universal or component-specific

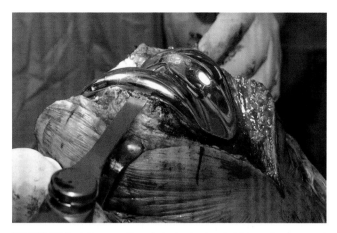

FIGURE 65-2 Intraoperative photograph showing femoral component removal with an oscillating saw.

instrument. If a cemented central stem is present, the stem often debonds from the cement, which allows extraction of the component and stems with minimal exertion. The remaining cement column can then be removed separately.[4] In situations where the stem does not disengage from the bone, care must be exercised to prevent a femoral fracture or severe bone damage. To directly access the stem–cement or stem–bone interface, it may be necessary to cut the prosthesis free from the stem with a metal-cutting high-speed saw either through the box or from the medial or lateral distal aspect of the knee.[4] The majority of the femoral component with its disrupted interfaces can then easily be removed, leaving the well-fixed stem behind. The stem can then be extracted by direct disruption of its interface by using instruments such as a fine-tipped burr, ultrasonic tools, or small osteotomes. As most stemmed constructs are modular, prior knowledge of the unique features of the implant being removed may be important. For example, some modular junctions are connected with a bolt that can be accessed through the notch using a component-specific screwdriver.[5] The ability to disengage the stem potentiates removal of the femoral articular component and subsequent focus on the well-fixed stem.

The techniques and instruments described earlier may be applied equally well to both cemented and uncemented femoral components to disrupt either the prosthesis–cement or prosthesis–bone interface. Although an uncemented porous stem is more likely to require a focused disruption of the stem–bone interface, removal requires that the prosthesis be cut free from the stem with a metal-cutting high-speed instrument, which allows direct access to the bone ingrown–stem interface in a similar manner as described for cemented stems.

In situations where a cone is used, the femoral component can be removed in a similar fashion as described above. However, unique to a revision with a cone, the interface may not be bone–cement implant, but cone–cement implant. In these cases, either metal–cement

interface can be debonded using a combination of osteotomes or saws.

Once the femoral component is removed, the cone implant should then be carefully assessed. If the implant is well ingrown with an appropriate diameter canal, it may be appropriate to retain it in aseptic scenarios and to build the reconstruction on this stable cone. If this is not appropriate, use of a fine pencil tip burr and osteotomes may be required to remove the porous metal cone by disrupting the implant–bone interface.[5] Certain porous cones can have the diameter increased by use of a metal-cutting burr to enable a revision implant to be used if the introitus is too restrictive.

However, the patient may need a distal femoral replacement if removal of a well-ingrown cone and complex femoral components would result in an incompetent distal femur.

Tibial Component

Removal of well-fixed tibial components tends to be somewhat easier than removal of well-fixed femoral components due to the simpler geometry of the tibial tray. This is occasionally balanced by the increased challenge in access to the posterolateral aspect of the tibia as well as the challenges in clearing the femoral condyles. The principles of adequate exposure to gain access to the component interfaces and subsequent disruption of those interfaces before any attempt at removal to minimize bone loss or fracture are the same.

As with the femoral component, the cement–implant interfaces can efficiently be disrupted using osteotomes (**Fig. 65-3**) or a power saw (**Fig. 65-4**) or both. Although challenging laterally, the periphery of the component interface should initially be defined as completely as the exposure allows to safely identifying the cement–implant interface. Disruption of this interface should proceed with caution to maintain the instrument adjacent to the component to minimize the amount of bone resected. The

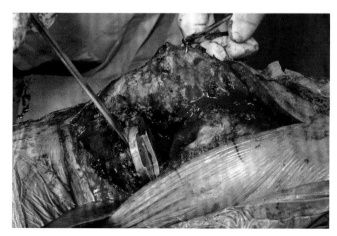

FIGURE 65-3 Intraoperative photograph showing the use of straight osteotomes for tibial component removal.

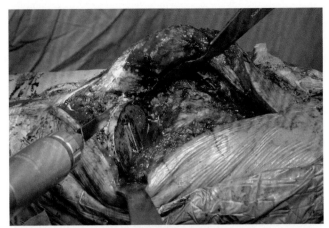

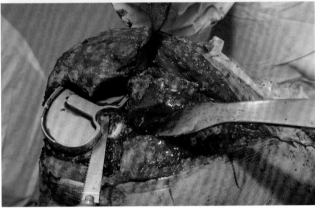

FIGURE 65-4 Intraoperative photographs showing removal of a tibial component with reciprocating saw.

most reproducible technique to debond the posterolateral corner is to carefully use an oscillating saw having the blade come from the posteromedial corner and advancing slowly laterally while protecting the posterior neurovascular structure with a retractor (**Fig. 65-4**). If one chooses to use osteotomes, he/she should also proceed in a medial to lateral direction to facilitate disruption of the less accessible lateral interface, both anterior and posterior to the central stem. At all times, the patellar tendon must be protected.

The "stacked" osteotome technique can be utilized to lift the prosthesis away from the bone surface (A). Multiple osteotomes are introduced into the interface on top of one another to gradually lift the implant. A broad osteotome should be used closest to bone to help distribute the forces over a larger surface area. However, the osteotomes should not be used to lever against the tibial plateau, as this may crush the underlying cancellous bone. The challenge with this technique is that often the surgeon is dealing with deficient and osteolytic bone and it can be very difficult to not inadvertently crush the bone. Once sufficiently loosened, the prosthesis allows easy removal with a bone tamp. Notably, care should be taken to access the area posterior to the fins of the tibial component and behind the stem. Finally, if an all-polyethylene component is in place, the tibial component

can be removed by using an oscillating saw at the poly-ethylene–cement interface, through the post and fins with subsequent removal of the cement.

Cemented central stems on the tibial prostheses are designed to debond from the surrounding cement when a reasonable amount of force is applied. If the circumstance should arise in which the stem does not debond from the cement without excessive force, despite adequate disruption of the tibial plateau interface, then the stem should be cut free from the tibial tray with a high-speed cutting device to allow direct access to the stem interface.[4]

Uncemented tibial components often have additional fixation with screws, and component-specific screwdrivers should be available. Bone-ingrown tibial components that cannot be removed with reasonable force should be approached in the same manner as well-fixed cemented stems by cutting the stem or keel free of the prosthesis and directly disrupting this interface. In implants with a porous keel, the implant may have areas designed to facilitate access to and enable the expedient disengagement of the tray from the porous keel. The keel then can be removed using a high-speed pencil tip burr.

As discussed for femoral cones, well-fixed tibial cones may be retained once the tibial component is removed. The aseptic cone should then be assessed if appropriate to retain for the reconstruction or removed. If the decision is to remove the cone, pencil tip burrs and osteotomes can facilitate its extraction. Canoe or "u"-curved osteotomes and narrow osteotomes may be helpful.

After removal of the tibial articular component, removal of the cone and stem can then be facilitated by accessing the cone–bone or cone–cement interface in situations of cementless or cemented constructs, respectively. Rarely, a proximal tibial replacement may also be necessary due to incompetent bone once tibial components are removed.

Patellar Component

The majority of the time in revision total knee arthroplasty cases, the patellar component does not need to be revised. However, removal of a well-fixed patella may be indicated in cases of malposition, maltracking, or infection. If removal is deemed indicated, this should be approached with care to avoid compromise of the extensor mechanism. The resurfaced patella is thin, and often the bone is soft. This is complicated by the fact that removal of the anchoring pegs can further compromise the bone of the patella. Poor technique risks removal of too much bone or fracture of the patella.[4] If the component is well-fixed and there is only cold-flow deformation of the polyethylene, then the patella should be retained when possible. If removal is required, then a careful and meticulous technique as outlined for the femoral and tibial components should be used. Débridement of the peripatellar soft tissue is performed to gain access to the prosthetic interface. If the component is made entirely of polyethylene, it is preferred to use an oscillating saw at the component–cement interface, erring toward slight polyethylene retention. Any excess polyethylene, the pegs and cement can then directly be accessed and removed with a fine-tipped burr. Use of osteotomes on the patella should be used with extreme caution and are best normally avoided.

Metal-backed patellar components often involve polyethylene wear and dissociation from the underlying well-fixed metal plate.[6] Use of an osteotome to disrupt the bone/metal interface or to pry the patellar component is likely to be ineffective when the fixation pegs are ingrown with bone and are bone destructive and increase the probability of creating an iatrogenic fracture. A simple technique has been described in which the pegs are cut free from the prosthetic plate using a metal-cutting wheel.[7] After adequate peripatellar soft-tissue débridement and definition of the bone–prosthesis interface, a metal-cutting circular saw is introduced circumferentially around the patella. This frees the bone–prosthesis interface as well as the peg–plate connection, and the well-fixed pegs are subsequently removed with a fine-tipped burr. Use of a wet sponge is recommended to reduce metal debris deposition.

REMOVAL OF CEMENT

The surgeon can choose to remove the cement as part of the bone preparation for the revision or fully remove the cement prior to bone preparation. If prior to bone preparation, surface cement can be removed with straight osteotomes or a rongeur, with minimal loss of underlying bone. Alternatively, power burrs can be used. On rare occasion, small pockets of extremely well-fixed cement, particularly in the tibia, can be retained at the time of aseptic revision.

When cement is present in the canals (femoral or tibial), removal techniques utilizing splitter osteotomes, straight osteotomes, and gouges can be used. Backward-directed gouges (crochet hooks) can also be used, however, with great caution as cortical disruption can occur. Ideally osteotomes are used to radially split the cement rather than at the bone–cement interface due to the potential

destruction of the softer bone. Ultrasonic tools are also very effective, particularly for removal of any well-fixed diaphyseal cement plugs. Care should be exercised to avoid perforation, particularly of the thin tibial cortices. Replacement of a patellar component may be required to optimize quadriceps function, but often it is not required. Revising a patellar button is technically challenging and risks fracturing the patella or compromising the fragile blood supply to the patella.

CONCLUSION

Surgeons about to embark on a revision knee replacement need to understand the surgical objectives as well as the surgical techniques, instruments, and tools needed prior to beginning the surgery. Having a good exposure is critical to the implant extraction and subsequent reconstruction of the knee. Efficient implant and cement removal needs to be performed with minimal soft tissue or bone damage. Knowing when alternative approaches and instruments are needed and how to perform them is also mandatory as revision knee arthroplasty often requires alternate plans beyond the initial approach. Only good exposure and minimally destructive implant extraction enable the surgeon to begin the reconstruction for a stable and durable total knee revision.

REFERENCES

1. Fehring TK, Odum S, Griffin WL, Mason JB. Patellar inversion method for exposure in revision total knee arthroplasty. *J Arthroplasty*. 2002;17:101-104.
2. Masri BA, Mitchell PA, Duncan CP. Removal of solidly fixed implants during revision hip and knee arthroplasty. *J Am Acad Orthop Surg*. 2005;13(1):18-27.
3. Klapper RC, Caillouette JT, Callaghan JJ, Hozack WJ. Ultrasonic technology in revision joint arthroplasty. *Clin Orthop Relat Res*. 1992;285:147-154.
4. Mason JB, Fehring TK. Removing well-fixed total knee arthroplasty implants. *Clin Orthop Relat Res*. 2006;446:76-82.
5. Martin JR, Watters TS, Levy DL, Jennings JM, Dennis DA. Removing a well-fixed femoral sleeve during revision total knee arthroplasty. *Arthroplasty Today*. 2016;2(4):171-175.
6. Bayley JC, Scott RD, Ewald FC, Holmes GB Jr. Failure of the metal-backed patellar component after total knee replacement. *J Bone Joint Surg Am*. 1988;70:668-674.
7. Dennis DA. Removal of well-fixed cementless metal-backed patellar components. *J Arthroplasty*. 1992;7(2):217-220.

chapter 66

Implant Selection in Revision Total Knee Arthroplasty

Douglas A. Dennis, MD | Jacob M. Elkins, MD, PhD

INTRODUCTION

Total knee arthroplasty (TKA) is one of the most successful and commonly performed orthopedic procedures. Despite its success, failures do occur. While failure mechanisms have varied based on the era of TKA, aseptic prosthetic loosening, infection, and instability have been predominate.[1] Additional failure mechanisms have included periprosthetic fracture, arthrofibrosis, polyethylene wear, component malposition, and extensor mechanism failure. Infection is typically the most common cause of failure for early (less than 2 years), while aseptic loosening dominates failure modalities for late revisions.[2] While revision TKA is the prescribed treatment for the majority of TKA failures, the specifics of the revision procedure and required prosthetic device must be carefully tailored to the individual circumstances of each patient.

In general, when performing revision TKA, the use of implants specifically designed for revision TKA is preferred as they have been shown to reduce the incidence for re-revision. Bugbee et al[3] compared outcomes of three groups of revision TKA patients. Group 1 consisted of revisions performed using primary TKA implants; group 2 consisted of revisions performed with modified primary components; and the final group consisted of revisions using specially designed revision implants. At a mean follow-up duration of 7 years, the re-revision rates of the three groups were 25%, 14%, and 6%. The scope of available revision implants is broad and continuing to expand. Correct selection of the appropriate implant is paramount to maximize the success of revision TKA.

PREOPERATIVE CLINICAL ASSESSMENT

An extensive preoperative patient evaluation is necessary to improve the outcome of revision TKA. This includes performing a thorough history taking and physical examination, laboratory assessment, and critical review of radiographs. Preoperative determination of the cause of the failed TKA is critical. Success rates of revision TKA procedures have clearly been unfavorable if the cause of failure is not identified preoperatively.[1,4] Infection, Charcot arthropathy, neuromuscular disease, or significant preoperative medical conditions which may contribute to adverse outcomes should be addressed preoperatively.

Knowledge of previous surgical procedures and the prosthetic devices implanted is necessary. Review of the previous surgical approach, soft-tissue releases performed, and the size and type of prosthetic components implanted enhance the likelihood of a successful revision procedure.

Clinical examination includes the assessment of range of motion, ligamentous stability, lower limb alignment, extensor mechanism integrity, and patellofemoral tracking. Evaluation of the hip and ankle to assess for any factors contributing to overall limb alignment is mandatory. Other causes of limb pain, such as vascular insufficiency, hip disease, and radicular pain should be evaluated and addressed before revision arthroplasty.

Ultimately, the final choice of revision implants will be dictated by the specific mode of failure of the previous construct.

Preoperative Assessment of the Existing Implant Design

Preoperative assessment of the existing implant aids the surgeon in selecting the appropriate revision implant. The revision total knee surgeon will encounter patients implanted with a myriad of different prosthetic devices. Some revision TKA procedures involve revising only a portion of the existing implant, and thorough knowledge of the implant system in place is necessary to prepare adequately for these cases. A thorough knowledge of the implant type with available modularity and revision options for the implant in place is necessary. In addition, awareness of the specific implant design in place allows the surgeon to order implant-specific extraction devices, should these be indicated. If the previous arthroplasty was performed by another surgeon, the operative note and purchasing order should be obtained to verify implant type and size.

INDICATIONS FOR REVISION TKA

Instability

Instability remains one of the most common causes leading to revision to primary and revision TKA.[1] As outlined by Vince et al,[5] there are seven causes of knee instability following TKA: (1) component loosening, (2) bone loss, (3) prosthetic breakage, (4) errors in component size or position, (5) fracture, (6) wear, and (7) collateral ligament failure. The authors emphasized that only incompetency of the collateral ligaments typically requires revision with an increased-constraint implant.

There are four recognized patterns of instability: recurvatum, varus–valgus (mediolateral or coronal), flexion, and global. The treatment for each frequently differs and is discussed below.

Recurvatum is the rarest form of instability[6] and may be the most challenging to properly treat. In fact, it has been argued that the best treatment for recurvatum is prevention, as the deformity seldom develops following knee replacement except in situations of neuromuscular dysfunction.[7] Intraoperatively, either an excessive extension gap or collateral ligament instability[8] may result in knee hyperextension. Recurvatum deformity in the preoperative patient is typically due to substantial quadriceps deficiency, frequently from neuromuscular disorders (classically poliomyelitis[9]), but may also be seen secondary to spinal stenosis, in patients with a fixed valgus deformity with a contracted iliotibial band, or associated with rheumatoid arthritis with marked collateral ligamentous laxity.[8] With quadriceps weakness, the knee displays compensatory hyperextension to stabilize the limb. This mechanism may also result in progressive recurvatum deformity following primary or revision TKA. Primary arthroplasty in patients with recurvatum deformity and quadriceps weakness should be approached with caution. One advocated surgical technique includes underresection of the distal femur, resulting in a deliberate slight flexion contracture.[7] A second surgical technique, recommended by Krackow and Weiss,[6] is to advance the femoral attachments of the collateral ligaments proximally, thereby attempting to recreate the normal tensioning effect of the collaterals during knee extension. Recurvatum presents with substantial treatment difficulty during revision TKA. Deformity secondary to true paralysis of the quadriceps is often best treated with arthrodesis rather than arthroplasty.[5] Arthroplasty treatment in the setting of quadriceps weakness frequently requires the use of rotating hinged constraint[9-11]; however, there is concern about excessive forces imposed with a hyperextension stop, potentially leading to early implant failure,[5] and a "three-step" revision arthroplasty technique has been advocated[5,12] which involves reestablishing the tibial platform, then stabilizing the knee in flexion, followed by stabilization in extension.

Instability in the coronal plane (varus–valgus instability) is a much more commonly encountered clinical entity following primary TKA. This is typically due to ligament imbalance, component malpositioning, excessive bone loss, or component failure. When performing a clinical assessment of knee balance, it is important to examine the knee in both extension and flexion. As varus–valgus instability is often associated with preoperative deformity, it is important to analyze the original preoperative imaging studies. Intraoperatively, technical errors in ligament balancing, asymmetric bone resection, iatrogenic ligament injury may all lead to an unstable knee in the coronal plane. Postoperative attenuation of ligamentous soft tissues may result in a delayed diagnosis.

Flexion instability is another commonly encountered complication following primary TKA, where laxity is felt to be due to an excessively loose flexion gap. Flexion instability has historically been associated with the use of cruciate-retaining (CL) components[13] and may have been underdiagnosed in patients with this construct.[7] This pattern of instability may be symmetric involving both the medial and lateral aspects of the flexion gap or asymmetric, often associated with malrotation of the femoral component. Patients will typically complain of pain while navigating stairs (especially descent), have point tenderness over the pes anserinus bursa, have a positive posterior drawer test (or lag test), and yet demonstrate excellent flexion upon range-of-motion testing.[5] Flexion instability may manifest with the knee positioned in 90° of flexion or in mid-flexion. As intuited from the descriptive title of this clinical complication, mid-flexion instability occurs at intermediate ranges of knee flexion between extension and 90°, with the knee perceived to be otherwise stable.

There is a paucity of outcome studies following revision arthroplasty for TKA instability. Functional improvement has been demonstrated to improve following revision for instability.[14] There are a few investigations which report good outcomes following revision of CL TKA to posterior-stabilized TKA.[13,15,16] However, the specific surgical treatment for instability must be carefully chosen. For example, polyethylene liner exchange alone has been reported to have a high incidence of postrevision failure.[13,16,17]

Bone Loss

Most of the causes of TKA failure will result in some degree of pathologic bone loss, whether it be from infection, osteolysis, osteonecrosis, aseptic loosening, stress shielding, or mechanical failure.[18] The management of bone loss in TKA is dictated by the extent and location of bone deficiency. In revision TKA, significant bone loss is often encountered, and the extent is usually more than preoperative radiographs would indicate.

While preoperative radiographs may provide some clues as to the extent of bone defect, accurate determination of bone deficiency typically occurs during revision TKA after the previous components have been removed, as the removal of well-fixed implants may accentuate the preoperative bone loss.

Infection

Infection following TKA is a devastating complication. As previously stated, it is the most common cause of early TKA failure, and one of the more common reasons for revision TKA at all time points.[1] Treatment for infection is nearly universally surgical. While acute infections may be appropriately treated with irrigation, débridement, and polyethylene liner exchange, this treatment strategy is inappropriate for more chronic infections. For these chronic infections, there remains no clear consensus supporting treatment with single- or two-stage revisions. Two-stage revision procedures typically employ the use of high-dose antibiotic-impregnated bone cement as part of either a static or articulating spacer. Articulating spacers are typically either fashioned using primary TKA components with a liberal use of antibiotic cement or with the use of systems which allow for molded acrylic implants. During both single- and two-stage procedures, preservation of bone stock is of paramount importance for future reconstructive efforts. In general, implant selection following eradication of infection in TKA is similar as for other indications for revision TKA.

PRINCIPLES OF IMPLANT SELECTION IN REVISION TKA

General Principles

Although the principles of revision TKA are similar to those of primary arthroplasty, numerous additional difficulties are often encountered, including soft-tissue scarring, bone loss, flexion–extension gap imbalance, ligamentous instability, and disturbance of the anatomic joint line. To deal with these difficulties, use of a revision implant system, which includes various levels of prosthetic constraint, augmentations, and diaphysis-engaging stems, is imperative.[3] The surgeon's experience with the implant design system selected is paramount in ensuring the success of the revision arthroplasty.

In choosing a revision implant system, the surgeon must consider multiple variables. The coronal and sagittal geometry of the implant must be appropriate to provide proper kinematic function. Prostheses with increasing levels of constraint, ranging from posterior cruciate retention to posterior cruciate substitution, varus–valgus constraint, and hinged designs must be available. A vast array of implant designs is available which may have differences in eventual kinematic function. For example, cam-and-post mechanisms of posterior cruciate–substituting (PS) designs vary widely in size, shape, and position of the cam and post in addition to the degree of flexion at which cam-post engagement occurs. These differences are reflected in variable levels of implant performance. The locking mechanism for polyethylene bearing fixation to the tibial tray should be evaluated. A thorough knowledge of each implant type allows the surgeon to choose the appropriate implant for each individual patient. Because of the complexity of each procedure, no single implant type can be used for all cases.

Single-Component Revision

In revision TKA, isolated single-component revision is typically reserved for situations of polyethylene liner exchange or patellar revision. Isolated polyethylene exchange has demonstrated good short-term success when performed for wear and early osteolysis. Griffin et al[19] reported on the short-term outcomes following isolated polyethylene exchange in 68 press-fit condylar TKAs (PFC; DePuy Synthes, J&J, Warsaw, IN). At a minimum of 24 months, there were 16% failures, the majority being due to aseptic loosening; however, 97% of subjects in this study did not demonstrate any perceivable progression of osteolytic lesions. There is some evidence to suggest that isolated polyethylene exchange for severe wear, however, is fraught with complications.[20] Furthermore, isolated polyethylene liner exchange for reasons other than wear are frequently associated with poor outcomes. Babis et al[17] demonstrated particularly poor outcomes of isolated polyethylene exchange in the setting of knee stiffness. All patients in this study where either severely painful or required revision at a mean follow-up of 4.2 years. Brooks et al[21] reported nearly a 30% failure rate for isolated polyethylene exchange for situations of knee instability. Additionally, it appears that time to revision plays a role in the success of isolated polyethylene exchange. Willson et al[22] demonstrated that patients with an isolated polyethylene exchange within 3 years of the primary procedure were 3.8 times more likely to undergo re-revision than patients with exchange occurring more than 3 years after the index procedure.

LEVELS OF CONSTRAINT IN REVISION TKA

Posterior Cruciate–Retaining Revision TKA

In broad terms, cruciate-retaining (CR) implants provide for the least amount of mechanical constraint in TKA. Their use in revision TKA is limited and requires a surgeon skilled in appropriate balance of the posterior cruciate ligament (PCL). Preoperative assessment of both flexion and extension stability and the competence of the PCL is essential to the use of this type of implant. Principles of posterior cruciate retention are the same in revision TKA as in primary TKA. If present, the PCL may be retained if the operative surgeon can achieve flexion and extension balance with maintenance and competence of the PCL and restoration of the anatomic joint line. Advantages of the use of CR designs in revision knee arthroplasty are the preservation of bone stock and the theoretic advantages for retention of the PCL found in primary TKA. Disadvantages of the use of CR designs are the difficulty of balancing the PCL, restoring the joint line to its anatomic position, and obtaining adequate flexion stability in revision cases in which the competency of the existing PCL may be difficult to evaluate. Therefore, retaining or using a CR implant at the time of revision TKA is infrequently indicated. One possible indication would

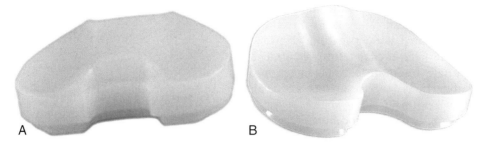

FIGURE 66-1 Standard **(A)** and ultracongruent **(B)** polyethylene inserts.

be for a simple isolated polyethylene exchange (which, as described above, already has a very narrow range of indication) in the setting of a well-functioning CR knee with an intact PCL. The PCL is frequently observed to be attenuated or grossly absent at the time of revision TKA, which necessitates the conversion to a cruciate-substituting construct. Of particular note, patients with inflammatory arthritis such as rheumatoid arthritis have demonstrated higher rates of complications following CR TKA, and such implants should be utilized with caution in this population in the revision setting.[23]

Considering the increased difficulty of determining PCL integrity (continuity, tension, and histologic damage) in revision TKA cases, surgeons favoring avoidance of conversion to a PCL-substituting design (cam and post) have utilized ultracongruent polyethylene inserts to enhance sagittal-plane stability[24] (**Fig. 66-1**). **While medial pivot designs have been utilized in revision TKA, meaningful reports documenting their clinical value in revision TKA is lacking in the literature.**

Posterior Cruciate–Substituting Revision TKA

PS devices remain the authors' implant choice for the majority of revision TKA cases. Advantages of these designs include reliable substitution for an absent or incompetent PCL, easier correction of deformity, increased flexion stability, and increased range of motion[25,26] secondary to forced posterior femoral rollback. This can be beneficial in those cases in which preoperative stiffness is problematic. PS TKA designs incorporate a cam-and-post mechanism to enhance flexion stability and posterior femoral rollback. There are multiple types of cam-and-post mechanisms available that differ in post size (height and width), shape, and sagittal-plane position. As mentioned earlier, these design variances are reflected in differing patterns of kinematic function. The surgeon must be aware of these differences and select a design that optimizes patient function while providing long-term durability. Historically, in the most commonly implanted PS designs, the cam and post do not engage until approximately 70° of knee flexion.[27] Therefore, the cam and post are not engaged during lesser flexion activities such as walking. Other PS TKA designs allow cam-and-post

engagement as early as 30° of knee flexion. Advocates of these designs report earlier posterior femoral rollback and enhanced quadriceps function due to an increased quadriceps lever arm.[28] Polyethylene post wear in traditional PS TKA designs has been limited. It is not yet known if post wear will become problematic in designs that permit earlier cam-post engagement.

Potential problems encountered with use of PS TKA implants include posterior dislocation of the cam relative to the post,[29,30] intercondylar fracture due to increased bone resection,[31] polyethylene post wear or fracture,[32,33] and an increased incidence of patellar clunk syndrome.[34,35] While mechanically enhancing flexion stability, the surgeon must still strictly adhere to the principle of obtaining flexion–extension gap balance to lessen the risk of dislocation. The risk of femoral condylar fracture is typically increased in the multiply revised TKA in which excessive distal femoral bone resection has previously been performed or in cases with substantial distal femoral osteolysis. The risk of condylar fracture is greatest medially because the medial metaphyseal contour transitions more abruptly to the diaphysis than the lateral contour. Because of this, the amount of bone remaining at the proximal margin of the intercondylar notch resection required for PS TKA designs is less medially. **The risk of condylar fracture is enhanced in smaller subjects with reduced bone mass and those with significant osteopenia or osteolysis. This is of particular importance in certain TKA designs in which the intercondylar box size is not proportionally reduced with smaller implant sizes.**

Zingde et al[36] analyzed the *in vivo* cam-post kinematics of both fixed and mobile-bearing PS designs using video fluoroscopy. In mobile-bearing designs, they observed the polyethylene insert rotates axially in accord with the rotating femur, maintaining central cam-post contact. This phenomenon was often not observed in the fixed-bearing TKAs. If femoral–tibial axial rotation occurred in fixed-bearing designs, eccentric contact of the cam on the post was seen, typically observed on the posteromedial aspect of the post. This may account for the eccentric wear observed on retrievals of fixed-bearing PS TKA. Excessive post wear can result in post fracture. Post fracture has been most commonly observed in cases associated with significant instability and with use of highly crosslinked polyethylene[37,38] (**Fig. 66-2**).

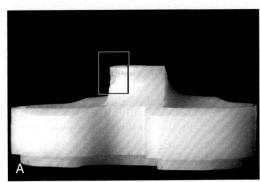
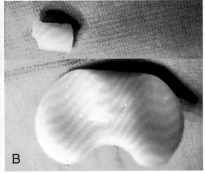

FIGURE 66-2 **A:** Wear is identified on the posteromedial aspect of the polyethylene post secondary to cam-post engagement. In some situations, this can result in further damage to the post mechanism, eventually causing fracture of the post **(B)**.

Although the incidence of patellar clunk syndrome has been higher in PS TKA, the incidence is clearly design related. Designs with a more "boxy" (rectangular) sagittal geometry and those with a higher (more proximal) margin of the intercondylar box are at greater risk. Martin et al[39] evaluated the incidence of patellar crepitus in a large series of two different modern PS TKA designs at 2 years postoperatively (1109 PFC Sigma; 600 Attune, Depuy Synthes, Warsaw, IN). The crepitus incidence was 9.4% in those implanted with the PFC Sigma design versus 0.83% in the Attune cohort.

Last, one must realize that traditional PS TKA designs do not provide stability in the presence of varus or valgus loads and therefore do not provide stability in cases of advanced collateral ligamentous laxity or loss. Varus–valgus constrained TKA devices must be considered in these cases.

Varus/Valgus Constrained TKA

The next level of constraint in revision TKA design is the unlinked varus–valgus constrained implant. These implants provide markedly more varus/valgus and rotational constraint than do traditional PS designs. These implants typically provide for a deeper femoral intercondylar box and a correspondingly taller polyethylene post which is often reinforced with a metal peg. The tighter fit between the post and box provides coronal stability in the setting of collateral ligament injury or laxity (**Fig. 66-3**). However, this tighter conformity may result in eventual failure of the post-cam mechanism in the setting of complete incompetency of the medial collateral ligament (MCL).[40] Another disadvantage of a varus–valgus constrained implant is the potential for increased interfacial strain due to increased implant constraint, leading

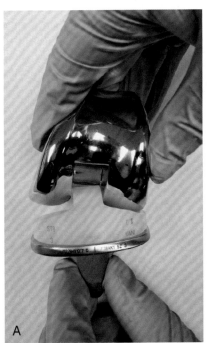
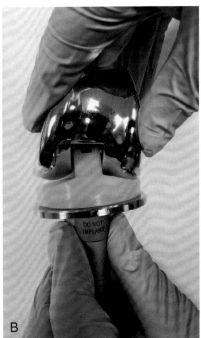

FIGURE 66-3 Differences between a standard posterior-stabilized polyethylene insert **(A)** and a varus/valgus constrained insert **(B)**. The varus/valgus stabilized insert is taller, allowing for peripheral engagement of the post with the box, increasing coronal plane stability.

to fixation failure. This mechanical stress can potentially be lessened with the use of mobile-bearing designs. Experimentally, the use of a mobile-bearing prosthesis has been demonstrated to reduce proximal tibial strain by as much as 73%.[41] While mid-term clinical and radiographic results of mobile-bearing revision TKA appears promising,[42] longer-term follow-up is required to further distinguish actualized benefits of mobile-bearing technology as regards to polyethylene wear, reduced interfacial stresses, and cam-post longevity.

Linked Hinge Constrained TKA

The linked hinge design represents the most constrained total knee implant. Curiously, the first hinged TKA was performed over 125 years ago, when Themistocles Gluck implanted a hinged and diaphyseal-engaging-stemmed ivory total knee implant in a 17-year-old girl inflicted with tuberculosis.[43] This design was remarkably similar to early linked hinged TKAs designed in the latter half of the 20th century such as the Stanmore, Walldius, Guepar, and Herbert devices. With linked constrained devices, the femoral and tibial components are linked, typically via an intercondylar locking pin. In the authors' practice, the use of these devices is uncommon and limited to patients with total MCL loss, severe flexion instability, uncontrolled hyperextension deformities, and massive bone loss from tumor resection or comminuted supracondylar femoral fractures.

Linked hinge designs are often excessively constrained and have the same problems (premature polyethylene wear and prosthetic loosening) as unlinked constrained devices. Early linked hinge implants allowed no rotational laxity and failed prematurely due to component loosening.[44-46] Most modern hinged designs incorporate a mobile polyethylene bearing that permits rotation and lessens loads to both the polyethylene bearing and the fixation interface. However, the early clinical results of mobile-bearing linked revision TKAs were disappointing,[47-49] further limiting their widespread adoption. The most recent generation of linked hinged revision TKA implants have addressed many of the previous mechanical limitations, such as improved patellofemoral articulation, more robust metaphyseal and diaphyseal fixation options, and

modifications of the hinge mechanism to permit lower stresses at this articulation.[10] Thus, these devices—assuming appropriate clinical indications—today enjoy favorable clinical results. In a study by Hossain et al[50] patients receiving a rotating hinge prosthesis demonstrated both higher patient satisfaction and implant survivorship at a mean follow-up duration of 5 years, compared to subjects implanted with PS and unlinked varus/valgus constrained revision devices. Nevertheless, owing to excessive kinematic constraint, these designs are favored only in the rare situation that a constrained hinged TKA is required.

To maximize the longevity of constrained devices, surgeons must still concentrate on restoration of normal limb alignment, balancing the remaining soft-tissue envelope, and not depending totally on implant constraint to provide knee stability.

AUGMENTATION IN REVISION TKA

Augments for Bone Loss

Treatment options for smaller defects include removing the bone defect with mild additional bony resection or shifting the components away from the defect. Additionally, small defects may be filled with morselized bone graft,[51,52] cement, or a combination of cement and screws[53] for a reinforced filler.

Modular metal augmentations have a rich clinical history in addressing bone loss.[54-56] They are particularly useful for moderate-sized (<15 mm), peripheral bony defects. Available peripheral augments historically have been provided in both angular and rectangular shapes for both unicondylar or bicondylar defects (**Fig. 66-4**). In substantial bicondylar tibial defects, use of medial and lateral block augments can bring the joint line up to a more appropriate level without having to use a polyethylene bearing with excessive thickness (**Fig. 66-5**). If the remaining supporting bone is poor or in cases with higher body mass index, the risk of osseous collapse increases and the addition of a stem extension is wise (**Fig. 66-6**). Disadvantages of use of peripheral augments include a potential for increased fretting at the modular interface and their limited size and shapes, which often preclude use in repairing massive defects. They also do not restore

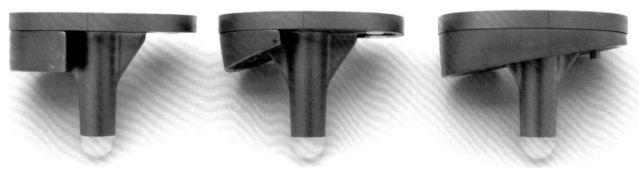

FIGURE 66-4 Tibial metal augments are available in several different geometries. Displayed here are block and wedge augments.

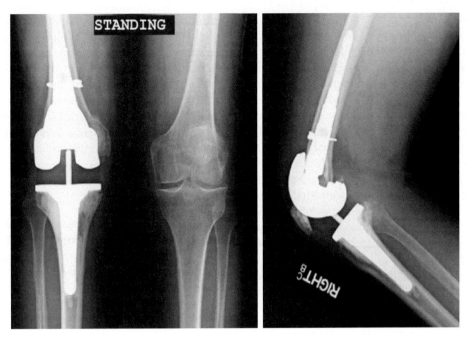

FIGURE 66-5   An alternative to block tibial augments would be the use of thicker polyethylene insert.

bone stock, which is of concern in younger patients. While long-term clinical data following metal augmentation are sparse, intermediate-term follow-up has demonstrated favorable results. Both Pagnano et al[55] and Lee et al[57] report good to excellent clinical outcomes following tibial metal augmentation. However, while both reported a high incidence of radiolucencies, these were early and did not appear to progress.

While traditionally treated with large structural allograft reconstructions, large metaphyseal defects are

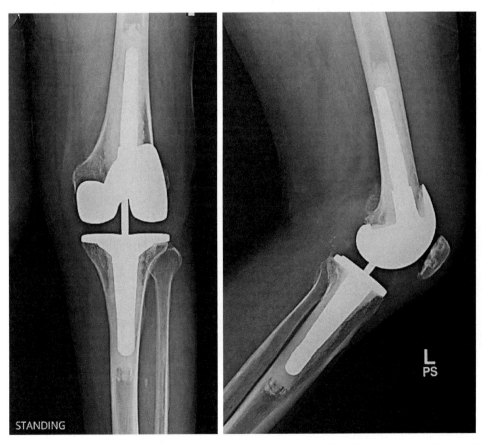

FIGURE 66-6   The use of a tibial stem can assist in transfer of the loading stress to the tibial diaphysis, decreasing the risk of tibial collapse.

increasingly treated with metaphyseal augments (sleeves and cones). These devices offer many widespread advantages, such as ease of use, and predictable long-term fixation. Many sizes and shapes are available, thereby being applicable for the majority of AORI type-II and many AORI type-III defects (**Fig. 66-7**—Sleeves and cones). Short and intermediate results have been promising.[10,5][8-64] Watters et al[65] reported on outcomes following 104 revision TKAs performed with metaphyseal sleeves. At a mean follow-up of 5.3 years, only two sleeves (1.5%) required removal due to recurrent infection and only one sleeve demonstrated failed osteointegration. Metaphyseal sleeves are typically implanted by cementing only the condylar surface and placement of the sleeve without bone cement to allow bone ingrowth into the porous portion of the sleeve (**Fig. 66-8**).

Like sleeves, porous metaphyseal cones have demonstrated favorable intermediate-term clinical results. Kamath et al[66] reported outcomes following 66 revision TKAs performed with porous tantalum metaphyseal cones. At a mean follow-up of 5.8 years, only three cones required revision, and only two cones demonstrated radiolucencies. While bone sleeves and cones have been used without additional stem extensions, it is the authors'

opinion that it is wise to add stem extensions to enhance fixation to bone that is typically compromised. Cones are placed into contact with host bone, allowing bone ingrowth into the peripheral surface of the cone. The condylar surface and stem are then cemented with the cone providing a cancellous structure into which the metaphyseal cement can interdigitate (**Fig. 66-9**). The major limitation of metal metaphyseal augmentation is the inability to restore bone stock and difficulties encountered with sleeve or cone removal.

Stem Fixation

Stems provide a valuable technique for adjuvant fixation in revision TKA. Their primary impact is in the ability to distribute load away from the articulating surface to the diaphyseal cortical bone, as well as to absorb and neutralize interfacial shear stress arising from increased constraint seen in many revision constructs. Controversy exists as to whether the stem should be fully cemented or press-fit.[67] Historically, equivalent results have been reported using both techniques.[68-70] Cementless stems should be canal filling[71] and provide rotational stability. Cemented stems should have rounded contours to facilitate removal if necessary. Modular locking mechanisms must be secure to prevent fretting or stem dissociation.[72,73] The use of press-fit stems provides better remaining bone stock should future revision TKA be necessary. Due to the canal-filling nature of press-fit stems, the condylar position of the femoral or tibial component is determined by the stem position within the medullary canal. This fact may preclude their use in patients with angular deformity, particularly in the metaphyseal or diaphyseal regions. Use of offset tibial trays or offset intramedullary stems can be helpful in these situations, assuming angular deformity is limited (**Fig. 66-10**). Cemented stems are favored in patients with anatomic deformity or severe osteopenia and in cases in which rigid fixation cannot be obtained with a press-fit design. Cemented stems provide immediate fixation, increased flexibility in the positioning of the stem, and the ability to provide local delivery of antibiotics.[67]

The required stem length for cemented stems is another debated topic. There is some evidence to suggest that 30-mm cemented stem extensions provide adequate fixation, even in the setting of metaphyseal bony defects and the use of constrained polyethylene.[74] However, in that study, Lachiewicz et al demonstrated the appearance of radiolucent lines in nearly all knees with this fixation technique. They note that the use of supplementary cones was associated with a significant reduction in radiolucencies.

Disadvantages and complications with the use of stems are frequently related to intraoperative fracture and cortical perforation—particularly with cementless diaphyseal-fitting stems—with a complication rate as high as 50%.[75] Additionally, difficulty with cemented stem extraction during subsequent procedures can result

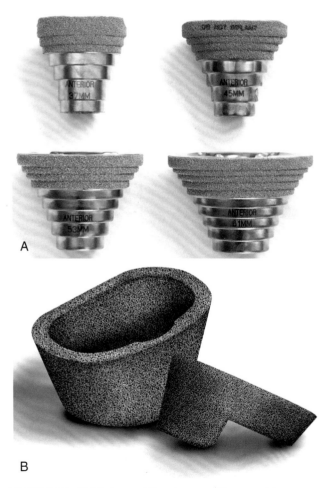

FIGURE 66-7 Tibial sleeves (**A**) and cones (**B**) are useful augments in the setting of metaphyseal bone loss.

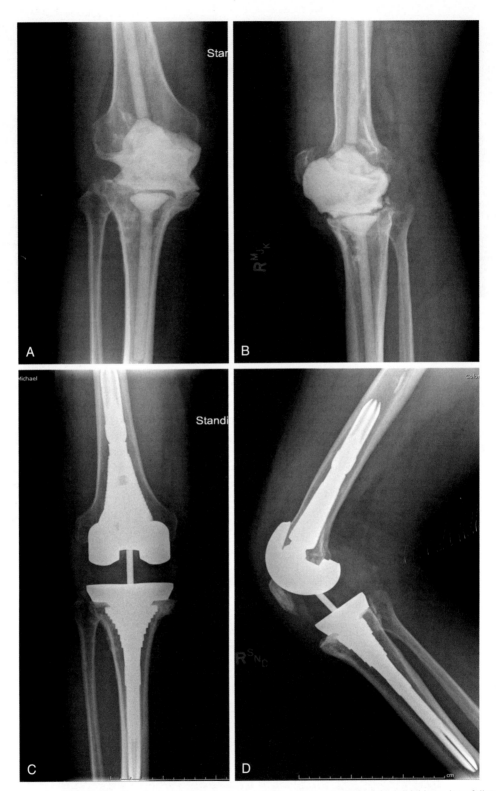

FIGURE 66-8   Case example of a 67-year-old patient with periprosthetic infection demonstrating marked tibial bone loss following removal of the primary implant and placement of an antibiotic spacer **(A** and **B)**. A tibial sleeve and block augment **(C** and **D)** was utilized to reestablish the joint line while providing for additional metaphyseal bony support.

in large bone loss. Transfer of the axial load away from the condyles may result in stress shielding, which may affect long-term fixation.[76] Additionally, pain at the tip of the stem, particularly with press-fit constructs, has been

reported. Barrack et al[77] described diaphyseal pain in 11% of patients with press-fit femoral stems, and in 14% of patients with press-fit tibial stems. They also noted a 19% rate of stem-tip pain in patients with cemented

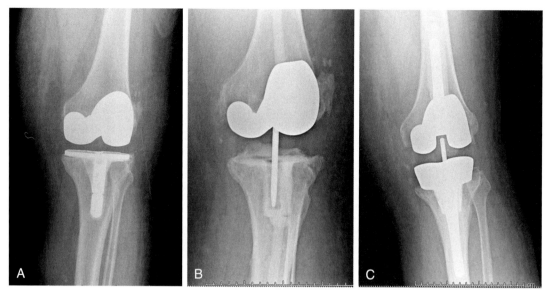

FIGURE 66-9 54-year-old male with posttraumatic osteoarthritis, who underwent unicompartmental arthroplasty of his right knee which was revised to a TKA **(A)** secondary to aseptic loosening. This unfortunately became infected, requiring placement of an antibiotic spacer **(B)**. At time of reimplantation **(C)**, a tibial cone and block augments were used to restore the joint line and to provide additional metaphyseal fixation due to bone loss.

tibial stems. In this series, however, patients with press-fit stems demonstrated poorer clinical outcome scores and were more dissatisfied with the procedure compared to patients with cemented stems. Stem-tip pain may resolve over 1 to 2 years, often associated with development of cortical hypertrophy at the stem tip which better withstands the increased stem-tip loads (**Fig. 66-11**). To lessen

the incidence of stem-tip pain, slotted stems tips are now available to lessen distal stem stiffness and subsequent load transfer (**Fig. 66-12**).

More recently, the use of the so-called "hybrid" technique has become increasingly popular. This technique consists of a combination of uncemented press-fit stems and cemented metaphyseal components.[78] Recent

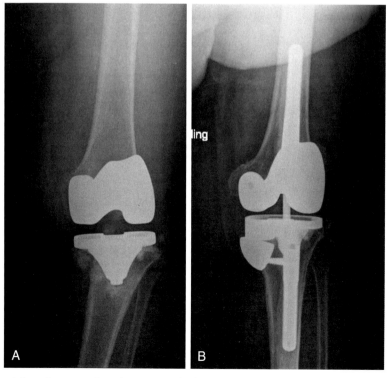

FIGURE 66-10 Offset intramedullary stems may be advantageous in the setting of bony angular deformity. Radiographs demonstrate severe medial osteolysis and subsequent varus collapse of the tibial base tray **(A)**. At the time of revision, the knee was reconstructed with a metal medial augment, wedge tibial augment, and an offset tibial stem **(B)**.

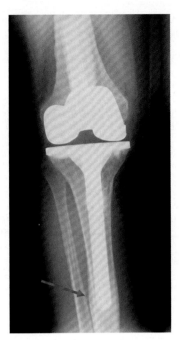

FIGURE 66-11 Cortical hypertrophy (red arrow) associated with a press-fit stem.

mid-term results of this technique has indeed demonstrated excellent fixation with low rates of loosening and high implant survivorship at a mean of 5 years.[79]

CONCLUSIONS

To successfully manage the myriad of problems faced in revision TKA, a modular revision TKA system is favored. A prosthetic system must provide multiple levels of prosthetic constraint, femoral and tibial augmentations, and fixation augmentation with stems. Use of an implant system allows the surgeon to assemble the desired prosthetic components based on intraoperative findings. One must realize that long-term durability of prosthetic components is inversely proportional to prosthetic constraint. Selection of the least-constrained prosthetic components that provide satisfactory stability is recommended. Stems are often required due to the weakened metaphyseal bone encountered in most cases of revision TKA.

IMPLANT SELECTION SUMMARY

The following is a brief algorithm for selection of components for revision TKA. Of course, proper diagnosis and surgical indication is of paramount importance to the long-term success of revision TKA.

Cruciate-Retaining Components

Few indications. Examples include isolated patellar component exchange or revision of a unicompartmental arthroplasty to TKA in the setting of a competent PCL.

Posterior-Stabilized Components

The workhorse of revision TKA. Appropriate for most revision situations. Must be able to achieve varus/valgus and flexion stability. Ligamentous function must be intact.

Unlinked Varus/Valgus Implants

Indicated for varus/valgus instability due to collateral attenuation. MCL must not be completely disrupted. Consider mobile-bearing/rotating platform construct to limit potential post-cam complications and to decrease interfacial shear.

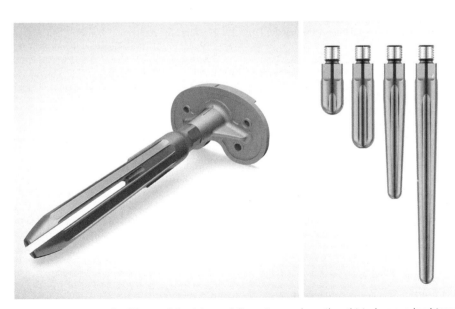

FIGURE 66-12 Slots decrease the overall stiffness of the intramedullary stem and are thought to improve load transfer and decrease the incidence of stem-tip pain.

Linked (Hinged) Implants

Rarely indicated. Examples include complete disruption of collateral ligamentous structure(s) and in the elderly patient with recurvatum.

Stem Augmentation

Indicated for the majority of TKA revisions (apart from simple polyethylene insert or patellar button replacement). No clear preference for press-fit diaphyseal-engaging stems versus cemented stems.

Modular Augments

Indicated for situations of bone loss that are not amendable to simple bone grafting. Examples include block augments for tibial base and distal/posterior femur. Large metaphyseal defects can be treated with structural allograft or increasingly with the use of metaphyseal sleeves and cones.

REFERENCES

1. Sharkey PF, Lichstein PM, Shen C, Tokarski AT, Parvizi J. Why are total knee arthroplasties failing today—has anything changed after 10 years? *J Arthroplasty.* 2014;29:1774-1778.
2. Anon. Australian Orthopaedic Association National Joint Replacement Registry. Annual Report 2018. Available at: https://aoanjrr.sahmri.com/documents/10180/576950/Hip%2C Knee %26 Shoulder Arthroplasty. Accessed January 25, 2019.
3. Bugbee WD, Ammeen DJ, Engh GA. Does implant selection affect outcome of revision knee arthroplasty? *J Arthroplasty.* 2001;16:581-585.
4. Mont MA, Serna FK, Krackow KA, Hungerford DS. Exploration of radiographically normal total knee replacements for unexplained pain. *Clin Orthop Relat Res.* 1996;331:216-220.
5. Vince KG, Abdeen A, Sugimori T. The unstable total knee arthroplasty: causes and cures. *J Arthroplasty.* 2006;21:44-49.
6. Krackow KA, Weiss AP. Recurvatum deformity complicating performance of total knee arthroplasty. A brief note. *J Bone Joint Surg Am.* 1990;72:268-271.
7. Parratte S, Pagnano MW. Instability after total knee arthroplasty. *J Bone Joint Surg Am.* 2008;90:184-194.
8. Meding JB, Keating EM, Ritter MA, Faris PM, Berend ME. Genu recurvatum in total knee replacement. *Clin Orthop Relat Res.* 2003;416:64-67.
9. Giori NJ, Lewallen DG. Total knee arthroplasty in limbs affected by poliomyelitis. *J Bone Joint Surg Am.* 2002;84:1157-1161.
10. Barrack RL. Evolution of the rotating hinge for complex total knee arthroplasty. *Clin Orthop Relat Res.* 2001;392:292-299.
11. Callaghan JJ, O'Rourke MR, Liu SS. The role of implant constraint in revision total knee arthroplasty: not too little, not too much. *J Arthroplasty.* 2005;20:41-43.
12. Vince K. Revision total knee arthroplasty and arthrodesis of the knee. 2001.
13. Pagnano MW, Hanssen AD, Lewallen DG, Stuart MJ. Flexion instability after primary posterior cruciate retaining total knee arthroplasty. *Clin Orthop Relat Res.* 1998;356:39-46.
14. Firestone TP, Eberle RW. Surgical management of symptomatic instability following failed primary total knee replacement. *J Bone Joint Surg Am.* 2006;88:80-84.
15. Schwab JH, Haidukewych GJ, Hanssen AD, Jacofsky DJ, Pagnano MW. Flexion instability without dislocation after posterior stabilized total knees. *Clin Orthop Relat Res.* 2005;440:96-100.
16. Waslewski GL, Marson BM, Benjamin JB. Early, incapacitating instability of posterior cruciate ligament-retaining total knee arthroplasty. *J Arthroplasty.* 1998;13:763-767.
17. Babis GC, Trousdale RT, Morrey BF. The effectiveness of isolated tibial insert exchange in revision total knee arthroplasty. *J Bone Joint Surg Am.* 2002;84:64-68.
18. Backstein D, Safir O, Gross A. Management of bone loss: structural grafts in revision total knee arthroplasty. *Clin Orthop Relat Res.* 2006;446:104-112.
19. Griffin WL, Scott RD, Dalury DF, Mahoney OM, Chiavetta JB, Odum SM. Modular insert exchange in knee arthroplasty for treatment of wear and osteolysis. *Clin Orthop Relat Res.* 2007;464:132-137.
20. Engh GA, Koralewicz LM, Pereles TR. Clinical results of modular polyethylene insert exchange with retention of total knee arthroplasty components. *J Bone Joint Surg Am.* 2000;82:516-523.
21. Brooks DH, Fehring TK, Griffin WL, Mason JB, McCoy TH. Polyethylene exchange only for prosthetic knee instability. *Clin Orthop Relat Res.* 2002;405:182-188.
22. Willson SE, Munro ML, Sandwell JC, Ezzet KA, Colwell CW. Isolated tibial polyethylene insert exchange outcomes after total knee arthroplasty. *Clin Orthop Relat Res.* 2010;468:96.
23. Laskin RS, O'Flynn HM. The Insall Award. Total knee replacement with posterior cruciate ligament retention in rheumatoid arthritis. Problems and complications. *Clin Orthop Relat Res.* 1997;345:24-28.
24. Hofmann AA, Tkach TK, Evanich CJ, Camargo MP. Posterior stabilization in total knee arthroplasty with use of an ultracongruent polyethylene insert. *J Arthroplasty.* 2000;15:576-583.
25. Stiehl JB, Komistek RD, Dennis DA, Keblish PA. Kinematics of the patellofemoral joint in total knee arthroplasty. *J Arthroplasty.* 2001;16:706-714.
26. Yoshiya S, Matsui N, Komistek RD, Dennis DA, Mahfouz M, Kurosaka M. In vivo kinematic comparison of posterior cruciate-retaining and posterior stabilized total knee arthroplasties under passive and weight-bearing conditions. *J Arthroplasty.* 2005;20:777-783.
27. Insall JN, Lachiewicz PF, Burstein AH. The posterior stabilized condylar prosthesis: a modification of the total condylar design. Two to four-year clinical experience. *J Bone Joint Surg Am.* 1982;64:1317-1323.
28. Lombardi AV, Mallory TH, Fada RA, Adams JB, Kefauver CA. Late vs. early engagement of posterior stabilized prostheses: effect on extensor moment arm and resulting patellofemoral loads. *J Bone Joint Surg Br.* 1999;81:165.
29. Hossain S, Ayeko C, Anwar M, Elsworth CF, McGee H. Dislocation of Insall-Burstein II modified total knee arthroplasty. *J Arthroplasty.* 2001;16:233-235.
30. Lombardi AV Jr, Mallory TH, Vaughn BK, et al. Dislocation following primary posterior-stabilized total knee arthroplasty. *J Arthroplasty.* 1993;8:633-639.
31. Lombardi AV, Mallory TH, Waterman RA, Eberle RW. Intercondylar distal femoral fracture: an unreported complication of posterior-stabilized total knee arthroplasty. *J Arthroplasty.* 1995;10:643-650.
32. Callaghan JJ, O'Rourke MR, Goetz DD, Schmalzried TP, Campbell PA, Johnston RC. Tibial post impingement in posterior-stabilized total knee arthroplasty. *Clin Orthop Relat Res.* 2002;404:83-88.
33. Puloski SKT, McCalden RW, MacDonald SJ, Rorabeck CH, Bourne RB. Tibial post wear in posterior stabilized total knee arthroplasty: an unrecognized source of polyethylene debris. *J Bone Joint Surg Am.* 2001;83:390-397.
34. Beight JL, Yao B, Hozack WJ, Hearn SL, Booth JRE. The patellar "clunk" syndrome after posterior stabilized total knee arthroplasty. *Clin Orthop Relat Res.* 1994;299:139-142.
35. Lucas TS, DeLuca PF, Nazarian DG, Bartolozzi AR, Booth JRE. Arthroscopic treatment of patellar clunk. *Clin Orthop Relat Res.* 1999;367:226-229.

36. Zingde SM, Leszko F, Sharma A, Mahfouz MR, Komistek RD, Dennis DA. In vivo determination of cam-post engagement in fixed and mobile-bearing TKA. *Clin Orthop Relat Res.* 2014;472:254-262.

37. Chiu Y-S, Chen W-M, Huang C-K, Chiang C-C, Chen T-H. Fracture of the polyethylene tibial post in a NexGen posterior-stabilized knee prosthesis. *J Arthroplasty.* 2004;19:1045-1049.

38. Diamond OJ, Howard L, Masri B. Five cases of tibial post fracture in posterior stabilized total knee arthroplasty using Prolong highly cross-linked polyethylene. *Knee.* 2018;25:657-662.

39. Martin JR, Jennings JM, Watters TS, Levy DL, McNabb DC, Dennis DA. Femoral implant design modification decreases the incidence of patellar crepitus in total knee arthroplasty. *J Arthroplasty.* 2017;32:1310-1313.

40. Dennis DA, Johnson DR, Kim RH. Revision total knee arthroplasty. In: Liberman JR, Berry DJ, Azar FM, eds. *Advanced Reconstruction: Knee.* American Academy of Orthopaedic Surgeons/Lippincott Williams & Wilkins; 2011.

41. Bottlang M, Erne OK, Lacatusu E, Sommers MB, Kessler O. A mobile-bearing knee prosthesis can reduce strain at the proximal tibia. *Clin Orthop Relat Res.* 2006;447:105-111.

42. Kim RH, Martin JR, Dennis DA, Yang CC, Jennings JM, Lee G-C. Midterm clinical and radiographic results of mobile-bearing revision total knee arthroplasty. *J Arthroplasty.* 2017;32:1930-1934.

43. Gluck T. Referat uber die durch das moderne chirurgische experiment gewonnenen positiven resultate, betreffend die naht und den ersatz von defecten hcherer gewebe, sowie uber die verwerthung vesorbirbarer und lebendiger tampons in der chirurgie. *Arch Klin Chir.* 1890;41:187-239.

44. Bargar WL, Amstutz HC. Results with the constrained total knee prosthesis in treating severely disabled patients and patients with failed total knee replacements. *J Bone Joint Surg Am.* 1980;62:504-512.

45. Deburge A. Guepar hinge prosthesis: complications and results with two years' follow-up. *Clin Orthop Relat Res.* 1976;120:47-53.

46. Hui FC, Fitzgerald RH Jr. Hinged total knee arthroplasty. *J Bone Joint Surg Am.* 1980;62:513-519.

47. Kester MA, Cook SD, Harding AF, Rodriguez RP, Pipkin CS. An evaluation of the mechanical failure modalities of a rotating hinge knee prosthesis. *Clin Orthop Relat Res.* 1988;228:156-163.

48. Rand JA, Chao EY, Stauffer RN. Kinematic rotating-hinge total knee arthroplasty. *J Bone Joint Surg Am.* 1987;69:489-497.

49. Shindell R, Neumann R, Connolly JF, Jardon OM. Evaluation of the Noiles hinged knee prosthesis. A five-year study of seventeen knees. *J Bone Joint Surg Am.* 1986;68:579-585.

50. Hossain F, Patel S, Haddad FS. Midterm assessment of causes and results of revision total knee arthroplasty. *Clin Orthop Relat Res.* 2010;468:1221-1228.

51. Lotke PA, Carolan GF, Puri N. Impaction grafting for bone defects in revision total knee arthroplasty. *Clin Orthop Relat Res.* 2006;446:99-103.

52. Lotke PA, Carolan GF, Puri N. Technique for impaction bone grafting of large bone defects in revision total knee arthroplasty. *J Arthroplasty.* 2006;21:57-60.

53. Ritter MA. Screw and cement fixation of large defects in total knee arthroplasty. *J Arthroplasty.* 1986;1:125-129.

54. Brand MG, Daley RJ, Ewald FC, Scott RD. Tibial tray augmentation with modular metal wedges for tibial bone stock deficiency. *Clin Orthop Relat Res.* 1989;248:71-79.

55. Pagnano MW, Trousdale RT, Rand JA. Tibial wedge augmentation for bone deficiency in total knee arthroplasty. A followup study. *Clin Orthop Relat Res.* 1995;321:151-155.

56. Rand JA. Bone deficiency in total knee arthroplasty. Use of metal wedge augmentation. *Clin Orthop Relat Res.* 1991;271:63-71.

57. Lee JK, Choi CH. Management of tibial bone defects with metal augmentation in primary total knee replacement: a minimum five-year review. *J Bone Joint Surg Br.* 2011;93:1493-1496.

58. Alexander GE, Bernasek TL, Crank RL, Haidukewych GJ. Cementless metaphyseal sleeves used for large tibial defects in revision total knee arthroplasty. *J Arthroplasty.* 2013;28:604-607.

59. Beckmann NA, Mueller S, Gondan M, Jaeger S, Reiner T, Bitsch RG. Treatment of severe bone defects during revision total knee arthroplasty with structural allografts and porous metal cones—a systematic review. *J Arthroplasty.* 2015;30:249-253.

60. Bugler KE, Maheshwari R, Ahmed I, Brenkel IJ, Walmsley PJ. Metaphyseal sleeves for revision total knee arthroplasty: good short-term outcomes. *J Arthroplasty.* 2015;30:1990-1994.

61. Dalury DF, Barrett WP. The use of metaphyseal sleeves in revision total knee arthroplasty. *Knee.* 2016;23:545-548.

62. Howard JL, Kudera J, Lewallen DG, Hanssen AD. Early results of the use of tantalum femoral cones for revision total knee arthroplasty. *J Bone Joint Surg Am.* 2011;93:478-484.

63. Long WJ, Scuderi GR. Porous tantalum cones for large metaphyseal tibial defects in revision total knee arthroplasty: a minimum 2-year follow-up. *J Arthroplasty.* 2009;24:1086-1092.

64. Villanueva-Martínez M, De la Torre-Escudero B, Rojo-Manaute JM, Ríos-Luna A, Chana-Rodriguez F. Tantalum cones in revision total knee arthroplasty. A promising short-term result with 29 cones in 21 patients. *J Arthroplasty.* 2013;28:988-993.

65. Watters TS, Martin JR, Levy DL, Yang CC, Kim RH, Dennis DA. Porous-coated metaphyseal sleeves for severe femoral and tibial bone loss in revision TKA. *J Arthroplasty.* 2017;32:3468-3473.

66. Kamath AF, Lewallen DG, Hanssen AD. Porous tantalum metaphyseal cones for severe tibial bone loss in revision knee arthroplasty: a five to nine-year follow-up. *J Bone Joint Surg Am.* 2015;97:216-223.

67. Shannon BD, Klassen JF, Rand JA, Berry DJ, Trousdale RT. Revision total knee arthroplasty with cemented components and uncemented intramedullary stems. *J Arthroplasty.* 2003;18:27-32.

68. Engh G. Treatment of major defects of bone with bulk allografts and stemmed components during total knee arthroplasty. *J Bone Joint Surg Am.* 1997;79:1030.

69. Haas SB, Insall JN, Montgomery W, Windsor RE. Revision total knee arthroplasty with use of modular components with stems inserted without cement. *J Bone Joint Surg Am.* 1995;77:1700-1707.

70. Murray PB, Rand JA, Hanssen AD. Cemented long-stem revision total knee arthroplasty. *Clin Orthop Relat Res.* 1994;309:116-123.

71. Fehring TK, Odum S, Olekson C, Griffin WL, Mason JB, McCoy TH. Stem fixation in revision total knee arthroplasty: a comparative analysis. *Clin Orthop Relat Res.* 2003;416:217-224.

72. Boe CC, Fehring KA, Trousdale RT. Failure of the stem-condyle junction of a modular femoral stem in revision total knee arthroplasty. *Am. J Orthop.* 2015;44:E401-E403.

73. Lim L-A, Trousdale RT, Berry DJ, Hanssen AD. Failure of the stem–condyle junction of a modular femoral stem in revision total knee arthroplasty: a report of five cases. *J Arthroplasty.* 2001;16:128-132.

74. Lachiewicz PF, Soileau ES. A 30-mm cemented stem extension provides adequate fixation of the tibial component in revision knee arthroplasty. *Clin Orthop Relat Res.* 2015;473:185-189.

75. Meek RMD, Garbuz DS, Masri BA, Greidanus NV, Duncan CP. Intraoperative fracture of the femur in revision total hip arthroplasty with a diaphyseal fitting stem. *J Bone Joint Surg Am.* 2004;86:480-485.

76. Bourne RB, Finlay JB. The influence of tibial component intramedullary stems and implant-cortex contact on the strain distribution of the proximal tibia following total knee arthroplasty. An in vitro study. *Clin Orthop Relat Res.* 1986;208:95-99.

77. Barrack RL, Rorabeck C, Burt M, Sawhney J. Pain at the end of the stem after revision total knee arthroplasty. *Clin Orthop Relat Res.* 1999;367:216-225.

78. Goldberg VM, Kraay M. The outcome of the cementless tibial component: a minimum 14-year clinical evaluation. *Clin Orthop Relat Res.* 2004;428:214-220.

79. Greene JW, Reynolds SM, Stimac JD, Malkani AL, Massini MA. Midterm results of hybrid cement technique in revision total knee arthroplasty. *J Arthroplasty.* 2013;28:570-574.

chapter 67

Stems in Revision Total Knee Arthroplasty

Denis Nam, MD, MSc | Wayne G. Paprosky, MD

INTRODUCTION

The goal in revision total knee arthroplasty (TKA) is to recreate a stable joint that is positioned and oriented close to the normal anatomic axis in all planes. This becomes a more difficult task in the revision setting secondary to bone and soft tissue loss. The abnormalities present during revision surgery may result from a combination of different factors: primary disease deformity, infection, osteolysis, aseptic loosening, implant removal complications, and concomitant systemic disease. To anatomically recreate the knee joint, the surgeon may be required to use augments of a biologic or mechanical nature to compensate for the bone or soft tissue loss.

In the normal tibia, the cancellous and cortical bone of the proximal tibia buttresses and supports the overlying articular cartilage. The stiffness of the cancellous bone decreases distally as the stiffness of the cortical shell increases.[1] The joint load is transmitted through the articular cartilage to the cancellous and cortical bone beneath. In the setting of primary knee arthroplasty, the combination of plastic, metal, and polymethylmethacrylate transmits the load directly to the underlying cancellous and cortical bone. In the revision setting, there is loss of the strongest supporting bone, and transmission of forces to the remaining subsurface could lead to early failure.[2]

Stems in primary TKA were introduced with early hinged prosthesis designs with the goals of resisting torsional and bending stresses at the bone–implant interface due to increased intraprosthetic constraint.[3] Revision TKA components are commonly stemmed to protect the limited autogenous bone stock that is remaining. This bone may be directly under the component or under the cement, metal augments, or structural bone graft. When one is using large volumes of morselized or structural grafts, one may want to protect the graft from significant load.[4] Conclusively, revision components without stems can place abnormal stresses on the normal bone by their constrained design nature. Joint loads are several times body weight. A stemmed component can transfer these loads if it is composed of materials that can withstand the stresses imposed on them.[5] If the stem fails to transfer the load, then the remaining cancellous bone experiences load beyond its ultimate strength, and this will lead to a loss in fixation.[6]

A stem's purpose, therefore, is to transmit force away from the joint line and, in so doing, lessen the stresses placed on the joint.[7,8] Stems perform this function by being rigid and by being attached to a solid femoral component or tibial base plate. Brooks et al have shown that, in the varus-deficient proximal tibia, the addition of a metal-backed component decreases stress and allows for a more uniform distribution of force across the proximal tibia.[9] Because these components are more rigid than the remaining cancellous bone, force is transmitted through them and onto the stem or onto the remaining tibial cortical rim. Bartel and associates have shown by finite element analysis that stresses on the cancellous bone beneath prostheses of conventional design can be diminished if a metal tray and a central peg are used.[5] Lewis et al found that tibial post designs provided the lowest stresses on host bone.[10] Once a stem (or post) length reaches 70 mm, the axial load at the joint line can be reduced by 23% to 39%.[7-9] The bending moment carried by the stem can be variable, as fixation of the stem occurs distally.[9] Addition of a central post and stem to the tray, however, increases the stiffness of the component and, in doing so, decreases the bending moment.[8] The force is then returned to the bone at the metadiaphyseal or diaphyseal area, depending on the geometry, size, length, position, and composition of the stem. Bourne and Finlay demonstrated in a fresh cadaveric strain gauge study that loss of proximal cortical tibial contact resulted in a 33% to 60% decrease in strain values.[11] When stems up to 15 cm long are evaluated, marked stress shielding of the proximal tibial cortex and doubling of the strain located at the tip is noted. Additional potential advantages of the use of stems in revision TKA include an increased surface area for fixation, assistance with component alignment, and delivery of antibiotic cement into the intramedullary canals.

Two traditional methods of stem insertion have been used. Use of a cemented stem results in transmission of load closer to the joint line, as the stems are shorter (often 30 to 100 mm) and the force is transmitted along the bone–cement interface. The use of cement can fill metaphyseal voids between the stem and bone and help eliminate micromotion. This should decrease severe stress shielding.[12] Additional proposed advantages of the use of cemented metaphyseal stems include an increased freedom of anteroposterior and mediolateral component placement, decreased end of stem pain, and the avoidance of anatomic abnormalities including a diaphyseal bow or deformity. Filling the intramedullary canal with cement can make future revisions more problematic, however, and may lead to further bone loss and destruction during cement removal.[13] With diaphyseal engaging cementless stems (often greater than 150 mm in length), forces are transmitted to the tip of the stem where cortical bone contact occurs.[13-15] Proposed advantages include their ease of removal (when using polished cementless stems lacking an ongrowth surface) and ability to assist with component alignment. Researchers have raised concern regarding possible proximal stress shielding with cementless stems; however, this is, more often than not, technique-dependent.[11] Stress shielding may actually be less if the stem is not anchored in cement.[14] Cementless stem insertion may actually weaken bone due to excessive reaming or may possibly promote early loosening if the stem is undersized.[15,16] Furthermore, there is the potential for increased end of stem pain.[17-19] End of stem pain has been reported to have an incidence of up to 11% on the femoral and 14% on the tibial sides with the use of a cobalt-chrome diaphyseal engaging cementless stem.[17] However, the development of titanium stems with slots or flutes has led to a decrease in end of stem pain due to a decrease in modulus of elasticity.[18] Concerns of stress shielding and end of stem pain are technique-related and should not be indications to avoid the use of cementless stems. Biomechanically, several studies have indicated similar improvements in implant stability and stress distribution when using either cemented metaphyseal engaging or cementless diaphyseal engaging stems.[20,21]

It is essential that the revision surgeon realize that stems are not a substitute for optimal component fit. They are simply an adjunct to relieve a portion of the excess stress seen by the components at the joint line. The type and size of stem are irrelevant if the juxtaarticular tissues are not adequately reconstructed. As stresses become greater or the soft tissues more compromised, the approach to stem fixation must be altered.[16]

There are a multitude of different stem geometries available. Use of larger diameter stems leads to increased load transmissions, but this is usually negated by the fact that most systems have a set diameter fixation point at the stem-component junction.[22] In addition, the bending moment of the base plate is determined at this junction.[23] Longer stems in the knee result in more proximal bone shielding.[8] This factor cannot be assessed in isolation, as shorter, wider stems impinge at their tips because of the conical shape of metaphyseal endosteum. The use of longer, thinner stems prevents tip impingement, as the stem can migrate in the sleeve of tubular diaphyseal endosteum. The contact area of the stem within the bone also determines how the load is transferred to the cortex. To complicate matters, the surface preparation of the stem may also alter fixation. Presently, most cementless stems

are smooth or blasted without a porous coating. Stem composition is often titanium to decrease the modulus of elasticity and potential for end of stem pain and proximal stress shielding. Flutes have been added to the stems to aid in fixation and decrease stem stiffness. Flutes or splines on the stem engage in endosteal bone and, it is hoped, function to decrease rotational stresses at the joint line. The flutes may also act to decrease the modulus of elasticity of the stems and thus decrease the severity of proximal stress shielding (**Fig. 67-1**).

PREOPERATIVE PLANNING

Preoperative planning is essential before knee revision arthroplasty. Full-length anteroposterior and lateral radiographs allow for complete assessment of the femur and tibia. Besides allowing determination of the position of the joint line, alignment of bony cuts, size and position of components, and need for augmentation, these radiographs permit assessment of the intramedullary canals to ensure that intramedullary alignment conforms to the mechanical axis orientation. It is critical to template the entry point of the femoral and tibial stem to optimize component alignment, to determine the ideal stem length

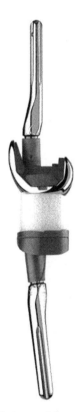

FIGURE 67-1 Example of stemmed femoral and tibial components for press-fit use. Stems are fluted, which helps to engage endosteal bone. This allows control of rotational forces. Press-fitting of the stems also controls bending forces. The smooth surface allows subsidence to maintain compression forces at the joint line. The stems are offset to compensate for asymmetric joint surfaces. (Courtesy of Zimmer, Warsaw, IN.)

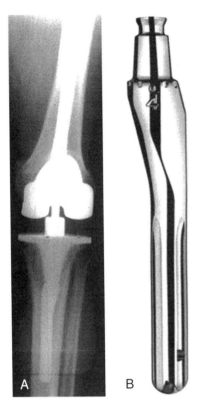

FIGURE 67-2 **A:** Offset stem allows displacement of the tibial base plate in the desired direction to prevent component overhang and allow for optimal coverage. **B:** Offset tibial stemmed component. (A, Courtesy of Zimmer, Warsaw, IN.)

and mode of fixation, and to determine whether offset stems are required. Eccentric joint surfaces may require the use of offset stems or tibial housings to ensure proper alignment of the component while optimizing tibial plateau coverage and preventing implant overhang (**Figs. 67-1** and **67-2**). Canal assessment ensures that straight-stemmed components may be inserted and possibly determine the need for an osteotomy secondary to severe deformity. Presence of a severe diaphyseal deformity may influence stem selection as use of a short cemented stem may be preferred in this scenario. For cementless stems, stem length and width are estimated to obtain adequate endosteal press-fit. Stem length must be estimated with the component to account for each component's respective housing. In general, longer stems are used to provide more rigid support, as their point of contact extends for a longer length along the endosteal diaphyseal surface. Length and degree of support cannot be assessed in isolation, as the extent of press-fit is a significant concomitant factor. Longer stems with tight diaphyseal endosteal cortical press-fit are chosen in cases of massive bony deficiencies (**Fig. 67-3**). Long stems may also be used to provide constrained component support when significant soft tissue imbalance or instability is present and more constrained implants are used (**Fig. 67-4**).

It is useful to template for at least two possible stem lengths with their corresponding different stem widths (**Fig. 67-5**). Commonly, a predetermined stem length

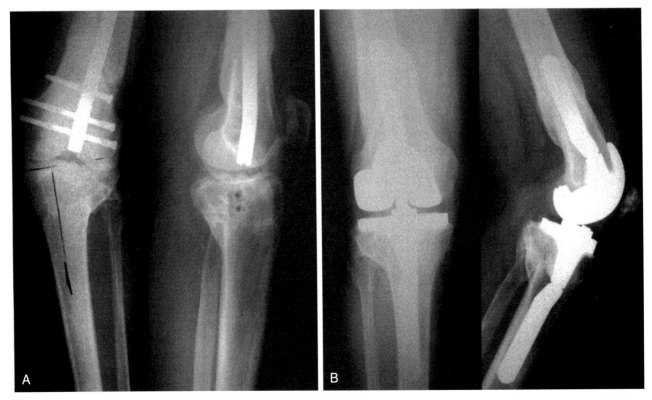

FIGURE 67-3 Radiographs of the knee of a 77-year-old man who experienced a fall 9 mo before assessment. Attempts at open reduction and internal fixation failed to achieve union. **A:** Anteroposterior and lateral radiographs of a supracondylar femur fracture with posttraumatic arthritis and failed internal fixation. **B:** Postoperative radiographs at 9 mo.

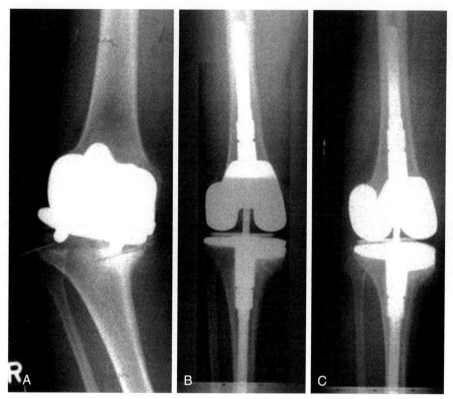

FIGURE 67-4 Radiographs of a 55-year-old woman with primary uncemented total knee arthroplasty for degenerative osteoarthritis. Patient was complaining of significant medial knee and lower leg pain. **A:** Anteroposterior radiograph of an unstable uncemented total knee prosthesis. Two-month **(B)** and 2-y **(C)** postoperative anteroposterior radiographs of a cemented constrained total knee prosthesis with press-fit stems. Incompetency of the medial collateral ligamentous complex prevented balancing of the joint and therefore required the use of constrained polyethylene to compensate for ligamentous laxity.

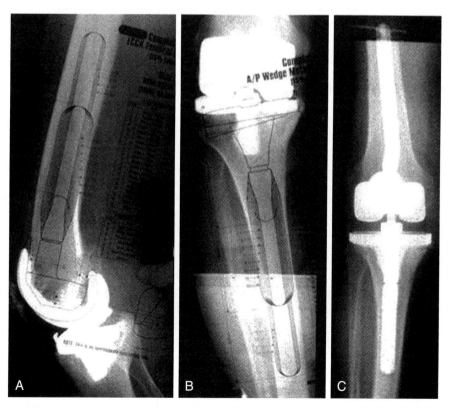

FIGURE 67-5 Radiographs of the knee of a 65-year-old man with severe osteolysis secondary to excessive polyethylene wear. The patient had previously undergone removal of a metal-backed patella. Preoperative anteroposterior **(B)** and lateral **(A)** radiographs with overlying templates. With severe osteolysis, reconstitution of bone stock with bulk allografting or impaction grafting must be considered. **C:** Postoperative radiograph.

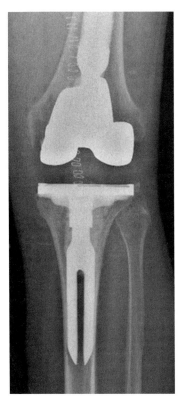

FIGURE 67-6 Revision total knee arthroplasty in which a cementless diaphyseal engaging stem was used for the tibia. This anteroposterior radiograph demonstrates unnecessary over-reaming and oversizing of the tibial stem with removal of endosteal bone.

relation to the intramedullary canal. With straight stems, placement of the component in the sagittal plane is dictated by the stem and therefore predetermines the flexion gap. To increase or decrease the flexion gap during the use of straight stems, the only option is to upsize or downsize the femoral component, respectively (**Fig. 67-5**). Shifting of the component position or addition of posterior femoral augments cannot be used to alter the flexion gap, as component position has been predetermined by the straight intramedullary stem. If available, an offset stem or a component with a different housing junction point is another viable option. On the tibial side, stem positioning tends to be a greater problem in the coronal plane, as the medial and lateral tibial plateaus are commonly asymmetric (**Fig. 67-7**). Ultimately, position of the component must correlate with both the bone of the joint line and the intramedullary canal alignment to prevent significant overhang of the component.

Many newer revision knee systems have a swivel joint at the tibial component-stem junction or are equipped with an offset stem that allows for adjustment of component position (**Figs. 67-1** and **67-2**). Curved stems allow for longer support on the femoral side and attempt to lessen the possibility of endosteal impingement. Offset stem options and presence of a swivel joint at the stem–implant junction have simplified the use of cementless diaphyseal engaging stems when the desired component position is not directly in line with the diaphysis.

may be too loose because of undersizing or the stem may impinge if it is oversized. Attempting to insert a stem of larger or smaller diameter, respectively, may then cause the reciprocal problem. Usually, the problem of impingement can be avoided by reaming away more endosteal bone. This helps lessen the impingement that occurs at the tip of the stem where the intramedullary canal begins to narrow. If the amount of bone removed is excessive, however, a stress riser may be created at the tip of the stem, which can lead to stem tip pain or fracture. Care should be taken in patients with osteoporotic bone as over-reaming can easily occur in which an excessive amount of endosteal bone is removed (**Fig. 67-6**). With the use of cementless, press-fit diaphyseal fixation, the intraoperative periprosthetic fracture risk has been reported to be 4.9% on the tibial and 1% on the femoral side (com bined incidence of 3.0%). These were nondisplaced fractures that were found to heal uneventfully without operative intervention.[24] An alternative is to change to a stem of shorter or longer length with a different diameter. Templating helps ensure that the stem length chosen is sufficient so that structural bone will support the stem.

Most stems attach to a fixed point on the revision arthroplasty component. Estimation of component position in the coronal and sagittal planes is therefore essential. Commonly, the femoral component sizing in the coronal plane is decided by the knee anatomy, as the medial and lateral condyles have a relatively symmetric width in

OPERATIVE TECHNIQUE

Before reconstruction of the knee joint, infection must be ruled out and the original components removed, with every attempt made to preserve the underlying host bone stock. The surrounding soft tissues must be adequately assessed and protected during the reconstruction.

In rare instances, a stemmed component may be considered during a primary arthroplasty because of severe deformity, significant bone loss, or severe ligamentous insufficiency. Conversion to a stemmed component cannot immediately proceed after implantation of a regular component if extramedullary alignment has been used. The possibility exists of mismatching the bone cuts to the intramedullary axes, which can cause impingement of the intramedullary stem on the endosteal surface. This can lead to malalignment of components, poor fit of components on the bone surfaces, or iatrogenic bone fractures from attempts to make the component fit with forceful impaction.

Preparation of the femoral and tibial bony surfaces is done with an intramedullary alignment guide. Rather than using the narrow intramedullary guide rods that attach to the cutting jigs of most systems, the authors prefer to use the intramedullary reamers from the cutting jig guide rod. The initial step is to minimally ream and push the largest diameter reamer past the isthmus. Reaming can be performed "by hand" or "with power" at the surgeon's

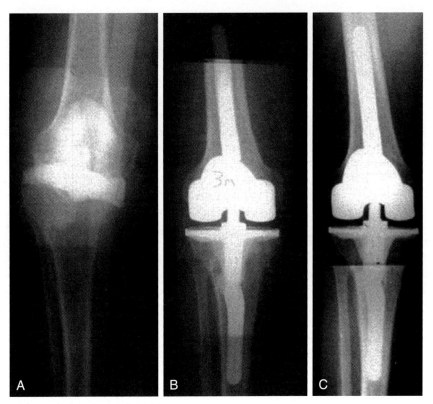

FIGURE 67-7   Revision total knee arthroplasty requiring a tibial offset stem as the patient had previously undergone a high tibial osteotomy and was left with a deficient medial tibial plateau. The patient underwent a two-staged revision because of previous infection. **A:** Preoperative radiograph. **B:** Three-month postoperative radiograph. **C:** Two-year postoperative radiograph. The offset stem allowed for better lateral coverage of the tibial surface with no significant medical overhang of the component.

discretion. Use of power reaming may decrease the surgical time, but it is critical to avoid potential cortical thinning, perforation, or fracture when reaming with power, especially when using a longer, diaphyseal fit stem. In most instances, straight reamers can be used to ream both the femoral and tibial canals. However, in a case in which long and possibly bowed stems are planned, flexible reamers may aid in canal preparation. If bypassing a cortical defect, a guidewire can be placed with the use of flexible reamers to avoid eccentric reaming. The initial reamer produces an entry point in the juxtaarticular bone and is rotated to enlarge the entry site. This removes ectatic and sclerotic bone that can lever the reamers away from the true longitudinal axes of the bones. In the revision setting, it is also critical to remove any well-fixed cement within the meta-diaphyseal region that may deflect the reamer and cause eccentric reaming. Cement can be removed with reverse curettes, but care must be taken to avoid cortical perforation with their use. An ultrasonic drive can also be considered to aid with removal of prior cement plugs deep within the canal. Reaming is then continued in millimeter increments until minimal endosteal cortical contact is felt or heard. As stated earlier, reaming is minimal, as the reamers are being used more as guide rods for cut alignment and stem position. Cutting blocks are then attached to this rod, and initial cuts are completed. By using the largest diameter rod in the canal and ensuring

that the rod passes the isthmus, one can better assure that the bony cuts for the component optimally correlate with the stem orientation and prevent impingement or malpositioning of the component-stem construct. A full-length reamer or a reamer of equal width throughout its length provides for the best alignment, as there is minimal toggle along its shaft. Once the entry site has been cleared of sclerotic bone, the reamer should be gently pushed up the canal rather than forcibly reamed into the canal. The reamer is acting as a guide rod at this point. Alternatively, based on the surgeon's comfort level, reaming for press-fit can be performed immediately based on templating and intraoperative feel. Then, a smaller diameter reamer may be placed even further distally to ensure appropriate alignment during preparation of the cut surfaces.

Balancing of the joint in the flexion–extension and varus–valgus planes proceeds in a routine manner once the initial cuts have been made. The initial bone cuts required are the proximal tibial cut and the distal and posterior femoral cuts. Cuts should resect minimal bone and are performed before assessing the flexion and extension spaces. The use of premeasured spacer blocks or a measurable tensioning device is essential at this stage. Joint line positioning is decided by this assessment and by preoperative templating. The size of the femoral component, the amount of femoral distal buildup, and the amount of tibial thickness can then be determined arithmetically.

The tibial component affects both the flexion and extension gaps. Its thickness is determined by an estimation of the position of the joint line. This measurement can be subtracted from the spacer block measurements of the flexion and extension gaps to determine the size of the femoral component required for flexion gap balance and the amount of distal femoral augment for extension gap balance. In our experience, the tendency in revision TKA is to elevate the joint line. Thus, use of preoperative templating and intraoperative assessment is critical to avoid joint line elevation and distal femoral augmentation is almost always utilized. To avoid a loose flexion gap, an offset or larger femoral component size may be necessary.

It is essential to reiterate that the position of the femoral and tibial components is dictated by the position of the press-fit stem if offset junctions are not available for use. The size of the tibial base plate determines not only the amount of coverage but also the amount of overhang on the tibia in the coronal plane. If the canal is eccentric or the tibial plateaus deficient, then a base plate with an offset housing or offset stem must be considered to correct this problem. A similar but less common problem occurs in the sagittal plane.

With the femoral component, there is an additional concern of altering the thickness in the sagittal plane. Preoperative planning is critical to determine whether increase or reduction of the flexion gap is desired during the revision procedure. It is useful to remove the prior femoral component and determine its anteroposterior size relative to the revision component to be implanted. This will determine the change in femoral size and potential impact on the flexion gap. Changing the femoral sizing alters the flexion gap thickness by predetermined amounts and is the only way to alter the flexion gap when assessing the femoral component in isolation. The extent that a smaller-sized femoral component increases the flexion gap is system-specific and must be known. Posterior femoral augments are used as a filler to ensure that the posterior aspect of the component is in bony contact and thus rotationally stable. Once the size of the femoral component is determined, chamfer cuts and housing resection can be completed. Final shaping for augments is also completed. All bone cuts should be performed in reference to an intramedullary alignment rod.

If bulk allograft is required, sizing, shaping, and fixation are now performed. Depending on defect size, grafting can be completed before gap assessment. Length estimates are performed with the calculations noted earlier if a complete structural allograft is required to replace the juxtaarticular bone. Completion of bony allograft resection is completed to accept the component and component housing. The cuts are performed on a satellite table with intramedullary alignment. The diameter of the intramedullary guide within the allograft is determined by the width of reaming required within the host bone. Appropriate graft size is required to ensure that excessive reaming of the graft does not occur and weaken the graft.

Femoral and tibial canals are then sequentially reamed to the appropriate length and width to accept the press-fit stem. As noted earlier, this can be performed as an initial step if the surgeon desires. Furthermore, reaming can again be performed either "by hand" or "with power" at the surgeon's discretion. A preoperative estimate along with the intraoperative assessment is required to determine the extent of press-fit required. With a wide variety of stems available, different permutations of stem length and width give adequate press-fit in most situations. Surgeons should note differences among implant systems as some will provide 1 mm diameter increments, while others will only provide even or odd sized diameters or larger intervals between stem sizes. For more severe defects, fewer stem choices exist, which emphasizes the need for preoperative templating to ensure appropriate stem availability. A greater degree of press-fit is required when there is greater structural bone loss or greater soft tissue imbalance or insufficiency. This translates to reaming to greater depths with removal of more endosteal bone to ensure that there is a sleeve of cortical endosteal bone supporting the stemmed component. It is important to adjust reamer depth based on the planned use of augments.

The width of reaming is templated preoperatively and correlates intraoperatively to the point at which cortical chatter is felt or heard with the reamer. Assessment of reaming is also of value in determining if endosteal cortical bone is being removed. Traditionally, the authors ream approximately 1 cm past the tip of the stem to ensure that there is no tip impingement with the possibility of cortical erosion. Some revision systems incorporate this into the etchings on the reamers and thus if reaming to a particular depth, the actual stem length for that depth will be 1 cm shorter to avoid tip impingement. Remaining depth must include the stem length and the length of the component housing. A shorter stem of a wider variety is indicated if reaming past the tip of the stem will remove excess bone. For routine revisions, reaming should not be overly aggressive and does not need to proceed to the point of significant cortical chatter. Stem insertion and reaming proceeds line to line. If the revision requires more support from the stem, then reaming can be more aggressive. It is difficult to absolutely quantitate the extent of reaming for each situation; this must be done with clinical judgment as determined preoperatively and intraoperatively. It is important to compare the integrity of the bone and soft tissues to the primary arthroplasty setting and then determine the extent of extra support required. For structural bulk allografts, stem fixation along the endosteal bone should have cortical contact and should occur over a longer extent (**Fig. 67-3**). Reaming should therefore continue at least a millimeter or two wider beyond the point at which cortical chatter is felt and heard.

Trial reduction of the femoral and tibial components is performed with the required augments but without the stem extensions to assess the accuracy of the bony cuts. Before any recutting is attempted, it is important to retrial the components with the stems. Failure to seat components then can be assessed. Failure to seat the components without the stem indicates inaccurate bone cuts that require refinement. Easy seating of components without the stem but failure to easily seat with the stem either means that the stem has been incorrectly sized and endosteal impingement is occurring or that bony cuts have not correlated with the intramedullary positioning of the stem. If stem impingement is occurring, then re-reaming of the canal or resizing of the stem is required. Cortication of the juxtaarticular bone occurs secondary to the osteolytic and loosening process in the revision setting. This bone can deflect the guide rod, reamer, stem, or component housing and lead to malpositioning. Ensuring adequate removal of bone for the component housing helps in alignment of the components. Failure to remove this bone or realize this problem leads to improper cut alignment and component malpositioning. At this stage, the only option is to replace the intramedullary guide rod and recut the femur.

Occasionally, when the relationship of the cut surfaces to the intramedullary alignment guide is reassessed, cuts are noted to be accurate; however, on upsizing reamers to accept a wider press-fit stem, cuts do not correlate with the stemmed component. This occurs because the bone is bowed or noncylindrical, with the wider stem seating in a position, in that segment of bone, different from the longitudinal axis as determined by the intramedullary guide. The choice is then to recut the bone to correlate with the wider press-fit stem or to accept a narrower stem with or without increased length. The latter option better relates the bone cuts to the longitudinal axis of the bone and, in the majority of cases, the latter option is accepted, as the risk of malalignment is prevented. Once components are inserted, final assessment of flexion and extension gaps is performed.

It is important to note that intraoperative imaging should be considered in cases where the surgical plan is not proceeding as would be expected based on preoperative planning. If there is concern about the size of the stems being used, cortical fit or perforation, or whether a prior defect is being bypassed accordingly, intraoperative imaging should be considered. Intraoperative imaging is a valuable tool to assess whether the desired reconstruction has been achieved.

In many revision situations, bulk allografting is not required for the contained cavitary defects that are present. Morselized autogenous or allogenic bone graft is useful in reconstituting bone stock in these situations. The trial stem, with or without the component, is inserted into the diaphysis but not fully seated. The stem acts as a mold for the actual component and a stopper to prevent graft from filling the intramedullary canal. Graft is placed around the stem and in the defects. The graft is then impacted, which gives it structure and more extensive contact with the host bone. The trial stem is then removed, with the graft maintaining its structural integrity.

Final components are then inserted in a routine manner. If components are cemented, cement should extend to but not include the stem-component junction. If cement extends to a point on the housing at which the taper of the component begins increasing in width, as in the junction of the component housing with a wider stem, removal of the component can be extremely difficult. The cement collar acts as an impediment to removal of the stem and can lead to fracturing at re-revision.

If complete juxtaarticular allografts are being used, attempts at trial reduction without the graft are performed to determine appropriate rotation of the component-allograft composite. Reduction of the joint should be possible, as the stemmed component will be stable in the host bone with the press-fit stem. Marking of the host bone and graft then allows for reproduction of the appropriate rotation and estimation of stem length. The graft-prosthesis composite is cemented, with the stem-graft junction kept void of cement. The composite is then impacted into the host, and final trimming of the junction is performed to ensure that host and graft cortical contact is maximized to minimize the stresses through the stem (**Fig. 67-8**).

RESULTS

The longest follow-up on revision TKAs with stemmed components has occurred with cemented stems. Results have been very successful at a follow-up of 58.2 months. This presently is the gold standard to follow. Forty stemmed arthroplasty revisions were performed. Only one femoral component was radiographically determined to be loose, and three femurs and five tibias developed incomplete, progressive radiolucent lines.[12] Lachiewicz et al retrospectively reviewed 58 revision TKAs with the use of a cemented 30 mm tibial stem extension at a mean follow-up of 5 years. They found no patients to require revision for tibial component loosening, but the vast majority had small metaphyseal defects at the time of revision.[25]

Bertin et al have reported early results of the use of uncemented stems in 53 patients.[1,13] Stems were of limited sizes and, although uncemented, were not always press-fit. Excluding four knees that had serious postoperative complications, 91% of patients had relief of pain, 84% had more than 90° of motion, and 80% were able to walk longer than 30 minutes. Eighty-eight percent of the stems were noted to have surrounding radiopaque lines, which were unrelated to degree of pain or failure rate. However, the results of this investigation are difficult to interpret as it is known that biomechanically an uncemented stem should be press-fit into the diaphysis to improve stability. In a review of 113 revision TKAs (107 cemented metaphyseal and 95 press-fit metaphyseal), Fehring et al found 93% of cemented stems to be radiographically stable at a

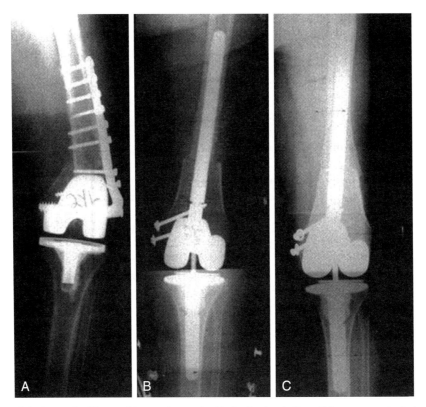

FIGURE 67-8 Radiographs of the knee of a 69-year-old man who required bulk structural allograft for severe osteolysis and failed internal fixation. **A:** Preoperative radiograph. **B:** Immediately postoperative radiograph. The structural allograft was cut on a satellite table with an intramedullary rod of equal width to the reamer in the host endosteal canal. The component-graft composite was cemented, which ensured adequate stem for press-fit into host bone. Ideally, no cement should extend beyond or into the host-graft junction. **C:** Two-year follow-up radiograph.

minimum of 2-years of follow-up versus 71% of cement-less stems. Thus, the authors cautioned against the use of cementless *metaphyseal* stem fixation.[26]

The Insall group has performed follow-up on 76 knees at 42 months, with only 3 failures occurring from loosening and 3 from infection.[15] Fluted diaphyseal stems were used in all patients. There was a 13% complication rate, with all complications being unrelated to the stems. Overall, 84% of patients had a good or excellent result according to the Hospital for Special Surgery rating scale. The procedure failed in six of the knees and another revision was required. In 67% of femoral rods and 69% of tibial rods, a 1- to 2-mm radiopaque line was noted to surround the stems completely or incompletely. These sclerotic lines usually appeared a few months after the procedure and had no correlation with outcome. In 4% of the femoral and 6% of the tibial rods, a progressive radiopaque line longer than 2 mm was present but again had no correlation to outcome.[27] This appearance was markedly different from that of stems that fail.[16] Sah et al reported on the use of hybrid stem fixation in 88 both-component revision TKAs at a mean follow-up of 5.5 years. In this technique, a cementless press-fit diaphyseal stem is used with cementation in the metaphyseal region only. They noted a Kaplan–Meier survivorship free of aseptic loosening to be 100% at 5 years and 90% at 10 years.[28]

Few direct comparisons are present in the literature comparing cemented metaphyseal and cementless diaphyseal engaging stems in revision TKA. Gililland et al performed a two-center retrospective review of aseptic revision TKAs using metaphyseal cemented stems with cement restrictors (48 cases, mean follow-up 76 months) versus 33 diaphyseal cementless stems (33 cases, mean follow-up 121 months). They found no differences in change in total KSS between the two cohorts from preoperatively to postoperatively (p = .7), or signs of radiographic failure of the femur or tibia between the two groups (p = .6 to .99).[29]

Paprosky reported on a select group of patients in whom stemmed components were used with distal femoral allografts.[30] This combination was used in cases of periprosthetic femoral fractures, fracture nonunion, and severe distal femoral bone loss. Distinctly absent from this patient population were patients with bone tumors. At an average follow-up of 32 months, seven of the nine patients had excellent or good results and the remaining two had fair results according to the Hospital for Special Surgery knee score. Complications were again unrelated to the stems. Soft tissue balancing was the greatest concern, with imbalance leading to patellar subluxation or genu recurvatum. Extreme emphasis was placed on protected weight-bearing and bracing until union of the allograft site was evident. Results from the study of Mnaymneh et al are similar, with union of allograft occurring in 86% of cases and motion averaging 92°.[31] Two patients experienced nonunion and fracture on the femoral side. These procedures were considered salvage procedures. Vince and Long reported on 44 revision knee arthroplasties using press-fit stems with 2 to 6 years of follow-up.[16] Three patients developed clinical or radiographic evidence of loosening despite adequate canal fill. It was concluded that, even with adequate canal fill, fixation is inadequate in poor-quality bone using a press-fit stem, and consideration should be given to cementing the stem in position. Significant radiolucencies completely surrounded the stems of those components that failed. In addition to the endosteal radiolucencies, a cortical reaction was evident.

CONCLUSION

As time progresses, as with hip revision arthroplasty, the number of revision knee arthroplasties increases. As the numbers increase, so do the severity of the defects and the complexity of the reconstructions. Use of a press-fit stem on revision components can protect the juxtaarticular bone and transfer the load to stronger diaphyseal bone. The balance between overshielding the juxtaarticular bone and overloading it to failure still needs to be determined. Presently, these stems provide for excellent structural protection of the abnormal bone with no substantial evidence of stress shielding. The stems provide protection from shear, bending, and rotational forces while still allowing compression of the bone. This requires the presence of bone with enough structural integrity to support these remaining forces. Medium-term findings for procedures using these components have demonstrated results that have been unparalleled, so that these stems are an essential adjunct to the revision arthroplasty procedure. They are not, however, a substitute for ensuring solid juxtaarticular support for the components.

REFERENCES

1. Behrens JC, Walker PS, Shoji H. Variations in strength and structure of cancellous bone at the knee. *J Biomech.* 1974;7(3):201-207.
2. Albrektsson BE, Ryd L, Carlsson LV, et al. The effect of a stem on the tibial component of knee arthroplasty. A roentgen stereophotogrammetric study of uncemented tibial components in the Freeman-Samuelson knee arthroplasty. *J Bone Joint Surg Br.* 1990;72(2):252-258.
3. Jones GB. Total knee replacement-the Walldius hinge. *Clin Orthop Relat Res.* 1973;94:50-57.
4. Dennis DA. Structural allografting in revision total knee arthroplasty. *Orthopedics.* 1994;17(9):849-851.
5. Bartel DL, Burstein AH, Santavicca EA, Insall JN. Performance of the tibial component in total knee replacement. *J Bone Joint Surg Am.* 1982;64(7):1026-1033.
6. Wright T. *Biomaterials and prosthesis design in total knee arthroplasty.* In: *Orthopaedic Knowledge Update: Hip and Knee Reconstruction.* Rosemont, IL: American Academy of Orthopaedic Surgeons; 1995.
7. Murase K, Crowninshield RD, Pedersen DR, Chang TS. An analysis of tibial component design in total knee arthroplasty. *J Biomech.* 1983;16(1):13-22.
8. Reilly D, Walker PS, Ben-Dov M, Ewald FC. Effects of tibial components on load transfer in the upper tibia. *Clin Orthop Relat Res.* 1982;165:273-282.
9. Brooks PJ, Walker PS, Scott RD. Tibial component fixation in deficient tibial bone stock. *Clin Orthop Relat Res.* 1984;184:302-308.
10. Lewis JL, Askew MJ, Jaycox DP. A comparative evaluation of tibial component designs of total knee prostheses. *J Bone Joint Surg Am.* 1982;64(1):129-135.
11. Bourne RB, Finlay JB. The influence of tibial component intramedullary stems and implant-cortex contact on the strain distribution of the proximal tibia following total knee arthroplasty. An in vitro study. *Clin Orthop Relat Res.* 1986;208:95-99.
12. Murray PB, Rand JA, Hanssen AD. Cemented long-stem revision total knee arthroplasty. *Clin Orthop Relat Res.* 1994;309:116-123.
13. Bertin KC, Freeman MA, Samuelson KM, Ratcliffe SS, Todd RC. Stemmed revision arthroplasty for aseptic loosening of total knee replacement. *J Bone Joint Surg Br.* 1985;67(2):242-248.
14. Elia EA, Lotke PA. Results of revision total knee arthroplasty associated with significant bone loss. *Clin Orthop Relat Res.* 1991;271:114-121.
15. Haas SB, Insall JN, Montgomery W, Windsor RE. Revision total knee arthroplasty with use of modular components with stems inserted without cement. *J Bone Joint Surg Am.* 1995;77(11):1700-1707.
16. Vince KG, Long W. Revision knee arthroplasty. The limits of press fit medullary fixation. *Clin Orthop Relat Res.* 1995;317:172-177.
17. Barrack RL, Rorabeck C, Burt M, Sawhney J. Pain at the end of the stem after revision total knee arthroplasty. *Clin Orthop Relat Res.* 1999;367:216-225.
18. Barrack RL, Stanley T, Burt M, Hopkins S. The effect of stem design on end-of-stem pain in revision total knee arthroplasty. *J Arthroplasty.* 2004;19(7 suppl 2):119-124.
19. Mihalko WM, Whiteside LA. Stem pain after cementless revision total knee arthroplasty. *J Surg Orthop Adv.* 2015;24(2):137-139.
20. Jazrawi LM, Bai B, Kummer FJ, Hiebert R, Stuchin SA. The effect of stem modularity and mode of fixation on tibial component stability in revision total knee arthroplasty. *J Arthroplasty.* 2001;16(6):759-767.
21. Heesterbeek PJ, Wymenga AB, van Hellemondt GG. No difference in implant micromotion between hybrid fixation and fully cemented revision total knee arthroplasty: a randomized controlled trial with radiostereometric analysis of patients with mild-to-moderate bone loss. *J Bone Joint Surg Am.* 2016;98(16):1359-1369.
22. Donaldson WF, Sculco TP, Insall JN, Ranawat CS. Total condylar III knee prosthesis. Long-term follow-up study. *Clin Orthop Relat Res.* 1988;226:21-28.
23. Askew MJ, Lewis JL, Jaycox DP. Interface stresses in a prosthesis-tibia structure with varying bone properties. *Trans Orthop Res Soc.* 1978;3(17).
24. Cipriano CA, Brown NM, Della Valle CJ, Moric M, Sporer SM. Intra-operative periprosthetic fractures associated with press fit stems in revision total knee arthroplasty: incidence, management, and outcomes. *J Arthroplasty.* 2013;28(8):1310-1313.
25. Lachiewicz PF, Soileau ES. A 30-mm cemented stem extension provides adequate fixation of the tibial component in revision knee arthroplasty. *Clin Orthop Relat Res.* 2015;473(1):185-189.
26. Fehring TK, Odum S, Olekson C, Griffin WL, Mason JB, McCoy TH. Stem fixation in revision total knee arthroplasty: a comparative analysis. *Clin Orthop Relat Res.* 2003;416:217-224.
27. Insall JN, Ranawat CS, Aglietti P, Shine J. A comparison of four models of total knee-replacement prostheses. *J Bone Joint Surg Am.* 1976;58(6):754-765.

28. Sah AP, Shukla S, Della Valle CJ, Rosenberg AG, Paprosky WG. Modified hybrid stem fixation in revision TKA is durable at 2 to 10 years. *Clin Orthop Relat Res.* 2011;469(3):839-846.

29. Gililland JM, Gaffney CJ, Odum SM, Fehring TK, Peters CL, Beaver WB. Clinical & radiographic outcomes of cemented vs. diaphyseal engaging cementless stems in aseptic revision TKA. *J Arthroplasty.* 2014;29(9 suppl):224-228.

30. Paprosky WG. Use of distal femoral allografts in revision total knee arthroplasty. In: Insall IN, Scott WN, Scuderi GR, eds. *Current Concepts in Primary and Revision Total Knee Arthroplasty.* New York, NY: Lippincott-Raven Publishers; 1996:217-226.

31. Mnaymneh W, Emerson RH, Borja F, Head WC, Malinin TI. Massive allografts in salvage revisions of failed total knee arthroplasties. *Clin Orthop Relat Res.* 1990;260:144-153.

chapter 68

Hinged Knee and Megaprosthesis

Nicholas A. Bedard, MD | Matthew P. Abdel, MD

INTRODUCTION

Hinged knee arthroplasty was first introduced in the 1950s.[1,2] This new prosthetic knee design allowed for management of more complex knee deformities and pathologies than was possible with other knee arthroplasty designs of the time. However, failure rates of initial hinge designs were quite high, and as further developments were made for standard condylar resurfacing implants, utilization of hinged knee arthroplasty designs dramatically declined. In the 1980s, the use of megaprostheses began to emerge as a technique for managing large bone defects after tumor resection. The term megaprosthesis includes distal femoral replacement and total femur replacement. The indications for megaprostheses have since expanded to include other causes of large bone defects around the knee such as fracture and prosthetic joint infection (PJI). This chapter reviews the evolution and clinical results of the various types of hinged knee prostheses and megaprostheses, as well as indications for these implants.

EVOLUTION AND CLINICAL RESULTS OF HINGED KNEE PROSTHESES

Clinical data regarding hinged prostheses should be interpreted carefully. Because of improvements in implant design, surgical technique, and patient selection, results with early hinged knee designs do not reflect current outcomes. Furthermore, many reports of hinged implants include results of combined analyses of both primary and revision procedures, with large variation among patients in terms of bone loss, soft tissue compromise, and number of previous operations.

Fixed-Hinge Designs

Initial hinged knee implants were metal-on-metal articulations with a fixed hinge that permitted motion only in flexion and extension.[3] Such implants included the Walldius[2] and the Shiers[1] prostheses. In the 1970s, the Stanmore[4] and the Guepar[5] all-metal fixed-hinge implants were also introduced.

Results with early metal-on-metal fixed-hinge implants were poor. In 1986, data from the Swedish arthroplasty registry showed that the 5- to 6-year survival rate of fixed-hinge knee implants for primary total knee arthroplasty (TKA) in osteoarthritic knees was only 65% compared to 87% for the two- or three-compartment designs used at that time.[6] Results for patients with rheumatoid arthritis were more favorable. However, in such patients, the 5- to 6-year survival rate of the hinge implant was 83% compared to 90% for two- or three-compartment prostheses. The most common reason for revision of the hinged prostheses were aseptic loosening of the components (16.4%) followed by infection (12.1%).[6]

It is likely many of the failures identified in these studies were a result of poor implant design. The fixed axis of rotation with these hinge designs resulted in stress transmission to the bone–cement interface, facilitating component loosening. It is also likely that the metal-on-metal implant design and resultant metal debris contributed to the high number of knees with postoperative effusions[7] and subsequent synovitis and osteolysis may have compounded the loosing problems with these implants.[8]

Even with modification of the metal-on-metal fixed Guepar hinge to include longer stem lengths, results were disappointing. At follow-up of 2 to 13 years in 45 patients with the Guepar II implant, Cameron et al[9] reported an aseptic loosening rate of only 7%, which they attributed to longer stem lengths and improved cementing technique. The percentage of good to excellent results, however, had declined to 38% from an earlier report of 67% at 1 to 7 years of follow-up,[10] and extensor mechanism problems and infection continued to be troublesome.

Poor results with metal-on-metal fixed hinges led to redesign of the Stanmore implant to include metal-polyethylene bushings to articulate with the metal implant. In a series of 103 cases in which Stanmore implants were used for both primary and revision procedures, Grimer et al[11] reported 80% prosthetic retention at an average follow-up of 68 months; only 64% of patients were enthusiastic about their knee implants, and 70% were free of pain. Since then, the Stanmore implant has been further modified to a rotating hinge with metal-on-plastic bearing surfaces.

In Germany, Blauth and Hassenpflug introduced a fixed-hinge implant that sought to improve upon deficiencies in previous fixed-hinged designs including non-anatomical positon of load-bearing axes, directed metal-to-metal transmission of load, and the need for massive bone resection.[3] The Blauth prosthesis had interposed polyethylene components that conform to the larger condylar surfaces of the femoral implant. The purpose of this design was to transfer the constrained forces through these large surfaces to adjacent bone and away from the hinge. Some gliding motion was possible, and the patella could be resurfaced. This prosthesis was evaluated at mean follow-up of 6 years in 422 consecutive primary TKA using this design.[12] Only three patients (0.7%) were revised for loosening and the overall deep infection rate was 3.8%. The 10- and 20-year survivorship for aseptic loosening was 98.4% and 96.0%, respectively. The cumulative rate of implant survival at 20 years was 87% for a worst-case definition of failure, including removal, infection, and patients lost to follow-up.[12] It is important to note that these results are for primary implants and do not include any revision procedures which likely explain their relatively successful results.

Other authors have also reported improved long-term results with fixed-hinge prosthesis in the setting of limb salvage surgery for tumors around the knee. Ruggieri et al[13] evaluated 699 consecutive patients with musculoskeletal tumors treated with limb salvage surgery and reconstruction using modular fixed-hinge megaprostheses (The Kotz Modular Femur-Tibia Reconstruction System (KMFTR; Stryker; UK) and the Howmedica Modular Reconstruction System (HMRS; Stryker; UK)) at a mean follow-up of 11 years. They reported an overall survival to failure of 80% and 55% at 10 and 20 years, respectively, with revisions occurring for breakage, aseptic loosening, and infection. They also reported an overall survival to aseptic loosening of 94% and 82% at 10 and 20 years, respectively.

Although this is an extremely different population of patients with more significant bone loss being replaced with the megaprostheses than previous studies discussed, these results do demonstrate improved survivorship compared to early fixed-hinge knee prostheses, especially in terms of aseptic loosening. Despite these results, the authors of this study do acknowledge the improvements associated with rotating-hinge designs and now use a rotating-hinge version of HMRS for the majority of their patients. However, Ruggieri et al[13] do recommend fixed-hinged megaprostheses for total femoral reconstructions, elderly patients with minimal muscle strength, and distal femoral resections with extensive quadriceps defects given the additional stability provided with a fixed-hinge arthroplasty.

Rotating Hinge

Development

Because of concerns about the contribution of a fixed axis of rotation and relatively poor results with these implants, rotating-hinge designs that allowed for rotation about axes other than flexion and extension were developed. Early designs included the spherocentric,[14] Sheehan,[15] and Herbert[16] knee implants. Many of the original rotating hinge designs did not have a trochlear flange or patella component which was a potential failure mechanism corrected in subsequent designs.

The first Noiles rotary-hinge arthroplasty was performed in 1976.[17] Unlike a fixed-hinge implant, this design incorporated a tibia-bearing component that fits into a cemented polyethylene tibial component. The tibia-bearing component was then fixed between the flanges of the femoral component by the axle. The tibia-bearing component could rotate within the cemented polyethylene tibial component up to 20° from neutral without significant prosthetic resistance. Some axial distraction of the tibia-bearing component within the cemented polyethylene component was also possible.[17] In theory, permitting rotation and axial distraction would reduce stress at the bone–cement interface.[17] Subsequently, several modifications were made, including redesign of the femoral component to a condylar-type implant to prevent subsidence of the femoral component.[18,19]

The Noiles rotating-hinge articulation has undergone many modifications over the years evolving into what is now known as the S-ROM Modular, Mobile-Bearing Hinged Prosthesis (Depuy, Inc Warsaw, IN) and such modifications have resulted in significantly improved midterm radiographic and clinical follow-up.[20] There have been many modifications to other rotating-hinge designs, and new rotating-hinge implant systems have been developed since these early designs. There are multiple rotating-hinge systems available on the market today.

Clinical Results

Although early results of rotating-hinged TKA seemed promising when compared to early results of metal-on-metal fixed-hinge designs, issues with component loosening and patellar instability remained a problem. Two studies reporting on the early results of the kinematic rotating-hinge implant for treatment of significant ligamentous instability and/or loss of bone reported satisfactory results in 80% of patients with a primary procedure[21,22] and in 61%[22] to 74%[21] of patients with revision surgery at a mean follow-up of approximately 50 months. Probable loosening observed on radiographs was a concern in 10% of knees in one study.[21] Progression of radiolucent lines occurred in 26% of knees in that study[21] and in 7% after primary and 20% after revision procedures in the other study.[22] The most common complication was instability of the non-resurfaced patella, which occurred in approximately 22% of primary knee arthroplasty[21,22] and 36% of revision procedures.[22] A slightly longer-term follow-up of this same implant design reported similar results at a mean follow-up of 75 months of 69 kinematic rotating-hinged knee replacements for non-neoplastic conditions.[23] Although these patients did have a significant improvement in their function, the complication rate was high (14.5% deep infection, 13% patellar complications, 10% component breakage), and at final follow-up, the incidence of component loosening was 13%.[23]

Seeking improved results, further develops were made with regard to implant design for multiple rotating-hinge knee systems. Design innovation along with improvements in cementing technique and metaphyseal fixation options lead to improved outcomes with more contemporary rotating-hinge designs at longer-term follow-up.

In 2017, Cottino et al[24] reported on the largest series to date of 408 contemporary rotating-hinge TKAs at a mean follow-up of 4 years performed for multiple different primary and revision indications (re-implantation after primary TKA infection [35%], aseptic loosing [13%], periprosthetic fracture [13%], fracture non-union [5%], mechanical failure [4%], arthrofibrosis [4%], component malposition [3%], neurologic conditions [4%], rheumatoid arthritis [2%], rickets, extensor mechanism failure, dwarfism, and congenital dislocation [0.2% each]). In this series, multiple contemporary rotating-hinge designs were utilized and metaphyseal fixation with cones was used in 28% of cases. The cumulative incidence of revision for aseptic loosening was excellent at 4.5% at 10 years. However, the authors reported a cumulative incidence of revision for any reason of 9.7% at 2 years and 22.5% at 10 years, with the most common reason for revision or reoperation being septic in nature (54% of all revision and reoperations). The authors hypothesized the high infection rate was likely due to high patient comorbidities, multiply operated on knees and most importantly many with history of prior joint infections in this cohort.[24]

Another relatively large series with a similar duration of follow-up identified lower survivorship and higher complications than Cottino et al[24] in their retrospective review of 142 rotating-hinge knees (all Orthopedic Salvage System [OSS]; originally the Finn Knee, Biomet Inc, Warsaw, Indiana) at a mean follow-up of 57 months.[25] This study included 11 primary procedure and 131 revisions, 42% of which were second stage of two-stage reimplantation for infection. They reported a 15% and 1.5% incidence of femoral and tibial aseptic loosening, respectively. Although difficult to directly compare, is important to note that no metaphyseal fixation, such as sleeve or cones, was utilized in this study, which may account for the differences in aseptic loosening rates when contrasted with the results of Cottino et al.[24] The cumulative survival analysis in this study by Farid et al[25] demonstrated a 73% overall implant survival without revision at 5 years and 51% at 10 years. Incidence of other complications identified in this series included 12 acute deep infection and 21 late deep infection (23% incidence of deep infection), 7% periprosthetic fracture, 5% extensor mechanism complications, 4% stem fracture, and 4% mechanical hinge failure.[25]

A systematic review published in 2018 attempted to summarize outcomes for contemporary rotating-hinge knee arthroplasties from studies with more than 50 procedures included.[26] Studies that only evaluated primary procedures, utilized megaprostheses, included oncologic diagnoses, or one-stage revisions for infection were excluded. The authors identified 10 studies that met criteria. The most common indications for rotating hinge in this review were infection, aseptic loosening, instability, and bone loss. Five-year survivorship varied dramatically between studies ranging from 51% to 90% for any revision procedures.[26] Deep infection was the most commonly reported postoperative complications for 7 of the 10 studies included with incidence of infection ranging from 3% to 24%. Similarly, rates of aseptic loosening varied from 1% to 16% at final follow-up, but five of the studies reported aseptic loosening rates of 5% or less.[26]

The variability in clinical outcomes and complications with rotating-hinge TKA identified in this systematic review and in the studies by Cottino et al[24] and Farid et al[25] highlights the difficulty in comparing studies of complex knee arthroplasty procedures which vary greatly in terms of indications, patient populations, soft tissue status, implant type, and modes of fixation. In general, it seems that substantial improvement has been made in terms of aseptic loosing of hinged knee implants when comparing contemporary rotating-hinged knees to fixed-hinged or earlier rotating-hinged designs. However, as pointed out by Farid et al,[25] despite rotating-hinge implants offering improved design and lower rates of complications such as loosening or mechanical failures, the profile of patients in need of hinged knee arthroplasty has changed dramatically in recent years.

Over the last 3 decades of rotating-hinge knee arthroplasties, this area of practice has evolved in opposing directions where improvement of mechanical features of the prostheses may be offset by unfavorable results due to expanded indications in more complex problems.[25] This may explain the relatively high infection rates associated with this procedure,[24-26] which is likely independent of prosthesis designs and more reflective of the complexity of patients in need of such a prosthesis.

Given the difficulty in comparing outcomes for a procedure performed for multiple different indications across studies, the following sections will evaluate clinical results relative to specific indications for rotating-hinged and megaprosthetic knee arthroplasty.

Megaprostheses

Rotating-hinge articulations are commonly used in implants designed for reconstruction after resection of bone tumors about the knee when marked loss of ligamentous structures has occurred. Such implants are designed to replace the large resected bone segment (e.g., distal femur) and are referred to as *megaprostheses*. Megaprostheses have evolved from non-modular implants to segmental modular systems with a porous coating at the shoulder of the implant to encourage extra-cortical bone bridging between the remaining host meta-diaphyseal bone and the adjacent portion of the implant. Modularity allowed for surgery to proceed without delay for prosthesis constructions and provided the surgeon with more intraoperative freedom to reconstruct bone defects different than the preoperative plan indicated.[27] The vast majority of megaprostheses are utilized in the reconstructions of bone loss after resection of malignant and aggressive benign bone tumors around the knee.

Pala et al[28] published on 247 rotating-hinge Global Modular Reconstruction Systems (GRMS; Stryker; Mahway, NJ, USA) knee megaprostheses implanted during the treatment of malignant and aggressive benign tumors around the knee at a mean of 4 years follow-up (range; 2 to 8 years). At this midterm follow-up, they identified an overall incidence of failure of 29.1% with the most common reason for implant failure being infec-tion (9.3%) followed by soft tissue failure (8.5%), aseptic loosening (5.7%), and tumor recurrence (5.7%). Overall implant survivorship at 4 and 8 years was 70% and 58%, respectively.[28] Survivorship was dramatically higher when considering only "classically" defined causes of failure (infection, aseptic loosening, and implant breakage) with survival of 84% and 69% at 4 and 8 years, respectively. No differences in implant survival were noted when com-paring sites of reconstruction (distal femur versus proxi-mal tibia).[28]

Longer-term follow-up for megaprosthetic reconstruc-tion for tumors of the distal femur and proximal tibia has been published by Myers et al.[29,30] In these series, the authors also contrasted survivorship based upon fixed-hinge versus rotating-hinge design in the setting of megaprosthesis reconstruction. At a mean follow-up of 15 years, 335 distal femoral replacements were evaluated and found to have an overall risk of revision surgery of 17% at 5 years, 33% at 10 years, and 58% at 20 years. Early rates of any failure were similar between fixed-hinge and rotating-hinge designs. However, the risk of revision for aseptic loosening of a fixed hinge was 35% at 10 years compared with 24% in the rotating-hinge design without a hydroxyapatite collar and 0% for rotating hinges with a hydroxyapatite collar. The overall risk of revision fell by 52% when the rotating-hinge implant was utilized.[29] Similar results were found when these authors analyzed megaprostheses implanted for reconstruction of tumors of the proximal tibia.[30] At a mean of 15 years follow-up for 194 proximal tibia replacements, Myers et al[30] reported an overall incidence of revision of 28% and similar risk of revision at 5, 10, and 20 years as the distal femur replacement cohorts with risks of 21%, 42%, and 59%, respectively.

Much like the distal femoral replacement cohort, rotating-hinge megaprostheses for proximal tibia tumors performed significantly better than fixed-hinge designs with over 50% decreased risk of any revision at both 10

and 20 years.[30] The majority of this decreased revision risk for rotating-hinge designs was due to less aseptic loosening with an incidence of aseptic loosening of 46% in the fixed-hinge design versus 3% in the rotating-hinge design at 10 years follow-up.[30] Despite relatively accept-able survivorship rates for both of these cohorts, espe-cially when only rotating-hinged designs are utilized, deep infection continues to be a problem for these large recon-structive procedures with a 10% infection rate for distal femoral replacements[29] and 31% and 14% for proximal tibia reconstructions before and after the introduction of gastrocnemius flaps, respectively.[30]

Despite the magnitude of surgery associated with megaprosthesis reconstructions after bone tumor resec-tions, patients tend to maintain an acceptable level of function. In 2015, Bernthal et al[31] published gait lab-oratory and activity monitor analysis of 69 patients with lower extremity tumor prosthesis at mean of 13.2 years after their reconstructions. Although one-third of these patients had proximal femoral replacements, the majority were patients with megaprosthetic reconstruc-tion for tumors around the knee. The authors reported slightly reduced knee strength for patients with prox-imal tibia replacements relative to distal or proximal femur reconstructions, but all groups had efficient gait and were equally active at home and in the community. Interestingly, patients with lower extremity megaprosthe-ses for tumor resections were found to be similarly active as patients after standard total hip arthroplasty.[31]

Although relatively high failure and complication rates are associated with megaprostheses for distal femur and proximal tibia tumors when compared to primary arthroplasty procedures,[32] reconstruction of the knee with megaprostheses after tumor resection has allowed for successful limb savage surgery with acceptable func-tion[31] and similar outcomes to hinged knee arthroplasty for other indications,[24,25] especially when rotating-hinge designs are utilized.[29,30] Given these results, utilization of megaprostheses has expanded from tumor reconstruction to include other causes of significant bone loss around the knee such as fracture, infection, and revision surgery.

Aseptic Revision Total Knee Arthroplasty

Although rotating-hinge prostheses are often utilized in revision TKAs, relatively little literature has been pub-lished focusing on the outcomes of rotating hinges for specific revision indications and rather, most studies include multiple different indications for revision TKA (i.e., instability, aseptic loosening, re-implantation after resection for infection, periprosthetic fracture, etc.) in a single cohort. Although these more inclusive studies are helpful for understanding the general outcomes of rotat-ing hinges in the revision setting, it is also important to evaluate indication-specific outcomes as results can vary dramatically based upon surgical indications.

A common indication for rotating-hinge knee arthro-plasty is instability following primary TKA; however, only a minority of unstable primary TKAs require a conversion to hinged knee prosthesis. Many cases of instability can be corrected with changes to implant position, component sizing, or valgus–varus constraint (VVC) implant designs. In cases of complete collateral ligament deficiency, extreme flexion and extension gap mismatch that is unable to be corrected with other techniques and/or instability of primary TKA that already has a relatively high degree of constraint (i.e., VVC), a rotating-hinged knee arthroplasty is often indicated. In 2015, the results of 96 elderly patients (age ≥75 years) who were treated with rotating-hinge prosthesis for gross instability following primary TKA were published with a mean follow-up of 7.3 years.[33] These authors reported significant improvement in Knee Society Scores (mean of 37 points preoperatively and 79 points postoperatively), 0% loosening and only one case of deep infection (1% incidence) at final follow-up.[33] A similar series of 26 rotating hinges performed for collateral ligament deficiency were evaluated at a mean of 46 months follow-up.[34] It is important to note this series did include five primary procedures and was also a relatively older cohort (mean age = 77 years). At final follow-up, there were no cases of aseptic loosening and only three revisions (one periprosthetic fracture and two deep infections).[34]

Joshi and Navarro-Quilis[35] published a series of 78 revision knees performed for aseptic failure to determine outcomes for rotating hinges in this population without confounding the results with primary hinges or those performed for infectious-related diagnoses. At a mean follow-up of 7.8 years, the authors reported excellent results in 73% of knees and good results in 9%. Seven knees (9%) were revised for instability/dislocation; there were four cases of radiographic aseptic loosening (5%) but no revisions for aseptic loosening and two revisions for septic loosening (2.6%).[35]

Although difficult to directly compare different studies, it does appear that rotating hinges performed for aseptic revision indications in older patient populations can perform quite well with acceptable midterm survivorship and substantially improved infectious outcomes compared to literature that includes cases of septic revisions procedures.

Another aseptic indication for revision TKA in which rotating-hinge prosthesis is becoming increasingly utilized is revision of TKAs with arthrofibrosis. Farid et al[36] performed preoperative irradiation and revision TKA with VVC or rotating-hinge implants for severe, idiopathic arthrofibrosis. About 9 of the 14 revision TKAs in their study had such severe capsular and collateral ligament scaring and/or heterotopic ossification that significant distal femoral shorten and collateral ligament resection was required to improve range of motion and thus a rotating hinge was utilized. At a mean follow-up of 34 months, 86% of patients had a mean improvement of 35° of flexion with at least 100° of flexion at final follow-up. Similar improvements in flexion contractures were seen

with these same 12 patients obtaining mean correction of flexion contracture of 28° and only 4 patients with residual flexion contracture (mean of 8°) at final follow-up.[36] One patient (7%) required further revision surgery for unsatisfactory motion and was revised from a VVC to rotating hinge and was able to obtain 5° to 120° range of motion at 2 years follow-up. The final patient was revised to a rotating hinge and unfortunately had a worsening of their flexion contracture but opted for no further surgery.[36] There were no deep infections in this cohort, but one hematoma required surgical excavation and one case of incisional cellulitis that resolved with antibiotics.

Similar outcomes were reported by van Rensch et al[37] in 2018 in their report of 38 patients with stiff primary TKA (defined as <70° of motion) revised to rotating-hinge prosthesis. Of the 38 stiff TKAs, underlying causes of stiffness were thought to be identified in 24 patients (malposition in 15, aseptic loosening in 7, and instability in 2) and infection was ruled out in all patients. At final follow-up the authors documented a significant increase in range of motion (median gain of 40°); however, 6 patients (16%) continued to have <70° of motion postoperatively. At 2 years follow-up, 79% of patients reported they would undergo the same procedure again. This procedure was not without complications as the authors reported two cases of aseptic loosening requiring revision (5%) and one deep infection that led to eventual amputation (2.6%).[37]

It has been hypothesized that rotating-hinge TKA can be helpful in revisions for arthrofibrosis because such prosthetic design allows for more aggressive capsuloligamentous débridement while maintaining a stable knee as compared to other less constrained knee arthroplasty designs. Hermans et al[38] investigated this hypothesis by retrospectively analyzing 40 patients revised for idiopathic arthrofibrosis to either a rotating hinge (55%) or a VVC prosthesis (45%). Despite similar preoperative data, the authors found that revision to a rotating hinge yielded significantly better Knee Society function scores, Knee Society pain score, knee pain improvement, greater maximal flexion and flexion gain, and better maximal extension and greater extension gain than knees revised to a VVC design.[38] Although there are obvious limitations from the retrospective nature of this study design, these results and those of other studies discussed seem to suggest that rotating-hinge knee arthroplasty can be helpful in the revision of TKAs with arthrofibrosis as they allow for aggressive débridement and optimal implant stability.[36-38]

Prosthetic Joint Infection

PJI and surgery to treat the infection can result in devastating loss of bone and soft tissue around the knee requiring hinged TKA for subsequent knee reconstruction of these patients. Many large series of rotating hinges and megaprostheses often include patients being reconstructed after two-stage exchanges for treatment of infection.[24-26]

However, most of these series also include primary and other revision procedures making it difficult to interpret the results of these prostheses specifically in the setting of PJI treatment.[24-26] However, in 2018, Alvand et al[39] published a series of megaprosthetic reconstruction specifically for management of hip and knee PJI. In this series, the authors reported on 29 knees and 40 hips with a minimum of 2 years follow-up. The majority of reconstructions were performed as a two-stage procedure (70%). Overall complication rate was 48%, with over half of complications being accounted for by recurrence of injection. Infection eradication was more successful in the hip (83% eradication) than in the knee (59% eradication). There was no difference in complication rate or implant survivorship between hip and knee reconstruction. The overall 5-year implant survival was 81%.[39]

In addition to utilizing rotating-hinged prostheses to reconstruct knees in a two-stage fashion for PJI, some authors have described one-stage exchange procedures consisting of radical débridement (complete synovectomy, excision of collateral, and cruciate ligaments to completely expose posterior capsule) and use of a rotating-hinge knee prosthesis along with standard PJI treatment principles (antibiotics in the cement, culture directed intravenous antibiotic therapy). In 2016, Zahar et al[40] published a 10-year follow-up of 70 one-stage revision TKAs for infection utilizing rotating-hinge arthroplasty for reconstruction. The indications for one-stage exchange were a diagnosis of PJI with a known causative organism. During the study period only 11 other patients were treated with techniques other than one-stage exchange for infection (8 two-stage exchanges due to culture negative infection and 3 knee arthrodesis due to damaged extensor mechanism). At final follow-up, 5 patients (7%) were re-infected and 10-year competing risk survival free of infection was 93%.[40] In this series there was a 10% rate of revision for aseptic loosening and survivorship free from any reoperation was 75% at 10 years.[40]

Rotating-Hinged TKA as a Primary Procedure

As described in earlier sections, in modern TKAs, the use of a rotating-hinge implant is usually reserved for patients with severe bony defects or significant ligamentous instability. Occasionally such indications may arise in the native knee and rotating-hinge prosthesis may need to be utilized in the primary setting. Kowalczewski et al[41] published a minimum 10-year follow-up for 12 primary rotating-hinge TKAs performed in the primary setting for medial collateral ligament (MCL) disruption or joint destruction requiring both MCL and lateral collateral ligament release in patients with end-stage arthritis of the knee. The authors reported no cases of PJI, aseptic loosening, or revision surgery at final follow-up.[41]

A larger series of primary rotating-hinge TKAs was published by Petrou et al,[42] in which they review 100 primary cemented Endo-model rotating-hinge knee replacements (Waldemar Link GMBG & Co, Hamburg, Germany) implanted for deformed or maligned knees with bony or ligamentous defects. The cohort was reported at a mean follow-up of 11 years and had acceptable outcomes with Knee Society Score of 93 and functional score of 70 at final follow-up. There were two cases of PJI (2%) and no reported cases of aseptic loosening. Survivorship at 15 years for the endpoint of revision for any reason was 96.1%, but decreased to 80.3% at 12 years if the 5 knees lost to follow-up were to have been revised.[42] The results of these studies demonstrate that rotating-hinged knee arthroplasty can perform well in the primary setting and seem to have lower risk of complications, such as PJI, when compared to rotating hinges implanted for aseptic or septic revision indications.

Another setting in which rotating-hinge TKA is often utilized in the primary setting is for patients with end-stage arthritis secondary to Charcot (neuropathic) arthropathy. The significant bony destruction and loss of protective sensation about the knee that is associated with this diagnosis has led many authors to advocate for increased levels of constraint when performing knee arthroplasty in this population.[43,44] Bae et al[43] reported on their 10- to 22-year results (mean follow-up of 12 years) of 11 rotating-hinge knee arthroplasties performed in 9 patients with Charcot joint secondary to neurosyphilis. They reported significant increases in function (mean knee and function scores both increased 45 points) at final follow-up. Of the 11 procedures, there was one deep infection (9%) and two component dislocations (18%). The rate of revision for any reason at 10 years follow-up was 27%.[43] Similar outcomes and relatively high complications rates for primary arthroplasty for patients with Charcot arthroplasty were described by Tibbo et al.[44] These authors reported on 37 primary TKAs in patients with Charcot from multiple causes and found a 10-year survivorship free of aseptic revision of 88% and free of any revision of 70%.[44] It is important to note that only 35% of cases in this study utilized a rotating-hinge prosthesis with the remainder being either posterior stabilized (19%) or VVC (46%).

Occasionally, congenital deformities of the knee that necessitate arthroplasty reconstruction may require use of rotating-hinge TKA if the magnitude of deformity or ligamentous instability is unable to be managed with lesser levels of constraint. In 2012, Sewell et al[45] reported on 11 primary custom-made rotating-hinge TKAs for advanced osteoarthritis secondary to skeletal dysplasia. At a mean of 7 years follow-up, patient had significantly improved Knee Society pain and function scores. There were four revisions (36%): one revision for aseptic loosening, two for periprosthetic fracture (patella fracture and tibia fracture), and one patellectomy for anterior knee pain.[45]

Distal Femur Fracture

With the relative success of megaprostheses for managing bone loss secondary to tumor resection, indication for these prostheses expanded and now some authors are advocating for use of distal femoral arthroplasty for the management of distal, communicated supracondylar femur fracture around well-fixed or lose implants, especially in elderly patients who can benefit from early mobilization and are often unable to comply with weight-bearing restrictions. Mortazavi et al[46] reported on 22 periprosthetic fractures of the distal femur treated with distal femoral replacement, 3 of which were non-unions after prior attempts at fixation. All patients received rotating-hinged distal femoral replacements. Of the 18 knees available at final follow-up (mean of 59 months), 5 knees underwent additional surgery (28%; 10 total procedures). There was one case of aseptic loosening and three periprosthetic fractures. Similar results were reported by Rahman et al[47] in their review of 17 distal femoral arthroplasty for periprosthetic supracondylar femoral fracture at a mean follow-up of 34 months. Overall there were 3 re-operations (18%). There were two periprosthetic fractures (one managed non-operatively and one with revision TKA) and one deep infection.[47] The results of these studies led both authors to conclude that although complication rates with this procedure are not insignificant, distal femoral arthroplasty can be a successful tool for managing distal femur periprosthetic fractures with similar complication and reoperation rates to other treatment options for these cases.

More recently, indications for distal femoral replacement have expanded to include comminuted distal femur fractures of native knees. Hart et al[48] reported on a cohort of 38 patients older than 70 years treated for intra-articular distal femur fracture with either open reduction and internal fixation (ORIF, $n = 28$) or distal femoral replacement ($n = 10$). The type of treatment patients received was at the discretion of the treating surgeon and patients had similar overall comorbidity status between cohorts. There were no significant differences in terms of postoperative complications between cohorts and only one deep infection in each cohort. Differences between groups with respect of all-cause reoperation (11% vs. 10%), need for ambulatory device at 1 year, and 1-year mortality did not reach statistical significance.[48] Although more data are needed, especially prospective studies, these results demonstrate that distal femoral replacement can be an equally effective option in the management of comminuted, intra-articular fractures in elderly patients.

INDICATIONS FOR HINGED KNEE ARTHROPLASTY

Fixed-Hinged Knee Arthroplasty

In the author's opinion, there are currently no indications for use of a fixed-hinge TKA. Some authors do recommend consideration of fixed-hinged TKA during total femoral reconstructions, elderly patients with minimal muscle strength and distal femoral resections with extensive quadriceps defects given the additional stability provided with a fixed hinge,[13] but the current authors have not found a fixed hinged to be particularly beneficial in these settings.

Rotating-Hinged Total Knee Arthroplasty

In general, rotating-hinged TKA should be considered in primary or revision arthroplasty settings with bone loss proximal to collateral ligament origins and ligamentous instability that is unable to be adequately managed with lesser constrained knee prostheses. When utilizing increasing levels of constraint in knee arthroplasty setting, the authors feel it is important to increase the level of fixation with use of stems and metaphyseal fixation (cones or sleeves) in order to counteract the increased forces transmitted to bone prosthesis interface from the increasing constraint. The following is a list of indications for which the authors will consider the use of a rotating-hinge or megaprostheses if it is felt that more conventional knee arthroplasty implants are unable to be utilized.

Tumor Resection of the Proximal Tibia or Distal Femur

Depending upon the degree of bony resection required for adequate margins, a rotating-hinge arthroplasty can be utilized for reconstruction of a knee after tumor resection (**Fig. 68-1**). This is particularly true if bony resection is needed proximal or distal to the collateral ligament attachments. If extensive bony resection is required, segmental modular rotating-hinge knee systems (megaprostheses) are helpful for rebuilding the segment of bone resected. With proximal tibia tumors, particular attention should be paid to the tibial tubercle and if this must be included in the resection, then recreating the extensor mechanism should be incorporated into the reconstruction procedure.

Severe Malalignment

Cases of severe malalignment in the primary or revision setting often is often associated with bone loss and may require significant ligamentous release to achieve appropriate alignment. Rotating-hinge TKA may be needed in such cases to help control residual instability after alignment is obtained.

Extensive Bone Loss

Bone loss proximal to the collateral ligament origins may be encountered when reconstructing a knee after prior revision arthroplasty procedures, surgical treatment of infection, and congenital or posttraumatic deformities (**Fig. 68-2**). Often the prior surgery or trauma and degree of bone loss have resulted in compromise of ligamentous stability of the knee, and rotating hinge or megaprostheses are required.

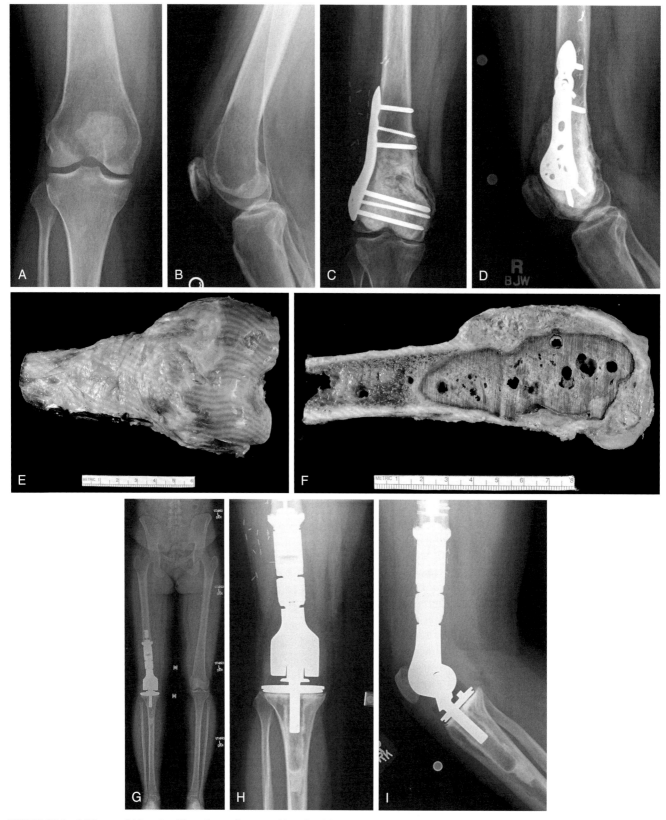

FIGURE 68-1 A 38-year-old female with a giant cell tumor of her distal femur initially managed with curettage, cementation, and stabilization with a lateral plate and subsequent revised to distal femoral replacement for local recurrence of giant cell tumor. **A** and **B:** Anterior–posterior and lateral radiographs of knee demonstrating giant cell tumor of the distal femur. **C** and **D:** Anterior–posterior and lateral radiographs of knee demonstrating recurrence of giant cell tumor after curettage, cementation, and stabilization with lateral plate. **E** and **F:** Photographs of resected distal femur. **G** to **I:** Standing long-leg, anterior–posterior, and lateral radiographs after distal femoral replacement.

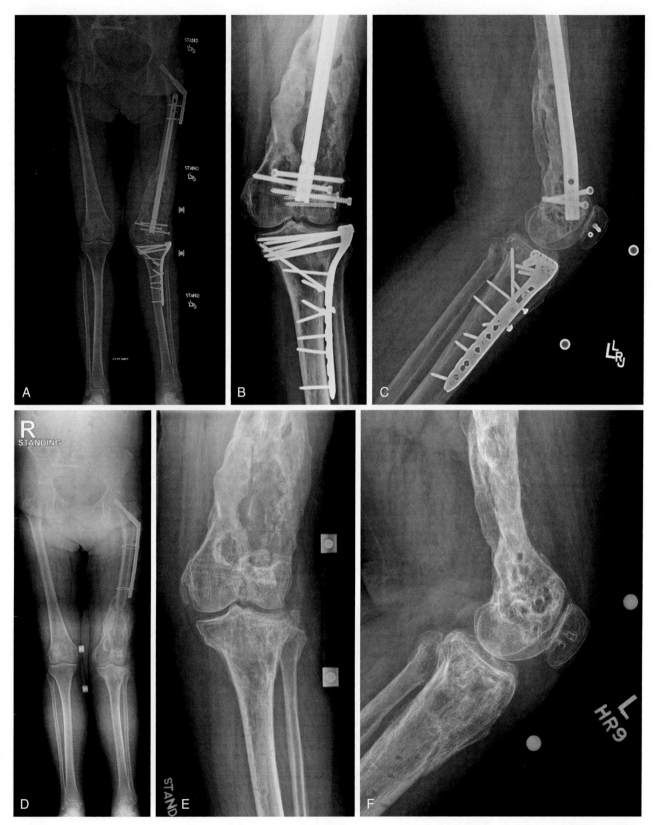

FIGURE 68-2   A 61-year-old female with posttraumatic deformity of the femur and tibia with sequent knee arthritis and a distal femoral osteomyelitis. **A** to **C:** Standing long-leg, anterior–posterior, and lateral radiographs prior to surgery. **D** to **F:** Standing long-leg, anterior–posterior, and lateral radiographs prior after hardware removal. **G:** Resected distal femur. This was resected for concerns of residual osteomyelitis and significant deformity. **H:** Resected distal femur was utilized to help size the distal femoral replacement. **I:** Intraoperative photograph of articulated rotating-hinge distal femoral replacement. **J** to **L:** Standing long-leg, anterior–posterior, and lateral radiographs at final follow-up.

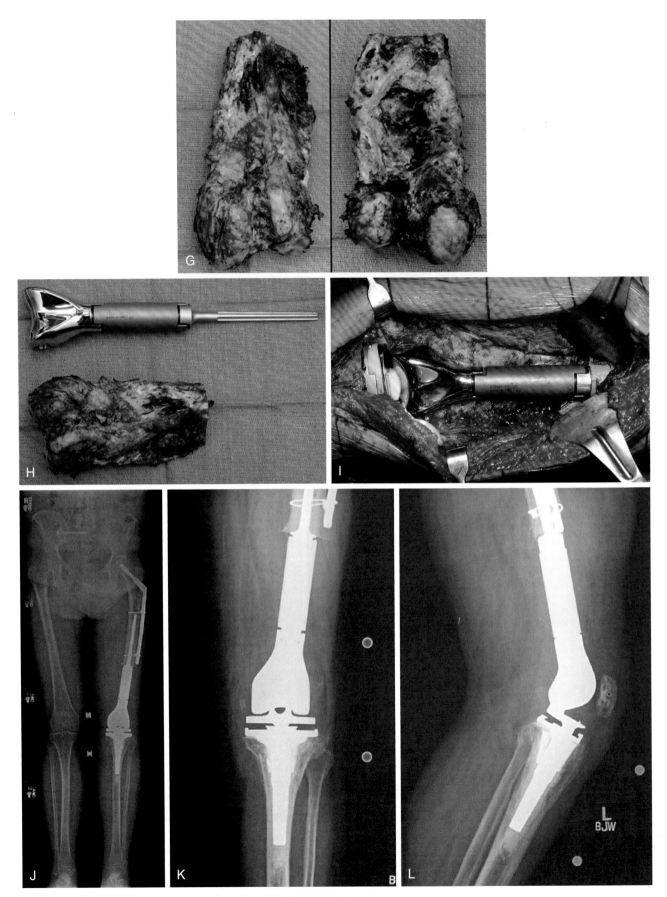

FIGURE 68-2 *Continued*

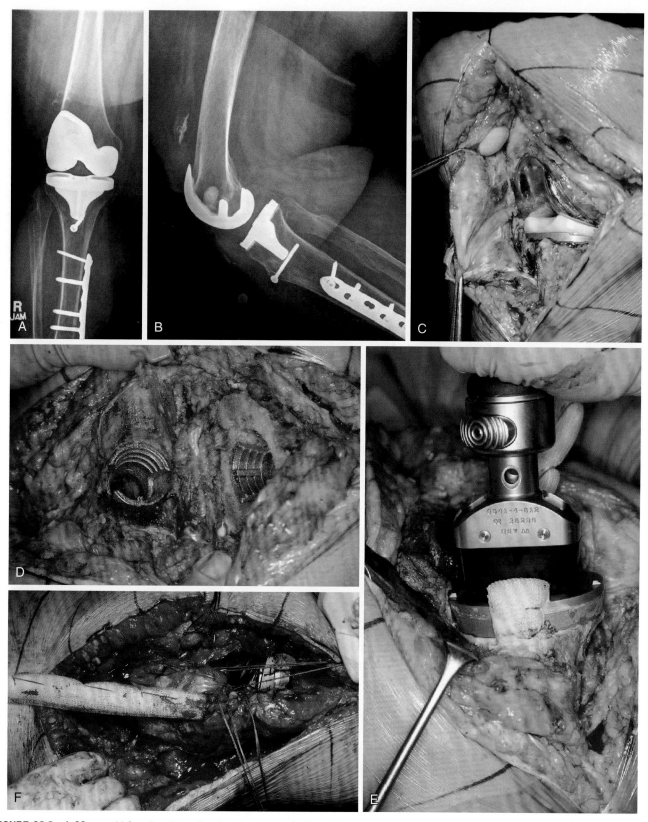

FIGURE 68-3 A 63-year-old female with a chronic extensor mechanism disruption after prior repair with 20° of recurvatum of her primary total knee arthroplasty (TKA) who underwent Marlex mesh extensor mechanism reconstruction and revision to rotating-hinged TKA. **A** and **B:** Preoperative anterior–posterior and lateral radiographs prior to revision surgery. **C:** Intraoperative photo of failure of extensor mechanism repair. **D:** Intraoperative photo of cones being utilized to optimize metaphyseal fixation for the rotating-hinge TKA. **E:** Mesh being cemented into the canal during the cementation of the tibial component. **F:** Mesh being passed through the quadriceps tendon and incorporated into the extensor mechanism. **G:** Intraoperative photo of final extensor mechanism repair. **H** to **J:** Standing long-leg, anterior–posterior, and lateral radiographs at final follow-up.

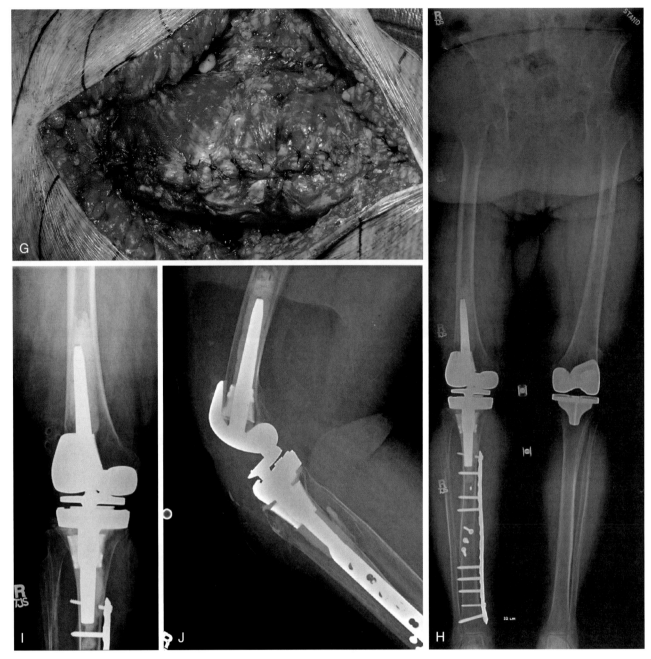

FIGURE 68-3 *Continued*

Severe Varus or Valgus Ligamentous Instability

If severe instability in the coronal plan is encountered and unable to be adequately controlled with ligamentous balancing and a VVC prosthesis, then a rotating-hinge TKA is often necessary.

Extreme Imbalance of the Flexion–Extension Gap

If flexion and extension gap imbalance is unable to be corrected with improved component placement, metal augmentation and polyethylene insert thickness than use of a rotating-hinge implant may need to be considered.

Absence of a Functional Extensor Mechanism

With loss of the extensor mechanism, the anteroposterior stability of the knee is markedly compromised and use of a hinged component should be considered (**Fig. 68-3**). This is particular common in cases of significant quadriceps weakness due to neurologic causes such as polio.

Management of Certain Fractures

Periprosthetic fractures in elderly patients with osteoporotic bone, failed internal fixation of periprosthetic or native distal femur fractures in elderly patients, and acute, comminuted intra-articular distal femur fractures in elderly patients (particularly when goals of immediate weight-bearing and early mobilization are important) are all situations in which consideration of a rotating-hinge arthroplasty is appropriate.

Arthrofibrosis

When revising patients with a diagnosis of idiopathic arthrofibrosis, the authors prefer to utilize rotating-hinge prosthesis to allow for aggressive débridement and necessary bony resection to achieve motion while maintaining optimal implant stability (**Fig. 68-4**).

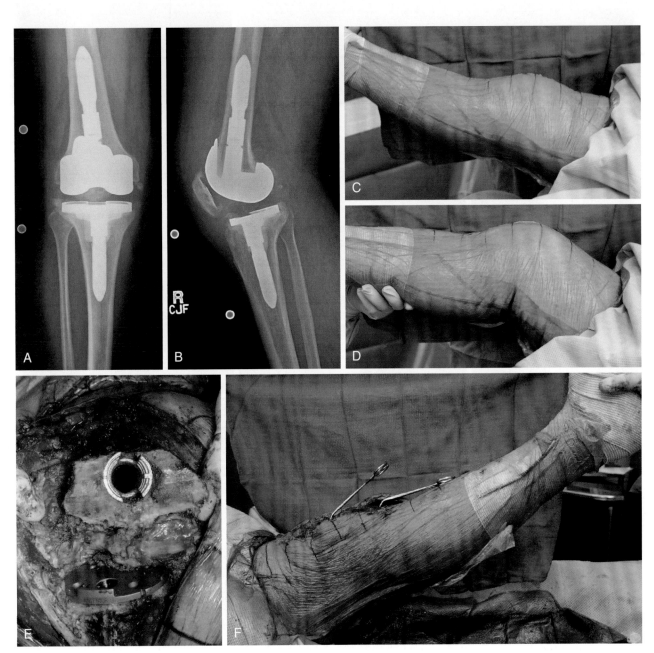

FIGURE 68-4 A 45-year-old male with arthrofibrosis and an arc of motion of 10°-25° treated with extensive débridement, revision to rotating-hinged total knee arthroplasty (TKA), and postoperative protocol of radiation and multiple antiinflammatory medications. At final follow-up, the patient had range of motion from 0° to 65°. **A** and **B:** Preoperative anterior–posterior and lateral radiographs prior to revision surgery. **C** and **D:** Intraoperative photos of prerevision extension and flexion. **E:** Intraoperative photo demonstrating extensive débridement and cones utilized for metaphyseal fixation for the rotating-hinge TKA. **F** and **G:** Intraoperative photos of extension and flexion after revision surgery. **H** to **J:** Standing long-leg, anterior–posterior, and lateral radiographs at final follow-up.

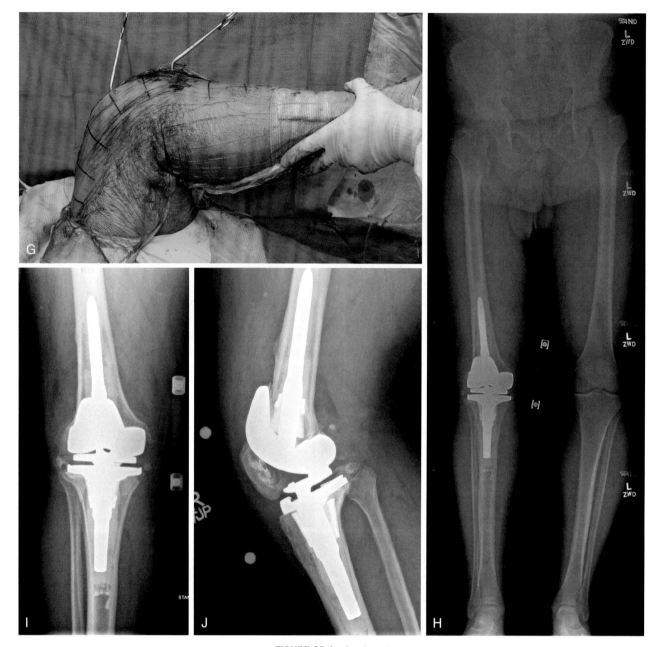

FIGURE 68-4 *Continued*

Neuropathic (Charcot) Arthropathy

The bony destruction and loss of protective sensation about the knee makes knee arthroplasty difficult in this patient population. Although increased constraint is not always required for these patients, one should be prepared for possibly needing a rotating-hinge prosthesis

when performing knee arthroplasty on patients with Charcot arthropathy.

Revision of Previous Hinged Knee Arthroplasty

Patients with a failed hinged knee arthroplasty typically require revision with another hinged prosthesis (**Fig. 68-5**).

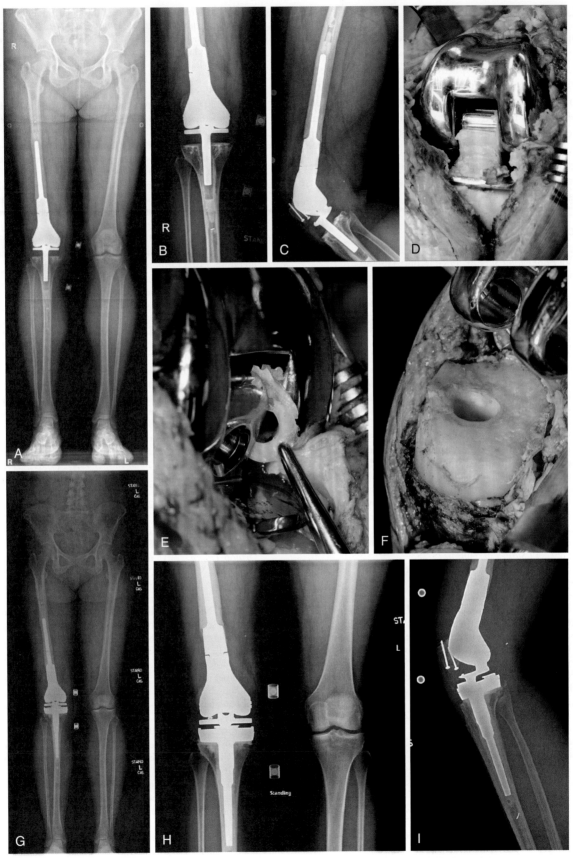

FIGURE 68-5   A 41-year-old male with a history of distal femoral resection for chondroplasty osteosarcoma of the distal femur 25 y prior now with pain and instability secondary to polyethylene wear. This patient was treated with tibia component revision and exchange of the femoral bushings. **A** to **C:** Preoperative standing long-leg, anterior–posterior, and lateral radiographs prior to revision surgery. **D** to **F:** Intraoperative photos of demonstrative extensive wear of the femoral bushings and all-polyethylene tibial component. **G** to **I:** Standing long-leg, anterior–posterior, and lateral radiographs at final follow-up.

CONCLUSION

Rotating-hinge knee TKA is an important tool in the armamentarium of the reconstructive knee surgeon. With improvement in implant design over the years, the indications for rotating-hinge knee and megaprostheses have expanded. Although design improvements have decreased the incidence of complications such as loosening or mechanical failures, reconstructions requiring this type of prosthesis design are inherently complex and are not without complication. However, satisfactory results are able to be achieved in these challenging cases.

REFERENCES

1. Shiers LG. Arthroplasty of the knee; preliminary report of new method. *J Bone Joint Surg Br.* 1954;36-B(4):553-560.
2. Walldius B. Arthroplasty of the knee using an endoprosthesis: 8 years' experience. *Acta Orthop Scand.* 1960;30:137-148.
3. Blauth W, Hassenpflug J. Are unconstrained components essential in total knee arthroplasty? Long-term results of the Blauth knee prosthesis. *Clin Orthop Relat Res.* 1990;258:86-94.
4. Lettin AW, Deliss LJ, Blackburne JS, et al. The Stanmore hinged knee arthroplasty. *J Bone Joint Surg Br.* 1978;60-B(3):327-332.
5. Deburge A, Guepar. Guepar hinge prosthesis: complications and results with two years' follow-up. *Clin Orthop Relat Res.* 1976;(120):47-53.
6. Knutson K, Lindstrand A, Lidgren L. Survival of knee arthroplasties. A nation-wide multicentre investigation of 8000 cases. *J Bone Joint Surg Br.* 1986;68(5):795-803.
7. Bargar WL, Cracchiolo A III, Amstutz HC. Results with the constrained total knee prosthesis in treating severely disabled patients and patients with failed total knee replacements. *J Bone Joint Surg Am.* 1980;62(4):504-512.
8. Cracchiolo A III, Revell P. Metal concentration in synovial fluids of patients with prosthetic knee arthroplasty. *Clin Orthop Relat Res.* 1982;170:169-174.
9. Cameron HU, Hu C, Vyamont D. Hinge total knee replacement revisited. *Can J Surg.* 1997;40(4):278-283.
10. Cameron HU, Jung YB. Hinged total knee replacement: indications and results. *Can J Surg.* 1990;33(1):53-57.
11. Grimer RJ, Karpinski MR, Edwards AN. The long-term results of Stanmore total knee replacements. *J Bone Joint Surg Br.* 1984;66(1):55-62.
12. Bohm P, Holy T. Is there a future for hinged prostheses in primary total knee arthroplasty? A 20-year survivorship analysis of the Blauth prosthesis. *J Bone Joint Surg Br.* 1998;80(2):302-309.
13. Ruggieri P, Mavrogenis AF, Pala E, et al. Long term results of fixed-hinge megaprostheses in limb salvage for malignancy. *Knee.* 2012;19(5):543-549.
14. Kaufer H, Matthews LS. Spherocentric knee arthroplasty. *Clin Orthop Relat Res.* 1979;(145):110-116.
15. Sheehan JM. Arthroplasty of the knee. *Clin Orthop Relat Res.* 1979;(145):101-109.
16. Murray DG, Wilde AH, Werner F, et al. Herbert total knee prosthesis: combined laboratory and clinical assessment. *J Bone Joint Surg Am.* 1977;59(8):1026-1032.
17. Accardo NJ, Noiles DG, Pena R, et al. Noiles total knee replacement procedure. *Orthopedics.* 1979;2(1):37-45.
18. Shindell R, Neumann R, Connolly JF, et al. Evaluation of the Noiles hinged knee prosthesis. A five-year study of seventeen knees. *J Bone Joint Surg Am.* 1986;68(4):579-585.
19. Kester MA, Cook SD, Harding AF, et al. An evaluation of the mechanical failure modalities of a rotating hinge knee prosthesis. *Clin Orthop Relat Res.* 1988;228:156-163.
20. Jones RE, Barrack RL, Skedros J. Modular, mobile-bearing hinge total knee arthroplasty. *Clin Orthop Relat Res.* 2001;392:306-314.
21. Rand JA, Chao EY, Stauffer RN. Kinematic rotating-hinge total knee arthroplasty. *J Bone Joint Surg Am.* 1987;69(4):489-497.
22. Shaw JA, Balcom W, Greer RB III. Total knee arthroplasty using the kinematic rotating hinge prosthesis. *Orthopedics.* 1989;12(5):647-654.
23. Springer BD, Hanssen AD, Sim FH, et al. The kinematic rotating hinge prosthesis for complex knee arthroplasty. *Clin Orthop Relat Res.* 2001;392:283-291.
24. Cottino U, Abdel MP, Perry KI, et al. Long-term results after total knee arthroplasty with contemporary rotating-hinge prostheses. *J Bone Joint Surg Am.* 2017;99(4):324-330.
25. Farid YR, Thakral R, Finn HA. Intermediate-term results of 142 single-design, rotating-hinge implants: frequent complications may not preclude salvage of severely affected knees. *J Arthroplasty.* 2015;30(12):2173-2180.
26. Kouk S, Rathod PA, Maheshwari AV, et al. Rotating hinge prosthesis for complex revision total knee arthroplasty: a review of the literature. *J Clin Orthop Trauma.* 2018;9(1):29-33.
27. Gkavardina A, Tsagozis P. The use of megaprostheses for reconstruction of large skeletal defects in the extremities: a critical review. *Open Orthop J.* 2014;8:384-389.
28. Pala E, Trovarelli G, Calabro T, et al. Survival of modern knee tumor megaprostheses: failures, functional results, and a comparative statistical analysis. *Clin Orthop Relat Res.* 2015;473(3):891-899.
29. Myers GJ, Abudu AT, Carter SR, et al. Endoprosthetic replacement of the distal femur for bone tumours: long-term results. *J Bone Joint Surg Br.* 2007;89(4):521-526.
30. Myers GJ, Abudu AT, Carter SR, et al. The long-term results of endoprosthetic replacement of the proximal tibia for bone tumours. *J Bone Joint Surg Br.* 2007;89(12):1632-1637.
31. Bernthal NM, Greenberg M, Heberer K, et al. What are the functional outcomes of endoprosthestic reconstructions after tumor resection? *Clin Orthop Relat Res.* 2015;473(3):812-819.
32. Houdek MT, Wagner ER, Wilke BK, et al. Long term outcomes of cemented endoprosthetic reconstruction for periarticular tumors of the distal femur. *Knee.* 2016;23(1):167-172.
33. Rodriguez-Merchan EC, Gomez-Cardero P, Martinez-Lloreda A. Revision knee arthroplasty with a rotating-hinge design in elderly patients with instability following total knee arthroplasty. *J Clin Orthop Trauma.* 2015;6(1):19-23.
34. Hernandez-Vaquero D, Sandoval-Garcia MA. Hinged total knee arthroplasty in the presence of ligamentous deficiency. *Clin Orthop Relat Res.* 2010;468(5):1248-1253.
35. Joshi N, Navarro-Quilis A. Is there a place for rotating-hinge arthroplasty in knee revision surgery for aseptic loosening? *J Arthroplasty.* 2008;23(8):1204-1211.
36. Farid YR, Thakral R, Finn HA. Low-dose irradiation and constrained revision for severe, idiopathic, arthrofibrosis following total knee arthroplasty. *J Arthroplasty.* 2013;28(8):1314-1320.
37. van Rensch PJH, Heesterbeek PJC, Hannink G, et al. Improved clinical outcomes after revision arthroplasty with a hinged implant for severely stiff total knee arthroplasty. *Knee Surg Sports Traumatol Arthrosc.* 2018;27(4):1043-1048.
38. Hermans K, Vandenneucker H, Truijen J, et al. Hinged versus CCK revision arthroplasty for the stiff total knee. *Knee.* 2018;26(1):222-227.
39. Alvand A, Grammatopoulos G, de Vos F, et al. Clinical outcome of massive endoprostheses used for managing periprosthetic joint infections of the hip and knee. *J Arthroplasty.* 2018;33(3):829-834.
40. Zahar A, Kendoff DO, Klatte TO, et al. Can good infection control be obtained in one-stage exchange of the infected TKA to a rotating hinge design? 10-year results. *Clin Orthop Relat Res.* 2016;474(1):81-87.
41. Kowalczewski J, Marczak D, Synder M, et al. Primary rotating-hinge total knee arthroplasty: good outcomes at mid-term follow-up. *J Arthroplasty.* 2014;29(6):1202-1206.

42. Petrou G, Petrou H, Tilkeridis C, et al. Medium-term results with a primary cemented rotating-hinge total knee replacement. A 7- to 15-year follow-up. *J Bone Joint Surg Br.* 2004;86(6):813-817.

43. Bae DK, Song SJ, Yoon KH, et al. Long-term outcome of total knee arthroplasty in Charcot joint: a 10- to 22-year follow-up. *J Arthroplasty.* 2009;24(8):1152-1156.

44. Tibbo ME, Chalmers BP, Berry DJ, et al. Primary total knee arthroplasty in patients with neuropathic (Charcot) arthropathy: contemporary results. *J Arthroplasty.* 2018;33(9):2815-2820.

45. Sewell MD, Hanna SA, Al-Khateeb H, et al. Custom rotating-hinge primary total knee arthroplasty in patients with skeletal dysplasia. *J Bone Joint Surg Br.* 2012;94(3):339-343.

46. Mortazavi SM, Kurd MF, Bender B, et al. Distal femoral arthroplasty for the treatment of periprosthetic fractures after total knee arthroplasty. *J Arthroplasty.* 2010;25(5):775-780.

47. Rahman WA, Vial TA, Backstein DJ. Distal femoral arthroplasty for management of periprosthetic supracondylar fractures of the femur. *J Arthroplasty.* 2016;31(3):676-679.

48. Hart GP, Kneisl JS, Springer BD, et al. Open reduction vs distal femoral replacement arthroplasty for comminuted distal femur fractures in the patients 70 years and older. *J Arthroplasty.* 2017;32(1):202-206.

chapter 69

Management of Bony Defects in Revision Total Knee Joint Replacement

Shankar Thiagarajah, MB ChB, FRCS (Tr&Orth), PhD I Allan E. Gross, MD, FRCSC, O.Ont I David Backstein, MD, MEd, FRCSC

Surgeons treating patients requiring revision total knee arthroplasty (TKA) commonly encounter bone stock deficiencies. Massive bone loss occurs as a result of several etiologies including osteolysis, septic loosening, stress shielding, aberrant intraoperative bone cuts, trauma, and iatrogenic bone loss when removing well-fixed components.

The management of bone defects is dependent upon several factors including their size, location, and whether they are contained or uncontained. The key to any successful strategy is achieving implant support and stable fixation. Small contained and uncontained defects may be amenable to repair with bone cement, morselized bone graft, or modular augments. The latter are an integral part of most contemporary knee revision systems. Moderate defects may be addressed using structural allografts, modular augments, or metaphyseal fixation devices (sleeves and cones). In the face of massive uncontained metaphyseal bone loss, particularly with damage to the adjacent collateral ligaments, allograft-prosthetic composites (APCs), or more commonly megaprostheses are credible options.

In this chapter, we present the classification of bony defects in revision TKA, review the pathogenesis of bone destruction, appraise the treatment options for bony defects, outline the techniques for the treatment of bone loss, and review the results of these treatment options.

CLASSIFICATIONS

Bone defects encountered in revision TKA have been classified to enable the surgeon to categorize the extent of the bone loss. Bone defects are better assessed once all components have been removed and preliminary cuts performed intraoperatively. Classifications aid the surgeon in deciding the appropriate revision procedure and the necessary implants required.

While there is no universally accepted classification system, the most widely adopted is the Anderson Orthopaedic Research Institute (AORI) classification that provides an algorithm for the surgeon in the management of bone loss (**Table 69-1**).[1] Type 1 bone defects are minor contained deficiencies of trabecular bone involving the bone–implant interface. The adjacent metaphyseal bone is intact, and thus, the joint line is typically maintained. Such defects may be resected with a thicker bone cut or filled with bone graft or cement. A type 2 defect has a damaged metaphysis in either (2A) or both (2B) the medial and lateral compartments. A type 3 defect represents significant deficiencies to the metaphyseal portions of the femur and/or tibia that may involve the collateral ligaments and/or the patella tendon also. Small type 2 defects can be treated with cement, morselized graft, or metal augments. More substantial metaphyseal type 2 and type 3 defects will require structural allograft or a metaphyseal fixation device. Type 3 defects involving the adjacent ligaments will require either an APC or more commonly a megaprosthesis.

An alternative, the Mount Sinai Toronto system, considers defects simply as either contained or uncontained (segmental or circumferential) (**Table 69-2**).[2] Contained defects possess an intact circumferential cortex, whereas an uncontained defect is deficient of adequate surrounding cortical bone to allow packing it with morselized bone graft.

Contained defects are subdivided into:

Type I defects, the metaphyseal bone is intact and no bone grafting or augmentation is required to restore a normal joint line. Small bone defects can be filled with cement or resected with a bone cut. While not always absolutely necessary, generally a stemmed, condylar prosthesis is recommended to be used in all revision TKA cases.

Type II defects have damaged metaphyseal bone. Small defects (<1.5 cm) may require bone grafting, a cement fill, or metal augments to restore a normal joint line. These defects are best treated with stemmed revision prostheses, particularly when augments are deployed. Larger defects will require a structural allograft or a metaphyseal fixation device (sleeve or cone).

TABLE 69-1   Anderson Orthopedic Research Institute (AORI) Classification of Bone Loss for the Distal Femur and Proximal Tibia

AORI Grade (Femur)	Defect	MCL/LCL	Bone Reconstruction Options
F1	Intact metaphyseal bone	Intact	Cement or morselized graft
F2a	Metaphyseal loss, single condyle	Intact	Metal augment or allograft
F2b	Metaphyseal loss, both condyles	Intact	Structural graft or metaphyseal fixation device
F3[a]	Deficient metaphysis	Compromised	Allograft-prosthetic composite or megaprosthesis
AORI Grade (Tibia)	**Defect**	**MCL/LCL**	**Bone Reconstruction Options**
T1	Intact metaphyseal bone	Intact	Cement or morselized graft
T2a	Metaphyseal loss, single plateau	Intact	Metal augment or allograft
T2b	Metaphyseal loss and lateral plateau	Intact	Metal augment, structural graft, or metaphyseal fixation device
T3[a]	Deficient metaphysis	Compromised	APC or segmental replacement

[a]Possible extensor mechanism compromise.
LCL, lateral collateral ligament; MCL, medial collateral ligament.

Uncontained defects have segmental bone loss with no remaining cortex. These defects are subdivided as:

Type III or noncircumferential defects. Small defects may be addressed using a structural allograft and/or modular augments, whereas larger deficiencies will require a structural allograft or a metaphyseal fixation device.

Type IV or circumferential defects. Massive defects involving the collateral ligaments require a megaprosthesis or APC.

PATHOGENESIS OF BONE DEFECTS IN TOTAL KNEE REPLACEMENT

The etiology of bony defects is multifactorial. In this section, we discuss mechanical bone loss, stress shielding, osteolysis, and infection.

Mechanical Bone Loss

Historically, bone excision at the time of the primary TKA was a common cause of bone loss. Due to the excessive constraints in many early designs, high rotational forces were distributed to the implant–bone interface, which led to premature loosening of the implant. Gross loosening resulted in a windshield-wiper–like action, often with dramatic bone loss.[3,4] The early 1980s witnessed a transition to resurfacing-style prostheses requiring minimal bone resection and using relatively thin polyethylene inserts. Paradoxically, this resulted in increased polyethylene wear, which led to particulate-mediated osteolysis.[5-8]

Iatrogenic bone loss can occur at the revision of well-fixed components, particularly in the case of cementless implants. The posterior femoral condyles are particularly at risk. Thus, great care must be taken to ensure that the bone–cement–implant interface is loosened adequately before implant removal.

Stress Shielding

The tibial component is the most common implant to fail in TKA surgery due to compressive failure of trabecular support.[9] Stress shielding may be an important factor in this mechanism of failure. Use of a metal tibial tray and stem has been shown to reduce maximum compressive stresses in underlying bone by up to 39%.[10]

The strength of the metaphyseal region of the distal femur is also reduced. Finite element analysis reveals that the rigid femoral component reduces stress to the anterior distal femur by a magnitude of 1.[11] Bone loss occurs primarily in the first year, however, can progress thereafter.[12] The effect of the type of fixation on stress shielding is controversial. Mintzer et al[13] showed that osteopenia was independent of implant design and fixation, whereas Seki et al[14] demonstrated a 57% decrease in bone density with a cemented implant compared with a 28% drop for a cementless implant of the same design. This area of stress shielding correlates with the clinically and radiographically observed area of osteopenia in the anterior distal femur.

Osteolysis

Wear particle generation is a significant factor in stimulating periprosthetic inflammation and subsequent bone loss in total joint arthroplasty.[15] Historically, osteolysis was common in TKA and could occur in the femur, tibia, and patella. Osteolysis would result in catastrophic failure of the construct when the bone is unable to support the implant.[9,16] Weakening of the subchondral bone could also lead to periprosthetic fractures.[17,18]

The etiology of wear particle generation is multifactorial. Finite element analysis has demonstrated much higher

TABLE 69-2	**Mount Sinai Classification of Bone Loss at the Knee**			
Type	**Type of Bone Loss**	**Description**	**MCL/LCL**	**Bone Reconstruction Options**
1	No notable loss of bone stock	There may be erosion of the endosteal bone, but no involvement of the cortex. No migration of the primary component has occurred, and bone is largely intact.	Intact	Cement or morselized graft
2	Contained loss of bone stock with cortical thinning	The canal is widened, but there still exists a sleeve of cortical bone.	Intact	Cement if <4 mm Metal augment if 4-15 mm Metaphyseal fixation device or structural allograft if >15 mm
3	Uncontained (segmental) loss of bone stock >50% of medial and/or lateral condyle	Uncontained bone loss represents less than 50% of the medial and/or lateral femoral and/or tibial condyle and is less than 15 mm in depth.	Intact	Metal augment if unicondylar Metaphyseal fixation device or structural allograft if involving both condyles
4	Uncontained (segmental) loss of bone stock >50% of medial and/or lateral condyle	Uncontained bone loss represents greater than 50% of the medial and/or lateral femoral and/or tibial condyle and is greater than 15 mm in depth.	Deficient	Megaprosthesis or APC

APC, allograft-prosthetic composite.

contact stresses in the nonconforming TKA than in the more conforming total hip arthroplasty.[5,19,20] Clinically, this is demonstrated from retrievals of tibial polyethylene inserts in less conforming TKAs.[5,6,8,21] Contact stresses in TKA can exceed the yield stress of polyethylene, particularly if the polyethylene is less than 6 mm. The nonarticulating surface of the polyethylene can also generate wear particles.[22,23] This has been termed *back-sided wear*. Studies by Engh et al[22] demonstrated a wide variation in the degree of wear between implants. Wear characteristics of the inner tray surface and integrity of the tibial implant locking mechanism are important factors.

The numbers of wear particles increases with applied load and number of cycles. Thus, greater osteolysis is expected in heavier and more active patients.[20,24,25] Limb malalignment causing increased contact stresses increases both wear and mechanical collapse, potentially leading to premature failure.[26] The polyethylene patella button is also a source of wear particles. The force across the patellofemoral joint can be in excess of 4600 N. This can be over a small area, particularly if there is patella maltracking or tilt.[27] Thus, the yield strength of polyethylene may be exceeded.[21]

Material-related causes of osteolysis include the use of poor-quality polyethylene,[7,21] heat-pressed polyethylene,[21,28] or gamma-irradiated polyethylene, which oxidizes[29]; the use of titanium as a bearing surface[30-32]; and screw fixation of tibial implants.[33] Some reports suggest that osteolysis is more common with cementless implants.[24,34] Extensive porous coating has been shown to decrease the incidence of osteolysis.[35] While highly cross-linked polyethylene has been reported to be as an effective material for decreasing polyethylene wear and osteolysis in TKA, this has not yet been shown to improve the clinical and radiographic outcomes in mid-term follow-up after TKA.[36] While relatively recently adopted, highly cross-linked polyethylene has contributed to a rapid decline in revision rates due to osteolysis. Consequently large bony defects secondary to polyethylene wear–associated osteolysis are now seldom encountered.

Infection

Infection causes an acute inflammatory reaction and the production of a purulent cytokine-rich inflammatory exudate that can result in rapid destructive bone loss. Low-virulence organisms such as *Staphylococcus epidermidis* can result in progressive periprosthetic radiolucencies without frank clinical signs of infection.

Further bone loss can occur at the time of implant removal during revision of an infected TKA. The two-stage revision approach may also lead to further mechanical bone loss from compression and abrasion due to the use of antibiotic spacers. One study quantified the loss as an average of 12.8 mm for the femur and 6.2 mm for the tibia.[37] No metal rods were inserted across the knee. The authors will typically use a poorly cemented condylar total knee prosthesis at the first stage if stability of the knee permits its use. If the knee is unstable (e.g., the medial collateral ligament is deficient), then either a cemented rotating hinged prosthesis or a tibial intramedullary nail is used to bridge the knee.

TREATMENT

Options

Commonly accepted options for the treatment of bony defects in revision TKA include bone cement, autograft, structural allograft, modular augmentation, metaphyseal fixation devices, megaprostheses, and APCs. The technique used depends on the degree of bone loss and the extent to which the defect is contained.

Bone Cement

Cement has a role in filling contained defects where the bone loss is minimal. The major advantage of bone cement is that it can be molded to fit an irregular defect. It is a nonphysiologic material, however, and therefore lacks biomechanical integrity in larger defects, even when used with screws. The author's indications for use of cement alone are therefore limited to cases with an uncontained defect which is less than 5 mm in depth. For contained defects with a solid surrounding rim of the bone, cement may be used when the deficiency involves less than 50% of the hemi tibial plateau or femoral condyle.[36]

Autograft

Autograft is the optimum material for grafting defects, as it is both osteoinductive and osteoconductive. However, bony defects are often too large to be repaired solely with autograft. It is the authors' experience that contained defects greater than 10 mm × 10 mm are difficult to fill with autologous bone alone, and generally speaking, autologous bone is not an option for contained defects in the revision context. Despite this, autograft is useful to augment and enhance allograft in contained defects, and its use is imperative at the host–allograft interface to ensure healing.

Allograft

Allograft is an appealing alternative to autograft as it also restores bone stock. It is available in unlimited quantities, and there is no donor site morbidity. While the graft can be tailored to match the geometry of the bony defect, the use of allograft size matching with the dimensions of the defect is advantageous as any modification

of the original allograft may theoretically weaken it. Allograft is osteoconductive but not osteoinductive; thus, the incorporation of cancellous bone and the healing of cortical bone are slower than with autogenous grafts.[38] Allograft incorporation varies with the clinical scenario. The most critical factor is the recipient host bed. Morselized allograft incorporation occurs through a combination of revascularization, osteoconduction, and remodeling. In contrast, a structural allograft unites to the host at the host–allograft interface, but there is limited internal remodeling of the allograft.[39] A structural allograft is defined as any allograft not composed of morselized bone that is used to fill a defect.[2] Revision TKA with structural allograft typically makes use of femoral heads, bulk tibia, or bulk distal femoral and proximal tibial allografts to achieve mechanical stability for the implants.

The most common techniques of allograft processing are freezing and freeze-drying. This enables long-term preservation of the graft. Bone frozen at −70°C has a shelf life of 5 years.[40] These techniques have been shown to decrease or eliminate the immunogenicity of allografts; however, they also decrease their biologic activity by killing any live cells. The major histocompatibility complex class I and II antigens on specialized antigen-presenting cells are responsible for the immune response to allograft bone.[41] Animal studies have shown a strong immune response if there are major histocompatibility differences; however, there is no difference in the biologic incorporation of the graft.[42,43] Similarly, the effect of human leukocyte antigen (HLA) matching in allografts has been evaluated. A multicenter study showed sensitization to HLA; however, no biologic or clinical effects were ascertained.[44] Other studies have shown better radiologically demonstrated incorporation with HLA matching; however, this effect was not statistically significant.[45,46] Thus, at present, no major histocompatibility complex or HLA matching is performed in revision joint arthroplasty using allograft bone.

A relative contraindication for the use of structural allograft is an actively smoking patient. All efforts ought to be made to ensure that smoking cessation prior to surgery takes place. Active infection is an absolute contraindication.

Modular Augmentation

Modern revision total knee systems are able to address moderate (<1.5 cm) contained and uncontained bone stock loss using metal augmentation on both the femoral and tibial sides. Metal augments offer the advantage of extensive modularity, while being readily available and technically easier than allograft implantation. In addition, it is not associated with disease transmission, nonunion, or resorption. Disadvantages include relative expense, inability to restore bone stock, and often the requirement to resect additional bone in order to seat the augment satisfactorily.

Tibial augments have been shown to be biomechanically superior to cement alone or screw-augmented cement.[47] Metal augments are also useful on the femoral side, as asymmetric bone loss is common. Medial and lateral augments are available for use distally and posteriorly. The use of distal augments enables the surgeon to accurately recreate the anatomic joint line, whereas posterior femoral augments are helpful to correct rotational errors resulting from the primary procedure or asymmetric bone loss. Posterolateral augments are routinely used to prevent femoral internal rotation, and medial tibial augments are effective at avoiding varus malalignment.

Utilizing finite element analysis, the use of a metal base plate and stem was found to significantly reduce metaphyseal stresses in the bone-deficient tibia.[10] Additionally, in the absence of a cancellous bed to support the component, the best solution is to transfer the load to the cortical rim. This work was supported by Brooks et al,[48] who showed that a 70-mm tibial stem will bear approximately 30% of the total load, unloading the deficient tibia.

Metaphyseal Fixation Devices

Metal metaphyseal cones and sleeves are designed to fill large (>2 cm) contained and uncontained defects that are too extensive to be managed by metal augments alone. Its primary constituent, tantalum, is an ideal material for providing rapid osseointegration due to its high porosity,[49] high coefficient of friction,[50] and its affinity for osteoblastic activity.[51,52] Once integrated, these devices share the transmitted axial loading forces and provide rotational stability, protecting the tibial and femoral component fixation interfaces. Metaphyseal sleeves are implant-specific, whereas a range of prostheses can be cemented into the inner, central surface of the majority of metaphyseal cone designs.[53]

Cones or sleeves are indicated when there is concern that implant fixation will be inadequate to resist rotational forces. On the tibial side, cones or sleeves are recommended when there is insufficient bone available to allow for purchase of the implant keel in the bone. On the femoral side, cones or sleeves are recommended when the box of femoral implant is not surrounded by any bone on the medial, lateral, or both sides.

Both sleeves and cones are acceptable methods of achieving this fixation; selection of implant is based on surgeon preference or the necessities of the particular revision TKA system being used.

Advantages over structural allograft include a reduction in the overall complexity of the reconstruction, long-term reliable biologic fixation, and enablement of early postoperative weight-bearing. Disadvantages include expense, the need to remove the host bone in order to appropriately position the device, and potential difficulty of later removal.[54] Long-term outcomes are also lacking.

Megaprostheses and Allograft-Prosthetic Composites

Massive uncontained defects that are also often circumferential and involving the collateral ligaments cannot be treated with structural allografts or metaphyseal fixation devices alone and instead require either a megaprosthesis or an APC.

Megaprostheses utilize metal to compensate for extensive bone loss and a rotating hinge for the inherent ligamentous deficiencies in such cases.

APCs entail preparation of a "back-table" stemmed implant cemented into a distal femur or proximal tibial allograft. This is then press-fit into the host via a step cut and cerclage wires. APCs are less frequently performed due to their prolonged surgical exposure, technical difficulty, and inferior ligamentous compensation when compared with megaprostheses. The authors' only current indication for APC is in the presence of a long total hip replacement femoral stem above the knee which makes it impossible to place the stem of a distal femoral replacement.

Techniques

In this chapter, we concentrate on the surgical technique for treatment of uncontained defects using either structural allograft or APCs. Excellent step-by-step technical instructions are provided by the implant companies for use of modular augments, metaphyseal fixation devices, and megaprostheses.

Preoperative Planning

Preoperative radiographs should be evaluated for bone loss. Computed tomography (CT) often provides a more detailed assessment of defect shape, location, dimensions, and detail regarding the presence or absence of cortical containment. The indication for CT imaging very much depends on the individual surgeon's experience and availability of bone graft, augments, and other equipment. Since defects are generally larger than they appear on plain X-ray, the authors recommend a CT for any surgeon that does not have the expertise or equipment to perform revision surgery that may require augments or allograft. In addition, if there is concern that bone loss may involve the origin or insertion of one of the collateral ligaments, CT should be performed to verify and insure that constrained or hinged implants are available.

These imaging modalities combined with a detailed clinical examination provide important information toward determining surgical approach, the potential need for extensile exposure maneuvers, the type of allograft likely to be required, and component selection. Frequently defects are encountered intraoperatively which are larger than originally anticipated from preoperative imaging, and more allograft tissue may be required than initially anticipated. As is the case with virtually all revision procedures, the use of stemmed implants is required in order to obtain satisfactory stability of the component at the host–allograft or host–augment interface. In the case of ligamentous instability, implants with increasing constraint may be required. If there is concern about the extensor mechanism, synthetic mesh or a proximal tibia with an extensor mechanism attached should be made available.

The major principles of revision are to recreate the true joint line, balance the knee in flexion and extension, and provide the appropriate level of constraint required for varus–valgus and anteroposterior stability.

Allograft Procurement

The allograft is procured under sterile conditions according to the protocol of the American Association of Tissue Banks.[48] The bone is deep-frozen at −70°C and treated with 25,000 Gy of radiation.

Surgical Technique

STRUCTURAL ALLOGRAFT

Structural allograft, in the form of a femoral head, partial distal femur, or proximal tibia, can be used for either large (>1.5 cm) contained or uncontained defects.

The preexisting implants are removed, and all nonviable host tissues are debrided. A geometric cut is made where the host bone is structurally sound (**Fig. 69-1**). A high-speed burr is then used to remove any sclerotic nonviable bone. The metaphyseal bone defect is then reamed to a hemispherical shape using a male-type reamer. Care is taken to ream to a bed of bleeding cancellous bone without creating an uncontained defect.

The structural allograft is then fashioned in an appropriate bone-holding device on the sterile back table to fit the bony defect. A female-type reamer, either the same size or one size larger than the male-type reamer used to prepare the host bone defect, is employed to prepare the allograft. Once decorticated, the allograft is pulse lavaged to remove all marrow rudiments.

Ideally, cancellous autograft is placed at the base of the prepared bone defect to enhance union. The prepared allograft is now either impacted (in the case of contained defects) or positioned and secured with Kirschner wires (in the case of uncontained defects). The K-wires should not be placed in a location in which they would interfere with the component stem. Dependant on its stability, the structural allograft can then be fixed to the bone with cancellous screws (**Fig. 69-2**). Additional fixation is obtained with long press-fit stems (**Fig. 69-3**). Care must be taken to ensure that the screws do not interfere with the press-fit stems. Two 6.5-mm AO screws are usually satisfactory. Morselized allograft is used to fill any contained bony defects. Cement is used to secure the allograft–implant and host–implant interfaces but is not used to enhance stem fixation in the diaphyseal region. Care should be taken to avoid cementing the host–allograft junction.

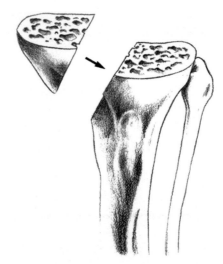

FIGURE 69-1 A geometric defect is made in the noncircumferential defect to accept the allograft.

In the event that screw fixation of the allograft is not required, the K-wires stabilizing the allograft are removed once the cement has fully cured.

ALLOGRAFT-PROSTHETIC COMPOSITE

For circumferential defects, the margins of the host bone are dissected out to reveal the extent of the bone loss. It is imperative to retain as much residual host bone with soft-tissue attachments as possible. The size and shape of the

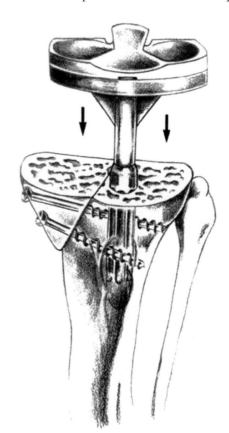

FIGURE 69-2 The allograft is screwed to the host bone.

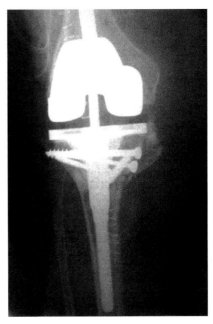

FIGURE 69-3 Press-fit stems are used to increase stability.

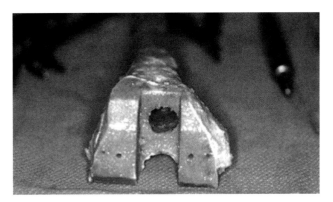

FIGURE 69-4 The allograft is fashioned on the back table using revision instruments.

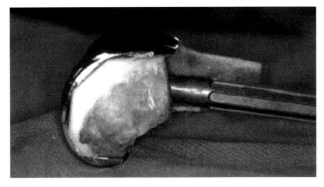

FIGURE 69-5 A step cut is made in the allograft for stability. The allograft–implant interface is cemented only.

bony defect are evaluated, and a replacement construct is fashioned on the sterile back table (**Fig. 69-4**).

The size and position of the tibial component is estimated based upon an appropriate position of the tibial

base plate in order to restore the anatomic joint line. The tibial height and femoral component size and position are chosen in order to balance the knee at 90° of flexion and full extension. An appropriately thick trial polyethylene liner is selected. The level of appropriate constrained required is assessed based upon the knee's collateral and anteroposterior stability.

A step cut is created in the host bone at the location of the prosthetic–composite interface (**Fig. 69-5**). Ideally, the longer limb ought to be on the host bone side. The step cut provides good rotational control of the allograft and increases the contact area between the host and allograft potentially optimizing the chances of incorporation. It is important to ensure that there is good approximation of bone at the allograft–host interface and that the allograft construct is satisfactorily externally rotated.

Appropriate cuts are made using revision total knee joint instrumentation. A trial reduction is then performed. The level of the joint line must be carefully assessed, as there is a tendency to translate the joint line with allograft constructs. With a femoral allograft, the tendency is to depress the joint line, whereas a tibial allograft tends to elevate the joint line.

The most accurate method to measure the joint line is to measure the distance from the proximal tip of the fibula to the joint line on the normal contralateral knee radiograph. If the patient has undergone a joint replacement on the contralateral knee, guidelines for the joint line are the following: 1.5 cm proximal to the tip of the fibula, 2.5 cm distal to the medial epicondyle, or the site of the residual meniscal rim scar. The surgeon must also ensure that the flexion and extension gaps are balanced, that the rotation of the components is correct, and that the alignment of the limb is acceptable. Rotational positioning of the implants is trialed with the epicondylar axis in the femur and the long axis of the tibia as a guide. It is important to ensure that the rotation is matched for the femoral and tibial components. We use patellar tracking as a guide to ensure that we have correct external rotation of the components.

Once the surgeon is satisfied that the aforementioned criteria for the allograft construct have been met, the components can be cemented to the allograft on the back table (**Fig. 69-5**). Cement is used at the implant–allograft interface and the stem–allograft interface; however, care is taken to ensure that no cement is present at the proposed allograft–host interface or in the host canal. Stability of the construct is gained from the step-cut and press-fit stems (**Fig. 69-6**). The stem is not cemented or porous coated, which makes the host canal available for further surgery. In the femur, the cortical shell of bone with the attached collateral ligaments is fixed with cerclage wires or screws to the construct to act as a vascularized graft at the host–allograft junction and to provide ligamentous support (**Fig. 69-7**). In the tibia, excellent stability is usually obtained with the step-cut and press-fit

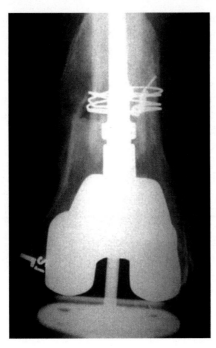

FIGURE 69-6 Stems are used to enhance stability.

stem; however, if there is any doubt, fixation can be augmented with cortical screws. Morselized autograft and allograft are laid around the allograft–host junction. We do not recommend plate fixation to enhance fixation of the allograft,[55,56] as the multiple drill holes produce channels in the allograft that may facilitate revascularization and fracture of the graft.[57] If there is concern regarding the stability of the construct, cortical struts or plates may be used as a last resort. Plates and screws should be avoided in the proximal tibia due to concerns regarding soft-tissue coverage.

Postoperative Management

Postoperative management varies according to the complexity of the surgery. Following grafting for contained defects, weight-bearing as tolerated may be possible while APCs should be protected from full weight-bearing for 6 to 12 weeks. Range of motion and strengthening

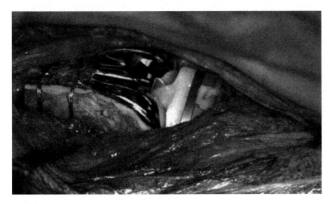

FIGURE 69-7 The host–graft interface is stabilized with cerclage wire.

exercises are commenced immediately postoperatively. Radiographs are recommended at 3, 6, and 12 months to check for graft integration. Union at the allograft–host interface usually takes approximately 3 months.

RESULTS OF TREATMENT

Cement

Murray et al[58] reported on a series of 40 long-stem knee revisions where cement alone was used to fill a contained defect. At an average follow-up of 58 months, clinical outcome as measured by the Knee Society Score was maintained at a mean of 83 points. Early radiolucent lines were seen but not progressive. Vince and Long[59] compared 31 patients with posterior stabilized implants and stems and 13 with constrained implants. Three of the 13 constrained implants failed; however, all these revisions were for infection. The investigators concluded that the press-fit technique with limited cement may not provide adequate fixation for the constrained condylar implant, especially when bone quality is poor.

Ritter[60] evaluated 57 TKAs with a minimum 3-year follow-up. Defects in the tibial plateau were filled with screw and cement. At 3 years, 15 had radiolucency between the cement and bone that was unchanged from that in the radiograph taken 2 months postoperatively. No radiolucency was noted at the stem bone–cement interface or between the screw and bone. Ten of the 27 knees followed longer than 4 years showed similar findings. There were no loose tibial components in any of the 57 cases.

Metal Augments

The use of modular metal augmentation in the management of bony deficiencies during revision TKA has demonstrated favorable outcomes for AORI type 2 defects in several studies.[61-64] Despite metal augments appearing to be a convenient and efficient method of filling bone defects, concerns regarding potential fretting corrosion at the augment–implant interface, as well as the appearance of radiolucent lines adjacent to the augment, have been described.

While the relationship between clinical outcome and radiological stability is not entirely clear, Kyung-Jae et al reported the greater the number of metal augments used in AORI 2 and 3 defects, the greater the area of radiolucency around the implants.[65]

Patel et al reported the outcomes of 79 AORI type 2 bone defects treated with modular metal augments in revision TKA. The survival of the components was 92% at 11 years (95% confidence interval [CI], 10.3 to 11.2).[63] The presence of nonprogressive radiolucent lines around the augment in 14% of knees was not associated with poorer knee scores, range of motion, or survival of the component or the type of insert that was used.

Hockman et al demonstrated a higher rate of loosening (59%) at a minimum 5-year follow-up, in those revision TKAs where metal augments alone were used to address AORI type 2 defects.[66] There was less loosening (16%) when a structural allograft was used in combination with metal augmentation for the more severe AORI type 3 defects.

We would advise the use of metal augments alone in unilateral deficiencies of 15 mm or less. With a greater extent of bone loss (severe type 2 or type 3 defects), we would advise the use of some form of metaphyseal fixation device rather than metallic augmentation alone.

Morselized Allograft

Whiteside and Bicalho[67] reported the use of morselized cancellous allograft to fill large contained femoral and/or tibial defects in 63 patients (63 revision TKAs). Stable seating of the components on a rim of viable bone and rigid fixation with an intramedullary stem was achieved in all. Only two patients required subsequent revision surgery. Evidence of healing, bone maturation, and formation of trabeculae was seen in all visible areas treated with allograft at 1 year following surgery. No significant bone graft loss was seen in any case. All biopsy specimens including those taken at 3-weeks post surgery showed evidence of active new bone formation in the allografted areas. Active bone formation was found in and around the allograft, and new osteoid formed directly on the dead allograft trabeculae. Vascular stroma was present between the bone fragments deep in the allograft mass. Older biopsy specimens demonstrated progressive maturation. Evidence of active osteoclastic activity was absent by 18 months following surgery. All but one patient had significant improvement in their pain scores. Despite a high complication rate (22%), all but one patient achieved lasting fixation to bone, adequate ligament balancing, and a good range of motion. The two patients that required revision surgery, both had greatly improved bone stock, so that new implants could be applied with minor additional grafting. The investigators concluded that this method of bone stock restoration is reliable when used in conjunction with firm rim implant seating and rigid intramedullary stem fixation.

Structural Allograft

The evidence supporting the short and mid-term outcomes of structural allograft in revision TKA is promising. The 5-year survivorship of the revision TKA implant/allograft construct ranges from 78.7% to 93%.[2,68-71] Ten-year survivorship ranges from 72% to 93%.[71-74] Revision specifically due to allograft-related complications only such as nonunion, fracture, and aseptic loosening, ranges from 3.3% to 11.5% at 10 years post surgery.[71-74]

Clatworthy et al[72] reported a series of 50 patients undergoing 52 revision TKAs with 66 structural grafts. In this complex cohort, all defects were large and uncontained. Noncircumferential defects were treated with femoral head, partial distal femurs, or partial proximal tibias rigidly fixed to the host bone. Circumferential defects were treated with APCs. Success was defined as radiological union, an increase of greater than 20 points in the modified Hospital for Special Surgery (HSS) knee score at the time of final review, and the absence of an additional operation related to the allograft. At an average of 8-years follow-up, overall success was 75%. Graft survivorship at 5 years was 92% (95% CI, 89% to 95%) and at 10-years, 72% (95% CI, 69% to 75%). The mean modified HSS knee score had improved from 32.5 points preoperatively to 75.6 points at the time of review, and the mean range of motion had improved from 60.5° preoperatively to 88.6° postoperatively.

Chun et al retrospectively reviewed the records of 27 patients who had undergone revision TKA between August 1997 and March 2003 using a fresh-frozen femoral head allograft.[74] In 26 out of 27 patients, union of the allograft was seen at an average of 7 months post surgery. With a minimum 8-year follow-up, only upon knee (infection) underwent a further operation. There were no revisions secondary to allograft-related complications.

Wang et al retrospectively reviewed 28 patients (30 knees) with AORI type 3 defects that underwent revision using femoral head structural allograft and stemmed components.[70] All grafts healed to host bone, at an average of 6.6 months postoperatively. Implant and allograft survivorship was 100% at an average follow-up of 6.3 years.

Bauman et al retrospectively reviewed the outcomes of 65 patients (70 knees) who underwent either femoral head allograft or an APC at the time of revision TKA.[68] Five-year revision-free survival was 80.7% (95% CI, 71.7–90.8) and 10-year survivorship was 75.9% (95% CI, 65.6–87.8).

Engh and Ammeen reviewed a single-surgeon series of revision arthroplasty in 47 patients (49 knees) with a severe tibial bone defect.[73] Structural allograft was used alone in 35 knees and in conjunction with a tibial metal augment in 14. At a mean of 8 years postoperatively, they found no instance of graft collapse or aseptic loosening associated with the structural allograft.

Richards et al compared the clinical outcomes of patients undergoing revision TKA with femoral head structural allograft (n = 24) to those without (n = 48).[75] Despite the presence of more significant bone loss in the allograft group, the allograft cohort had significantly better patient-related outcome scores.

Most recently, Sandiford et al found no difference in survivorship, pain, and function when comparing trabecular metal cones (n = 15 patients) and femoral head allografts (n = 30 patients) for severe bone defects in revision TKA, at a minimum of 5-year follow-up.[71] Five- and 10-year survivorship of the allografts was 93% (95% CI, 77–98) and 93% (95% CI, 77–99), respectively. Union of the allograft was noted from 3 months post surgery and was complete in all cases at 6 months. Five-year survivorship of the trabecular metal cones was 91% (95% CI 56-98).

In summary, structural allograft combined with stemmed, press-fit revision components is a viable method for dealing with bone loss in the setting of revision TKA with the added benefit of restoring bone stock. This surgery, however, can be technically challenging and requires careful preoperative preparation.

Metaphyseal Fixation Devices

Studies reporting the outcomes of metaphyseal cones and sleeves in revision TKA are limited to case series' with relatively short-term follow-up.

A recent review of the literature by Bonanzinga et al included 16 studies with a total of 442 patients that had undergone revision TKA (447 implants and 523 tantalum cones).[76] At a mean follow-up of 42 months (range 5-105 months), signs of loosening were found in 1.3% of the 523 cones implanted. It was noted that the majority of these loose cones were on the femoral side (5 out of 7) indicating that special attention be placed on preparation of the femoral metaphysis during implantation. The overall infection rate was 7.38%; however, the vast majority were in preexisting septic cases. The incidence of new infection was only 0.99%.

Zanirato et al performed a recent systematic review of the outcomes of metaphyseal sleeves in the management of bony deficiencies in revision TKA.[77] From the 13 included Level IV studies, a total of 1079 revision TKAs (1554 sleeves) were analyzed. At a mean follow-up of 4 years, the implant and sleeve aseptic survival rates were 97.7% and 99.2%, respectively. The incidence of deep infection was 2.7%.

Despite the need for a greater level of evidence with longer-term follow-up, current data appear to suggest that metaphyseal cones and sleeves both represent credible options for management of bone deficiency (AORI type 2b and 3 defects) in the setting of revision TKA.

Megaprostheses

To date, several small case series have evaluated the outcome of mega modular prosthesis implantation in the setting of revision TKA.

Berend et al retrospectively reviewed 39 rotating hinged distal femoral replacements in 37 patients. Indications for surgery included 35 as revision procedures (including 13 for periprosthetic fractures). The knee society scores improved from 39 preoperatively to 87, with a low short-term reoperation rate and an implant survivorship of 87% at 46 months.[78]

Barry et al report a 100% (95% CI, 100%-100%) survivorship at 2 years and 90% (95% CI, 75%-100%) at 5-year survivorship in their retrospectively collected cohort of 17 distal femoral replacements performed in the revision setting.[79] When compared with $n = 15$ diaphyseal femoral replacements, the deep infection rate (25% vs. 90%) was significantly higher in the diaphyseal replacement group. Five-year survivorship of the diaphyseal femoral replacements was unsurprisingly inferior also at only 30% (95% CI, 12%-73%).

Kostuj et al compared the mid-term outcomes of megaprostheses used in the setting of malignant tumor versus those implanted for bone stock deficiency at revision. While deep infection rates were higher in the revision group (29.5% vs. 9.1%), clinical outcome scores were equivalent.[80]

A recent literature review by Kouk et al reported on the outcome of rotating hinge knee implants for complex revision TKA. From the 10 included studies, the devices had a good survivorship ranging from 51% to 92.5% at 10 years. Complication rates ranged from 9.2% to 63% with infection and aseptic loosening as the most common complications.[81]

CONCLUSION

Revision TKA is increasing in frequency, therefore the need to treat significant bony deficiencies is becoming more important. Today's revision surgeon's armamentarium includes a number of viable treatment options that yield good medium-term results.

The authors recommend cement use alone for a AORI type 1 contained defect if the bone loss is minimal (<4 mm); however, we have a low threshold for packing the defect with morselized allograft, augmented with autograft where possible, to restore bone.

For a noncircumferential (medial or lateral compartment) uncontained AORI type 2a defect in which the bone loss is 1.5 cm or less in the femur or tibia, we recommend the use of modular augments and wedges. However, if the bone loss is present in both medial and lateral compartments (AORI type 2b), we would strongly advise the use of a metaphyseal fixation device to provide additional rotational stability which augments alone would lack. In the face of more significant noncircumferential or circumferential contained AORI type 3 bone loss with sufficient collateral stability, we favor metaphyseal fixation devices and/or structural allografts, used in conjunction with a stemmed constrained condylar prosthesis. If the bone deficiency is combined with collateral ligament insufficiency (particularly the medial collateral ligament), a prosthesis with rotating hinge constraint is preferred. If the metaphyseal bone loss is massive and uncontained, a megaprosthesis is favored over an APC.

REFERENCES

1. Engh GA, Ammeen DJ. Bone loss with revision total knee arthroplasty: defect classification and alternatives for reconstruction. *Instr Course Lect.* 1999;48:167-175.
2. Backstein D, Safir O, Gross A. Management of bone loss. *Clin Orthop Relat Res.* 2006;446:104-112.
3. Grimer RJ, Karpinski MR, Edwards AN. The long-term results of Stanmore total knee replacements. *J Bone Joint Surg Br.* 1984;66(1):55-62.
4. Rand JA, Chao EY, Stauffer RN. Kinematic rotating-hinge total knee arthroplasty. *J Bone Joint Surg Am.* 1987;69(4):489-497.
5. Bartel DL, Bicknell VL, Wright TM. The effect of conformity, thickness, and material on stresses in ultra-high molecular weight components for total joint replacement. *J Bone Joint Surg Am.* 1986;68(7):1041-1051.
6. Bartel DL, Rawlinson JJ, Burstein AH, Ranawat CS, Flynn WF. Stresses in polyethylene components of contemporary total knee replacements. *Clin Orthop Relat Res.* 1995;317:76-82.
7. Collier JP, Mayor MB, Surprenant VA, Surprenant HP, Dauphinais LA, Jensen RE. The biomechanical problems of polyethylene as a bearing surface. *Clin Orthop Relat Res.* 1990;261:107-113.
8. Engh GA. Failure of the polyethylene bearing surface of a total knee replacement within four years. A case report. *J Bone Joint Surg Am.* 1988;70(7):1093-1096.
9. Hvid I, Bentzen SM, Jørgensen J. Remodeling of the tibial plateau after knee replacement. CT bone densitometry. *Acta Orthop Scand.* 1988;59(5):567-573.
10. Bartel DL, Burstein AH, Santavicca EA, Insall JN. Performance of the tibial component in total knee replacement. *J Bone Joint Surg Am.* 1982;64(7):1026-1033.
11. Angelides M, Shirazi-Adl A, Shrivastava SC, Ahmed AM. A stress compatible finite element for implant/cement interface analyses. *J Biomech Eng.* 1988;110(1):42-49.
12. Van Lenthe GH, de Waal Malefijt MC, Huiskes R. Stress shielding after total knee replacement may cause bone resorption in the distal femur. *J Bone Joint Surg Br.* 1997;79(1):117-122.
13. Mintzer CM, Robertson DD, Rackemann S, Ewald FC, Scott RD, Spector M. Bone loss in the distal anterior femur after total knee arthroplasty. *Clin Orthop Relat Res.* 1990;260:135-143.
14. Seki T, Omori G, Koga Y, Suzuki Y, Ishii Y, Takahashi HE. Is bone density in the distal femur affected by use of cement and by femoral component design in total knee arthroplasty? *J Orthop Sci.* 1999;4(3):180-186.
15. Goldring SR, Clark CR, Wright TM. The problem in total joint arthroplasty: aseptic loosening. *J Bone Joint Surg Am.* 1993;75(6):799-801.
16. Robinson EJ, Mulliken BD, Bourne RB, Rorabeck CH, Alvarez C. Catastrophic osteolysis in total knee replacement. A report of 17 cases. *Clin Orthop Relat Res.* 1995;321:98-105.
17. Morrey BF, Chao EY. Fracture of the porous-coated metal tray of a biologically fixed knee prosthesis. Report of a case. *Clin Orthop Relat Res.* 1988;228:182-189.
18. Scott RD, Ewald FC, Walker PS. Fracture of the metallic tibial tray following total knee replacement. Report of two cases. *J Bone Joint Surg Am.* 1984;66(5):780-782.
19. Levitz CL, Lotke PA, Karp JS. Long-term changes in bone mineral density following total knee replacement. *Clin Orthop Relat Res.* 1995;321:68-72.
20. Wright TM, Bartel DL. The problem of surface damage in polyethylene total knee components. *Clin Orthop Relat Res.* 1986;205:67-74.
21. Collier JP, Mayor MB, McNamara JL, Surprenant VA, Jensen RE. Analysis of the failure of 122 polyethylene inserts from uncemented tibial knee components. *Clin Orthop Relat Res.* 1991;273:232-242.
22. Engh GA, Dwyer KA, Hanes CK. Polyethylene wear of metal-backed tibial components in total and unicompartmental knee prostheses. *J Bone Joint Surg Br.* 1992;74(1):9-17.

23. Wasielewski RC, Parks N, Williams I, Surprenant H, Collier JP, Engh G. Tibial insert undersurface as a contributing source of polyethylene wear debris. *Clin Orthop Relat Res.* 1997;345:53-59.
24. Cadambi A, Engh GA, Dwyer KA, Vinh TN. Osteolysis of the distal femur after total knee arthroplasty. *J Arthroplasty.* 1994;9(6):579-594.
25. Hirakawa K, Bauer TW, Stulberg BN, Wilde AH, Borden LS. Characterization of debris adjacent to failed knee implants of 3 different designs. *Clin Orthop Relat Res.* 1996;331:151-158.
26. Lotke PA, Ecker ML. Influence of positioning of prosthesis in total knee replacement. *J Bone Joint Surg Am.* 1977;59(1):77-79.
27. Leblanc JM. Patellar complications in total knee arthroplasty. A literature review. *Orthop Rev.* 1989;18(3):296-304.
28. Bloebaum RD, Nelson K, Dorr LD, Hofmann AA, Lyman DJ. Investigation of early surface delamination observed in retrieved heat-pressed tibial inserts. *Clin Orthop Relat Res.* 1991;269:120-127.
29. Sutula LC, Collier JP, Saum KA, et al. The Otto Aufranc Award. Impact of gamma sterilization on clinical performance of polyethylene in the hip. *Clin Orthop Relat Res.* 1995;319:28-40.
30. La Budde JK, Orosz JF, Bonfiglio TA, Pellegrini VD. Particulate titanium and cobalt-chrome metallic debris in failed total knee arthroplasty. A quantitative histologic analysis. *J Arthroplasty.* 1994;9(3):291-304.
31. Milliano MT, Whiteside LA. Articular surface material effect on metal-backed patellar components. A microscopic evaluation. *Clin Orthop Relat Res.* 1991;273:204-214.
32. Milliano MT, Whiteside LA, Kaiser AD, Zwirkoski PA. Evaluation of the effect of the femoral articular surface material on the wear of a metal-backed patellar component. *Clin Orthop Relat Res.* 1993;287:178-186.
33. Lewis PL, Rorabeck CH, Bourne RB. Screw osteolysis after cementless total knee replacement. *Clin Orthop Relat Res.* 1995;321:173-177.
34. Peters PC, Engh GA, Dwyer KA, Vinh TN. Osteolysis after total knee arthroplasty without cement. *J Bone Joint Surg Am.* 1992;74(6):864-876.
35. Whiteside LA. Effect of porous-coating configuration on tibial osteolysis after total knee arthroplasty. *Clin Orthop Relat Res.* 1995;321:92-97.
36. Yu B-F, Yang G-J, Wang W-L, Zhang L, Lin X-P. Cross-linked versus conventional polyethylene for total knee arthroplasty: a meta-analysis. *J Orthop Surg Res.* 2016;11(1):39.
37. Calton TF, Fehring TK, Griffin WL. Bone loss associated with the use of spacer blocks in infected total knee arthroplasty. *Clin Orthop Relat Res.* 1997;345:148-154.
38. Goldberg VM, Stevenson S. The biology of bone grafts. *Semin Arthroplasty.* 1993;4(2):58-63.
39. Enneking WF, Mindell ER. Observations on massive retrieved human allografts. *J Bone Joint Surg Am.* 1991;73(8):1123-1142.
40. Czitrom AA. Principles and techniques of tissue banking. *Instr Course Lect.* 1993;42:359-362.
41. Stevenson S, Horowitz M. The response to bone allografts. *J Bone Joint Surg Am.* 1992;74(6):939-950.
42. Bos GD, Goldberg VM, Zika JM, Heiple KG, Powell AE. Immune responses of rats to frozen bone allografts. *J Bone Joint Surg Am.* 1983;65(2):239-246.
43. Stevenson S, Li XQ, Davy DT, Klein L, Goldberg VM. Critical biological determinants of incorporation of non-vascularized cortical bone grafts. Quantification of a complex process and structure. *J Bone Joint Surg Am.* 1997;79(1):1-16.
44. Strong DM, Friedlaender GE, Tomford WW, et al. Immunologic responses in human recipients of osseous and osteochondral allografts. *Clin Orthop Relat Res.* 1996;326:107-114.
45. Muscolo DL, Ayerza MA, Calabrese ME, Redal MA, Santini Araujo E. Human leukocyte antigen matching, radiographic score, and histologic findings in massive frozen bone allografts. *Clin Orthop Relat Res.* 1996;326:115-126.

46. Muscolo DL, Caletti E, Schajowicz F, Araujo ES, Makino A. Tissue-typing in human massive allografts of frozen bone. *J Bone Joint Surg Am.* 1987;69(4):583-595.

47. Brand MG, Daley RJ, Ewald FC, Scott RD. Tibial tray augmentation with modular metal wedges for tibial bone stock deficiency. *Clin Orthop Relat Res.* 1989;248:71-79.

48. Brooks PJ, Walker PS, Scott RD. Tibial component fixation in deficient tibial bone stock. *Clin Orthop Relat Res.* 1984;184:302-308.

49. Cohen R. A porous tantalum trabecular metal: basic science. *Am J Orthop.* 2002;31(4):216-217.

50. Levine B, Sporer S, Valle Della CJ, Jacobs JJ, Paprosky W. Porous tantalum in reconstructive surgery of the knee: a review. *J Knee Surg.* 2007;20(3):185-194.

51. Howard JL, Kudera J, Lewallen DG, Hanssen AD. Early results of the use of tantalum femoral cones for revision total knee arthroplasty. *J Bone Joint Surg Am.* 2011;93(5):478-484.

52. Lachiewicz PF, Bolognesi MP, Henderson RA, Soileau ES, Vail TP. Can tantalum cones provide fixation in complex revision knee arthroplasty? *Clin Orthop Relat Res.* 2012;470(1):199-204.

53. Vasso M, Beaufils P, Cerciello S, Schiavone Panni A. Bone loss following knee arthroplasty: potential treatment options. *Arch Orthop Trauma Surg.* 2014;134(4):543-553.

54. Mabry TM, Vessely MB, Schleck CD, Harmsen WS, Berry DJ. Revision total knee arthroplasty with modular cemented stems: long-term follow-up. *J Arthroplasty.* 2007;22(6 suppl 2):100-105.

55. Harris AI, Poddar S, Gitelis S, Sheinkop MB, Rosenberg AG. Arthroplasty with a composite of an allograft and a prosthesis for knees with severe deficiency of bone. *J Bone Joint Surg Am.* 1995;77(3):373-386.

56. Mnaymneh W, Emerson RH, Borja F, Head WC, Malinin TI. Massive allografts in salvage revisions of failed total knee arthroplasties. *Clin Orthop Relat Res.* 1990;260:144-153.

57. Burchardt H. The biology of bone graft repair. *Clin Orthop Relat Res.* 1983;174:28-42.

58. Murray PB, Rand JA, Hanssen AD. Cemented long-stem revision total knee arthroplasty. *Clin Orthop Relat Res.* 1994;309:116-123.

59. Vince KG, Long W. Revision knee arthroplasty. The limits of press fit medullary fixation. *Clin Orthop Relat Res.* 1995;317:172-177.

60. Ritter MA, Keating EM, Faris PM. Screw and cement fixation of large defects in total knee arthroplasty. A sequel. *J Arthroplasty.* 1993;8(1):63-65.

61. Panni AS, Vasso M, Cerciello S. Modular augmentation in revision total knee arthroplasty. *Knee Surgery, Sports Traumatol Arthrosc.* 2013;21(12):2837-2843.

62. Pagnano MW, Trousdale RT, Rand JA. Tibial wedge augmentation for bone deficiency in total knee arthroplasty. A followup study. *Clin Orthop Relat Res.* 1995;321:151-155.

63. Patel JV, Masonis JL, Guerin J, Bourne RB, Rorabeck CH. The fate of augments to treat type-2 bone defects in revision knee arthroplasty. *J Bone Joint Surg Br.* 2004;86(2):195-199.

64. Rand JA. Modular augments in revision total knee arthroplasty. *Orthop Clin North Am.* 1998;29(2):347-353.

65. Lee K-J, Bae K-C, Cho C-H, Son E-S, Jung J-W. Radiological stability after revision of infected total knee arthroplasty using modular metal augments. *Knee Surg Relat Res.* 2016;28(1):55-61.

66. Hockman DE, Ammeen D, Engh GA. Augments and allografts in revision total knee arthroplasty: usage and outcome using one modular revision prosthesis. *J Arthroplasty.* 2005;20(1):35-41.

67. Whiteside LA, Bicalho PS. Radiologic and histologic analysis of morselized allograft in revision total knee replacement. *Clin Orthop Relat Res.* 1998;357:149-156.

68. Bauman RD, Lewallen DG, Hanssen AD. Limitations of structural allograft in revision total knee arthroplasty. *Clin Orthop Relat Res.* 2009;467(3):818-824.

69. Lyall HS, Sanghrajka A, Scott G. Severe tibial bone loss in revision total knee replacement managed with structural femoral head allograft: a prospective case series from the Royal London Hospital. *Knee.* 2009;16(5):326-331.

70. Wang J-W, Hsu C-H, Huang C-C, Lin P-C, Chen W-S. Reconstruction using femoral head allograft in revision total knee replacement: an experience in Asian patients. *Bone Joint J.* 2013;95-B(5):643-648.

71. Sandiford NA, Misur P, Garbuz DS, Greidanus NV, Masri BA. No difference between trabecular metal cones and femoral head allografts in revision TKA: minimum 5-year followup. *Clin Orthop Relat Res.* 2016;475(1):118-124.

72. Clatworthy MG, Ballance J, Brick GW, Chandler HP, Gross AE. The use of structural allograft for uncontained defects in revision total knee arthroplasty. A minimum five-year review. *J Bone Joint Surg Am.* 2001;83-A(3):404-411.

73. Engh GA, Ammeen DJ. Use of structural allograft in revision total knee arthroplasty in knees with severe tibial bone loss. *J Bone Joint Surg Am.* 2007;89(12):2640-2647.

74. Chun C-H, Kim JW, Kim SH, Kim BG, Chun K-C, Kim KM. Clinical and radiological results of femoral head structural allograft for severe bone defects in revision TKA–a minimum 8-year follow-up. *Knee.* 2014;21(2):420-423.

75. Richards CJ, Garbuz DS, Pugh L, Masri BA. Revision total knee arthroplasty: clinical outcome comparison with and without the use of femoral head structural allograft. *J Arthroplasty.* 2011;26(8):1299-1304.

76. Bonanzinga T, Gehrke T, Zahar A, Zaffagnini S, Marcacci M, Haasper C. Are trabecular metal cones a valid option to treat metaphyseal bone defects in complex primary and revision knee arthroplasty? *Joints.* 2018;6(1):58-64.

77. Zanirato A, Cavagnaro L, Basso M, Divano S, Felli L, Formica M. Metaphyseal sleeves in total knee arthroplasty revision: complications, clinical and radiological results. A systematic review of the literature. *Arch Orthop Trauma Surg.* 2018;138(7):993-1001.

78. Berend KR, Lombardi AV. Distal femoral replacement in nontumor cases with severe bone loss and instability. *Clin Orthop Relat Res.* 2009;467(2):485-492.

79. Barry JJ, Thielen Z, Sing DC, Yi PH, Hansen EN, Ries M. Length of endoprosthetic reconstruction in revision knee arthroplasty is associated with complications and reoperations. *Clin Orthop Relat Res.* 2017;475(1):72-79.

80. Kostuj T, Streit R, Baums MH, Schaper K, Meurer A. Midterm outcome after mega-prosthesis implanted in patients with bony defects in cases of revision compared to patients with malignant tumors. *J Arthroplasty.* 2015;30(9):1592-1596.

81. Kouk S, Rathod PA, Maheshwari AV, Deshmukh AJ. Rotating hinge prosthesis for complex revision total knee arthroplasty: a review of the literature. *J Clin Orthop Trauma.* 2018;9(1):29-33.

chapter 70

Cementless Revision Total Knee Arthroplasty

Leo A. Whiteside, MD

Implant fixation, bone reconstruction, and ligament balancing are the three primary goals of revision total knee arthroplasty (**Fig. 70-1**). After failure occurs one or more times, fixation is difficult to achieve with cement because the cancellous bone has been depleted, so it is tempting to cement the implant to diaphyseal cortical bone. Use of cement leads to compromise of even more bone stock, and if removal is necessary as in cases of infection, diaphyseal osteotomy and extensive exposure almost certainly will be required. This complex set of circumstances may produce a situation that only can be salvaged by amputation in cases of repeat failure. A more reliable and durable surgical technique uses an uncemented stem to engage the isthmus and rim contact to engage the metaphyseal cortical bone. This technique creates a stable construct around which the bone can be rebuilt.[1-3] In almost all cases of revision, the implant can be fixed to available bone stock, which obviates massive allografts that do not reconstitute the lost bone stock and often fail due to late collapse and infection.[4] Two major concerns with massive bone grafting—vascularization and incorporation—remain significant issues in the knee,[4] and bone grafting with allograft still raises the questions of immune compatibility. Bone tissue itself is not highly immunogenic, whereas the marrow cells do incite a vigorous immune response[5] and can create an inflammatory process that blocks ossification and incorporation of the graft.[6]

An effort has been made since 1984 to reconstruct clean or infected failed total knee arthroplasty with cementless techniques and to fix the implants directly to the patient's remaining bone structure. Durability of the construct and reliability of fixation of the implants have been very good, and repeated revision due to mechanical failure has been rare.[1-3,7,8]

In cases of infection around a total knee prosthesis, the standard treatment has been to remove the implants, treat with antibiotics for 6 weeks, and finally perform revision arthroplasty with antibiotic-loaded cement.[9-12] Cementless reconstruction, however, is attractive for these revision cases because further bone destruction is avoided and bone stock also can be restored.[1,2,13,14] In the early series, the implants were removed and the knee was thoroughly debrided and then the patient was treated with parenteral antibiotics for 6 weeks. Three months after the final débridement, the joint was reconstructed

using stemmed implants and morselized allograft. After obtaining nearly uniform success in eradicating the infection and achieving successful fixation with cementless reconstruction of the joint, an infusion technique was developed to deliver antibiotics in high concentration directly into the joint.[15,16] With this innovation, a direct exchange single-stage revision was done and the 3-month waiting period was eliminated. In these cases, no bone graft was used, and the implants were fixed firmly to diaphyseal cortical bone with either a fluted or fully porous-coated stem and the metaphyseal rim was seated directly on the remaining cortical shell.[16-18] Despite the absence of grafting of substantial defects in the metaphyseal bone, fixation was uniformly successful in these early series, and eradication of the infection was achieved in more than 95% of cases infected with resistant organisms.[16-18]

GRAFTING TECHNIQUE

Block allografts traditionally have been used for massive bone deficiency, but complication rates with their use are high, and the destructive effects of allograft rejection can limit their long-term success.[2,6] Because marrow is immunogenic, rejection can be a major problem with allograft.[6,18] Marrow elements, however, can be thoroughly removed from morselized allograft to minimize the inflammatory response and loss of graft and to capitalize on the osteoconductive potential of the allograft. Washing and soaking the components in an antibiotic solution have the added benefit of making available a reservoir of antibiotic that is released slowly during the postoperative period.[19] Large segments of allograft also heal slowly, are never replaced by new bone, and weaken as the ossification and vascularization front proceeds.[20,21] In contrast, morselized allograft, if protected initially by stem and rim fixation of the implants, has proven reliable both for small and large defects while supporting new bone formation.[22,23] Morsels that are 1 cm in diameter maintain their integrity long enough to act as a substrate for new bone formation. Morsels that are smaller than 0.5 to 1.0 cm in diameter tend to be resorbed, whereas those larger than 1 cm incorporate slowly, if ever, and tend to collapse under weight-bearing stress.

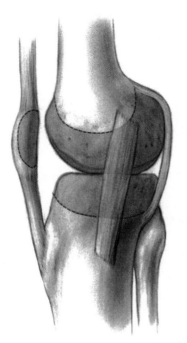

FIGURE 70-1 Bone loss from the femur, tibia, and patella may be extensive in failed total knee arthroplasty, but the ligaments and capsule usually are competent. Cancellous bone stock rarely is intact. The shaded area represents loss of cortical wall and cancellous structure. (From Whiteside LA. Results: cementless. In: Rorabeck CH, Engh GA, eds. *Revision Total Knee Arthroplasty*. Baltimore: Williams & Wilkins; 1997, with permission.)

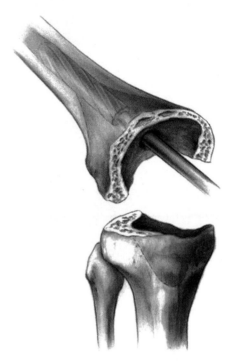

FIGURE 70-2 Intramedullary alignment provides the only reliable landmark for minimal resection. Recognizing that severe bone loss has occurred, the surgeon should resect only a small amount of bone to allow firm footing for the implant. (From Whiteside LA. Results: cementless. In: Rorabeck CH, Engh GA, eds. *Revision Total Knee Arthroplasty*. Baltimore: Williams & Wilkins; 1997, with permission.)

The allograft is not osteoinductive but acts as scaffolding for new bone growth. Demineralized bone, which is mildly osteoinductive, can be added to the allograft to enhance bone formation. The surrounding bone structure supplies most of the osteoinductive activity because metaphyseal bone has a rich blood supply and maintains the capacity to heal even after repeated failure of arthroplasty.

BONE PREPARATION TECHNIQUE

Minimal bone should be resected during preparation (**Fig. 70-2**). Bone erosion already present makes complete seating of the component nearly impossible, but side-to-side and front-to-back toggle of the implants can be eliminated by placing a stem rigidly in the medullary canal. The implant seats on the remaining rim of metaphyseal bone. Seating the implant on the patient's own bone stock controls axial migration, and the stem prevents the implant from tilting into the defect. Screw and peg fixation may be used to add stability to the construct, but usually it is not needed if the stem is firmly fixed in the diaphysis. This technique results in substantial uncontained cavitary defects that may be filled with morselized bone. This bone-grafting technique promotes rapid healing and reconstitution of bone stock without the technical difficulty and late collapse associated with massive allograft replacement.

Tibial Preparation

Reconstruction of massive tibial defects relies on rim support for axial loading and stem fixation for toggle control. Screws can be used in the tibial component to augment fixation, combined with the use of nonstructural allograft to fill central and peripheral defects, and massive block allografting also may be used for these defects. However, when a long stem is used to engage the diaphyseal cortical bone, morselized cancellous allograft can reconstruct the proximal tibial bone without screws or structural allograft with low failure and complication rates.[3]

The lateral tibial cortex usually is relatively well preserved. The fibular head almost always is present and can be used for proximal seating of the tibial component if the rest of the tibial architecture is destroyed (**Fig. 70-3**). In the worst cases, all cancellous bone is gone, which leaves a large cavitary defect and substantial deficiency of the tibial rim. Long-stem fixation is advised in these cases regardless of whether block or morselized allograft is used. When morselized graft is used, the tibial tray should seat on the intact portion of the tibial rim, and the stem should engage the isthmus of the tibia. As with the femoral component, the tightly fit diaphyseal stem maintains stability and prevents tilting of the component, so that massive defects may be filled with allograft and protected until healing and bone formation occurs in the grafted area (**Fig. 70-4**). When the entire proximal tibial

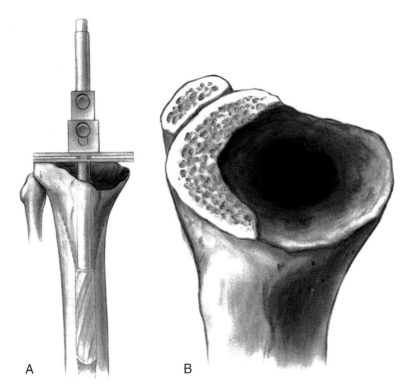

FIGURE 70-3   **A:** Intramedullary instruments allow accurate alignment. Here, a tibial cutting guide is used to trim the upper tibial rim. Minimal resection should be done, which may leave large rim defects. **B:** With long-stem support of the tibial component, one-fourth of the rim of the proximal tibia can be used to support the implant. The fibular head also may be used for tibial support. (From Whiteside LA. Results: cementless. In: Rorabeck CH, Engh GA, eds. *Revision Total Knee Arthroplasty.* Baltimore: Williams & Wilkins; 1997, with permission.)

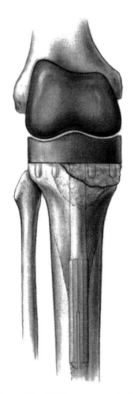

FIGURE 70-4   Fixation of the tibial component with rim contact on viable bone, screw fixation into the cortical shell, peg fixation into intact bone structure, and stem fixation into the diaphysis allow adequate stabilization until the grafted area can be incorporated. (From Whiteside LA. Results: cementless. In: Rorabeck CH, Engh GA, eds. *Revision Total Knee Arthroplasty.* Baltimore: Williams & Wilkins; 1997, with permission.)

metaphysis has been destroyed (**Fig. 70-5**), porous metal augments are used to substitute for deficient bone. This often requires more than one augment on both sides of the tibia to achieve maximum medial and lateral support. These augments are placed against the remaining metaphyseal rim medially and laterally, and a diaphysis-engaging stem is fixed into the distal cortical bone to achieve the stability necessary for bone ingrowth (**Fig. 70-6**).

Femoral Preparation

When bone destruction is assessed, the medial and lateral condyles usually are found to be at least partially intact. With intramedullary instrumentation as a guide, the distal surface of the femur should be resected just enough to achieve firm seating of the femoral component on one side of the bone. Both sides may be engaged by the implant in some cases, but often only one of the two condyles can afford firm seating for the femoral component without excessive resection of the distal femur (**Fig. 70-7**). Adequate fixation of the femoral component requires seating of the posterior flange surfaces to prevent anteroposterior translation of the component in flexion and to augment torsional fixation. The posterior surfaces also are minimally resected, with as much bone stock as possible left on which to seat the surfaces of the femoral component. In many cases, the posterior bone erosion leaves little or nothing of the posterior femoral condyles and the posterior femoral cuts are flush with the posterior cortex of the femur (**Figs. 70-8** and **70-9**).

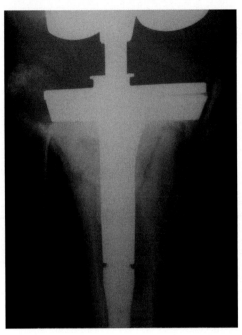

FIGURE 70-5 Preoperative radiograph of a patient in which multiple surgical revisions and infections have destroyed the proximal tibial metaphyseal cancellous and cortical bone, leaving reasonably good cortical rims medially and laterally further down the metaphysis. The radiolucent line around the cement mantle defines the extent of bone loss.

The deficient bone is replaced with posterior surface augments, and these posterior femoral surfaces are aligned with the epicondylar axis of the femur to achieve correct varus–valgus alignment of the femoral implant in flexion. Posterior and distal femoral bone deficiency can be reconstructed with stacked augments to achieve distal and

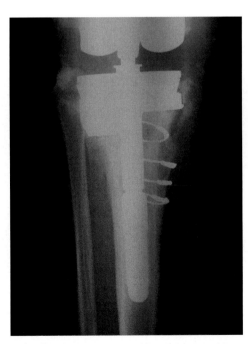

FIGURE 70-6 Radiograph of the tibia in **Fig. 70-5** after reconstruction with a tibial component and porous augments stabilized with a diaphysis-engaging fluted stem.

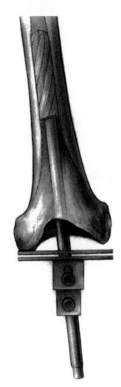

FIGURE 70-7 An intramedullary reamer is used to align the femoral cutting guide. The guide is set at 5° of valgus alignment and positioned to resect minimal bone from the most prominent distal surface of the femur. (From Whiteside LA. Results: cementless. In: Rorabeck CH, Engh GA, eds. *Revision Total Knee Arthroplasty*. Baltimore: Williams & Wilkins; 1997, with permission.)

posterior bone contact, and this construct is stabilized with a diaphysis-engaging stem using three-point fixation technique (**Figs. 70-10** and **70-11**). After the implant has been fully seated, more bone graft can be packed into the distal and posterior cavitary defects.

In some cases the entire distal femoral structure, including the metaphysis, is missing or deficient and must be replaced by a component that is stabilized only by the diaphyseal stem (**Fig. 70-12**). In these cases, a fully porous stem can be press-fit with adequate stability to accept axial, torsional, and anterior and posterior offset loads that occur in knee flexion (**Fig. 70-13**). Prolonged protection from weight-bearing usually is not necessary because the implants are supported well on viable bone, but protection from weight-bearing in flexion is necessary for 6 to 8 weeks when the posterior surfaces of the femoral condyles are not supported by bone.

Graft Preparation and Placement

Fresh frozen cancellous allograft in morsels measuring 0.5 to 1.0 cm in diameter is soaked for 5 to 10 minutes in normal saline solution that contains polymyxin B sulfate 500,000 U and vancomycin 2 g/L. The fluid is removed and 10 cm³ of powdered demineralized cancellous bone is added to each 30 cm³ of the cancellous morsels. To improve the osteoinductive potential, autogenous bone

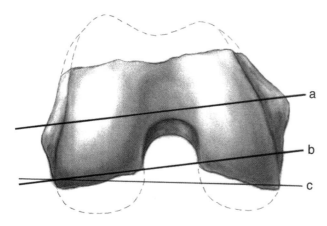

FIGURE 70-8 A straight line through the medial and lateral femoral epicondyles provides correct rotational alignment. The dotted lines represent the original contours of the distal femur before total knee failure. Line a passes through the epicondyles. Line b represents the proper resection line for the posterior femoral condyles. If line c is followed, severe internal rotation of the femoral component will occur. (From Whiteside LA. Results: cementless. In: Rorabeck CH, Engh GA, eds. *Revision Total Knee Arthroplasty*. Baltimore: Williams & Wilkins; 1997, with permission.)

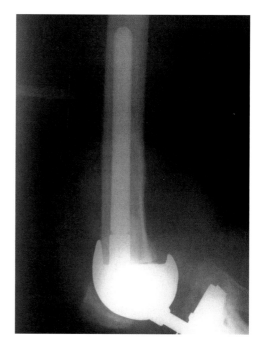

FIGURE 70-10 Radiograph of a patient whose femoral component is grossly loose and the posterior condylar bone stock is missing. However, the posterior femoral cortex is intact and available for engagement with the femoral component.

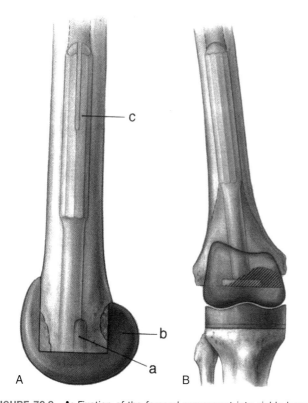

FIGURE 70-9 **A:** Fixation of the femoral component into viable bone is achieved by means of pegs driven into the distal femoral surface (a), a thickened posterior surface (b), and a long stem (c), which allow soft bone graft to be used. **B:** Tight fixation of the stem in the diaphysis in combination with rim seating prevents the implant from migrating proximally and tilting into the defect. (From Whiteside LA. Results: cementless. In: Rorabeck CH, Engh GA, eds. *Revision Total Knee Arthroplasty*. Baltimore: Williams & Wilkins; 1997, with permission.)

fragments and diaphyseal reamings are added. This mixture is packed loosely into the bone defects and then the implants are impacted so as to seat on the remnant of viable bone while compacting the morselized bone graft. Remaining cavitary defects are filled with bone graft, but the bone is not compacted so that early vascularization and healing will not be impeded.

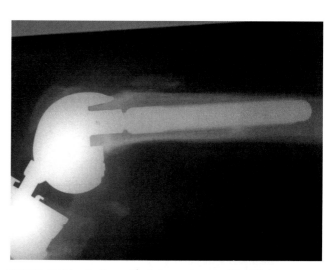

FIGURE 70-11 Radiograph of the patient in **Fig. 70-10** who was reconstructed by using stacked porous augments on the posterior femoral condylar flange surfaces. The construct is stabilized by a stem fixed with three-point fixation technique which is capable of accepting weight-bearing in flexion early in the postoperative period.

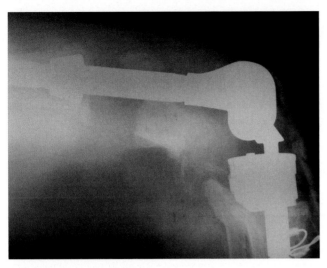

FIGURE 70-12 Radiograph of a patient whose knee has been reconstructed with a distal femoral replacement prosthesis, so no posterior bone remains to accept torsional loads or anterior–posterior offset loading on the femoral component.

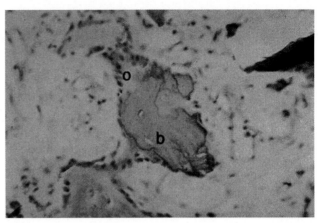

FIGURE 70-14 Histologic section from the 3-week biopsy specimen. Granules of demineralized bone (b) are visible and are surrounded by plump osteoblasts (o) and new osteoid. Vascular stroma is present throughout the allografted area. There is no histologic evidence of bone resorption. (From Whiteside LA. Results: cementless. In: Rorabeck CH, Engh GA, eds. *Revision Total Knee Arthroplasty*. Baltimore: Williams & Wilkins; 1997, with permission.)

CLINICAL EXPERIENCE

Since 1984, a cementless fixation technique has been used at the author's institution in aseptic and infected cases of revision total knee arthroplasty.[2,3,7,8,14] Clean revision cases followed for 2 to 10 years had a failure rate of 3% due to loosening.[14] The remainder had radiographic evidence of stable fixation. Biopsy results for 17 knees showed early, vigorous bone formation, and late maturation throughout the grafts (**Figs. 70-14 to 70-17**). Thirty-three infected knees underwent revision using this technique 6 to 12 weeks after débridement.[7] Four knees required repeated débridement and revision due

to recurrent infection but currently are functioning well. One had repeated infection that required amputation.

Clinical experience has shown that migration of the tibial component after reconstruction with morselized allograft is rare during the first 2 to 5 years after surgery.[4] These results are remarkably good in light of reported experience with structural allograft in the acetabulum. Jasty and Harris[24] reported loosening of acetabular components after 4 years in 32% of their cases. The biologic behavior of morselized allograft differs from that of block allograft, however. Vascularization and ossification are rapid, and a permanent, competent load-bearing structure is achieved by filling large deficient areas[1,2] (**Figs. 70-18 to 70-21**). The biologic

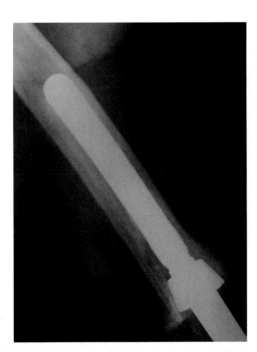

FIGURE 70-13 Radiograph of the patient in **Fig. 70-12** in which a porous-coated femoral component with wedge augment was used to accept axial, torsional, and offset loading of the component.

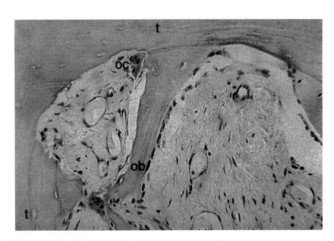

FIGURE 70-15 Histologic section from the 3-mo biopsy specimen. Dead trabeculae (t) are still abundant. Osteoclasts (oc) and new osteoid with osteoblasts (ob) are evident adjacent to the allograft. The allografted area contains multiple sites of bone resorption. New osteoid is often found on one surface of a trabecula and osteoclastic resorption on the opposite surface. Osteoblasts at this time are flatter and less numerous than in the 3-wk biopsy specimen. (From Whiteside LA. Results: cementless. In: Rorabeck CH, Engh GA, eds. *Revision Total Knee Arthroplasty*. Baltimore: Williams & Wilkins; 1997, with permission.)

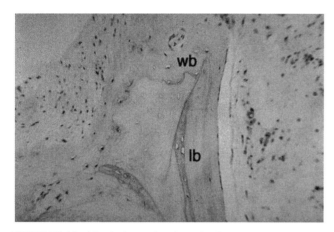

FIGURE 70-16 Histologic section from the 21-mo biopsy specimen. Mature lamellar bone (lb) and disorganized woven bone (wb) surround the allograft. The bone remodeling rate in the allografted area has decreased significantly. Trabeculae now are completely entombed by mature or woven bone. Bone remodeling has decreased, and osteoblastic or osteoclastic activity is directed toward new bone, not toward allograft. (From Whiteside LA. Results: cementless. In: Rorabeck CH, Engh GA, eds. *Revision Total Knee Arthroplasty*. Baltimore: Williams & Wilkins; 1997, with permission.)

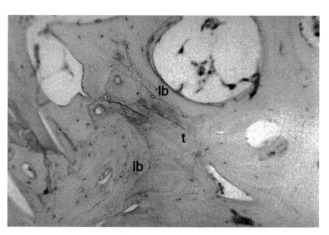

FIGURE 70-17 Histologic section from the 37-mo biopsy specimen. Entombed trabeculae (t) are present throughout the biopsied allograft. The visible allograft is completely encased by mature lamellar bone (lb). Bone remodeling continues at normal levels; few osteoclasts are found, and there is minimal evidence of osteoblastic activity. (From Whiteside LA. Results: cementless. In: Rorabeck CH, Engh GA, eds. *Revision Total Knee Arthroplasty*. Baltimore: Williams & Wilkins; 1997, with permission.)

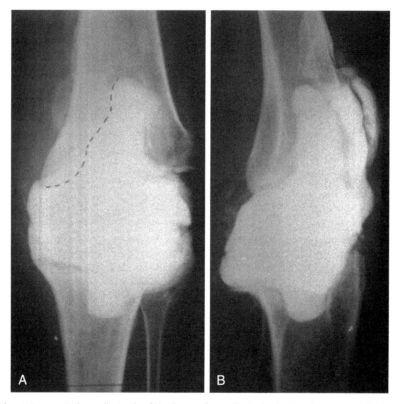

FIGURE 70-18 **A:** Preoperative anteroposterior radiograph of the knee of a patient who had undergone a total knee replacement with a history of two previous infections. The dotted line indicates the interface between the cement spacer and bone. The medial and lateral femoral condyles are severely deficient; the medial and lateral tibial plateaus, the upper half of the fibular head, and the tibiofibular joint have been destroyed. **B:** Preoperative lateral radiograph of the same case as in **(A)**. The anterior femoral bone stock and posterior femoral condyles have been destroyed.

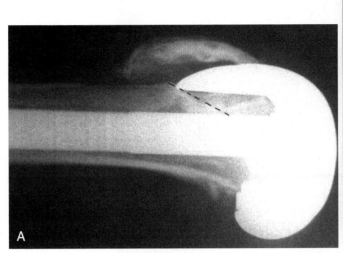
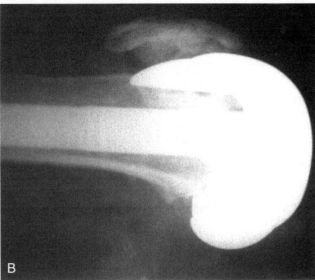

FIGURE 70-19   A: Postoperative lateral view of the same knee as in **Fig. 70-14** 1 mo after surgery. The dotted line indicates the distal extent of the patient's own anterior femoral bone stock. The material under the femoral flange is morselized cancellous allograft and demineralized allograft bone. The posterior surfaces of the femoral component are seated against the remaining portion of the femoral diaphysis. **B:** Postoperative lateral radiograph of the same knee 2 y after surgery. The bone graft has consolidated.

response obtained with the correct technique appears to be early and vigorous. It does not seem likely that progressive collapse will occur after remodeling and healing have been established.

Bone graft handling is crucial to the success of grafting the knee. Antibiotic soaking and washing, removal of bone marrow, and adequate support of the implants are all necessary for consistent success with this technique. The results

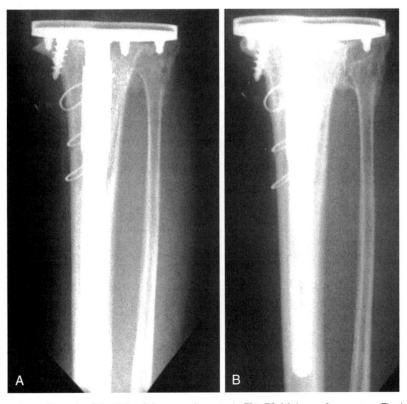

FIGURE 70-20   A: Anteroposterior radiograph of the tibia of the same knee as in **Fig. 70-14** 1 mo after surgery. The long stem engages the diaphysis of the tibia, and the distal slot is closed. Fresh graft is visible in the tibiofibular joint. The medial edge of the tibia and upper surfaces of the fibular head support the tibial component until healing is complete. **B:** Anteroposterior radiograph of the tibia of the same knee, taken 2 y after surgery. The slot in the stem is still closed, and the tibiofibular joint appears to be solidly healed.

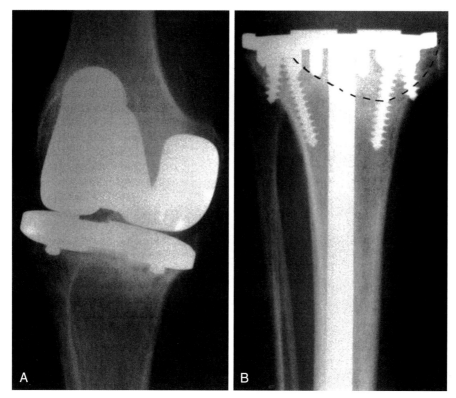

FIGURE 70-21   **A:** Anteroposterior radiograph of a cemented total knee replacement 5 y after surgery. The tibial component has loosened and migrated into a varus position, destroying much of the medial tibial plateau. **B:** Anteroposterior radiograph of the same knee as in (A) 1 y after surgery. The dotted line indicates the previous bony defect. The lateral rim and diaphyseal stem have supported the tibial component as bone grew and healed under the medial side of the tibial component. The bone graft has healed, producing supporting bone stock for the medial side of the tibial component.

of this salvage procedure have been encouraging. The grafting technique appears to provide long-term support for the implant so that repeat revision likely will be uncommon.

The success with cementless fixation in cases of infection that do not incorporate allograft suggests that the rim and stem fixation technique is not dependent on the graft, but it is more dependent on direct attachment of viable bone to the porous metal surfaces, especially those of the stem. This implies that the implants themselves must have strength characteristics that would support a lifetime of service without fatigue fracture.

REFERENCES

1. Samuelson K. Bone grafting and noncemented revision arthroplasty of the knee. *Clin Orthop Relat Res.* 1988;226:93-101.
2. Whiteside LA. Cementless reconstruction of massive tibial bone loss in revision total knee arthroplasty. *Clin Orthop Relat Res.* 1989;248:80-86.
3. Whiteside LA, Ohl M. Tibial tubercle osteotomy for exposure of the difficult knee arthroplasty. *Clin Orthop Relat Res.* 1990;260:6-9.
4. Wilde A, Schickendantz M, Stulberg B, et al. The incorporation of tibial allografts in total knee arthroplasty. *J Bone Joint Surg Am.* 1990;72:815-824.
5. Goldberg V, Powell A, Shaffer J, et al. Bone grafting: role of histocompatibility in transplantation. *J Orthop Res.* 1985;3:389-404.
6. Muscolo D, Caletti E, Schajowicz F, et al. Tissue-typing in human massive allografts of frozen bone. *J Bone Joint Surg Am.* 1987;69:583-595.
7. Whiteside L. Treatment of infected total knee arthroplasty. *Clin Orthop Relat Res.* 1994;299:169-172.
8. Whiteside L, Bicalho PS. Radiologic and histologic analysis of morselized allograft in revision total knee replacement. *Clin Orthop Relat Res.* 1998;357:149-156.
9. Booth R Jr, Lotke P. The results of spacer block technique in revision of infected total knee arthroplasty. *Clin Orthop Relat Res.* 1989;248:57-60.
10. Freeman M, Sudlow R, Casewell M, et al. The management of infected total knee replacements. *J Bone Joint Surg Br.* 1985;67:764-768.
11. Jacobs M, Hungerford D, Krackow K, et al. Revision of septic total knee replacement. *Clin Orthop Relat Res.* 1989;238:159-166.
12. Windsor R, Miller D, Insall J, et al. Two-stage reimplantation for the salvage of total knee arthroplasty complicated by infection. *J Bone Joint Surg Am.* 1990;72:272-278.
13. Whiteside LA. Bone grafting in revision cementless total knee arthroplasty. *Tech Orthop.* 1992;7:39-46.
14. Whiteside LA. Cementless revision total knee arthroplasty. *Clin Orthop Relat Res.* 1993;286:160-167.
15. Roy ME, Peppers MP, Whiteside LA, LaZear RM. Vancomycin concentration in synovial fluid: direction injection into the knee v intravenous infusion. *J Arthroplasty.* 2014;29:564-568.
16. Whiteside LA, Roy ME, Nayfeh TA. Intra-articular infusion: a direct approach to treatment of infected total knee arthroplasty. *Bone Joint J.* 2016;98(suppl A):31-36.
17. Whiteside LA, Nayfeh TA, LaZear R, Roy ME. Reinfected revised TKA resolves with an aggressive protocol and antibiotic infusion. *Clin Orthop Relat Res.* 2012;470:236-243.
18. Whiteside LA, Peppers M, Nayfeh TA, Roy ME. Methicillin resistant *Staphylococcus aureus* in TKA treated with revision and direct intra-articular antibiotic infusion. *Clin Orthop Relat Res.* 2011;269:26-33.
19. Friedlaender G. Current concepts review: bone grafts. *J Bone Joint Surg Am.* 1987;69:786-790.

20. McLaren A. Antibiotic bone graft: early clinical results. Paper presented at: 57th Annual Meeting of the American Academy of Orthopaedics Surgeons; February 8-13, 1990; New Orleans.

21. Gitelis S, Helgimen D, Quill G, et al. The use of large allografts for tumor reconstruction and salvage of the failed total hip arthroplasty. *Clin Orthop Relat Res.* 1988;231:62-70.

22. Head W, Malinn T, Berklacich F. Freeze-dried proximal femur allografts in revision total hip arthroplasty. *Clin Orthop Relat Res.* 1987;215:109-120.

23. Gerber S, Harris W. Femoral head autografting to augment acetabular deficiency in patients requiring total hip replacement. *J Bone Joint Surg Am.* 1986;68:1241-1248.

24. Jasty M, Harris WH. Salvage total hip reconstruction in patients with major acetabular bone deficiency using structural femoral head allografts. *J Bone Joint Surg Br.* 1990;72:63-67.

chapter 71

Management of the Patella in Revision Total Knee Arthroplasty

Kevin I. Perry, MD | Arlen D. Hanssen, MD

Historically there has been a relative rarity of published literature regarding the management of the patella during revision total knee arthroplasty (TKA). One of the primary reasons for this phenomenon is that during the majority of revision TKA, the existing patellar component can be retained if it is well-fixed, has only slight wear, and tracks well.[1-7] By definition, all patellar components should be removed in cases of revision TKA associated with deep periprosthetic infection. In aseptic revision TKA, patellar component retention occurs in approximately 60% to 70% of cases.[7,8] Retention of a well-fixed patellar prosthesis that is of an unmatched design with the femoral trochlea has been shown to be clinically acceptable as long as the mismatch is not severe and the patella tracks well in the new femoral trochlea.[3,8] The purpose of this chapter is to briefly review the surgical principles of management of the patella during revision TKA and in particular to emphasize the surgical techniques available for the bone-deficient patella.

It is critically important to recognize that a successful clinical outcome for patellar function and long-term durability of the patellar construct are highly dependent on proper axial and rotational positioning of the femoral and tibial components.[9,10] This concept is most often overlooked when attempting an isolated revision of the patellar component and is one of the reasons that isolated patellar revision has been associated with an increased incidence of lateral retinacular release, suboptimal clinical outcomes, and an increased risk of postoperative complications.[11-13] In most cases, the reason that a patella has maltracking, aseptic loosening, prosthesis fracture, or excessive wear is because of associated femoral and/or tibial component malposition. Therefore, it is essential to ensure proper femoral and tibial component position before proceeding with patellar component revision and recognize that isolated patellar component revision is almost never warranted.

SURGICAL CONSIDERATIONS

During revision TKA, it is imperative that extensor mechanism disruption is avoided at all costs. Traditionally it has been common practice to evert the patella during surgical exposure; however, it is quite evident that lateral subluxation of the extensor mechanism with concomitant anterior subluxation on external rotation of the tibia from beneath the femur provides excellent exposure of the knee joint during revision TKA. It is the authors' opinion that patellar eversion is never required during revision TKA except when the knee is fully extended. Release of all adhesions in the lateral gutter facilitates lateral subluxation of the extensor mechanism. Occasionally in particularly stiff knees, extensile exposures such as a rectus snip or tibial tubercle osteotomy may be required to safely expose the knee.

The primary indications for revision of a patellar component are listed in **Table 71-1**. If patellar component revision is deemed necessary, the quality and quantity of remaining patellar bone stock will determine the choice of the new implant or a variety of alternative surgical techniques. Reasons for patellar bone loss include over-resection of the patella at the primary procedure, patellar osteolysis, infection, or iatrogenic bone loss associated with removal of the existing patellar implant, particularly with removal of well-fixed metal-backed patellar components. In patellar components with metal lugs, a diamond wheel cutting tool is used to side cut the lugs at junction of the baseplate.[14] In the aseptic revision, it is reasonable to simply leave these lugs in place and cover them when implanting the new patellar prosthesis. Certain metal-backed patellar component designs are extremely difficult to remove without loss of significant patellar bone. In these circumstances and if the other criteria for patellar component retention are met, it seems reasonable to retain these metal-backed patellar components for the alternative of treating a patella with severe bone loss or fracture after their removal is much less desirable.

Once the prior patellar component has been removed, the patella should be prepared by removing fibrous tissue and any remaining cement deemed necessary for removal. If cement or metal lugs are well-fixed and will not interfere with fixation and positioning of another patellar implant, it is acceptable in the absence of infection to retain this material rather removing any additional patellar bone. Patellar bone stock should then be assessed with regard to quality, quantity, and location of remaining bone to determine whether there is enough bone stock to provide adequate fixation for the new component. Whenever possible, it is most desirable to implant another patellar prosthesis.

TABLE 71-1 Indications for Patellar Component Revision
Aseptic Loosening
Severe patellar osteolysis
Patellar component fracture
Moderate to severe patellar component damage
Malposition or mismatch affecting patellar tracking
Removal required due to presence of active infection

In general, remaining patellar bone stock of >8 to 10 mm occurs in approximately 85% to 90% of revision patellar procedures, and implantation of standard pegged or biconvex polyethylene patellar components can be successfully performed.[6,7,15-21] However, if the remaining patellar bone stock measures <8 to 10 mm, the bone-deficient patella, alternative implants, or reconstructive techniques are usually required (**Table 71-2**). The location and quality of remaining patellar bone, particularly the absence of peripheral rim support, dictate the choice of any given surgical technique used to address the bone-deficient patella. It is the authors' opinion that patellectomy is never indicated during revision TKA with the sole exception being resection of a grossly necrotic and osteomyelitic patella.

TREATMENT OPTIONS AFTER PATELLAR COMPONENT REMOVAL

Adequate Remaining Patellar Bone Stock

Standard three-Pegged Polyethylene Patellar Components

With 10 to 15 mm of remaining bone, it is usually possible to prepare the patella by creating new lug holes in areas of retained cancellous bone and by using any small areas of cavitary bone loss as additional areas of cement fixation. It is preferable that there are only minimal areas of peripheral segmental bone loss, and in the remaining areas of sclerotic bone, small drill holes or ridges created with a saw or burr can be also created for additional fixation.

TABLE 71-2 Treatment Options for the Bone-Deficient Patella
Techniques Without Patellar Component Implantation
Patellar resection arthroplasty
Gull-wing osteotomy
Cancellous impaction bone grafting
Techniques With Patellar Component Implantation
Screw or pinning with cement augmentation
Transcortical wiring
Structural bone grafting
Three-pegged porous metal monoblock patella
Porous metal baseplate

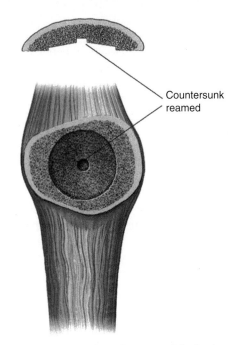

Countersunk reamed

FIGURE 71-1 Schematic of patella prepared for implantation of an inset biconvex patellar component.

Biconvex Polyethylene Patellar Components

If the patella has enough generalized cavitary bone loss to preclude support for a traditional pegged patellar button, the patella can be prepared to accept a polyethylene biconvex patellar component (**Fig. 71-1**). It has been shown that the use of a biconvex patellar component is possible for patellae with as little as 5 mm of central bone provided that there is good peripheral support of the patellar implant.[20] The primary disadvantage of this technique is that the overall patellar composite height is less than the normal patellar height or other techniques that restore the anatomic thickness of the patella (**Fig. 71-2**).[20] In a clinical series of 89 biconvex patellar components implanted during revision TKA, 10- and 14-year survivorship using aseptic loosening as an end point were 98% and 86%, respectively.[16] In this revision series and an adjacent report using this implant during primary TKA, patellar fracture was associated with a radiographical measurement of central patellar thickness of <6 mm.[16,17] Aseptic failure was associated with patellar osteonecrosis and absence of a superior rim of supporting bone.[16,17]

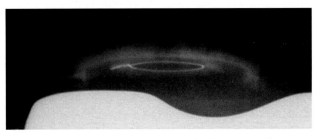

FIGURE 71-2 Merchant view radiograph of a biconvex patellar component with resultant decrease in anteroposterior patellar height.

The Bone-Deficient Patella

In approximately 10% of cases, when patellar component revision has been deemed necessary, patellar bone stock is insufficient enough that alternative treatment strategies are required.[19] Severe patellar bone deficiency, i.e., <8 to 10 mm of remaining bone, has historically been a difficult problem that has adversely affected clinical outcomes of revision TKA. In the decades of the 1980s and 1990s, the most common approach was to simply remove the patellar component also known as patelloplasty or patellar resection arthroplasty.[8,22] Over the past several decades, a variety of alternative treatment options have emerged to address patellar bone deficiency during revision TKA. These alternative reconstructive options can be classified as those that include implantation of a patellar button or those that do not include implantation of another patellar implant.

Techniques Without Patellar Component Implantation

Patellar Resection Arthroplasty (Patelloplasty)

Historically, simple removal of the patellar component was an easy and often used treatment option.[23,24] Typically this technique consists of contouring the patellar remnant to remove eccentric or sharp bone edges and to facilitate central patellar tracking within the femoral trochlea. Although this alternative is attractive because of its simplicity, the clinical outcomes of this approach were often suboptimal due to persistent anterior knee pain, patellar fragmentation, and patellar subluxation over the lateral femoral trochlea at mid-term follow-up (**Fig. 71-3A** and **B**).[24] These results were almost certainly influenced by the lack of understanding about the need to ensure proper rotational position of the femoral and tibial components.[23]

In several more recent studies, when attention to proper femoral and tibial component rotational position was universally realized, the clinical results of patellar resection have been more promising.[25,26] The primary disadvantage of a patellar resection arthroplasty is that reconstruction of the normal anteroposterior patellar height, which optimizes patellar kinematics and quadriceps extensor forces, does not occur. In the authors' opinion, there are only several times when patellar resection arthroplasty is preferable. One is when the soft tissues and capsule are so tight, as in the second stage of reimplantation for infection, that capsular closure is facilitated by avoiding patellar resurfacing.[23,27] An additional reason to avoid patellar resurfacing is in cases of severe patella baja, often associated with conflict between the patellar button and tibial prosthesis.[28,29]

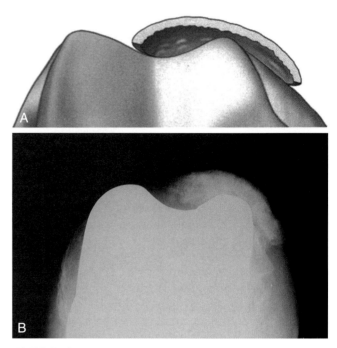

FIGURE 71-3   A: Schematic and **B:** Merchant view radiograph of a patellar resection arthroplasty, 6 years postoperatively, that has subluxed over the lateral femoral trochlea.

Gull-Wing Osteotomy

Rather than only removing the patellar component, this technique was proposed as a way to optimize the remaining patellar bony shell and facilitate central tracking of the patellar remnant within the femoral trochlea.[30] In this surgical procedure, the patellar remnant is purposely osteotomized in the sagittal plane to create medial and lateral "wings" (**Fig. 71-4**). Hence, the patellar remnant when viewed on a Merchant or patellar view radiograph appears as "gull-wings." The purpose of this technique is to create patellar fragments that are oriented so that the undersurface of the fragments become opposed against the sides of the femoral trochlea which theoretically facilitates central patellar tracking.

Subsequent reports on this technique have been relatively satisfactory.[2,31] In a consecutive series of 12 patients, gull-wing osteotomy accomplished centralized patellar tracking and no lateral subluxation with satisfactory clinical results at follow-up.[31] In a recent series of 17 (15%), gull-wing osteotomies out of 115 revised patellae, patients with <12 mm of remaining bone stock were selected for this technique.[2] Of the 13 patients with radiographic follow-up, 12 healed radiographically in a central trochlear position, and one had a solid fibrous union. While none of these had a fracture, one developed avascular necrosis and fragmentation. The 13th patient had lateral patellar subluxation at 3 years follow-up.

As such, gull-wing osteotomy may be considered as a treatment option for management of the bone-deficient patella; however, it also has the distinct disadvantage of a reduced patellar height which likely affects optimal

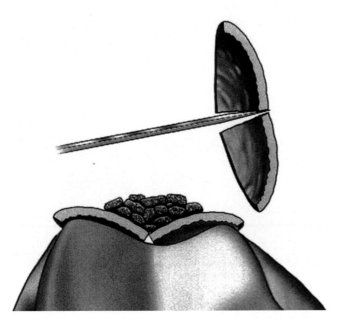

FIGURE 71-4 Schematic of the "gull-wing osteotomy" created by a sagittal patellar osteotomy to facilitate central patellar tracking within the femoral trochlea combined with the concomitant cancellous bone graft placed ventral to the osteotomy site.

tissue, and the remaining patellar rim with multiple interrupted nonabsorbable size-0 sutures. A small purse-string opening is left in one portion of the tissue flap repair to facilitate delivery of the bone graft into the patellar defect.

Cancellous autograft is usually harvested from the metaphyseal portion of the femur during femoral preparation of the revision implant. In the absence of locally available cancellous autograft, cancellous allograft bone has been used successfully. The bone graft is prepared by morseling the bone into small fragments of approximately 5 to 8 mm in height and width. The bone graft is tightly impacted through the opening of the fascial flap into the patellar bone defect, with enough volume so that the final patellar construct has a height of approximately 25 mm. The tissue flap is then closed completely to contain the bone graft within the patellar shell to provide a watertight closure (**Fig. 71-5C**). If there is inadequate local soft-tissue available, a free tissue flap obtained from either the suprapatellar pouch or the fascia lata in the lateral gutter of the knee joint can be used. The adequacy of the suture repair is examined to ensure that the tissue flap securely contains the impacted bone graft. The peripatellar arthrotomy site is provisionally repaired with several sutures or towel clips to mold the patellar construct in the femoral trochlea as the knee is placed through the full range of motion. Postoperative rehabilitation is the same as the usual protocol following revision knee arthroplasty.

In the initial report describing this technique in nine knees (eight patients), all patellae measured <9 mm and at average 36 months follow-up, the radiographic patellar height measured on average 19.7 mm (range, 17-22.5 mm).[19] This review has led to the recommendation of achieving at least 25 mm of anteroposterior patellar height initially as the bone graft compresses approximately 3 to 5 mm over time (**Fig. 71-6A and B**).[19] In a subsequent experience at the authors' institution, 93 knees with a bone-deficient patella were managed with this procedure between 1997 and 2014 (*unpublished data, 2018*). In these patients, 10-year survivorship free of patellar revision was 96%. The primary advantages of this simple surgical procedure include the potential for restoration of patellar bone stock and marked improvement of anteroposterior patellar height. The primary disadvantage is the need for cancellous allograft if local autograft is not available.

In a small case series of three patients, a modification of this technique has been described to be used when there is concern for the strength and integrity of the patellar tendon and/or quadriceps attachment to the remaining patellar bony shell.[32] Under these circumstances, the extensor mechanism is augmented by securing an Achilles tendon allograft to the distal part of the quadriceps tendon and the proximal portion of the patellar tendon.[32] Although it is difficult to estimate when imminent patellar fracture

extensor mechanism function. In some instances, it may be possible to add some cancellous bone graft on the ventral aspect of the osteotomy beneath the fibrous tissue and the patellar osteotomy (**Fig. 71-4**). If contained, this bone graft may potentially facilitate successful healing of the osteotomy, and once incorporated may impart partial restoration of patellar bone stock.

Cancellous Impaction Patellar Bone Grafting

This technique (**Video**) is based on the use of a soft-tissue flap to contain cancellous bone chips within the residual patellar shell.[19] The tissue flap acts as a fascial interposition arthroplasty against the femoral trochlea allowing the contained bone graft to undergo molding and compression within the trochlea during range of motion. There are several important technical aspects when performing this procedure. During exposure of the revision knee, it is helpful to retain the pseudomeniscus of scar tissue and most of the peripatellar fibrotic tissue on the undersurface of the quadriceps tendon and on the periphery of the remaining patellar rim. This local tissue constitutes the basis of this technique and as such one should resist the temptation to remove this peripatellar tissue during exposure.

The patellar shell is prepared by removing all fibrous membrane in the crevices of the remaining patellar bone. The most reliable tissue for a local soft-tissue flap lies on the undersurface of the quadriceps tendon (**Fig. 71-5A**). The flap is created by elevating the tissue from proximal to distal, leaving the base of the tissue firmly attached to the superior aspect of the patella (**Fig. 71-5B**).

The tissue flap is then turned down and sewn into the periphery of the pseudomeniscus, peripatellar fibrous

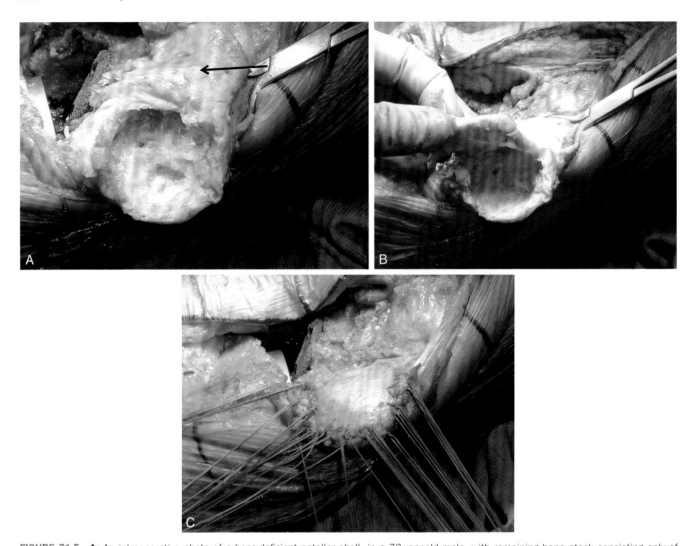

FIGURE 71-5   **A:** An intraoperative photo of a bone-deficient patellar shell, in a 72-year-old male, with remaining bone stock consisting only of anterior cortex and some areas of patellar rim. The arrow designates the fibrotic tissue on the undersurface of the quadriceps tendon that will be elevated to create an *in situ* tissue flap. **B:** Intraoperative photo of the tissue flap after elevation from undersurface of the quadriceps tendon. **C:** Intraoperative photo of patella after closure of tissue flap with interrupted sutures to provide a watertight closure containing the cancellous bone graft.

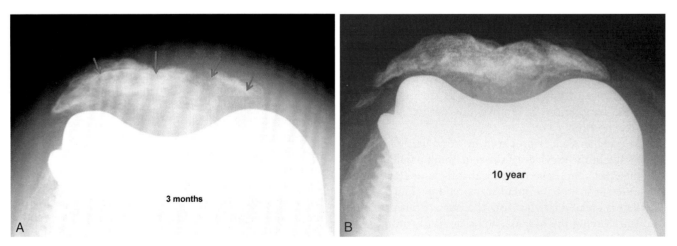

FIGURE 71-6   **A:** Merchant radiograph view at 3 months postoperatively of the patellar bone grafting performed in the same 72-year-old male. The arrows depict the interface between the patellar shell and contained cancellous bone graft. **B:** Merchant radiograph view at 10 years postoperatively, demonstrating excellent incorporation of bone graft and 4 mm of reduced patellar height as compared with immediate postoperative radiographs.

may be present, this technique modification may also be beneficial in these circumstances or when there is a small pole fracture present at the time of bone grafting.

TECHNIQUES WITH PATELLAR COMPONENT IMPLANTATION

Screw or Wire With Cement Augmentation

Based on a case report,[33] in a patella with a unilateral segmental bone defect of either half of the patella, in a manner similar to fixing small tibial bone defects, a transverse bone screw placed into the bone of the patella can allow the screw head to support a standard three-pegged all polyethylene patellar component. In a slight variation, for patellae with primarily cavitary bone loss precluding lug fixation of a patellar component and retained patellar rim, the use of crossed transcortical K-wires inserted through the rims across the defect can augment the cement fixation within the central bone defect.

Transcortical Wiring

A novel approach, also using the standard three-pegged all polyethylene patellar component has been described.[34] In this series of 28 patients (30 knees), all patellae were <8 mm. After preparation of the patellar bony bed, three 24-gauge wires are secured around the three pegs of the polyethylene patellar component (**Fig. 71-7**). These wires are then placed through three corresponding holes of the anterior cortex of the patella so that bone cement placed into the interval between the patella and patellar component can be adequately compressed and cured by tension tightening of the wires on the anterior patellar surface. These authors recommend careful contouring and in setting of these wires to avoid a postoperative patellar fracture. The main disadvantage of this technique is that the average patellar construct height often averages <15 mm.

Structural Bone Grafting of the Patella

An autologous monocortical iliac bone graft, harvested from the medial cortex of the anterior iliac crest, is shaped to accommodate the patellar shell.[35] The cancellous surface of the graft is opposed to the patella bone and fixed with four 1.5 mm cortical screws. Any remaining defects are filled with cancellous bone chips. The new patellar button is then cemented into the cortical surface of the bone graft. Requirements for this procedure include (1) the patellar shell is not fractured and can accommodate or accept the graft, (2) the patellar bone is of sufficient quality to allow good screw purchase, and (3) the extensor mechanism is in continuity. Autologous bone is recommended to increase the chances of union in a poor-quality bony bed.[35] This procedure has the disadvantage that there is donor site morbidity at the iliac wing and the fact that this area of the pelvis is not always flat. Additionally, the new patellar button is cemented directly into the cortical surface of the bone graft, rather than a cancellous bony bed, and postoperative radiolucencies at this interface are common.[35]

Three-Pegged Porous Metal Monoblock Patella

In a unique application of a 3-D printed titanium monoblock patellar component, the patella is prepared to create as much flat surface area as is possible (personal communication, Victor Krebs, 2016). The patella remnant is then prepared for three lug holes that correspond with the intended implant. These lug holes often perforate the anterior cortex of the patellar remnant, and the patellar fixation lugs often protrude through the cortex by several millimeters. In most cases, these fixation lugs protrude through the anterior cortex by several millimeters. In the authors' experience of five cases, this technique has been useful for patellae that are relatively flat

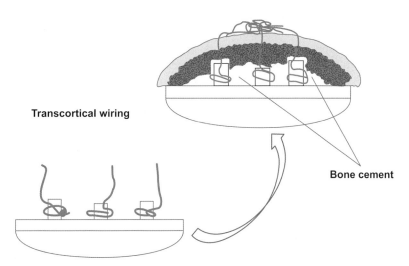

FIGURE 71-7 Schematic demonstrating the application of wires to the three pegs of a standard polyethylene component. The wires are passed through drill holes created in the anterior patellar cortex and then are tightened during the curing of the bone cement

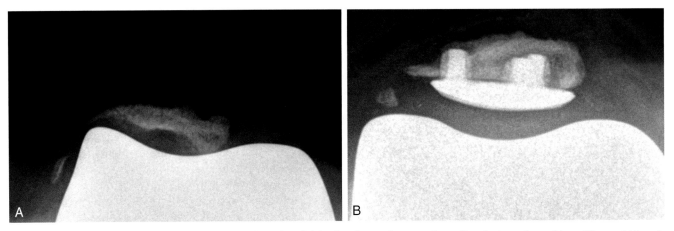

FIGURE 71-8 **A:** Merchant radiograph view of a persistently painful sclerotic patellar resection arthroplasty performed in a 53-year-old female with flexion instability. **B:** Merchant view radiograph of same patient 3 years postoperatively, following femoral and tibial component revision with implantation of a 3-D titanium porous metal monoblock patellar component.

patellar remnants of 8 to 12 mm and are quite sclerotic (**Fig. 71-8A** and **B**) *(unpublished data, 2018)*. It is recognized that, in many of these patients, other techniques such as a biconvex patellar component may have been implanted. However, unlike an inset patella, use of this cementless metal-backed patellar component produces an anterior patellofemoral height of 18 to 22 mm which likely improves extensor mechanism function.

Porous Metal Augmentation Baseplate

A unique porous metal implant was designed to specifically address severe patellar bone loss and correspondingly reconstruct the anteroposterior patellar height. In a cadaveric study of an augmentation patella versus a patellar resection arthroplasty, the baseplate reconstruction with normal anteroposterior patellar height had superior patellar kinematics and quadriceps extensor force.[36]

The surgical technique for implantation of this prosthesis is quite straightforward. The bone-deficient patella is prepared with spherical reamers to prepare a concave patellar remnant that can accept the dome-shaped porous metal baseplate (**Fig. 71-9**). Once apposed, interrupted sutures are passed through the suture portals of the baseplate into the extensor mechanism and surrounding soft tissues to maintain implant position and apposition. A polyethylene component is then cemented onto the porous metal baseplate.

In the initial report on 20 patients with a bone-deficient patella, results were good or excellent in 17 (85%) at 32-months follow-up with three patients experiencing pole fractures.[37] In a similar report, all 11 patients had excellent incorporation of the baseplate into the patellar bony shell at average 32-months follow-up.[38] In 23 revision patellae of <10 mm, at an average follow-up of 7.7 years, an 83% survivorship was observed with failures observed when the patellar shell was avascular or when the baseplate was secured into soft tissues only.[39]

In a comparative study in 16 patients (18 knees), all seven baseplates sewn into soft tissue only ultimately loosened and failed.[22] Others have reported failure in all patients when using this baseplate in patients with a prior patellectomy.[26,40] Therefore it seems important to emphasize the need for adequate patellar bone stock when using this implant. The primary advantage of this implant is the accurate reconstitution of anteroposterior patellar height in an effort to optimize patellar kinematics and quadriceps extensor forces. The primary disadvantage of this implant is the extremely high cost of this implant in relationship to other treatment alternatives.

DISCUSSION

Revision of the patella during revision knee arthroplasty remains an important area of treatment as evidenced by the multiple different approaches proposed to solve this problem. The prevention of patellar maltracking with the use of current prosthetic designs and better understanding of the proper positioning of prosthetic components will hopefully reduce the incidence of patellar implant failure. When a patellar implant fails, an isolated patellar revision should be done rarely as it is likely that femoral and/or tibial revision to correct rotational position will be required to alleviate the underlying source of stresses that led to patellar failure.

With sufficient patellar bone stock present, insertion of a standard three-pegged or biconvex polyethylene prosthesis is relatively straightforward. In the face of severe patellar bone deficiency, there are many treatment options available. It is likely that any isolated patellar revision procedure in the setting of severe patellar bone deficiency is prone to recurrent failure if the underlying etiology resulting in patellar tracking is not adequately addressed. Patellectomy is strongly discouraged and although patellar resection arthroplasty may occasionally be deemed appropriate, inferior clinical results often occur. Many of

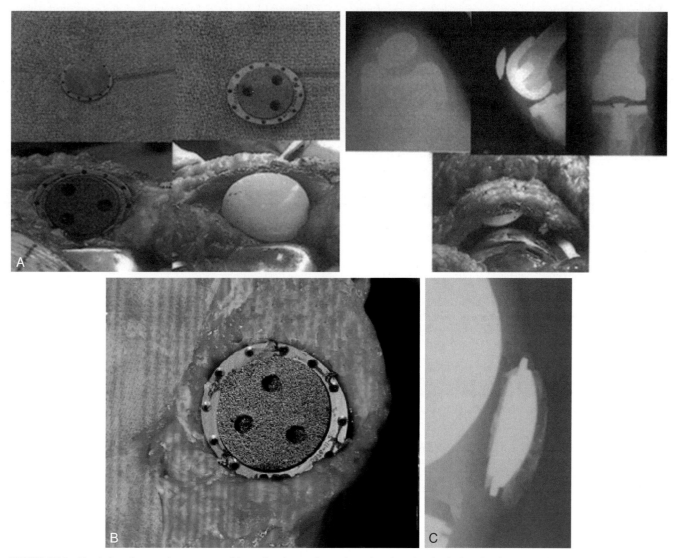

FIGURE 71-9 The trabecular metal porous metal baseplate has a dome-shaped surface that is designed to be apposed against the patellar shell. The opposite surface of the baseplate has three lug holes that accept the all polyethylene patellar component, which is fixed with bone cement. The patellar shell is prepared with domed reamers to mate with the domed metal baseplate **(A)**. The external titanium ring has suture anchor holes to fix the baseplate to the surrounding soft tissues and remaining patellar rim **(B)**. Postoperative lateral radiograph at 18 months shows integration of the baseplate into the patellar shell **(C)**.

the described techniques do not restore anteroposterior patellar height or the potential for restoration of patellar bone stock. Bone grafting procedures impart the potential for restoration of both. Newer technologies, like the porous metal baseplate, emphasize the underlying principle of attaining anatomic patellar height and offer the presence of a polyethylene articular surface.

REFERENCES

1. Barrack RL, Rorabeck C, Partington P, et al. The results of retaining a well-fixed patellar component in revision total knee arthroplasty. *J Arthroplasty*. 2000;15:413-417.
2. Gililland JM, Swann P, Pelt CE, Erickson J, Hamad N, Peters CL. What is the role for patelloplasty with gullwing osteotomy in revision TKA? *Clin Orthop Relat Res*. 2016;474:101-106.
3. Lewis PL, Gamboa AE, Campbell DG, et al. Outcome of prosthesis matched and unmatched patella components in primary and revision total knee replacement. *Knee*. 2017;24:1227-1232.
4. Lonner JH, Mont MA, Sharkey PF, et al. Fate of the unrevised all-polyethylene patellar component in revision total knee arthroplasty. *J Bone Joint Surg*. 2003;85A:56-59.
5. Maheshwari AV, Tsailas PG, Ranawat AS, et al. How to address the patella in revision total knee arthroplasty. *Knee*. 2009;16:92-97.
6. Rorabeck CH, Mehin R, Barrack RL. Patellar options in revision total knee arthroplasty. *Clin Orthop Relat Res*. 2003;416:84-92.
7. Tetreault MW, Gross CE, Yi PH, et al. A classification-based approach to the patella in revision total knee arthroplasty. *Arthroplast Today*. 2017;3:264-268.
8. Patil N, Lee K, Huddleston JI, et al. Patellar management in revision total knee arthroplasty: is patellar resurfacing a better option? *J Arthroplasty*. 2010;25:589-593.
9. Bhattee G, Moonot P, Govindaswamy R, et al. Does malrotation of components correlate with patient dissatisfaction following secondary patellar resurfacing? *Knee*. 2014;21:247-251.
10. Vanbiervliet J, Bellemans J, Verlinden C, et al. The influence of malrotation and femoral component material on patellofemoral wear during gait. *J Bone Joint Surg*. 2011;93B:1348-1354.

11. Berry DJ, Rand JA. Isolated patellar component revision of total knee arthroplasty. *Clin Orthop Relat Res.* 1993;286:110-115.

12. Garcia RM, Kraay MJ, Goldberg VM. Isolated all-polyethylene patellar revisions for metal-backed patellar failure. *Clin Orthop Relat Res.* 2008;466:2784-2789.

13. Leopold SS, Silverton CD, Barden RM, et al. Isolated revision of the patellar component in total knee arthroplasty. *J Bone Joint Surg.* 2003;85A:41-47.

14. Dalury DF, Adams MJ. Minimum 6-year follow-up of revision total knee arthroplasty without patella reimplantation. *J Arthroplasty.* 2012;27(8 suppl):91-94.

15. Barrack RL, Matzkin E, Ingraham R, et al. Revision knee arthroplasty with patella replacement versus bony shell. *Clin Orthop Relat Res.* 1998;356:139-143.

16. Erak S, Bourne RB, MacDonald SJ, et al. The cemented inset biconvex patella in revision knee arthroplasty. *Knee.* 2009;16:211-215.

17. Erak S, Rajgopal V, Macdonald SJ, et al. Ten-year results of an inset biconvex patella prosthesis in primary knee arthroplasty. *Clin Orthop Relat Res.* 2009;467:1781-1792.

18. Garcia RM, Kraay MJ, Conroy-Smith PA, et al. Management of the deficient patella in revision total knee arthroplasty. *Clin Orthop Relat Res.* 2008;466:2790-2797.

19. Hanssen AD. Bone-grafting for severe patellar bone loss during revision knee arthroplasty. *J Bone Joint Surg.* 2001;83A:171-176.

20. Ikezawa Y, Gustilo RB. Clinical outcome of revision of the patellar component in total knee arthroplasty. A 2- to 7-year follow-up study. *J Orthop Sci.* 1999;4:83-88.

21. Maheshwer CB, Mitchell E, Kraay M, et al. Revision of the patella with deficient bone using a biconvex component. *Clin Orthop Relat Res.* 2005;440:126-130.

22. Ries MD, Cabalo A, Bozic KJ, et al. Porous tantalum patellar augmentation: the importance of residual bone stock. *Clin Orthop Relat Res.* 2006;452:166-170.

23. Pagnano MW, Scuderi GR, Insall JN. Patellar component resection in revision and reimplantation total knee arthroplasty. *Clin Orthop Relat Res.* 1998;356:134-138.

24. Parvizi J, Seel MJ, Hanssen AD, et al. Patellar component resection arthroplasty for the severely compromised patella. *Clin Orthop Relat Res.* 2002;397:356-361.

25. Chen AF, Tetreault MW, Levicoff EA, et al. Increased incidence of patella baja after total knee arthroplasty revision for infection. *Am J Orthop.* 2014;43:562-566.

26. Lavernia CJ, Alcerro JC, Drakeford MK, et al. Resection arthroplasty for failed patellar components. *Int Orthop.* 2009;33:1591-1596.

27. Glynn A, Huang R, Mortazavi J, et al. The impact of patellar resurfacing in two-stage revision of the infected total knee arthroplasty. *J Arthroplasty.* 2014;29:1439-1442.

28. Dennis DA. Removal of well-fixed cementless metal-backed patellar components. *J Arthroplasty.* 1992;7:217-220.

29. Kaneko T, Kono N, Mochizuki Y, et al. Use of porous monoblock patella component should avoid for patient with patella baja. *J Orthop.* 2018;15:432-437.

30. Vince KG, Roidis N, Blackburn D. Gull-wing sagittal patellar osteotomy in total knee arthroplasty. *Tech Knee Surg.* 2002;1:106-112.

31. Klein GR, Levine HB, Ambrose JF, et al. Gull-wing osteotomy for the treatment of the deficient patella in revision total knee arthroplasty. *J Arthroplasty.* 2010;25:249-253.

32. Boettner F, Bou Monsef J. Achilles tendon allograft for augmentation of the Hanssen patellar bone grafting. *Knee Surg Sports Traumatol Arthrosc.* 2015;23:1035-1038.

33. Jayasekera N, Lakdawala A, Toms AD, et al. Screw and cement augmentation of patella defects in knee arthroplasty. *Ann R Coll Surg Engl.* 2014;96:78-79.

34. Seo JG, Moon YW, Lee BH, Kim SM. Reconstruction of a deficient patella in revision total knee arthroplasty: results of a new surgical technique using transcortical wiring. *J Arthroplasty.* 2015;30:254-258.

35. Tabutin J. Osseous reconstruction of the patella with screwed autologous graft in the course of repeat prosthesis of the knee. *Rev Chir Orthop Reparatrice Appar Mot.* 1998;84:363-367.

36. Mountney J, Wilson DR, Paice M, et al. The effect of an augmentation patella prosthesis versus patelloplasty on revision patellar kinematics and quadriceps tendon force: an ex vivo study. *J Arthroplasty.* 2008;23:1219-1231.

37. Nelson CL, Lonner JH, Lahiji A, et al. Use of a trabecular metal patella for marked patella bone loss during revision total knee arthroplasty. *J Arthroplasty.* 2003;18:37-41.

38. Nasser S, Poggie RA. Revision and salvage patellar arthroplasty using a porous tantalum implant. *J Arthroplasty.* 2004;19:562-572.

39. Kamath AF, Gee AO, Nelson CL, et al. Porous tantalum patellar components in revision total knee arthroplasty minimum 5-year follow-up. *J Arthroplasty.* 2012;27:82-87.

40. Tigani D, Trentani P, Trentani F, et al. Trabecular metal patella in total knee arthroplasty with patella bone deficiency. *Knee.* 2009;16:46-49.

Management of the Infected Total Knee Replacement

HANY S. BEDAIR

Prevalence, Prevention, and Economic Implications of Infection After Total Knee Arthroplasty

Stephen J. Nelson, MD | Patrick K. Strotman, MD | James A. Browne, MD

INTRODUCTION

Periprosthetic joint infection (PJI) is one of the most dreaded complications following total knee arthroplasty (TKA). The combination of increasingly drug-resistant pathogens with a large foreign body in a capacious potential space makes these infections particularly difficult to fully eradicate, requiring intense intervention—both surgical and antibiotic. Even when treated appropriately, PJI carries a significant risk factor for mortality.[1] Such outcomes are distressing to both the patient and surgeon. With such weighty consequences, the old adage rings true, "An ounce of prevention is worth a pound of cure." This chapter will comment on the prevalence of infection following TKA and then discuss risk factors, steps for prevention, and the economic implications associated with PJI.

PREVALENCE

While PJI is a relatively uncommon complication, it has supplanted polyethylene wear and aseptic loosening as the most common reason for revision TKA.[2-4] Bozik et al evaluated the national inpatient sample and found that 25.2% of revision procedures were performed for infection. Its incidence has been reported to be in a range from 0.7% to 2.2%.[5-7] Kurtz evaluated the Medicare 5% national sample administrative data and noted that the incidence of infection within 2 years of surgery was 1.55%.[7] Crowe examined 3419 primary TKA procedures performed at NYU Lagone Medical Center between 2009 and 2011 and noted an infection rate of 0.76%.[5] Pulido evaluated their rates of PJI at Thomas Jefferson University Hospital in a series of 4185 patients prospectively gathered between 2001 and 2006. They also reported an infection rate of 1.1%.[6] Despite increasing attempts at prevention, there is some evidence that the incidence of PJI may be slowly increasing given the increase in life expectancies and higher volumes of joint arthroplasty procedures.[8,9]

Though acute postoperative infection is of primary concern for the orthopedic surgeon, Kurtz and colleagues found that the risk of infection extends beyond the 2-year mark postoperatively, as 0.46% of patients developed an infection between 2 and 10 years.[7] In an evaluation of the Finnish health registry, Huotari noted that the incidence rate of late PJI (after 2 years) after hip or knee arthroplasty was approximately 0.07% per prosthesis year.[10]

Infection rates are exponentially higher following total knee revision procedures, with Frank et al reporting a rate of 7%.[11] If the reason for revision TKA is infection, Cochran et al report risk of reinfection being 24.6% for 1-stage and 19% for 2-stage revision patients, respectively, at 1 year postoperatively. In their study, the cumulative risk of revision at 6 years was 38.3% and 29.1% for 1- and 2-stage revision patients, respectively.[12] It is unclear whether the higher risk of infection after revision procedures is due to the increased length and complexity of surgery, the incomplete eradication of the infection which indicated the revision procedure in the first place, or the failure to diagnose implant failure as an infectious process. It is likely all of these factors drive the higher infection rate in patients who have undergone multiple revisions.

PREVENTION

The prevention of infection in TKA can be broken down into three phases: preoperative prevention, intraoperative prevention, and postoperative prevention. Efforts during each of these periods are aimed at either increasing the immunocompetence of the patient or decreasing the bioburden of surgery.

Preoperative Prevention

Appropriate patient selection and optimization cannot be overemphasized in the battle to decrease the incidence of infection. There have been several patient-specific risk factors for infection identified in TKA, including inflammatory arthritis, male gender, age, ASA >2, lower socioeconomic status, and hepatitis C.[7,13-16] Season of the year has also been implicated in the likelihood of surgical site infection (SSI).[17] Such risk factors may or may not be modifiable. Modifiable risk factors include malnutrition, diabetes, obesity, depression, smoking, opiate dependence, methicillin-resistant *Staphylococcus aureus*

(MRSA) colonization, and recent arthroscopic surgery or steroid injection. Each of these modifiable risk factors will be addressed individually. It should be noted that there is little prospective data supporting optimization of patient risk factors to decrease PJI rates available at this point in time.

Optimal nutritional status to facilitate appropriate wound healing is a requisite for PJI prevention. Saleh et al[18] observed that patients who have 5 days or more of postoperative wound drainage were 12.5 times more likely to develop infection than those without drainage. Malnutrition impedes synthesis of collagen-derived peptides and causes immune system dysfunction. Greene noted that preoperative nutritional status was strongly correlated with the likelihood of a postoperative wound complication.[19] A preoperative lymphocyte count of less than 1500 cells/mm was associated with a fivefold greater frequency of developing a major wound complication, and an albumin level of less than 3.5 g/dL had a seven times greater frequency.[19] Jaberi and colleagues also examined patients who experienced prolonged wound drainage and found that malnourished patients (serum transferrin <200 mg/dL, serum albumin <3.5 g/dL, or total lymphocyte count <1500/mm^3) undergoing total joint arthroplasty are more likely to develop deep infection.[20] Yi et al found that having one or more of the three laboratory parameters outlined above is independently associated with both chronic septic failure and acute postoperative infection complicating an aseptic revision arthroplasty.[21]

Diabetes has been associated with mixed outcomes following TKA. Marchant et al evaluated the Nationwide Inpatient Sample and found that patients with uncontrolled diabetes exhibited significantly increased odds of surgical and systemic complications, higher mortality, and increased length of stay during index hospitalization following lower extremity total joint arthroplasty.[22] The authors also found an increased risk for wound infection (OR = 2.28; 95% CI = 1.36 to 3.81; P = .002). Conversely, Adams et al[23] evaluated the Kaiser Permanente Total Joint Replacement Registry and were unable to identify an increased risk of revision arthroplasty or deep infection in patients with diabetes. Despite this apparent discrepancy, Cancienne was able to identify an association between perioperative HbA1c and the rates of deep postoperative infection requiring surgical intervention after TKA.[15,16] The analysis indicated that the inflection point where the risk of infection increased was an HbA1c of 8.0 mg/dL (**Fig. 72-1**). The authors caution that the A1c should be interpreted in the context of the patient's other risk factors for PJI.[15,16] An attempt at reducing the A1c prior to surgery seems warranted but may not serve as a good cutoff to recommend against surgery.

Obese patients have been found to have an increased risk of infection following TKA. The exact pathophysiology is unknown but may be related to increased surface tension at the incision site or the need to perform a more involved dissection for exposure that results in hematoma formation, seroma collection, or prolonged drainage. Jämsen performed a single center series study of 7181 patients in Finland undergoing lower extremity arthroplasty and demonstrated that the infection rate increased from 0.37% in patients with a normal body mass index (BMI) to 4.66% in the morbidly obese group.[24] Nunez et al performed a case control study of 60 patients with

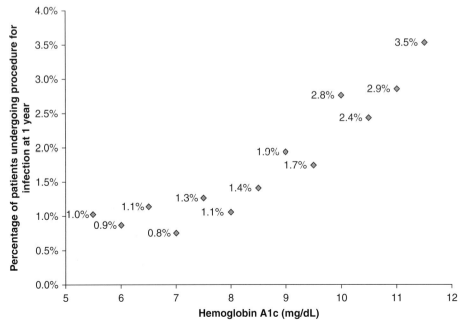

FIGURE 72-1 The rate of deep infection within 1 year after primary total knee arthroplasty stratified by HbA1C within 3 months of surgery. (From Cancienne JM, Werner BC, Browne JA. Is there an association between hemoglobin A1C and deep postoperative infection after TKA? *Clin Orthop Relat Res.* 2017;475(6):1642-1649.)

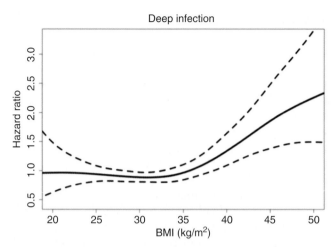

FIGURE 72-2 The risk of periprosthetic joint infection after total knee arthroplasty as a function of body mass index (BMI) at the time of surgery from the Mayo Clinic database. The dashed lines represent the 95% CI. (Reproduced from Wagner ER, Kamath AF, Fruth K, Harmsen WS, Berry DJ. Effect of Body Mass Index on Reoperation and Complications After Total Knee Arthroplasty. *J Bone Joint Surg Am.* 2016;98(24):2052-2060.)

an average BMI of 39.9 who underwent primary TKA. The authors demonstrated nearly twice the risk (11.6% vs. 6.6%) of in-hospital wound problems and three times the rate of PJI compared to controls (5.0% vs. 1.6%).[25] A recent study from the Mayo Clinic found a striking association between BMI and risk for deep wound infection (**Fig. 72-2**). The smoothing spline analysis demonstrated that beginning at a BMI threshold of 35 kg/m^2, there was a 7% increased risk of superficial or deep infection per unit increase in BMI above 35 kg/m^2 (HR, 1.07; $P <$ .001).[26]

Whether or not weight loss prior to TKA reduces the risks of infection remains unclear. A number of authors have examined whether or not bariatric surgery prior to arthroplasty improves clinical outcomes in obese patients; Smith et al performed a meta-analysis of five studies to this end.[27] The authors noted that the incidence of wound infection and overall medical complications was lower in the bariatric surgery group.[27]

Depression has also been associated with poor outcomes following TJA. Gold et al performed a retrospective study utilizing the all-payer California Healthcare Cost and Utilization Project database and found depression was more prevalent in those readmitted at the 90-day time point in their multivariable analysis.[28] Ricciardi et al demonstrated a similar finding at the 30-day time point after reviewing 10,759 total knee replacements performed over a 5-year period between 2010 and 2014. In a separate multivariate analysis of the National Inpatient Sample, the rate of diagnosis of depression was 10%, and among those patients, there was a higher risk of infection (OR = 1.33).[29] While identifying and treating patients with depression and those with other psychiatric diagnoses which result in poor coping skills may result in improved rates of satisfaction, it is unclear if this will impact rates of PJI.

Tobacco smoking is a modifiable risk factor and has been associated to several adverse postoperative outcomes, including infection and need for revision. Nicotine alters perfusion within the microvasculature system, decreases wound bed oxygen tension, and impairs epithelialization.[30] In an evaluation of the Mayo database, tobacco users undergoing total hip arthroplasty (THA) or TKA were found to have higher hazard ratios for deep infection (2.37; 95% CI, 1.19 to 4.72; P = .01) and implant revision (1.78; 95% CI 1.01, 3.13; P = .04).[31] Sahota et al looked at complications in smokers undergoing total hip or knee replacement in the acute postoperative period. After utilizing propensity matching to limit confounding variables often observed in this population, they noted that a smoker is twice as likely to experience a surgical complication which was primarily driven by an SSI diagnosis.[32] In 2002, Møller et al conducted a randomized controlled trial to demonstrate that smoking cessation 6 to 8 weeks before total hip or knee arthroplasty led to a significant decrease in wound complications and need for secondary surgery.[33] A meta-analysis by Bedard et al demonstrated a significantly increased risk of any wound complication (OR, 1.36 [1.16 to 1.60]) and PJI (OR, 1.52 [1.07 to 2.14]) for current tobacco users relative to former tobacco users showing that some smoking-mediated changes may be reversible.[34]

Opiates have immunosuppressive properties, and preoperative opioid consumption has been found to increase the risk of PJI (adjusted OR, 1.53 [95% CI, 1.14 to 2.05], P = .005).[35] A large database study by Cancienne et al examined patients who underwent primary TKA between 2007 and 2015. Their results demonstrated that the most significant risk factor for prolonged postoperative opiate use was filling a preoperative narcotic prescription (OR 5.74). Infection was associated independently with preoperative narcotic use (OR = 1.16) and postoperative narcotic use (OR = 1.33).[36] It is important to utilize caution when prescribing opioids in patients with degenerative joint disease who may be candidates for arthroplasty and identify patients via state-wide prescription monitoring programs filling narcotic prescriptions in the preoperative and postoperative periods.

In a recent study, previous steroid injection into a native knee has also been identified as a possible risk factor for infection. Papavasiliou et al[37] evaluated three PJIs in a series of 144 patients who underwent TKA. The authors noted that the patients who developed PJI all received an intra-articular steroid in the months before surgery. This finding was confirmed in the evaluation of a medical record database where the incidence of infection was found to be significantly higher in those patients who had a steroid injection within 3 months of surgery.[38] There was no significant difference in patients who underwent TKA more than 3 months after injection, suggesting that a window of at least 3 months be maintained between corticosteroid injection and arthroplasty.

Knee arthroscopy within 6 months of arthroplasty has also been identified as a risk factor for postoperative infection. Compared to an age-matched group of control patients also undergoing TKA, there were higher incidences of infection (OR 2.0, $P = .004$), stiffness (OR 2.0, $P = .001$), and venous thromboembolism (VTE) (OR 1.6, $P = .047$) in patients who underwent TKA within 6 months after knee arthroscopy.[39,40] There were no increased risks of complications when a waiting period was maintained beyond 6 months. If a patient has recently undergone an invasive procedure about the knee joint, it may be prudent to delay elective TKA to mitigate risk of PJI.

Each of the previously mentioned modifiable risk factors has focused on attempting to increase the immunocompetence of the patient; however, there is also a place for decreasing the bioburden of the host. Asymptomatic colonization with MRSA has been described as a risk factor for subsequent MRSA infection. In a series of 758 patients, MRSA colonization at admission has been found to increase the risk of subsequent MRSA infection, compared with methicillin-sensitive *S. aureus* (MSSA) colonization (RR, 13; 95% CI, 2.7 to 64) or no staphylococcal colonization (RR, 9.5; 95% CI, 3.6 to 25) at admission suggesting that asymptomatic MRSA hosts should be identified for preoperative MRSA intervention. Rao et al screened patients for nasal carriage of *S. aureus* and decolonized those patients with mupirocin ointment to the nares twice daily and chlorhexidine bath once daily for 5 days before surgery.[41] The authors noted that of all 164 of 636 participants who tested positive for *Staphylococcus* and completed the decolonization protocol, none had a postoperative infection at 1-year follow-up.[41] Kim also evaluated the implementation of a prescreening program for MSSA and MRSA and found that treatment of carriers with an eradication protocol consisting of intranasal mupirocin and chlorhexidine showers decreased infection rates to 0.19%, which was significantly lower than the infection rate observed prior to the decolonization protocol (0.45%, $P = .0093$).[42]

Preoperative bathing with chlorhexidine has also been found to decrease the incidence of wound infection following knee arthroplasty. In a meta-analysis of four clinical trials, use of preoperative chlorhexidine was associated with a reduced total incidence of infection (RR = 0.22; 95% CI = 0.12 to 0.40; $P = .000$).[43] Banerjee et al noted that preoperative chlorhexidine multiple showers or topical applications of chlorhexidine may lead to more substantial reduction in colony counts of pathogenic organisms.[44] The authors argue that whole-body cleaning rather than site-specific application may confer additional advantages.[44]

Intraoperative Prevention

Anesthesia appears to have an impact on the infection rate following arthroplasty. Chang et al conducted a database study comparing outcomes of patients who underwent THA and TKA under general anesthesia versus those who had neuraxial anesthesia only. The odds ratio of SSI after adjusting for type of surgery, age, sex, comorbidities, and teaching status of the hospital was found to be 2.21 for general anesthesia compared to neuraxial.[45] Zorrilla-Vaca performed a meta-analysis of 13 studies and also found a beneficial impact on the rate of SSI for TKA if neuraxial anesthesia was used (OR = 0.75; 95% CI, 0.68 to 0.84; $P < .001$) as compared with general anesthesia.[46] Of note, peripheral nerve block procedures have been found to not influence the incidence of SSI.[47] In addition, maintaining physiologic normothermia decreases risk of postoperative complication. Inadvertent hypothermia may result in vasoconstriction and decreased oxygen tension at the surgical site. Awareness and communication between multidisciplinary teams in the operating room is critical to decreasing patient risk.

The perioperative administration of antibiotics significantly impacts the rates of SSI following arthroplasty. In a meta-analysis of seven studies it was found that antibiotic prophylaxis reduced the absolute risk of wound infection by 8% and the relative risk by 81% compared with no prophylaxis ($P < .00001$).[48] The National Surgical Infection Prevention Project recommends that infusion of the first antimicrobial dose should begin within 1 hour before incision and that prophylactic antimicrobials should be discontinued within 24 hours after the end of surgery.[49] The appropriate timing of such antibiotic prophylaxis can be a challenge in a busy perioperative area. Rosenburg et al found that when antibiotic administration was incorporated into the surgical "time out," the compliance rate of appropriate antibiotic administration went from 65% to 99.1%.[50] The authors advocate incorporating antibiosis into the time out in order to facilitate communication and appropriate care. The common practice of continuing antibiotics postoperatively for 24 hours has recently come under scrutiny, with the CDC recommending against additional prophylactic antimicrobial agent doses after the surgical incision is closed in the operating room, even in the presence of a drain.[51]

The optimal surgical skin preparation to decrease infection rates has long been debated. Darouiche performed a prospective, randomized controlled trial comparing chlorhexidine–alcohol versus povidone–iodine for surgical site antisepsis of clean contaminated surgery (i.e., colorectal, small intestinal, gastroesophageal, biliary, thoracic, gynecologic, or urologic operations performed under controlled conditions without substantial spillage or unusual contamination).[52] The authors found that chlorhexidine–alcohol was protective against both superficial incisional infections (4.2% vs. 8.6%, $P = .008$) and deep incisional infections (1% vs. 3%, $P = .05$). Some authors have advocated for an iodine-based skin prep due to the better adherence of plastic adhesive drapes in these patients.[53,54] These authors argue that residual skin flora after surgical skin preparation may be exposed if uncovered and have demonstrated that DuraPrep solution had significantly greater drape adhesion compared with skin prepared with ChloraPrep.[54] However, the merit of plastic adhesive drapes during surgery for preventing SSI has yet to be established.[55] Current CDC guidelines state that skin preparation in the operating room should be performed using an alcohol-based agent unless contraindicated.[51]

Regardless of the preferred chemical prep for the surgical site, the technique and meticulousness with which skin preparation is performed is likely important. Often, the leg is held in extension during aseptic preparation for TKA despite the more relaxed tension of the anterior skin when in that position. When a leg is prepped in extension and then brought into flexion, close examination shows asymmetries in the prep and missed spots in the natural creases of the leg (**Fig. 72-3**). As such, skin preparation of the knee in flexion instead of extension may provide superior coverage of the skin surface and has no clear downside.[56]

A second surgical skin prep after draping has been suggested as a way to decrease the incidence of SSI. Morrison et al[57] investigated the effect of performing an additional surgical skin prep with iodine povacrylex and isopropyl alcohol before application of the final adhesive drape and found a significant reduction in the incidence of superficial SSI for the intervention group (1.8%, 5 of 283) compared to the control group (6.5%, 19 of 294, P = .02).

Within the operating room there have been numerous studies and strategies to decrease bacterial counts and infection rates. Permeable cotton gowns and drapes have been found to be inferior to impervious gown and drape

materials for the prevention of SSI.[58] In terms of surgical attire, there has been no evidence that scrubs, head covering, arm covering for nonscrubbed personnel, or masks have any effect on infection rates.[58] The regular changing of surgical gloves has been shown to decrease glove contamination rates; however, there has been no clear association with SSI.[59]

Though body exhaust suits have been found to decrease the air count of bacteria, they have not been shown to decrease wound contamination.[60] Despite their failure to reduce infection rates, some have argued that body exhaust suits and surgical helmet systems may provide the surgeon additional comfort and splash protection, which may justify their higher cost over conventional gowns and masks.[61]

Laminar air flow has been widely used in an effort to decrease counts of airborne bacteria, but its actual effect on SSI remains controversial. Miner et al investigated the effect of laminar airflow and outcomes in the acute postoperative period in a series of 8288 total knee replacements. The authors did not find a difference in the incidence of infection.[62] Similarly, in a German cohort study of 33,463 patients undergoing THA, laminar air flow was not found to have any effect on infection rates.[63] This is a difficult variable to study in a controlled fashion with important cofounders related to operating room traffic, number of staff in the room, and tray exposure.

The use of antibiotic-impregnated bone cement is another strategy by which some surgeons have sought to lower infection rates. Though there may be some evidence that gentamicin-impregnated antibiotic bone cement decreases deep infection rates,[64] a recent systematic review

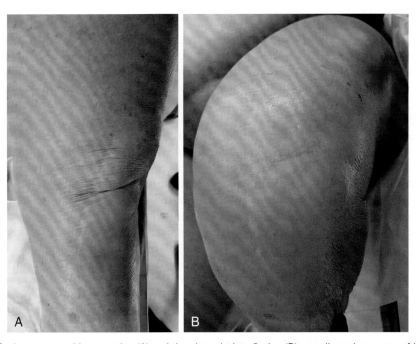

FIGURE 72-3 Example of a knee prepped in extension (A) and then brought into flexion (B) revealing a large area of inadequate prep within the skinfold. (Reproduced from Knoll PA, Browne JA. Prepping the knee in maximal flexion: getting into every nook, cranny, and fold. *Arthroplast Today.* 2016;3(2):99-103.)

and meta-analysis have shown no significant difference in the rate of deep or superficial SSI in patients receiving antibiotic-impregnated bone cement compared with plain bone cement during primary TKA.[65,66] Ultimately, there is a lack of randomized clinical trials and retrospective series with long-term follow-up which examine the efficacy of antibiotic cement in primary TKA.

Irrigation with dilute betadine before wound closure may be an effective means of decreasing SSI rates. Brown et al compared 1862 consecutive THA or TKA cases where dilute betadine lavage was not used in 688 consecutive cases where the protocol was employed. The authors noted only one infection in the group treated with a 3-minute rinse with 0.35% betadine lavage compared to 18 infections in the pretreatment group (P = .14).[67] However, concerns remain regarding the safe use of this irrigant, and dilute chlorhexidine gluconate irrigation may offer similar benefits.[68]

When closing the arthrotomy, there has been no difference in infection associated with barbed suture or interrupted conventional sutures.[69] However, Fowler demonstrated that barbed sutures had significantly less bacterial adherence than conventional braided sutures (48,000 vs. 299,000 CFU/cm^2; P = .04).[70] With regard to superficial wound closure, staples have been demonstrated to provide the fastest closure[71] and subcuticular suture closures have resulted in the greatest perfusion of the wound edges.[72] However, no sutures, staples, or adhesives have demonstrated superiority with regard to infection.[69,73]

Prolonged operative time may have an association with a higher rate of PJI. George et al[74] evaluated the National Surgical Quality Improvement Program database and found that longer operative times were associated with higher risks reoperation (P < .001), SSI (P < .001), and wound dehiscence (P < .001) among other adverse outcomes. Willis-Owen et al[75] found that a longer tourniquet time was associated with a higher incidence of infection. Naranje et al reviewed 9973 primary TKAs collected between 2000 and 2012. After controlling for confounding variables related to age and sex, there was no significant effect of operative time on risk for septic revision.[76] As with many of the aforementioned risk factors previously listed, surgical time is a variable with a complex interaction between others. Ultimately, steps should be taken to decrease intraoperative delays in order to limit prolonged exposure to microorganisms.

Postoperative Prevention

Several different dressing materials are available for TKA incisions; however, it remains unclear whether one material is superior in the prevention of PJI. Sharma et al[77] performed a meta-analysis for wound care following hip and knee arthroplasty, evaluating 12 randomized controlled trials, and found that wounds managed with film dressings (OR, 0.35; 95% CI, 0.21 to 0.57) or with hydrofiber dressings (OR, 0.28; 95% CI, 0.20 to 0.40) were significantly less likely to have wound complications than those managed with passive dressings. No dressing significantly reduced SSI or PJI rates compared with any other dressing.

In the era of short hospitalizations following TKA, routine indwelling urinary catheter use has decreased in frequency. Such management has decreased nosocomial infection, as postoperative catheterization longer than 2 days has been associated with an increased likelihood of in-hospital urinary tract infection (HR, 1.21; 95% CI, 1.04 to 1.41).[78] Miller et al demonstrated that spinal anesthetic is not an indication for indwelling urinary catheterization.[79] The authors randomized 200 patients undergoing THA with spinal anesthetic to treatment with or without insertion of an indwelling catheter and found no difference in urinary retention, the prevalence of urinary tract infection, or the length of stay.[79]

Allogeneic blood transfusions have also been associated with increased risk for SSI. Kim et al performed a meta-analysis of six studies including data on 21,770 patients and found that allogeneic blood exposure increased SSI rates from 1.74% to 2.88% (OR = 1.71, 95% CI, 1.23 to 2.40, P = .002).[80] Some authors have advocated for preoperative autologous blood donation as autologous recipients do not seem to have the same allogeneic susceptibility to SSI[81,82]; however, with the utility of appropriate transfusion triggers and antifibrinolytics, blood transfusion has been dramatically decreasing in frequency and preoperative autologous donation appears unnecessary with modern blood conservation strategies.[83] Use of a tourniquet has not been shown to reduce the transfusion rate.[84]

Poor postoperative glycemic control is associated with infection in both the diabetic and nondiabetic population. Acute hyperglycemia affects cellular recruitment and action, thereby decreasing innate immunity potential to prevent infection.[85] Jämsen et al examined a series of 1565 primary total knee replacements for osteoarthritis and was the first to demonstrate a link between elevated glucose levels identified preoperatively and PJI. This remained significant even after adjustment for BMI.[86] Mraovic et al also demonstrated that patients with PJI had significantly higher perioperative blood glucose values, including nonfasting preoperative and postoperative day 1 blood glucose levels. The authors reported postoperative morning hyperglycemia greater than 200 mg per deciliter (mg/dL) increased the risk of PJI twofold.[87] Kheir et al investigated perioperative blood glucose control and performed a retrospective review of nearly 25,000 arthroplasty cases. The authors found that the rate of PJI was associated with high blood glucose levels on the morning of the first postoperative day. They demonstrated a linear association with glucose levels

≥115 mg/dL.[88] The study highlighted the importance of perioperative blood glucose control and noted that the optimal blood glucose threshold to reduce the likelihood of PJI was 137 mg/dL.[88]

The extended use of oral antibiotics of prophylaxis for arthroplasty patients beyond the typical 24 hours is a subject of controversy. Inabathula performed a retrospective cohort study where patients at high risk of PJI were prescribed an extended oral antibiotic prophylaxis for 7 days after discharge. High-risk patients without extended antibiotics were 4.9 (P = .009) times more likely to develop infection compared to those high-risk patients discharged on extended oral antibiotic prophylaxis.[89] Further studies are necessary before the routine use of extended oral antibiotic prophylaxis can be recommended.

Attempts to limit wound drainage after surgery may reduce the risk of infection. Patel et al investigated factors associated with prolonged wound drainage following THA and TKA in the perioperative period.[90] The authors found that morbid obesity, increased drain output, and patients who received low-molecular-weight heparin for prophylaxis against deep venous thrombosis had a longer time until the postoperative wound was dry than did those treated with aspirin or Coumadin.[90] While no definitive evidence exists to show that certain medications used for VTE prophylaxis result in increased rates of PJI, an association between TKA infection and anticoagulant use with higher bleeding risk has been reported.[91]

During extended postoperative follow-up, the use of prophylactic antibiotics for the patient undergoing a dental procedure has been a subject of controversy. There is concern that normal dental flora can lead to transient bacteremia after routine cleanings or more invasive procedures. Though the 2009 AAOS Information Statement advocated for the consideration of antibiotic prophylaxis in arthroplasty patients who are undergoing dental procedures, the 2013 AAOS-ADA clinical practice guideline advises against the long-standing practice of prescribing prophylactic oral antibiotics.[92] No concrete link between the bacteremia associated with dental work and PJI has been established.

ECONOMIC IMPLICATIONS

The appropriate treatment of PJI is an expensive endeavor. Patients admitted for the treatment of PJI have been shown to have increased costs associated with pharmaceuticals, operating room services, laboratory costs, diagnostic and radiographic evaluations, blood products, anesthesia services, and physical therapy.[93] The mean annual cost for treatment of a PJI at a tertiary care center was recently reported to be $116,383 (range, $44,416 to $269,914).[93] This price tag is noted to be four times the cost of a matched patient undergoing a primary TKA ($28,249; range, $20,454 to $47,957).[93]

The costs associated with the treatment of drug-resistant organisms are dramatically more expensive than caring for those with drug-sensitive strains. Parvizi noted that the cost associated with treatment of a methicillin-resistant infection was $107,264 per case compared to $68,053 for treating PJI caused by sensitive strains (P < .0001).[94]

The economic implications of this problem should be expected to increase as the incidence and prevalence of PJI is on the rise. In an evaluation of the Nationwide Inpatient Sample, Kurtz noted that the relative incidence of PJI increased during their study period from 2001 to 2009.[8] The authors noted that the annual cost of infected revisions to US hospitals increased from $320 million to $566 million during their study period (**Fig. 72-4**). When fully accounting for the increased costs associated with treatment of PJI and the increased frequency of TKA in the aging US population, the cost associated with its treatment was projected to exceed $1.62 billion for the US healthcare system by 2020.[8]

With such expense associated with treatment, several healthcare organizations and companies have been incentivized to participate in infection prevention. Stambough demonstrated the cost-effectiveness of a universal staphylococcus decolonization protocol.[95] Fornwalt[96] instituted a number of quality improvement initiatives and room disinfection strategies which also demonstrated cost-effectiveness. Siegel advocated for the use of single-use instrumentation to decrease surgical infection rates.[97] With such a variety of approaches to infection control, the optimal cost-effective bundle has yet to be discovered.

In the current drive to bundle episodes of care, the financial risk of caring for infections falls to the physician, hospital, or accountable care organization. Healthcare organizations may therefore be disincentivized to care for high-risk patients. Maintaining care for these individuals who are of high risk for PJI is a concern,[98] and the future of TKA in these patients will be of great interest. The economic burden associated with treatment of PJI may continue to drive efforts at medical optimization of high-risk patients and standardize infection prevention protocols; however, it may also simply block arthroplasty care to these patients entirely.

CONCLUSION

Infection following TKA is a devastating and costly complication. While relatively uncommon, its increased incidence over time and the steep cost associated with its treatment are of utmost concern to patients, surgeons, and society as a whole. Prevention strategies should be employed in order to optimize patients preoperatively and provide appropriate care throughout their course such that this complication may be diminished.

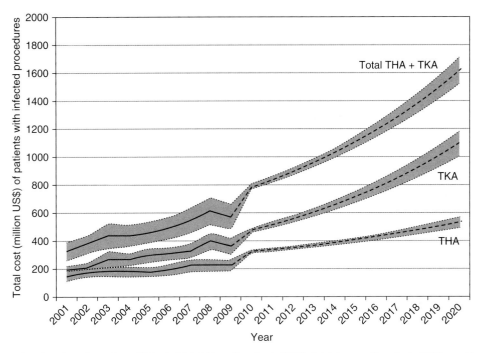

FIGURE 72-4   Historical and projected number of infected total hip arthroplasty (THA), total knee arthroplasty (TKA), and total (THA + TKA) procedures in the United States. The dashed lines represent the projected values per surgery type, and the dotted lines represent the 95% CI of the historical estimates (2001-2009) and the statistical projections (2010-2020). (Reproduced from Kurtz SM, Lau E, Watson H, Schmier JK, Parvizi J. Economic burden of periprosthetic joint infection in the United States. *J Arthroplasty.* 2012;27(8 suppl):61-65.e1.)

REFERENCES

1. Zmistowski B, Karam JA, Durinka JB, Casper DS, Parvizi J. Periprosthetic joint infection increases the risk of one-year mortality. *J Bone Joint Surg Am.* 2013;95(24):2177-2184.

2. Abdel MP, Ledford CK, Tauton MJ, et al. Contemporary failure aetiologies of the primary, posterior-stabilised total knee arthroplasty. *Bone Joint J.* 2017;99-B(5):647-652.

3. Postler A, Lützner C, Beyer F, Tille E, Lützner J. Analysis of total knee arthroplasty revision causes. *BMC Musculoskelet Disord.* 2018;19(1):55-60. doi:10.1186/s12891-018-1977-y.

4. Bozic KJ, Kurtz SM, Lau E, et al. The epidemiology of revision total knee arthroplasty in the United States. *Clin Orthop Relat Res.* 2010;468(1):45-51. doi:10.1007/s11999-009-0945-0.

5. Crowe B, Payne A, Evangelista P, et al. Risk factors for infection following total knee arthroplasty: a series of 3,836 cases from one institution. *J Arthroplasty.* 2015;30:2275-2278.

6. Pulido L, Ghanem E, Joshi A, Purtill JJ, Parvizi J. Periprosthetic joint infection: the incidence, timing, and predisposing factors. *Clin Orthop Relat Res.* 2008;466(7):1710-1715.

7. Kurtz SM, Ong KL, Lau E, Bozic KJ, Berry D, Parvizi J. Prosthetic joint infection risk after TKA in the Medicare population. *Clin Orthop Relat Res.* 2010;468(1):52-56.

8. Kurtz SM, Lau E, Watson H, Schmier JK, Parvizi J. Economic burden of periprosthetic joint infection in the United States. *J Arthroplasty.* 2012;27(8 suppl):61-65.e1.

9. Patel A, Pavlou G, Mújica-Mota RE, et al. The epidemiology of revision total knee and hip arthroplasty in England and Wales: a comparative analysis with projections for the United States. A study using the national joint registry dataset. *Bone Joint J.* 2015;97-B:1076-1081. doi:10.1302/0301-620X.97B8.35170.

10. Huotari K, Peltola M, Jämsen E. The incidence of late prosthetic joint infections: a registry-based study of 112,708 primary hip and knee replacements. *Acta Orthop.* 2015;86(3):321-325. doi:10.31 09/17453674.2015.1035173.

11. Frank RM, Cross MB, Della Valle CJ. Periprosthetic joint infection: modern aspects of prevention, diagnosis, and treatment. *J Knee Surg.* 2015;28(2):105-112. doi:10.1055/s-0034-1396015.

12. Cochran AR, Ong KL, Lau E, Mont MA, Malkani AL. Risk of reinfection after treatment of infected total knee arthroplasty. *J Arthroplasty.* 2016;31(9 suppl):156-161.

13. Kong L, Cao J, Zhang Y, Ding W, Shen Y. Risk factors for periprosthetic joint infection following primary total hip or knee arthroplasty: a meta-analysis. *Int Wound J.* 2017;14(3):529-536.

14. Chen J, Cui Y, Li X, et al. Risk factors for deep infection after total knee arthroplasty: a meta-analysis. *Arch Orthop Trauma Surg.* 2013;133(5):675-687. doi:10.1007/s00402-013-1723-8.

15. Cancienne JM, Kandahari AM, Casp A, et al. Complication rates after total hip and knee arthroplasty in patients with hepatitis C compared with matched control patients. *J Am Acad Orthop Surg.* 2017;25(12):e275-e281.

16. Cancienne JM, Werner BC, Browne JA. Is there an association between Hemoglobin A1C and deep postoperative infection after TKA? *Clin Orthop Relat Res.* 2017;475(6):1642-1649.

17. Anthony CA, Peterson RA, Sewell DK, et al. The seasonal variability of surgical site infections in knee and hip arthroplasty. *J Arthroplasty.* 2018;33(2):510-514.e1. doi:10.1016/j.arth.2017.10.043.

18. Saleh K, Olson M, Resig S, et al. Predictors of wound infection in hip and knee joint replacement: results from a 20 year surveillance program. *J Orthop Res.* 2002;20(3):506-515.

19. Greene KA, Wilde AH, Stulberg BN. Preoperative nutritional status of total joint patients: relationship to postoperative wound complications. *J Arthroplasty.* 1991;6(4):321-325.

20. Jaberi FM, Parvizi J, Haytmanek CT, Joshi A, Purtill J. Procrastination of wound drainage and malnutrition affect the outcome of joint arthroplasty. *Clin Orthop Relat Res.* 2008;466(6):1368-1371.

21. Yi PH, Frank RM, Vann E, Sonn KA, Moric M, Della Valle CJ. Is potential malnutrition associated with septic failure and acute infection after revision total joint arthroplasty? *Clin Orthop Relat Res*. 2015;473(1):175-182.

22. Marchant MH Jr, Viens NA, Cook C, Vail TP, Bolognesi MP. The impact of glycemic control and diabetes mellitus on perioperative outcomes after total joint arthroplasty. *J Bone Joint Surg Am*. 2009;91(7):1621-1629.

23. Adams AL, Paxton EW, Wang JQ, et al. Surgical outcomes of total knee replacement according to diabetes status and glycemic control, 2001 to 2009. *J Bone Joint Surg Am*. 2013;95(6):481-487.

24. Jämsen E, Nevalainen P, Eskelinen A, Huotari K, Kalliovalkama J, Moilanen T. Obesity, diabetes, and preoperative hyperglycemia as predictors of periprosthetic joint infection: a single center analysis of 7181 primary hip and knee replacements for osteoarthritis. *J Bone Joint Surg Am*. 2012;94(14):e101.

25. Núñez M, Lozano L, Núñez E, Sastre S, Luis Del Val J, Suso S. Good quality of life in severely obese total knee replacement patients: a case-control study. *Obes Surg*. 2011;21(8):1203-1208.

26. Wagner ER, Kamath AF, Fruth K, Harmsen WS, Berry DJ. Effect of body mass index on reoperation and complications after total knee arthroplasty. *J Bone Joint Surg Am*. 2016;98(24):2052-2060.

27. Smith TO, Aboelmagd T, Hing CB, MacGregor A. Does bariatric surgery prior to total hip or knee arthroplasty reduce postoperative complications and improve clinical outcomes for obese patients? Systematic review and meta-analysis. *Bone Joint J*. 2016;98-B(9):1160-1166. doi:10.1302/0301-620X.98B9.38024.

28. Gold HT, Slover JD, Joo L, Bosco J, Iorio R, Oh C. Association of depression with 90-day hospital readmission after total joint arthroplasty. *J Arthroplasty*. 2016;31:2385-2388.

29. Browne JA, Sandberg BF, D'Apuzzo MR, Novicoff WM. Depression is associated with early postoperative outcomes following total joint arthroplasty: a nationwide database study. *J Arthroplasty*. 2014;29(3):481-483.

30. Porter SE, Hanley EN Jr. The musculoskeletal effects of smoking. *J Am Acad Orthop Surg*. 2001;9:9-17.

31. Singh JA, Schleck C, Harmsen WS, Jacob AK, Warner DO, Lewallen DG. Current tobacco use is associated with higher rates of implant revision and deep infection after total hip or knee arthroplasty: a prospective cohort study. *BMC Med*. 2015;13:283. doi:10.1186/s12916-015-0523-0.

32. Sahota S, Lovecchio F, Harold RE, Beal MD, Manning DW. The effect of smoking on thirty-day postoperative complications after total joint arthroplasty: a propensity score-matched analysis. *J Arthroplasty*. 2018;33(1):30-35.

33. Møsller AM, Villebro N, Pedersen T, Tønnesen H. Effect of preoperative smoking intervention on postoperative complications: a randomised clinical trial. *Lancet*. 2002;359(9301):114-117.

34. Bedard NA, DeMik DE, Owens JM, Glass NA, DeBerg J, Callaghan JJ. Tobacco use and risk of wound complications and periprosthetic joint infection: a systematic review and meta-analysis of primary total joint arthroplasty procedures. *J Arthroplasty*. 2018;34(2):385-396.e4.

35. Bell KL, Shohat N, Goswami K, Tan TL, Kalbian I, Parvizi J. Preoperative opioids increase the risk of periprosthetic joint infection after total joint arthroplasty. *J Arthroplasty*. 2018;33(10):3246-3251.e1.

36. Cancienne JM, Patel KJ, Browne JA, Werner BC. Narcotic use and total knee arthroplasty. *J Arthroplast*. 2018;33(1):113-118. doi:10.1016/j.arth.2017.08.006.

37. Papavasiliou AV, Isaac DL, Marimuthu R, Skyrme A, Armitage A. Infection in knee replacements after previous injection of intra-articular steroid. *J Bone Joint Surg Br*. 2006;88(3):321-323.

38. Cancienne JM, Werner BC, Luetkemeyer LM, Browne JA. Does timing of previous intra-articular steroid injection affect the post-operative rate of infection in total knee arthroplasty?. *J Arthroplasty*. 2015;30(11):1879-1882.

39. Werner BC, Burrus MT, Novicoff WM, Browne JA. Total knee arthroplasty within six months after knee arthroscopy is associated with increased postoperative complications. *J Arthroplasty*. 2015;30(8):1313-1316.

40. Werner BC, Kurkis GM, Gwathmey FW, Browne JA. Bariatric surgery prior to total knee arthroplasty is associated with fewer postoperative complications. *J Arthroplasty*. 2015;30(9 suppl):81-85.

41. Rao N, Cannella B, Crossett LS, Yates AJ Jr, McGough R III. A preoperative decolonization protocol for staphylococcus aureus prevents orthopaedic infections. *Clin Orthop Relat Res*. 2008;466(6):1343-1348.

42. Kim DH, Spencer M, Davidson SM, et al. Institutional pre-screening for detection and eradication of methicillin-resistant *Staphylococcus aureus* in patients undergoing elective orthopaedic surgery. *J Bone Joint Surg Am*. 2010;92(9):1820-1826.

43. Wang Z, Zheng J, Zhao Y, et al. Preoperative bathing with chlorhexidine reduces the incidence of surgical site infections after total knee arthroplasty: a meta-analysis. *Medicine (Baltimore)*. 2017;96(47):e8321.

44. Banerjee S, Kapadia BH, Mont MA. Preoperative skin disinfection methodologies for reducing prosthetic joint infections. *J Knee Surg*. 2014;27(4):283-288. doi:10.1055/s-0034-1371771.

45. Chang CC, Lin HC, Lin HW, et al. Anesthetic management and surgical site infections in total hip or knee replacement: a population-based study. *Anesthesiology*. 2010;113:279-284.

46. Zorrilla-Vaca A, Grant MC, Mathur V, Li J, Wu CL. The impact of neuraxial versus general anesthesia on the incidence of postoperative surgical site infections following knee or hip arthroplasty: a meta-analysis. *Reg Anesth Pain Med*. 2016;41(5):555-563.

47. Kopp SL, Berbari EF, Osmon DR, et al. The impact of anesthetic management on surgical site infections in patients undergoing total knee or total hip arthroplasty. *Anesth Analg*. 2015;121(5):1215-1221.

48. AlBuhairan B, Hind D, Hutchinson A. Antibiotic prophylaxis for wound infections in total joint arthroplasty: a systematic review. *J Bone Joint Surg Br*. 2008;90(7):915-919.

49. Bratzler DW, Houck PM, Surgical Infection Prevention Guidelines Writers Workgroup, et al. Antimicrobial prophylaxis for surgery: an advisory statement from the National Surgical Infection Prevention Project. *Clin Infect Dis*. 2004;38(12):1706-1715.

50. Rosenberg AD, Wambold D, Kraemer L, et al. Ensuring appropriate timing of antimicrobial prophylaxis. *J Bone Joint Surg Am*. 2008;90(2):226-232.

51. Berríos-Torres SI, Umscheid CA, Bratzler DW, et al. Centers for disease control and prevention guideline for the prevention of surgical site infection, 2017. *JAMA Surg*. 2017;152(8):784-791.

52. Darouiche RO, Wall MJ Jr, Itani KM, et al. Chlorhexidine-alcohol versus povidone iodine for surgical-site antisepsis. *N Engl J Med*. 2010;362(1):18-26.

53. Jacobson C, Osmon DR, Hanssen A, et al. Prevention of wound contamination using DuraPrep solution plus Ioban 2 drapes. *Clin Orthop Relat Res*. 2005;439:32-37.

54. Grove GL, Eyberg CI. Comparison of two preoperative skin antiseptic preparations and resultant surgical incise drape adhesion to skin in healthy volunteers. *J Bone Joint Surg Am*. 2012;94(13):1187-1192.

55. Webster J, Alghamdi AA. Use of plastic adhesive drapes during surgery for preventing surgical site infection. *Cochrane Database Syst Rev*. 2007;(4):CD006353.

56. Knoll PA, Browne JA. Prepping the knee in maximal flexion: getting into every nook, cranny, and fold. *Arthroplast Today*. 2016;3(2):99-103.

57. Morrison TN, Chen AF, Taneja M, Küçükdurmaz F, Rothman RH, Parvizi J. Single vs repeat surgical skin preparations for reducing surgical site infection after total joint arthroplasty: a prospective, randomized, double-blinded study. *J Arthroplasty*. 2016;31(6):1289-1294.

58. Salassa TE, Swiontkowski MF. Surgical attire and the operating room: role in infection prevention. *J Bone Joint Surg Am.* 2014;96(17):1485-1492.

59. Al-Maiyah M, Bajwa A, Mackenney P, et al. Glove perforation and contamination in primary total hip arthroplasty. *J Bone Joint Surg Br.* 2005;87(4):556-559.

60. Der Tavitian J, Ong SM, Taub NA, Taylor GJ. Body-exhaust suit versus occlusive clothing: a randomised, prospective trial using air and wound bacterial counts. *J Bone Joint Surg Br.* 2003;85(4):490-494.

61. Young SW, Zhu M, Shirley OC, Wu Q, Spangehl MJ. Do 'surgical helmet systems' or 'body exhaust suits' affect contamination and deep infection rates in arthroplasty? A systematic review. *J Arthroplasty.* 2016;31(1):225-233. doi:10.1016/j.arth.2015.07.043.

62. Miner AL, Losina E, Katz JN, Fossel AH, Platt R. Deep infection after total knee replacement: impact of laminar airflow systems and body exhaust suits in the modern operating room. *Infect Control Hosp Epidemiol.* 2007;28(2):222-226.

63. Breier AC, Brandt C, Sohr D, Geffers C, Gastmeier P. Laminar airflow ceiling size: No impact on infection rates following hip and knee prosthesis. *Infect Control Hosp Epidemiol.* 2011;32(11):1097-1102.

64. Wang J, Zhu C, Cheng T, et al. A systematic review and meta-analysis of antibiotic-impregnated bone cement use in primary total hip or knee arthroplasty. *PLoS One.* 2013;8(12):e82745. doi:10.1371/journal.pone.0082745. eCollection 2013.

65. Schiavone Panni A, Corona K, Giulianelli M, Mazzitelli G, Del Regno C, Vasso M. Antibiotic-loaded bone cement reduces risk of infections in primary total knee arthroplasty? A systematic review. *Knee Surg Sports Traumatol Arthrosc.* 2016;24(10):3168-3174.

66. Zhou Y, Li L, Zhou Q, et al. Lack of efficacy of prophylactic application of antibiotic-loaded bone cement for prevention of infection in primary total knee arthroplasty: results of a meta-analysis. *Surg Infect.* 2015;16(2):183-187. doi:10.1089/sur.2014.044.

67. Brown NM, Cipriano CA, Moric M, Sporer SM, Della Valle CJ. Dilute betadine lavage before closure for the prevention of acute postoperative deep periprosthetic joint infection. *J Arthroplasty.* 2012;27(1):27-30.

68. Frisch NB, Kadri OM, Tenbrunsel T, Abdul-Hak A, Qatu M, Davis JJ. Intraoperative chlorhexidine irrigation to prevent infection in total hip and knee arthroplasty. *Arthroplast Today.* 2017;3(4):294-297.

69. Krebs VE, Elmallah RK, Khlopas A, et al. Wound closure techniques for total knee arthroplasty: an evidence-based review of the literature. *J Arthroplasty.* 2018;33(2):633-638.

70. Fowler JR, Perkins TA, Buttaro BA, Truant AL. Bacteria adhere less to barbed monofilament than braided sutures in a contaminated wound model. *Clin Orthop Relat Res.* 2013;471(2):665-671. doi:10.1007/s11999-012-2593-z. Epub 2012 Sep 22.

71. Khan RJ, Fick D, Yao F, et al. A comparison of three methods of wound closure following arthroplasty: a prospective, randomized, controlled trial. *J Bone Joint Surg Br.* 2006;88(2):238-242.

72. Wyles CC, Jacobson SR, Houdek MT, et al. The Chitranjan Ranawat Award: running subcuticular closure enables the most robust perfusion after TKA: a randomized clinical trial. *Clin Orthop Relat Res.* 2016;474(1):47-56.

73. Eggers MD, Fang L, Lionberger DR. A comparison of wound closure techniques for total knee arthroplasty. *J Arthroplasty.* 2011;26(8):1251-1258.e1-4.

74. George J, Mahmood B, Sultan AA, et al. How fast should a total knee arthroplasty be performed? An analysis of 140,199 surgeries. *J Arthroplasty.* 2018;33(8):2616-2622.

75. Willis-Owen CA, Konyves A, Martin DK. Factors affecting the incidence of infection in hip and knee replacement: an analysis of 5277 cases. *J Bone Joint Surg Br.* 2010;92(8):1128-1133.

76. Naranje S, Lendway L, Mehle S, et al. Does operative time affect infection rate in primary total knee arthroplasty? *Clin Orthop Relat Res.* 2015;473:64-69.

77. Sharma G, Lee SW, Atanacio O, Parvizi J, Kim TK. In search of the optimal wound dressing material following total hip and knee arthroplasty: a systematic review and meta-analysis. *Int Orthop.* 2017;41(7):1295-1305. doi:10.1007/s00264-017-3484-4.

78. Wald HL, Ma A, Bratzler DW, Kramer AM. Indwelling urinary catheter use in the postoperative period: analysis of the national surgical infection prevention project data. *Arch Surg.* 2008;143(6):551-557.

79. Miller AG, McKenzie J, Greenky M, et al. Spinal anesthesia: should everyone receive a urinary catheter? A randomized, prospective study of patients undergoing total hip arthroplasty. *J Bone Joint Surg Am.* 2013;95(16):1498-1503.

80. Kim JL, Park JH, Han SB, Cho IY, Jang KM. Allogeneic blood transfusion is a significant risk factor for surgical-site infection following total hip and knee arthroplasty: a meta-analysis. *J Arthroplasty.* 2017;32(1):320-325. doi:10.1016/j.arth.2016.08.026.

81. Friedman R, Homering M, Holberg G, Berkowitz SD. Allogeneic blood transfusions and postoperative infections after total hip or knee arthroplasty. *J Bone Joint Surg Am.* 2014;96(4):272-278.

82. Innerhofer P, Klingler A, Klimmer C, Fries D, Nussbaumer W. Risk for postoperative infection after transfusion of white blood cell-filtered allogeneic or autologous blood components in orthopedic patients undergoing primary arthroplasty. *Transfusion.* 2005;45(1):103-110.

83. Yang ZG, Chen WP, Wu LD. Effectiveness and safety of tranexamic acid in reducing blood loss in total knee arthroplasty: a meta-analysis. *J Bone Joint Surg Am.* 2012;94(13):1153-1159.

84. Zhang W, Li N, Chen S, Tan Y, Al-Aidaros M, Chen L. The effects of a tourniquet used in total knee arthroplasty: a meta-analysis. *J Orthop Surg Res.* 2014;9(1):13. doi:10.1186/1749-799X-9-13.

85. Turina M, Fry DE, Polk HC Jr. Acute hyperglycemia and the innate immune system: clinical, cellular, and molecular aspects. *Crit Care Med.* 2005;33:1624-1633. doi:10.1097/01.CCM.0000170106.61978.D8.

86. Jämsen E, Nevalainen P, Kalliovalkama J, et al. Preoperative hyperglycemia predicts infected total knee replacement. *Eur J Intern Med.* 2010;21(3):196-201.

87. Mraovic B, Suh D, Jacovides C, Parvizi J. Perioperative hyperglycemia and postoperative infection after lower limb arthroplasty. *J Diabetes Sci Technol.* 2011;5:412-418. doi:10.1177/193229681100500231.

88. Kheir MM, Tan TL, Kheir M, Maltenfort MG, Chen AF. Postoperative blood glucose levels predict infection after total joint arthroplasty. *J Bone Joint Surg.* 2018;100(16):1423-1431.

89. Inabathula A, Dilley JE, Ziemba-Davis M, et al. Extended oral antibiotic prophylaxis in high-risk patients substantially reduces primary total hip and knee arthroplasty 90-day infection rate. *J Bone Joint Surg Am.* 2018;100(24):2103-2109.

90. Patel VP, Walsh M, Sehgal B, Preston C, DeWal H, Di Cesare PE. Factors associated with prolonged wound drainage after primary total hip and knee arthroplasty. *J Bone Joint Surg Am.* 2007;89(1):33-38.

91. Wang Z, Anderson FA Jr, Ward M, Bhattacharyya T. Surgical site infections and other postoperative complications following prophylactic anticoagulation in total joint arthroplasty. *PLoS One.* 2014;9(4):e91755.

92. Jevsevar DS, Abt E. The new AAOS-ADA clinical practice guideline on prevention of orthopaedic implant infection in patients undergoing dental procedures. *J Am Acad Orthop Surg.* 2013;21(3):195-197.

93. Kapadia BH, McElroy MJ, Issa K, Johnson AJ, Bozic KJ, Mont MA. The economic impact of periprosthetic infections following total knee arthroplasty at a specialized tertiary-care center. *J Arthroplasty.* 2014;29(5):929-932.

94. Parvizi J, Pawasarat IM, Azzam KA, Joshi A, Hansen EN, Bozic KJ. Periprosthetic joint infection: the economic impact of methicillin-resistant infections. *J Arthroplasty.* 2010;25(6 suppl):103-107.

95. Stambough JB, Nam D, Warren DK, et al. Decreased hospital costs and surgical site infection incidence with a universal decolonization protocol in primary total joint arthroplasty. *J Arthroplasty.* 2017;32(3):728-734.e1. doi:10.1016/j.arth.2016.09.041. Epub 2016 Oct 8.

96. Fornwalt L, Ennis D, Stibich M. Influence of a total joint infection control bundle on surgical site infection rates. *Am J Infect Control.* 2016;44(2):239-241. doi:10.1016/j.ajic.2015.09.010.

97. Siegel GW, Patel NN, Milshteyn MA, Buzas D, Lombardo DJ, Morawa LG. Cost analysis and surgical site infection rates in total knee arthroplasty comparing traditional vs. Single-use instrumentation. *J Arthroplasty.* 2015 Dec;30(12):2271-2274.

98. McLawhorn AS, Buller LT. Bundled payments in total joint replacement: keeping our care Affordable and high in quality. *Curr Rev Musculoskelet Med.* 2017;10(3):370-377. doi:10.1007/s12178-017-9423-6.

SECTION 10 / MANAGEMENT OF THE INFECTED TKR

chapter 73

Diagnosing Infection

Karim G. Sabeh, MD | Hany S. Bedair, MD

CASE

A 59-year-old female who underwent bilateral total knee arthroplasty (TKA) 12 years ago for advanced osteoarthritis presents with atraumatic, increasing right knee pain associated with fever, malaise, and nausea for the past 4 days. She reported that she had symptoms consistent with an upper respiratory tract infection 10 days prior, which is now resolved. On physical examination, the incision is clean, dry, and intact with no drainage. The knee is warm to touch with evidence of a large effusion. Knee range of motion is 5° to 98° with pain at terminal flexion (range of motion was 0 to 110 the week before). Plain X-rays demonstrate well-aligned TKA components with subtle radiolucency around the bone-cement-implant interface without large areas of osteolysis. The erythrocyte sedimentation rate (ESR) was 86 mm/h (normal <30 mm/h) and the C-reactive protein (CRP) was 16 mg/L (normal <8 mg/L). Aspiration of the knee joint reveals a synovial WBC count of 369K nucleated cells/μL and 99% PMNs. Gram stain shows gram-positive cocci in clusters. Cultures eventually grew methicillin-susceptible *Staphylococcus aureus*.

DEFINITION

The definition of periprosthetic joint infection (PJI) has been refined in recent decades. The Musculoskeletal Infection Society (MSIS) established a definition of PJI in 2011,[1] which was later modified by the International Consensus Meeting (ICM) in efforts to standardize the criteria for the diagnosis of PJI.[2] Standardization of the infection criteria based on a validated and evidence-based system has provided guidelines to aid the clinicians in accurately diagnosing PJI after TKA. More recently, evidence-based and validated criteria were published in 2018, which were an extension of the original MSIS criteria based on a multicenter, formally validated study.[3] The new criteria (**Table 73-1**) demonstrates a higher sensitivity of 97.7% compared to the MSIS (79.3%) and International Consensus Meeting definition (86.9%), with a similar specificity of 99.5%.

BACKGROUND

PJIs and surgical site infections (SSIs) after TKA are extremely problematic and have been associated with significant morbidity. Given the degree of medical, emotional, and financial impact on the patients, surgeons, and health care systems, substantial efforts have been put forth by the orthopedic community in attempts to limit the risk of infection after elective total joint replacement. Furthermore, the recent implementation of the bundled payment initiatives aiming to improve patient care while reducing costs has put considerable pressure on surgeons and health care systems to minimize complications such as PJIs, which have been shown to have a significant impact in the setting of a value-based system.[4]

The diagnosis of infection after TKA is often challenging and sometimes requires complex decision-making. The ability of the surgeon to make an accurate diagnosis is paramount, given that the treatment algorithms are often vastly different from those of other failure mechanisms. Early steps to diagnosing infection begin with the understanding of risk factors and a focused history with attention to the patient's relevant medical, surgical, and social history followed by a physical examination. An index of suspicion is then established which will help interpret subsequent testing in accordance with Bayesian theory.

When evaluating a painful TKA, it is important for the clinician to have a high index of suspicion for infection based upon the patient's risk factors, history, and examination and to ensure that proper workup is established to rule out or diagnose infection. Diagnosis of infection, especially in the acute postoperative period, can be particularly challenging, given that most tests evaluate systemic inflammatory measures and not infection directly. Acute PJI is defined as an infection that occurs within 90 days of surgery, whereas chronic PJIs occur at 90 days or later after surgery. Laffer et al proposed that 45% of infections present early, 23% delayed, and 32% represent late infections.[5,6] Infections originate from bacterial contamination of the implant either during surgery for acute infections or later through hematogenous transfer or local dissemination.[7] In the early postoperative period, symptoms can be confused with normal healing and inflammatory markers are usually elevated due to the systemic inflammatory response of surgery.[8,9] All patients with a suspected PJI should have a physical examination, appropriate imaging, and inflammatory markers including ESR and CRP. Positive values in the setting of a high clinical suspicion merit an aspiration for further evaluation.

TABLE 73-1   The 2018 Musculoskeletal Infection Society (MSIS) Criteria for Diagnosing Prosthetic Joint Infection (PJI)

Major criteria (At least one of the following = Infected)	Two positive cultures of the same organism Sinus tract with evidence of communication to the joint or visualization of the prosthesis	
Minor criteria ≥6 Infected 2-5 Possibly infected (warrants further intraoperative evaluation) 0-1 Not infected	**Minor criteria (serum or synovial markers)**	**Score**
	Elevated serum CRP *or* D-dimer	2
	Elevated serum ESR	1
	Elevated synovial WBC count or leukocyte esterase	3
	Positive α-defensin	3
	Elevated synovial PMN (%)	2
	Elevated synovial CRP	1
Inconclusive (if minor criteria score 2-5) *or* dry tap	**Intraoperative factors**	**Score**
	Minor criteria score	-
	Positive histology	3
	Positive purulence	3
	Single positive culture	2

CRP, C-reactive protein; ESR, erythrocyte sedimentation rate; PMN, polymorphonuclear; WBC, white blood cell. If minor criteria score is 2-5 refer to intraoperative factors to fulfill the definition for PJI.[3]

RISK FACTORS

A number of factors that can alter the risk of infection after TKA have been identified; some are associated with increased risk while some may be protective. The use of antibiotic prophylaxis in addition to modern surgical and sterilization techniques has helped reduce the incidence of PJI tremendously over the past few decades.[9-11] However, PJIs remain a major problem. Factors that appear to reduce the rate of PJI include shorter duration of surgery, prophylactic antibiotics given within 60 minutes of the surgical incision, skin/nasal decolonization, use of antibiotic-impregnated methylmethacrylate fixation cement, preoperative chlorhexidine wash, and directed laminar airflow in the operating room.[10-14] On the other hand, multiple studies have identified risk factors that are associated with increased risk of PJI. Pulido et al identified higher American Society of Anesthesiologists (ASA) score, morbid obesity, bilateral arthroplasty, allogenic transfusion, postoperative atrial fibrillation, myocardial infarction, urinary tract infection, and longer hospitalization as independent predictors for PJI based on a 9245 patient analysis study.[15] Similarly, Namba et al identified a number of risk factors associated with deep surgical site infection after primary TKA based on an analysis of 56,216 knees.[16] Their study showed that body mass index (BMI) of ≥35 (hazard ratio [HR] = 1.47), diabetes mellitus (HR = 1.28), male sex (HR = 1.89), an American Society of Anesthesiologists (ASA) score of ≥3 (HR = 1.65), and a diagnosis of posttraumatic arthritis (HR = 3.23) all had an increased incidence of

PJI. Furthermore, inflammatory arthritis, sickle cell disease, psoriasis, malnutrition, a compromised immune system, and previous surgery to the limb have all been linked to PJI postoperatively[17-21] (**Table 73-2**).

In addition to the recognition of obesity and diabetes being linked to PJI, nutritional status has become increasingly important in optimizing surgical outcomes and preventing postoperative infections and wound complications. Serum albumin, prealbumin, and transferrin levels are well-recognized biologic markers of the patient's nutritional status, with serum transferrin levels having been shown to be more sensitive than both lymphocyte counts and albumin levels in predicting postoperative infection rates.[22-25] Patients with low nutritional markers should raise the index of suspicion for infection, and malnourished patients should be nutritionally optimized prior to surgery.[26]

Inflammatory arthritis is also recognized as a well-known risk factor for the development of infection after TKA.[17,27] Rheumatoid arthritis (RA) patients have been shown to be twice at risk of developing infection, regardless of the site, than the non-RA population.[27] Comparing osteoarthritis with RA in more than 2000 total knee arthroplasties, the rate of infection was 2.4 times greater in patients with RA with conventional designs and 2.5 times greater for hinged total knee designs.[28,29] Wilson et al reviewed 4171 total knee arthroplasties performed between 1973 and 1987 and found that 67 (1.6%) developed PJI. The incidence of infection was significantly higher for knees affected by RA (45 [2.2%] of 2076) than those affected by osteoarthritis (16[1%] of 1857).[30] Similarly, patients with psoriatic arthritis

TABLE 73-2 Risk factors and Associated Increased Risk for Prosthetic Joint Infection (PJI)

Risk Factors for PJI	Odds Ratio
Obesity (BMI > 35)	1.37
BMI > 40	6.7
BMI > 50	21.3
Posttraumatic arthritis	3.23
American Society of Anesthesiologists (ASA) score > 3	1.65
Diabetes mellitus	1.28-3.1
Knee injection within 3 months	2.0
Rheumatoid arthritis	1.81
Alcohol abuse	2.95
Tobacco use	2.02
Malnutrition	5-7
Depression	1.5

have an increased infection rate after TKA. Twenty-four arthroplasties performed in 16 patients with established long-standing psoriatic arthritis were reviewed. Four (17%) subsequently developed a deep infection. Two of the infections occurred at 1 and 6 months postoperatively; the other two occurred 3 and 5 years postoperatively.[31] Recent studies are showing better results with the emergence of biologics and new psoriasis treatment modalities.[32] Diagnosis of infection can be more difficult in patients with inflammatory arthritis, given the clinical picture, symptomatology, and presence of elevated inflammatory markers at baseline. However, Della Valle et al found that the utility of all serum and synovial tests for predicting chronic periprosthetic joint infection was similar for patients with noninflammatory and inflammatory arthritis and therefore advocate for using similar ESR, CRP, and synovial fluid white blood cell count with differential cutoff values in patients with inflammatory arthritis for the diagnosis of PJI.[17]

A history of old infection in the knee prior to TKA has demonstrated an increased susceptibility to the development of deep infection after TKA. In a review of 65 total knee arthroplasties with a history of infection, deep infection occurred in five (7.7%) overall. In 20 of these 65 patients who demonstrated prior history of both bone and joint infection, three (15%) developed deep infection. In the other 45 patients who had a prior history of only joint sepsis, two (4%) developed deep infection.[33] Moreover a history of PJI in a different joint, despite being adequately treated, increases the risk of PJI after TKA.[34]

Timing of intra-articular steroid injections in the knee has been linked to postoperative infection. Browne et al showed that there was no significant difference in patients who underwent TKA more than 3 months after injection

based on a national database study.[35] The incidence of infection within 3 months (2.6%, OR 2.0 [1.6-2.5], $P < .0001$) and 6 months (3.41%, OR 1.5 [1.2-1.8], $P < .0001$) after TKA within 3 months of knee injection was significantly higher than the control cohort. Meanwhile there was no significant difference in patients who underwent TKA more than 3 months after injection.[36,37] In contrast, another large database study performed by Bedard et al showed that there is an increased risk of PJI if the knee injection occurred within 7 months (OR 1.38-1.88; $P < .05$), but the risk returns to baseline after 7 months.[38]

Numerous additional endogenous or host risk factors have been identified that may predispose certain patients to postoperative septic complications. These include smoking, alcohol abuse, opiates use disorder, psychiatric illnesses, substance abuse disorder, chronic renal failure, infection at a remote site from TKA, malignancy, oral steroid use, and development of postoperative hematoma, as well as increased operative time >121 minutes.[18,39-45]

Patient risk factors can be classified as modifiable and nonmodifiable risk factors. Many preoperative risk factors for the development of PJI are related to patient comorbidities and are, therefore, modifiable. Many studies to date highlight the need for preoperative optimization of modifiable risk factors to further reduce the risk of complications after surgery.[20,46-48]

HISTORY AND PHYSICAL EXAMINATION

Patients often present with nonspecific symptoms of knee pain following TKA. Though this is a common complaint, particularly in the postoperative period, symptoms concerning for PJI include constitutional symptoms (fevers, chills, malaise), drainage, and/or new or progressive pain and decline in function.

A patient history should include the types of prostheses, date of implantation, past surgeries on the joint or limb, history of wound healing problems following surgery, remote infections, current clinical symptoms, comorbid conditions, prior and current microbiology results from aspirations and surgeries if applicable, and antimicrobial therapy for the PJI including local antimicrobial therapy. While being febrile is traditionally associated with infection, it is important to distinguish fever resulting from infection from a normal postoperative course.[49,50] A recent study of 100 patients undergoing total hip arthroplasty (THA) and 100 patients undergoing TKA showed that the normal postoperative febrile response peaked on the first postoperative day and normalized by the fifth day. In 19% of patients, the maximum body temperature was between 39°C and 39.8°C.[51] Febrile episodes can be a sign of other complications with significant morbidity and mortality, such as atelectasis, hematoma, urinary tract infection, fat emboli, or venous thromboembolism (deep vein thrombosis/pulmonary embolism).[49]

Unremitting pain with or without swelling and fever in the acute (within 90 days) postoperative period is uncommon, and it should suggest the possibility of deep infection. Similarly, new-onset pain with or without swelling and fever, preceded by a quiescent period, is suggestive of late hematogenous infection. In either case, AAOS clinical practice guidelines recommend against initiating antibiotic treatment in patients with suspected periprosthetic joint infection until after an appropriate workup, including cultures from the joint, has been obtained.[52]

Subclinical infections, with no overt physical findings of inflammation, swelling, or drainage, are more diagnostically challenging. Host factors, the infecting organism, or previous administration of antibiotics may contribute to the maintenance of a subclinical infection. Although certain mechanical factors may be excluded by physical examination, pain may be the only consistent finding in the presence of deep joint infection. In a study of 52 patients with infection after total knee replacement, pain was present in 100% of the patients. Seventy-seven percent had swelling of the knee, whereas 27% had active drainage.[53,54]

Prolonged drainage or delayed wound healing may also aid in the diagnosis of infection as they are recognized as a risk factor for the development of deep periprosthetic infection.[55] In the acute postoperative period, a small amount of drainage is not uncommon. However, prolonged wound drainage can effectively serve as a conduit through which bacteria can enter the wound. Drainage occurs in approximately 25% of knee arthroplasty cases and may be further classified culture-negative or culture-positive.[54] Cultures taken from wound drainage are generally unreliable, and it is not recommended to base antibiotic treatment solely on this result.

Tetreault et al investigated 55 patients with draining wounds after total joint arthroplasty with wound swabs and found that only 47% of the wound swabs correlated with deep cultures.[56] The superficial cultures were typically polymicrobial and would have resulted in an antibiotic regimen change in 41.8% of cases. More importantly, superficial cultures yielded microbial growth in 80% of cases deemed negative for deep infection. The authors thus recommended against wound or sinus swabs for diagnosis due to possible overtreatment.[56,57] However, the onset of newly observable drainage in a healed wound after TKA can be diagnostic of infection and joint aspiration should follow.

IMAGING MODALITIES

PLAIN RADIOGRAPHY

New radiographs should be obtained and when possible compared to previous radiographs when evaluating a patient with a painful TKA. In the acute phase of PJI, X-rays are unlikely to reveal any signs suggestive of infection. Chronic infections, however, may include signs indicative of implant loosening, osteolysis of subchondral bone, progressive radiolucency, focal osteopenia, and periosteal reaction. Progressive prosthetic loosening is the most consistent radiographic finding associated with deep periprosthetic infection[58], although it is important to note that not all progressive periprosthetic loosening is caused by an infection (**Fig. 73-1**).

RADIOACTIVE ISOTOPE SCANNING (SCINTIGRAPHY)—BONE SCAN

Nuclear medicine tests may be helpful in the diagnosis of infection in TKA. Triple-phase technetium-99 bone scan (TPBS) is a widely available test which is very sensitive to detecting bone remodeling changes around TKA components making it a potentially useful test.[59] However, it has low specificity such that it may not distinguish between aseptic loosening and infection. It is also important to recognize that an increased uptake of radiopharmaceuticals may be seen in normal prostheses for up to 1 year after surgery, reflecting induced marginal osteoblastic activity.[60] Indium-111-labeled white cell scans have a much higher sensitivity in infection, which has been found to be 77%, with specificity of 86%, a positive predictive value of 54%, and a negative predictive value of 95%.[63] However, this test is expensive and time consuming, and its utility in the acute postoperative period is unknown.[61] Combining an indium[111] WBC scan with a technetium-99m bone scan improves the accuracy for detecting deep infection up to 95%[62] (**Fig. 73-2**).

Fluorodeoxyglucose positron emission tomography (FDG-PET) scans have been recently evaluated for diagnosis of PJI in TKA. FDG-PET detects increased intracellular accumulation of deoxyglucose secondary to increased expression of glucose transporters by inflammatory cells. One study found 91% sensitivity and 72% specificity for diagnosis of TKA infections.[63] However, PET scans are not widely available, are expensive, and can still produce false positives secondary to uptake of FDG in aseptic inflammation around implants.[64] Reinartz et al reported that the accuracy of the TPBS, WBC imaging, and FDG-PET scan in diagnosing infection around TKA was 81%, 84%, and 83%, respectively.[65]

To improve on the limitations regarding specificity, sequential imaging with complementary techniques has been advocated to provide the most accurate and reliable information to assist in the diagnosis of infection. Wukich et al reported an 85% sensitivity and specificity using sequential technetium-99m and indium-111 in a retrospective examination of 24 patients with osteomyelitis or infection around a total joint prosthesis.[63] Johnson et al reported a sensitivity of 88% and a specificity of 95% using sequential technetium-99m and indium-111 leukocyte imaging.[66] The study included 28 patients, 9 of whom had a surgically confirmed infection. Palestro et al reported a sensitivity of 67% and a specificity of 78% in 41 patients, with 9 surgically confirmed infections using

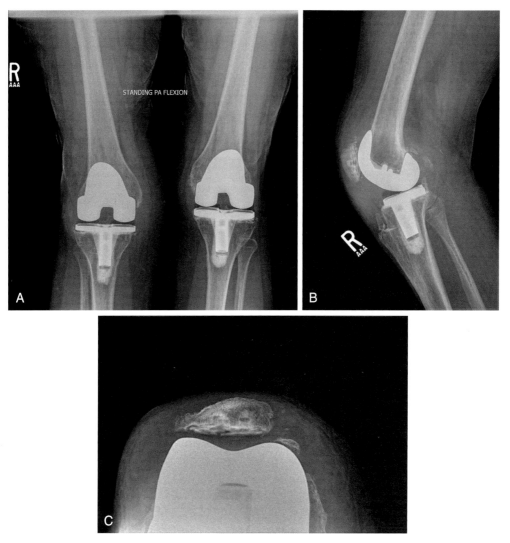

FIGURE 73-1 AP **(A)**, lateral **(B)**, and sunrise **(C)** views of the right knee after total knee arthroplasty (TKA). Imaging showed well-aligned TKA components. There are subtle areas of radiolucency in the cement–bone interface mainly appreciated on the lateral view under the femoral component without periosteal reaction or osteolysis. There is a large effusion.

sequential technetium-99m and indium-111 scans.[67] In a large study of 166 cases with 22 infected hip and knee arthroplasties, sequential use of technetium-99m and indium-111 leukocyte imaging was 64% sensitive and 78% specific.[68] New techniques such as indium-111-labeled immunoglobulin G and technetium-99m monoclonal antibody continue to be developed in an effort to improve on the diagnostic accuracy of infection.

Despite encouraging findings with advanced imaging testing, they have not proven to be superior to standard radiographs combined with the laboratory testing protocol outlined below.

LABORATORY STUDIES

SEROLOGICAL TESTS

Serology can assist the surgeon in accurately diagnosing PJIs. Traditionally used hematologic tests in the workup of infection include white blood cell (WBC) count, ESR,

and CRP. These tests are acute-phase reactants and are therefore naturally elevated postoperatively. However, inflammatory markers have a well-characterized curve in the postoperative period.[69]

The white blood cell count is rarely elevated and has been shown to have little or no value in predicting deep prosthetic infection.[70,71] Grogan et al identified 14 deep knee infections over a 10-year period.[70] Although the peripheral leukocyte count ranged from 5100 to 41,600 per mL at the time of diagnosis of the sepsis, the WBC count was higher than 10,000 per mL in only four patients. Hanssen et al reviewed 86 patients with 89 infected total knee arthroplasties. The leukocyte count averaged 8440 (range of 3800 to 19,200) and was elevated greater than 9500 in only 17 patients.[72]

Beligen et al described the normal distribution of CRP and ESR in total hip and knee patients.[69] CRP was found to be highest on day 2 postoperatively, with a rapid decrease over the first 3 weeks, and a return to baseline

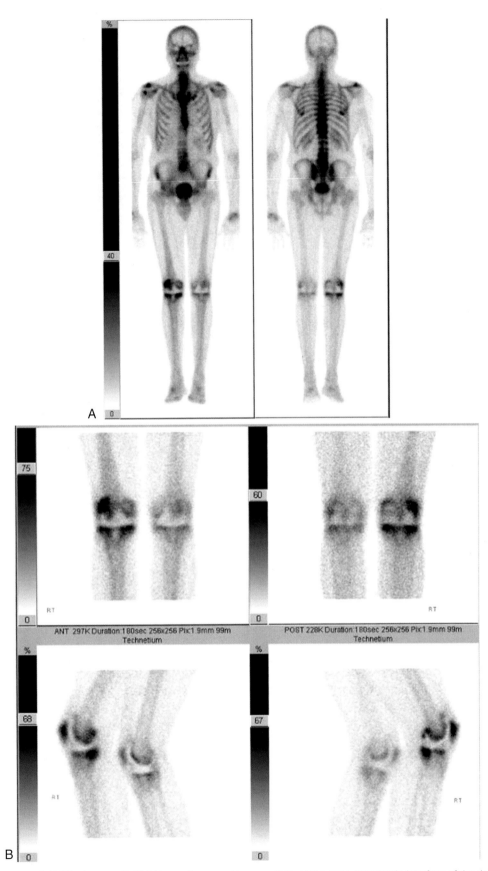

FIGURE 73-2   Bone scan. **A:** Full body scan. **B:** Right knee. Increased tracer activity at the bone/prosthesis interface of the right knee consistent with expected inflammation.

by 3 months. Meanwhile, average ESR levels were the highest on day 5 after surgery and show a rapid decline over the first month but can remain elevated for up to 1 year after surgery. CRP levels are therefore more helpful in diagnosing acute PJIs, and any reversal of downtrend in inflammatory markers should raise concern for an infection.[73,74]

Inflammatory markers values can be difficult to interpret in the acute postoperative period. Several studies have attempted to quantify a cutoff value to accurately diagnose PJI in the acute postoperative period. Bedair et al[75] evaluated 11,964 primary TKAs and identified 146 knee aspirations within 6 weeks of surgery. Deep PJI was diagnosed in 19 out of the 146 based on frank purulence and positive cultures. The mean CRP values were significantly elevated in the infected patients compared to the noninfected group, while mean ESR values were not. They identified a cutoff value of 95 mg/L (normal < 10 mg/L) which provides a negative predictive value of 91% and is therefore more helpful in *ruling out* infection. They concluded that serum CRP is an excellent screening test, and that values near or above 93 to 95 mg/L should prompt an aspiration of the knee. For chronic PJIs (90 days after surgery), on the other hand, the MSIS criteria identify an ESR cutoff value of 30 mm/h and a CRP value of 10 mg/L as normal, and therefore any values greater than these should prompt an aspiration in the setting of a suspected deep infection.[1-3,76]

INTERLEUKIN-6 (IL-6)

IL-6 is an inflammatory cytokine produced by stimulated monocytes and macrophages. It induces the production of acute-phase proteins and acts as an activating factor for T-lymphocytes and differentiating factor for B-lymphocytes. Attraction to the value of IL-6 in diagnosing infections was first drawn to clinicians after a meta-analysis published in 2010 comparing the efficacy of IL-6 to ESR and CRP levels.[77] In their meta-analysis, Barberi et al found that IL-6 had a sensitivity of 97% and specificity of 91% in diagnosing PJI, which is higher than ESR and CRP. However, Glehr et al[78] performed a prospective study of 124 patients who underwent revision arthroplasties for PJI based on the MSIS criteria. In their study, IL-6 had a sensitivity of 81% and specificity of 68%. Furthermore, Gollwitzer et al[79] prospectively evaluated 35 patients undergoing revision THA and TKA for PJI and found that serum IL-6 had a sensitivity of 48% and specificity of 95%. Similarly, Randau et al[80] performed a prospective study of 120 patients who underwent revision TKA and THA and reported a sensitivity of IL-6 ranging from 49% to 79% and specificity of 58% to 88%. Therefore, this variability in the results has limited its application as a screening tool to replace serum ESR and CRP.

D-Dimer

Serum D-dimer is a widely available blood test that detects fibrinolysis. Recent studies have demonstrated its effectiveness in detecting fibrinolytic activities that occur during infection and therefore, its benefit in detecting PJI. Shahi prospectively evaluated 245 patients and concluded that the median D-dimer level was significantly higher (*P* < .0001) for the patients with PJI (1110 ng/mL [range, 243-8,487 ng/mL]) than for patients with aseptic loosening (299 ng/mL [range, 106-2571 ng/mL]). In their study, serum D-dimer outperformed serum CRP and ESR, with 89% sensitivity and 93% specificity. They also concluded that serum D-dimer test may be helpful in determining the optimal timing of reimplantation.[81]

JOINT ASPIRATION

Knee arthrocentesis is considered an essential tool in establishing a PJI diagnosis. The synovial fluid white blood cell count, differential, Gram stain, and culture may help the clinician establish a diagnosis. Furthermore, identifying a bacterial culture and antibiotic susceptibility can help focus on the specific antimicrobial treatment.

In the setting of a chronic or delayed infection, the MSIS has determined a synovial fluid WBC cutoff value of 3000 WBC/μL and a differential of higher than 80% polymorphonuclear (PMN) cells are suggestive of infection.[1-3] In the early postoperative period, in contrast, synovial fluid WBC levels are expected to be elevated due to normal postoperative inflammation and hematoma around the knee. The MSIS criteria suggest that acute PJIs (within 90 days) should have a synovial fluid WBC cutoff value of 10,000 cells with 90% PMNs. However, to better determine the value of synovial fluid WBC count and differential within the first 6 weeks of undergoing TKA, Bedair et al[75] reviewed 11,964 primary TKAs of which 146 knees had undergone an arthrocentesis based on clinical symptoms suggestive of infection. They found that synovial fluid WBC count was the best test for establishing the diagnosis of infection in the early postoperative period. This study demonstrated that most noninfected patients had a WBC count of less than 27,800 cells/μL, while most infected patients had a WBC cell count of greater than 10,700 cells/μL. Therefore, using 10,700 cells/μL as the threshold for infection diagnosis yielded a 95% sensitivity and 91% specificity. Meanwhile, a cutoff synovial fluid WBC count of 27,800 cell/μL yielded 84% sensitivity and 99% specificity. A differential PMN percentage of 89% yielded 84% sensitivity and 69% specificity.

If the suspicion of infection remains high and the aspiration is negative or inconclusive, repeat aspiration in 3 to 4 weeks is highly advised before completely ruling out infection.[71] Barrack et al evaluated 69 knees in 67 patients and found an overall sensitivity of 75%, specificity of 96%, and accuracy of 90%.[71] They found the sensitivity of the knee aspiration to improve with multiple knee aspirations specifically if the patient had stopped antibiotics treatment. They concluded that multiple aspirations are prudent for two reasons: (1) Repeat aspirations may yield an organism if cultures from earlier aspirations were negative and (2) subsequent aspirations may be confirmatory if the original aspiration yielded growth of an organism and a contaminant or false-positive result is suspected. In any case, it is important to note that the administration of antibiotics is highly discouraged if PJI is suspected until proper evaluation has been performed.[52]

α-Defensin

α-Defensin is a human antimicrobial peptide that is secreted into the synovial fluid by neutrophils in response to pathogen presence. This peptide causes rapid killing of the pathogen by integrating into the pathogen's cell membrane, thus providing antimicrobial support to the immune system.[82] The α-defensin test is an immunoassay that can measure the concentration of the α-defensin peptide in human synovial fluid. Bonanzinga et al[83] prospectively studied 156 patients (65 knees and 91 hips) who had undergone fluid aspiration and α-defensin assay preoperatively before undergoing revision surgery. Of that cohort, 29 of the 156 were found to meet the International Consensus Group criteria for PJI. They found a 97% sensitivity and 97% specify of the α-defensin immunoassay, with a positive predictive value of 88% and a negative predictive value of 99%. In another study by Parvizi et al[84] evaluating 23 patients with PJI and 23 with aseptic failure, they found that the α-defensin immunoassay demonstrated 100% sensitivity and specificity. A recent systemic review and meta-analysis by Lee et al in 2017 assessing synovial biomarkers for the diagnosis of PJI showed that synovial fluid WBC count, CRP, α-defensin, leukocyte esterase (LE), IL-6, IL-8, and PMN% all demonstrated high sensitivity for diagnosing PJI, with α-defensin being the best synovial marker based on the highest diagnostic odds ratio.[85]

LEUKOCYTE ESTERASE

The utilization of LE in the diagnosis of PJI has also been of interest in recent years. LE is an enzyme that is secreted by neutrophils that have been recruited to the site of infection that has traditionally been used to help diagnose urinary tract infections. LE is a simple, inexpensive test that can be measured easily and quickly using a colorimetric strip (urinalysis dipstick).[86] One drawback to its use, however, is that the presence of blood within the synovial fluid can interfere with color change. Therefore, the clinician must be aware of this finding and ensure that blood contamination is removed from the synovial fluid sample by centrifuging the sample prior to using it.[87,88] A meta-analysis by Wyatt et al showed a sensitivity of 81% with a specificity of 97% using a (++) reading as a threshold for PJI.[89]

Synovial CRP

Recent studies by Parvizi et al suggested a superiority of synovial fluid CRP over serum CRP for the diagnosis of PJI.[84,90] However, a follow-up study by Tetreault et al[91] demonstrated that synovial CRP does not offer any diagnostic advantage over serum CRP in detection of PJI and that further studies are needed to confirm this conclusion. Nonetheless, the most recent 2018 International Consensus Meeting Criteria for PJI included synovial CRP levels as a minor criterion in the detection of PJI (**Table 73-3**).

INTRAOPERATIVE ANALYSIS

Despite multiple attempts at aspiration, even in the absence of antibiotics, cultures may fail to yield an offending organism. False-positive cultures secondary to contamination from skin flora occasionally complicate the diagnosis. For this reason, many surgeons reserve the final diagnosis of infection until after intraoperative histopathologic analysis and tissue culture results.

TABLE 73-3 Lab Values and Corresponding Sensitivity and Specificity for Total Knee Arthroplasty (TKA) Prosthetic Joint Infection (PJI) Diagnosis.[1-3]

Lab Value	Sensitivity	Specificity
ESR > 30 mm/h	42%-94.3%	33%-87%
CRP > 10 mg/L	74%-94%	20%-100%
Combining elevated ESR/CRP	97.6%	93%
Leukocyte esterase (If ++ is used)	81%	97%
Interleukin-6 (IL-6)	48%	95%
D-dimer	89%	93%
α-defensin	97%	97%
The 2018 International Congress meeting PJI Criteria	97.7%	99.5%

The intraoperative use of Gram staining (GS) alone is inadequate for excluding the diagnosis of infection. Della Valle et al[92] reviewed the results of 413 intraoperative Gram stains compared with the results of operative cultures, permanent histology, and the surgeon's intraoperative assessment to determine the ability of Gram stains to identify periprosthetic infection. They found GS correctly identified the presence of infection in only 10 of the 68 cases that met the study criteria for infection (sensitivity of 14.7%). They concluded that Gram stains alone do not have adequate sensitivity to be helpful in identifying periprosthetic infection and should not be performed on a routine basis. GS may aid in cases in which gross purulence is encountered to assist in the selection of initial antibiotic therapy.

Current consensus recommendations suggest that at least three but not more than six intraoperative samples should be sent for culture.[93,94] In order to achieve optimal yield from traditional cultures, these should be incubated for a minimum of 14 days, with a longer duration (up to 21 days) in cases of suspected culture-negative PJI or where indolent and fastidious organisms such as *Propionibacterium acnes* are suspected.[95,96]

Previous studies have demonstrated intraoperative frozen sections to be a reliable and accurate means of differentiating infection from a loose total joint prosthesis.[97-99] Feldman et al performed a retrospective analysis of 33 consecutive total hip and knee revision arthroplasties.[99] To assess the usefulness of intraoperative frozen sections, they compared (1) the results of analyses of frozen sections with those of analyses of permanent histologic section; (2) the results of analyses of frozen sections with those of intraoperative cultures; (3) the results of clinical and radiographic follow-up with the final diagnosis; (4) the surgeon's operative impression regarding infection with the final pathologic result; and (5) the findings on preoperative radiographs, nuclear scans, laboratory studies, and intraoperative GS with the final pathologic result. Frozen sections were considered positive for infection if there were more than five PMN leukocytes per high-power field in at least five distinct fields. Comparing the results of frozen sections (both positive and negative) with those of permanent sections of similar tissue was 100% sensitive, 100% specific, and 100% accurate. In patients with positive intraoperative cultures, all had positive frozen sections. Of the 24 patients who had negative intraoperative cultures, 23 had negative frozen sections (specificity, 96%). Of the nine positive intraoperative cultures, only two were found to have infection on intraoperative GS. The surgeon's operative assessment regarding the presence of infection compared with the final pathologic diagnosis demonstrated a sensitivity of 70%, a specificity of 87%, and an accuracy of 82%.[99] In a follow-up study, Lonner et al performed a prospective study of 175 consecutive revision joint surgeries and found that frozen sections have a sensitivity of 84% and a specificity of 96%

for correctly distinguishing between infection and aseptic loosening when the index five PMN leukocytes per high-power field were used.[100] The positive predictive value of the frozen sections increased significantly from 70% to 89% when the index increased from 5 to 10 PMN leukocytes per high-power field.[100]

MOLECULAR-BASED TESTING

Polymerase chain reaction (PCR) is another method that has recently been used to ascertain evidence of infection. There are messenger DNA strands that can identify particular species of bacteria, allowing for the precise identification of the organism present in the joint. However, the PCR technique is expensive and has an approximately 2-hour turnaround time, which may be prohibitively long for practical use in the operating room setting. Additionally, observations of false-positive results have been reported recently.[101] PCR technology is still developing, and this technique may become an extremely powerful tool in aiding the surgeon in both evaluation of infection and exact identification of the offending organism in the imminent future.

Other molecular-based technologies such a next-generation sequencing (NGS) has demonstrated utility in the setting of diagnosing PJI. NGS refers to a collection of DNA sequencing method that can produce large amounts of data in shorter time and lower costs than PCR.[102] Unlike PCR, NGS can be used in "open" mode which does not rely on a set of preidentified primers. It is therefore capable of providing a complete picture of the microbial profile by characterizing all DNA present within the sample. NGS searches all known microbial databases for a match—including bacteria, viruses, yeast, fungi, and parasites—without the need for additional individual testing. It also has the potential to suggest antimicrobial resistance through identification of known resistance genes.[103] However, these modalities are emerging technologies and are yet to be validated. Further work is needed to establish their benefits and cost-effectiveness while addressing their limitations.

FUTURE TESTS AND BIOMARKERS

The need for improved diagnostic modalities to aid in accurately diagnosing PJI has led to the emergence of new technologies in recent years. Recent studies suggest that these tests may help reach a diagnosis of PJI when conventional tests are negative or equivocal. Biomarkers have been shown to offer potentially promising results in this arena. Parvizi et al identified several biomarkers including human α-defensin, neutrophil elastase 2, bactericidal/permeability-increasing protein, neutrophil gelatinase–associated lipocalin, lactoferrin, and LE that correctly predicted PJI with 100% sensitivity and specificity in 95 patients who met the MSIS criteria for PJI.[91]

Furthermore, in another study, Deirmengian et al[92] identified that the combined measurement of synovial fluid α-defensin and synovial CRP levels correctly diagnosed 99% of PJIs based on 112 patients (37 PJIs). They found that these results were achieved despite the inclusion of patients with systemic inflammatory disease and those receiving treatment with antibiotics. While these new biomarkers and technologies are exciting as they offer new methods to aid the clinician in accurately diagnosing PJI, further studies are needed to validate their effectiveness and utilization in this patient population.[104]

CONCLUSION

Accurately diagnosing PJI and TKA can be a challenging for the clinician and patient. The diagnosis of infection is usually facilitated by obtaining a thorough clinical history, physical examination, and laboratory tests. Imaging modalities can aid in the overall assessment of infection, while joint aspiration is needed to confirm the diagnosis. If the presence of infection is confirmed, the surgeon should rapidly initiate definitive treatment using a variety of available options. Antibiotic suppression alone, surgical débridement with retention of the components plus antibiotic suppression, and one- or two-stage exchange of the total knee replacement should be done depending on the clinical situation. Salvage procedures such as arthrodesis, excision arthroplasty, and amputation should be considered only in the most difficult and extenuating circumstances.

REFERENCES

1. Parvizi J, Zmistowski B, Berbari EF, et al. New definition for periprosthetic joint infection. From the workgroup of the Musculoskeletal Infection Society. *Clin Orthop Relat Res.* 2011;469:2992-2994. doi:10.1007/s11999-011-2102-9.
2. Parvizi J, Gehrke T, Chen AF. Proceedings of the international consensus on periprosthetic joint infection. *Bone Joint J.* 2013;95-B:1450-1452. doi:10.1302/0301-620X.95B11.33135.
3. Parvizi J, Tan TL, Goswami K, et al. The 2018 definition of periprosthetic hip and knee infection: an evidence-based and validated criteria. *J Arthroplast.* 2018;33(5):1309-1314.e2. doi:10.1016/j.arth.2018.02.078.
4. Sabeh KG, Rosas S, Buller LT, Freiberg AA, Emory CL, Roche MW. The impact of medical comorbidities on primary total knee arthroplasty reimbursements. *J Knee Surg.* 2019;32(6):475-482. doi:10.1055/s-0038-1651529. PubMed PMID: 29791928.
5. Laffer RR, Graber P, Ochsner PE, Zimmerli W. Outcome of prosthetic knee-associated infection: evaluation of 40 consecutive episodes at a single centre. *Clin Microbiol Infect.* 2006;12(5):433-439. PubMed PMID: 16643519.
6. Tsukayama DT, Estrada R, Gustilo RB. Infection after total hip arthroplasty. A study of the treatment of one hundred and six infections. *J Bone Joint Surg Am.* 1996;78(4):512-523. PubMed PMID: 8609130.
7. Trampuz A, Widmer AF. Infections associated with orthopedic implants. *Curr Opin Infect Dis.* 2006;19(4):349-356. Review. PubMed PMID: 16804382.
8. Della Valle C, Parvizi J, Bauer TW, et al. Diagnosis of periprosthetic joint infections of the hip and knee. *J Am Acad Orthop Surg.* 2010;18(12):760-770. PubMed PMID: 21119142.
9. Yi PH, Cross MB, Moric M, et al. The 2013 Frank Stinchfield Award: diagnosis of infection in the early postoperative period after total hip arthroplasty. *Clin Orthop Relat Res* 2014;472:424-429.
10. Rao N, Cannella BA, Crossett LS, et al. Preoperative screening/decolonization for Staphylococcus aureus to prevent orthopedic surgical site infection: prospective cohort study with 2-year follow-up. *J Arthroplasty.* 2011;26:1501.
11. Matthews PC, Berendt AR, McNally MA, Byren I. Diagnosis and management of prosthetic joint infection. *BMJ.* 2009;338:b1773.
12. Momohara S, Kawakami K, Iwamoto T, et al. Prosthetic joint infection after total hip or knee arthroplasty in rheumatoid arthritis patients treated with nonbiologic and biologic disease-modifying antirheumatic drugs. *Mod Rheumatol.* 2011;21:469.
13. Berbari EF, Osmon DR, Lahr B, et al. The Mayo prosthetic joint infection risk score: implication for surgical site infection reporting and risk stratification. *Infect Control Hosp Epidemiol.* 2012;33:774.
14. Tande AJ, Palraj BR, Osmon DR, et al. Clinical presentation, risk factors, and outcomes of hematogenous prosthetic joint infection in patients with *Staphylococcus aureus* bacteremia. *Am J Med.* 2016;129:221.e11.
15. Pulido L, Ghanem E, Joshi A, Purtill JJ, Parvizi J. Periprosthetic joint infection: the incidence, timing, and predisposing factors. *Clin Orthop Relat Res.* 2008;466(7):1710-1715. doi:10.1007/s11999-008-0209-4. Epub 2008 Apr 18. PubMed PMID: 18421542; PubMed Central PMCID: PMC2505241.
16. Namba RS, Inacio MC, Paxton EW. Risk factors associated with deep surgical site infections after primary total knee arthroplasty: an analysis of 56,216 knees. *J Bone Joint Surg Am.* 2013;95(9):775-782. doi:10.2106/JBJS.L.00211. PubMed PMID: 23636183.
17. Cipriano CA, Brown NM, Michael AM, Moric M, Sporer SM, Della Valle CJ. Serum and synovial fluid analysis for diagnosing chronic periprosthetic infection in patients with inflammatory arthritis. *J Bone Joint Surg Am.* 2012;94(7):594-600. doi:10.2106/JBJS.J.01318. PubMed PMID: 22488615.
18. Peersman G, Laskin R, Davis J, Peterson M. Infection in total knee replacement: a retrospective review of 6489 total knee replacements. *Clin Orthop Relat Res.* 2001;(392):15-23. PubMed PMID: 11716377.
19. Chun KC, Kim KM, Chun CH. Infection following total knee arthroplasty. *Knee Surg Relat Res.* 2013;25(3):93-99.
20. Ratto N, Arrigoni C, Rosso F, et al. Total knee arthroplasty and infection: how surgeons can reduce the risks. *EFORT Open Rev.* 2016;1(9):339-344. doi:10.1302/2058-5241.1.000032.
21. Chen J, Cui Y, Li X, et al. Risk factors for deep infection after total knee arthroplasty: a meta-analysis. *Arch Orthop Trauma Surg.* 2013;133:675-687.
22. Greene KA, Wilde AH, Stulberg BN. Preoperative nutritional status of total joint patients. Relationship to postoperative wound complications. *J Arthroplasty.* 1991;6:321-325.
23. Dreblow DM, Anderson CF, Moxness K. Nutritional assessment of orthopaedic patients. *Mayo Clin Proc.* 2001;56:51-54.
24. Smith TK. Nutrition: its relationship to orthopaedic infections. *Orthop Clin.* 1991;22:373-377.
25. Jensen JE, Jensen TG, Smith TK, et al. Nutrition in orthopaedic surgery. *J Bone Joint Surg Am.* 1982;64:1263-1272.
26. Roche M, Law TY, Kurowicki J, et al. Albumin, prealbumin, and transferrin may Be predictive of wound complications following total knee arthroplasty. *J Knee Surg.* 2018;31(10):946-951. doi:10.1055/s-0038-1672122. Epub 2018 Oct 3. PubMed PMID: 30282102.
27. Doran MF, Crowson CS, Pond GR, O'Fallon WM, Gabriel SE. Frequency of infection in patients with rheumatoid arthritis compared with controls: a population-based study. *Arthritis Rheum.* 2002;46(9):2287-2293.

28. Poss R, Thornhill TS, Ewald FC, et al. Factors influencing the incidence and outcome of infection following total joint arthroplasty. *Clin Orthop.* 1984;182:117-126.

29. Hsieh PH, Huang KC, Shih HN. Prosthetic joint infection in patients with rheumatoid arthritis: an outcome analysis compared with controls. *PLoS One.* 2013;8(8):e71666. doi:10.1371/journal.pone.0071666. eCollection 2013. PubMed PMID: 23990969; PubMed Central PMCID: PMC3753295.

30. Wilson MG, Kelly K, Thornhill TS. Infection as a complication of total knee-replacement arthroplasty. Risk factors and treatment in 67 cases. *J Bone Joint Surg Am.* 1990;72:878-883.

31. Stern SH, Insall JN, Windsor RE, et al. Total knee arthroplasty in patients with psoriasis. *Clin Orthop.* 1989;248:108-111.

32. Iofin I, Levine B, Badlani N, Klein GR, Jaffe WL. Psoriatic arthritis and arthroplasty: a review of the literature. *Bull NYU Hosp Joint Dis.* 2008;66(1):41-48. Review. PubMed PMID: 18333827.

33. Jerry GJ, Rand JA, Ilstrup D. Old sepsis prior to total knee arthroplasty. *Clin Orthop.* 1988;236:135-140.

34. Bedair H, Goyal N, Dietz MJ, et al. A history of treated periprosthetic joint infection increases the risk of subsequent different site infection. *Clin Orthop Relat Res.* 2015;473(7):2300-2304. doi:10.1007/s11999-015-4174-4. PubMed PMID: 25670654; PubMed Central PMCID: PMC4457745.

35. Cancienne JM, Werner BC, Luetkemeyer LM, Browne JA. Does timing of previous intra-articular steroid injection affect the postoperative rate of infection in total knee arthroplasty? *J Arthroplasty.* 2015;30(11):1879-1882. doi:10.1016/j.arth.2015.05.027. Epub 2015 May 23. PubMed PMID: 26071248.

36. Papavasiliou AV, Isaac DL, Marimuthu R, Skyrme A, Armitage A. Infection in knee replacements after previous injection of intra-articular steroid. *J Bone Joint Surg Br.* 2006;88-B:321-323.

37. Desai A, Ramankutty S, Board T, Raut V. Does intraarticular steroid infiltration increase the rate of infection in subsequent total knee replacements?. *Knee.* 2009;16:262-264.

38. Bedard NA, Pugely AJ, Elkins JM, et al. The John N. Insall Award: do intraarticular injections increase the risk of infection after TKA? *Clin Orthop Relat Res.* 2017;475(1):45-52. doi:10.1007/s11999-016-4757-8. PubMed PMID: 26970991; PubMed Central PMCID: PMC5174022.

39. D'Ambrosia RD, Shoji H, Heater R. Secondarily infected total joint replacements by hematogenous spread. *J Bone Joint Surg Am.* 1976;58:450-453.

40. Hall AJ. Late infections about a total knee prosthesis. *J Bone Joint Surg Br.* 1974;56:144-147.

41. Stinchfield FE, Bigliani LV, Nere HC, et al. Late hematogenous infections of total joint replacements. *J Bone Joint Surg Am.* 1980;62:1345-1350.

42. Thomas BJ, Moreland JR, Amstutz HC. Infection after total joint arthroplasty from distal extremity sepsis. *Clin Orthop.* 1983;181:121-125.

43. Klement MR, Nickel BT, Penrose CT, et al. Psychiatric disorders increase complication rate after primary total knee arthroplasty. *Knee.* 2016;23(5):883-886. doi:10.1016/j.knee.2016.05.007. Epub 2016 Jun 7. PubMed PMID: 27288068.

44. Bell KL, Shohat N, Goswami K, Tan TL, Kalbian I, Parvizi J. Preoperative opioids increase the risk of periprosthetic joint infection after total joint arthroplasty. *J Arthroplasty.* 2018;33(10):3246-3251.e1. doi:10.1016/j.arth.2018.05.027. Epub 2018 May 29. PubMed PMID: 30054211.

45. Anis HK, Sodhi N, Klika AK, et al. Is operative time a predictor for post-operative infection in primary total knee arthroplasty? *J Arthroplasty.* 2019;34(7S):S331-S336. pii: S0883-5403(18)31150-1. doi:10.1016/j.arth.2018.11.022. PubMed PMID: 30545655.

46. DeFroda SF, Rubin LE, Jenkins DR. Modifiable risk factors in total joint arthroplasty: a pilot study. *R I Med J.* 2016;99(5):28-31. PubMed PMID: 27128514.

47. Maoz G, Phillips M, Bosco J, et al. The Otto Aufranc Award: modifiable versus nonmodifiable risk factors for infection after hip arthroplasty. *Clin Orthop Relat Res* 2015;473(2):453-459. doi:10.1007/s11999-014-3780-x. PubMed PMID: 25024028; PubMed Central PMCID: PMC4294894.

48. Jiranek W. Modifiable risk factors in total joint arthroplasty. *J Arthroplasty.* 2016;31(8):1619. doi:10.1016/j.arth.2016.06.017. PubMed PMID: 27449557.

49. Athanassious C, Samad A, Avery A, Cohen J, Chalnick D. Evaluation of fever in the immediate postoperative period in patients who underwent total joint arthroplasty. *J Arthroplasty.* 2011;26(8):1404-1408.

50. Bindelglass DF, Pellegrino J. The role of blood cultures in the acute evaluation of postoperative fever in arthroplasty patients. *J Arthroplast.* 2007;22(5):701-702.

51. Shaw JA, Chung R. Febrile response after knee and hip arthroplasty. *Clin Orthop Relat Res.* 1999;(367):181-189.

52. Parvizi J, Della Valle CJ. AAOS Clinical Practice Guideline: diagnosis and treatment of periprosthetic joint infections of the hip and knee. *J Am Acad Orthop Surg.* 2010;18(12):771-772. PubMed PMID: 21119143.

53. Windsor RE, Insall JN, Urs WK, et al. Two-stage reimplantation for the salvage of total knee arthroplasty complicated by infection. *J Bone Joint Surg Am.* 1990;72:272-278.

54. Hanssen AD, Rand JA. Evaluation and treatment of infection at the site of a total hip or knee arthroplasty. *J Bone Joint Surg Am.* 1998;80:910-922.

55. Weiss AP, Krackow KA. Persistent wound drainage after primary total knee arthroplasty. *J Arthroplasty.* 1993;8:285-289.

56. Tetreault MW, Wetters NG, Aggarwal VK, et al. Should draining wounds and sinuses associated with hip and knee arthroplasties be cultured?. *J Arthroplasty.* 2013;28(8):133-136.

57. Cuñé J, Soriano A, Martínez JC, García S, Mensa J. A superficial swab culture is useful for microbiologic diagnosis in acute prosthetic joint infections. *Clin orthop Relat Res.* 2009;467(2):531-535.

58. Rand JA, Bryan RS, Morrey BF, et al. Management of infected total knee arthroplasty. *Clin Orthop.* 1986;205:75.

59. Love C, Marwin SE, Palestro CJ. Nuclear medicine and the infected joint replacement. *Semin Nucl Med.* 2009;39(1):66-78.

60. Eustace S, Shah B, Mason M. Imaging orthopedic hardware with an emphasis on hip prostheses. *Orthop Clin.* 1998;29:67-84.

61. Scher DM, Pak K, Lonner JH, et al. The predictive value of indium-111 leukocyte scans in the diagnosis of infected total hip, knee, or resection arthroplasties. *J Arthroplasty.* 2000;15:295-300.

62. Tehranzadeh J, Gubernick I, Blaha D. Prospective study of sequential technetium-99m phosphate and gallium imaging in painful hip prostheses (comparison of diagnostic modalities). *Clin Nucl Med.* 1988;13(4):229-236.

63. Wukich DK, Abren SH, Callaghan JJ, et al. Diagnosis of infection by preoperative scintigraphy with indium-labeled white blood cells. *J Bone Joint Surg Am.* 1987;69:1353-1360.

64. Stumpe KD, Notzli HP, Zanetti M, et al. FDG PET for differentiation of infection and aseptic loosening in total hip replacements: comparison with conventional radiography and three-phase bone scintigraphy. *Radiology.* 2004;231(2):333-341.

65. Reinartz P. FDG-PET in patients with painful hip and knee arthroplasty: technical breakthrough or just more of the same. *Q J Nucl Med Mol Imaging.* 2009;53(1):41-50.

66. Johnson JA, Christie MJ, Sandler MP, et al. Detection of occult infection following total joint arthroplasty using sequential technetium-99m HDP bone scintigraphy and indium-111 WBC imaging. *J Nucl Med.* 1988;29:1347-1353.

67. Palestro CJ, Swyer AJ, Kim CK, et al. Infected knee prosthesis: diagnosis with In-111-leukocyte, Tc-99m sulfur colloid, and Tc-99m MDP imaging. *Radiology.* 1991;179:645-648.

68. Teller RE, Christie MJ, Martin W, et al. Sequential indium-labeled leukocyte and bone scans to diagnose prosthetic joint infection. *Clin Orthop.* 2000;373:241-247.

69. Bilgen O, Atici T, Durak K, Karaeminoğullari, Bilgen MS. C-reactive protein values and erythrocyte sedimentation rates after total hip and total knee arthroplasty. *J Int Med Res* 2001;29(1):7-12. PubMed PMID: 11277348.

70. Grogan TJ, Dorey F, Rollins J, et al. Deep sepsis following total knee arthroplasty. *J Bone Joint Surg Am.* 1987;69:489-497.

71. Barrack RL, Jennings RW, Wolfe MW, et al. The value of preoperative aspiration before total knee revision. *Clin Orthop.* 1997;345:8-16.

72. Hanssen AD, Rand JA, Osmon DR. Treatment of the infected total knee arthroplasty with insertion of another prosthesis: the effect of antibiotic-impregnated bone cement. *Clin Orthop.* 1994;309:44-54.

73. White J, Kelly M, Dunsmuir R. C-reactive protein level after total hip and total knee replacement. *J Bone Joint Surg Br.* 1998;80(5):909-911. PubMed PMID: 9768908.

74. Yi PH, Cross MB, Moric M, Sporer SM, Berger RA, Della Valle CJ. The 2013 Frank Stinchfield Award: diagnosis of infection in the early postoperative period after total hip arthroplasty. *Clin Orthop Relat Res.* 2014;472(2):424-429. doi:10.1007/s11999-013-3089-1. PubMed PMID: 23884798; PubMed Central PMCID: PMC3890203.

75. Bedair H, Ting N, Jacovides C, et al. The Mark Coventry Award: diagnosis of early postoperative TKA infection using synovial fluid analysis. *Clin Orthop Relat Res.* 2011;469(1):34-40. doi:10.1007/s11999-010-1433-2. PubMed PMID: 20585914; PubMed Central PMCID: PMC3008895.

76. Diaz-Ledezma C, Lichstein PM, Dolan JG, Parvizi J. Diagnosis of periprosthetic joint infection in Medicare patients: multicriteria decision analysis. *Clin Orthop Relat Res.* 2014;472(11):3275-3284. doi:10.1007/s11999-014-3492-2. PubMed PMID: 24522385; PubMed Central PMCID: PMC4182413.

77. Berbari E, Mabry T, Tsaras G, et al. Inflammatory blood laboratory levels as markers of prosthetic joint infection: a systematic review and meta-analysis. *J Bone Joint Surg Am.* 2010;92-A:2102-2109.

78. Glehr M, Friesenbichler J, Hofmann G, et al. Novel biomarkers to detect infection in revision hip and knee arthroplasties. *Clin Orthop Relat Res.* 2013;471:2621-2628.

79. Gollwitzer H, Dombrowski Y, Prodinger PM, et al. Antimicrobial peptides and proinflammatory cytokines in periprosthetic joint infection. *J Bone Joint Surg Am.* 2013;95-A:644-651.

80. Randau TM, Friedrich MJ, Wimmer MD, et al. Interleukin-6 in serum and in synovial fluid enhances the differentiation between periprosthetic joint infection and aseptic loosening. *PLoS One.* 2014;9:e89045.

81. Shahi A, Kheir MM, Tarabichi M, Hosseinzadeh HRS, Tan TL, Parvizi J. Serum D-dimer test is promising for the diagnosis of periprosthetic joint infection and timing of reimplantation. *J Bone Joint Surg Am.* 2017;99(17):1419-1427. doi:10.2106/JBJS.16.01395. PubMed PMID: 28872523.

82. Ganz T, Selsted ME, Szklarek D, et al. Defensins. Natural peptide antibiotics of human neutrophils. *J Clin Invest.* 1985;76:1427-1435.

83. Bonanzinga T, Zahar A, Dütsch M, Lausmann C, Kendoff D, Gehrke T. How reliable is the alpha-defensin immunoassay test for diagnosing periprosthetic joint infection? A prospective study. *Clin Orthop Relat Res.* 2017;475(2):408-415. doi:10.1007/s11999-016-4906-0. PubMed PMID: 27343056; PubMed Central PMCID: PMC5213924.

84. Deirmengian C, Kardos K, Kilmartin P, et al. The alpha-defensin test for periprosthetic joint infection outperforms the leukocyte esterase test strip. *Clin Orthop Relat Res.* 2015;473(1):198-203. doi:10.1007/s11999-014-3722-7. PubMed PMID: 24942960; PubMed Central PMCID: PMC4390923.

85. Lee YS, Koo KH, Kim HJ, et al. Synovial fluid biomarkers for the diagnosis of periprosthetic joint infection: a systematic review and meta-analysis. *J Bone Joint Surg Am.* 2017;99(24):2077-2084. doi:10.2106/JBJS.17.00123. Review. PubMed PMID: 29257013.

86. Parvizi J, Jacovides C, Antoci V, Ghanem E. Diagnosis of periprosthetic joint infection: the utility of a simple yet unappreciated enzyme. *J Bone Joint Surg Am.* 2011;93:2242-2248. doi:10.2106/JBJS.J.01413.

87. Wetters NG, Berend KR, Lombardi AV, Morris MJ, Tucker TL, Della Valle CJ. Leukocyte esterase reagent strips for the rapid diagnosis of periprosthetic joint infection. *J Arthroplast.* 2012;27:8-11. doi:10.1016/j.arth.2012.03.037.

88. Aggarwal VK, Tischler E, Ghanem E, Parvizi J. Leukocyte esterase from synovial fluid aspirate: a technical note. *J Arthroplasty.* 2013;28:193-195. doi:10.1016/j.arth.2012.06.023.

89. Wyatt MC, Beswick AD, Kunutsor SK, Wilson MJ, Whitehouse MR, Blom AW. The alpha-defensin immunoassay and leukocyte esterase colorimetric strip test for the diagnosis of periprosthetic infection: a systematic review and meta-analysis. *J Bone Joint Surg Am.* 2016;98(12):992-1000. doi:10.2106/JBJS.15.01142. Review. PubMed PMID: 27307359; PubMed Central PMCID: PMC4901182.

90. Parvizi J, Jacovides C, Adeli B, Jung KA, Hozack WJ. Mark B. Coventry Award: synovial C-reactive protein: a prospective evaluation of a molecular marker for periprosthetic knee joint infection. *Clin Orthop Relat Res.* 2012;470(1):54-60. doi:10.1007/s11999-011-1991-y. PubMed PMID: 21786056; PubMed Central PMCID: PMC3237977.

91. Tetreault MW, Wetters NG, Moric M, Gross CE, Della Valle CJ. Is synovial C-reactive protein a useful marker for periprosthetic joint infection?. *Clin Orthop Relat Res.* 2014;472(12):3997-4003. doi:10.1007/s11999-014-3828-y. Epub 2014 Jul 29. PubMed PMID: 25070920; PubMed Central PMCID: PMC4397770.

92. Della Valle CJ, Scher DM, Yong YH, et al. The role of intraoperative Gram stain in revision total joint arthroplasty. *J Arthroplasty.* 1999;14:500-504.

93. Mikkelsen DB, Pedersen C, Højbjerg T, Schønheyder HC. Culture of multiple peroperative biopsies and diagnosis of infected knee arthroplasties. *APMIS Acta Pathol Microbiol Immunol Scand.* 2006;114:449-452. doi:10.1111/j.1600-0463.2006.apm_428.x.

94. Schäfer P, Fink B, Sandow D, Margull A, Berger I, Frommelt L. Prolonged bacterial culture to identify late periprosthetic joint infection: a promising strategy. *Clin Infect Dis.* 2008;47:1403-1409. doi:10.1086/592973.

95. Kamme C, Lindberg L. Aerobic and anaerobic bacteria in deep infections after total hip arthroplasty: differential diagnosis between infectious and non-infectious loosening. *Clin Orthop.* 1981;(154):201-207.

96. Atkins BL, Athanasou N, Deeks JJ, et al. Prospective evaluation of criteria for microbiological diagnosis of prosthetic-joint infection at revision arthroplasty. The OSIRIS Collaborative Study Group. *J Clin Microbiol.* 1998;36:2932-2939.

97. Charosky CB, Bullough PG, Wilson PD Jr. Total hip replacement failures. A histological evaluation. *J Bone Joint Surg Am.* 1973;55:49-58.

98. Mirra JM, Amstutz HC, Matos M, et al. The pathology of the joint tissues and its clinical relevance in prosthesis failure. *Clin Orthop.* 1976;117:221-240.

99. Feldman DS, Lonner JH, Desai P, et al. The role of intraoperative frozen sections in revision total joint arthroplasty. *J Bone Joint Surg Am.* 1995;77:1807-1813.

100. Lonner JH, Desai P, DiCesare PE, et al. The reliability of analysis of intraoperative frozen sections for identifying active infection during revision hip or knee arthroplasty. *J Bone Joint Surg Am.* 1996;78:1553-1558.

101. Mariani BD, Martin DS, Levine MJ, et al. Polymerase chain reaction detection of bacterial infection in total knee arthroplasty. *Clin Orthop*. 1996;331:11-22.

102. Goldberg B, Sichtig H, Geyer C, Ledeboer N, Weinstock GM. Making the leap from research laboratory to clinic: challenges and opportunities for next-generation sequencing in infectious disease diagnostics. *mBio*. 2015;6:e01888-e01815. doi:10.1128/mBio.01888-15.

103. Dunne WM, Westblade LF, Ford B. Next-generation and whole-genome sequencing in the diagnostic clinical microbiology laboratory. *Eur J Clin Microbiol Infect Dis*. 2012;31:1719-1726. doi:10.1007/s10096-012-1641-7.

104. Goswami K, Parvizi J, Maxwell Courtney P. Current recommendations for the diagnosis of acute and chronic PJI for hip and knee—cell counts, alpha-defensin, leukocyte esterase, next-generation sequencing. *Curr Rev Musculoskelet Med*. 2018;11(3):428-438. doi:10.1007/s12178-018-9513-0.

chapter 74

Microbes and Antibiotics

Sandra B. Nelson, MD | Laura K. Certain, MD, PhD

MICROBIOLOGY OF PERIPROSTHETIC KNEE INFECTIONS

Many bacterial species and some nonbacterial pathogens have been implicated as causes of periprosthetic infection (Table 74-1). Most organisms that cause periprosthetic joint infection (PJI) are organisms that reside commensally either on or within the human host but take advantage of breaches of mucosal integrity to gain access to the joint space. As the clinician faces decisions about empiric antibiotic selection and local antibiotic delivery, understanding which organism is likely to be infective is of paramount importance. Notably, few studies report on the specific microbiology of total knee arthroplasty infections; most literature combines data on both hip and knee arthroplasty infections. When available, studies that focus on the microbiology of only periprosthetic knee infections will be prioritized in this chapter.

Taken all together, the majority of organisms causing PJI are Gram-positive, with staphylococcal infections comprising most of these.[1-5] Depending on the study, 5% to 12% of infections are Gram-negative,[1,3,6-8] 3% to 36% are polymicrobial,[1,2,4,6,7] and 7% to 25% are culture-negative.[1,4,7,8] Summary statistics do not always account for differences in the prevalence of certain organisms according to the timing of the PJI (early, delayed, or late hematogenous)[3] or to host risk factors, both of which influence the likelihood of certain organisms causing PJI. Further differences in the proportions of various organisms between studies likely represent important differences in both patient populations along with differences in local microbiology. Studies that included more early postsurgical infections in general reported a higher proportion of polymicrobial and culture-positive infection, with referral centers seeing more monomicrobial and culture-negative infections.

Most PJIs are monomicrobial, but some periprosthetic knee infections are caused by more than one organism. Depending on the series, between 3% and 17% of infections are polymicrobial.[1,2,7] Polymicrobial infections are more commonly associated with early infection[6,9] and in the presence of soft-tissue defects, wound dehiscence, and wound drainage.[9] Staphylococcal organisms remain the most common organisms recovered in polymicrobial infections[2]; in particular, methicillin-resistant *Staphylococcus aureus* (MRSA)[6,9] and anaerobic organisms[9] may be more frequently represented in polymicrobial infections.

Early Periprosthetic Infections

Early periprosthetic infections (generally defined as those occurring within the first 3 months after surgery) are due to organisms that are inoculated during surgery or in the postoperative window prior to skin and soft tissue healing. Prolonged drainage, hematoma, and seroma may contribute to this risk by impairing skin closure and facilitating the introduction of organisms from the cutaneous microbiome. Although the likelihood of such infection is reduced by surgical antibiotic prophylaxis and by optimal cutaneous antisepsis, some organisms survive and are not effectively cleared by surgical antisepsis.[10] Further, organisms may be inoculated in the perioperative window after surgical antimicrobial prophylaxis has completed. Most early periprosthetic infections are caused by virulent organisms, as these organisms replicate more rapidly and induce a more robust inflammatory response, leading to their manifesting earlier. For example, *S. aureus* comprises over 50% of early periprosthetic knee infections[3]; other organisms include streptococci, Gram-negative bacilli, and enterococci. Notably, the cutaneous microbiome varies between different regions of the body.[11] As early postoperative infections are primarily due to organisms that reside at the surgical site, the microbiology of early infections differs between hip and knee arthroplasty infections. Infections due to organisms that comprise enteric flora are more common on perineal skin than about the knee; these organisms (including Gram-negative bacilli and enterococci) are therefore seen less commonly in the knee than the hip in early infection.[1] Notably, the type of antibiotic prophylaxis may influence the types of organisms seen in early PJIs. In one series, patients who received vancomycin for surgical antimicrobial prophylaxis were more likely to suffer infection due to Gram-negative organisms than those who received cefazolin; however, they were less likely to develop infection due to MRSA.[12]

Delayed Periprosthetic Infections

Delayed periprosthetic infections may also be caused by organisms introduced in the perioperative window but present in a more subacute to chronic fashion. These infections are caused by organisms that grow more slowly and are of lower virulence and are therefore less likely to be identified in the early perioperative window. Patients

TABLE 74-1   Organisms Causing Periprosthetic Knee Infections[a]

Organisms	Prevalence in Periprosthetic Joint Infection[b]
Gram-positive organisms	60%-72%
Staphylococci	44%-51%
Staphylococcus aureus	12%-35%
Coagulase-negative staphylococci	16%-37%
Streptococci	9%-13%
Enterococci	4%-9%
Gram-negative organisms	5%-12%
Enteric Gram-negatives (e.g., *Escherichia coli*)	7%-10%
Pseudomonas species	1%-3%
Anaerobes	1%-5%
Cutibacterium acnes	3%
Candida species	0%-1%
Polymicrobial infections	3%-7%
Culture-negative infections	16%-25%

[a]Only publications reporting microbiology specific to knee arthroplasty infections were included.[1,3,7,8]

[b]As polymicrobial infections were included, the total percentages add up to more than 100%.

with infections caused by these organisms often achieve an early clinical response after arthroplasty, before presenting with increasing pain 3 to 6 months after surgery. While virulent organisms such as *S. aureus* and *Staphylococcus lugdunensis* can present this way, in many studies nonvirulent organisms including coagulase-negative staphylococci are more common. Gram-negative organisms are less common causes of delayed arthroplasty infections.[3] One way that organisms causing chronic periprosthetic infection are able to survive the host immune response is by producing biofilm. Biofilms are comprised of clusters of microorganisms that adhere to the surface of the device and elaborate a polymer matrix.[13] Organisms within biofilms often replicate more slowly and are protected from the host immune response and antimicrobial therapies by mechanical and electrostatic barriers. Due both to their growth characteristics and the impenetrability of the biofilm matrix, sessile organisms within biofilms may be 10 to >500 times less susceptible to antimicrobials than their planktonic counterparts (those organisms that have left the biofilm).[14]

Late Periprosthetic Infections

Late infections are primarily due to hematogenous spread of organisms, i.e., due to virulent organisms that gain access to the bloodstream. Organisms can translocate

into the bloodstream through weaknesses or loss of integrity of epidermal and mucosal surfaces, including breaks in the skin, oropharyngeal and nasopharyngeal mucosa, bladder endothelium, and gut mucosal surfaces. The types of organisms causing hematogenous infection may be inferred based on the portal of entry. Organisms that enter through breaks in the skin are those that reside on the skin surface, including *S. aureus*, *S. lugdunensis*, *Streptococcus agalactiae* (Group B streptococcus) and pyogenic streptococci such as *Streptococcus pyogenes* (Group A), and *Streptococcus dysgalactiae* (Groups C/G). These may be more common in the setting of cutaneous diseases like eczema, psoriasis, and ulcers caused by venous and/or arterial insufficiency. Overall, compared with early and delayed infections, streptococcal species are more common causes of hematogenous PJI, in some series causing up to 37% of late hematogenous PJI.[15] Similarly, coagulase-negative staphylococci are less common causes of late hematogenous infection.[5,16]

Antecedent dental infection and gingivitis may contribute to infection with viridans streptococci and other mouth flora, including organisms collectively grouped by the HACEK acronym (*Haemophilus aphrophilus*, *Actinobacillus actinomycetomcomitans*, *Cardiobacterium hominis*, *Eikenella corrodens*, and *Kingella kingae*). Urinary tract infection and bacteriuria are a risk for later PJI.[17] Although still less common than Gram-positive organisms as a cause of PJI, Gram-negative infections are more commonly seen in patients with a history of bacteriuria.[18]

Injection drug use is unfortunately an increasing source of hematogenous infection, though still not as common among patients who have undergone arthroplasty. Bacteria may be introduced because of inadequate skin preparation (e.g., skin organisms such as *S. aureus* and *S. pyogenes*) because of the practice of needle-licking (oral streptococci and oral anaerobes such as *E. corrodens*) or because of contamination of the drug itself. Other organisms seen more commonly in the setting of injection drug use include *Pseudomonas aeruginosa* (because of the use of tap water for preparation) and *Candida* species.[19]

Rarely, the organisms causing late periprosthetic infections may be introduced directly into the joint, primarily in the setting of trauma. In addition to the organisms that reside on the host's skin, organisms associated with traumatic inoculation include environmental organisms: Gram-negative bacilli, mycobacteria, fungal species, and environmental anaerobes such as *Clostridia*. Organisms that reside within water sources (e.g., *P. aeruginosa* and other nonenteric Gram-negative bacilli, nontuberculous mycobacteria) may be seen after marine trauma.

With advances in microbiologic diagnostic techniques, the spectrum of organisms capable of causing periprosthetic infection is expanding. While still rare, fungal and mycobacterial infections are increasingly being reported.[20-23] These organisms should be considered in the setting of prior antibiotic exposure (*Candida*), injection drug use (*Candida*), and environmental trauma. As diagnostic techniques improve, many additional organisms that do not grow well in culture and were not previously thought to be pathogens in the setting of arthroplasty (e.g., *Mycoplasma* and Lyme) are being identified.[24-26] We anticipate that the spectrum of organisms capable of causing PJI will continue to expand as our diagnostic modalities improve.

Despite advancements in microbiologic diagnostics, the organisms causing some periprosthetic knee infections remain elusive. Depending on the study, between 7% and 25% of infections are culture-negative.[1,4,7,8] Culture negativity may be more common in chronic biofilm-associated infections, as the organisms may be encapsulated within the biofilm matrix and less adapted to growth in culture media.[13] Prior antibiotic exposure (defined as antibiotic treatment within 3 months) increases the likelihood that an infection may be culture-negative.[27,28] Fastidious organisms or those that require special growth media (e.g., nutritionally deficient streptococci, HACEK organisms) are often implicated as causes of culture negativity. Mycoplasma, fungi, and mycobacteria do not always grow in routine bacterial cultures and therefore suspicion of their presence is important to ensure that the correct culture media are utilized. Newer non–culture-based diagnostic modalities (discussed later in the chapter) may ultimately reduce the proportion of infections for which the causative pathogen is unknown.

With the expanding use of antimicrobial therapies worldwide, more infections are being caused by antibiotic-resistant organisms, including MRSA and methicillin-resistant coagulase-negative staphylococci, ampicillin- and vancomycin-resistant enterococci, and Gram-negative organisms with extended-spectrum beta-lactamases (ESBL). Some studies have also identified an increasing prevalence of resistant organisms causing PJI over time.[1,8] Predicting the likelihood of resistance is important in empiric antimicrobial management and also in considering different surgical strategies, as resistant organisms have been more commonly associated with treatment failure.[29,30] Patients with prior antimicrobial exposure and those with comorbidities may be more likely to harbor resistant organisms.[31] The prevalence of certain resistant organisms differs geographically and institutionally as well: MRSA is more commonly found as a cause of PJI in the United States than at European Centers.[7] As clinicians, understanding the local microbiology is paramount.

MICROBIOLOGIC DIAGNOSIS

Culture-based Diagnostics

In order to treat PJIs with optimal antibiotic therapy, one must identify the causative pathogen, and the mainstay for this identification remains standard microbiological culture. Synovial fluid may be aspirated prior to surgery and sent for culture, and periprosthetic tissue should always be sent intraoperatively when a surgery is done out of concern for infection. In addition, the prosthesis—if removed—can itself be sonicated and sent for culture.[28] Regardless of how they are obtained, all samples should be sent for aerobic and anaerobic bacterial culture. Fungal and mycobacterial cultures should not be sent routinely, as they are rarely the cause of PJI, and therefore the increased cost for their analysis is not justified. However, in cases where the history suggests an atypical cause (immunocompromised, prior antibiotic treatment without improvement, unusual exposures; see above section on Microbiology), these special cultures should also be performed.

In a stable patient, common practice is to hold antibiotics until after tissue samples are collected, since the administration of antibiotics prior to surgery is thought to reduce the yield of tissue cultures. Indeed, patients who have received systemic antibiotics in the weeks to months prior to revision arthroplasty are more likely to have culture-negative PJIs.[27,28,32] Therefore, if a PJI is suspected, one should not treat with antibiotics alone; rather, plans must be made for surgical treatment of the infection and antibiotics withheld until surgery. It is worth noting, however, that the single dose of standard perioperative antibiotics appears to cause little if any reduction in culture yield.[33-38] A reasonable approach, therefore, is to hold antibiotics prior to surgery, give standard perioperative prophylaxis at the standard time (30 to 60 minutes prior to skin incision), and then postoperatively start empiric antibiotic therapy for PJI based on the most likely causative pathogens (see section on Empiric Treatment).

Because the microbial burden in periprosthetic infections is often low, multiple tissue samples should be collected intraoperatively, typically three to five.[39,40] When collecting tissue samples, a new instrument should be used to obtain each sample. This practice avoids cross-contamination, leading to greater interpretability and reliability of results.[41] Because many of the pathogens in PJIs (*Staphylococcus epidermidis*, *Cutibacterium acnes*) are also common contaminants, it is exceedingly useful to note how many of the intraoperative tissue cultures yield the same pathogen. For example, if only one colony of *C. acnes* grows from only one of five tissue samples sent for culture, it is likely to represent a contaminant rather than a true pathogen. Using new instruments to take each sample decreases the likelihood of a contaminant growing from multiple cultures and thus reduces false-positive results. Tissue samples are always favored over swabs, as they have much higher sensitivity.[42]

Despite obtaining multiple tissue samples, many PJIs remain culture-negative. One practice that may increase the yield of cultures is sonication of the removed prosthesis.[28,43,44] Sonication refers to the practice of placing the removed prosthesis in a bath of sterile saline (or other fluid) and applying high-frequency sound waves to the solution. The resulting vibration causes particles to break apart. Since the bacteria causing a PJI can exist in a biofilm on the prosthesis, sonication disrupts the biofilm, thereby releasing the bacteria into the surrounding fluid, which can then be inoculated onto a culture plate or into liquid culture media. While not all studies have found sonication to increase culture yield,[45,46] the bulk of data thus far does suggest that sonication increases the detection of bacteria, and that it can be a useful adjunct to standard culture techniques.[47] However, sonication is not widely available and where available the techniques have not been standardized across institutions. Further, some institutions have found it challenging to create a reliable pathway for processing samples in this way, especially if the microbiology lab is not located on-site. In addition to sonication, inoculating samples directly into blood culture bottles may increase yield, though it is not part of standard procedures.[48]

Standard bacterial cultures are typically held for 5 to 7 days, at which point they are considered negative if no bacterial growth is observed. However, some pathogens in PJI—particularly in chronic or otherwise indolent presentations of PJI—take longer than 1 week to grow. Studies have shown that increasing the culture incubation period to 10 to 14 days will increase detection of fastidious or slow-growing organisms, in particular *C. acnes*.[49,50] Therefore, particularly in cases of chronic periprosthetic infections, it is recommended to hold the cultures for 10 to 14 days to increase yield of slow-growing organisms. However, this will also increase detection of contaminants and thus decrease specificity. Again, sending multiple distinct samples for culture can help clinicians interpret the results.

Molecular Diagnostics

The unacceptably high prevalence of culture-negative PJI has led to the exploration of using sequence-based diagnostics to identify the causative pathogen. Three main methods have been applied to PJI (**Table 74-2**): 16S ribosomal sequencing, multiplex polymerase chain reaction (PCR), and next-generation shotgun sequencing (metagenomics). In the case of the first, universal primers are used in a PCR to amplify the 16S ribosomal genes from any bacteria present in the sample. Any amplicons are then sequenced, and those sequences are compared against a reference database to identify the microbes present in the sample. While this offers the possibility of identifying pathogens that failed to grow by conventional culture methods, in practice it is not clear that this is more sensitive than routine culture.[51-53] For example, one large study found that in cases of culture-negative PJI, 16S sequencing was able to identify a pathogen in 8 of 16 patients who had received antibiotics prior to sample collection, thus demonstrating the potential of this technique to detect noncultured pathogens. However, the same study found that 16S sequencing failed to identify any pathogen in one-quarter of known culture-positive PJIs.[51]

A different molecular approach is to use multiplex PCR, in which primers specific for a chosen set of potential pathogens are used. This approach was established first for blood cultures and cerebral spinal fluid samples and has since been applied to synovial fluid. Results are mixed regarding whether it is an improvement over standard culture.[54-58] Since culture can detect a single bacterium, it is not surprising that for most infections it remains the most sensitive test. In addition, when a low-virulence organism is detected by PCR (e.g., *C. acnes*, *S. epidermidis*), it is difficult to judge whether it represents a true infection or simply the expected presence of genetic material from commensal bacteria. Unlike culture, which gives a quantitative description of how many colonies grew from a given sample, PCR-based results are generally reported as present versus not present. While the use of real-time PCR can give a quantitative result, the clinical relevance of this value is unknown. Finally, while

TABLE 74-2	Sequence-Based Diagnostics for Periprosthetic Joint Infection			
Technique	**Description**	**Advantages**	**Disadvantages**	**References**
16S Ribosomal sequencing	Universal primers amplify the 16S ribosomal gene of any bacteria in the sample. The resulting amplicons (if any) are sequenced and compared to a reference database for identification.	Can detect nonculturable bacteria.	In practice, not more sensitive than culture. Done at only a few reference laboratories, so results take days to weeks to return.	51-53
Multiplex polymerase chain reaction (PCR)	A set of primer pairs for a predetermined set of pathogens is used in a PCR to determine if those pathogens are present in the sample.	Builds on existing commercially available technology in use for blood and cerebrospinal fluid samples. Results can be available within hours.	Only detects the pathogens in the panel, not all pathogens. Sensitivity and specificity unknown for joint infections.	54-58
Metagenomics	All genetic materials in the sample are sequenced and then compared against reference sequences.	Unbiased approach to detecting pathogens. Can give semi-quantitative data about pathogen abundance.	Contamination remains an unsolved problem. Sensitivity and specificity unknown for joint infections.	59-61

the multiplex PCR assays can be designed to look for specific antibiotic resistance genes, they cannot give phenotypic antibiotic resistance information, and thus standard bacterial culture remains necessary for full susceptibility profiling.

More recently, metagenomic techniques have become available, in which all the genetic material in a sample are sequenced and compared against reference databases ("next-generation" or "shotgun" sequencing). In case reports, this technique has been used to identify an otherwise elusive pathogen (e.g., *Mycoplasma*).[26] Metagenomics offers an advantage over multiplex PCR in that it makes no *a priori* assumptions about which organisms are likely to be present. In addition, by measuring the proportion of DNA that is from a given organism and by determining if the entire genome of the organism is present, this technique can give semi-quantitative data about the amount of pathogen present and therefore how likely it is to be a true pathogen rather than a contaminant. However, exactly how to define analyses to determine if the organism(s) identified represent a true pathogen or simply a contaminant (sensitivity versus specificity) is not yet known.[59-61] For example, in one study, next-generation sequencing identified a pathogen in 9 of 11 culture-negative PJIs, but it also detected a "pathogen" in 6 of 17 primary arthroplasties.[62] In addition, because this analysis is done only at a few reference or research laboratories, the results may not be available quickly enough to be useful for patient management. Sequence-based diagnostics remain an area of active and promising research, but it has not yet been shown that acting on the results of these tests improves patient outcomes, and thus they are not part of standard practice. If they are used, we recommend consulting with an infectious disease specialist or a microbiologist for assistance with interpreting the results.

SYSTEMIC ANTIMICROBIAL TREATMENT

Once the diagnosis of prosthetic joint infection is suspected and/or confirmed, patients should be considered for surgical management. For most patients, antimicrobial therapy should be withheld prior to surgery, as prior antibiotic therapy interferes with the yield of surgical cultures, as outlined above.[27,28,32] Patients who are clinically unstable due to acute infection (either early or late hematogenous) should be started on empiric antibiotics after blood cultures are collected.

Empiric Antibiotics

After surgical samples have been obtained, the patient should be started on empiric antibiotic therapy while awaiting culture results, and these antibiotics should target the most likely organisms. If a preoperative joint aspirate has identified a likely pathogen, then empiric antibiotics can be targeted to that microbe, while

recognizing that surgical cultures may provide additional information. (For example, a single colony of coagulase-negative staphylococcus from a joint aspirate may or may not be the cause of the PJI.) As discussed above, the most likely pathogens at all stages are Gram-positive bacteria, with staphylococci being the most common. In most institutions, a glycopeptide (e.g., vancomycin) is the typical empiric choice for treating the Gram-positive bacteria, given the prevalence of MRSA and methicillin-resistant coagulase-negative staphylococci such as *S. epidermidis*. While Gram-positive bacteria remain the most common cause of PJIs, Gram-negative bacteria cause PJI often enough at all stages that empiric coverage should include an antibiotic active against Gram-negative bacteria.

The exact choice of agents should be guided by local antibiotic resistance profiles; developing institution-specific guidelines in consultation with the Infectious Disease division and/or the Microbiology lab can help to standardize practices and to ensure that the most common pathogens in the local milieu are being covered with the empiric antibiotics. In general, a combination of a glycopeptide and a third-generation cephalosporin (e.g., vancomycin plus ceftriaxone) will cover the most common causes of PJI and is a reasonable first-approximation antibiotic regimen for the typical patient. Broader empiric coverage (e.g., for *Pseudomonas*, ESBL Gram-negatives, or *Candida*) may be appropriate in select patients, as discussed above in the Microbiology section. If a specific pathogen is not identified, then the treatment course can be completed with the empiric regimen.

Definitive Antibiotic Selection

Once the culprit pathogen has been identified, antibiotics should be narrowed to target that pathogen. In general, beta-lactams are preferred for streptococcal, enterococcal, and staphylococcal infections, assuming the organism is susceptible. For example, penicillin is preferred for sensitive streptococcal infections, ampicillin is preferred for sensitive enterococcal infections, and cefazolin, nafcillin, or oxacillin is preferred for methicillin-sensitive staphylococcal infections. For Gram-negative infections, a later-generation cephalosporin, carbapenem, or fluoroquinolone is typically used, with the exact choice depending on the susceptibility profile of the infecting organism. Regardless of the choice of antibiotic or the duration, either intravenous antibiotics or highly bioavailable oral antibiotics should be used, to ensure adequate penetration of the antibiotic into the bone (**Tables 74-3** and **74-4**).

In addition to the identified or suspected organisms, host factors impact the selection of antimicrobials for empiric and definitive management. For example, patients with underlying renal disease are at higher risk of nephrotoxicity due to glycopeptides.[63] Patients with congestive heart failure or chronic renal disease may develop volume overload when administered antimicrobials with high salt content (e.g., piperacillin sodium). Many

TABLE 74-3   Recommended Antimicrobial Treatment of Common Microorganisms Causing Periprosthetic Joint Infection(PJI)

Microorganism	Preferred Treatment[a]	Alternative Treatment[a]
Staphylococci, oxacillin-susceptible	Nafcillin[b] sodium 1.5-2 g IV q4-6h or cefazolin 1-2 g IV q8h or ceftriaxone[c] 1-2 g IV q24h	Vancomycin IV 15 mg/kg q12h or daptomycin 6 mg/kg IV q24h or linezolid 600 mg PO/IV every 12 h
Staphylococci, oxacillin-resistant	Vancomycin[d] IV 15 mg/kg q12h	Daptomycin 6 mg/kg IV q24h or linezolid 600 mg PO/IV q12h
Enterococcus spp., penicillin-susceptible	Penicillin G 20-24 million units IV q24h continuously or in 6 divided doses or ampicillin sodium 12 g IV q24h continuously or in 6 divided doses	Vancomycin 15 mg/kg IV q12h or daptomycin 6 mg/kg IV q24h or linezolid 600 mg PO or IV q12h
Enterococcus spp., penicillin-resistant	Vancomycin 15 mg/kg IV q12h	Linezolid 600 mg PO or IV q12h or daptomycin 6 mg IV q24h
Pseudomonas aeruginosa	Cefepime 2 g IV q12h or meropenem[e] 1 g IV q8h	Ciprofloxacin 750 mg PO bid or 400 mg IV q12h or ceftazidime 2 g IV q8h
Enterobacter spp.	Cefepime 2 g IV q12h or ertapenem 1 g IV q24h	Ciprofloxacin 750 mg PO or 400 mg IV q12h
Enterobacteriaceae	IV β-lactam based on *in vitro* susceptibilities or ciprofloxacin 750 mg PO bid	
β-Hemolytic streptococci	Penicillin G 20-24 million units IV q24h continuously or in 6 divided doses or ceftriaxone 2 g IV q24h	Vancomycin 15 mg/kg IV q12h
Cutibacterium acnes	Penicillin G 20 million units IV q24h continuously or in 6 divided doses or ceftriaxone 2 g IV q24h	Clindamycin 600-900 mg IV q8h or clindamycin 300-450 mg PO qid or vancomycin 15 mg/kg IV q12h

bid, twice daily; IV, intravenous; PO, per oral; q, every; qid, 4 times daily.

[a]Antimicrobial dosage needs to be adjusted based on patients' renal and hepatic function. Antimicrobials should be chosen based on *in vitro* susceptibility as well as patient drug allergies, intolerances, and potential drug interactions or contraindications to a specific antimicrobial. Clinical and laboratory monitoring for efficacy and safety should occur based on prior IDSA guidelines.[88] The possibility of prolonged QTc interval and tendinopathy should be discussed and monitored when using fluoroquinolones. The possibility of *Clostridium difficile* colitis should also be discussed when using any antimicrobial.

[b]Flucloxacillin may be used in Europe. Oxacillin can also be substituted.

[c]There was not a consensus on the use of ceftriaxone for methicillin-susceptible staphylococci (see text).

[d]Target troughs for vancomycin should be chosen with the guidance of a local infectious disease physician based on the pathogen, its *in vitro* susceptibility, and the use of rifampin or local vancomycin therapy. Recent guidelines[89,90] for the treatment of methicillin-resistant *Staphylococcus aureus* (MRSA) infections have been published. (These guidelines suggest that dosing of vancomycin be considered to achieve a vancomycin trough at steady state of 15-20. Although this may be appropriate for MRSA PJI treated without rifampin or without the use of local vancomycin spacer, it is unknown if these higher trough concentrations are necessary when rifampin or vancomycin impregnated spacers are utilized. Trough concentrations of at least 10 may be appropriate in this situation. It is also unknown if treatment of oxacillin-resistant, coagulase-negative staphylococci require vancomycin dosing to achieve these higher vancomycin levels.)

[e]Other antipseudomonal carbapenems can be utilized as well.

From Osmon DR, Berbari EF, Berendt AR, et al. Diagnosis and management of prosthetic joint infection: clinical practice guidelines by the Infectious Diseases Society of America. *Clin Infect Dis*. 2013;56(1):1-25.

TABLE 74-4   Antibiotics With Good Oral Bioavailability

Oral Antibiotic	Spectrum of Activity	Comments
Amoxicillin	Streptococci *Cutibacterium acnes*	Only for bacteria highly susceptible to penicillin.
Clindamycin	Gram-positives	Must be taken 3-4 times daily.
Fluoroquinolones	Gram-negatives Staphylococci (in combination with rifampin)	Adverse effects—a growing concern.
Rifampin	Staphylococci (Streptococci, *C. acnes*—unclear benefit)	Many drug interactions. Always used in combination, never alone.
Tetracyclines	Staphylococci	Susceptibility can differ between agents in this class.
Trimethoprim-sulfamethoxazole	Staphylococci Gram-negatives	Significant side effects at higher doses.
Linezolid	Gram-positives	Not safe for long-term use.

antimicrobials interact with other medications; potential drug–drug interactions should be reviewed prior to starting any antimicrobials. These are most relevant for drugs that impact hepatic metabolism, including rifampin and azoles (e.g., fluconazole). Some drug–drug interactions in frail patients may preclude the use of certain antimicrobials (e.g., rifampin in a patient receiving warfarin or other oral anticoagulant therapies). Allergy histories should be reviewed prior to antimicrobial prescription. Approximately 10% of patients in the United States report a penicillin allergy; however, the vast majority of these patients are nonallergic when penicillin allergy testing is conducted.[64] When beta-lactam therapy is indicated, patients who receive alternative therapy based on allergy history have a higher likelihood of poor outcome including readmission for infection.[65] Therefore, in these patients referral for penicillin skin testing and/or test dose administration should be strongly considered.

While it has long been considered that intravenous antimicrobial therapy is optimal for treatment of infections involving osteoarticular sites, the data to support this practice are limited.[66] Experience in European centers suggests that many orthopedic infections can be managed with oral antimicrobials (often after 1 to 2 weeks of intravenous therapy). A large randomized controlled trial (RCT) conducted among patients with a variety of musculoskeletal infections did not identify a treatment advantage to intravenous antibiotic therapy over oral therapy.[67] When oral antimicrobials are considered, in general, those with high bioavailability and reliable bone penetration, such as tetracyclines, trimethoprim-sulfamethoxazole, fluoroquinolones, and linezolid, are preferred.[68] Among available oral agents, retrospective studies suggest that the combination of rifampin and levofloxacin is most effective for PJI due to *S. aureus*.[69,70] Ability to comply with antibiotic-specific dietary restrictions and to adhere to an oral regimen also need to be considered and discussed with patients when oral antimicrobials are employed.

Logistical factors also may impact the choice of definitive antimicrobial therapy. For patients who will complete a course of intravenous therapy after discharge, regimen simplicity is often a factor. Once daily intravenous antimicrobials, including ceftriaxone, daptomycin, and ertapenem, are appealing for use after hospital discharge. However, these options may come at the expense of an unnecessarily broad antimicrobial spectrum, thereby raising the risk of gastrointestinal side effects and *Clostridium difficile* colitis. Ultimately, the choice of antimicrobial therapy is best guided by a specialist in Infectious Diseases.

Duration of Antibiotic Treatment

The optimal duration of antibiotic treatment for PJI is not known, but anywhere from 6 weeks to 6 months is typical. Definitive management of periprosthetic knee infections depends upon the surgical management of the infection, the culprit organism, and patient characteristics. There are guidelines from the Infectious Disease Society of America[71] and from the European Society of Clinical Microbiology and Infectious Diseases[13] regarding management of prosthetic joint infections; however, it should be noted that there were very few high-quality clinical trials available to inform these guidelines.

Patients managed with débridement, antibiotics, and implant retention (DAIR) should be treated with antibiotics for at least 6 weeks and potentially for as long as 6 months if the infection is caused by staphylococci. The practice of using 6 months of treatment for staphylococcal knee PJI managed with DAIR comes from a small RCT done more than 20 years ago, which demonstrated the benefit of using rifampin in combination with a fluoroquinolone for these infections.[71] However, duration of treatment was not tested in this trial: it simply showed good clinical outcomes with 6 months of antibiotic treatment. More recently, another RCT demonstrated that 8 weeks of antibiotic treatment had equivalent outcomes to 6 months for staphylococcal PJI treated with DAIR, again using a quinolone plus rifampin.[72] Observational studies including PJI caused by a variety of organisms have likewise found that shorter treatment courses (1.5 to 3 months rather than 6) do not adversely affect outcome.[73,74] Thus, treating for 6 months is likely unnecessary for the majority of patients, though for now it remains common practice.

Regardless of treatment duration, for patients managed by DAIR treatment, success is likely to be higher if a "biofilm-active" agent is used, such as rifampin for staphylococci or a fluoroquinolone for Gram-negative bacteria.[13,71] The principle is that the retained prosthesis is likely to have a biofilm of bacteria still on it, and therefore an antibiotic known to be active against biofilms should be used to increase the likelihood of cure. However, rifampin should never be used alone because resistance develops rapidly. Likewise, quinolones should not be used alone for staphylococcal infections due to concerns about the emergence of resistance on therapy. The benefit of rifampin for staphylococcal PJI is long-established.[71] Rifampin may also have a role in treating infections caused by streptococci and *C. acnes*; however, the data are less clear and it is not yet part of standard treatment of PJI caused by these organisms.[75-77]

For patients who have the implant removed and replaced in a single surgery (a one-stage approach), 6 to 12 weeks of antibiotic therapy is recommended, with the addition of rifampin in the case of staphylococcal infections.[78] In general, patients infected with staphylococci should receive longer courses of treatment, and their treatment should include rifampin unless the infected prosthesis was completely removed and a new one was not implanted until several months later (two-stage exchange). In cases of a two-stage exchange, guidelines recommend 4 to 6 weeks of antibiotic therapy after the implant was removed, regardless of the causative pathogen.[78] After completion of therapy, it is common practice to observe patients off antibiotics for several weeks to monitor for any signs of recrudescent infection. The goal is for the patient to be infection-free prior to the implantation of a new prosthesis.

Suppressive Antimicrobial Therapy

Regardless of surgical strategy and antimicrobial regimen, a significant minority of patients treated for knee arthroplasty infection is not cured and is therefore at risk of relapse; the likelihood of noncure is higher with DAIR procedures and with certain organisms, including methicillin-resistant staphylococci.[79-81] There is no reliable laboratory or imaging test that can be employed at the time of antibiotic completion that confirms the infection is microbiologically cured. The decision to stop antibiotic therapy after a defined treatment duration versus transition to a long-term suppression approach (generally for the life of the implant) is important but often challenging for patients and physicians to navigate.

No randomized controlled studies report on the optimal use of long-term antimicrobial therapy, though the strategy has been employed when the risk or consequences of recurrence are felt to be high. Factors known to reduce the likelihood of treatment success, including nonsurgical management, use of DAIR procedures for chronic infections, infection with resistant organisms, and inability to use rifampin for staphylococcal infections when DAIR is utilized, might lead the clinician to favor long-term suppression. The impact of recurrent infection on the patient should also be considered; those infections that would be life- or limb-threatening may be considered for suppression. Medically frail patients who may not tolerate reoperation for PJI are often considered for suppression.[82] The risk of recurrent infection needs to be balanced against the risks of chronic antimicrobial use. These risks include direct toxicities of the drug, antimicrobial intolerances (particularly chronic gastrointestinal symptoms), and the impact on host flora (including risk of resistant infections and *C. difficile* colitis). While some of these risks are difficult to quantify, multiple retrospective studies suggest that most patients (in the range of 80%) tolerate long-term suppression with few discontinuations for side effects.[82-85]

It is important to note that suppression does not guarantee freedom from recurrence—even with antimicrobial suppression, about one-third of patients require reoperation for infection within 5 years.[86,87] In the largest series to report on outcomes of long-term suppression,

patients with PJI who underwent DAIR or two-stage exchange were more likely to achieve infection-free survival when long-term antimicrobial suppression was maintained (69% vs. 41%).[87] The greatest benefit to long-term suppression was seen in those with *S. aureus* infections and those undergoing DAIR procedures.[87] Nonetheless, when infection recurs despite long-term antimicrobial suppression, in some cases the infection is more resistant, complicating later efforts to provide a definitive cure.[84]

SUMMARY

The effective antimicrobial management of PJIs requires integrated knowledge of the likely pathogens, the host, and antibiotic efficacy. Identifying the culprit pathogen is crucial to management, and therefore taking appropriate cultures is key to caring for patients with these infections. Unfortunately, a sizable minority of PJI remain culture-negative. Sequence-based diagnostics may improve diagnosis, but these techniques have not yet been shown to improve patient outcomes. Ultimately, choosing an antibiotic regimen and duration is based on published guidelines but tailored to individual patients and their microbes.

REFERENCES

1. Bjerke-Kroll BT, Christ AB, McLawhorn AS, Sculco PK, Jules-Elysée KM, Sculco TP. Periprosthetic joint infections treated with two-stage revision over 14 years: an evolving microbiology profile. *J Arthroplasty*. 2014;29(5):877-882.
2. Holleyman RJ, Baker P, Charlett A, Gould K, Deehan DJ. Microorganisms responsible for periprosthetic knee infections in England and Wales. *Knee Surg Sport Traumatol Arthrosc*. 2016;24(10):3080-3087.
3. Wang YP, Chen CF, Chen HP. Wang FD. The incidence rate, trend and microbiological aetiology of prosthetic joint infection after total knee arthroplasty: a 13 years' experience from a tertiary medical center in Taiwan. *J Microbiol Immunol Infect*. 2018;51(6):717-722.
4. Peel TN, Cheng AC, Buising KL, Choong PFM. Microbiological aetiology, epidemiology, and clinical profile of prosthetic joint infections: are current antibiotic prophylaxis guidelines effective? *Antimicrob Agents Chemother*. 2012;56(5):2386-2391.
5. Fulkerson E, Valle CJ, Wise B, Walsh M, Preston C, Di Cesare P. Antibiotic susceptibility of bacteria infecting total joint arthroplasty sites. *J Bone Joint Surg Am*. 2006;88:1231-1237.
6. Moran E, Masters S, Berendt AR, McLardy-Smith P, Byren I, Atkins BL. Guiding empirical antibiotic therapy in orthopaedics: the microbiology of prosthetic joint infection managed by debridement, irrigation and prosthesis retention. *J Infect*. 2007;55(1):1-7.
7. Aggarwal VK, Bakhshi H, Ecker NU, Parvizi J, Gehrke TKD. Organism profile in periprosthetic joint infection: pathogens differ at two arthroplasty infection referral centers in Europe and in the United States. *J Knee Surg*. 2014;27(5):399-406.
8. Rosteius T, Jansen O, Fehmer T, et al. Evaluating the microbial pattern of periprosthetic joint infections of the hip and knee. *J Med Microbiol*. 2018;67:1608-1613.
9. Marculescu CE, Cantey JR. Polymicrobial prosthetic joint infections: risk factors and outcome. *Clin Orthop Relat Res*. 2008;466(6):1397-1404.

10. Boe E, Sanchez HB, Kazenske FM, Wagner RA. Efficacy of skin preparation in eradicating organisms before total knee arthroplasty. *Am J Orthop.* 2014;43(12):E309-E312.

11. Kong HH, Segre JA. The molecular revolution in cutaneous biology: investigating the skin microbiome. *J Invest Dermatol.* 2017;137(5):e119-22.

12. Tan TL, Springer BD, Ruder JA, Ruffolo MR, Chen AF. Is vancomycin-only prophylaxis for patients with penicillin allergy associated with increased risk of infection after arthroplasty? *Clin Orthop Relat Res.* 2016;474(7):1601-1606.

13. Høiby N, Bjarnsholt T, Moser C, et al. ESCMID* guideline for the diagnosis and treatment of biofilm infections 2014. *Clin Microbiol Infect.* 2015;21(S1):S1-S25.

14. Donlan RM. Biofilm formation: a clinically relevant microbiological process. *Clin Infect Dis.* 2001;33(8):1387-1392.

15. Konigsberg BS, Valle CJD, Ting NT, Qiu F, Sporer SM. Acute hematogenous infection following total hip and knee arthroplasty. *J Arthroplasty.* 2014;29(3):469-472.

16. Fink B, Schuster P, Schwenninger C, Frommelt L, Oremek D. A standardized regimen for the treatment of acute postoperative infections and acute hematogenous infections associated with hip and knee arthroplasties. *J Arthroplasty.* 2017;32(4):1255-1261.

17. Weale R, El-Bakri F, Saeed K. Pre-operative asymptomatic bacteriuria: a risk factor for prosthetic joint infection? *J Hosp Infect.* 2019;101(2):210-213.

18. Sousa R, Muñoz-Mahamud E, Quayle J, et al. Is asymptomatic bacteriuria a risk factor for prosthetic joint infection? *Clin Infect Dis.* 2014;59(1):41-47.

19. Allison DC, Holtom PD, Patzakis MJ, Zalavras CG. Microbiology of bone and joint infections in injecting drug abusers. *Clin Orthop Relat Res.* 2010;468(8):2107-2112.

20. Azzam K, Parvizi J, Jungkind D, et al. Microbiological, clinical, and surgical features of fungal prosthetic joint infections: a multi-institutional experience. *J Bone Joint Surg Am.* 2009;91(suppl 6):142-149.

21. Cobo F, Rodríguez-Granger J, Sampedro A, Aliaga-Martínez L, Navarro-Marí JM. *Candida* prosthetic joint infection. A review of treatment methods. *J Bone Joint Infect.* 2017;2(2):114-121.

22. Jakobs O, Schoof B, Klatte TO, et al. Fungal periprosthetic joint infection in total knee arthroplasty: a systematic review. *Orthop Rev.* 2015;7(1). doi:10.4081/or.2015.5623.

23. Eid AJ, Berbari EF, Sia IG, Wengenack NL, Osmon DR, Razonable RR. Prosthetic joint infection due to rapidly growing mycobacteria: report of 8 cases and review of the literature. *Clin Infect Dis.* 2007;45(6):687-694.

24. Collins KA, Gotoff JR, Ghanem ES. Lyme Disease: a potential source for culture-negative prosthetic joint infection. *J Am Acad Orthop Surg Glob Res Rev.* 2017;1(5):e023.

25. Wright WF, Oliverio JA. First case of Lyme arthritis involving a prosthetic knee joint. *Open Forum Infect Dis.* 2016;3(2):1-3.

26. Thoendel M, Jeraldo P, Greenwood-Quaintance KE, et al. A novel prosthetic joint infection pathogen, Mycoplasma salivarium, identified by metagenomic shotgun sequencing. *Clin Infect Dis.* 2017;65(2):332-335.

27. Malekzadeh D, Osmon DR, Lahr BD, Hanssen AD, Berbari EF. Prior use of antimicrobial therapy is a risk factor for culture-negative prosthetic joint infection. *Clin Orthop Relat Res.* 2010;468(8):2039-2045. https://doi.org/10.1007/s11999-010-1338-0.

28. Trampuz A, Piper KE, Jacobson MJ, et al. Sonication of removed hip and knee prostheses for diagnosis of infection. *N Engl J Med.* 2007;357(7):654-663. http://www.nejm.org/doi/abs/10.1056/NEJMoa061588.

29. Salgado CD, Dash S, Cantey JR, Marculescu CE. Higher risk of failure of methicillin-resistant *Staphylococcus aureus* prosthetic joint infections. *Clin Orthop Relat Res.* 2007;461:48-53.

30. Parvizi J, Azzam K, Ghanem E, Austin MS, Rothman RH. Periprosthetic infection due to resistant staphylococci: serious problems on the horizon. *Clin Orthop Relat Res.* 2009;467(7):1732-1739.

31. Tan TL, Gomez MM, Kheir MM, Maltenfort MG, Chen AF. Should preoperative antibiotics Be tailored according to patient's comorbidities and susceptibility to organisms? *J Arthroplasty.* 2017;32(4):1089-1094.e3.

32. Shahi A, Deirmengian C, Higuera C, et al. Premature therapeutic antimicrobial treatments can compromise the diagnosis of late periprosthetic joint infection. *Clin Orthop Relat Res.* 2015;473(7):2244-2249. http://dx.doi.org/10.1007/s11999-015-4142-z.

33. Wouthuyzen-Bakker M, Benito N, Soriano A. The effect of preoperative antimicrobial prophylaxis on intraoperative culture results in patients with a suspected or confirmed prosthetic joint infection: a systematic review. *J Clin Microbiol.* 2017;55(9):2765-2774.

34. Anagnostopoulos A, Bossard DA, Ledergerber B, et al. Perioperative antibiotic prophylaxis has no effect on time to positivity and proportion of positive samples: a cohort study of 64 Cutibacterium acnes bone and joint infections. *J Clin Microbiol.* 2018;56(2): e01576-17.

35. Burnett RSJ, Aggarwal A, Givens SA, McClure JT, Morgan PM, Barrack RL. Prophylactic antibiotics do not affect cultures in the treatment of an infected TKA: a prospective trial. *Clin Orthop Relat Res.* 2010;468(1):127-134.

36. Pérez-Prieto D, Portillo ME, Puig-Verdié L, et al. Preoperative antibiotic prophylaxis in prosthetic joint infections: not a concern for intraoperative cultures. *Diagn Microbiol Infect Dis.* 2016;86(4):442-445.

37. Tetreault MW, Wetters NG, Aggarwal V, Mont M, Parvizi J, Della Valle CJ. The Chitranjan Ranawat Award: should prophylactic antibiotics be withheld before revision surgery to obtain appropriate cultures? *Clin Orthop Relat Res.* 2014;472(1):52-56.

38. Bedenčič K, Kavčič M, Faganeli N, et al. Does preoperative antimicrobial prophylaxis influence the diagnostic potential of periprosthetic tissues in hip or knee infections? *Clin Orthop Relat Res.* 2016;474(1):258-264.

39. Peel TN, Spelman T, Dylla BL, et al. Optimal periprosthetic tissue specimen number for diagnosis of prosthetic joint infection. *J Clin Microbiol.* 2017;55(1):234-243.

40. Bémer P, Léger J, Tandé D, et al. How many samples and how many culture media to diagnose a prosthetic joint infection: a clinical and microbiological prospective multicenter study. *J Clin Microbiol.* 2016;54(2):385-391.

41. Makki D, Abdalla S, El Gamal T, Harvey D, Jackson G, Platt S. Is it necessary to change instruments between sampling sites when taking multiple tissue specimens in musculoskeletal infections? *Ann R Coll Surg Engl.* 2018;100(7):563-565. https://publishing.rcseng.ac.uk/doi/10.1308/rcsann.2018.0097.

42. Aggarwal VK, Higuera C, Deirmengian G, Parvizi J, Austin MS. Swab cultures are not as effective as tissue cultures for diagnosis of periprosthetic joint infection. *Clin Orthop Relat Res.* 2013;471(10):3196-3203.

43. Rothenberg AC, Wilson AE, Hayes JP, O'Malley MJ, Klatt BA. Sonication of arthroplasty implants improves accuracy of periprosthetic joint infection cultures. *Clin Orthop Relat Res.* 2017;475(7):1827-1836.

44. Dudareva M, Barrett L, Figtree M, et al. Sonication versus tissue sampling for diagnosis of prosthetic joint and other orthopaedic device-related infections. *J Clin Microbiol.* 2018;56(12):e00688-18.

45. Van Diek FM, Albers CGM, Van Hooff ML, Meis JF, Goosen JHM. Low sensitivity of implant sonication when screening for infection in revision surgery. *Acta Orthop.* 2017;88(3): 294-299.

46. Grosso MJ, Frangiamore SJ, Yakubek G, Bauer TW, Iannotti JP, Ricchetti ET. Performance of implant sonication culture for the diagnosis of periprosthetic shoulder infection. *J Shoulder Elbow Surg.* 2018;27(2):211-216. https://doi.org/10.1016/j.jse.2017.08.008.

47. Liu H, Zhang Y, Li L, Zou HC. The application of sonication in diagnosis of periprosthetic joint infection. *Eur J Clin Microbiol Infect Dis.* 2017;36(1):1-9.

48. Peel TN, Dylla BL, Hughes JG, et al. Improved diagnosis of prosthetic joint infection by culturing periprosthetic tissue specimens in blood culture bottles. *mBio*. 2016;7(1):e01776-15. http://mbio.asm.org/lookup/doi/10.1128/mBio.01776-15.

49. Butler-Wu SM, Burns EM, Pottinger PS, et al. Optimization of periprosthetic culture for diagnosis of Propionibacterium acnes prosthetic joint infection. *J Clin Microbiol*. 2011;49(7):2490-2495.

50. Schäfer P, Fink B, Sandow D, Margull A, Berger I, Frommelt L. Prolonged bacterial culture to identify late periprosthetic joint infection: a promising strategy. *Clin Infect Dis*. 2008;47(11):1403-1409. https://academic.oup.com/cid/article-lookup/doi/10.1086/592973.

51. Bémer P, Plouzeau C, Tande D, et al. Evaluation of 16S rRNA gene PCR sensitivity and specificity for diagnosis of prosthetic joint infection: a prospective multicenter cross-sectional study. *J Clin Microbiol*. 2014;52(10):3583-3589.

52. Marín M, Garcia-Lechuz JM, Alonso P, et al. Role of universal 16S rRNA gene PCR and sequencing in diagnosis of prosthetic joint infection. *J Clin Microbiol*. 2012;50(3):583-589.

53. Gomez E, Cazanave C, Cunningham SA, et al. Prosthetic joint infection diagnosis using broad-range PCR of biofilms dislodged from knee and hip arthroplasty surfaces using sonication. *J Clin Microbiol*. 2012;50(11):3501-3508.

54. Renz N, Feihl S, Cabric S, Trampuz A. Performance of automated multiplex PCR using sonication fluid for diagnosis of periprosthetic joint infection: a prospective cohort. *Infection*. 2017;45:877-884.

55. Morgenstern C, Cabric S, Perka C, Trampuz A, Renz N. Synovial fluid multiplex PCR is superior to culture for detection of low-virulent pathogens causing periprosthetic joint infection. *Diagn Microbiol Infect Dis*. 2018;90(2):115-119. https://doi.org/10.1016/j.diagmicrobio.2017.10.016.

56. Suda AJ, Tinelli M, Beisemann ND, Weil Y, Khoury A, Bischel OE. Diagnosis of periprosthetic joint infection using alpha-defensin test or multiplex-PCR: ideal diagnostic test still not found. *Int Orthop*. 2017;41(7):1307-1313.

57. Portillo ME, Salvadó M, Sorli L, et al. Multiplex PCR of sonication fluid accurately differentiates between prosthetic joint infection and aseptic failure. *J Infect*. 2012;65(6):541-548.

58. Prieto-Borja L, Rodriguez-Sevilla G, Auñon A, et al. Evaluation of a commercial multiplex PCR (Unyvero i60®) designed for the diagnosis of bone and joint infections using prosthetic-joint sonication. *Enferm Infecc Microbiol Clin*. 2017;35(4):236-242. http://linkinghub.elsevier.com/retrieve/pii/S0213005X16302877.

59. Thoendel MJ, Jeraldo PR, Greenwood-Quaintance KE, et al. Identification of prosthetic joint infection pathogens using a shotgun metagenomics approach. *Clin Infect Dis*. 2018;67:1333-1338. https://academic.oup.com/cid/advance-article/doi/10.1093/cid/ciy303/4965775.

60. Ivy MI, Thoendel MJ, Jeraldo PR, et al. Direct detection and identification of prosthetic joint infection pathogens in synovial fluid by metagenomic shotgun sequencing. *J Clin Microbiol*. 2018;56(9):1-11.

61. Thoendel M, Jeraldo PR, Greenwood-Quaintance KE, et al. Impact of contaminating DNA in whole-genome amplification kits used for metagenomic shotgun sequencing for infection diagnosis. *J Clin Microbiol*. 2017;55(6):1789-1801.

62. Tarabichi M, Shohat N, Goswami K, et al. Diagnosis of periprosthetic joint infection: the potential of next-generation sequencing. *J Bone Joint Surg Am*. 2018;100:147-154.

63. Carreno JJ, Kenney RM, Lomaestro B. Vancomycin-associated renal dysfunction: where are we now? *Pharmacotherapy*. 2014;34(12):1259-1268.

64. Sakoulas G, Geriak M, Nizet V. Is a reported penicillin allergy sufficient grounds to forgo the multidimensional antimicrobial benefits of β-lactam antibiotics? *Clin Infect Dis*. 2018;68:157-164.

65. MacFadden Derek R, LaDelfa A, Leen J, et al. Impact of reported beta-lactam allergy on inpatient outcomes: a multicenter prospective cohort study. *Clin Infect Dis*. 2016;63(7):904-910.

66. Conterno LO, Turchi MD. Antibiotics for treating chronic osteomyelitis in adults (review) cochrane library. *Cochrane Database Syst Rev*. 2013;(9):CD004439.

67. Li H-K, Rombach I, Zambellas R, et al. Oral versus intravenous antibiotics for bone and joint infection. *N Engl J Med*. 2019;380(5):425-436. http://www.nejm.org/doi/10.1056/NEJMoa1710926.

68. Spellberg B, Lipsky BA. Systemic antibiotic therapy for chronic osteomyelitis in adults. *Clin Infect Dis*. 2012;54(3):393-407.

69. Senneville E, Joulie D, Legout L, et al. Outcome and predictors of treatment failure in total hip/knee prosthetic joint infections due to *Staphylococcus aureus*. *Clin Infect Dis*. 2011;53(4):334-340.

70. Lora-Tamayo J, Murillo O, Iribarren JA, et al. A large multicenter study of methicillin-susceptible and methicillin-resistant *Staphylococcus aureus* prosthetic joint infections managed with implant retention. *Clin Infect Dis*. 2013;56(2):182-194.

71. Zimmerli W, Widmer AF, Blatter M, Frei R, Ochsner PE. Role of rifampin for treatment of orthopedic implant – related staphylococcal infections a randomized controlled trial. *J Am Med Assoc*. 1998;279(19):1537-1541.

72. Lora-Tamayo J, Euba G, Cobo J, et al. Short- versus long-duration levofloxacin plus rifampicin for acute staphylococcal prosthetic joint infection managed with implant retention: a randomised clinical trial. *Int J Antimicrob Agents*. 2016;48(3):310-316. http://dx.doi.org/10.1016/j.ijantimicag.2016.05.021.

73. Puhto AP, Puhto T, Syrjala H. Short-course antibiotics for prosthetic joint infections treated with prosthesis retention. *Clin Microbiol Infect*. 2012;18(11):1143-1148. http://dx.doi.org/10.1111/j.1469-0691.2011.03693.x.

74. Chaussade H, Uçkay I, Vuagnat A, et al. Antibiotic therapy duration for prosthetic joint infections treated by Debridement and Implant Retention (DAIR): similar long-term remission for 6 weeks as compared to 12 weeks. *Int J Infect Dis*. 2017;63:37-42. http://dx.doi.org/10.1016/j.ijid.2017.08.002.

75. Lora-Tamayo J, Senneville É, Ribera A, et al. The not-so-good prognosis of streptococcal periprosthetic joint infection managed by implant retention: the results of a large multicenter study. *Clin Infect Dis*. 2017;64(12):1742-1752.

76. Huotari K, Vuorinen M, Rantasalo M. High cure rate for acute streptococcal prosthetic joint infections treated with debridement, antimicrobials, and implant retention in a specialized tertiary care center. *Clin Infect Dis*. 2018;67(8):1288-1290. https://academic.oup.com/cid/article/67/8/1288/4976482.

77. Jacobs AME, Van Hooff ML, Meis JF, Vos F, Goosen JHM. Treatment of prosthetic joint infections due to Propionibacterium. *Acta Orthop*. 2016;87(1):60-66.

78. Osmon DR, Berbari EF, Berendt AR, et al. Diagnosis and management of prosthetic joint infection: clinical practice guidelines by the Infectious Diseases Society of America. *Clin Infect Dis*. 2013;56(1):1-25.

79. Koyonos L, Zmistowski B, Della Valle CJ, Parvizi J. Infection control rate of irrigation and débridement for periprosthetic joint infection. *Clin Orthop Relat Res*. 2011;469(11):3043-3048.

80. Kurd MF, Ghanem E, Steinbrecher J, Parvizi J. Two-stage exchange knee arthroplasty: does resistance of the infecting organism influence the outcome? *Clin Orthop Relat Res*. 2010;468(8):2060-2066.

81. Mortazavi SMJ, Vegari D, Ho A, Zmistowski B, Parvizi J. Two-stage exchange arthroplasty for infected total knee arthroplasty: predictors of failure. *Clin Orthop Relat Res*. 2011;469(11):3049-3054.

82. Prendki V, Ferry T, Sergent P, et al. Prolonged suppressive antibiotic therapy for prosthetic joint infection in the elderly: a national multicentre cohort study. *Eur J Clin Microbiol Infect Dis*. 2017;36(9):1577-1585.

83. Rao N, Crossett LS, Sinha RK, Le Frock JL. Long-term suppression of infection in total joint arthroplasty. *Clin Orthop Relat Res*. 2003;414(414):55-60.

84. Pradier M, Robineau O, Boucher A, et al. Suppressive antibiotic therapy with oral tetracyclines for prosthetic joint infections: a retrospective study of 78 patients. *Infection*. 2018;46(1):39-47.

85. Keller SC, Cosgrove SE, Higgins Y, Piggott DA, Osgood G, Auwaerter PG. Role of suppressive oral antibiotics in orthopedic hardware infections for those not undergoing two-stage replacement surgery. *Open Forum Infect Dis.* 2016;3(4):1-9.
86. Weston JT, Mabry TM, Hanssen AD, Berry DJ, Abdel MP, Watts CD. Irrigation and debridement with chronic antibiotic suppression for the management of infected total knee arthroplasty: a contemporary analysis. *Bone Joint J.* 2018;100B(11):1471-1476.
87. Siqueira MBP, Saleh A, Klika AK, et al. Chronic suppression of periprosthetic joint infections with oral antibiotics increases infection-free survivorship. *J Bone Joint Surg Am.* 2014;97(15): 1220-1232.
88. Tice AD, Rehm SJ, Dalovisio JR, et al. Practice guidelines for outpatient parenteral antimicrobial therapy. IDSA guidelines. *Clin Infect Dis.* 2004;39:1651-1672.
89. Rybak M, Lomaestro B, Rotschafer JC, et al. Therapeutic monitoring of vancomycin in adult patients: a consensus review of the American Society of Health System Pharmacists, the Infectious Diseases Society of America, and the Society of Infectious Diseases Pharmacists. *Am J Health Syst Pharm.* 2009;66:82-98.
90. Liu C, Bayer A, Cosgrove SE, et al. Clinical practice guidelines by the Infectious Diseases Society of America for the treatment of methicillin-resistant Staphylococcus aureus infections in adults and children. *Clin Infect Dis.* 2011;52:e18-55.

chapter 75

Débridement and Implant Retention and Nonsurgical Options for Implant Salvage

Darin J. Larson, MD | Kevin L. Garvin, MD

INTRODUCTION

Total knee arthroplasty (TKA) has been one of the most successful procedures in the field of orthopedics over the course of the last several decades. High rates of patient satisfaction and ever-increasing implant survivorship have resulted in a substantial increase in demand for the operation. Although these operations have had a significant positive impact, complications still exist. As the volume of primary TKA continues to trend upward, rates of revision TKA due to a variety of causes have been projected to increase as well. Periprosthetic joint infections remain one of the most difficult of all of the complications to manage. While certain causes of revision have been decreasing, the relative rate of periprosthetic infections as a cause of revision has been increasing, now accounting for approximately 15% to 25% of all revision TKA procedures.[1-4] Current rates of prosthetic joint infection after primary TKA range from 0.4% to 2%, which has largely remained stable over the last decade.[5-12]

The goals of treatment of TKA infections are threefold: elimination of infection, provision of a functional limb in order to allow the patient to perform their daily activities, and alleviation of pain. In order to accomplish these goals, multiple techniques have been described utilizing a combination of surgical intervention with a course of culture-specific antibiotics. These techniques include (a) irrigation and débridement with implant retention, (b) one-stage reimplantation, (c) two-stage reimplantation, (d) arthrodesis, and (e) amputation. Chronic antibiotic suppression may also be considered, although this treatment option does not eradicate infection. Indications for antibiotic suppression will be discussed later in this chapter. In the United States, the current gold standard for treatment of most TKA infections is a two-stage arthroplasty with placement of an antibiotic cement spacer. Success rates have been in the range of 72% to 100%.[4-8,13-15] However, the potential for severe bone loss following explant and significant difficulties with mobility prior to reimplantation are causes for concern. This is even more troubling when considering the typical demographics of patients undergoing these large, staged procedures with a prolonged recovery, as these patients are more likely to be older with multiple medical comorbidities (i.e., diabetes, cancer, obesity). Two-stage reimplantation involves resection of all prosthetic components during the initial débridement with placement of an antibiotic-laden cement spacer, followed by a period of intravenous antibiotic administration, and eventually a return to the operating room for removal of the spacer, débridement, and reimplantation of new prosthetic components if there is evidence that the previous infection has been cleared.[5-7]

Prosthetic component retention, also known as débridement and implant retention (DAIR), has been studied as an alternative to two-stage reimplantation TKA. Indications for DAIR include clinically and radiographically well-fixed components, acute postoperative infections, or acute hematogenous infections as described by Tsukayama and Segawa,[16,17] absence of a draining sinus tract, and infection with a single, low-virulence organism that is susceptible to antibiotics.[18] These specific criteria will be discussed in depth later in this chapter. By retaining implants, bone stock may be preserved and the lengthy period of restricted weight-bearing and other functional limitations may be avoided. Management of periprosthetic infections involving component retention includes the following: (a) open irrigation and débridement with or without modular component exchange, (b) arthroscopic irrigation and débridement, (c) long-term antibiotic suppression without surgical intervention, and (d) serial joint aspirations combined with antibiotic administration (**Table 75-1**). While certain levels of success have been documented in the literature with component retention, these techniques have not matched the success rate of two-stage reimplantation. Outcomes with component retention can be improved if stringent indications for treatment are used.[16-21]

OPEN IRRIGATION AND DÉBRIDEMENT

Open irrigation and débridement with modular component exchange (including placement of a new polyethylene tibial implant) is the most frequently described method of component retention in the management of TKA infections. This is accomplished with an arthrotomy, typically

TABLE 75-1 Component Retention Methods and Indications in Periprosthetic Infections of the Knee

Treatment	Success Rate (%)	Indications	Comments
Open irrigation and débridement with or without polyethylene exchange	17.9%-100%	• Symptom duration under 4 wk • Low-virulence organism, susceptible to antibiotics • Absence of draining sinus tract • No evidence of radiographic or clinical loosening • No radiographic or clinical evidence of infection	• Combined with a postoperative course of culture-specific antibiotics • Failure to exchange the polyethylene component is a predictor of failure
Arthroscopic irrigation and débridement	38%-100%	• Same as open • Consider in patients with coagulopathies or those with high potential for wound healing problems	• Polyethylene component cannot be removed
Long-term suppressive antibiotics	18%-25%	• Refusal of further surgery • Patients unable to undergo an operation due to significant medical comorbidities • Infection with low-virulence organism • Ability to tolerate antibiotic side effects	• Potential for issues with compliance • May lead to antibiotic resistance • Contraindicated in presence of other noninfected implants
Serial aspirations	10%-15%	• Similar to suppressive antibiotics	• Limited data available regarding its use

utilizing the prior skin incision. Following the arthrotomy, a radical synovectomy of the knee including the medial and lateral gutters and posterior capsule as well as extensive lavage of the retained components is then undertaken. Care must be taken to perform a comprehensive débridement of all necrotic and infected tissues, as this can be a nidus for persistent infection. Removal of the polyethylene liner allows for improved exposure and subsequent débridement of the posterior capsule. Although a postoperative course of intravenous antibiotics for several weeks is a necessary part of treatment following débridement, antibiotics alone or in the setting of an insufficient synovectomy will be unable to eradicate the infection (**Fig. 75-1**). Thus, a thorough débridement is the essential component of this technique. No violation of the bone-prosthesis, cement-prosthesis, or bone-cement interfaces is necessary. However, these interfaces must be directly visualized to ensure that there is no evidence of loosening.[4,22]

Historically, open irrigation and débridement with polyethylene exchange has not been as successful at eradicating infection as two-stage reimplantation. A wide range of success rates with this technique has been described in the literature (**Table 75-2**).[23,24] Burger et al[25] followed 39 periprosthetic knee infections for an average of 4 years; only 7 of the 39 (17.9%) infections were successfully eliminated. Meehan and colleagues[26] reported a 100% retention rate in 13 patients with a mean follow-up of 5.8 years. The evidence is somewhat conflicting, as there is no standardized definition of "success" and "failure." Multiple studies have considered a case to be successful after multiple débridements as long as the prosthetic components are retained, whereas others have recorded failures if more than one surgical procedure is required.[4,7,24-26]

Certain cohorts do appear to be more amenable to irrigation and débridement with component retention. Multiple studies have discussed duration of symptoms prior to undergoing surgical intervention as the most important predictor of success. In general, the maximum amount of time allowed when considering retention of the prosthesis after symptom onset is 2 to 4 weeks. However, the true duration of infection may be difficult to ascertain, specifically within the first month following the index procedure. Thus, the duration of infection in the early postoperative period is typically quantified as the amount of time since the procedure was performed.[4,7,22,24,27,28]

When discussing the duration of symptoms, it is essential to differentiate infections in the early postoperative period and those that occur months to years after the initial arthroplasty. Tsukayama, Segawa, and colleagues have proposed a classification system based on the clinical presentation of periprosthetic joint infections. They describe four types of infections: (a) type-I infections are identified from positive cultures at the time of revision arthroplasty; (b) type-II infections are acute postoperative infections; (c) type-III infections are acute hematogenous infections; and (d) type-IV infections are chronic indolent infections that have been present for over 1 month. Acute postoperative knee infections occur within the first month following the index TKA; acute hematogenous infections are usually the result of a bacteremic event followed by acute symptom onset in the affected prosthetic joint within 48 hours. These acute hematogenous infectious can manifest after months to years without prior complication.[16,17,29] The duration of symptoms is of utmost importance in these situations. Gehrke et al[4] reported a failure rate exceeding 60% for late-presenting cases. Triantafyllopoulos et al[24] evaluated 78 periprosthetic knee infections with successful retention in 43 of the 78 knees (55.1%) at final follow-up. Symptom

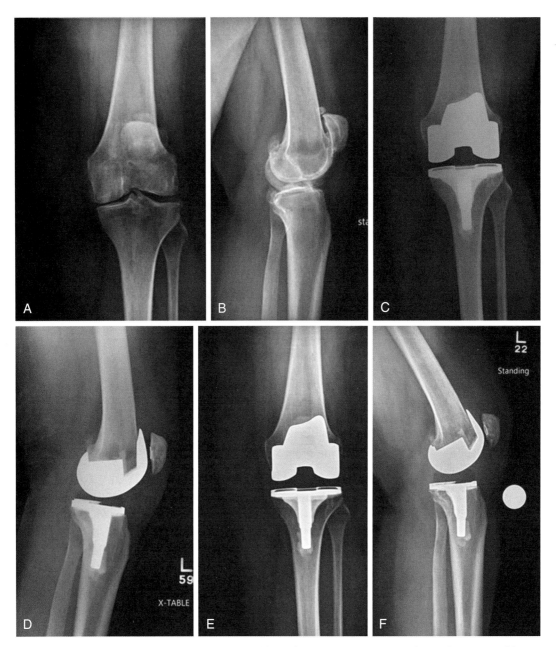

FIGURE 75-1   A 65-year-old woman with osteoarthritis was treated with a left total knee arthroplasty. She had an uneventful recovery for 4½ mo postoperatively until she suddenly developed a fever and left knee pain. Inflammatory markers were mildly elevated (erythrocyte sedimentation rate of 26, C-reactive protein of 1.1). The knee was aspirated and sent for cell count and culture. Gross purulence was noted during the aspiration. Synovial white blood cell count of 15,000 with 93% neutrophils was reported. Cultures grew methicillin-sensitive *Staphylococcus aureus*. **A** and **B:** Radiographs of the left knee prior to the index arthroplasty. **C** and **D:** Radiographs taken within 24 h of developing symptoms. No evidence of osteomyelitis, osteolysis, progressive radiolucent lines, or loosening is noted. The patient underwent open irrigation and débridement with extensive synovectomy and polyethylene exchange. All metallic components were retained. Dakin's solution irrigation was utilized. **E** and **F:** Postoperative radiographs obtained at 16-mo follow-up following the open débridement with no signs of recurrent infection.

present for longer than 5 days was an independent risk factor for failure. Urish et al[27] noted a higher risk of failure with symptoms for longer than 4 weeks compared to those with symptoms present for less than 1 week. In this study, an overall failure rate of 57.4% following irrigation and débridement with component retention was noted at 4 years, with most of the failures (89.9%) occurring within the first year following DAIR. Failure was defined as the need for any subsequent operation. In a study by Wasielewski

and colleagues,[30] seven acutely infected knees (defined as symptoms present for less than 2 weeks) were treated with open débridement and component retention. Eradication of infection was reported in five of seven knees (29% failure rate). The authors also reported failure of infection control in one of two chronically infected knees (symptoms present for longer than 2 weeks) treated with open débridement, noting that chronic infections were significantly less likely to be successful with attempted component retention.

Continued

TABLE 75-2   Summary of Studies on Irrigation and Débridement for Periprosthetic Infections of the Knee

Study	Number of Cases With PJI of the Knee	Mean Age of Patients (y)	Type of I&D	Pathogens	Follow-Up	Success Rate	Predictive Factors	Notes
Aboltins et al[52]	7	72.1 (range, 58-81)	Open with exchange of the polyethylene liner when possible	MRSA, MSSA, CNS	29 mo (6-65)	71.4%	n/a	One patient died at 6 mo due to causes unrelated to infection.
Azzam et al[36]	53	65 (range, 17-88)[a]	Open with exchange of polyethylene liner in 26 patients and reimplantation of preexisting liner in 27 patients after immersion in betadine solution	Methicillin-resistant staphylococci, methicillin-sensitive staphylococci, polymicrobial infections[a]	5.7 (2.4-10.4) y[a]	45.3%	Adjusted analysis: staphylococcal infections, ASA score, and purulence around the joint. Unadjusted analysis: urinary tract infections during hospital stay and persistent drainage after débridement.[a]	
Barberan et al[53]	28	74.6 ± 8.4	Not specified	Staphylococcus aureus, CNS	>1 y	57.2%	Duration of symptoms >6 mo, MRSA infection.[a]	
Bradbury et al[34]	19	n/a	Open with polyethylene exchange	MRSA	43 (27-55) mo	16%	n/a	Prosthesis retention under chronic suppressive treatment with antibiotics was considered successful outcome.
Brandt et al[54]	26	n/a	Not specified	S. aureus	Success group: 2345.5 (55-5221) d, failure group: 81 (15-614) d[a]	38.5%	I&D performed >2 d after onset of symptoms and primary arthroplasty related with negative outcomes.[a]	
Buller et al[55]	247	65 (range 12-94)[a]	Open with polyethylene exchange	Four groups: (1) MRSA, vancomycin-resistant Enterococcus, and MRSE; (2) methicillin-sensitive CNS or MSSA; (3) other Gram-positive organisms or fungus; and/or (4) Gram-negative organisms[a]	34 mo (range, 8 d-12.9 y)[a]	50.6%	Duration of symptoms, preoperative ESR, pathogen (group 1), previous infection.[a]	

TABLE 75-2   Summary of Studies on Irrigation and Débridement for Periprosthetic Infections of the Knee—Continued

Study	Number of Cases With PJI of the Knee	Mean Age of Patients (y)	Type of I&D	Pathogens	Follow-Up	Success Rate	Predictive Factors	Notes
Burger et al[25]	39	n/a	Open (fate of liner not specified)	Staphylococcal species, streptococcal species, Gram-negative bacteria, enterococci, polymicrobial	4.1 (1-13) y	17.9%	Duration of symptoms <2 wk, susceptible pathogens, absence of prolonged drainage or sinus tract, and absence of loosening were correlated with positive outcomes.	No clear statistical method reported for defining predictive factors.
Byren et al[32]	51	n/a	Open with polyethylene liner exchange or arthroscopic	MRSA, MSSA, CNS[a]	2.3 y[a]	74.5%	S. aureus infection, previous revision, and arthroscopic washout related with negative prognosis.[a]	
Chiu et al[56]	40	72.7 (range, 59-85)	Open with polyethylene liner exchange	MRSA, MSSA, CNS, Staphylococcus epidermidis, Gram-negative bacteria, streptococci, polymicrobial, Candida species	79 (36-143) mo	30%	Early postoperative (type I) and hematogenous (type III) infections correlated with better outcomes.	Only infected revision TKAs were studied. Chronic infections (n = 20) included in this cohort.
Chung et al[46]	16	70 (56-78)	Arthroscopic	Streptococci, MSSA, MRSA, CNS, Mycoplasma hominis, negative cultures	47 (24-86) mo	62.5%	n/a	Only patients with duration of symptoms less than 72 h, previously well-functioning prosthesis, and no radiographic signs of loosening were included.
Duque et al[49]	67	64.5 (36-82)	Open with polyethylene exchange and lavage with normal saline, betadine, Dakin's solution, and bacitracin	Non-MRSA Staphylococcus, MRSA, Enterococcus, Streptococcus, Pseudomonas, Peptostreptococcus, Escherichia sp., Serratia sp., Proteus sp., Prevotella sp., Granulicatella sp., Enterobacter sp., Citrobacter sp., Aerococcus sp.	4.81 (2.04-9.40) y	68.66%	All MRSA and Pseudomonas infections failed.	100% success rate with Streptococcus sp. and anaerobes.

Study	N	Mean age (range)	Procedure	Organisms	Follow-up	Success rate	Comments
Estes et al[22]	16	67 (range, 28-91)[a]	Staged open procedure with use of antibiotic impregnated cement beads[a]	MRSA, MSSA, CNS, Escherichia coli, streptococcal species, polymicrobial, Enterococcus faecalis, negative cultures	3.5 (1.2-7.5) y[a]	87.5%	n/a
Fehring et al[57]	46	61 (range, 17-89)[a]	Open with polyethylene liner exchange in 98% of cases	Susceptible and resistant staphylococci, others[a]	46 (24-106) mo[a]	37%	n/a
Fink et al[28]	39 (early periprosthetic) and 28 (acute hematogenous)	67.8 (30.0-80.0)	Open with modular component exchange and irrigation with octenidine	S. aureus, S epidermidis, other Staphylococcus species, Propionibacterium acnes, Streptococcus sp., others	41.8 (24-132) mo	71.6% overall, (82.1% early infections, 57.1% acute hematogenous)	Negative factors: longer time between procedure and first appearance of symptoms (>2 d), higher number of previous operations, higher ASA classification, and nicotine abuse.
Gardner et al[58]	44	70 (range, 48-94)	Open with polyethylene liner exchange	S. aureus, S. epidermidis, other Gram-positive bacteria, Gram-negative bacteria	5 (1-9) y	43.2%	n/a
Geurts et al[59]	20	69 (range, 27-93)[a]	Staged open procedure with use of gentamicin-PMMA beads and without exchange of polyethylene liner	S. aureus, CNS, streptococci, Enterobacter, Pseudomonas aeruginosa, P. acnes, polymicrobial, negative cultures	52 (3-202) mo	85%	Interval between symptom onset and treatment (cutoff 4 wk).[a]
Ilahi et al[43]	5	60.2 (range, 49-70)	Arthroscopic	Streptococci, CNS	41 (36-43) mo	100%	Very small case series.
Konigsberg et al[29]	22	60 (range, 25-86)[a]	Open with exchange of polyethylene liner	Staphylococcal species, streptococcal species, others[a]	56 (25-124) mo[a]	77.3%	Staphylococcal infection was the only negative predictive factor.[a]
Koyonos et al[60]	78	64 (range, 18-89)[a]	Open with exchange of polyethylene liner	Staphylococcal species, Gram-negative organisms, negative cultures[a]	54 (12-115) mo[a]	38.5%	Only staphylococcal infection independently predicted failure.[a]

(Continued)

TABLE 75-2   Summary of Studies on Irrigation and Débridement for Periprosthetic Infections of the Knee—Continued

Study	Number of Cases With PJI of the Knee	Mean Age of Patients (y)	Type of I&D	Pathogens	Follow-Up	Success Rate	Predictive Factors	Notes
Kuiper et al[61]	29	70 (success group), 69 (failure group)	Open with or without exchange of polyethylene liner and with or without the use of gentamicin sponges or beads	CNS, S. aureus, streptococcal species, E. coli, Enterobacter cloacae, E. faecalis, others[a]	35 (0-79) mo[a]	75.9%	Rheumatoid arthritis, symptoms >1 wk, late infection (>2 y from index procedure), ESR >60 mm, and CNS infection were correlated with negative outcome.	
Löwik et al[50]	86	73.2 y (standard deviation ± 11.5)	Open with optional exchange of modular components, gentamicin-impregnated beads, or sponges were inserted	S. aureus, Cutibacterium acnes, Bacteroides fragilis, Finegoldia magna, Proteus, Corynebacterium, others	Final follow-up not specified	62.8%	KLIC score used to predict failure in débridement and implant retention.	
Marculescu et al[31]	52 cases	74 (range, 23-95)[a]	Open with or without exchange of polyethylene liner[a]	Staphylococci, streptococci, enterococci, Gram-positive bacilli, Gram-negative bacilli, anaerobic, polymicrobial, negative cultures, fungi, others[a]	700 (1-2779) d[a]	60% at 2 y[a]	Univariate analysis: S. aureus, presence of sinus tract, and duration of symptoms ≥8 d correlated with adverse outcomes. Multivariate analysis: presence of sinus tract and duration of symptoms ≥8 d correlated with adverse outcomes.[a]	
Martinez-Pastor et al[62]	32	70.7 ± 11.3[a]	Open with exchange of polyethylene liner	Gram-negative bacilli	463 (344-704) d[a]	75%	Negative predictors: CRP >15 mg/dL, treatment not including fluoroquinolones.[a]	
Meehan et al[26]	13	70 (range, 44-86)[a]	Open. Liner exchange was performed in four patients	Streptococcal species	2120 (672-4015) d	100%	n/a	
Mont et al[38]	24 joints in 22 patients	66 (range, 46-80)	Open with exchange of polyethylene liner in 21 cases and reimplantation of preexisting liner in 3 cases after immersion in betadine solution	Staphylococcal species, streptococci, Gram-negative bacteria, Aspergillus	45.1 (24-140) mo	83.3%	n/a	

Study	No. of patients	Mean age (y)	Procedure	Organisms	Minimum 1-y follow-up	Success rate	Comments
Narayanan et al[51]	55	60.7 (success group), 58.7 (failure group)	Open with exchange of polyethylene liner	S. aureus, S. epidermidis, Staphylococcus lugdunensis, Actinomyces meyeri, Group B Streptococcus, P. acnes, P. granulosum, Pseudomonas, polymicrobial		82% (if treated within 2 wk), 50% after 2 wk	I&D after 2 wk was significantly more likely to fail.
Segawa et al[17]	17	n/a	Open with polyethylene liner exchange	Staphylococci, streptococci, enterococci	n/a	58.8%	n/a
Teeny et al[63]	21	58 (30-74)[b]	Open (fate of liner not specified)	Staphylococci, streptococci, Gram-negative bacteria, polymicrobial[b]	4 (2-12) y[b]	28.5%	n/a
Urish et al[27]	216	65.9 ± 12.2	Open with exchange of polyethylene liner	Culture-negative, S. aureus, others	31.5 (IQR 14.4-67.0) mo	49.5%	Culture-negative infection had highest risk of failure, followed by infection with S. aureus.
Vilchez et al[64]	35	70 ± 10.8[b]	Open with exchange of polyethylene liner	S. aureus	879.3 ± 205 d[b]	68.6%	Negative predictive factors: onset of infection ≤25 d after joint arthroplasty, CRP at admission >22 mg/dL, documented bacteremia and the need for a second débridement.[b]
Waldman et al[45]	16	72 (range, 57-82)	Arthroscopic	Staphylococci, streptococci, E. coli	64 (36-151) mo	38%	n/a
Zurcher-Pfund et al[65]	21	80	Open in 11 patients, arthroscopic in 10 patients	MRSA, MSSA, CNS, streptococci, E. coli, Clostridium septicum, Pasteurella multocida	7 (4-20) y	33%	Only patients with symptoms ≤7 d and without radiographic evidence of loosening were included.[b]

[a]Data include patients with PJI of the hip.
[b]Data include patients subjected to 2-stage revision.

ASA, American Society of Anesthesiologists; CNS, coagulase-negative staphylococci; CRP, C-reactive protein; ESR, erythrocyte sedimentation rate; MRSA, methicillin-resistant Staphylococcus aureus; MRSE, methicillin-resistant Staphylococcus epidermidis; MSSA, methicillin-sensitive Staphylococcus aureus; n/a, not available; TKA, total knee arthroplasty.

Updated from Triantafyllopoulos GK, Poultsides LA, Zhang W, Sculco PK, Ma Y, Sculco TP. Periprosthetic knee infections treated with irrigation and débridement: outcomes and preoperative predictive factors. J Arthroplasty. 2015;30(4):649-657.

Outcomes following urgent irrigation and débridement with polyethylene exchange in 22 infected prosthetic knees in the setting of acute hematogenous infection were studied by Konigsberg et al.[29] Of the 22 knees, 5 had recurrent infection at a follow-up of a minimum of 2 years. Following the procedure, culture-specific parenteral antibiotics were administered for 6 weeks under the direction of the Infectious Disease service. A high mortality rate (25%) was noted in the study, but the authors postulated that this was due to poor overall patient health and not directly related to the infection. In a study by Gardner et al,[7] 44 patients were evaluated with an average duration of symptoms of 8.4 days prior to operative intervention and followed for a minimum of 1 year. Open débridement with component retention was considered a failure if a second procedure or long-term antibiotic suppression was necessary. Failure was reported in 25 of 44 (56.8%) knees at an average of 167 days following the procedure. Marculescu et al[31] reviewed 99 prosthetic joint infections and concluded that symptoms persisting longer than 8 days correlated with a higher rate of failure. Fink et al[28] looked at outcomes after acute periprosthetic infections occurring after the index procedure compared to outcomes after treatment for an acute hematogenous infection. Irrigation and débridement with component retention was much more successful for the acute postoperative group (82.1%) than the hematogenous infection group (57.1%). This raises the question of whether the symptoms originated from a new infection or, in the case of the hematogenous group, if a subacute indolent infection became recently symptomatic. In this study, a higher failure rate was reported with symptom duration longer than 2 days. The authors of this study associated this higher failure rate to the rapid formation of biofilm.

Biofilm production can make eradication of bacteria difficult. Certain types of bacteria can collect on protein-coated surfaces and produce a glycocalyx or polysaccharide film. Bacteria within a biofilm exhibit characteristics that increase resistance to antibiotics including gene transfer, altered local environment resulting in increased acidity, and production of protective enzymes. As time after symptom onset increases, the risk of biofilm maturation also increases, making treatment exponentially more difficult. Gehrke et al[4] have suggested that biofilm formation can occur within a matter of hours, not days. Rifampin has been identified as being bactericidal against biofilm-producing *Staphylococcal* species, but rapidly develops resistance if it is used in isolation.[15,22]

As mentioned earlier, several studies have reported failure of the initial débridement, but eventual control of the infection (**Fig. 75-2**). Choi and colleagues[5] evaluated 32 prosthetic knees treated with débridement and retention. Infection control after a single procedure was found in only 31% after an initial débridement, but did improve to 81% at final follow-up after undergoing an average of 1.7 additional procedures. Two independent predictors for failure were reported: *Staphylococcus aureus* infection and failure to exchange polyethylene. The authors stated that correct identification of a pathogen is essential for successful treatment. Byren et al[32] reported a 75% success rate

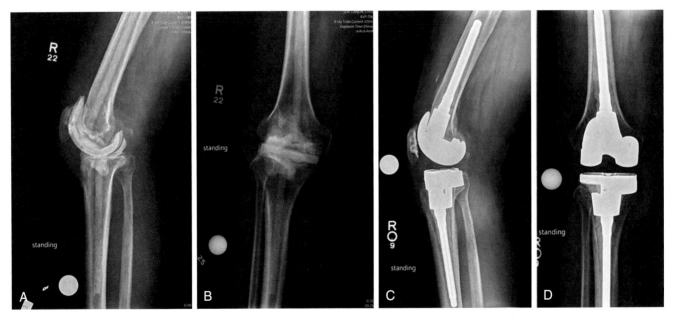

FIGURE 75-2 A 61-year-old male who underwent a right total knee arthroplasty. Postoperatively, his course was complicated by persistent wound issues. He was eventually taken back to the operating room approximately 6 mo later for open irrigation and débridement with polyethylene exchange. His components were well-fixed at that time. Tissue was obtained at the time of débridement; Gram stain was positive for mixed Gram-positive cocci, but all cultures were initially negative. He received a 6-wk course of antibiotics. His infection persisted, and he eventually underwent resection of his components 2 mo later. An antibiotic spacer was placed, and a gastrocnemius muscle flap was performed. He required multiple débridements prior to reimplantation. Cultures eventually grew *Propionibacterium acnes*. He eventually underwent successful reimplantation. No evidence of recurrence was noted 4 y postoperatively. **A** and **B:** Placement of a static antibiotic spacer. **C** and **D:** After successful reimplantation of total knee arthroplasty components.

with débridement and component retention in 51 knees over a 2-year follow-up period. In this study, repeat irrigation and débridement was not considered to be a failure. Symptom duration was not specified. Although many early postoperative infections and acute hematogenous infections can be successfully treated with open débridement and component retention, multiple operations may occasionally be necessary. Each subsequent débridement will theoretically decrease the bacterial load.[6]

Although timing of treatment has been identified as the most important factor in treatment as evidenced by Tsukayama, Segawa, and colleagues,[16,17] other factors predicting success of débridement with component retention play a role as well, including (a) correct identification of the offending low-virulence organism with institution of culture-specific antibiotics, (b) absence of component loosening (radiographically or based on intraoperative findings), (c) absence of a draining sinus tract, (d) acceptable condition of bone and soft tissues surrounding the implant, and (e) absence of radiographic/clinical signs of persistent infection (osteolysis or osteomyelitis) (**Fig. 75-3**).[7,15,19,33,34]

According to the majority of studies, certain bacteria are more prone to cause treatment failure than others. *S. aureus* is cited as one of the most common offenders.[6] Urish et al[27] reported that culture-negative infection had the highest risk of failure, followed by *S. aureus*. Even in the acute setting, a higher failure rate (65%) in attempted implant retention was noted with Gram-positive bacteria in a study by Deirmengian et al.[35] They concluded that this was likely due to biofilm produced by *Staphylococcus*. A 92% failure rate was found in knees infected with *S. aureus* compared to 44% in knees infected with other

Gram-positive bacteria. Of the Gram-positive failures, 40% had subsequent infection with the same organism. Bradbury et al[34] evaluated 19 prosthetic knee infections in the setting of methicillin-resistant *S. aureus*. Secondary procedures were required in 16 of the 19 cases (84% failure rate). Symptom duration did not seem to be predictive of failure in this study; the 3 successful cases underwent débridement and polyethylene exchange after an average of 11.6 days, and the 16 failures underwent surgery at an average of 4.4 days following the onset of symptoms. In the study by Gardner and colleagues,[7] 71% of infections caused by *S. aureus* failed compared to failure in 29% of cases as a result of *Staphylococcus epidermidis*. However, no difference in failure rate was noted between methicillin-sensitive *S. aureus* and methicillin-resistant *S. aureus* (MRSA) infections. Azzam et al[36] reported on 104 patients with a mean follow-up of 5.7 years. Failure was noted in 56% of all cases, but a higher proportion of failures were associated with periprosthetic infections caused by *S. aureus*. Triantafyllopoulos[24] identified failure of component retention in 54.5% of cases due to MRSA. In contrast to the aforementioned studies, others have demonstrated no significant difference in failure rates with regard to species of bacteria.[28]

Progressive radiolucent lines or intraoperative findings of component loosening are contraindications to component retention. These findings are typically noted late in the infectious process and necessitate component removal and two-stage reimplantation. Loosening of the components creates a potential space at the interfaces between the bone, cement, and implants. Bacteria can become sequestered in this potential space, rendering attempts at component retention futile.[4,19]

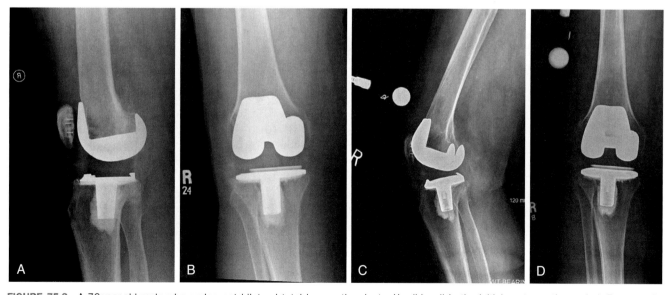

FIGURE 75-3 A 76-year-old male who underwent bilateral total knee arthroplasty. He did well in the initial postoperative period. Four months following his index procedure, he developed acute-onset pain in his right knee. His right knee was aspirated and a synovial white blood cell count of 68,000 was reported. Cultures revealed group G streptococcus. He was taken to the operating room the following day for open irrigation and débridement with polyethylene exchange. He remained on suppressive oral antibiotics following his procedure. No evidence of recurrent infection was noted at final follow-up 14 y postoperatively. **A** and **B:** 1 y status post irrigation and débridement with polyethylene exchange. **C** and **D:** Final follow-up, 14 y postoperatively, with no radiographic evidence of loosening or recurrent infection.

Presence of a draining sinus tract following TKA is an ominous finding suggestive of soft-tissue compromise.[31,36,37] In a retrospective review of 60 periprosthetic knee infections, Burger et al[25] attempted débridement with component retention in 39 cases. Of these 39 cases, a draining sinus tract was noted in 17 knees. None of these 17 knees were salvageable at the completion of the study.

Radiographic evidence of osteomyelitis noted preoperatively, usually in the form of periprosthetic osteolysis, or clinical evidence found at the time of surgery is another contraindication to attempts at implant retention. As mentioned previously, abnormal radiographic findings are not typically seen until the more advance stages of a prosthetic joint infection, indicating more extensive involvement of the bone and surrounding soft tissues. Mont et al[38] reported a high success rate (83%) after irrigation and débridement with implant retention in periprosthetic knee infections. In the four failed cases, pathologic changes in the bone consistent with chronic osteomyelitis were documented at the time of surgery. Successful treatment in these cases would necessitate significant bony débridement, potentially destabilizing implanted components.

Additional factors contributing to the success of attempted implant retention have also been described, some of which are controversial. Successful procedures are more likely in young and healthy patients,[36] whereas failures can be predicted by advanced age.[35] Purulence around the joint at the time of débridement has also been reported as a negative risk factor.[36] Silva et al[39] report poor outcomes with hinged prostheses and immunocompromised patients. Gehrke et al[4] also agree that these procedures should not be attempted in patients with diabetes mellitus, rheumatoid arthritis, or other immunocompromising conditions. However, in a retrospective multicenter review of 216 infected TKA, Urish et al[27] discussed that, when adjusted, American Society of Anesthesiologists score, diabetes mellitus, and rheumatoid arthritis do not predict failure of irrigation and débridement with component retention.

Poor outcomes have been reported following failed open irrigation and débridement with implant retention. Studies report inferior outcomes of subsequent procedures.[4,27] Sherrell et al[40] noted failure in 28 of 83 (34%) infected TKA following two-stage reimplantation procedures in patients who had previously undergone irrigation and débridement with attempted implant retention. In contrast, others have documented successful treatment with two-stage reimplantation or arthrodesis following failure of open débridement with retention.[30,38]

ARTHROSCOPIC IRRIGATION AND DÉBRIDEMENT

When performing arthroscopic irrigation and débridement, the technique involves flushing a copious amount of fluid through the classically described anterolateral and anteromedial portals. Accessory portals, including superolateral, superomedial, posteromedial, and posterolateral portals, may be utilized as needed if further visualization or access is necessary. Many studies advocate irrigating the infected joint with at least 12 L of fluid. During the procedure, an extensive synovectomy is performed with a motorized shaver. Thorough débridement of the suprapatellar pouch, medial and lateral gutters, intercondylar notch, bone-implant interface, and posterior capsule is essential. At the end of the procedure, all implants are left in place. Postoperatively, as with open procedures, a course of culture-directed antibiotics is indicated, typically for a period of 6 weeks or more. Indications for arthroscopic procedures are essentially identical to those listed for open procedures: short duration of symptoms, no evidence of loosening or osteomyelitis clinically or radiographically, absence of a draining sinus tract, and presence of a low-virulence organism.[41-43]

Multiple studies have described lower rates of success with arthroscopic débridement compared to open treatment. While minimally invasive, modular component removal is not achievable. This may result in incomplete eradication of bacteria, particularly if a biofilm has already formed. If the accessory portals are not used, full access to the posterior capsule is nearly impossible; this may also contribute to an incomplete débridement.[28,32,44] As previously noted, failure to exchange the polyethylene insert has been identified as an independent factor for failure.[5] Although success rates may be lower than open procedures, these less-invasive operations may be an option for patients with significant medical comorbidities, coagulopathies, or those patients who are at higher risk for wound healing complications with larger incisions.

Results from the literature regarding arthroscopic débridement and retention must be interpreted with caution, as many of these studies are based on small numbers of patients. Wasielewski et al[30] reported successful arthroscopic treatment in a single patient (100%) with an acute prosthetic knee infection. This patient was included within a larger cohort of patients treated with an open procedure. Ilahi et al[43] similarly noted a high level of success in a small series. All five knees treated with arthroscopic débridement had successfully retained their components without evidence of recurrent infection at a mean follow-up of 41 months. As in other studies, these patients were treated after a short duration of symptoms (under 7 days) and had been infected with a single, low-virulence organism that was susceptible to antibiotics.

Not all studies investigating arthroscopic débridement have had high levels of success. Waldman et al[45] reported failures in 10 of 16 infected TKA (38% success rate). In this study, indications for arthroscopic management included symptom duration of 1 week or less, no signs of loosening, and patients who were anticoagulated or medically unfit for open procedures. Byren and colleagues[32] compared the results of arthroscopic and open débridement. Success was noted in 88% of the open cases, but only 47% of the patients managed with arthroscopy. Further complicating interpretation of these studies, techniques and postoperative treatment regimens have not been standardized. Liu et al[42] reported successful treatment in 15 of 17 (88%) infected TKA with arthroscopic débridement. In their series, a continuous antibiotic irrigation and suction system was utilized for several days following the procedure. Chung et al[46] evaluated outcomes of arthroscopic débridement guided by C-reactive protein (CRP) levels. Initially, 10 of 16 knees (62.5%) successfully retained their implants after an arthroscopic débridement. In the remaining six infected TKA with persistently elevated CRP levels, all eventually underwent open irrigation and débridement with polyethylene exchange resulting in eradication of the infection.

LONG-TERM ANTIBIOTIC SUPPRESSION

Long-term antibiotic suppression without operative intervention has also been described as an implant retention method in the setting of an infected TKA. Although the infection cannot be completely eliminated without surgical débridement, the goal is infection control while maintaining function of the knee. This treatment should only be used in certain situations. Indications for antibiotic suppression include (a) significant medical comorbidities precluding operative intervention, (b) single, low-virulence organism that is susceptible to oral antibiotics, (c) side effects of the medication must be tolerable, (d) no radiographic evidence of loose components, and (e) patient refusal of any further surgical procedure. Garcia-Ramos Garcia et al discussed severe bone loss and poor quality of surrounding soft tissues as additional indications for antibiotic suppression. However, monitoring is essential due to the potential for negative effects on multiple organ systems.[47] Contraindications include the presence of other noninfected implants, such as artificial heart valves or other total joint prostheses.[4,19,44] As in any situation requiring long-term antibiotic use, concerns of bacteria developing antibiotic resistance exist.

Success rates of long-term suppression with antibiotics have been abysmal. In a multicenter study, Bengtson and Knutson reported successful treatment in only 40 of 225 infected total knees (18%).[48] Other sources have reported a success rate of 25%.[19] To our knowledge, no other large-scale studies evaluating the outcomes of antibiotic suppression in infected TKA have been performed.

SERIAL ASPIRATIONS

Multiple aspirations have been proposed as a method of implant retention. The technique involves repetitive aspirations of an infected TKA in order to reduce bacterial load. Parenteral antibiotics are given in addition to the serial aspirations. A paucity of data regarding outcomes of serial aspirations in the setting of periprosthetic knee infections is available. Low bacterial clearance rates have been noted in the literature (10% to 15%).[20] In fact, complete eradication may be impossible due to a lack of a thorough débridement. This treatment should be reserved for patients unable to undergo any surgical procedure. Other indications for this technique are comparable to those listed for long-term antibiotic use listed previously.

CONCLUSION

TKA is one of the most successful operations for patients suffering from knee arthritis. However, complications have not been completely eliminated. Of the known complications after TKA, periprosthetic infection is arguably the most difficult to manage. Two-stage reimplantation has been well-documented as the gold standard in the treatment of these infections. However, retention of the implants has been studied as an option to reduce the morbidity and prolonged functional limitations produced by these staged procedures. Multiple strategies to retain the implants have been described. Of these strategies, open irrigation and débridement with exchange of the modular components has had a variable success rate.

Open débridement with polyethylene exchange is best reserved for patients meeting specific criteria. The duration of infection has been listed as the most important predictor of success or failure in cases of débridement. Treatments occurring when symptoms have been present for 4 weeks or less have had the best results. Other factors predicting success include (a) absence of a draining sinus tract, (b) no evidence of radiographic or clinical loosening of components, (c) infection with a single, low-virulence organism that is susceptible to antibiotics, and (d) lack of radiographic evidence of infection. Following a thorough débridement, a course of antibiotics is administered. If all of the above criteria are met, further surgical procedures and component explant may potentially be avoided.

Arthroscopic irrigation and débridement, long-term antibiotic suppression, and serial aspirations have also been discussed as potential techniques for implant retention. However, a limited amount of data is available supporting their utilization.

REFERENCES

1. Khan M, Osman K, Green G, Haddad FS. The epidemiology of failure in total knee arthroplasty: avoiding your next revision. *Bone Joint J.* 2016;98-B(1 suppl A):105-112.
2. Bozic KJ, Kurtz SM, Lau E, et al. The epidemiology of revision total knee arthroplasty in the United States. *Clin Orthop Relat Res.* 2010;468(1):45-51.
3. Delanois RE, Mistry JB, Gwam CU, Mohamed NS, Choksi US, Mont MA. Current epidemiology of revision total knee arthroplasty in the United States. *J Arthroplasty.* 2017;32(9):2663-2668.
4. Gehrke T, Alijanipour P, Parvizi J. The management of an infected total knee arthroplasty. *Bone Joint J.* 2015;97-B(10 suppl A):20-29.
5. Choi HR, von Knoch F, Zurakowski D, Nelson S, Malchau H. Can implant retention be recommended for treatment of infected TKA? *Clin Orthop Relat Res.* 2011;469:961-969.

6. Garvin KL, Konigsberg BS. Infection following total knee arthroplasty: prevention and management. *Instr Course Lect.* 2012;61:411-419.

7. Gardner J, Gioe TJ, Tatman P. Can this prosthesis be saved? Implant salvage attempts in infected primary TKA. *Clin Orthop Relat Res.* 2011;469:970-976.

8. Namba RS, Inacio MC, Paxton EW. Risk factors associated with deep surgical site infections after primary total knee arthroplasty: an analysis of 56,216 knees. *J Bone Joint Surg Am.* 2013;95(9):775-782.

9. Mahomed NN, Barrett J, Katz JN, Baron JA, Wright J, Losina E. Epidemiology of total knee replacement in the United States Medicare population. *J Bone Joint Surg Am.* 2005;87(6):1222-1228.

10. Kurtz SM, Ong KL, Lau E, Bozic KJ, Berry D, Parvizi J. Prosthetic joint infection risk after TKA in the Medicare population. *Clin Orthop Relat Res.* 2010;468(1):52-56.

11. Khatod M, Inacio M, Paxton EW, et al. Knee replacement: epidemiology, outcomes, and trends in Southern California: 17,080 replacements from 1995 through 2004. *Acta Orthop.* 2008;79(6):812-819.

12. Inacio MC, Paxton EW, Chen Y, et al. Leveraging electronic medical records for surveillance of surgical site infection in a total joint replacement population. *Infect Control Hosp Epidemiol.* 2011;32(4):351-359.

13. Mortazavi SM, Vegari D, Ho A, Zmistowski B, Parvizi J. Two-stage exchange arthroplasty for infected total knee arthroplasty: predictors of failure. *Clin Orthop Relat Res.* 2011;469:3049-3054.

14. Haddad FS, Sukeik M, Alazzawi S. Is single-stage revision according to a strict protocol effective in treatment of chronic knee arthroplasty infections? *Clin Orthop Relat Res.* 2015;473:8-14.

15. Trebse R, Pisot V, Trampuz A. Treatment of infected retained implants. *J Bone Joint Surg Br.* 2005;87(2):249-256.

16. Tsukayama DT, Estrada R, Gustilo RB. Infection after total hip arthroplasty. A study of the treatment of one hundred and six infections. *J Bone Joint Surg Am.* 1996;78:512-523.

17. Segawa H, Tsukayama DT, Kyle RF, Becker DA, Gustilo RB. Infection after total knee arthroplasty. A retrospective study of the treatment of eighty-one infections. *J Bone Joint Surg Am.* 1999;81(10):1434-1445.

18. Garvin KL, Miller RE, Gilbert TM, White AM, Lyden ER. Late reinfection may recur more than 5 years after reimplantation of THA and TKA: analysis of pathogen factors. *Clin Orthop Relat Res.* 2018;476(2):345-352.

19. Severson EP, Perry KI, Hanssen AD. The infected total knee replacement. In: Scott WN, ed. *Insall & Scott Surgery of the Knee.* 6th ed. Philadelphia: Elsevier; 2018:1916-1926.

20. Mulvey TJ, Thornhill TS, Kelly MA, Healy WL. Complications associated with total knee arthroplasty. In: Pellicci PM, Tria AJ, Garvin KL, eds. *Orthopaedic Knowledge Update. Hip and Knee Reconstruction 2.* Rosemont, IL: American Academy of Orthopaedic Surgeons, 2000:323-329.

21. Krebs VE, Malkani AL, Ulrich SD, et al. Complications of knee arthroplasty. In: Mont MA, Tanzer M, eds. *Orthopaedic Knowledge Update. Hip and Knee Reconstruction 5.* Rosemont, IL: American Academy of Orthopaedic Surgeons, 2017:233-266.

22. Estes CS, Spangehl MJ, Clarke HD. Irrigation and débridement with component retention for acute periprosthetic total knee arthroplasty infections. In: Scuderi GR, ed. *Techniques in Revision Hip and Knee Arthroplasty.* 1st ed. Philadelphia, PA: Elsevier Saunders: 2015:271-279.

23. Haleem AA, Berry DJ, Hanssen AD. Mid-term to long-term followup of two-stage reimplantation for infected total knee arthroplasty. *Clin Orthop Relat Res.* 2004;428:35-39.

24. Triantafyllopoulos GK, Poultsides LA, Zhang W, Sculco PK, Ma Y, Sculco TP. Periprosthetic knee infections treated with irrigation and débridement: outcomes and preoperative predictive factors. *J Arthroplasty.* 2015;30(4):649-657.

25. Burger RR, Basch T, Hopson CN. Implant salvage in infected total knee arthroplasty. *Clin Orthop Relat Res.* 1991;273:105-112.

26. Meehan AM, Osmon DR, Duffy MC, Hanssen AD, Keating MR. Outcome of penicillin-susceptible streptococcal prosthetic joint infection treated with débridement and retention of the prosthesis. *Clin Infect Dis.* 2003;36(7):845-849.

27. Urish K, Bullock A, Kreger A, et al. A multicenter study of irrigation and débridement in total knee arthroplasty periprosthetic joint infection: treatment failure is high. *J Arthroplasty.* 2018;33(4):1154-1159.

28. Fink B, Schuster P, Schwenninger C, Frommelt L, Oremek D. A standardized regimen for the treatment of acute postoperative infections and acute hematogenous infections associated with hip and knee arthroplasties. *J Arthroplasty.* 2017;32(4):1255-1261.

29. Konigsberg BS, Della Valle CJ, Ting NT, Qiu F, Sporer SM. Acute hematogenous infection following total hip and knee arthroplasty. *J Arthroplasty.* 2014;29(3):469-472.

30. Wasielewski RC, Barden RM, Rosenberg AG. Results of different surgical procedures on total knee arthroplasty infections. *J Arthroplasty.* 1996;11:931.

31. Marculescu CE, Berbari EF, Hanssen AD, et al. Outcome of prosthetic joint infections treated with débridement and retention of components. *Clin Infect Dis.* 2006;42:471-478.

32. Byren I, Bejon P, Atkins BL, et al. One hundred and twelve infected arthroplasties treated with 'DAIR' (débridement, antibiotics and implant retention): antibiotic duration and outcome. *J Antimicrob Chemother.* 2009;63:1264-1271.

33. Deirmengian C, Greenbaum J, Stern J, et al. Open débridement of acute Gram-positive infections after total knee arthroplasty. *Clin Orthop Relat Res.* 2003;416:129-134.

34. Bradbury T, Fehring TK, Taunton M, et al. The fate of acute methicillin-resistant *Staphylococcus aureus* periprosthetic knee infections treated by open débridement and retention of components. *J Arthroplasty.* 2009;24(6 suppl):101-104.

35. Deirmengian C, Greenbaum J, Lotke PA, Booth RE Jr, Lonner JH. Limited success with open débridement and retention of components in the treatment of acute *Staphylococcus aureus* infections after total knee arthroplasty. *J Arthroplasty.* 2003;18(7 suppl 1):22-26.

36. Azzam KA, Seeley M, Ghanem E, Austin MS, Purtill JJ, Parvizi J. Irrigation and débridement in the management of prosthetic joint infection: traditional indications revisited. *J Arthroplasty.* 2010;25:1022-1027.

37. Parvizi J, Jacovides C, Zmistowski B, Jung KA. Definition of periprosthetic joint infection: is there a consensus? *Clin Orthop Relat Res.* 2011;469:3022-3030.

38. Mont MA, Waldman B, Banerjee C, Pacheco IH, Hungerford DS. Multiple irrigation, débridement, and retention of compartments in infected total knee arthroplasty. *J Arthroplasty.* 1997;12:426-433.

39. Silva M, Tharani R, Schmalzried TP. Results of direct exchange or débridement of the infected total knee arthroplasty. *Clin Orthop Relat Res.* 2002;404:125-131.

40. Sherrell JC, Fehring TK, Odum S, et al. The Chitranjan Ranawat Award: fate of two-stage reimplantation after failed irrigation and débridement for periprosthetic knee infection. *Clin Orthop Relat Res.* 2011;469:18-25.

41. Miles J, Parratt MT. Arthroscopic débridement of infected total knee arthroplasty. In: Rodríguez-Merchán E, Oussedik S, eds. *The Infected Total Knee Arthroplasty.* 1st ed. Cham, Switzerland: Springer: 2018:127-131.

42. Liu CW, Kuo CL, Chuang SY, et al. Results of infected total knee arthroplasty treated with arthroscopic débridement and continuous antibiotic irrigation system. *Indian J Orthop.* 2013;47:93-97.

43. Ilahi OA, Al-Habbal GA, Bocell JR, Tullos HS, Huo MH. Arthroscopic débridement of acute periprosthetic septic arthritis of the knee. *Arthroscopy.* 2005;21(3):303-306.

44. Leone JM, Hanssen AD. Management of infection at the site of a total knee arthroplasty. *Instr Course Lect.* 2006;55:449-461.

45. Waldman BJ, Hostin E, Mont MA, Hungerford DS. Infected total knee arthroplasty treated by arthroscopic irrigation and débridement. *J Arthroplasty.* 2000;15(4):430-436.

46. Chung JY, Ha CW, Park YB, Song YJ, Yu KS. Arthroscopic débridement for acutely infected prosthetic knee: any role for infection control and prosthesis salvage? *Arthroscopy.* 2014;30:599-606.

47. Garcia-Ramos Garcia JA, Rico-Nieto A, Rodriguez Merchan E. Antibiotic suppression in the infected total knee arthroplasty. In: Rodríguez-Merchán E, Oussedik S, eds. *The Infected Total Knee Arthroplasty.* 1st ed. Cham, Switzerland: Springer; 2018:123-126.

48. Bengtson S, Knutson K. The infected knee arthroplasty. A 6-year follow-up of 357 cases. *Acta Orthop Scand.* 1991;62:301-311.

49. Duque AF, Post ZD, Lutz RW, Orozco FR, Pulido SH, Ong AC. Is there still a role for irrigation and débridement with liner exchange in acute periprosthetic total knee infection? *J Arthroplasty.* 2017;32(4):1280-1284.

50. Löwik CAM, Jutte PC, Tornero E, et al. Predicting failure in early acute prosthetic joint infection treated with débridement, antibiotics, and implant retention: external validation of the KLIC score. *J Arthroplasty.* 2018;33(8):2582-2587.

51. Narayanan R, Anoushiravani AA, Elbuluk AM, Chen KK, Adler EM, Schwarzkopf R. Irrigation and débridement for early periprosthetic knee infection: is it effective? *J Arthroplasty.* 2018;33(6):1872-1878.

52. Aboltins CA, Page MA, Buising KL, et al. Treatment of staphylococcal prosthetic joint infections with debridement, prosthesis retention and oral rifampicin and fusidic acid. *Clin Microbiol Infect.* 2007;13(6):586.

53. Barberan J, Aguilar L, Carroquino G, et al. Conservative treatment of staphylococcal prosthetic joint infections in elderly patients. *Am J Med.* 2006;119(11):993.e7.

54. Brandt CM, Sistrunk WW, Duffy MC, et al. *Staphylococcus aureus* prosthetic joint infection treated with debridement and prosthesis retention. *Clin Infect Dis.* 1997;24(5):914.

55. Buller LT, Sabry FY, Easton RW, et al. The preoperative prediction of success following irrigation and debridement with polyethylene exchange for hip and knee prosthetic joint infections. *J Arthroplasty.* 2012;27(6):857.

56. Chiu FY, Chen CM. Surgical debridement and parenteral antibiotics in infected revision total knee arthroplasty. *Clin Orthop Relat Res.* 2007;461:130.

57. Fehring TK, OdumSM, Berend KR, et al. Failure of irrigation and debridement for early postoperative periprosthetic infection. *Clin Orthop Relat Res.* 2013;471(1):250.

58. Gardner J, Gioe TJ, Tatman P. Can this prosthesis be saved? Implant salvage attempts in infected primary TKA. *Clin Orthop Relat Res.* 2011;469(4):970.

59. Geurts JA, Janssen DM, Kessels AG, et al. Good results in postoperative and hematogenous deep infections of 89 stable total hip and knee replacements with retention of prosthesis and local antibiotics. *Acta Orthop.* 2013;84(6):509.

60. Koyonos L, Zmistowski B, Della Valle CJ, et al. Infection control rate of irrigation and debridement for periprosthetic joint infection. *Clin Orthop Relat Res.* 2011;469(11):3043.

61. Kuiper JW, Vos SJ, Saouti R, et al. Prosthetic joint-associated infections treated with DAIR (debridement, antibiotics, irrigation, and retention): analysis of risk factors and local antibiotic carriers in 91 patients. *Acta Orthop.* 2013;84(4):380.

62. Martinez-Pastor JC, Munoz-Mahamud E, Vilchez F, et al. Outcome of acute prosthetic joint infections due to gram-negative bacilli treated with open debridement and retention of the prosthesis. *Antimicrob Agents Chemother.* 2009;53(11):4772.

63. Teeny SM, Dorr L, Murata G, et al. Treatment of infected total knee arthroplasty. Irrigation and debridement versus two-stage reimplantation. *J Arthroplasty.* 1990;5(1):35.

64. Vilchez F, Martinez-Pastor JC, Garcia-Ramiro S, et al. Outcome and predictors of treatment failure in early post-surgical prosthetic joint infections due to *Staphylococcus aureus* treated with debridement. *Clin Microbiol Infect.* 2011;17(3):439.

65. Zurcher-Pfund L, Uckay I, Legout L, et al. Pathogen-driven decision for implant retention in the management of infected total knee prostheses. *Int Orthop.* 2013;37(8):1471.

chapter 76

Reimplantation After Infection

Charles S. Carrier, MD | Antonia F. Chen, MD, MBA

INTRODUCTION

Reimplantation during a two-stage exchange arthroplasty performed for periprosthetic-joint infection (PJI) is a pivotal step and can often help to resolve pain and restore function. Preoperatively, the surgeon must evaluate the patient and address modifiable risk factors to decrease the likelihood for reinfection. Prior to reimplantation, surgeons must confirm successful infection treatment to the best of their abilities, which unfortunately remains an imperfect science. Serum markers of inflammation and synovial fluid analysis may help determine if a patient should undergo reimplantation or requires repeat débridement. Intraoperatively, thorough débridement strategies should be employed, and bone and soft tissue defects, joint contracture and scar, implant and cement options, wound closure, and dressing management should all be addressed for each reimplantation patient. Postoperatively, weight bearing progression, antibiotic therapy, antibiotic prophylaxis, and patient monitoring must be tailored for each PJI case.

PREOPERATIVE PATIENT OPTIMIZATION

After a patient has undergone implant removal, thorough irrigation and débridement, and placement of an antibiotic spacer for PJI during the first stage, the surgeon must evaluate a patient's risk factors and determine if any of the risk factors can be modified to improve the likelihood of successful PJI treatment (**Table 76-1**). This approach is useful as it may prompt closer monitoring, more aggressive surgical and nonsurgical management, and guide the discussion of considering alternate surgical treatments, such as fusion or amputation.

Inflammatory Arthropathy

Rheumatoid arthritis (RA) and other closely associated inflammatory arthropathies are well established as independent risk factors for failure following reimplantation.[1,2] Compared to osteoarthritis (OA) patients, RA patients have a much higher risk of PJI following reimplantation with a hazard ratio of 5.5.[3] Disease-modifying antirheumatic drugs (DMARDs) are likely to play a prominent role in this increased PJI risk and are an established risk factor for PJI in primary total knee arthroplasty (TKA) patients.[4] Current American College of

Rheumatology (ACR) and American Association of Hip and Knee Surgeons (AAHKS) recommendations state that some DMARDs should be continued during the perioperative timeframe for elective total joint arthroplasty (TJA), while biologics should be held for one dosing cycle prior to surgery and 2 weeks postoperatively.[5] In patients undergoing reimplantation who were on DMARDs prior to explantation, it may be beneficial to withhold reimplantation until the dosing cycle of biologics is completed to minimize the risk of reinfection. It is not recommended to administer DMARDs between stages, if possible.

Diabetes

Diabetes is another well-established risk factor that contributes to increased reinfection after reimplantation, as Hoell et al found that diabetes was associated with an odds ratio of 6.65 for reinfection.[2,6] Thus, we advocate that reimplantation patients establish proper glycemic control prior to reimplantation, including a hemoglobin A1C of <7.7% and a blood glucose of <200 mg/dL, which is similar to values for patients undergoing elective primary TJA.[7]

Body Mass Index

Body mass index (BMI) currently has mixed literature with regard to its role in the success of two-stage exchange arthroplasty. Some studies have demonstrated it as an independent risk, with 1 kg/m² increase in BMI leading to a 22% increase in risk of reinfection.[6] Conversely, other studies have shown no difference in two-stage exchange arthroplasty success between high and low BMI patients.[8] If clinically possible, it is recommended that reimplantation follow primary TJA guidelines, with a recommendation of BMI < 40 kg/m², but reimplantation should not be withheld waiting for weight loss.

Malnutrition

Malnutrition is often overlooked and inadequately worked up, despite being an established risk factor for PJI. Although sometimes visibly evident in elderly and frail patients, many patients do not show physical signs of malnutrition. In fact, obese patients often demonstrate paradoxical malnutrition, accounting for 42.9% of malnourished patients in one study of TJA patients.[9] Several

TABLE 76-1 Modifying Patient Risk Factors Prior to Reimplantation

Inflammatory arthropathy[3]
  DMARDs: continue perioperatively[5]
  Biologics: hold 1 cycle preoperatively, continue 2 wk
    postoperatively[5]
Diabetes
  HbA1c <7.7%[7]
  Glucose <200 mg/dL[7]
BMI[6] <30 kg/m[2]
Malnutrition
  Serum albumin >3.5 g/dL[11]
  Serum prealbumin >18 mg/dL
  Total protein >6 g/dL
  Total lymphocyte count[11] >1500 cells/mm[3]
  Transferrin >200 mg/dL[11]
Smoking
  Cessation 4–8 weeks prior to surgery[14,15]
Others: Cardiac optimization, correcting anemia to hemoglobin
  >10 g/dL, screen and decolonize S. aureus colonization

BMI, body mass index; DMARDs, disease-modifying antirheumatic drugs; HbA1c, hemoglobin A1c.

serum markers are well established as useful proxies for malnutrition. They include serum albumin less than 3.5 g/dL, prealbumin less than 18 mg/dL, total protein less than 6 g/dL, total lymphocyte count less than 1500 cells/mm[3], and transferrin less than 200 mg/dL.[10] Yi et al found that serum markers below the above-threshold values were independent risk factors for PJI in the revision setting.[11] As such, patients found to be preoperatively malnourished should work with a dietitian to improve their nutritional status prior to reimplantation.

Smoking

There are many studies linking tobacco product use to an increased risk of PJI in primary TJA. Similarly, smoking has been shown to be a risk factor for recurrent PJI after two-stage exchange arthroplasty. One study demonstrated a 71% risk of infection with a 21.5 odds ratio of infection in patients who smoke.[6] Smoking has been shown not only to increase the risk of reoperation for infection within 90 days of performing TJA, but also does so in a dose-dependent manner.[12] It is important to note that both current and former smokers have been shown to have increased postoperative complication risks, including PJI.[13] Smoking cessation at least 4 to 6 weeks prior to reimplantation is necessary to restore immune function to decrease the likelihood of postoperative complications.[14,15]

Other Contributing Factors

Individual studies have found associations with a wide variety of additional patient risk factors that can broadly be grouped as either patient health factors (cardiac disease, anemia, chronic *Staphylococcus* carrier, culture negative PJI,

and methicillin-resistant *Staphylococcus aureus* [MRSA] PJI) or surgical factors (postoperative hematoma, wound dehiscence, and number of previous surgeries).[1,2,6,8] Optimizing patients prior to surgery by collaborating with consulting specialists, including cardiologists, hematologists, endocrinologists, and infectious disease specialists, can be beneficial to patients prior to undergoing reimplantation surgery. Additional screening and decolonization of MRSA and methicillin-sensitive *Staphylococcus aureus* (MSSA) may decrease the likelihood of a subsequent *S. aureus* PJI.[16] Modifiable surgical risk factors, such as reducing blood loss, ensuring blood salvage, and reducing transfusions, may also reduce the risk of reinfection.

CONFIRMING INFECTION ERADICATION: PREOPERATIVE WORKUP

Once the decision has been made to proceed with reimplantation, a workup must be initiated to investigate the success of infection treatment as effective reimplantation is dependent on preventing PJI recurrence (**Table 76-2**). Testing should be performed after an antibiotic holiday; however, the duration of the antibiotic holiday is debatable but is often a minimum of 2 weeks.[17] The first step in this workup is an appropriate history and physical exam. Red flags in the patient's history mirror the presentation of PJI after primary TKA and include fevers, chills, sweats, pain, warmth, erythema, wound drainage, or dehiscence.[18] The physical exam is also similar to that for a primary PJI, with the exception that range of motion testing may be precluded by a nonarticulating antibiotic spacer. The skin and surgical site should be carefully inspected for drainage, dehiscence, sinus tracts, fluctuance, or overlying cellulitis.

Serologic Testing

Once a careful history and physical exam has been completed, serologic testing should be pursued. In contrast to

TABLE 76-2 Confirming Successful Infection Treatment Prior to Reimplantation

History
Exam
Serologic testing
  ESR: limited utility[8,19,20]
  CRP: limited utility[8,19,20]
  CBC with differential
  IL-6: >13 pg/mL reinfected, <8 pg/mL not reinfected[24]
  D-Dimer: >850 ng/mL predicts PJI[27]
  Fibrinogen: >4.01 g/L predicts PJI[28]
Synovial fluid testing—negative for reinfection
  Synovial WBC <3000[22]
  % polymorphonucleocytes <80%[22]
  Alpha-defensin = negative (sensitivity 1.00, specificity 0.96)[51]
  Leukocyte esterase = negative (sensitivity 0.81, specificity 0.97)[51]

CBC, complete blood count; CRP, C-reactive protein; ESR, erythrocyte sedimentation rate; IL-6, interleukin-6; WBC, white blood cell.

the workup for primary PJI, erythrocyte sedimentation rate (ESR) and C-reactive protein (CRP) have not been shown to be predictive of infection recurrence prior to reimplantation in a two-stage exchange arthroplasty.[8,19,20] Fu et al demonstrated a high specificity of ESR and CRP for diagnosing infection, but these same laboratory values show poor sensitivity and have limited utility for ruling out infection, which is necessary prior to reimplantation.[21] These labs are often persistently elevated prior to reimplantation, even if the infection has been controlled.[22] Stambaugh et al evaluated whether the percent change of ESR and CRP between resection and reimplantation would be more useful than an absolute threshold value, but unfortunately, no percentage of ESR/CRP reduction was predictive of recurrent PJI after reimplantation.[23] However, a combination of elevated preoperative serum ESR (>99 mm/h), synovial fluid WBC (>60,000 cells/µL), and synovial fluid polymorphonucleocytes (>92%) are predictors of failure of two-stage exchange arthroplasty, and reimplantation is not recommended if these laboratory values are present.[18]

Interleukin-6 (IL-6) is a systemic inflammatory marker that appears to be a useful biomarker for predicting persistent infection after the first stage of two-stage exchange arthroplasty. IL-6 values greater than 13pg/mL showed a positive predictive value of 90.9% for persistent PJI, whereas values less than 8pg/mL showed a negative predictive value of 92.1% for persistent PJI.[24]

D-dimer, a serum biomarker of fibrinolytic activity that has been utilized as a screening test for venous thromboembolism, has recently shown utility for diagnosing PJI, particularly in patients awaiting reimplantation. Two studies have demonstrated an increase in fibrinolytic activity in the setting of infection.[25,26] A study by Shahi et al demonstrated that when using a threshold of 850 ng/mL, serum D-dimer was predictive of PJI both in patients with primary TKA as well as in patients awaiting reimplantation.[27] Fibrinogen has also shown promise as another coagulation-related indicator of PJI. Li et al showed that plasma fibrinogen outperformed the classic biomarkers of ESR and CRP along with outperforming D-dimer in both sensitivity and specificity of diagnosing primary PJI.[28] While it was historically important to observe trends in ESR and CRP values throughout the treatment course, IL-6, D-dimer, and fibrinogen may be more reliable biomarkers for patients awaiting reimplantation.

Synovial Fluid Testing

Joint aspiration is an additional diagnostic modality to utilize when evaluating the persistence of infection prior to reimplantation. Contrary to primary PJI, synovial fluid testing for reimplantation is more nuanced and less predictable. There is a high risk of sampling error in the setting of antibiotic spacer placement, as there may be infected pockets of fluid that are not continuous with the aspirated fluid pocket.[29] Synovial white blood cell (WBC) count and

differential may be useful for predicting persistent infection, although the results in literature are variable, with recurrent infection as synovial fluid WBC >3000 WBC/µL and polymorphonucleocyte (PMN) percentage >80%.[22] However, other studies have demonstrated that repeat synovial fluid testing prior to reimplantation is not reliable for determining reinfection.[30]

Alpha-defensin is an antimicrobial peptide released by activated neutrophils and can be detected via an immunoassay as evidence of PJI. Bingham et al demonstrated the utility of alpha-defensin for diagnosing PJI in both primary TKA and reimplantation patients. The sensitivity of alpha-defensin for PJI was 100% with a specificity of 95%, although it should be noted that primary infection and pre-reimplantation patients were grouped together in this analysis.[31]

TIMING FOR SECOND-STAGE REVISION

Assuming that the preoperative workup for infection does not yield any indication of persistent infection or reinfection, the surgeon must consider the timing of reimplantation. Most two-stage exchange arthroplasty protocols are heavily based on the initial report by Insall in 1983, where the implant was removed and the patient was placed on a 6-week course of antibiotics, followed by several weeks of an antibiotic hiatus to allow for clinical, serologic, and synovial testing to rule out recurrent infection.[32] Recently, the time between stages of greater than 16 weeks demonstrated an increased risk for failure after reimplantation.[21]

INTRAOPERATIVE CONSIDERATIONS

Intraoperative Tests for Infection

The first and most important decision at the time of surgery is whether to proceed with reimplantation. Additional intraoperative testing including intraoperative cultures and intraoperative histology can be performed to confirm infection eradication or reinfection (**Table 76-3**). Intraoperative cultures, which are often sent by surgeons in every infection case, may be unreliable in the setting of reimplantation given the presence of an antibiotic spacer and the potential for isolated pockets of infection.[33] Additionally, cultures often require at least 24 to 48 hours of incubation. Sonication of explanted spacers has been trialed for predicting failure and reinfection following reimplantation; however, the utility of this practice is currently unclear.[34,35] Although no guidelines currently exist regarding the use of antibiotics until intraoperative cultures have finalized, a 3-month course of oral antibiotics after two-stage revision has been shown to decrease the risk of failure due to reinfection.[36] If a patient has a positive culture from reimplantation, this is a poor prognostic sign, and the patient may be a candidate for receiving additional postoperative antibiotics.[37]

TABLE 76-3 Surgical Considerations During Reimplantation

Timing: Antibiotic spacer duration <16 wk[21]
Intraoperative testing
  Intraoperative culture: unreliable[33]
  Intraoperative frozen sections:
    5 PMN/HPF × 5 samples, 400× high-power microscopic fields[38]
    10 PMN/HPF × 5 samples, 400× high-power microscopic fields[38]
Débridement
  Methylene blue: improves débridement efficacy[43]
  Povidone-iodine lavage[44]
Exposure
  TTO > Quadriceps snip[41]

HPF, high-power field; PMN, polymorphonucleocytes; TTO, tibial tubercle osteotomy.

Histology is another method of intraoperative testing for persistent infection. A sample of tissue can be sent to the histology lab, frozen, sectioned, and evaluated at 400× magnification for the number of neutrophils per high-power field. The Clinical Practice Guidelines from the American Academy of Orthopaedic Surgeons (AAOS) gave strong support for two separate thresholds for confirming primary infection with histologic samples: (1) five neutrophils in each of five, 400× high-power microscopic fields (of maximum tissue concentration) or (2) ten neutrophils in each of five, 400× high-power microscopic fields.[38] Unfortunately, current literature on frozen section histology is variable between stages prior to reimplantation. Utilizing the criteria of 10 neutrophils per high-power field, Della Valle et al identified only one of four persistent PJI cases during two-stage exchange arthroplasty.[39] Additionally, George et al found that while frozen section is highly specific for PJI and an excellent tool for confirming infection on the day of reimplantation, poor sensitivity limits the ability to rule out infection or predict failure.[40] On the other hand, Fu et al found frozen section to be reliable with an accuracy of 74%, a sensitivity of 90%, and a specificity of 83% for reimplantation.[21]

Surgical Exposure in Reimplantation

When performing reimplantation surgery for PJI, the joint often has soft-tissue contractures and excessive scar tissue that develops after antibiotic spacer placement that can preclude access to the joint. Surgical exposure is important to adequately debride the bone and soft tissues, as well as for reconstruction. An extensile approach should be utilized when performing reimplantation. In order to protect the extensor mechanism while providing adequate access, a quadriceps snip or a tibial tubercle osteotomy can be performed. The tibial tubercle osteotomy has gained support in the literature for providing improved functional scores over the quadriceps snip, which has an increased risk of extensor lag.[41] Additional considerations

to improve exposure include release of the posterior cruciate ligament (PCL) if present, posterior capsule, and suprapatellar scar.[29]

Débridement

With the primary goal of preventing reinfection, an adequate second débridement of all potential infection sources is of paramount importance. Due to its inherent antibiotic resistance, bacterial biofilm confers a high risk of reinfection.[42] Due to significant scarring and potential tissue discoloration from prolonged immobilization and antibiotic spacer placement, identifying these tissues can be a significant challenge even for veteran surgeons. Dilute methylene blue has demonstrated the ability to bind and stain devitalized cells, as well as bacterial biofilm. This is prepared by combining 20 mL of 1% methylene blue with 180 mL normal saline to create 200 mL of 0.1% methylene blue. This solution is instilled into the joint cavity immediately following capsulotomy for a period of 60 seconds after which the knee is copiously irrigated with pulse lavage. Biofilm and devitalized tissue will remain stained blue, allowing for their identification and removal.[43] To this point, methylene blue stained tissue had a ninefold greater bioburden than unstained tissue.[43]

With regard to irrigation during reimplantation, dilute povidone-iodine lavage prior to wound closure has been shown to reduce the risk of deep surgical site infection in primary total joint arthroplasty.[44] Povidone-iodine has also been shown to have more potent and broader bactericidal activity than either chlorhexidine or vancomycin powder, regardless of exposure time.[45] *In vitro* studies evaluating alternative lavage solutions, such as acetic acid to address biofilms, have not yet identified a clinically useful methodology.[46] Several new technologies have recently been developed to improve tissue débridement by utilizing an ultrasonic scalpel (Misonix, Farmingdale NY) or a hydroscalpel (Versajet, Smith and Nephew, London, England). Although there is currently no arthroplasty literature assessing these devices in debriding biofilm *in vivo*, they may play a role in future PJI débridements.

POSTOPERATIVE CONSIDERATIONS

Postoperative decision-making includes duration of postoperative intravenous antibiotic administration, whether or not chronic suppressive oral antibiotics should be prescribed, as well as the mode and duration of antibiotic prophylaxis for dental and gastrointestinal procedures (**Table 76-4**). Current recommendations encourage intravenous antibiotic administration for the standard 24 hours in the perioperative period, but not prolonged intravenous antibiotics.[47] Some authors propose following patients clinically and trending ESR and CRP to monitor for infection, and do not initiate prolonged antibiotics in the absence of objective concern for chronic or recurrent infection.[29] On the other hand, one prospective,

TABLE 76-4 Postoperative Considerations After Reimplantation

Postoperative antibiotic duration
  24-h perioperative antibiotics[47]
  Consider 3 mo oral antibiotics[36]
Intervals and methodology for monitoring
  Consider ESR and CRP[29]
  Intervals for monitoring is patient-dependent
Dental and gastrointestinal procedure prophylaxis
  Dependent on comorbidities and risk factors[49,50]

CRP, C-reactive protein; ESR, erythrocyte sedimentation rate.

randomized controlled trial demonstrated that 3 months of tailored oral antibiotic administration decreased the risk of reinfection after performing two-stage exchange arthroplasty for PJI.[36]

The AAOS and the American Dental Association do not recommend antibiotic prophylaxis before dental procedures in patients with prosthetic joints.[48] However, appropriate use criteria may recommend the utilization of antibiotics prior to these procedures in very select circumstances, such as patients who are undergoing dental procedures involving oral mucosa perforation or tissue manipulation in the periapical or gingival tissue, are severely immunocompromised, have known active diabetes (blood glucose >200 mg/dL and hemoglobin A1C >8), and have a history of PJI.[49,50] Revisiting patient risk factors for failure is useful for determining the intervals for monitoring of reinfection and the need for antibiotic prophylactic treatment.

SUMMARY

Reimplantation in the setting of two-stage exchange arthroplasty is the gold standard management for chronic PJI. It is essential that arthroplasty surgeons develop systematic means of progressing through preoperative patient risk assessment and optimization; investigation of infection eradication via serologic, synovial, and histologic testing; and ultimately, management of the intraoperative and postoperative challenges posed by this complex problem. Literature directly addressing the appropriateness and timing of reimplantation is currently sparse; however, it is a topic of rapid growth and investigation. New technologies and improved academic inquiry will continue to improve our understanding of PJI and outcomes after reimplantation.

REFERENCES

1. Sakellariou VI, Poultsides LA, Vasilakakos T, Sculco P, Ma Y, Sculco TP. Risk factors for recurrence of periprosthetic knee infection. *J Arthroplasty*. 2015;30(9):1618-1622.
2. Sabry FY, Buller L, Ahmed S, Klika AK, Barsoum WK. Preoperative prediction of failure following two-stage revision for knee prosthetic joint infections. *J Arthroplasty*. 2014;29(1):115-121.
3. Bongartz T, Halligan CS, Osmon DR, et al. Incidence and risk factors of prosthetic joint infection after total hip or knee replacement in patients with rheumatoid arthritis. *Arthritis Rheum*. 2008;59(12):1713-1720.
4. Momohara S, Kawakami K, Iwamoto T, et al. Prosthetic joint infection after total hip or knee arthroplasty in rheumatoid arthritis patients treated with nonbiologic and biologic disease-modifying antirheumatic drugs. *Mod Rheumatol*. 2011;21(5):469-475.
5. Goodman SM, Springer B, Guyatt G, et al. 2017 American College of Rheumatology/American association of hip and knee surgeons guideline for the perioperative management of antirheumatic medication in patients with rheumatic diseases undergoing elective total hip or total knee arthroplasty. *J Arthroplasty*. 2017;32(9):2628-2638.
6. Hoell S, Sieweke A, Gosheger G et al. Eradication rates, risk factors, and implant selection in two-stage revision knee arthroplasty: a mid-term follow-up study. *J Orthop Surg Res*. 2016;11(1):93.
7. Tarabichi M, Shohat N, Kheir MM, et al. Determining the threshold for HbA1c as a predictor for adverse outcomes after total joint arthroplasty: a multicenter, retrospective study. *J Arthroplasty*, 2017. 32(9 suppl):S263-S267.e1.
8. Mortazavi SM, Vegari D, Ho A, et al. Two-stage exchange arthroplasty for infected total knee arthroplasty: predictors of failure. *Clin Orthop Relat Res*. 2011;469(11):3049-3054.
9. Huang R, Greenky M, Kerr GJ, Austin MS, Parvizi J. The effect of malnutrition on patients undergoing elective joint arthroplasty. *J Arthroplasty*. 2013;28(8 suppl):21-24.
10. Ellsworth B, Kamath AF. Malnutrition and total joint arthroplasty. *J Nat Sci*. 2016;2(3):e179.
11. Yi PH, Frank RM, Vann E, et al. Is potential malnutrition associated with septic failure and acute infection after revision total joint arthroplasty? *Clin Orthop Relat Res*. 2015;473(1):175-182.
12. Tischler EH, Matsen Ko L, Chen AF, et al. Smoking increases the rate of reoperation for infection within 90 Days after primary total joint arthroplasty. *J Bone Joint Surg Am*. 2017;99(4):295-304.
13. Duchman KR, Gao Y, Pugely AJ, et al. The effect of smoking on short-term complications following total hip and knee arthroplasty. *J Bone Joint Surg Am*. 2015;97(13):1049-1058.
14. Tonnesen H, Nielsen PR, Lauritzen JB, Moller AM. Smoking and alcohol intervention before surgery: evidence for best practice. *Br J Anaesth*. 2009;102(3):297-306.
15. Moller AM, Villebro N, Pedersen T, Tonnesen H, Effect of preoperative smoking intervention on postoperative complications: a randomised clinical trial. *Lancet*. 2002;359(9301):114-117.
16. Jeans E, Holleyman R, Tate D, Reed M, Malviya A, Methicillin sensitive staphylococcus aureus screening and decolonisation in elective hip and knee arthroplasty. *J Infect*. 2018;77(5):405-409.
17. Tan TL, Kheir MM, Rondon AJ, et al. Determining the role and duration of the "antibiotic holiday" period in periprosthetic joint infection. *J Arthroplasty*. 2018;33(9):2976-2980.
18. Dwyer MK, Damsgaard C, Wadibia J, et al. Laboratory tests for diagnosis of chronic periprosthetic joint infection can help predict outcomes of two-stage exchange. *J Bone Joint Surg Am*. 2018;100(12):1009-1015.
19. Ghanem E, Azzam K, Seeley M, Joshi A, Parvizi J., Staged revision for knee arthroplasty infection: what is the role of serologic tests before reimplantation? *Clin Orthop Relat Res*. 2009;467(7):1699-1705.
20. Saleh A, George J, Faour M, Klika AK, Higuera CA. Serum biomarkers in periprosthetic joint infections. *Bone Joint Res*. 2018;7(1):85-93.
21. Fu J, Ni M, Li H, et al. The proper timing of second-stage revision in treating periprosthetic knee infection: reliable indicators and risk factors. *J Orthop Surg Res*. 2018;13(1):214.
22. Kusuma SK, Ward J, Jacofsky M, Sporer SM, Della Valle CJ. What is the role of serological testing between stages of two-stage reconstruction of the infected prosthetic knee? *Clin Orthop Relat Res*. 2011;469(4):1002-1008.
23. Stambough JB, Curtin BM, Odum SM. Does change in ESR and CRP guide the timing of two-stage arthroplasty reimplantation? *Clin Orthop Relat Res*. 2019;477(2):364-371.
24. Hoell S, Borgers L, Gosheger G, et al. Interleukin-6 in two-stage revision arthroplasty: what is the threshold value to exclude persistent infection before re-implanatation? *Bone Joint J*. 2015;97-b(1):71-75.

25. Gando S. Role of fibrinolysis in sepsis. *Semin Thromb Hemost.* 2013;39(4):392-399.

26. Ribera T, Monreal L, Armengou L, Ríos J, Prades M. Synovial fluid D-dimer concentration in foals with septic joint disease. *J Vet Intern Med.* 2011;25(5):1113-1117.

27. Shahi A, Kheir MM, Tarabichi M, et al. Serum D-dimer test is promising for the diagnosis of periprosthetic joint infection and timing of reimplantation. *J Bone Joint Surg Am.* 2017;99(17):1419-1427.

28. Li R, Shao HY, Hao LB, et al. Plasma fibrinogen exhibits better performance than plasma D-dimer in the diagnosis of periprosthetic joint infection: a multicenter retrospective study. *J Bone Joint Surg Am.* 2019;101(7):613-619.

29. Burnett RS, Kelly MA, Hanssen AD, Barrack RL. Technique and timing of two-stage exchange for infection in TKA. *Clin Orthop Relat Res.* 2007;464:164-178.

30. Frangiamore SJ, Siqueira MB, Saleh A, et al. Synovial cytokines and the MSIS criteria are not useful for determining infection resolution after periprosthetic joint infection explantation. *Clin Orthop Relat Res.* 2016;474(7):1630-1639.

31. Bingham J, Clarke H, Spangehl M, et al. The alpha defensin-1 biomarker assay can be used to evaluate the potentially infected total joint arthroplasty. *Clin Orthop Relat Res.* 2014;472(12):4006-4009.

32. Insall JN, Thompson FM, Brause BD. Two-stage reimplantation for the salvage of infected total knee arthroplasty. *J Bone Joint Surg Am.* 1983;65(8):1087-1098.

33. Boelch SP, Roth M, Arnholdt J, Rudert M, Luedemann M. Synovial fluid aspiration should not be routinely performed during the two-stage exchange of the knee. *BioMed Res Int.* 2018;2018:6720712.

34. Olsen AS, Wilson A, O'Malley MJ, Urish KL, Klatt BA. Are sonication cultures of antibiotic cement spacers useful during second-stage reimplantation surgery for prosthetic joint infection?. *Clin Orthop Relat Res.* 2018;476(10):1986-1992.

35. Rothenberg AC, Wilson AE, Hayes JP, O'Malley MJ, Klatt BA. Sonication of arthroplasty implants improves accuracy of periprosthetic joint infection cultures. *Clin Orthop Relat Res.* 2017;475(7):1827-1836.

36. Frank JM, Kayupov E, Moric M, et al. The Mark Coventry, MD, Award: oral antibiotics reduce reinfection after two-stage exchange: a multicenter, randomized controlled trial. *Clin Orthop Relat Res.* 2017;475(1):56-61.

37. Tan TL, Gomez MM, Manrique J, Parvizi J, Chen AF. Positive culture during reimplantation increases the risk of subsequent failure in two-stage exchange arthroplasty. *J Bone Joint Surg Am.* 2016;98(15):1313-1319.

38. Della Valle C, Parvizi J, Bauer TW, et al. American Academy of Orthopaedic Surgeons clinical practice guideline on: the diagnosis of periprosthetic joint infections of the hip and knee. *J Bone Joint Surg Am.* 2011;93(14):1355-1357.

39. Della Valle CJ, Bogner E, Desai P, et al. Analysis of frozen sections of intraoperative specimens obtained at the time of reoperation after hip or knee resection arthroplasty for the treatment of infection. *J Bone Joint Surg Am.* 1999;81(5):684-689.

40. George J, Kwiecien G, Klika AK, et al. Are frozen sections and MSIS criteria reliable at the time of reimplantation of two-stage revision arthroplasty? *Clin Orthop Relat Res.* 2016;474(7):1619-1626.

41. Bruni D, Iacono F, Sharma B, Zaffagnini S, Marcacci M. Tibial tubercle osteotomy or quadriceps snip in two-stage revision for prosthetic knee infection? A randomized prospective study. *Clin Orthop Relat Res.* 2013;471(4):1305-1318.

42. Stewart PS, Costerton JW. Antibiotic resistance of bacteria in biofilms. *Lancet.* 2001;358(9276):135-138.

43. Shaw JD, Miller S, Plourde A, et al. Methylene blue-guided débridement as an intraoperative adjunct for the surgical treatment of periprosthetic joint infection. *J Arthroplasty.* 2017;32(12):3718-3723.

44. Ruder JA, Springer BD. Treatment of periprosthetic joint infection using antimicrobials: dilute povidone-iodine lavage. *J Bone Jt Infect.* 2017;2(1):10-14.

45. Cichos KH, Andrews RM, Wolschendorf F, et al. Efficacy of intraoperative antiseptic techniques in the prevention of periprosthetic joint infection: superiority of betadine. *J Arthroplasty.* 2019;34(7S):S312-S318.

46. Tsang STJ, Gwynne PJ, Gallagher MP, Simpson AHRW. The biofilm eradication activity of acetic acid in the management of periprosthetic joint infection. *Bone Joint Res.* 2018;7(8):517-523.

47. AlBuhairan B, Hind D, Hutchinson A. Antibiotic prophylaxis for wound infections in total joint arthroplasty: a systematic review. *J Bone Joint Surg Br.* 2008;90(7):915-919.

48. Watters W III, Rethman MP, Hanson NB, et al. Prevention of orthopaedic implant infection in patients undergoing dental procedures. *J Am Acad Orthop Surg.* 2013;21(3):180-189.

49. Rees HW. AAOS appropriate use criteria: management of patients with orthopaedic implants undergoing dental procedures. *J Am Acad Orthop Surg.* 2017;25(7):e142-e143.

50. Quinn RH, Murray JN, Pezold R, Sevarino KS. Management of patients with orthopaedic implants undergoing dental procedures. *J Am Acad Orthop Surg.* 2017;25(7):e138-e141.

51. Wyatt MC, Beswick AD, Kunutsor SK, et al. The alpha-defensin immunoassay and leukocyte esterase colorimetric strip test for the diagnosis of periprosthetic infection: a systematic review and meta-analysis. *J Bone Joint Surg Am.* 2016;98(12):992-1000.

chapter 77

Soft-Tissue Coverage for Infected Total Knee Arthroplasty

Kevin A. Raskin, MD

Soft-tissue competency is critical toward the success in the surgical management of infected total knee arthroplasty. The unfortunate nature of the infected knee replacement often implies compromised anterior soft tissues. Like the elbow and the ankle, there is a paucity of adequate, well-vascularized soft tissues overlying the knee joint. Commonly, surgeons must rely on tenuous soft tissues to protect and defend a revision or replanted arthroplasty against pathogens eager to reinfect from the skin or the external environment. Recognizing patients at risk for soft-tissue compromise, understanding their soft-tissue coverage options, and employing the appropriate resources to provide adequate coverage will prove critical to the outcome of infected total knee arthroplasty.

PATIENT FACTORS

Systemic factors play an important role in predictable soft-tissue healing. Smoking, obesity, and malnutrition are primary drivers toward poor outcomes. Additionally, poorly controlled diabetes mellitus, peripheral vascular disease, kidney failure, bleeding dyscrasias, and rheumatologic disorders all potentially contribute to poor anterior tissue quality and reliable soft-tissue coverage for the infected total knee replacement.

Further, the use of suction drains in the postoperative period and the need to evacuate postoperative blood and fluid accumulations collectively serve to decompress the anterior soft tissue to afford a more tension-free closure. Postoperative hematoma applies untoward tension to the suture line and deprives the healing surgical site of much needed microvascular blood supply. The diminished oxygen tension at the incision can predictably result in areas of wound necrosis and require surgical débridement.

MAKING COVERAGE DECISIONS

The surgeon must appreciate the patient factors described above and the end goal of robust, durable soft-tissue coverage over an infected or replanted knee arthroplasty. The process of identifying the myriad factors contributing to the coverage problem, in combination with choosing the appropriate closure modality, is patient specific but should be as thoughtful and as algorithmic as possible.

Generally, this simplest closure is often the best. If a patient's soft tissues can be approximated and healed primarily, this should be the optimal choice. When patients cannot be closed primarily a methodical approach toward closure should be undertaken-taking into consideration the balance between surgical morbidity and a durable result. The approach to durable soft-tissue coverage in infected total knee arthroplasties lies in a balance between the simplest and the most complicated of methods as deemed most appropriate, given the state of the patient and the character of the wound, surrounding soft tissues, and defect.

CLOSURE BY PRIMARY AND SECONDARY INTENTION

Primary closure remains the workhorse and preferred choice among surgeons when faced with a wound that can be closed without undue tension along the suture line. The choice of skin staples versus nondissolvable monofilament suture has yet to be determined. Both are viable options for primary closure. If the wound edges cannot be opposed tension-free or if after primary sutures have been placed, wound ischemia is observed (white edges along the suture line) a second-line option is necessary. In other surgical scenarios, healing by secondary intention (allowing for granulation tissue to populate a defect) is an acceptable option. However, in the setting of joint replacement surgery especially involving the knee, prolonged exposure of the fascia to dressing changes persists as an ongoing vulnerability that may undermine the sterility of the joint and increase the risk of deep infection. For this reason, healing by secondary intention is not advisable.

Negative-pressure wound therapy (NPWT) can be used as a temporary measure to aid in the formation of granulation tissue in preparation for skin grafting. Prolong use of NPWT can lead to increased risk of deep periprosthetic infection. The decision to either skin graft or perform definitive coverage should be in place before committing a patient to prolonged NPWT. NPWT should be brief.

Along the spectrum of soft-tissue closure methods, split-thickness skin grafting is the next most logical choice for coverage. A healthy bed of granulation tissue is mandatory for predictable "take" of the skin grafts. NPWT is quite helpful in creating a healthy bed of granulation tissue and can be used temporarily for this purpose. Overall, split-thickness skin grafts serve to cover small areas subserved by healthy granulation tissue. STSGs can contract and limit range of motion. Skin grafts are best targeted for the proximal portions of knee arthroplasty incisions and less so for the distal aspect overlying the proximal tibia.

FLAPS

Local Flaps

Flap options for infected total knee arthroplasty are dictated by the geometry of the defect, health of the surrounding soft tissue, regional blood supply, and donor-site morbidity. Like the spectrum of soft-tissue coverage options addressed in this chapter, within the options for flap coverage are a variety of local, regional, and distant flap options. Determining which flap option is most suitable depends on the size and orientation of the defect and the ease by which healthy soft tissues can be retrieved and repurposed to close a defect.

Fasciocutaneous or perforator flaps utilize local angiosomes, vascular supply from perforating arteries through the underlying fascia to the overly skin. These flaps, compromised of skin, fat, and fascia, are raised in juxtaposition to a wound defect and rotated in a propeller-type fashion over the defect covering it. A second defect is inherently created after raising the fasciocutaneous flap. This defect is typically closed primarily. In areas where tissue bulk is not needed, fasciocutaneous propeller flaps are reasonable choices for soft-tissue coverage. Exposed prosthesis would be a relative contraindication for this type of flap. Where metal is exposed, it is preferred to have muscle or at minimum very well-perfused tissue overlying a prosthesis.

Local muscle flaps around the knee are first-line choices for coverage. The well-vascularized nature of the muscle is frequently sufficient when searching for healthy soft-tissue coverage. The medial gastrocnemius muscle is an easy, reliable, and robust local flap and frequently a first choice among reconstructive surgeons. The medial sural artery serves as its main arterial blood supply and takes origin from the popliteal artery. Positioned posteriorly, the muscle can be harvested either through an extension of an anterior knee arthrotomy incision or via a second, parallel incision and tunneled under an anterior skin bridge. The medial gastrocnemius muscle has a robust tendinous attachment to the Achilles tendon. When harvested carefully, should not alter the biomechanics of the triceps surae as they attach to the calcaneus. Skin overlying a newly positioned medial gastrocnemius rotational flap is frequently stented open and cannot be closed in a tension-free manner. In this setting, a split-thickness skin graft is indicated to cover the flap.

Lateral gastrocnemius rotational muscle flaps also exist as a local soft-tissue choice for anterior coverage in infected total knee arthroplasty. The lateral gastrocnemius is a small-caliber muscle and should be chosen if the preferential defect is either lateral or anterolateral geographically about the knee. Careful consideration of the peroneal nerve is required when rotating the lateral gastrocnemius anteriorly. The nerve is precariously positioned at the point of rotation, proximally between the lateral femoral condyle and the fibular head. If not dissected free, the peroneal nerve can be compressed by a newly rotated lateral gastrocnemius resulting in a nerve palsy. Positioning the muscle deep to the peroneal nerve has been described as an effort to avoid compression by the muscle flap.

Both the medial and lateral gastrocnemius flaps are limited in the cranial reach. Wounds occurring in the distal one-third are easily managed by gastrocnemius rotations flaps; however, central or proximal wounds are often left untreated by gastrocnemius rotations flaps. The vastus lateralis muscle can serve as a local rotations flap option for proximal wound defects. The distal arterial perforating anastomosis can maintain adequate blood supply to the vastus lateralis if rotated distally to cover a proximal and anterior wound defect.

CONCLUSION

Soft-tissue management in the setting of an infected total knee arthroplasty is critical to a successful outcome. Without a competent soft-tissue envelope and durable soft-tissue coverage, deep prosthetic implants cannot survive. A stepwise, algorithmic approach is suggested. For small superficial breaches in the wound, local wound care or NPWT is recommended. As the soft-tissue defect becomes more sinister, engagement of plastic surgical colleagues and consideration of local- and free-tissue transfer is necessary to obtain adequate, reliable coverage.

BIBLIOGRAPHY

1. Galat DD, McGovern SC, Larson DR, Harrington JR, Hanssen AD, Clarke HD. Surgical treatment of early wound complications following primary total knee arthroplasty. *J Bone Joint Surg Am.* 2009;91(1):48-54.
2. Vince KG, Abdeen A. Wound problems in total knee arthroplasty. *Clin Orthop Relat Res.* 2006;452:88-90.
3. Laing JH, Hancock K, Harrison DH. The exposed total knee replacement prosthesis: a new classification and treatment algorithm. *Br J Plast Surg.* 1992;45(1):66-69.
4. Nahabedian MY, Orlando JC, Delanois RE, Mont MA, Hungerford DS. Salvage procedures for complex soft tissue defects of the knee. *Clin Orthop Relat Res.* 1998;356:119-124.
5. Menderes A, Demirdover C, Yilmaz M, Vayvada H, Barutcu A. Reconstruction of soft tissue defects following total knee arthroplasty. *Knee.* 2002;9(3):215-219.
6. Ries MD, Bozic KJ. Medial gastrocnemius flap coverage for treatment of skin necrosis after total knee arthroplasty. *Clin Orthop Relat Res.* 2006;446:186-192.
7. Auregan JC, Bégué T, Tomeno B, Masquelet AC. Distally-based vastus lateralis muscle flap: a salvage alternative to address complex soft tissue defects around the knee. *Orthop Traumatol Surg Res.* 2010;96(2):180-184.
8. Louer CR, Garcia RM, Earle SA, Hollenbeck ST, Erdmann D, Levin LS. Free flap reconstruction of the knee: an outcome study of 34 cases. *Ann Plast Surg.* 2015;74(1):57-63.

chapter 78

Salvage Procedures: Knee Arthrodesis, Resection Arthroplasty, Amputation

James B. Stiehl, MD, MBA

INTRODUCTION

Complex problems of the knee such as severe trauma, chronic infection, or failed total joint arthroplasty require salvage techniques. This chapter considers current trends and experience with amputation, resection, and knee arthrodesis. My prior chapter discussed the introduction of new surgical techniques to improve the outcomes of knee arthrodesis, and while numbers were small, most series showed successful fusion in over 85% of cases.[1-6] It seemed that we were on the verge of eliminating amputations as few were being reported in the literature. However, Big Data has changed all that, and while I can show that we are performing more secondary revision arthroplasties and fewer salvage procedures, arthrodesis, amputation, and resection arthroplasty, all have important roles. The major advance has been to understand our patient's overall health, and that guides our choice of treatment. Effort will be made to include many of those concepts. We can now profile high-risk and extraordinary-risk patients where the best options may be the unspoken "A" words. Discussion of surgical technique has changed little, but I will try to include as many "pearls" as possible.

INDICATIONS

Primary Arthrodesis

With the evolutionary success of total knee arthroplasty, primary arthrodesis of the arthritic knee has become an unusual operation; however, there are several settings where primary fusion remains an attractive or at least a reasonable option.[7] The first is a young patient with severe extremity trauma to the knee joint complicated with chronic sepsis and extensor mechanism loss. In this instance, the consideration is to prevent the poor outcome of a potentially functional young male from becoming "depressed, divorced, and destitute." Knee arthrodesis has been shown by numerous authors to be durable in the long term even if interposing grafts are needed. Wolf et al followed up patients with arthrodesis following tumor limb salvage finding independent ambulation in 86%.

At a mean follow-up of 17 years, the majority continued to have satisfactory function.[8] Bensen et al compared failed knee arthroplasty arthrodesis with primary total knee arthroplasty finding nearly identical SF 36 scores. Physical mobility was better with knee arthroplasty but pain was better with arthrodesis.[9]

Other indications include serious general conditions such as neuropathic Charcot joint. The limb may be insensible, and the patient often has very poor control of knee function due to severe spinal cord involvement or a myelopathic process.[10,11] Knee arthrodesis for treatment of primary malignant bone tumors may be the best option using such augments as autologous grafts or vascularized fibular transplants. Chronic poliomyelitis syndrome is another neurological condition where there is severe instability in extension. For virtually all other circumstances, primary arthrodesis has been displaced by total knee arthroplasty. The functional outcome is significantly inferior with arthrodesis and most older patients will require ambulatory aids such as a cane or crutches, and lifestyle compromise for some may be severe.

Secondary Arthrodesis

The most common current circumstance for arthrodesis is chronic sepsis following total knee arthroplasty in a patient who is not a candidate for reimplantation. This is typically a type B or C host, where the risk of infection recurrence is high, especially when combined with extensor mechanism problems such as patellar tendon rupture. Type B hosts have significant local and systemic factors that impair the normal immune processes. Local factors include chronic lymphedema, major vessel disease, venous stasis, extensive scarring, or radiation fibrosis. Systemic problems include malnutrition, malignancy, extremes of age, hepatic or renal failure, diabetes mellitus, and alcohol abuse. Type C hosts are sufficiently fragile such that undertaking aggressive treatment could endanger the patient. We are particularly concerned about patients who have evidence of chronic malnutrition; become infected from a chronic source such as a stoma, urine, or diverticulum; have multiple organism infections; have chronic infections that respond poorly to débridement and antibiotic therapy with persistent signs of inflammation; or have life-threatening infections from methicillin-resistant *Staphylococcus aureus* (MRSA) or vancomycin-resistant *Enterococcus* (VREC). Inflammatory/nutrition markers such as serum prealbumin, serum albumin, sedimentation rate, C-reactive protein, and depressed lymphocyte counts offer clear estimation of chronic risks. A recent study has shown that there is at least a 50% chance of recurrence following an attempted two-stage débridement and reimplantation of a previously revised total knee for chronic sepsis. Careful judgment is needed for each patient, especially for multiple failed revisions, and close consultation with medical infectious disease specialists is required to balance the risk of long-term antibiotic treatment or suppressive antibiotic therapy versus the surgical choices of fibrous resection arthroplasty, total knee reimplantation, arthrodesis, or amputation. With chronic infections, surgical débridement may create the best end point to eradicate biofilm-forming bacteria, and this may include amputation.

Another important total knee complication that should be considered for knee arthrodesis is the failed extensor mechanism. When combined with periprosthetic joint infection, the balance clearly tips to salvage knee arthrodesis. Friederich et al evaluated the results of 37 such cases, finding that 87% were infection free as follow-up. However, persistent problems with the fusion site required implant removals and the 6-year survivorship table revealed that 74% of implants remained intact. However, the overall clinical results were acceptable considering factors of pain and functional outcome.[12]

Amputation

There are severe circumstances where amputation becomes the best option. Patients with recalcitrant infection, high risk reconstructive options, and serious comorbidities are considered for amputation. The decision is usually multifactorial, but serious skin deficiency problems, arterial calcifications that rule out free tissue transfer, and bone defects that limit bone healing point toward amputation. Patients with morbid obesity, chronic diabetes and other medical issues, multiple failed knee revisions, and deep vein thrombosis should be considered for amputation. Son et al demonstrated that the Charlson comorbidity score was substantially higher in those undergoing amputation versus arthrodesis (hazard ratio for score of 5+ was 2.56 [confidence interval: 2.12-3.14]).[13] Also, patients undergoing amputation had a higher risk of death from amputation versus arthrodesis, again confirming the fact that these patients are sicker and more fragile.

There is a discussion that most surgeons dread, and that is the need for amputation following a popliteal vessel injury. First, the surgeon should always consider the potential injury to these vessels as they lay directly behind the posterior cruciate ligament that may be incised. Anatomical studies show that the distance is about 10-11 mm from the posterior ledge of the proximal tibia. Placing a Hohmann or Chandler retractor on this ledge virtually eliminates the potential of damaging the vessels but there is no place for saws, drills, or surgical dissection beyond the posterior tibia. If there is a sudden "flood of blood," quick action is needed including putting up the tourniquet, packing the wound, and calling a vascular surgical consult. That surgeon will usually perform intraoperative arteriograms and will solve the vessel problem. If pulses return and the possibility of compartment syndrome is slight, the surgeon may complete the surgical procedure. Otherwise, the wound should be closed over packing and the leg be observed. Prompt restoration of blood flow is highly effective, but delay beyond 2 hours may lead to a poor outcome. Vigilance, anticipation, and expedient action are the solutions to this problem.

TECHNIQUE

External Fixation[7,14]

A publication now 20 years old demonstrated 100% solid fusion using an anterior unilateral frame for arthrodesis. This contrasts to the 40% to 80% failure of earlier methods that attempted something near the Charnley compression technique. Inadequate stability, which is the key element, probably explained the large failure rates. I would hesitate to recommend external fixators particularly in older patients with soft osteopenic bone. The best construct is a double frame technique where two or three threaded pin groups are applied proximally and distally in sound cortical bone of the femur and tibia. Optimum apposition with a good degree of compression is desired. Careful pin site care is desired and late bone osteomyelitis is a risk of long-term pin use. Patients are best kept non–weight-bearing for extended periods of 3 to 5 months (**Fig. 78-1**).

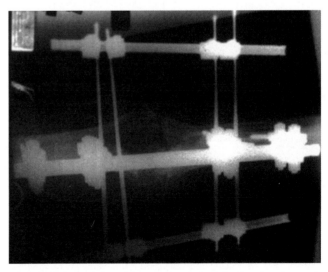

FIGURE 78-1 Failed total knee arthroplasty following chronic sepsis and extensor mechanism loss treated with a double plane external fixation device.

Double Plate Fixation (Nichols)[15]

This technique uses two broad AO DCP plates with 10 to 18 holes (average 12 holes). Bone cuts are made such that the normal femorotibial valgus of 7° is restored. One plate is placed anteromedial while the other is anterolateral. Careful contouring of the plates is usually needed. The patella may be osteotomized and applied to the anterior surface of the femur and tibia as a graft. Sepsis requires a two-stage technique with fusion done after 6 weeks of antibiotics. Postoperative management includes a long leg cast until the fusion is ascertained to be solid (average 5.6 months; range 3 to 10). The biggest liability is the fairly extensive amount of dissection that is needed (**Fig. 78-2**).

Intramedullary Nail Fixation (Stiehl)[3]

Several different rod configurations have been developed with particular advantages noted with each. My original experience was with a simple Kuntscher nail that was inserted anterograde through a separate incision with the use of a medial AO DCP 10-hole compression plate. This technique is particularly valuable if a long interposing allograft is required as rigid fixation of the graft is essential for union. The patient is placed supine on a fluoroscopic imaging operating table with 45° bump under the affected buttock. The pelvis and lower extremity are draped such that proximal hip exposure

will allow entry, and reaming of the femur anterograde is done under fluoroscopic view. It is important to have the fluoroscope placed such that one can follow the nail insertion all the way down the leg, especially distal as rods have passed out of the soft distal tibia. A sterile tourniquet is used to minimize blood loss. The fusion site is entered with a longitudinal anterior knee incision. The knee implant is removed or the previously debrided infected knee is assessed and the fusion site is prepared. At this point, incision is made over the greater trochanter with split of the gluteus medius muscle to expose the piriformis fossa. The proximal femoral canal is entered as for a femoral fracture and a guidewire is passed down to the knee joint. At this point, the surfaces may be cut using the axis of the guide pin to create maximally abutting surfaces. Anterograde reaming is done over the guidewire. Generally, this can be done to 12 or 13 mm which is the nominal size of the tibial reaming and provides a suitable nail size for strength. The guide pin is passed down the tibia and fluoroscopic control is used to make certain that the center of the ankle joint is reached. Depending on the nail used, one may overream 0.5 mm on the tibial side and 1 mm on the femoral side. Nail dimension is determined on the tibial size. Length of the nail is based on guide pin measurement from the tip of the greater trochanter to a point 2 cm above the ankle joint. The bowed fusion nail is then carefully inserted over the guide pin down to the knee joint and passed across to the tibia with an assistant holding the fusion site opposed. The anterior bow of the femoral shaft will determine the position of the nail and tends to direct the nail out the very anterior cortex of the distal femur. One must carefully assess insertion distally into the tibia to prevent perforation and to ensure distal positioning about 2 cm above the ankle joint. The proximal end of the nail should be within 1 cm of the tip of the greater trochanter (**Fig. 78-3**). At this point, adjunct fixation

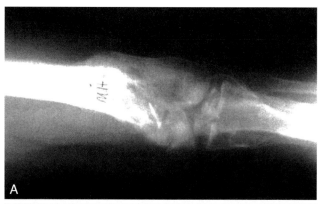
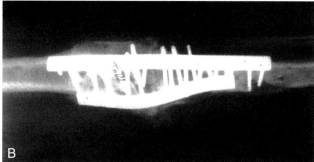

FIGURE 78-2 **A:** Healed intra-articular distal femoral and proximal tibial 3C open fracture complicated with extensor mechanism loss and chronic sepsis in a 22-year-old male factory worker. **B:** Successful double plate fixation after failed attempt at external fixation.

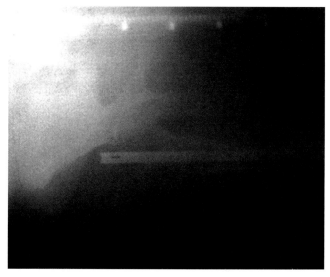

FIGURE 78-3 Prominent and symptomatic intramedullary nail inserted 2 cm above the tip of the greater trochanter which required removal.

may be considered. This may include a 10-hole medial AO neutralization plate, crossed cancellous screws, or proximal and distal locking screws in the nail. Additional bone graft and enhancing substances may be added to the fusion site. Closure of the wound may be problematic because of the shortening of the leg and chronic scar tissue, hence a consideration for avoiding additional plates. Postoperatively, no external splints or casts are needed, but the patient must be non–weight-bearing for 6 to 10 weeks, depending on the progression of healing (**Fig. 78-4**). I would add that there are many makers of suitable nails, including international groups who may favor the SIGN nail.[16] Importantly, the surgeon must consider specific details of the nail design, and the SIGN nail actually should be inserted through the greater trochanter. Again, I consider this an evolution from earlier methods, and still relevant, but combining intramedullary nailing with an intrinsic compression method that does not add surgical dissection is most desirable.

Intramedullary Nail (Neff)[1]

This titanium modular nail was developed for insertion retrograde of the femoral side with anterograde insertion of the tibial side. The implant comes in sizes of 11, 13, and 15 mm with a bowed segment on the femoral side and straight rod on the tibial side. The rods are locked with a conical taper locking mechanism supplemented with small engaging screws that add additional compression and prevent separation if the nail becomes disengaged. The nail is fluted and designed to engage the isthmus segments of the tibia and femur and then extend about 4 to 6 cm beyond this region. The rods may be cut off intraoperatively to provide the appropriate length. Finally, preparation requires reaming of 1.5 mm over the nominal size to be used. With slight rotation of the femoral side, a valgus alignment of the femur can be developed. The particular advantages of this knee are that it can be inserted through the knee joint, allows for different sizes of the nails applied to the femur and tibia, avoids the hip joint if concurrent hip arthroplasty is required, and over many years, has an extremely successful overall experience. Use with segmental allografts has been reported with the use of supplemental plates. The nail may require the use of a high-speed burr to transect the implant for removal.[1,15]

Intramedullary Nail (Wichita)[2,17]

The modular knee arthrodesis nail known as the Wichita nail has relatively short femoral and tibial segments that are fixed with interlocking screws at each end. Reaming is done using fixed dimension reamers. Adjustment of tibial placement allows for eventual engagement of a locking segment that can be screwed together creating longitudinal compression. This requires specific instrumentation to

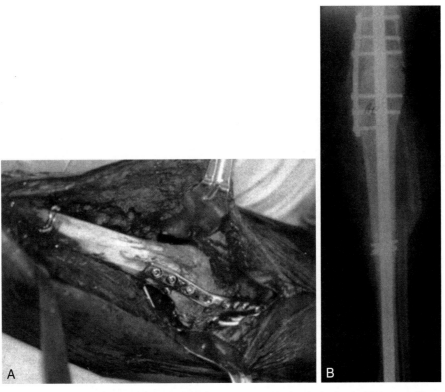

FIGURE 78-4 **A:** Intramedullary nail and AO compression plate fixation of a knee arthrodesis done with interposition of 20 cm proximal tibial allograft for severe osteomyelitis following motor vehicle trauma. Note that distal fusion site has a step-cut osteotomy with cerclage fixation. **B:** Satisfactory fusion of both allograft junctions at 6-month follow-up.

precisely place the nails, such that with opposition of the cut bone surfaces, the nail engages, and the locking turnbuckle screw is tightened to compress the fusion surfaces. The particular advantage of this system is that excellent compression of the fusion site is possible and blood loss is minimal which can be a problem if intramedullary reaming is needed. Another advantage is the ability to dissemble the locking turnbuckle screw, take down the fusion site, and remove the nail. I have used this system for many years, but I confess that the details of guide assembly are somewhat complicated. For that reason, I show the system which is quickly understood by looking at pictures (**Fig. 78-5**).

One of the perplexing problems with operative knee arthrodesis technique is what to do with the extra skin and soft tissues when you close over a significant implant absent the joint space. I do not have good answers, except to say that the problem is seen in most cases, and wound closure with minimal tension of skin edges is possible in most cases. As these wounds are basically put at rest with the fusion technique, good wound suction drainage and careful observation will suffice in most.

After many years of performing these procedures, regardless of implants chosen, I believe the key goal is rigid fixation of the fusion bone surfaces. One of the tricks commonly understood is to use your favorite proximal tibial cut guide to make a proximal tibia but that is absolutely perpendicular to the mechanical axis of the tibia. One of the attributes of the Wichita nail is the very significant compression possible at the fusion site. For some reason, peroneal palsy has been commonly seen. The dissection does not go near this structure, but manipulation of the leg during the procedure may place the nerve on stretch. My recommendation is to be mindful of the problem and careful.

Finally, the issue of bone preparation and débridement is critical to the success of this operation. As most of these cases are caused by chronic infection, débridement to bleeding and viable tissue is the goal, and this must be radical. We understand that biofilm production is a key feature of bacteria that can cause late and chronic infection. It would seem that biofilm, though permeable, can protect bacteria in deep knee wounds leading to late infection recurrence. It is more complicated, and biofilm production is one of many functions of bacteria, that have become "persistors" in this extremely hostile human environment. Additionally, we have some bacteria like *Pseudomonas* and MRSA that seem to be better at it than others. Radical surgical débridement, even to the level of transfemoral amputation, must be the limit that any surgeon will go to for resolution of this problem. Antibiotics and antiseptics are only helpful in the context of removing planktonic bacteria that have not morphed into the biofilm forming state. Pressurized irrigation is the most important element of this surgical method as biofilm bacteria have been shown to be quite vulnerable to this approach.

Amputation

Transfemoral amputation should be done as described in Campbell's *Operative Orthopaedics* (**Fig. 78-6**). In general, most of these cases are performed in compromised patients and should be considered as ischemic limbs. The salient points are that the resection level must be at least 10 cm above the joint line to accommodate prosthetics that have a typical knee joint, and a special myodesis or separating the muscle from the overlying fascia is not recommended. The incisions are a fish mouth shape starting at the level of bone cut, and gently extending distally about one-half the diameter of the thigh at this level. The quadriceps incision starts at the distal incision cut and gently curves to the midpoint of the incisions. The posterior muscle incision of hamstrings and the adductors is resected closer to the bone cut, such that they retract to the level of the bone cut. The vascular bundle and sciatic nerve are double ligated and distally resected. The sciatic nerve should be cut well proximal to the bone level. The bone is cut with a saw, and the anterior distal cut surface is beveled to decrease pressure with the overlying muscles. The posterior muscles should stabilized with bone holes in the distal femur. The anterior myodesis is then folded over the bone and attached to the posterior muscle group under slight tension. Closure is done in standard fashion over suction drains.

RESULTS

For knee arthrodesis for all methods and patient groups, the fusion rate ranges from 60% to 100%.[7,14] External fixators mirror this experience but clearly have lower rates of fusion in more complex and desperate cases (**Table 78-1**). The method is clearly safer with high risk recalcitrant bacteria like MRSA. Double frame constructs with three pin fixations have shown the best results. The other problems with this approach include pin tract infections and stress fractures through old hole sites. A recent series utilized the Ilizarov method, with 93% fusion with a mean leg length discrepancy of 4 cm. The authors cite the ability of the Ilizarov method to enhance bone quality and improve microcirculation that could reduce infection.[18] Intramedullary fixation and double plate fixation have revealed healing rates of 85% to 100% including cases with severe bone loss requiring allografts or vascularized fibular transplants. While this technique has good experience, the amount of dissection required about the knee joint may not be optimal in older and higher risk patients.

From literature review, postfusion complications include delayed union, recurrence of infection, wound healing problems, stress fracture, reflex dystrophy, and partial peroneal palsy and rates have ranged from 38% to 50% in selected series.[1,3,7,14,15,19] The last problem has been noted by multiple authors and no obvious explanation is offered other than stretching of the nerve may result from positioning of the knee during the operative procedure.

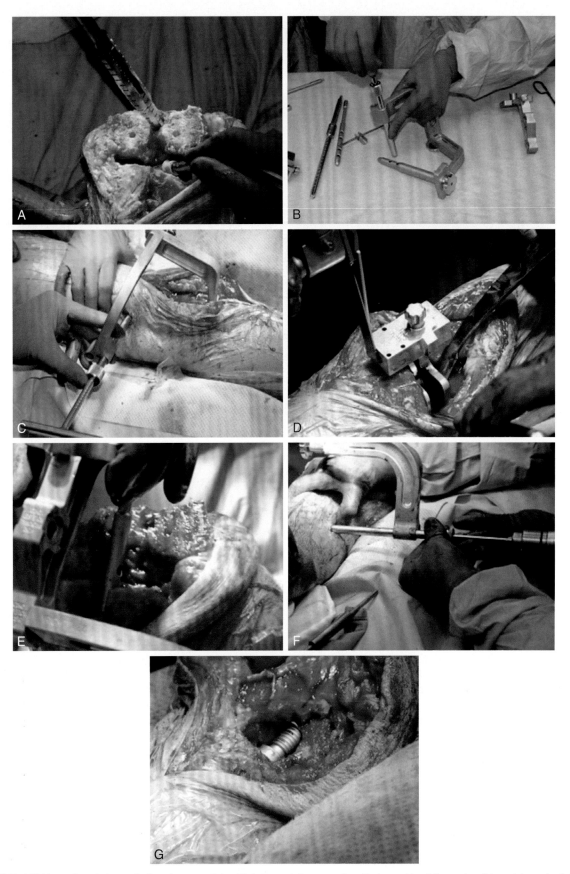

FIGURE 78-5 Wichita nail technique. **A:** Canal preparation with intramedullary reaming. **B:** Assembly of femoral nail to outrigger for interlocking screws insertion. **C:** Insertion of femoral intramedullary nail and proximal interlocking screws. **D:** Tibial slot is cut with slot cutting jig. **E:** Tibial nail is inserted with the target frame assembled to the proximal nail. **F:** Using jig, screws are inserted into the tibial nail. **G:** Demonstration of nail assembly, noting the tibial nail is assembled to femoral nail with the turnbuckle compression screw that is advanced with wrench. **G:** Compression screw is tightened into the femoral nail and gap closure is done with turnbuckle effect. Simple practice on the back table makes this device intuitive. As the screw has open slot to allow assembly, placing suture around the assembled device is helpful.

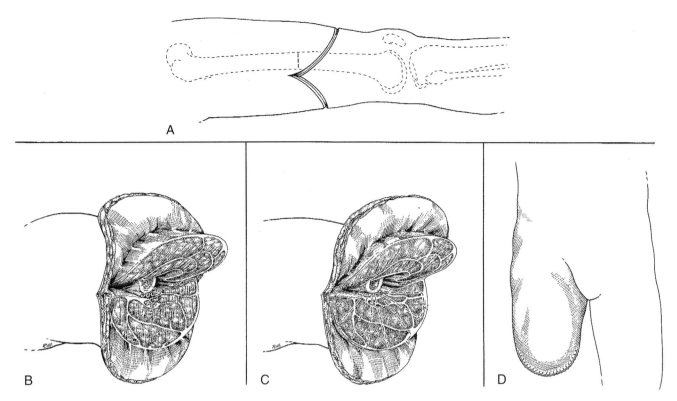

FIGURE 78-6 **A:** The amputation is at the middle third of the thigh but must be at least 10 cm above the knee joint. **B:** The incisions are fish mouth extending distally from bond level at the corners to about one half the diameter of the thigh. The quadriceps starts at the distal incision and tapers back to the corners. **C:** The distal hamstring and the adductors are cut distal to the bone cut to retract back to the bone cut level. They are attached to the distal bone through drill holes. The quadriceps are folded over the bone and the myodesis is attached to the posterior muscles under slight tension. **D:** Completed amputation. (Reprinted from Campbell WC, Crenshaw AH, Daugherty K. *Campbell's Operative Orthopaedics*. 8th ed. St. Louis: Mosby Year Book; 1992. Copyright © 1992 Elsevier. With permission.)

Most of these described resolved in time and there were no cases where direct surgical trauma has been described. Treatment of recurrent sepsis has included débridement of the site and eventual nail removal in certain cases. This is an example where resection arthroplasty may be considered. If there is a small joint space of no more than 20 mm, resection arthroplasty may be done by stabilizing the knee with splint or immobilizer for several months to allow soft-tissue scarring and modest stability. This option could be applied in elderly patients with minimal expectations for ambulation. It will never approach Girdlestone arthroplasty of the hip, where I have seen a patient with no limp and normal gait after that operation.

Authors recently have discussed the possibility of late takedown of fusions after failed total knee arthroplasty. In general, patients have been satisfied with this approach, the majority stating that they would consider having the operation again if offered.[19-22]

Kemkays et al reviewed 123 patients where a prior knee arthrodesis was converted to a total knee replacement finding the subsequent knee flexion increased to 80° on average, but significant complications occurred in 65% of cases. Skin necrosis (25%), arthrofibrosis (13%), re-infection (11%), and recurrent revision (11%) were the most frequent complications and death occurred in 5%.

The greatest disadvantage of knee arthrodesis is the resultant complete stiffness. If the knee is fused in extension, walking is effective and generally smooth. Unfortunately, sitting is inconvenient and the attendance in social circumstances with crowded seating such as movies, sporting events, church, etc. can be particularly difficult. Stiehl et al noted that an optimal amount of shortening for clearance of the shoe on gait swing through ambulation was 1.5 to 2.5 cm. Patients would choose shoe lift adjustments to this level. Most older patients required a cane or walker for community ambulation.[23]

Dr David Green, while a resident, carefully assessed a large group of patients following successful knee arthrodesis. Automobile driving did not prove any problem, particularly if the car had an automatic transmission. Most patients avoided theater seats unless an aisle seat could be reserved. Household chores posed special problems, but most patients could bend to the floor resulting from stretching of the hamstrings and hypermobility of the lumbar spine. Patients were capable of engaging in virtually every type of sport or recreational activity including tennis, golf, bowling, baseball, handball, and even horseback riding. However, no patient was known to have attempted snow skiing.[14]

DISCUSSION

The use of intramedullary nail techniques offered satisfactory solution to difficult problems following sepsis and bone loss in failed total knee arthroplasty. White et

TABLE 78-1	Results After Knee Arthrodesis			
Author	N	Rate of Fusion	Year	Technique
Arroyo	21	90%	1997	Neff Nail
Cheng	2	100%	1995	Short IM Nail
Donley	20	85%	1991	IM Nail
Hak	19	58%	1995	Single Plane Ex Fix
Hak	17	61%	1995	Double Plane Ex Fix
Hessmann	19	100%	1996	External Fixator
Nichols	11	100%	1996	Double Plate
Rasmussen	13	92%	1995	IM Rod, Fibula
Stiehl	8	100%	1993	IM Rod, Plate
Robinson	23	87%	2018	Mixed methods
McQuail	23	60%	2018	Wichita Modular
Friederich	37	86%	2017	Modular Nail
Gottfried	165	65%	2016	IM Nail, Ex Fix
Bruno	16	93%	2017	Ilizarov

al demonstrated a significantly higher ratio of fusions with intramedullary nailing versus external fixators (odds ratio: 5.1 [95% confidence interval: 2.7-9.7]).[24] Gathen et al evaluated the ability of knee arthrodesis to solve periprosthetic joint infection after total knees, noting the rate of revision to be much lower after arthrodesis ($P < .02$) though there were clearly no advantages with functional outcome.[25] Robinson et al showed that salvage knee arthrodesis was successful in 87% of cases to handle a failure of a two-stage total knee revision, though 3 of 23 cases ultimately required an amputation.[26]

With chronic sepsis after total knee arthroplasty, a staged reconstruction seems appropriate with a delay of 6 to 8 weeks combined with appropriate adjunctive antibiotic therapy. The choice of nail does not seem to affect the rate of fusion, but certain advantages accrue with each particular nail. The simple bowed femoral nail allows straightforward anterograde insertion but has the possibility of migrating, bone perforation, and proximal femoral fracture if reaming is inadequate. Adjunct fixation such as crossed cancellous screws or neutralization bone plate may be needed at the fusion site. The addition of interlocking screws can add rotational stability at the fusion site. The modular knee arthrodesis nail such as the Wichita nail is a significant improvement. This nail is inserted at the fusion site, has an excellent external jig for insertion of interlocking screws and has an articulating turnbuckle that assembles at the fusion site. Compression at the fusion site is optimal with the turnbuckle, and the design may be taken apart and the nail removed at a later point. While fusion rates with this nail have been comparable to other nails, McQuail et al recently reported a fusion rate of 60%. Most likely this reflects the choice of more complicated patients.[17]

Recent authors have compared outcomes of knee arthrodesis versus amputation following failed total knee revisions. Hungerer et al noted that the infection recurrence after arthrodesis was 22% while 36% of amputations had chronic infection. An interesting finding of function was that amputees fitted with a microprocessor-controlled knee joint prosthesis had a significantly better functional outcome.[27]

Several authors consider an interesting trend of treatment after prosthetic removal for chronic prosthetic joint infection. Using US Medicare database, Cancienne et al found that after treatment of periprosthetic joint infection in 18,533 patients, 61% underwent implant reimplantation, 4.5% underwent knee arthrodesis, 3.1% underwent amputation, 14% underwent repeat débridement without being re-implanted, and 12.5% retained the initial spacer. Importantly, with large numbers, 38% were not undergoing secondary revision with a significant group having a resection arthroplasty.[28] Gottfried et al studied knee arthrodesis trends using the Danish National patient registry noting that the 15-year cumulative arthrodesis rate was 0.26%. However, the rate decreased from 0.32% in 2002 to 0.09% in 2013. Knee arthrodesis was utilized with infection in 93%, extensor mechanism disruption in 28%, and soft tissue deficiency in 15%. Solid fusion occurred in 65% of patients, being highest in the intramedullary procedures. Repeat arthrodesis was done in 21% of cases and 14% ultimately underwent transfemoral amputation.[29] Matar et al reviewed the outcomes of patients classified as McPherson Type C host, finding that 40% to 50% of patients failed treatment regardless of technique.[30] Warren et al noted that soft-tissue deficiency is extremely challenging following prosthetic joint infection with 69% of patients who had rotational flap procedures having recurrent infection. Of this group, 19% required knee arthrodesis, and 23% required amputation.[31]

My conclusion after this review is that knee arthrodesis and amputation will continue to be utilized by tertiary level experts with decreasing numbers overall. This will drive up the complication rates, and patients will tend to have higher Charlson comorbidity rates being at higher risk for treatment failure. This is an important fact and must be considered carefully by those in the political and legal business, who independently review poor surgical outcomes.

REFERENCES

1. Aroyo JS, Garvin KL, Neff JR. Arthrodesis of the knee with a modular titanium intramedullary nail. *J Bone Joint Surg.* 1997;79: 26-35.
2. Cheng SL, Gross AE. Knee arthrodesis using a short locked intramedullary nail. A new technique. *Am J Knee Surg.* 1995;8:56-59.
3. Hessman M, Gotzen L, Boumgaertal F. Knee arthrodesis with a unilateral external fixator. *Acta Chir Belg.* 1995;96:123-127.
4. Nichols SJ, Landon GC, Tullos HS. Arthrodesis with dual plates after failed total knee arthroplasty. *J Bone Joint Surg.* 1991;73:1020-1024.
5. Rassmussen MR, Bishop AT, Wood MB. Arthrodesis of the knee with a vascularized fibular rotatory graft. *J Bone Joint Surg.* 1995;77A:751-759.
6. Donley BG, Matthews LS, Kaufer H. Arthrodesis of the knee with and intremedullary nail. *J Bone Joint Surg Am.* 1991;73:907-913.
7. Deldycke J, Rommens P, Reynders P, Claes P, Broos P. Primary arthrodesis of the injured knee: still a solution in 1994? Case Report. *J Trauma.* 1994;37:862-866.
8. Wolf RE, Scarborough MT, Enneking WF. Long-term follow-up of patients with autogenous resection arthrodesis of the knee. *Clin Orthop Relat Res.* 1999;358:36-40.
9. Benson ER, Resine ST, Lewis CG. Functional outcome of arthrodesis for failed total knee arthroplasty. *Orthopaedics.* 1998;21:875-879.
10. Figueiredo A, Ferreira R, Alegre C, Fonseca F. Charcot osteoarthropathy of the knee secondary to neurosyphilis; a rare condition managed by a challenging arthrodesis. *BMJ Case Rep.* 2018. doi:10.1136/bcr-2018-225337.
11. Rebelo T, Morais J, Agostinho F, et al. Knee arthrodesis in a patient with Charcot neuroarthropathy secondary to familial amyloid polyneuropathy: a case report. *JBJS Case Connect.* 2017. doi:10.2106/JBJS.17.00110. Epub ahead of print.
12. Friederich MJ, Schmolders J, Wimmer MD, et al. Two-stage knee arthrodesis with a modular intramedullary nail due to septic failure of revision total knee arthroplasty with extensor mechanism deficiency. *Knee.* 2017;24:1240-1246.
13. Son MS, Lau E, Parvizi J, Mont MA, et al. What are the frequency, associated factors, and mortality of amputation and arthrodesis after a failed infected TKA. *Clin Orthop Relat Res.* 2017;475:2905-2913.
14. Green DP, Parkes JC, Stinchfield FE. Arthrodesis of the knee: A followup study. *J Bone Joint Surg.* 1967;49A:1065-1074.
15. Hak DJ, Lieberman JR, Finerman GA. Single plane and biplane external fixators for knee arthrodesis. *Clin Orthop Relat Res.* 1995;316:134-144.
16. Anderson DR, Anderson LA, Haller JM, et al. The SIGN nail for knee fusion: technique and clinical results. *SICOT J.* 2016;2:6.
17. McQuail P, McCartney B, Baker J, et al. Radiographic and functional outcomes following knee arthrodesis using the Wichita fusion nail. *J Knee Surg.* 2018;31:479-484.
18. Bruno AA, Kirienko A, Peccati A, et al. Knee arthrodesis by the Ilizarov method in the treatment of total knee arthroplasty failure. *Knee.* 2017;24:91-99.
19. Henkel TR, Boldt JG, Drobny TK, Munzinger UK. Total knee arthroplasty after formal knee fusion using unconstrained and semiconstrained components: a report of 7 cases. *J Arthroplasty.* 2001;16:768-776.
20. Cameron HU. Results of total knee arthroplasty following takedown of formal knee fusion. *J. Arthroplasty.* 1996;11:732-737.
21. Kim JH, Kim JS, Cho SH. Total knee arthroplasty after spontaneous osseous ankylosis and takedown of formal knee fusion. *J Arthroplasty.* 2000;15:453-460.
22. Kernkamp WA, Verra WC, Pijls BG, et al. Conversion from knee arthrodesis to arthroplasty: systematic review. *Int Orthop.* 2016;40:2069-2074.
23. Stiehl JB, Hanel DP. Knee arthrodesis using combined intramedullary rod and plate fixation. *Clin Orthop Relat Res.* 1993;294:238-241.
24. White CJ, Palmer AJR, Rodriguez-Merchan EC. External fixation vs intramedullary nailing for knee arthrodesis after failed infected total knee arthroplasty: a systematic review and meta-analysis. *J Arthroplasty.* 2018;33:1288-1295.
25. Gathen M, Wimmer MD, Ploeger MM, et al. Comparison of two-stage revision arthroplasty and intramedullary arthrodesis in patients with failed infected knee arthroplasty. *Arch Orthop Trauma Surg.* 2018;138:1443-1452.
26. Robinson M, Piponov HI, Ormseth A, et al. Knee arthrodesis outcomes after infected total knee arthroplasty and failure of two-stage revision with antibiotic cement spacer. *J Am Acad Orthop Surg Global Res Rev.* 2018;2:77.
27. Hungerer S, Kiechle M, von Ruden C, et al. Knee arthrodesis versus above-the-knee amputation after septic failure of revision total knee arthroplasty: comparison of functional outcome and complication rates. *BMC Musculoskeletal Disord.* 2017;18:443.
28. Cancienne JM, Granadillo VA, Patel KJ, et al. Risk factors for repeat débridement, spacer retention, amputation, arthrodesis, and mortality after removal of an infected total knee arthroplasty with spacer placement. *J Arthroplasty.* 2018;33:515-520.
29. Gottfriedsen TB, Schroder BM, Odgaard A. Knee arthrodesis after failure of knee arthroplasty: a nationwide register-based study. *J Bone Joint Surg Am.* 2016;98:1370-1377.
30. Matar HE, Stritch P, Emms N. Higher failure rate of two stage-revision for infected knee arthroplasties in significantly compromised (host C) patients. *Knee Surg Sports Traumatol Arthrosc.* 2018;27(7):2206-2210.
31. Warren SI, Murtaugh TS, Lakra A, et al. Treatment of periprosthetic knee infection with concurrent rotational muscle flap coverage is associated with high failure rates. *J Arthorplasty* 2018;33(10):3263-3267.

INDEX